MEDICAL~ SURGICAL NURSING

Critical Thinking
for Collaborative Care

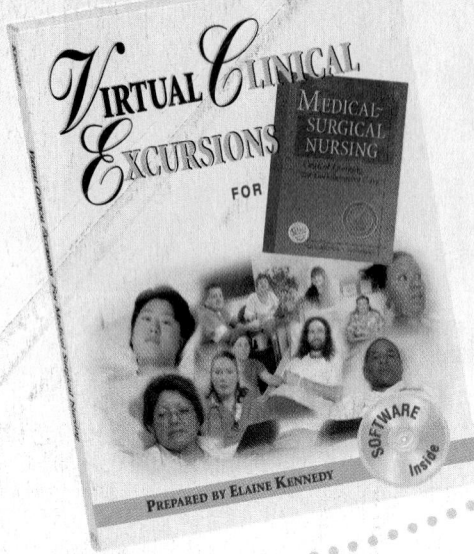

MEDICAL~ SURGICAL NURSING

Critical Thinking for Collaborative Care

Donna D. Ignatavicius, MS, RN, Cm
President, DI Associates, Inc.
Hughesville, Maryland;
Former Professor,
Charles County Community College,
La Plata, Maryland

M. Linda Workman, PhD, RN, FAAN
Gertrude Perkins Oliva Professor of Oncology,
Frances Payne Bolton School of Nursing,
Case Western Reserve University,
Cleveland, Ohio

with 689 illustrations

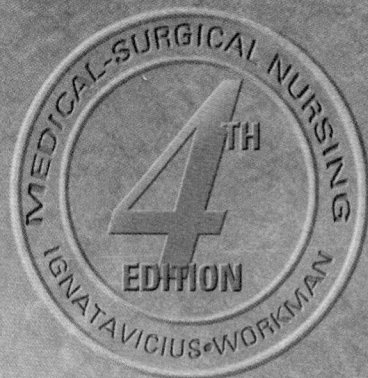

SAUNDERS
An Imprint of Elsevier

SAUNDERS
An Imprint of Elsevier

The Curtis Center
Independence Square West
Philadelphia, Pennsylvania 19106

NOTICE

Pharmacology is an ever-changing field. Standard safety precautions must be followed, but as new research and clinical experience broaden our knowledge, changes in treatment and drug therapy may become necessary or appropriate. Readers are advised to check the most current product information provided by the manufacturer of each drug to be administered to verify the recommended dose, the method and duration of administration, and contraindications. It is the responsibility of the licensed prescriber, relying on experience and knowledge of the patient, to determine dosages and the best treatment for each individual patient. Neither the publisher nor the editor assumes any liability for any injury and/or damage to persons or property arising from this publication.

Library of Congress Cataloging-in-Publication Data

Medical-surgical nursing: critical thinking for collaborative care / [edited by] Donna D. Ignatavicius, M. Linda Workman.—
4th ed.
    p. ; cm.
Rev. ed. of: Medical-surgical nursing across the health care continuum. 3rd ed. c1999.
Includes bibliographical references and index.
ISBN 0-7216-8762-8 (1 v.) — ISBN 0-7216-8763-6 (2 v. set)
 1. Nursing. 2. Surgical nursing. I. Ignatavicius, Donna D. II. Workman, M. Linda. III. Medical-surgical nursing across the health care continuum.
[DNLM: 1. Perioperative Nursing. WY 161 M489 2001]
RT41 .I36 2001
610.73—dc21

2001042655

Vice President and Publishing Director: Sally Schrefer
Executive Editor: Robin Carter
Managing Editor: Lee Henderson
Project Manager: Deborah L. Vogel
Project Specialist: Jodi M. Willard
Book Designer: Teresa Breckwoldt

MEDICAL-SURGICAL NURSING: CRITICAL   Single Volume 0–7216–8762–8
THINKING FOR COLLABORATIVE CARE, 4th edition   2-Volume Set 0–7216–8763–6

Printed in the United States of America.

Last digit is the print number: 9   8   7   6

About the Authors

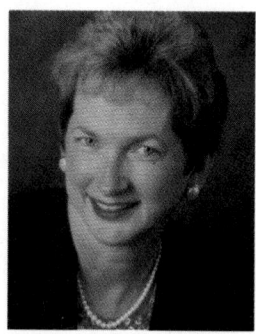

Donna D. Ignatavicius received her diploma in nursing from the Peninsula General School of Nursing in Salisbury, Maryland. After working as a staff and charge nurse in medical-surgical nursing, she became an instructor in Staff Development at the University of Maryland Medical Center. She then received her BSN from the University of Maryland School of Nursing. For 5 years she taught in several schools of nursing while working toward her MS in Nursing, which she received in 1981. Ms. Ignatavicius then taught in the BSN program at the University of Maryland for 6 years, after which she continued to pursue her interest in gerontology and accepted the position of Director of Nursing of a major skilled nursing facility in her home state of Maryland. She has been a certified gerontologic nurse since 1989 and was certified in nursing case management by the American Nurses Credentialing Center in 1998. Recently, she has taught in both diploma and associate-degree nursing programs. Through her consulting and seminar business, Ms. Ignatavicius has gained national recognition in nursing education and critical thinking. She is currently the President of DI Associates, Inc. (http://www.diassociates.com/), a company dedicated to improving health care through education and consultation.

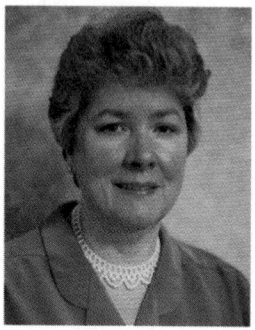

M. Linda Workman received her BSN from the University of Cincinnati College of Nursing and Health. After serving in the U.S. Army Nurse Corps and working as an Assistant Head Nurse and Head Nurse in civilian hospitals, Dr. Workman, a native of Canada, earned her MSN from the University of Cincinnati College of Nursing and Health and a PhD in Developmental Biology from the University of Cincinnati College of Arts and Sciences. Dr. Workman's 22 years of academic experience include teaching at the diploma, associate-degree, baccalaureate, and master's levels. Her areas of teaching expertise include medical-surgical nursing, physiology, pathophysiology, genetics, oncology, and immunology. Dr. Workman has been recognized nationally for her teaching expertise and was inducted into the American Academy of Nursing in 1992. She is a former American Cancer Society Professor of Oncology Nursing and is currently the Gertrude Perkins Oliva Professor of Oncology at the Frances Payne Bolton School of Nursing, Case Western Reserve University.

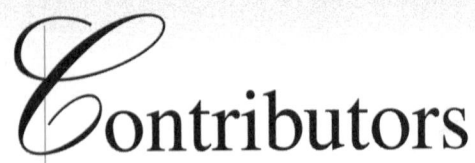ontributors

ROBIN L. BARANOWSKI, BSN, RN
Infusion Therapy Nurse; PICC Line Specialist
Calvert Memorial Hospital
Prince Frederick, Maryland

MARCIA CHORBA, RN, MSN
Education Coordinator, Critical Care
Veterans Administration Pittsburgh Healthcare System
Pittsburgh, Pennsylvania

CAROLYN CORAZZA, BSN, RN, CWOCN
Private Practice ET Nurse
E.T. Consultants, Inc.
Rockville, Maryland

JANICE CUZZELL, MA, RN, CNS
Vice President of Staff Development
Island Health Care, Inc.
Savannah, Georgia

LUCILLE SANZERO ELLER, PhD, RN
Assistant Professor, College of Nursing
Rutgers University
Newark, New Jersey

KATHLEEN ELLSTROM, PhD, RN, CNS
Clinical Nurse Manager, Critical Care Services
Kaiser Foundation Hospitals—Riverside
Grand Terrace, California

DOROTHY J. HAMILTON, MSN, RN, CNP, CCRN
Nurse Practitioner
University Hospitals of Cleveland
Cleveland, Ohio

E. JEAN HAYES, MS, RN
Associate Professor
Purdue University—North Central
Westville, Indiana

DEBORAH H. HEATHERLY, BSN, MA
Healthcare Consultant
Moncks Corner, South Carolina

MARY KAZANOWSKI, PhD, ARNP, AOCN, CRNH
Professor, Saint Anselm College;
Palliative Care Nurse, Visiting Nurses Association Hospice
Manchester, New Hampshire

ANNE KEANE, EdD, CRNP, FAAN
Associate Professor, School of Nursing
University of Pennsylvania
Philadelphia, Pennsylvania

ELAINE BISHOP KENNEDY, EdD, RN
Professor, Nursing
Wor-Wic Community College
Salisbury, Maryland

LORI KLINGMAN, MSN, RN
UPMC Passavant Hospital
Pittsburgh, Pennsylvania

DEITRA L. LOWDERMILK, PhD, RNC, FAAN
Clinical Professor
University of North Carolina at Chapel Hill
Chapel Hill, North Carolina

ANN BUTLER MAHER, MS, RN, APNC, ONC
Family Nurse Practitioner
Sussex Family Practice
Sussex, New Jersey

JUDY MALKIEWICZ, PhD, RN
School of Nursing
University of Northern Colorado
Greeley, Colorado

ERIC MARSH, MSN, RN
Trauma Program Manager
Rainbow Pediatric Trauma Center
University Hospitals of Cleveland;
Trauma Nurse Coordinator
University Hospitals Health System
Cleveland, Ohio

JAN HOOT MARTIN, PhD, RN, GNP
Professor, School of Nursing
University of Northern Colorado
Greeley, Colorado

ELIZABETH McCLURE, MS, RN
Instructor, Adult-Health Nursing Department
University of Cincinnati College of Nursing
Cincinnati, Ohio

M. ELAINE McLEOD, MSN, APRN, BC, CDE
Clinical Nurse Specialist
Veterans Administration Tennessee Valley Healthcare
    System
Nashville, Tennessee

ERIN M. McMENAMIN, MSN, CRNP, AOCN
Pain Medicine Nurse Practitioner/Program Manager
University of Pennsylvania
Philadelphia, Pennsylvania

DONNA McMULLEN, RN, CWOCN
Private Practice ET Nurse
E.T. Consultants, Inc.
Rockville, Maryland

MARJORIE G. MORGAN, PhD, RN
Certified Nurse-Midwife, Certified Transcultural Nurse
South Carolina Department of Health
    and Environmental Control
Myrtle Beach, South Carolina

AMY NICHOLS, EdD, RN
Associate Professor, School of Nursing
San Francisco State University
San Francisco, California

REBECCA M. PATTON, MSN, RN, CNOR
Director of Nursing
Richmond Heights Hospital
University Hospitals Health System
Cleveland, Ohio

KATHLEEN OUIMET PERRIN, PhD(c), RN, CCRN
Associate Professor of Nursing
Saint Anselm College
Manchester, New Hampshire

TOMMIE WRIGHT PNIEWSKI, MSN, RN, CNAA
Associate Professor of Nursing
Hopkinsville Community College
Hopkinsville, Kentucky

ROSEMARY C. POLOMANO, PhD, RN, FAAN
Assistant Professor, Department of Anesthesiology
Penn State Milton S. Hershey Medical Center
Pennsylvania State University College of Nursing
Hershey, Pennsylvania

SUSAN M. SCHNEIDER, PhD, RN, CS, AOCN
Director, Graduate Oncology Nursing Program
Duke University
Durham, North Carolina

DEBORAH WRIGHT SHPRITZ, PhD, RN, CCRN
Assistant Professor, Department of Adult Health
University of Maryland School of Nursing
Baltimore, Maryland

JUDITH P. STURGIS, RN, BSN, CIC
Infection Control Director
Calvert Memorial Hospital
Prince Frederick, Maryland

JANICE TAZBIR, RN, MS, CCRN
Assistant Professor of Nursing
Purdue University—Calumet
Hammond, Indiana

SHIRLEY E. VAN ZANDT, MSN, MPH, CRNP
Instructor, School of Nursing
Johns Hopkins University
Baltimore, Maryland

CONSTANCE VISOVSKY, RN, PhD(c), ACNP
Research Nurse/Nurse Practitioner
Case Western Reserve University
University Hospitals of Cleveland;
Research Nurse, CHANGE Exercise Study
Frances Payne Bolton School of Nursing
Case Western Reserve University
Cleveland, Ohio

CHRIS WINKELMAN, PhD, RN, CCRN
Assistant Professor, Frances Payne Bolton School
    of Nursing
Case Western Reserve University
Cleveland, Ohio

Reviewers

OLGA E. HENRY, BSN, MBA, RN, C
Broward Community College
Davie, Florida

LAWRENCE "BUDDY" HERRINGTON, MSN, RN
Tarrant County College
Fort Worth, Texas

MIMA M. HORNE, RN, MS, CDE
New Hanover Regional Medical Center
Wilmington, North Carolina

SUSAN J.W. HSIA, RN, PhD
Washburn University
Topeka, Kansas

CAROL A. HUNTER, RN, MSN
The Christ Hospital School of Nursing
Cincinnati, Ohio

PAULA S. JOHNSON, BSN, CCRN
Nash Health Care Systems
Rocky Mountain, North Carolina

TAMARA M. KEAR, MSN, RN, CNN
Thomas Jefferson University Hospital
Philadelphia, Pennsylvania

LEA KEESEE, RN, BSN
South Plains College
Levelland, Texas

ELAINE BISHOP KENNEDY, EdD, RN
Wor-Wic Community College
Salisbury, Maryland

NANCY L. GINDELE KRANZLEY, MS, RN
The Christ Hospital
Cincinnati, Ohio

DARLENE LACY, MSN, RNC
University of Mary Hardin-Baylor
Belton, Texas

PATRICK J. LILLEY, MBA, MSN, RN
North Central Texas College
Gainsville, Texas

BRENDA LOHRI-POSEY, RN, EdD
Wheeling Jesuit University
Wheeling, West Virginia

EDWINA A. McCONNELL, RN, PhD, ERCNA
Independent Nurse Consultant
Gorham, Maine

MARY ANN SICILIANO McLAUGHLIN, MSN, RN
Independent Nurse Consultant
Magnolia, New Jersey

MICHELLE M. MONTPAS, RN, MSN, OCN
C.S. Mott Community College
Flint, Michigan

JAY K. OBER, RN, BS, CCRN, CEN
Bay State Medical Center
United States Air Force Reserves
Springfield, Massachusetts

PATRICIA A. PADAMS, RN, BSN, CEN
Thomas Jefferson University Hospital
Philadelphia, Pennsylvania

TOMMIE W. PNIEWSKI, MSN, RN, CNAA
Hopkinsville Community College
Hopkinsville, Kentucky

JANE RENFRO, PhD, ANP (C)
Kaiser Permanente
Arlington Free Clinic
Arlington, Virginia

ANNE RATH RENTFRO, MSN, RN, CS
University of Texas at Brownsville
Brownsville, Texas

DOTTIE ROBERTS, MSN, MACI, RN, C, ONC, CNS
Penrose-St. Francis Health Services
Colorado Springs, Colorado

MARY B. SCOTT, RN, PhD, CNN
University of California—San Francisco
San Francisco, California

SUSAN SEMB, RN-CS, MSN, CDE, PHN
Sun Plus Home Health Services
San Diego, California

AMY B. SHARRON, MS, RN, CS, GNP
Roger Williams Medical Center
Providence, Rhode Island

GAIL JANET SMITH, RN, MSN
Miami Dade Community College
Miami, Florida

TERESA E. KELLY SNYDER, MN, RN
Montana State University
Missoula, Montana

CHRIS STEWERT-AMIDEI, RN, MSN, CNRN, CCRN
University of Chicago Hospitals
Chicago, Illinois

KATHLEEN G. STILLING, MS, RN, C
The Community College of Baltimore County, Essex,
Baltimore, Maryland

JUDITH P. STURGIS, RN, BSN, CIC
Calvert Memorial Hospital
Prince Frederick, Maryland

DAVID TILTON, RN, BSN, ACLS, BCLS
Western State Hospital
Tacoma, Washington

SUZANNE M. VANET, BSN, CMSN
Louis A. Johnson VA Medical Center
Clarkburg, West Virginia

CATHERINE R. VAN SON, RN, MSN
Oregon Geriatric Education Center
Portland, Oregon

NANCY CLARKE VERDIRAME, RN, BSN, MSN
Louise Obici School of Nursing
Suffolk, Virginia

JANIS WAITE, EdD, RN
St. Francis Medical Center College of Nursing
Peoria, Illinois

TERRY WOOD, RN, MSN
Jewish Hospital College of Nursing
St. Louis, Missouri

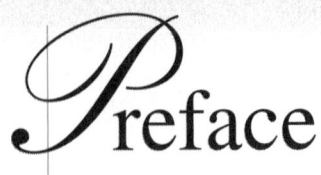

Preface

The first edition of this text, entitled *Medical-Surgical Nursing: A Nursing Process Approach,* found widespread acclaim as *the* medical-surgical nursing text of the 1990s. The second and third editions built on that achievement and further solidified the book's position as a compass for the practice of adult nursing. Now in its fourth edition, just 3 years since the previous edition, the book maps a fresh course for the future of adult nursing—a course reflected in the book's new title: *Medical-Surgical Nursing: Critical Thinking for Collaborative Care.*

This title was carefully chosen to reflect this edition's fresh emphasis on developing and enhancing critical thinking skills to help today's nursing students function in interdisciplinary teams in a variety of health care settings, including both acute care and community-based settings.

In addition to this focus on critical thinking, *Medical-Surgical Nursing: Critical Thinking for Collaborative Care,* 4th edition, provides expanded coverage of women's health issues, cultural considerations, complementary and alternative (integrative) therapies, and the special needs of older adults. Also, concepts of case management and community-based care are interwoven throughout to help the reader understand these new and growing roles and trends.

New to this edition are Critical Thinking Challenges, which are interspersed throughout the text. These case-based exercises provide a safe and effective means of practicing the on-the-spot decision making that students will face in the fast-paced world of medical-surgical nursing. Suggested answer guidelines for these Critical Thinking Challenges are provided on the book's SIMON website.

But these answer guidelines are just the beginning of the integrated multimedia learning experience provided in the fourth edition. For each of the Learning Objectives now provided at the start of each chapter, students will find corresponding Self-Assessment Questions on the SIMON website, written by co-author M. Linda Workman. Also on the SIMON site are web-based Learning Activities that correspond to the collaborative management of major diseases and disorders. These activities stimulate and validate critical thinking to help students understand and apply the material covered in the text. Internet Resources and annotated Suggested Readings are also found on the SIMON website.

CLINICAL CURRENCY AND ACCURACY

To ensure the text's currency and accuracy, we listened to the readers of the first three editions—their impressions of and experiences with the text. Based on this input, we formulated our revision plan. We assembled a team of clinical experts to revise, rewrite and, in some cases, draft entirely new chapters. We then commissioned in-depth reviews of each chapter by clinicians and instructors from across the United States and Canada and used their reviews to guide us in revising the chapters into their final form. We even enlisted the assistance of an enterostomal therapist and an infection control nurse to review every clinical chapter.

The results are reflected in the fourth edition's strong, consistent focus on critical thinking, collaborative care, pathophysiology, and community-based care; its foundation of relevant research; and its emphasis on the critical "need to know" information that nurses must master in order to provide safe, effective care based on solid scientific evidence. This base of scientific evidence is emphasized throughout the text and is highlighted in our new "Best Practice" charts.

OUTSTANDING READABILITY

With the assistance of a team of writing experts who conducted reading level analyses of each and every chapter, the fourth edition has been carefully revised from cover to cover to ensure a consistent reading level ideally suited for today's nursing students. To achieve this consistency, our writing experts evaluated the readability of the first draft of each chapter. We revised the chapters based on those results and then tested the revised chapters for readability. Those chapters that tested above our target threshold were carefully edited once again to reduce the reading level still further. These chapters were tested a third time to confirm that the editing resulted in exactly the right level of readability. The result is a med-surg text of consistently outstanding readability.

EASE OF ACCESS

To make the text as easy to use as possible, we have maintained the third edition's approach of smaller chapters of more uniform length. The fourth edition has 77 chapters, including new introductory chapters on substance abuse (Chapter 8) and cultural aspects of health (Chapter 6). Based on faculty input, we have condensed the content on stress and adaptation, body image, and sexuality—formerly separate chapters—and have incorporated this material as appropriate into other chapters.

We also have maintained the third edition's unit structure, with vital body systems (cardiovascular, respiratory, and neurologic) appearing earlier in the book. In these three units, we have continued to provide critical care content in separate chapters on managing critically ill clients with coronary artery disease, respiratory problems, and neurologic problems. To help break up long blocks of text and also to highlight key information, we have included numerous headings, bulleted lists, tables, charts, and in-text highlights. We end each chapter with a Selected Bibliography (with classic sources noted with an asterisk [*]). Key Terms are now in boldface type and are defined in the text to foster learning of need-to-know vocabulary.

A COLLABORATIVE APPROACH

As in the previous three editions, we take a collaborative approach to client care. We believe that in the real world of health care, nurses, clients, and other health care providers (including physicians, respiratory and physical therapists, advanced-practice nurses, and physician's assistants) *share* responsibility for the management of client problems. Thus we present client care in a collaborative management framework. In this framework we make no artificial distinctions between medical treatment and nursing care. Instead, under each Collaborative Management heading we cover the entire range of approaches taken by health care practitioners of all disciplines when dealing with client problems.

New to this edition are eight Concept Maps that underscore this collaborative approach. Also known as *clinical correlation maps,* these Concept Maps address eight complex health problems and visually organize the steps of the nursing process and related concepts to illustrate the relationships among disease processes, medical treatments, nursing interventions, and more. Identifying these relationships not only underscores the collaborative nature of health care but also stimulates critical thinking and fosters learning.

Although our approach is collaborative, the text is first and foremost a *nursing* text. We therefore use a nursing process approach to organize discussions of client health problems and their management. Discussions of key health problems follow a full nursing process format, with the following structure:

Health Problem
 Overview
  Pathophysiology
  Etiology
  Incidence/Prevalence
 Collaborative Management
  Assessment
  Analysis
   Common Nursing Diagnoses and Collaborative Problems
   Additional Nursing Diagnoses and Collaborative Problems
  Planning and Implementation
   Nursing Diagnosis/Collaborative Problem
    Planning: Expected Outcomes
    Interventions
  Community-Based Care
   Health Teaching
   Home Care Management
   Health Care Resources
  Evaluation: Outcomes
The nursing diagnoses used in this edition are the very latest 2001-2002 NANDA-approved diagnoses, making "Iggy" the

first med-surg text to incorporate the sweeping changes of NANDA's Taxonomy II.

Discussions of less common or less complex disorders, although not given this complete subhead structure, nonetheless follow the same basic format: a discussion of the problem itself (including pertinent information on pathophysiology, etiology, and incidence) followed by a section on collaborative care of clients with the disorder.

Integral to this collaborative management approach is a clear delineation of just who is responsible for what. When a responsibility is primarily the nurse's, the text says so. When a decision must be made jointly by the client, nurse, health care provider, and therapist, this is clearly stated. When different health care practitioners in different care settings might be involved in the client's care, this also is stated.

To further emphasize the nurse's role, we have integrated pertinent components of the Nursing Interventions Classification (NIC) system and the Nursing Outcomes Classification (NOC) system. These systems were developed by the Center for Nursing Classification to standardize nursing interventions and outcomes and the terminology used to describe them. Where appropriate for health problems that receive full nursing process coverage, NIC interventions are clearly identified with a NIC symbol (NIC). Selected activities associated with each identified intervention are listed in NIC Intervention Activities charts.

The expected outcomes for client care in this edition are consistent with the NOC system. However, NOC continues to be developed and refined to ensure that outcomes are evidence-based. We have therefore included outcome statements that use NOC language when appropriate, as well as other outcome statements validated empirically by clinical practice. Those statements that are particularly consistent with NOC language are identified with a NOC symbol (NOC).

ORGANIZATION

The 77 chapters of *Medical-Surgical Nursing: Critical Thinking for Collaborative Care* are grouped into 16 units. A Core Concepts Grid introduces each unit of content and highlights the essential information that the student needs to learn in the chapters that follow. These Core Concepts Grids play an integral part in linking the textbook and several of its companion publications.

Unit 1, Health Promotion and Illness, lays the foundation for the health care concepts incorporated throughout the text. Unit 2 covers important biopsychosocial concepts related to health care, including pain and rehabilitation. In addition to the new chapters on culture and substance abuse, Chapter 7 now reflects the emerging view of pain as the "fifth vital sign," and Chapter 9 has been revised to focus on end-of-life care. Unit 3 consists of six chapters on the management of clients with fluid, electrolyte, and acid-base imbalances. This unit now includes an expanded chapter on infusion therapy (Chapter 14).

Unit 4 presents the perioperative nursing content that medical-surgical nurses need to know. This content provides a solid foundation to help the student better understand the specific surgeries covered throughout the remainder of the text. Unit 5 provides core content on health problems related to immune system function. This content includes normal inflammation and the immune response, altered cell growth and cancer development, and interventions for clients with connective tissue disease, HIV infection, and other immunologic disorders, cancers, and infections. A new chapter (Chapter 23) focuses on interventions for clients with immune function excess (hypersensitivity and autoimmunity).

The remaining 11 units cover medical-surgical content by body system. Each of these units begins with an Assessment chapter and continues with one or more Interventions chapters for clients with specific health problems in that body system.

MULTINATIONAL, MULTICULTURAL, MULTIGENERATIONAL FOCUS

To reflect the increasing diversity of our society, *Medical-Surgical Nursing: Critical Thinking for Collaborative Care* takes a multinational, multicultural, and multigenerational focus. Addressing the needs of both U.S. and Canadian readers, we have included examples of trade names of drugs available in the United States and those available in Canada. A maple leaf icon (✦) identifies the Canadian trade names.

To help nurses provide quality care for clients whose cultural background differs from their own, numerous Cultural Considerations boxes highlight important aspects of culturally competent care throughout the text. A new introductory chapter on the cultural aspects of health (Chapter 6) is also included in this edition. Also new to this edition and located inside the back cover is an innovative Communication Quick Reference for Spanish-Speaking Clients. This Quick Reference helps ensure clear communication between native English speakers and the rapidly growing population of Spanish-speaking people.

Increases in life expectancy and the "graying" of the baby-boom generation add up to a steadily increasing older adult population. To help equip nurses for this challenge, the fourth edition features expanded coverage of the care of older adults. It includes a greater number of Nursing Focus on the Older Adult charts and highlights laboratory values and drug dosages typical for older clients. Charts specifying normal physiologic changes to expect in the older population are included in each Assessment chapter. In addition, Considerations for Older Adults boxes are highlighted throughout the text to emphasize key points to keep in mind when caring for these clients.

Also appearing throughout the text are Women's Health Considerations boxes, which address topics of concern to female clients and their health care providers. These in-text highlights alert the reader to gender-related differences in assessment parameters and in the incidence, severity, and treatment of common health problems.

ADDITIONAL PEDAGOGIC FEATURES

The fourth edition includes a wealth of pedagogic features to help the student quickly identify and understand key information and to serve as study aids:

- Written in "client-friendly" language, Client Education Guide charts provide the types of instructions that nurses must learn to provide to clients and their families to help them cope with life changes caused by illness.
- Laboratory Profile charts summarize important information on laboratory tests commonly ordered to evaluate health problems. Information typically includes normal ranges of laboratory values (including differences for older adults,

when appropriate) and the possible significance of abnormal findings.
- Drug Therapy charts summarize important information about commonly used drugs. These charts include both U.S. and Canadian trade names, usual dosages (including dosages for older clients, as appropriate), and nursing interventions with rationales.
- Key Features charts highlight the clinical manifestations of important disorders.
- Evidence-Based Practice for Nursing boxes, provided in nearly every chapter, give synopses of recent nursing research articles and other scientific articles applicable to nursing. Each box provides a summary of the article, a brief critique, and a summary of implications for nursing practice. The goal of this feature is to help students identify the strengths and weaknesses of the research and see how research can help guide nursing practice.
- Client Care Plans and Clinical Pathways—although declining somewhat in importance in today's streamlined health care environment—remain significant tools with which the student nurse must be familiar. The fourth edition therefore includes selected examples of these care planning tools. Client Care Plans now include a distinctive icon to signal tasks that can be delegated to assistive nursing personnel.
- Focused Assessment charts serve as a convenient summary of essential assessment points for selected conditions.
- Assessment Using Gordon's Functional Health Patterns charts provide a convenient one-stop list of relevant questions to ask clients regarding the impact of health conditions on everyday function.
- Meeting Healthy People 2010 Objectives boxes suggest specific activities that nurses can undertake to promote achievement of the specific numbered objectives of the Healthy People 2010 program.
- Cost of Care: Implications for Nursing boxes provide an important financial context for medical-surgical nursing, in which nurses must increasingly understand cost factors in order to help clients work toward wellness despite financial limitations.
- Legal/Ethical Issues in Health Care boxes introduce students to some of the dilemmas they will face in the increasingly high-tech world of medical-surgical nursing.
- To help students keep pace with the constantly changing landscape of health care, each chapter concludes with a link to Online Resources—including Suggested Readings and Internet Resources—found on the book's companion SIMON website.

AN INTEGRATED MULTIMEDIA RESOURCE BASED ON PROVEN LEARNING STRATEGIES

Medical-Surgical Nursing: Critical Thinking for Collaborative Care, 4th edition, is more than a web-linked textbook. It is the hub of a comprehensive package of electronic and print publications that break new ground in the application of proven learning strategies and evidence-based educational practice. This integrated multimedia resource actively engages the student in problem-solving and critical thinking. Every effort has been made to correlate content among the text and its companion publications and to focus the content on the Core Concepts Grids developed specifically for this purpose. Unlike many textbook authors, we have personally been involved in the development of each of the companion publications to ensure consistency and cohesion between the textbook and the companion publications.

RESOURCES FOR INSTRUCTORS

Resources for instructors include an Instructor's Manual, a Test Bank, and a LectureView Image/Slide Collection.

The Instructor's Manual, written by Susan Behmke, Sharon Souter, and Donna D. Ignatavicius, continues to be a groundbreaking educational ancillary. It provides content on how to promote collaborative or cooperative learning with features never before presented in any comparable instructor's manual. It includes critical learning outcomes, suggested learning activities, and a list of supplemental resources arranged in a practical three-column format. Learning activities that involve group work are included, as are time frames for learning and strategies for promoting active learning, including aspects of teaching/learning via distance education. Supplemental resources, which foster independent exploration, include transparency masters, Internet resources, and materials from community organizations. Numerous graphic organizers—including concept maps, algorithms, team concept maps, and sequence chains—are provided to help faculty to teach students how to make connections among isolated pieces of information and to encourage them to assemble the puzzle of today's complex health care system. The focus of content is on the Core Concepts Grids, which are provided for each unit and serve as content organizers for the teaching strategies and learning activities that follow.

A high-caliber Test Bank—delivered on CD-ROM together with the LectureView—provides instructors with more than 2000 test questions. Of these 2000 questions, 900 are completely new for this edition, and each question is coded for Correct Answer, Rationale, Cognitive Type, NCLEX Client Needs Category, and Nursing Process Step. The questions, prepared by M. Linda Workman and Constance Visovsky, have been written in response to feedback from faculty to be both more challenging and more reflective of the scope of questions on the NCLEX examination. Most are application-based questions, and only about 10% are knowledge- or comprehension-level questions. Questions were written focusing on the Core Concepts Grids presented in the *Instructor's Manual,* the *Critical Thinking Study Guide,* and the textbook.

LectureView is a CD-ROM lecture resource that includes 400 full-color images from the text along with 480 text slides for projection in the classroom. This PowerPoint-compatible ancillary allows instructors to prepare customized lecture presentations with ease using their own PowerPoint software.

RESOURCES FOR STUDENTS

Resources for students include the Critical Thinking Study Guide, the Clinical Companion, and the new Virtual Clinical Excursions workbook/CD-ROM.

The newly redesigned and reformatted *Critical Thinking Study Guide* provides material to enhance learning to promote mastery of the text. Echoing one of the text's core themes, the study guide emphasizes questions aimed at *enhancing critical thinking skills.* The study guide was written by a team of authors, led by Carol Dignon, in conjunction with the *Instructor's Manual* to ensure consistency. As with the *Instructor's Manual,* its focus is on the Core Concepts Grids, which are included in the *Critical Thinking Study Guide* to help students internalize the textbook material.

The pocket-sized *Clinical Companion,* authored by Kathy Hausman with Donna D. Ignatavicius, retains the alphabetical organization that proved so popular in the first three editions. Its newly streamlined format makes it easy to find essential information in seconds. The *Clinical Companion* is a pocket-sized "Iggy" written for students going into clinicals by an author who actively supervises clinicals and who knows first-hand what students in clinicals are being asked to know about their clients.

An exciting addition to the ancillary package for this edition—and a groundbreaking learning tool in its own right—is the *Virtual Clinical Excursions* workbook/CD-ROM package. This package guides the student through a computer-generated virtual clinical environment and helps the student apply textbook content to "virtual clients" in that environment. The clinical simulations and workbook, the latter authored by Elaine Kennedy, represent the next generation of research-based learning tools that promote critical thinking and meaningful learning.

For more information on any of these innovative companion publications, contact your Harcourt Health Sciences sales representative, visit http://www.harcourthealth.com/, or call Harcourt Health Sciences Faculty Support at 1-800-222-9570.

• • •

In summary, *Medical-Surgical Nursing: Critical Thinking for Collaborative Care,* 4th edition, together with its fully integrated multimedia ancillary package, provides the tools you will need to meet the challenge of nursing in the first decade of the 21st century and beyond. The only elements that remain to be added to this package are those that you alone can provide—your diligence, your commitment, your innovation, *your nursing care.*

Donna D. Ignatavicius
M. Linda Workman

Acknowledgments

Publishing a textbook of this depth and breadth would not be possible without the combined efforts of many people. Our contributing authors once again provided consistently excellent manuscripts in a timely fashion. Our reviewers—expert clinicians and instructors from around the United States and Canada—provided invaluable suggestions and encouragement throughout the book's development.

The staff of W.B. Saunders/Harcourt Health Sciences once again provided us with crucial guidance and support throughout the planning, writing, revision, and production of the fourth edition. In particular, Executive Editor Robin Carter and Developmental Editor Jeanne Allison worked closely with us in the early stages of this edition to help us hone and focus our revision plan. Jeanne Allison and Managing Editor Lee Henderson then worked with us step by step—with wise insights from Robin Carter—to bring the fourth edition from vision to publication. Special thanks to Senior Editor's Assistant Marie Thomas, who handled the countless administrative details associated with a project of this size. She is without peer among editorial assistants.

Project Specialist Jodi Willard was a joy to work with. Her attention to detail, flexibility, and conscientiousness not only helped to make this edition the most consistently readable ever, but also made the entire production process incredibly smooth and headache-free. Thanks, too, to Copyeditor Judi Bange, who worked closely with Jodi in copyediting the entire text and supported Jodi's own work with diligence and painstaking attention to detail.

Special thanks also to Project Manager Debbie Vogel. Debbie's quiet leadership and personal commitment to the project were exemplary. Without fail, she exercised her role as collaborator and problem solver to help bring this edition to publication precisely on schedule.

Designer Teresa Breckwoldt worked tirelessly and with good humor to create a completely new interior design for this edition. Her sophisticated design treatment of this edition is easy on the eye—making long study sessions more tolerable—and it brings into appropriately sharp focus those pedagogic elements that required a distinctive look.

Thanks also to Donna Macaluso of MacArt Design and to photographer Rick Brady, whose full-color illustrations and photographs play an important part in conveying the content and context of medical-surgical nursing in the new millennium.

Our acknowledgments would not be complete without recognizing Joyce Owen, Teresa Hajdu, and other key members of the Sales and Marketing staff who helped to put this book into your hands.

Finally, we wish to thank Vice President and Nursing Editorial Director Sally Schrefer. Sally's personal leadership style creates a unique publishing environment in which authors and editors have the freedom to interact creatively to produce the best books in the field.

Donna D. Ignatavicius
M. Linda Workman

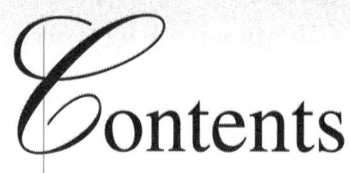

Contents

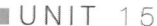

Guide to Special Features

EVIDENCE-BASED PRACTICE FOR NURSING

FOCUSED ASSESSMENT of

$\mathcal{L}$EGAL/$\mathcal{E}$THICAL $\mathcal{I}$SSUES IN HEALTH CARE

$\mathcal{M}$EETING HEALTHY PEOPLE 2010 OBJECTIVES

 INTERVENTION ACTIVITIES *for*

NURSING FOCUS *on the* OLDER ADULT

PROBLEMS OF SENSATION

Management of Clients with Problems of the Sensory System

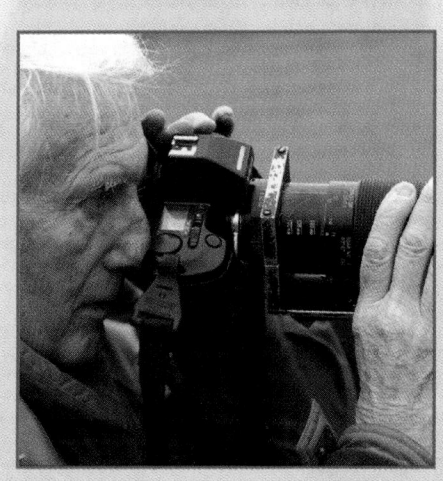

UNIT 10 — PROBLEMS OF SENSATION: EYES AND EARS ■ Core Concepts Grid

Anatomy	Physiology	Pathophysiology	History	Physical Exam	Diagnostic Tests	Interventions	Pharmacology
Cranial nerves Optic (II) Oculomotor (III) Trochlear (IV) Trigeminal (V) Abducens (VI) Facial (VII) Vestibulo-cochlear (VIII) **Ears** External canal Tympanic membrane Middle ear Ossicles Eustachian tube Inner ear Semicircular canals Cochlea Endolymph Perilymph Organ of Corti **Eyes** Eyelids/eyeballs Conjunctiva Lacrimal glands Cornea Uvea Iris/lens/retina Canal of Schlemm Aqueous/vitreous humor	• **Sound transmission** • **Light transmission** • **Color discrimination** • **Refraction** • **Accommodation** • **Coordination**	• **Inflammation** • **Obstruction** • **Tinnitus** • **Vertigo** • **Dizziness** • **Hearing loss** • **Hyperopia** • **Myopia** • **Astigmatism** • **Increased intraocular pressure (IOP)** • **Opacity of lens** • **Retinal detachment** • **Hemorrhage** • **Vision loss**	• **Client past medical history** Systemic medical conditions Past injuries • **Family history** • **Social history** Medications Occupation Gender Diet history Leisure activities Age	**Ear** Otoscopic examination Light reflex Voice test Watch test Tuning fork Rinne test Weber test **Eye** Exophthalmos Ptosis Scleral color Anisocoria Pupillary reaction Snellen chart Visual fields Jaeger card Six cardinal positions of gaze Corneal light reflex Cover/uncover test	• **Cultures** • **Computed tomography (CT)** • **Audiometry** Bone conduction Pure tone Speech • **Tympanometry** • **Slit-lamp examination** • **Corneal staining** • **Tonometry** • **Ophthalmoscopy** • **Gonioscopy**	• **Ear medication installations** • **Removal of cerumen** • **Removal of foreign objects from ear canal** • **Ear medication installation** • **Care for the deaf** • **Communication with the deaf** Signing Speech reading • **Eye care** Eye glasses Artificial eyes Contact lenses • **Care for the blind** • **Communication with the blind** Clock TTY Braille	• **Systemic antibiotics** • **Ear medications** Antibiotic Antifungal Anti-inflammatory • **Antivertigo agents** • **Antiemetics** • **Artificial tears** • **Eye medications** Antibiotic Antifungal Anti-inflammatory • **Midriatics** • **Miotics** Beta blockers Pilocarpine Carbonic anhydrase inhibitors

Assessment of the Eye and Vision

M. LINDA WORKMAN

Learning Objectives

After studying this chapter, you should be able to:

1. Explain the concept of refraction in relation to how the cornea, lens, aqueous humor, and vitreous humor contribute to vision.
2. Describe age-related changes in the eye, eyelids, and vision.
3. List five systemic disorders that have an impact on the eye and vision.
4. Discuss which elements of a client's history might predict visual impairment later in life.
5. Discuss the educational needs of a client undergoing fluorescein angiography.
6. Explain the relationship between intraocular pressure and eye health.
7. Use proper technique to instill eyedrops.

SIMON

Go to http://www.wbsaunders.com/SIMON/Iggy/ for self-assessment questions related to these Learning Objectives.

Many people consider vision to be their most important sense and the major way to communicate with the world. Vision begins with the eye and is fully perceived in the brain. Many conditions can affect the eye and alter vision temporarily or permanently. Changes in the eye and vision can provide important data regarding the client's general health status and the problems that might be encountered in self-care.

ANATOMY AND PHYSIOLOGY REVIEW

Structure

The eyeball, a ball-shaped or spherical organ about 2.5 cm in length and 2.3 cm in diameter, is located in the anterior portion of the orbit. The **orbit** is the bony socket of the skull that surrounds and protects the eye and the attached muscles, nerves, vessels, and tear-producing glands.

LAYERS OF THE EYEBALL

The eye has three layers, or coats (Figure 46-1). The external layer is the **sclera** (the opaque tissue making up the "whites" of the eye) and the transparent cornea on the front of the eye.

The middle layer, or **uvea,** is heavily pigmented. This layer consists of the choroid, the ciliary body, and the iris. The **choroid,** a dark brown membrane between the sclera and the retina, lines most of the sclera. The choroid has many blood vessels that supply nutrients to the retina.

The **ciliary body** connects the choroid with the iris and secretes **aqueous humor.** The **iris** is the colored portion of the external eye; its center opening is the **pupil.** The muscles of the iris contract and relax to control pupil size and the amount of light entering the eye.

The innermost layer is the **retina,** a thin, delicate structure through which the sensory fibers that transmit impulses to the optic nerve are distributed. The retina contains blood vessels and two types of photoreceptors called **rods** and **cones.** The rods work at low levels of light and provide peripheral vision. The cones are active at bright levels of light and provide color and central vision.

The **optic fundus** is the area at the inside back of the eye that can be seen with an ophthalmoscope. This area contains the **optic disk,** a creamy pink to white depressed area in the retina (Figure 46-2). The optic nerve enters the eyeball at this point. The optic disk is sometimes called the **blind spot** because it contains only nerve fibers and no photoreceptor cells. To one side of the optic disk is a small, yellowish-pink area called the **macula lutea.** The center of the macula is the **fovea centralis,** where vision is the most acute.

REFRACTIVE STRUCTURES AND MEDIA

Light waves pass through the following structures on the way to the retina: cornea, aqueous humor, lens, and vitreous humor. Each of these structures has a different density, which causes the light waves to bend, or **refract,** to some degree and focus images on the retina. These structures are the **refracting media** of the eye.

The **cornea** is the clear layer that forms the external coat on the front of the eye (see Figure 46-1). The **aqueous humor** is a clear, watery fluid that fills the anterior and posterior chambers of the eye. Aqueous humor is continually produced

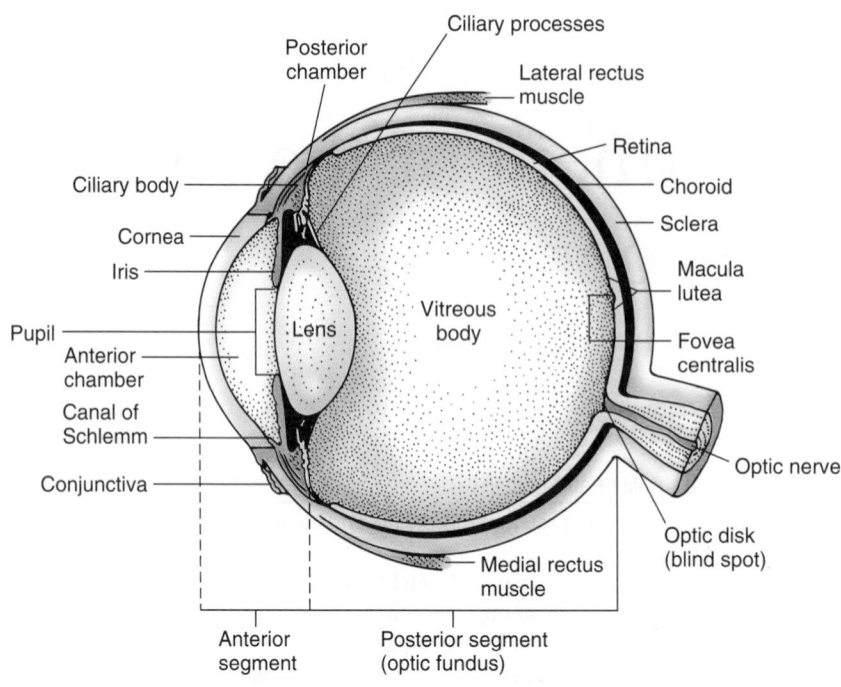

Figure 46-1 ● Anatomic features of the eye.

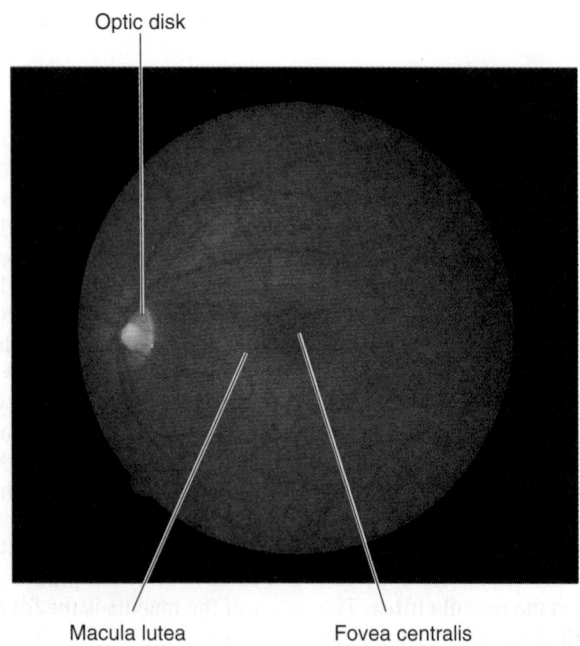

Figure 46-2 ● A normal optic fundus.

by the ciliary processes and passes from the posterior chamber, through the pupil, and into the anterior chamber. This fluid drains through the **canal of Schlemm** into the blood to maintain a balanced intraocular pressure (IOP, or the pressure within the eye).

The **lens** is a circular, convex structure that lies behind the iris and in front of the vitreous body. It is normally transparent. The lens bends the rays of light entering through the pupil so they focus properly on the retina. The curve of the lens changes to focus on near or distant objects.

The **vitreous body** is a gelatinous substance that fills the vitreous chamber (the space between the lens and the retina). This gelatin-like body transmits light and shapes the eye.

■ EXTERNAL STRUCTURES

The eyelids are thin, movable folds of skin that protect the eyes, shut out light during sleep, and keep the cornea moist. The upper eyelid is larger than the lower one. The **canthus** is the place at which the two eyelids meet at the corner of the eye.

The **conjunctivae** are the mucous membranes of the eye. The **palpebral conjunctiva** is a thick, vascular membrane that lines the under surface of each eyelid. Located over the sclera is the thin, transparent **bulbar conjunctiva.**

Tears are produced by a small **lacrimal gland,** which is located in the upper outer part of each orbit (Figure 46-3). Tears flow across the front of the eye, toward the nose, and into the inner canthus. They drain out through the **punctum** (found at the nasal side of the lid edges), into the **lacrimal duct** and **sac,** and then into the nose through the nasolacrimal duct.

■ MUSCLES

Six voluntary muscles rotate the eye and coordinate eye movements (Figure 46-4). Table 46-1 summarizes the functions of these muscles. Coordinated eye movements ensure that the retina of each eye receives an image at the same time so only a single image is seen.

■ NERVES

The extraocular muscles are innervated by the following cranial nerves: oculomotor (cranial nerve III), trochlear (cranial nerve IV), and abducens (cranial nerve VI). The **optic nerve** (cranial nerve II) is the nerve of sight, connecting the optic

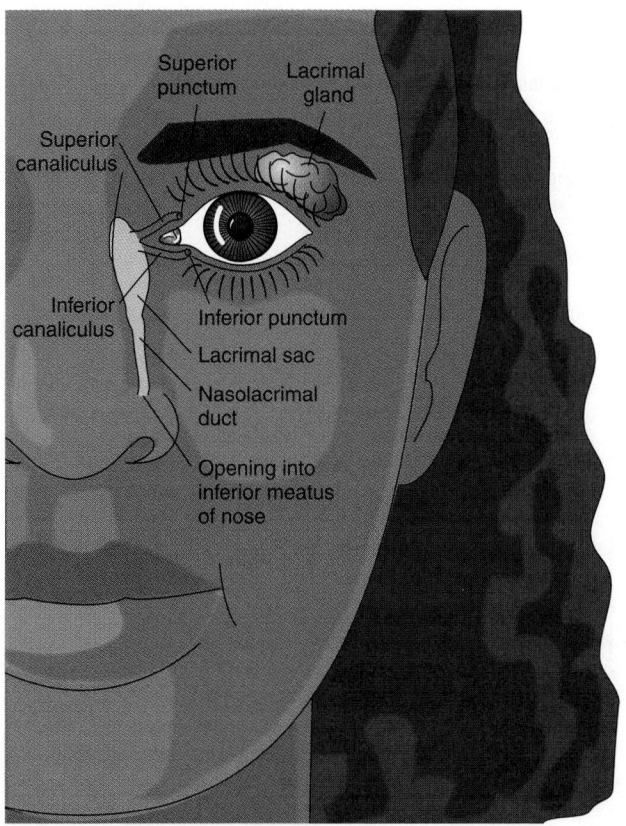

Figure 46-3 ● Anterior view of the eye and adjacent struc-

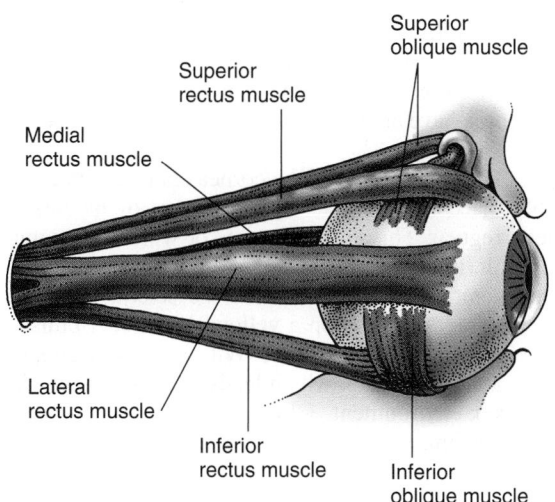

Figure 46-4 ● The extraocular muscles.

disk to the brain. Part of the trigeminal nerve (cranial nerve V) causes the sensory portion of the blink reflex and is stimulated when the cornea is touched. The facial nerve (cranial nerve VII) innervates the lacrimal glands and muscles controlling lid closure.

BLOOD VESSELS

The ophthalmic artery brings oxygenated blood to the structures in the orbit. This artery branches to supply blood to the

TABLE 46-1 • FUNCTIONS OF OCULAR MUSCLES
SUPERIOR RECTUS MUSCLE   • Together with the lateral rectus, this muscle moves the eye diagonally upward toward the side of the head.   • Together with the medial rectus, this muscle moves the eye diagonally upward toward the middle of the head.   **LATERAL RECTUS MUSCLE**   • Together with the medial rectus, contraction of this muscle holds the eye in a straight position.   • Contracting alone, this muscle turns the eye toward the side of the head.   **MEDIAL RECTUS MUSCLE**   • Contracting alone, this muscle turns the eye toward the nose.   **INFERIOR RECTUS MUSCLE**   • Together with the lateral rectus, this muscle moves the eye diagonally downward toward the side of the head.   • Together with the medial rectus, this muscle moves the eye diagonally downward toward the middle of the head.   **SUPERIOR OBLIQUE MUSCLE**   • Contraction pulls the eye downward.   **INFERIOR OBLIQUE MUSCLE**   • Contraction pulls the eye upward.

retina. The ciliary arteries supply the sclera, choroid, ciliary body, and iris. Venous drainage is through the two ophthalmic veins.

Function

Three functions of the eye provide clear images of near and far objects: refraction, pupillary constriction, and accommodation.

REFRACTION

The different curved surfaces and refractive media of the eye allow light to pass through to the retina. Each surface and media bends (refracts) light differently to focus an image on the retina. **Emmetropia** is the ideal refraction of the eye: with the lens at rest, light rays from a distant source (6 m or more) are focused into a sharp image on the retina. Figure 46-5 shows the normal refraction of light within the eye. Images fall on the retina inverted and reversed left to right. For example, an object in the lower nasal visual field strikes the upper outer area of the retina.

Errors of refraction are common. **Hyperopia** (also called hypermetropia or farsightedness) is a condition in which the eye does not refract light enough. As a result, images actually fall (converge) behind the retina (see Figure 46-5). Vision beyond 20 feet is normal, but near vision is poor. Hyperopia is corrected with a convex lens in eyeglasses or contact lenses.

Myopia (nearsightedness) is a condition in which the eye overrefracts or overbends the light. As a result, images are focused in front of the retina (see Figure 46-5). Near vision is normal, but distance vision is poor. Myopia is corrected with a biconcave lens in eyeglasses or contact lenses.

Astigmatism is a refractive error caused by unevenly curved surfaces on or in the eye, which results in visual distortion. Astigmatism is usually caused by uneven corneal surfaces.

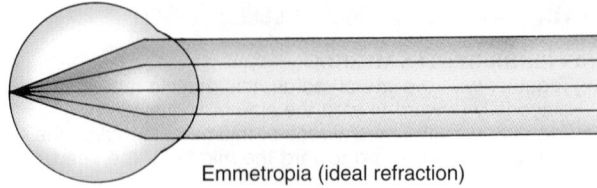

Emmetropia (ideal refraction)

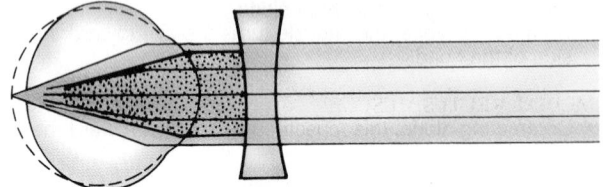

Hyperopia (hypermetropia, or farsightedness)

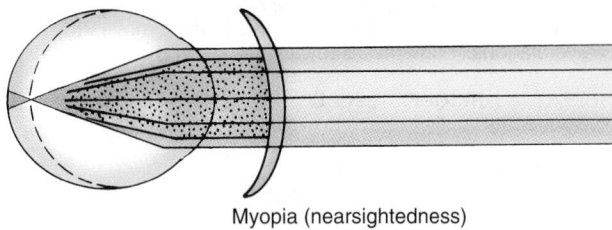

Myopia (nearsightedness)

Figure 46-5 ● Refraction and correction in emmetropia, hyperopia, and myopia.

■ PUPILLARY CONSTRICTION

The pupil controls the amount of light that enters the eye. If the level of light to one or both eyes is increased, both pupils constrict (become smaller). The amount of constriction depends on how much light is available and how well the retina can adapt to light changes. Pupillary constriction is called **miosis,** and pupillary dilation is called **mydriasis.** Medications can alter pupillary constriction.

■ ACCOMMODATION

The healthy eye can focus sharp images on the retina whether the image is close to the eye or more distant. The process of maintaining a clear visual image when the gaze is shifted from a distant to a near object is known as **accommodation.** The eye is able to adjust its focus by changing the curve of the lens.

■ Eye Changes Associated with Aging

Changes directly within the eye cause visual acuity to decrease with age. Age-related changes within the nervous system and in the structures supporting the eye also contribute to decreasing visual function (Chart 46-1).

■ AGE-ASSOCIATED STRUCTURAL CHANGES

In the older adult, decreased eye muscle tone reduces the ability to maintain an upward gaze and to keep focused on a single object. The lower eyelid may relax and fall away from the eye **(ectropion),** exposing more of the eye and leading to dry eye symptoms.

CHART 46-1

nursing focus *on the* **Older adult**
Changes in the Eye Related to Aging

Structure/Function	Change
Appearance	Eyes appear to be sunken. Arcus senilis forms. Sclera yellows.
Cornea	Cornea flattens, which causes blurring of vision.
Ocular muscles	Muscle strength is reduced, which results in a diminished capacity to maintain an upward gaze and to maintain a single image.
Lens	Elasticity is lost, which increases the near point of vision. Lens hardens and becomes compact. Cataracts form.
Iris	Decrease in ability to dilate results in small pupil size and poor adaptation to darkness.
Pupil	Pupil size is smaller. Aperture size takes longer to change, which reduces ability to see in dim light.
Color vision	Discrimination among colors of short wavelength (green, blue, violet) decreases.
Tears	Diminished tear production results in dry eyes, increasing discomfort and risk for infection.

Arcus senilis, an opaque ring formed within the circumference of the cornea, is caused by the deposition of fatty globules (Figure 46-6). Although it is very common, not all older people have arcus senilis. This condition does not affect vision.

The clarity and shape of the cornea change with age. After age 65, the cornea flattens and the curve of its surface becomes irregular. This change causes or worsens astigmatism. As a result, images are distorted and blurred.

Degenerative changes occur in the sclera; fatty deposits cause the sclera to develop a yellowish tinge. A bluish color may be noted as the sclera thins. With increasing age, the iris has less ability to dilate, which leads to difficulty in adapting to a darker environment. Older adults may need additional light for reading.

■ AGE-ASSOCIATED FUNCTIONAL CHANGES

The lens yellows with aging, which affects the ability of the eye to transmit and focus light. The aging lens hardens, shrinks, and loses elasticity. As the lens loses elasticity, the ability of the eye to accommodate is gradually lost. The **near point of vision** (the closest distance at which the eye can see an object clearly) increases. Near objects (especially reading material) must be placed farther from the eye to be seen clearly. This age-related change is called **presbyopia.** In addition, the **far point** (farthest point at which an object can be distinguished) decreases. Thus the older person has a narrower visual field.

As a person ages, general color sensitivity decreases, as does discrimination among the colors of green, blue, and vio-

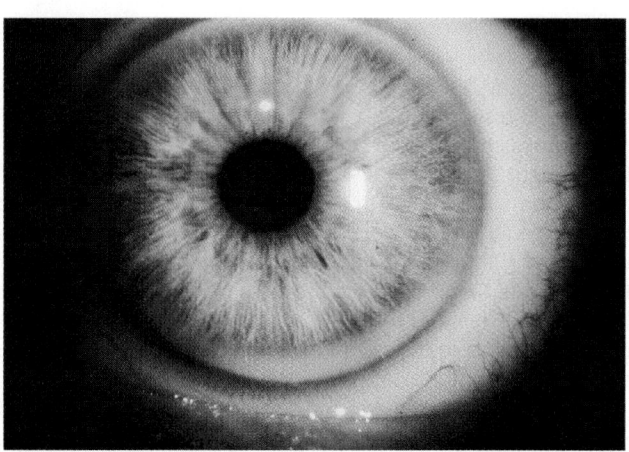

Figure 46-6   ● Arcus senilis of the iris.

let. More light is needed to stimulate the visual receptors. Intraocular pressure (IOP) is slightly higher in older than in younger adults.

ASSESSMENT TECHNIQUES

History

The nurse collects subjective information from the client to determine whether problems with the eye or vision have an impact on daily functioning. Chart 46-2 suggests some questions to ask when assessing eye and vision history.

■ DEMOGRAPHIC DATA

Age is an important factor to consider when assessing the visual processes and eye structure. The incidence of glaucoma and cataract formation increases with aging. Presbyopia commonly begins in the 40s.

Gender also may be important. For example, retinal detachments are more common in men, and dry eye symptoms are more common in women.

■ PERSONAL AND FAMILY HISTORY

The nurse asks the client about a family history of eye problems. Some conditions, such as a refractive error, show a familial tendency. The nurse also asks about any systemic medical conditions that could have ocular involvement or cause complications (Table 46-2).

The client is asked about past accidents, injuries, surgeries, or blows to the head that may have led to the present problem. The nurse asks specifically about previous laser surgeries, because clients often do not classify laser treatment as surgery. The nurse asks about the types of sports the client plays; some injuries are more common to specific sports.

The client is asked about medications, particularly decongestants and antihistamines. The ocular effects of these drugs are well documented. Many clients do not consider over-the-counter eyedrops to be medication. The name, strength, dose, and scheduling for all ophthalmic medications are recorded. Many systemic drugs can cause eye disturbances (see Table 46-2). Clinical manifestations of ocular drug effects include

TABLE 46-2 ● EXTRAOCULAR CONDITIONS AFFECTING THE EYE AND VISION	
SYSTEMIC DISORDERS	**DRUGS**
• Diabetes mellitus	• Antihistamines
• Hypertension	• Decongestants
• Lupus erythematosus	• Antibiotics
• Sarcoidosis	• Opioids
• Thyroid dysfunction	• Anticholinergics
• Acquired immunodeficiency syndrome	• Cholinergic agonists
• Cardiac disease	• Sympathomimetics
• Multiple sclerosis	• Oral contraceptives
	• Antineoplastic agents
	• Corticosteroids
	• Carbonic anhydrase inhibitors
	• Beta blockers

pruritus (itching), foreign body sensation, redness, tearing, sensitivity to light **(photophobia),** and the development of cataracts or glaucoma.

■ DIET HISTORY

Because some ocular problems are caused by or made worse with vitamin deficiencies, the nurse asks the client about his or her food choices. For example, vitamin A deficiency can cause conjunctival dryness, keratomalacia, and blindness.

■ SOCIOECONOMIC STATUS

The nurse asks the client about his or her work and specifically how the eyes are used. In some occupations, such as computer programming, constant exposure to monitor screens may lead to eyestrain and the need for eyeglasses. Machine operators are at risk for eye injury because of the high speeds at which particles can be thrown at the eye. The client who works in industrial settings is asked about the use of protective eyewear, such as goggles. Chronic exposure to infrared or ultraviolet light may cause photophobia and cataract formation.

■ CURRENT HEALTH PROBLEMS

The nurse asks the client about the onset of visual changes. Has the change occurred rapidly or slowly? *A client with a sudden or persistent loss of vision within the past 48 hours should be seen immediately by an ophthalmologist, as should the client experiencing trauma, a foreign body in the eye, sudden ocular pain, or sudden redness.* The client is asked whether the same symptoms are present to the same degree in both eyes.

The following questions are asked if ocular injury or eye trauma is involved:

- How long ago did the injury occur?
- What was the client doing when it happened?
- If a foreign body was involved, what was its source?
- Was any first aid administered at the scene? If so, what actions were taken?

Physical Assessment

■ INSPECTION

The nurse looks for head tilting, squinting, or other noticeable actions that offer clues to compensatory stances for attaining clear vision. For example, clients with double vision may cock the head to the side in an attempt to focus the two images into one, or they may close one eye to see more clearly.

The nurse observes for symmetry in the appearance of the eyes. The eyes are checked to determine if they are an equal distance from each other, of the same size, and of the same degree of prominence. The eyes also are assessed for their placement in the orbits and for symmetry of movement. **Exophthalmos** (proptosis) is a condition in which the eyes protrude; in **enophthalmos,** the eyeballs are sunken.

The nurse assesses the eyebrows and eyelashes for hair distribution. The direction of the eyelashes is determined. Eyelashes normally point outward and away from the eyelid. The eyelids are assessed for **ptosis** (drooping), redness, lesions, or swelling. The lids normally close completely, with the upper and lower lid edges touching. When the eyes are open, the upper lid covers a small portion of the iris. The edge of the lower lid lies below the line between the cornea and sclera. No sclera should be visible between the eyelid and the iris.

■ Scleral and Corneal Assessment

The sclera is examined for color; it is usually white. A yellow color may indicate jaundice or systemic problems. In dark-skinned people the normal sclera may appear yellow, and small, pigmented dots may be visible (Jarvis, 2000).

The nurse can best observe the cornea by directing a light at it from the side using several angles. The cornea should be transparent, smooth, shiny, and bright. Any cloudy areas or specks may be the result of accidents or injuries.

The blink reflex is assessed by bringing a fist quickly toward the client's face; clients with vision will blink. Alternatively, a syringe full of air can be expelled toward the eyes. The client blinks if the reflex is intact.

■ Pupillary Assessment

The pupils are usually round and of equal size. Approximately 5% of people normally have a slight but noticeable difference in the size of their pupils (**anisocoria**). Pupil size varies in people exposed to the same amount of light. Pupils are smaller in older adults. People with myopia have larger pupils; people with hyperopia have smaller pupils. The normal pupil diameter is between 3 and 5 mm.

The nurse observes the pupils for their response to light. Increasing light causes pupillary constriction, whereas decreasing light causes dilation. Constriction of both pupils is the normal response to direct light. Pupils also constrict in response to accommodation. The nurse assesses pupillary reaction to light by asking the client to look straight ahead while quickly bringing the beam of a penlight in from the side and directing it at the right (**oculus dexter [OD]**) pupil. Constriction of the right pupil is a direct response to shining the penlight into that eye. Constriction of the left (**oculus sinister [OS]**) pupil when light is shined at the right pupil is known as a **consensual response.** Direct and consensual responses are assessed for each eye.

Each pupil is evaluated for speed of reaction. The pupil should immediately constrict when a light is directed at it. This rapid response is termed **brisk.** If the pupil takes more than 1 second to constrict, the response is termed **sluggish.** Pupils that fail to react are termed **nonreactive** or **fixed.** The reactivity speed of right and left pupils is compared, and any discrepancy is noted.

In assessing for accommodation, the nurse holds the index finger about 18 cm from the client's nose and moves it toward the nose. The client's eyes normally converge during this movement, and the pupils constrict equally. When accommodation stops, the pupils begin to enlarge and return to their normal size.

■ MEASUREMENT OF VISION

Vision is measured by various tests. Each eye is tested separately, and then both eyes are tested together. Clients who routinely wear corrective lenses are tested both without and with their corrective lenses.

■ Acuity

Visual acuity tests measure both distance and near vision. The Snellen chart, or "eye chart," is a simple tool to measure distance vision. This chart has letters, numbers, pictures, or a single letter presented in various positions (Figure 46-7). The client stands 20 feet from the chart, covers one eye, and uses the other eye to read the line that appears most clear. If the client can do this accurately, he or she is asked to read the next lower line. This sequence is repeated to the last line on which the client can correctly identify most characters. The procedure is repeated for the other eye. Findings are recorded as a comparison between what the client can read at 20 feet and the distance at which a person with normal vision can read the same line. For example, 20/50 means that the client is able to see at 20 feet from the chart what a "healthy eye" can see at 50 feet.

For clients who are in a confined space that does not permit a 20-foot distance to the eye chart or who cannot see the 20/400 character, visual acuity is assessed by holding fingers in front of their eyes and asking them to count (Figure 46-8). This procedure is repeated five times. Acuity is recorded as "count fingers vision at 5 feet," or the farthest distance at which the client can count the fingers correctly.

Clients who cannot count fingers are tested for **hand motion (HM) acuity.** The nurse stands about 2 to 3 feet in front of the client. The eye not being tested is covered. A light is directed onto the hand from behind the client. The nurse demonstrates the three possible directions in which the hand can move during the test (stationary, left-right, or up-down).

LETTER CHART FOR 20 FEET
Snellen Scale

E — 200 ft

H N — 100 ft

D F N — 70 ft

P T X Z — 50 ft

U Z D T F — 40 ft

D F N P T H — 30 ft

P H U N T D Z — 20 ft

N P X T Z F H — 15 ft

Figure 46-7 ● A typical Snellen chart. (Courtesy National Society to Prevent Blindness, Schaumburg, IL.)

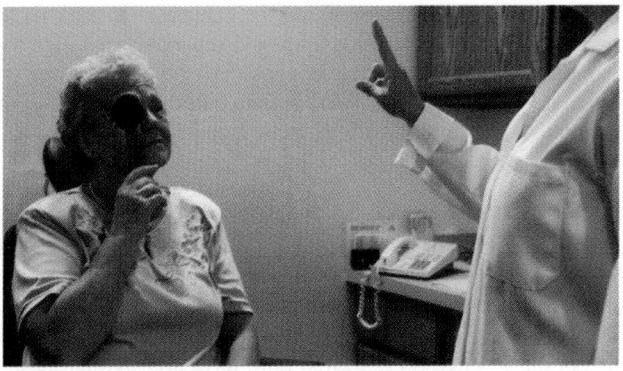

Figure 46-8 ● Client counting fingers during determination of visual acuity.

The nurse moves the hand slowly (1 second per motion) and asks the client, "What is my hand doing now?" This procedure is repeated at least five times. Visual acuity is recorded as HM at the farthest distance at which the client correctly identifies most of the hand motions.

If the client cannot detect hand movement, the nurse tests acuity by measuring **light perception (LP).** The client is first asked to cover the left eye (OS). In a darkened room, the beam of a penlight is directed at the right eye (OD) from a distance of 2 to 3 feet for 1 to 2 seconds. Clients are instructed to say "on" when the beam of light is perceived and "off" when it is no longer detected. This procedure is repeated five times. If the client identifies the presence or absence of light three times correctly, acuity is recorded as LP.

■ Near-Vision Testing

Near vision is tested for clients who have difficulty reading and in clients older than 40 years of age. The nurse uses a small, handheld Snellen chart called a Jaeger card (Figure 46-9) or a Rosenbaum Pocket Vision Screener. The client holds the card

ROSENBAUM POCKET VISION SCREENER

					Point	Jaeger	distance equivalent
95							20/800
874							20/400
2843					26	16	20/200
638	E Ш Ǝ	X O O			14	10	20/100
8745	Ǝ M Ш	O X O			10	7	20/70
63925	M E Ǝ	X O X			8	5	20/50
428365	Ш E M	O X O			6	3	20/40
374258	Ǝ Ш Ǝ	X X O			5	2	20/30
937826	Ш M E	X O O			4	1	20/25
428739	E Ш M	O O X			3	1+	20/20

Card is held in good light 14 inches from eye. Record vision for each eye separately with and without glasses. Presbyopic patients should read thru bifocal segment. Check myopes with glasses only.

DESIGN COURTESY J. G. ROSENBAUM, M.D., CLEVELAND, OHIO

PUPIL GAUGE (mm.)

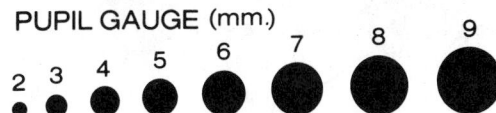

2 3 4 5 6 7 8 9

Figure 46-9 ● A typical Jaeger card. (Courtesy of SMP Division, Cooper Laboratories [P.R.], San German, Puerto Rico.)

14 inches away from the eyes, and the nurse asks him or her to read the characters. The eyes are tested separately and then together. The nurse records the Jaeger value of the lowest line on which the client can identify more than half the characters. For example, acuity might read "J2 at 14 inches."

Assessment of Visual Fields

A **confrontation test** is used to examine the client's visual fields, or peripheral vision. During the test, the nurse and the client sit facing each other and look directly into each other's eyes. The nurse covers his or her right eye (OD) and the client covers the left eye (OS) so that both have approximately the same visual field. The nurse moves a finger or an object from a nonvisible area into the client's line of vision.

This test provides only a crude estimate of the client's visual fields but can reveal large-field defects such as **hemianopia** (blindness in one half of the field of vision), **quadrantanopia** (blindness in one fourth of the field of vision), or large **scotomas** (blind spots in the visual field).

Assessment of Extraocular Muscle Function

Assessment of extraocular muscle function includes three components: the corneal light reflex, the six cardinal positions of gaze, and the cover-uncover test. The nurse also observes for parallelism of the eyes and smoothness of ocular movements.

The corneal light reflex determines alignment of the two eyes. After asking the client to stare straight ahead, the nurse shines a penlight at both corneas from a distance of 12 to 15 inches. The bright dot of light reflected from the shiny surface of the cornea should be in a symmetric position (e.g., at the 1 o'clock position in the right eye and at the 11 o'clock position in the left eye). An asymmetric reflex indicates a deviating eye and possible muscle imbalance.

The six cardinal positions of gaze are used to assess muscle function (Figure 46-10). The eye will not turn to a particular position if the muscle is weak or if the controlling nerve is affected. The nurse asks the client to hold his or her head still and to move the eyes to follow a small object such as a pen. The nurse moves the object to the client's right (lateral), upward and right (temporal), down and right, left (lateral), upward and left (temporal), and down and left (see Figure 46-10). While the client moves the eyes to these positions, the nurse observes for parallel eye movements and any deviation of movement. **Nystagmus,** an involuntary, rhythmic, and rapid twitching of the eyeball, is a normal finding for the far lateral gaze. It may also be caused by abnormal innervation or prolonged reduced vision.

A different method of assessing muscle function is the cover-uncover test. The nurse asks the client to use both eyes to look at a specific fixed point, such as the nurse's nose. One of the client's eyes is covered with a card. The nurse observes the un-

covered eye to see if it moves to fix on the object; if the eye moves, it was not focused on the fixed point before the other eye was covered. The nurse then removes the cover and observes for any movement in the eye just uncovered. The presence and direction of any deviations of eye movement are recorded.

Assessment of Color Vision

Several methods are available for testing color vision. The most commonly used tool is the **Ishihara chart,** which shows numbers composed of dots of one color within a circle of dots of a different color (Figure 46-11). Testing each eye separately, the examiner asks the client what numbers he or she sees on the chart. The ability to read the numbers correctly depends on the normal functioning of color vision.

Psychosocial Assessment

Clients undergoing changes in visual perception may be anxious or fearful about a possible loss of vision. Clients with severe visual defects may be unable to perform normal activities of daily living and may need to change their leisure activities. The sense of dependency resulting from reduced vision can affect self-esteem. The nurse investigates the client's feelings about the visual disturbances and assesses the effectiveness of his or her coping techniques. The nurse also discusses the client's concerns with family members or significant others to determine whether support is available. The client's current knowledge and use of available services for the visually impaired are assessed.

Diagnostic Assessment
LABORATORY TESTS

Cultures and smears of corneal or conjunctival swabs and scrapings aid in the diagnosis of infections. A sample of the exudate is obtained for culture before antibiotics or topical

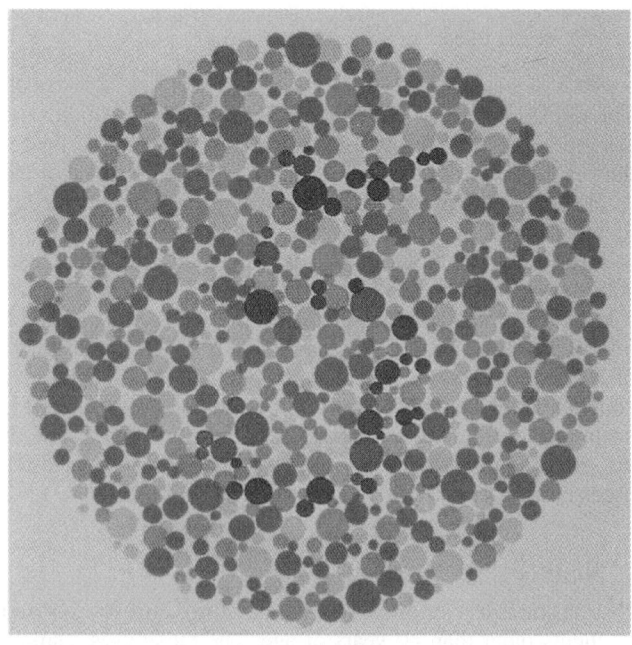

Figure 46-11 ● An Ishihara chart for testing color vision.

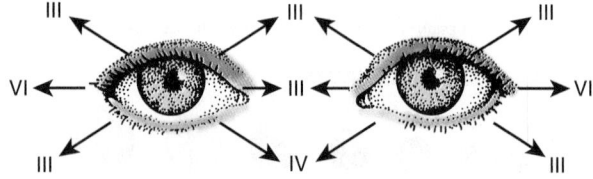

Figure 46-10 ● Checking extraocular movements in the six cardinal positions indicates the functioning of cranial nerves III, IV, and VI.

anesthetics are instilled. Swabs are taken from the conjunctivae and any ulcerated or inflamed areas.

RADIOGRAPHIC EXAMINATIONS

Computed Tomography

Computed tomography (CT) is a radiographic diagnostic method in which computers form a cross-sectional image. It is valuable in visualizing the eyes, extraocular muscles, and optic nerves. It is a sensitive method for detecting tumors in the orbital space. Data are obtained by scanning the skull and orbits with beams of low-intensity x-rays. Because contrast material is not usually administered, no special client preparation or follow-up care is required. The nurse informs the client that this test is not painful. However, the client must be positioned in a confined space and keep the head still during the procedure.

Radioisotopic Scanning

Radioisotopes are used to locate tumors and lesions in various body organs. Isotope studies differentiate an intraocular tumor from a hemorrhage, especially in the choroid layer.

CLIENT PREPARATION. After the informed consent process, the client receives a tracer dose of the radioactive isotope, either orally or by injection.

PROCEDURE. The client is asked to lie still and breathe normally. The scanner measures the radioactivity emitted by the radioactive atoms concentrated in the area being studied. Clients who are restless, anxious, or agitated may require sedation.

FOLLOW-UP CARE. The nurse assures the client that the amount of radioisotope used as a tracer is extremely small and that he or she is not radioactive. No other special follow-up care is required.

OTHER DIAGNOSTIC TESTS

A variety of techniques are used to examine specific eye structures. Such techniques are not necessary in the routine visual assessment of all people but may be indicated for those with special risks, symptoms, or exposures. Such techniques require special skill and are used only by physicians, optometrists, or advanced practice nurses.

Slit-Lamp Examination

The slit lamp permits the examination of anterior ocular structures under microscopic magnification (Figure 46-12). The client leans on a chin rest to stabilize the head. A narrow beam (slit) of light is aimed so that it brightly illuminates only a narrow segment of the eye. This technique allows the examiner to locate accurately the position of any abnormality in the cornea, lens, or anterior vitreous humor. The slit beam also may help identify the abnormal presence of cells in the aqueous humor.

Corneal Staining

Corneal staining consists of placing fluorescein or other topical dye into the conjunctival sac. The dye outlines irregularities of the corneal surface that are not easily visible. Corneal staining is indicated in cases of corneal trauma, problems caused by a contact lens, or the presence of foreign bodies, abrasions, ulcers, or other corneal disorders.

This procedure is noninvasive and is performed under aseptic conditions. The dye is applied topically to the eye, and the eye is then viewed through a blue filter. Nonintact areas of the cornea stain a bright green color.

Tonometry

A **tonometer** is an instrument for measuring **intraocular pressure (IOP).** Normal IOP readings are 10 to 21 mm Hg. About 5% of clients with healthy eyes have a slightly higher pressure. Tonometer readings are indicated for all clients older than 40 years of age. Adults with a family history of glaucoma should have their IOP measured once or twice a year.

IOP varies throughout the day. It tends to be highest in the morning but may peak at any time of the day, depending on the individual. Therefore the time of IOP measurement is always documented.

Several methods and instruments are available to measure IOP (Figure 46-13). Some involve direct contact with the eye, whereas others use a noncontact technique. Table 46-3 compares the advantages and disadvantages of each method.

Ophthalmoscopy

The direct ophthalmoscope allows viewing of the eye's external structures and interior. It is easiest to examine the fundus when the room is dark because the pupil will dilate. When performing direct ophthalmoscopy, the nurse holds the instrument with the right hand when examining the right eye and with the left hand when examining the left eye. The nurse stands on the same side as the eye being examined. The client is instructed to look straight ahead at an object on the wall behind the nurse. A thumb can be placed on the client's eyebrow to assist in knowing the distance from the ophthalmoscope to the client. The ophthalmoscope is held firmly against the examiner's face and is aligned so that the examiner's eye sees through the sight hole (Figure 46-14).

When using the ophthalmoscope, the nurse comes toward the client's eye from about 12 to 15 inches away and about

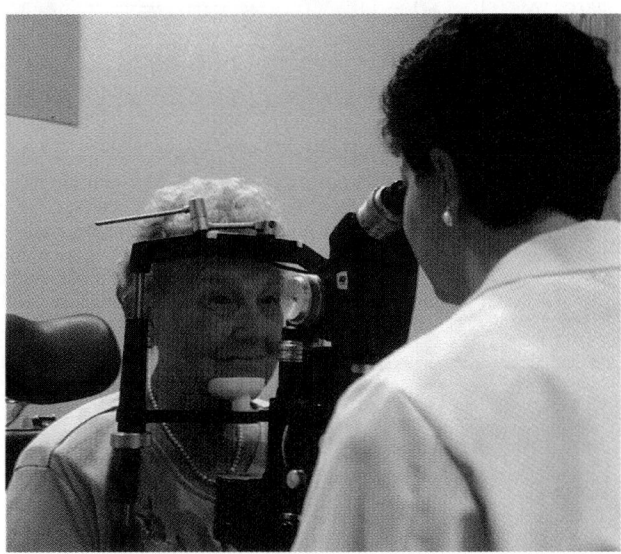

Figure 46-12 ● Slit-lamp ocular examination.

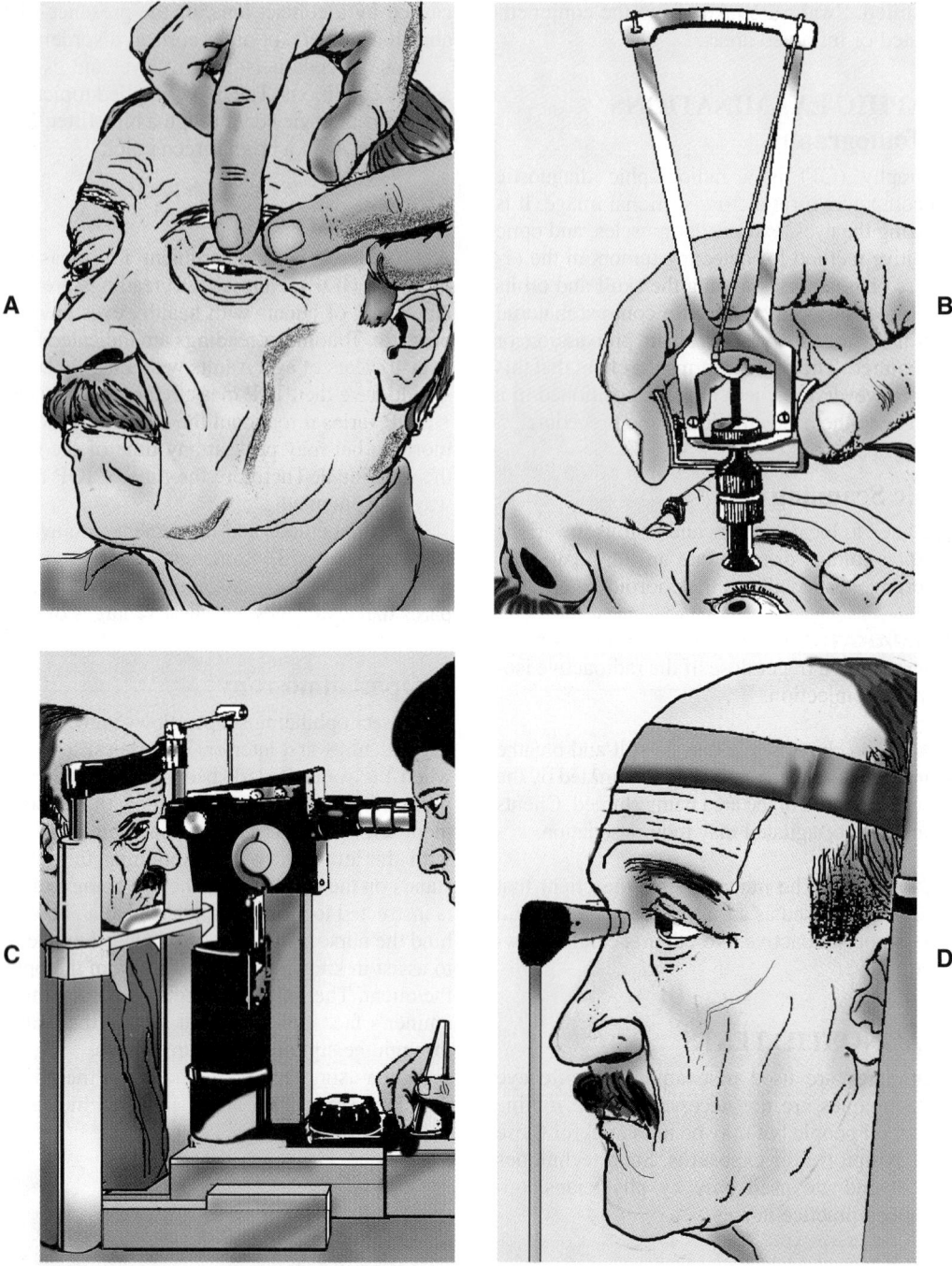

Figure 46-13 ● Methods of intraocular pressure estimation. **A,** Finger palpation is useful only when a large difference exists between the intraocular pressure of the two eyes, as in unilateral angle-closure glaucoma. **B,** Schiötz tonometry can be learned readily. Because the tonometer is relatively inexpensive, it can be used in every physician's office to screen for chronic simple glaucoma. **C,** The air-puff tonometer can be used for screening large numbers of clients but is far more expensive than Schiötz's tonometer. **D,** Goldman's applanation tonometer, used with a slit lamp, is the standard instrument for glaucoma diagnosis and management for most ophthalmologists. It is expensive and requires considerable skill.

TABLE 46-3 • TYPES OF TONOMETRY

Type of Tonometry	Advantages	Disadvantages
Noncontact (air-puff) tonometer A puff of air indents the cornea	No direct contact with the client's cornea No anesthesia needed Very rapid	Less accurate than direct contact methods The puff of air is unpleasant and may startle the client
Schiötz tonometer A small pressure gauge is placed on the cornea, and a weighted plunger is depressed	Reliable readings Portable Low cost	Touches the client's cornea Requires topical anesthetic May abrade or infect the cornea
Goldman's applanation tonometer The machine exerts a force against the cornea	Highly accurate Rapid	Touches the client's cornea Requires topical anesthetic Danger of infection Machine is expensive
Tono-Pen XL A penlight-sized appliance is placed against the cornea and exerts a force against the cornea	Rapid Portable Accurate Uses a sleeve to prevent infection	Touches the client's cornea Requires topical anesthetic

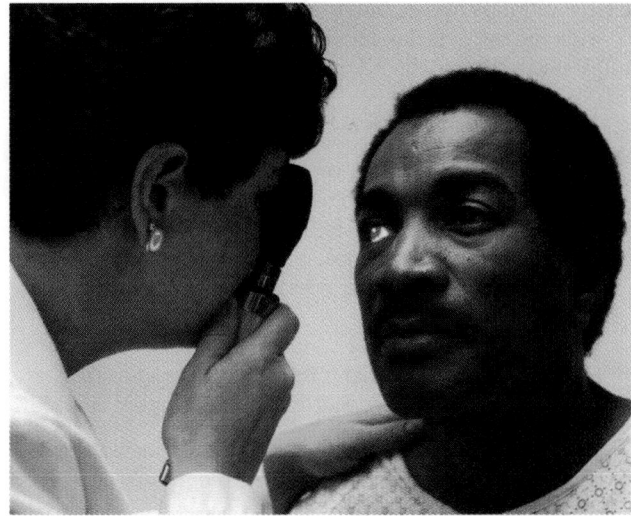

Figure 46-14 ● Proper technique for direct ophthalmoscopic visualization of the retina.

TABLE 46-4 • STRUCTURES TO ASSESS BY DIRECT OPHTHALMOSCOPY

RED REFLEX
- Presence or absence

OPTIC DISK
- Color
- Margins (sharp or blurred)
- Cup size
- Presence of rings or crescents

OPTIC BLOOD VESSELS
- Size
- Color
- Kinks or tangles
- Light reflection
- Narrowing
- Nicking at arteriovenous crossings

FUNDUS
- Color
- Tears or holes
- Lesions
- Bleeding

MACULA
- Presence of blood vessels
- Color
- Lesions
- Bleeding

15 degrees lateral to the client's line of vision. As the ophthalmoscope is directed at the pupil, a red glare **(red reflex)** is seen in the pupil. The red reflex is a reflection of the light on the retina. An absent red reflex may indicate an opacity in the lens or cloudiness of the vitreous. The nurse, who has both eyes open, moves toward the client's pupil while following the red reflex. The retina should then be visible through the ophthalmoscope. Structures examined with the ophthalmoscope include the optic disk, optic vessels, fundus, and macula. Table 46-4 lists the features that should be observed in each structure.

Ultrasonography

Ultrasonography is used to examine the orbit and eye with high-frequency sound waves. This noninvasive test aids in the diagnosis of trauma, intraorbital tumors, proptosis, and choroidal or retinal detachments. It is also used to determine gross outline changes in the eye and the orbit in clients with cloudy corneas or lenses, which prevents examination of the fundus. Ultrasonography helps calculate the length of the eye, one of the measurements used to determine the strength of the intraocular lens implant needed after cataract surgery.

CLIENT PREPARATION. The nurse explains the test to the client and instills anesthetic drops into the lower lid. The client is cautioned to avoid rubbing the eye. Clients are seated upright with the chin in the chin rest.

PROCEDURE. The probe is touched against the client's anesthetized cornea, and sound waves are bounced through the eye. The sound waves return to the transducer when they strike a non–fluid-filled structure. The anatomic structures that reflect sound waves are the cornea, anterior and posterior lens capsule, and retina. When these reflected sound waves return to the transducer, a characteristic "spike" pattern appears on the screen.

FOLLOW-UP CARE. The nurse reminds the client not to rub or bump the eye until the effects of the anesthetic drops have worn off.

Magnetic Resonance Imaging

Magnetic resonance imaging (MRI) has many ophthalmic uses and avoids exposing the client to radiation. *It is not used with an actual or suspected metallic foreign body, because the magnetic pull can move the metal fragment and damage the eye.*

The nurse explains to the client that the MRI study may be performed in an enclosed space (although MRI units with open sides are becoming more available). Sedation may be necessary. If the client is sedated, pulse oximetry is performed during the procedure because direct observation of respiratory status is not possible. All metallic jewelry is removed until the procedure is completed.

Fluorescein Angiography

Fluorescein angiography provides a detailed image and permanent record of eye circulation. Photographs are taken in rapid succession after the intravenous (IV) administration of dye. This test is useful for the diagnosis of conditions affecting the circulation of the retina (e.g., diabetic retinopathy and macular degeneration) or for the diagnosis of intraocular tumors.

CLIENT PREPARATION. The nurse explains the procedure to the client, asks about allergies and previous reactions to dyes, and instills mydriatic eyedrops (cause pupil dilation) approximately 1 hour before the test. Chart 46-3 describes the best practice patterns for the correct instillation of eyedrops. The nurse checks that the informed consent has been signed by the client or responsible person. The nurse warns that the dye may cause the skin to appear yellow for several hours after the test. The stain is gradually eliminated through the urine, which changes color.

PROCEDURE. IV access must be obtained. After the catheter is in the vein, 5 mL of a 10% solution of fluorescein is injected into the client's peripheral vein. A camera is set up with ophthalmologic equipment to photograph retinal and choroidal blood vessels as the dye passes through them. The procedure takes only minutes because the vessels fill quickly.

FOLLOW-UP CARE. After the test, the client may feel weak and nauseated. After the nausea resolves, clients are encouraged to drink fluids to help eliminate the dye. The nurse encourages rest and emphasizes that any yellow staining of the skin will disappear in a few hours. After the test, the urine will be bright green until the dye is excreted. The client is instructed to avoid direct sunlight until pupil dilation returns to normal.

Electroretinography

Electroretinography is the process of graphing the retina's response to light stimulation. An electroretinogram is obtained by placing a contact lens electrode on an anesthetized cornea. Lights at varying speeds and intensities are flashed, and the neural response is graphed. The measurement from the cornea is identical to the response that would be obtained if electrodes were placed directly on the retina.

Preparation includes instilling an anesthetic into the eye. Afterward, the client is reminded to avoid rubbing the eye until the effects of the anesthetic have disappeared.

This procedure is especially helpful in detecting and evaluating retinal blood vessel changes such as diabetic or hypertensive retinopathy; trauma to the retinal blood supply, such as with retinal detachment; toxic changes from the use of drugs; and systemic disorders, such as vitamin A deficiency.

CRITICAL THINKING CHALLENGE

The client is a 60-year-old Hispanic woman who speaks no English. She is scheduled to have a slit-lamp evaluation and measurement of intraocular pressure by the Schiötz method. As she comes into the examination area, she begins to cry and cover her eyes. There is no one who can speak Spanish in the clinic.
• What is your first priority?
• How will you explain what is involved in these tests?
• How will you reduce her concerns about pain or eye damage?

For suggested answer guidelines, go to http://www.wbsaunders.com/SIMON/Iggy/.

ONLINE RESOURCES

For suggested readings and Internet resources, go to http://www.wbsaunders.com/SIMON/Iggy/.

SELECTED BIBLIOGRAPHY

Asterisk indicates a classic or definitive work on this subject.

Bron, A. (2001). The architecture of the corneal stroma. *British Journal of Ophthalmology, 85*(4), 379-381.

Cleary, B. (1997). Age-related changes in the special senses. In M. Matteson, E. McConnell, & A. Linton (Eds.), *Gerontological nursing: Concepts and practice* (2nd ed., pp. 384 405). Philadelphia: W.B. Saunders.

*Cleary, M. (1995). Helping the person who is visually impaired: Concerns, questions, remedies, and sources. *Journal of Ophthalmic Nursing and Technology, 14*(5), 205-211.

Cohen, S., & Kawasaki, A. (1999). Introduction to formal visual field testing: Goldman and Humphrey perimeter. *Journal of Ophthalmic Nursing and Technology, 18*(1), 7-11.

Cotran, R., Kumar, V., & Collins, T. (1999). *Robbins pathologic basis of disease* (5th ed.). Philadelphia: W.B. Saunders.

Garber, N. (1999). Applanation tonometry. *Journal of Ophthalmic Nursing and Technology, 18*(6), 270-279.

Garber, N. (1999). Iris and pupil evaluation: Key considerations. *Journal of Ophthalmic Nursing and Technology, 18*(5), 207-218.

CHART 46-3

BEST PRACTICE *for*
Instillation of Ophthalmic Drops

• Wash your hands.
• Don gloves if secretions are present.
• Explain the procedure to the client.
• Check the name, strength, and expiration date of the solution.
• Stand behind the client.
• Instruct the client to tilt the head backward, open the eyes, and look up.
• Have the client's head rest against your body.
• Pull the lower lid downward against the cheekbone.
• Hold the medication bottle like a pencil, with the tip down.
• Rest the wrist holding the bottle on the client's cheek.
• Without touching the tip of the bottle to the client's conjunctiva, squeeze the bottle gently and release the correct number of drops into the conjunctival pocket.
• Gently release the lower eyelid.
• Instruct the client to close the eyes gently, without squeezing the lids together.

Garber, N. (2000). A guide to performing basic manifest refractometry. *Journal of Ophthalmic Nursing and Technology, 19*(2), 84-95.

Garber, N. (2000). Performing direct ophthalmoscopy. *Journal of Ophthalmic Nursing and Technology, 19*(3), 120-133.

Gordon, M. (2000). *Manual of nursing diagnosis* (9th ed.). St. Louis: Mosby.

Guyton, A., & Hall, J. (2000). *Textbook of medical physiology* (10th ed.). Philadelphia: W.B. Saunders.

Jarvis, C. (2000). *Physical examination and health assessment* (3rd ed.). Philadelphia: W.B. Saunders.

Ramos, M. (1999). Prevention of work-related injuries: A look at eye protection use and suggested prevention strategies. *Journal of Ophthalmic Nursing and Technology, 18*(3), 117-119.

Segal, W., et al. (2001). Disinfection of Goldman tonometers after contamination with hepatitis C virus. *American Journal of Ophthalmology, 131*(2), 184-187.

Shoemaker, J. (1997). Adult vision screening by nonphysicians. *Journal of Ophthalmic Nursing & Technology, 16*(5), 244-250.

*Sullivan, N. (1983). Vision in the elderly. *Journal of Gerontological Nursing, 9*(4), 228-235.

*Vaughan, D., Asbury, T., & Riordan-Eva, P. (Eds.). (1995). *General ophthalmology* (14th ed.). Norwalk, CT: Appleton & Lange.

Interventions for Clients with Eye and Vision Problems

M. LINDA WORKMAN

Learning Objectives

After studying this chapter, you should be able to:

1. Describe how to correctly instill ophthalmic drops and ointment into the eye.
2. Explain the consequences of increased intraocular pressure (IOP).
3. Identify common practices that increase IOP.
4. Prioritize educational needs for the client after cataract surgery with and without lens replacement.
5. Compare and contrast myopia and hyperopia and the correction needed for each.
6. Describe the pathologic bases, symptoms, and nursing care priorities for primary open-angle glaucoma and acute angle-closure glaucoma.
7. Identify the nursing care priorities for the donor when corneal donation is planned.
8. Explain how diabetes mellitus and hypertension affect vision.
9. Prioritize educational needs for the client after corneal transplantation.
10. Describe the common visual deficits for the client with dry macular degeneration.
11. Identify nursing interventions to promote home safety for the client with impaired vision.

Go to http://www.wbsaunders.com/SIMON/Iggy/ for self-assessment questions related to these Learning Objectives.

Vision is affected by many conditions. Some conditions occur gradually, such as cataracts, and others can result from an acute insult or illness. Even temporary visual impairment causes the client distress and necessitates some changes in function or lifestyle.

EXTERNAL EYE DISORDERS: EYELID DISORDERS

The eyelid is composed of small muscles and thin skin. The eyelid protects the external eye surface and is responsible for the spread of tears. Disorders can be related to changes in the structure, function, or position of the eyelid. Lid structure may also be altered by age (Figures 47-1 and 47-2).

Blepharitis

OVERVIEW

Blepharitis, an inflammation of the eyelid edges, is most common in the older adult and is often associated with *dry eye syndrome* (see Keratoconjunctivitis Sicca, p. 1027). The lack of sufficient tears with this disorder may lead to bacterial invasion of the eye structures, because tears are bacteriostatic.

▶ COLLABORATIVE MANAGEMENT

Clients usually have itchy, red, and burning eyes. **Seborrhea** (greasy, itchy scaling) of the eyebrows and eyelids is often present. On slit-lamp examination, greasy scales and mattering may be seen on the eyelid-eyelash margin.

Blepharitis is best controlled by a regimen of eyelid care using warm, moist compresses followed by gentle scrubbing with dilute baby shampoo. The nurse instructs the client to avoid rubbing the eyes, because this action can spread the infection to other eye structures.

Entropion

OVERVIEW

An **entropion** is an inversion of the eyelid causing the eyelashes to rub against the eye. The condition usually develops after age 40 years. Entropion can be caused by eyelid muscle spasms or by scarring and deformity of the eyelid itself as a result of trauma. Older clients are susceptible to entropion because of a loss of tissue support with aging.

▶ COLLABORATIVE MANAGEMENT

The client usually reports "feeling something in my eye." Pain and tearing may also be present. On inspection, the eyelid is turned inward, and the conjunctiva appears inflamed. Corneal abrasion may result from constant irritation.

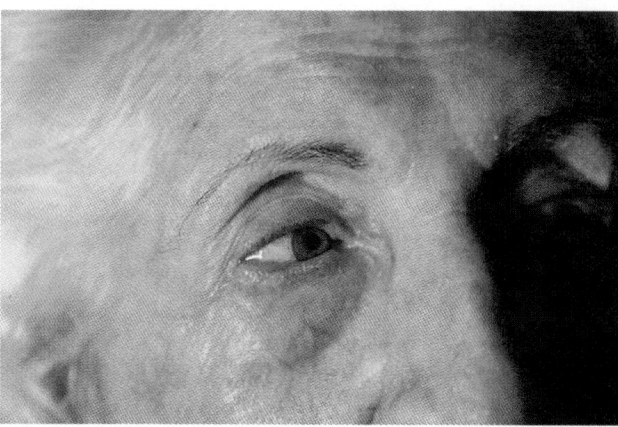

Figure 47-1 ● Eyelid eversion (ectropion).

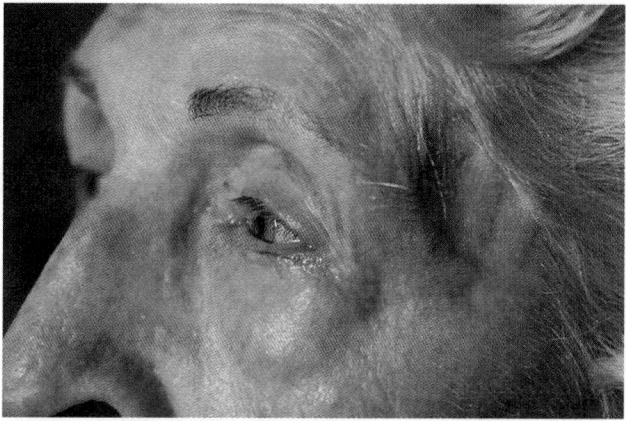

Figure 47-2 ● "Bags" under the eyes.

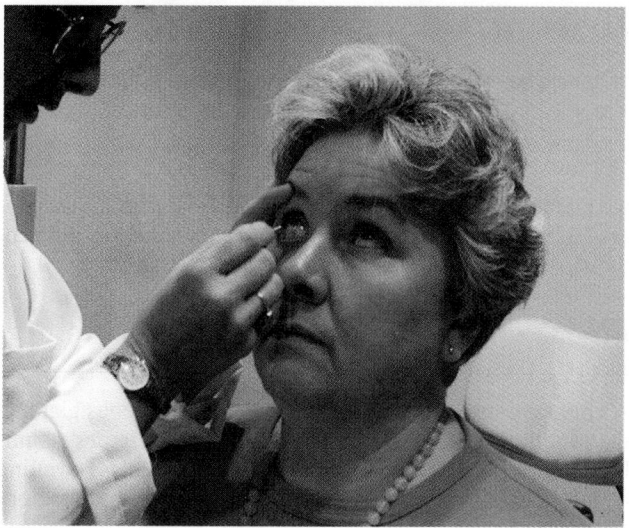

Figure 47-3 ● Application of ophthalmic ointment.

Surgery may correct the position of the eyelid by either tightening the orbicular muscle (thus moving the eyelid to a normal position) or directly preventing inward rotation of the eyelid margin. After surgery, the eye is usually covered with a patch, and the client is discharged a few hours later.

CHART 47-1

BEST PRACTICE *for*
Instillation of Ophthalmic Ointments

- Wash your hands.
- Wear gloves.
- Explain the procedure to the client.
- Check the name, strength, and expiration date of the medication.
- Instruct the client to tilt the head backward, open the eyes, and look up.
- Pull the client's lower lid downward, toward the cheekbone, creating a "pocket" in the lower lid.
- Hold the tube like a pencil, with the tip downward.
- Rest the wrist holding the tube on the client's cheek.
- Do not touch the tip of the tube to the conjunctiva.
- Squeeze the tube gently until a small amount of ointment is in the pocket.
- Release the lower eyelid.
- Instruct the client to close the eye gently.
- Tell the client that vision may be blurred by the ointment.
- Instruct the client to remove the ointment before driving or operating equipment.
- Remove ointment by closing the eye and wiping the closed lid from the inner canthus outward with a clean tissue.

The nurse demonstrates instillation of eyedrops and evaluates the client's ability to instill the drops. The client is instructed to leave the patch in place until he or she is seen by the ophthalmologist and to inform the ophthalmologist of any pain or drainage under the patch. The nurse teaches the client or significant other how to clean the suture line with a cotton swab and the prescribed solution. A small amount of antibiotic ointment may be applied (Figure 47-3). Chart 47-1 describes best practices for applying ophthalmic ointment; Chart 47-2 summarizes important information on ophthalmic drugs.

Ectropion

▮ OVERVIEW

An **ectropion** is the outward sagging and eversion of the eyelid (see Figure 47-1) that is usually associated with aging. Ectropion is caused by relaxation of the orbicular muscle. This lid position does not permit tears to wash adequately over the anterior surface of the eye, leading to corneal drying and ulceration.

► COLLABORATIVE MANAGEMENT

Clients frequently have complaints of constant tearing and outward deviation of the eyelid. Surgery is required to restore proper lid alignment. After surgery, the eye is covered with a patch and the client is discharged. Nursing interventions are the same as those for an entropion.

Hordeolum

▮ OVERVIEW

A **hordeolum,** or **stye,** can be external or internal. An external hordeolum is an infection of the sweat glands in the eyelid, occurring near the emergence of the eyelashes from the eyelid (called the **eyelid-eyelash margin**). A red, swollen, tender area is noted on the skin surface side of the eyelid. An internal hordeolum is caused by an infection of the eyelid sebaceous glands. The most common causative organisms are *Staphylo-*

CHART 47-2

DRUG THERAPY *for* **Eye Problems**

Drug	Nursing Interventions	Rationale
TOPICAL ANESTHETICS Proparacaine HCl, or proxymetacaine (AK-Taine, Alcaine, Ocu-Caine, Ophthetic) Tetracaine HCl, cocaine HCl (Pontocaine)	Use nasal punctal occlusion. Remind the client not to rub or touch the eye while it is anesthetized. Patch the eye if the client leaves the facility before the anesthetic wears off. Do not use discolored solution. Store the bottle tightly closed.	This technique decreases systemic absorption and side effects. Touching may injure the eye. The use of a patch prevents injury, such as corneal abrasion. Discoloration is a sign of altered drug composition. Air may cause drug contamination and oxidation.
TOPICAL STEROIDS Prednisolone acetate (Ocu-Pred, Ophtho-Tate✦) Prednisolone phosphate (Inflamase) Dexamethasone (Dexair, Dexotic, Maxidex) Betamethasone (Betnesol) Fluorometholone (Fluor-Op, Liquifilm)	Shake vigorously before use. Monitor the client for signs of corneal ulceration. Advise the client not to share eyedrops with others.	Medication is a suspension; shaking is required to distribute the medication evenly in the solution. Steroid use predisposes the client to local infection. Disease transmission is possible when sharing eyedrops.
ANTI-INFECTIVE AGENTS Gentamicin (Alcomicin✦, Garamycin, Genoptic) Tobramycin (Tobrex) Ciprofloxacin (Ciloxan) Erythromycin (Ilotycin) Chlortetracycline (Aureomycin) Sulfisoxazole (Gantrisin) Ofloxacin (Ocuflox)	Be sure to obtain a specimen for culture before use. Clean exudate from the eyes before administering drops. Reinforce the importance of completing the prescribed medication regimen.	Use of an antibiotic before a culture specimen is obtained may alter culture results. Cleansing decreases the risk of contaminating the medication and increases contact of the conjunctiva with the medication. Compliance is critical to maintain a therapeutic level of medication.
ANTIBIOTIC-STEROID COMBINATIONS Tobramycin with dexamethasone (TobraDex) Neomycin sulfate with polymyxin B sulfate and dexamethasone (Maxitrol)	This is the same as for each component alone.	This is the same as for each component alone.
TOPICAL ANTIVIRAL AGENTS Idoxuridine (Herplex, Stoxil) Trifluridine (Viroptic) Vidarabine (Vira-A)	Refrigerate and protect from light. Monitor the client for itching lids and burning eyes.	Cool temperatures and absence of light ensures medication stability. Sensitivity to this drug is common.

coccus aureus, Staphylococcus epidermidis, and *Streptococcus.* The hordeolum usually affects only one eyelid at a time. Vision is not affected.

▶ **COLLABORATIVE MANAGEMENT**

Small, beady, edematous areas may be seen on the skin side of the eyelid or on the conjunctival side of the eyelid-eyelash margin. As the hordeolum forms, it fills with purulent material, causing pain.

Treatment includes the use of warm compresses four times a day and an antibacterial ointment. When the lesion opens, either spontaneously or after application of the warm compresses, the purulent material drains and the pain subsides.

Nursing interventions include applying a clean washcloth compress and instructing the client in this application. Chart 47-3 describes the proper technique for applying ocular compresses.

After the compresses have been applied for the prescribed time, the nurse instills antibiotic ointment. The client is advised that ointments may cause blurred vision and is taught to remove

the ointment from the eyes before driving or operating machinery. To remove the ointment, the client closes the eye and gently wipes the closed eyelid from the inner canthus outward.

Chalazion

■ **OVERVIEW**

A **chalazion** is a sterile inflammation of a sebaceous gland in the eyelid. It begins with inflammation and tenderness (similar to the hordeolum), followed by a gradual painless swelling at the gland. In its fully developed state, no inflammatory signs are present.

▶ **COLLABORATIVE MANAGEMENT**

Most chalazia protrude on the conjunctival side of the eyelid. The client has eye fatigue, sensitivity to light, and possibly excessive tearing (**epiphora**).

Treatment includes the use of warm compresses for 15 minutes four times a day, followed by instillation of ophthalmic ointment. The physician excises the chalazion if it is

CHART 47-2

DRUG THERAPY *for* **Eye Problems—cont'd**

Drug	Nursing Interventions	Rationale
ADRENERGICS Dipivefrin HCl (Propine)	Instruct the client to use nasal punctal occlusion during administration. Monitor the client's heart rate and blood pressure.	Nasal punctal occlusion decreases systemic absorption and side effects. Systemic absorption increases the heart rate and blood pressure.
BETA BLOCKERS Carteolol (Ocupress) Levobunolol (Betagan) Timolol (Timoptic, Apo-Timop♣)	Instruct the client to use nasal punctal occlusion during administration. Monitor the client's heart rate and blood pressure.	Nasal punctal occlusion decreases systemic absorption and side effects. Systemic absorption slows the heart rate and may decrease blood pressure, causing orthostatic hypotension.
MIOTICS Carbachol (Isopto Carbachol, Miostat) Pilocarpine HCl (Isopto Carpine, Miocarpine♣, Pilocar, Spersacarpine♣)	Warn the client that visual acuity is decreased in low-light environments. Use with caution in clients who have urinary tract obstruction.	This drug causes severe pupillary constriction. This drug mimics the parasympathetic system and can cause urinary retention.
MYDRIATICS AND CYCLOPLEGICS Atropine (Atropair, Minims Atropine♣, Ocu-Tropine) Cyclopentolate (Cyclogyl, Minims Cyclopentate♣) Phenylephrine (Minims Phenylephrine♣, Neo-Synephrine, Ocu-Phrin, Spersaphrine♣) Tropicamide (Minims Tropicamide♣, Mydriacyl, Tropicacyl)	Instruct the client to wear sunglasses until the drug wears off. Instruct the client to avoid driving or operating hazardous machinery until the drug wears off. Instruct the client to use nasal punctal occlusion during administration.	This drug causes photophobia. *dilates* This drug causes blurred vision. This technique decreases systemic absorption and side effects.
NONSTEROIDAL ANTI-INFLAMMATORY AGENTS Flurbiprofen (Ocufen) Diclofenac (Voltaren) Ketorolac (Acular)	Monitor the client for bleeding in the eye. Instruct the client not to wear soft contact lenses during therapy with these drugs.	These drugs disrupt platelet aggregation. These drugs interact with contact lens materials and increase the risk for infection.

CHART 47-3

CLIENT EDUCATION GUIDE
Application of an Ocular Compress

1. Wash your hands.
2. Fold a clean washcloth into fourths.
3. Soak the washcloth with running tap water that is warm to your inner wrist. (If cool compresses are needed, follow the same steps using cold running tap water.)
4. Place the cloth over your *closed* eye.
5. Keep the cloth in place with minimal pressure until the cloth cools.
6. Refold the washcloth so that a different "fourth" will be held against the eye.
7. Resoak the cloth with running tap water.
8. Repeat applications three times for as many times each day as are ordered by your physician.

large enough to affect vision, is cosmetically displeasing to the client, or recurs frequently.

After excision, antibiotic ointment is instilled and the eye is covered with a patch. Best practices for proper application of a nonpressure eyepatch are described in Chart 47-4.

The client is instructed to leave the eyepatch intact for 4 to 6 hours and then remove the patch and begin applying warm, moist compresses. Antibiotic eyedrops are instilled after use of the compresses. The nurse instructs the client to report any evidence of infection, increasing redness, purulent drainage, or reduced vision to the ophthalmologist immediately.

LACRIMAL APPARATUS DISORDERS: KERATOCONJUNCTIVITIS SICCA

■ OVERVIEW

The lacrimal system moistens the external eye with tears and removes tears from the external surface of the eye. Problems can arise from insufficient tear production or from infection or inflammation in any part of the lacrimal system.

Keratoconjunctivitis sicca, or dry eye syndrome, results from changes in the composition of tears, lacrimal gland malfunction, or altered tear distribution. Decreased tear production can also occur during antihistamine, beta-adrenergic blocking agent, or anticholinergic drug therapy. Diseases associated with decreased tear production include rheumatoid arthritis, leukemia, sarcoidosis, multiple sclerosis, mumps, and lymphoma. Radiation or chemical burns can also decrease lacrimal system function. Injury to the facial nerve (cranial nerve VII) can inhibit tearing. Eye dryness may follow vision-enhancing surgery.

CHART 47-4

BEST PRACTICE *for*
Application of an Eyepatch

Nonpressure Eyepatch
1. Assemble the equipment:
   - Eyepatch
   - Skin preparation
   - Nonallergenic paper tape
2. Explain the procedure to the client.
3. Wash your hands.
4. Apply a skin preparation to the client's forehead and cheek.
5. Instruct the client to close both eyes gently.
6. Place a patch over the closed eyelid.

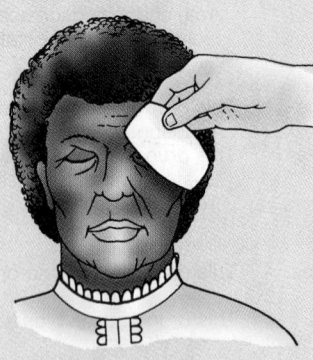

7. Apply tape from the cheek to the middle of the forehead in a diagonal line.

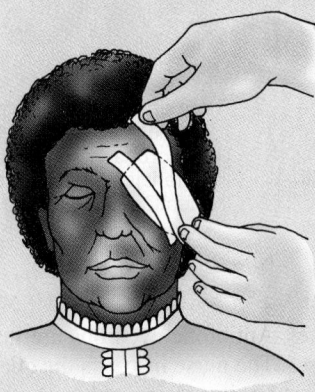

8. Cover the patch with overlapping pieces of tape.

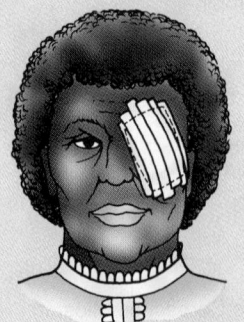

Pressure Eyepatch
1. Assemble the equipment:
   - Two eyepatches for each eye requiring treatment
   - Skin preparation pad
   - Nonallergenic paper tape
2-5. Follow corresponding steps under Nonpressure Eyepatch.
6. Fold one eyepatch in half, place it over the closed eyelid, and apply a second eyepatch (unfolded) over the folded one.

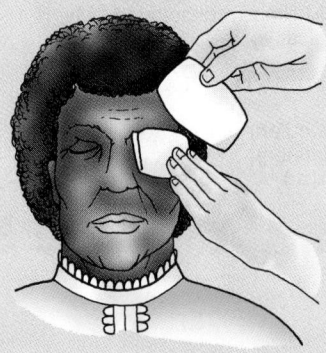

7, 8. Follow corresponding steps under Nonpressure Eyepatch.

► COLLABORATIVE MANAGEMENT

The client has the sensation of a foreign body in the eye, burning and itching eyes, and photophobia (increased sensitivity to light). The corneal light reflex is dulled or distorted. The tear film may contain strands of mucus.

Treatment depends on the severity of the symptoms. Artificial tears (HypoTears, Refresh) are prescribed for daytime use to reduce dryness and can be used as often as necessary. A lubricating ointment (Lacri-Lube S.O.P., Refresh P.M.) is used at night. If the dry eye syndrome is caused by an abnormal eyelid position or function, surgery may be required.

CONJUNCTIVAL DISORDERS

The conjunctiva is a thin mucous membrane that covers and protects the eye. Because of its location, the conjunctiva is subject to trauma and exposure to noxious gases; it is also susceptible to infection.

Subconjunctival Hemorrhage
■ OVERVIEW

Subconjunctival blood vessels are fragile and can break after increased pressure resulting from sneezing, coughing, or vomiting. These hemorrhages may also be associated with hypertension, trauma, or blood dyscrasias.

► COLLABORATIVE MANAGEMENT

The small, well-defined area of hemorrhage is bright red under the conjunctiva. The client is usually quite concerned about its appearance. No pain or visual impairment accompanies the hemorrhage, and it resolves gradually within 10 to 14 days without treatment.

Conjunctivitis
▌OVERVIEW

Conjunctivitis is an inflammation or infection of the conjunctiva. Inflammatory conjunctivitis results from exposure to allergens or irritants and is not contagious. Infectious conjunctivitis occurs as a result of bacterial or viral infection and is readily transmitted from person to person.

▶ COLLABORATIVE MANAGEMENT

Symptoms of allergic conjunctivitis include conjunctival edema, a sensation of burning, **vascular injection** (engorgement of blood vessels—"bloodshot" appearance), excessive tearing, and itching.

Treatment includes the instillation of vasoconstrictors and corticosteroid eyedrops. The client is instructed to avoid using makeup until all symptoms of conjunctivitis subside.

Bacterial conjunctivitis, or "pink eye," is caused by *Staphylococcus aureus, Haemophilus influenzae,* or *Pseudomonas aeruginosa.* Symptoms include blood vessel dilation, mild conjunctival edema, tearing, and discharge. The discharge is watery at first and then gradually becomes thicker, with shreds of mucus.

Cultures of the drainage are obtained to identify the causative microorganism. Treatment is aimed at controlling the infection. Appropriate topical antibiotics are administered.

Nursing interventions focus on preventing the spread of the disease. For example, cross-contamination may spread the infection to the other eye. The amount, color, and type of drainage are noted. The nurse reviews hygienic principles with the client, including handwashing after touching the eye and before instilling eyedrops. The client is warned not to touch the unaffected eye without first washing the hands and to avoid sharing washcloths and towels with others.

Trachoma
▌OVERVIEW

Trachoma is a chronic, bilateral scarring form of conjunctivitis caused by *Chlamydia trachomatis.* Trachoma is the chief cause of blindness in the world. The incidence is highest in warm, moist climates where hygienic practices are substandard.

▶ COLLABORATIVE MANAGEMENT

The incubation period is 5 to 14 days. Initially, trachoma resembles bacterial conjunctivitis. Symptoms include tearing, photophobia, edema of the eyelids, and conjunctival edema. Follicles form on the upper eyelid conjunctiva. As the disease progresses, the eyelid scars and turns inward, causing the eyelashes to damage the cornea.

Specimens are obtained for culture to identify the causative organism. A 4-week course of oral tetracycline (Achromycin, Apo-Tetra✤) or erythromycin (Apo-Erythro-EC✤, E-Mycin, E.E.S.) is given. These drugs may be applied topically if the systemic forms are unavailable.

Nursing interventions focus on infection control. The client is instructed to wash the hands before and after touching the eyes. The nurse advises the client to keep washcloths

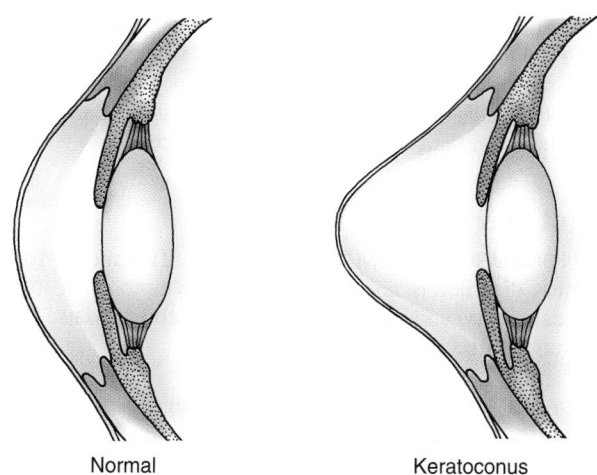

Figure 47-4 ● Profiles of a normal eyeball and one with keratoconus.

TABLE 47-1 · COMMON CAUSES OF CORNEAL DISORDERS	
KERATOCONUS • Autosomal recessive trait • Down syndrome • Aniridia • Marfan syndrome • Atopic allergy • Retinitis pigmentosa **KERATITIS (EXPOSURE)** • Ectropion/entropion • Exophthalmos • Neurologic deficits	**KERATITIS** **(ACANTHAMOEBA)** • Protozoal infection **CORNEAL ULCERS** • Mechanical injury • Chemical injury • Drying • Infection

separate from those of unaffected people and to launder them separately. The nurse also emphasizes the importance of completing the prescribed course of antibiotics.

CORNEAL DISORDERS
▌OVERVIEW

For a sharp image to be focused on the retina, the cornea must be transparent and intact. Corneal problems are the leading cause of visual impairment in the United States and Canada. Corneal disorders may be caused by degeneration of the cornea (keratoconus) (Figure 47-4); deposition of substances in the cornea, altering its refracting power (dystrophies); inflammation from either irritation or infection (keratitis); or ulceration of the corneal surface. Table 47-1 lists common causes of corneal disorders.

▶ COLLABORATIVE MANAGEMENT
▌ Assessment

The client with a corneal disorder usually has pain, reduced vision, photophobia, and eye secretions. Cloudy or purulent (pus-filled) fluid may be present on the eyelids or eyelashes. Gloves are worn during the examination when secretions are noted.

The cornea may look hazy or cloudy. An altered corneal light reflex may be noted. The cornea may no longer be intact, and patchy areas may be visible on examination. When fluorescein is used, these areas appear green.

No definitive tests confirm corneal disease, although microbial culture and corneal scrapings can help determine which organism is causing a corneal ulcer. For culture, swabs from the ulcer and its edges are obtained to identify microorganisms. For corneal scrapings, the cornea is anesthetized with a topical agent, and a sterile spatula is used to remove samples from the center and edge of the ulcer.

▶ Interventions

NONSURGICAL MANAGEMENT. Treatment for a corneal disorder is aimed at reducing symptoms, restoring corneal clarity, and enhancing the client's ability to use his or her remaining vision.

DRUG THERAPY. Antibiotics, antifungals, and antivirals are prescribed to reduce or eliminate microorganisms. Clients are first started on a regimen of a broad-spectrum antibiotic,

---

CHART 47-5

BEST PRACTICE *for*
Eyedrop Administration

- Administer drugs at frequent, precise intervals. *The timing of administration is critical.* Clients with eye problems are often given several broad-spectrum antibiotics. If each drug is administered every hour, create separate dosage schedules. For example, give antibiotic A at 7:00, 8:00, 9:00, and 10:00. Then give antibiotic B at 7:30, 8:30, 9:30, and 10:30.
- If two medications must be administered *at the same time, separate the instillation by 5 minutes.* For example, a client with glaucoma and a bacterial ulcer receives timolol (Apo-Timop✦, Timoptic) at 7:00 and tobramycin (Tobrex) at 7:05.
- If the same medication is required for both eyes and one eye is infected, use *separate* bottles of medication.
- Clearly label each bottle for the appropriate eye (OS for the left eye, OD for the right eye).
- Wear gloves when ocular drainage is present.
- Wash your hands before and after administering eyedrops.

---

which may be changed when the results of the culture are known. Steroids may be used with antibiotics to reduce the inflammatory response in the eye. Drugs can be administered topically as eyedrops, injected subconjunctivally, or administered intravenously. Chart 47-5 describes best practices for eyedrop administration.

VISION ENHANCEMENT. The nurse assists clients in using their functional vision, suggesting sunglasses and indirect lighting if glare creates difficulties. The nurse also informs clients about assistive devices, such as magnifiers and special light fixtures.

SURGICAL MANAGEMENT. Keratoplasty, or corneal transplant, is the surgical removal of diseased corneal tissue and replacement with tissue from a human donor cornea. Transplantation restores vision by removing corneal deformities and replacing them with healthy corneal tissue.

PREOPERATIVE CARE. Corneal transplantation is performed as a scheduled surgical procedure or when donor tissue becomes available. Usually the client is quite anxious. The nurse's calm approach is helpful during discussions. The nurse assesses the client's knowledge of the surgery and of preoperative and postoperative routines, providing information as needed.

The client's eyes are examined for signs of infection, and any redness, drainage, or edema around the eye is reported to the ophthalmologist. Antibiotic drops are instilled into the eye to reduce the risk for infection. Intravenous (IV) access is placed before surgery.

OPERATIVE PROCEDURE. The surgeon removes the center 7 to 8 mm of the diseased cornea (Figure 47-5) with a **trephine,** a circular knife that operates much like a cookie cutter. The same trephine is used to cut the tissue graft from

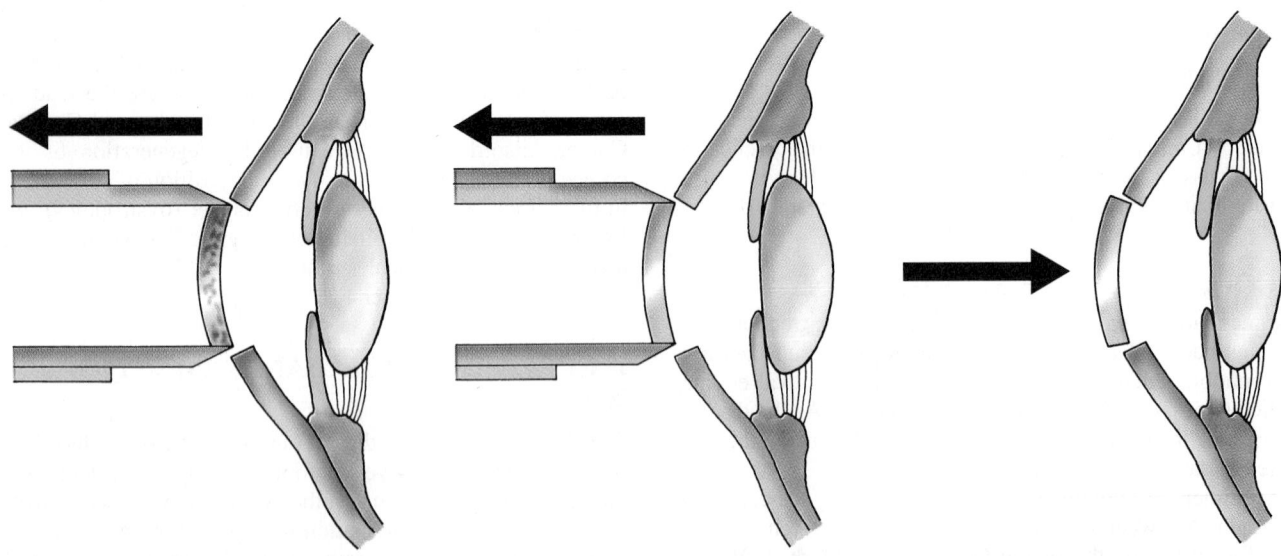

The diseased cornea is removed with a trephine.

A button, or graft, of donor cornea is removed with the same trephine so that the cuts are identical.

The donor cornea is placed on the eye and stitched into place with suture material that is finer than a human hair.

Figure 47-5 ● The steps involved in corneal transplantation (penetrating keratoplasty).

the donor cornea. The donor corneal graft is positioned on the eye and sutured into place. Figure 47-6 shows the eye after corneal transplantation.

During a keratoplasty, the client is usually under regional anesthesia. The nerves around and behind the eye are numbed so that the client cannot move or see out of the eye.

POSTOPERATIVE CARE. After the procedure is completed, a subconjunctival antibiotic injection is given and an antibiotic ointment instilled. The eye is covered with a pressure patch and a protective shield. This initial dressing is left in place until the next day. The nurse does not remove or change the dressing without a specific order from the ophthalmologist.

The nurse notifies the ophthalmologist of changes in vital signs or of drainage on the dressing. The client is instructed to lie on the nonoperative side to reduce intraocular pressure (IOP). During the immediate postoperative period, he or she cannot see out of the affected eye because of the eyepatch and shield.

If the client is to maintain the patches after discharge, the nurse shows him or her how to apply a patch and obtains a return demonstration. For the first postoperative month, the client is instructed to wear the shield at night and whenever he or she is around small children or pets. Complications after corneal transplant surgery include bleeding, wound leakage, infection, and graft rejection.

Although the cornea has no blood supply, graft rejection is possible. The inflammatory process starts in the donor cornea near the graft edge and moves centrally. Vision is reduced, and the cornea becomes cloudy. The client is treated with frequent applications of topical corticosteroids. If the rejection process continues, the graft becomes opaque, and blood vessels may begin to branch into the opaque tissue.

EYE DONATION. Tissue for a keratoplasty is obtained from a local eye or tissue bank. An eye bank obtains its supply of corneal tissue from volunteer donors. These donors must be free of infectious disease or cancer at the time of death.

If a deceased client is a potential eye donor, the nurse:
* Raises the head of the bed 30 degrees
* Instills antibiotic eyedrops, such as Neosporin or tobramycin
* Closes the eyes and applies a *small* ice pack to the closed eyes
* Contacts the family and physician to discuss eye donation

INTRAOCULAR DISORDERS: LENS DISORDERS
Cataract
■ OVERVIEW
The lens is a biconvex, transparent, refractive elastic structure suspended behind the iris. A cataract is an opacity of the lens that distorts the image projected onto the retina (Figure 47-7). The degree of reduced vision created by the cataract is determined by the location and density of the opacification. Intervention is indicated when visual acuity has been reduced to a level that the client finds unacceptable or that adversely affects lifestyle.

■ Pathophysiology
With aging, the lens gradually loses water and increases in density. This increased density results from the compression of older lens fibers and the production of new fibers in the outer layers. Opacities can develop in any part of the lens or capsule. A cataract forms as compaction of fibers reduces lens water content, causing lens proteins to precipitate and form crystals. Over time, a progressive and painless loss of lens transparency occurs. Both eyes may have cataracts; however, the rate of progression in each eye is usually different.

■ Etiology
Cataracts are classified by nature or by onset. They may be present at birth or develop at any time. Cataracts may be age related or result from trauma or exposure to toxic substances. Cataract formation is also associated with specific diseases and other ocular disorders (Table 47-2).

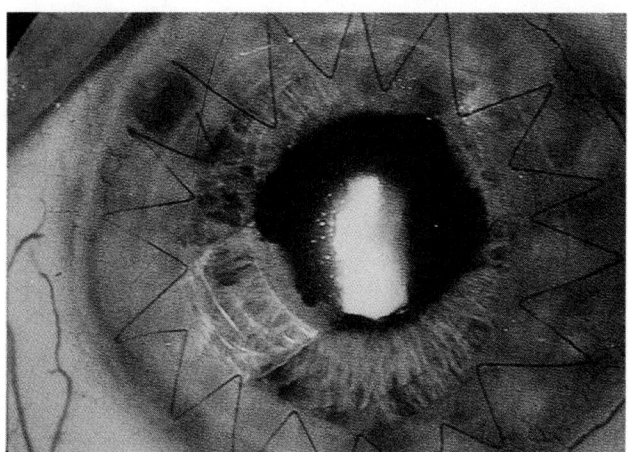
Figure 47-6 ● The appearance of the eye with sutures in place after corneal transplantation. (Courtesy John A. Costin, MD.)

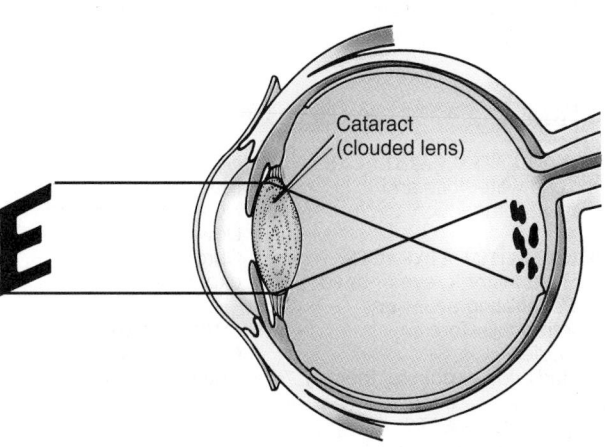
Figure 47-7 ● The visual impairment produced by the presence of a cataract.

■ Incidence/Prevalence

Cataracts develop in approximately 5 to 10 million people worldwide every year. The age-related cataract is the most common type. Some degree of cataract formation is expected in all people older than 70 years of age (Vaughan, Asbury, & Riordan-Eva, 1995).

► COLLABORATIVE MANAGEMENT
■ Assessment
■ HISTORY

When taking a history from a client with cataracts, the nurse notes his or her age, because cataracts are most prevalent in the older adult. The nurse asks about other predisposing factors, including the following:

- Recent or past trauma to the eye
- Exposure to radioactive materials or x-rays
- Systemic disease (such as diabetes mellitus, hypoparathyroidism, Down syndrome, or atopic dermatitis)
- Use of medications (such as corticosteroids, chlorpromazine, or miotic drugs)
- Intraocular disease (such as recurrent uveitis)

The nurse asks the client to describe his or her vision. For example, the nurse might say, "Tell me what you can see well and what you have difficulty seeing." This technique helps the nurse determine the impact of visual deficits on the client.

■ PHYSICAL ASSESSMENT/CLINICAL MANIFESTATIONS

Early manifestations of cataract development include slightly blurred vision and decreased color perception (Chart 47-6). As lens cloudiness continues, the client may complain of a decrease in vision adversely affecting daily activities. Blurred and double vision may occur. Without surgical intervention, visual impairment can progress to blindness. *No pain or eye redness is associated with age-related cataract formation.*

Visual acuity is significantly reduced. Vision is tested using a Snellen chart and brightness acuity testing (see Chapter 46). The nurse evaluates the client's acuity under various lighting conditions, which can help determine the degree of visual disability.

The nurse examines the lens with the direct ophthalmoscope and describes any observed densities by size, shape, and loca-

tion. As the cataract matures, the opacity makes visualization of the retina increasingly difficult. Eventually, the red reflex is absent. When this occurs, the pupil is white (Figure 47-8); this is the most easily detected symptom of a cataract.

■ PSYCHOSOCIAL ASSESSMENT

Loss of vision is gradual, and the client may not be aware of the change until activities such as reading, meal preparation, and driving are affected. Fear of losing one's eyesight can be overwhelming, and the client may exhibit great anxiety during an ocular evaluation.

■ Analysis
■ COMMON NURSING DIAGNOSES AND COLLABORATIVE PROBLEMS

The most common nursing diagnosis for clients with cataracts is Disturbed Sensory Perception (Visual) related to ocular lens opacity.

■ ADDITIONAL NURSING DIAGNOSES AND COLLABORATIVE PROBLEMS

In addition to the most common nursing diagnosis, clients with cataracts may have one or more of the following:

- Fear related to loss of eyesight, scheduled surgery, or inability to regain eyesight
- Risk for Injury related to decreased vision, age, or presence in an unfamiliar environment

---

CHART 47-6

KEY FEATURES of Cataracts

Early
- Blurred vision
- Decreased color perception

Late
- Diplopia
- Reduced visual acuity progressing to blindness
- Absence of red reflex
- Presence of white pupil

TABLE 47-2 • COMMON CAUSES OF CATARACTS

AGE-RELATED CATARACTS	ASSOCIATED CATARACTS
• Lens water loss and fiber compaction	• Diabetes mellitus
	• Hypoparathyroidism
TRAUMATIC CATARACTS	• Down syndrome
• Blunt injury to eye or head	• Chronic sunlight exposure
• Penetrating eye injury	
• Intraocular foreign bodies	**COMPLICATED CATARACTS**
• Radiation exposure, therapy	• Retinitis pigmentosa
	• Glaucoma
TOXIC CATARACTS	• Retinal detachment
• Corticosteroids	
• Phenothiazine derivatives	
• Miotic agents	

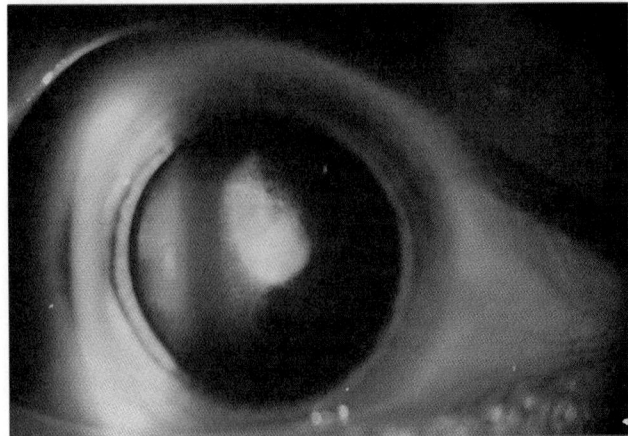

Figure 47-8 ● The appearance of an eye with a mature cataract. (Courtesy John A. Costin, MD.)

- Social Isolation related to reduced visual acuity, fear of injury, decreased ability to navigate in the community, or fear of embarrassment
- Self-Care Deficit related to visual impairment
- Deficient Knowledge (Cataract Pathophysiology and Treatment) related to lack of information or misinterpretation of previously acquired information
- Impaired Home Maintenance related to age, limited vision, or activity restrictions imposed by surgery

> ### CRITICAL THINKING CHALLENGE
> The client is a 75-year-old woman with changes in vision that have taken place over the past 3 years. She tells you that her glasses always seem dirty; she can no longer tell blue, green, and purple apart; she cannot distinguish shapes at night; and when car headlights approach, she sees "sparklers." You suspect that she has cataracts.
> - What additional assessment questions should you ask to distinguish cataracts from glaucoma?
> - What physical findings would you expect?
> - How would cataracts affect her visual fields?

For suggested answer guidelines, go to SIMON http://www.wbsaunders.com/SIMON/Iggy/.

● Planning and Implementation
■ DISTURBED SENSORY PERCEPTION (VISUAL)

PLANNING: EXPECTED OUTCOMES. The client with cataracts is expected to have improved vision.

INTERVENTIONS. Surgery and a variety of nursing interventions facilitate the client's recovery of vision.

PREOPERATIVE CARE. The health care provider gives the client accurate information so that he or she can make informed decisions about treatment. The nurse teaches about the nature of cataracts, their progression, and their treatment.

Because cataract surgery is usually an outpatient procedure and most clients are older, adequate preoperative teaching is problematic. The nurse assesses how the client's vision affects the activities of daily living, especially dressing, eating, and ambulating.

An IV infusion is usually started in the operating room. A sedative is given preoperatively, and oral acetazolamide (Acetazolam✤, Diamox) may be given on the morning of surgery to reduce intraocular pressure (IOP). The nurse instills a series of sympathomimetic drugs, such as phenylephrine (Neo-Synephrine, Spersaphrine✤), preoperatively to achieve mydriasis and vasoconstriction. Parasympatholytic drops, such as tropicamide (Minims Tropicamide✤, Mydriacyl) or cyclopentolate hydrochloride (Cyclogyl, Minims Cyclopentolate✤), are also administered to induce paralysis to prevent lens movement.

After the client is in the surgical area, a local anesthetic is administered into the muscle cone behind the eye to achieve anesthesia and ensure eye paralysis. The client may receive an IV injection of midazolam (Versed) to create a few minutes of light anesthesia during the administration of local anesthesia.

> ### CRITICAL THINKING CHALLENGE
> Your 75-year-old client has been diagnosed with cataracts and is scheduled to have surgery for removal of one cataract, to be followed immediately with an intraocular lens implant.
> - What is your teaching priority for this client?

For suggested answer guidelines, go to SIMON http://www.wbsaunders.com/SIMON/Iggy/.

OPERATIVE PROCEDURE. Extraction of the cataractous lens can be extracapsular or intracapsular (Figure 47-9). The most common procedure is extracapsular cataract extraction (ECCE). The anterior portion of the capsule is opened and removed. The ophthalmologist then removes the lens cortex and nucleus. Any remaining lens material is carefully removed from the eye. The posterior lens capsule is left inside the eye.

In intracapsular cataract extraction, the ophthalmologist removes the lens and capsule completely. A disadvantage of this approach is that the protective posterior capsule is removed, placing the eye at greater risk for retinal detachment and resulting in the loss of a supportive structure for the intraocular lens (IOL) implant.

After the lens with the cataract is removed, the eye has no accommodative power and has lost most of its refractive ability (**aphakia**). A replacement lens is required to focus light rays in the retina. Most often, a small, clear, high-density plastic lens is implanted at the same time that the cataract is removed. Replacement lenses can be selected to allow correction of a specific refractive error. Some clients have distant vision restored to 20/20 and may need glasses only for reading or close work. A newer replacement lens with multiple focal planes may correct all vision for a client to the extent that glasses or contact lenses are either no longer needed or are only minimally needed.

POSTOPERATIVE CARE. Immediately after surgery, the nurse administers an antibiotic subconjunctivally and instills an antibiotic plus steroid ointment. The eye may or may not be covered with a patch and a protective shield. The client is positioned in semi-Fowler's position or on the nonoperative

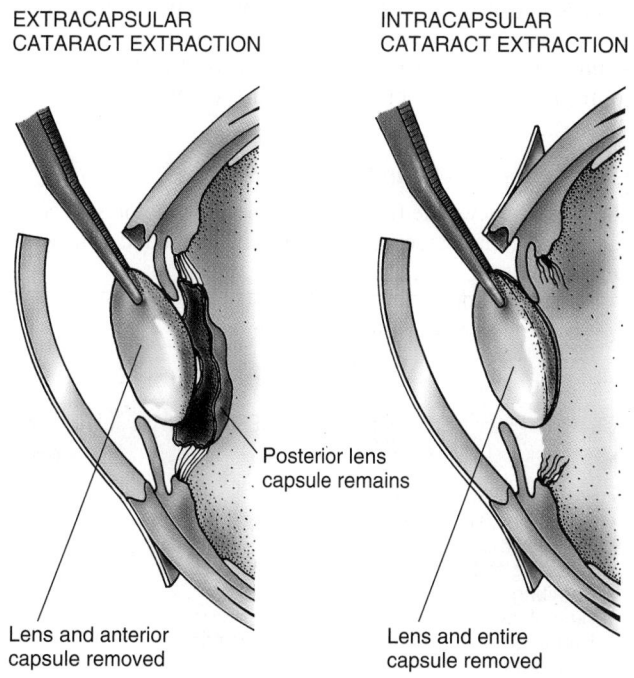

EXTRACAPSULAR
CATARACT EXTRACTION

INTRACAPSULAR
CATARACT EXTRACTION

Posterior lens
capsule remains

Lens and anterior
capsule removed

Lens and entire
capsule removed

Figure 47-9 ● Surgical approaches to lens removal for cataracts.

side. The nurse observes the dressing for evidence of drainage and reports any drainage to the surgeon.

If a dressing is used, the ophthalmologist usually performs the first dressing change and examines the eye with a slit-lamp microscope the next day. Antibiotic-steroid eyedrops, such as tobramycin combined with dexamethasone (TobraDex), are instilled.

Mild itching caused by the small stitches used to close the incision is normal. Cool compresses may be beneficial. Discomfort at the site is controlled by a mild analgesic such as acetaminophen (Abenol✤, Tylenol) or acetaminophen with oxycodone (Endocet✤, Percocet, Tylox). Aspirin is avoided because of its effects on blood coagulation.

Pain in the early postoperative period may indicate a serious complication, such as increased IOP or hemorrhage. The nurse instructs the client to contact the ophthalmologist if pain accompanied by nausea or vomiting is present.

To minimize increases in IOP (the major complication during the postoperative period), the nurse enforces and teaches the client and family about activity restrictions. Activities that can cause a sudden rise in IOP are listed in Table 47-3.

Another major complication is infection. The client is instructed to observe for increasing redness of the eye, a change in visual acuity, tearing, and photophobia. Creamy white, dry, crusty drainage on the eyelids and lashes is normal. Yellow or green drainage must be reported, however.

Bleeding into the anterior chamber of the eye also may occur, usually several days after surgery. Blood may come from the incision, iris, or ciliary body. The client is instructed to report any change in vision immediately to the ophthalmologist.

Most clients experience a dramatic improvement in vision as early as the day of surgery. The nurse cautions, however, that final best vision will not be present until 4 to 6 weeks after surgery.

● Community-Based Care

The client is usually discharged within 2 hours after cataract surgery. Because of early discharge, the nurse is essential in helping the client and family with plans for return to the home, assisted living, or extended care setting.

■ HEALTH TEACHING

The nurse reviews the following signs and symptoms of complications after cataract surgery with the client and family before discharge:
- Sharp, sudden pain
- Bleeding or increased discharge

TABLE 47-3 ●	ACTIVITIES THAT INCREASE INTRAOCULAR PRESSURE

- Bending from the waist
- Sneezing, coughing
- Blowing the nose
- Straining to have a bowel movement
- Vomiting
- Sexual intercourse
- Keeping the head in a dependent position
- Wearing tight shirt collars

- Lid swelling
- Decreased vision
- Flashes of light or floating shapes

The nurse also tells the client to avoid activities that might increase IOP (see Table 47-3). The client may wash his or her hair a day or two after surgery, but only with the head tilted back, such as in a beauty salon or barber shop, to avoid getting water in the eye. For the immediate postoperative period, the client is advised to stand in the shower with the face held away from the shower head.

Cooking and light housekeeping are permitted, but vacuuming should be avoided for several weeks because of the forward flexion involved and the rapid, jerky movements required. The client is also advised to refrain from driving, operating machinery, and participating in certain sports, such as golf, until given specific permission from the ophthalmologist.

> **CRITICAL THINKING CHALLENGE**
>
> Your 75-year-old client, who just underwent cataract surgery with intraocular lens replacement, cleans her own house, does her own shopping, eats lunch out with her friends once each week, volunteers in a soup kitchen one day per week, plays cards once each week, plays golf once each week, and plays bingo three times each week. She also drinks one glass of wine with dinner each day and bakes her own bread.
>
> - Which activities may she continue, and which activities should she avoid for the first week following surgery?

For suggested answer guidelines, go to ⟨SIMON⟩ http://www.wbsaunders.com/SIMON/Iggy/.

NIC MEDICATION ADMINISTRATION: EYE. The nurse reviews the procedure for instilling eyedrops with the client or caretaker. If the client is concerned that the drops may not be correctly instilled, the nurse may advise him or her to refrigerate the eyedrops. Then, when the eyedrop falls into the conjunctival sac, the client will experience a cool feeling. Eyedrops are typically prescribed for 4 to 6 weeks after cataract surgery (Chart 47-7).

CHART 47-7

NIC INTERVENTION ACTIVITIES for
The Client Requiring Topical Eye Medication

Medication Administration: Eye: *Preparing and instilling ophthalmic medications*
- Wash hands before preparing or administering medication.
- Follow the five rights of medication administration.
- Note client's medical history and history of allergies.
- Determine client's knowledge of medication and understanding of method of administration.
- Position client supine with neck slightly hyperextended; ask client to look at ceiling.
- Instill medication into the conjunctival sac using aseptic technique.
- Apply gentle pressure to nasolacrimal sac if medication has systemic effects.
- Instruct client to close eye gently to help distribute medication.
- Wash hands after eye medication administration.

NIC intervention activities selected from McCloskey, J.C., & Bulechek, G.M. (2000). *Nursing interventions classification (NIC)* (3rd ed.). St. Louis: Mosby. No part of this work is to be altered without prior written permission from the Publisher.

◼ HOME CARE MANAGEMENT

If the client has difficulty instilling eyedrops, a supportive neighbor, friend, or family member can be taught the procedure. Adaptive equipment that positions the bottle of eyedrops directly over the eye can also be purchased. Chart 47-8 lists items to cover in the focused assessment of a client in the home environment after cataract surgery.

◼ HEALTH CARE RESOURCES

If the client lives alone and has no family or significant others, the nurse arranges for a home care nurse to assess the client and the home situation. If the client is unable to instill eyedrops independently, a friend, neighbor, or family member can be taught this technique.

> **CRITICAL THINKING CHALLENGE**
>
> About 8 hours after cataract surgery and intraocular lens replacement, your 75-year-old client calls and tells you that her pupil on the operative side is twice as large as the pupil in the nonoperative eye and that the operative eye itches.
> • What additional information should you obtain?
> • Should this client be seen tonight, or should she keep her morning appointment?

For suggested answer guidelines, go to SIMON http://www.wbsaunders.com/SIMON/Iggy/.

◉ Evaluation: Outcomes

The nurse evaluates the care of the client with cataracts on the basis of the identified nursing diagnoses and collaborative problems. The expected outcomes include that the client will:
- Have improved vision
- Recognize signs and symptoms of complications
- Instill eyedrops correctly
- State activities that might increase IOP
- Remain free from injury

Glaucoma

◼ OVERVIEW

Glaucoma is a group of ocular diseases resulting in increased IOP. When IOP is greater than the tissues can tolerate, the cells of the retina and the optic nerve are damaged. If the condition progresses, blindness results. In most common forms of glaucoma, vision is lost gradually and painlessly, without the person's awareness.

◼ Pathophysiology

Intraocular pressure (IOP) is the fluid (aqueous humor) pressure within the eye. A normal IOP of 10 to 21 mm Hg is maintained when there is a balance between production and outflow of aqueous humor. IOP can be raised by decreasing the outflow of aqueous fluid through the anterior chamber or by overproducing aqueous humor. In people with glaucoma, aqueous humor builds up inside the eye, and the increased pressure reduces blood flow to the optic nerve and retina. The sensitive nerve tissue becomes ischemic and dies. Tissue damage usually starts in the periphery and moves inward toward the fovea centralis. Left untreated, glaucoma can result in blindness.

There are several causes and types of glaucoma (Table 47-4). Glaucoma is classified as primary, secondary, or associated. In primary glaucoma, the most common form, the structures involved in circulation and reabsorption of the aqueous humor undergo direct pathologic change.

Primary open-angle glaucoma (POAG), the most common form of primary glaucoma, is usually bilateral and asymptomatic in the early stages. There is reduced outflow of aqueous humor through the chamber angle. Because the fluid cannot leave the eye at the same rate at which it is produced, IOP gradually increases.

Angle-closure glaucoma (also called closed-angle glaucoma, narrow-angle glaucoma, or acute glaucoma) is much less common, has a sudden onset, and is treated as an emergency. The basic problems are a narrowed angle and forward displacement of the iris. Displacement of the iris against the cornea narrows or closes the chamber angle, obstructing the

---

CHART 47-8

FOCUSED ASSESSMENT of
Home Care Clients After Cataract Surgery

Assess the eye and vision, including:
- Visual acuity in both eyes using a Jaeger card
- Visual fields of both eyes
- Compare operative eye with nonoperative eye for presence or absence of:
  Redness
  Tearing
  Drainage

Ask the client about:
- Pain in or around the operative eye
- Any change in visual acuity (decreased or improved) in the operative eye
- Whether any of the following has been noticed in the operative eye:
  Dark spots
  Increase in the number of floaters
  Bright flashes of light

Assess the home environment for:
- Safety hazards (especially tripping and falling hazards)
- Kitchen hazards
- Level of room lighting

Assess client compliance with and understanding of treatment and limitations, including:
- Signs and symptoms to report
- Medication regimen
- Activity restrictions

Assess functional ability, including:
- Activities of daily living
- Compliance with medication regimen

TABLE 47-4 • COMMON CAUSES OF GLAUCOMA

PRIMARY GLAUCOMA	ASSOCIATED GLAUCOMA
• Aging	• Diabetes mellitus
• Heredity	• Hypertension
• Central retinal vein occlusion	• Severe myopia
	• Retinal detachment
SECONDARY GLAUCOMA	
• Uveitis	
• Iritis	
• Neovascular disorders	
• Trauma	
• Ocular tumors	
• Degenerative disease	
• Eye surgery	

outflow of aqueous humor. This can happen suddenly and without warning.

Secondary glaucoma results from ocular diseases that cause a narrowed angle or an increased volume of fluid within the eye. These diseases or conditions indirectly disrupt the activity of the structures involved in circulation and reabsorption of aqueous humor. This can happen suddenly and without warning.

▪ Incidence/Prevalence

Glaucoma is a common cause of blindness in industrialized countries. Incidence is age related, with as many as 10% of people older than 80 years of age affected (Vaughan, Asbury, & Riordan-Eva, 1995).

▶ COLLABORATIVE MANAGEMENT

Primary open-angle glaucoma develops slowly, usually without symptoms. The gradual loss of visual fields associated with this disease may go unnoticed because central vision is unaffected. At times, the client may have foggy vision, reduced accommodation, mild aching in the eyes, or headaches and may require frequent changes in eyeglass prescriptions. Late symptoms of glaucoma occur after irreversible damage to optic nerve function and include visual field losses, decreased visual acuity not correctable with eyeglasses, and the appearance of halos around lights. Chart 47-9 lists common clinical manifestations of glaucoma.

● Assessment

▪ PHYSICAL ASSESSMENT/CLINICAL MANIFESTATIONS

Ophthalmoscopic examination of the client with glaucoma reveals cupping and atrophy of the optic disk. The disk becomes wider and deeper and turns white or gray (Figure 47-10).

To determine the extent of peripheral field losses, visual fields are measured. A visual field examination (to detect blind spots) maps the areas seen by the eye while it fixates on a central point. In chronic open-angle glaucoma, the visual fields initially show a small crescent-shaped defect that gradually progresses to a larger field defect. In acute angle-closure glaucoma, the visual fields can quickly decrease.

The clinical manifestations of acute angle-closure glaucoma differ from those of open-angle glaucoma. The onset of symptoms is acute, and the client complains of sudden, excruciating pain around the eyes that radiates over the sensory distribution of the fifth cranial nerve. Headache or brow ache, nausea, vomiting, and abdominal discomfort also may occur. Other symptoms may include seeing colored halos around lights and sudden blurred vision with decreased light perception.

On examination, the sclera may appear reddened and the cornea foggy. Ophthalmoscopic examination reveals a shallow anterior chamber, cloudy aqueous humor, and a moderately dilated, nonreactive pupil.

▪ OTHER DIAGNOSTIC ASSESSMENT

TONOMETRY. Intraocular pressure (IOP), as measured by tonometry, is elevated in glaucoma. If an elevated reading is found during routine screening examination, the nurse takes several readings over a period of time at various times of the day to determine a pattern, because IOP varies during the day. In open-angle glaucoma, the tonometry reading is between 22 and 32 mm Hg (normal is 10 to 21 mm Hg). In angle-closure glaucoma, the tonometry reading may be 30 mm Hg or higher.

TONOGRAPHY. Tonography combines the use of an electronic indentation tonometer with a recording device. The outflow of aqueous humor from the eye is measured while a weight rests on the globe. The slope of the graph is significant. A flat tracing indicates a reduced rate of outflow, as in glaucoma. A steep downhill tracing indicates adequate drainage.

GONIOSCOPY. A special lens that eliminates the corneal curve facilitates the view of the drainage angle in the anterior chamber of the eye. The entire 360-degree circumference of the iridocorneal angle is examined. Adhesions, abnormal blood vessels, sites of trauma, and other data are noted as possible causes of secondary glaucoma.

● Interventions

NONSURGICAL MANAGEMENT. Blindness from glaucoma can be prevented by early detection, lifelong treatment, and a commitment to close monitoring and follow-up care. Usually some degree of vision loss is experienced. Chart 47-10 provides information that the nurse can use to help the older client with impaired vision to remain as independent as possible.

CHART 47-9

KEY FEATURES *of*
Glaucoma

Early
- Increased intraocular pressure
- Diminished accommodation

Late
- Diminished visual fields (loss of peripheral vision)
- Decreased visual acuity not correctable with glasses
- Halos around lights
- Headache or eye pain (acute closed-angle glaucoma)
- Increased cup-disk ratio
- Pale optic disk

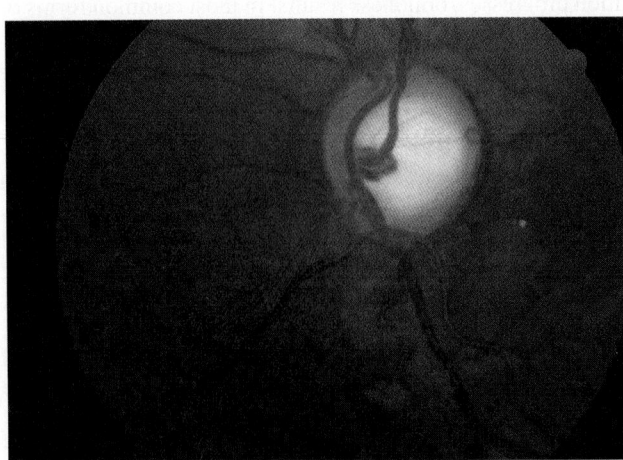

Figure 47-10 ● The optic fundus of a client with glaucoma.

DRUG THERAPY. Drug therapy for glaucoma focuses on reducing IOP through two mechanisms:

- Physically constricting the pupil so that the ciliary muscle is contracted, which allows better circulation of the aqueous humor to the site of absorption
- Inhibiting the production of aqueous humor

Pupillary Constriction. Drugs that constrict the pupil and contract the ciliary muscle **(miotics),** such as pilocarpine hydrochloride (Isopto Carpine, Pilocar, Spersacarpine❦), are commonly used to treat glaucoma. In acute angle-closure glaucoma, constriction of pupil size is also desired, because it stretches the iridocorneal angle and enhances aqueous outflow. Carbachol (Isopto Carbachol, Miostat) may be used with or in place of pilocarpine. Echothiophate iodide (Phospholine Iodide) produces miosis and increases outflow. The nurse reminds the client that miotics may cause blurred vision for 1 to 2 hours after use and that adaptation to dark environments is difficult because of the pupillary constriction.

Inhibition of Aqueous Humor. Beta blockers such as timolol (Apo-Timop❦, Timoptic) and levobunolol (Betagan) are the drug of choice for decreasing IOP. When used as eye-drops, beta blockers reduce aqueous humor production without causing pupillary constriction.

Carbonic anhydrase inhibitors, such as acetazolamide (Acetazolam❦, Diamox) and methazolamide (Neptazane), reduce aqueous humor production to help maintain a lowered IOP. Epinephrine 0.5% to 2% and dipivefrin hydrochloride (Propine) also reduce aqueous humor production. Epinephrine-containing agents are not used in angle-closure glaucoma because of the pupillary dilation caused by their sympathomimetic action.

Osmotic agents may be administered systemically for a client with angle-closure glaucoma as part of emergency treatment to rapidly reduce IOP. Such agents include oral glycerin (Osmoglyn) and IV mannitol (Osmitrol).

SURGICAL MANAGEMENT

LASER SURGERY. When a medical regimen for the client with open-angle glaucoma has been ineffective at controlling IOP, laser surgery is indicated.

Preoperative Care. Nursing interventions include informing the client about laser technology, expected sights and

---

CHART 47-10

NURSING FOCUS *on the* OLDER ADULT
Promote Independent Living in Clients with Impaired Vision

MEDICATIONS
- Having a neighbor, relative, friend, or visiting nurse visit once a week to measure the proper medications for each day may be helpful.
    If the client is to take medications more than once each day, it is helpful to use a container of a different shape (with a lid) each time. For example, if the client is to take medication at 9 AM, 1 PM, and 9 PM, the 9 AM medications would be placed in a round container, the 1 PM medications in a square container, and the 9 PM medications in a triangular container.
    It is helpful to place each day's medication containers in a separate box with raised letters on the side of the box spelling out the day.
- "Talking clocks" are available for the client with low vision.

COMMUNICATION
- Telephones with large, raised block numbers may be helpful. The best models are those with black numbers on a white phone or white numbers on a black phone.
- Telephones that have a programmable, automatic dialing feature are very helpful. Programmed numbers should include those for the fire department, police, relatives, friends, neighbors, and 911.

SAFETY
- It is best to leave furniture the way the client wants it and not move it.
- Throw rugs are best eliminated.
- Appliance cords should be short and kept out of walkways.
- Lounge-style chairs with built-in footrests are preferable to footstools.
- Nonbreakable dishes, cups, and glasses are preferable to breakable ones.
- Cleansers and other toxic agents should be labeled with large, raised letters.
- Hook-and-loop (Velcro) strips at hand level may help to mark the locations of switches and electrical outlets.

FOOD PREPARATION
- Meals on Wheels is a service that many older adults find helpful. This service brings meals at mealtime, cooked and ready to eat. The cost of this service varies, depending on the client's ability to pay.

- Many grocery stores offer a "shop by telephone" service. The client can either complete a computer booklet indicating types, amounts, and brands of items desired, or the store will complete this booklet over the telephone by asking the client specific information. The store then delivers groceries to the client's door (many stores also offer a "put away" service) and charges the client's bank card.
- A microwave oven is a safer means of cooking than a standard stove, although many older clients are afraid of microwave ovens. If the client has and will use a microwave oven, others can prepare meals ahead of time, label them, and freeze them for later use. Also, many complete, microwavable frozen dinners that comply with a variety of dietary restrictions are available.
- Friends or relatives may be able to help with food preparation. Often relatives do not know what to give an older person for birthdays or other gift-giving occasions. One suggestion is a homemade prepackaged frozen dinner that the client enjoys.

PERSONAL CARE
- Handgrips should be installed in bathrooms.
- The tub floor should have a nonskid surface.
- Male clients should use an electric shaver rather than a razor.
- Choosing a hairstyle that is becoming but easy to care for (avoiding parts) will help in independent living.
- Home hair care services may be available.

DIVERSIONAL ACTIVITY
- Some clients are able to use large-print books, newspapers, and magazines (available through local libraries and vision services).
- Books, magazines, and some newspapers are available on audiotape.
- Clients experienced in knitting or crocheting may be able to create items fashioned from straight pieces, such as afghans.
- Card games, dominoes, and some board games that are available in large, high-contrast print may be helpful for clients with low vision.

sounds commonly heard during this procedure, and expected outcomes.

Operative Procedure. A laser **trabeculoplasty** burns the trabecular meshwork, scarring it and causing the meshwork fibers to tighten. This tightening of the fibers increases the size of the spaces between the fibers, allowing outflow of aqueous humor and a reduction in IOP. Topical or local anesthesia is used. Clients commonly experience a temporary increase in IOP immediately after this procedure.

Laser surgery is also indicated for clients with angle-closure glaucoma. The laser makes a hole near the edge of the iris, allowing aqueous humor to flow from the posterior chamber to the anterior chamber and then into the trabecular meshwork.

Postoperative Care. The client is instructed to arrange for transportation home because driving is prohibited immediately after the surgery. Because laser procedures can sometimes increase IOP, the pressure should be re-evaluated 1 hour after surgery and before discharge. The ophthalmologist may prescribe an ocular steroid, such as prednisolone acetate (Ocu-Pred, Ophtho-Tate✦).

STANDARD SURGICAL THERAPY. In open-angle glaucoma that fails to respond to drug and laser therapy and in selected cases of angle-closure glaucoma, surgical intervention is required. This surgery either creates a new drainage channel for aqueous humor or destroys the structures responsible for its production.

Glaucoma surgery is performed either in a hospital or on an outpatient basis. The usual length of stay is several hours to several days.

After surgery, the ophthalmologist administers an antibiotic subconjunctivally. The eye is covered with a patch after an antibiotic-steroid ointment is inserted, and a protective shield is applied over it. The client is instructed to avoid taking aspirin, to avoid lying on the operative side, and to report any brow pain, severe eye pain, or nausea.

The most serious complication after glaucoma surgery is choroidal hemorrhage. If IOP is too low, fluid may enter the suprachoroid space and cause a choroidal detachment. The accumulation of fluid in this space may break blood vessels located there. Symptoms of choroidal hemorrhage include the following:

- Acute pain deep in the eye
- Decreased vision
- Vital sign changes

OCULAR CHAMBER DISORDERS: VITREOUS HEMORRHAGE

▌OVERVIEW

The vitreous is the gelatinous body that makes up the posterior two thirds of the eye and provides the eye's shape. Vitreous hemorrhage (bleeding into the vitreous cavity) may result from aging, systemic diseases, or trauma, or it may occur spontaneously. With aging, the vitreous may spontaneously detach from the retina. If blood vessels are torn, bleeding into the vitreous results. Diseases that disrupt the retinal blood vessels, such as hypertensive retinopathy and proliferative diabetic retinopathy, also may cause blood leakage into the vitreous.

▶ COLLABORATIVE MANAGEMENT

The primary symptom of vitreous hemorrhage is reduced visual acuity; the degree of reduction varies with the severity of the hemorrhage. A mild hemorrhage may cause the client to see a red haze or series of vitreous "floaters." The client experiencing a moderate hemorrhage may graphically describe seeing "black streaks" or "tiny black dots." Severe hemorrhage may cause visual acuity to be reduced to hand motion. Eye examination shows a reduced red reflex because light rays are blocked from reaching the retina. Ultrasonography is used to determine the location and extent of the hemorrhage.

A vitreous hemorrhage may absorb slowly with no treatment. If the hemorrhage is still present several weeks to months later, a **vitrectomy** (surgical removal of the vitreous) is indicated.

UVEAL TRACT DISORDERS: UVEITIS

▌OVERVIEW

The uveal tract is composed of three distinct but related parts: the iris, the ciliary body, and the choroid. The most common problem associated with these structures is inflammation, or **uveitis.** Uveitis may occur in the anterior or posterior portion of the eye.

Anterior uveitis can include inflammation of the iris, inflammation of the ciliary body, or both. The cause of anterior uveitis is unknown, but the condition is associated with exposure to allergens, infectious agents, trauma, or systemic disease (rheumatoid arthritis, ankylosing spondylitis, herpes simplex, herpes zoster). It can follow any local or systemic bacterial infection. Symptoms include aching around the eye; tearing; blurred vision; photophobia; a small, irregular, nonreactive pupil; and a "bloodshot" appearance of the sclera.

Posterior uveitis is the common term for **retinitis** (inflammation of the retina) and **chorioretinitis** (inflammation of both the choroid and the retina). Posterior uveitis is associated with tuberculosis, syphilis, and toxoplasmosis.

The onset of symptoms is slow and insidious. Visual impairment in the affected eye, the primary symptom, results from protein-rich fluid, fibrin, and cells leaking into the vitreous cavity. The pupil is small, nonreactive, and irregularly shaped. Black dots are visible against the red background of the fundus. Chorioretinal lesions appear as grayish yellow patches on the retinal surface.

▶ COLLABORATIVE MANAGEMENT

Treatment of the client with anterior or posterior uveitis includes resting the ciliary body with a cycloplegic agent. The pupil is dilated to prevent adhesions between the iris and the lens. Steroid drops are administered every hour to decrease the inflammatory response of the eye and to prevent adhesions of the iris to the cornea and lens. Subconjunctival injections of steroids may be used in posterior uveitis or when topical steroids have been ineffective. Analgesics that contain neither aspirin nor opioids are ordered for pain. Antibiotic therapy may be started for the client with posterior uveitis or when infection is present with anterior uveitis.

Cool or warm compresses are applied for ocular pain. Darkening the room and wearing sunglasses reduce the discomfort of photophobia. Because of blurred vision from the cycloplegic drops, the nurse instructs the client not to drive or operate machinery. The nurse reviews the signs and symptoms of bacterial and fungal ulcers and the indications of increased intraocular pressure (IOP).

RETINAL DISORDERS

Hypertensive Retinopathy

■ OVERVIEW

Many Americans have hypertension. Hypertension causes blood vessel changes in the eyes that lead to retinal damage and decreased vision.

Hypertensive retinopathy is classified by grades. With each increasing grade, progressive changes are noted in the retina. A direct relationship exists between narrowing of the retinal arterioles and elevation of the diastolic blood pressure.

▶ COLLABORATIVE MANAGEMENT

As blood pressure increases, retinal arterioles narrow and take on a characteristic "copper wire" appearance (Figure 47-11). Nicking, or narrowing, of the vessel at arteriovenous crossings is apparent. If blood pressure remains elevated, areas of localized ischemia, known as soft exudates or "cotton wool" spots, develop as a result of occlusion of the arteriole. Small hemorrhages may be noted. The client may also have headaches and vertigo. Left untreated, hypertensive retinopathy can cause retinal detachment.

Treatment focuses primarily on management of the systemic hypertension (see Chapter 36) and controlling IOP.

Diabetic Retinopathy

■ OVERVIEW

Diabetic retinopathy is the vascular complication of diabetes in the retina. The longer the person has diabetes, the greater is the incidence and severity of retinopathy (Cotran, Kumar, & Collins, 1999). Another factor influencing the severity of retinopathy is blood glucose control. Good control lessens the severity of the disease. There are two types of diabetic retinopathy: background diabetic retinopathy and proliferative diabetic retinopathy.

In **background diabetic retinopathy,** the supporting cells of the retinal vessels die, and the capillary walls of the retina allow fluid to leak. As this fluid is absorbed, thick yellow-white deposits, or hard exudates, are formed. The retinal capillaries become diseased and lose their ability to transport needed oxygen and nutrients. Outpouches in the walls of capillaries (**microaneurysms**) are formed. These fragile capillaries bleed easily and cause intraretinal hemorrhages in the nerve fiber layer of the retina (Figure 47-12). Visual acuity is diminished by reduction of the capillary blood supply to the retina or by macular edema.

In clients with **proliferative diabetic retinopathy,** a network of fragile new blood vessels develops, leaking blood and protein into the surrounding tissue. Development of these blood vessels is stimulated by the hypoxic state of the retina that results from poor capillary perfusion of retinal tissues. New blood vessels grow in the retina, encroach onto the iris, and grow into the posterior face of the vitreous. The vitreous contracts and pulls away from the retina, causing blood vessels to break and bleed into the vitreous.

▶ COLLABORATIVE MANAGEMENT

Treatment of the client with diabetic retinopathy depends on the degree of retinal involvement. Laser therapy can be used to seal microaneurysms, resulting in decreased bleeding. Scattering of laser burns across the retina can also decrease the retina's need for oxygen and control the growth of new blood vessels.

A vitrectomy is performed if frequent bleeding into the vitreous occurs and the body is unable to reabsorb it or if fibrin bands threaten to detach the retina. Fibrin bands within the vitreous are severed and removed. An endolaser may be used in the eye during surgery to seal leaking or bleeding blood vessels.

Macular Degeneration

■ OVERVIEW

Macular degeneration (deterioration of the macula, the area of central vision) can be atrophic (age related, or *dry*) or exudative *(wet).* Atrophic degeneration is characterized by scle-

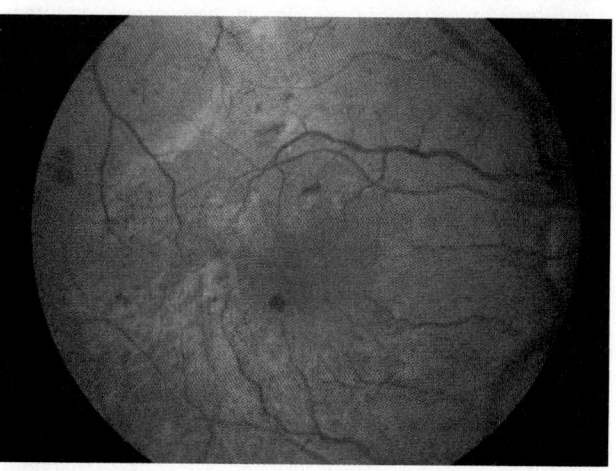

Figure 47-11 ● The optic fundus of a client with hypertension.

Figure 47-12 ● The optic fundus of a client with diabetes.

rosing of retinal capillaries, causing macular cells to become ischemic and necrotic. Rod and cone photoreceptors die. Central vision declines, and clients describe "mild blurring and distortion." This type of degeneration is more common and progresses at a faster rate among smokers than among non-smokers. Current research into nutrition therapy suggests that the risk for atrophic macular degeneration can be reduced by increasing long-term dietary intake of antioxidants and the carotenoids lutein and zeaxanthin (see the Evidence-Based Practice for Nursing box below).

Clients with exudative degeneration experience a sudden decrease in vision after a serous detachment of pigment epithelium in the macula. Blood vessels invade this injured area and cause fluid and blood to accumulate under the macula (like a blister), resulting in scar formation and progressive distortion of vision.

► COLLABORATIVE MANAGEMENT

Treatment of atrophic macular degeneration aims to help the client maximize remaining vision. The associated loss of central vision may interfere with the ability to read, write, recognize safety hazards, and drive. The nurse suggests alternative strategies (such as large-print books and public transportation) and referrals to community organizations that provide a wide range of adaptive equipment.

Management of clients with exudative macular degeneration is geared toward slowing the process and identifying further changes in visual perception. Fluid and blood may resorb

in a small percentage of clients with exudative degeneration. Laser therapy to seal the leaking blood vessels in or near the macula can limit the extent of the damage.

Retinal Holes, Tears, and Detachments
▌OVERVIEW

A retinal hole is a break in the integrity of the peripheral sensory retina. Retinal holes can be caused by trauma or can occur with aging.

A retinal tear is a more jagged and irregularly shaped break in the retina. It can result from traction on the retina.

A retinal detachment is the separation of the sensory retina from the pigmented epithelium. Retinal detachments are classified by the nature of their development.

Rhegmatogenous detachments occur following a hole or tear in the retina caused by mechanical force, creating an opening for the vitreous to filter into the subretinal space. When sufficient fluid collects in this space, the retina detaches.

Traction detachments are created when the retina is pulled away from the epithelium by bands of fibrous tissue in the vitreous.

Exudative detachments are caused by fluid accumulation in the subretinal space; they occur in association with a systemic disease or with ocular tumors. No retinal break occurs.

► COLLABORATIVE MANAGEMENT

The onset of a retinal detachment is usually sudden and painless because no pain fibers are located in the retina. Clients may suddenly see bright flashes of light (**photopsia**) or floating dark spots in the affected eye. During the initial phase of the detachment or if the detachment is partial, the client may describe the sensation of a curtain being pulled over part of the visual field. The visual field loss corresponds to the area of detachment.

▐● Assessment

On ophthalmoscopic examination, detachments appear as gray bulges or folds in the retina that quiver with movement. This appearance is in marked contrast to the flat pink-orange color of the choroid as it shows through the transparent retina. Depending on the cause of the detachment, a hole or tear also may be seen at the edge of the detachment.

▐● Interventions

If a retinal hole or tear is discovered before it causes a detachment, the ophthalmologist may elect to close or seal the break. Closure prevents the accumulation of fluid under the retina, reducing the likelihood of a detachment. Treatment aims to create an inflammatory response that will bind the retina and choroid together around the break. This inflammatory response can be created through external application of **cryotherapy** (a freezing probe), **photocoagulation** (laser), or **diathermy** (high-frequency current).

Spontaneous reattachment of the retina is rare. Surgical repair is required to place the retina in contact with the underlying structures. A common repair procedure is scleral buckling.

PREOPERATIVE CARE. Clients requiring retinal surgery are anxious and fearful about a possible permanent loss of vision. The nurse provides information and reassurance to allay fears.

Depending on the location and size of the retinal break, activity restrictions may be necessary immediately to prevent further tearing or detachment and to promote drainage of any subretinal fluid.

The nurse places an eyepatch over the client's affected eye to reduce eye movement. Topical medications to inhibit accommodation and constriction of the pupil are administered before surgery.

OPERATIVE PROCEDURE. The surgery is performed with the client under general anesthesia. In scleral buckling, the ophthalmologist repairs wrinkles or folds in the retina so that the retina can assume its normal smooth position, and the sclera flattens against the retina. To promote reattachment, a small piece of silicone is placed against the sclera and held in place by an encircling band (Figure 47-13). These devices keep the retina in contact with the choroid and sclera to promote attachment. Any subretinal fluid present is drained.

To further encourage retinal reattachment, a gas such as sulfahexafluoride (SF6) or silicone oil can be used. These agents float up against the retina to hold it in place until healing occurs.

POSTOPERATIVE CARE. After retinal reattachment surgery, an eyepatch and shield are applied. The nurse monitors the client's vital signs and checks the eyepatch and shield for any drainage.

Activity status varies. If gas or oil has been used, the nurse positions the client on his or her abdomen to allow the gas to float against the retina. The client lies with the head turned so that the operative eye is facing up, for several days or until the gas has been absorbed. As an alternative, he or she can sit on the side of the bed and place the head on an over-the-bed table. Bathroom privileges are allowed once the client is fully awake.

The client may experience nausea and pain postoperatively. The nurse administers analgesics and antiemetics as prescribed. Any complaint of a sudden increase in pain or pain accompanied by nausea is reported to the ophthalmologist because these symptoms may indicate the development of complications. The nurse also instructs the client to avoid activities that increase intraocular pressure (IOP) (see Table 47-3).

In the first week after retinal detachment surgery, the client must avoid reading, writing, and close work, such as sewing, because these activities cause rapid eye movements. The nurse teaches the client about the signs and symptoms associated with infection and detachment. The client is instructed to notify the nurse or physician if any signs or symptoms occur.

Retinitis Pigmentosa

▮ OVERVIEW

Several types of bilateral retinal disorders with progressive degeneration of the retina and a loss of visual receptors lead to blindness. Retinitis pigmentosa is a condition in which retinal nerve cells degenerate and the pigmented cells of the retina grow and move into the sensory areas of the retina, causing further degeneration. Different forms of this disorder can be inherited as an autosomal dominant trait, an autosomal recessive trait, or an X-linked recessive trait (Cotran, Kumar, & Collins, 1999).

▶ COLLABORATIVE MANAGEMENT

The most common early clinical manifestation experienced by a person with retinitis pigmentosa is night blindness. Over time, decreased visual acuity progresses to total blindness. Ophthalmoscopic examination of the retina shows excessive pigmentation in a lattice-like pattern. Cataracts may accompany this disorder.

No current therapy has proved effective in preventing or slowing the degenerative process. Because some retinal destruction resembles that seen with vitamin A deficiency, a regimen of vitamin A, along with decreased exposure of the retina to bright light, is being tried.

REFRACTIVE ERRORS

▮ OVERVIEW

The ability of the eye to focus images on the retina depends on the length of the eye from front to back and the refractive power of the lens system. **Refraction** is the bending of light rays. Problems in either eye length or refraction can result in refractive errors.

▮ Myopia

In **myopia** (nearsightedness), the refractive ability of the eye is too strong for the eye length. Images are bent and fall in front of, not on, the retina.

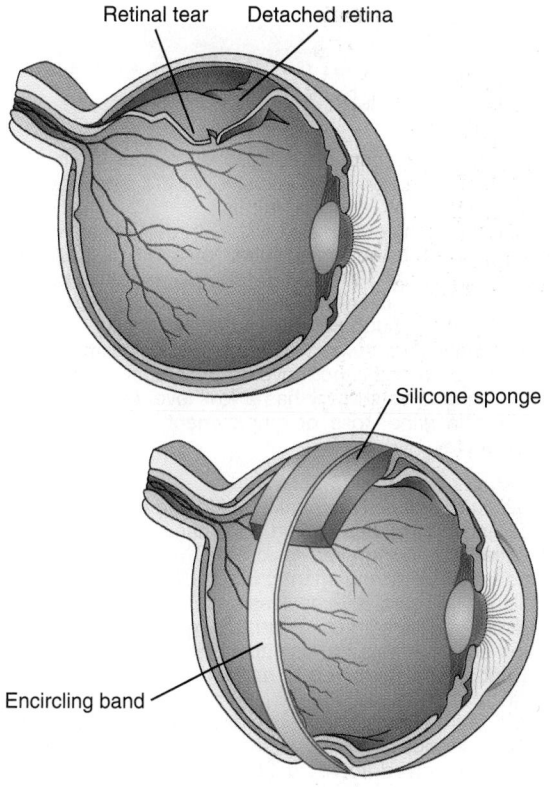

Retinal tear   Detached retina

Silicone sponge

Encircling band

Figure 47-13 ● The scleral buckling procedure for repair of retinal detachment.

Hyperopia

In **hyperopia,** or **hypermetropia** (farsightedness), the refractive ability of the eye is too weak, causing images to be focused behind the retina. A shorter length of the eye may contribute to the development of hyperopia.

Presbyopia

As people age, the crystalline lens loses its elasticity and is less able to alter its shape to focus the eye for close work **(presbyopia).** As a result, images fall behind the retina. Presbyopia usually occurs in people in their 30s and 40s.

Astigmatism

Astigmatism occurs when the curve of the cornea is uneven. Because light rays are not refracted equally in all directions, a focus point on the retina is not achieved.

► COLLABORATIVE MANAGEMENT

● Assessment

Refractive errors are diagnosed through a process known as **refraction.** The client is asked to view an eye chart while lenses of different strengths are systematically placed in front of the eye, and is then asked whether the lenses sharpen or worsen vision. The power or strength of the lens necessary to permit focusing of the image on the retina is expressed in measurements called **diopters.**

● Interventions

NONSURGICAL MANAGEMENT. Errors of refraction must be corrected through the use of a lens to permit light rays to focus on the retina (see Figure 46-5). Myopic vision is corrected to bring the image forward onto the retina with a concave lens. Hyperopic vision is corrected with a convex lens to move the focused image back to the retina.

EYEGLASSES. Eyeglasses commonly correct errors of refraction. Advantages of eyeglasses, when compared with other refractive error corrections, include ease of use, durability, availability, and low cost. Disadvantages include a change in physical appearance, the weight of the frame on the nose, and reduced peripheral vision (vision is corrected only when the client looks through the center of the lens).

CONTACT LENSES. Contact lenses can also correct refractive errors. Round plastic disks rest against the cornea and fit under the eyelid.

Hard Lenses. Hard contact lenses correct refractive errors by changing the shape of the cornea, which increases its refracting ability, and by placing the specific refractive power and shape needed in front of the eye so that light rays can be correctly focused onto the retina.

Complications of hard contact lens wear include corneal edema, which occurs when the lenses are worn for an extended period. Corneal abrasions can result from overwear, which dries the epithelium and causes minute breaks, or from the irritation of the contact lens against the cornea.

Soft Lenses. Soft contact lenses are larger but better tolerated than hard contact lenses. They resemble the thickness of plastic wrap and can be worn for longer periods because the lenses' hydrophilic character allows greater corneal access to moisture and oxygen. Most problems with wearing soft lenses are related to lens deterioration, deposits in the lens, and lack of compliance with lens care practices.

There are two types of soft contact lenses: daily-wear lenses (worn during waking hours) and extended-wear lenses. Extended-wear contact lenses can be worn continuously for several days to several weeks, depending on the client's environment, activities, and tolerance of the lenses.

SURGICAL MANAGEMENT. Surgery is becoming a popular alternative for the treatment of refractive errors. Such vision-enhancing surgeries include radial keratotomy, photorefractive keratectomy, laser in-situ keratomileusis, and placement of Intacs corneal ring segments. All surgical procedures are much more expensive than eyeglasses or any type of contact lens. These procedures are rarely covered by insurance (see the Cost of Care box below).

RADIAL KERATOTOMY. **Radial keratotomy (RK)** is an outpatient surgical procedure for the treatment of mild to moderate myopia. Eight to 16 diagonal incisions are made through 90% of the peripheral cornea. Because the central cornea is not incised, vision is not diminished. These incisions flatten the cornea, which decreases the length of the eye and allows the image to be focused closer to the retina.

Slight overcorrection or undercorrection of the refractive error is possible, in which case the client still must wear some form of visual correction after the surgery. Other complications include corneal scarring and chronic dry eyes.

COST OF CARE
IMPLICATIONS FOR NURSING

VISION-ENHANCING SURGERY

Cost of Care
- The cost of prescription eyeglasses ranges from $50 to $500, depending on the complexity of the prescription, the quality of the lens, and the frames.
- The cost of contact lenses (hard, soft, daily wear, extended wear) represents an initial outlay of $100 to $300 and a yearly expense of $80 to $150 for consumable supplies.
- The cost of any vision-enhancing surgical procedure ranges from $2000 to $5000 per eye (varies regionally).
- Vision-enhancing surgery is considered cosmetic rather than indicated and is not covered by insurance.
- Vision-enhancing surgery has a low level of complications resulting in either loss of employment time or increased hospital stay.

Implications for Nursing
Poor vision decreases the quality of life and vocational opportunities and contributes to injury in many ways. In addition, some clients with impaired vision may require assistance or dependent living arrangements. Enhancing vision can be accomplished with assistive devices such as eyeglasses or contact lenses and by surgical means. Surgical procedures result in vision enhancement that is superior to that of assistive devices. Long-term follow-up is needed to determine whether the high cost of vision-enhancing surgery may be offset by decreased lifetime costs of assistive devices or by decreased incidence of serious injury. Currently, nurses need to help clients weigh the perceived and actual benefits against the costs related to different types of vision enhancement.

PHOTOREFRACTIVE KERATECTOMY. **Photorefractive keratectomy (PRK)** is an alternative for people with mild to moderate stable myopia and low astigmatism. PRK is not a laser version of radial keratotomy but a completely different procedure. An excimer laser pulses a brief but powerful beam of ultraviolet light on the central superficial cornea. This beam removes small portions of the tissue surface, reshaping the cornea to properly focus an image on the retina.

Photorefractive keratectomy is performed as an outpatient procedure with the client under local anesthesia. One eye is treated at a time, usually at least 3 months apart. The eye is patched after surgery. Complete healing to best vision may take up to 6 months.

Most people do not need corrective lenses for distance vision after PRK but may still need reading glasses. Expected side effects of PRK in the postoperative period include pain, hazy vision, light sensitivity, tearing, and pupil enlargement. Possible complications include difficulty with night vision, corneal clouding, undercorrection, far-sightedness, increased intraocular pressure (IOP), chronic dry eyes, and glare.

LASER IN-SITU KERATOMILEUSIS. **Laser-in-situ keratomileusis (LASIK)** is a newer procedure for correcting near-sightedness, far-sightedness, and astigmatism using the excimer laser. With this procedure, the superficial layers of the cornea are lifted temporarily as a flap and brief but powerful laser pulses reshape the deeper corneal layers. After reshaping the deeper layers, the superficial cornea is placed back into its original position.

LASIK is performed as an outpatient procedure with the client under local anesthesia. Usually both eyes are treated at the same time, although some clients prefer separate surgeries. Most clients have improved functional vision within an hour after surgery; complete healing to best vision may take up to 4 weeks.

This procedure is thought to be superior to PRK because the outer corneal layer is not damaged. Pain is reportedly less than for PRK, and the time to best vision is reduced. Most clients require less postoperative medication, and a wider variety of refractive errors can be treated with LASIK than with PRK.

After LASIK correction of refractive errors, many clients no longer require eyeglasses or contact lenses. Overcorrection or undercorrection is possible, however, and some clients may need a mild prescription for a refractive error. The risk for complications is reportedly less than for other types of vision-enhancing surgery and includes corneal clouding and chronic dry eyes.

INTACS CORNEAL RING. Intacs corneal ring placement is the most recent vision-enhancing procedure for near-sightedness. This surgery does not involve the use of a laser and has the advantage of being reversible. With this procedure, the shape of the cornea is changed by placing a polymeric ring in the outer edges of the cornea (outside of the optical zone).

Intacs ring placement is performed as an outpatient procedure with the client under local anesthesia. Healing to best vision is immediate. Overcorrection or undercorrection of refraction is possible; however, removal, replacement, or adjustment of ring tightness can enhance satisfaction. In addition, replacements can be made if the client's vision changes further as a result of aging. Because the ring is applied to the cornea outside of the optical zone, the risk for corneal clouding or scarring is lower than with other surgical procedures.

TRAUMATIC DISORDERS

Trauma to the eye or periorbital area can result from almost any activity. Care varies depending on the area of the eye affected and whether the globe of the eye has been penetrated.

Hyphema

▌ OVERVIEW

A **hyphema** is a hemorrhage in the anterior chamber. It occurs when a force is applied to the eye and breaks the blood vessels.

► COLLABORATIVE MANAGEMENT

If the hyphema is large, it may block the pupil and reduce vision, possibly causing pain and photophobia. Hemolysis of the blood occurs, and the blood is filtered out of the eye through the trabecular meshwork. If the hemolyzed blood obstructs the trabecular meshwork, increased intraocular pressure (IOP) results.

The client with a hyphema is treated by bedrest in semi-Fowler's position to use gravity as an aid in keeping the hyphema away from the optical center of the cornea. Minimal or no sudden eye movements are permitted for 3 to 5 days to decrease the risk for rebleeding. Cycloplegic eyedrops may be ordered to place the eye at rest, and the eye is protected by a patch and shield. Television and reading are restricted. A hyphema usually resolves in 5 to 7 days.

Contusion

▌ OVERVIEW

A contusion of the eyeball and surrounding tissue is caused by traumatic contact with a blunt object. The force of the blow pushes the eye back in the socket. The globe is compressed, and stretching of the ocular soft tissues occurs, which can produce damage and possibly rupture the globe.

Results of the injury may not be seen immediately. These results include edema of the eyelids, subconjunctival hemorrhage, corneal edema, and hyphema.

► COLLABORATIVE MANAGEMENT

Periorbital ecchymosis, or "black eye," a common contusion injury, is usually caused by blunt trauma. Bleeding into the soft tissue occurs, creating the characteristic purple bruise. The color fades gradually and disappears in approximately 10 days. Visual acuity is usually not affected, although orbital pain, photophobia, eyelid edema, and diplopia may be present.

Treatment begins at the time of injury. Ice is applied immediately. The client should receive a thorough eye examination to rule out any other eye injuries.

Foreign Bodies

▌ OVERVIEW

Eyelashes, dust, fingernails, dirt, and airborne particles can come in contact with the conjunctiva or cornea and irritate or abrade the surface. If nothing is seen on the cornea or conjunctiva, the eyelids are everted to examine the palpebral and bulbar conjunctivae.

▶ COLLABORATIVE MANAGEMENT

The client complains of "feeling something in my eye" or of blurry vision. Pain is a common symptom if the corneal epithelium is injured. Tearing and photophobia may be present.

Evaluation of vision is done before treatment. The nurse examines the eye of any client with a suspected or known corneal abrasion with fluorescein, followed by ocular irrigation with normal saline (0.9%) to gently remove the particles. Best practices for ocular irrigation are described in Chart 47-11.

After the foreign body is removed and the eyepatch applied, the nurse tells the client how long the patch must be left in place (usually overnight). The client is reminded to seek follow-up care to have the patch removed and the eye examined.

Lacerations
■ OVERVIEW

Lacerations are wounds caused by sharp objects and projectiles. Lacerations can occur to any part of the eye, but the most common areas of involvement are the eyelids and the cornea.

▶ COLLABORATIVE MANAGEMENT

Initially, the eye is closed and a small ice pack is applied to decrease bleeding. The client receives medical attention as soon as possible.

CHART 47-11

BEST PRACTICE *for*
Ocular Irrigation

1. Assemble equipment:
   - Normal saline IV (1000-mL bag)
   - Macrodrip IV tubing
   - IV pole
   - Eyelid speculum
   - Topical anesthetic (proparacaine hydrochloride)
   - Gloves
   - Collection receptacle (emesis basin works well)
   - Towels
   - pH paper
2. Quickly obtain a history from the client while flushing the tubing with normal saline:
   - Nature and time of the injury
   - Type of irritant or chemical (if known)
   - Type of first aid administered at the scene
   - Any allergies to the "caine" family of medications
3. Evaluate the client's visual acuity *before* treatment:
   - Ask the client to read your name tag with the affected eye while covering the good eye.
   - Ask the client to "count fingers" with the affected eye while covering the good eye.
4. Put on gloves.
5. Place a strip of pH paper in the cul-de-sac of the client's affected eye.
6. Instill proparacaine hydrochloride eyedrops as ordered.
7. Place the client in a supine position with the head turned slightly toward the affected eye.
8. Have the client hold the affected eye open, or position an eyelid speculum.
9. Direct the flow of normal saline across the affected eye from the nasal corner of the eye toward the outer corner of the eye.
10. Assess the client's comfort during the procedure.
11. If both eyes are affected, irrigate them simultaneously using separate personnel and equipment.

If the client can open the eye, the nurse checks visual acuity and cleans the eyelids. Minor lacerations of the eyelid can be sutured in an emergency department, an urgent care center, or an ophthalmologist's office. A microscope is necessary in the operating room if the client has a laceration that involves the eyelid margin, affects the lacrimal system, involves a large area, or has jagged edges.

Corneal lacerations are considered an ocular emergency because ocular contents may prolapse through the laceration. Symptoms include severe eye pain, photophobia, tearing, decreased visual acuity, and inability to open the eyelid. If the laceration is the result of a penetrating injury, an object may be noted protruding from the eye. *This object must never be removed except by the ophthalmologist, because it may be holding ocular structures in place.*

Antibiotics are initiated to reduce the likelihood of an infection. Depending on the depth of the laceration, scarring may develop. If the scar alters vision, a corneal transplant may be needed later. If the ocular contents have prolapsed through the laceration or if the injury is severe, enucleation (surgical eye removal) may be indicated.

Penetrating Injuries
■ OVERVIEW

Clients with penetrating ocular injuries have the poorest chance of retaining vision in the injured eye. Glass, high-speed metallic or wood particles, BB pellets, and bullets are common causes of penetrating injuries. The particles can enter the eye through the eyelid, sclera, or cornea and can lodge in or behind the eyeball.

▶ COLLABORATIVE MANAGEMENT

The client usually complains of some eye pain and relates a history of "suddenly feeling hit in the eye." An entrance wound may be visible. Depending on the location of the entrance and the resting place of the projectile, vision may be affected.

X-ray studies and computed tomography (CT) scans of the orbit are obtained. Ultrasonography of the globe and orbit may also be performed. *Magnetic resonance imaging (MRI) is contraindicated because the procedure may move any metal-containing projectile and cause more injury.*

Surgery is usually required to remove the foreign object. In some cases, foreign bodies need to be removed by a vitrectomy. IV antibiotics are started before surgery to reduce the chance of an infection or endophthalmitis. A tetanus booster is administered if necessary.

Visual acuity is assessed and documented. If the client cannot see print, the nurse determines whether he or she can count fingers or see directional movement of the nurse's hand. If the client cannot see movement, the nurse assesses his or her ability to see light.

OCULAR MELANOMA
■ OVERVIEW

Melanoma is the most common intraocular malignant tumor in adults. This tumor occurs most often in the uveal tract among people in their 30s and 40s.

Because of its rich blood supply, an ocular melanoma can spread easily. Common pathways for metastatic spread are extension through the sclera or through invasion of other intraocular structures into surrounding tissue and the brain.

► COLLABORATIVE MANAGEMENT
● Assessment

Symptoms of malignant melanoma may not be readily apparent; the tumor may be discovered during a routine examination. Blurring of vision may occur if the macular area is invaded. Visual acuity is reduced if the tumor grows inward toward the center of the eye from the choroid and alters the visual pathway. Increased intraocular pressure (IOP) can result if the tumor invades the canal of Schlemm and obstructs outflow of aqueous humor. A change in iris color may occur if the tumor infiltrates the iris. Sudden loss of a portion of the visual field may result from tumor invasion of the subretinal space, producing retinal detachment.

Diagnostic tests for a malignant melanoma depend on the size and growth rate of the tumor. Ultrasonography is performed to determine the tumor's location and size.

● Interventions

Treatment also depends on the tumor's size and growth rate, as well as the condition of the other eye. Small lesions of the iris not affecting the iris root are monitored until growth is observed. Tumors of the choroid can be treated by surgical enucleation or by radiation therapy with a radioactive cobalt plaque.

SURGERY. Enucleation (surgical removal of the entire eyeball) is performed with the client under general anesthesia. After the eye is removed, a ball implant is inserted to provide a base for the socket prosthesis and to ensure the best cosmetic result.

The implant is covered with surrounding tissue, muscles, and conjunctiva. A plastic conformer is placed over the conjunctiva to maintain the shape of the eyelids until a prosthesis can be fitted. After the dressing is removed, a pressure patch is placed over the eye for 24 hours.

Until the prosthesis is fitted (usually 1 month after surgery), an antibiotic-steroid ointment is inserted into the cul-de-sac once a day. Best practices for the insertion and removal of the prosthesis are presented in Chart 47-12.

RADIATION THERAPY. Radiation therapy can reduce the size and thickness of malignant melanomas. The radioactive plaque, a round, flat disk about the size of a dime and containing a radioactive material, such as cobalt-60 or iodine-125, is sutured to the sclera overlying the tumor site. The length of time the plaque remains sutured to the sclera depends on the size of the tumor and the dose of radiation to be delivered.

Complications of radiation therapy include vascular changes, retinopathy, glaucoma, necrosis of the sclera, and cataract formation. Vitreous hemorrhage may develop as the tumor becomes smaller and pulls or breaks blood vessels.

While the plaque is in place, the eye may or may not be covered with a patch. Cycloplegic eyedrops and an antibiotic-steroid combination are administered. The nurse teaches the client how to instill eyedrops.

BLINDNESS
■ OVERVIEW

Different forms of blindness exist and may affect any or all aspects of vision, including color, light, image, movement, and acuity. Clients are classified as legally blind if their best visual acuity with corrective lenses is 20/200 or less in the better eye or if the widest diameter of the visual field in that eye is no greater than 20 degrees.

Blindness can occur in one or both eyes. When one eye is affected, the field of vision is narrowed and depth perception is impaired.

Central vision can be impaired by diseases involving the macula, such as macular edema or macular degeneration. Loss of peripheral vision is associated with glaucoma. The loss of side vision affects the client's ability to drive and his or her awareness of hazards in the periphery.

► COLLABORATIVE MANAGEMENT

The nurse teaches the client techniques to make better use of existing vision. Moving the head slightly up and down can enhance a three-dimensional effect. When shaking hands or pouring water, the client can line up the object and move toward it. He or she should choose a position that favors the good eye; for example, people with vision in the right eye should position people and items on their right.

Nursing interventions for the client with reduced sight fall into four areas: orientation, ambulation, self-care, and support.

ORIENTATION. Most clients seen in health care settings have varied degrees of sight. Most clients categorized as "blind" had sight at some time and thus have a background knowledge regarding size and shape on which the nurse can rely when providing information. When talking with a client who has limited sight or is blind, the nurse always uses a normal tone of voice.

The nurse first orients the client to the immediate environment, including the approximate size of the room. One object in the room, such as an examination chair or hospital bed, serves as the focal point during the nurse's description. The nurse guides the client to the focal point and orients him or her to the environment from that point. For example, the nurse might say, "To the left of the bed is a chair." The nurse then describes all other objects in relation to the focal point. The nurse accompanies the client to other important areas, such as the bathroom, so that the client can learn their locations. The nurse highlights the location of the toilet, sink, and toilet paper holder. The client with limited sight is never left in the center of an unfamiliar room.

Clients with limited sight prefer to establish the location of important objects, such as the call bell, water pitcher, and clock. Once their location has been fixed, these items are not moved without the client's consent. The location of movable items, such as chairs, stools, and wastebaskets, are not disturbed without consulting him or her.

At mealtime, the nurse or assistive nursing personnel sets up food on the tray using clock placement. For example, "There is sliced ham at 6 o'clock; peas are located at 3 o'clock; to the right of the plate is coffee; salt and pepper are next to the coffee."

CHART 47-12

BEST PRACTICE *for*
Insertion and Removal of an Ocular Prosthesis

Insertion
1. Assemble equipment:
   - Prosthesis
   - Gloves
   - Towel
2. Explain the procedure to the client.
3. Wash your hands.
4. Cover the work area with a cloth or towel.
5. Don gloves.
6. Remove the prosthesis from its container and rinse it with tepid water.
7. Lift the client's upper lid using your nondominant hand.

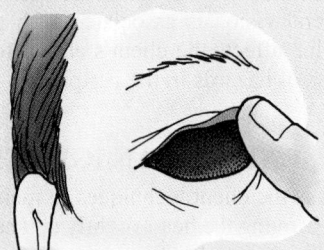

8. Place the prosthesis between the thumb and forefinger of your dominant hand. The notched end of the prosthesis should be closest to the client's nose.

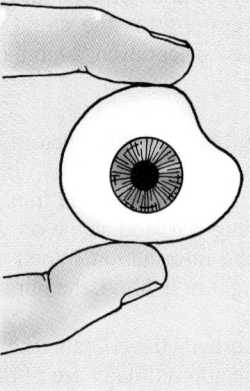

9. Insert the prosthesis with the top edge slipping under the upper lid. Continue until most of the iris is covered by the upper lid.

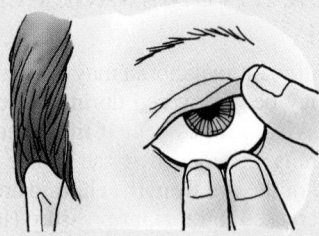

10. Gently release the upper eyelid.
11. Retract the lower lid slightly until the bottom edge of the prosthesis slips behind it.

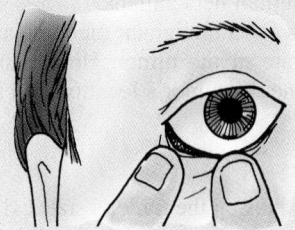

12. Release your hands slowly.

Removal
1. Assemble equipment:
   - Normal saline-filled labeled container
   - Gloves
2. Explain the procedure to the client.
3. Wash your hands.
4. Don gloves.
5. Instruct the client to sit up and tilt the head slightly downward.
6. Place your hand against the client's cheek, palm side up.
7. Pull the lower lid slightly down and laterally.
8. Allow the prosthesis to slide out onto your hand, or pull gently if necessary.
9. Place the prosthesis in a container filled with normal saline labeled with the client's name. Cover the container.

AMBULATION. When helping a client with limited sight to ambulate, the nurse allows him or her to grasp the nurse's arm at the elbow. The arm is kept close to the nurse's body so that the client can detect the direction of movement. When obstacles are noted in the path ahead, the nurse alerts the client.

Clients may use a cane to detect obstacles, such as furniture, walls, or curbs. The cane is held in the dominant hand several inches off the floor and sweeps the ground where the client's foot will be placed next. The laser cane sends out signals to help a blind client detect obstacles.

SELF-CARE. The ability to control the environment is important to the client with a visual impairment. The nurse knocks on the door before entering the hospital room or any other environment of a client with limited sight. The nurse

states his or her name and reason for visiting when entering the room.

SUPPORT. Clients' reaction to the loss of sight is similar to the reaction to loss of a body part. Newly blind clients may experience a period of physical or psychologic immobility. A period of grieving is needed for the "dead" (nonseeing) eye. Clients often experience hopelessness and denial. With time, anger usually gives way to acceptance. The ability to cope may begin within days, but some clients mourn for months or years.

Clients benefit from the honest, empathetic support that nurses can provide. They need to hear that it is normal to mourn, to cry, and to feel the loss. Nurses help clients move toward acceptance by encouraging the mastery of one task at a time and by providing positive reinforcement for each success.

ONLINE RESOURCES

For suggested readings and Internet resources, go to http://www.wbsaunders.com/SIMON/Iggy/.

SELECTED BIBLIOGRAPHY

Asterisk indicates a classic or definitive work on this subject.

*Bass, S., & Giovinazzo, V. (1996). Laser treatment of macular disease. *Optometry Clinics, 5*(1), 161-173.

*Cleary, M. (1995). Helping the person who is visually impaired: Concerns, questions, remedies, and sources. *Journal of Ophthalmic Nursing and Technology, 14*(5), 205-211.

Cohen, S., & Kawasaki, A. (1999). Introduction to formal visual field testing: Goldman and Humphrey perimeter. *Journal of Ophthalmic Nursing and Technology, 18*(1), 7-11.

Collins, M., et al. (2001). Effect of laser in situ keratomileusis (LASIK) on the corneal endothelium three years postoperatively. *American Journal of Ophthalmology, 131*(1), 1-6.

Cotran, R., Kumar, V., & Collins, T. (1999). *Robbins pathologic basis of disease* (5th ed.). Philadelphia: W.B. Saunders.

DuBosar, R. (1999). Age-related macular degeneration: New treatments show promise. *Journal of Ophthalmic Nursing and Technology, 18*(2), 60-70.

Gilbard, J. (1999). Dry eye, blepharitis, and chronic eye irritation: Divide and conquer. *Journal of Ophthalmic Nursing and Technology, 18*(3), 109-115.

Jarvis, C. (2000). *Physical examination and health assessment* (3rd ed.). Philadelphia: W.B. Saunders.

Kearney, K. (1997). Emergency! Retinal detachment. *American Journal of Nursing, 97*(8), 50.

McCloskey, J.C., & Bulechek, G.M. (2000). *Nursing interventions classification (NIC)* (3rd ed.). St. Louis: Mosby.

Moore, L. (2000). Severe visual impairment in older women. *Western Journal of Nursing Research, 22*(5), 571-595.

Noecker, R., & Golightly, S. (1999). Pharmacology of ocular surgery. *Journal of Ophthalmic Nursing and Technology, 18*(3), 101-108.

Pratt, S. (1999). Dietary prevention of age-related macular degeneration. *Journal of the American Optometric Association, 70*(1), 39-47.

Rakow, P. (1999). Making miracles with prosthetic soft lenses. *Journal of Ophthalmic Nursing and Technology, 18*(3), 120-122.

Ramos, M. (1999). Prevention of work related injuries: A look at eye protection use and suggested prevention strategies. *Journal of Ophthalmic Nursing and Technology, 18*(3), 117-119.

Ramponi, D. (2000). Go with the flow during an eye emergency. *Nursing2000, 30*(8), 54-56.

Rapaport, M. (2000). Eyelid dermatitis. *Dermatology Nursing, 12*(5), 352-354.

Shoemaker, J. (1997). Adult vision screening by nonphysicians. *Journal of Ophthalmic Nursing and Technology, 16*(5), 244-250.

Smith, S. (1999). The role of antioxidants in AMD: Ongoing research. *Journal of Ophthalmic Nursing and Technology, 18*(2), 68-70.

*Sullivan, N. (1983). Vision in the elderly. *Journal of Gerontological Nursing, 9*(4), 228-235.

United States Pharmacopeia Dispensing Information (USP DI): Vol. I. Drug information for the health care professional (20th ed.). (2000). Englewood, CO: Micromedix.

*Vader, L. (1992). Vision and vision loss. *Nursing Clinics of North America, 27*(3), 705-714.

*Vaughan, D., Asbury, T., & Riordan-Eva, P. (Eds.). (1995). *General ophthalmology* (14th ed.). Norwalk, CT: Appleton & Lange.

Whitaker, R., Whitaker, V., & Dill, C. (1999). Glaucoma: What the ophthalmic nurse should know. *Insight: The Journal of the American Society of Ophthalmic Registered Nurses, 24*(3), 86- 91.

Assessment of the Ear and Hearing

JUDY MALKIEWICZ

Learning Objectives

After studying this chapter, you should be able to:

1. Describe the key elements to inspect when performing assessment of the external ear.
2. Describe age-related changes in the structure of the ear and hearing.
3. Identify 10 drugs that have an impact on hearing.
4. Demonstrate the correct use of an otoscope.
5. Describe the landmarks of the tympanic membrane.
6. Compare and contrast air conduction and bone conduction of sound.
7. Demonstrate the correct use of a tuning fork in performing the Weber and Rinne tests for hearing.
8. Prioritize educational needs for the client about to undergo pure tone audiometry and electronystagmography.

Go to http://www.wbsaunders.com/SIMON/Iggy/ for self-assessment questions related to these Learning Objectives.

Ear and hearing assessment are important skills for nurses caring for clients of all ages. Many difficulties with the ear and hearing develop over a long period of time, and hearing may also be affected by several medications. An understanding of the anatomy and physiology of the ear is essential. Table 48-1 defines terms commonly used in assessing the ear and hearing.

ANATOMY AND PHYSIOLOGY REVIEW

Structure

The ear consists of three structural parts: the external ear, the middle ear, and the inner ear; each is important to the hearing process.

EXTERNAL EAR

The external ear develops in the embryo at the same time as the kidneys and urinary tract. Therefore any person with a defect of the external ear must also be examined for possible problems or defects of the renal and urinary systems.

The external ear (**pinna**), which is composed of cartilage covered by skin, is embedded in the temporal bone bilaterally at the level of the eyes, attached to the head by skin and cartilage at approximately a 10-degree angle. The external ear extends from the pinna through the external canal to the **tympanic membrane,** or eardrum (Figure 48-1). The external ear canal is slightly S-shaped and lined with **cerumen** (wax)–

producing glands (which help protect and lubricate the ear canal), sebaceous glands, and hair follicles. The hair follicles and cerumen protect the tympanic membrane and the middle ear. In the adult, the distance from the opening of the external canal to the tympanic membrane is approximately 1 to 1½ inches (2.5 to 3.75 cm). The external ear includes the **mastoid process,** the bony ridge located over the temporal bone behind the pinna.

MIDDLE EAR

The middle ear begins at the medial side of the tympanic membrane. It consists of the **epitympanum,** a compartment containing the three bony **ossicles** (Figure 48-2): the malleus, the incus, and the stapes. The proximal end of the eustachian tube also opens in the middle ear.

The tympanic membrane is a thick, transparent sheet of tissue providing a barrier between the external ear and the middle ear. The landmarks on the tympanic membrane include the annulus, the pars flaccida, and the pars tensa. The tympanic membrane is attached to the first bony ossicle, the **malleus** (hammer), at the **umbo** (Figure 48-3). The bony ossicles behind the tympanic membrane are joined, although not rigidly, allowing vibratory movement.

The pars flaccida and pars tensa are parts of the tympanic membrane. The pars flaccida is that portion of the tympanic membrane above the short process of the malleus; the pars tensa is that portion surrounding the long process of the malleus. It is usually transparent, opaque, or pearly gray and moves when air is injected into the external canal. The umbo is seen through the tympanic membrane as a white dot at the end of the long process of the malleus. The short process of the malleus, the long process of the malleus, and the umbo are structures seen through the transparent tympanic membrane.

The middle ear is separated from the inner ear by the round window and the oval window. The eustachian tube originates from the floor of the middle ear at the proximal end and opens at the distal end in the nasopharynx. The distal opening in the nasopharynx is surrounded by adenoid lymphatic tissue (Figure 48-4). The eustachian tube allows equalization of pressure on both sides of the tympanic membrane. Secretions from the middle ear drain through it.

TABLE 48-1 • TERMINOLOGY COMMONLY USED IN EAR AND HEARING ASSESSMENT
cerumen   Waxlike secretion of the external ear canal
conductive hearing loss   Hearing loss resulting from a physical disruption in the transmission of sound waves
decibel   A unit of sound for expressing loudness
masking   The process of hiding a specific sound from one ear while the other ear is tested for its ability to hear that sound
Meniere's disease   An intermittent but progressive deterioration of hearing and balance
otitis media   Inflammation/infection of the middle ear
otosclerosis   Formation of spongy bone around structures of the middle and inner ear, leading to low-tone hearing impairment
ototoxic   Damaging to the structures important for hearing
presbycusis   Age-related degenerative changes in the ear, leading to decreased hearing acuity
sensorineural   Hearing loss resulting from neural defects
spondee   Words of two syllables on which equal stress is placed during pronunciation
vestibular hearing loss   Relating to the functions of the ear for the sense of balance and position

■ INNER EAR

The inner ear, lying on the other side of the oval window, contains the semicircular canals, the cochlea, and the distal end of the eighth cranial nerve (see Figure 48-2). The **semicircular canals** contain fluid and hair cells connected to the sensory nerve fibers of the vestibular portion of the eighth cranial nerve; fluid and hair cells help to maintain the sense of balance.

The **cochlea,** the spiral organ of hearing, is divided into the scala tympani and the scala vestibuli. Reissner's membrane stretches across the scala vestibuli and forms the duct of the cochlea, or the scala media. The scala media is filled with **endolymph,** a fluid similar to intracellular fluid. The scala tympani and scala vestibuli are filled with **perilymph.** Endolymph and perilymph are fluids that protect the cochlea and the semicircular canals; these structures literally float in the fluids and are thus cushioned against abrupt movements of the head.

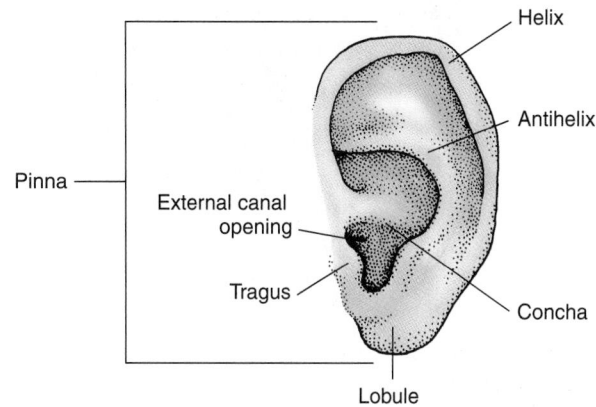

Figure 48-1 ● Anatomic features of the external ear.

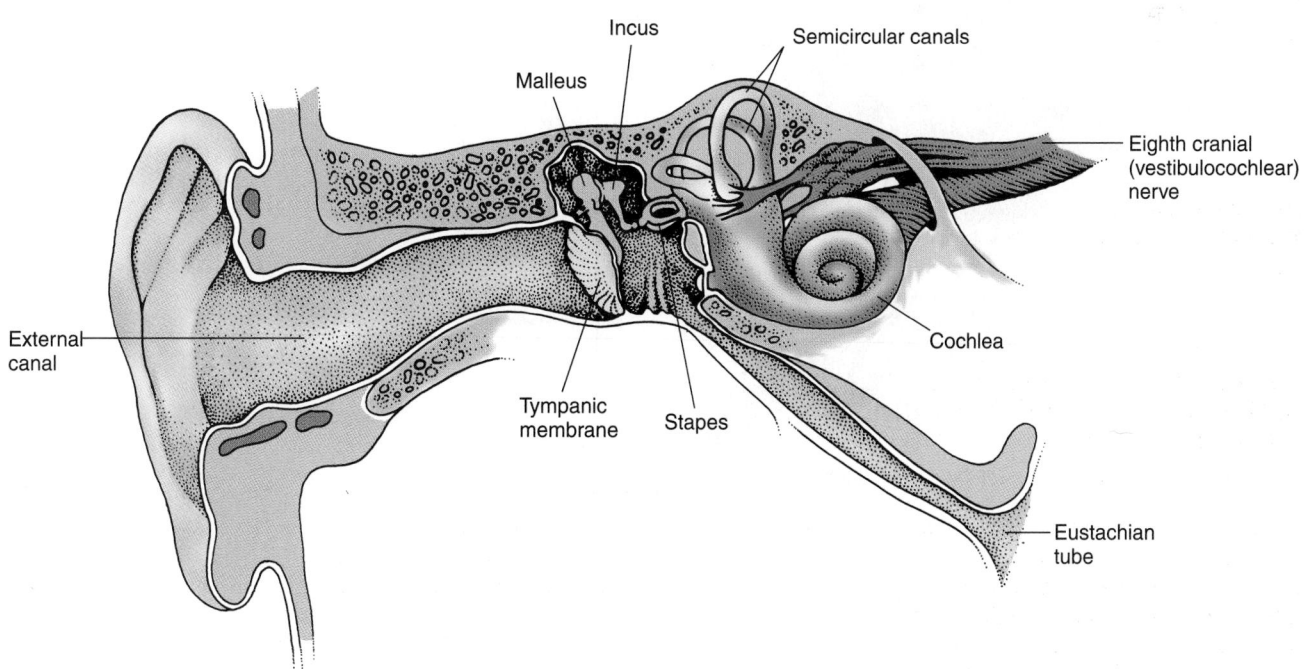

Figure 48-2 ● Anatomic features of the internal ear.

The **organ of Corti** is the receptor end-organ of hearing located on the basilar membrane of the cochlea. The cochlea contains hair cells that detect vibration from sound and stimulate the eighth cranial nerve.

Function

The ear's main function is hearing, which is accomplished when sound is delivered through the air to the external ear

RIGHT TYMPANIC MEMBRANE

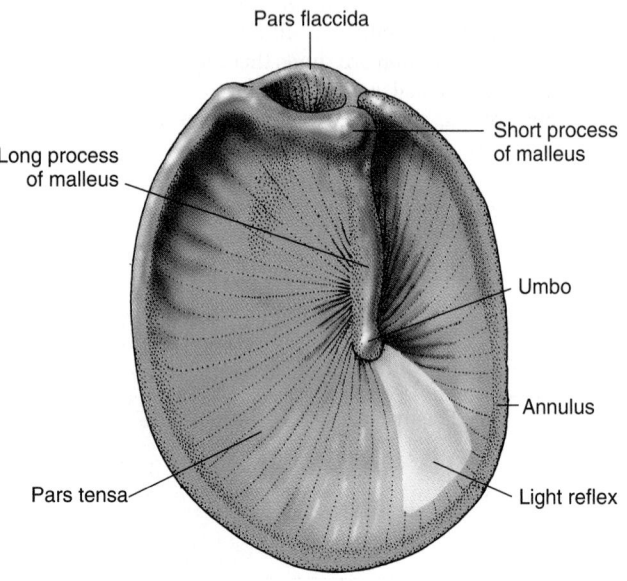

Figure 48-3 ● Landmarks on the tympanic membrane.

canal and the temporal bone covering the mastoid air cells. The sound waves strike the mastoid and the movable tympanic membrane, which is connected to the first bony ossicle, the malleus, at the umbo. The sound wave vibrations are transferred from the tympanic membrane to the malleus, the incus, and the stapes. From the stapes the vibrations are transmitted to the cochlea. Receptors there **transduce** (change) the vibrations into action potentials, conducted to the brain as neural impulses by the cochlear portion of the eighth cranial (or auditory) nerve. Sound is processed and interpreted by the brain.

Ear and Hearing Changes Associated with Aging

Ear and hearing changes related to aging are summarized in Chart 48-1. Some of these changes are harmless (see the Evidence-Based Practice for Nursing box on p. 1052); others pose serious threats to the hearing ability of older clients and call for nursing interventions.

ASSESSMENT TECHNIQUES
History

The nurse obtains a thorough history from the client. Informal hearing assessment begins as the nurse observes the client listening to and answering questions. The client's posture and appropriateness of responses provide additional information about his or her hearing acuity.

During the interview, the nurse sits in adequate light, facing the client, which allows the client to see the nurse speaking. The nurse is careful to use ordinary language. The nurse also assesses demographic data, personal and family history, socioeconomic status, and current health problems. Chart

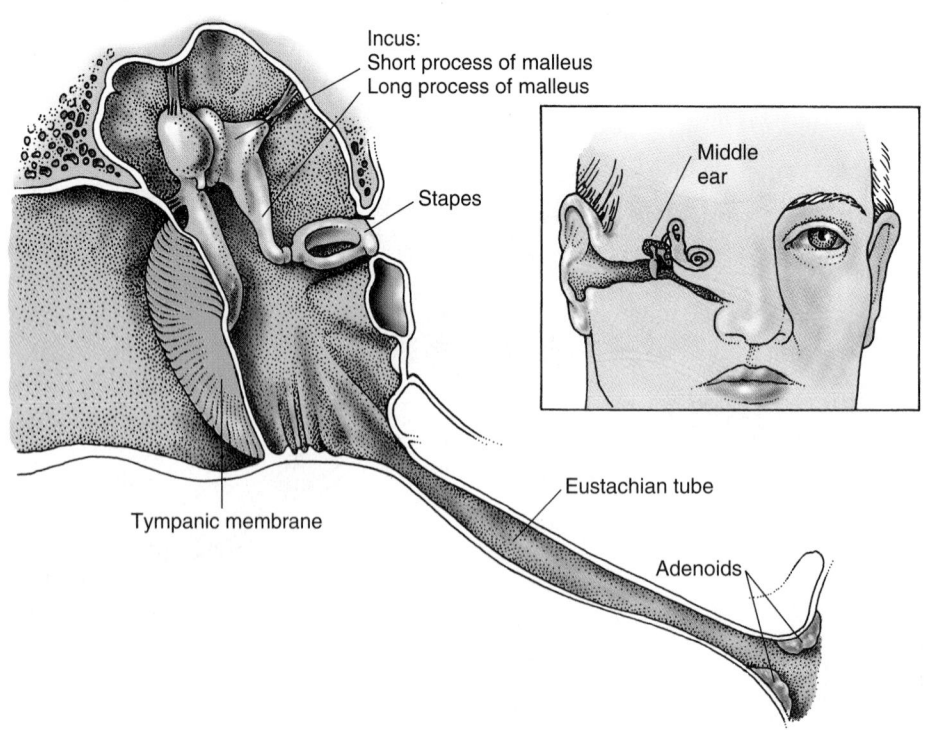

Figure 48-4 ● Anatomic features and attached structures of the middle ear.

48-2 lists important questions to ask regarding ear and hearing assessment.

DEMOGRAPHIC DATA

The gender of the client is important. Some auditory disorders, such as otosclerosis, are more common in women; others, such as Meniere's disease, are more common in men. Age is also a significant factor in hearing loss.

PERSONAL AND FAMILY HISTORY

Personal history includes information on past or current signs and symptoms of ear pain, ear discharge, vertigo, tinnitus, decreased hearing, and difficulty understanding people when they talk or difficulty hearing environmental noises. The nurse asks the client about the following:

- Ear trauma
- Ear surgery
- Past infections

- Excessive cerumen
- Ear itch
- Any invasive instruments routinely used to clean the ear
- Type and pattern of ear hygiene
- Exposure to loud noise or music
- Air travel (especially in unpressurized aircraft)
- Swimming habits and the use of protective ear devices for swimming
- History of hereditary factors and health conditions causing changes in the blood supply to the ear (heart disease, hypertension, diabetes)
- History of vitiligo (a pigment disorder in which there may be a loss of melanin-containing cells [and their protective function] in the inner ear, resulting in hearing loss)
- History of smoking (nicotine increases the carboxyhemoglobin in the blood, resulting in a decreased oxygen supply to the cochlea, possibly increasing sensory cell damage)
- History of vitamin B_{12} and folate deficiency (appears to be associated with age-related hearing loss)

CHART 48-1

NURSING FOCUS *on the* **OLDER ADULT**
The Ear and Hearing

Physiologic Change	Nursing Implications	Rationale
The pinna becomes elongated because of normal loss of subcutaneous tissue and decreased tissue elasticity.		
Hair becomes coarser and longer, especially in men.		
Cerumen-producing glands decrease in number and function.	Irrigate ear canal weekly.	Irrigation removes excess cerumen, preventing impaction and enhancing transmission of sound waves.
Cerumen tends to be drier in older clients; it becomes impacted, which causes hearing loss.	Place 1-2 drops of oil into ear canal 8 hr before irrigation.	Oil softens impacted cerumen, facilitating removal.
The tympanic membrane loses elasticity; it may normally appear dull and retracted.		
Bony ossicles have decreased movement.		
The cochlea undergoes degenerative changes.		
Disturbed vestibular function results in occasional dizziness, vertigo, and sensations of unsteadiness in 50%–60% of older clients.	Assist the client with standing and initial ambulation.	The nurse provides a stable point of reference. Assistance decreases the risk of falling as a result of vestibular disorientation.
Hearing acuity diminishes with advancing age.	Establish that a hearing deficiency exists.	Determine whether interventions are needed. Not all older clients have diminished hearing acuity.
The ability to hear high-frequency sounds is nearly gone by age 60, which affects speech reception and increases auditory reaction time greatly. Clients have particular difficulty with the *f, s, sh,* and *pa* sounds. Some older clients hear a persistent noise (tinnitus). Presbycusis (a sensorineural type of hearing loss) is common in older adults.	When speaking to an older client with a hearing deficiency: • Provide a quiet environment. • Face the client. • Speak slowly in a deeper voice.	This makes it easier for the client to hear and communicate. • Extraneous noise may interfere with the client's auditory perception. • The client can benefit by being able to see lip movement. • The client may be able to discern lower frequencies more easily.

EVIDENCE-BASED PRACTICE FOR NURSING

Ear size as a predictor of chronologic age

Tan, R., Osman, V., & Tan, G. (1997). Ear size as a predictor of chronological age. *Archives of Gerontology and Geriatrics, 25*(2), 187-191.

This study examined the external ear circumference in 100 Caucasian men (n=79) and women (n=21) between the ages of 21 and 98 years. It was found that the external ear circumference increased in size an average of 0.51 mm/year.

Critique. External ear circumference was found to be predictive of chronologic age in the population studied. Since the external ear is composed of elastic cartilage covered by skin, it was thought that the increases in external ear circumference with age were due to changes in collagen.

Implications for Nursing. Older clients can be reassured that increasing external ear circumference is common.

CHART 48-2

EAR AND HEARING ASSESSMENT
Using Gordon's Functional Health Patterns

Cognitive-Perceptual Pattern
Do you notice that you have the volume of the television or radio set at an increased level?
Are you sitting closer to the television or radio in order to hear more clearly?
Do you have difficulty in your ability to hear or follow conversations in a noisy environment, such as a restaurant?
Do you have difficulty hearing high-pitched sounds like the doorbell?

Health Perception/Health Management Pattern
Have you had your hearing checked?
If you are or were exposed to environmental noise, have you consistently used appropriate hearing protection?
Do you avoid cleaning your ear canals with foreign objects such as toothpicks or paper clips?
Have you discussed with your health care provider the side effects of any drugs you may be taking that might affect your ear and hearing?

Based on Gordon, M. (2000). *Manual of nursing diagnosis* (9th ed.). St. Louis: Mosby.

TABLE 48-2 • IMPACT OF OTOTOXIC SUBSTANCES ON AUDITORY FUNCTION

Drug	Auditory Effects
ANTIBIOTICS	
Amikacin (Amikin)	++
Chloramphenicol (Chloromycetin, Novochlorocap✦)	+ to ++
Erythromycin (Apo-Erythro E-C✦, E.E.S., E-Mycin, Novorythro✦)	+ to ++
Gentamicin (Cidomycin✦, Garamycin)	++
Kanamycin (Kantrex)	++
Neomycin	++
Streptomycin	++
Tobramycin (Nebcin)	++
Vancomycin (Lyphocin, Vancocin)	++
DIURETICS	
Acetazolamide (Apo-Acetazolamide✦, Diamox)	++
Ethacrynic acid (Edecrin)	++
Furosemide (Apo-Furosemide✦, Lasix, Furoside✦)	++
NONSTEROIDAL ANTI-INFLAMMATORY AGENTS	
Ibuprofen (Advil, Amersol✦, Motrin, Novoprofen✦)	+
Indomethacin (Indocid✦, Indocin)	+
Naproxen (Anaprox, Apo-Napro-Na✦, Naprosyn, Novonaprox✦)	+
Salicylates (Apo-ASA✦, Ascriptin, Bufferin, Entrophen✦)	++
MISCELLANEOUS	
Carbamazepine (Tegretol)	++
Cisplatin (Abiplatin✦, Platinol)	++
Mechlorethamine (Mustargen)	+
Quinine (Legatrin, NovoQuinine✦, Quinamm)	+
Quinidine (Apo-Quinidine✦, Cardioquin, Quinidex)	+

+, Slight impact; ++, significant impact.

If the client uses a hearing aid, the nurse determines how well it works, the date of the last hearing test, the type of test given, and the results. The client is asked about other conditions that may impair hearing, such as allergies, upper respiratory tract infection, hypothyroidism, arteriosclerosis, head trauma, and recent head, facial, or dental surgery.

A thorough medication history is crucial because many drugs are ototoxic (Table 48-2).

The client is asked about his or her occupation and any hobbies involving exposure to excessive environmental noise or music. The nurse also investigates the use of protective ear devices or any devices inserted into the ear, such as a telephone operator headset or a stethoscope. Information about hearing loss among family members is important because some types of hearing loss are hereditary or have a genetic component.

SOCIOECONOMIC STATUS

The nurse assesses the client's socioeconomic status to determine the availability of health care. Clients of lower socioeconomic status often do not seek health care for ear-related problems until hearing damage is extensive. Clients at any socioeconomic level, however, might hesitate to have their hearing loss diagnosed because of the fear of wearing a hearing amplification device.

CURRENT HEALTH PROBLEMS

The nurse assesses current ear-related health problems, asking whether the client has noticed any "trouble with" his or her ears, ear pain, or discharge, including any earwax. The client is asked about any change in hearing, such as an intolerance for sound levels that do not bother other people (hyperacusis), or associated problems, such as ringing in the ears. If a change in hearing is reported, the nurse asks whether one or both ears are involved and whether the change was sudden or gradual. The client is also asked about any problems with dizziness (an off-balance feeling or lightheadedness) or **vertigo** (spinning sense of movement).

Physical Assessment

Inspection and palpation are the only examination techniques used to assess the ear. The nurse begins the examination by placing the client in either a sitting or a supine position. Uncooperative clients are carefully restrained to prevent injury to the external canal. Any hearing aids should be removed during the examination. After the otoscopic examination, the nurse inspects the hearing aid for cracks, debris, and a proper fit. Ear examination is divided into external ear and mastoid assessment, otoscopic assessment, and auditory assessment.

EXTERNAL EAR AND MASTOID ASSESSMENT

The mastoid process is inspected for redness and swelling, which indicate inflammation. To assess for tenderness, the nurse gently taps with one finger over the mastoid process, compresses the tragus with one finger, and gently manipulates the pinna forward and backward. Any tenderness suggests an inflammatory process in either the external ear or the mastoid.

The entire external ear is inspected for shape, location of attachment to the head, and condition of the visible external canal. The normal pinna is uniformly shaped without additional skin tags or deformity. The pinna should be attached vertically to the side of the head at a posterior angle of no greater than 10 degrees. It should fall within or touch the eye-occiput line, an imaginary line drawn from the greatest protuberance on the occiput to the lateral canthus of the eye. Any variation from the normal ear shape and attachment is recorded.

Abnormalities of the pinna include swelling, nodules, and lesions. In chronic gout, accumulations of uric acid crystals result in hard, irregular, painless nodules called tophi on the helix and antihelix portions of the pinna. Other painless nodules on the pinna might be due to basal cell carcinoma or rheumatoid arthritis. Small, crusted, ulcerated, or indurated lesions on the pinna that fail to heal could be squamous cell carcinoma.

The normal external canal is free from lesions, dry, clean, and not reddened. The nurse assesses for the following abnormalities:

- Furuncles
- Large accumulations of cerumen
- Scaliness
- Redness
- Swelling of or drainage from the ear associated with a foreign object (insects or inanimate substances), trauma, or infection

The nurse also notes any other drainage (blood, cerebrospinal fluid, pus, or serous fluid) and its character.

OTOSCOPIC ASSESSMENT

An instrument called an otoscope is used to examine the ear. Many types are available. An otoscope (Figure 48-5) consists of a light, a handle, a magnifying lens, and a pneumatic attachment for injecting air into the external canal to test mobility of the tympanic membrane.

Specula of various diameters attach to the head of the otoscope; the largest that most comfortably fits the client's external canal is selected for the examination. *The speculum is never blindly introduced into the external canal because of the risk of perforating the tympanic membrane.*

If the client experiences any pain during external ear examination, the nurse attempts a cautious otoscopic examina-

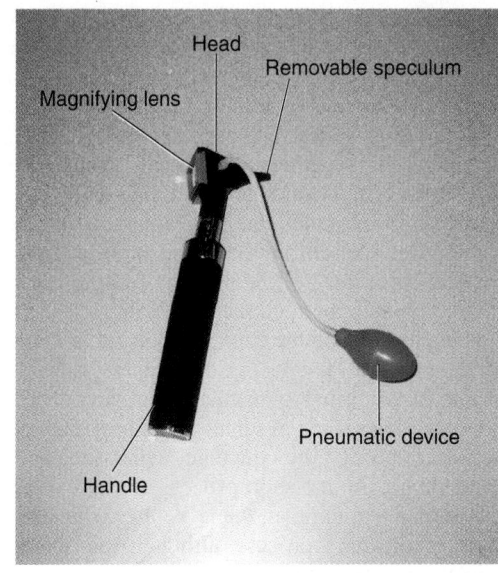

Figure 48-5 ● Functional components of an otoscope.

Labels: Head; Removable speculum; Magnifying lens; Pneumatic device; Handle

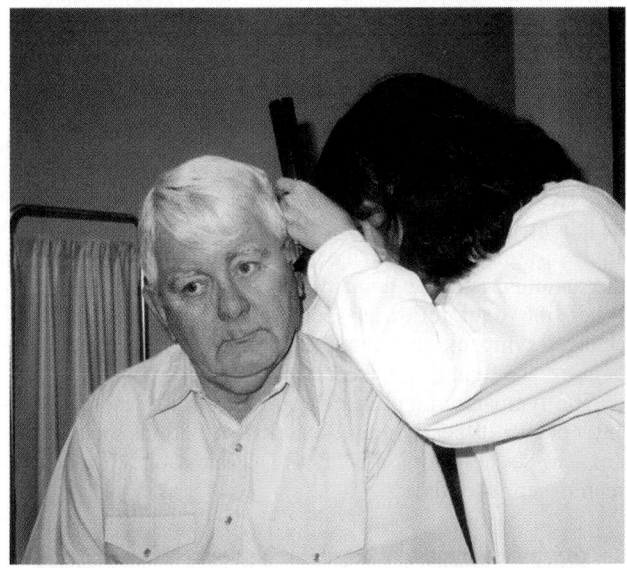

Figure 48-6 ● Proper technique for an otoscopic examination.

tion. (The speculum will cause extreme pain if it comes in contact with inflamed tissue in the external canal.) The nurse must become familiar with and memorize all of the structures of the tympanic membrane and middle ear before attempting to visualize them with an otoscope.

When performing an otoscopic examination, the nurse tilts the client's head slightly away and holds the otoscope upside down, like a large pen (Figure 48-6). This position permits the nurse's hand to lie against the client's head for support. If the client moves, both the nurse's hand and the otoscope move as well, preventing damage to the external canal or tympanic membrane. The nurse holds the otoscope in the dominant hand and gently pulls the pinna up and back with the nondominant hand. The external canal is visualized while the speculum is slowly inserted. The examiner uses caution and avoids jamming the speculum into the walls of the external canal, which causes pain.

After the pinna is correctly displaced and the otoscope is comfortably introduced in the external canal, the tympanic membrane is observed for color, intactness, and shape. The nurse further assesses for lesions and the amount and consistency of cerumen and hair. The normal external canal is skin colored, intact, and without lesions; it contains various amounts of soft cerumen and has small, fine hairs.

Next, the tympanic membranes are assessed for intactness, normal structures seen through the tympanic membrane (the long and short processes of the malleus and the umbo), portions of the tympanic membrane itself (light reflex, pars flaccida, and pars tensa), and the color, shape, and mobility of the membrane, as well as any lesions. Figure 48-7 shows an otoscopic view of a normal tympanic membrane. The normal tympanic membrane is always intact. The long process of the malleus is seen through the tympanic membrane as a whitish streak extending from the short process of the malleus to the umbo. A normal variation in some people with allergies is vascularity of the long process, although this might be an early indication of otitis media.

The short process of the malleus is seen through the tympanic membrane as a white structure that seems more three-dimensional (projecting out toward the otoscope) than the other structures on the tympanic membrane. The umbo appears as a round, white dot.

The long and short processes of the malleus, in addition to the umbo, are always easily identified in the normal ear. Abnormal variations are caused by serous otitis and otitis media, among other disorders.

Reflection of the otoscope's light off of the tympanic membrane reveals the **light reflex,** a clearly demarcated triangle of light in the normal ear. The base of the triangle is on the annulus, and the point of the triangle is on the umbo. When the light reflex is spotty or multiple because of a changed tympanic membrane shape from either retraction or bulging, the light reflex is termed **diffuse.**

The tympanic membrane is normally shiny and transparent, opaque, or pearly gray. Abnormal variations include redness (as seen in otitis media) and dullness or retraction (as seen in serous otitis).

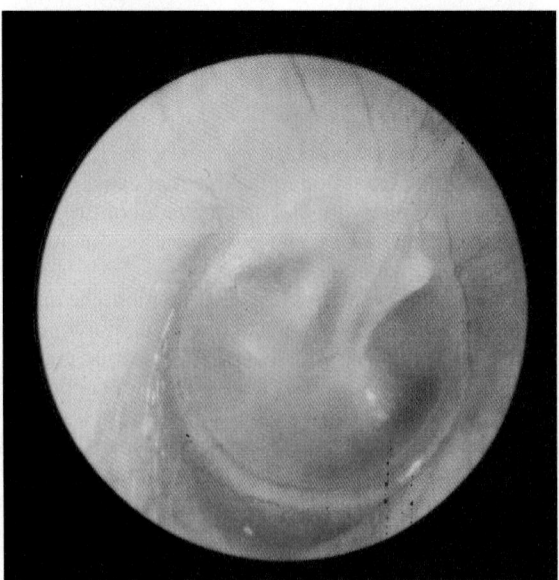

Figure 48-7 ● Otoscopic view of a normal tympanic membrane.

The normal tympanic membrane is slightly concave, allowing the pars tensa portion to move gently on testing with a puff of air from the pneumatic device on the otoscope.

The normal tympanic membrane is free of lesions. The most common lesion is scarring caused by previous ear infection and perforation. A scar thickens the tympanic membrane, which makes it difficult or impossible to see through the membrane at the point of the scar and reduces the mobility of the tympanic membrane.

The nurse tests the mobility of the tympanic membrane by gently injecting a small puff of air through the pneumatic device into the external canal and watching the pars tensa portion for movement. The normal tympanic membrane moves gently. Decreased or absent mobility results from scarring, retraction, bulging, the presence of fluid in the middle ear, and decreased mobility of the ossicles associated with aging.

CULTURAL CONSIDERATIONS

Cerumen is generally moist and tan or brown in Caucasian and African-American clients. It is dry and light brown to gray in Asians and Native Americans. The color of the lining of the external ear canal varies with the client's skin tone.

CRITICAL THINKING CHALLENGE

The client is an older nursing home resident who speaks no English. The staff, who do not understand her native language, have noticed that her right external ear is red with peeling skin on the inner aspect. You are to perform an external and otoscopic examination on her.

- How will you explain these procedures to the client (you also do not speak her native language)?
- Describe how you will proceed with the inspection of the external ear.
- How will you select the proper-size speculum for the otoscopic examination?

For suggested answer guidelines, go to SIMON http://www.wbsaunders.com/SIMON/Iggy/.

■ AUDITORY ASSESSMENT

After completing bilateral external ear and otoscopic examinations, the nurse assesses the client's hearing acuity. Sound is transmitted by air conduction and bone conduction. Air conduction of sound is normally more sensitive than bone conduction. If hearing acuity is decreased, the hearing loss is categorized as follows:

- **Conductive hearing loss,** resulting from any physical obstruction of sound wave transmission (such as a foreign body in the external canal, a retracted or bulging tympanic membrane, or fused bony ossicles)
- **Sensorineural hearing loss,** resulting from a defect in the cochlea, the eighth cranial nerve, or the brain itself
- **Mixed conductive-sensorineural hearing loss,** a profound hearing loss

Each of the auditory function tests determines the degree of hearing loss and differentiates the type of loss.

■ Voice Test

A simple hearing acuity test can be conducted by asking the client to block one external ear canal while standing 1 to 2 feet (30 to 60 cm) away. The examiner quietly whispers a statement and asks the client to repeat it. Each ear is tested separately. If the client does not respond correctly, a louder whisper is used. If the client is suspected of lip-reading, the examiner's hand can be used to block his or her view of the examiner's mouth.

Watch Test

A ticking watch is used to test hearing acuity for high-frequency sounds. The nurse holds a ticking watch about 5 inches (12.7 cm) from each of the ears and asks whether the ticking is heard. The client with normal hearing should be able to hear it.

Audioscopy

The lightweight audioscope allows the examiner to visualize the external ear and tympanic membrane. Hearing can be measured at a 40-decibel (dB) intensity at frequencies of 500, 1000, 2000, and 4000 cycles per second (cps), or hertz (Hz). The audioscope is larger than a conventional otoscope, and nurses can easily use it to assess hearing.

Tuning Fork Tests

Hearing acuity can be tested by the Weber and Rinne tuning fork tests. Tuning fork tests are useful, although limited, in differentiating between conductive and sensorineural hearing losses. The frequency range of the tuning fork used for these tests corresponds to that of normal speech: 512 or 1024 Hz. To perform this assessment, the nurse stands in front of the sitting client.

WEBER TUNING FORK TEST

To perform the Weber tuning fork test, the nurse places the vibrating tuning fork on the middle of the client's head, at the midline of the forehead, or above the upper lip over the teeth. Many clients object to the vibration over the upper lip, so the

preferred site is the midline of the skull (Figure 48-8). The nurse takes care to hold the vibrating tuning fork by the stem only, not by the vibrating fork. The nurse asks the client in which ear the sound is louder. The normal test result is sound heard equally in both ears. If the client hears the sound louder in one ear, the term *lateralization* describes the side on which the sound is the loudest.

RINNE TUNING FORK TEST

The Rinne tuning fork test compares hearing by air conduction with hearing by bone conduction. Sound is normally heard two to three times longer by air conduction than by bone conduction. The nurse performs the Rinne tuning fork test by placing the vibrating tuning fork stem on the client's mastoid process. The client indicates when he or she no longer hears the sound, and the nurse quickly brings the tuning fork in front of the pinna without touching the client, asking whether he or she still hears the sound (Figure 48-9). The nurse records the duration of both phases, bone conduction followed by air conduction, and compares the times. The client normally continues to hear the sound two times longer in front of the pinna after not hearing it with the tuning fork touching the mastoid process.

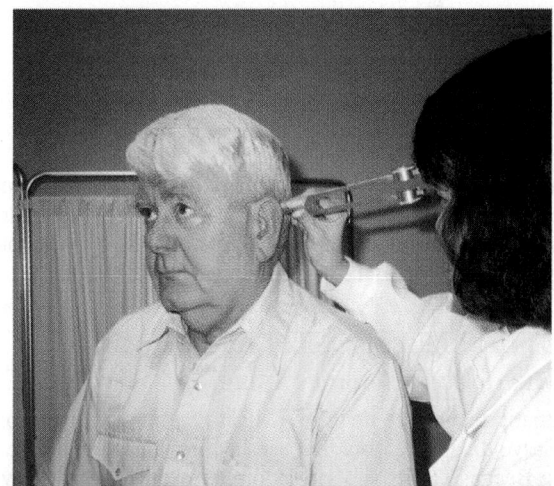

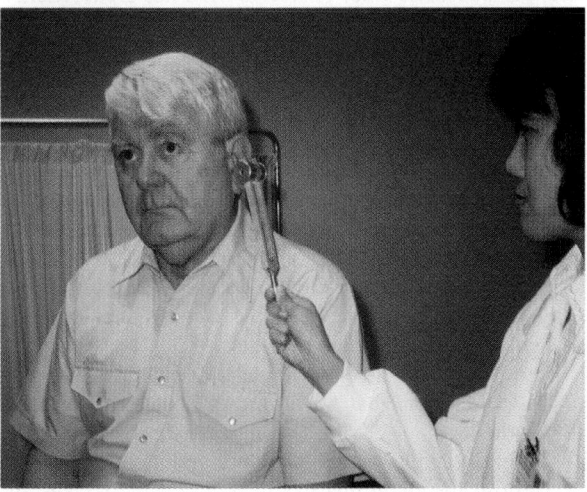

Figure 48-9 ● Correct placement of the tuning fork for the Rinne test.

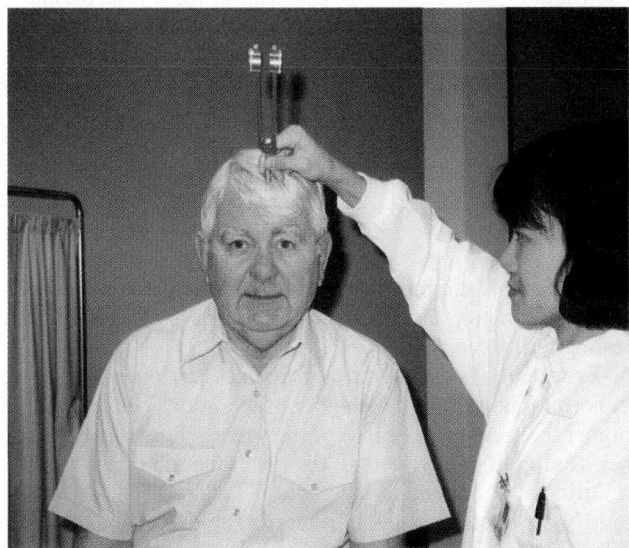

Figure 48-8 ● Correct placement of the tuning fork for the Weber test.

Psychosocial Assessment

The client may become irritable, frustrated, and depressed by an inability to hear and respond appropriately. The inability to hear results in frustrating experiences and often isolates the client from the world. Depression may result from the sensory isolation of hearing loss. The nurse is sensitive to the client and conducts the interview at a pace appropriate for that individual.

The nurse investigates the social and work relationships to determine whether the client experiences isolation because of hearing problems. In addition, the client is encouraged to express feelings related to hearing loss and discuss changes in daily living activities for coping. The nurse also obtains information from family members, especially if the client denies having a hearing problem. Throughout the assessment, the nurse remains patient and empathetic.

Diagnostic Assessment

LABORATORY TESTS

Laboratory tests are not of value in determining hearing acuity except for determinations of cholesterol (low-density liprotein–high-density lipoprotein [LDL/HDL]) ratios in older women. Women with high LDL/HDL ratios have better hearing (by 5 dB) than women with low LDL/HDL ratios. For an external ear infection, microbial culture and antibiotic sensitivity tests can determine the causative organism and the most appropriate antibiotic.

RADIOGRAPHIC EXAMINATIONS: COMPUTED TOMOGRAPHY

Computed tomography (CT), with or without contrast enhancement, reveals the structures of the ear in great detail by multiple x-ray scans of the head, which are then averaged by a computer. CT is especially helpful in diagnosing acoustic tumors.

OTHER DIAGNOSTIC ASSESSMENT
Magnetic Resonance Imaging

Magnetic resonance imaging (MRI) is a noninvasive, nonradioactive diagnostic tool that uses a computer to generate images. Because of its superior contrast resolution, no bony artifacts can obscure tissue. Therefore MRI has great sensitivity to soft-tissue changes. Clients with internal metal vascular clips cannot have MRI.

Auditory Brainstem-Evoked Response

Auditory brainstem-evoked response (ABR) is done to assess hearing in clients who are unable to indicate, or are unreliable in indicating, recognition of sound stimuli during hearing testing. This test helps diagnose both conductive and sensorineural hearing losses. Electrodes are placed on the scalp during the test. After the test, the client's hair should be cleansed to remove the electrode gel.

To prepare the client for ABR testing, the nurse:
- Tells the client that no fasting or sedation is necessary for the test
- Carefully explains the procedure and its purpose
- Informs the client that the procedure usually takes about 30 minutes

Electronystagmography

Electronystagmography (ENG) is a cost-effective test that is sensitive in detecting both central and peripheral disease of the vestibular system in the ear. The ENG detects **nystagmus** (involuntary eye movements) that can be recorded. Electrodes are taped to the skin near the eyes, and one or more procedures (caloric testing, changing gaze position, or changing head position) are done to stimulate nystagmus. Failure of nystagmus to occur with cerebral stimulation suggests an abnormality in the vestibulocochlear apparatus, the cerebral cortex, the auditory nerve, or the brainstem.

To prepare the client for ENG, the nurse:
- Carefully explains the procedure and its purpose
- Tells the client to fast for several hours before the test and to avoid caffeine-containing beverages for 24 to 48 hours before the test
- Tells clients with pacemakers that they should not have the test
- Carefully introduces fluids after the test to prevent nausea and vomiting

Caloric Testing

Caloric testing is performed to evaluate the vestibular (inner-ear) portion of the auditory nerve. Water warmer or cooler than body temperature is infused into the ear. A normal response is demonstrated by the onset of **vertigo** (spinning sensation) and nystagmus (involuntary eye movements) within 20 to 30 seconds. To prepare the client for caloric testing, the nurse:
- Carefully explains the procedure and its purpose
- Tells the client to fast for several hours before the test
- Tells the client that the affected side will be tested first
- Explains that the client will be maintained on bedrest after the procedure with careful introduction of fluids to prevent nausea and vomiting

Dix-Hallpike Test for Vertigo

The Dix-Hallpike test for vertigo is performed by assisting the client to a sitting position on an examination table. The nurse stands to the side of the client and quickly repositions him or her from sitting to supine with the head extending beyond the end of the table. This change of position is done first to one side and then to the other side. A client with benign positional vertigo will have a burst of nystagmus after a delay of 5 to 10 seconds.

To prepare the client for the Dix-Hallpike test, the nurse:
- Carefully explains the procedure and its purpose
- Explains that double vision may occur during the test

Audiometry

Audiometry is the measurement of hearing acuity. To understand audiometry, the nurse must first understand audiometric testing terminology.

Frequency is the highness or lowness of tones (expressed in hertz). The greater the number of vibrations per second, the higher the frequency (pitch) of the sound; the fewer the number of vibrations per second, the lower the pitch.

Intensity of sound is expressed in decibels. The lowest intensity at which a young, normal ear can detect sound (about 50% of the time) is 0 dB. Sound at 110 dB is so intense (loud) that it is painful for most people with normal hearing. Conversational speech is generally around 60 dB, and a soft whisper is around 20 dB (Table 48-3). A hearing loss of 45 to 50 dB renders the person unable to hear speech without a hearing aid. A person with a hearing loss of 90 dB may not be able to hear speech even with a hearing aid.

Threshold is the lowest level of intensity at which pure tones and speech are heard by a client (about 50% of the time). **Pure tones** are generated by an **audiometer** (Figure 48-10) to determine hearing acuity. There are two types of audiometry: pure tone audiometry and speech audiometry.

PURE TONE AUDIOMETRY

Tones generated by an audiometer are presented to the client at frequencies for hearing speech, music, and other common sounds. Pure tone audiometry is performed by air conduction testing or bone conduction testing. The results of pure tone audiometry are plotted on an **audiogram** (Figure 48-11). For some clients, the hearing of one ear is "masked" while the hearing of the other ear is tested.

AIR CONDUCTION TEST. Pure tone air conduction testing determines whether a client hears normally or has a hearing loss. It is designed to test air conduction hearing sensitivity (through earphones) at frequencies of 125, 250, 500, 750, 1000, 1500, 2000, 3000, 4000, 6000, and 8000 Hz, but thresholds are usually confined to the frequencies of 250, 500, 1000, 2000, 4000, and 8000 Hz. The intensities for the pure tones generally range from 10 to 110 dB.

CLIENT PREPARATION. The client is placed in a sound-isolated room in which ambient noise does not exceed American National Standards Institute noise standards. The nurse sits facing the client because his or her facial expressions are frequently helpful in evaluating responses. Hearing-impaired clients may benefit from lip-reading the nurse's instructions. The nurse instructs the client as follows:

"I am going to test your hearing. The object of the test is to find the point at which you can just barely hear the tones. The tones will sound like soft bells or tuning forks. Every time you hear one, no matter how soft, signal by raising your hand (or pushing the button) on the side you hear the tone." (If the client cannot raise a hand or push a button because of physical or motor disabilities, a yes-no verbal response is appropriate.)

"When you no longer hear the tone, lower your hand (or release the button). This lets me know when you hear the tone and when it goes away."

PROCEDURE. The ear with the better hearing is tested first. Before beginning the test, the nurse adjusts the audiometric equipment by:

1. Setting the frequency control at 1000 Hz and the hearing level control at 40 dB

Sound	Decibel Intensity (dB)	Safe Exposure Time*
Threshold of hearing	0	
Whispering	20	
Average residence or office	40	
Conversational speech	60	
Car traffic	70	>8 hr
Motorcycle	90	8 hr
Chain saw	100	2 hr
Rock concert, front row	120	3 min
Jet engine	140	Immediate danger
Rocket launching pad	180	Immediate danger

TABLE 48-3 • DECIBEL INTENSITY AND SAFE EXPOSURE TIME FOR COMMON SOUNDS

*For every 5-dB increase in intensity, the safe exposure time is cut in half.

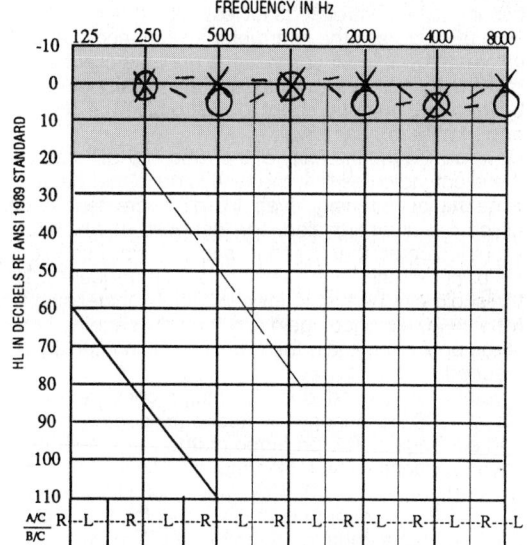

AUDIOGRAM

Audiogram Key	Left	Right		Left	Right
AC Unmasked	x	o	AC Masked	□	△
BC Unmasked	>	<	BC Masked	]	[
No Response	↓	↙	SF		S

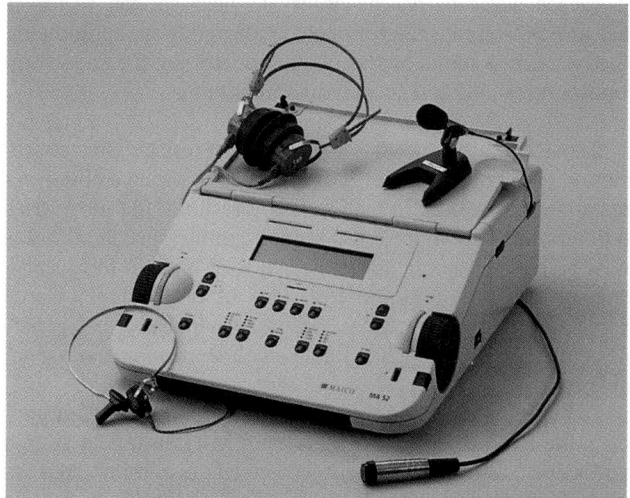

Figure 48-10 ● A pure tone audiometer. (Courtesy Maico, Inc., Minneapolis, MN.)

Figure 48-11 ● Audiogram pattern depicting normal hearing. (Courtesy Cleveland Hearing and Speech Center, Cleveland, OH.)

2. Putting on the earphones and listening to the tone while switching from one ear to the other
3. In each earphone, listening to the tone while gradually turning the hearing level control toward 0 dB
4. Testing the signal cord and light to make sure they are working

Best practices for conduction audiometry to obtain a profile of the client's hearing for pure tones across the frequencies tested, from low to high frequencies, are presented in Chart 48-3. No special follow-up care is needed.

BONE CONDUCTION TEST. Pure tone bone conduction testing determines whether the hearing loss detected by air conduction testing is due to conductive or sensorineural factors, or to a combination of the two. It is used only when the results of air conduction testing are abnormal. There are restrictions on both the frequency and the intensity of the sound produced by the device. The frequencies are usually restricted to those between 250 and 4000 Hz. Because a bone conduction oscillator requires great power to vibrate the skull, maximal outputs for bone conduction are also lower.

CLIENT PREPARATION. The nurse explains that hearing sensitivity for bone conduction is going to be checked. The sounds and how the client should respond are the same as those for the air conduction test.

PROCEDURE. The ear with greater acuity is tested first. If neither ear is "better," it makes no difference which is tested first.

The bone conduction vibrator is placed behind the pinna, firmly on the mastoid process. The nurse then follows steps 4 through 9 of Chart 48-3. Remember that restrictions are placed on both the intensity and the frequency used in bone conduction testing. Restrictions are usually described on the face of the audiometer. No special follow-up care is needed.

INTERPRETATION OF RESULTS. Audiometric evaluation determines whether the client's hearing is within normal limits or, with a hearing impairment, whether the hearing loss is conductive, sensorineural, or mixed. The type of loss can be determined by the configuration of the audiogram after completion of pure tone air and bone conduction audiometry.

In the hands of an experienced clinician, the audiometer is a useful tool for evaluating the extent and type of hearing loss. For interpreting the results of a hearing test, the expertise of the person who performed the test and the reliability of the client's responses must be considered. In reality, the audiogram is the diagnostician's best estimate of hearing, based on observations of the client's auditory behavior in the testing situation.

Figure 48-11 is an audiogram showing normal results of air and bone conduction tests. Hearing is generally considered normal when the pure tone thresholds are at 10 dB or better. The line at 0 dB on the audiogram represents the hearing thresholds of a young person with normal hearing. Figure 48-12 depicts audiogram representations of various types of hearing loss.

◼ SPEECH AUDIOMETRY

In speech audiometry, the ability to hear spoken words is measured through a microphone connected to an audiometer. The two components of speech audiometry are the speech reception threshold and speech discrimination.

SPEECH RECEPTION THRESHOLD. Speech reception threshold is the level of intensity at which a client can repeat simple words. In testing this threshold, the nurse tries to determine how intense (or loud) a simple speech stimulus must be before the client can hear it well enough to repeat it correctly. In one common test, lists of two-syllable words called **spondee** are used (i.e., words in which there is generally equal stress on each syllable, such as *airplane, railroad,* and *cowboy*).

The speech reception threshold measured by the audiometer is the hearing level at which the client can repeat simple words correctly 50% of the time. The test is administered essentially in the same manner as for the pure tone tests, but the microphone is activated through the audiometer. The intensity dial on the audiometer regulates word level intensity.

CHART 48-3

BEST PRACTICE *for*
Pure Tone Air Conduction Audiometry

1. After explaining the procedure to the client, place the earphones on the client. Make sure that the side marked *left* is on the left ear and the side marked *right* is on the right ear. The earphones must cover the ears.
2. If the client reports a hearing difference between the two ears, test the ear with better hearing first.
3. Begin the testing at 1000 Hz. This frequency is near the middle of the ear's sensitivity spectrum, and it has been demonstrated to have good test-retest reliability.
4. Adjust the audiometer so that the tone is inaudible unless the interrupter switch is depressed. Start with the hearing level control at its lowest setting, either 0 or −10 dB. Depress the interrupter switch, and gradually increase the intensity of the tone until the client signals that the tone is heard. Increase the intensity of the tone beyond this point by about 20 dB to give the client an opportunity to hear it well.
5. Now reduce the intensity of the tone in 5-dB steps until the client indicates that the tone is no longer heard. Note the last intensity level, in 5-dB decrement steps, at which the client signaled. The last point at which the client indicated that the tone was still heard should be his or her threshold for hearing for that frequency. The threshold can be tested for reliability by increasing the tone by 20 dB once again and then descending in 5-dB steps until once again the lowest point in intensity is reached.
6. If you have succeeded in obtaining a consistent threshold at 1000 Hz, change the frequency control to 500 Hz and start again. The preferred method is to test the lower frequencies first (500 and 250 Hz) and then move higher, usually to 2000, 4000, and 8000 Hz. At each frequency, the procedure is the same as for 1000 Hz.
7. After you have completed the threshold measurements on the first ear, switch the output selector to the opposite earphone. Proceed in the same manner to obtain thresholds for the other ear, also beginning at 1000 Hz.
8. If the thresholds of the second ear seem to differ by 40 dB or more from those of the first ear, masking of the better-hearing ear is indicated to rule out its participation in the test.
9. In operating the interrupter switch, make sure that you do not fall into rhythmic patterns that the client can follow. The pattern of tonal presentations should be irregular so that the client cannot predict when the tone will be presented.

SPEECH DISCRIMINATION. Speech discrimination testing establishes the ability to discriminate among similar sounds or among words that contain similar sounds. The ability to understand speech is considered the most important measurable aspect of human auditory function. Speech discrimination testing assesses understanding of speech. A hearing loss may not only decrease sensitivity to sound but also impair understanding of what is being said.

A standard format contains lists of 25 to 50 **monosyllabic** (one-syllable) words, such as *carve, day, toe,* and *ran,* phonemically balanced (designed to include the phonemes of Amer-

ican English in the proper proportion) and with equal word difficulty between lists. The lists are presented to the client through earphones at a selected loudness level, generally about 30 to 40 dB above the speech reception threshold, or at the client's most comfortable listening level. A percentage score is derived from the number of words repeated correctly.

■ Tympanometry

Tympanometry assesses compliance (mobility) of the tympanic membrane and structures of the middle ear as a function

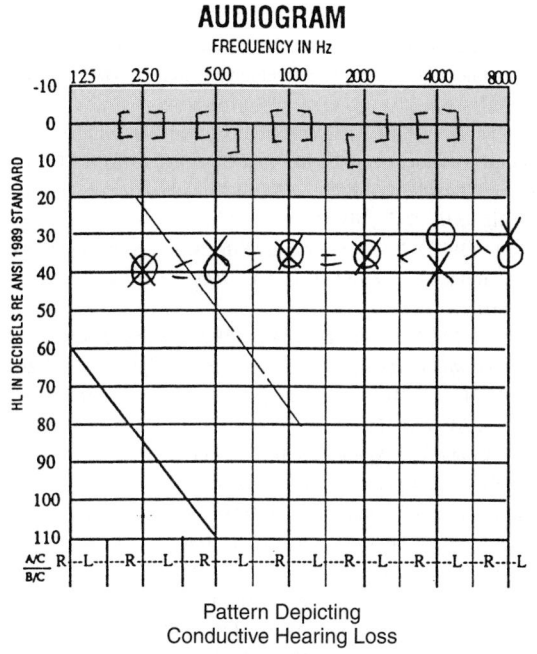
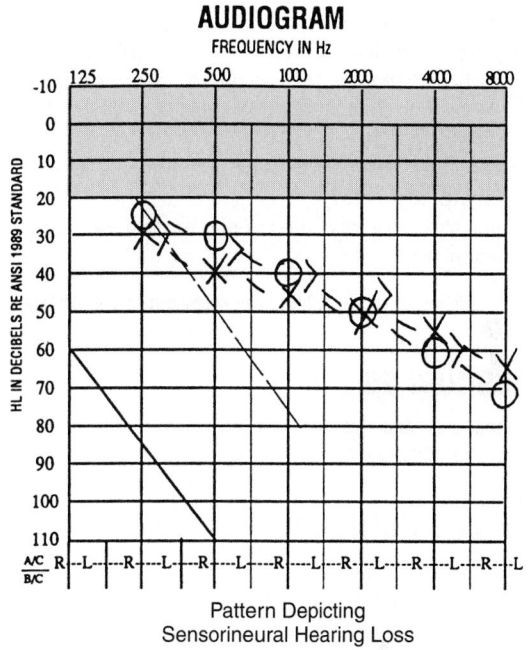

Figure 48-12 ● Audiogram patterns depicting various types of hearing loss. (Courtesy Cleveland Hearing and Speech Center, Cleveland, OH.)

of systematically varied air pressure in the external auditory canal. The progression or resolution of serous otitis and otitis media can be accurately monitored with this procedure.

Tympanometry is helpful in distinguishing middle-ear pathologic conditions, such as otosclerosis, ossicular disarticulation, otitis media, and perforation of the tympanic membrane. It is also valuable for assessing patency of the eustachian tube and for observing postsurgical recovery of middle-ear function.

CRITICAL THINKING CHALLENGE

Your client is an 86-year-old woman who lives at home and is scheduled to have pure tone audiometry performed next week. She drives herself and performs all of her own housekeeping responsibilities. In addition, she cooks meals for a neighbor who is blind. She is concerned about pain and whether she will be able to attend her art class later that night after the audiometry.

- What should you tell her regarding the preparation and actual audiometry procedures?
- What activities should be restricted during the first 24 hours following audiometry?

For suggested answer guidelines, go to http://www.wbsaunders.com/SIMON/Iggy/.

ONLINE RESOURCES

For suggested readings and Internet resources, go to http://www.wbsaunders.com/SIMON/Iggy/.

SELECTED BIBLIOGRAPHY

Asterisk indicates a classic or definitive work on this subject.

Ardic, F.N., et al. (1998). High-frequency hearing and reflex latency in patients with pigment disorder. *American Journal of Otolaryngology, 19*(6), 365-369.

Bagley, M. (1998). Helping older adults to live better with hearing and vision losses. *Journal of Case Management, 7*(4), 147-152.

Baloh, R.W. (1998). Decision making in medicine: Dizzy patients: The varieties of vertigo. *Hospital Practice, 33*(6), 55-58, 61-63, 67-68.

*Benjamin, B., et al. (1994). *A color atlas of otorhinolaryngology.* Philadelphia: Lippincott-Raven.

*Bess, F.H., & Humes, L.E. (1995). *Audiology: The fundamentals.* Baltimore: Williams & Wilkins.

Cavendish, R. (1998). Clinical snapshot: Adult hearing loss. *American Journal of Nursing, 98*(8), 50-51.

Chaimoff, M., et al. (1999). Sudden hearing loss as a presenting symptom of acoustic neuroma. *American Journal of Otolaryngology, 20*(3), 157-160.

de la Cruz, M., & Bance, M. (1999). Carbamazepine-induced sensorineural hearing loss. *Archives of Otolaryngology–Head and Neck Surgery, 125*(2), 225-227.

Friedman, E.M., et al. (1997). When and how to retrieve foreign bodies. *Patient Care, 31*(13), 186-190, 193-194, 197-200.

Gates, G.A., Couropmitree, N.N., & Myers, R.H. (1999). Genetic associations in age-related hearing thresholds. *Archives of Otolaryngology–Head and Neck Surgery, 125*(6), 654-659.

Guyton, A., & Hall, J. (2000). *Textbook of medical physiology* (10th ed.). Philadelphia: W.B. Saunders.

Houston, D.K., et al. (1999). Age-related hearing loss, vitamin B-12, and folate in elderly women. *American Journal of Clinical Nutrition, 69*(3), 564-571.

Hsu, R., & Levine, S.C. (1998). Sudden hearing loss: How to identify the cause promptly. *Consultant, 38*(1), 23-26, 31-32.

Hull, R.H. (1997). *Aural rehabilitation: Serving children and adults* (3rd ed.). San Diego: Singular Publishing.

Jarvis, C. (2000). *Physical examination and health assessment* (3rd ed.). Philadelphia: W.B. Saunders.

Larson, P.D., Hazen, S.E.; & Martin, J.L.H. (1997). Assessment and management of sensory loss in elderly patients. *AORN Journal, 65*(2), 432-437.

Lee, F.S., et al. (1998). Analysis of blood chemistry and hearing levels in a sample of older persons. *Ear and Hearing, 19*(3), 180-190.

Lucas, L. & Matthews-Flint, L. (2001). Sound advice about hearing aids. *Nursing2001, 31*(2), 59-61.

Lusk, S.L. (1997). Noise exposures: Effects of hearing and prevention of noise induced hearing loss. *AAOHN Journal, 45*(8), 397-405, 409-410.

Malarkey, L.M., & McMorrow, M.E. (1999). *Nurse's manual of laboratory tests and diagnostic procedures.* Philadelphia: W.B. Saunders.

Martin, F.N. (2000). *Introduction to audiology* (7th ed.). Needham Heights: Allyn & Bacon.

National Council on Aging. (2000). The consequences of untreated hearing loss in older persons. *ORL–Head and Neck Nursing, 18*(1), 12-16.

Noorhassim, I., & Rampal, K.G. (1998). Multiplicative effect of smoking and age on hearing impairment. *American Journal of Otolaryngology, 19*(4), 240-243.

Ota, Y., & Oda, M. (1999). Lesion site in sudden deafness: Study with electrocochleography and transiently evoked otoacoustic emission. *Acta Oto-Laryngologica, 119*(1), 33-41.

Pagana, K.D., & Pagana, T.J. (1999a). *Diagnostic testing and nursing implications: A case study approach* (5th ed.). St. Louis: Mosby.

Pagana, K.D., & Pagana, T.J. (1999b). *Mosby's diagnostic and laboratory test reference* (4th ed.). St. Louis: Mosby.

Shaw, L. (1997). Protocol for detection and follow-up of hearing loss. *Clinical Nurse Specialist, 11*(6), 240-247.

Sheehan, J. (2000). Caring for the deaf: Do you do enough? *RN, 63*(3), 69-72.

Stewart, M.G., et al. (1999). Cost-effectiveness of the diagnostic evaluation of vertigo. *Laryngoscope, 109*(4), 600-605.

Stone, C.M. (1999). Clinical outlook: Preventing cerumen impaction in nursing facility residents. *Journal of Gerontological Nursing, 25*(5), 43-45.

Tan, R., Osman, V., & Tan, G. (1997). Ear size as a predictor of chronological age. *Archives of Gerontology and Geriatrics, 25*(2), 187-191.

Thobaden, M. (1998). Helping clients with presbycusis. *Home Care Provider, 3*(4), 186-188.

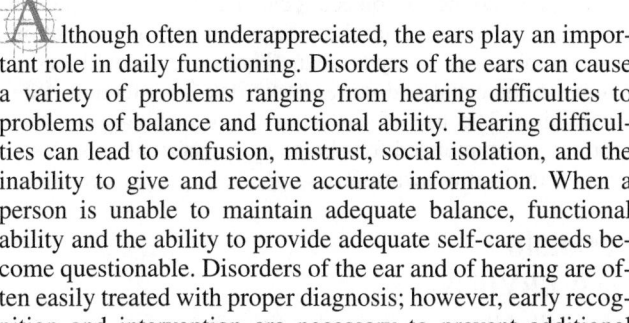

Interventions for Clients with Ear and Hearing Problems

JAN HOOT MARTIN

Learning Objectives

After studying this chapter, you should be able to:

1. Compare and contrast the clinical manifestations and interventions for external otitis and otitis media.
2. Describe how to correctly instill medications into the ear.
3. Explain the procedures to safely remove impacted cerumen from the ear canal of an older client.
4. Prioritize educational needs for the client with Meniere's disease.
5. Compare and contrast the causes and interventions for conductive versus sensorineural hearing loss.
6. Prioritize nursing care needs for the client after tympanoplasty.
7. Prioritize educational needs for the client after stapedectomy.
8. Identify an appropriate method for communicating with a client who has recently become hearing impaired.
9. Develop a teaching plan for a client who is learning to use a hearing aid.

Go to http://www.wbsaunders.com/SIMON/Iggy/ for self-assessment questions related to these Learning Objectives.

Although often underappreciated, the ears play an important role in daily functioning. Disorders of the ears can cause a variety of problems ranging from hearing difficulties to problems of balance and functional ability. Hearing difficulties can lead to confusion, mistrust, social isolation, and the inability to give and receive accurate information. When a person is unable to maintain adequate balance, functional ability and the ability to provide adequate self-care needs become questionable. Disorders of the ear and of hearing are often easily treated with proper diagnosis; however, early recognition and intervention are necessary to prevent additional damage and to promote a maximal level of wellness.

CONDITIONS AFFECTING THE EXTERNAL EAR

The external ear is the outermost part of the ear structures and, as such, is subject to outside forces that can cause problems. Disorders of the external ear include **congenital malformation** (birth defects), trauma, and infectious or noninfectious lesions of the pinna, auricle, or auditory canal. Ear structures (external, middle, and inner ear) develop at different times during fetal development; thus the presence of birth defects in one area does not necessarily mean that other areas will be affected similarly. Abnormalities of the external ear range from crumpling or falling forward of the pinna to absence **(atresia)** of the auditory canal. In addition, trauma can damage or destroy the auricle and external canal. Surgi-

cal reconstruction, generally completed in phases, can re-form the pinna with skin grafts and plastic prostheses. Trauma to the auricle resulting in a hematoma necessitates the removal of blood via needle aspiration to prevent calcification and hardening, which is often referred to as a **cauliflower** or **boxer's ear.**

Benign cysts or polyps of the auricle or external canal are surgically removed if they grow large enough to block the canal and affect hearing. Malignant cells, most commonly basal cell carcinoma, can also be found on the pinna. In general, treatment consists of simple excision. As the lesion becomes larger, its proximity to the skull and facial nerve makes treatment more difficult.

External Otitis

▮ OVERVIEW

External otitis is a painful condition caused when irritating or infective agents come into contact with the skin of the external ear. The result to the external auditory canal or auricle is either an allergic response or inflammation with or without infection. Affected skin becomes red, swollen, and tender to touch or movement. Swelling of the auditory canal can lead to hearing loss due to canal obstruction. Allergic external otitis is commonly caused by contact with cosmetics, hair sprays, earphones, earrings, or hearing aids. The most common infectious organisms, usually bacterial or fungal, are *Pseudomonas aeruginosa,*

Streptococcus, Staphylococcus, and *Aspergillus.* Table 49-1 compares external otitis and otitis media.

External otitis occurs more often in hot, humid environments, especially in the summer, and is commonly referred to as **swimmer's ear** because of the high incidence in people involved in water sports. In addition, clients who have traumatized and opened lesions in their external auditory canal with sharp or small objects (such as hairpins or cotton-tipped applicators) or through headphones are more susceptible to external otitis.

Necrotizing or **malignant external otitis** is the most virulent form of external otitis; the organism spreads beyond the external auditory canal into the adjacent structures of the ear and skull. The high mortality rate seen with malignant external otitis results from complicating disorders such as meningitis, brain abscess, and destruction of cranial nerves, especially the facial nerve (cranial nerve VII).

➤ COLLABORATIVE MANAGEMENT
◗ Assessment

Clinical manifestations of external otitis include a variety of complaints, ranging from mild itching to pain with movement of the pinna or tragus. Clients have pain with physical manipulation of the pinna and tragus or when upward pressure is applied to the external canal. They report feeling as though the ear is plugged and hearing is reduced.

The nurse uses extreme caution during otoscopic examination to avoid exerting pressure on the walls of the external canal, which causes excessive pain. Drainage from the ear, when present, is often greenish white. To prevent cross-contamination, the nurse is careful to dispose of the otoscope tip and wash his or her hands thoroughly before examining the opposite ear. Hearing loss can be severe on the affected side when inflammation causes obstruction of the auditory canal and reduces access of sounds to the tympanic membrane.

◗ Interventions

Treatment of external otitis focuses on reducing local inflammation, edema, and pain. The nurse or assistive nursing personnel applies heat locally for 20 minutes three times a day, using towels warmed with water and then wrapped in a plastic bag, or heating pads placed on a low setting. Bedrest is often helpful in limiting head movements, thereby reducing pain.

Topical antibiotic and steroid therapies are the most effective means of decreasing inflammation and pain. The nurse reviews best practices for instilling eardrops with the client, as shown in Chart 49-1. The nurse observes the client to make sure that he or she uses proper technique. If edema has caused an obstruction of the external canal, an earwick is inserted past the blockage, with medicated drops applied to the outside end (Figure 49-1). A long piece of gauze dressing serves as an earwick, which the physician or nurse practitioner inserts using forceps to push carefully through the blocked external auditory canal to the tympanic membrane. The earwick may be removed when medication can flow freely into the canal. Thorough handwashing is strictly enforced. Systemic oral or intravenous antibiotics are used in severe cases, especially when cellulitis is present or the auricular lymph nodes are enlarged.

Analgesics, including opioids, may be necessary for pain relief during the initial days of therapy. Acetylsalicylic acid (aspirin, Entrophen✢) or acetaminophen (Tylenol, Abenol✢) can be given to relieve less severe pain.

After the inflammation has subsided, diluted alcohol may be dropped into the ear to keep it clean and dry and to prevent recurrence. The nurse teaches the client not to use cotton-tipped applicators to dry the ears, because use could lead to trauma to the canal and increase the risk for infection or inflammation. The use of ear plugs when engaging in water sports is recommended for clients with recurrent episodes of external otitis after swimming.

Furuncle
▮ OVERVIEW

Often called localized external otitis, a **furuncle** is caused by bacterial infection, usually *Staphylococcus,* of a hair follicle. A furuncle is located on the outer half of the external canal.

TABLE 49-1 • COMPARISON OF FEATURES BETWEEN EXTERNAL OTITIS AND OTITIS MEDIA		
Etiology	**Clinical Manifestations**	**Treatment**
EXTERNAL OTITIS		
Allergic reactions	Pain	Topical antibiotics
Bacterial or fungal infection	Itching	Corticosteroids
Swimming	Hearing loss	Oral analgesics
Local trauma	Plugged feeling in ear	Local heat
	Redness and edema	
	Exudate	
OTITIS MEDIA		
Bacterial or viral infection	Pain	Systemic antibiotics
Accumulation of fluid	Pressure in ear	Analgesics
	Hearing loss	Local heat
	Tinnitus	Antipyretics
	Fever	Antihistamines
	Malaise	Decongestants
	Nausea or vomiting	Myringotomy
	Bulging tympanic membrane	
	Fluid behind tympanic membrane	

CHART 49-1

BEST PRACTICE *for*
Instillation of Eardrops

1. Gather the solutions to be administered.
2. Check the labels to ensure correct dosage and time.
3. Remove and discard any ear packing.
4. Irrigate the ear if the tympanic membrane is intact.
5. Place the bottle of eardrops (with the top on tightly) in a bowl of warm water for 5 minutes.
6. Tilt the client's head in the opposite direction of the affected ear and place the drops in the ear.
7. With the head tilted, gently move the head back and forth five times.
8. Insert a cotton ball into the opening of the ear canal to act as packing.

COLLABORATIVE MANAGEMENT

The clinical manifestations of a furuncle include intense local pain to light touch. The area is swollen and red, with tight skin covering the area, possibly with a purulent head. No drainage is noted unless the furuncle has ruptured. Hearing is impaired if the lesion occludes the canal.

Treatment is similar to that of other types of external otitis: local and systemic antibiotic administration and localized heat application. An earwick may be used with one-half strength Burow's solution to relieve pain. The furuncle might need to be incised and drained if it does not resolve with the use of antibiotics.

Cerumen or Foreign Bodies

▌ OVERVIEW

Many objects can enter or be placed in the external auditory canal. Cerumen, or wax, is the most common cause of an impacted canal. Vegetables, beads, pencil erasers, and insects are other common items that may also enter the ear, with or without the client's help. Although uncomfortable, these are rarely true emergencies, and the nurse takes care when removing cerumen or foreign bodies.

COLLABORATIVE MANAGEMENT

● Assessment

Clients have a sensation of fullness in the ear, with or without associated hearing loss, and may have ear pain, itching, and/or bleeding from the ear. The object may or may not be visible with direct inspection.

● Interventions

When the occluding material is cerumen, the nurse irrigates the canal with a mixture of water and hydrogen peroxide at body temperature (Figure 49-2), following best practices for proper irrigation (Chart 49-2). Removal of wax by irrigation is a slow process and may take more than one sitting. When cerumen obstruction is the cause of hearing loss, however, removal results in increased hearing. Between 50 and 70 mL of solution is the maximum amount that the client can tolerate at one sitting. Irrigation is contraindicated in clients who have tympanic membrane perforation or otitis media.

If the cerumen is thick and dry or cannot be removed easily, the health care provider may prescribe a ceruminolytic product such as Cerumenex to soften the wax before trying to remove it. Another way to soften cerumen is to add 3 drops of glycerin or mineral oil to the ear at bedtime and 3 drops of hydrogen peroxide twice a day. After several days of this treatment, the cerumen is more easily removed through irrigation. In some cases, a small curette or cerumen spoon may be used to scoop out the wax. Only trained health care providers should use this method, because damage to the canal or the tympanic membrane is likely with improper technique. Refer to Chart 49-3 for nursing care considerations of older adult clients with cerumen impaction.

Irrigation is *not* used when the foreign object is vegetable matter, because this material expands with hydration, worsening the impaction. The object needs to be physically removed by an experienced health care provider.

Insects are killed before removal unless they can be coaxed out by a flashlight or a humming noise. Mineral oil or diluted alcohol is instilled into the ear to suffocate the insect, which is then removed with ear forceps.

If the client has local irritation, an antibiotic or steroid ointment may be applied to prevent infection and reduce local irritation. Hearing acuity is tested if hearing loss is not resolved by removal of the object.

In rare cases, surgical removal of the foreign object is necessary. The object is removed through the transcanal route using a wire bent at a 90-degree angle. The wire is looped around the object, and the object is pulled out. Because this procedure is painful, general anesthesia is necessary.

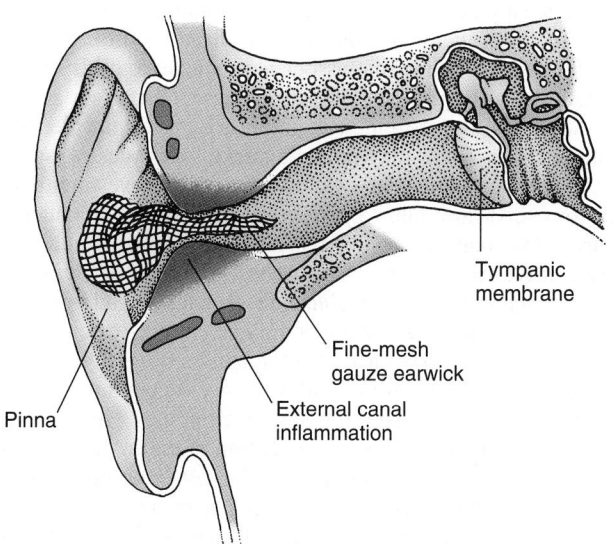

Figure 49-1 ● Earwick for instillation of antibiotics into the external canal. When edema occludes the external auditory canal, it is difficult for antibiotic solutions to enter the canal adequately. An earwick is placed through the meatus. Solutions placed on the external portion of the earwick are absorbed through the canal.

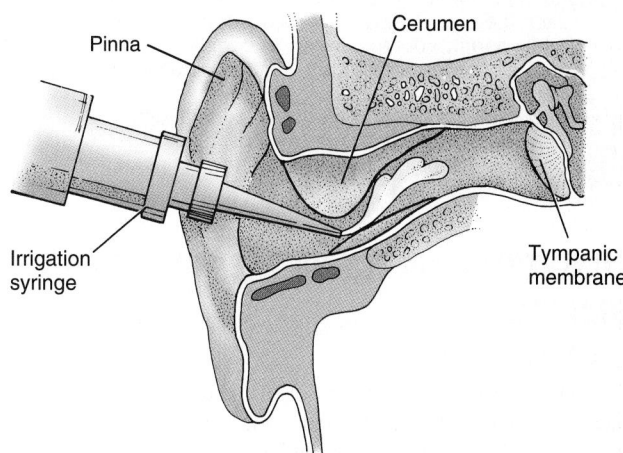

Figure 49-2 ● Irrigation of the external canal. Cerumen and debris can be removed from the ear by irrigation with warm water. The stream of water is aimed above or below the impaction to allow backpressure to push it out rather than further down the canal.

CHART 49-2

BEST PRACTICE *for*
Ear Irrigation

1. Gather the proper equipment: basin, syringe, otoscope, towel.
2. Warm tap water to body temperature.
3. Fill a syringe with warm water.
4. Place a towel around the client's neck.
5. Place a basin under the ear to be irrigated.
6. Use an otoscope to check the location of the impacted cerumen; ascertain that the tympanic membrane is intact and that the client does not have otitis media.
7. Place the tip of the syringe at an angle so that the fluid pushes on one side and not directly on the impaction (this helps to loosen the impaction instead of forcing it further into the canal).
8. Watch the fluid return for signs of cerumen plug removal.
9. Continue to irrigate the ear with approximately 70 mL of fluid.
10. If the cerumen does not drain out, wait 10 minutes and repeat the irrigation procedure.
11. Monitor the client for signs of nausea.
12. If the client becomes nauseated, stop the procedure.
13. If the cerumen cannot be removed by irrigation, the client may place mineral oil into the ear three times a day for 2 days to soften dry, impacted cerumen, after which irrigation may be repeated.

CHART 49-3

NURSING FOCUS *on the* **OLDER ADULT**
Cerumen Impaction

- Assess the hearing of all older clients using simple voice tests (see Chapter 48).
- Perform a gentle otoscopic inspection of the external canal and tympanic membrane of any older client who has a problem with hearing acuity, especially the client who wears a hearing aid.
- Use ear irrigation to remove any impacted cerumen.
- Make certain that the irrigating fluid is approximately 98° F (37° C) to reduce the chance of stimulating the vestibular sense.
- Use no more than 5 to 10 mL of irrigating fluid at a time.
- If nausea, vomiting, or dizziness develops, stop the irrigation immediately.
- Teach the client how to irrigate his or her own ears.
- Obtain a return demonstration of ear irrigation from the client, observing for specific areas in which the client may need assistance.
- Encourage the client to wash the external ears daily using a soapy, wet washcloth over the index finger (best done in the shower or while washing the hair).

CONDITIONS AFFECTING THE MIDDLE EAR
Otitis Media
■ OVERVIEW

The three most common forms of otitis media are acute otitis media, chronic otitis media, and serous otitis media. Each affects the middle-ear structures but has slightly different causes, incidences, and pathologic changes. If otitis progresses or remains untreated, permanent conductive hearing loss may occur. Otitis media is less common in adults than in children but does occur.

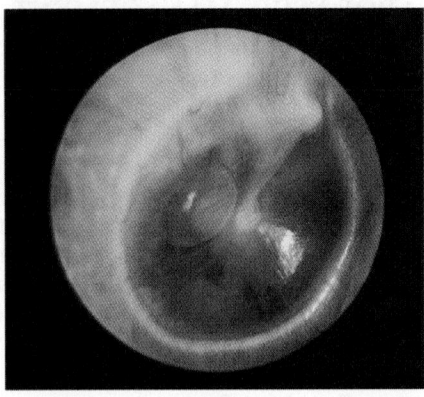

Figure 49-3 ● Otoscopic view of otitis media.

Acute otitis media and chronic otitis media, also known as suppurant or purulent otitis media, are similar in pathophysiology. An infecting agent introduced into the middle ear causes an inflammation within the mucosa, leading to swelling and irritation of the ossicles within the middle ear. This process is followed by a purulent inflammatory exudate. Acute disease has a sudden onset and a relatively short duration of 3 weeks or less. Chronic otitis media usually follows repeated acute episodes, has a longer duration, and can be associated with greater morbidity or injury to the middle ear.

The eustachian tube and mastoid, connected to the middle ear by a continuation of cells, are also affected by the infection. If the tympanic membrane perforates and infective materials spill into the external ear, external otitis also develops, which, untreated, thickens and scars the middle ear. Necrosis of the ossicles leads to destruction of the middle-ear structures.

➤ COLLABORATIVE MANAGEMENT
▶ Assessment

The chief complaint of the client with acute or chronic otitis media is ear pain with or without manipulation of the external ear structures. Pain associated with chronic otitis media is much less severe than that associated with acute otitis media. As the pressure in the middle ear increases, there is a greater sensation of fullness in the ear, and hearing is diminished and distorted. The client may notice a sticking or cracking sound in the ear on yawning or swallowing or may have tinnitus in the form of a low hum or a low-pitched sound. Conductive hearing loss may occur as a result of physical obstruction in sound wave transmission. Headaches are common, and systemic symptoms such as malaise, fever, nausea, and vomiting can occur. As the pressure on the middle ear presses on the inner ear, the client may have slight dizziness or vertigo.

Otoscopic examination findings vary, depending on the stage of the disease. The tympanic membrane is initially retracted, which allows clear visualization of the ear landmarks. At this early stage, the client has only vague ear discomfort; however, as the disease progresses, the tympanic membrane's blood vessels dilate and appear red (Figure 49-3). In the third stage, the tympanic membrane becomes red, thickened, and bulging, with loss of landmarks. Decreased membrane mobility is evident on inspection with a pneumatic otoscope. Exudate behind the membrane may be visible.

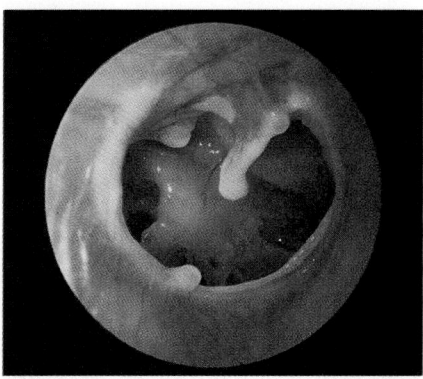

Figure 49-4 ● Otoscopic view of a perforated tympanic membrane.

If the disease progresses, the tympanic membrane spontaneously **perforates** (breaks open) and pus or blood drains from the ear (Figure 49-4). This discharge may be pulsating when viewed through the otoscope. When the membrane ruptures, the client notices a marked decrease in pain as the pressure on middle-ear structures is relieved (Figure 49-5). Tympanic perforations from any cause may heal if the underlying problem is controlled. The membrane covering initially appears thinner over the healed perforation. A simple central perforation does not interfere with hearing unless the ossicles of the middle ear are damaged or the perforation is large. However, repeated perforations with extensive scarring can cause hearing loss.

Cultures of drainage after a perforation from uncontrolled otitis media may reveal the infecting agent. Cultures are rarely taken unless previous treatment has been ineffective. When the tympanic membrane is not perforated, a needle aspiration or myringotomy draws fluid for culture.

● Interventions

NONSURGICAL MANAGEMENT. Treatment can be as simple as putting the client in a quiet environment without distractions. Bedrest limits head movements that intensify the pain. Localized heat may be applied by using a heating pad adjusted to a low setting. Application of cold may occasionally relieve pain.

Systemic antibiotic therapy can decrease pain by reducing inflammation. Topical antibiotics are not used to treat otitis media. Analgesics such as acetylsalicylic acid (aspirin, Entrophen♣) and acetaminophen (Tylenol, Abenol♣) aid in pain relief, and their antipyretic effects help the client feel better by relieving an elevated temperature. When the client has severe pain, opioid analgesics such as codeine and meperidine hydrochloride (Demerol) also may be used.

Antihistamines and decongestants are prescribed to decrease mucus production in the nasopharynx and to decrease fluid in the middle ear. The body can then reabsorb the fluid, reducing pressure and pain.

SURGICAL MANAGEMENT. If the pain persists after initial antibiotic therapy and the tympanic membrane continues to bulge, a **myringotomy** (surgical opening of the pars tensa of the tympanic membrane) is performed. Myringotomies drain middle-ear fluids and almost immediately relieve pain.

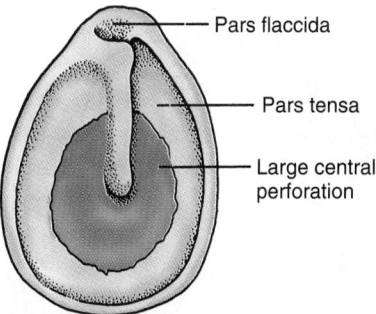

With a **large central perforation,** clients complain of significant hearing loss.

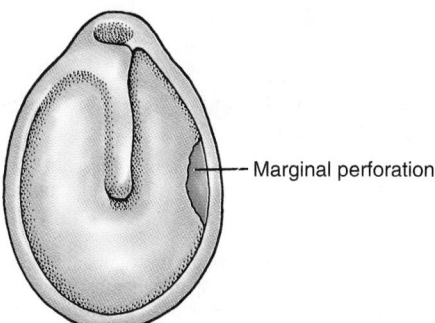

With a **marginal perforation,** clients might complain of significant hearing loss.

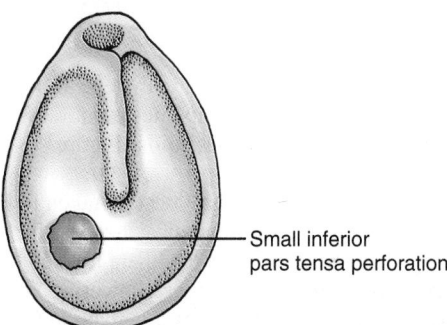

With a **small inferior pars tensa perforation,** clients do not complain of much interference with hearing.

Figure 49-5 ● Perforations of the tympanic membrane. Central perforations heal more quickly than marginal perforations. Marginal perforations that do not heal allow cholesteatoma formation.

PREOPERATIVE CARE. The nurse reassures the client that the myringotomy will relieve pain and is usually performed without anesthesia. Many people are apprehensive about a perforation and its effect on hearing. To relieve some of this anxiety, the nurse discusses the reasons for the procedure with the client and encourages relaxation techniques such as deep breathing before and during the procedure. Systemic antibiotic therapy continues before and after this procedure. The nurse cleans the external canal with a bacteriostatic solution such as povidone-iodine (Betadine) before the myringotomy.

OPERATIVE PROCEDURE. The small surgical incision can be performed in an office or clinic setting and heals rapidly. An alternative is the removal of fluid from the middle ear via needle aspiration. For relief of pressure caused by serous

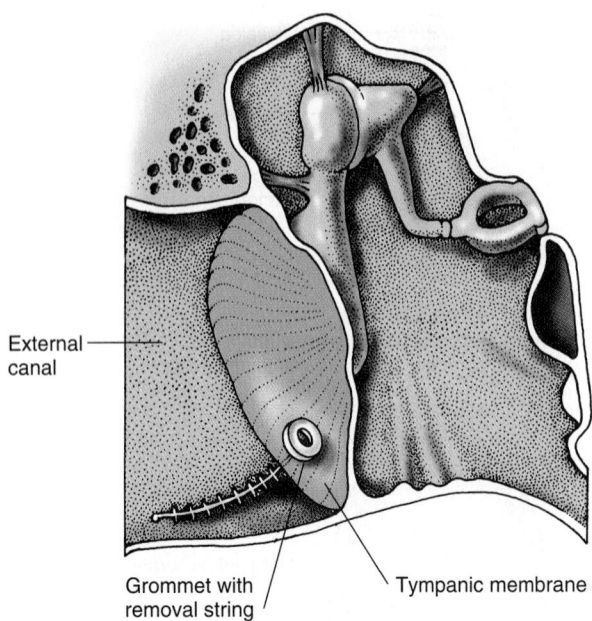

Figure 49-6 ● Grommet through the tympanic membrane. A small grommet is placed through the tympanic membrane away from the margins, which allows prolonged drainage of fluids from the middle ear. The grommet can be removed later, and the tympanic membrane can be allowed to heal naturally or be patched with a small piece of homogenous tissue.

otitis media, a small **grommet** (polyethylene tube) may be surgically placed through the tympanic membrane to allow continuous drainage of middle-ear fluids (Figure 49-6).

POSTOPERATIVE CARE. Care must be taken to keep the external ear and canal free of other substances while the incision is healing. The nurse instructs the client to keep his or her head dry by not washing the hair or showering for several days. Other postoperative instructions are given in Chart 49-4.

CRITICAL THINKING CHALLENGE

You are assigned to care for a 28-year-old man who has been admitted with diabetic ketoacidosis. During the course of his hospitalization, he tells you that he thinks he has an ear infection.

- What assessment information will you need before notifying the health care provider?
- What nursing interventions would you perform regardless of the location of the infection?
- If otitis media is diagnosed, what is the proper route for antibiotic therapy, and why?

For suggested answer guidelines, go to [SIMON] http://www.wbsaunders.com/SIMON/Iggy/.

Mastoiditis

OVERVIEW

The epithelial lining of the middle ear is continuous with the epithelial lining of the mastoid air cells, which are embedded in the temporal bone. **Mastoiditis** is a secondary disorder resulting from untreated or inadequately treated otitis media and can be acute or chronic. Before antibiotic therapy, mastoiditis

---

CHART 49-4

CLIENT EDUCATION GUIDE
Recovery from Ear Surgery

- Avoid straining when you have a bowel movement.
- Do not drink through a straw for 2 to 3 weeks.
- Avoid air travel for 2 to 3 weeks.
- Avoid excessive coughing for 2 to 3 weeks.
- Stay away from people with colds.
- If you need to blow your nose, blow gently, one side at a time, with your mouth open.
- Avoid getting your head wet, washing your hair, and showering for 1 week.
- Keep your ear dry for 6 weeks by placing a ball of cotton coated with petroleum jelly (such as Vaseline) in your ear. Change the cotton ball daily.
- Avoid rapidly moving the head, bouncing, and bending over for 3 weeks.
- Change your ear dressing every 24 hours as directed.
- Report excessive drainage immediately to your physician.

---

was a leading cause of death in children and of hearing loss in adults. Today, antibiotic therapy is aimed at treating the middle-ear infection before it progresses to mastoiditis.

▶ COLLABORATIVE MANAGEMENT

▶ Assessment

The clinical manifestations of mastoiditis include swelling behind the ear and pain with minimal movement of the tragus, the pinna, or the head. Pain is not relieved by myringotomy. **Cellulitis** (infection spreading laterally through the tissues of the skin) develops on the skin or external scalp over the mastoid process. Otoscopic examination reveals a red, dull, thick, immobile tympanic membrane with or without perforation. Postauricular lymph nodes are tender and enlarged. Clients with mastoiditis also have low-grade fever, malaise, and anorexia.

▶ Interventions

NONSURGICAL MANAGEMENT. Antibiotic therapy aims to prevent the continued spread of infection from the otitis media or mastoiditis but has limited use in actual mastoiditis treatment because of the difficulty of achieving effective antibiotic levels within the bony structure of the mastoid. Cultures obtained from the ear drainage or myringotomy determine the sensitivities of infecting organisms to specific antibiotics.

SURGICAL MANAGEMENT. Surgical removal of the infected tissue is necessary if the client does not respond to antibiotic administration within a few days. A simple or modified radical mastoidectomy with tympanoplasty is the most common treatment. All infected tissue must be removed so that the infection does not spread to other structures. A tympanoplasty is then performed to reconstruct the ossicles and the tympanic membrane to restore hearing. Client preparation, the operative procedure, and follow-up care for tympanoplasty are discussed on pp. 1073 and 1074.

Complications arise when infective material has not been removed completely or when other structures outside the mastoid and middle ear are contaminated. Complications of mastoiditis include damage to the abducens and facial cranial nerves (cranial nerves VI and VII), decreasing the client's ability to look laterally (cranial nerve VI) and causing a drooping of the mouth on the affected side (cranial nerve VII). Other complications include vertigo, meningitis, brain abscess, chronic purulent otitis media, and wound infection.

Trauma
▌ OVERVIEW

Trauma and damage may occur to the tympanic membrane and ossicles by infection, by direct damage to the structures, or through rapid changes in the middle-ear cavity pressure. Foreign objects placed in the external canal may exert pressure on the tympanic membrane and cause perforation. If the objects continue through the canal, the bony structure of the stapes, incus, and malleus may be damaged. Blunt injury to the basal skull and ears can also damage middle-ear structures through fractures extending to the middle ear. Slapping of the external ear increases the pressure in the external auditory canal, tearing the eardrum when the pressure is great enough. The tympanic membrane has a limited stretching ability and gives way under high pressure. Excessive nose blowing and rapid changes of pressure that occur with nonpressurized air flight (**barotrauma**) can cause an increase in pressure within the middle ear. High pressure damages the ossicles and can cause outward perforation of the eardrum.

▶ COLLABORATIVE MANAGEMENT

Tympanic membrane perforations usually heal within 24 hours. Repeated perforations, especially from chronic otitis media, heal slower, with tympanic scarring. Depending on the amount of damage to the ossicles, hearing may or may not return. Hearing aids can improve hearing in this type of hearing loss. Surgical reconstruction of the ossicles and tympanic membrane through a tympanoplasty or a myringoplasty may also improve hearing (see later discussion of nursing care under Tympanoplasty, pp. 1073-1074).

Preventive measures should be taken to avoid trauma. The nurse instructs clients to avoid inserting objects into the external canal. Ear protectors can be used when blunt trauma is likely, especially in sports such as boxing.

Neoplasms
▌ OVERVIEW

Tumors of the middle ear are rare. The most common type of tumor is the glomus jugulare, a highly vascular benign lesion arising from the jugular vein. Extremely rare malignant tumors include primary adenocarcinoma, adenoid cystic carcinoma, and mucoepidermoid carcinoma. The growth of any lesion within the middle-ear fossa disrupts conductive hearing, erodes the ossicles, and has the potential to involve the inner ear and adjacent cranial nerves.

▶ COLLABORATIVE MANAGEMENT

Clients experience progressive hearing loss and tinnitus. Infection and pain are rarely associated with glomus jugulare tumors. A physical examination reveals bulging of the tympanic membrane or a mass extending to the external auditory canal. The highly vascular nature of the glomus jugulare tumor gives it a reddish color and a visible pulsation when seen through the eardrum.

Diagnosis is made by physical examination, tomography, and angiography. Neoplasms are removed by surgery, which generally sacrifices hearing in the affected ear. If all of the margins of the tumor can be seen clearly through the tympanic membrane, a transcanal approach is used to remove the lesion. When the tumor margins extend past the tympanic membrane, further diagnostic tests are necessary to determine the extent of growth and vascular involvement. Radiation therapy is used to decrease the vascularity of the glomus jugulare tumor but is not the preferred method of treatment. Benign lesions are removed because, with continued growth of the neoplasm, cranial structures other than the middle ear can be affected, further damaging the facial or trigeminal nerve. When possible, reconstructive surgery of the middle ear structures is performed later to restore conductive hearing.

CONDITIONS AFFECTING THE INNER EAR
Tinnitus
▌ OVERVIEW

Tinnitus (continuous ringing or noise perception in the ear) is one of the most common complaints of clients with ear or hearing disorders. The health care provider cannot use diagnostic testing to confirm tinnitus, nor does the disorder have observable characteristics, but tinnitus can lead to particularly disturbing emotional consequences for the person afflicted with this disorder.

▶ COLLABORATIVE MANAGEMENT

Symptoms of tinnitus range from mild ringing, which can go unnoticed during the day, to a loud roaring in the ear, which can interfere with thinking and attention span. When clients report tinnitus, the nurse is alert to the wide variety of pathologic disorders and other factors that cause tinnitus: presbycusis, **otosclerosis** (irregular bone growth around ossicles), Meniere's disease, certain drugs, exposure to loud noise, and other inner-ear abnormalities.

The exact pathophysiology and treatment of tinnitus vary with the underlying cause. When no underlying cause can be found or the disorder is untreatable, therapy focuses on ways to mask the tinnitus with background sound, noisemakers, and music during sleeping hours. Ear mold hearing aids can amplify sounds to drown out the tinnitus during the day. The American Tinnitus Association assists clients in coping with tinnitus when other therapy is unsuccessful.

Vertigo and Dizziness
▌ OVERVIEW

Vertigo and dizziness are common clinical manifestations of many ear disorders. Dizziness is a disturbed sense of a person's proper relationship to space. Clients vary greatly in defining dizziness. Vertigo is often used interchangeably with dizziness, but the definition, as well as the cause, is somewhat different. True **vertigo** is a real sense of whirling or turning in space.

The visual system, the vestibular system (cochlea, semicircular canals), and the proprioceptive system (muscles and nerve endings) combine to give input to the cerebellum about balance. Dysfunction in any of these areas leads to a disturbed sense of balance or motion. Common factors affecting the ear that cause vertigo include Meniere's disease, labyrinthitis, acoustic neuromas, benign paroxysmal vertigo, trauma, motion sickness, and drug or alcohol ingestion.

➤ COLLABORATIVE MANAGEMENT

Associated symptoms of vertigo include nausea, vomiting, falling, nystagmus, hearing loss, and tinnitus. Until the underlying cause of the vertigo can be treated, each clinical manifestation is treated. Clients are advised to:
- Restrict head motions and move more slowly
- Maintain adequate hydration, especially after vomiting
- Take medications with antivertiginous effects, such as dimenhydrinate (Dramamine, Gravol✤), diazepam (Valium, Apo-Diazepam✤), and scopolamine (Transderm Scop, Transderm-V✤).

Many clients are dissatisfied with treatment because side effects of the medications, especially drowsiness, can be worse than the vertigo. The nurse cautions clients to maintain a safe, uncluttered environment to prevent accidents during periods of vertigo and to use a cane or walker to maintain balance. The nurse further instructs clients not to drive or operate machinery when taking antivertiginous drugs.

Labyrinthitis
■ OVERVIEW

Labyrinthitis is an infection of the labyrinth, which occasionally occurs as a complication of acute or chronic otitis media. Infection results from an erosion of the bony capsule, allowing infective materials to invade the inner ear. Labyrinthitis often results from the growth of a **cholesteatoma** (benign overgrowth of squamous cell epithelium) from the middle ear into the lateral semicircular canal. Labyrinthitis may follow middle-ear or inner-ear surgery when infection is present. When the infecting organism is viral, the labyrinthitis may be part of a systemic viral infection such as an upper respiratory tract infection or infectious mononucleosis.

➤ COLLABORATIVE MANAGEMENT

Clinical manifestations include hearing loss, tinnitus, spontaneous nystagmus to the affected side, and vertigo with associated nausea and vomiting. **Meningitis** (infection of the brain covering) is the most common complication of labyrinthitis.

Treatment of labyrinthitis includes the use of systemic antibiotics such as ampicillin (Omnipen, Apo-Ampi✤). Clients are advised to stay in bed in a darkened room until clinical manifestations have diminished. Antiemetics, such as chlorpromazine hydrochloride (Thorazine, Novo-Chlorpromazine✤), and antivertiginous medications, such as dimenhydrinate (Dramamine, Gravol✤), relieve symptoms.

The client also needs psychosocial support. Hearing loss on the affected side may be permanent, although vertigo sub-sides as the inflammation resolves. Persistent balance problems may improve with gait training and physical therapy.

Meniere's Disease
■ OVERVIEW

Meniere's disease has three distinct characteristics—tinnitus, unilateral sensorineural hearing loss, and vertigo—occurring in attacks that can last for several days. Clients are almost totally incapacitated during an attack, and several days are needed for full recovery. The pathologic changes of Meniere's disease are either overproduction or decreased reabsorption of endolymphatic fluid, causing a distortion of the entire inner-canal system. This distortion leads to decreased hearing from dilation of the cochlear duct, vertigo because of damage to the vestibular system, and tinnitus from unknown cause. Involvement is generally unilateral. The initial hearing loss is reversible, but repeated damage to the cochlea, caused by increased fluid pressure, leads to permanent hearing loss.

The cause of Meniere's disease is unknown but is associated with viral or bacterial infections, allergic reactions, and biochemical disturbances that increase fluid imbalances. Mild long-term stress also seems to be associated with Meniere's disease.

➤ COLLABORATIVE MANAGEMENT
● Assessment

The onset of Meniere's disease symptoms usually occurs in people between the ages of 20 and 50 years, with a greater prevalence in men and Caucasians. Times of severe, debilitating attacks alternate with almost symptom-free periods. Clients often have certain clinical manifestations before an attack of vertigo, such as headaches, increasing tinnitus, and a feeling of fullness in the affected ear. Clinical manifestations are unilateral in 60% to 70% of the cases.

Clients describe the tinnitus as a continuous, low-pitched roar or a humming sound, which worsens just before and during a severe attack. Hearing loss is initially of the low-frequency tones but worsens to include all levels after repeated episodes. Hearing loss is worse during an attack. In the early stages of Meniere's disease, periods of remission are marked by normal or nearly normal hearing, but permanent hearing loss develops as the attacks increase.

Clients describe the vertigo as periods of whirling, which might even cause them to fall. The vertigo is so intense that even while lying down, clients hold the bed or ground to prevent the whirling. The severe vertigo usually lasts 3 to 4 hours, but clients continue to feel dizzy long after the attack. Nausea and vomiting are common. Other clinical manifestations include rapid eye movements and severe headaches.

● Interventions

NONSURGICAL MANAGEMENT. The nurse instructs clients to make slow head movements to prevent worsening of the vertigo. Dietary and lifestyle changes, such as salt and fluid restrictions that reduce the amount of endolymphatic fluid, are recommended. Clients are advised to stop smoking because of the vasoconstrictive effects.

Drug therapy aims to control the vertigo and vomiting and restore normal balance. Mild diuretics are prescribed to decrease endolymph volume. Nicotinic acid has been found to be useful because of its vasodilatory effect. Antihistamines such as diphenhydramine hydrochloride (Benadryl, Allerdryl✸) and dimenhydrinate (Dramamine, Gravol✸) help reduce the severity of or stop an acute attack. Antiemetics such as chlorpromazine hydrochloride (Thorazine, Novo-Chlorpromazine✸), droperidol (Inapsine), and trimethobenzamide hydrochloride (Arrestin, Tigan) help control the nausea and vomiting. Diazepam (Valium, Apo-Diazepam✸) calms the anxious client; controls vertigo, nausea, and vomiting; and allows the client to rest quietly during an attack.

SURGICAL MANAGEMENT. Surgical treatment of Meniere's disease remains controversial because the hearing in the affected ear is often sacrificed. When medical therapy is ineffective and the client's functional hearing level has decreased significantly, surgery is performed. The most radical procedure involves resection of the vestibular nerve or total removal of the labyrinth **(labyrinthectomy),** performed via the transcanal route. The footplate of the stapes is moved aside, and the labyrinth is removed through the oval window with fine forceps.

Another procedure performed early in the course of the disease is **endolymphatic decompression** with drainage and a shunt. The endolymphatic sac is drained, and a small tube is inserted to enhance fluid drainage. Some clients report relief of vertigo and preservation of their hearing.

If an endolymphatic decompression has been performed, manipulation of the vestibular structures of the inner ear causes postoperative vertigo. The nurse reassures the client that the vertigo is temporary as a result of the surgical procedure, not the disease.

Acoustic Neuroma
OVERVIEW

An **acoustic neuroma** is a benign tumor of cranial nerve VIII. The location makes it destructive because of the frequent involvement of the cerebellum. Depending on the size and exact location of the tumor, damage to hearing, facial movements, and sensation can occur. Also, other neurologic-pathologic disorders associated with a lesion occupying intracranial space may result.

➤ COLLABORATIVE MANAGEMENT

Clinical manifestations begin with tinnitus and progress to gradual sensorineural hearing loss in more than 90% of clients. Later, clients experience constant mild vertigo. As the tumor enlarges, adjacent cranial nerves are damaged.

Acoustic neuromas are diagnosed with computed tomography (CT) scanning and magnetic resonance imaging (MRI). Audiograms diagnose sensorineural hearing loss. Cerebrospinal fluid assays show increased pressure and positive results for protein.

Surgical removal via a craniotomy is necessary, and the remaining hearing is sacrificed. Extreme care is taken to preserve the function of the facial nerve (cranial nerve VII). Routine postcraniotomy care is discussed in Chapter 45. Acoustic neuromas rarely recur after surgical removal.

HEARING LOSS
OVERVIEW
Pathophysiology

Hearing loss is one of the most common physical handicaps in North America. Hearing loss may be conductive, sensorineural, or a combination of the two (Figure 49-7). Conductive hearing loss occurs when sound waves are blocked from contact with inner-ear nerve fibers because of external-ear or middle-ear disorders. If the inner-ear nerve, or sensory, fibers that lead to the cerebral cortex are damaged, the hearing loss is termed sensorineural. Combination hearing loss is known as mixed conductive-sensorineural.

The differences in conductive and sensorineural hearing loss are summarized in Table 49-2. Disorders that lead to conductive hearing loss can often be corrected with no or minimal permanent damage. Sensorineural hearing loss is often permanent, and measures must be taken to prevent further damage or to amplify sounds as a means to improve hearing.

Etiology
COMMON CAUSES OF CONDUCTIVE HEARING LOSS

Any inflammatory process or obstruction of the external or middle ear by cerumen or foreign objects leads to conductive hearing loss. Changes in the tympanic membrane such as bulges, retractions, and perforations may indicate damage to middle-ear structures, which leads to conductive hearing loss. Tumors, scar tissue buildup, and overgrowth of soft bony tissue (otosclerosis) on the ossicles from previous middle-ear surgery also lead to conductive hearing loss.

COMMON CAUSES OF SENSORINEURAL HEARING LOSS

When the inner ear or auditory nerve (cranial nerve VIII) is damaged, sensorineural hearing loss develops. Prolonged exposure to loud noise can damage the hair cells of the cochlea. Many drugs are toxic **(ototoxic)** to the inner-ear structures, and their effects on hearing can be transient or permanent, unilateral or bilateral, dose related, or non–dose related. When ototoxic drugs (such as those listed in Table 48-2) are given to clients with reduced renal function, increased ototoxicity can result because drug elimination takes longer. Older clients are especially susceptible to ototoxicity because of reduced kidney function.

Presbycusis is a common cause of sensorineural hearing loss associated with the process of aging. This hearing loss is commonly caused by degeneration or atrophy of the ganglion cells in the cochlea, loss of elasticity of the basilar membrane, or a decreased vascular supply to the inner ear. Recent research findings suggest that deficiencies of vitamin B_{12} and folic acid may play a role in presbycusis (see the Evidence-Based Practice for Nursing box on p. 1071). Other causes of sensorineural hearing loss include inherited disorders, circulatory disorders (such as arteriosclerosis and hypertension), bacterial or viral infections, prolonged fever, Meniere's disease, diabetes mellitus, and ear surgery. Each is thought to accelerate degenerative changes of the cochlea. Trauma to the ear or the head also contributes to sensorineural hearing loss.

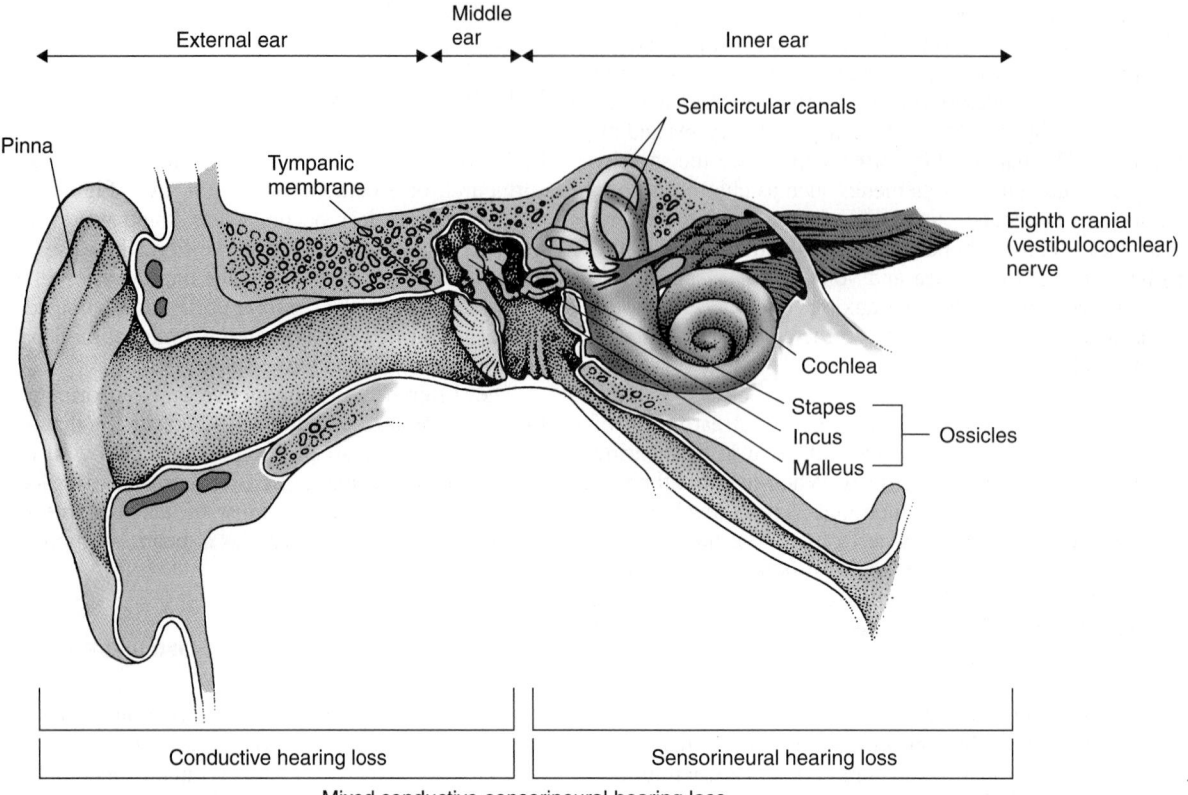

Figure 49-7 ● Anatomy of hearing loss. Hearing loss can be divided into three types: (1) conductive loss (difficulty in the external or the middle ear), (2) sensorineural loss (difficulty in the inner ear or the acoustic nerve), and (3) mixed conductive-sensorineural loss (a combination of the two).

TABLE 49-2 ● DIFFERENTIAL FEATURES OF CONDUCTIVE AND SENSORINEURAL HEARING LOSS

Conductive Hearing Loss	Sensorineural Hearing Loss
CAUSES	
Cerumen	Prolonged exposure to
Foreign body	noise
Perforation of the tympanic	Presbycusis
membrane	Ototoxic substances
Edema	Meniere's disease
Infection of the external or	Acoustic neuroma
middle ear	Diabetes mellitus
Tumors	Labyrinthitis
Otosclerosis	Infection
	Myxedema
ASSESSMENT FINDINGS	
Evidence of obstruction with	Normal appearance of
otoscope	external canal and
Abnormality in tympanic	tympanic membrane
membrane	Tinnitus common
Speaking softly	Occasional dizziness
Hearing best in a noisy envi-	Speaking loudly
ronment	Hearing poorly in loud
Rinne test: air conduction	environment
greater than bone conduction	Rinne test: air conduc-
Weber test: lateralization to	tion less than bone
affected ear	conduction
	Weber test: lateralization
	to unaffected ear

▇ Incidence/Prevalence

Because hearing loss may be gradual and affect only some aspects of hearing, many adults are unaware that their hearing is impaired. The actual incidence of hearing loss is not known exactly; however, approximately 30% to 35% of people ages 65 to 75 years have a hearing loss, and as many as half of the people older than 85 years of age have some degree of hearing loss (National Institute on Deafness and Other Communications Disorders).

► COLLABORATIVE MANAGEMENT
● Assessment

▇ HISTORY

The nurse asks clients how long they have noticed a difference in their hearing and whether the changes occurred suddenly or gradually. Age is an important factor, because some ear and hearing changes occur with advanced age; also, chronic otitis media is diagnosed more often in the older adult. The nurse notes occupational exposure to loud or continuous noises, as well as current or previous use of ototoxic drugs. Clients are also asked about any history of external-ear or middle-ear infection and whether tympanic membrane perforation accompanied the infection. The nurse questions clients about any history of direct trauma to the ears. Because some types of hearing loss have a genetic predisposi-

EVIDENCE-BASED PRACTICE
FOR NURSING

Can dietary modification reduce age-related hearing loss?

Houston, D., et al. (1999). Age-related hearing loss, vitamin B-12, and folate in elderly women. *American Journal of Clinical Nutrition, 69*(3), 564-571.

The authors undertook this study to examine possible causes of presbycusis, or age-related hearing loss. As the title suggests, the hypothesis was that deficiencies in vitamin B_{12} and folate might play a role in the hearing loss so common in older adults. For analysis, subjects were recruited and included or excluded depending on criteria that suggested they either had or could have hearing loss due to specific causes such as infections, ototoxicity, trauma, or conductive hearing loss. Data collections included blood counts, hematologic measures, and serum tests for hepatic, renal, and thyroid function. In addition, serum vitamin B_{12}, red blood cell folate, and serum folate levels were determined. Auditory examinations were conducted, and hearing function was categorized using criteria similar to those of the National Health and Nutrition Examination Survey. Correlation coefficients and chi-square analysis were used for analysis demonstrating poor vitamin B_{12} and folate status associated with greater hearing loss.

Critique. The investigators used a very complex methodology to examine this question. Much was done to ensure close control over the variables. This study was conducted with a larger study examining bone health and auditory functioning and included only white women ages 60-71 years. These demographics limit generalization of the findings, but the notion of a vitamin deficiency leading to age-related hearing loss is unique.

Implications for Nursing. Nurses are educated to pay attention to the nutritional status of clients. This study suggests an additional reason for the importance of proper nutrition. Although serum vitamin and red blood cell folate levels are not measured often in general practice, the nurse can become an advocate for instituting supportive nutrition when necessary.

tion, the nurse asks whether any family members are hearing impaired.

When pain accompanies acute-onset hearing loss, the nurse asks about recent upper respiratory tract infection and possible allergies affecting the upper respiratory system.

■ PHYSICAL ASSESSMENT/CLINICAL MANIFESTATIONS

Chart 49-5 presents focused assessment techniques for clients with suspected hearing loss. Hearing loss may be sudden or gradual and is often bilateral. The ability to hear high-frequency soft, discriminating consonants—especially *s, sh, f, th,* and *ch* sounds—is lost first. Clients often state that they have no problem with hearing but cannot understand specific words. They might think that the speaker is mumbling. They often experience high-pitched, continuous bilateral tinnitus. Vertigo may be present, depending on the extent of inner-ear involvement.

TUNING FORK TESTS. Tuning fork tests help diagnose hearing loss (see Chapter 48). With the Weber test, the client can usually hear sounds well in the ear with a suspected conductive hearing loss because of the preserved bone conduction. With the Rinne test, the client reports that sound transmitted by bone conduction is louder and more sustained than that transmitted by air conduction.

OTOSCOPIC EXAMINATION. The nurse performs an otoscopic examination to assess the external auditory canal,

---

CHART 49-5

FOCUSED ASSESSMENT *of*
The Client with Suspected Hearing Loss

Assess whether the client has any of the following ear complaints:
- Pain
- Feeling of fullness or congestion
- Dizziness or vertigo
- Tinnitus
- Difficulty understanding conversations, especially in a noisy room
- Difficulty hearing sounds
- Needing to strain to hear
- Needing to turn the head to favor one ear or needing to lean forward to hear

Assess visible ear structures, particularly the external canal and tympanic membrane:
- Position and size of the pinna
- Patency of the external canal; presence of cerumen or foreign bodies, edema, or inflammation
- Condition of the tympanic membrane: intact, edema, fluid, inflammation

Assess functional ability, including:
- Frequency of asking people to repeat statements
- Withdrawal from social interactions or large groups
- Shouting in conversation
- Failing to respond when not looking in the direction of the sound
- Answering questions incorrectly

---

the tympanic membrane, and structures of the middle ear visible through the tympanic membrane (see Chapter 48). Physical findings from examination vary, depending on the cause of the hearing loss.

Obstruction of the external auditory canal can result in hearing loss. The nurse inspects the canal and notes the following:
- Whether the canal is open
- The amount and character of cerumen present
- The integrity of the skin lining the canal
- The presence of redness, exudates, lesions, or foreign objects

Middle-ear infections can also diminish hearing. In infection or inflammation, the tympanic membrane appears red, thickened, and bulging, with a loss of landmarks. Loss of mobility of the membrane is evident with inspection through a pneumatic otoscope. The nurse notes the presence of any scars or perforations on the tympanic membrane. With close observation, the nurse may be able to see exudate behind the membrane.

■ PSYCHOSOCIAL ASSESSMENT

For persons with a hearing loss, communication can become a struggle, and they may isolate themselves because of the difficulty in talking and listening. Social isolation can lead to depression, fear, and despair. The nurse is sensitive to emotional changes that may be related to reduced hearing and a decline in conversational skills.

■ LABORATORY ASSESSMENT

No laboratory tests can definitively diagnose hearing loss. However, some laboratory findings can indicate pathologic problems that might affect hearing.

White blood cell counts are elevated in the client with acute or chronic otitis media. Microbial culture and antibiotic sensitivity tests can determine the causative organism and the most appropriate antibiotic therapy when infection causes hearing loss.

The client with hearing loss associated with peripheral neuropathy may have other systemic diseases, including poorly controlled diabetes mellitus. The fasting blood glucose level may be elevated, and the blood, even when diluted, may be positive for serum acetone.

RADIOGRAPHIC ASSESSMENT

Radiographic assessment can determine nonauditory problems affecting hearing ability. Some auditory problems can be diagnosed using radiographic techniques: skull x-ray films to determine bony involvement in otitis media and the location of otosclerotic lesions, and computed tomography (CT) and magnetic resonance imaging (MRI) to determine soft-tissue involvement and the presence and location of tumors.

OTHER DIAGNOSTIC ASSESSMENT

Audiometry can assist in the diagnosis and determine the extent and type of hearing loss. An audiogram shows whether hearing loss is only conductive or whether it has a sensorineural component. This is important in determining possible causes of the hearing loss and in planning appropriate interventions.

CRITICAL THINKING CHALLENGE

You are assigned treatment of an 85-year-old woman who is admitted for congestive heart failure, hypertension, type 2 diabetes mellitus, and degenerative joint disease with a history of bilateral hip replacements. She reports that she has been losing some of her hearing for the past few years, but that since being admitted to the hospital her hearing has become much worse.

- What physical assessment findings are needed to gain additional information?
- Considering the woman's admitting diagnoses, what factors associated with treatment of these other disorders may play a role in her hearing loss?

For suggested answer guidelines, go to SIMON http://www.wbsaunders.com/SIMON/Iggy/.

● Analysis

COMMON NURSING DIAGNOSES AND COLLABORATIVE PROBLEMS

The following are common nursing diagnoses for clients with any degree of hearing impairment:

1. Disturbed Sensory Perception (Auditory) related to obstruction, infection, damage to the middle ear, or damage to the auditory nerve
2. Anxiety related to an inability to communicate

ADDITIONAL NURSING DIAGNOSES AND COLLABORATIVE PROBLEMS

In addition to the common nursing diagnoses, clients with hearing loss or impairment may have one or more of the following:

- Deficient Knowledge related to treatment and prevention
- Activity Intolerance related to pain

- Social Isolation related to pain and decreased hearing
- Risk for Injury related to altered auditory perception and infection
- Acute Pain related to an inflammatory process and fluid in the middle ear
- Impaired Physical Mobility related to vertigo

● Planning and Implementation

DISTURBED SENSORY PERCEPTION (AUDITORY)

PLANNING: EXPECTED OUTCOMES. The client with hearing loss or impairment is expected to either experience an increase in auditory sensory perception to a functional level or maintain existing levels of hearing.

INTERVENTIONS. Interventions aim at identifying the problem, halting the pathologic processes, and improving auditory sensory perception.

NIC EAR CARE. For most people, hearing is accepted as an important factor in social interactions and to gain knowledge. With special care to the ears, hearing can be preserved at maximal levels (Chart 49-6).

NONSURGICAL MANAGEMENT. Nonsurgical interventions include early detection of hearing impairment, use of drug therapy and comfort measures, and use of assistive devices to amplify or augment the client's auditory perception.

CHART 49-6

NIC INTERVENTION ACTIVITIES for Care of the Ears

Ear Care: *Prevention or minimization of threats to ear or hearing*

- Monitor for drainage from ears, as appropriate.
- Irrigate the ear, as appropriate.
- Avoid placing sharp objects in the ear.
- Administer eardrops, as appropriate.
- Explain the relationship between balance and the inner ear, as appropriate.
- Monitor for episodes of dizziness associated with ear problems, as appropriate.
- Determine if cerumen in the ear canal is causing pain or hearing loss.
- Instill mineral oil in the ear to soften impacted cerumen before irrigation.
- Irrigate the ear canal with a Water Pik (or similar device) on low setting using warm water (80° to 90° F), as appropriate.
- Demonstrate proper technique for ear irrigation to caregiver, as appropriate.
- Monitor frequency of ear infections.
- Instruct how to monitor and regulate high-volume noise exposure.
- Instruct client to wear hearing protection for exposure to high-intensity noise.
- Instruct client concerning the potential danger of exposure to high-volume music, especially with headphones.
- Instruct client with pierced ears how to avoid infection at the insertion site.
- Encourage use of earplugs for swimming, if client is susceptible to ear infections.

NIC intervention activities selected from McCloskey, J.C., & Bulechek, G.M. (Eds.). (2000). *Nursing interventions classification (NIC)* (3rd ed.). St. Louis: Mosby. No part of this work is to be altered without prior written permission from the Publisher.

EARLY DETECTION. Early detection helps correct the problem causing the hearing loss. When hearing loss is gradual, the client can compensate. The nurse assesses for indications of hearing loss, as listed in Chart 49-6.

DRUG THERAPY. Drug therapy is aimed at either correcting the underlying pathologic change or reducing the side effects of disorders associated with hearing loss. Local (topical) antibiotics are administered to clients with external otitis. Systemic antibiotics are necessary when clients have other auditory infections. By treating the infection, antibiotics resolve local edema and improve hearing. When pain accompanies hearing disorders, local or systemic analgesics are often used, depending on the type and location of the pain. Many ear disorders disturb equilibrium, causing vertigo and dizziness with nausea and vomiting. Antiemetic, antihistamine, antivertiginous, and benzodiazepine drugs can help correct nausea, vertigo, and dizziness.

ASSISTIVE DEVICES. Many devices are useful for clients with permanent, progressive hearing loss. Telephone amplifiers increase telephone volume, allowing the caller to speak in a normal voice. Flashing lights activated by the ringing telephone or doorbell alert clients visually. In some cases, clients may be referred for the use of a specially trained dog to help them be aware of sounds (ringing telephones or doorbells, cries of other people, and potential dangers), in much the same way that a seeing eye dog assists a blind person.

Small, portable audio amplifiers can assist the nurse in communicating with clients experiencing hearing loss but who have chosen not to use a hearing aid. The use of audio amplifiers or allowing clients to use a stethoscope helps nurses to communicate with elders and others who require additional volume to hear speech.

Hearing Aids. A hearing aid is a miniature electronic amplifier that is usually used for clients with conductive hearing loss. Hearing aids are less effective for sensorineural hearing loss and may make functional hearing worse by amplifying background noise. The amplifier can be worn in one or both ears. Local agencies offer special rehabilitation classes for the hearing impaired that will help the wearer obtain the most benefit from this device.

The nurse offers some special tips to help the client adjust to the hearing aid. Hearing with a hearing aid can be different from natural hearing. The client is encouraged to start using the hearing aid slowly, initially wearing it only at home and only during part of the day. Listening to television and the radio and reading aloud can help the client get used to new sounds. The tone or volume of the hearing aid can be adjusted. The most important and difficult aspect of a hearing aid is the amplification of background noise, as well as voices. The client must learn to concentrate and filter out background noises.

The client must also learn to care for the hearing aid (Chart 49-7). Hearing aids are delicate electronic devices that should be handled only by people who know how to care for them properly. The cost of the aids varies greatly but represents a significant investment.

Cochlear Implants. Cochlear implantation may help clients with sensorineural hearing loss. A small computer converts sound waves into electronic impulses. Electrodes are placed by the internal ear, with the computer attached to the external ear. The electronic impulses then directly stimulate

nerve fibers. Some clients have a 50% return of their hearing with this method.

SURGICAL MANAGEMENT. Many surgical interventions are available for clients with specific disorders leading to hearing loss.

TYMPANOPLASTY. Tympanoplasty reconstructs the middle ear to improve hearing caused by conductive hearing loss. The procedures vary from simple reconstruction of the tympanic membrane (**myringoplasty**) to replacement of the ossicles within the middle ear. A type I tympanoplasty is used for a myringoplasty; a type II tympanoplasty is used in cases of greater damage and to provide more extensive reconstruction (Figure 49-8).

Preoperative Care. The nurse gives specific instructions to the client scheduled for a tympanoplasty. Systemic antibiotics reduce the numbers of infecting organisms. Before surgery, the nurse irrigates the ear with a solution of equal parts of vinegar and sterile water to restore normal ear pH. The client follows other measures to decrease the chances of postoperative infection, such as avoiding people with upper respiratory tract infections, getting adequate rest, eating a balanced diet, and maintaining an adequate fluid intake.

The nurse assures the client that initial hearing loss after surgery is normal because of the packing in the canal, and that hearing will improve on packing removal. The nurse explains the importance of deep breathing and coughing postoperatively but emphasizes that forceful coughing increases pressure in the middle ear and must be avoided.

Operative Procedure. Surgical treatment is performed only if the middle ear is free of infection and if the condition of the eustachian tube does not promote continued infection. If an infection is present, the graft is more likely to become infected and not heal properly. Surgery of the tympanic membrane and

---

CHART 49-7

CLIENT EDUCATION GUIDE
Hearing Aid Care

- Keep the hearing aid dry.
- Clean the ear mold with mild soap and water while avoiding excessive wetting.
- Clean debris from the hole in the middle of the part that goes into your ear with a toothpick or a pipe cleaner.
- Turn off the hearing aid and remove the battery when not in use.
- Check and replace the battery frequently.
- Keep extra batteries on hand.
- Keep the hearing aid in a safe place.
- Avoid dropping the hearing aid or exposing it to temperature extremes.
- Adjust the volume to the lowest setting that allows you to hear, to prevent feedback squeaking.
- Avoid using hair spray, cosmetics, oils, or other hair and face products that might come into contact with the receiver.
- If the hearing aid does not work:
  Change the battery.
  Check the connection between the ear mold and the receiver.
  Check the on/off switch.
  Clean the sound hole.
  Adjust the volume.
  Take the hearing aid to an authorized service center for repair.

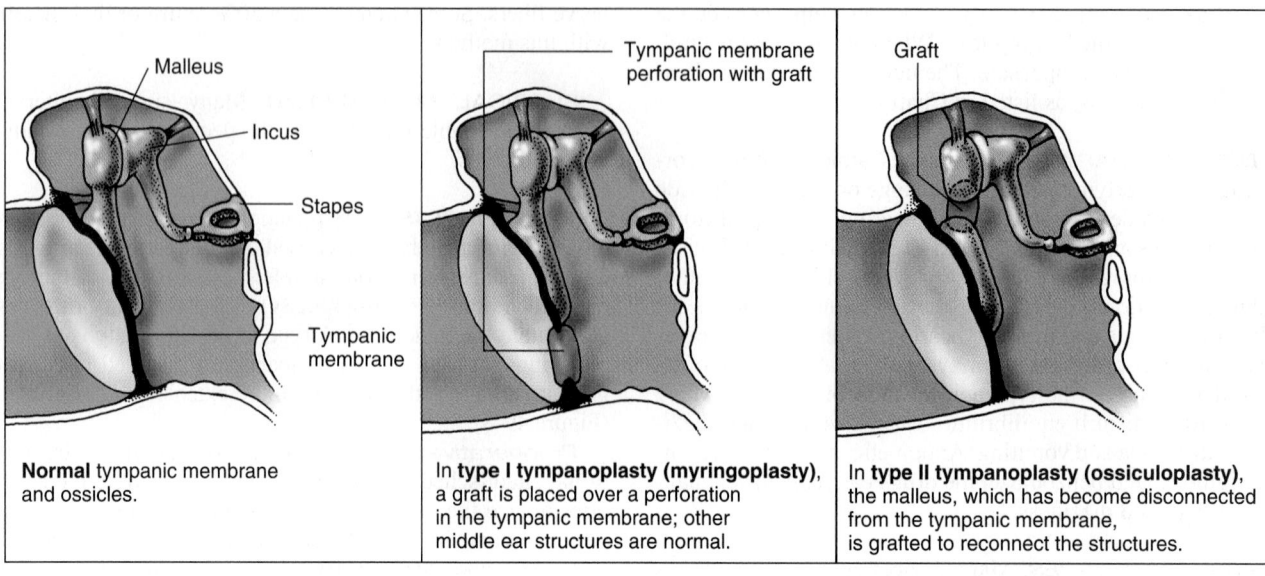

Figure 49-8 ● A normal tympanic membrane and two types of tympanoplasties.

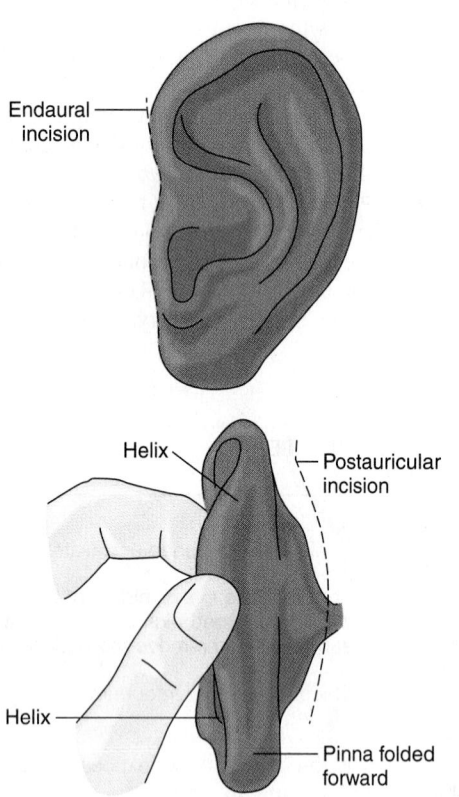

Figure 49-9 ● Surgical approaches for the ear. The endaural approach is used when the external canal is too small to use for a transcanal approach (not shown because no external incision is used). The postauricular approach is used for more extensive repair of the middle-ear and inner-ear structures.

ossicles requires the use of a microscope and is a delicate procedure. Local anesthesia can be used, although general anesthesia is often chosen to prevent the client from moving.

The surgeon can repair the tympanic membrane with a variety of materials, including temporal muscle fascia, a split-thickness skin graft, and venous tissue. If the ossicles are damaged, more extensive measures must be taken to repair or replace them. The surgeon reaches the ossicles via a transcanal approach, an endaural incision, or the postauricular route with a mastoidectomy (Figure 49-9).

The surgeon then removes diseased tissue and cleans the middle-ear cavity. The ossicles are assessed for damage and the extent to which repair or replacement is necessary. The surgeon uses autogenous cartilage or bone, cadaver ossicles, stainless steel wire, or polytetrafluoroethylene (Teflon) to repair or replace the ossicles.

Postoperative Care. An antiseptic-soaked gauze, such as iodoform gauze (Nu Gauze), is packed in the auditory canal. If the postauricular or endaural incision is used, an external dressing is placed over the operative site. Dressings are kept clean and dry, and the nurse uses sterile technique when changing them. The client is kept flat, with the head turned to the side and the operative ear facing up for at least 12 hours postoperatively. Antibiotic therapy is used to prevent infections from recurring.

Clients generally report hearing improvement after the canal packing is removed. Until that time, the nurse communicates as with a hearing-impaired client, directing conversation to the unaffected ear. The nurse also instructs the client in postoperative care and activity restrictions (see Chart 49-4).

STAPEDECTOMY. A partial or complete stapedectomy with a prosthesis effectively corrects hearing loss. This procedure is most effective for clients with hearing loss related to otosclerosis.

Preoperative Care. To prevent the introduction of infective material to the middle-ear structures, no signs or symptoms of external otitis can be present at surgery. The nurse instructs the client to follow measures that prevent middle-ear or external-ear infections (Chart 49-8).

The nurse reviews the expected outcomes and possible complications of the surgery. Hearing is initially worse after a stapedectomy. The success rate of this procedure is high; however, as with all ear procedures, it carries a risk of failure

CHART 49-8

CLIENT EDUCATION GUIDE
Prevention of Ear Infection or Trauma

- Do not use small objects, such as cotton-tipped applicators, matches, toothpicks, or hairpins, to clean your external ear canal.
- Wash your external ear and canal daily in the shower or while washing your hair.
- Blow your nose gently.
- Do not occlude one nostril while blowing your nose.
- Sneeze with your mouth open.
- Wear sound protection around loud or continuous noises.
- Avoid activities with high risk for head or ear trauma, such as wrestling, boxing, motorcycle riding, and skateboarding.
- Wear head and ear protection when engaging in these activities.
- Keep the volume on head receivers at the lowest setting that allows you to hear.
- Frequently clean objects that come into contact with your ear (headphones, telephone receivers, and so on).
- Avoid environmental conditions with rapid changes in air pressure.

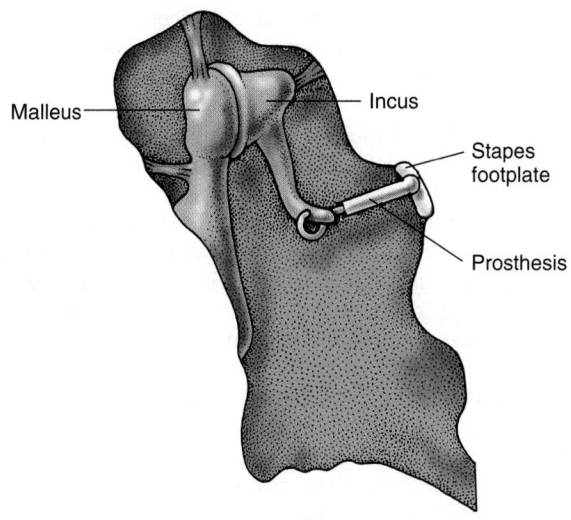

Figure 49-10 ● Prosthesis used with stapedectomy. The stapes is removed, leaving the footplate. After a hole is drilled in the footplate, a metal or plastic prosthesis is connected to the incus and inserted through the hole to act as a vibration device, much as the stapes worked before the development of otosclerosis.

that might lead to total deafness on the affected side. Other possible complications include prolonged vertigo, infection, and facial nerve damage. A decision to proceed with surgery should be made with the client's full knowledge and understanding of these complications.

Operative Procedure. A stapedectomy is usually performed through the external auditory canal with the client under local anesthesia. The head and neck of the stapes and, less often, the footplate are removed. After removal of the immobile bone, a small hole is drilled in the footplate; a metal or plastic prosthesis in the shape of a piston is connected between the incus and the footplate (Figure 49-10). Sounds cause the prosthesis to vibrate as the stapes did. After stapedectomy, up to 90% of clients experience restoration of practical hearing.

Postoperative Care. The nurse informs the client that noticeable improvement in hearing may not occur until 6 weeks after surgery. Initially, the ear packing interferes with hearing. Postoperative swelling in the ear continues to affect hearing until the edema has resolved. Medications for pain help reduce discomfort, and antibiotics are given to reduce the risk for infection at the surgical site. The nurse instructs the client to follow the postoperative procedures in Chart 49-4.

The surgical procedure is performed in an area where cranial nerves VII, VIII, and X might be damaged by direct trauma or by postoperative swelling. The nurse observes for complications of surgery by assessing for facial nerve damage or muscle weakness and changes in tactile sensation or taste. Vertigo, nausea, and vomiting are common complaints because of the proximity to inner-ear structures.

Antivertiginous drugs, such as meclizine hydrochloride (Antivert, Bonamine✦), and antiemetic medications, such as droperidol (Inapsine), are given. Care is taken to prevent injury, especially during times of increased vertigo. The nurse assists the client with ambulating during the first 1 to 2 days after surgery. Siderails on the bed are kept up, and the nurse reminds the client to move the head slowly when changing position, to avoid vertigo.

CHART 49-9

BEST PRACTICE *for*
Communicating with a Hearing-Impaired Client

- Position yourself directly in front of the client.
- Make sure that the room is well lighted.
- Get the client's attention before you begin to speak.
- Move closer to the better-hearing ear.
- Speak clearly and slowly.
- Do not shout (shouting raises the frequency of the sound and often makes understanding more difficult).
- Keep hands and other objects away from your mouth when talking to the client.
- Attempt to have conversations in a quiet room with minimal distractions.
- Have the client repeat your statements rather than just indicating assent.
- Rephrase sentences and repeat information to aid in understanding.
- Use appropriate hand motions.
- Write messages on paper if the client is able to read.

■ ANXIETY

PLANNING: EXPECTED OUTCOMES. The client with hearing loss or impairment is expected to state that anxiety about communication is reduced and become proficient in alternative communication techniques.

INTERVENTIONS. Interventions focus on facilitating communication and reducing anxiety.

Best practices for communicating with a hearing-impaired client are listed in Chart 49-9. Shouting to the client is of little benefit, because the sound may be projected at a higher frequency, making him or her less able to understand. The most obvious means of communicating with such a client is by the written word (if he or she is able to see, read, and write) or with pictures of familiar phrases and objects. Many television programs are now closed captioned (subtitled) for the hearing impaired.

ASSISTIVE DEVICES. Assistive devices, described on p. 1073, can greatly increase communication for the client with a hearing impairment.

LIP-READING. Lip-reading and sign language can also enhance communication. In a formal lip-reading class, clients are taught the special cues to look for when lip-reading and how to understand body language. However, the best lip-reader still misses more than 50% of what is being said. Because hearing is assisted by even minimal lip-reading, clients are encouraged to wear their eyeglasses when talking with someone to see subtle movements of the lips.

SIGN LANGUAGE. For clients with more severe hearing loss, special languages have been developed, including American Sign Language (ASL). Such languages combine speech with hand movements that signify letters, words, and phrases. These languages take time and effort to learn, and many people are unable to learn them, just as many people cannot learn foreign languages. However, as the hearing-impaired person become less able to function, motivation to learn may increase.

MANAGING ANXIETY. A major source of anxiety is the possibility of permanent hearing loss. The nurse provides honest and accurate information about the likelihood of hearing returning. When the hearing impairment is likely to be permanent or become more profound, the nurse reassures clients that communication and social interaction can be maintained.

To reduce anxiety and prevent social isolation, clients use remaining resources to make social contact satisfying. The most obvious way to decrease social isolation is by improving communication (as previously described). The nurse asks about past or present diversional activities to identify the client's most satisfying activities and social interactions and determine the amount of effort necessary to continue them. Activities can be altered to maximize client satisfaction. Someone accustomed to large gatherings might choose smaller groups instead. A quiet evening meal at home with friends might substitute for dinner in a noisy restaurant.

● Community-Based Care

Lengthy hospitalization is rare for most clients with ear and hearing disorders. If surgical repair is necessary and the procedure is completed without complications, the procedure may be completed as an outpatient or the hospital stay is usually only a day.

▓ HEALTH TEACHING

The nurse gives clients written instructions about how to take medications and when to return for follow-up care. If the client cannot read, the nurse gives these instructions to a family member who may assist with care. The nurse teaches clients how to instill eardrops (see Chart 49-1) and irrigate the ears (see Chart 49-2), and asks for a return demonstration.

To promote health and prevent late postoperative infections, clients are instructed to follow the suggestions in Chart 49-8. For clients who use a hearing aid, the nurse teaches them how to use it effectively.

COST OF CARE
IMPLICATIONS FOR NURSING

HEARING LOSS

Cost of Care
- The cost of assistive devices for hearing-impaired individuals can be staggering.
- Hearing aids are available in a variety of styles and vary greatly, depending on the style and circuitry options available. Prices for hearing aids range from $700 to $2400 for one device, with the cost doubling if two devices are needed.
- Batteries for hearing aids must be changed as often as every few days to once a week, depending on the volume settings. Batteries cost about $1 to $2 per battery, depending on how many are purchased at the same time.
- Telephone devices for the deaf (TDD) also vary in cost and options. These devices cost from $300 to $600 per unit. Portable amplifiers cost approximately $25.
- In addition to the cost of hearing aids and telephone devices, there are a variety of devices that are needed to either improve the quality of life for hearing-impaired individuals or aid in their safety needs. Examples include alert systems, doorbells, baby alarms, fire alarms, and alarm clocks. A special alarm clock called the Sonic Boom cost $90. Complete security systems for hearing-impaired individuals range from $377 to $775.

Implications for Nursing
People with severe hearing loss require devices that people with normal hearing would never need. Hearing aids are generally used by the individual at all times when he or she is awake. However, they are removed at night for sleeping, and given their small size, these devices can be easily misplaced or broken if care is not taken to secure them in the institutional setting. Nurses need to familiarize themselves with how to replace batteries and how to turn hearing aids on and off to preserve battery life.

Data from Department of Speech and Communication Disorders, Audiology Section, University of Northern Colorado, Greeley, CO.

▓ HOME CARE MANAGEMENT

Clients who experience persistent vertigo, either in association with the disorder or as a side effect of surgery, remain in danger of falling. The home must therefore be assessed for potential hazards and to determine whether family members or significant others are available to assist with meal preparation and other activities of daily living. A nurse case manager can, in collaboration with the home care nurse, assist clients and their families in determining the best ways to maintain adequate self-care abilities, maintain a safe environment, decide about assistance needs, and provide needed care.

▓ HEALTH CARE RESOURCES

If clients do not have family or friends to help during the postoperative period, a referral to a home care agency is necessary. Assistance with meal preparation, cleaning, and personal hygiene can be contracted for with the hospital discharge planners.

Follow-up hearing tests are scheduled for clients when the lesions are well healed, in about 6 to 8 weeks. Audiograms done before and after treatment are compared, and evaluation for further intervention to improve hearing begins. A complication of an unsuccessful surgery is continued disability or complete loss of hearing in the affected ear. Surgery is performed on the ear with the greatest hearing loss. If the surgery does not improve hearing, clients

TABLE 49-3 • AGENCIES OFFERING SERVICES FOR EAR AND HEARING DISORDERS

HOUSE EAR INSTITUTE
2100 West Third Street, Fifth Floor
Los Angeles, CA 90057
Voice: (800) 352-8888
TTY: (213) 484-2642
Internet: http://www.hei.org

NATIONAL INFORMATION CENTER ON DEAFNESS
Gallaudet University
800 Florida Avenue NE
Washington, DC 20002
Voice: (202) 651-5051
TTY: (202) 651-5000
E-mail: nidc@gallux.gallaudet.edu
Internet: http://www.gallaudet.edu

AMERICAN ACADEMY OF OTOLARYNGOLOGY/HEAD AND NECK SURGERY
One Prince Street
Alexandria, VA 22314
Voice: (703) 519-1589
TTY: (703) 836-4444
Internet: http://www.entnet.org

AMERICAN SPEECH-LANGUAGE-HEARING ASSOCIATION
10801 Rockville Pike
Rockville, MD 20852
Voice/TTY: (301) 897-5700
Voice: (800) 638-8255
Internet: http://www.asha.org

SELF HELP FOR HARD OF HEARING PEOPLE, INC. (SHHH)
7910 Woodmont Avenue, Suite 1200
Bethesda, MD 20814
Voice: (301) 657-2248
TTY: (301) 657-2249
Fax: (301) 913-9413
Internet: http://www.shhh.org

must decide to either attempt surgical correction of the other ear or continue to use an amplification device. When the underlying disorder causing the hearing impairment is progressive, this decision is difficult. The nurse supports clients by listening to their concerns and giving additional information when needed.

Costs to the individual with a hearing impairment can be extensive (see the Cost of Care box on p. 1076). Information and support can come from several organizations that publish informative articles to help clients reduce hearing loss (Table 49-3). Many public and private institutions offer hearing evaluations, as well as supplying information and counseling for clients with hearing disorders.

Evaluation: Outcomes

NOC The nurse evaluates the care of the client with hearing loss or impairment on the basis of the identified nursing diagnoses and collaborative problems. The expected outcomes include that the client will:

- State that the hearing is at least partially improved
- State that anxiety is reduced
- Demonstrate proper technique for using assistive devices
- Identify potential postoperative hazards
- State the importance of follow-up hearing assessments
- Be able to communicate effectively with family, friends, co-workers, and health care professionals

- Have receptive ability for communication
- Acknowledge messages received
- Maintain satisfactory social contacts
- State that the pain is reduced or alleviated
- Describe the proper use of antibiotic therapy
- Demonstrate proper techniques when using eardrops, ointments, powders, or irrigation liquids
- Identify and avoid potential causes of otitis media
- Seek assistance with activities of daily living until vertigo and dizziness have subsided

ONLINE RESOURCES

For suggested readings and Internet resources, go to http://www.wbsaunders.com/SIMON/Iggy/.

SELECTED BIBLIOGRAPHY

Asterisk indicates a classic or definitive work on this subject.

Bagley, M. (1998). Helping older adults to live better with hearing and vision losses. *Journal of Case Management, 7*(4), 147-152.

Baloh, R. (1998a). *Dizziness, hearing loss, and tinnitus.* Philadelphia: F.A. Davis.

Baloh, R. (1998b). Dizzy patients: The varieties of vertigo. *Hospital Practice, 33*(6), 55-63.

Barry, B., et al. (1999). Otogenic intracranial infections in adults. *Laryngoscope, 109*(3), 483-487.

Bellenir, K., & Shin, L. (1998). *Ear, nose, and throat disorders sourcebook.* Detroit: Omnigraphics.

Berger, M. (Ed.). (1998). *Ear, nose and throat disorders.* Philadelphia: W.B. Saunders.

Billue, J. (1998). Subjective idiopathic tinnitus. *Clinical Excellence for Nurse Practitioners, 2*(2), 73-82.

Bumby, A., & Stephens, S. (1997). Clonazepam in the treatment of tinnitus—A pilot study. *Journal of Audiological Medicine, 6*(2), 98-104.

Cavendish, R. (1998). Clinical snapshot: Adult hearing loss. *American Journal of Nursing, 98*(8), 50-51.

Chaimoff, M., et al. (1999). Sudden hearing loss as a presenting symptom of acoustic neuroma. *American Journal of Otolaryngology, 20*(3), 157-160.

*Clinical guidelines: Adult screening for hearing. (1996). *Nurse Practitioner, 21*(6), 106, 108, 115.

Cook, R. (1998). Ear syringing. *Nursing Standard, 13*(13-15), 56-61.

de la Cruz, M., & Bance, M. (1999). Carbamazepine-induced sensorineural hearing loss. *Archives of Otolaryngology–Head and Neck Surgery, 125*(2), 225-227.

Dhillon, R., & East, C. (1999). *Ear, nose, and throat, and head and neck surgery: An illustrated colour text.* New York: Churchill Livingstone.

Doyle, W., et al. (1999). Illness and otological changes during upper respiratory virus infection. *Laryngoscopy, 109*(2), 324-328.

Erber, N., Holland, J., & Osborn, R. (1998). Communicating with elders: Effects of speaker-listener distance. *British Society of Audiology, 32*(3), 135-138.

Flatau, E., et al. (1998). Hearing impairment in residents of a long-term care facility: Prevalence and relationship to cognitive dysfunction. *Annals of Long Term Care, 6*(13), 410-413.

Garstecki, D., & Erler, S. (1998). Hearing and aging. *Topics in Geriatric Rehabilitation, 14*(2), 1-17.

Gates, G., Couropmitree, N, & Myers, R. (1999). Genetic association in age-related hearing thresholds. *Archives in Otolaryngology–Head and Neck Surgery, 125*(6), 654-659.

Gelfand, S. (1998). *Hearing: An introduction to psychological and physiological acoustics* (3rd ed.). New York : Marcel Dekker.

Hagnebo, C., et al. (1997). The influence of vertigo, hearing impairment and tinnitus on the daily life of Meniere's patients. *Scandinavian Audiology, 26*(2), 69-76.

Heath, H. (1997). Sensory function in older people. *Community Nurse, 3*(11), 13-14.

Herdman, S. (1997). Advances in the treatment of vestibular disorders. *Physical Therapy, 77*(6), 602-618.

Hope, B. (1999). Create sensitivity to the elderly's sensory changes. *Homecare Education Management, 2,* 26-27.

Houston, D., et al. (1999). Age-related hearing loss, vitamin B-12, and folate in elderly women. *American Journal of Clinical Nutrition, 69*(3), 564-571.

Hsu, R., & Levine, S. (1998). Sudden hearing loss: How to identify the cause promptly. *Consultant, 38*(1), 23-26.

Kaufman, G. (1998). Ear problems: Care and prevention. *Practice Nurse, 15*(6), 338-342.

Kendrick, J. (1997). New strategies for hearing protection. *Occupational Health and Safety, 66*(10), 134-138.

Kujdychy, N. (1999). Prescribing trends in the treatment of acute otitis media. *ADVANCE for Nurse Practitioners, 7*(8), 30-35.

LaRosa, S. (1998). Primary care management of otitis externa. *Nurse Practitioner, 23*(6), 125-128.

Larsen, P., Hazen, S., & Martin, J. (1997). Assessment and management of sensory loss in elderly patients. *AORN Journal, 65*(2), 432-437.

Leblanc, A. (1999). *Atlas of hearing and balance organs : a practical guide for otolaryngologists.* New York: Springer.

Lorentine, M., et al. (1998). On the behavioral characteristics of loud-music listening. *Ear and Hearing, 19*(6), 420-428.

Lucas, L., & Matthews-Flint, L. (2001). Sound advice about hearing aids. *Nursing2001, 31*(2), 59-61.

Lucente, F., & Har-El, G. (1999). *Essentials of otolaryngology* (4th ed.). Philadelphia: Lippincott, Williams, & Wilkins.

Ludman, H., & Wright, T. (1998). *Diseases of the ear* (3rd ed.). New York: Oxford University Press.

Lusk, S. (1997). Noise exposures. *AAOHN Journal, 45*(8), 397-409.

Luxon, L. (1998). Disorders of hearing and balance. *Reviews in Clinical Gerontology, 8*(1), 31-43.

Martin, R. (1998). Nuts and bolts: What to do when the patient "can't understand the words." *Hearing Journal, 51*(6), 70-72.

Mostafapour, S., Lahargoue, K., & Gates, G. (1998). Noise-induced hearing loss in young adults: The role of personal listening devices and other sources of leisure noise. *Laryngoscope, 108*(12), 1832-1839.

National Council on the Aging. (2000). The consequences of untreated hearing loss in older persons. *ORL–Head and Neck Nursing, 18*(1), 12-16.

National Institute on Deafness and Other Communication Disorders. (1999). What is presbycusis? NIH Pub. No. 97-4233; http://www.nidcd.nih.gov/.

Noorhassin, I., & Rampal, K. (1998). Multiplicative effect of smoking and age on hearing impairment. *American Journal of Otolaryngology, 19*(4), 240-243.

Nusbaum, N. (1999). Aging and sensory senescence. *Southern Medical Journal, 92*(3), 267-275. Also available at http://www.medscape.com/SMA/SMJ/1999/v92.n03/smj9203.02.nusb/smj9203.02.nusb-01.html.

Ramsay, H., Karkainen, J., & Palva, T. (1997). Success in surgery for otosclerosis: Hearing improvement and other indicators. *American Journal of Otolaryngology, 18*(1), 23-28.

*Ross, V., Echevarria, K., & Robinson, B. (1991). Geriatric tinnitus: Causes, clinical treatment, and prevention. *Journal of Gerontological Nursing, 17*(10), 6-11.

Sanna, M. (1999). *Color atlas of otoscopy: From diagnosis to surgery.* New York: Thieme.

Shaw, L. (1997). Protocol for detection and follow-up of hearing loss. *Clinical Nurse Specialist, 11*(6), 240-247.

Sheehan, J. (2000). Caring for the deaf: Do you do enough? *RN, 63*(3), 69-72.

Silverstein, H., et al. (1999). Direct round window membrane application of gentamicin in the treatment of Meniere's disease. *Archives of Otolaryngology–Head and Neck Surgery, 120*(5), 649-655.

Simpson, J., Donaldson, I., & Davies, W. (1998). Use of homeopathy in the treatment of tinnitus. *British Journal of Audiology, 32*(4), 227-233.

Singhal, S., et al. (1999). Genetic correlation in otosclerosis. *American Journal of Otolaryngology, 20*(2), 102-105.

Stone, C. (1999). Preventing cerumen impaction in nursing facility residents. *Journal of Gerontological Nursing, 25*(5), 43-45.

Thobaben, M. (1998). Helping clients with presbycusis. *Home Care Provider, 3*(4), 186-188.

Tolson, D. (1997). Age-related hearing loss: A case for nursing intervention. *Journal of Advanced Nursing, 26*(6), 1150-1157.

Tolson, D., & Stephens, D. (1997). Age-related hearing loss in the dependent elderly population: A model for nursing care. *International Journal of Nursing Practice, 3*(4), 224-230.

Vilholm, O., Moller, K., & Jorgensen, K. (1998). Effect of traditional Chinese acupuncture on severe tinnitus: A double-blind placebo-controlled, clinical investigation with open therapeutic control. *British Journal of Audiology, 32*(3), 197-204.

Waddinton, C., McKennis, A., & Goodlett, A. (1997). Treatment of conductive hearing loss with ossicular chain construction procedures. *AORN Journal, 65*(3), 511-518.

Walker, J., & Barnes, B. (1998). Dizziness. *Emergency Medicine Clinics of North America, 16*(4), 845-875.

Wazen, J., et al. (1998). Long-term hearing results following vestibular surgery in Meniere's disease. *Laryngoscope, 108*(10), 1470-1473.

Weimert, T. (1997). The acute ear. *Emergency Medicine, 29*(12), 34-45.

*Winslow, E.H. (1994). Hearing loss? Check for impacted cerumen. *American Journal of Nursing, 94*(10), 55.

PROBLEMS OF MOBILITY

*Management of Clients
with Problems of the
Musculoskeletal System*

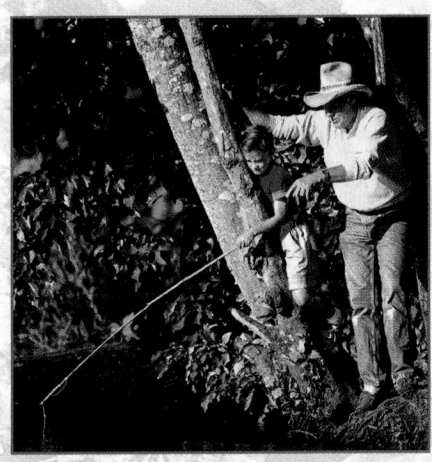

UNIT 11 — PROBLEMS OF MOBILITY: MUSCULOSKELETAL SYSTEM ■ Core Concepts Grid

Anatomy	Physiology	Pathophysiology	History	Physical Exam	Diagnostic Tests	Interventions	Pharmacology
• **Skeletal system** Bones Cartilage Tendons Ligaments Joints • **Muscular system**	• **Calcium storage** • **Hematopoesis** • **Protection** • **Form/framework** • **Motion** • **Joint articulation**	• **Fracture** • **Sprain** • **Contusion** • **Trauma** • **Osteoporosis** • **Infection**	• **Client medical history** Injury Illness Musculo- skeletal Systemic • **Family history** Congenital problems • **Social history** Occupation Sports Nutrition Age Race Gender • **Risk factors** Diet Exercise	• **Joint appearance** • **Gait** • **Range of motion** • **Flexion** • **Extension** • **Hyperextension** • **Abduction** • **Adduction** • **Pronation** • **Supination** • **Circumduction** • **Rotation** • **Inversion** • **Eversion** • **Alignment** • **Bruising/skin trauma** • **Kyphosis**	• **Radiologic studies** • **Arthroscopy** • **Magnetic resonance imaging (MRI)** • **Bone scan** • **Serum calcium** • **Serum phosphorus**	• **Cast care** • **Traction** • **Neurovascular checks** • **Braces/splints** • **Pin tract care** • **Skin assessment** • **Positioning** • **Logroll turning** • **Range-of-motion exercises** • **Body alignment** • **Lifestyle modifications** Diet Exercise • **Rest** • **Physical rehabilitation** • **Preventing immobility complications**	• **Analgesics** • **Muscle relaxants** • **Nonsteroidal anti-inflammatory drugs (NSAIDs)** • **Antibiotics** • **Calcium** • **Vitamin D** • **Selective estrogen receptor modulators** • **Anticoagulants**

Assessment of the Musculoskeletal System

DONNA D. IGNATAVICIUS

Learning Objectives

After studying this chapter, you should be able to:

1. Recall the anatomy and physiology of the musculoskeletal system.
2. Perform a musculoskeletal assessment using Gordon's Functional Health Patterns.
3. Evaluate important assessment findings in a client with a musculoskeletal health problem.
4. Explain the use of laboratory testing for a client with a musculoskeletal health problem.
5. Identify the use of radiography in diagnosing musculoskeletal health problems.
6. Plan follow-up care for clients undergoing musculoskeletal diagnostic testing.

Go to http://www.wbsaunders.com/SIMON/Iggy/ for self-assessment questions related to these Learning Objectives.

The musculoskeletal system is the second largest body system; it includes the bones, joints, and skeletal muscles, as well as their supporting structures. Disease, surgery, and trauma often affect one or more parts of this system, yet its assessment is often overlooked by nurses. This chapter does not include diagnostic testing related to arthritis or specific tests for osteoporosis. Descriptions of those tests are found in Chapters 21 and 51 under discussions of those diseases.

ANATOMY AND PHYSIOLOGY REVIEW
Skeletal System

The skeletal system consists of 206 bones and multiple joints. The growth and development of these structures occur during childhood and adolescence and are not discussed in this text.

▌ BONES
▌ Types

Bones may be classified by their shape. *Long bones,* such as the femur, are cylindric with rounded ends; they often bear weight. *Short bones,* such as the phalanges, are small and bear little or no weight. *Flat bones,* such as the scapula, protect vital organs and often contain blood-forming cells. Bones that have unique shapes are known as *irregular bones* (e.g., the carpal bones in the wrist). The *sesamoid bone* is the least common type and develops within a tendon; the patella is a typical example.

▌ Structure

As shown in Figure 50-1, the outer layer of bone, or cortex, is composed of dense, compact bone tissue. The inner layer, in the medulla, contains spongy, cancellous tissue. Almost every bone has both tissue types but in varying quantities. The long bone typically has a shaft, or diaphysis, and two knoblike ends, or epiphyses.

The structural unit of the cortical, compact bone is the haversian system, as detailed in Figure 50-1. The haversian system is a complex canal network containing microscopic blood vessels, which supply nutrients and oxygen to bone, and lacunae, which are small cavities that house osteocytes (bone cells). The canals run longitudinally within the hard, cortical bone tissue.

The softer, cancellous tissue contains large spaces, or trabeculae, which are filled with red and yellow marrow. Hematopoiesis (production of blood cells) occurs in the red marrow. The yellow marrow contains fat cells, which can be dislodged and enter the bloodstream to cause fat embolism syndrome (FES), a life-threatening complication. Volkmann's canals connect bone marrow vessels with the haversian system and periosteum, the outermost covering of the bone. Osteogenic cells, which later differentiate into **osteoblasts** (bone-forming cells) and **osteoclasts** (bone-destroying cells), are found in the deepest layer of the periosteum.

Bone also contains a matrix (also called *osteoid*) consisting chiefly of collagen, mucopolysaccharides, and lipids. Deposits of inorganic calcium salts (carbonate and phosphate) in the matrix provide the hardness of bone.

Bone is a very vascular tissue; its estimated total blood flow is between 200 and 400 mL/min. Each bone has a principal nutrient artery, which enters near the middle of the shaft and branches into ascending and descending vessels. These vessels supply the cortex, the marrow, and the haversian system. Sympathetic and afferent (sensory) fibers constitute the sparse nerve supply to bone. Dilation of blood vessels is controlled by the sympathetic nerves. The afferent fibers transmit

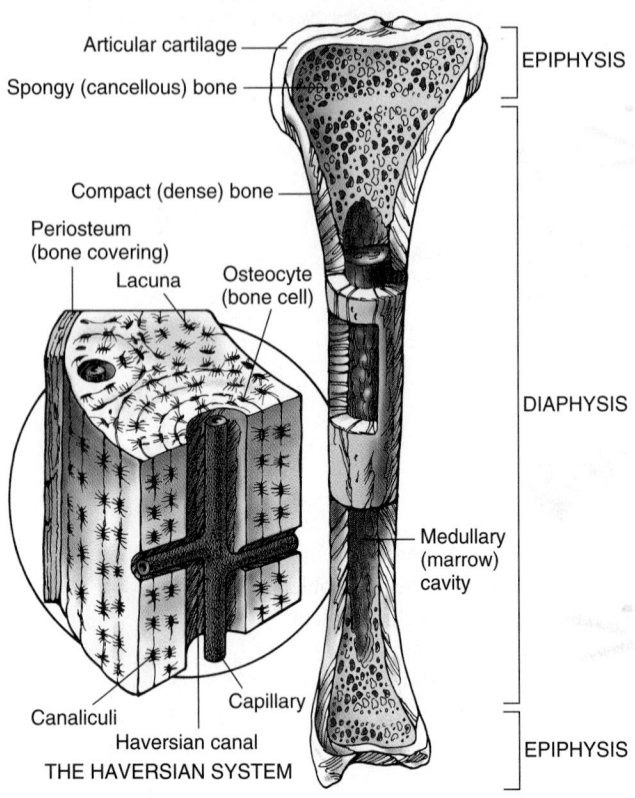

Articular cartilage
Spongy (cancellous) bone
EPIPHYSIS

Compact (dense) bone
Periosteum (bone covering)
Lacuna
Osteocyte (bone cell)

DIAPHYSIS

Medullary (marrow) cavity

Canaliculi
Capillary
Haversian canal
EPIPHYSIS
THE HAVERSIAN SYSTEM

Figure 50-1 ● The structure of a typical long bone. The cortex, or outer layer, is composed of dense, compact tissue. The microscopic structure of this compact cortical tissue is the haversian system.

the pain experienced by clients who have primary lesions of the bone.

Growth and Metabolism

After puberty, bone reaches its maturity and maximal growth. Bone is a dynamic tissue, however, that undergoes a continuous process of formation and resorption, or destruction, at equal rates until the age of 35 years. In later years, bone resorption accelerates, decreasing bone mass and predisposing clients to injury. (See Chapter 51 for a discussion of the effects of aging on bone metabolism.)

Bone growth and metabolism are affected by numerous minerals and hormones, including the following:

- Calcium
- Phosphorus
- Calcitonin
- Vitamin D
- Parathyroid hormone (PTH)
- Growth hormone
- Glucocorticoids
- Estrogens and androgens
- Thyroxine
- Insulin

■ CALCIUM AND PHOSPHORUS

Bone accounts for approximately 99% of the calcium in the body and 90% of the phosphorus. The serum concentrations

of calcium and phosphorus maintain an inverse relationship; for example, when calcium levels rise, phosphorus levels decrease. When serum levels of calcium and phosphorus are altered, calcitonin and PTH work to maintain equilibrium. If the calcium level of the blood is decreased, for example, the bone (which stores calcium) releases calcium into the vascular system in response to PTH stimulation.

■ CALCITONIN

Calcitonin is produced by the thyroid gland and *decreases* the serum calcium concentration if it is increased above its normal level. Calcitonin inhibits bone resorption and increases renal excretion of calcium and phosphorus as needed.

■ VITAMIN D

Vitamin D and its metabolites are produced in the body and transported in the blood to promote the absorption of calcium and phosphorus from the small intestine. They also seem to enhance PTH activity in the release of calcium from the bone. A decrease in the body's vitamin D level can result in osteomalacia in the adult. An external source of vitamin D may be given to clients at risk for or diagnosed with osteomalacia. Vitamin D metabolism and osteomalacia are detailed in Chapter 51.

■ PARATHYROID HORMONE

When serum calcium levels are lowered, parathyroid hormone (PTH, or parathormone) secretion increases and stimulates bone to promote osteoclastic activity and *donate* calcium to the blood. PTH reduces the renal excretion of calcium and facilitates its absorption from the intestine. Conversely, when serum calcium levels increase, PTH secretion diminishes to preserve the bone calcium supply; this is an example of the feedback loop system of the endocrine system.

■ GROWTH HORMONE

Growth hormone secreted by the anterior lobe of the pituitary gland is responsible for increasing bone length and determining the amount of bone matrix formed before puberty. During childhood, an increased secretion results in gigantism, and a decreased secretion results in dwarfism. In the adult, an increase causes acromegaly, which is characterized by bone and soft-tissue deformities (see Chapter 63).

■ GLUCOCORTICOIDS

Adrenal glucocorticoids regulate protein metabolism, either increasing or decreasing catabolism to reduce or intensify the organic matrix of bone. They also aid in regulating intestinal calcium and phosphorus absorption.

■ ESTROGENS AND ANDROGENS

Estrogens stimulate osteoblastic activity and inhibit PTH. When estrogen levels decline at menopause, women are susceptible to low serum calcium levels with subsequent bone loss (osteoporosis). Androgens, such as testosterone, promote anabolism and increase bone mass. External sources of estrogen and testosterone may be prescribed for clients at risk for or diagnosed with osteoporosis.

■ THYROXINE

Thyroxine is one of the principal hormones secreted by the thyroid gland. Its primary function is to increase the rate of protein synthesis in all types of tissue, including bone.

■ INSULIN

Insulin works together with growth hormone to build and maintain healthy bone tissue.

■ Function

The skeletal system:
- Provides a framework for the body
- Supports the surrounding tissues (e.g., muscle and tendons)
- Assists in movement through muscle attachment and joint formation
- Protects vital organs, such as the heart and lungs
- Manufactures blood cells in red bone marrow
- Provides storage for mineral salts (e.g., calcium and phosphorus)

■ JOINTS

A **joint** is a space in which two or more bones come together. The primary function of a joint is to provide movement and flexibility in the body.

■ Types

There are three types of joints in the body:
- Synarthrodial, or completely immovable, joints (e.g., in the cranium)
- Amphiarthrodial, or slightly movable, joints (e.g., in the pelvis)
- Diarthrodial (synovial), or freely movable, joints (e.g., the elbow and knee)

Although any of these joints can be affected by disease or injury, the diarthrodial joints are most commonly involved.

■ Structure and Function

The **diarthrodial,** or **synovial, joint** is the most common type of joint in the body. Synovial joints are so named because they are the only type lined with synovium, a membrane that secretes synovial fluid for lubrication and shock absorption. As illustrated in Figure 50-2, the synovium lines the internal portion of the joint capsule but does not normally extend onto the surface of the cartilage at the spongy bone ends. Articular cartilage consists of a collagen fiber matrix impregnated with a complex ground substance. Bursae, small sacs located at joints to prevent friction, are also lined with synovial membrane.

Synovial joints are subtyped by their anatomic structures. *Ball-and-socket* joints (shoulder, hip) permit movement in any direction. *Hinge* joints (elbow) allow motion in one plane, flexion, and extension. The knee is often classified as a hinge

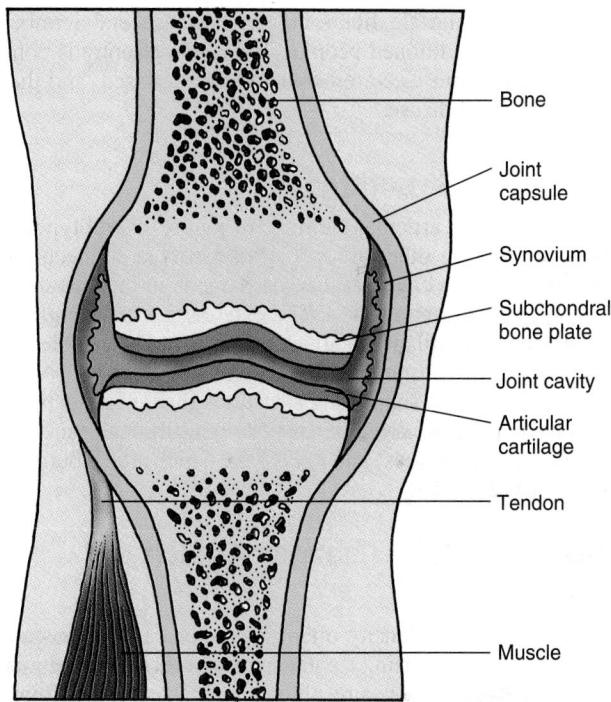

Figure 50-2 ● The structure of a diarthrodial joint. Synovium lines the joint capsule but does not extend into the articular cartilage.

Labels: Bone; Joint capsule; Synovium; Subchondral bone plate; Joint cavity; Articular cartilage; Tendon; Muscle

joint, but it rotates slightly, as well as flexes and extends. It is best described as a *condylar* type of synovial joint. The gliding movement of the wrist is characteristic of the *biaxial* joint. *Pivot* joints permit rotation only, as in the radioulnar area.

Muscular System

There are three types of muscle in the body: smooth muscle, cardiac muscle, and skeletal muscle. Smooth, or nonstriated, involuntary muscle is responsible for contractions of organs and blood vessels and is controlled by the autonomic nervous system. Cardiac muscle, or the myocardium, is also controlled by the autonomic nervous system. The smooth and cardiac muscles are discussed with the body systems to which they belong in the assessment chapters.

■ Structure

In contrast to smooth and cardiac muscle, skeletal muscle is voluntarily controlled by the central and peripheral nervous systems. The junction of a peripheral motor nerve and the muscle cells that it supplies is sometimes referred to as a motor end plate. Muscle fibers are held in place by connective tissue in bundles, or fasciculi. The entire muscle is surrounded by dense, fibrous tissue (fascia) containing the muscle's blood, lymph, and nerve supply.

■ Function

The primary function of skeletal muscle is movement of the body and its parts. When bones, joints, and supporting structures are adversely affected by injury or disease, the adjacent muscle tissue is often involved, limiting mobility. During the aging process, muscle fibers decrease in size and number, even in well-conditioned people. This senile atrophy is compounded when muscles are not regularly exercised, and they deteriorate from disuse.

Supporting Structures

In addition to the articular cartilage of joints, several types of cartilage occur in other areas. *Costal* cartilage connects the sternum to the rib cage. *Hyaline* cartilage is in the septum of the nose, larynx, and trachea. The external ear and epiglottis contain *yellow* cartilage. In all areas, the tissue is flexible and elastic and can withstand enormous tension.

Other important supporting structures that are susceptible to injury include *tendons* (bands of tough, fibrous tissue that attach muscles to bones) and *ligaments,* which attach bones to other bones at joints.

Musculoskeletal Changes Associated with Aging

As one ages, bone density often decreases, causing postural changes and predisposing a person to fractures. Synovial joint cartilage degenerates as a result of the repeated use of joints, especially weight-bearing joints such as the hips and knees. The result is often degenerative joint disease. Muscle tissue atrophy occurs, but its rate may be slowed by increased activity and exercise. Collectively, these changes cause decreased coordination, gait changes, and predisposition to falls with injury. Chart 50-1 lists the major anatomic and physiologic changes and suggested nursing interventions.

ASSESSMENT TECHNIQUES

History

In the assessment of a client with an actual or potential musculoskeletal problem, a detailed history aids the nurse in identifying diagnoses and subsequent interventions (Chart 50-2).

■ DEMOGRAPHIC DATA

Young men are at the greatest risk for trauma related to motor vehicle crashes. Older adults are at the greatest risk for falls that result in fractures and soft-tissue injury (see Chapter 5).

> **WOMEN'S HEALTH CONSIDERATIONS**
> The age and sex of the client are important indicators in musculoskeletal disorders. Older women, for example, are most likely to have metabolic bone disease, such as osteoporosis. Women of any age are at the highest risk for most types of arthritis.

■ PERSONAL AND FAMILY HISTORY

Accidents, illnesses, and medications may relate to a client's current problem. When taking a personal health history, the nurse questions the client about all traumatic incidents, regardless of the date of occurrence. An injury to the lumbar spine 30 years previously may contribute to a client's current complaint of low back pain. A motor vehicle crash can be the cause of traumatic arthritis years after the event.

Previous or concurrent diseases may affect musculoskeletal status. For example, a client with diabetes who is treated for a foot ulcer is at high risk for acute or chronic osteomyelitis (bone infection). In addition, diabetes slows the healing process. Certain disorders have a familial or genetic tendency. Osteoporosis (age-related bone loss), for instance, often occurs in several generations of a family, and bone cancer tends to be genetically linked. It is also important for the nurse to determine a history of previous hospitalizations and illnesses or complications.

The nurse also asks about previous and current use of medications. Some drugs, such as steroids, can affect calcium metabolism and promote bone loss. Other drugs may be taken to relieve musculoskeletal pain. The client should also be asked about herbal or biologic compounds that may be used for arthritis, such as chondroitin. Complementary and alternative therapies are commonly employed by clients with various types of arthritis (see Chapter 21).

CHART 50-1

NURSING FOCUS *on the* OLDER ADULT
Changes in the Musculoskeletal System Related to Aging

Physiologic Change	Nursing Implications	Rationale
Decreased bone density	Teach safety tips to prevent falls. Reinforce need to exercise, especially weight-bearing exercise.	Porous bones are more likely to fracture. Exercise slows bone loss.
Increased bone prominence	Prevent pressure on bone prominences.	There is less soft tissue to prevent skin breakdown.
Kyphotic posture: widened gait, shift in the center of gravity	Teach proper body mechanics; instruct the client to sit in supportive chairs with arms.	Correction of posture problems prevents further deformity; the client should have support for bony structures.
Cartilage degeneration	Provide moist heat, such as a shower or warm, moist compresses.	Moist heat increases blood flow to the area.
Decreased ROM	Assess the client's ability to perform ADLs and mobility.	The client may need assistance with self-care skills.
Muscle atrophy, decreased strength	Teach isometric exercises.	Exercises increase muscle strength.
Slowed movement	Do not rush the client; be patient.	The client may become frustrated if hurried.

ROM, Range of motion; *ADLs,* activities of daily living.

DIET HISTORY

An evaluation of the client's diet history helps determine the cause of inadequate nutrition. For example, most people, especially women, do not consume adequate amounts of calcium. People who cannot afford to buy food are especially at risk for undernutrition.

> **CONSIDERATIONS FOR OLDER ADULTS**
> An inadequate intake of calcium or protein or insufficient exposure to sunlight predisposes the older adult to loss of bone and lean muscle. Homebound or institutionalized older clients are particularly at risk if they are not exposed to sunlight.

Inadequate protein or insufficient vitamin C in the diet inhibits healing of bone and tissue. Obesity places excess stress and strain on bones and joints, with resultant fractures and degeneration of cartilage. In addition, obesity inhibits mobility in clients with musculoskeletal problems, which predisposes them to complications such as respiratory and circulatory problems.

SOCIOECONOMIC STATUS

When assessing a client with a possible musculoskeletal alteration, the nurse inquires about lifestyle. A person's occupation can cause or contribute to an injury. For instance, fractures are not uncommon in clients whose jobs require manual labor, such as carpenters and mechanics. Certain occupations, such as computer-related jobs, may predispose a person to carpal tunnel syndrome (entrapment of the median nerve in the wrist). Construction workers may experience back injury from prolonged standing and excessive lifting. Amateur and professional athletes often experience acute musculoskeletal injuries, such as joint dislocations and fractures, or chronic disorders, such as degenerative joint disease.

CHART 50-2

MUSCULOSKELETAL ASSESSMENT
Using Gordon's Functional Health Patterns

Activity-Exercise Pattern
Do you have sufficient energy for desired/required activities?
What is your exercise pattern? Type of exercise? Regularity?
What spare time (leisure) activities do you engage in?
What is your perceived ability for (code for level according to key below):

Feeding?	Level 0: Full self-care
Bathing?	Level I: Requires use of equipment
Toileting?	or device
Bed mobility?	Level II: Requires assistance or su-
Dressing?	pervision of another person
Grooming?	Level III: Requires assistance or
General mobility?	supervision of another person
Cooking?	and equipment or device
Home maintenance?	Level IV: Is dependent and does
Shopping?	not participate

Cognitive-Perceptual Pattern
Do you experience any discomfort?
Do you have pain? If so, how do you manage it?
What is the easiest way for you to learn things?
Do you have any difficulty learning?

Based on Gordon, M. (2000). *Manual of nursing diagnosis* (9th ed.). St. Louis: Mosby.

Socioeconomic status may be related to the client's occupation and therefore affect the likelihood of musculoskeletal problems. For example, an executive working in an office is less likely to sustain a musculoskeletal injury than is a painter or roofer engaged in manual labor and activities such as climbing ladders.

> **CULTURAL CONSIDERATIONS**
> The body proportions of African Americans differ from those of Caucasians, Asian Americans, and Native Americans. African Americans have shorter trunks and longer legs than do other groups. Their long bones are significantly longer and narrower than those of Caucasians. All bones are denser, and African-American men have denser bones than do African-American women. Caucasian women have the least amount of bone density of any group, which makes them the most susceptible to osteoporosis and fractures (Ignatavicius, 1998).
>
> Many African Americans also have a lactose intolerance (i.e., an inability to convert lactose to glucose and galactose). Because milk and dairy products are good sources of calcium for bone building but are rich in lactose, African Americans may need to obtain their calcium from other food sources, such as dark green, leafy vegetables. Inuits also have a low tolerance for milk, and the adult diet is low in calcium.
>
> A client's ethnic and cultural background may also be helpful in ascertaining his or her tolerance to pain. There may be differences in reactions to pain among cultural populations, as discussed in Chapter 7. The nurse uses this information to aid in pain assessment.

CURRENT HEALTH PROBLEM

The nurse gathers data pertinent to the client's presenting complaint as follows:

- Date and time of onset
- Factors that cause or exacerbate (worsen) the problem
- Course of the problem (e.g., intermittent or continuous)
- Clinical manifestations (as expressed by the client) and the pattern of their occurrence
- Measures that improve clinical manifestations (e.g., heat)

The most common complaint of people with musculoskeletal problems is pain. The pain may be acute or chronic, depending on its onset and duration. The nurse may use the PQRST model to elicit a complete assessment of the client's pain:

P   Provoking incident? (Was there a certain incident or event that precipitated the pain or caused an exacerbation of the pain?)

Q   Quality of pain? (What does the pain feel like in descriptive terms? Is it burning, throbbing, stabbing?)

R   Region, radiation, and relief? (Exactly where is the pain located? Does the pain travel or radiate? Does anything help relieve the pain?)

S   Severity of the pain? (How severe is the pain? The client may use a pain scale [see Chapter 7] or describe how the pain has interfered with his or her ability to function.)

T   Time? (How long does the pain last? When does it occur? Is it worse at night or during the day? If the pain awakens a person at night, the source of the pain is most likely inflammatory, not degenerative.)

With any pain assessment, it is always best if the client describes the pain in his or her own words and points to its location, if possible.

Physical Assessment

Although bones, joints, and muscles are usually assessed simultaneously in a head-to-toe approach, each subsystem is described separately for emphasis and understanding. For physical assessment of the musculoskeletal system, the nurse incorporates inspection, palpation, active range of motion (ROM), and special techniques for specific problems. A general assessment is described in this chapter. More specific assessment techniques are discussed in the interventions chapters that follow for each musculoskeletal problem.

ASSESSMENT OF THE SKELETAL SYSTEM
General Inspection

The nurse observes the client's posture, gait, and mobility for gross deformities and impairment.

POSTURE

Posture includes the person's body build and alignment when standing and walking. The nurse observes the curvature of the spine and the length, shape, and symmetry of extremities. Figure 50-3 illustrates some common spinal deformities. Muscle mass is also inspected for size and symmetry.

GAIT

Most clients with musculoskeletal problems eventually have a problem with gait. The two phases of normal, automatic gait (Figure 50-4) are the stance phase and the swing phase.

The nurse or therapist evaluates the client's balance, steadiness, and ease and length of stride; any limp or other asymmetric leg movement or deformity is noted. An abnormality in the stance phase of gait is called an *antalgic* gait. When part of one leg is painful, the person shortens the stance phase on the affected side. An abnormality in the swing phase is called a *lurch*. This abnormal gait occurs when the muscles in the but-

tocks and/or legs are too weak to allow the person to change weight from one foot to the other. In this case, the shoulders are moved either side to side or front to back for help in shifting the weight from one leg to the other. Some clients, such as those with chronic hip pain and muscle atrophy from arthritic disorders, have a combination of an antalgic gait and lurch.

MOBILITY

In collaboration with the physical or occupational therapist, the nurse observes the client's need for or use of ambulatory devices, such as canes and walkers, during transfer from bed to chair and while walking and climbing stairs. The nurse also assesses mobility by asking the client to perform activities of daily living (ADLs) such as dressing and bathing. Pain and deformity may limit physical mobility and function. A complete discussion of functional assessment is found in Chapter 10.

After performing a functional assessment, the nurse assesses major bones, joints, and muscles by inspection, palpation, and determination of ROM. A goniometer (used by physical therapists and clinical specialists) provides an exact measurement of ROM, but the degree of joint mobility can be estimated by having the client put each joint through its ROM. The nurse uses the movements shown in Figure 50-5. As long as the client can function to meet personal needs, a limitation in ROM may not be significant. For each anatomic location, the skin is observed for color, elasticity, and lesions that may relate to musculoskeletal dysfunction.

Assessment of the Head and Neck

The nurse inspects and palpates the skull for shape, symmetry, tenderness, and masses. The temporomandibular joints (TMJs) are best evaluated by palpation. The client is asked to open his or her mouth while the nurse palpates the TMJs. Common abnormal findings are tenderness or pain, crepitus (a grating sound), and a spongy swelling caused by excess synovium and fluid.

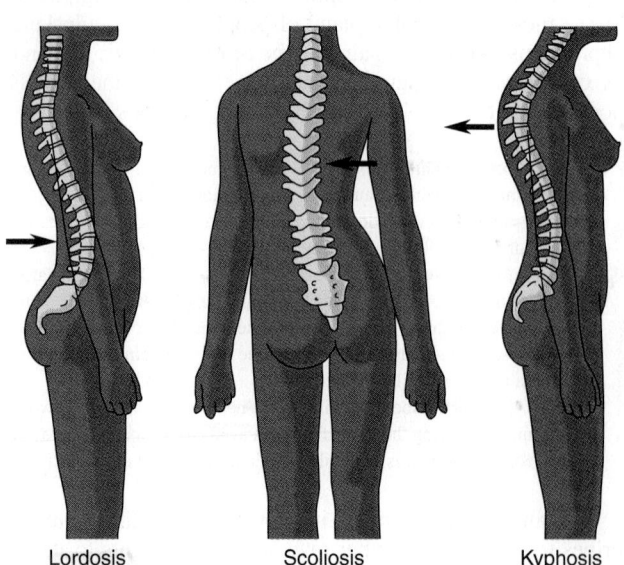

Lordosis   Scoliosis   Kyphosis

Figure 50-3 Common spinal deformities.

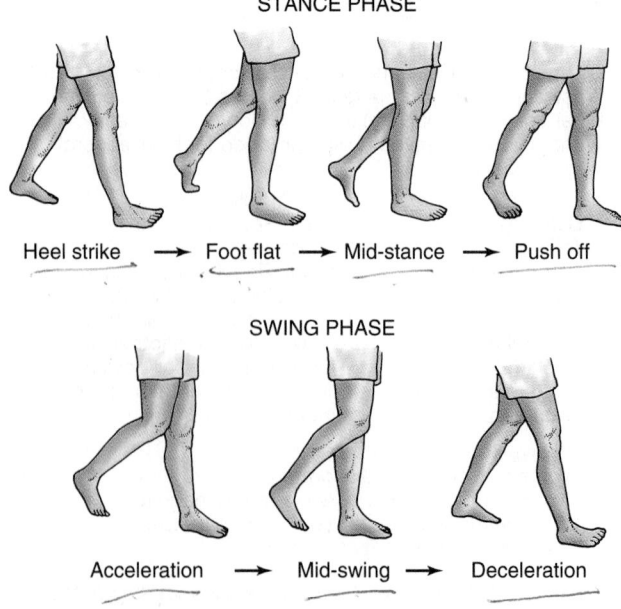

STANCE PHASE

Heel strike → Foot flat → Mid-stance → Push off

SWING PHASE

Acceleration → Mid-swing → Deceleration

Figure 50-4 The phases of gait.

The nurse then inspects and palpates each vertebra of the spine in the neck. Clinical findings may include malalignment; tenderness; or inability to flex, extend, and rotate the neck as expected.

Assessment of the Spine

The thoracic spine, lumbar spine, and sacral spine are evaluated in the same manner as the neck. Spinal alignment problems are common (see Figure 50-3). In addition, the nurse places both hands over the lumbosacral area and applies pressure with the thumbs to elicit tenderness. Many clients do not complain of discomfort until the area is palpated.

Assessment of the Upper Extremities

The nurse assesses both extremities concurrently. For example, both shoulders are inspected and palpated for size, swelling, deformity, malalignment, tenderness or pain, and mobility. A shoulder injury may prevent the client from combing his or her hair with the affected arm, but severe arthritis may inhibit movement in both arms. The elbows and wrists are assessed in a similar way.

Because the hand has multiple joints in a single digit, assessment of hand function is perhaps the most critical part of the examination. The nurse inspects and palpates the metacarpophalangeal (MCP), proximal interphalangeal (PIP), and distal interphalangeal (DIP) joints. The same digits are compared on the right and left hands (Figure 50-6). The nurse also determines range of motion (ROM) for each joint by observing active movement, if such movement is possible. For a quick and easy assessment of ROM, the client is asked to make a fist and then appose each finger to the thumb. If he or she can perform these maneuvers, ROM of the hand is not seriously restricted.

Assessment of the Lower Extremities

Evaluation of the hip joint relies primarily on determination of its degree of mobility, because the joint is deep and difficult to inspect or palpate. The client with hip pain usually experiences pain in the *groin* area, or the pain may radiate to the knee. The knee is readily accessible for nursing assessment, particularly when the client is sitting and the knee is flexed. Fluid accumulation, or effusion, is easily detected in the knee joint; limitations in movement with accompanying pain are common findings. The knees may be malaligned, as in genu valgum ("knock-knee") or genu varum ("bowlegged") deformities.

The ankles and feet are often neglected in the physical examination; however, they contain multiple bones and joints that can be affected by disease and injury. The nurse observes and palpates each joint and tests for ROM.

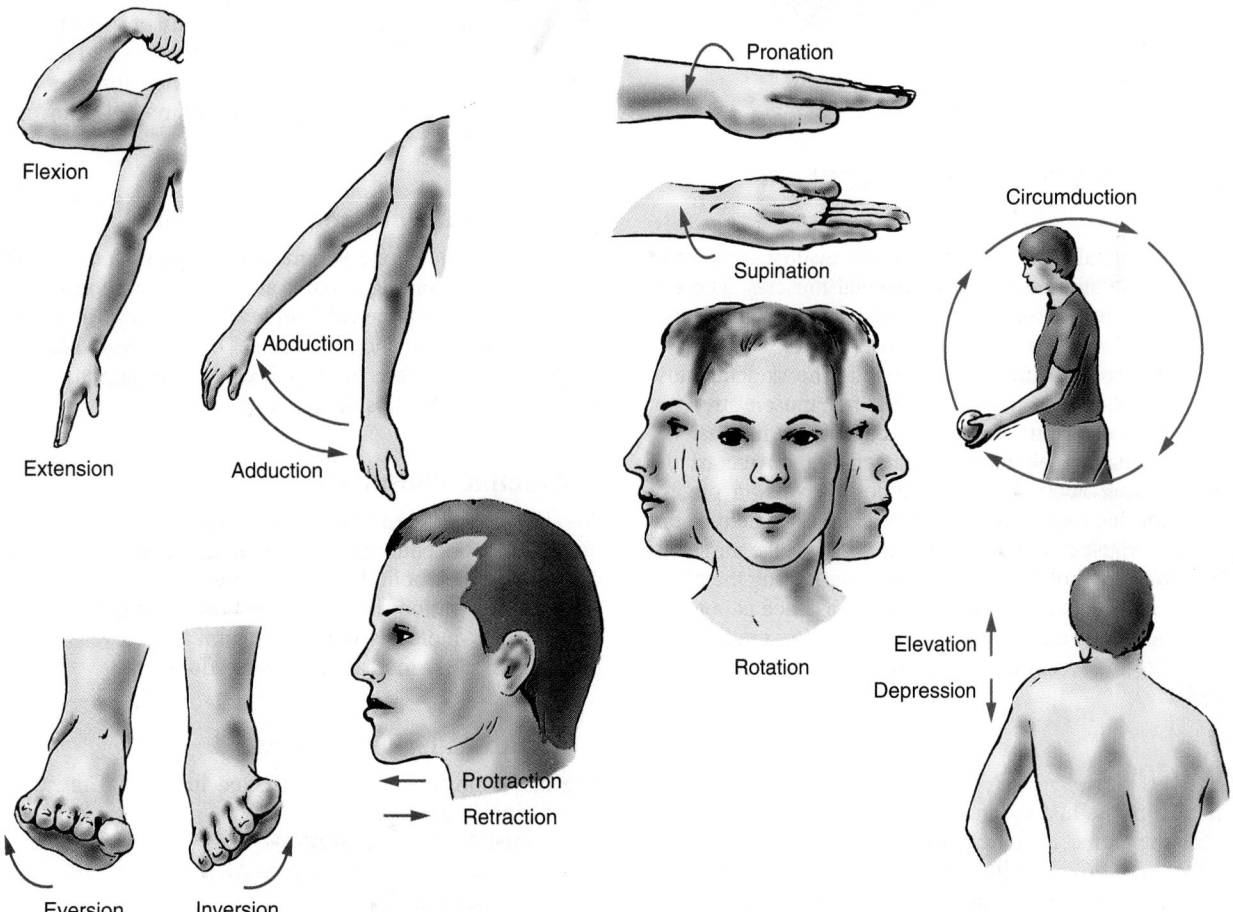

Figure 50-5 ● Movements of the skeletal muscles. (Modified from Jarvis, C. [2000]. *Physical examination and health assessment* [3rd ed.]. Philadelphia: W.B. Saunders.)

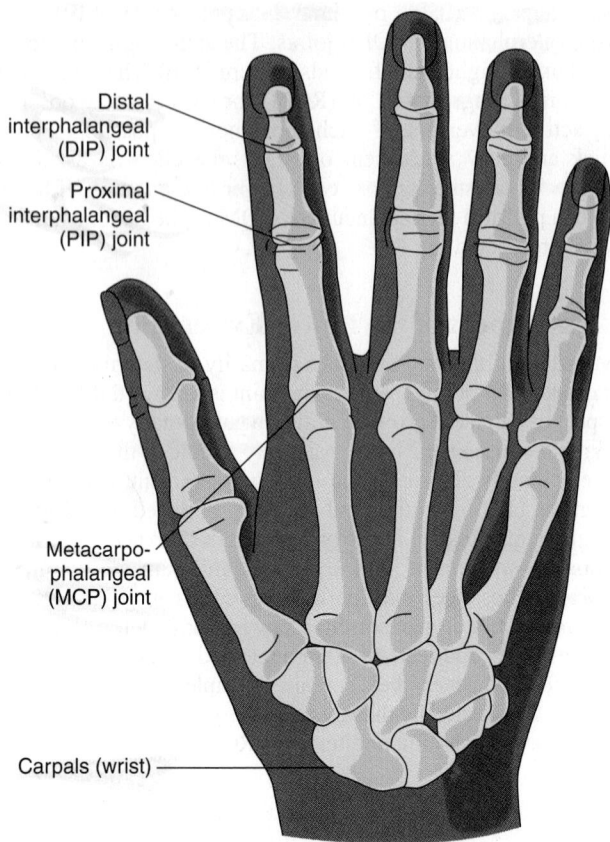

Distal
interphalangeal
(DIP) joint

Proximal
interphalangeal
(PIP) joint

Metacarpo-
phalangeal
(MCP) joint

Carpals (wrist)

Figure 50-6 ● The small joints of the hand.

▊ ASSESSMENT OF THE MUSCULAR SYSTEM

During the skeletal assessment, the nurse evaluates the size, shape, tone, and strength of major skeletal muscles. The circumference of each muscle may be measured and compared symmetrically for an estimation of muscle mass.

In addition to inspecting and palpating the skeletal muscles, the nurse asks the client to demonstrate muscle strength. For instance, to determine grip strength, the nurse may ask the client to squeeze a sphygmomanometer bulb to record the level of pressure achieved. This method provides a precise measurement that can be used to observe improvement or deterioration of muscle ability. In another method, the nurse applies resistance by holding the extremity and asking the client to move it. Although movement against resistance is not easily quantified, several scales are available for grading the client's strength. A commonly used scale is delineated in Table 50-1.

Psychosocial Assessment

The data from the history and physical examination provide clues for the nurse in anticipating psychosocial problems. For instance, the client with multiple fractures who requires extensive immobilization and therapy is at high risk for sensory deprivation. Prolonged absence from employment or permanent disability may cause the client to lose his or her job or occupation. Further stress may be experienced if

TABLE 50-1 • LOVETT'S SCALE FOR GRADING MUSCLE STRENGTH

Rating	Description
5	Normal: ROM unimpaired against gravity with full resistance
4	Good: can complete ROM against gravity with some resistance
3	Fair: can complete ROM against gravity
2	Poor: can complete ROM with gravity eliminated
1	Trace: no joint motion and slight evidence of muscle contractility
0	Zero: no evidence of muscle contractility

ROM, Range of motion.

chronic pain ensues and he or she cannot cope with numerous stressors simultaneously. Deformities resulting from musculoskeletal disease or injury can affect a person's body image and self-concept.

Diagnostic Assessment

▊ LABORATORY TESTS

Chart 50-3 lists the major laboratory tests used in assessing clients with musculoskeletal disorders. There is no special client preparation or follow-up care for any of these tests. The nurse teaches the client the purpose of the test and the procedure that can be expected. Tests performed for clients with connective tissue diseases, such as rheumatoid arthritis, are described in Chapter 21.

▊ Serum Calcium and Phosphorus

The concentrations of calcium and phosphorus, or phosphate (inorganic phosphorus), have an inverse relationship. In a healthy state, when the calcium level decreases, the phosphorus level increases, and vice versa. Disorders of bone and the parathyroid gland are often reflected in an alteration of the serum calcium or phosphorus level.

▊ Alkaline Phosphatase

Alkaline phosphatase (ALP) is an enzyme normally present in blood. The concentration of ALP increases with bone or liver damage. In metabolic bone disease and bone cancer, the enzyme concentration rises in proportion to the osteoblastic activity, which indicates bone formation. The level of ALP is normally slightly increased in older adults.

▊ Serum Muscle Enzymes

The major muscle enzymes affected in skeletal muscle disease or injury are as follows:
- Creatine kinase (CK-MM)
- Aspartate aminotransferase (AST)
- Aldolase (ALD)
- Lactate dehydrogenase (LDH)

As a result of damage, the muscle tissue releases additional amounts of these enzymes, which increases serum levels.

CHART 50-3

LABORATORY PROFILE
Musculoskeletal Assessment

Test	Normal Range for Adults	Significance of Abnormal Findings
Serum calcium	8.6-10.0 mg/dL (2.15-2.50 mmol/L) >60 yr: Slightly lower >90 yr: 8.2-9.6 mg/dL	*Hypercalcemia* (increased calcium) • Metastatic cancers of the bone • Paget's disease • Bone fractures in healing stage *Hypocalcemia* (decreased calcium) • Osteoporosis • Osteomalacia
Serum phosphorus	2.7-4.5 mg/dL (0.87-1.45 mmol/L) >60 yr: 2.3-3.7 mg/dL (M) 2.8-4.1 mg/dL (F)	*Hyperphosphatemia* (increased phosphorus) • Bone fractures in healing stage • Bone tumors • Acromegaly *Hypophosphatemia* (decreased phosphorus) • Osteomalacia
Alkaline phosphatase (ALP)	25-100 units/L	*Elevations* may indicate: • Metastatic cancers of the bone • Paget's disease • Osteomalacia
Serum muscle enzymes Creatine kinase (CK$_3$)	Total CK: • Men: 38-174 units/L • Women: 26-140 units/L >90 yr: 21-203 (M) 22-99 (F)	*Elevations* may indicate: • Muscle trauma • Progressive muscular dystrophy • Effects of electromyography
Lactate dehydrogenase (LDH)	Total LDH: 140-280 units/L 60-90 yr: 110-210 units/L >90 yr: 99-284 units/L LDH$_5$: 0%-5%	*Elevations* may indicate: • Skeletal muscle necrosis • Extensive cancer • Progressive muscular dystrophy
Aspartate aminotransferase (AST)	8-10 units/L (slightly lower in women) >60 yr: 11-26 units/L (M) 10-20 units/L (F)	*Elevations* may indicate: • Skeletal muscle trauma • Progressive muscular dystrophy
Aldolase (ALD)	1.0-7.5 units/L	*Elevations* may indicate: • Polymyositis and dermatomyositis • Muscular dystrophy

M, Males; *F,* females.

The serum CK level begins to rise 2 to 4 hours after muscle injury and is elevated early in muscle disease, such as muscular dystrophy. The CK molecule has two subunits: M (muscle) and B (brain). Three isoenzymes have been identified. Skeletal muscle CK (CK-MM, or CK$_3$) is the only isoenzyme that rises in concentration with damage to skeletal muscle.

AST is moderately elevated (three to five times normal) in certain muscle diseases, such as muscular dystrophy and dermatomyositis. The levels of the isoenzymes aldolase A (ALD-A) and LDH$_5$ also increase in clients with these disorders.

RADIOGRAPHIC EXAMINATIONS
Standard Radiography

The skeleton is readily visible on standard x-ray films. Anteroposterior and lateral projections are the initial screening views. Other approaches, such as oblique or stress views, depend on the part of the skeleton to be evaluated and the necessity of the x-ray study.

Observations of bone density, alignment, swelling, and intactness are made. The conditions of joints can be determined, including the size of the joint space, the smoothness of articular cartilage, and synovial swelling. Soft-tissue involvement may be evident but not clearly differentiated.

The nurse informs the client that the x-ray table is hard and cold and instructs him or her to remain still during the filming process.

Tomography and Xeroradiography

Whereas standard x-ray studies superimpose one structure on another, tomography produces planes, or slices, for focus and blurs the images of other structures. This procedure is helpful in detailing the musculoskeletal system, because the many close structures make visualization difficult.

Xeroradiography highlights the contrast between structures. Margins and edges can be clearly seen (edge enhancement). Disadvantages of xeroradiography are the higher radiation dose to the client and inability of xeroradiography to determine tissue densities.

Myelography

Myelography involves the injection of contrast medium, or dye, into the subarachnoid space of the spine, usually by spinal puncture. The vertebral column, intervertebral disks, spinal nerve roots, and blood vessels can be visualized. Although this test is still performed, it is far less popular; computed tomography (CT) and magnetic resonance imaging

(MRI) have often replaced such invasive, and potentially painful, diagnostic techniques. Further discussion of myelography is found in Chapter 43.

Arthrography

An arthrogram is an x-ray study of a joint after contrast medium (air or solution) has been injected to enhance its visualization. Double-contrast arthrography, which uses both air and contrast, may be performed when a traumatic injury is suspected. The physician can often determine bone chips, torn ligaments, or other loose bodies within the joint.

CLIENT PREPARATION. The most common joints studied are the knee and the shoulder. The client is questioned about allergy to shellfish or iodine.

The radiology nurse or technician informs the client that the test may be uncomfortable because of pressure at the needle insertion site. The joint may be swollen for several days after the test, and strenuous physical activity should be avoided for 12 to 24 hours. The joint may be wrapped, and ice may be applied at intervals for the first few hours after the test to decrease swelling.

PROCEDURE. If the knee is examined, the client is supine while the knee is flexed. After a local anesthetic is applied, the physician injects an iodine-based contrast medium directly into the joint through a medial or lateral approach. The client feels pressure but should not experience pain. X-ray images are then taken of the joint, which may be put through range of motion (ROM) during the test.

FOLLOW-UP CARE. Because the contrast medium mixes with synovial fluid, it is not withdrawn after the procedure. As a result, the client's joint is enlarged and slightly uncomfortable. Some clients state that they feel the solution moving in the joint and hear "swishing" noises for several days until the solution is absorbed by the body. If these sensations continue, the health care provider should be contacted.

In most cases, the client can resume usual activities but should avoid strenuous exercise, such as participating in contact sports, for at least 12 hours after the test. If the client has an identified joint injury, he or she may require a longer period of immobilization. An elastic support bandage may be worn around the joint for several days. The application of ice may reduce some of the swelling.

Computed Tomography

Computed tomography (CT) has gained wide acceptance for the detection of musculoskeletal problems, particularly those of the vertebral column. It may be used with or without a contrast medium, which is given orally or intravenously. If the administration of a contrast agent is planned, the radiology nurse or technician checks that the client has been allowed nothing by mouth (NPO) for at least 4 hours and is not allergic to iodine.

As a noninvasive procedure, the CT scan requires minimal nursing intervention except for client education. During the procedure, the client must remain still for 30 to 60 minutes on a hard table while the affected part is encased in the machine. Complaints of claustrophobia and annoyance from the clicking sounds made by the scanner on rotation are common, but the client is reassured that there is no danger from the machine.

OTHER DIAGNOSTIC TESTS

Bone Biopsy

In a bone biopsy, the physician extracts a specimen of bone for microscopic examination. This invasive test may confirm the presence of infection or neoplasm. One of two techniques may be used to retrieve the specimen: needle (closed) biopsy or incisional (open) biopsy.

CLIENT PREPARATION. The nurse teaches the client about the procedure and post-test care. The open technique is more invasive and requires more care.

PROCEDURE. The health care provider may perform bone biopsy in the client's room, in a special procedures room in the radiology department, or in the operating room with the use of local or general anesthesia. If the client is not given a general anesthetic, this procedure is quite painful. After anesthesia is induced, the health care provider inserts a long needle into the bone cortex or makes a small incision to reveal the bone tissue. A sterile dressing is applied after extraction of the osseous tissue. If an incision is made, a pressure dressing is applied.

FOLLOW-UP CARE. The nurse inspects the biopsy site for bleeding, swelling, and hematoma formation, which are the most common complications of bone biopsy during the first 24 hours after the procedure. Because the pressure dressing inhibits observation, the nurse monitors the client's level of pain. If internal bleeding or marked swelling occurs, the client complains of severe pain instead of the mild to moderate discomfort usually associated with the procedure. For decreasing the likelihood of bleeding, he or she is taught to immobilize the affected extremity for 12 to 24 hours. If bone infection occurs as a complication of bone biopsy, the client's temperature may be elevated 1 to 3 days after the procedure.

A mild analgesic often relieves the discomfort resulting from the procedure. After an open biopsy, the nurse teaches the client to reapply the dressing daily over the incision site while inspecting the wound for signs of inflammation or infection, such as redness, warmth, and tissue swelling.

Muscle Biopsy

Muscle biopsy is done for the diagnosis of atrophy (as in muscular dystrophy) and inflammation (as in polymyositis). The procedure and care for clients undergoing muscle biopsy are the same as those for clients undergoing bone biopsy.

Electromyography

Electromyography (EMG) is usually accompanied by nerve conduction studies for determining the electrical potential generated in an individual muscle. EMG helps in the diagnosis of neuromuscular, lower motor neuron, and peripheral nerve disorders.

CLIENT PREPARATION. The nurse informs the client that EMG may cause temporary discomfort, especially when the client is subjected to episodes of electrical current. For selected clients, mild sedation is ordered. The physician may also order a temporary discontinuation of skeletal muscle relaxants several days before the procedure to prevent medication from having effects on the test results.

PROCEDURE. The test may be performed at the bedside or in an EMG laboratory. When both EMG and nerve conduction studies are done, nerve conduction is usually tested first. Flat electrodes are placed along the nerve to be evaluated, and low electrical currents are passed through the electrodes to the nerve and muscle innervated. If nerve conduction is accomplished, the muscle contracts.

For testing muscle potential, multiple needle electrodes varying from $\frac{1}{2}$ to 3 inches (1.3 to 7.5 cm) are inserted. The client may be asked to perform activities for measurement of muscle potential during minimal and maximal contraction. The degree of nerve and muscle activity is recorded on an oscilloscope, which provides a graphic readout for later interpretation.

FOLLOW-UP CARE. A few medical complications are associated with EMG. The nurse provides comfort measures and inspects the needle sites for hematoma formation. The application of ice can prevent this complication. The client may also complain of increased pain and anxiety after the test.

Arthroscopy

An arthroscope is a fiberoptic tube inserted into a joint for direct visualization; the knee and shoulder are most commonly evaluated. In addition, synovial biopsy and surgical procedures to repair traumatic injury can be accomplished through the arthroscope.

CLIENT PREPARATION. Because the knee is most commonly "scoped," the care described for the client undergoing arthroscopy relates to that joint. Arthroscopy is performed on an ambulatory basis or as same-day surgery. Clients who cannot flex their knees at least 40 degrees or who have infected knees are not candidates for the procedure. The client must be able to flex the knee, and joint infection may worsen from the mechanical trauma of arthroscope insertion.

If possible, the client should have a physical therapy consultation before arthroscopy to learn the leg exercises that are necessary after the test, especially if the procedure will be surgical. Straight-leg raises (SLRs) and quadriceps setting exercises (isometrics with the leg extended) are practiced in sets of 10 each. Range-of-motion (ROM) exercises are also taught but may not be allowed immediately after arthroscopic surgery. The nurse in the surgeon's office or at the surgical center can teach these exercises or reinforce the information provided by the physical therapist. The nurse also explains the procedure and post-test care.

PROCEDURE. The client is usually given local, light general, or epidural anesthesia, depending on the purpose of the procedure. In some settings, a large pneumatic tourniquet is used around the thigh to minimize bleeding during the procedure. Medications promoting vasoconstriction for control of bleeding may be used alone or in conjunction with the tourniquet.

The knee is flexed to at least 40 degrees, and saline or lactated Ringer's solution is used to irrigate the knee. As shown in Figure 50-7, the arthroscope is inserted through a small incision less than $\frac{1}{4}$ inch (0.6 cm) long. Multiple incisions may be required to allow inspection at a variety of angles. After the procedure, a bulky pressure dressing and an elastic bandage may be applied, depending on the amount of manipulation during the test or surgery.

FOLLOW-UP CARE. The nurse evaluates the neurovascular status of the client's affected limb frequently, in accordance with the nursing standard of care. Initially, the typical protocol is every hour. The technique for this assessment is described in detail in Chapter 52 and includes monitoring distal pulses, warmth, color, capillary refill, pain, movement, and sensation of the affected extremity.

The nurse encourages the client to perform exercises as taught before the examination. For the mild discomfort experienced after the diagnostic arthroscopy, the physician prescribes a mild analgesic, such as acetaminophen (Tylenol, Ace-Tabs✤). The client has short-term activity restrictions, depending on the musculoskeletal problem. Ice is often used for 24 hours, and the extremity should be elevated for 24 to 48 hours. When arthroscopic surgery is performed, the health care provider usually prescribes an opioid-analgesic combination, such as oxycodone and acetaminophen (Percocet, Tylox).

Although complications are not common, the nurse monitors and teaches the client to monitor for the following:

- Swelling
- Hypothermia (decreased body temperature) resulting from the use of the tourniquet during the procedure
- Increased joint pain attributable to mechanical injury
- Thrombophlebitis
- Infection

Severe joint or limb pain after discharge may indicate a possible complication and warrants that the client contact the

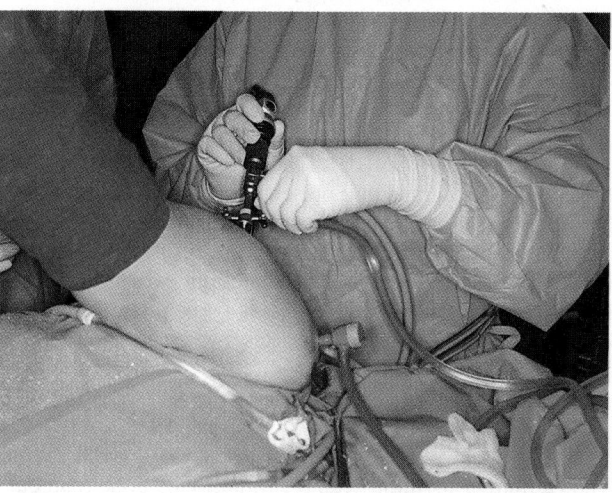

Figure 50-7 ● An arthroscope is used in the diagnosis of pathologic changes in the joints. This client is undergoing arthroscopy of the shoulder.

physician immediately. The health care provider may see the client about 1 week after the test to check for complications.

CRITICAL THINKING CHALLENGE
A young male client complains of severe left knee pain following a ski trip last weekend. The orthopedic surgeon suspects damage to the meniscus and schedules the client for an arthroscopy.
• As his office nurse, what health teaching will you need to provide to prepare the client for this procedure?
• What immediate post-test care will the client require? What discharge instructions will the postanesthesia care unit (PACU) nurse need to review?

For suggested answer guidelines, go to SIMON http://www.wbsaunders.com/SIMON/Iggy/.

Bone Scan

The bone scan is a radionuclide test in which radioactive material is injected for visualization of the entire skeleton. It is used primarily to detect tumors, arthritis, osteomyelitis, osteoporosis, vertebral compression fractures, and unexplained bone pain.

CLIENT PREPARATION. A nuclear medicine physician or technician injects the client intravenously with the radioactive isotope of technetium (^{99m}Tc) several hours before the scanning procedure. As a bone-seeking substance, the isotope migrates to bone. The nurse assures the client that the dose is minimal and that no complications will result from receipt of the material. He or she is asked to void immediately before the scan to prevent an obliterated view of the pelvis by the urinary bladder.

PROCEDURE. The client is taken to the nuclear medicine department and placed on the scanning table. For an accurate image, the client must be able to lie still for 30 to 60 minutes during scanning. Clients who are older, restless, or in pain may find this test uncomfortable and may need mild sedation. The examiner looks for areas of bone in which there is increased uptake, or concentration, of the isotope. These hot lesions indicate abnormal bone metabolism, a sign of bone disease. Cold lesions, in which there is decreased uptake, indicate poor blood flow to bone, as in severe arteriosclerosis.

FOLLOW-UP CARE. The amount of radioactivity in the isotope is minimal and presents no hazard to the client or the nurse. The substance is excreted in urine and stool. Because the substance rapidly deteriorates in the body, no special precautions are required for handling excreta. The nurse encourages the client to push fluids to facilitate urinary excretion. Repeated scans may be taken, but no additional injection of the radioisotope is required.

Gallium/Thallium Scans

The gallium or thallium scan is similar to the bone scan but is more specific and sensitive in detecting bone problems. Gallium citrate (^{67}Ga) is the radioisotope most commonly used. This substance also migrates to brain, liver, and breast tissue and therefore is used in examination of these structures when disease is suspected.

For clients with osteosarcoma, thallium (^{201}Tl) is better than gallium or technetium for diagnosing the extent of the disease. Thallium has traditionally been used for the diagnosis of myocardial infarctions but is now also used for evaluation of cancers of the bone.

CLIENT PREPARATION. Because bone takes up gallium slowly, the nuclear medicine physician or technician administers the isotope 1 to 2 days before scanning. Other tests that require contrast media or other isotopes cannot be given during this time.

The nurse instructs the client that the radioactive material poses no threat because it readily deteriorates in the body. Because gallium is excreted through the intestinal tract, it tends to collect in feces before the scanning procedure.

PROCEDURE. Depending on the tissue to be examined, the client is taken to the nuclear medicine department 1 to 2 days after injection. The procedure takes 30 to 60 minutes, during which time the client must lie still for accurate test results to be achieved. Mild sedation may be necessary to facilitate relaxation and cooperation during the procedure for confused older clients or those in severe pain.

FOLLOW-UP CARE. No special care is required after the test. The radioisotope is excreted in stool and urine, but no precautions are taken in handling the excreta. The nurse encourages the client to push fluids to facilitate urinary excretion.

Magnetic Resonance Imaging

Magnetic resonance imaging (MRI), with or without the use of contrast media, can be used to diagnose musculoskeletal disorders. Its use is expanding and replacing some of the more traditional tests, such as bone scans. The MRI is more accurate than computed tomography (CT) and myelography for many spinal and knee problems (Patel & Lauerman, 1997).

The image is produced through the interaction of magnetic fields, radio waves, and atomic nuclei showing hydrogen density. Simply put, the radio waves "bounce" off the body tissues being examined. Because each tissue has its own density, the computer image clearly distinguishes normal and abnormal tissues. For some tissues, the cross-sectional image is better than that produced by radiography or CT. The lack of hydrogen ions in cortical bone makes it easily distinguishable from soft tissues. The test is particularly useful in identifying problems with muscles, tendons, and ligaments.

The nurse ensures that the client removes all metal objects and checks for clothing zippers and metal fasteners. Although joint implants made of titanium or stainless steel are safe, pacemakers and surgical clips are not. Chart 50-4 lists questions that the nurse or technician should consider in preparing the client for MRI. Open MRIs prevent the claustrophobia that occurs with the older, encased machines.

Gadolinium-DTPA (diethylenetriamine-pentaacetic acid) is the only contrast agent approved for MRI. It is most commonly used to diagnose degenerative vertebral disease and recurrent disk herniation—sometimes referred to as the failed back surgery syndrome (Patel & Lauerman, 1997).

CHART 50-4

BEST PRACTICE *for*
The Client Preparing for Magnetic Resonance Imaging

- Is the client pregnant?
- Does the client have magnetic metal fragments or implants, such as an aneurysm clip?
- If the client has an IV catheter, can it be converted to a heparin lock temporarily?
- Does the client have a pacemaker or electronic implant?
- Can the client be without supplemental oxygen for an hour?
- Can the client tolerate the supine position for 20 to 30 minutes?
- Can the client lie still for 20 to 30 minutes?
- Does the client need life support equipment?
- Can the client communicate clearly and understand verbal communication?

Ultrasonography

Sound waves produce an image of the tissue in ultrasonography. An ultrasound procedure may be used to visualize the following:

- Soft-tissue disorders, such as masses and fluid accumulation
- Traumatic joint injuries
- Osteomyelitis
- Surgical hardware placement

A jelly-like substance applied to the skin over the site to be examined promotes the movement of a metal probe. No special preparation or post-test care is necessary. A quantitative ultrasound (QUS) may be done for determining fractures or bone density.

ONLINE RESOURCES

For suggested readings and Internet resources, go to http://www.wbsaunders.com/SIMON/Iggy/.

SELECTED BIBLIOGRAPHY

Asterisk indicates a classic or definitive work on this subject.

Burke, M.M., & Walsh, M.B. (1997). *Gerontologic nursing: Wholistic care of the older adult* (2nd ed.). St. Louis: Mosby.

Corbett, J.V. (1998). Laboratory tests and diagnostic procedures in orthopaedic nursing practice. *Nursing Clinics of North America, 33*(4), 685-700.

Eliopoulos, C. (1997). *Gerontological nursing* (4th ed.). Philadelphia: J.B. Lippincott.

*Guyton, A.C. (1995). *Textbook of medical physiology.* Philadelphia: W.B. Saunders.

Ignatavicius, D.D. (1998). *Introduction to long-term care.* Philadelphia: F.A. Davis.

Jarvis, C. (2000). *Physical examination and health assessment* (3rd ed.). Philadelphia: W.B. Saunders.

Mangini, M. (1998). Physical assessment of the musculoskeletal system. *Nursing Clinics of North America, 33*(4), 643-652.

Martsolf, D.S. (1999). Cultural aspects of orthopaedic nursing. *Orthopaedic Nursing, 18*(2), 65-71.

Matteson, M.A., McConnell, E.S., & Linton, A.D. (1997). *Gerontological nursing: Concepts and practice* (2nd ed.). Philadelphia: W.B. Saunders.

Neal, L. (1997). Basic musculoskeletal assessment: Tips for the home health nurse. *Home Healthcare Nurse, 15*(4), 227-235.

O'Hanlon-Nichols, T. (1998). Basic assessment series: A review of the adult musculoskeletal system. *American Journal of Nursing, 98*(6), 48-52.

Pagana, K.D., & Pagana, T.J. (1999). *Mosby's diagnostic and laboratory test reference* (4th ed.). St. Louis: Mosby.

Patel, P.R., & Lauerman, W.C. (1997). The use of magnetic resonance imaging in the diagnosis of lumbar disc disease. *Orthopaedic Nursing, 16*(1), 59-65.

Scura, K.W., & Whipple, B. (1997). How to provide better care for the postmenopausal woman. *American Journal of Nursing, 97*(4), 36-44.

Interventions for Clients with Musculoskeletal Problems

DONNA D. IGNATAVICIUS

Learning Objectives

After studying this chapter, you should be able to:

1. Explain the risk factors for primary and secondary osteoporosis.
2. Describe ways to decrease the risk for osteoporosis.
3. Discuss the role of drug therapy in the prevention and management of osteoporosis.
4. Compare and contrast osteoporosis and osteomalacia.
5. Identify common assessment findings in clients with Paget's disease of the bone.
6. Differentiate acute and chronic osteomyelitis.
7. Analyze assessment data to determine common nursing diagnoses and collaborative problems for the client with a malignant bone tumor.
8. Discuss the psychosocial aspects associated with a diagnosis of bone cancer.
9. Develop a community-based plan of care for a client with a malignant bone tumor.
10. Evaluate the nursing care of a client with a bone tumor using expected outcome criteria.
11. Explain the pathophysiology and risk factors for carpal tunnel syndrome.
12. Discuss treatment options for the client diagnosed with carpal tunnel syndrome.
13. Describe common disorders of the foot, including hallux valgus and plantar fasciitis.
14. Explain the role of the nurse when caring for a client with muscular dystrophy.

Go to http://www.wbsaunders.com/SIMON/Iggy/ for self-assessment questions related to these Learning Objectives.

Musculoskeletal disorders include metabolic bone diseases, bone tumors, and a variety of deformities and syndromes. The older adult is at the greatest risk for the development of most of these health problems. The incidence of bone cancer is increasing in both the young and the older population. As technologic advances occur and clients survive longer with primary lesions, metastatic cancer becomes more prevalent. This chapter focuses on selected disorders not covered in Chapter 21 on connective tissue diseases.

METABOLIC BONE DISEASES

Osteoporosis

■ OVERVIEW

Osteoporosis is a metabolic disease in which bone demineralization results in decreased density and subsequent fractures. The wrist, hip, and vertebral column are most often affected.

The World Health Organization (WHO) has developed a standard for osteoporosis diagnosis based on **bone mineral density (BMD)** values using T-scores. A T-score is the number of standard deviations above or below the average BMD. Low bone mass **(osteopenia)** is present when the T-score is between -1 and -2.5. Osteoporosis in postmenopausal women is defined as a BMD T-score at or below -2.5 (Ott, 1999).

Osteoporosis is a major health problem in many countries. Therefore a World Congress on Osteoporosis was convened in 2000 to explore how to best prevent and treat this costly health problem. The estimated cost for osteoporosis-related health care in the United States alone is more than \$14 billion each year (Cutson & Meuleman, 2000).

■ Pathophysiology

Bone is a dynamic tissue. Throughout a person's life span, new bone is formed by osteoblastic activity, whereas old bone is resorbed through osteoclastic activity; this process is known as bone modeling. BMD determines bone strength and peaks between 30 and 35 years of age. After the peak years, bone resorption activity exceeds bone-building activity, and bone density decreases. Trabecular, or cancellous (spongy), bone is lost first, followed by loss of cortical (compact) bone.

BMD decreases rapidly in postmenopausal women as serum estrogen levels diminish. Approximately 40% to 45% of a woman's bone mass is lost during her life span. It is estimated that 50% of all women older than 65 years of age have symptomatic osteoporosis.

More than half of all Caucasian women have at least one osteoporotic fracture during their lifetime. Men also develop osteoporosis and resulting fractures. Studies have shown that although men are less likely than women to experience a fracture, the lifetime risk of fracture in men is 13% to 25% (Bilezikian, 1999).

CLASSIFICATION OF OSTEOPOROSIS

Osteoporosis is an irreversible osteopenia. There are two major types: primary osteoporosis and secondary osteoporosis. **Primary osteoporosis** is more common and is not associated with an underlying pathologic condition. It occurs in both genders at any age but most often affects women after menopause and men in their later years. **Secondary osteoporosis** results from an associated medical condition, such as hyperparathyroidism; long-term drug therapy, such as with corticosteroids; or prolonged immobility, such as that seen with spinal cord injury (Table 51-1). Treatment of the secondary type is directed toward the cause of the osteoporosis when possible.

Primary osteoporosis can be divided into two subtypes. *Type I* (postmenopausal) osteoporosis occurs in women between the ages of 55 and 65 years. Estrogen presumably prevents or decreases the rate of bone resorption in women and is unavailable in sufficient quantities after menopause. Vertebral and wrist fractures are common in postmenopausal women because the predominant bone type in the vertebrae and wrists is cancellous.

Type II (senile) osteoporosis occurs in those older than 65 years of age and affects women twice as often as men. Hip and vertebral fractures are often seen in clients with type II disease.

THEORIES OF OSTEOPOROSIS DEVELOPMENT

The exact pathophysiology of osteoporosis is unclear, but two theories of disease development have been advocated. First, osteoporosis may result from decreased osteoblastic activity. The osteoblasts, or bone-forming cells, may have a shortened life span or may be less efficient in the client with osteoporosis. The second, and more popular, theory suggests an increase in osteoclastic (bone resorption) activity. The latter theory has gained increased recognition over the past decade and has resulted in treatment directed toward measures to prevent rapid bone resorption.

Etiology

The exact cause of primary osteoporosis is unknown; however, numerous risk factors have been identified (Chart 51-1). In view of the high cost of osteoporosis in both health care dollars and quality of life, young women need to be aware of appropriate health and lifestyle practices that can prevent this potentially disabling disease (see the Meeting Healthy People 2010 Objectives box on p. 1096). A nursing study by Berarducci et al. (2000) found that most health care providers focus on the risk of osteoporosis in women over 50 years of age and do not assess risk as often in women age 49 years and younger (see the Evidence-Based Practice for Nursing box on p. 1096).

Primary osteoporosis most often occurs in women after menopause as a result of decreased estrogen levels. Women lose approximately 2% of their bone mass every year in the first 5 years after menopause. For women who cannot take estrogen replacement, such as breast cancer survivors, the risk of osteoporosis increases.

In addition, body build seems to predict the occurrence of the disease. Osteoporosis occurs more often in thin, lean-built Caucasian and Asian women, particularly those who do not exercise regularly. Obese women can store estrogen in their tissues for use as necessary to maintain a normal level of serum calcium. Exercise decreases bone resorption and stimulates bone formation. Immobilization, such as prolonged bedrest, produces rapid bone loss.

The relationship of osteoporosis to dietary factors is not as well established. A diet deficient in calcium and vitamin D stimulates the parathyroid gland to produce parathyroid hormone (PTH). PTH triggers the release of calcium from the bony matrix. Malabsorption, caused by disease or drugs, also contributes to low serum calcium levels. Institutionalized or homebound people who are not exposed to sunlight may be at a higher risk because they do not receive adequate vitamin D for the metabolism of calcium.

Protein deficiency may contribute to the incidence of bone demineralization, although this theory is controversial. Be-

---

TABLE 51-1 • CAUSES OF SECONDARY OSTEOPOROSIS

DISEASES/CONDITIONS
- Diabetes mellitus
- Hyperthyroidism
- Hyperparathyroidism
- Cushing's syndrome
- Growth hormone deficiency
- Metabolic acidosis
- Female hypogonadism
- Paget's disease
- Osteogenesis imperfecta
- Rheumatoid arthritis
- Prolonged immobilization
- Marfan's syndrome
- Bone cancer
- Cirrhosis
- Chronic airway limitation

DRUGS (CHRONIC USE)
- Corticosteroids
- Heparin
- Anticonvulsants
- Ethanol (alcohol)
- Drugs that induce hypogonadism (decreased levels of sex hormones)
- High levels of exogenous (external) thyroid hormone

CHART 51-1

BEST PRACTICE *for*
Assessing Risk Factors for Primary Osteoporosis

Assess for the following:
- Client's age greater than 60
- Family history of osteoporosis
- Caucasian or Asian race
- Thin, lean body build
- Low, lifetime calcium intake
- Estrogen deficiency
- Androgen deficiency
- Smoking history
- High alcohol intake
- Lack of physical exercise or prolonged immobility

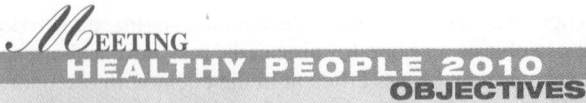

OSTEOPOROSIS

Objective 2.10:   Reduce the proportion of adults who are hospitalized for vertebral fractures associated with osteoporosis.

- Teach women of all ages about osteoporosis as a disease and cause of potentially life-threatening fractures.
- Teach young and middle-aged women the need to practice a lifestyle that reduces the risk factors for osteoporosis (e.g., no smoking, increased exercise, increased calcium intake).
- Teach middle-aged and older adults to have bone mineral density screening tests to determine their bone loss percentage (often available at no or minimal cost at local health fairs or pharmacies).
- Remind clients to use proper body mechanics, such as using large leg muscles rather than back muscles for lifting.
- If clients are at high risk for osteoporosis, tell them to avoid jarring activities such as jogging or horseback riding.
- If clients are at high risk for osteoporosis, tell them to consult with a health care provider and comply with preventive treatment.

EVIDENCE-BASED PRACTICE
FOR NURSING

Do health care providers assess knowledge of osteoporosis in young women?

Berarducci, A., et al. (2000). Health-promoting educational practices related to osteoporosis. *Applied Nursing Research, 13*(4), 173-180.

This descriptive study was designed to determine if health care providers educate women of all ages about osteoporosis, including assessing risk factors for the disease. The researchers surveyed 90 health care providers in southwest Florida. Forty-nine surveys were returned, and 47 were usable. The responses of the providers showed significant differences between women 49 years of age and younger and women over 50 years of age. Health care providers routinely assessed risk factors in older women and educated these women, but they did not identify risk factors or provide education for younger women.

Critique. Although the sample size was small and the subjects constituted a convenience sample, this research is one of the few studies that address the issue of health promotion to prevent osteoporosis in young women. The study cannot be generalized and needs to be repeated using a larger sample in a larger geographic area.

Implications for Nursing. Nurses and other health care professionals in any setting have a responsibility to educate all women, regardless of age, about the risk factors for osteoporosis and how to reduce them. Other studies have supported the belief that lifestyle changes in young adulthood can prevent or minimize the risk for osteoporosis as women age.

cause 50% of serum calcium is protein bound, protein is needed for calcium utilization; however, excessive protein intake may increase calcium loss in the urine. Protein is needed, however, for bone healing when a fracture occurs.

Alcohol consumption and cigarette smoking are other possible risk factors. Although the exact mechanisms are not known, these substances may promote acidosis, which in turn increases bone loss. Alcohol also has a direct toxic effect on bone tissue, resulting in decreased bone formation and increased bone resorption (Leslie, 2000). Excessive caffeine intake can increase calcium loss in the urine.

Hereditary factors may play a role for both men and women, but this hypothesis has not been confirmed (Orwell, 2000). Several of the suspected risk factors, such as body build, are determined in part by heredity; however, heredity or a genetic influence alone probably is not predictive for osteoporosis.

CONSIDERATIONS FOR OLDER ADULTS
Aging is a major risk factor for osteoporosis. As aging occurs, serum concentrations of 1,25-dihydroxycholecalciferol, a vitamin D metabolite, decrease. Osteoporosis is often accompanied by low levels of serum calcitonin, a hormone secreted by the thyroid gland that helps maintain a normal serum calcium level. In addition, some older adults living at home or in health care settings are undernourished and deficient in calcium and protein.

Incidence/Prevalence

Between 25 and 35 million Americans, 80% of whom are women, have osteoporosis. The incidence of the disease is greater in women than in men (at least 5:1) because men usually have larger bones and protection provided by bone-building testosterone. Ninety percent of men and women over age 75 suffer from osteoporosis.

Osteoporosis results in more than 1.5 million fractures each year, 300,000 of which are hip fractures. In people older than 90 years of age, one third of women and one fifth of men experience at least one hip fracture. The mortality for older clients with hip fractures is very high, especially within the first 6 months, and the debilitating effects can be devastating (McClung, 2000).

CULTURAL CONSIDERATIONS
Caucasian women are affected more often than African-American women. It is well documented that African-American women have 10% more bone mass than Caucasian women. Northern European and Asian-American women are at a higher risk than Caucasian women (McClung, 2000).

▶ COLLABORATIVE MANAGEMENT

● Assessment

Typically, a diagnosis of osteoporosis is made after the client sustains a vertebral, wrist, or hip fracture. The client may be asymptomatic before admission with one or more bone fractures. When taking a history, the nurse determines the risk factors for osteoporosis, as described under Etiology, p. 1095.

PHYSICAL ASSESSMENT/CLINICAL MANIFESTATIONS

When performing a musculoskeletal assessment, the nurse inspects and palpates the vertebral column. The classic "dowager's hump," or kyphosis of the dorsal spine, is usually present (Figure 51-1). The client often states that height has been shortened, perhaps as much as 2 to 3 inches (5 to 7 cm) within the previous 20 years. Height and weight should be measured and compared with previous measurements if they are available.

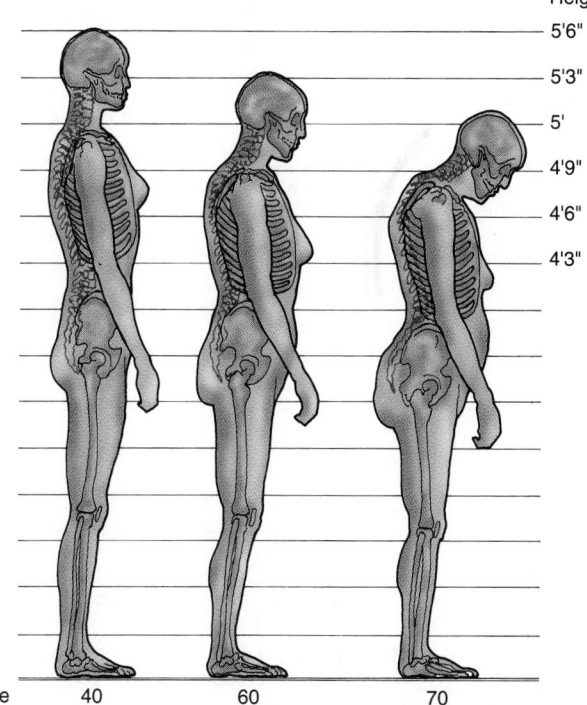

Height
5'6"
5'3"
5'
4'9"
4'6"
4'3"

Age   40   60   70

Figure 51-1 ● A normal spine at age 40 years and osteoporotic changes at ages 60 and 70 years. These changes can cause a loss of as much as 6 inches in height and can result in the so-called dowager's hump *(far right)* in the upper thoracic vertebrae.

Accompanying the spinal deformity is the complaint of back pain, which often occurs after lifting, bending, or stooping. The pain may be sharp and acute in onset. Pain is worse with activity and is relieved by rest. Palpation of the vertebrae, particularly the lower thoracic and lumbar vertebrae, usually increases the client's discomfort. Therefore palpation should be gentle.

Back pain accompanied by tenderness and voluntary restriction of spinal movement suggests one or more compression vertebral fractures, the most common type of osteoporotic fracture. Movement restriction and spinal deformity may result in constipation, abdominal distention, reflux esophagitis, and respiratory compromise in severe cases. The most likely area for fracture occurrence is between T8 and L3.

Fractures are also common in the distal end of the radius and the upper third of the femur (hip). The nurse directs special attention to these areas as part of the physical assessment.

■ PSYCHOSOCIAL ASSESSMENT

Women often associate osteoporosis with menopause, getting older, and becoming less independent. The disease can result in suffering, deformity, and disability that can affect the client's well-being and life satisfaction. The quality of life may be further impacted by pain, insomnia, depression, and **fallophobia** (fear of falling).

The nurse assesses the client's concept of body image, especially if the client is severely kyphotic. For example, the client may have difficulty finding clothes that fit properly. Social interactions may be curtailed because of a change in appearance or the physical limitations of being unable to sit in chairs in restaurants, movie theaters, and other places. Alterations in sexuality may occur as a result of poor self-esteem or the discomfort imposed by positioning during intercourse.

Because osteoporosis readily predisposes a client to fractures, the client must be extremely cautious about activities. As a result, the threat of fracture can create anxiety and fear and result in further limitation of social or physical activities. The nurse assesses for the presence of these feelings because they may affect the response to health care. For instance, the client may be anxious to the point that he or she will not exercise as prescribed for fear that a fracture will occur.

■ LABORATORY ASSESSMENT

There are no definitive laboratory tests that confirm a diagnosis of primary osteoporosis; however, a number of biochemical markers can provide information about bone modeling. A battery of tests can be performed to rule out secondary osteoporosis or other metabolic bone diseases, such as osteomalacia and Paget's disease. These include determination of serum calcium, vitamin D, phosphorus, and alkaline phosphatase levels.

Urinary calcium levels may also be assessed. Serum protein measurements and thyroid function tests are performed to exclude hyperthyroidism.

A simple, more specific and sensitive test to evaluate bone resorption is being used with clients with spinal cord injury and others at risk. The Upyr Crosslinks assay measures urinary concentrations of pyridinium, a collagen substance found in bone and cartilage. An increase in urinary levels indicates increased bone resorption (loss). The advantage of this test is its ability to detect bone loss early. In addition, no special client preparation is required. The disadvantage of the test is its cost, which is high because the test is relatively new. However, pyridinium and other biochemical markers of bone modeling may be used in the future as a routine screening test (Hunt, Civitelli, & Halstead, 1995).

■ RADIOGRAPHIC ASSESSMENT

X-ray studies of the spine and long bones show loss of bone density and the presence of fractures. However, radiographic findings of bone density changes are evident only after a 25% to 40% bone loss has occurred.

In the search for a more sensitive diagnostic test to detect early bone changes, computed tomography (CT) has been used extensively, particularly for the spine. CT allows better visualization of changes in the cancellous bone than in the cortical bone. Because the vertebral column consists primarily of cancellous bone, the test is helpful in the early diagnosis of osteoporosis. Quantitative CT (QCT) measures the bone density of vertebral bone.

In the past decade, technologic advances have enabled the detection of early changes in bone density. One of the newer diagnostic tools is dual photon absorptiometry, sometimes called **dual energy x-ray absorptiometry (DEXA)**. DEXA is a painless scan that measures bone mineral density (BMD) in the hip, wrist, or vertebral column. It is the best tool currently available for diagnosis. In July 1998, Medicare began covering the cost of bone density studies for high-risk clients. No special client preparation or follow-up care is required.

CLIENT CARE PLAN • THE CLIENT WITH OSTEOPOROSIS

NURSING DIAGNOSIS NO. 1 • Risk for Falls related to trivial accidents

Expected Outcomes	Nursing Interventions	Rationale
The client will not experience falls or fractures resulting from falls.	Create a hazard-free environment for the client while he or she is in the hospital or other setting. **D** Get the client out of bed with the bed height in the lowest position. **D** Teach the client to wear nonskid slippers. **D** Inspect the floor for spills and the room for equipment that may cause tripping or stumbling. **D** Provide additional lighting for an older client. **D** Place necessary items close to the bed within easy reach (e.g., water pitcher and call bell). **D** Keep two siderails up, especially for older adults who are confused. **D** Teach the importance and use of handrails in the bathroom. **D**	Creating a hazard-free environment reduces the risk of falls and subsequent fracture.
	Provide ambulatory support as needed. **D** Assess the need for a cane or a walker. Consult with a physical therapist. Teach the client to call for assistance. **D** Teach the client to take his or her time when getting out of bed and walking. **D**	Ambulatory aids provide additional support when walking and help prevent rushing, which contributes to falls. Older clients often hurry to the bathroom to prevent incontinence.
	When helping with activities of daily living (ADLs), prevent the client from accidentally hitting siderails, door frames, and so on. **D**	Striking hard surfaces can cause bone fracture, since bones are porous from calcium loss.
	Teach the client to bend or stoop slowly and not to lift or move heavy objects, such as hospital furniture.	Quick body movements can easily lead to vertebral compression fractures in the client with osteoporosis.
	Monitor side effects for any drugs the client may be taking for concurrent medical conditions.	Diuretics, phenothiazines, and tranquilizers can cause dizziness, drowsiness, and weakness, predisposing the client to falls.
	Teach the importance of diet in preventing further osteoporosis. Refer to dietary consultation. Teach the client which foods are high in calcium content. Teach the need to decrease caffeine and alcohol intake.	Dietary calcium is needed to maintain the serum level, thus preventing additional loss from bone. Caffeine excess can increase calcium loss in urine; alcohol excess can promote acidosis, which increases bone resorption.
	Teach the effect of cigarette smoking on bone remodeling (if the client is a smoker).	Cigarette smoking can promote acidosis.

D Indicates tasks that can be delegated to assistive nursing personnel.

■ OTHER DIAGNOSTIC ASSESSMENT

Magnetic resonance imaging (MRI) is sometimes used instead of the CT scan to detect the presence of bone density changes, especially in the spine. Ultrasound has recently been approved to detect osteoporotic bone changes. Although not as precise as DEXA, it is less expensive and more available, making it a good screening tool for the disorder.

● Interventions

Because the client is predisposed to fractures, drugs and diet therapy are used to retard bone resorption and form new bony tissue. Exercise and education can prevent osteoporosis or slow its progress. These measures help to reduce the chance of fracture and subsequent complications (see the Client Care Plan above).

DRUG THERAPY. The health care provider may prescribe estrogen, calcium supplements, vitamin D, biphosphonates (BPs), selective estrogen receptor modulators, calcitonin, or a combination of several drugs to treat osteoporosis, as well as to prevent it (Chart 51-2). Other agents have been given, but with limited success. Estrogen is the least expensive of the drugs used for osteoporosis.

ESTROGEN. Estrogen blocks bone resorption by inhibiting cytokines, which are chemicals that stimulate osteoclastic activity. Therefore estrogen replacement (ERT) is effective in slowing bone loss and treating established disease. Studies have shown a remarkable reduction of fractures in women undergoing estrogen therapy (Capriotti, 2000). It is recommended, however, that the drug be initiated shortly after menopause and continued on a long-term basis.

The health care provider may prescribe low doses, such as 0.625 mg, of conjugated estrogens (Premarin, C.E.S.♣) because the side effects of the drug, such as endometrial or breast cancer, are potentially serious. Some providers do not use the drug for preventive purposes. Others believe that the

CLIENT CARE PLAN • THE CLIENT WITH OSTEOPOROSIS—cont'd

NURSING DIAGNOSIS NO. 2 • Impaired Physical Mobility related to decreased muscle tone, dysfunction secondary to previous fractures, or pain secondary to recent fractures

Expected Outcomes	Nursing Interventions	Rationale
The client will increase mobility to the level of ADL independence.	Consult with the physical therapist regarding an exercise program to include strengthening and weight-bearing exercises. Assist the client as necessary with exercises **D** Teach the client that ADLs do not replace prescribed exercises. Teach the importance of exercises.	Strengthening exercises increase joint movement, increase muscle tone, and stimulate blood circulation to bone and muscle tissue. Weight-bearing exercises decrease the rate of bone loss and increase bone formation.
	Assist with ADLs as necessary, allowing the client to be as independent as possible. **D**	Pain and poor muscle tone may limit the client's ability to be independent, especially after a fracture.
	Assess the need for assistive and adaptive devices in order to perform ADLs; consult with the occupational therapist to obtain appropriate equipment.	Devices may be needed for the client to be independent in ADLs. Overuse and reliance, however, should be discouraged.

NURSING DIAGNOSIS NO. 3 • Acute Pain and Chronic Pain related to effects of vertebral fracture

The client will experience alleviation or reduction of pain so that he or she can be independent in care.	Assess the need for pain medication: opioid or non-opioid analgesics, muscle relaxants, or anti-inflammatory drugs.	Clients usually receive pain medication on a prn schedule. Older clients often do not request pain medication even if needed; therefore the nurse must anticipate this need.
	Maintain orthotic devices for vertebral fracture. Check that the brace or corset fits properly. Inspect the skin where the device causes pressure. **D** Apply the device for use when the client gets out of bed. **D**	Orthotic devices maintain spine alignment and provide spinal column support.
	Apply moist heat to the back (heat packs or hot compresses) as needed to reduce pain. (The physical therapist may do this.) (See also Chapter 7.)	Heat increases blood circulation to affected areas, thus relieving muscle spasms, which cause pain.

D Indicates tasks that can be delegated to assistive nursing personnel.

benefit of estrogen in preventing potentially debilitating and life-threatening fractures outweighs its risks. The health care provider often prescribes progesterone along with the estrogen (hormone replacement therapy [HRT]) to minimize cancer occurrence. For middle-aged women, especially those in their 40s and early 50s (sometimes referred to as the "transition years"), birth control pills may be used to provide these supplements. However, some clients do not want to have uterine bleeding and breast tenderness.

A newer form of estrogen, the estrogen patch (Estraderm, Estrace, Femogex✤), delivers an even, continuous amount of estrogen when applied several times each week. These patches are available in several doses, from 4 mg/10 cm (0.05 mg/24 hr) to 8 mg/10 cm (0.1 mg/24 hr).

CALCIUM. If a person cannot ingest sufficient quantities of calcium in the diet, calcium supplements are used. Natural calcium sources, such as oyster shells, are preferable. Supplements should be started in the high-risk population in young adulthood, because bone resorption accelerates after age 30 to 35 years. Calcium carbonate, found in over-the-counter (OTC) drugs such as Tums, is one of the most cost-effective and is best taken with food, since gastric acid is needed to absorb it. Calcium citrate does not require gastric acid for absorption and

is therefore most often recommended as a calcium supplement (Capriotti, 2000). Forty percent of calcium carbonate is elemental calcium that can be used by the body. For example, a 600-mg tablet contains about 240 mg of elemental calcium.

The client should take calcium supplements under the supervision of a health care provider. **Hypercalcemia** (excess serum calcium) can cause serious damage to the urinary system. The amount of calcium prescribed is affected by the addition of estrogen therapy and the presence of risk factors for osteoporosis.

In the United States the typical daily intake of dietary calcium is between 450 and 550 mg. The recommended daily allowance (RDA) of calcium is 1200 mg. Many clinicians and researchers believe that the RDA is insufficient to meet the calcium requirements of postmenopausal women, who may require as much as 1500 mg or more daily to prevent osteoporosis. An increased calcium intake may prevent bone loss in men as well. The nurse teaches the client to consume foods rich in calcium, such as milk and dairy products and dark green, leafy vegetables (see Chapter 11 for a list of foods high in calcium).

VITAMIN D. Vitamin D supplementation may be necessary for the institutionalized or homebound client or for those

CHART 51-2

DRUG THERAPY *for* Osteoporosis

Drug	Usual Dosage	Nursing Interventions	Rationale
Calcium (e.g., Os-Cal, Tums, Caltrate-600, Citracal)	1.0-1.5 g in divided doses PO	Give a third of daily dose at bedtime. Push fluids.	Calcium is most readily utilized by the body when the client is fasting and immobile. Increased fluid intake aids in preventing the formation of calcium-based urinary stones.
		Assess for a history of urinary stones.	Calcium supplements are not given to clients who are susceptible to urinary stone formation.
		Monitor serum calcium level.	Hypercalcemia, or calcium excess, is a side effect of calcium supplementation.
		Monitor urinary calcium level (no more than 4 mg/kg in 24 hr).	The kidneys attempt to excrete excess calcium.
		Observe for signs of hypercalcemia.	Hypercalcemia can result in urinary stones, cardiac arrhythmias, and an increase or decrease in skeletal muscle tone.
Estrogen (e.g., Premarin, Estinyl, Estrace C.E.S.✦, Transderm) may be given with progesterone on days 16-25	0.425-1.25 mg PO for 25 days/mo 0.05 mg/24 hr or 0.1 mg/24 hr transdermally	Assess for history of tumors, hypertension, thromboembolytic disease, or liver or gallbladder disease.	Estrogen therapy is withheld from clients with susceptibility to an exacerbation of one or more of these problems.
		Teach the importance of gynecologic examinations every 6 months.	Endometrial and breast cancer can result from estrogen therapy.
		Teach breast self-examination.	Clients can detect potentially malignant lesions early so that treatment can begin immediately.
		Observe for vaginal bleeding.	Vaginal bleeding is a side effect of estrogen therapy and a sign of possible endometrial cancer.
		Monitor blood pressure.	Hypertension and other cardiovascular complications may result from combined estrogen-progesterone therapy.
		Observe for thrombus formation.	Deep vein thrombosis is a complication of combined estrogen-progesterone therapy.
		Monitor serum liver enzyme and cholesterol levels.	An elevation of liver enzyme levels may be indicative of liver involvement resulting from estrogen. An elevated cholesterol level can result in hypertension and thrombus formation.
Alendronate (Fosamax)	5 mg/day PO	Take early in AM with 8 oz water; do not lie down until after breakfast.	Although not common, esophagitis or esophageal ulcers may result from alendronate therapy.
Raloxifene (Evista)	60 mg qd	Teach client to monitor weight and BP frequently.	Drug causes increased water and sodium retention.
		Monitor liver function tests (LFTs) in collaboration with health care provider.	Raloxifene can cause increased LFTs or worsen hepatic disease (should not be given to client who has liver disease).
Calcitonin (e.g., Calcimar [salmon], Cibacalcin [human], Miacalcin [salmon; nasal spray])	100 IU/day SC or IM 200 IU/day intranasally, alternating nostrils	Rotate injection sites for parenteral administration.	Injection sites become irritated and reddened.
		Monitor for flushing, headache, nausea, and vomiting.	These are common side effects of calcitonin.
		Monitor renal function, calcium, and vitamin D levels.	Toxicity from calcitonin can cause renal problems.

who do not meet daily requirements. An adequate level of vitamin D is needed for optimal calcium absorption in the intestines. The prescribed dosage is usually 400 to 800 international units (IU)/day. Higher doses can produce toxic effects, such as hypercalcemia and hyperphosphatemia.

BIPHOSPHONATES. Biphosphonates (BPs) inhibit bone resorption by binding with crystal elements in bone, especially spongy, trabecular bone tissue. Two BPs, alendronate (Fosamax) and etidronate (Didronel) have been approved for the prevention and management of osteoporosis, Paget's disease, and hypercalcemia associated with cancer.

Although side effects are not common, when they do occur, they tend to be serious. Esophagitis and esophageal ulcers have been reported with the use of Fosamax, especially when the pill is not completely swallowed. The nurse teaches clients taking this drug to take it early in the morning with 8 ounces of water. They should not lie down until after breakfast. If chest pain occurs, a symptom of esophageal irritation, they should discontinue the drug and contact their health care provider. Clients with poor renal function, hypocalcemia, or gastrointestinal reflux disease (GERD) should not take BPs.

Other BPs, such as risedronate, are being investigated. Because of poor gastrointestinal absorption of most BPs, parenteral administration is also being studied. Clodronate may be given every 2 weeks intramuscularly to enhance bone mineral density (BMD), but the injection is very painful. Ibandronate, given intravenously every 3 months, has shown increases in vertebral bone mass (Capriotti, 2000).

SELECTIVE ESTROGEN RECEPTOR MODULATORS.
Selective estrogen receptor modulators (SERMs), a newer class of drugs, are designed to mimic estrogen in some parts of the body while blocking its effect elsewhere. Raloxifene (Evista) is used for prevention and management of osteoporosis in postmenopausal women. It increases BMD, reduces bone resorption, and lowers serum cholesterol. The recommended dose is 60 mg/day. The drug should not be given to women who have a history of thromboembolitic disease (Leslie, 2000).

CALCITONIN.
Calcitonin is a thyroid hormone that inhibits osteoclastic activity, thus decreasing bone loss. It is used for the treatment of osteoporosis, Paget's disease, and hypercalcemia associated with cancer. The drug also has an analgesic effect after vertebral fracture, thereby promoting early recovery.

Calcitonin (salmon) can be given intramuscularly, subcutaneously, or intranasally (Miacalcin). Nasal administration is preferred because it improves compliance, minimizes side effects, and is convenient. The nurse teaches the client to alternate nostrils to prevent nasal mucosal irritation, a common side effect.

OTHER AGENTS.
Androgens, such as testosterone propionate (Testex, Malogen♣), have been successful in decreasing bone resorption and increasing bone growth. When given to postmenopausal women, however, androgens cause masculine traits and may lead to liver disease. Androgens may decrease bone resorption in men, however, particularly older men.

DIET THERAPY.
The dietary considerations for the treatment of a client with a diagnosis of osteoporosis are the same as those for preventing the disease. Adequate amounts of protein, magnesium, vitamin K, and trace minerals are needed for bone formation. Calcium and vitamin D intake needs to be increased, and alcohol and caffeine consumption should be discouraged. For the client who has sustained a fracture, intake of protein, vitamin C, and iron is increased to promote bone healing.

PREVENTION OF FALLS.
The client must be careful to prevent falls and other activities that can cause a fracture. A hazard-free environment is necessary to meet this goal, and the nurse must teach the client about its importance.

Many hospitals and long-term care facilities have risk management programs in which clients are assessed for their risk for falls. For those at high risk, programs such as the Falling Star protocol have reduced falls by making the staff aware of the client's high risk. In this program, a star is placed at the head of the bed to designate a person at high risk. Chap-

ter 5 discusses fall prevention in health care agencies and at home in more detail.

Hip protectors are inexpensive devices that can prevent hip fracture if the client experiences a fall. A hip protector is a pad that is worn while ambulating. If the client falls onto his or her trochanter, the probability of hip fracture is lessened.

EXERCISE.
Exercise is important in the prevention and management of osteoporosis. It also plays a vital role in pain management, cardiovascular function, and an improved sense of well-being.

In collaboration with the health care provider, the physical therapist prescribes exercises for strengthening the abdominal and back muscles. These exercises improve posture and provide an improved support for the spine. Abdominal isometrics, deep breathing, and pectoral stretching are stressed in order to increase pulmonary capacity. Exercises for the extremity muscles include isometric, resistive, and range-of-motion (ROM) exercises. The nurse encourages active ROM exercises, which improve joint mobility and increase muscle tone.

In addition to exercises for muscle strengthening, a general weight-bearing exercise program is implemented. Walking for 30 minutes three times a week, swimming, or bicycling are recommended activities. The nurse teaches the client that certain high-impact recreational activities, such as bowling and horseback riding, may cause vertebral compression and should be avoided.

PAIN MANAGEMENT.
The pain management program depends on the intensity and duration of the pain. With treatment, pain from spinal fractures often resolves 6 to 8 weeks after injury; treatment usually includes drug therapy and orthotic devices. The health care provider prescribes analgesics (opioid and nonopioid) during the acute phase of the pain (i.e., from the time of injury to as long as several weeks afterward). Muscle relaxants, which ease the discomfort associated with muscle spasms, are often used for spinal fractures. Nonsteroidal anti-inflammatory drugs (NSAIDs) are beneficial for pain relief and for decreasing spinal nerve root inflammation from crushed vertebrae. The nurse is alert to the problems associated with NSAIDs, such as gastrointestinal bleeding and congestive heart failure, particularly in older adults.

ORTHOTIC DEVICES.
Known as dorsolumbar orthoses, orthotic devices immobilize the spine during the acute pain phase and provide spinal column support (Figure 51-2). The physical therapist or orthotist custom fits the client for this lightweight device. The client is taught to inspect the skin for irritation and report tolerance to the device.

CRITICAL THINKING CHALLENGE
You are working in a nursing home where one of your older female residents has fallen three times this week. When you review her chart, you note that she has been diagnosed with osteoporosis for about 10 years but has not been treated. The resident ambulates independently without an assistive device.
- What assessments will you want to perform on this resident?
- What options might the resident have for medical management of her osteoporosis?
- What health teaching should you plan for her?

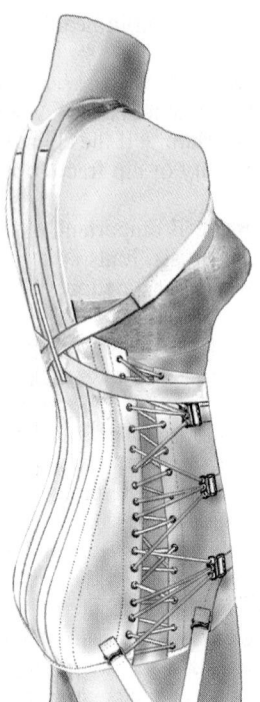

Figure 51-2 ● A dorsolumbar orthosis. (Courtesy Truform Orthotics and Prosthetics, Cincinnati, OH.)

● Community-Based Care

Clients with osteoporosis are usually managed at home. However, some experience fractures that may require hospitalization.

The client with osteoporosis who has one or more fractures can be discharged to the home setting. In some instances, the client is discharged to a long-term care facility for rehabilitation or permanent residence when support systems are not available.

■ HOME CARE MANAGEMENT

If the client is discharged to the home setting, the nurse must assess the environment for potential hazards before discharge. The nurse uses the database completed by the nurse or occupational therapist at the time of admission to ascertain whether alterations in the home environment are necessary. For example, if scatter rugs are used in the home, the client is advised to have these removed to reduce the chance of falling.

A two-story house or apartment may be a problem if physical mobility is limited or if an adequate support railing is not available to assist with stair climbing. The social worker, discharge planner, or case manager, in conjunction with the nurse, helps the client identify adaptations that may have to be made to create as hazard free an environment as possible.

Assistive or adaptive devices for personal use may be needed, if only for a short time. Devices to assist with activities of daily living (ADLs), such as a dressing stick to put on pants, are helpful in maintaining the client's independence. The occupational therapist works with the nurse to determine the need for assistive devices. Chapter 10 describes the promotion of ADL independence in detail.

The nurse and physical therapist assess the need for ambulatory aids in the home. A walker or cane may provide the additional support necessary to prevent falls.

■ HEALTH TEACHING

The teaching plan for the client with osteoporosis includes prevention of falls (see the Meeting Healthy People 2010 Objectives box on p. 1096), exercise, diet therapy, and drug therapy. Psychosocial support is also important to help the client maintain the highest quality of life possible.

PREVENTION OF FALLS. Clients must be extremely careful to prevent falls. Ambulatory aids should be used for additional support, although some clients refuse to be seen in public with a cane or walker. Similarly, clients may not want to wear orthotic devices because of embarrassment or discomfort. The nurse and physical therapist provide a thorough explanation of the necessity and the proper method for using these devices.

EXERCISE. The physical therapist prescribes a structured exercise program, which the nurse reinforces. Strengthening, ROM, and weight-bearing exercises are taught. Follow-up physical therapy visits ensure that clients have learned the exercises and are compliant.

DIET THERAPY. The nurse emphasizes the importance of a diet rich in calcium-containing foods. A diet consultation before discharge can help clients select foods they like and that are high in the essential nutrients. If a fracture has occurred, the nurse encourages clients to eat foods rich in vitamin C, protein, and iron. The nurse also instructs them to decrease caffeine and alcohol consumption and to stop smoking.

DRUG THERAPY. For clients who will be homebound or institutionalized, sunlight exposure should be promoted as an essential source of vitamin D. The importance of sunlight should be stressed to the long-term care facility where the client may be transferred. The nurse teaches about the therapeutic and adverse effects associated with drug therapy for osteoporosis (see Chart 51-2).

PSYCHOSOCIAL SUPPORT. Because clients are often afraid that they will sustain a fracture, it is extremely important to allay their fears to the extent possible. The degree of osteoporosis determines the likelihood of injury. The more severe the osteoporosis, the more limited the activities should be. For example, a woman with severe osteoporosis may sustain vertebral compression fractures from stooping or bending. For most clients, an aggressive treatment plan prevents fractures from trivial trauma.

Explaining the importance of orthotic and ambulatory aids in the prevention of injury increases compliance and decreases reluctance to use the devices. A supportive spouse, family member, or significant other can encourage clients to adhere to the treatment plan.

✥ CONSIDERATIONS FOR OLDER ADULTS

Because most clients with osteoporosis are older, they may not comply with the diet or exercise. Often the older adult is used to eating less than the required daily nutrients. Consumption of milk and dairy products is usually minimal. As a result, the health care provider prescribes calcium supplements for long-term maintenance. The nurse instructs clients to take only the prescribed amount; too much calcium can lead to hypercalcemia. Exercise compliance may also be a problem for older adults.

Clients who are receiving estrogen therapy need to have frequent gynecologic checkups to detect early signs of endometrial cancer. The nurse teaches clients how to monitor for side effects. Follow-up visits to the health care provider are scheduled frequently to monitor calcium blood levels and determine further progression of osteoporosis.

■ HEALTH CARE RESOURCES

If the client cannot return home after a fracture, placement in a nursing home may be necessary, at least for a short time. The hospital nurse or case manager documents the client's needs on the transfer record and communicates the special considerations required.

If returning to a home environment, the client may need equipment for ADLs and ambulation. Financial resources are assessed before equipment is obtained. If the client's insurance or other third-party payer will not reimburse him or her, other sources are explored. Religious and support organizations are possible resources for free materials. Items are often donated to these groups for use as needed in the community. Rental of equipment is also an option. The hospital or local medical supplier can provide cost estimates of renting versus purchasing the needed equipment. The equipment should be accessible before the client returns home.

A home care nurse may be needed for follow-up in the home environment. The nurse in this setting can be contacted to assist in the discharge planning for the client, to assess potential environmental hazards, and to obtain equipment and supplies. The home care nurse determines the need for physical or occupational therapy, social work, and homemaking personnel in the home.

In addition to home care resources, the Osteoporosis Foundation provides information to clients and health care professionals regarding the disease and its treatment. Large metropolitan hospitals often have osteoporosis specialty clinics and support groups for clients with osteoporosis.

Osteomalacia
■ OVERVIEW

Osteomalacia is a reversible metabolic disease in which there is a defect in the mineralization of bone. Unlike in osteoporotic tissue, the amount and quality of bone matrix (osteoid) in osteomalacia are normal but mineralization is delayed or inadequate (Table 51-2).

■ Pathophysiology

Osteomalacia is the adult equivalent of rickets, or vitamin D deficiency, in children. In its natural form, vitamin D is obtained from the ultraviolet radiation of the sun and from certain foods. In combination with calcium and phosphorus, the vitamin is necessary for bone formation.

Vitamin D is actually a group of vitamins, including vitamins D_2 and D_3. The naturally occurring substance is D_3 (cholecalciferol), which is manufactured by photochemical activation in the skin, which is triggered by the sun's ultraviolet light. As illustrated in Figure 51-3, the D_3 from either the skin or food is carried to the liver bound to an alpha globulin as transcalciferin. There, part of the substance is converted to 25-hydroxycholecalciferol, or calcidiol.

Characteristic	Osteoporosis	Osteomalacia
Definition	Decreased bone mass	Demineralized bone
Pathophysiology	Lack of calcium	Lack of vitamin D
Radiographic findings	Osteopenia, fractures	Pseudofractures, Looser's zones, fractures
Calcium level	Normal	Low or normal
Phosphate level	Normal	Low or normal
Parathyroid hormone	Normal	High or normal
Alkaline phosphatase	Normal	High

TABLE 51-2 ● DIFFERENTIAL FEATURES OF OSTEOPOROSIS AND OSTEOMALACIA

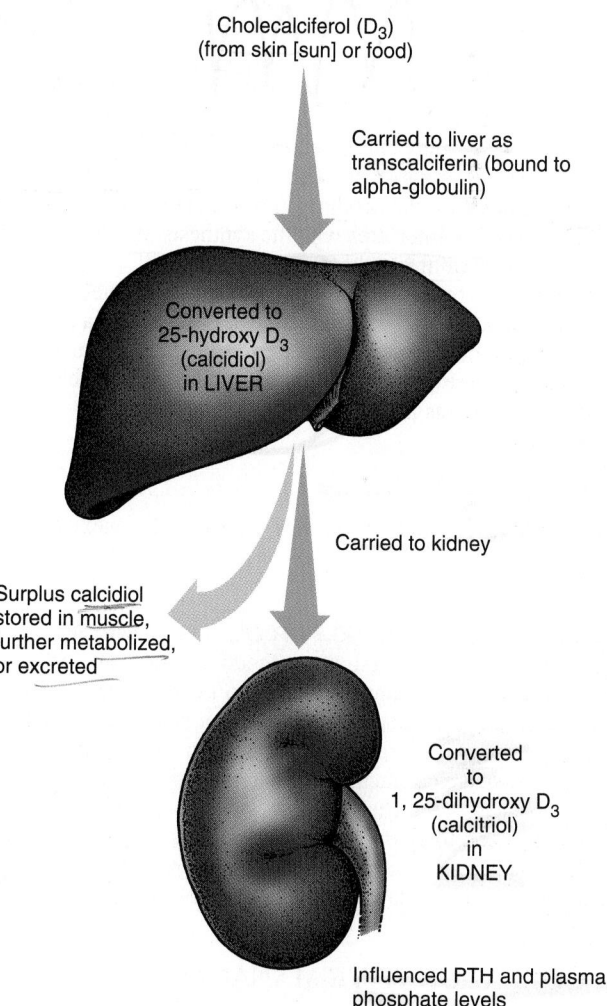

Figure 51-3 ● Process of vitamin D metabolism in the body. (*PTH*, Parathyroid hormone.)

Calcidiol is then transported to the kidney for transformation into the major active vitamin D metabolite, 1,25-dihydroxycholecalciferol, or calcitriol. The amount of calcitriol produced is regulated by parathyroid hormone (PTH) and the blood level of phosphate, the inorganic form of phosphorus. Calcitriol production increases when there is an increase in PTH or a decrease in serum phosphate levels.

Calcitriol is needed for optimal intestinal absorption of calcium and works in combination with PTH for the release of calcium from bone to assist in serum calcium regulation. Consequently, calcitriol or vitamin D deficiency results in decreased calcium absorption from the gut, which in turn leads to PTH stimulation and a decrease in both serum phosphate and calcium levels.

In osteomalacia, a primary or secondary vitamin D deficiency causes insufficient bone mineralization. Nonmineralized or poorly mineralized osteoid accumulates over the surfaces of both cortical and cancellous bone.

◼ Etiology

In addition to primary vitamin D deficiency related to lack of sunlight exposure or dietary intake, vitamin D deficiency attributable to various pathologic conditions may result in osteomalacia (Table 51-3). Malabsorption of the vitamin from the small bowel is a common postsurgical complication of partial or total gastrectomy and bypass or resection surgery of the small intestine. Disease of the small bowel, such as Crohn's disease, may cause decreased vitamin absorption. Liver and pancreatic disorders interrupt vitamin D metabolism and decrease the production of usable substance. Renal failure or disease interferes with the synthesis of calcitriol, the most active vitamin metabolite.

Conditions that contribute to phosphate depletion (hypophosphatemia) lead to osteomalacia. Osteomalacia is also a complication of the intake of certain drugs, particularly anticonvulsants, barbiturates, and fluoride. The exact mechanism for the drug effects is not known.

◼ Incidence/Prevalence

Until recently, osteomalacia was considered nonexistent in Western countries.

> **✿ CONSIDERATIONS FOR OLDER ADULTS**
> Although the disease is not thought to be common, researchers and clinicians are exploring its incidence in older adults. In the older population, significant numbers of people are deprived of sun exposure, maintain poor diets, or both. Although there are no statistical data to indicate the incidence of osteomalacia in the United States, health care professionals are continuing to study its occurrence in nursing homes and other residences for older adults. As a result, osteomalacia is recognized as a health problem for the older population.

▶ COLLABORATIVE MANAGEMENT
◼ Assessment

The important data for the nurse to obtain for a client with osteomalacia or suspected osteomalacia include age, exposure to sunlight, and skin pigmentation. The older adult who has been homebound or chronically institutionalized is at the greatest risk. People who have dark skin and consume minimal protein are more at risk than light-skinned people with the same dietary habits. The nurse also takes a thorough diet history to determine the intake of foods containing vitamin D and calcium.

◼ PHYSICAL ASSESSMENT/CLINICAL MANIFESTATIONS

Osteomalacia is easily confused with osteoporosis. Many of the clinical manifestations are similar, and both disorders may occur at the same time.

In the early stages of osteomalacia, the manifestations are nonspecific. Muscle weakness and bone pain are often misdiagnosed as arthritis or rheumatism. In some cases, proximal muscle weakness in the shoulder and pelvic girdle areas is the only complaint.

Muscle weakness in the lower extremities may cause a waddling and unsteady gait, which contributes to falls and subsequent fractures. Hypophosphatemia leads to an inadequate production of muscle cell adenosine triphosphate, thus resulting in a decrease in muscle cell energy. If hypocalcemia is present, muscle cramping may accompany the weakness.

The nurse assesses muscle strength and observes the client's gait. The nurse records complaints of muscle cramps and bone pain. The skeletal discomfort is often vague and generalized. The spine, ribs, pelvis, and lower extremities are most often affected. The client usually describes the pain as aggravated by activity and worse at night.

In addition to the client's subjective complaint of pain, the nurse palpates the affected bones for tenderness. Bone tenderness can be elicited by pressure on the tibia or rib cage. The nurse observes skeletal malalignment as long-bone bowing or spinal deformity, similar to that seen in osteoporosis. In extreme cases, the pelvis narrows, so that vaginal childbirth is difficult.

If osteomalacia is untreated, vertebral, rib, and long-bone fractures may occur. The client may be misdiagnosed as having bone cancer or osteoporosis.

◼ DIAGNOSTIC ASSESSMENT

Table 51-2 shows the changes in laboratory values that help to support the diagnosis of osteomalacia. X-ray studies of bone tissue with osteomalacia show a decrease in the trabeculae of cancellous bone and lack of osteoid sharpness. The classic diagnostic finding specific to the disease, however, is the presence of radiolucent bands (Looser's lines or zones). Looser's zones are pseudofractures; they represent stress fractures that have not mineralized. They often appear symmetrically in the inner femora, ribs, and inferior pubic rami and may progress to complete fractures with minimal trauma.

TABLE 51-3 • CAUSES OF OSTEOMALACIA

VITAMIN D DISTURBANCE	KIDNEY DISEASE
Inadequate production	Chronic renal failure
Lack of sunlight exposure	Renal tubular disorders
Dietary deficiency	• Acidosis
Abnormal metabolism	• Hypophosphatemia
Drug therapy	
• Phenytoin (Dilantin)	**FAMILIAL METABOLIC**
• Fluoride	**ERROR**
• Barbiturates	Hypophosphatemia
Liver disease	
Renal disease	
Inadequate absorption	
• Postgastrectomy	
• Malabsorption syndrome	
Inflammatory bowel disease	

● Interventions

Because the nursing diagnoses for osteomalacia are the same as those for osteoporosis, the client goals are also similar. An increase in vitamin D through dietary intake, sun exposure, and drug supplementation is promoted. The nurse teaches about foods high in vitamin D and the importance of frequent sun exposure for the manufacture of the vitamin.

The recommended daily allowance (RDA) of vitamin D is 10 μg, or 400 international units (IU). Because older adults are at risk for bone demineralization from aging, as well as for osteomalacia, a safe and adequate daily requirement may be as high as 15 to 20 g, or 600 to 800 IU. Chart 51-3 lists interventions for helping older clients meet the daily requirement of vitamin D.

Paget's Disease of the Bone

■ OVERVIEW

Paget's disease, or osteitis deformans, is a metabolic disorder of bone remodeling, or turnover, in which increased resorption or loss results in bone deposits that are weak, enlarged, and disorganized. First described in 1876 by Sir James Paget, an English surgeon, the disease was thought to be an inflammatory process, infectious in origin. Until the 1960s, Paget's disease was considered a medical curiosity and given little attention. With the growing number of affected older adults in Western countries, interest in the disease has increased and treatment has improved.

Three pathophysiologic phases of the disorder have been described: active, mixed, and inactive. In the first phase (the active phase), a prolific increase in osteoclasts (cells that break down bone) causes massive bone destruction and deformity. The osteoclasts of pagetic bone are large and multinuclear, unlike the osteoclasts of normal bone tissue.

In the mixed phase, the osteoblasts (bone-forming cells) react in a compensatory manner to form new bone. The result is bone that is disorganized and chaotic in structure. The new trabecular bone has a mosaic pattern with a volume twice that of normal bone.

When the osteoblastic activity exceeds the osteoclastic activity, the inactive phase occurs. The newly formed bone becomes sclerotic and Ivory hard. The number of osteoclasts begins to return toward normal.

As a result of the metabolic bone process, the vascularity of the newly formed bone tissue is increased. The arterial capillaries of pagetic bone become hypertrophied, causing marrow sinus and venous system distention. Paget's disease occurs in one bone or in multiple sites. The most common areas of involvement are the vertebrae, the femur, the skull, the sternum, and the pelvis.

The exact cause of Paget's disease is unknown, but it may be the result of a latent viral infection contracted in young adulthood and manifesting as a disease 20 to 40 years later. Bone biopsy specimens have revealed an antigen from a respiratory virus and measles. Because the disorder is present in monozygotic twins, a familial autosomal dominant pattern has been suggested. The disease has been noted in up to 30% of people with a positive family history for Paget's disease.

> **CONSIDERATIONS FOR OLDER ADULTS**
> Approximately 1 to 3 million people in the United States suffer from Paget's disease. It is primarily a disease of the older age-group. It occurs in a very small percentage of people younger than 40 years of age.

> **CULTURAL CONSIDERATIONS**
> Because Paget's disease occurs more often in Europe and less often in Asia and Scandinavia, there may be a possible link between the disease and ethnic origin.

▶ COLLABORATIVE MANAGEMENT
● Assessment

■ PHYSICAL ASSESSMENT/CLINICAL MANIFESTATIONS

Of clients with Paget's disease, 80% are asymptomatic. The disease may be confined to one bone. The disease is often accidentally discovered during a routine laboratory or radiographic examination. In more severe disease, the manifestations are diverse and potentially fatal (Chart 51-4).

MUSCULOSKELETAL AND NEUROLOGIC ASSESSMENT. Bone pain causes the client to seek medical attention. The pain is aching, poorly described, deep, and worsened by pressure and weight bearing. It is most noticeable at night or when the client is resting, and the pain is typically mild to moderate. Back pain and headache are common complaints.

CHART 51-3

NURSING FOCUS *on the* OLDER ADULT
Meeting the Daily Requirement for Vitamin D

- Advise clients to get sun exposure for at least 5 minutes weekly, even in the summer and winter.
- Recommend that clients eat food high in calcium to promote vitamin D absorption and utilization in the small intestines.
- Suggest that clients eat natural and fortified foods containing vitamin D, including milk and dairy products, such as ice cream (or ice milk), yogurt, and cheese.
- Recommend that clients exercise on a regular basis (at least three times a week for 20 to 30 minutes) to prevent bone loss.

CHART 51-4

KEY FEATURES *of*
Paget's Disease of the Bone

Musculoskeletal Manifestations
- Bone and joint pain (may be in a single bone) that is aching, poorly described, and aggravated by walking
- Low back and sciatic nerve pain
- Bowing of long bones
- Loss of normal spinal curvature
- Enlarged, thick skull
- Pathologic fractures
- Osteogenic sarcoma

Skin Manifestations
- Flushed, warm skin

Other Manifestations
- Apathy, lethargy, fatigue
- Hyperparathyroidism
- Gout
- Urinary or renal stones
- Heart failure from fluid overload

The pain associated with the disorder may result from metabolic bone activity, secondary arthritis, impending fracture, or nerve impingement. Arthritis occurs at the joints of the affected bones, but its relationship to Paget's disease is unclear. Nerve impingement is particularly common in the lumbosacral area of the vertebral column, presenting as back pain that radiates along one or both lower extremities.

The nurse assesses the location and extent of the client's pain to determine the areas involved. Posture, stance, and gait are also observed to identify gross bony deformities. Because of the enlargement of the vertebrae, loss of normal spinal curvature, and lower extremity malalignment, the client is usually short. Long-bone bowing in the arms and legs with subsequent varus deformity of the elbows and knees is often symmetric. Flexion contractures of the hips are often present.

When performing a musculoskeletal assessment in a client with Paget's disease, the nurse pays particular attention to the size and shape of the skull, which is typically soft, thick, and enlarged. Involvement of the temporal bone may lead to deafness and vertigo, whereas basilar complications can compress any of the cranial nerves and result in neurologic compromise. Platybasia, or basilar invagination, causes brainstem manifestations that threaten life. In some cases, the bony enlargement of the skull blocks cerebrospinal fluid (CSF), resulting in hydrocephalus.

Pathologic fractures may be the presenting clinical manifestation of the disorder. As many as 30% of clients with Paget's disease sustain at least one incomplete or complete fracture. The femur and the tibia are most often affected, and fracture of these bones can result from minimal trauma. The fracture line is usually perpendicular to the long axis of the bone, and healing is unpredictable because of abnormal metabolic activity within the bone.

The most dreaded complication of Paget's disease is neoplasm, most commonly osteogenic sarcoma (see the discussion under Malignant Bone Tumors, p. 1112). Sarcomas occur in about 1% of clients with pagetic bone. They appear primarily in the pelvis, the femur, and the humerus and carry a grave prognosis because of early metastasis to the lung or extensive local invasion. They are often multifocal, and they occur more often in men. When severe bone pain is present in a client with Paget's disease, neoplasm is suspected.

SKIN ASSESSMENT. The nurse assesses the skin for its color and temperature. In people with Paget's disease, the skin is typically flushed and warm because of increased vascularity. In addition, the nurse assesses the client's energy level. The client usually complains of apathy, lethargy, and fatigue.

OTHER MANIFESTATIONS. Other, less common manifestations of Paget's disease include hyperparathyroidism and gout. Secondary hyperparathyroidism leads to an increase in serum and urinary calcium levels. In severe cases, calcium excess results from prolonged immobilization. Calcium deposits occur in joint spaces or as stones in the urinary tract. Hyperuricemia (serum uric acid excess) and gout occur because the increased metabolic activity of bone creates an increase in nucleic acid catabolism.

In a few cases, increased vascularity causes an increase in cardiac output, resulting in congestive heart failure. Cardiac complications tend to occur only when more than a third of the skeleton is involved.

■ LABORATORY ASSESSMENT

Increases in serum alkaline phosphatase (ALP) and urinary hydroxyproline levels are the primary laboratory findings indicating the probability of Paget's disease. Overactive osteoblasts cause the alteration in ALP level. An evaluation of the 24-hour urinary hydroxyproline level reflects an increase in bone collagen turnover and indicates the degree of the disease process. The higher the value of hydroxyproline, the greater the severity of Paget's disease.

The calcium levels in blood and urine are normal or elevated. The immobilized client is more likely to have an increase in calcium levels as a result of calcium moving from bone into the blood.

Paget's disease often causes an elevation of uric acid because nucleic acid from overactive bone metabolism increases. This finding may be misinterpreted as primary gout.

■ RADIOGRAPHIC ASSESSMENT

X-ray studies of pagetic bone reveal radiolucent, or punched-out, areas indicative of increased bone resorption. Depending on the phase of the disease, the overall bone mass is enlarged and the cortices are thickened. Malalignment deformities, fractures, and secondary arthritic changes may be present.

Computed tomography (CT) is useful in the detection of sarcomas, changes in the skull, and spinal cord or nerve compression.

■ OTHER DIAGNOSTIC ASSESSMENT

Bone scans using radioactive isotopes are only slightly more sensitive than routine x-ray studies in delineating the bone changes of Paget's disease. When the diagnosis is difficult, the physician may perform a bone biopsy. Magnetic resonance imaging (MRI) may also be used for the same purpose as the CT scan.

● Interventions

Nonsurgical or surgical management may be necessary to reduce pain. Nonsurgical interventions are used initially.

NONSURGICAL MANAGEMENT. Drug therapy is the primary intervention used for pain relief. Not only can drugs relieve pain, but also they may cause the disease to go into remission for a period of time by reducing pagetic bone resorption. Other pain relief measures are also used.

DRUG THERAPY. The purpose of drug therapy in Paget's disease is to relieve pain and to decrease bone resorption. Mild to moderate pain may be alleviated by aspirin or nonsteroidal anti-inflammatory drugs (NSAIDs), such as ibuprofen (Motrin, Apo-Ibuprofen✦). When the calcium level is more than twice the normal value and multisystem disease is present, the physician usually prescribes more potent drugs, such as calcitonin, etidronate disodium (EHDP), mithramycin, or one of the new biphosphonates (BPs).

Calcitonin. Calcitonin is a thyroid hormone that is 75% effective in initiating a remission of Paget's disease. It seems to retard bone resorption and, subsequently, relieve pain. The drug often causes a dramatic decrease in the alkaline phosphatase level in a few weeks. Given intramuscularly, subcutaneously, or intranasally (Miacalcin), calcitonin (salmon) is a fairly safe medication but has side effects, including nausea, flushing, and rash. Intranasal administration can cause nasal mucosal irritation. Most of these effects occur within 1 hour of drug administration. The usual duration of therapy is 6 months, followed by a 6-month course of etidronate.

Etidronate. Etidronate (Didronel), an older BP, is prescribed orally in a dosage range of 5 to 20 mg/kg/day and tends to have a longer-lasting effect on Paget's disease as compared with calcitonin. The dosage is kept to a minimum because high dosages may cause osteomalacia or vitamin D deficiency. Its major disadvantage is that the drug is poorly absorbed from the small intestine. Therefore etidronate should be taken on an empty stomach 1 to 2 hours after breakfast or at bedtime with water or juice. Milk or milk products inhibit the drug's absorption as well. Diarrhea may occur in a few clients, but this problem is treated with an antidiarrheal medication.

Calcitonin and Didronel are often the first drugs prescribed and are often used in combination. If repeated courses of these drugs are not effective, mithramycin or other BPs may be added to the drug regimen.

Mithramycin. Mithramycin (plicamycin, Mithracin) is a potent antineoplastic and antibiotic with many side effects. It is reserved for clients with marked hypercalcemia or severe disease with neurologic compromise. By suppressing both osteoblast and osteoclast activity, the drug can relieve bone pain in 4 to 5 days. The usual dosage range is 10 to 25 $\mu g/kg/day$ IV, with 15 $\mu g/kg$ being the most commonly administered dosage. The nurse observes for signs of toxicity to the liver, gastrointestinal tract, and kidneys. Liver and kidney function test results and intake and output are monitored daily. Because mithramycin also suppresses platelets, daily platelet counts and bleeding precautions are taken. When liver enzyme levels become extremely high, drug therapy is interrupted temporarily.

Biphosphonates. Calcitonin and etidronate typically reduce pain and achieve a 50% reduction in bone resorption. Newer and more potent biphosphonates (BPs) achieve a greater reduction and promote disease remission. The duration of remission may exceed 1 year or more after a single course of drug therapy (Siris, 1999).

BPs work by binding with crystal elements in the bone to inhibit bone resorption. A number of BPs have been established in many countries as effective treatment for Paget's disease of the bone, myeloma, and bone metastases. Examples include tiludronate, alendronate, and risedronate. Short-term therapy with oral olpadronate has been successful for treatment of clients with Paget's disease in countries other than the United States.

The nurse and health care provider monitor the client's alanine phosphatase levels periodically to determine drug effectiveness. Periodic x-ray studies may also be ordered to assess bone changes during and after drug therapy.

OTHER PAIN RELIEF INTERVENTIONS. In addition to administering medication, the nurse uses physical measures to reduce pain. These measures may include application of heat, massage, and institution of an exercise program, and they are performed in conjunction with a physical therapist. The client may be fitted for an orthotic device to immobilize and provide support for the vertebrae or long bones. Additional interventions for pain relief, such as relaxation techniques, are discussed in Chapter 7.

The nurse provides the client with the address for the Paget's Disease Foundation and the local chapter of the Arthritis Foundation. These resources provide information and support for the client and family or significant others.

SURGICAL MANAGEMENT. When a client with Paget's disease has secondary arthritis and pain relief is not achieved, he or she may undergo a partial or total joint replacement (see Chapter 21).

OSTEOMYELITIS

OVERVIEW

Osteomyelitis is the term used to describe any infection of the bone. Even with current antibiotic treatment options, osteomyelitis continues to be a common problem and a difficult challenge for the health care team.

Pathophysiology

Osteomyelitis is divided into two major types: acute osteomyelitis and chronic osteomyelitis. An infection lasting less than 4 weeks is acute; an infection lasting longer than that time is chronic.

Regardless of the type of osteomyelitis, the pathophysiologic process is the same. On invasion by one or more pathogenic microorganisms, the bone, and often the surrounding soft tissues, becomes inflamed. The resulting increased vascularity promotes edema. Within several days, vessel thromboses develop, causing ischemia (decreased blood flow) to the involved bone, which consequently dies. The presence of necrotic bone (sequestrum) retards bone healing and causes superimposed infection, often in the form of bone abscess. As shown in Figure 51-4, the cycle repeats itself as the superimposed infection

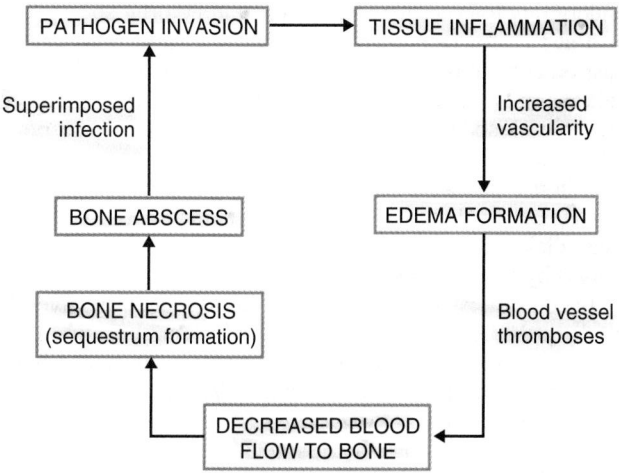

Figure 51-4 ● Infection cycle of osteomyelitis.

leads to further inflammation, vessel thromboses, and necrosis. Increased attention has been given to the mechanisms by which pathogens invade bone tissue: hematogenous spread, direct inoculation, or contiguous spread.

ACUTE OSTEOMYELITIS

Acute hematogenous osteomyelitis occurs more often in children, but it is becoming increasingly common in adults, particularly older adults. An infection occurring in another part of the body moves to and invades bone tissue, particularly the long bones (such as the femur) and the vertebrae. Pathogenic microbes favor bone that has a rich vascular supply and a marrow cavity.

Osteomyelitis resulting from direct inoculation often occurs in adults. The client experiences penetrating trauma, which allows the offending organism direct access to bone tissue. The microbe may originate from the client's skin or from a penetrating object, such as a nail.

Contiguous spread of microorganisms occurs when surrounding soft tissue becomes infected. This mechanism is common in adults who have vascular compromise, as in those with diabetes or peripheral vascular disease. The client with vascular insufficiency is typically older than 50 years of age and has soft-tissue infections of the small bones in the feet or hands. Many different types of microbes invade the adjacent bone simultaneously.

CHRONIC OSTEOMYELITIS

Chronic osteomyelitis may result from any of the acute types. The adult with a compromised vascular supply is at greatest risk for chronic infection. Advanced age and concurrent disease may prolong the course of the infection for as long as a year or more.

Etiology

Each type of bone infection has its own causative factors. Acute hematogenous spread results from bacteremia, underlying disease, or nonpenetrating trauma. Urinary tract infections, particularly in older men, tend to spread to the lower vertebrae. Long-term intravenous (IV) catheters, such as Hickman catheters, are primary sources of infection. Clients undergoing long-term hemodialysis and IV drug abusers are also at risk for osteomyelitis. *Salmonella* infections of the gastrointestinal tract may spread to bone. Clients with sickle cell anemia and other hemoglobinopathies often experience multiple episodes of salmonellosis, which can cause bone infection.

Minimal trauma of the nonpenetrating type can cause hemorrhages or small-vessel occlusions, leading to bone necrosis. Regardless of the source of infection, many infections are caused by *Staphylococcus aureus.*

In contrast, penetrating trauma leads to acute osteomyelitis by direct inoculation. A concurrent soft-tissue infection may be present as well. Animal bites, puncture wounds, and bone surgery can result in bone infection. The most common offending organism is *Pseudomonas aeruginosa,* but other gram-negative bacteria may be found.

Contiguous spread occurs when adjacent soft tissues are infected. Poor dental hygiene and radiation therapy can predispose the mandible to infection.

> **CONSIDERATIONS FOR OLDER ADULTS**
> Malignant external otitis media involving the base of the skull and mastoid bones is seen in older clients with diabetes. The most common case of contiguous spread is found in the client with diabetes or peripheral vascular disease who has a slow-healing foot ulcer. Multiple organisms are responsible for the subsequent osteomyelitis.

If bone infection is misdiagnosed or inadequately treated, chronic osteomyelitis occurs. Inadequate treatment results when the treatment period is too short or when the treatment is delayed or inappropriate. Gram-negative bacteria alone or mixed with gram-positive organisms account for nearly 50% of all chronic bone infections.

COLLABORATIVE MANAGEMENT

Assessment

The client with acute osteomyelitis manifests fever, usually above 101° F (38° C). The area around the infected bone swells and is tender when palpated. Erythema (redness) and heat may also be present.

When vascular insufficiency is suspected, the nurse assesses circulation in the distal extremities. Draining ulcers may be present on the feet or hands, indicating inadequate healing ability as a result of poor circulation.

Bone pain, with or without other manifestations, is a common complaint of clients with bone infection. The pain is described as a constant, localized, pulsating sensation that intensifies with movement. When there is severe vascular compromise, clients may not feel discomfort because of nerve damage from lack of blood supply.

Fever, swelling, and erythema are less common in those with chronic osteomyelitis. Ulceration resulting in sinus tract formation, localized pain, and drainage are more characteristic of chronic infection (Chart 51-5).

The client with osteomyelitis usually has an elevated white blood cell (leukocyte) count, often double the normal value. In chronic infection, normal or slight elevations are not uncommon.

The erythrocyte sedimentation rate (ESR) may be normal early in the course of the disease but rises as the condition progresses. The rate may remain elevated for as long as 3 months after drug therapy is discontinued.

If bacteremia is present, a blood culture identifies the offending organisms to determine which antibiotics should be

CHART 51-5

KEY FEATURES *of* Acute and Chronic Osteomyelitis

Acute Osteomyelitis
- Fever, temperature usually above 101° F (38° C)
- Swelling around the affected area
- Erythema of the affected area
- Tenderness of the affected area
- Bone pain that is constant, localized, and pulsating; intensifies with movement

Chronic Osteomyelitis
- Ulceration of the skin
- Sinus tract formation
- Localized pain
- Drainage from the affected area

used in treatment. Approximately 50% of clients with acute hematogenous infection have positive blood cultures.

Although bone changes cannot be detected early with standard x-ray studies, changes in blood flow can be seen early in the course of the disease by radionuclide scanning. A bone scan, using technetium or gallium, is extremely helpful in the diagnosis of osteomyelitis and identifies most cases. In some cases, magnetic resonance imaging (MRI) may be more sensitive than traditional bone scanning in the diagnosis of osteomyelitis.

The definitive diagnosis of osteomyelitis may be made by bone biopsy. A culture of soft tissue or of the sinus tract may not identify the offending microbes invading the bone. Often the organisms affecting soft tissue and bone are different, and each must be treated.

● Interventions

The specific treatment protocol depends on the type and number of microbes present in the infected tissue. If other measures fail to resolve the infectious process, surgical management may be needed.

NONSURGICAL MANAGEMENT. To reverse osteomyelitis, the health care provider initiates antibiotic therapy as soon as possible. Contact precautions prevent the spread of the offending organism to other clients and health care personnel (see Chapter 26 for a discussion of contact precautions).

DRUG THERAPY. IV antibiotic therapy is usually prescribed for several weeks for acute osteomyelitis. More than one antibiotic may be needed to combat the presence of multiple types of organisms. The hospital or home care nurse gives the drugs at specifically ordered times so that therapeutic serum levels are achieved. The nurse must become familiar with the drugs' actions, side effects, toxicity, interactions, and precautions for administration. Family members in the home setting are taught how to administer the antibiotics.

The optimal drug regimen for clients with chronic osteomyelitis is not well established. Prolonged therapy for more than 3 months may be needed to eliminate the infection. Because of the cost of lengthy hospital stays, clients are typically discharged to the home setting with central IV catheters, such as the Hickman catheter, for medication administration. After discontinuation of IV drugs, oral antibiotic therapy may be needed for weeks or months. A cost-saving alternative to IV drug therapy is the use of newer and more potent oral antibiotics, such as fleroxacin (Megalone).

In addition to parenteral or oral drug administration, the wound may be irrigated, either continuously or intermittently, with one or more antibiotic solutions. The nurse is responsible for drug administration and uses sterile technique at all times. A technique in which beads are impregnated with an antibiotic and packed into the wound provides direct contact of the antibiotic with the offending organism.

INFECTION CONTROL. If an open wound or ulcer is present in the hospital or long-term care setting, the client's treatment usually includes standard precautions for limited infections in which the wound is covered, but this practice varies according to health care agency policy. Contact precautions are reserved for more severe infections, particularly when the purulent material cannot be adequately contained by a dressing. The open area is covered, and strict aseptic technique is used

when dressings are changed to prevent further contamination. Wounds may be managed through the window of a cast, which must remain dry during dressing or irrigation procedures.

HYPERBARIC OXYGEN THERAPY. One fairly new treatment to increase tissue perfusion for clients with chronic, unremitting osteomyelitis is the use of a hyperbaric chamber or portable device to administer hyperbaric oxygen (HBO) therapy. These devices are usually available in large teaching hospitals and may not be accessible to all clients who might benefit from them. With HBO therapy, the affected area is exposed to a high concentration of oxygen that diffuses into the tissues to promote healing. In conjunction with high-dose antibiotic therapy and surgical debridement, HBO has proved very useful in treating a number of anaerobic infections.

SURGICAL MANAGEMENT. Antibiotic therapy alone may not be sufficient to meet the goals of treatment. Surgical techniques are used to minimize the disfigurement that heretofore has been a devastating result of severe osteomyelitis. Most often, surgery is reserved for clients with chronic osteomyelitis.

SEQUESTRECTOMY. Because bone cannot heal in the presence of necrotic tissue, a sequestrectomy is performed to debride the infected bone and allow revascularization of tissue.

BONE GRAFTS. The excision of devitalized and infected bone often results in a sizable cavity, or bone defect. The use of cancellous bone grafts to obliterate bone defects began in the 1940s and is still widely used today. One of the most popular surgical techniques is the Papineau procedure, or open cancellous bone graft, which is used primarily with large bone and soft-tissue defects.

As a three-step procedure, the surgeon excises necrotic bone, grafts the bone, and covers the skin, if necessary (Figure 51-5). The donor bone is most often taken from the client's posterior ileum. The surgeon tightly packs small chips of bone into the cavity and applies a pressure dressing. In 4 or 5 days, the first postoperative dressing is applied in the operating room under sterile conditions. Daily sterile dressings are applied until about 2 weeks later, when the graft stabilizes. If needed, the surgeon performs a skin graft, usually a simple split-thickness graft, between 8 and 16 weeks after the bone graft.

BONE SEGMENT TRANSFERS. When infected bone is extensively resected, reconstruction with microvascular bone transfers may be useful. In general, a bone transfer is reserved for larger skeletal defects.

The most common donor sites are the client's fibula and iliac crest. The bone graft may have an attached muscle or skin flap, if necessary. The steps of the procedure are similar to those of cancellous grafting in that debridement precedes bone transfer.

MUSCLE FLAPS. If the bony defect is relatively small, a muscle flap may be the only surgery required. Local muscle flaps are used in the treatment of chronic osteomyelitis when soft tissue does not obliterate the dead space, or cavity, resulting from bone debridement. The flap provides wound coverage and enhances blood flow to promote healing. A split-thickness skin graft is often applied several days after the muscle flap.

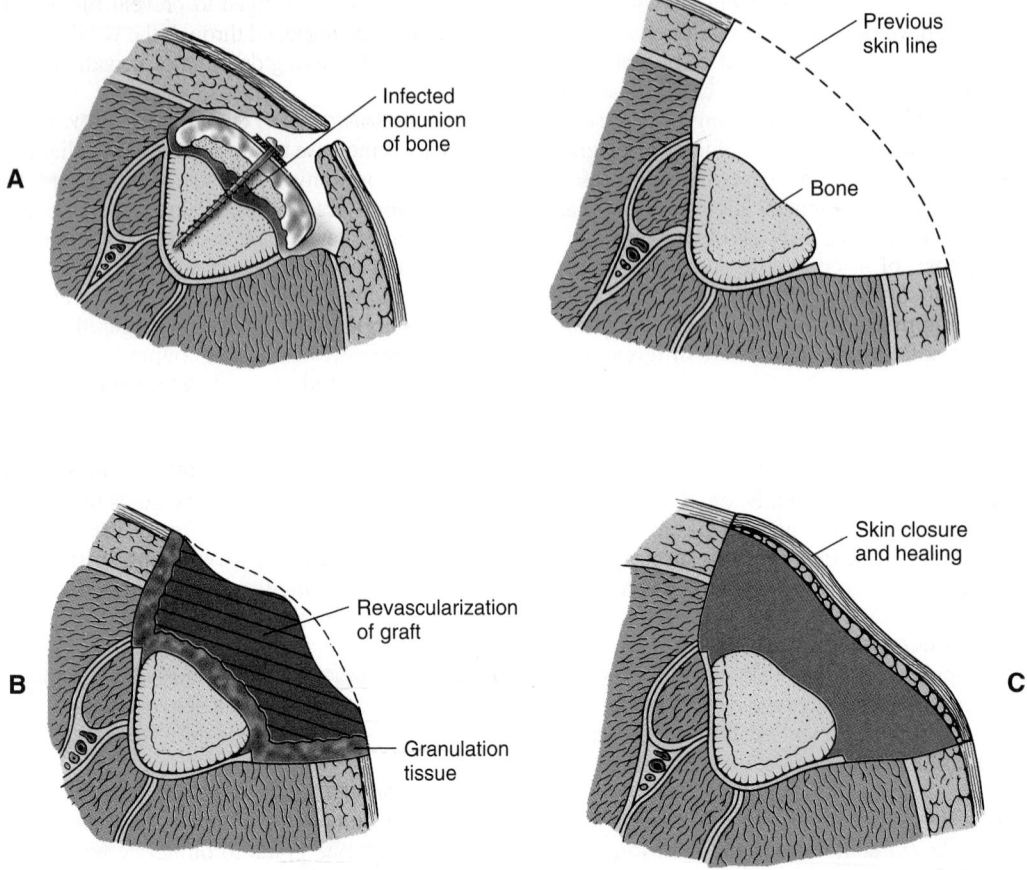

Figure 51-5 ● The three stages of the Papineau procedure. **A,** Stage 1: excision and stabilization, allowing tissue to granulate. **B,** Stage 2: open cancellous bone graft showing vascularization. **C,** Stage 3: skin coverage if not spontaneous.

AMPUTATION. When the previously described surgical procedures are not appropriate or successful, the affected limb may need to be amputated. The physical and psychologic care for a client who has undergone an amputation is discussed in Chapter 52.

For all of the surgical procedures and their recovery phases, long-term antibiotic treatment is necessary. The preoperative and postoperative nursing care is similar to that for repair of musculoskeletal trauma.

> ### CRITICAL THINKING CHALLENGE
>
> A 58-year-old man with a history of diabetes mellitus, coronary artery disease, hypertension, and pulmonary emphysema comes with a foot wound to the clinic where you work. He states that he attempted to cut out an ingrown toenail last week, but his "little knife" slipped and entered the soft tissue around the nail. On inspection, the area is red, warm, and slightly tender. He has a temperature of 101.8° F (39° C).
> * What other physical assessment should be performed at this time?
> * What laboratory tests will the nurse practitioner most likely order?
> * Based on his probable diagnosis, what treatments may the client have?

For suggested answer guidelines, go to [SIMON] http://www.wbsaunders.com/SIMON/Iggy/.

BONE TUMORS
Benign Bone Tumors
▇ OVERVIEW

Benign bone tumors are often asymptomatic and may be discovered on routine x-ray examination or as the cause of pathologic fractures. The cause of benign bone tumors is not known.

Tumors may arise from several types of tissue. The major classifications include chondrogenic tumors (from cartilage), osteogenic tumors (from bone), and fibrogenic tumors (from fibrous tissue and found most often in children) (Table 51-4). The cause of bone tumors, like other neoplasms, is unknown. Although many specific benign tumors have been identified, only the common ones are described here.

▇ Chondrogenic Tumors
▇ OSTEOCHONDROMA

PATHOPHYSIOLOGY/ETIOLOGY. The most common benign bone tumor is the osteochondroma. Although its onset is usually in childhood, the tumor grows until skeletal maturity and may not be diagnosed until adulthood. The tumor may be a single growth or multiple growths and can occur in any bone. The femur and the tibia are most often involved.

TABLE 51-4 • CLASSIFICATION OF PRIMARY BONE TUMORS	
BENIGN	**MALIGNANT**
Chondrogenic	*Chondrogenic*
Osteochondroma	Chondrosarcoma
Chondroma	
	Osteogenic
Osteogenic	Osteosarcoma
Osteoid osteoma	
Osteoblastoma	*Fibrogenic*
Giant cell tumor	Fibrosarcoma
	Unknown Origin
	Ewing's sarcoma

On gross appearance, the tumor has a large cartilaginous cap with a bony stalk protruding from the bone. As the cap grows, the tumor ossifies and may become malignant. About 10% of osteochondromas change into sarcomas.

INCIDENCE/PREVALENCE. Osteochondromas account for about 40% of all benign bone tumors and typically affect males more often than females.

■ CHONDROMA

PATHOPHYSIOLOGY/ETIOLOGY. The chondroma, or endochondroma, is closely related to the osteochondroma in histologic (cellular) presentation. Unlike the osteochondroma, however, the chondroma is a lesion of mature hyaline cartilage affecting primarily the hands and the feet. The ribs, the sternum, the spine, and the long bones may also be involved. Chondromas are slow growing and often cause pathologic fractures after trivial injury.

INCIDENCE/PREVALENCE. Chondromas are found in people of all ages, occur in both males and females, and can affect any bone.

■ Osteogenic Tumors
■ OSTEOID OSTEOMA

PATHOPHYSIOLOGY/ETIOLOGY. The osteoid osteoma is distinguished by its pinkish, granular appearance, resulting from the proliferation of osteoblasts. Unlike other tumors, a single lesion is usually less than 0.4 inch (1 cm) in diameter. Any bone can be affected, but the femur and the tibia are most often involved. When the osteoid osteoma occurs in the spinal column and sacrum, the clinical manifestations resemble those of the lumbar disk syndrome. The client complains of unremitting bone pain, probably attributable to the increase in prostaglandin levels associated with the tumor.

INCIDENCE/PREVALENCE. Approximately 10% of all benign bone tumors are osteoid osteomas. The lesion occurs in children and young adults, with a predominance among males.

■ OSTEOBLASTOMA

PATHOPHYSIOLOGY/ETIOLOGY. Often called *giant osteoid osteoma,* the osteoblastoma affects the vertebrae and long bones. The tumor is larger than the osteoid osteoma

and lies in cancellous bone. Its reddish, granular appearance facilitates diagnosis.

INCIDENCE/PREVALENCE. The lesion accounts for fewer than 1% of primary bone tumors and affects adolescent boys and young adults of both sexes.

■ GIANT CELL TUMOR

PATHOPHYSIOLOGY/ETIOLOGY. The origin of the giant cell tumor remains uncertain. This lesion is aggressive and can be extensive. On gross examination, the lesions are gray to reddish brown and may involve surrounding soft tissue. Although classified as benign, giant cell tumors can metastasize to the lung.

INCIDENCE/PREVALENCE. Unlike most other benign bone tumors, giant cell tumors affect women older than 20 years of age; the peak incidence occurs in clients in their 30s. Approximately 18% of all benign bone tumors are giant cell tumors.

► COLLABORATIVE MANAGEMENT
● Assessment
■ PHYSICAL ASSESSMENT/CLINICAL MANIFESTATIONS

If a client experiences clinical manifestations of a benign bone tumor, pain is the most frequent complaint. The pain can range from mild to moderate, as seen with chondromas, to unremitting and intense, as is typical with osteoid osteomas. Pain can be caused by direct tumor invasion into soft tissue, compressing peripheral nerves, or by a resulting pathologic fracture.

In addition to collecting information regarding the nature of the client's pain, the nurse observes and palpates the suspected involved area. When the tumor affects the lower extremities or the small bones of the hands and feet, local swelling may be detected as the neoplasm enlarges. In some cases, muscle atrophy or muscle spasm may be present. The nurse palpates the bone and muscle to detect these changes and elicit tenderness.

■ DIAGNOSTIC ASSESSMENT

Routine radiography and conventional tomography are extremely beneficial in localizing and visualizing neoplasms of the bone. Benign tumors are characterized by sharp margins, intact cortices, and smooth, uniform periosteal bone.

Computed tomography (CT) is less useful, except in complex anatomic areas, such as the spinal column and sacrum. The test is helpful in evaluating the extent of soft-tissue involvement.

When the diagnosis of a benign tumor is uncertain, an open or needle biopsy of the bone is performed. The open, surgical method is preferred in order to obtain a sufficient amount of tissue.

A bone scan is not specific in distinguishing a benign tumor from a malignant one, but it allows the extent of the lesions to be better visualized as compared with most radiographic examinations.

Magnetic resonance imaging (MRI) may be helpful in viewing problems of the spinal column.

▶ Interventions

NONSURGICAL MANAGEMENT. The physician uses drug therapy and surgery in combination when possible. Nondrug pain relief measures are also used. Depending on the client's preference and tolerance, measures such as application of heat or cold may be helpful to relieve pain.

In addition to ordering analgesics to reduce pain, the health care provider usually prescribes one or more nonsteroidal anti-inflammatory drugs (NSAIDs) to inhibit prostaglandin synthesis and thus relieve pain in the client with an osteoid osteoma. The nurse observes for drug actions and side effects, administering the drug after meals or with milk and crackers.

SURGICAL MANAGEMENT. The most common surgical procedure used for clients with benign bone tumors is curettage, or simple excision of the tumor tissue. If the tumor is small, surgery may not be indicated. When the lesion is extremely extensive, as in a giant cell tumor, the neoplasm is removed with care to restore or maintain the function of the adjacent joint, most often the knee. In some cases, the knee is replaced with a prosthetic device or is fused (arthrodesis). Bone grafting may be needed. The nursing care for clients undergoing these surgical procedures is discussed in Chapter 21.

Malignant Bone Tumors

▮ OVERVIEW

Malignant bone tumors may be primary (those that originate in bone; see Table 51-4) or secondary (those that originate in other tissues and metastasize to bone). Primary tumors occur most often in people between 10 and 30 years of age and make up a small percentage of bone cancers. As for other forms of cancer, the exact cause of bone cancer is unknown. Metastatic lesions most often occur in the older age-group and account for most bone cancers.

▮ Primary Tumors

▮ OSTEOSARCOMA

PATHOPHYSIOLOGY/ETIOLOGY. Osteosarcoma, or osteogenic sarcoma, is the most common type of primary malignant bone tumor. More than 50% occur in the distal femur, followed, in decreasing order of occurrence, by the proximal tibia and humerus. Flat-bone and long-bone incidence is about equal in people older than 25 years of age.

The lesion is relatively large, causing pain and swelling of short duration. The involved area is usually warm, since the vascularity to the site increases. The central portion of the mass is sclerotic from increased osteoblastic activity; the periphery is soft, extending through the bone cortex in the classic sunburst appearance associated with the neoplasm. An inward expansion into the medullary canal is also common.

Osteosarcoma may be osteoblastic, chondroblastic, or fibroblastic, depending on the tissue of origin. Regardless of its source, the lesion typically metastasizes to the periphery of the lung within 2 years of treatment; metastasis usually results in death.

INCIDENCE/PREVALENCE. Osteosarcoma occurs more often in males than in females (2:1), between ages 10 and 30 years, and in older clients with Paget's disease. Clients who have received radiation for other forms of cancer or who have benign lesions are also at high risk.

▮ EWING'S SARCOMA

PATHOPHYSIOLOGY/ETIOLOGY. Although Ewing's sarcoma is not as common as other tumors, it is the most malignant. Like other primary tumors, it causes pain and swelling. In addition, systemic manifestations, particularly low-grade fever, leukocytosis, and anemia, characterize the lesions. The pelvis and the lower extremity are most often affected. Pelvic involvement is a poor prognostic sign.

On a cellular level the tumor is similar to bone lymphoma. On x-ray examination the characteristic mottled destructive pattern and "onion skin" appearance of the bone surface distinguish the neoplasm as Ewing's sarcoma. Like other malignant tumors, it is not encapsulated and often extends into soft tissue. Death results from metastasis to the lungs and other bones.

INCIDENCE/PREVALENCE. Five percent of all malignant bone tumors are Ewing's sarcoma. Although the tumor can be seen in clients of any age, it usually occurs in children and young adults in their 20s. Men are affected more often than women.

▮ CHONDROSARCOMA

PATHOPHYSIOLOGY/ETIOLOGY. In contrast to the client with osteosarcoma, the client with chondrosarcoma experiences dull pain and swelling for a long period. The tumor typically affects the pelvis and proximal femur near the diaphysis. Arising from cartilaginous tissue, the lesion destroys bone and often calcifies. The client with chondrosarcoma has a better prognosis than the client with osteogenic sarcoma.

INCIDENCE/PREVALENCE. Chondrosarcoma occurs in middle-aged and older people, with a slight predominance in men, and accounts for fewer than 10% of all malignant bone tumors.

▮ FIBROSARCOMA

PATHOPHYSIOLOGY/ETIOLOGY. Arising from fibrous tissue, fibrosarcomas can be divided into subtypes, of which malignant fibrous histiocytoma (MFH) is the most malignant. Most often, the clinical presentation of MFH is slow and insidious, without specific manifestations. Local tenderness, with or without a palpable mass, occurs in the long bones of the lower extremity. Like other bone cancers, the lesion can metastasize to the lungs.

INCIDENCE/PREVALENCE. Although MFH affects people of all ages, it typically occurs in middle-aged men. Fortunately, the lesion is not common.

▮ Metastatic Bone Disease

PATHOPHYSIOLOGY/ETIOLOGY. Primary tumors of the prostate, breast, kidney, thyroid, and lung are called *bone-seeking* cancers; they metastasize to the bone more often than other primary tumors. The vertebrae, pelvis, femur, and ribs are the bone sites commonly affected. Simply stated, primary tumor cells, or seeds, are carried to bone through the bloodstream. Almost all metastatic lesions are of epithelial origin and begin in the bone marrow.

Pathologic fractures, which occur in 10% to 15% of cases, are a major concern in management. The most commonly affected areas for fracture are the acetabulum and the proximal femur.

INCIDENCE/PREVALENCE. Metastatic bone tumors greatly outnumber primary malignant neoplasms. Metastatic bone disease primarily affects people older than 40 years of age. In clients with a history of cancer and local pain, metastasis is suspected. The incidence of bone metastasis ranges from 20% to 70%, depending on the statistical reporting source. It is suspected that the reported incidence of metastasis is grossly understated.

► COLLABORATIVE MANAGEMENT

Activity
Link

● Assessment

■ HISTORY

The data collected for the client suspected of having a malignant tumor are similar to the data required for the client with a benign growth. In addition, the nurse asks whether the client has had previous radiation therapy for cancer and elicits information about the client's general health.

■ PHYSICAL ASSESSMENT/CLINICAL MANIFESTATIONS

The clinical manifestations seen in the client with a primary malignant tumor or metastatic disease vary, depending on the specific type of lesion. Most often, the client has a group of nonspecific complaints, including pain, local swelling, and a tender, palpable mass. Marked disability may be present in advanced metastatic bone disease.

In a client with Ewing's sarcoma, a low-grade fever may occur because of the systemic features of the neoplasm. For this reason, Ewing's sarcoma is often confused with osteomyelitis. Fatigue and pallor resulting from anemia are also common.

In performing a musculoskeletal assessment, the nurse inspects the involved area and palpates the mass for size characteristics and tenderness. The client's ability to perform mobility tasks and activities of daily living (ADLs) is also determined. The nurse observes the client performing mobility tasks and may record the results on a functional assessment tool (see Chapter 10). The degree of disability can then be determined for comparison with later measurements after medical and nursing intervention.

■ PSYCHOSOCIAL ASSESSMENT

Often, clients with malignant bone tumors are young adults whose socially productive lives are just beginning. They need support systems to help cope with the diagnosis and its treatment. Family, significant others, and health care professionals are major components of the needed support. The nurse assesses the systems available to clients.

Clients often experience a loss of control over their lives when a diagnosis of malignancy is made. As a result, they become anxious and fearful about the outcome of their illness. Coping with the diagnosis becomes a challenge. They go through the grieving process; initially, there is denial. The nurse identifies the anxiety level and assesses the stage or stages of the grieving process. The nurse also identifies any maladaptive behavior, indicating ineffective coping mechanisms. Chapter 25 further elaborates on the psychosocial assessment for clients with malignancy.

■ LABORATORY ASSESSMENT

The client with a primary malignant or metastatic bone tumor typically shows elevated serum alkaline phosphatase (ALP) levels, indicating the body's attempt to form new bone by increasing osteoblastic activity.

The client with Ewing's sarcoma or metastatic bone lesions often has normocytic anemia. In addition, leukocytosis is common with Ewing's sarcoma.

In some clients with bone metastasis from the breast, kidney, or lung, the serum calcium level is elevated. Massive bone destruction stimulates release of the mineral into the bloodstream.

In clients with Ewing's sarcoma and bone metastasis, often the erythrocyte sedimentation rate (ESR) is elevated, which is probably attributable to secondary tissue inflammation.

■ RADIOGRAPHIC ASSESSMENT

As with benign bone tumors, routine x-ray studies and computed tomography (CT) allow for adequate visualization of malignant lesions. Although each tumor type has its own characteristic radiographic pattern, certain findings are common to all. Malignant tumors typically show poor margination, bone destruction, irregular periosteal new bone, and cortical breakthrough.

Metastatic lesions may increase or decrease bone density, depending on the amount of osteoblastic and osteoclastic activity. CT is helpful in determining the extent of soft-tissue damage.

■ OTHER DIAGNOSTIC ASSESSMENT

BONE BIOPSY. A bone biopsy may be performed to diagnose the tumor type. A needle biopsy is usually done when metastasis to the bone is suspected. An open method, through a surgical incision, is preferred for primary lesions. The surgeon keeps the incision as small as possible. The biopsy scar is removed during bone cancer surgery to eliminate a possible source of tumor seeds.

After biopsy, the cancer is staged according to the grade of the tumor. One popular method is the TNM staging system, which uses determinations of *t*umor size, *n*odal involvement, and evidence of *m*etastasis.

Another surgical staging method is to correlate the tumor grade (high or low), tumor site (intracompartmental or extracompartmental), and presence of metastatic disease (positive or negative). Staging guides the health care team in their decision regarding treatment.

BONE SCAN. Although a bone scan is not helpful in determining the type of tumor, it allows the extent of the cancer to be visualized. A scan is almost always ordered when bone metastasis is suspected.

▶ Analysis

▨ COMMON NURSING DIAGNOSES AND COLLABORATIVE PROBLEMS

The following are common nursing diagnoses for clients with malignant bone tumors:

1. Acute Pain and Chronic Pain related to direct tumor invasion into soft tissue
2. Anticipatory Grieving related to a change in body image or impending death
3. Disturbed Body Image related to the effects of chemotherapy, radiation therapy, or surgery

A common collaborative problem is Potential for Fractures.

▨ ADDITIONAL NURSING DIAGNOSES AND COLLABORATIVE PROBLEMS

In addition to the common nursing diagnoses and collaborative problems, clients with malignant bone tumors may have one or more of the following:

- Fear and Anxiety related to the medical diagnosis, possible disfiguring surgery, or impending death
- Ineffective Coping related to nonacceptance of the medical diagnosis
- Compromised Family Coping related to nonacceptance of the medical diagnosis
- Dysfunctional Grieving related to an inability to cope with the medical diagnosis
- Impaired Physical Mobility related to the size and extent of the tumor, weakness, and/or the effects of terminal metastatic disease
- Imbalanced Nutrition: Less Than Body Requirements related to an increased metabolic process secondary to cancer
- Disturbed Sleep Pattern related to pain
- Self-Care Deficit (Total) related to impaired physical mobility and weakness
- Ineffective Role Performance related to a temporary or permanent inability to maintain the family or community role
- Spiritual Distress related to fear of death

▶ Planning and Implementation

▨ ACUTE PAIN; CHRONIC PAIN

NOC PLANNING: EXPECTED OUTCOMES. The client with a malignant bone tumor is expected to experience a reduction or alleviation of pain associated with the bone lesion as indicated by self-report.

INTERVENTIONS. Because the pain is often due to direct tumor invasion, treatment is aimed at reducing the size of or removing the tumor. A combination of nonsurgical and surgical management is often used to promote client comfort and eliminate the complications of bone cancer.

NONSURGICAL MANAGEMENT. In addition to analgesics for local pain relief, chemotherapeutic agents and radiation therapy are often administered in an attempt to cause tumor regression. In clients with vertebral metastatic disease,

bracing and immobilization with cervical traction reduce back pain.

DRUG THERAPY. The physician may prescribe chemotherapy to be given alone or in combination with radiation or surgery. Certain proliferating tumors, such as Ewing's sarcoma, are sensitive to cytotoxic medications. Others, such as chondrosarcomas, are often totally drug resistant. Chemotherapy seems to work best for small, metastatic lesions and may be administered before or after surgery. For most tumors, the physician orders a combination of agents. At present, there is no universally accepted protocol of chemotherapeutic agents. The drugs selected are determined in part by the primary source of the cancer in metastatic disease. For example, when metastasis occurs from breast cancer, estrogens and progesterones may be used.

The nurse observes the client carefully for side and toxic effects and monitors laboratory tests diligently. Chapter 25 discusses the nursing care associated with the administration of cytotoxic agents.

RADIATION THERAPY. Radiation is used for selected types of malignant tumors. For clients with Ewing's sarcoma and early osteosarcoma, radiation may be the treatment of choice in reducing tumor size and thus pain.

For clients with metastatic disease, radiation is given primarily for palliation. The therapy is directed toward the painful sites in an attempt to provide a more comfortable life span. One or more treatments are given, depending on the extent of disease. With precise planning, radiation therapy can be used with minimal complications. The nursing care for clients receiving radiation therapy is described in Chapter 25.

SURGICAL MANAGEMENT. The treatment of primary bone tumors is surgery, often combined with radiation or chemotherapy.

PREOPERATIVE CARE. Preoperatively, the nurse thoroughly evaluates the client to assist the physician in the selection of the surgical procedure to be performed. In addition to the nature, progression, and extent of the tumor, the client's age and general health state are taken into consideration. Chemotherapy may be administered preoperatively.

As for any client preparing for cancer surgery, the client with bone cancer needs psychologic support from the nurse and other members of the health care team. The nurse assesses the level of understanding of the client and the family or significant others. As a client advocate, the nurse encourages the expression of concerns and questions and provides information regarding hospital routines and procedures. Spiritual support is important to some clients, who may prefer to contact their own clergy, rabbi, or spiritual leader or talk with the clergy affiliated with the hospital. The nurse helps to arrange for spiritual assistance if needed.

Postoperative needs are anticipated and planned for as much as possible before the client undergoes surgery. The nurse informs the client what to expect postoperatively and how to help ensure adequate recovery.

OPERATIVE PROCEDURES. Wide or radical resection procedures are commonly performed for clients with bone sarcomas. Wide excision is removal of the lesion surrounded by an intact cuff of normal tissue and leads to cure of low-grade tumors only. A radical resection includes removal of the lesion, the entire muscle, bone, and other tissues directly involved. It is the only procedure adequate for high-grade tumors.

In the past, limb amputation was commonly performed for bone tumors, with or without disarticulation (joint removal). Today, advances in reconstructive surgery allow for resection of the tumor and repair of the resulting bony defect to salvage the limb. The following are used to correct bone defects:

- Total joint replacements with prosthetic implants, either whole or partial
- Custom metallic implants
- Allografts from the iliac crest, rib, or fibula

In a few cases, arthrodesis (joint fusion) may be the procedure of choice. Total joint replacements are discussed in Chapter 21.

As an alternative to total replacement, an allograft may be implanted with internal fixation for those clients who do not have metastases. This is a common procedure for sarcomas of the proximal femur. Allograft procedures for the knee are also performed, particularly in young adults. Preoperative chemotherapy is given to enhance the likelihood of success. Allografts with adjacent tendons and ligaments are harvested from cadavers and can be frozen or freeze-dried for a prolonged period. The graft is fixed with a series of bolts, screws, or plates. The nurse observes for signs of hemorrhage, infection, or fracture.

For clients with metastatic disease, intractable pain is surgically treated with percutaneous cordotomy (cutting of the spinal nerve roots). Cryosurgery (cold application) may reduce pain and tumor size.

POSTOPERATIVE CARE. The surgical incision for a limb salvage procedure is often extensive. A pressure dressing with wound suction is typically maintained for up to 5 days.

The client who has undergone a limb salvage procedure has resulting impaired physical mobility and a self-care deficit. The nature and extent of the alterations depend on the location and extent of the surgery.

Promotion of Physical Mobility. Usually, muscle strengthening and range-of-motion (ROM) exercises begin immediately postoperatively and continue for at least a year. After upper extremity surgery, the client can engage in active-assistive exercises by using the opposite hand to help achieve motions such as forward flexion and abduction of the shoulder. Continuous passive motion (CPM) using a CPM machine may be initiated as early as the first postoperative day for either upper extremity or lower extremity procedures.

After lower extremity surgery, the emphasis is on strengthening the quadriceps muscles by using passive and active motion when possible. Maintaining muscle tone is an important prerequisite to weight bearing, which progresses from toe touch or partial weight bearing to full weight bearing by 3 months postoperatively.

The client who has had a bone graft has a plaster cast that remains in place for several months. Weight bearing is prohibited until there is evidence that the graft is incorporated into the adjacent bone tissue.

During the recovery phase, the client also needs assistance with activities of daily living (ADLs), particularly if the surgery involves the upper extremity. The nurse assists if needed, but at the same time tries to encourage the client to do as much as possible unaided.

Neurovascular Assessment. Surrounding tissues, including nerves and blood vessels, may be sacrificed during surgery. Vascular grafting is common, but the lost nerve is usually not replaced. The nurse assesses the neurovascular status of the affected extremity and its digits thoroughly and frequently. Splinting or casting of the limb may also cause neurovascular compromise and needs to be checked for proper placement.

Pelvic lesions, although not commonly seen, are also excised. Reconstruction generally entails bone fusion with muscle and nerve preservation. A hip spica cast or brace may be necessary until graft incorporation has occurred. The client may need a cane for ambulation.

The major complications peculiar to reconstructive surgery for which the nurse should observe are superficial and deep wound infection, dislocation or loosening of the implants, and rapid neurovascular compromise.

An increase in pain or temperature or a rapid deterioration in circulatory status alerts the nurse to notify the physician promptly.

Psychologic Support. In addition to needing psychologic help in coping with physical disabilities, the client may need help coping with the surgery and its effects postoperatively. Having identified the available support systems preoperatively, the nurse helps to mobilize them for use after surgery.

As a result of most of the surgical procedures, the client experiences an alteration in body image. The nurse can suggest ways to minimize cosmetic changes. For example, a shoulder droop can be covered by a custom-made pad worn under clothing. The client can cover lower extremity defects with pants.

▨ ANTICIPATORY GRIEVING

NOC PLANNING: EXPECTED OUTCOMES. The client with a malignant bone tumor is expected to work through the grieving process by taking action to manage stressors and accept the prognosis.

INTERVENTIONS. The nurse's most important role is to be an active listener and to encourage the client and family or significant others to verbalize their feelings. Counselors and members of the clergy or spiritual leaders may provide additional assistance in promoting acceptance of the diagnosis, treatment, or possibly, impending death. Chapter 9 provides information about death and dying.

NIC GRIEF WORK FACILITATION. Regardless of the prognosis, a diagnosis of bone cancer is a major stressor that causes the client and family or significant others to grieve. The nurse helps the client and others to cope with the loss and resolve the grief (Chart 51-6).

ADVOCACY. The nurse also acts as an advocate for the client and the family and often promotes the physician-client relationship. For instance, the client may not completely understand the medical or surgical treatment plan but may be hesitant to question the physician. The nurse's intervention increases communication, which is essential in successful management of the client with cancer.

▨ DISTURBED BODY IMAGE

NOC PLANNING: EXPECTED OUTCOMES. The client with a malignant bone tumor is expected to experience a positive perception of, and adjust to changes in, his or her body appearance.

CHART 51-6

NIC INTERVENTION ACTIVITIES *for*
The Client with Bone Cancer (Psychosocial Care)

Grief Work Facilitation: *Assistance with the resolution of a significant loss*
- Identify the loss.
- Assist the client to identify the nature of the attachment to the lost object or person.
- Assist the client to identify the initial reaction to the loss.
- Encourage expression of feelings about the loss.
- Instruct in phases of the grieving process, as appropriate.
- Support progression through personal grieving stages.
- Identify significant others in discussion and decisions, as appropriate.
- Assist to identify personal coping strategies.
- Communicate acceptance of discussing loss.
- Identify sources of community support.
- Reinforce progress made in the grieving process.
- Assist in identifying modifications needed in lifestyle.

Body Image Enhancement: *Improving a client's conscious and unconscious perceptions and attitudes toward his/her body*
- Assist client to discuss changes caused by illness or surgery, as appropriate.
- Help client determine the extent of actual changes in the body or its level of functioning.
- Assist to determine the influence of a peer group on the client's perception of present body image.
- Identify the significance of the client's culture, religion, race, sex, and age on body image.
- Monitor whether client can look at the changed body part.
- Determine if a change in body image has contributed to increased social isolation.
- Assist client to identify actions that will enhance appearance.
- Identify support groups available to client.

NIC intervention activities selected from McCloskey, J.C., & Bulechek, G.M. (2000). *Nursing interventions classification (NIC)* (3rd ed.). St. Louis: Mosby. No part of this work is to be altered without prior written permission from the Publisher.

INTERVENTIONS. The client's self-perception of body image is closely associated with his or her ability to accept the illness. The nurse recognizes and accepts the client's view about the body image alteration. A trusting nurse-client relationship allows the client freedom to verbalize negative feelings. The client's strengths and remaining capabilities are emphasized. Realistic mutual goals regarding lifestyle are established (see Chart 51-6).

POTENTIAL FOR FRACTURES

PLANNING: EXPECTED OUTCOMES. As with other bone diseases in which pathologic fracture is a possible complication (e.g., osteoporosis), the client with a malignant bone tumor is expected to avoid falls and minimize trauma to prevent fractures. In people with metastatic bone disease, fractures occur more readily and are not as preventable because of resulting destructive bone changes. A more realistic outcome for people with metastatic disease, then, may be that the client's pain will be minimized through treatment of the fracture.

INTERVENTIONS. Radiation or surgery may be required to reinforce or replace the diseased bone to prevent fracture. In recent years, surgical techniques have also been improved for fracture fixation.

NONSURGICAL MANAGEMENT. Newer techniques in radiation therapy have improved the incidence of bone healing for actual and impending pathologic fractures. To improve muscle tone and, consequently, to reduce the risk for fracture, the client performs strengthening exercises. Physical therapy on an ambulatory basis is commonly prescribed.

SURGICAL MANAGEMENT. The principles of surgery for metastatic fractures include the following:
- Replacing as much defective bone as possible
- Being thorough in technique to avoid a second procedure
- Aiming to return the client to a functional state with a minimum of hospitalization and immobilization

Fractures of the proximal femur are very common. Prosthetic replacement reinforced with polymethylmethacrylate is preferred over open reduction with internal fixation (ORIF) when feasible. The surgeon uses intramedullary rods and compression screws for more distal fractures. Prophylactic fixation may be indicated for microscopic fractures that cause chronic pain. Chapter 52 discusses the nursing management for clients undergoing repair of a fractured hip.

> **CRITICAL THINKING CHALLENGE**
> You are caring for a young adult who has had reconstructive surgery for tibial bone carcinoma. Before his diagnosis, he had been very active in sports, especially skiing and snowmobiling. He tells you that he is very concerned that the cancer diagnosis and surgery will markedly change his life, particularly his relationship with his long-time girl friend.
> - What questions might you ask the client as part of a psychosocial assessment?
> - What nursing diagnoses might you anticipate?
> - What realistic outcomes should he expect to achieve?
> - What health teaching will you need to provide?

For suggested answer guidelines, go to SIMON http://www.wbsaunders.com/SIMON/Iggy/.

Community-Based Care

After medical treatment for a primary malignant tumor, the client is usually managed at home with follow-up care. The client with metastatic disease may remain in the home or, when home support is not available, may be admitted to a long-term care facility for extended or hospice care. His or her care may be managed by a case manager.

HEALTH TEACHING

For the client receiving intermittent chemotherapy on an ambulatory basis, the nurse emphasizes the importance of keeping appointments. The nurse reviews the side effects and toxic effects of the medications. The client is taught how to treat minor side effects and when to alert the health care provider. If the drugs are administered at home via long-term IV catheter, the nurse explains the care involved with daily dressing changes and potential catheter complications. Chapter 14 describes the health teaching required for a client receiving infusion therapy at home.

The client receiving radiation therapy is also taught the importance of keeping appointments and recognizing the complications of treatment. The nurse reviews interventions that can be used at home for minor complications.

If the client has undergone surgery, he or she has a wound and limited mobility. The nurse teaches how to care for the wound and perform activities of daily living (ADLs) and mobility activities independently. Physical and occupational therapists assist in ADL teaching and provide or recommend assistive and adaptive devices if necessary. The physical therapist also teaches the proper use of ambulatory aids, such as crutches, and exercises.

Pain management can be a major problem, particularly in the client with metastatic bone disease. The nurse reviews nondrug pain relief measures, including relaxation and music therapy. The nurse emphasizes those techniques that worked during hospitalization.

The client with bone cancer typically fears that the malignancy will return. The nurse acknowledges this possibility but reinforces confidence in the health care team and medical treatment chosen.

Realistic goals regarding return to work, recreational activities, and so forth are mutually established. The nurse encourages the client to resume a functional lifestyle but cautions that it should be gradual. Certain activities, such as participating in sports, may be prohibited.

The client with advanced metastatic bone disease needs to prepare for death. The nurse and other support personnel assist the client through the stages of death and dying and identify resources that can help the client write a will, visit with distant family members, or do whatever he or she thinks is needed to die in peace.

■ HOME CARE MANAGEMENT

In collaboration with the occupational therapist, the nurse evaluates the client's home environment for structural barriers that may hinder mobility. The client may be discharged with a cast, crutches, or a wheelchair.

Accessibility to eating and toileting facilities is essential to promote independence. Because the client with metastatic disease is susceptible to pathologic fractures, potential hazards that may contribute to falls or injury should be removed.

■ HEALTH CARE RESOURCES

In addition to family and significant others, cancer support groups are helpful to the client with bone cancer. Some organizations, such as I Can Cope, provide information and emotional support; others, such as CanSurmount, are geared more toward client and family education.

The hospital staff nurse, discharge planner, or case manager also ensures that follow-up care, including nursing care and physical or occupational therapy, is available in the home. The client with terminal cancer may choose to become part of a hospice program (see Chapter 9).

● Evaluation: Outcomes

NOC The nurse evaluates the care of the client with a malignant bone tumor on the basis of the identified nursing diagnoses and collaborative problems. The expected outcomes may include that the client will:

- State that pain is reduced or alleviated
- Perform ADLs and ambulation activities independently
- Seek health care resources as needed, including cancer support groups
- State that body image perception is improved

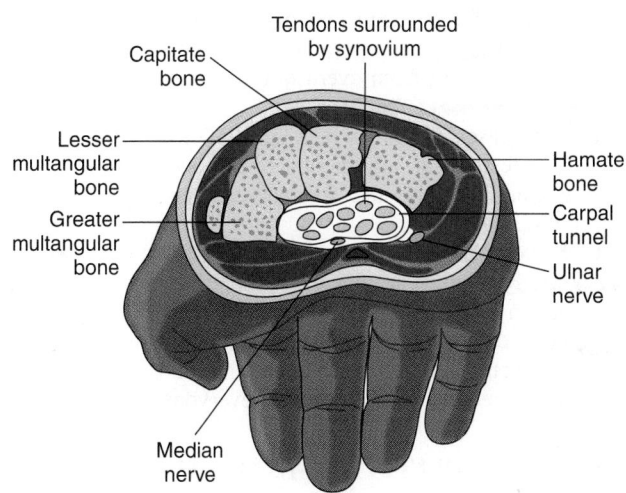

Figure 51-6 ● Anatomy of the carpal tunnel.

- Return to a functional lifestyle (or accept impending death in the case of advanced metastasis)
- State that anxiety regarding medical diagnosis and treatment is decreased

DISORDERS OF THE HAND
Carpal Tunnel Syndrome
■ OVERVIEW

Carpal tunnel syndrome (CTS) is a common condition in which the median nerve in the wrist becomes compressed, causing pain and numbness. The carpal tunnel is a rigid canal lying between the carpal bones and a fibrous tissue sheet called the flexor retinaculum. As seen in Figure 51-6, a group of nine tendons enveloped by synovium share space with the median nerve in the carpal tunnel. When the synovium becomes swollen or thickened, the nerve is compressed.

The median nerve supplies the motor, sensory, and autonomic function for the first three digits of the hand and the palmar aspect of the fourth digit. Because of the median nerve's proximity to other structures, wrist flexion causes nerve impingement against the flexor retinaculum; extension causes increased pressure in the distal portion of the carpal tunnel.

CTS usually manifests as a chronic problem; acute cases are rare. Excessive hand exercise, edema or hemorrhage into the carpal tunnel, or thrombosis of the median artery can lead to acute CTS. Clients with a Colles' fracture of the wrist or hand burns are particularly at risk for rapid CTS development.

In most cases, however, the causative factors may not result in neurologic deficit for years. CTS is a common complication of certain metabolic and connective tissue diseases. For example, synovitis (inflammation of the synovium) occurs in clients with rheumatoid arthritis. The hypertrophied synovium compresses the median nerve. In other chronic disorders such as diabetes mellitus, inadequate blood supply can cause median nerve neuropathy, or dysfunction, resulting in CTS.

CTS is the most common repetitive strain injury (RSI)—the fastest growing type of occupational injury. People whose jobs require repetitive hand activities involving pinch or grasp during wrist flexion, such as factory workers, computer operators, and jackhammer operators, are predisposed to CTS. CTS can also result from overuse in sports activities such as golf, tennis, or racquetball.

In a few cases, CTS may be a familial or congenital problem, manifesting in adulthood. Space-occupying lesions, such as ganglia, tophi, and lipomas, can also result in nerve compression.

CTS occurs in adults of all ages but peaks between ages 30 and 60 years. Women are five times more likely to experience the problem than men. Most often, CTS affects the dominant hand, but it can occur in both hands simultaneously. Children and adolescents are beginning to experience CTS as a result of the increased use of computers in everyday life.

➤ COLLABORATIVE MANAGEMENT

● Assessment

On the basis of the client's history and complaint of hand pain and numbness, a medical diagnosis is often made without further assessment. The nurse questions clients regarding the nature, intensity, and location of the pain. Clients often state that the pain is worse at night as a result of flexion or direct pressure during sleep. The pain may radiate to the arm, the shoulder and neck, or the chest.

In addition to the complaint of numbness, clients with carpal tunnel syndrome (CTS) may also experience paresthesia (painful tingling). Sensory changes usually precede motor manifestations by weeks or months.

■ PHYSICAL ASSESSMENT/CLINICAL MANIFESTATIONS

The health care provider performs several tests to elicit abnormal sensory findings. Phalen's wrist test, sometimes called **Phalen's maneuver,** produces paresthesia in the median nerve distribution within 60 seconds. The client is asked to relax the wrist into flexion or place the backs of the hands together and flex both wrists simultaneously (Figure 51-7). Of clients with CTS, 80% have a positive Phalen's test result.

The same sensation can be elicited by tapping lightly over the area of the median nerve in the wrist (**Tinel's sign**). If the test is unsuccessful, a blood pressure cuff can be placed on the upper arm and inflated to the client's systolic pressure. The result is often pain and tingling.

Motor changes begin with a weak pinch, clumsiness, and difficulty with fine movements and then progress to muscle weakness and wasting. The nurse may test for pinching ability and ask the client to perform a fine-movement task, such as threading a needle. Strenuous hand activity worsens the subjective complaints.

In addition to inspecting for muscle atrophy and task performance, the nurse observes the wrist for swelling. The area is palpated, and characteristics are described. Autonomic changes may be evidenced by skin discoloration; nail changes, such as brittleness; and increased or decreased palmar sweating.

■ DIAGNOSTIC ASSESSMENT

Routine x-ray studies are ordered to visualize bone changes, space-occupying lesions, and synovitis. If these causative fac-

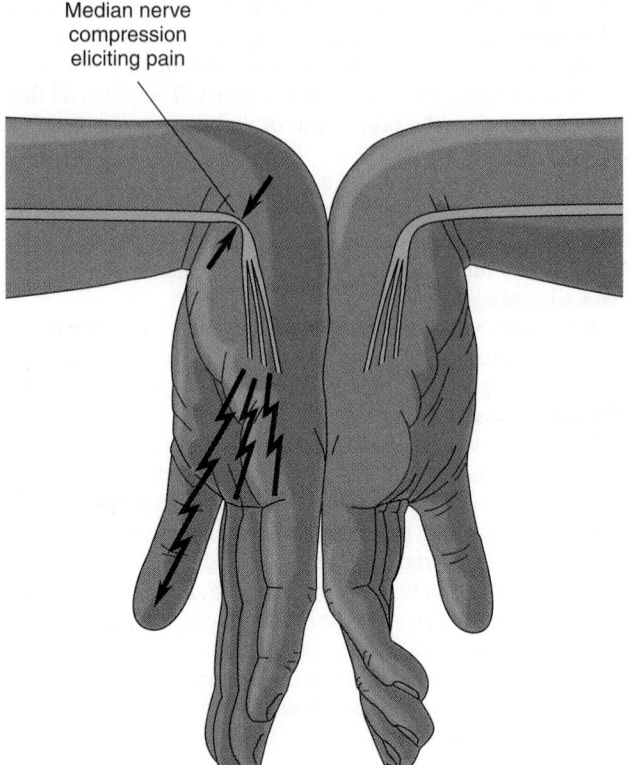

Median nerve compression eliciting pain

Figure 51-7 ● Phalen's maneuver for detection of carpal tunnel syndrome.

tors are not suspected, a client with CTS may not have x-ray studies done.

The health care provider may order electromyography (EMG), magnetic resonance imaging (MRI), or ultrasonography when a definitive diagnosis is uncertain. Problems of the cervical spine and spinal nerves can mimic the clinical manifestations of CTS. EMG testing reveals nerve dysfunction before muscle atrophy is observed. More recently, MRI has been used to help diagnose CTS. The most common finding is an enlarged median nerve within the carpal tunnel. The newest technique for diagnosis is the use of ultrasound.

● Interventions

The health care provider uses conservative measures before surgical intervention. With either type of treatment, however, CTS can recur.

NONSURGICAL MANAGEMENT. Drug therapy and immobilization of the wrist are the major components of nonsurgical management. The nurse teaches the client the importance of these modalities in the hope of preventing surgical intervention.

DRUG THERAPY. The most commonly prescribed drugs for the relief of pain and inflammation, if present, are aspirin and other nonsteroidal anti-inflammatory drugs (NSAIDs).

In addition to or instead of systemic medications, the physician may inject corticosteroids directly into the carpal tunnel. If the client responds to the medication, several additional weekly or monthly injections are given.

As with any medication, the nurse monitors the effects of drug therapy. Aspirin and NSAIDs are given with or after meals to reduce gastric irritation.

IMMOBILIZATION. A splint may be used to immobilize the wrist during the day, during the night, or both. Many clients experience temporary relief with splinting. The occupational therapist places the wrist in the neutral position or in slight extension. Even when a splint is not used, the nurse instructs the client to minimize hand activities, at least temporarily.

PREVENTION OF CARPAL TUNNEL SYNDROME. Many businesses have recognized the hazards of repetitive motion as a primary cause of occupational injury and disability. Young men and women in the labor force are experiencing increasing numbers of repetitive strain injuries (RSIs). Occupational health nurses have played an important role in the development of ergonomically appropriate furniture and other aids to decrease CTS and other musculoskeletal injuries. Federal and state legislation has been passed to ensure that businesses provide ergonomically appropriate workstations for their employees.

SURGICAL MANAGEMENT. Surgery is necessary in about 50% of clients with CTS. Surgery can relieve the pressure on the median nerve by providing nerve decompression.

PREOPERATIVE CARE. The nurse in the physician's office or same-day surgical center reinforces the teaching provided by the surgeon regarding the nature of the surgery. Postoperative care is reviewed so that the client knows what to expect.

OPERATIVE PROCEDURES. The two most common surgeries are the open carpal tunnel release (OCTR) and the newer endoscopic carpal tunnel release (ECTR). When CTS is a complication of rheumatoid arthritis, a synovectomy (removal of excess synovium via incision) through an inner-wrist incision may resolve the problem. Removal of a space-occupying lesion, if present, also decompresses the nerve. Whatever the cause of nerve compression, the physician removes it either by cutting or by the newer laser technique. In some cases, CTS recurs months to years after surgery.

An alternative to OCTR is the endoscopic release. The surgeon makes a very small incision (less than ½ inch [1.2 cm]) through which the endoscope is inserted. The surgeon then uses special instruments, which may include a laser, to free the trapped median nerve.

POSTOPERATIVE CARE. Although ECTR is less invasive and costs less than the open procedure, the client may experience pain and numbness for a longer time postoperatively as compared with recovery from OCTR. Major surgical complications are rare following CTS surgery.

In addition to monitoring vital signs, the nurse checks the pressure dressing carefully for drainage and tightness. If the endoscopic procedure has been performed, the dressing is very small. The surgeon may require that the client's hand and arm be elevated above heart level for 1 or 2 days to reduce swelling from surgery. The nurse checks the neurovascular status of the digits every hour during the immediate postoperative period, encouraging the client to move all fingers of the affected hand frequently. The nurse offers pain medication and assures the client that he or she will be given a prescription for analgesics for use at home during recovery.

After surgery, the client's wrist is placed in a splint that allows thumb and finger movements. The splint is usually applied after the sutures have been removed and may be used for up to 2 weeks.

Hand movements, including lifting heavy objects, may be restricted for 4 to 6 weeks. The client can expect weakness and discomfort for weeks or perhaps months. The nurse teaches how to assess for neurovascular status.

The client must realize that the surgical procedure might not be a cure. For instance, synovitis may recur in the client with rheumatoid arthritis and may recompress the median nerve. Multiple operations and other treatments are not uncommon with CTS.

The client may need assistance with routine daily tasks or even self-care activities during recovery. The nurse ensures that assistance in the home is available; this is usually provided by the family or significant others.

Dupuytren's Contracture

Dupuytren's contracture, or deformity, is a slowly progressive contracture of the palmar fascia, resulting in flexion of the fourth or fifth digit of the hand. The third digit is occasionally affected. Although Dupuytren's contracture is a fairly common problem, the cause is unknown. It usually occurs in older men, tends to be familial, and can be bilateral.

When function becomes impaired, surgical release is required. A partial or selective fasciectomy (removal of fascia) is performed. After removal of the dressing and drain, a splint may be used. Nursing care is similar to that for the client with carpal tunnel repair.

Ganglion

A **ganglion** is a round, cystlike lesion, often overlying a wrist joint or tendon. The synovium surrounding the tendon degenerates, allowing the tendon sheath tissue to become weak and distended. Ganglia are painless on palpation, but they can cause joint discomfort after prolonged joint use or minor trauma, such as a strain. The lesion can disappear and then recur. Ganglia are most likely to develop in people between 15 and 50 years of age.

Although the fluid within the lesion can be aspirated, total excision is preferred. The postoperative care is the same as that for the client undergoing other hand surgery.

DISORDERS OF THE FOOT
Hallux Valgus

The **hallux valgus** deformity, sometimes referred to as a bunion, is a common foot problem. The great toe deviates laterally at the metatarsophalangeal (MTP) joint (Figure 51-8). Although hallux valgus is often congenital, it can occur as a result of arthritis or poorly fitted shoes. As the deviation worsens, the bony prominence enlarges and causes pain, particularly when shoes are worn. Women are affected more often than men.

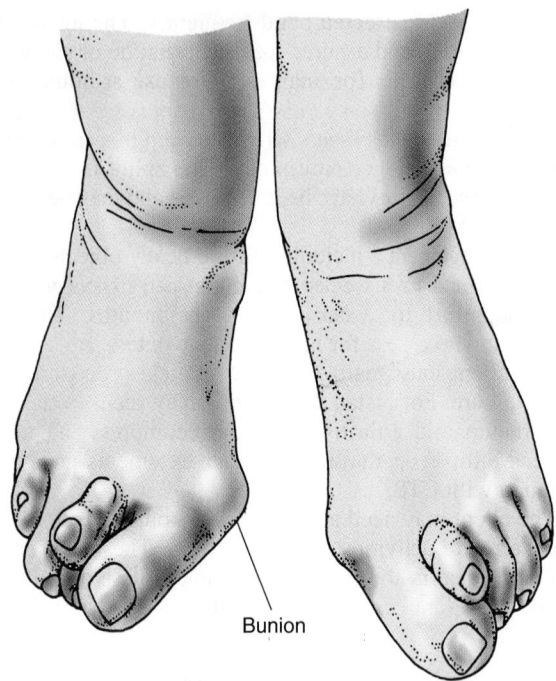

Figure 51-8 ● Appearance of hallux valgus with a bunion.

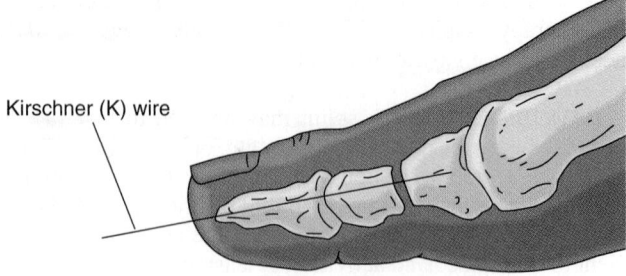

Figure 51-9 ● Use of Kirschner wires to repair hallux valgus and other toe deformities.

The surgical procedure, a simple bunionectomy, involves removal of the bony overgrowth and bursa. When other toe deformities accompany the condition or if the bony overgrowth is large, several osteotomies, or bone resections, may be performed. In this case, Kirschner wires are inserted vertically through the toes until healing occurs (Figure 51-9). If both feet are affected, one foot is treated at a time.

Hammertoe

Often clients have hammertoes and hallux valgus deformities simultaneously. As shown in Figure 51-10, a **hammertoe** is the dorsiflexion of any MTP joint with plantar flexion of the adjacent proximal interphalangeal (PIP) joint. The second toe is most often affected. As the deformity worsens, corns may develop on the dorsal side of the toe and calluses may appear on the plantar surface. Clients are uncomfortable when wearing shoes and walking.

Hammertoe is treated by surgical correction of the deformity with osteotomies and the insertion of Kirschner wires for fixation (see Figure 51-9). The postoperative course is similar to that for the client with hallux valgus repair. The client uses crutches until full weight bearing is allowed 3 to 4 weeks postoperatively.

Morton's Neuroma

In the client with **Morton's neuroma,** or plantar digital neuritis, a small tumor grows in a digital nerve of the foot. The client usually describes the pain as an acute, burning sensation in the web space. The pain involves the entire surface of the third and fourth toes.

Treatment involves surgical removal of the neuroma and application of a pressure dressing. Ambulation is usually permitted immediately after surgery.

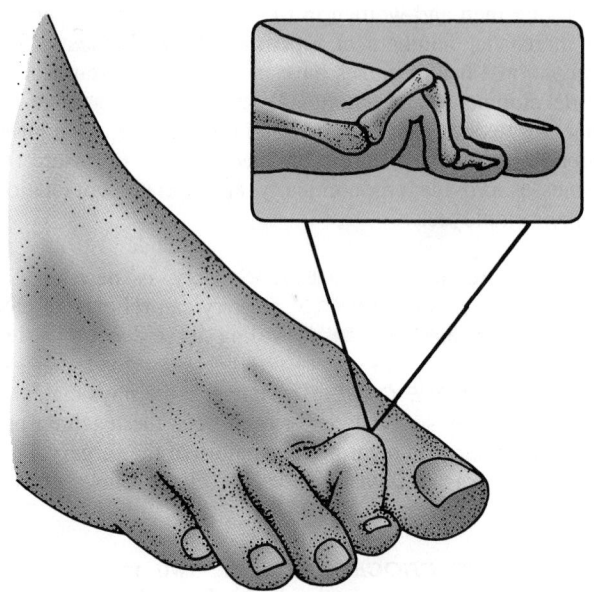

Figure 51-10 ● Hammertoe of the second metatarsophalangeal joint.

Tarsal Tunnel Syndrome

Tarsal tunnel syndrome is the ankle version of carpal tunnel syndrome (CTS). The posterior tibial nerve in the ankle becomes compressed, resulting in loss of sensation and pain in a portion of the foot. Typically, the median and lateral plantar branches, which supply the sole of the foot and the distal phalanges, are affected by the nerve compression. Diagnosis and treatment are similar to those for CTS.

Plantar Fasciitis

Plantar fasciitis is an inflammation of the plantar fascia, which is located in the area of the arch of the foot. It is often seen in middle-aged and older adults, as well as athletes, especially runners. In ambulatory care settings, plantar fasciitis accounts for 10% of running injuries. Obesity is also a contributing factor.

Clients complain of pain in the arch of the foot, especially when getting out of bed. The pain is worsened with weight bearing. Although most clients experience unilateral plantar fasciitis, the problem can affect both feet.

More than 90% of clients respond to conservative management, which includes rest, ice, stretching exercises, strapping of the foot to maintain the arch, shoes with good support, and or-

TABLE 51-5 • TREATMENT OF COMMON FOOT PROBLEMS

Description/Cause	Treatment
CORN Induration and thickening of the skin caused by friction and pressure, painful conical mass	Surgical removal by podiatrist
CALLUS Flat, poorly defined mass on the sole over a bony prominence caused by pressure	Padding and lanolin cremes; overall good skin hygiene
INGROWN NAIL Nail sliver penetration of the skin, causing inflammation	Removal of sliver by podiatrist; warm soaks; antibiotic ointment
HYPERTROPHIC UNGUAL LABIUM Chronic hypertrophy of nail lip caused by improper nail trimming; results from untreated ingrown nail	Surgical removal of necrotic nail and skin; treatment of secondary infection

thotics. Nonsteroidal anti-inflammatory drugs (NSAIDs) or steroids may be needed to control pain and inflammation. If conservative measures are unsuccessful, endoscopic surgery to remove the inflamed tissue may be required.

Nursing care involves teaching the client about the importance of complying with the treatment plan and coordinating care with the physical therapist for instruction in exercise.

Other Problems of the Foot

Table 51-5 cites other common foot problems. Although clients are usually not hospitalized for these conditions, the nurse may recognize a foot disorder and alert the physician.

OTHER DISORDERS OF THE SKELETON
Scoliosis
■ OVERVIEW

Scoliosis is a C- or S-shaped lateral curvature of the vertebral spine (see Figure 50-3). Many individuals with scoliosis are diagnosed and treated before adolescence. Children are typically screened for scoliosis during their middle school years. Information about caring for children with scoliosis is presented in most pediatric nursing texts.

➤ COLLABORATIVE MANAGEMENT
● Assessment

In the adult with scoliosis, the impairment is usually cosmetic, although severe deviations of more than 50 degrees can compromise cardiopulmonary function. The abnormal curvature can cause low back pain, for which treatment is initiated. Women are affected more often than men.

Methods of treating adult scoliosis differ from those used for children. The adult spinal column is less flexible and

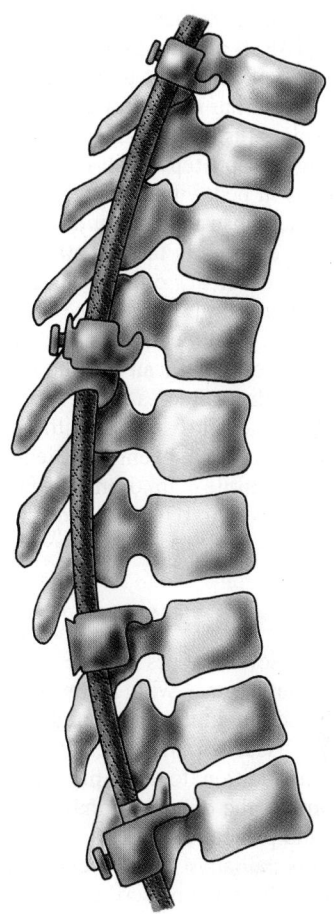

Figure 51-11 ● Correction of the lateral spine contour with Cotrel-Dubousset instrumentation and spinal fusion.

therefore less likely to respond to exercises, weight reduction, bracing, and casting for correction of the deformity. In the adult, the disorder is progressive and can result in an additional 1 degree of deviation each year.

Clients who underwent scoliosis surgery 20 to 25 years previously are returning with progressive, debilitating back pain from degenerative disk disease below the fusion and with "flat back" syndrome (loss of lumbar curvature). In some of these clients, fusion was not accomplished with instrumentation, and surgery may be necessary to resolve the pain.

● Interventions

Surgical intervention is the most common treatment for adults. The procedure consists of surgical fusion and insertion of instrumentation. The surgeon performs one or more spinal fusions by packing cancellous bone chips, usually from the iliac crest, between the affected vertebrae for support and stabilization. Both an anterior and a posterior approach may be needed. If so, the surgeon may perform both procedures during the same operative day or may stage them 7 to 10 days apart.

The metal instrumentation straightens the spine and immobilizes the fused area during healing (Figure 51-11). The earlier instrumentation systems include those by Harrington, Dwyer, and Luque. In the 1980s, Cotrel-Dubousset (CD) implants became popular and are still used today. Other systems similar to the CD implant include the Texas Scottish Rite Hospital system (TSRH) and the ISOLA system.

The nursing care of the client undergoing corrective surgery for scoliosis is similar to that for the client undergoing a laminectomy or spinal fusion (see Chapter 43). The major difference is the length of postoperative immobilization, which can be several days in bed with Harrington or Dwyer procedures. Luque and CD instrumentation allow the client to be out of bed the same evening or the day after surgery. A thoracolumbosacral (dorsolumbar) orthosis (TLSO) is typically used to support the vertebral column (see Figure 51-2).

With the newer surgical techniques, the client may return to work in about 3 weeks and can resume activities such as swimming and bicycling. Recreational sports, such as tennis, are usually resumed in 6 weeks with CD implant surgery, but other surgery may prevent the client from performing these activities until 3 to 6 months postoperatively. Many clients are allowed to return to contact sports within a year or less.

Osteogenesis Imperfecta

Although there are several types of osteogenesis imperfecta (OI), the milder tarda form with autosomal inheritance is more prevalent in adults. In this rare hereditary disease, a defect of connective tissue formation results in fragile and deformed bones. In addition to multiple fractures and poor skeletal development, the client may have blue sclerae; soft, brownish teeth; and presenile deafness.

The treatment is palliative, and the client's life span is often shortened. The physician prescribes steroids, calcium, vitamin C, and sodium fluoride. Physical therapy, casting or bracing, and intramedullary rodding are used to maintain mobility and promote ambulation if possible. The nurse refers the client to the Osteogenesis Foundation in the United States or to the "Brittle Bones" society in other countries for information and support.

MUSCULAR DISEASES
Progressive Muscular Dystrophies
■ OVERVIEW

At least nine types of **muscular dystrophy (MD)** have been clinically identified. They can be broadly categorized as slowly progressive or rapidly progressive. The slowly progressive types are most commonly seen in adults.

Five forms of MD are often seen in adults. Each type has its own distinct characteristics and causes, but all are progressive (Table 51-6).

The exact pathophysiologic mechanisms are unknown, but three theories have been advocated. The vascular theory suggests that a lack of blood flow causes the typical degeneration of muscle tissue seen in MD. Microscopic necrotic areas in dystrophied muscle tissue support this hypothesis, although this finding does not explain the marked degree of degeneration often seen in the disease.

The neurogenic theory proposes a disturbance in nerve-muscle interaction. Research has failed, however, to locate the nature of the disturbance.

The most popular belief is the membrane theory. This theory suggests that cell membranes are genetically altered,

TABLE 51-6 • DIFFERENTIAL FEATURES OF COMMON MUSCULAR DYSTROPHIES

Onset	Genetics	Clinical Manifestations	Progression
DUCHENNE (SEVERE X-LINKED) DYSTROPHY			
18 mo-4 yr	Sex-linked recessive, expression in males	Symmetric pelvic and shoulder girdle muscle weakness; waddling gait; cardiac involvement common; mental retardation in one third	Severely progressive, leading to inability to walk between 7 and 11 yr of age; death from cardiac or respiratory failure in 20s or 30s
BECKER (BENIGN X-LINKED) DYSTROPHY			
5-25 yr	Sex-linked recessive, expression in males	Wasting of pelvic and shoulder muscles; normal cardiac and mental function	Gradual progression; inability to walk 25 yr after onset; usually normal life span
LIMB-GIRDLE DYSTROPHY			
Usually 20s or 30s	Usually autosomal dominant, expression in either sex	Upper extremity and neck muscles and lower extremity and hip muscle weakness	Extremely variable; severe disability within 10-20 yr after onset; life span shortened by 10-20 yr
FACIOSCAPULOHUMERAL (LANDOUZY-DEJERINE) DYSTROPHY			
Usually in 20s	Autosomal dominant, expression in either sex	Facial and shoulder girdle muscle involvement	Usually benign; normal life span
MYOTONIC (STEINERT) DYSTROPHY			
Birth to 40s	Autosomal dominant, expression in either sex	Muscle atrophy with multiple organ involvement (e.g., heart, lungs, smooth muscle, and endocrine system)	Usually gradual if onset in adulthood

causing a compromise in cell integrity. An increase in the activity of muscle proteolytic enzymes may accompany the membrane alteration, leaving the muscle cell vulnerable to degeneration. Increased enzyme activity has been documented in the client with dystrophied muscles.

The cause of MD is unknown, but there may be a genetic influence for most of the major types. Some forms of MD are transmitted as autosomal dominant or recessive traits, whereas others are sex linked.

The most commonly occurring type of MD is the severe X-linked recessive variety initially described by Guillaume Duchenne in 1868. Each year, 20 to 33 cases are reported per 100,000 live male births. In an X-linked recessive disorder, one half of the male children of an unaffected mother, or carrier, manifest the disease. Becker's dystrophy is also inherited in an X-linked recessive manner, but it is less common than Duchenne's dystrophy. The other types of MD seen in adults can occur in either sex.

► COLLABORATIVE MANAGEMENT

Diagnosis of MD is often difficult because the clinical manifestations are similar to those of other muscular disorders. Muscle biopsy often confirms the diagnosis. Muscle weakness and trophic changes are characteristic of all types of MD. Serum muscle enzyme values may be elevated, and electromyographic (EMG) findings are often abnormal.

Management of the client with MD is supportive and involves the entire health care team. Physical and occupational therapy helps the client maintain as much function and independence as possible. Major organ or body system involvement is medically managed, but the life span is often shortened from these manifestations of the disease. With the exception of prednisone, no drug has been found to slow the progression of the disorder, although immunosuppressive agents, anabolic steroids, and growth factors have been tried.

An experimental treatment called myoblast transfer therapy (MTT) has been supported by the Food and Drug Administration (FDA). MTT involves injections of healthy muscle cells (myoblasts) taken from a donor and multiplied in a laboratory. The cells are then given to the client with MD, where they theoretically fuse with each other and the recipient's unhealthy muscle cells. Effective gene therapy may also be an option for curing MD in the future.

Nursing interventions focus on making the client as comfortable as possible and reinforcing techniques and exercises taught in the physical therapy program. The nurse's role in caring for a client with cardiac or other organ involvement is the same as for any client with dysfunction of these areas.

Other Muscular Disorders

Most muscular disorders are classified as neuromuscular disorders, such as myasthenia gravis, or as connective tissue diseases, such as polymyositis. Therefore these disorders are discussed in Chapters 44 and 21, respectively.

ONLINE RESOURCES

For suggested readings and Internet resources, go to http://www.wbsaunders.com/SIMON/Iggy/.

SELECTED BIBLIOGRAPHY

Asterisk indicates a classic or definitive work on this subject.

Ailinger, R.L., & Emerson, J. (1998). Women's knowledge of osteoporosis. *Applied Nursing Research, 11*(3), 111-114.

Ashworth, L. (1997). Can alendronate help my osteoporosis? *Home Care Provider, 2*(1), 37-39.

Bayles, C.M., Cochran, K., & Anderson, C. (2000). The psychosocial aspects of osteoporosis in women. *Nursing Clinics of North America, 35*(1), 279-286.

Berarducci, A., et al. (2000). Health-promoting educational practices related to osteoporosis. *Applied Nursing Research, 13*(4), 173-180.

Bilezikian, J.P. (1999). Osteoporosis in men. *Journal of Endocrinology and Metabolism, 84*(10), 3431-3434.

Capriotti, T. (2000). Pharmacologic prevention and treatment of osteoporosis in women. *MEDSURG Nursing, 9*(2), 86-90.

Cutson, T.M., & Meuleman, E. (2000). Managing menopause. *American Family Physician, 61*(5), 1391-1400.

Dowd, R., & Cavalieri, R.J. (1999). Help your patient live with osteoporosis. *American Journal of Nursing, 99*(4), 55, 57-60.

Hall, J., & Riley, R.E. (1999). Nutritional strategies to reduce the risk of osteoporosis. *MEDSURG Nursing, 8*(5), 281-293.

*Hunt, A.H. (1996). The relationship between height change and bone mineral density. *Orthopaedic Nursing, 15*(3), 57-71.

*Hunt, A.H., Civitelli, R., & Halstead, L. (1995). Evaluation of bone resorption: A common problem during impaired mobility. *SCI Nursing, 12*(3), 90-94.

*Kessenich, C.R., & Rosen, C.J. (1996). Vitamin D and bone status in elderly women. *Orthopaedic Nursing, 15*(3), 67-71.

LeBoff, M.S. (1997). Metabolic bone disease. In W.N. Kelley et al. (Eds.), *Textbook of rheumatology* (5th ed., pp. 1563-1580). Philadelphia: W.B. Saunders.

Leslie, M. (2000). Issues in the nursing management of osteoporosis. *Nursing Clinics of North America, 35*(1), 189-197.

Lewis, T., et al. (1999). Caring for the patient with Paget's disease of the bone. *Nurse Practitioner, 24*(7), 53, 57-58.

Maher, A.B., Salmond, S.W., & Pellino, T.A. (1999). *Orthopaedic nursing* (2nd ed.). Philadelphia: W.B. Saunders.

Mahon, S.M. (1998). Osteoporosis: A concern for cancer survivors. *Oncology Nursing Forum, 25*(5), 843-851.

Marchigiano, G. (1997). Osteoporosis: Primary prevention and intervention strategies for women at risk. *Home Care Provider, 2*(2), 76-82.

Matteson, M.A., McConnell, E.S., & Linton, A.D. (1997). *Gerontological nursing: Concepts and practice* (2nd ed.). Philadelphia: W.B. Saunders.

McClung, B.L. (2000). *Nursing practice guideline: Clinical management of patients at risk for or diagnosed with osteoporosis.* New York: Medical Information Services.

*National Osteoporosis Foundation. (1995). *Position paper: Current perspective on diagnosis, prevention, and treatment of osteoporosis.* Washington, DC: Author.

Orwell, E. (2000). Men with osteoporosis. Presented at the World Congress on Osteoporosis 2000, June 17, 2000, Chicago.

Ott, S.M. (1999). Osteoporosis and osteomalacia. In W.R. Hazzard et al. (Eds.), *Principles of geriatric medicine and gerontology* (4th ed., pp. 1057-1084). New York: McGraw-Hill.

Peterson, J.A. (2001). Osteoporosis overview. *Geriatric Nursing, 22*(1), 17-23.

*Piasecki, P.A. (1996). Nursing care of the patient with metastatic bone disease. *Orthopaedic Nursing, 15*(4), 25-33.

*Quaschnick, M.S. (1996). The diagnosis and management of plantar fasciitis. *Nurse Practitioner, 21*(4), 50-63.

Sedlak, C.A., et al. (1998). Osteoporosis prevention in young women. *Orthopaedic Nursing, 17*(3), 53-60.

Siris, E.S. (1999). Goals of treatment for Paget's disease of bone. *Journal of Bone and Mineral Research, 14*(Suppl. 2), 49-52.

Solomon, J. (1998). Osteoporosis: When support weakens. *RN, 61*(5), 37-40.

Tawil, R. (1999). Outlook for therapy in the muscular dystrophies. *Seminars in Neurology, 19*(1), 81-86.

Vanderford, V. (1999). Using bone density measurements in the detection and treatment of osteoporosis. *Geriatric Nursing, 20*(4), 211.

Wright, A. (1998). Nursing interventions with advanced osteoporosis. *Home Healthcare Nurse, 16*(3), 145-151.

52

Interventions for Clients with Musculoskeletal Trauma

ANN BUTLER MAHER

Learning Objectives

After studying this chapter, you should be able to:

1. Compare and contrast common types of fractures.
2. Discuss the usual healing process for bone.
3. Identify common complications of fractures.
4. Explain the typical clinical manifestations that are seen in clients with one or more fractures.
5. Analyze common nursing diagnoses for the client with a fracture.
6. Describe the nursing care of the client with a cast, including client education.
7. Describe the nursing care of the client in traction.
8. Discuss pain management for the client with a fracture.
9. Prioritize nursing care for the postoperative client who has undergone open reduction with internal fixation of the hip.
10. Evaluate the nursing care of a client with a fracture.
11. Identify common types of amputations.
12. Explain the psychosocial aspects related to amputations.
13. Develop a community-based teaching plan for a client who has undergone an elective amputation.
14. Describe the collaborative management for the client with complex regional pain syndrome.
15. Identify the common types of sports-related injuries and their management.

Go to http://www.wbsaunders.com/SIMON/Iggy/ for self-assessment questions related to these Learning Objectives.

Musculoskeletal injury is one of the primary causes of disability in the United States. Trauma to the musculoskeletal system ranges from simple muscle strain to multiple bone fractures with severe soft-tissue damage. With advancing age, a person is more likely to develop decreased bone mass (osteoporosis), which causes fractures. Hip, wrist, vertebral, and pelvic fractures are common in late adulthood.

FRACTURES

OVERVIEW

A **fracture** is a break or disruption in the continuity of a bone. Fractures can occur anywhere in the body and at any age. All fractures have the same basic pathophysiologic mechanism and nursing management, regardless of fracture type or location.

Pathophysiology

CLASSIFICATION OF FRACTURES

A fracture is classified by the extent of the break as follows:

- *Complete fracture.* The break is across the entire width of the bone in such a way that the bone is divided into two distinct sections.

- *Incomplete fracture.* The fracture does not divide the bone into two portions, because the break is through only part of the bone.

A fracture is described by the extent of associated soft-tissue damage as **open** (or **compound**) or **closed** (or **simple**). The skin surface over the broken bone is disrupted in a compound fracture, which causes an external wound. These fractures are often graded to define the extent of tissue damage. Grade I is the least severe injury, and skin damage is minimal. In grade II, an open fracture is accompanied by skin and muscle contusions. The most severe injury is grade III, in which there is damage to skin, muscle, nerve tissue, and blood vessels; the wound is more than 2.4 to 3.2 inches (6 to 8 cm) in diameter. A closed (simple) fracture does not extend through the skin. Therefore there is no visible wound.

Figure 52-1 illustrates common types of fractures. The nurse needs to be familiar with the differences in these types because they often dictate the specific nursing care required for the client.

In addition to being identified by type, fractures are characterized by their cause. A **pathologic (spontaneous) fracture** occurs after minimal trauma to a bone that has been weakened by disease. For example, a client with bone cancer or osteoporosis can easily sustain a pathologic fracture. A **fatigue or**

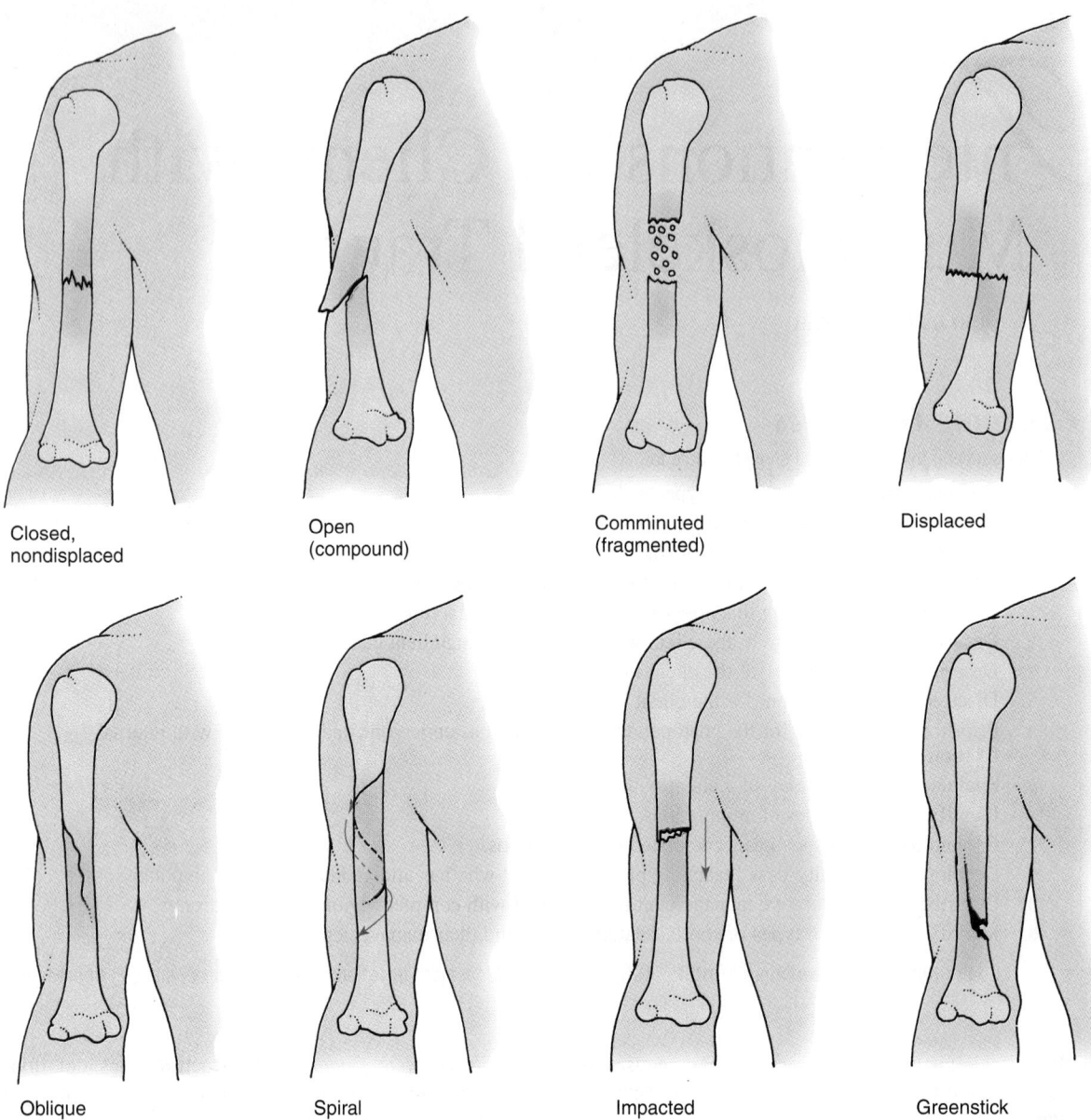

Closed,
nondisplaced

Open
(compound)

Comminuted
(fragmented)

Displaced

Oblique

Spiral

Impacted

Greenstick

Figure 52-1 ● Common types of fractures.

stress fracture results from excessive strain and stress on the bone. **Compression fractures** are produced by a loading force applied to the long axis of cancellous bone. They commonly occur in the vertebrae of clients with osteoporosis.

■ STAGES OF BONE HEALING

When a bone is broken, the body immediately begins the healing process to repair the injury and restore the body's equilibrium. Within 48 to 72 hours after the injury, a hematoma forms at the site of the fracture because bone is extremely vascular. Blood supply to and within the bone usually diminishes because of the injury, which causes an area of bone necrosis. The dead cells prompt migration of fibroblasts and osteoblasts to the fracture site as part of the inflammatory process. This prompts the formation of fibrocartilage, providing the foundation for bone healing (within 3 days to 2 weeks).

As a result of vascular and cellular proliferation, the fracture site is surrounded by new vascular tissue known as a callus (within 2 to 6 weeks). Callus formation is the beginning of a nonbony union. As healing continues, the callus is transformed from a loose, fibrous tissue into bone (within 3 weeks to 6 months). Excess callus is resorbed. During the final phase of healing, consolidation, and remodeling, bone continues to be resorbed and deposited in response to stress, reshaping to meet mechanical demands. This process may start as early as 6 weeks after fracture and can continue for up to 1 year. Figure 52-2 summarizes the stages of bone healing.

In young, healthy adult bone, healing takes about 6 weeks. In the older person who has reduced bone mass, healing time is lengthened; complete healing often takes 3 to 6 months. Other factors that affect healing include the severity of the trauma, the type of bone injured, inadequate immobilization, infections at the fracture site, and avascular necrosis (AVN).

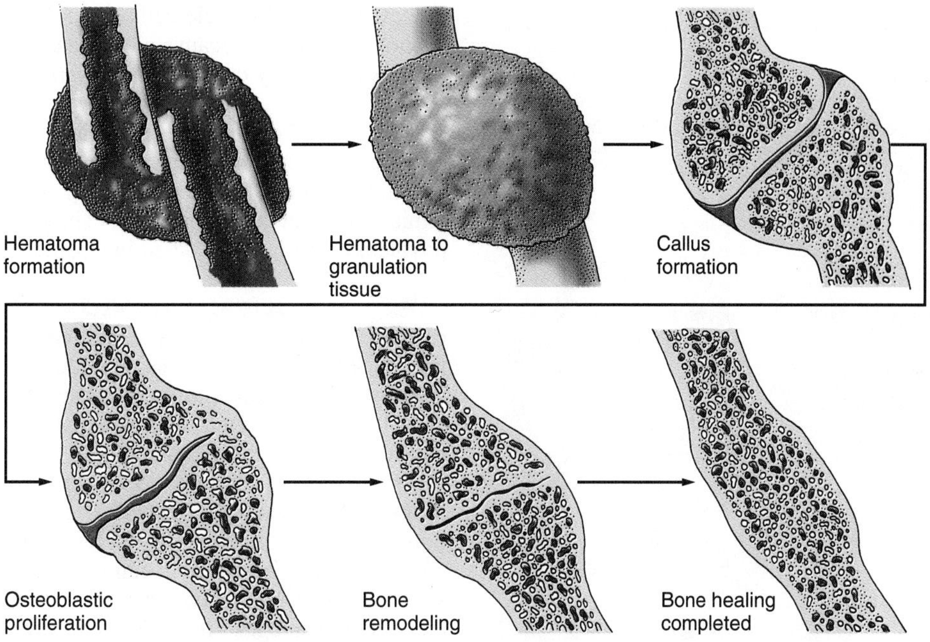

Figure 52-2 ● The stages of bone healing.

Hematoma formation

Hematoma to granulation tissue

Callus formation

Osteoblastic proliferation

Bone remodeling

Bone healing completed

CONSIDERATIONS FOR OLDER ADULTS

Healing can be affected by a number of factors in addition to the aging process. Bone formation and strength rely on adequate nutrition. Calcium, phosphorus, vitamin D, and protein are necessary for the production of new bone (see Chapter 53). For women, the loss of estrogen after menopause is detrimental to the body's ability to form new bone tissue. Concurrent diseases can also affect the rate at which bone heals. For instance, peripheral vascular diseases, such as arteriosclerosis, reduce arterial circulation to bone; thus the bone receives less oxygen and lesser amounts of nutrients, both of which are needed for repair.

■ COMPLICATIONS OF FRACTURES

Regardless of the type or location of the fracture, several limb and life-threatening complications can result from the injury. The nurse must be able to recognize the clinical manifestations of impending complications so that treatment can be started immediately. In some cases, careful monitoring and assessment can prevent these complications.

ACUTE COMPARTMENT SYNDROME. Compartments are sheaths of inelastic fascia that support and partition muscles, blood vessels, and nerves in the body. **Acute compartment syndrome (ACS)** is a serious condition in which increased pressure within one or more compartments causes massive compromise of circulation to the area. The most common sites for ACS are the compartments in the lower leg and the dorsal and volar compartments of the forearm.

The pressure to the compartment can be from an external or internal source. Tight, bulky dressings and casts are examples of external pressure. Blood or fluid accumulation is a common source of internal pressure. ACS is not limited to clients with musculoskeletal problems; clients with severe burns, extensive insect bites, or massive infiltration of intra-venous (IV) fluids are also susceptible to compartment syndrome. In these situations, edema increases pressure in one or more compartments.

PATHOPHYSIOLOGIC CHANGES. The primary pathophysiologic changes of increased compartment pressure are sometimes referred to as the ischemia-edema cycle. Capillaries within the viable muscle dilate, which raises capillary pressure. Capillaries become more permeable because of the release of histamine by the ischemic muscle tissue. As a result, plasma proteins leak into the interstitial fluid space, and edema occurs. Edema causes pressure on nerve endings and subsequent pain. Blood flow to the area is reduced, and further ischemia results. Sensory deficits (e.g., paresthesia) generally appear before changes in vascular or motor signs. The color of the tissue pales, and pulses begin to weaken but rarely disappear; the affected area is usually palpably tense, and pain can be elicited with passive motion of the extremity. If the condition is not treated, cyanosis, tingling, numbness, paresis, and severe pain occur. Chart 52-1 summarizes the sequence of pathophysiologic events in compartment syndrome and the associated clinical assessment findings.

ACS is not common, but it creates an emergency situation when it does occur. Within 4 to 6 hours after the onset of compartment syndrome, neuromuscular damage is irreversible. The limb can become useless in 24 to 48 hours.

In some cases, clients at especially high risk for ACS are monitored by an invasive procedure. Compartment pressures can be monitored on a one-time basis with a handheld device with a digital display, or they can be monitored continuously. Continuous monitoring requires placement of a wick or slit-tip catheter connected to a transducer and is recommended for comatose or unresponsive at-risk clients.

If ACS is verified, the surgeon may perform a **fasciotomy** by making an incision through the skin and subcutaneous tissues into the fascia of the affected compartment. This proce-

CHART 52-1

KEY FEATURES *of*
Compartment Syndrome

Physiologic Change	Clinical Findings
Increased compartment pressure	No change
Increased capillary permeability	Edema
Release of histamine	Increased edema
Increased blood flow to area	Pulses present Pink tissue
Pressure on nerve endings	Pain
Increased tissue pressure	Referred pain to compartment
Decreased tissue perfusion	Increased edema
Decreased oxygen to tissues	Pallor
Increased production of lactic acid	Unequal pulses Flexed posture
Anaerobic metabolism	Cyanosis
Vasodilation	Increased edema
Increased blood flow	Tense muscle swelling
Increased tissue pressure	Tingling Numbness
Increased edema	Paresthesia
Muscle ischemia	Severe pain unrelieved by medication
Tissue necrosis	Paresis/paralysis

dure relieves the pressure in order to restore circulation to the affected area. No consensus exists on what pressure requires fasciotomy (normal = 0 to 8 mm Hg); compartment pressures must be considered in relation to the client's hemodynamic status. After fasciotomy, the nurse packs and dresses the open wound on a regular basis until secondary closure occurs, usually in 4 to 5 days. At that time, the surgeon usually debrides the wound and may apply a skin graft to promote healing.

POSSIBLE RESULTS OF COMPARTMENT SYNDROME. Specific problems resulting from compartment syndrome include infection, persistent motor weakness in the affected extremity, contracture, and myoglobinuric renal failure. In extreme cases, amputation may be necessary.

Infection from the necrotic tissue may become severe enough that amputation of the limb is warranted. *Motor weakness* from injured nerves is not reversible, and the client may require braces or other orthotic devices for assistance in movement. Volkmann's *contractures,* which can begin within 12 hours of the pressure increase, result from shortening of the ischemic muscle and from nerve involvement.

Myoglobinuric renal failure (rhabdomyolysis) is a potentially fatal complication of compartment syndrome. It commonly occurs when large or multiple compartments are involved. Injured muscle tissues release myoglobulin (muscle protein) into the circulation, where it can occlude the distal convoluted tubule and precipitate acute renal failure. Although the exact pathophysiologic mechanisms are unknown, it is suspected that myoglobulin has a direct toxic effect on the

kidney. Damaged muscle cells also release potassium, which cannot be excreted because of the renal failure. The resulting hyperkalemia may cause cardiac dysrhythmias.

SHOCK. Bone is quite vascular; therefore there is a risk of bleeding with bone injury. In addition, trauma can sever adjacent arteries and cause hemorrhage; consequently, hypovolemic shock can develop rapidly. (The pathophysiology of hypovolemic shock is described in Chapter 37.)

FAT EMBOLISM SYNDROME. Fat embolism syndrome **(FES)** is a serious complication, usually resulting from a fracture, in which fat globules are released from the yellow bone marrow into the bloodstream. FES may also occur, although less often, with pancreatitis, diabetic coma, osteomyelitis, or sickle cell anemia.

The release of fat emboli is most likely with fractures of long bones or multiple fractures, although a break in any bone with sufficient bone marrow content can cause the complication. The problem can occur at any age or in either sex, but young men between ages 20 and 40 years and older adults between ages 70 and 80 years are at the greatest risk. The older client with a fractured hip has the highest risk, but FES is also common in clients with fractures of the pelvis.

Several theories have been offered to explain how fat is released from the bone marrow. The metabolic theory proposes that the elevated concentration of catecholamines as a result of trauma causes mobilization of free fatty acids, which leads to platelet aggregation and the formation of fat globules. The mechanical theory suggests that the pressure within yellow bone marrow is greater than capillary pressure, and therefore fats are released directly from the bone. In either case, the fat globules are deposited in small blood vessels that supply the major organs of the body, most commonly the lungs.

The *earliest* manifestation of FES is altered mental status, which is caused by a low arterial oxygen level. The client then typically experiences respiratory distress, tachycardia, tachypnea, fever, and petechiae (a macular, measles-like rash over the neck, upper arms, and/or chest and abdomen). Petechiae are characteristic of fat emboli, but the physiologic basis for their development is not known.

Laboratory findings in FES include the following:
- Increased erythrocyte sedimentation rate (ESR)
- Decreased serum calcium levels
- Decreased red blood cell and platelet counts
- Increased serum lipase level

These changes in blood values are poorly understood, but they aid in diagnosis of the condition.

Fat embolism usually occurs within 48 hours of the fracture and can result in respiratory failure or death, often from pulmonary edema. When the lungs are affected, the complication may be misdiagnosed as a pulmonary embolism from a blood clot (Chart 52-2).

THROMBOEMBOLITIC COMPLICATIONS. Deep vein thrombosis (DVT) often develops in people who are immobile because of trauma, surgery, or disability. It is the most common complication of lower extremity surgery or trauma and the most often fatal complication of musculoskeletal surgery. A person who smokes, is obese, has heart disease, or has

CHART 52-2

KEY FEATURES *of*
Pulmonary Emboli: Fat Embolism Versus Blood Clot Embolism

Fat Embolism	Blood Clot Embolism
Definition	
Obstruction of the pulmonary vascular bed by fat globules	Obstruction of the pulmonary artery by a blood clot or clots
Origin	
95% from fractures of the long bones; occurs usually within 48 hr	85% from deep vein thrombosis in the legs or pelvis; can occur anytime
Assessment Findings	
Altered mental status (earliest sign)	Same as for fat embolism, except no petechiae
Increased respirations, pulse, temperature	
Chest pain	
Dyspnea	
Crackles	
Decreased Sao₂	
Petechiae (50%-60%)	
Retinal hemorrhage (not common)	
Mild thrombocytopenia	
Treatment	
Bedrest	Preventive measures (e.g., leg exercises, antiembolism stockings, SCDs)
Gentle handling	
Oxygen	Bedrest
Hydration (IV fluids)	Oxygen
Possibly steroid therapy	Possibly mechanical ventilation
Fracture immobilization	Anticoagulants
	Thrombolytics
	Possible surgery: pulmonary embolectomy, vena cava umbrella

Sao₂, Arterial oxgen saturation; *SCD*, Sequential compression device.

a history of thromboembolitic complications is at an increased risk for DVT. The incidence of life-threatening embolic conditions is highest in older adults, particularly during the first 2 to 3 days after musculoskeletal surgery.

Certain fracture sites are more often associated with life-threatening thrombi. For example, DVT that leads to pulmonary embolism is more likely to develop in clients with fractures of the lower extremities and pelvis. Local venous stasis secondary to trauma or surgical procedures (e.g., use of tourniquets in lower extremity injuries) increases the chance of DVT in clients with musculoskeletal trauma. A further discussion of DVT is found in Chapter 36.

INFECTION. Any time there is trauma to tissues, the body's defense system is disrupted. Wound infections are the most common type of infection resulting from orthopedic trauma; they range from superficial skin infections to deep wound abscesses. Infection can also be caused by implanted hardware used to repair a fracture surgically, such as pins, plates, or rods. Clostridial infections can result in gas gangrene or tetanus and can prevent the bone from healing properly.

Bone infection, or osteomyelitis, is most common with open fractures in which skin integrity is lost and after surgical repair of a fracture (see Chapter 53). For clients experiencing this type of trauma, the risk of hospital-acquired (nosocomial) infections is increased.

AVASCULAR NECROSIS. **Avascular necrosis (AVN)** is sometimes referred to as aseptic or ischemic necrosis or osteonecrosis. Blood supply to the bone is disrupted, which results in the death of bone tissue. AVN is most often a complication of hip fractures, or any fracture in which there is displacement of bone. Surgical repair of fractures also can lead to AVN because the hardware can interfere with circulation.

FRACTURE BLISTERS. Fracture blisters are associated most commonly with high-energy fractures and twisting injuries in the lower extremities. Extensive tissue edema allows fluid to move into the weakened space between the epidermis and the dermis. The increased colloidal osmotic pressure then pulls more fluid into the space. Fracture blisters can lead to wound infection and delayed fracture treatment, which may then contribute to potential nonunion. Nursing measures that can assist in preventing or minimizing fracture blisters include maintaining proper immobilization before definitive treatment, and elevation to limit edema.

DELAYED UNION, NONUNION, AND MALUNION. Delayed union describes a fracture that has not healed within 6 months of injury. Some fractures never achieve union; that is, they never completely heal (nonunion); others heal incorrectly (malunion). These problems are most common in clients with tibial fractures, fractures for which a number of different treatment techniques have been used (e.g., cast, traction), and pathologic fractures. Union may also be delayed or not achieved in the older client. If bone does not heal, the client typically experiences pain and immobility from deformity.

Etiology

The primary cause of a fracture is trauma from a motor vehicle accident or fall. The trauma experienced may be a direct blow to the bone or an indirect force from muscle contractions or pulling forces on the bone. Sports, vigorous exercise, and malnutrition are contributing factors. Bone diseases, such as osteoporosis, increase the risk of a fracture in older adults.

Incidence/Prevalence

The incidence of fractures depends on the location of the injury. Rib fractures are the most common type in the adult population. Femoral shaft fractures occur most often in young and middle-aged adults. The incidence of proximal femur (hip) fractures is highest in older adults. Humeral fractures are common in adults; the older the person, usually the more proximal the fracture. Wrist (Colles') fractures are typically seen in middle and late adulthood.

WOMEN'S HEALTH CONSIDERATIONS
It is estimated that more than 1 million fractures occur annually in the United States as a result of osteoporosis, and most occur in middle-aged and older women. By age 80, 1 in 5 women has suffered a hip fracture.

> ≋ **CULTURAL CONSIDERATIONS**
> Hip fractures occur less often in African Americans or in men of any race than in Caucasian and Asian women because of a lower incidence of osteoporosis. This is due in some degree to the denser bone mass in African Americans and in men of any race.

▶ COLLABORATIVE MANAGEMENT

● Assessment

▦ HISTORY

The nurse collects data to determine the cause of the fracture, which helps in developing an individualized plan of care for the client.

PRECEDING EVENTS. The nurse asks the client to recall the specific events up to the time of the injury. Some type of force, such as incisional, crush, acceleration or deceleration, shearing, or friction, leads to most musculoskeletal injuries. As a result, several body systems are often affected.

Incisional (as from a knife wound) and crush injuries cause hemorrhage and disrupt blood flow to major organs. Acceleration or deceleration injuries cause direct trauma to the spleen, brain, and kidneys when these organs are moved from their fixed locations in the body. Shearing and friction damage the skin and cause a high level of wound contamination.

By asking about the events leading to the injury, the nurse can determine which forces have been experienced and therefore which body systems or parts of the body to assess. For example, a forward fall often results in Colles' fracture of the wrist because the person tries to catch himself or herself with an outstretched hand. Knowing the mechanism of injury also helps the nurse determine whether other types of injury, such as head and spinal cord injury, may be present.

OTHER HISTORY. A medication history, including substance abuse (recreational drug use), is important regardless of age. For example, a young adult may have had an excessive amount of alcohol, which contributed to a motor vehicle accident or to a fall at the work site. Many older adults also consume alcohol and an assortment of prescribed and over-the-counter drugs, which can cause dizziness and loss of balance.

A medical history elicits possible causes of the fracture and gives clues as to how long it will take for the bone to heal. Certain diseases, such as bone cancer and Paget's disease, cause pathologic fractures that often do not achieve union.

The nurse asks about the client's occupation and recreational activities. Some occupations are more hazardous than others; for instance, construction work is potentially more physically dangerous than office work. Certain hobbies and recreational activities are also extremely hazardous (e.g., skiing and in-line skating). Contact sports, such as football and ice hockey, often result in musculoskeletal injuries, including fractures. Other activities do not have such an obvious potential for injury but can cause fractures nonetheless. For instance, daily jogging and frequent marching in a band can lead to fatigue fractures.

Because inadequate nutrition contributes to fractures and can inhibit bone healing, the nurse takes a complete diet history. Health promotion counseling is a major focus for comprehensive health care today.

> ✿ **CONSIDERATIONS FOR OLDER ADULTS**
> A diet history is especially important for older adults. For example, some older clients eat poorly because of loss of companionship and poor finances. They may be unable to prepare meals and thus rely on others for proper nutrition. Inadequate exposure to sunlight in many older adults may contribute to vitamin D deficiency.

▦ PHYSICAL ASSESSMENT/CLINICAL MANIFESTATIONS

BODY SYSTEM ASSESSMENT. The client with a fracture often sustains trauma to other body systems. Consequently, the nurse assesses all major body systems *first* for life-threatening complications, including head, thoracic, and abdominal injuries. The assessment of these areas is described elsewhere in this text.

MUSCULOSKELETAL ASSESSMENT. When inspecting the site of a possible fracture, the nurse observes for a change in bone alignment. The bone may appear deformed, or a limb may be internally or externally rotated. Accompanying these deviations may be an alteration in the length of the extremity (usually a shortening) or a change in bone shape. The nurse asks the client to move the involved body part. If pain is elicited, the movement is stopped immediately. Range of motion (ROM) is typically decreased. When the affected part is moved, the nurse may hear **crepitation,** a continuous grating sound created by bone fragments.

The nurse also observes the skin for integrity. If the skin is intact (closed fracture), the area over the fracture may be ecchymotic (bruised) from bleeding into the underlying soft tissues. Subcutaneous emphysema, the appearance of bubbles under the skin because of air trapping, is not uncommon but is seen later.

Swelling at the fracture site is rapid and can result in marked neurovascular compromise. Therefore the nurse performs a thorough neurovascular assessment and compares the injured area with its symmetric counterpart. Skin color and temperature, sensation, mobility, pain, and pulses are assessed distal to the fracture site. If the fracture involves an extremity, the nurse checks the nails for capillary refill by applying pressure to the nail and observing for the speed of blood return. If nails are brittle or thick, the skin adjacent to the nail is assessed. Chart 52-3 describes the procedure for a neurovascular assessment, which evaluates circulation, movement, and sensation.

For an open fracture, the nurse determines the degree of soft-tissue damage and the amount of overt bleeding. The area may be lightly palpated for tenderness, but a sterile glove is worn if the skin is disrupted.

Clients often complain of moderate to severe pain at the site of the fracture or in an adjacent or distal area. For example, clients with a fractured hip may have groin pain or pain referred to the back of the knee. Pain is usually due to muscle spasm and edema, which result from the fracture. In clients with one or more fractured ribs, severe pain occurs when deep

CHART 52-3

BEST PRACTICE *for*
Assessment of Neurovascular Status in Clients
with Musculoskeletal Injury

ASSESSMENT TECHNIQUE	NORMAL FINDINGS
Skin Color Inspect the area distal to the injury.	No change in pigmentation compared with other parts of the body.
Skin Temperature Palpate the area distal to the injury (the dorsum of the hands is most sensitive to temperature).	The skin is warm.
Movement Ask the client to move the affected area or the area distal to the injury (active motion). Move the area distal to the injury (passive motion).	The client can move without discomfort. No difference in comfort compared with active movement.
Sensation Ask the client if numbness or tingling is present (paresthesia). Palpate with a paper clip (especially the web space between the first and second toes or the web space between the thumb and forefinger).	No numbness or tingling. No difference in sensation in the affected and unaffected extremities. (Loss of sensation in these areas indicates perineal nerve or median nerve damage.)
Pulses Palpate the pulses distal to the injury.	Pulses are strong and easily palpated; no difference in the affected and unaffected extremities.
Capillary Refill Press the nail beds distal to the injury until blanching occurs (or the skin near the nail if nails are thick and brittle).	Blood returns (return to usual color) within 3 seconds (5 seconds for older clients).
Pain Ask the client about the location, nature, and frequency of the pain.	Pain is usually localized and is often described as stabbing or throbbing. (Pain out of proportion to the injury and unrelieved by analgesics might indicate compartment syndrome.)

breaths are taken. The nurse assesses respiratory status, which may be severely compromised from pain or pneumothorax (air in the pleural cavity).

SPECIAL ASSESSMENT CONSIDERATIONS. For fractures of the shoulder and upper arm, the physical assessment is best done with the client in a sitting or standing position, if possible, so that shoulder drooping or other abnormal positioning can be seen. The nurse supports the affected arm and flexes the elbow to promote comfort during the assessment. For more distal areas of the arm, the assessment is done with the client in a supine position so that the extremity can be elevated to reduce swelling.

The nurse places the client in a supine position for assessment of the lower extremities and pelvis. A client with an impacted hip fracture may be able to walk for a short time after injury, although this is not recommended. The client with any type of hip fracture has pain and decreased ROM in the hip.

Some fractures can cause internal organ damage, resulting in hemorrhage. When a pelvic fracture is suspected, the nurse assesses vital signs, skin color, and the level of consciousness for indications of possible hypovolemic shock. The urine is checked for blood, which indicates damage to the urinary system, often the bladder. If the client is unable to void, the nurse suspects damage to the urethra.

■ **PSYCHOSOCIAL ASSESSMENT**

The psychosocial status of a client with a fracture depends on the extent of the injury and other complications. Hospitalization is usually not required for a single, uncomplicated fracture, and the client may return to usual daily activities within a few days. Healing is usually complete in a young adult in 4 to 6 weeks.

In contrast, a client suffering multiple trauma can be hospitalized for weeks and may undergo many surgical procedures and other treatments. For these clients, disruptions in lifestyle can create a high level of stress.

The stresses that result from a chronic condition affect relationships between the client and family members or significant others. The nurse assesses the client's feelings about himself or herself as a person and asks about how he or she coped with previously experienced stressful events. Body image and sexuality may be altered by deformity, treatment modalities for fracture repair, and/or long-term immobilization.

■ **LABORATORY ASSESSMENT**

No special laboratory tests are available for assessment of fractures. The client's hemoglobin level and hematocrit are often low because of bleeding caused by the injury. If extensive soft-tissue damage accompanies the fracture, the erythrocyte sedimentation rate (ESR) may be elevated, which indicates the expected inflammatory response. If the ESR increases during fracture healing, the client may have a bone infection. During the healing stages, serum calcium and phosphorus levels are often increased as the bone releases these elements into the blood.

■ **RADIOGRAPHIC ASSESSMENT**

The health care provider orders standard x-ray studies and tomograms to confirm a diagnosis of fracture. These reveal the bone disruption, malalignment, or deformity. If the x-ray film does not show a fracture but the client is symptomatic, the x-ray study is usually repeated with additional views.

The computed tomography (CT) scan is useful in detecting fractures of complex structures, such as the hip and pelvis. It also identifies compression fractures of the spine.

■ **OTHER DIAGNOSTIC ASSESSMENT**

The health care provider may order a bone scan (with technetium or gallium) for help in detecting certain types of fractures, particularly pathologic fractures. It is impossible for fractures of small bones or occult fractures to be visualized by conventional x-ray studies as early as by a bone scan. In addition, the bone scan can better determine fracture complications, such as delayed bone healing, nonunion, infection, and avascular necrosis (AVN).

Magnetic resonance imaging (MRI) is useful in determining the amount of soft-tissue damage that may have occurred with the fracture. It is also helpful in visualizing vertebral and skull fractures.

● Analysis

■ COMMON NURSING DIAGNOSES AND COLLABORATIVE PROBLEMS

The following are common nursing diagnoses for clients with fractures:

1. Risk for Peripheral Neurovascular Dysfunction related to bone and soft-tissue trauma and immobility
2. Acute Pain related to bone disruption, soft-tissue damage, muscle spasm, and edema
3. Risk for Infection related to bone trauma and soft-tissue damage
4. Impaired Physical Mobility related to pain
5. Imbalanced Nutrition: Less Than Body Requirements related to additional metabolic need for healing of bone and soft tissues

■ ADDITIONAL NURSING DIAGNOSES AND COLLABORATIVE PROBLEMS

In addition to the common nursing diagnoses, clients with fractures may have one or more of the following:

- Activity Intolerance related to pain and impaired mobility
- Constipation related to prolonged immobility (particularly in older adults)
- Ineffective Coping related to prolonged immobility, hospitalization, and/or lifestyle changes
- Compromised Family Coping related to prolonged hospitalization and/or lifestyle changes
- Deficient Diversional Activity related to prolonged hospitalization and rehabilitation
- Anticipatory Grieving related to altered lifestyle
- Self-Care Deficit related to pain and immobility
- Disturbed Body Image related to deformity and/or treatment modality
- Sexual Dysfunction related to pain and immobility
- Disturbed Sleep Pattern related to chronic pain and/or prolonged hospitalization
- Fear related to possible nursing home placement and/or death (particularly in older adults)
- Impaired Skin Integrity and Impaired Tissue Integrity related to bone injury

The following collaborative problems may be appropriate for clients with severe fractures:

- Potential for Acute Compartment Syndrome
- Potential for Hypovolemic Shock
- Potential for Fat Embolism Syndrome
- Potential for Thromboembolitic Complications
- Potential for Avascular Necrosis
- Potential for Delayed Healing, Malunion, or Nonunion

● Planning and Implementation

■ RISK FOR PERIPHERAL NEUROVASCULAR DYSFUNCTION

NOC PLANNING: EXPECTED OUTCOMES. The client with a fracture is expected to have sufficient blood flow for adequate oxygen and nutrient delivery to tissues, especially distal to the fracture site, as indicated by strong distal peripheral pulses, brisk capillary refill, normal skin color, and intact muscle function.

INTERVENTIONS. A fracture can occur anywhere. The nurse provides emergency interventions until medical treatment in a hospital is available.

EMERGENCY CARE. A fracture may be accompanied by multiple injuries to vital organs. Therefore the nurse *first* assesses the client for respiratory distress, bleeding, and head injury. If any of these is present, the nurse provides lifesaving care before being concerned about the fracture.

The fracture injury is then assessed (Chart 52-4). If the person is clothed, the nurse or another person trained in first aid cuts away clothing from the fracture site for best visualization. Bleeding is controlled by direct pressure on the area and digital pressure over the proximal artery nearest the fracture. At the same time, to prevent shock, the nurse checks vital signs, places the client in a supine position, and keeps him or her warm with coverings.

The nurse also:

- Inspects the fracture site for intactness of skin, swelling, and deformity (e.g., shortening and rotation)
- Palpates the area *lightly* to determine temperature (coolness), decreased sensation, and blanching
- Assesses distal pulses by comparing affected and unaffected extremities, if applicable
- Assesses for motor function by asking the client to move an area distal to the fracture (e.g., if a femoral fracture is suspected, he or she is asked to move the ankle and foot on the affected side; the upper portion of the leg remains immobilized)

To prevent further damage, reduce pain, and increase circulation, the nurse immobilizes the area of the fracture by splinting. Any object or device that extends to the joints above and below the fracture can be used as a splint. At the scene of an accident, the nurse may need to improvise by using avail-

---

CHART 52-4

BEST PRACTICE *for*
Emergency Care of the Client with an Extremity Fracture

1. Remove the client's clothing (cut, if necessary) to inspect the affected area while supporting the injured area above and below the injury. Do not remove shoes, since this can cause increased trauma.
2. Apply direct pressure on the area if there is bleeding and pressure over the proximal artery nearest the fracture.
3. Keep the client warm and in a supine position.
4. Check the neurovascular status of the area distal to the extremity: temperature, color, sensation, movement, and capillary refill. Compare affected and unaffected limbs.
5. Immobilize the extremity by splinting; include joints above and below the fracture site. Recheck circulation after splinting.
6. Cover the affected area with a dressing (preferably sterile).

able materials, such as a board. If the skin is broken, the nurse loosely applies a clean (preferably sterile) cloth to prevent further contamination of the wound. Neurovascular assessment is rechecked following splinting.

In the emergency department, physician's office, or clinic, fracture management begins with reduction and immobilization of the fracture:

- Reduction, or realignment of the bone ends for proper healing, is accomplished by a closed method (e.g., traction) or an open (surgical) procedure.
- Immobilization is achieved by the use of bandages, casts, traction, internal fixation, or external fixation.

The health care provider selects the treatment method on the basis of the type, location, and extent of the fracture. These interventions prevent further injury and reduce discomfort. The nurse is responsible for maintaining these devices and for assessing, preventing, and intervening for complications that can result from their use.

> ### CRITICAL THINKING CHALLENGE
> A 30-year-old man arrives at your emergency department via ambulance. He was the driver of a motorcycle involved in a collision with a sport utility vehicle (SUV). Paramedics report that the client was hit from the side; the bike fell on him, and he was trapped underneath the SUV. Initial reports from the ambulance en route describe an individual in shock with a mangled left leg below the knee and a left wrist fracture. The client was wearing a helmet at the time of the crash.
> - What information given above is helpful in predicting other injuries this client may have sustained?
> - What are the priority assessments you should perform when he arrives at the hospital?
> - What assessments of the leg injury will determine the type and grade of the fracture?
> - What initial assessments of the injured leg should you perform?
>
> For suggested answer guidelines, go to [SIMON] http://www.wbsaunders.com/SIMON/Iggy/.

NEUROVASCULAR MONITORING. The nurse performs a neurovascular assessment (Chart 52-5) at frequent intervals if the client is admitted to the hospital, depending on the severity and extent of the fracture and agency policy. The nurse pays particular attention to *early* signs and symptoms of acute compartment syndrome (ACS) by doing a thorough pain assessment. The client with early ACS typically complains of severe, diffuse pain that is not relieved by analgesics; pain during passive motion is greater than pain during active motion. If the client presents with this complaint, the nurse notifies the health care provider *immediately*.

NONSURGICAL MANAGEMENT. Nonsurgical management typically involves closed reduction and immobilization with a bandage, splint, cast, or traction. For each modality, the nurse's primary concern is assessment and prevention of neurovascular dysfunction or compromise.

CLOSED REDUCTION. **Closed reduction** is the most common nonsurgical method for managing a simple fracture. While applying a manual pull, or traction, on the bone, the health care provider manipulates the bone ends so that they realign. Anesthesia or analgesia may be used during this procedure to minimize pain. An x-ray verifies that the bone ends are approximated before the bone is immobilized.

Bandages and Splints. For certain areas of the body, such as the scapula and clavicle, an elastic bandage or commercial mobilizer may be used to immobilize the bone during healing. Because upper extremity bones do not bear weight, splints may be sufficient to keep bone fragments in place. Figure 52-3 illustrates the use of a wrist splint for fracture immobilization. Thermoplast, a durable, flexible material for splinting, allows custom fitting to the client's body part.

The nurse's primary responsibility is to assess the area distal to the bandage or splint for neurovascular compromise. The client usually complains of increased discomfort that is not relieved by analgesics if the splint or bandage is too tight. The nurse reinforces the need for elevation as appropriate and teaches how to assess for circulatory changes. The client is reminded to keep the device as dry and clean as possible to prevent skin breakdown and infection.

Casts. For more complex fractures or fractures of the lower extremity, the physician or orthopedic technician ap-

---

> **CHART 52-5**
>
> ### INTERVENTION ACTIVITIES *for*
> ### The Client at Risk for Peripheral Neurovascular Dysfunction
>
> **Circulatory Care (Arterial Insufficiency/Venous Insufficiency):** *Promotion of arterial and venous circulation.*
> - Perform a comprehensive appraisal of peripheral circulations (e.g., check peripheral pulses, edema, capillary refill, color, and temperature).
> - Monitor degree of discomfort or pain.
> - Palpate limb with caution.
> - Place extremity in a dependent position, as appropriate.
>
> **Peripheral Sensation Management:** *Prevention or minimization of injury or discomfort in the client with altered sensation.*
> - Monitor for paresthesia: numbness, tingling, hyperesthesia, and hypoesthesia.
> - Monitor fit of bracing devices, prosthesis, shoes, and clothing.
> - Administer analgesics, as necessary.
> - Discuss or identify causes of abnormal sensations or sensation changes.

NIC intervention activities selected from McCloskey, J.C., & Bulechek, G.M. (2000). *Nursing interventions classification (NIC)* (3rd ed.). St. Louis: Mosby. No part of this work is to be altered without prior written permission from the Publisher.

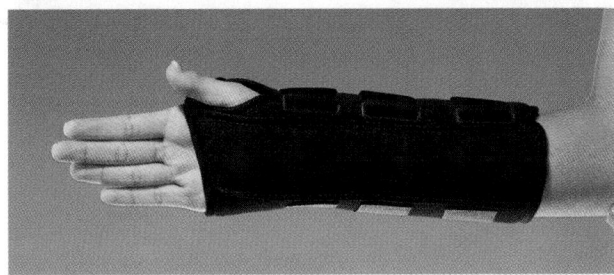

Figure 52-3 ● A universal wrist and forearm splint used for immobilization. (Courtesy Smith & Nephew, Inc., Orthopaedics Division, Memphis, TN.)

plies a cast to hold bone fragments in place after reduction. A **cast** is a rigid device that immobilizes the affected body part while allowing other body parts to move. A cast also allows early mobility and reduces pain. Although its most common use is for fractures, a cast may be applied for correction of deformities (such as clubfoot) or for prevention of deformities (such as those seen in some clients with rheumatoid arthritis).

Cast Materials. Several types of materials are used to make casts. The traditional plaster of Paris (anhydrous calcium sulfate) cast requires application of a well-fitted stockinette under the material. If the stockinette is too tight, it may impair circulation; if it is too loose, wrinkles can lead to the development of pressure ulcers and subsequent skin breakdown. Padding is applied over the stockinette, followed by wet plaster rolls wrapped around the extremity or other body part. The cast feels hot because an immediate chemical reaction occurs, but it soon becomes damp and cool. This type of cast takes 24 to 72 hours to dry, depending on the size and location of the cast. A wet cast feels cold, smells musty, and is grayish. The cast is dry when it feels hard and firm, is odorless, and has a shiny white appearance.

On occasion, the plaster cast may have rough edges, which can crumble and cause skin irritation. To resolve this problem, the nurse petals the cast if the underlying stockinette does not cover the edges of the cast. Small strips of tape are placed over the rough edges to protect the skin. If the skin under the cast was disrupted, the health care provider, orthopedic technician, or specially trained nurse cuts a window into the cast so that the wound can be observed and cared for. A window is also an access for taking pulses, removing wound drains, or relieving abdominal distention when the client is in a body or spica cast.

If the cast is too tight, it may be cut with a cast cutter to relieve pressure or allow tissue swelling. The physician may choose to bivalve the cast (cut it lengthwise into two equal pieces) if bone healing is almost complete. The nurse can remove either half of the cast for inspection or for provision of care. The two pieces are then reunited by an elastic bandage wrap.

Synthetic materials for casts include fiberglass and polyester–cotton knit (Figure 52-4). These materials are lighter than plaster and require minimal drying time. Fiberglass casts are dry in 10 to 15 minutes and can bear weight 30 minutes af-

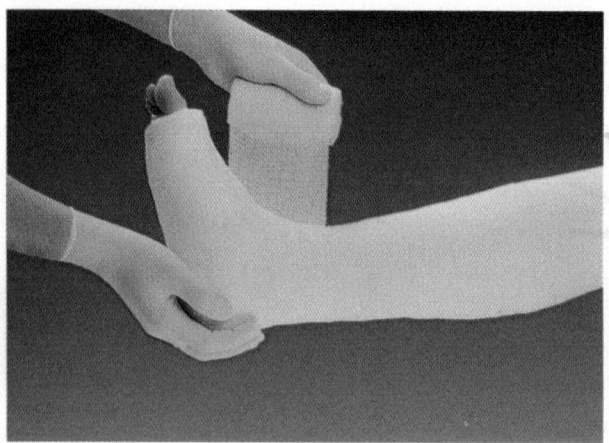

Figure 52-4 ● Application of a fiberglass synthetic cast. (Courtesy Smith & Nephew, Inc., Orthopaedics Division, Memphis, TN.)

ter application. Polyester–cotton knit casts take 7 minutes to dry and can withstand weight bearing in approximately 20 minutes. Some health care providers use synthetic casts for upper extremities and plaster of Paris casts for lower extremities because plaster casts can bear more weight for a longer time.

Types of Casts. Casts can be generally divided into four main groups: arm casts, leg casts, cast braces, and body or spica casts. Table 52-1 describes specific casts that are used for various parts of the body.

When a client is in bed with an *arm cast,* a sling is used to elevate the arm above the heart to reduce swelling. The hand should be higher than the elbow. Ice may be ordered for the first 24 to 48 hours. When the client is out of bed, the arm is supported with a sling placed around the neck to alleviate fatigue caused by the weight of the cast. The sling should distribute the weight over a large area of the shoulders and trunk, not just the neck. Some health care providers prefer that after the first few days in an arm cast, particularly a short-arm cast, the client not use a sling, to encourage normal movement of the mobile joints and enhance bone healing.

A *leg cast* permits mobility and requires the client to use ambulatory aids, such as crutches. A cast shoe, sandal, or boot that attaches to the foot or a rubber walking pad attached to the sole of the cast assists in ambulation (if weight bearing is allowed) and helps prevent damage to the cast. The affected leg is elevated on several pillows to reduce swelling, and ice is applied for the first 24 hours or as ordered.

A *cast brace* enables the client to bend unaffected joints while the fracture is healing. The fracture must show signs of healing and minimal tissue edema before application of this cast. Two cylindric casts are made and connected by a hinge to allow joint movement. As healing occurs, the casts may be removed and replaced with a soft brace. Commercial immobilizers, which serve the same function as a cast brace, are available and may be used in some cases.

A *body cast* encircles the trunk of the body; a *spica cast* encases a portion of the trunk and one or two extremities. A client with either of these casts presents a special challenge for nursing care. Potential complications related to severe impairment in mobility include the following:

* Skin breakdown
* Respiratory dysfunction, such as pneumonia and atelectasis
* Constipation
* Joint contractures

Cast syndrome (superior mesenteric artery syndrome), an uncommon but serious complication, is most often seen in orthopedic clients who have been placed in a hip spica or body cast. Partial or complete upper intestinal obstruction results in classic symptoms: abdominal distention, epigastric pain, nausea, and vomiting. The vomiting often occurs after meals, and clients may have normal bowel sounds. Partial obstruction occurs initially from compression of the third portion of the duodenum between the superior mesenteric artery and the aorta. This progresses to complete obstruction from duodenal edema caused by continued vomiting and distention. Placing a window in the abdominal portion of the cast or bivalving the cast may be sufficient to relieve pressure on the duodenum. Management of intestinal obstruction is the same as for any client with this complication (see Chapter 57).

Cast Care. Before the cast is applied, the nurse explains the purpose of the cast and the procedure for its application.

With a plaster cast, it is particularly important for the nurse to warn the client about the heat that will be felt immediately after the wet cast is applied. The new cast is not covered; this facilitates air-drying.

When a client with a wet plaster cast is moved and turned, the nurse handles the cast with the palms of the hands to prevent indentations and resultant areas of pressure on the skin. The client is turned every 1 to 2 hours to allow air to circulate and dry all parts of the cast. If the client is hospitalized, the nurse or assistive nursing personnel places a sign at the head of the bed as a reminder that the cast is wet and requires special handling. If the health care provider orders that the cast be elevated to reduce swelling, a cloth-covered pillow is used instead of one encased in plastic, which could cause the cast to retain heat and prevent drying. Elevation of the casted extremity reduces edema but may impair arterial circulation to the affected limb. Uniform support is needed while the cast is drying to prevent development of pressure points.

For preventing contamination by urine or feces, the perineal area of a dry long leg or body cast is encased in a plastic, protective covering. Fracture pans are preferred over traditional bedpans because they are smaller and more comfortable for the client. Care is taken to prevent spillage onto the cast.

The nurse checks to ensure that the cast is not too tight and frequently monitors the client's neurovascular status, usually every hour for the first 24 hours after application (see Chart 52-3 for a description of the procedure and normal findings). The nurse should be able to insert a finger between the cast and the skin. Ice may be applied for the first 24 to 36 hours to reduce swelling and inflammation.

Once the plaster cast is dry, it is inspected at least once every 8 hours for drainage, cracking, crumbling, alignment, and fit. Areas of drainage on the cast should be measured and documented, although there is no direct relationship between the amount of cast drainage and the amount of drainage from the wound. Plaster casts act like sponges and absorb drainage, whereas synthetic casts act like a wick, pulling drainage away from the drainage site. Padding can also absorb wound drainage. Drainage on any cast should always be measured and documented in the client record; however, sources disagree on whether drainage should be circled on the cast, because it may increase anxiety. The nurse immediately reports sudden increases in the amount of drainage or a change in the integrity of the cast to the health care provider. After swelling decreases, it is not uncommon for the cast to become too loose and need replacement. If the client is not admitted to the hospital, he or she is given instructions regarding cast care, as discussed later under Community-Based Care, p. 1141.

Cast Complications. During hospitalization, the nurse assesses for other complications resulting from casting that can

TABLE 52-1 • TYPES OF CASTS USED FOR MUSCULOSKELETAL TRAUMA	
Type and Characteristics of Cast	**Use**
UPPER EXTREMITY CASTS	
Short-arm cast (SAC) (extends from below the elbow to and including part of the hand)	Stable fractures of the wrist (metacarpals, carpals, or distal radius)
Long-arm cast (LAC) (includes the upper arm to and including part of the hand)	Unstable fractures of the wrist, distal humerus, radius, or ulna
Hanging-arm cast (same as LAC but heavier, with added loop at the mid-forearm)	Fractures of the humerus that cannot be aligned by LAC (Light traction is possible while the client is in bed or by an attached strap that extends around the neck.)
Thumb spica (gauntlet) cast (similar to SAC with the thumb casted in abduction)	Fractures of the thumb
Shoulder spica cast (the shoulder is casted in abduction with the elbow flexed)	Unstable fractures of the shoulder girdle or humerus; dislocations of the shoulder
LOWER EXTREMITY CASTS	
Short-leg cast (SLC) (from below the knee to the base of the toes)	Fractures of the ankle, metatarsals, or foot
Long-leg cast (LLC) (from the mid-upper thigh to the base of the toes)	Unstable fractures of the tibia, fibula, or ankle
Walking cast (a walking device on the bottom of SLC or LLC)	Same as for SLC or LLC
Leg cylinder (similar to SLC, but the ankle and foot are not casted)	Stable fractures of the tibia, fibula, or knee
Long-leg cylinder (similar to LLC, but the ankle and foot are not casted)	Stable fractures of the distal femur, proximal tibia, or knee
CAST BRACES (OR BRACE CASTS)	
Patellar weight-bearing cast (similar to SLC or leg cylinder)	Midshaft or distal shaft fractures of the femur
External polycentric knee hinge cast (a hinge connects the lower and upper leg and allows 90 degrees of knee flexion)	Same as for the patellar weight-bearing cast
BODY CASTS	
Hip spica (extends from below the nipple line down the affected leg [single], down the leg and half of the unaffected leg [1½], or down both legs [double])	Dislocation of the hip; pelvic or hip injuries
Risser's cast (the body jacket extends from the shoulders to beyond the iliac crests and hips, with a large opening over the anterior chest)	Scoliosis; thoracic spinal fractures
Halo cast (the body jacket contains a halo brace)	Fractures of the cervical spine

be serious and life threatening, such as infection, circulation impairment, and peripheral nerve damage. If the client returns home after cast application, the client and family are taught how to monitor for these complications and when to notify the health care provider.

Infection most often results from the breakdown of skin under the cast (pressure necrosis). If pressure necrosis occurs, the client typically complains of a very painful "hot spot" under the cast, and the cast may feel warmer in the affected area. The nurse smells the area for mustiness or an unpleasant odor that would indicate infected material. If the infection progresses, a fever may develop.

Circulation impairment and peripheral nerve damage can result from constriction of the cast. The nurse performs frequent neurovascular assessments, as described in Chart 52-3. A client with a new cast may require hourly assessments. A client with a cast that is 3 or 4 days old usually requires assessments every 4 to 8 hours.

The client with a cast may be immobilized for a prolonged period, depending on the extent of the fracture and the type of cast. The nurse assesses for complications of immobility, such as skin breakdown, pneumonia, atelectasis, thromboembolism, and constipation. Before the cast is removed, the nurse informs the client that the cast cutter will not injure the skin but that heat may be felt during the procedure.

Because of prolonged immobilization, a joint may become contracted, usually in a fixed state of flexion, or degenerative arthritis may develop from lack of weight bearing, which is necessary for cartilage viability. Muscle can also atrophy from lack of exercise during prolonged immobilization of the affected body part, usually an extremity.

CRITICAL THINKING CHALLENGE

Following initial assessment in the emergency department, your client who was injured in the motorcycle accident has a closed reduction of the wrist fracture and application of a long-arm cast. He is alert and oriented when he arrives on the orthopedic unit.

• What assessment should you perform to evaluate the neurovascular status of the client's injured arm?

• What is a potential cause of compartment syndrome in this client's fractured arm?

• What symptoms would raise suspicion of compartment syndrome?

For suggested answer guidelines, go to [SIMON] http://www.wbsaunders.com/SIMON/Iggy/.

Traction. **Traction** is the application of a pulling force to a part of the body to provide reduction, alignment, and rest. Traction can also decrease muscle spasm (thus relieving pain) and prevent or correct deformity and tissue damage. A client in traction is usually hospitalized longer, but in some cases home care is possible even for skeletal traction.

Mechanical traction can be either of the following:

• Continuous, as in fracture treatment
• Intermittent, for relief of muscle spasm in other types of musculoskeletal/neurologic trauma, such as cervical nerve root compression

Traction may also be classified as running traction or balanced suspension. In running traction, the pulling force is in one direction and the client's body acts as countertraction.

Moving the body or bed position can alter the countertraction force. Balanced suspension provides the countertraction, so that the pulling force of the traction is not altered when the bed or client is moved. This allows for increased client movement and facilitates care.

Types of Traction. Traction is typically one of five types: skin traction, skeletal traction, plaster traction, brace traction, or circumferential traction. Skin traction involves the use of a Velcro boot (Buck's traction) (Figure 52-5), belt, or halter, which is secured around a body part. The primary purpose of skin traction is to decrease painful muscle spasms that accompany fractures. The weight used as a pulling force is limited (5 to 10 pounds [2.3 to 4.5 kg]) to prevent injury to the skin.

In skeletal traction, pins (e.g., Steinmann), wires (e.g., Kirschner), tongs (e.g., Crutchfield), or screws are surgically inserted directly into bone. These allow the use of longer traction time and heavier weights (usually 15 to 30 pounds [6.8 to 13.6 kg]). Skeletal traction aids in bone realignment.

Plaster traction combines skeletal traction and a plaster cast. A brace traction device exerts a pull for correction of alignment deformities. Circumferential traction uses a belt around the body, such as pelvic traction for low back problems. Table 52-2 describes commonly used types of traction for various parts of the body.

Traction Care. The nurse may set up or assist in the setup of traction. In larger or specialty hospitals or units, orthopedic technicians may set up traction. Once traction is applied, the nurse is responsible for maintaining the correct balance between traction pull and countertraction force. Weights are not usually removed without an order; they are not usually lifted manually or allowed to sit on the floor. Weights should be freely hanging at all times. The nurse teaches this important point to staff members on the unit and to other personnel, such as in the radiology department.

The skin should be inspected at least every 8 hours for signs of irritation or inflammation. When possible, the nurse removes the belt or boot that is used for skin traction every 8 hours to inspect under the device.

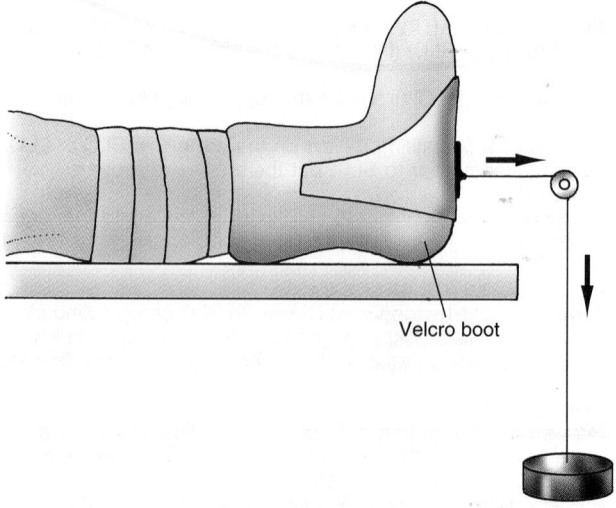

Velcro boot

Figure 52-5 ● Buck's traction with a hook-and-loop fastener (Velcro) boot, commonly used for hip fractures.

When skeletal traction is used, the nurse pays particular attention to the points of entry of pins, wires, or screws for signs of inflammation or infection. A small amount of clear fluid drainage ("weeping") is expected. Most health care providers prefer that the nurse perform pin care every day. No standardized method or protocol for pin care has been established throughout the United States. Some health care providers and nurse specialists believe that cleaning the pins disrupts the skin's natural barrier to infection and advise against this practice. In any case, the nurse observes pin sites at least every 8 hours for drainage, color, odor, and severe redness, which indicate inflammation and possible infection. Infection of the pin tract may result in osteomyelitis.

The nurse is responsible for checking traction equipment to ensure its proper functioning. All ropes, knots, and pulleys are inspected at least every 8 hours for loosening, fraying, and positioning. The nurse checks the weight for consistency with the health care provider's order. At times, the health care provider or qualified technician changes the weight without notifying the nurse or modifying the written order; the nurse contacts the person responsible for a new order for confirmation of the change. Sometimes one of the weights is accidentally displaced by a staff member or visitor who bumps into it. The nurse replaces the weights if they are not correct and notifies the health care provider or orthopedic technician.

If the client complains of severe pain from muscle spasm, the weights may be too heavy or the client may need realignment. The nurse reports the pain to the health care provider if body realignment fails to reduce the discomfort. The nurse also assesses the neurovascular status of the affected body part to detect circulatory compromise and subsequent tissue damage. For clients with casts, circulation is usually monitored every hour for the first 24 hours after traction is applied and every 4 hours thereafter (see Chart 52-3).

CONSIDERATIONS FOR OLDER ADULTS

Older clients often have peripheral vascular disease, connective tissue disease, and/or diabetes. Therefore they are at high risk for problems caused by skin or skeletal traction because of inadequate circulation and sensation. Traction of any type is not the ideal treatment for the older client, because it necessitates a prolonged period of immobilization; serious complications can result, such as pneumonia and pulmonary emboli. Abrasions, ulcers, and other skin problems should be reported to the health care provider. Care must be taken to avoid pressure on the bony prominences and superficial nerves. Pressure on the peroneal nerve at the point where it passes around the neck of the fibula must also be avoided, or footdrop could occur.

SURGICAL MANAGEMENT. For some types of fractures, casts and traction are not appropriate or sufficient treatment techniques. Surgical intervention may be needed to realign the bone for the healing process.

PREOPERATIVE CARE. For stabilizing the fracture, the client may be placed in traction before surgery. This procedure is typical for managing a fractured hip when Buck's traction may be used preoperatively (see Figure 52-5). The nurse teaches the client and family or significant others what to expect during and after the surgery. The preoperative care for a client undergoing musculoskeletal surgery is similar to that for any client preparing for surgery with general or epidural anesthesia. (See Chapter 17 for a thorough discussion of preoperative nursing care.)

TABLE 52-2 • TYPES OF TRACTION USED FOR MUSCULOSKELETAL TRAUMA	
Type and Characteristics of Traction	**Use**
UPPER EXTREMITY TRACTION	
Sidearm skin or skeletal traction (the forearm is flexed and extended 90 degrees from the upper part of the body)	Fractures of the humerus with or without involvement of the shoulder and clavicle
Overhead or 90-90 traction, skin or skeletal (the elbow is flexed and the arm is at a right angle to the body over the upper chest)	Same as above (depends on the physician's preference)
Plaster traction (pins inserted through the bone are fixed in the cast)	Fractures of the wrist
LOWER EXTREMITY TRACTION	
Buck's extension traction (skin) (the affected leg is in extension)	Fractures of the hip or femur preoperatively Prevention of hip flexion contractures Hip dislocation
Russell's traction (similar to Buck's traction, but a sling under the knee suspends the leg)	Fractures of the hip or end of the femur
Balanced skin or skeletal traction (the limb is usually elevated in a Thomas splint with Pearson's attachment, or a Böhler-Braun splint is used)	Fractures of the femur or pelvis (acetabulum)
SPINAL COLUMN AND PELVIC TRACTION	
Cervical halter (a strap under the chin)	Cervical muscle spasms, strain/sprain, or arthritis
Cervical skeletal (e.g., halo brace, Crutchfield tongs)	Cervical fractures of the spine Muscle spasms
Pelvic belt (a strap around the hips at the iliac crests is attached to weights at the foot of the bed)	Pain, strain, sprain, or muscle spasms, in the lower back
Pelvic sling (a wide strap around the hips is attached to an overhead bar to keep the pelvis off the bed)	Pelvic fractures; other pelvic injuries

OPERATIVE PROCEDURES. **Open reduction with internal fixation (ORIF)** is a common method of reducing and immobilizing a fracture. When this method is not feasible, **external fixation with closed reduction** is used. Although the nurse does not decide which surgical technique is used, the nurse's understanding of the procedures enhances client teaching and care.

Open Reduction with Internal Fixation. ORIF permits early mobilization. Consequently, it is often the preferred surgical method for an older adult who is susceptible to the complications of immobility.

Open reduction allows the surgeon direct visualization of the fracture site. Internal fixation uses pins, screws, rods, plates, and/or prostheses to immobilize the fracture during healing. The surgeon makes an incision to gain access to the broken bone and implants the device. After the bone achieves union, the hardware may be removed, depending on the location and type of fracture (e.g., fractured ankle). Specific types of internal fixation devices are discussed later under Fractures of Specific Sites, p. 1142.

External Fixation. An alternative modality for the initial management of fractures is the external fixation apparatus, as shown in Figure 52-6. After fracture reduction, the physician makes small percutaneous incisions so that pins may be implanted into the bone. All pins are self-drilling. The pins are held in place by an external metal frame to prevent bone movement.

Advantages and Disadvantages. External fixation has several advantages over other immobilization techniques:
- There is minimal blood loss in comparison with internal fixation.
- The device allows early ambulation and exercise of the affected body part while relieving pain.

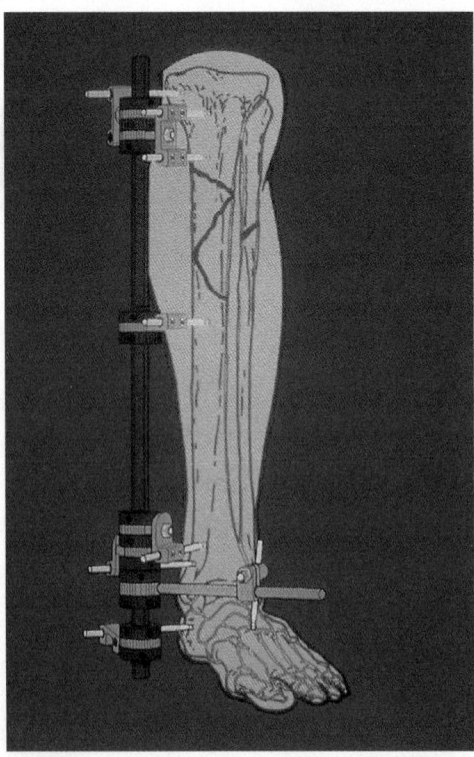

Figure 52-6 ● The Hex-Fix external fixation system for tibial fractures. (Courtesy Smith & Nephew, Inc., Orthopaedics Division, Memphis, TN.)

- The device maintains alignment in closed fractures that will not maintain position in a cast and stabilizes comminuted fractures that require bone grafting.
- In open fractures, in which skin and tissue trauma accompanies the fracture, the device permits easy access to the wound and promotes healing. This method is often preferred over the use of a window in a cast for wound care.

A disadvantage of external fixation is pin tract infection. Pin tract infections can lead to osteomyelitis, which is serious and difficult to treat (see Chapter 51). For prevention of these infections, some agencies have a pin care procedure that is performed several times a day. The procedure is similar to that described earlier for skeletal traction pins (see Traction Care, p. 1136). As with skeletal traction, the need for special cleaning of the pins and the area around the pins is controversial. Regardless of whether pin care is done, the nurse inspects the pin sites at least daily for severe redness, swelling, and purulent drainage.

Care of the Client with an External Fixator. As with any fracture treatment, the nurse assesses the neurovascular status of the extremity distal to the fracture. External fixators may be used for an extremity or for fractures of the pelvis. External fixation is not definitive treatment for fractures. After a fixator is removed, the client may be placed in a cast until healing is complete.

The client with an external fixator may experience a disturbed body image. The frame may be large and bulky, and the affected area may have massive tissue damage with dressings. The nurse is sensitive to this possibility in planning care.

> ### CRITICAL THINKING CHALLENGE
> Following evaluation in the emergency department, the client injured in the motorcycle accident is sent to the operating room for removal of his ruptured spleen, ORIF of an unstable pelvic fracture, and application of an external fixator to the grade III comminuted fracture of his left tibia and fibula.
> - What are the advantages of external fixation for treating fractures of the tibia and fibula?
> - What assessments of the external fixator should you perform frequently?
> - Your client tells you that when the fixator is removed, his leg will be completely healed and he will be able to bear weight completely. What does this statement indicate about the client's understanding of the role of external fixation in fracture management?

For suggested answer guidelines, go to $\boxed{\text{SIMON}}$ http://www.wbsaunders.com/SIMON/Iggy/.

Circular External Fixation. The Ilizarov technique of circular external fixation is sometimes used to treat new fractures (closed, comminuted fractures and open fractures with bone loss), as well as malunion or nonunion of fractures. It may also be used to treat congenital bone deformities, especially in children. This procedure originated in Russia about 50 years ago and was introduced in the United States in 1986.

A circular external fixation device stimulates bone growth. Unlike the traditional fixator, the Ilizarov external fixator promotes rotation, angulation, shortening, lengthening, and/or widening of bone while allowing healing of the soft-tissue defect. The nursing care of the client with this device is similar to the care of the client with other external fixation systems except in one major regard: if the device is being used for filling bone gaps, using bone transport or distraction, the client must be taught how to manually turn the four-sided nuts (clickers), usually four times a day, unless he or she has an automated device. Daily distraction rates vary among clients, but 1 mm/day is common. Screening and teaching are particularly important because the client adjusts and cares for the apparatus for a prolonged time.

POSTOPERATIVE CARE. The postoperative care for a client undergoing ORIF or external fixation is similar to that provided for any client undergoing surgery (see Chapter 19). However, because bone is a vascular, dynamic body tissue, the client is at risk for certain complications specific to fractures and musculoskeletal surgery. These problems (e.g., fat embolism and deep vein thrombosis [DVT]) are discussed earlier under Complications of Fractures, pp. 1127-1129.

PROCEDURES FOR NONUNION. Some surgical repairs are not successful, because the bone does not heal. Several additional options are available to the surgeon to promote bone union, such as electrical bone stimulation, bone grafting, and the newest therapy, ultrasound fracture treatment.

For selected clients, electrical bone stimulation may be successful. This procedure is based on research showing that bone has inherent electrical properties that are used in healing. The exact mechanism of action is unknown. Several types of devices have been developed. A noninvasive system uses magnetic coils applied on the skin or over a cast to deliver a pulsed magnetic field. There are no known risks with this system, although clients with pacemakers cannot use this device on an upper extremity. Implanted direct-current stimulators are placed directly in the fracture site and have no external apparatus. Both systems require about 6 months of treatment, and weight bearing is at the discretion of the health care provider.

Another method of treating nonunion is bone grafting. A bone graft may also replace diseased bone or increase bone tissue for joint replacement. In most cases, chips of bone are taken from the client's iliac crest or other site and are packed or wired between the bone ends to facilitate union. Allografts from cadavers may also be used. These grafts are frozen or freeze-dried and stored under sterile conditions in a bone bank, usually in a hospital.

Bone banking from living donors is becoming increasingly popular. If qualified, clients undergoing total hip replacement may donate their femoral heads to the bank for later use as bone grafts for other clients. Careful screening ensures that the bone is healthy and that the donor has no communicable disease. The bone cannot be donated without the client's written consent.

One of the newest modalities for fracture healing is low-intensity pulsed ultrasound (also called Exogen therapy). Used for slow-healing fractures or for new fractures as an alternative to surgery, ultrasound treatment has yielded excellent results. The client applies the treatment for about 20 minutes each day. It has no contraindications or adverse effects.

ACUTE PAIN

NOC **PLANNING: EXPECTED OUTCOMES.** The client with a fracture is expected to experience a reduction or alleviation of pain as indicated by the absence of or a decrease in reported pain, no changes in vital signs, and no facial expressions of pain.

INTERVENTIONS. The nonsurgical or surgical management of fractures through reduction and immobilization helps reduce pain and prevents neurovascular injury. The client often requires drug therapy and other pain relief measures.

DRUG THERAPY. Musculoskeletal pain related to soft-tissue damage, bone disruption, and muscle spasm is one of the most severe types of pain that can be experienced. The client often has the pain for a prolonged time, which makes pain management difficult. The health care provider commonly prescribes opioid analgesics, anti-inflammatory drugs, and muscle relaxants.

For clients with chronic, severe pain, opioid and nonopioid drugs are alternated or given together to manage pain both centrally and peripherally. The nurse and client mutually decide on the best times for the strong pain relievers to be administered (e.g., before a complex dressing change and at bedtime). The nurse observes the client carefully for the effectiveness of the medication and its side effects. An early sign of acute compartment syndrome (ACS) is often the sudden inability of pain medication to relieve pain. Chapter 7 discusses the various methods of pain management, including epidural analgesia and patient-controlled analgesia.

COMPLEMENTARY AND ALTERNATIVE THERAPIES. With chronic, severe pain, the client cannot depend solely on drugs for relief. The nurse uses temporary pain relief measures, such as ice or heat, depending on the cause of the pain. If swelling causes pressure on the affected area, ice and elevation of the affected body part may be appropriate. Muscle spasms are best relieved by application of heat and massage. Other physical measures include a warm, soothing bath, a back rub, and the use of therapeutic touch.

If these measures are not effective in reducing pain, the nurse may use distraction, imagery, or music therapy as alternatives. The nurse teaches relaxation techniques, such as deep breathing, for use during periods of severe pain. Chapters 4 and 7 discuss these techniques in detail.

RISK FOR INFECTION

PLANNING: EXPECTED OUTCOMES. The client with a fracture is expected to be free of a wound or bone infection.

INTERVENTIONS. When caring for a client with a fracture, particularly an open fracture, the nurse uses strict aseptic technique for dressing changes and wound irrigations. Signs and symptoms of local inflammation with purulent drainage are reported immediately to the physician. Other infections, such as pneumonia and urinary tract infection, may occur days after the fracture. The nurse or assistive nursing personnel monitors the client's vital signs every 4 to 8 hours; increases in temperature and pulse often indicate systemic infection.

For most clients with an open fracture, the health care provider prescribes one or more broad-spectrum antibiotics prophylactically. This treatment is especially important for fractures requiring surgical repair.

■ IMPAIRED PHYSICAL MOBILITY

NOC PLANNING: EXPECTED OUTCOMES. The client with a fracture is expected to be free of consequences of impaired mobility and independent in ambulation and mobility, such as transferring from bed to chair.

INTERVENTIONS. The interventions necessary for this diagnosis can be grouped into two types: those that help prevent complications of impaired mobility and those that help increase mobility.

PREVENTION OF COMPLICATIONS. The nurse plays a vital role in preventing and assessing complications in immobilized clients with fractures. Additional information about nursing care for preventing problems associated with immobility is found in Chapter 10 and earlier in this chapter in the discussion of specific complications under Complications of Fractures, pp. 1127-1129.

> **🌱 CONSIDERATIONS FOR OLDER ADULTS**
> The risk of each complication related to impaired mobility is dramatically increased if surgery is performed. Older clients are at the greatest risk; physiologic changes and prolonged immobility predispose them to these complications.

PROMOTION OF MOBILITY. The use of crutches or a walker increases mobility and assists in ambulation. The client may progress to use of a cane.

CRUTCHES. Crutches are the most commonly used ambulatory aid for many types of musculoskeletal trauma (e.g., fractures, sprains, and amputations). In most agencies, the physical therapist fits the client for crutches and teaches him or her how to ambulate with them on flat surfaces and stairs. The nurse's role may be to reinforce the instructions and evaluate whether the client is using the crutches correctly. However, in emergency department and ambulatory settings nurses routinely teach clients how to use crutches.

Walking with crutches requires strong upper extremities, balance, and coordination. For this reason, crutches are not used as often for older adults.

The therapist pads the tips and axillary bars of the crutches; padding prevents the tips from slipping and the bars from damaging the axillae. To prevent pressure on the axillary nerve, there should be two to three finger breadths between the axilla and the top of the crutch when the crutch tip is at least 6 inches (15 cm) diagonally in front of the foot. The crutch is adjusted by the therapist so that the elbow is flexed no more than 30 degrees when the palm is on the handle (Figure 52-7).

There are several types of gaits for walking with crutches. The most common one for musculoskeletal injury is the three-point gait, which allows minimal weight bearing on the affected leg.

WALKER. A walker is most often used by the older client who needs additional support for balance. The physical therapist assesses the strength of the upper extremities and the unaffected leg. Strength is improved with exercise as needed.

CANE. A cane is sometimes used if the client needs only minimal support for an affected leg. The straight cane offers

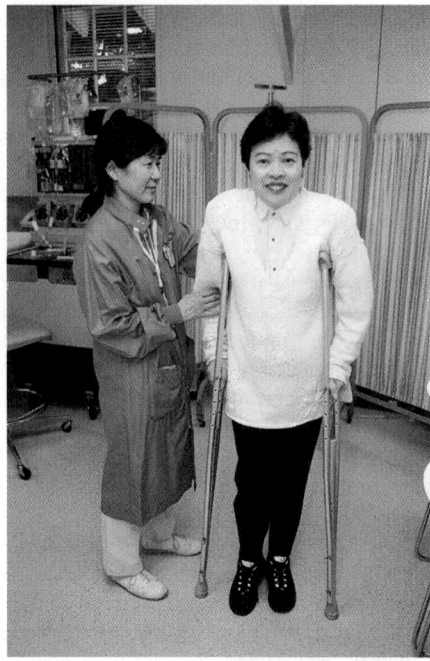

Figure 52-7 ● Assisting the client with crutch walking. Note how the therapist guards the client and how the client's elbows are at no more than 30 degrees of flexion.

the least support. A hemi-cane or quad-cane provides a broader base for the cane and therefore more support. The cane is placed on the *unaffected* side and should create no more than 30 degrees of flexion of the elbow. The top of the cane should be parallel to the greater trochanter of the femur.

■ IMBALANCED NUTRITION: LESS THAN BODY REQUIREMENTS

PLANNING: EXPECTED OUTCOMES. The client with a fracture is expected to maintain an adequate dietary intake to promote healing and prevent complications.

INTERVENTIONS. Nursing interventions focus on meeting the client's nutritional needs. The dietitian assesses the client's food likes and dislikes and collaborates with him or her to plan meals that are both appealing and nutritional. For promotion of bone and tissue healing, the client needs a high-protein, high-calorie diet. Supplements of vitamins B and C are also required for tissue nutrition. Clients with fractures may be immobilized for extended periods; thus they are predisposed to hypocalcemia, which results in loss of calcium from bone and in subsequent bone fragility. The nurse teaches the client to increase intake of foods high in calcium, particularly milk and milk products if they are tolerated.

A negative nitrogen balance can develop 7 to 10 days after injury in an immobilized client because of an increase in catabolism without compensatory protein intake. The nurse offers frequent small feedings and supplements of high-protein liquids, such as Ensure or Carnation Instant Breakfast preparations. Milk shakes are an excellent protein and calorie supplement, as well as a source of calcium.

Because of less weight bearing on long bones, the immobilized client with a fracture often becomes anemic. Blood loss from the injury or reparative surgery contributes to the anemic state. The nurse encourages intake of foods high in iron content. The health care provider may prescribe an oral iron supplement. It is not uncommon for the client to receive a daily multivitamin with iron.

● Community-Based Care

The client with an uncomplicated fracture is usually discharged to home from the emergency department. Older adults with hip or other fractures or clients with multiple trauma are hospitalized and then often transferred to a rehabilitation setting or to a long-term care facility for rehabilitation or permanent residence. To ensure continuity of care, the case manager or the discharge planner in the hospital communicates the plan of care to the health care agency receiving the client.

▩ HEALTH TEACHING

The client with a fracture may be discharged from the hospital, emergency department, office, or clinic with a bandage, splint, cast, or external fixator. The nurse provides verbal and written instructions on the care of these devices. Chart 52-6 describes care of the affected extremity after removal of the cast.

The client may also need to continue wound care at home. The nurse teaches the client and caregiver how to assess and dress the wound to promote healing and prevent infection. The client is taught how to recognize complications (see Complications of Fractures, p. 1127) and when and where to seek professional health care should complications occur.

Additional educational needs depend on the type of fracture and fracture repair. Care of external fixators and casts is discussed earlier under Cast Care (p. 1134) and External Fixation (p. 1138).

▩ HOME CARE MANAGEMENT

If the client is discharged to home, the nurse or case manager assesses the home environment for structural barriers to mobility, such as stairs.

> ### ❖ CONSIDERATIONS FOR OLDER ADULTS
> A home assessment is particularly important for older clients. A cast is bulky and requires room for maneuvering and ambulating. In collaboration with the therapy team, the nurse instructs the client and family or significant others to remove scatter rugs and other items that can contribute to falls. The rooms should not be cluttered with furniture, so that the client can maneuver with crutches, a walker, or a cane. An elevated toilet seat or shower chair may be needed to promote independence in toileting.

▩ HEALTH CARE RESOURCES

The nurse identifies potential or actual problems in the hospital and arranges for follow-up care at home. For example, professional counseling for depression may need to continue after discharge from the hospital. A social worker may need to help the client apply for funds to pay medical bills. If there is severe bone and tissue damage, the nurse must be realistic and help the client understand the long-term nature of the recov-

> ### CHART 52-6
> ### CLIENT EDUCATION GUIDE
> ### Care of the Extremity After Cast Removal
>
> - Remove scaly, dead skin carefully by soaking—do not scrub.
> - Move the extremity carefully. Expect discomfort, weakness, and decreased range of motion.
> - Support the extremity with pillows or your orthotic device until strength and movement return.
> - Exercise slowly as instructed by your physical therapist.
> - Wear support stockings or elastic bandages to prevent swelling (for lower extremity).

ery period, particularly if he or she experiences a major complication, such as infection, while in the hospital. Multiple treatment techniques and surgical procedures required for complications can be mentally and emotionally draining for the client and family. A vocational counselor may be needed to help the client seek a different type of job, depending on the nature of the fracture.

The client with a severe injury and multiple treatment modalities may need follow-up care in the home by a home care nurse. An older or incapacitated client may need assistance with activities of daily living (ADLs), which is provided by home care aides. The nurse in the hospital anticipates the client's needs and arranges for these services, usually with the assistance of the case worker or discharge planner.

It is extremely important for the hospital nurse to communicate the client's needs to the nurse or aide who will care for the client at home. A physical therapist may come to the home, or the client may go to a clinic, hospital, or private office for follow-up physical therapy after discharge from the hospital. An occupational therapist assists with retraining in the home environment for ADLs; adaptations in the home enable the client to be independent.

In addition to individual follow-up, it is the nurse's responsibility to participate in community education about injury prevention. Injury ranked fifth as the leading cause of death in 1996 and since 1980 has remained the leading cause of death between ages 1 and 44.

The cost to individuals and society at large is enormous (see the Cost of Care box on p. 1142). For every death due to injury, there are 16 hospitalizations and 400 outpatient visits. Each year, about 90,000 people sustain injuries serious enough to cause long-term disability. Injury is a definable, correctable event with specific identifiable risks. It is imperative that nurses be active in educating the public on prevention of injury through programs that highlight the major risk factors: alcohol, illicit drugs, and firearms among the young, and falls in older adults (see also Chapter 51).

● Evaluation: Outcomes

NOC The nurse evaluates the care of the client with a fracture on the basis of the identified nursing diagnoses and collaborative problems. The expected outcomes include that the client:

- Maintains adequate tissue perfusion as indicated by strong distal peripheral pulses, brisk capillary refill, normal skin color, and intact muscle formation
- Reports that pain is reduced or alleviated
- Does not acquire an infection of the bone or soft tissues

COST OF CARE
IMPLICATIONS FOR NURSING

MUSCULOSKELETAL TRAUMA

Cost of Care
- The cost of fractures due to osteoporosis could escalate to approximately $62 billion by the year 2020.
- The cost of hip fracture includes not only the cost of the fracture during hospitalization but also the cost of associated morbidities and posthospital care. Annual costs in the year following hip fracture have been estimated at $37,250 per person.
- Estimates place the lifetime cost of injury at more than $250 billion. The majority of this sum is related to the indirect cost of productivity—loss from death or disability. The direct cost of medical services accounts for approximately 30%.

Implications for Nursing
Injuries are the primary cause of musculoskeletal trauma. Injuries are not accidents; injuries have identifiable risk factors and patterns. Nurses can play a major role in injury prevention by educating the community about these risks. Prevention is a key factor in reducing costs related to musculoskeletal trauma.

Data from American College of Surgeons, Committee on Trauma. (1999). Injury prevention slide presentation; Anderson, E.G. (1997). Osteoporosis: Epidemic of the 21st century? *Geriatrics, 52*(6), 76-78; and Brainsky, A., et al. (1997). The economic cost of hip fractures in community-dwelling older adults: A prospective study. *Journal of the American Geriatrics Society, 45*(3), 281-287.

- Independently ambulates with or without ambulatory aids and provides self-care
- Does not experience consequences of immobility
- Maintains an adequate nutritional intake, as evidenced by bone and soft-tissue healing

Fractures of Specific Sites

UPPER EXTREMITY FRACTURES

Fractures of the Clavicle

Fractures of the clavicle typically result from a fall on an outstretched hand, a fall on the shoulder, or a direct injury. Most clavicular fractures are self-healing; a splint or bandage is used for immobilization. Complicated fractures, although uncommon, may require open reduction with internal fixation (ORIF) by pins, wires, or screws.

Fractures of the Scapula

Scapular fractures are not common and are usually caused by direct impact to the area. Serious internal trauma, including pneumothorax, pulmonary contusion, and fractured ribs, can accompany these fractures.

The shoulder is immobilized with a sling and swathe or a shoulder immobilizer until the fracture heals, usually in 2 to 4 weeks. Intra-articular neck and glenoid fractures may require surgical intervention with plate and screw fixation.

Fractures of the Humerus

Fractures of the proximal humerus, particularly impacted or displaced fractures, are common in the older adult. An impacted injury is usually treated conservatively, with a sling for immobilization. A displaced fracture often requires ORIF with pins or a prosthetic device.

Humeral shaft fractures are generally corrected by closed reduction and application of a hanging-arm cast or splint. If necessary, the fracture is repaired surgically (with an intramedullary rod or metal plate and screws) or with external fixation. Nonunion of the bone and radial nerve palsy are frequent complications of this fracture. Bone grafting facilitates union; prolonged splinting is necessary while the radial nerve regenerates.

A direct blow to the condyles of the distal humerus can cause either or both condyles to fracture, usually in a T- or Y-shaped configuration. The most serious complication is damage to the brachial or median nerve. Condylar fracture is usually treated by ORIF with a series of screws, although skeletal traction and casting can be used.

Fractures of the Olecranon

Fractures of the olecranon are relatively common in adults and typically result from a fall on the elbow. Many are successfully treated by closed reduction and application of a cast. The healing process usually takes more than 2 months, and several additional months may be needed before full use of the elbow is achieved. ORIF is performed for displaced fractures, and a splint is worn during the healing phase.

Fractures of the Radius and Ulna

Forearm fractures of the ulna without accompanying injury to the radius are rare. As with other fractures of long bones, closed reduction with casting may be the appropriate treatment. If the fracture is displaced, ORIF with intramedullary rods or plates and screws is required.

WOMEN'S HEALTH CONSIDERATIONS

Colles' fracture, or distal radius fracture, is common among older adults (particularly women); it results most often from a fall on an open hand. The distal radius has a large percentage of cancellous bone, the type that is initially affected by osteoporosis. Chapter 51 describes osteoporosis, or loss of bone mass, in detail. The options for reduction and immobilization include splinting, casting, plaster-and-pin fixation, or external fixation with a frame. External fixation may be used even with soft tissue damage.

Fractures of the Wrist and Hand

One or more of the bones in the wrist and hand can break, but the most common fracture is of the carpal scaphoid bone in young adult men. This is also one of the most misdiagnosed fractures because it is poorly visualized on an x-ray film. Closed reduction and casting for 6 to 12 weeks is the treatment of choice. If the bone does not heal, open reduction and bone grafting are performed.

Fractures of the metacarpals and phalanges are usually not displaced, which makes their treatment less difficult than that of other fractures. Metacarpal fractures are immobilized for 3 to 4 weeks. Phalangeal fractures are immobilized in finger splints for 10 to 14 days.

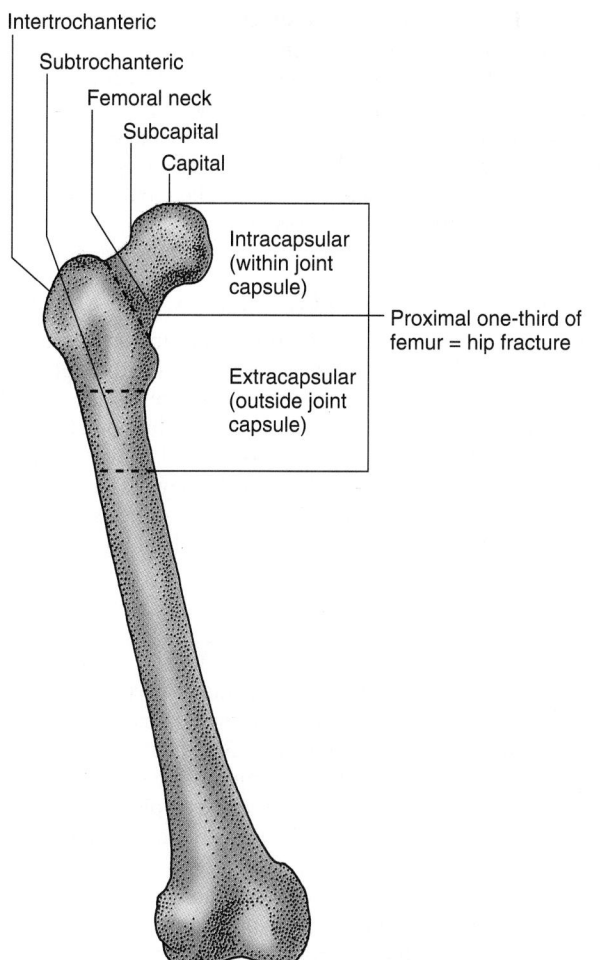

Intertrochanteric

Subtrochanteric

Femoral neck

Subcapital

Capital

Intracapsular
(within joint
capsule)

Extracapsular
(outside joint
capsule)

Proximal one-third of
femur = hip fracture

Figure 52-8 ● The types of hip fractures.

LOWER EXTREMITY FRACTURES
Fractures of the Hip

Hip fractures include those involving the upper third of the femur and are classified as intracapsular (within the joint capsule) or extracapsular (outside the joint capsule). These types are further divided according to fracture location (Figure 52-8).

CONSIDERATIONS FOR OLDER ADULTS

Hip fractures occur most often in older persons, particularly women who have osteoporosis. Repair of hip fracture is rapidly becoming the most common surgical procedure for people older than 85 years of age. As many as one third of older clients who sustain a hip fracture die within 1 year of injury from medical complications caused by the fracture or by immobility that occurs after the fracture. Approximately 50% cannot return home or live independently after the fracture (Lappe, 1998). Because of the poor prognosis of clients experiencing hip fractures, public education on osteoporosis and fracture prevention is crucial. Studies suggest that older, thin, Caucasian women are at the most risk for hip fracture (see the Evidence-Based Practice for Nursing box above).

EVIDENCE-BASED PRACTICE
FOR NURSING

Preventing hip fractures due to osteoporosis

Turner, L.W., Faile, P.A., & Tomlinson, R., Jr. (1999). Osteoporosis diagnosis and fracture. *Orthopaedic Nursing, 18*(5), 21-27.

This study examined correlates for osteoporosis diagnosis and hip fracture among a national sample of women over 50 years of age using data extracted from the Third National Health and Nutrition Examination Survey (NHANES III). Correlates for screening and diagnosis of osteoporosis included advancing age and race. Risk factors predicting hip fracture included age, race, low body mass index, and inactivity.

Critique. Randomly selected data from a large sample (n = 2336) confirmed prior research results. The NHANES III survey from which the data were derived included an oversampling of African Americans, Hispanics, and individuals over 60 years of age.

Implications for Nursing. Results of the present study combined with information from prior research can be used to formulate nursing guidelines for prevention of osteoporosis and related fractures among older women. Nurses should (1) screen and target high-risk women: those who are older, Caucasian, and underweight; (2) focus on helping clients to achieve and maintain a healthy body weight; (3) encourage safe physical activity two or more times per week consistent with the client's lifestyle and health status; and (4) promote public education regarding osteoporosis.

Falls cause most hip fractures; impaction or displacement, especially of the femoral neck, often results. If the degree of osteoporosis is so severe that it prevents surgical intervention, the client may be incapacitated for the remainder of his or her life.

The treatment of choice is surgical repair, when possible, to allow the older client to get out of bed. Buck's traction may be applied before surgery, which should be scheduled within 24 hours of injury if at all possible. Depending on the exact location of the fracture, open reduction with internal fixation (ORIF) may include an intramedullary rod, pins, a prosthesis, or a fixed sliding plate (such as a compression screw). The client with a compression screw can usually ambulate a few days after surgery and has a decreased chance of infection and nonunion, in comparison with clients for whom other procedures are used. If the femoral neck or head is fractured, a prosthetic device is implanted. Depending on the age of the client and prior mobility status, the surgeon replaces the femoral head only (Moore prosthesis) or performs a total hip replacement. Figures 52-9 and 52-10 illustrate examples of these devices used for ORIF of the hip. Nonsurgical options are Buck's traction and skeletal traction, followed by use of a cast brace (Taggart, 1999).

Hip fractures are common. Nurses in all health care settings need to know how to care for the special needs of the older adult with a hip fracture (see the Client Care Plan on p. 1145). The care is similar to that needed by older clients undergoing total hip replacement (see Chapter 21).

Fractures of the Femur

Fractures of the lower two thirds of the femur usually result from trauma (often from a motor vehicle accident). A femoral fracture is seldom immobilized by casting, because the powerful muscles of the thigh become spastic, which causes displacement of bone ends. Extensive hemorrhage is associated with femoral fracture.

Skeletal traction, followed by a cast brace or hip spica cast, is the typical nonsurgical treatment. Surgical treatment is ORIF with nails, rods, or a compression screw. In a few cases, external fixation may be employed. Healing time for a femoral fracture may be 6 months or longer.

Fractures of the Patella

Like most other fractures, patellar fractures result from direct impact. The surgeon typically repairs the fracture by closed reduction and casting or internal fixation with screws.

Fractures of the Tibia and Fibula

Trauma to the lower leg most often causes fractures of both the tibia and the fibula, particularly the lower third ("tib-fib" fractures). The three basic treatment techniques are closed reduction with casting, internal fixation, and external fixation. If closed reduction is used, the client wears a cast for at least 8 to 10 weeks. Delayed union is not unusual with this type of fracture. Internal fixation with nails or a plate and screws, followed by a long leg cast for 4 to 6 weeks, is another option. When the fractures cause extensive skin and soft-tissue damage, the initial treatment may be external fixation, often for 6 to 10 weeks. This is usually followed by application of a cast until the fracture is completely healed.

Fractures of the Ankle and Foot

Ankle fractures are described by their anatomic place of injury. For example, a bimalleolar (Pott's) fracture involves the medial malleolus of the tibia and the lateral malleolus of the fibula. Because of the instability of the ankle joint, the fracture can result from supination and eversion, pronation and abduction, or pronation and eversion. These forces generally create spiral, transverse, or oblique breaks, which are often

difficult to treat and present problems in healing. A combination of closed and open techniques may be used, depending on the severity and extent of the fracture. An arthrodesis (fusion) may be needed if the bone does not heal.

Treatment of fractures of the foot or phalanges is similar to that of other fractures, with either closed or open reduction. Phalangeal fractures are more painful than, but not as serious as, most other types of fractures.

FRACTURES OF THE RIBS AND STERNUM

Chest trauma may cause fractures of the ribs or sternum; the most commonly fractured ribs are numbers 4 through 8. The major concern with rib and sternal fractures is the potential for puncture of the lungs, heart, or arteries by bone fragments or ends. Fractures of the lower ribs may damage underlying organs, such as the liver, spleen, or kidneys. These fractures tend to heal spontaneously without surgical intervention. The client is often uncomfortable during the healing process and requires analgesia.

FRACTURES OF THE PELVIS

Because the pelvis is very vascular and close to major organs and blood vessels, associated internal damage is the chief concern in fracture management. After head injuries, pelvic fractures are the second most common cause of death from trauma. In young adults, pelvic fractures typically result from motor vehicle accidents or falls from buildings; falls are the most common cause in older adults. The major concern related to pelvic injury is venous oozing or arterial bleeding. Loss of blood volume leads to hypovolemic shock.

Internal abdominal trauma is assessed by checking for the presence of blood in the urine and stool and by watching the

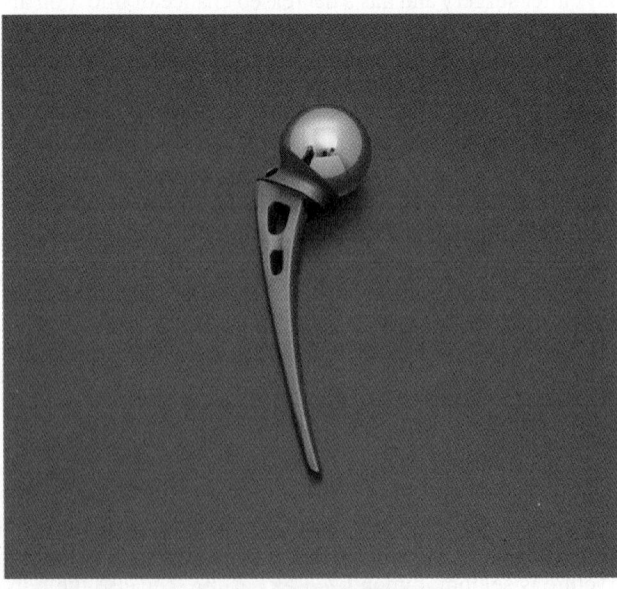

Figure 52-9 ● The Moore prosthesis, which is used for hip fractures. (Courtesy Smith & Nephew, Inc., Orthopaedics Division, Memphis, TN.)

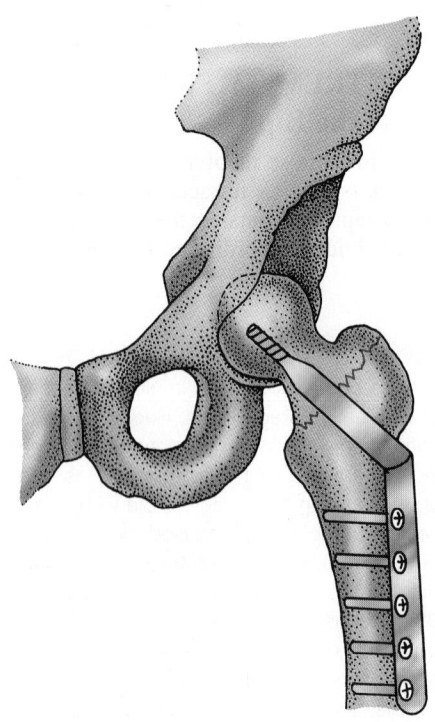

Figure 52-10 ● A compression hip screw used for open reduction with internal fixation (ORIF) of the hip.

CLIENT CARE PLAN • THE CLIENT UNDERGOING OPEN REDUCTION WITH INTERNAL FIXATION FOR A FRACTURED HIP

NURSING DIAGNOSIS NO. 1 • Risk for Injury related to subluxation or dislocation

Expected Outcomes	Nursing Interventions	Rationale
The client will not experience subluxation or dislocation of the operative hip during the hospital stay.	Place an abduction pillow, a splint, or a bed pillow between the client's legs in bed. **D**	Adduction of the affected leg beyond the body's midline can cause dislocation of the hip.
	Use a leg cradle or similar device to align the affected leg. **D**	These devices help prevent internal or external rotation of the affected hip, which could result in dislocation.
	Turn the client carefully toward either side to prevent adduction (check the physician's order). **D**	Adduction of the leg can cause dislocation of the hip.
	Do not flex the operative hip beyond 90 degrees. **D**	Hyperflexion of the operative hip can cause dislocation.
	Use an elevated toilet seat. **D**	
	Have the client sit in a supporting chair with a straight back and seat. **D**	
	Teach the client not to cross the legs.	Crossing the legs causes adduction.

NURSING DIAGNOSIS NO. 2 • Acute Pain related to surgical incision

The client will experience alleviation or reduction of surgical pain.	Give pain medication as needed; anticipate the client's need if the client cannot verbalize (epidural or patient-controlled analgesia [PCA] may be used).	Relieving the client's pain helps the client to participate more fully in the plan of care.
	Give pain medication before the physical therapy session (if it does not cloud the client's sensorium) or other periods of increased activity.	
	Use a fracture pan instead of a traditional bedpan. **D**	A fracture pan does not require as much lifting by the client; lifting increases pain.
	Use nondrug pain relief measures, such as distraction, music, and relaxation exercises as needed.	These measures work synergistically with medications; they may reduce the use of opioids and their side effects.

NURSING DIAGNOSIS NO. 3 • Risk for Infection related to impaired skin integrity

The client will not experience surgical wound infection.	Inspect the surgical dressing for drainage, and document the type and amount.	Purulent drainage indicates wound infection.
	Monitor and measure the drainage collected in a surgical drain, such as a Hemovac. Empty and compress only if there is an order (opening to remove drainage increases the risk of contaminating the surgical site).	Drains allow the removal of exudate, which can be a medium for bacterial growth.
	After removal of the surgical dressing, inspect the incision for redness, swelling, and warmth, as well as approximation of wound edges.	Signs of inflammation may indicate an infectious process.
	If a dressing is used, change the dressing by using sterile technique.	Sterile conditions reduce the chance of infection.
	Monitor vital signs every 4 hr for 1-3 days. **D**	Elevated pulse and temperature may indicate wound infection.

NURSING DIAGNOSIS NO. 4 • Impaired Physical Mobility related to hip precautions and surgical pain

The client will experience increased physical mobility.	Reinforce transfer and ambulation techniques (walker or crutches) as taught by the physical therapist.	Increasing mobility promotes the client's independence and return to society as a functional member.
	Have the trapeze and overhead frame on the bed before surgery and teach the client to use the device.	
	Teach the client to bear weight to tolerance (or to bear weight partially for at least 6 wk postoperatively).	
	Assess the client's need for assistive/adaptive devices to perform activities of daily living (ADLs) independently; consult with an occupational therapist.	
	Assess for and prevent complications of prolonged immobility, such as deep vein thrombosis, skin breakdown, or hypostatic pneumonia. (See Chapter 10 and earlier portions of this chapter for nursing assessment and prevention of complications.)	Complications of immobility cause the client discomfort and prolonged hospitalization.

D Indicates tasks that can be delegated to assistive nursing personnel.

abdomen for the development of rigidity or swelling. The trauma team may use peritoneal lavage, computed tomography (CT) scanning, or ultrasound (the newest diagnostic modality) for assessment of hemorrhage. Ultrasound is non-invasive, rapid, reliable, and cost-effective, and it can be done at the bedside in real time.

There are many classification systems for pelvic fractures. A system that is particularly useful for nurses divides fractures of the pelvis into two broad categories: non–weight-bearing fractures and weight-bearing fractures.

When a non–weight-bearing part of the pelvis is fractured, such as one of the pubic rami or the iliac crest, treatment can be as minimal as bedrest on a firm mattress or bed board. This type of fracture can be quite painful, and the client may need stool softeners to facilitate defecation because of hesitancy to move. Well-stabilized fractures usually heal in 2 months.

A weight-bearing fracture, such as multiple fractures of the pelvic ring creating instability or a fractured acetabulum, necessitate external fixation and/or open reduction with internal fixation (ORIF). Less commonly used now are skeletal traction or double-hip spica casts. Progress to weight bearing depends on the stability of the fracture following fixation. Some clients may fully bear weight within days of surgery, whereas others managed with traction may not bear weight for as long as 12 weeks.

■ FRACTURES AT OTHER SITES

Because the skull and vertebral column protect the brain and spinal cord, these fractures are described in Chapter 43. The nurse must be aware of the special care required for these clients because of possible neurologic damage resulting from these fractures. Fractures of the mandible or nose and other facial trauma are discussed elsewhere in the text.

AMPUTATIONS

■ OVERVIEW

An **amputation** is the removal of a part of the body. The nurse recognizes that the psychosocial ramifications of the procedure are often more devastating than the physical impairment that results. The loss experienced is complete and permanent and causes a change in body image and often in self-esteem. As with other types of loss, the client can be expected to progress through phases of the grieving process.

■ Pathophysiology

■ SURGICAL AMPUTATION

Amputations range from removal of part of a digit to removal of nearly half the entire body. The surgeon performs an amputation by one of two methods: open (or guillotine) method or closed (or flap) method.

The open method is used for clients who have, or are likely to develop, an infection. The wound remains open, and drains allow exudate to escape from the site until the infection clears. The surgeon may suture the skin flaps over the wound at a later time. In the closed technique, the surgeon pulls the skin flaps over the bone end and sutures them in place as part of the amputation procedure. One or more drains are typically inserted.

In either the closed or open method, the surgeon attempts to preserve as much of the part as possible and to keep major joints intact for maximal postoperative mobility.

■ TRAUMATIC AMPUTATION

Not all amputations are surgically planned. Some, classified as traumatic amputations, occur when a body part is severed unexpectedly (e.g., by a chain saw). Because the amputated part in these clients is usually healthy, attempts to replant it may be made.

One of the most likely replantations involves one or more digits. The current recommendation for prehospital care is that the severed digit be wrapped in a cool, dry cloth and moistened with normal saline, if possible, or bottled water. The digit should then be placed in a sealed plastic bag. The bag is placed in ice water, never directly on ice. Contact between the digit and the water is avoided to prevent tissue damage. Any semi-detached parts of the digit should not be removed.

■ LEVELS OF AMPUTATION

LOWER EXTREMITY. Lower extremity amputations are performed much more frequently than upper extremity amputations. Five types of lower extremity amputations may be performed (Figure 52-11).

The loss of any or all of the small toes presents a minor disability. Loss of the great toe is significant because it affects balance, gait, and "push off" ability during walking. Midfoot amputations (e.g., the Lisfranc amputation and the Chopart amputation) and the Syme amputation are common procedures for peripheral vascular disease. In the Syme amputation, most of the foot is removed but the ankle remains. The

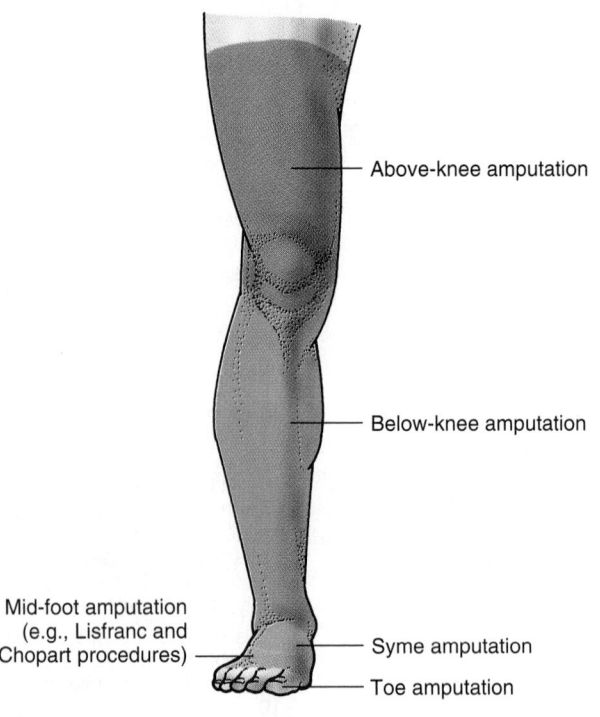

Above-knee amputation

Below-knee amputation

Mid-foot amputation (e.g., Lisfranc and Chopart procedures)

Syme amputation

Toe amputation

Figure 52-11 ● Common levels of lower extremity amputation.

advantage of this surgery over traditional amputations below the knee is that weight bearing can be accomplished without use of a prosthesis and without pain.

An intense effort is made to preserve knee joints with below-knee amputation (BKA) rather than above-knee amputation (AKA). When the cause for the amputation extends beyond the knee, however, above-knee or higher amputations are performed. Hip disarticulation, or removal of the hip joint, and hemipelvectomy procedures are more common in younger clients than in older clients, who cannot easily handle the cumbersome prostheses required for ambulation. The higher the level of amputation, the more energy is required for ambulation. These higher-level procedures are typically done for cancer of the bone, osteomyelitis, or trauma. Hemicorporectomy (hemipelvectomy and translumbar amputation) is a rare radical procedure performed as a last resort for cancer.

UPPER EXTREMITY. Fewer than 10% of all amputations are upper extremity amputations. An amputation of any part of the upper extremity is generally more incapacitating than one of the leg. The arms and hands are necessary for activities of daily living (ADLs), such as feeding, bathing, dressing, and driving a car. As much length as possible is saved to maintain function. Early replacement with a prosthetic device is vital for the client with this type of amputation.

■ COMPLICATIONS OF AMPUTATIONS

The following are common complications of elective or traumatic amputations:

- Hemorrhage
- Infection
- Phantom limb pain
- Problems associated with immobility
- Neuroma
- Flexion contractures

HEMORRHAGE. When a person loses part or all of an extremity either by surgery or by trauma, major blood vessels are severed, which causes bleeding. If the bleeding is uncontrolled, the client is at risk for hypovolemic shock and possibly death.

INFECTION. As with any surgical procedure or trauma, infection can occur in the wound or the bone (osteomyelitis). The older adult who is debilitated and confused is at the greatest risk because excreta may soil the wound, or the client may remove the dressing and pick at the incision.

PHANTOM LIMB PAIN. **Phantom limb pain (PLP)** is a frequent complication of amputation. Most clients experience phantom limb sensation in the early postoperative period. Sensation is perceived in the phantom foot or hand and diminishes over time. When phantom limb sensation persists and is unpleasant or painful, it is referred to as PLP. PLP is more common in clients who have experienced chronic limb pain before surgery and rare in those who experience traumatic amputations.

No one theory explains or predicts PLP. Three theories are being researched:

- Peripheral nervous system theory
- Central nervous system theory
- Psychologic theory

The peripheral nervous system theory implies that sensations remain as a result of severing peripheral nerves during the amputation. The central nervous system theory states that PLP results from a loss of inhibitory signals that are usually generated through afferent impulses from the amputated limb. When many sensory fibers are destroyed by amputation, the loss of inhibitory influences allows repetitive neural activity, which results in pain. Neither of these physiologic theories completely explains PLP. Most likely, a psychologic component helps predict and explain this phenomenon. Stress, anxiety, and depression often worsen or trigger an episode of PLP but are not likely to be the causative factors.

When experiencing PLP, the client complains of pain in the removed body part, most often shortly after surgery. The pain is often described either as an intense burning or crushing sensation or as cramping. Some clients say they feel as if the removed part is in a distorted, uncomfortable position; they experience numbness and tingling (sometimes called phantom limb sensation), as well as pain.

Some clients report that the most distal area of the removed part feels as if it is retracted into the residual limb end. For most clients, the pain is triggered by touching the residual limb, by temperature or barometric pressure changes, by concurrent illness, by fatigue, or by emotional stress. Routine activities, such as urination, can trigger the pain in other clients. If pain is long-standing, especially if it existed before the amputation, any stimulus can cause it, including touching any part of the body.

PROBLEMS ASSOCIATED WITH IMMOBILITY. Because the client experiences reduced mobility as a result of surgery, the complications of atelectasis, pneumonia, thromboembolism, and skin breakdown can readily occur. These problems are discussed earlier under Complications of Fractures, p. 1127.

NEUROMA. Neuroma—a sensitive tumor consisting of nerve cells found at severed nerve endings—forms most often in amputations of the upper extremity but can occur anywhere.

FLEXION CONTRACTURES. Flexion contractures of the hip or knee are seen in clients with amputations of the lower extremity. This complication must be avoided so that the client can ambulate with a prosthesis.

■ Etiology

Most knowledge about amputations was obtained during World War II, when trauma often necessitated a loss of one or more body parts. Today, with highly sophisticated microsurgery for revascularization of tissues, amputations related to trauma are less likely to be needed. Limb salvage procedures, such as those described in Chapter 51 (under Surgical Management in the section on malignant bone tumors), have reduced the need for amputation.

Traumatic amputations most often result from accidents. A person may be cleaning lawn mower blades or a snow blower without disconnecting the machine. A motor vehicle or industrial machine accident may also cause an amputation.

> ### CONSIDERATIONS FOR OLDER ADULTS
> The primary indication for surgical amputation is *ischemia* from peripheral vascular disease in the older client (see Chapter 36). The rate of lower extremity amputation, for example, is much greater among clients with diabetes than among other clients because of peripheral neuropathy and peripheral vascular disease (Spollett, 1998). In addition, these older diabetic clients have visual, cardiac, and kidney problems. A client with an amputation of one leg because of poor circulation will often have an amputation of the other leg within 5 years. Older adults of advanced age may not be candidates for prostheses because of the energy required for ambulation. The more proximal the amputation in the lower extremity, the more energy required for ambulation.

Incidence/Prevalence

Surgical amputations are not as common as they were in the past, because the success rates of revascularization and limb salvage techniques have improved over the last 30 years. However, more than 100,000 amputations are performed yearly in the United States, about half of these in clients with coexisting diabetes.

The typical client undergoing the procedure is a middle-aged or older man with diabetes and a lengthy history of smoking. The client most likely has failed to care for his feet properly, which has resulted in a nonhealing, infected foot ulcer and possibly gangrene.

The second largest group with amputations consists of young men who experience motorcycle or other vehicular accidents or who are injured at work by industrial equipment. These men may either experience a traumatic amputation or undergo a surgical amputation because of a severe crushing injury and massive soft-tissue damage.

> ### CULTURAL CONSIDERATIONS
> The incidence of lower extremity amputations is greater in the African-American and Hispanic populations because the incidence of major diseases leading to amputation, such as diabetes and arteriosclerosis, is greater in this population. Limited access to care for these minority groups may also play a major role in limb loss (Spollett, 1998).

► COLLABORATIVE MANAGEMENT

● Assessment

PHYSICAL ASSESSMENT/CLINICAL MANIFESTATIONS

When the client has peripheral vascular disease, the nurse's primary concern preoperatively is to assess circulation in other parts of the body The nurse assesses skin color, temperature, sensation, and pulses in both affected and unaffected extremities. Capillary refill is evaluated by applying pressure to the nail bed and waiting for the brisk return of normal color. In the older adult, however, this test may be difficult to do because the nails may be thick and opaque. In this situation, the skin near the nail bed can be assessed (see Chart 52-3).

PSYCHOSOCIAL ASSESSMENT

People react differently to the loss of a body part. The nurse needs to be aware that an amputation of a portion of one finger can be traumatic to the client; therefore the loss must not be underestimated. The client undergoing an amputation faces a complete, permanent loss. The nurse assesses the client's psychologic preparation for a planned amputation and expects him or her to experience the grieving process. Adjustment to a traumatic, unexpected amputation is often more difficult than accepting a planned one. The young client may be bitter, hostile, and uncooperative. In addition to loss of a body part, the client may lose a job, the ability to participate in favorite recreational activities, or a social relationship if the other person cannot accept the body change. Chapter 9 discusses the nursing assessment for a client experiencing loss.

The client is faced with an altered self-concept. The physical alteration that results from an amputation affects body image and self-esteem. For example, a client may think that an intimate relationship with a mate is no longer possible. An older adult may feel a loss of independence. The nurse assesses the client's feelings about himself or herself to identify areas in which he or she needs emotional support.

The nurse tries to determine the client's willingness and motivation to withstand prolonged rehabilitation after the amputation. Asking questions about how the client has dealt with previous life crises can provide clues. The client's willingness to change careers or other activities is also determined. Adjustment to the amputation and rehabilitation is less difficult if the client is willing to make necessary changes.

In addition to assessing the client's psychosocial status, the nurse assesses the family's or significant others' reaction to the surgery. The family's response usually correlates directly with the client's progress during recovery and rehabilitation. The family can be expected to grieve for the loss and must be allowed to adjust to the change in the client.

The nurse also assesses the client's coping abilities and helps him or her to identify personal strengths and weaknesses. The nurse ascertains that the client's religious or spiritual beliefs have been determined, because certain groups require that the amputated body part be stored for later burial with the rest of the body or be buried now.

DIAGNOSTIC ASSESSMENT

Routine preoperative x-ray studies, such as a chest x-ray, are done as appropriate for any client undergoing surgery. The surgeon determines which tests are performed to assess for viability of the limb. A large number of noninvasive techniques are available to assist the physician in this evaluation. For complete accuracy, the health care provider does not rely on any single test.

One procedure is measurement of segmental limb blood pressures, which can also be used by the nurse at the bedside. In this test, an ankle-brachial index (ABI) is calculated by dividing ankle systolic pressure by brachial systolic pressure. A normal ABI is greater than or equal to 1.

Blood flow in an extremity can also be assessed by many other noninvasive tests, including Doppler ultrasonography, laser Doppler flowmetry, and transcutaneous oxygen pressure ($TcPO_2$). The ultrasonography measures the velocity of blood flow in the limb. The $TcPO_2$ measures oxygen pressure to indicate blood flow in the limb. Angiography is the most commonly used invasive method; however, it is not helpful in predicting healing of amputations. Transcutaneous oxygen pressure has proved reliable for predicting healing.

◖ Interventions

Clients undergoing amputation today are not confined to a wheelchair. Advancements in the design of prosthetics have enabled clients to become independent in ambulation. Therefore complications from extended bedrest are not common, even for older adults.

ASSESSMENT OF TISSUE PERFUSION. The nurse's primary focus is to monitor for signs indicating that there is sufficient tissue perfusion but no hemorrhage. The skin flap at the end of the residual limb should be pink in a light-skinned person and not discolored (lighter or darker than other skin pigmentation) in a dark-skinned client. The area should be warm but not hot. The nurse assesses the closest proximal pulse for strength and compares it with that in the other extremity. If the client has bilateral vascular disease, however, comparison of limbs is not an accurate way of measuring blood flow.

MANAGEMENT OF PAIN. Phantom limb pain (PLP) must be distinguished from stump pain, since they are managed differently. Pain management related to stump pain is not unlike that for any client in pain (see Chapter 7). If the client complains of PLP, the nurse recognizes that the pain is real. It is not therapeutic for the nurse to remind the client that the limb cannot be hurting, because it is missing. To prevent increased pain, the nurse handles the residual limb carefully when assessing the site or changing the dressing.

DRUG THERAPY. Some studies have shown that opioids are not as effective for PLP as they are for residual limb pain. The health care provider prescribes medication on the basis of the type of PLP the client experiences. For instance, beta-blocking agents such as propranolol (Inderal, Apo-Propranolol✦, Detensol✦) are used for constant, dull burning. Anticonvulsants, such as phenytoin (Dilantin) and carbamazepine (Tegretol), may be used for knifelike pain; antispasmodics such as baclofen may be prescribed for muscle spasms or cramping.

COMPLEMENTARY AND ALTERNATIVE THERAPIES. More than 50 treatments for PLP have been used worldwide. Transcutaneous electrical nerve stimulation (TENS) has had the most consistent pain relief rates. Other treatment measures include the following:
- Ultrasound therapy
- Massage
- Exercises
- Biofeedback
- Distraction therapy
- Hypnosis
- Psychotherapy

PREVENTION OF INFECTION. The surgeon typically prescribes broad-spectrum prophylactic antibiotics for several days postoperatively. The initial pressure dressing and drains are usually removed by the surgeon 48 to 72 hours after surgery. The nurse:
- Inspects the wound site for signs of inflammation (e.g., redness and swelling)
- Monitors the healing process
- Records the characteristics of drainage, if present
- Changes the soft dressing every day until the sutures are removed

The below-the-knee limb may be casted in the operating room for protection, prevention of edema, and prevention of knee contractures. On the third postoperative day, a window is opened in the distal end of the cast to inspect the suture line.

PROMOTION OF AMBULATION. The nurse or health care provider consults with a physical therapist to initiate exercises as soon as possible after surgery. If the amputation is a planned one, the therapist often works with the client before surgery to start muscle strengthening exercises and to evaluate the need for aids, such as crutches. If the client can be instructed preoperatively in the use of these devices, learning how to ambulate after surgery is facilitated.

EXERCISE. For clients with above-knee amputations (AKAs) or below-knee amputations (BKAs), the nurse teaches range-of-motion (ROM) exercises for prevention of flexion contractures, particularly of the hip and knee. A trapeze and an overhead frame, as shown in Figure 52-12, aid in strengthening the upper extremities and allow the client to move independently in bed.

A firm mattress is essential for preventing contractures with a lower extremity amputation. The nurse assists the client into a prone position every 3 to 4 hours for 20- to 30-minute periods. This position may be uncomfortable initially, but it is necessary to prevent hip flexion contractures. The nurse instructs the prone client to pull the residual limb close to the other leg and contract the gluteal muscles of the buttocks. For BKAs, the nurse also teaches the client to push the residual limb down toward the bed while supporting it on a pillow. After the sutures are removed, the physical therapist may begin resistive exercises with a "sling-and-spring" apparatus, which can also be used at home.

Elevation of a lower leg residual limb on a pillow while the client is in a supine position is controversial. Some practitioners advocate avoiding this procedure at all times because it promotes hip or knee flexion contracture. Others allow ele-

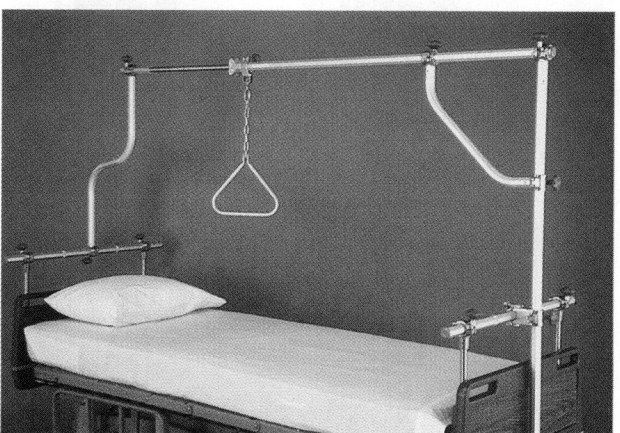

Figure 52-12 ● The placement of an overhead frame and trapeze on a bed.

vation for the first 24 hours to reduce swelling and subsequent discomfort. The nurse inspects the residual limb daily to ensure that it lies completely flat on the bed.

PROSTHESES. For an elective amputation, the nurse arranges for the client to see a certified prosthetist-orthotist (CPO) so that planning can begin for the client's postoperative needs. Arrangements for replacing an upper extremity are especially important so that the client can provide self-care. Some clients are fitted with a temporary prosthesis at the time of surgery. Other clients, particularly older clients with vascular disease, are fitted after the residual limb has healed.

The client being fitted with a lower extremity prosthesis should bring a sturdy pair of shoes to the fitting. The prosthesis will be adjusted to that heel height.

PREPROSTHETIC CARE. Several devices help shape and shrink the residual limb in preparation for the prosthesis. Rigid, removable dressings are preferred because they decrease edema, protect and shape the limb, and allow easy access to the wound for inspection. The Jobst air splint, a plastic inflatable device, is sometimes used for this purpose. This device is usually inflated to 20 mm Hg for 22 out of every 24 hours. One of its disadvantages is air leakage.

Wrapping with elastic bandages can be effective in reducing edema, shrinking the limb, and holding the wound dressing in place. Most surgeons prefer elastic bandages over a shrinker sock, although it is easier for the client to apply a sock than to wrap elastic bandages.

For wrapping to be effective, the nurse reapplies the bandages every 4 to 6 hours or more often if they become loose. Figure-eight wrapping prevents restriction of blood flow. The

nurse decreases the tightness of the bandages while wrapping in a distal-to-proximal direction. After wrapping, the nurse anchors the bandages to the most proximal joint, such as above the knee for BKAs (Figure 52-13).

PROSTHESIS APPLICATION. The design of and materials for prostheses have improved dramatically over the years. Computer-assisted design and manufacturing (CAD-CAM) is now available for a custom fit. One of the biggest developments in lower extremity prosthetics is the ankle-foot prosthesis. The Flex-Foot is used by more active amputees.

PROMOTION OF BODY IMAGE. The client often experiences feelings of inadequacy as a result of losing a body part, especially the older adult who was in poor health before surgery. If possible, the nurse arranges for the client to meet with a rehabilitated amputee. If the client is older, an older amputee is the ideal person with whom the client should interact.

Use of the word *stump* for referring to the remaining portion of the limb is controversial. Clients have reported feeling as if they were part of a tree when the term was used. However, some rehabilitation specialists who routinely work with amputees believe the term is appropriate because it forces the client to realize what has happened and enhances adjustment to the amputation. This discussion uses *residual limb* instead.

The nurse assesses the client's verbal and nonverbal references to the affected area. Some clients behave euphorically and seem to have accepted the loss. The nurse should not jump to the conclusion that acceptance has occurred. The client is asked to describe his or her feelings about changes in body image and self-esteem. The client may verbalize acceptance but refuse to look at the area during a dressing change.

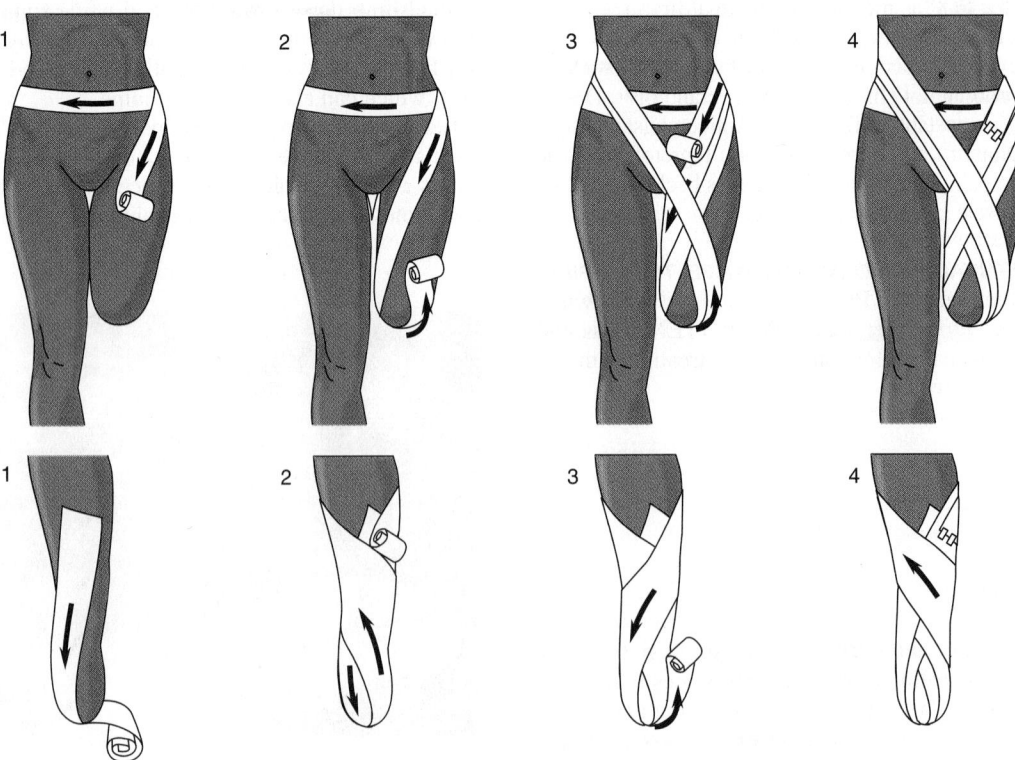

Figure 52-13   A common method of wrapping an amputation stump. *Top,* Wrapping for above-knee amputation. *Bottom,* Wrapping for below-knee amputation.

This inconsistent behavior is not unusual and should be noted by the nurse.

PROMOTION OF LIFESTYLE ADAPTATIONS. The client may believe that it will be impossible to return to a previous lifestyle, including intimate relationships, his or her job, and recreational activities. With advancements in prostheses, many clients can return to their jobs and other activities. Professional athletes who use prostheses are quite successful in sports. Clients with amputations ski, hike, bowl, and participate in other physically demanding activities. More than 20,000 amputees in the United States currently participate actively in sports; about a fourth of these individuals are engaged in organized competition.

If a job or career change is necessary, the nurse consults with a social worker for evaluation of the client's other skills that could be used in another capacity. A supportive family or significant other is important for the client's adjustment to this change. The client may also think that an intimate relationship is no longer possible because of physical changes. The nurse works with the sexual partner to help in the client's adjustment to the amputation. Professional assistance from a sex counselor or psychologist may be needed.

The nurse helps the client to set realistic goals and to take one day at a time. He or she is helped to recognize personal strengths, which are emphasized and taken into account in setting goals. If the goals are not realistic, frustration and disappointment may dampen the client's motivation during rehabilitation. Basic principles of rehabilitation are discussed in Chapter 10.

● Community-Based Care

The client is discharged directly to home or to a rehabilitation facility, depending on the extent of the amputation. In the few cases in which rehabilitation is not feasible (e.g., for a debilitated, confused older client), he or she may be discharged to a long-term care facility. The case manager or discharge planner coordinates this transfer.

▦ HEALTH TEACHING

After the sutures are removed (several weeks after surgery), the client begins residual limb care. The home care nurse teaches the client how to care for the residual limb and how to care for the prosthesis if it is available. The limb should be rewrapped three times a day with an elastic bandage applied in a figure-eight manner (see Figure 52-13) by the client or family member. After the residual limb is healed, it is cleaned each day with the rest of the body during bathing with soap and water, and it is inspected for signs of inflammation or skin breakdown.

Prostheses require special care for ensuring their reliability and proper function, and the prosthetist plays an important role in the rehabilitation team effort. Prostheses are custom made, taking into account the client's level of amputation, lifestyle, and occupation. Proper teaching regarding correct cleansing of the socket and inserts, wearing the correct liners, assessing shoe wear, and a schedule of follow-up care is essential before discharge.

A client who seemed to adjust to the amputation during hospitalization may realize that it is difficult to cope with the loss after discharge from the hospital. The nurse in the hospital setting should tell the client that this can happen. During the hospital stay, the nurse helps the client to identify strong support systems on which he or she can rely after discharge. The home care or rehabilitation nurse reinforces this supporting information.

▦ HOME CARE MANAGEMENT

The client with a lower extremity amputation needs to have enough room at home to maneuver a wheelchair if the leg prosthesis is not yet available. He or she must be able to use toileting facilities and have access to areas necessary for self-care, such as the kitchen. Structural changes may be required before the client goes home.

▦ HEALTH CARE RESOURCES

For the older adult or for the client with an extensive amputation, such as a hemipelvectomy, the case manager or discharge planner arranges for follow-up care in the home by a home care nurse (Chart 52-7). Physical therapy may continue in the home or on an ambulatory care basis.

The client with an upper extremity amputation may need occupational therapy to relearn activities of daily living (ADLs). The nurse or case manager also makes arrangements for vocational or family counseling, as needed. Some clients are discharged to a rehabilitation facility for 2 to 3 weeks for these services. Chapter 10 describes the rehabilitation phase of health care in detail. The nurse teaches the client to explore support groups for amputees that may be available in the client's community.

CRUSH SYNDROME

When multiple compartments in the leg or arm are injured, crush syndrome (CS) can occur. CS is a potentially life-threatening, systemic complication after a severe crush injury. Its pathophysiologic mechanism is similar to that of acute compartment syndrome (see p. 1127).

Specific causes of CS include the following:

- Prolonged use of a pneumatic antishock garment (PASG) or military antishock trousers (MAST) (For this reason, these devices are seldom used today.)
- Wringer-type injuries
- Natural disasters, such as earthquakes
- Work-related injuries, such as being trapped under heavy equipment or material

---

CHART 52-7

FOCUSED ASSESSMENT *of*
The Client with a Lower Extremity Amputation in the Home

Assess the residual limb for:
- Adequate circulation
- Infection
- Healing
- Flexion contracture
- Dressing/elastic wrap

Assess the client's ability to perform activities of daily living (ADLs) in the home.
Evaluate the client's ability to use ambulatory aids and care for the prosthetic device (if available).
Assess the client's nutritional status.
Assess the client's ability to cope with body image change.

- Drug/alcohol overdose, when one or more limbs may be compressed by body weight for a prolonged time

Regardless of the cause, CS is characterized by the following:

- Acute compartment syndrome
- Hypovolemia
- Hyperkalemia
- Rhabdomyolysis (myoglobulin release from skeletal muscle into the bloodstream)
- Acute tubular necrosis (ATN) resulting from hypovolemia and rhabdomyolysis

Nursing assessments include signs and symptoms of hypovolemia, hyperkalemia, and compartment syndrome. Treatments focus on preventing acute tubular necrosis secondary to myoglobin release and cardiac dysrhythmias related to hyperkalemia. Adequate IV fluids, diuretics, and low-dose dopamine to enhance renal perfusion may be ordered. An output of 100 to 200 ml/hr is the goal. Sodium bicarbonate is given to treat acidosis. Kayexalate may reduce serum potassium adequately, but hemodialysis may be required if potassium levels remain high or renal failure occurs.

COMPLEX REGIONAL PAIN SYNDROME

Complex regional pain syndrome (CRPS) (less commonly called **reflex sympathetic dystrophy syndrome [RSDS]**) is a poorly understood complex disorder that includes pain, trophic changes, autonomic dysfunction, and motor impairment (most notably muscle paresis). It is probably caused by an abnormally hyperactive sympathetic nervous system. It most often results from traumatic injury and commonly occurs in the feet and hands (Aprile, 1998).

The syndrome tends to progress through three classic stages. In stage 1, which lasts 1 to 3 months, the client complains of locally severe, burning pain; edema; vasospasm; and muscle spasm. Over the next 3 months, clients in stage 2 have more severe, diffuse pain and edema, muscle atrophy, and spotty osteoporosis, as shown on x-ray examination. In stage 3, the final stage, the client presents with marked muscle atrophy, intractable (unrelenting) pain, severely limited mobility of the affected area, contractures, and marked, diffuse osteoporosis. Timing of diagnosis is important, since the syndrome is more difficult to treat when diagnosed in the later stages.

The first priority of management is pain relief. Nurses play an important role in pain management, which includes drug therapy and an array of nonpharmacologic modalities. Chapter 7 discusses pain management in detail.

In collaboration with the physical and occupational therapist, the nurse also assists in maintaining adequate range of motion (ROM). The skin of a client with CRPS tends to alternate between warm, swollen, and red to cool, clammy, and bluish. Skin care needs to be gentle, with minimal stimulation.

The nurse assists the client in coping with CRPS. Psychotherapy may be indicated. The RSDS Association is available to help clients organize or locate support groups and other resources for clients with this syndrome.

SPORTS-RELATED INJURIES

In addition to the bone and muscle problems already discussed, trauma can cause cartilage, ligament, and tendon injury. Many musculoskeletal injuries are the result of participation in sports or other strenuous physical activities. These injuries have become so common that large metropolitan hospitals have sports medicine clinics and physicians who specialize in this field.

Although the specific types of injury are numerous, this chapter includes only the most common ones seen by the nurse in a hospital or ambulatory care setting. The principles of injury to one part of the body are analogous to those of similar injuries in other parts. For example, a tendon rupture in a knee is cared for in the same manner as a tendon rupture in the wrist. Chart 52-8 lists general emergency measures for sports-related injuries.

Because the knee is most often injured, it is discussed as a typical example of other areas of the body. Trauma to the knee results in internal derangement, a broad term for disturbances of an injured knee joint. When surgery is required to resolve the problem, most surgeons prefer to perform the procedure through an arthroscope when possible. A general description of arthroscopy is presented in Chapter 50.

Knee Injuries: Meniscus

■ OVERVIEW

There are two semilunar cartilaginous structures, or menisci, in the knee joint: the medial meniscus and the lateral meniscus. These pads act as shock absorbers, but they can tear. Tearing is usually a result of twisting the leg when the knee is flexed and the foot is placed firmly on the ground. The medial meniscus is much more likely to tear than the lateral meniscus because it is less mobile. Internal rotation causes a tear in the medial meniscus; external rotation causes a tear in the lateral meniscus.

Tears can be anterior or posterior, longitudinal or transverse. In the medial meniscus, a longitudinal tear, or "bucket handle" injury, often causes the knee to lock; that is, the torn cartilage jams between the femur and the tibia and prevents extension of the knee. Surgery is often required for this type of injury. In transverse tears, the knee does not lock, and surgery may not be required.

► COLLABORATIVE MANAGEMENT

The client with a torn meniscus typically has pain, swelling, and tenderness in the knee. A clicking or snapping sound can often be heard when the knee is moved.

A common diagnostic technique is the **McMurray test.** The examiner flexes and rotates the knee and then presses on

---

CHART 52-8

BEST PRACTICE *for*
Emergency Care of Sports-Related Injuries

- Do not move the victim until spinal cord injury is ascertained (see Chapter 45 for assessment of spinal cord injury).
- Immobilize the injured part; immobilize the joint above and below the injury by applying a splint.
- Apply ice intermittently for the first 24-48 hours (heat may be used thereafter).
- Elevate the affected limb to decrease swelling.
- Always assume the area is fractured until x-ray studies are done.
- Assess neurovascular status in the area distal to the injury.

the medial aspect while slowly extending the leg. The test result is positive if clicking is palpated or heard. A negative finding, however, does not rule out a tear.

For a locked knee, the treatment may be manipulation followed by casting for 3 to 6 weeks. If the problem recurs, a partial or total **meniscectomy** is performed. An open meniscectomy requires a surgical incision for removal of all or part of the meniscus and is rarely performed. Most surgeons prefer to remove only the affected portion, which can be accomplished through an arthroscope during a closed meniscectomy as a same-day surgical procedure. As described in Chapter 50, an arthroscope is a metal tubular instrument used for examination or surgery of joints. One or more small incisions (less than ¼ inch [0.6 cm] long) are made in the knee for insertion of the arthroscope. The surgeon threads a cutting device through the arthroscope for removal of the torn cartilage while the knee is irrigated with saline or lactated Ringer's solution, depending on the type of equipment used. The surgeon may use a laser during the procedure, depending on the type and severity of the injury. A bulky pressure dressing is applied after the procedure, and the affected leg is wrapped in elastic bandages.

As for any postoperative client, the nurse checks the surgical dressing for bleeding and monitors vital signs after the client is readmitted to the unit. The nurse performs circulation checks, as outlined in Chart 52-3, usually every hour for the first few hours and then every 4 hours.

The client begins leg exercises immediately after surgery to strengthen the leg, prevent thrombophlebitis, and reduce swelling. Quadriceps setting, in which the client straightens the leg while pushing the knee against the bed, is done in sets of 10 or more. Straight-leg raises are also performed as soon as the client awakens from anesthesia. Range-of-motion (ROM) exercises are usually not started for several days.

To prevent the client from bending the affected knee, the physician may order a knee immobilizer, such as the one shown in Figure 52-14. The nurse elevates the leg on one or two pillows according to the physician's preference and applies ice to reduce postoperative swelling. Full weight bearing is restricted for several weeks, depending on the amount of cartilage removed. The client is usually discharged from the hospital with crutches in less than 23 hours.

Knee Injuries: Ligaments

■ OVERVIEW

The cruciate and collateral ligaments in the knee are predisposed to injury, often from sports or vehicular accidents. The anterior cruciate ligament (ACL) is the most commonly torn ligament in the knee. Athletes often experience ACL injuries during skiing or gymnastics.

When the ACL is torn, the person feels a snap; the knee gives way because of ACL laxity. Within hours, the knee is swollen, stiff, and painful.

► COLLABORATIVE MANAGEMENT

Physical examination by the health care provider shows positive ligamentous laxity. The diagnosis of ACL deficiency is confirmed by x-ray studies, magnetic resonance imaging (MRI), or assessment with an arthrometer (an instrument for measuring the amount of tibial displacement).

Treatment may be nonsurgical or surgical, depending on the severity of the injury and the anticipated activity of the client. Exercises, bracing, and limits on activities while the ligament heals may be sufficient. If medical management is not effective, surgery may be needed.

The surgeon repairs the tear by reattaching the torn portions of the ligament, and the leg is placed in a cast. If the ligament cannot be repaired, reconstructive surgery may be performed with the use of autologous grafts. Since the early 1980s, the Food and Drug Administration (FDA) has approved several artificial knee ligaments. The Gore-Tex ligament is a permanent implant. A ligament augmentation device is used temporarily while the autograft heals. Both of these materials can be implanted through an arthroscope.

Complete healing of knee ligaments after surgery can take 6 to 9 months or longer. Nursing management is similar to the care of any client in a cast, which is described earlier in this chapter under Cast Care, p. 1134.

Tendon Ruptures

Rupture of the Achilles tendon is common in adults who participate in strenuous sports. In the older adult, quadriceps tendon rupture may occur from a fall down several steps. For severe damage, the tendon is surgically repaired and the leg is immobilized in a cast for 6 to 8 weeks. If the tendon is beyond repair, a tendon transplant (also known as tendon reconstruction) is performed. A tendon is removed from one part of the body and transplanted to the affected area. The nursing care for these clients is similar to that discussed earlier for a client with a cast (see Cast Care, p. 1134).

Dislocations and Subluxations

Dislocation of a joint occurs when the articulating surfaces are no longer in proximity. If the dislocation is not complete,

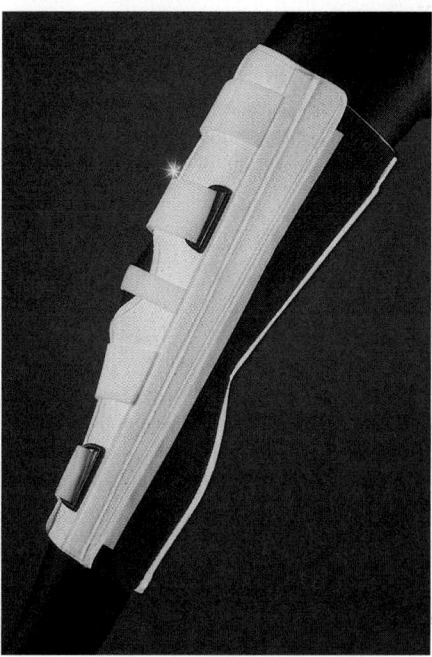

Figure 52-14 ● A knee immobilizer. (Courtesy Zimmer, Inc., Warsaw, IN.)

the joint is partially dislocated, or subluxed. Dislocation can occur in any diarthrodial (synovial) joint but is common in the shoulder, hip, knee, and fingers. This injury is most often the result of trauma but can be congenital or pathologic (resulting from joint disease, such as arthritis).

The typical manifestations of dislocation are as follows:
- Pain
- Immobility
- Alteration in contour of the joint
- Deviation in length of the extremity
- Rotation of the extremity

The health care provider performs a closed manipulation, or reduction, of the joint and forces it back into its original position while the client is anesthetized or under conscious sedation. The joint is immobilized by a cast or immobilizer until healing occurs.

Recurrent dislocations are common in the knee and shoulder. For this problem, the joint is fixed with wires to prevent further displacement; a cast, splint, or traction is applied for 3 to 6 weeks.

Strains

A strain is excessive stretching of a muscle or tendon when it is weak or unstable. Strains are sometimes referred to as muscle pulls. Falls, lifting of heavy items, and exercise often cause this injury.

Strains are classified according to their severity:
- A first-degree (mild) strain causes mild inflammation but little bleeding. Swelling, ecchymosis, and tenderness are usually present.
- A second-degree (moderate) strain involves tearing of the muscle or tendon fibers without complete disruption. Muscle function may be impaired.
- A third-degree (severe) strain involves a ruptured muscle or tendon with separation of muscle from muscle, tendon from muscle, or tendon from bone. Severe pain and disability result from severe strains.

Management usually involves cold and heat applications, exercise, and activity limitations. The health care provider may prescribe anti-inflammatory drugs to decrease inflammation and pain. Muscle relaxants may also be used. In third-degree strains, surgical repair of the ruptured muscle or tendon may be necessary.

Sprains

A sprain is excessive stretching of a ligament. Twisting motions from a fall or sports activity typically precipitate the injury. Sprains are classified according to severity:
- A first-degree (mild) sprain involves tearing of a few fibers of a ligament. Function of the joint is not impaired.
- In a second-degree (moderate) sprain, more fibers are torn, but stability of the joint remains intact.
- A third-degree (severe) sprain causes marked instability of the joint.

Pain and swelling characterize ligament injuries. The treatment for mild (first-degree) sprains is minimal:
- Rest
- Use of ice for the first 24 to 48 hours
- Application of a compression bandage for a few days to reduce swelling and provide joint support
- Elevation

Second-degree sprains require immobilization (elastic bandage and Air Stirrup ankle brace, splint, or cast) and partial weight bearing while the tear heals. For severe ligament damage (third-degree sprain), immobilization for 4 to 6 weeks is necessary. Surgery may be recommended, particularly for chronic instability, as discussed earlier under Knee Injuries: Ligaments, p. 1153.

For more specific client education, refer to the Clinical Pathway on p. 1833.

Rotator Cuff Injuries

The musculotendinous, or rotator, cuff of the shoulder functions to stabilize the head of the humerus in the glenoid cavity during shoulder abduction. The rotator cuff typically undergoes degenerative changes as one gets older. Young adults usually sustain a tear of the cuff by substantial trauma, such as may occur during a fall, while throwing a ball, or with heavy lifting. Older adults tend to have small tears related to aging, repetitive motions, or falls.

Clients with a torn rotator cuff have shoulder pain and cannot initiate or maintain abduction of the arm at the shoulder. When the arm is abducted, the client usually drops the arm because abduction cannot be maintained (drop arm test).

The health care provider usually treats the client conservatively with nonsteroidal anti-inflammatory drugs (NSAIDs), physical therapy, sling support, and ice/heat applications while the tear heals.

For clients who do not respond to conservative treatment or for those who have a complete tear, the surgeon repairs the cuff. After surgery, the affected arm is usually immobilized in a sling for several weeks. Pendulum exercises are started on the third or fourth postoperative day and progress to active exercises in about 2 weeks. If the surgery is extensive, the client's arm may be immobilized for a longer time before exercises begin.

ONLINE RESOURCES

For suggested readings and Internet resources, go to http://www.wbsaunders.com/SIMON/Iggy/.

SELECTED BIBLIOGRAPHY

Aprile, A.E. (1998). Complex regional pain syndrome. *Journal of the American Association of Nurse Anesthetists, 65*(6), 557-560.

Boulanger, B.R., Rozycki, G.S., & Rodriquez, A. (1999). Sonographic assessment of traumatic injury. *Surgical Clinics of North America, 79*(6), 1297-1316.

Browner, B.D., Alberta, F.G., & Mastrella, D.J. (1999). A new era in orthopedic trauma care. *Surgical Clinics of North America, 79*(6), 1431-1448.

Byrne, T. (1999). The set-up and care of a patient in Buck's traction. *Orthopaedic Nursing, 18*(2), 79-83.

Childs, S.G. (Ed.). (1999). *The upper extremity: Traumatic injuries and conditions.* Pitman, NJ: National Association of Orthopaedic Nurses.

Childs, S.G., & Holmes, S.B. (1998). *Guidelines for orthopaedic nursing: Adult trauma.* Pitman, NJ: National Association of Orthopaedic Nurses.

Church, V. (2000). Staying on guard for DVT and PE. *Nursing2000, 30*(2), 35-42.

Hager, C.A., & Brncick, N. (1998). Fat embolism syndrome. *Orthopaedic Nursing, 17*(2), 41-46, 58.

Hoover, T.J., & Seifert, J.A. (2000). Soft tissue complications of orthopedic emergencies. *Emergency Medicine Clinics of North America, 18*(1), 115-139.

Lappe, J.M. (1998). Prevention of hip fractures: A nursing imperative. *Orthopaedic Nursing, 17*(3), 15-26.

Ludwick, R., Dieckman, B., & Snelson, C.M. (1999). Assessment of geriatric orthopaedic trauma. *Orthopaedic Nursing, 18*(6), 13-20.

Maher, A.B. (2001). Trauma. In D.C. Schoen (Ed.), *Core curriculum for orthopaedic nursing* (4th ed.) Pitman, NJ: National Association of Orthopaedic Nurses.

Maher, A.B., Salmond, S.W., & Pellino, T.A. (Eds.). (1998). *Orthopaedic nursing.* Philadelphia: W.B. Saunders.

McCann, S., & Gruen, G. (1997). Fracture blisters: A review of the literature. *Orthopaedic Nursing, 16*(2), 17-23.

Plociak, B.J., Lato, A., & Palumbo, M. (1999). Case study: Fractured ankle. *Orthopaedic Nursing, 18*(4), 21-26.

Roberts, D. (1999). Introduction to bone: Structure and function, fractures, and osteoporosis. In C.M. Ceccio, J.A. Deuschle, D.R. Eckhouse-Ekeberg (Eds.), *An introduction to orthopaedic nursing* (2nd ed., pp. 3-16). Pitman, NJ: National Association of Orthopaedic Nurses.

Rudman, N., & McIlmail, D. (2000). Emergency department evaluation and treatment of hip and thigh injuries. *Emergency Medicine Clinics of North America, 18*(1), 29-66.

Spollett, G.R. (1998). Preventing amputations in the diabetic population. *Nursing Clinics of North America, 33*(4), 629-641.

Sprague, J. (1998). Cast syndrome: The superior mesenteric artery syndrome. *Orthopaedic Nursing, 17*(4), 12-15.

Taggart, H. (1999). Caring for the elderly hip fracture patient. In C.M. Ceccio, J.A. Deuschle, D.R. Eckhouse-Ekeberg (Eds.), *An introduction to orthopaedic nursing* (2nd ed., pp. 113-122). Pitman, NJ: National Association of Orthopaedic Nurses.

Turner, L.W., Faile, P.A., & Tomlinson, R., Jr. (1999). Osteoporosis diagnosis and fracture. *Orthopaedic Nursing, 18*(5), 21-27.

Williamson, V.C. (Ed.). (1998). *Management of lower extremity fractures.* Pitman, NJ: National Association of Orthopaedic Nurses.

PROBLEMS OF DIGESTION, NUTRITION, AND ELIMINATION

Management of Clients with Problems of the Gastrointestinal System

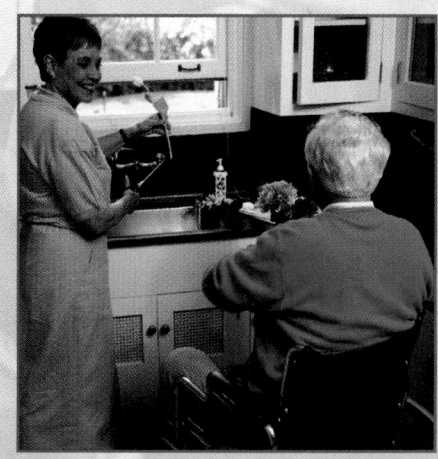

UNIT 12 — PROBLEMS OF DIGESTION, NUTRITION, AND ELIMINATION: GI SYSTEM ■ Core Concepts Grid

Anatomy	Physiology	Pathophysiology	History	Physical Exam	Diagnostic Tests	Interventions	Pharmacology
• Oropharynx	• Absorption	• Inflammation	• **Client history of**	• **Mouth**	• **Upper/lower GI series**	• **Therapeutic diets**	• Antacids
• Esophagus	• Specialized secretions	• Infection	Past problems	• **Skin**	• **Endoscopy**	• Saline lavage	• Histamine blockers
• Stomach	• **Digestion**	• Obstruction	Pain	Striae	• **Esophagastro-duodenoscopy (EGD)**	• Sclerotherapy	• Vasocontrictors
• Small intestine	Hydrochloric acid	• Hemorrhage	• **Family history of digestive system problems**	Cullen's sign	• **Endoscopic retrograde cholangiopancreatography (ERCP)**	• Tamponade	• Corticosteroids
• Large intestine	Lipase	• Perforation	• **Social history**	Grey-Turner's sign	• **Ultrasonography**	• Extracorporeal shock wave lithotripsy (ESWL)	• Anticholinergics
• Liver	Amylase	• **Dumping syndrome**	Alcohol	Color	• CAT scan	• **Rest**	• Chenodeoxycholic acid
• Gallbladder	• Phagocytosis	• Erosion	Drugs	• Peristalsis	• Liver biopsy	• **Tube**	• Urodeoxycholic acid
• Pancreas	• Coagulation	• Ascites	Stress management	• Bowel sounds	• Gastric analysis	Blakemore	• Immune serum globulin
• Rectum	• **Synthesis of**		Occupation	• Bruits	• Fecal analysis	Nasogastric	• **Hepatitis A vaccine (HAV)**
• Anus	Proteins		Age	• Tympany	• Serum bilirubin	Nasoenteric	• **Hepatitis B vaccine (HBV)**
	Carbohydrates		Race	• Masses	• **Aspartate aminotransferase (AST)**	Gastrostomy	• **Bowel stimulants**
	Fats		Gender	• **Abdominal distention**	• **Alanine aminotransferase (ALT)**	• **Ostomies**	• Antidiarrheals
	Vitamins		• **Bowel habits**	• Swallowing	• **Lactate dehydrogenase (LDH)**	Colostomy	• Antibiotics
	• Detoxification		• **Diet**	• Intake	• Amylase	Ileostomy	• Lactulose
				• Vital signs	• Lipase	• **Postoperative care**	• Chemotherapeutic agents
					• **Culture *Helicobacter pylori***	• **Rest**	
						• **Fluid replacement**	
						• **Blood transfusion**	
						• **Health teaching**	

53

Assessment of the Gastrointestinal System

CONSTANCE VISOVSKY

Learning Objectives

After studying this chapter, you should be able to:

1. Recall the anatomy and physiology of the gastrointestinal (GI) system.
2. Perform a GI assessment using Gordon's Functional Health Patterns.
3. Evaluate important assessment findings in a client with a GI health problem.
4. Explain the use of laboratory testing for a client with a GI health problem.
5. Identify the use of radiography in diagnosing GI health problems.
6. Plan follow-up care for clients having endoscopic procedures.

Go to http://www.wbsaunders.com/SIMON/Iggy/ for self-assessment questions related to these Learning Objectives.

The gastrointestinal (GI) system includes the GI tract, consisting of the mouth, esophagus, stomach, small and large intestines, and rectum. The salivary glands, liver, gallbladder, and pancreas secrete substances into the GI tract by connecting ducts (Figure 53-1). The adult GI tract is approximately 15 feet long. The main function of the GI tract, with the aid of organs such as the pancreas and the liver, is the digestion of food. Nutritional assessment is discussed in Chapter 61. The GI tract is susceptible to many pathologic conditions, including structural problems, impairments in motility, infection, and cancer.

ANATOMY AND PHYSIOLOGY REVIEW

Overview of the Gastrointestinal Tract

Structure

The GI tract consists of a hollow tube—the lumen—surrounded by a layer of surface and epithelial cells called the mucosa. The mucosa includes a thin layer of smooth muscle and some exocrine gland cells. This layer is surrounded by the submucosa, which is made up of connective tissue. The outermost layer is composed of both circular and longitudinal smooth muscles, which work to keep contents moving through the tract. Although the GI tract is continuous from the mouth to the anus, it is divided into specialized regions. The mouth, pharynx, esophagus, stomach, and small and large intestines each perform a specific function. In addition, the secretions of the salivary, gastric, and intestinal glands; liver; and pancreas empty into the GI tract to aid digestion.

Function

The functions of the GI tract include secretion, digestion, absorption, and motility. Food and fluids are ingested, swallowed, and propelled along the lumen to be eliminated. Contractions of the smooth muscles in the GI tract move food from the mouth to the anus. Before food can be absorbed, it must be dissolved and broken down. Digestion is a mechanical and chemical process whereby complex foodstuffs are broken down into simpler forms that can be used by the body. During digestion, the stomach secretes hydrochloric acid, the liver secretes bile, and digestive enzymes are released, aiding in food breakdown. After the digestive process is complete, absorption takes place. Absorption is carried out as the nutrients produced by digestion move from the lumen of the GI tract into the body's circulatory system for uptake by individual cells (Figure 53-2).

Nerve Supply

Innervation of the GI tract occurs in two ways. First, intrinsic contractile stimulation is provided by two internal nerve plexuses: the *myenteric* plexus (an outer plexus found in the longitudinal and circular smooth muscle) and the *submucosal* plexus (an inner nerve plexus in the submucosa). These nerve plexuses connect with each other along the entire length of the GI tract to maintain the tone of the smooth muscle and to stimulate movements.

The second type of innervation is provided by the autonomic nervous system, which connects with nerve fibers from the intrinsic nerve plexuses. Parasympathetic stimulation is provided primarily by the vagus nerve (cranial nerve X), which innervates the esophagus, the stomach, and to a lesser extent, the small intestine, the gallbladder, and part of the large intestine. This stimulation causes increased motor and secretory activity and relaxation of sphincters. Sympathetic stimulation via the thoracic and lumbar splanchnic nerves is provided to all parts of the GI tract; it slows movement, inhibits secretions, and contracts sphincters.

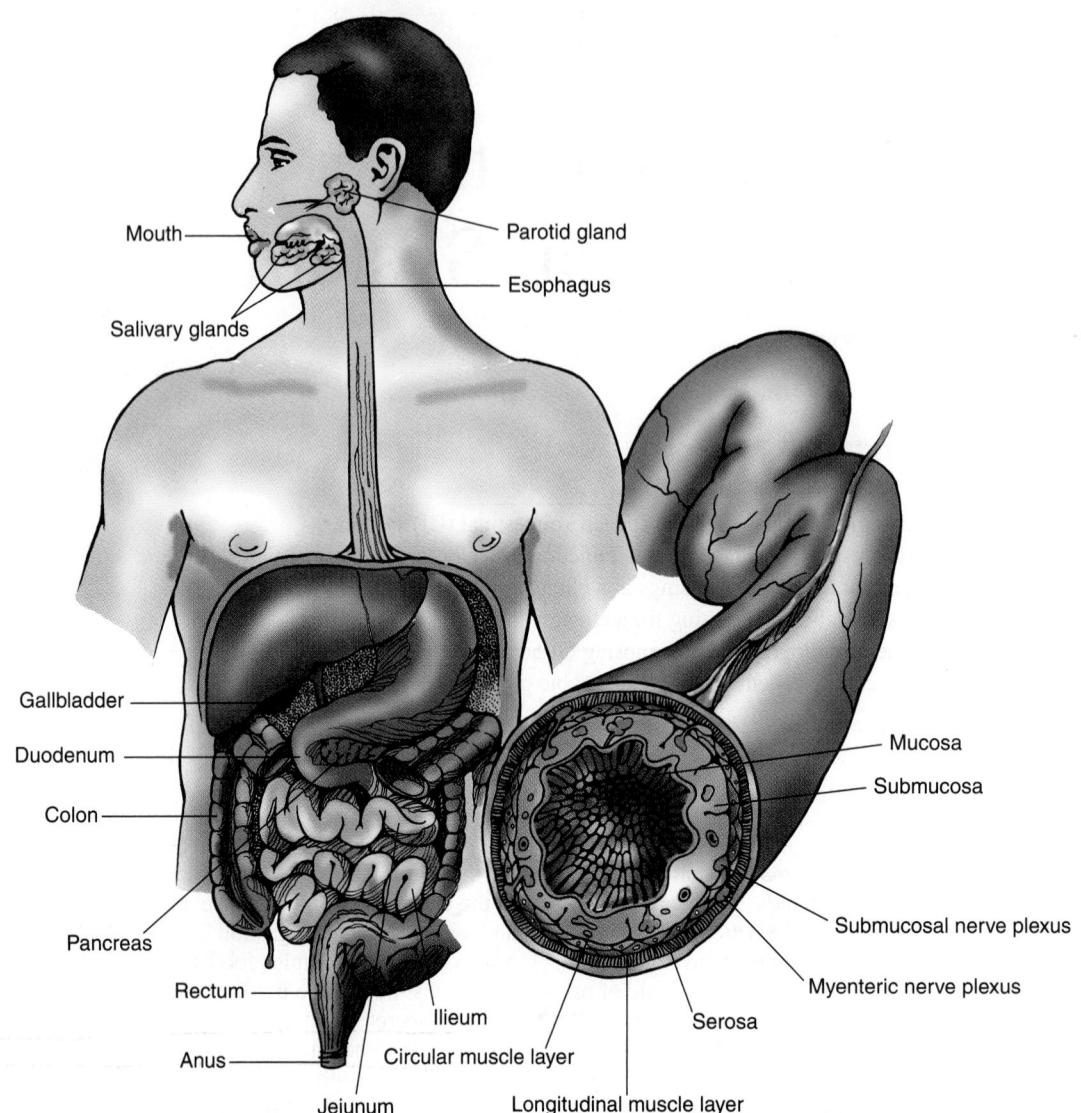

Figure 53-1 ● The gastrointestinal system (GI tract) can be thought of as a tube (with accessory structures) extending from the mouth to the anus for a 25-foot length. The structure of this tube (shown enlarged) is basically the same throughout its length.

Blood Supply

The blood supply to the GI tract originates from the aorta and branches to the many arteries throughout the length of the tract: the celiac, gastric, splenic, common hepatic, internal and external iliac, and superior and inferior mesenteric arteries. The venous system that carries absorbed nutrients away from the lumen of the GI tract consists of the gastric vein, the splenic vein, and other veins that drain into the portal vein of the liver. This blood circulates through the liver to the hepatic vein and returns to the heart via the inferior vena cava.

Oral Cavity

Structure

The oral cavity includes the buccal mucosa, lips, tongue, hard palate, soft palate, teeth, and salivary glands. The buccal mucosa is the mucous membrane lining the inside of the oral cavity. The lips are external to the oral cavity and are pink-red. The tongue lies on the floor of the mouth, anchored to the hy-

oid bone. The tongue is involved in speech, taste, and **mastication** (chewing). The mucous membrane covering the tongue consists of small projections, called papillae, that house the taste buds and provide a roughened surface, permitting the movement of food in the mouth during chewing. The hard palate and the soft palate together form the roof of the mouth.

Adults have 32 permanent teeth: 16 in each arch. The teeth are composed of a hard, calcified substance called dentin, which is then covered by enamel. There are four types of teeth: incisors, canines, premolars, and molars. The oral cavity contains three major salivary glands: the parotid glands, the submandibular glands, and the sublingual glands. These glands produce 1 to 1.5 L of saliva per day to assist in digestion by moistening food, thus enabling it to be formed into a bolus for swallowing.

The pharynx (throat) extends from the soft palate to the esophagus. It is lined with mucous membrane and contains three pairs of organs: the adenoids, the lingual tonsils (at the base of the tongue), and the tonsils.

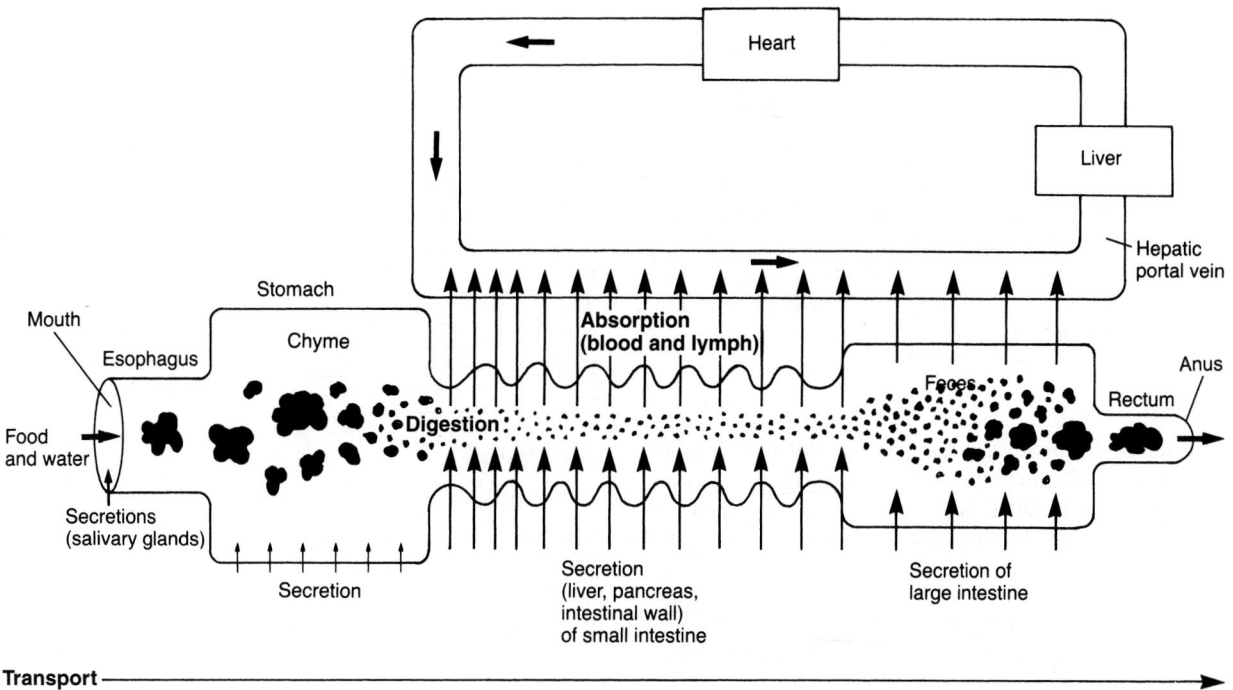

Figure 53-2 ● A conceptual view of the gastrointestinal system. (From Vander, A.J., Sherman, J.H., & Luciano, D.S. [1990]. *Human physiology* [5th ed.]. New York: McGraw-Hill. Used with permission.)

Function

The different types of teeth function to prepare food for digestion by cutting, tearing, crushing, or grinding the food. Swallowing begins after food is taken into the mouth and chewed. Saliva is secreted in response to the presence of food in the mouth and begins to soften the food. Saliva contains mucin and an enzyme, salivary amylase (also known as ptyalin), which begins the breakdown of carbohydrates.

The four phases of swallowing are oral preparatory, oral, pharyngeal, and esophageal. The *oral preparatory* phase begins with the intake of food into the mouth. The mandible, teeth, and tongue work to soften the food and form a bolus. The tongue acts to move the bolus toward the back of the mouth. The *oral* phase begins with the movement of the bolus toward the back of the mouth. The tongue presses the bolus against the hard palate, toward the anterior faucial arches, triggering the swallowing reflex.

The *pharyngeal* phase begins as the swallowing reflex is triggered. As the bolus is forced into the pharynx, the soft palate elevates, which seals the nasal cavity. At this time, the swallowing reflex also inhibits respiration and allows the opening of the esophagus so that the food can enter. The oral and pharyngeal phases are extremely rapid, usually taking less than 1 second.

The *esophageal* phase begins when the bolus enters the esophagus at the cricopharyngeal juncture. A peristaltic wave passes the food to the stomach, which takes about 9 seconds.

Esophagus

Structure

The esophagus is a muscular canal approximately 10 inches (24 cm) long; it extends from the pharynx to the stomach and passes through the hiatus in the center of the diaphragm. The wall of the esophagus consists of mucosa, submucosa, and muscularis propria. The mucosal layer is composed of squamous epithelial cells. The submucosa is composed of loose connective tissue containing blood vessels, lymphatics, and nerve fibers. The muscularis propria consists of smooth and striated muscle fibers. The portion of the esophagus proximal to the gastroesophageal junction is referred to as the lower esophageal sphincter (LES).

Function

The primary function of the esophagus is to propel food and fluids from the pharynx to the stomach and to prevent reflux of gastric contents into the esophagus. The propulsive function is the result of coordinated contractions of the muscular layers of the esophagus. The esophageal walls secrete mucus to lubricate the food and aid in the transport of the bolus to the stomach. As peristalsis pushes the bolus along the esophagus, the cardiac sphincter relaxes to allow the bolus to enter the stomach. The activity of the LES is regulated by smooth muscle, as well as neural and hormonal influences.

Stomach

Structure

The stomach is a glandular digestive and endocrine organ located in the midline and left upper quadrant (LUQ) of the abdomen. The stomach has four anatomic regions. The *cardia* is the narrow portion of the stomach that is distal to the gastroesophageal junction. The *fundus* is the area to the left above the gastroesophageal junction. The main area of the stomach is referred to as the *body* or *corpus.* The *antrum* is the distal portion of the stomach and is separated from the duodenum by the pyloric sphincter. Both ends of the stomach are guarded by sphincters (cardiac and pyloric), which aid in the transport of food through the gastrointestinal (GI) tract and also prevent backflow (Figure 53-3).

The surface of the stomach is covered with *rugae*, or folds of mucosa and submucosa that extend longitudinally. Smooth muscle cells that line the stomach are responsible for gastric motility. The stomach is also richly innervated with intrinsic and extrinsic nerves. Parietal cells lining the wall of the stomach secrete hydrochloric acid, whereas chief cells secrete pepsinogen (a precursor to pepsin, a digestive enzyme). Parietal cells also produce intrinsic factor, which works to facilitate the absorption of vitamin B_{12}.

Function

The stomach performs several functions. Following ingestion of food, the stomach functions as a food reservoir. The stomach serves a secretory function that aids digestion. Gastric secretion can be divided into three phases: cephalic, gastric, and intestinal.

The cephalic phase begins with the sight, smell, and taste of food and is regulated by the vagus nerve. Sympathetic nerve fibers activate neurons in the GI nerve plexus, which then serve to initiate secretory and contractile activity. The gastric phase begins with the presence of food in the stomach. The G-cells in the antrum secrete the hormone gastrin, which promotes the secretion of hydrochloric acid and pepsinogen.

Hydrochloric acid transforms inactive pepsinogen into active pepsins, which aid in the digestion of proteins. The secretion of mucus and bicarbonate protect the stomach from mechanical and chemical damage. The fluids secreted into the stomach are collectively referred to as gastric juice (Table 53-1). Intrinsic factor is secreted by parietal cells, which bind vitamin B_{12} to enhance its absorption in the ileum.

The stomach also mixes or churns the food, breaking apart the large food molecules and mixing them with gastric secretions to form chyme, which then empties into the duodenum. The intestinal phase begins as the chyme passes from the stomach into the duodenum, causing distention. The intestinal phase is mediated by secretin, a hormone that inhibits further acid production and decreases gastric motility.

Pancreas

Structure

The pancreas lies retroperitoneally in the upper abdominal cavity behind the stomach and extends horizontally from the duodenal C-loop to the spleen. The pancreas is divided into portions known as the head, the body, and the tail (Figure 53-4).

Function

Two major cellular bodies within the pancreas have separate functions: exocrine and endocrine. The *exocrine* part of the pancreas constitutes approximately 80% of the organ and consists of acinar cells, which secrete the enzymes that are necessary for the digestion of carbohydrates, fats, and proteins (trypsin, chymotrypsin, amylase, and lipase) (Table 53-2). The *endocrine* part of the pancreas is made up of the islets of Langerhans, with alpha cells producing glucagon and beta cells producing insulin. Although the islet cells account for less than 2% of the volume of the pancreas, the hormones produced are essential in the regulation of metabolism. Chapter 62 describes the endocrine function of the pancreas.

Liver

Structure

The liver is the largest organ in the body and is mainly located in the right upper quadrant (RUQ) of the abdomen. The liver is divided into two major regions: a larger right lobe and a smaller left lobe. The lobes are divided by the falciform ligament, which attaches the liver to the diaphragm. The liver is made up of functioning units called lobules (Figure 53-5). The organ has a connective tissue covering, called the Glisson capsule, which protects it. Hepatocytes, or liver cells, are arranged

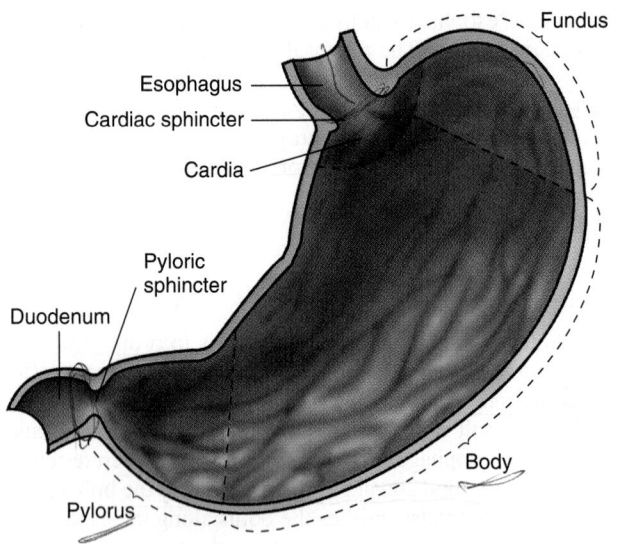

Fundus
Esophagus
Cardiac sphincter
Cardia
Pyloric sphincter
Duodenum
Body
Pylorus

Figure 53-3 ● The anatomy of the stomach.

TABLE 53-1 • GASTROINTESTINAL HORMONES		
Hormone	**Source**	**Effect**
Gastrin	Secreted by the gastric mucosa in the presence of peptides	Stimulates gastric motility and secretion of hydrochloric acid
Secretin	Secreted by the duodenum in the presence of hydrochloric acid	Stimulates the secretion of pancreatic juice and bile from the liver
Pancreozymin	Secreted by the duodenum in the presence of hydrochloric acid and peptides	Stimulates the secretion of pancreatic juice
Cholecystokinin	Secreted by the duodenum in the presence of amino acids and fatty acids	Stimulates the secretion of pancreatic enzymes and bile from the gallbladder

into cellular plates, which radiate from a central vein. Small bile channels fit between the plates and empty into terminal bile ducts. The right and left hepatic ducts transport bile from the liver. The liver receives its blood supply from the hepatic artery and the hepatic portal vein. Approximately 1500 mL of blood flows through the liver every minute.

Function

The liver performs more than 400 functions in three major categories: storage, protection, and metabolism. The liver stores several minerals and vitamins: copper, iron, magnesium, vitamin B_{12}, folic acid, vitamin B_6, niacin, and the fat-soluble vitamins A, D, E, and K.

The protective function of the liver involves phagocytic Kupffer's cells, which are part of the body's reticuloendothelial system. They engulf harmful bacteria and anemic red blood cells. The liver also detoxifies potentially harmful compounds (such as drugs, chemicals, and alcohol) that are ingested.

The liver functions in the metabolism of proteins considered vital for human survival. It breaks down amino acids to remove ammonia, which is then converted to urea and is excreted via the kidneys. In addition, the liver synthesizes several plasma proteins, including albumin, prothrombin, and fibrinogen. The liver's role in carbohydrate metabolism involves storing and releasing glycogen as the body's energy requirements change. The liver synthesizes, breaks down, and temporarily stores fatty acids and triglycerides.

TABLE 53-2 • MAJOR DIGESTIVE ENZYMES AND BILE

Substance	Source	Substrate	End Product
Salivary amylase (ptyalin)	Salivary glands	Starch	Dextrins, maltose
Gastric pepsin (protease)	Stomach	Proteins	Polypeptides
Gastric lipase	Stomach	Emulsified fats	Fatty acids* and glycerol*
Bile (contains no enzymes)	Liver; stored and released from the gallbladder	Unemulsified fats	Emulsified fats
Trypsin	Pancreas	Proteins and polypeptides	Polypeptides and amino acids*
Chymotrypsin	Pancreas	Proteins and polypeptides	Polypeptides and amino acids*
Carboxypeptidase	Pancreas	Polypeptides	Smaller polypeptides
Amylase	Pancreas	Starch	Maltose, lactose, and sucrose
Lipase	Pancreas	Bile and emulsified fats	Glycerol* and fatty acids*
Enterokinase	Duodenal mucosa	Trypsinogen	Trypsin
Peptidases	Intestine	Peptides	Amino acids*
Lactase	Intestine	Lactose (milk sugar)	Glucose* and galactose*
Maltase	Intestine	Maltose (malt sugar)	Glucose*
Sucrase	Intestine	Sucrose (cane sugar)	Glucose* and fructose*

*End product ready for digestion.

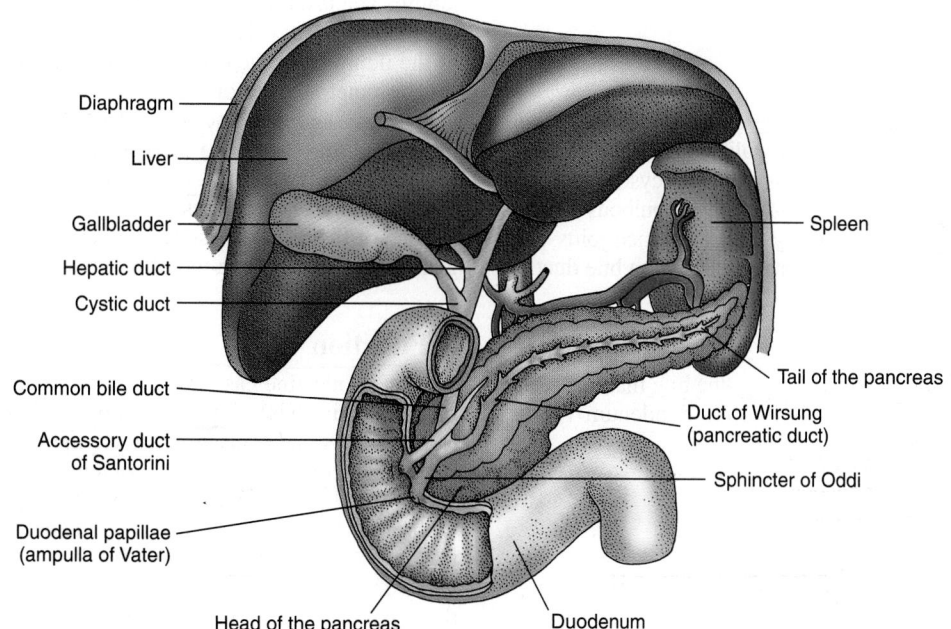

Figure 53-4 ● The anatomy of the pancreas, the liver, and the gallbladder.

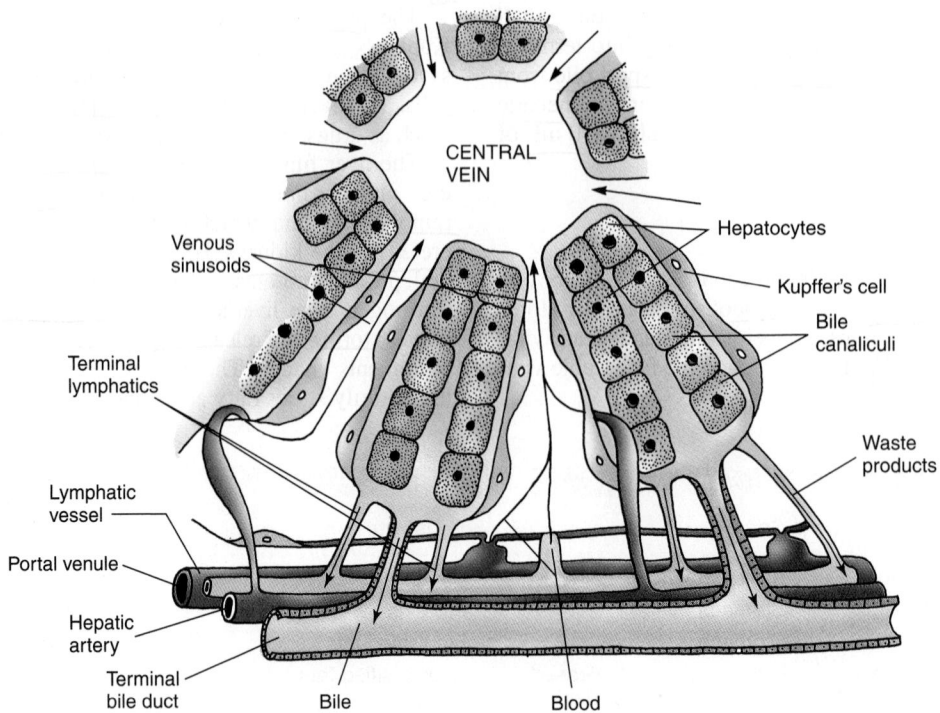

Figure 53-5 ● The anatomy and physiology of the liver lobule. Blood flows from the portal vein and hepatic artery to the central vein. As blood passes through the sinusoids, waste products are removed from the blood and excreted via the lymphatics. Bile is manufactured by the hepatocytes (liver cells) and is secreted into the bile canaliculi. From there, it flows into the bile ducts and then to the gallbladder.

The liver forms and continually secretes bile. Bile is essential for the emulsification of fat. The constituents of bile are bile salts, cholesterol, phospholipids (lecithin), water, electrolytes, and bile pigments (bilirubin). The secretion of bile increases in response to gastrin, secretin, and cholecystokinin. Bile is secreted into small ducts that empty into the common bile duct and into the duodenum at the sphincter of Oddi. However, if the sphincter is closed, the bile goes to the gallbladder for storage.

Gallbladder

■ Structure

The gallbladder is a pear-shaped bulbous sac that is located on the inferior surface of the liver. The gallbladder has three portions: the neck, which is continuous with the cystic duct; the body, or main portion; and the fundus, the lower bulbous section. The gallbladder is drained by the cystic duct, which joins with the hepatic duct from the liver to form the common bile duct.

■ Function

The gallbladder concentrates and stores the bile that has come from the liver. It releases the bile into the duodenum via the common bile duct when fat is present.

Small Intestine

■ Structure

The small intestine is the longest and most convoluted portion of the digestive tract. It is composed of three different regions: the duodenum, the jejunum, and the ileum. The duodenum is the first 10 inches (25 cm) of the small intestine and is at-

tached to the distal end of the pylorus. It is C-shaped, curving left around the head of the pancreas and bending behind the transverse portion of the large intestine. The common bile duct and pancreatic duct join to form the ampulla of Vater, emptying into the duodenum at the duodenal papilla. This papillary opening is surrounded by sphincter muscle known as the sphincter of Oddi. The 8-foot (2.5-m) portion of the small intestine that follows the sphincter of Oddi is the jejunum. The last 8 to 12 feet (2.5 to 4 m) of the small intestine is called the ileum. The ileocecal valve separates the entrance of the ileum from the cecum of the large intestine.

The inner surface of the small intestine has circular folds of mucosa and submucosa called plicae circulares, which project into the lumen to increase the surface area for digestion and absorption. Villi, microscopic finger-like projections, cover the plicae circulares to further increase the absorptive surface of the small intestine. The mucosa contains intestinal glands located between the villi.

■ Function

The small intestine has three main functions: movement (mixing and peristalsis), digestion, and absorption. The small intestine mixes and transports the chyme by movements called segmental contractions. The contents are moved back and forth over short distances, thereby allowing the chyme to mix with many digestive enzymes. The ileocecal valve opens only to allow the passage of chyme. It takes an average of 3 to 10 hours for the contents to be propelled by peristalsis through the small intestine. The intestinal glands secrete intestinal juice containing epithelial cells that are used to replace surface epithelial cells of the villi as they are lost. The intestinal

CHART 53-1

NURSING FOCUS *on the* **OLDER ADULT**
Changes in the Gastrointestinal System Related to Aging

Physiologic Change	Disorders Related to Change	Nursing Implications	Rationale
STOMACH Atrophy of the gastric mucosa is characterized by a decrease in the ratio of gastrin-secreting cells to somatostatin-secreting cells. This change leads to decreased hydrochloric acid levels (hypochlorhydria).	Decreased hydrochloric acid levels lead to decreased absorption of iron and vitamin B_{12} and to proliferation of bacteria. Atrophic gastritis occurs as a consequence of bacterial overgrowth.	Encourage frequent feedings of bland foods high in vitamins and iron. Assess for epigastric pain.	Frequent feedings help prevent gastritis. Assessment helps detect gastritis.
LARGE INTESTINE Peristalsis decreases, and nerve impulses are dulled.	Decreased sensation to defecate can result in postponement of bowel movements, which leads to constipation and impaction.	Encourage a high-fiber diet and 1500 mL of fluid intake daily (if not contraindicated). Encourage as much activity as tolerated.	These interventions increase the sensation of needing to defecate.
PANCREAS Distention and dilation of pancreatic ducts change. Calcification of pancreatic vessels occurs with a decrease in lipase production.	Decreased lipase level results in decreased fat absorption and digestion. Steatorrhea, or excess fat in the feces, occurs because of decreased fat digestion.	Encourage small, frequent feedings. Assess for diarrhea.	Small, frequent feedings help prevent steatorrhea. Diarrhea may be steatorrhea.
LIVER A decrease in the number and size of hepatic cells leads to decreased liver weight and mass. This change and an increase in fibrous tissue lead to decreased protein synthesis and changes in liver enzymes. Enzyme activity and cholesterol synthesis are diminished.	Decreased enzyme activity depresses drug metabolism, which leads to accumulation of drugs—possibly to toxic levels.	Assess all clients for adverse effects of all drugs, even those administered in normal doses.	Assessment detects drug toxicity.

cells also produce cells that contain enzymes aiding in the digestion of proteins, carbohydrates, and lipids.

Many digestive hormones and enzymes aid in the digestion of the chyme, each having a specific function (see Tables 53-1 and 53-2). Carbohydrates, fats, proteins, vitamins, water, and electrolytes are absorbed by both diffusion and active transport.

Large Intestine
■ Structure

The large intestine extends approximately 5 to 6 feet in length from the ileocecal valve to the anus and is lined with columnar epithelium that has absorptive and mucous cells. It begins with the cecum, with the appendix forming a narrow tube extending down from the cecum. The large intestine then extends upward from the cecum as the colon. The colon consists of four divisions: the ascending colon, the transverse colon, the descending colon, and the sigmoid colon. The sigmoid colon empties into the rectum.

Following the sigmoid colon, the large intestine bends downward to form the rectum. The last 3 to 4 cm of the large intestine is called the anal canal, which opens to the exterior of the body through the anus. The anal canal is surrounded by sphincter muscles.

■ Function
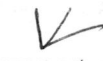

The large intestine's functions are movement, absorption, and elimination. Movement in the large intestine consists mainly of segmental contractions, like those in the small intestine, to allow enough time for the absorption of water. In addition, three or four strong peristaltic contractions per day are triggered by colonic distention in the proximal large intestine to propel the contents toward the rectum, where the material is stored until the urge to defecate occurs.

Absorption of water and some electrolytes occurs in the large intestine to reduce the fluid volume of the chyme, which creates a more solid material, the feces, for elimination. GI changes associated with aging are summarized in Chart 53-1.

ASSESSMENT TECHNIQUES
History

One method of assessing gastrointestinal (GI) functioning is to use the nutritional-metabolic and elimination patterns found in Gordon's Functional Health Patterns (Chart 53-2). The goal of the health history is to determine the events related to the current health problem.

GASTROINTESTINAL ASSESSMENT
Using Gordon's Functional Health Patterns

Nutritional-Metabolic Pattern
What is your typical daily food intake? Describe a day's meals, snacks, and vitamins.
How much salt do you typically add to your food? Do you use salt substitutes?
How is your appetite? Any recent change?
Do you have any difficulty chewing or swallowing?
Do you wear dentures? How well do they fit?
Do you ever experience indigestion or "heartburn"? How often? What seems to cause it? What helps it?
Do you have pain, diarrhea, gas, or any other problems? Do any specific foods cause this for you?
What is your typical daily fluid intake? What types of fluids (water, juices, soft drinks, coffee, tea)? How much?
Have you had any recent change in your weight? Weight gain? Weight loss? How much?
Have you noticed a change in the tightness of your rings or shoes? Tighter? Looser?
Have you noticed any difference in the size of your abdomen?

Elimination Pattern
What is your usual bowel elimination pattern? Frequency? Character? Discomfort? Laxatives?
Do you have any pain or bleeding associated with bowel movements?
Have you experienced any changes in your usual bowel pattern?
When was your last rectal examination?
Have you ever had an endoscopy or a colonoscopy?
What is your usual urinary elimination pattern? Frequency? Amount? Color? Odor? Control?
Have you noticed a change in the amount of urine?

Based on Gordon, M. (2000). *Manual of nursing diagnosis* (9th ed). St. Louis: Mosby.

DEMOGRAPHIC DATA

The nurse or assistive nursing personnel collects demographic data about the client, such as age, gender, culture, and occupation. This information can provide information regarding predispositions to particular GI tract disorders. For example, familial adenomatous polyposis (FAP) is an inherited autosomal dominant disorder that predisposes the client to colon cancer.

CONSIDERATIONS FOR OLDER ADULTS
The majority of GI tract cancers occur in adults age 50 and older. In addition, the incidence of hiatal hernia increases with each decade of life. Diverticulosis and gallstones are also seen increasingly in people older than 40 years of age.

CULTURAL CONSIDERATIONS
Inflammatory bowel diseases are more common in Caucasians than in African Americans or Asians. Ulcerative colitis is three to six times more prevalent among people of Jewish descent (Glickman, 1998). The incidence of GI cancers also varies among ethnic groups. For example, gastric cancer is prevalent in Japan, Korea, and southern China. Colon cancer is more prevalent among African-American men (Garlick Roll, 1999; Hawkins, 1999).

PERSONAL AND FAMILY HISTORY

A thorough review of the client's overall health status is an important part of every history. The nurse questions the client about previous GI disorders or abdominal surgery.

The client is asked about prescription medications being taken, including how much, when the drugs are administered, and why they have been prescribed. The nurse also explores whether the client takes over-the-counter medications, which he or she may use independently. In particular, the nurse asks whether aspirin, nonsteroidal anti-inflammatory drugs (NSAIDs) (such as ibuprofen), laxatives, or enemas are routinely taken. Large amounts of aspirin or NSAIDs can predispose the client to peptic ulcer disease and GI bleeding. Long-term use of laxatives or enemas can cause dependence on such stimulation and result in constipation.

Finally, the nurse investigates the client's travel history. The nurse asks the client whether he or she has traveled outside of the country recently. This information may provide clues as to the origin of symptoms such as diarrhea.

DIET HISTORY

A diet history is important when assessing GI tract function. Many conditions of the GI tract manifest themselves as a result of alterations in dietary intake and absorption of nutrients. The goals of a nutritional assessment are to gather information about ingestion, digestion, absorption, and metabolism (Hammond, 1999). The nurse inquires about any special diet and whether there are any known food allergies. The nurse also asks the client to describe the usual foods that are eaten daily and the times meals are taken.

The nurse explores with the client any changes that have occurred in eating habits as a result of illness. Anorexia (loss of appetite for food) can occur with GI disease. The nurse also asks about changes in taste and any difficulty or pain with swallowing (dysphagia) that could be associated with esophageal disorders. The nurse ascertains if abdominal pain or discomfort accompanies eating, and if the client has experienced any nausea, vomiting, or dyspepsia (indigestion or heartburn). Unknown food allergies often cause these symptoms. The nurse inquires about any unintentional weight loss, since some cancers of the GI tract may present in this manner. It is also important to assess alcohol and caffeine consumption, because both substances are associated with many GI disorders, such as gastritis and peptic ulcer disease.

CULTURAL CONSIDERATIONS
Cultural and religious patterns are important in obtaining a complete diet history. The nurse determines if culturally based foods pose a problem for the client. For example, the spices or hot pepper used in cooking in many cultures can aggravate or precipitate GI tract complaints, such as indigestion. The nurse should also note religious patterns such as fasting or abstinence.

Approximately 80% to 90% of African Americans are lactose intolerant (Greenberger & Isselbacher, 1998). A much smaller percentage of Caucasians also have this problem. Lactose intolerance causes bloating, cramping, and diarrhea as a result of lack of the enzyme lactase. Lactase is needed to convert lactose in milk and other dairy products to glucose and galactose.

SOCIOECONOMIC STATUS

Knowledge of the client's socioeconomic status can give the nurse valuable clues for determining his or her ability to obtain food, medications, and medical care. People who have limited budgets, such as elders or the unemployed, may not be able to purchase foods required for a balanced diet. In addition, they may substitute less expensive, and perhaps less effective, over-the-counter medications for prescription medications. Necessary medical care may be delayed, and clients may not seek health care until conditions are well advanced. Clients who are financially restricted may benefit from suggestions for managing nutrition while on a budget.

CURRENT HEALTH PROBLEMS

GI tract clinical manifestations are often vague and difficult for the client to describe. The nurse obtains a chronologic account of the current problem, symptoms, and any treatments taken. Furthermore, the nurse explores the characteristics associated with each symptom, including the location, quality, quantity, timing (onset, duration), and factors that may aggravate or alleviate the symptom (see Chart 53-2). The following examples are topics to explore with clients about specific GI tract symptoms.

A change in bowel habits is a significant complaint. The nurse explores the following with the client:

- Pattern of bowel movements
- Color and consistency of the feces
- Occurrence of diarrhea or constipation
- Effective action taken to relieve diarrhea or constipation
- Presence of frank blood or tarry stools
- Presence of abdominal distention or gas

An unintentional weight gain or loss is a symptom that warrants further investigation. The nurse assesses the client concerning the following:

- Normal weight
- Weight gain or loss
- Period of time for weight change
- Changes in appetite or oral intake

Smoking predisposes the client to several types of cancer, especially oral cancer, because nicotine is a GI irritant. The nurse obtains a smoking history, including the number of packs of cigarettes smoked per day per number of years. The nurse also asks about any history or current use of cigars, pipe tobacco, or chewing tobacco.

Pain is a common complaint in clients with GI tract disorders. The nurse asks about pain in relation to the following:

- Presence
- Location
- Radiation to another site
- Factors that make the pain better or worse
- Intensity

Abdominal pain is often vague and difficult to evaluate. Asking the client to apply descriptors to the type of pain, such as burning, gnawing, or stabbing, is often helpful. The location of the pain can be determined by asking the client to point to the involved site. The nurse also asks about the relationship of food intake to the onset or worsening of pain. For example, a high-fat meal often triggers gallbladder pain.

Changes in the skin can result from several GI tract disorders, such as liver and biliary system obstruction. The nurse asks the client about the following:

- Skin discolorations or rashes
- Itching
- Jaundice
- Increased susceptibility to bruising
- Increased tendency to bleed

Physical Assessment

Physical assessment of the gastrointestinal (GI) system involves a comprehensive examination of the client's nutritional status, the mouth and pharynx, the abdomen, and the extremities. Nutritional assessment is discussed in detail in Chapter 61.

MOUTH AND PHARYNX

Assessment of the mouth involves inspection and palpation. To begin the examination of the mouth, the nurse puts on gloves, faces the client, and inspects the lips for color, moisture, cracking, or lesions. To continue, the nurse needs a penlight and a tongue depressor. The medical-surgical nurse inspects the inner surfaces of the lips and the oral mucosa, starting on the client's left side and moving in a clockwise fashion. The advanced-practice nurse (APN) carefully palpates the U-shaped area under the tongue for nodules, since oral malignancies are most likely to develop in this area. The tongue is inspected for color, coating, ulcers, and variations in size and shape.

The nurse examines the teeth for evidence of dental caries and notes the absence of teeth. Tooth discoloration may be the result of excessive tobacco use. Referral to a dentist is appropriate if the nurse detects abnormalities or decay.

The gums should be pink, moist, and smooth. African-American clients may have a dark line on the margins of the gingiva. If the client wears dentures, they are removed. Throughout this examination, the nurse is alert to any significant mouth odors that suggest disease. For instance, a fruity smell may indicate uncontrolled diabetes mellitus.

Oral lesions or nodules are noted. For example, lesions from Kaposi's sarcoma may be seen in clients with acquired immunodeficiency syndrome (AIDS).

ABDOMEN

In preparation for examination of the abdomen, the client is instructed to empty his or her bladder and then to lie in a supine position with the knees bent, keeping the arms at the sides to prevent inadvertent tensing of the abdominal muscles.

During the abdominal examination, the nurse usually begins at the client's right side and proceeds in a systematic fashion (Figure 53-6):

- Right upper quadrant (RUQ)
- Left upper quadrant (LUQ)
- Left lower quadrant (LLQ)
- Right lower quadrant (RLQ)

Table 53-3 lists the organs that lie in each of these topographic areas.

If areas of pain or discomfort are noted from the history, the nurse places this area last in the examination sequence. This

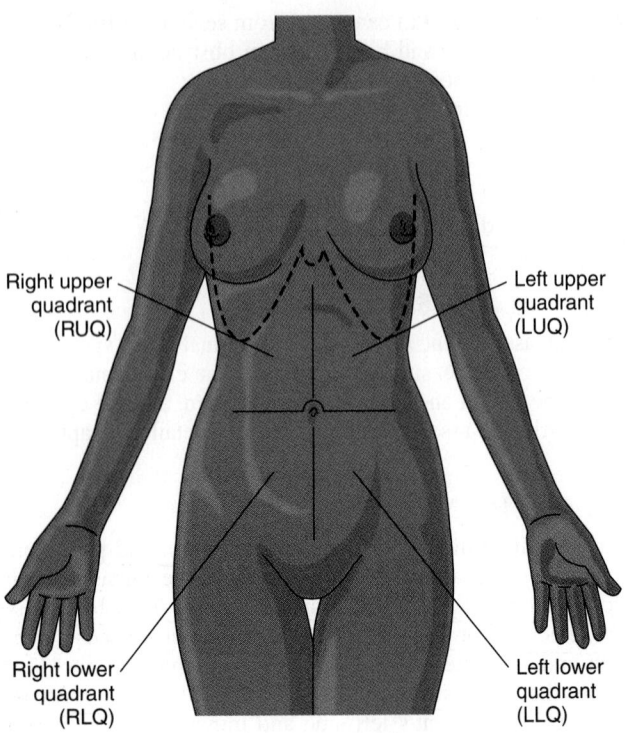

Figure 53-6 ● A topographic division of the abdomen into quadrants.

TABLE 53-3 ● LOCATION OF BODY STRUCTURES IN EACH ABDOMINAL QUADRANT	
RIGHT UPPER QUADRANT (RUQ) • Most of the liver • Gallbladder • Duodenum • Head of the pancreas • Hepatic flexure of the colon • Part of the ascending and transverse colon	**LEFT LOWER QUADRANT (LLQ)** • Part of the descending colon • Sigmoid colon • Left ureter • Left ovary and fallopian tube • Left spermatic cord
LEFT UPPER QUADRANT (LUQ) • Left lobe of the liver • Stomach • Spleen • Body and tail of the pancreas • Splenic flexure of the colon • Part of the transverse and descending colon	**RIGHT LOWER QUADRANT (RLQ)** • Cecum • Appendix • Right ureter • Right ovary and fallopian tube • Right spermatic cord **MIDLINE** • Abdominal aorta • Uterus (if enlarged) • Bladder (if distended)

sequence should prevent the client from tensing abdominal muscles because of the pain, which would make the examination difficult. The nurse examines any area of tenderness cautiously and instructs the client to state whether it is too painful. His or her face is observed for signs of distress or pain.

The nurse assesses the abdomen by using the four techniques of examination, but in a sequence different from that used for other body systems: inspection, auscultation, percussion, and then palpation. This sequence is preferred so that palpation and percussion do not increase intestinal activity and hence increase bowel sounds. Palpation is not performed if appendicitis or an abdominal aneurysm is suspected.

■ Inspection

The nurse inspects the skin and notes the following:
- Overall symmetry of the abdomen
- Presence of discolorations (rashes, lesions, striae, petechiae, scars, distended superficial veins, jaundice, and any other pigmentation changes)
- Abdominal distention
- Bulging flanks
- Taut, glistening skin

The nurse assesses the architecture of the abdomen by observing its contour and symmetry. The contour of the abdomen is the abdominal profile and can be rounded, flat, concave, or distended. The contour is best seen if one stands at the side of the bed. The nurse notes whether the contour is symmetric or asymmetric. Asymmetry in the upper quadrants can be indicative of a tumor, pancreatic cyst, or gastric dilation. Asymmetry in the lower quadrants can be caused by ovarian tumors, fibroid tumors, pregnancy, or bladder distention (O'Hanlon-Nichols, 1998). The nurse inspects the shape and position of the umbili-

cus for any deviations. The presence of ecchymosis around the umbilicus (Cullen's sign) is also noted as an indication of intraperitoneal hemorrhage (Wrobleski, Barth, & Oyen, 1999).

Finally, the nurse inspects the client's abdominal movements, including the normal rising and falling with inspiration and expiration, and notes any distress during movement. Occasionally, pulsations may be visible, particularly in the area of the abdominal aorta. Peristaltic movements are rarely seen on inspection unless the client is thin and has markedly increased peristalsis. If such movements are observed, the nurse notes the quadrant of origin and the direction of peristaltic flow. This finding is reported to the health care provider, since it may indicate an intestinal obstruction.

■ Auscultation

The nurse performs auscultation of the abdomen with the diaphragm of the stethoscope, since bowel sounds are usually high pitched. The stethoscope is placed lightly on the abdominal wall while the nurse listens for bowel sounds in all four quadrants, beginning in the RLQ at the ileocecal valve area.

Bowel sounds are created as air and fluid move through the GI tract. They are normally heard as relatively high pitched gurgles every 5 to 15 seconds, with a normal frequency range of 5 to 30 per minute. Bowel sounds are characterized as normal, hypoactive, or hyperactive. The nurse listens for the character and frequency of the sounds. Bowel sounds may be irregular, so the nurse must listen for *at least* 1 full minute in each quadrant to confirm the absence of bowel sounds. Bowel sounds are diminished or absent after abdominal surgery or in the client with peritonitis or paralytic ileus. Increased bowel sounds, especially loud gurgling sounds, result from hypermotility of the bowel (borborygmus). These sounds are usually heard in the client with diarrhea or gastroenteritis or above a complete intestinal obstruction.

The nurse also auscultates the abdomen for vascular sounds or bruits ("swooshing" sounds) over the abdominal aorta, the renal arteries, and the iliac arteries. A bruit heard over the aorta usually indicates the presence of an aneurysm. If this sound is heard, the nurse discontinues the examination and notifies the health care provider immediately.

The nurse may auscultate for two other abnormal circulatory sounds: friction rubs and venous hums. A friction rub, which sounds like two pieces of leather rubbing together, can be heard over the spleen or the liver and indicates the presence of a splenic infarct or a hepatic tumor. A continuous venous hum is heard in the periumbilical region in the presence of engorged liver circulation, as in hepatic cirrhosis.

Percussion

Percussion may be used during the abdominal assessment to determine the size of solid organs; to detect the presence of masses, fluid, and air; and to estimate the size of the liver and spleen. This part of the physical assessment is usually performed by a physician or advanced-practice nurse (APN). The examiner elicits percussion notes by placing the middle finger of the nondominant hand over the abdominal area to be percussed, striking his or her finger lightly with the tip of the middle finger of the dominant hand several times. Each quadrant is systematically assessed by comparing sounds over different areas. The **percussion notes** normally heard in the abdomen are termed **tympanic** (the high-pitched, loud, musical sound of an air-filled intestine) or **dull** (the medium-pitched, softer, thudlike sound over a solid organ, such as the liver).

To percuss the size of the liver span, the physician or APN begins from below the right nipple in the midclavicular line and is careful to percuss between ribs. The percussion note should change from resonance of the lung tissue to dullness of the liver when the upper liver border is reached. The examiner marks the area where percussion tones change, then percusses up from the iliac crest in the midclavicular line until the percussion note changes from tympany of the bowel to dullness of the liver at the lower border. Again, this area is marked. The distance between the two marks is the approximate liver span, which is normally 2.4 to 5 inches (6 to 12 cm). An enlarged liver span indicates **hepatomegaly** (liver enlargement).

The examiner may use percussion techniques to determine the size and position of the spleen at the tenth intercostal space in the left midaxillary line. Dullness heard forward of the midaxillary line or in the left anterior axillary line indicates enlargement of the spleen (splenomegaly). Mild to moderate splenomegaly can be detected before the spleen becomes palpable. Percussion can also be used to detect a distended bladder.

Palpation

The purpose of palpation is to determine the size and location of abdominal organs and to assess for the presence of masses or tenderness. Palpation of the abdomen consists of two types: light palpation and deep palpation. Only physicians and APNs, such as clinical nurse specialists and nurse practitioners, should perform deep palpation.

LIGHT PALPATION

The technique of light palpation is used to detect large masses and areas of tenderness and to help the client achieve muscular relaxation. The nurse places the first four fingers of the palpating hand close together and then places them lightly on the abdomen and proceeds smoothly and systematically from quadrant to quadrant. The abdomen is depressed to a depth of 0.5 to 1 inch (1.25 to 2.5 cm), and the assessment proceeds with a rotational movement of the palpating hand. Any areas of tenderness or guarding are noted, because these areas are examined last and cautiously during deep palpation. While performing light palpation, the nurse is alert to signs of rigidity, which, unlike voluntary guarding, is a sign of peritoneal inflammation. Areas of pain should be evaluated for rebound tenderness (Blumberg's sign). With fingers placed at a 90-degree angle in relation to the abdomen, the examiner pushes slowly and deeply, releasing quickly. Pain felt on release is a positive sign for rebound tenderness and should be reported to the health care provider.

DEEP PALPATION

Deep palpation is used to further determine the size and shape of abdominal organs and masses. The APN uses the palm and fingers of one or both hands and proceeds deliberately around the abdominal wall to a maximal depth. If both hands are used (bimanual palpation), one hand is placed on top of the other for palpation of a deep organ. This technique may be required in order to overcome the resistance felt by a large, obese abdomen.

There are two techniques that can be used for palpating the liver. For the first technique, the examiner stands at the client's right side and places the left hand under the client's back parallel to the eleventh and twelfth ribs. The right hand is placed in the right upper quadrant (RUQ) parallel to the midline. The client is then instructed to take a deep breath as the examiner presses the hand inward and upward under the rib cage until a maximal depth is reached. The liver may or may not be palpable, but the edge of the liver may be felt over the fingertips of the palpating hand as the client breathes.

The second technique for palpating the liver is the *hooking technique*. The examiner stands at the client's right side behind the shoulder and places both hands, next to one another, below the lower border of the liver. The client is instructed to take a deep breath while the nurse presses in with the fingers of both hands at the costal margin. The examiner attempts to feel the lower border of the liver as it descends.

Palpation is also used to detect an enlarged spleen; however, the spleen must be three times its original size before it is palpable. The same two techniques for palpating the liver are used for the spleen, but on the left side. The pancreas, the gallbladder, and the left kidney are not usually palpable in most healthy adults.

Psychosocial Assessment

Psychosocial assessment focuses on how the current complaint affects the client's lifestyle. The nurse asks whether there has been any interruption of, or disturbance to, usual activities, including employment. The nurse questions about recent stressful events experienced. Emotional stress has been associated with the development or exacerbation of irritable bowel syndrome (IBS).

CRITICAL THINKING CHALLENGE
A male client has been admitted to your unit complaining of RUQ pain and fever for the last 2 days. His usual dietary pattern consists of eating at restaurants several times weekly. The symptoms began 2 hours after eating a dinner of fried foods at a local restaurant.

- What specific areas of the history should you seek further information or clarification about?
- What physical assessment findings would you be most likely to find during the abdominal examination?

For suggested answer guidelines, go to SIMON http://www.wbsaunders.com/SIMON/Iggy/.

Diagnostic Assessment

LABORATORY ASSESSMENT

To make an accurate assessment of the many possible causes of gastrointestinal (GI) tract abnormalities, laboratory testing of blood, urine, and stool specimens can be performed.

Blood Tests

COMPLETE BLOOD COUNT

A complete blood count (CBC) aids in the diagnosis of anemia and infection; it also detects changes in the blood's formed elements. In adults, GI bleeding is the most frequent cause of anemia.

CLOTTING FACTORS

Because the liver is the main site of all proteins involved in coagulation, the prothrombin time is useful in evaluating the levels of these clotting factors. Prothrombin time measures the rate at which prothrombin is converted to thrombin, a process that is dependent on most of the vitamin K–associated clotting factors. Severe acute or chronic liver damage leads to prolongation of the prothrombin time secondary to impaired synthesis of clotting proteins.

SERUM ELECTROLYTES

Many electrolytes are altered in GI tract dysfunction. For example, calcium is absorbed in the GI tract and may be measured to detect malabsorption. Excessive vomiting or diarrhea causes electrolyte depletion, requiring replacement.

SERUM ENZYME ASSAYS AND LIVER FUNCTION TESTS

Assays of serum enzymes are important in the evaluation of liver damage. **Aspartate aminotransferase (AST)** and **alanine aminotransferase (ALT)** are two enzymes found in the liver and other organs. These enzymes are elevated in most liver disorders, but they are highest in conditions that cause necrosis, such as severe viral hepatitis.

Elevations in serum **amylase** and **lipase** are indicative of acute pancreatitis. In acute pancreatitis, serum amylase levels begin to elevate within 24 hours of onset and remain elevated for up to 5 days unless extensive pancreatic necrosis, obstruction, or a pseudocyst is present. Serum amylase and lipase measurements are the best indicators of the presence of acute pancreatitis, with elevations corresponding to pancreatitis in 75% to 80% of cases (Toskes & Greenberger, 1998; Wrobleski, Barth, & Oyen, 1999).

Bilirubin is the primary pigment in bile, which is normally conjugated and excreted by the liver and biliary system. It is measured as total serum bilirubin, conjugated (direct) bilirubin, and unconjugated (indirect) bilirubin. These measurements are important in the evaluation of jaundice and in the evaluation of liver and biliary tract functioning (Hass, 1999). Elevations in direct and indirect bilirubin levels can indicate impaired secretion or conjugation.

The serum level of ammonia is also measured to evaluate hepatic function. Ammonia is normally used to rebuild amino acids or is converted to urea for excretion. Elevated ammonia levels are seen in conditions that cause hepatocellular injury, such as cirrhosis of the liver.

TUMOR MARKERS

Two **oncofetal antigens**—CA19-9 and CEA—are evaluated to monitor the success of cancer therapy and to assess for the recurrence of cancer in the GI tract. These antigens may also be increased in benign GI conditions. Chart 53-3 lists blood tests commonly used by the health care provider in the diagnosis of GI disorders.

URINE TESTS

The presence of amylase can be detected in the urine. In acute pancreatitis, there is increased renal clearance of amylase. Amylase levels in the urine remain high even after serum levels return to normal; therefore there may be false-positive findings associated with this particular test.

Urine urobilinogen is a form of bilirubin that is converted by the intestinal flora and excreted in the urine. Its measurement is useful in the evaluation of hepatic and biliary obstruction, since the presence of bilirubin in the urine often precedes the development of jaundice (Chart 53-4).

STOOL TESTS

Several stool examinations are used in the evaluation of GI tract dysfunction (see Chart 53-4). Stool testing for occult blood is called the **fecal occult blood test (FOBT).** The FOBT measures the presence of blood in the stool from GI bleeding, a common finding associated with colorectal cancer.

Stool samples are collected to test for ova and parasites to aid in the diagnosis of parasitic infection. Stool samples tested for fecal fats are evaluated for steatorrhea and malabsorption. Fat is normally absorbed in the small intestine in the presence of biliary and pancreatic secretions. In malabsorption, fat is abnormally excreted in the stool.

WOMEN'S HEALTH CONSIDERATIONS
Compared with women of lower socioeconomic status, women of higher socioeconomic status are more likely to have regular physical examinations that include an annual FOBT and a proctosigmoidoscopy every 3 to 5 years after the age of 50. An annual FOBT reduces mortality from colorectal cancer in women (Allen & Phillips, 1997).

CHART 53-3

LABORATORY PROFILE
Gastrointestinal Assessment

Test	Normal Range for Adults	Significance of Abnormal Findings

Calcium (total)	*18-60 yr:* 8.6-10.0 mg/dL or 2.15-2.50 mmol/L
	60-90 yr: 8.8-10.2 mg/dL or 2.20-2.55 mmol/L
	>90 yr: 8.2-9.6 mg/dL or 2.15-2.40 mmol/L
		Decreased values indicate possible:
		    Malabsorption
		    Renal failure
		    Acute pancreatitis

Potassium	*Male:* 3.5-4.5 mEq/L or 3.5-4.5 mmol/L
	Female: 3.4-4.4 mEq/L or 3.4-4.4 mmol/L
		Decreased values indicate possible:
		    Vomiting
		    Gastric suctioning
		    Diarrhea
		    Drainage from intestinal fistulas

Albumin	*18-60 yr:* 3.4-4.8 g/dL *60-90 yr:* 3.2-4.6 g/dL	*Decreased* values indicate possible: Hepatic disease

Alanine aminotransferase (ALT)	*18-60 yr, male:* 10-40 units/L
	        female: 7-35 units/L
	60-90 yr, male: 13-40 units/L
	        female: 10-28 units/L
	>90 yr, male: 6-38 units/L
	        female: 5-24 units/L
		Increased values indicate possible:
		    Liver disease
		    Hepatitis
		    Cirrhosis

Aspartate aminotransferase (AST)	*18-60 yr:* 8-20 units/L
	>60 yr, male: 11-26 units/L
	        female: 10-20 units/L
		Increased values indicate possible:
		    Liver disease
		    Hepatitis
		    Cirrhosis

Lactate dehydrogenase (LDH)	140-280 units/L	*Increased* values indicate possible
		    damaged liver caused by hepatitis
		    and other hepatocellular disorders

Alkaline phosphatase	25-100 units/L or 0.43-1.70 μKat/L	*Increased* values indicate possible:
		    Hepatic disease
		    Biliary obstruction

Bilirubin
    Total serum
	18-60 yr: 0.3-1.2 mg/dL or 5-21 μmol/L
	60-90 yr: 0.2-1.1 mg/dL or 3-19 μmol/L
	>90 yr: 0.2-0.9 mg/dL or 3-15 μmol/L
		Increased values indicate possible:
		    Hemolysis
		    Biliary obstruction
		    Hepatic damage

Conjugated (direct)	<0.2 mg/dL or 3.4 μmol/L	*Increased* values indicate possible biliary obstruction

Unconjugated (indirect)	<1.1 mg/dL or 19 μmol/L	*Increased* values indicate possible:
		    Hemolysis
		    Hepatic damage

Ammonia	19-60 μg/dL or 11-35 μmol/L	*Increased* values indicate possible hepatic disease such as cirrhosis
Xylose absorption	*5-g dose in 2 hr:* >20 mg/dL or >1.3 mmol/L *25-g dose in 2 hr:* >25 mg/dL or >1.7 mmol/L	*Decreased* values in blood and urine indicate possible malabsorption in the small intestine
Serum amylase	*18-60 yr:* 27-131 IU/L or 0.46-2.23 μKat/L *60-90 yr:* 24-151 IU/L or 0.41-2.57 μKat/L	*Increased* values indicate possible acute pancreatitis
Serum lipase	13-141 units/L or 0.22-2.40 μKat/L *>60 yr:* 0-302 units/L or 0.0-5.13 μKat/L	*Increased* values indicate possible acute pancreatitis

Cholesterol	<200 mg/dL or 5.18 mmol/L	*Increased* values indicate possible:
		    Pancreatitis
		    Biliary obstruction
		Decreased values indicate possible liver cell damage

Carbohydrate antigen 19-9 (CA19-9)	<37 units/mL	*Increased* values indicate possible:
		    Cancer of the pancreas, stomach, colon
		    Acute pancreatitis
		    Inflammatory bowel disease

Carcinoembryonic antigen (CEA)	*Nonsmoker:* <2.5 ng/mL
	Smoker: up to 5 ng/mL
		Increased values indicate possible:
		    Colorectal, stomach, pancreatic cancer
		    Ulcerative colitis
		    Crohn's disease
		    Hepatitis
		    Cirrhosis

CHART 53-4

LABORATORY PROFILE
Common Urine and Stool Tests Used in Gastrointestinal Assessment

Test	Normal Range for Adults	Significance of Abnormal Findings
Urine bilirubin	Negative	*Increased* values indicate possible: Biliary obstruction Cirrhosis Hepatitis
Urobilinogen	Urine: 0.1-1.0 Ehrlich unit/mL	*Increased* values indicate possible: Hepatitis Cirrhosis *Absence* indicates possible obstructive jaundice
Urine amylase	Various levels, depending on unit of measure	*Increased* values indicate possible: Acute pancreatitis Pancreatic obstruction
Stool for occult blood	Negative	*Presence* indicates possible: Carcinoma Peptic ulcer Ulcerative colitis
Ova and parasites	Negative	*Presence* is diagnostic of infection
Fecal fat	<7 g/24 hr with normal diet	*Increased* values indicate possible: Crohn's disease Malabsorption syndrome Pancreatic disease

RADIOGRAPHIC EXAMINATIONS

Radiographic examinations and similar diagnostic procedures are useful in detecting structural and functional disorders of the gastrointestinal (GI) tract. The role of the nurse is to properly prepare the client for the examination, to provide an explanation of the procedure, and to provide the necessary postprocedure care. As with most invasive procedures, many of the diagnostic tests outlined here require a witnessed and signed informed consent.

Flat-Plate Film of the Abdomen

A flat-plate film of the abdomen is generally the first x-ray study that the health care provider orders when diagnosing a GI problem. A flat-plate film visualizes organs in the abdomen. This simple film has the ability to reveal abnormalities such as masses, tumors, and strictures or obstructions to normal movement. Patterns of bowel gas appear light on the abdominal film and can be useful in detecting ileus from obstruction. There is no required client preparation except to wear a hospital gown and remove any jewelry or belts, which may interfere with the film.

Upper Gastrointestinal Series and Small-Bowel Series

An upper GI radiographic series is an x-ray visualization from the oral part of the pharynx to the duodenojejunal junction. The upper GI series is used to detect disorders of structure or function of the esophagus (barium swallow), stomach, or duodenum. An extension of the upper GI series, the small-bowel follow-through (SBFT), continues the tracing of the barium through the small intestine up to and including the ileocecal junction to detect disorders of the jejunum or ileum.

CLIENT PREPARATION. The client is instructed to abstain from foods or liquids for 8 hours before the test. If possible, opioid analgesics and anticholinergic medications are withheld for 24 hours before the test, since they decrease intestinal tract motility.

The client is instructed about the barium preparation and the need to drink approximately 16 ounces of the barium. The radiology nurse or technician explains that a rotating examination table will be used to assist the client in assuming the vertical, supine, prone, and lateral positions required for this test.

PROCEDURE. The client drinks a mixture of barium sulfate, and fluoroscopy is used to trace the barium through the esophagus and stomach. The client stands against the x-ray table for this part of the test. The table then moves the client to a lying position for more views of the stomach and duodenum. Lying in a prone position, the client drinks more barium as quickly as possible while x-ray films are taken. To attempt to make the client as comfortable as possible, a pillow for the head and a sheet to prevent chilling are supplied whenever possible. The position changes help to coat the mucosa and identify gastroesophageal reflux and hiatal hernia.

If a small-bowel radiographic series is included, the client drinks additional barium, and more x-ray films are taken at intervals. This series can take several hours, depending on how long it takes the barium to reach the cecum.

FOLLOW-UP CARE. After either of these series, the nurse teaches the client to drink plenty of fluids to help eliminate the barium. The client may be given a mild laxative or stool softener to assist in elimination of the barium. The radiology nurse or technician instructs the client that stools may be chalky white for 24 to 72 hours as barium is excreted. The client is informed that when all barium is passed, brown stools return. If the client is at home, he or she is instructed to report abdominal fullness, pain, or a delay in return to brown stools.

Barium Enema

A barium enema examination, also known as a lower GI series, is a radiographic visualization of the large intestine. This test is usually ordered for a client with a complaint of blood or mucus in the stool or a change in bowel pattern, such as diarrhea or constipation. A barium enema can also detect bowel obstruction from volvulus (Korsten & Abittan, 1999). This test is usually contraindicated in clients when colon perforation or fistula is suspected, since there is the potential for barium to enter the venous circulation, causing cardiac arrest.

CLIENT PREPARATION. Adequate client preparation for a barium enema study is very important. The client consumes clear liquids 12 to 24 hours before the examination to reduce the amount of fecal matter in the bowel. The client is allowed nothing by mouth (NPO) after midnight on the night before the test. In addition, the health care provider orders a potent laxative, such as magnesium citrate, and possibly an oral liquid preparation, such as GoLYTELY, for cleaning the bowel the evening before the examination. In some cases, a cleansing enema is needed or required according to the agency's procedure.

PROCEDURE. To begin the barium enema examination, a rectal catheter with an inflatable balloon is inserted. Approximately 500 to 1500 mL of barium is instilled slowly by gravity, and the client is instructed to hold the barium. Films are taken with the client in supine, prone, and lateral positions. He or she may experience abdominal cramps and the urge to defecate as the barium enema is given. This procedure can be extremely uncomfortable, especially for older adults. The client is instructed to take slow, deep breaths and to hold the anal sphincter as tightly closed as possible. The test takes about 45 minutes to 1 hour. In some cases, a double-contrast study is ordered. In this study, air is instilled to enhance the contrast and outline small lesions.

FOLLOW-UP CARE. After the study is completed, the client is allowed to expel the barium. The radiology nurse or technician teaches the client to drink plenty of fluids to assist in eliminating the barium. A laxative is given to help remove the barium from the intestinal tract. The client is informed that the stools will be chalky white for about 24 to 72 hours, until all barium is expelled.

Percutaneous Transhepatic Cholangiography

Percutaneous transhepatic cholangiography is an x-ray study of the biliary duct system using an iodinated dye instilled via a percutaneous needle inserted into the hepatic ducts of the liver. This procedure is usually performed when a client has jaundice or persistent upper abdominal pain even after cholecystectomy.

CLIENT PREPARATION. A laxative is usually given to the client the evening before the procedure. He or she is on NPO status for 12 hours before the test, and the nurse asks about allergies to iodine or seafood. If the client has either of these allergies, the nurse informs the health care provider. Coagulation tests are monitored, since impaired clotting is a contraindication to this procedure. Before the procedure begins, an intravenous (IV) infusion is started for the administration of sedatives.

PROCEDURE. The client is placed in a supine position on the fluoroscopy table. The site is prepared and draped, and a local anesthetic is injected into the skin. During the test, the client is instructed to hold his or her breath on expiration while a needle is inserted into the liver under x-ray visualization. The dye is injected slowly until the biliary tree is filled. X-ray images are taken as the dye reaches the biliary duct system. A tilt table may be used to place the client in various positions to visualize the entire biliary tree. At the end of the test, the biliary ducts are aspirated of contrast medium. The procedure usually takes 30 minutes to 1 hour.

FOLLOW-UP CARE. After a percutaneous transhepatic cholangiography, the client is confined to bed for 6 hours. The nurse checks vital signs frequently, since there is a risk of hemorrhage and sepsis. The client is placed on the right side with a firm pillow or sandbag placed against the lower ribs and abdomen. The nurse inspects the lower right rib cage area for signs of bleeding, hematoma, ecchymosis, or bile leakage.

Gallbladder Series

A gallbladder radiographic series, or oral cholecystography, is an x-ray visualization of the gallbladder after oral ingestion of radiopaque, iodine-based contrast medium. It is not commonly performed today because of the availability and accuracy of gallbladder ultrasound. After the contrast medium is ingested, it is eventually cleared from the blood by the liver, and it is then deposited into the hepatic and biliary ducts and gallbladder. The test may be performed to identify causes of obstruction, such as stones, but gallbladder ultrasonography is more commonly done for this purpose. A gallbladder radiographic series should be done before any barium studies.

CLIENT PREPARATION. Before the gallbladder radiographic series, the nurse checks with the client about any allergies to iodine or seafood. On the day before the test, the client eats a fat-free or low-fat diet and takes 6 radiopaque iodine tablets (iopanoic acid [Telepaque]) approximately 2 hours after the evening meal. One tablet is taken with water every 5 minutes until all 6 tablets are consumed. The nurse instructs the client that the tablets can cause diarrhea. The client is on NPO status from midnight on the night before the test until after the test is completed.

PROCEDURE. The client is usually in the radiology department for about 60 minutes while several views of the gallbladder are taken. These films will identify any stones present in the gallbladder. The client is then given a fatty meal, or synthetic substitute, to cause contraction of the gallbladder within 10 to 30 minutes. A second series of films helps to confirm the presence of contrast material in the cystic duct, common duct, and duodenum.

FOLLOW-UP CARE. The nurse remains alert for allergic reaction to the contrast material.

Intravenous Cholangiography

Intravenous cholangiography (IVC) is an x-ray study of the gallbladder and biliary ducts. This test may be performed if the gallbladder is not visualized by a gallbladder radiographic series or gallbladder ultrasonography, or if biliary symptoms occur in a client who has had a cholecystectomy. It may also be done during surgery.

CLIENT PREPARATION. Before the test, the nurse checks with the client about any allergies to iodine or seafood and reports allergies to the physician. The client is on NPO status after midnight on the night before the test. Some agencies may require a bowel preparation. The nurse notifies the client that a sensation of warmth or flushing may be felt with the injection of the contrast medium.

PROCEDURE. The client may be in the radiology department for 2 to 4 hours for IVC. The client is given an IV injection of a contrast material, and x-ray films are taken at 20-minute intervals for 1 hour, or until the biliary ducts are visualized. The gallbladder should be visualized in 1 to 2 hours.

FOLLOW-UP CARE. The radiology personnel and nurse monitor the client for allergic reaction to the contrast material so that emergency measures can be instituted if necessary.

Computed Tomography of the Gastrointestinal Tract

Computed tomography (CT), also referred to as a CT scan, is a cross-sectional x-ray visualization that can detect tissue densities and abnormalities in the abdomen, liver, pancreas, spleen, and biliary tract. CT may be performed with or without contrast media.

CLIENT PREPARATION. The client is instructed that he or she will need to lie still in a rather enclosed space of the machine. The client is instructed to remove jewelry or metal from the x-ray field. If the use of a contrast medium is scheduled, the nurse asks about allergies to seafood and iodine. The client is on NPO status for 4 to 8 hours before the test if a contrast medium is to be used. IV access will be required for injection of the contrast medium. The client is advised that a warm, flushing feeling may be felt on injection.

PROCEDURE. The radiologic technician instructs the client to lie still and to hold his or her breath when asked. The client is placed on the examining table, and a series of x-ray images are taken. The contrast medium may be given by IV injection for a second set of images. The test takes approximately 1 to 2 hours to complete.

FOLLOW-UP CARE. No particular follow-up care is needed after a CT scan unless sedatives were administered. If the client was sedated, the nurse monitors vital signs until the client is alert and fully awake.

CRITICAL THINKING CHALLENGE
The health care provider suspects that your client may have an inflammation of the gallbladder as a result of gallstones.
- What diagnostic procedure will probably be ordered for this client to confirm the diagnosis?
- What information should the nurse ask the client about before the test is scheduled?

For suggested answer guidelines, go to SIMON http://www.wbsaunders.com/SIMON/Iggy/.

OTHER DIAGNOSTIC TESTS
Endoscopy

Endoscopy is direct visualization of the gastrointestinal (GI) tract by means of a flexible fiberoptic endoscope. Endoscopes of various sizes are used for different areas of the GI tract. Visualization of the esophagus, stomach, biliary system, and bowel is possible. Endoscopy is usually ordered to evaluate bleeding, ulceration, inflammation, masses, tumors, and cancerous lesions. Obtaining specimens for biopsy and cytologic studies is also possible through the endoscope. There are several types of endoscopic examinations.

ESOPHAGOGASTRODUODENOSCOPY

Esophagogastroduodenoscopy (EGD), a visual examination of the esophagus, stomach, and duodenum, is accomplished using a fiberoptic endoscope. The distal end of the endoscope is flexible, allowing visualization of the entire area.

CLIENT PREPARATION. The client preparing for an upper GI endoscopic examination is usually on NPO status after midnight on the night before the test, or 8 to 12 hours before the procedure. The nurse explains that during the test a flexible tube is passed down the esophagus with the client under conscious sedation. The physician usually orders medication, such as midazolam hydrochloride (Versed), meperidine (Demerol), or diazepam (Valium, E-Pam✦), to sedate the client. Atropine may be administered to dry secretions. In addition, a local anesthetic is sprayed to inactivate the gag reflex and facilitate passage of the tube. The nurse explains that this anesthetic will calm the gag reflex and that swallowing will be difficult. If the client has dentures, they are removed.

PROCEDURE. After the medications are administered, the client is usually placed in the left lateral decubitus (Sims') position with a towel or basin at the mouth for secretions. The physician passes the tube through the mouth and into the esophagus (Figure 53-7). The procedure takes approximately 30 minutes.

FOLLOW-UP CARE. The nurse checks vital signs frequently as ordered (usually every 30 minutes) until the sedation wears off. The siderails of the bed are raised during this time. The client remains on NPO status until the gag reflex returns (usually in 2 to 4 hours). The nurse monitors for signs of perforation, such as pain, bleeding, or fever. The client is instructed not to drive for 12 hours following the test. He or she is informed that a hoarse voice or sore throat may persist for several days following the test. Throat lozenges can be used to relieve throat discomfort.

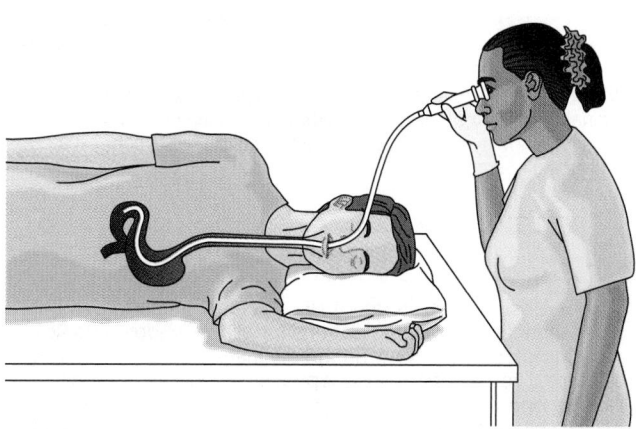

Figure 53-7 ⦿ Esophagogastroduodenoscopy allows visualization of the esophagus, the stomach, and the duodenum. If the esophagus is the focus of the examination, the procedure is called esophagoscopy. If the stomach is the focus, the procedure is called gastroscopy.

ENDOSCOPIC RETROGRADE CHOLANGIOPANCREATOGRAPHY

Endoscopic retrograde cholangiopancreatography (ERCP) includes visual and radiographic examination of the liver, gallbladder, and pancreas to identify the cause and location of obstruction. After the cannula is inserted into the main duct, a radiopaque dye is inserted, followed by several x-ray images. The physician may perform a papillotomy, a small incision in the sphincter around the ampulla of Vater, to remove gallstones.

CLIENT PREPARATION. The client is prepared in the same manner as for an EGD, including being on NPO status after midnight on the night before the test. The client will require IV access for the administration of sedation. The nurse asks about prior exposure to x-ray dye and any sensitivities or allergies.

PROCEDURE. The endoscopic portion of an ERCP is similar to that of an EGD, except that the endoscope is advanced farther, to the duodenum and into the biliary tract. Once the cannula is in the common duct, the radiologist or the radiologic technician injects contrast medium, and x-ray films are taken to evaluate the biliary tract. A tilt table assists in distributing the contrast medium to all branches of the biliary tree. Following examination of the biliary tree, the cannula is directed into the pancreatic duct for examination. The ERCP lasts from 30 minutes to 2 hours.

FOLLOW-UP CARE. The nurse assesses vital signs frequently, usually every 15 minutes, until the client is stable. The nurse observes for several postprocedure complications, including cholangitis, perforation, sepsis, and pancreatitis. These problems do not occur immediately after the procedure but may take several hours to 2 days to develop. Colicky abdominal pain can occur secondary to the air instilled during the procedure. The client is instructed to report abdominal pain, fever, nausea, or vomiting that fails to resolve. He or she remains on NPO status until the gag reflex returns. Once the gag reflex is intact, the client can begin taking clear fluids.

COLONOSCOPY

Colonoscopy is an endoscopic examination of the entire large bowel. The physician may also obtain tissue biopsy specimens or remove polyps through the colonoscope. A colonoscopy is also used to evaluate the cause of chronic diarrhea or locate the source of GI bleeding.

CLIENT PREPARATION. The client should have a liquid diet for at least 24 hours before a colonoscopy and is usually on NPO status after midnight on the night before the procedure.

> ### CONSIDERATIONS FOR OLDER ADULTS
> A complete bowel preparation ("prep") is necessary to enable the physician to visualize the entire colon. For many clients, especially older adults, the "prep" is the worst part of the procedure, resulting in weakness and fatigue.

An oral liquid preparation for cleaning the bowel (e.g., polyethylene glycol electrolyte solution [GoLYTELY]) is given to the client the evening before the examination. The solution should be chilled to make it more palatable. Even though it has a salty taste, the solution should not be diluted with water or ice. The nurse instructs the client to drink the preparation quickly—8 ounces (240 mL) every 10 minutes until all 4 L are consumed. This solution produces a watery diarrhea that begins in approximately 1 hour. The bowel clears in 4 to 5 hours. In some cases, the client may require laxatives, suppositories (e.g., bisacodyl [Dulcolax]), or one or more cleansing enemas. IV access is necessary for the administration of conscious sedation.

PROCEDURE. The physician orders medication to aid in relaxation, usually midazolam hydrochloride (Versed) or meperidine (Demerol). Initially, the client is placed on the left side with the knees drawn up while the endoscope is passed into the rectum to the cecum. Air may be instilled for better visualization. The entire procedure lasts approximately 60 minutes. Atropine sulfate is kept available in case of bradycardia resulting from vasovagal response.

FOLLOW-UP CARE. The nurse checks vital signs every 15 minutes until the client is stable. Siderails are kept up until sedation wears off. The client is observed for signs of perforation and hemorrhage. The nurse instructs the client that a feeling of fullness, cramping, and passage of flatus are expected for several hours after the test. If a polypectomy or tissue biopsy was performed, there may be a small amount of blood in the first stool after the colonoscopy. Excessive bleeding should be reported immediately to the health care provider (Chart 53-5). If the procedure was performed in an ambulatory care setting, the client will need another person to provide transportation home. The client should avoid driving for 8 to 12 hours after the procedure because of the effects of sedation.

PROCTOSIGMOIDOSCOPY

Proctosigmoidoscopy is an endoscopic examination of the rectum and sigmoid colon using a flexible or rigid scope. The

CHART 53-5

BEST PRACTICE *for*
Care of the Client After a Colonoscopy

- Do not allow the client to take anything by mouth until sedation wears off and the client is alert.
- Take vital signs every 15 to 30 minutes until the client is alert.
- Keep the siderails up until the client is alert.
- Assess for rectal bleeding or blood clots.
- Remind the client that fullness and mild abdominal cramping are expected for several hours.
- Assess for manifestations of bowel perforation, including *severe* abdominal pain and guarding. Fever may occur later.
- Assess for manifestations of hypovolemic shock, including dizziness, lightheadedness, decreased blood pressure, tachycardia, pallor, and altered mental status (may be the first sign).
- If the procedure is performed in an ambulatory care setting, arrange for another person to drive the client home.

purpose of this test is to screen for colon cancer, investigate the source of GI bleeding, or diagnose or monitor inflammatory bowel disease. If proctosigmoidoscopy is used as an alternative to colonoscopy for colorectal cancer screening, it is recommended that screening begin at 50 to 55 years of age (Levin et al., 1999).

CLIENT PREPARATION. The client should have a liquid diet for at least 24 hours before a sigmoidoscopy; a cleansing enema or sodium biphosphate (Fleet's) enema is usually given the morning of the procedure. A laxative may also be ordered the evening before the test (see the Evidence-Based Practice for Nursing box at right).

PROCEDURE. For a proctosigmoidoscopy, the client is placed on the left side in the knee-chest position or on a special table in the proctoscopic position. No sedation is required. The scope is lubricated and inserted into the anus to the required depth for visualization. Tissue biopsy may be performed during this procedure. The examination usually lasts about 30 minutes.

FOLLOW-UP CARE. The client is informed that mild gas pain and flatulence may be experienced from air instilled into the rectum during the examination. If a biopsy was obtained, a small amount of bleeding may be observed.

Gastric Analysis

Gastric analysis measures the hydrochloric acid and pepsin content for evaluation of gastric and duodenal disorders. There are two tests in gastric analysis: basal gastric secretion and gastric acid stimulation. Basal gastric secretion measures the secretion of hydrochloric acid between meals. If only small amounts of secretion are collected, a follow-up gastric stimulation test is given.

CLIENT PREPARATION. The client is on NPO status for at least 12 hours before the test. Alcohol, tobacco, and medications that may affect gastric secretion are avoided for 24 hours before the test. The nurse inserts a nasogastric (NG) tube and removes and discards the residual contents of the stomach.

EVIDENCE-BASED PRACTICE
FOR NURSING

Which of the following bowel preparations is best for flexible sigmoidoscopy: oral magnesium citrate combined with oral bisacodyl, one hypertonic phosphate enema, or two hypertonic phosphate enemas?

Fincher, R., et al. (1999). A comparison of bowel preparations for flexible sigmoidoscopy: Oral magnesium citrate combined with oral bisacodyl, one hypertonic phosphate enema, or two hypertonic phosphate enemas. *American Journal of Gastroenterology, 94*(8), 2122-2127.

The purpose of this randomized clinical trial was to compare three differing bowel preparations for clients undergoing flexible sigmoidoscopy. Two hundred ninety-one clients scheduled for a routine sigmoidoscopy were randomly assigned to receive one of three bowel preparations given with oral magnesium citrate: oral bisacodyl and magnesium citrate the night before the procedure, one hypertonic phosphate enema 1 hour before the procedure, or two hypertonic enemas given at 2 hours and 1 hour before the procedure. The physicians performing the endoscopy were blinded to the type of preparation the client received and were asked to rate the quality of the preparation. Clients were asked to rate their comfort and overall satisfaction.

There was no statistical difference in the bowel preparation quality between the three methods, and clients preferred the oral regimen, even though it was associated with more diarrhea.

Critique. Despite the lack of statistical differences in bowel preparations, this study builds on previous work by the same authors examining routine practices for their scientific basis and application to clinical practice. The rating scale of bowel preparation by the physicians may not have been clear enough to differ between excellent and good ratings.

Implications for Nursing. Proper bowel preparation is critical to an accurate procedure. No previous studies have identified a superior means of providing bowel preparation. An oral bowel preparation that is well tolerated may have implications for decreasing the number of repeat procedures needed because of lack of visualization, thereby decreasing test-associated costs. A completely oral regimen could reduce nursing time associated with administering enemas.

PROCEDURE. The NG tube is attached to suctioning equipment for collecting the contents at 15-minute intervals for 1 hour. The nurse collects each sample and labels the time and volume of each specimen.

For the gastric acid stimulation test, the NG tube is left in place, and a drug that stimulates gastric acid secretion (e.g., pentagastrin or betazole dihydrochloride [Histalog]) is given subcutaneously. Fifteen minutes after injection of the drug, specimens are again collected at 15-minute intervals for 1 hour. The nurse collects, labels, and measures the specimens. Depressed levels of gastric secretion suggest the presence of gastric carcinoma. Increased levels of gastric secretion indicate Zollinger-Ellison syndrome and duodenal ulcers (see Chapter 56).

FOLLOW-UP CARE. After the test is completed, the NG tube is removed and the client can resume normal eating patterns. No other follow-up is necessary.

Ultrasonography

Ultrasonography is a technique in which high-frequency, inaudible vibratory sound waves are passed through the body via a transducer; the echoes of the sound waves created are then recorded. The echoes are then converted into images and photographed for analysis. Ultrasound testing is commonly used to image soft tissues, such as the liver, the spleen, the pancreas, the gallbladder, and the biliary system.

CLIENT PREPARATION. The client is usually on NPO status for 8 to 12 hours before ultrasonography of the abdomen. The nurse informs the client that it will be necessary to lie still during the study. He or she instructed to drink 1 to 2 L of fluid just before the test, because a full bladder is necessary for accurate visualization.

PROCEDURE. The client is placed in a prone or supine position. The technician applies insulating gel to the end of the transducer and on the area of the abdomen under study. This gel allows airtight contact of the transducer with the skin. The technician moves the transducer back and forth over the skin until the desired images are obtained. The study takes about 15 to 30 minutes.

FOLLOW-UP CARE. No follow-up care is necessary after ultrasonography.

Endoscopic Ultrasonography

Endoscopic ultrasonography (EUS) provides images of the gastrointestinal (GI) wall and high-resolution images of the digestive organs. The ultrasonography is performed through the endoscope. This procedure is useful in diagnosing the presence of lymph node tumors, mucosal tumors, and tumors of the pancreas, stomach, and rectum. The client preparation and follow-up care are similar to the preparation and follow-up care for both endoscopy and ultrasonography.

Liver-Spleen Scan

A liver-spleen scan uses IV injection of a radioactive colloid that is taken up primarily by the liver and secondarily by the spleen. The scan evaluates the liver and the spleen for tumors or abscesses, organ size and location, and vascularity. This scan is useful in evaluating hepatocellular disease.

CLIENT PREPARATION. The nurse instructs the client about the need to lie still during the scanning. The client is assured that the colloid injection has only small amounts of radioactivity and is not dangerous. The nurse should ask female clients of childbearing age if they may be pregnant or are currently breastfeeding. The radionuclide can be found in breast milk, and radiation from x-ray studies should be avoided in pregnancy.

PROCEDURE. The technician or the physician gives the radioactive injection through an IV line, and a wait of about 15 minutes is necessary for uptake. The client is placed in many different positions while the scanning takes place. No follow-up care is necessary after a liver scan.

FOLLOW-UP CARE. The client should be instructed that the radionuclide is eliminated from the body through the urine in 24 hours. Careful handwashing following toileting will decrease the exposure to any radiation present in the urine.

ONLINE RESOURCES

For suggested readings and Internet resources, go to http://www.wbsaunders.com/SIMON/Iggy/.

SELECTED BIBLIOGRAPHY

Allen, K.M., & Phillips, J.M. (1997). *Women's health across the lifespan.* Philadelphia: Lippincott-Raven.

Berne, R.M., & Levy, M.N. (1998). *Physiology* (4th ed.). St. Louis: Mosby.

Chai, C., & Blackington, E. (2000). Colorectal cancer. *ADVANCE for Nurse Practitioners, 8*(4), 34-39.

Dammel, T. (1997). Fecal occult blood testing: Looking for hidden danger. *Nursing97, 27*(7), 44-45.

Fincher, R., et al. (1999). A comparison of bowel preparations for flexible sigmoidoscopy: Oral magnesium citrate combined with oral bisacodyl, one hypertonic phosphate enema, or two hypertonic phosphate enemas. *American Journal of Gastroenterology, 94*(8), 2122-2127.

Garlick Roll, M. (1999). Colon cancer. In C. Miaskowski & P. Buchsel (Eds.), *Oncology nursing: Assessment and clinical care* (pp. 863-887). St. Louis: Mosby.

Glickman, R. (1998). Inflammatory bowel disease: Ulcerative colitis and Crohn's disease. In A.S. Fauci, E. Braunwald, & K.J. Isselbacher (Eds.), *Harrison's principles of internal medicine* (14th ed., pp. 1633-1648). New York: McGraw-Hill.

Gordon, M. (2000). *Manual of nursing diagnosis* (9th ed.). St. Louis: Mosby.

Greenberger, N., & Isselbacher, K. (1998). Disorders of absorption. In A.S. Fauci, E. Braunwald, & K.J. Isselbacher (Eds.), *Harrison's principles of internal medicine* (14th ed., pp. 1616-1633). New York: McGraw-Hill.

Hammond, K. (1999). Nutrition-focused physical assessment. *Home Healthcare Nurse, 17*(6), 354-355.

Hass, P. (1999). Differentiation and diagnosis of jaundice. *AACN Clinical Issues: Advanced Practice in Acute and Critical Care, 10*(4), 433-441.

Hawkins, B. (1999). Stomach cancer. In C. Miaskowski & P. Buchsel (Eds.), *Oncology nursing: Assessment and clinical care* (pp. 863-887). St. Louis: Mosby.

Korsten, M., & Abittan, C. (1999). Obstipation and lower abdominal pain. *The Clinical Advisor, 2*(6), 68-70.

Levin, T.R., et al. (1999). Predicting advanced proximal colonic neoplasia with screening sigmoidoscopy. *Journal of the American Medical Association, 281*(17), 1611-1617.

Linton, A.D. (1997). Age-related changes in the gastrointestinal system. In M.A. Matteson, E.S. McConnell, & A.D. Linton (Eds.), *Gerontological nursing: Concepts and practice* (2nd ed., pp. 317-335). Philadelphia: W.B. Saunders.

Malarkey, L.M., & McMorrow, M.E. (1998). *Nurse's manual of laboratory tests and diagnostic procedures.* Philadelphia: W.B. Saunders.

O'Hanlon-Nichols, T. (1998). Basic assessment series: Gastrointestinal system. *American Journal of Nursing, 98*(4), 48-53.

Toskes, P., & Greenberger, N. (1998). Disorders of the pancreas. In A.S. Fauci, E. Braunwald, & K.J. Isselbacher (Eds.), *Harrison's principles of internal medicine* (14th ed., pp. 1737-1740). New York: McGraw-Hill.

Wellman, N. (1997) A case manager's guide to nutrition screening and intervention. *The Journal of Care Management, 3*(2), 12-27.

Wrobleski, D., Barth, M. & Oyen, L. (1999). Necrotizing pancreatitis: Pathophysiology, diagnosis, and acute care management. *AACN Clinical Issues: Advanced Practice in Acute and Critical Care, 10*(4), 464-477.

Interventions for Clients with Oral Cavity Problems

CONSTANCE VISOVSKY

Learning Objectives

After studying this chapter, you should be able to:

1. Develop a teaching plan for clients who have stomatitis.
2. Explain the common causes of malignant oral tumors.
3. Identify common nursing diagnoses for clients with oral cancer.
4. Prioritize postoperative care for clients undergoing surgery for oral cancer.
5. Develop a teaching plan for community-based care of clients with oral cancer.

Go to http://www.wbsaunders.com/SIMON/Iggy/ for self-assessment questions related to these Learning Objectives.

Oral cavity disorders can severely impact speech, nutrition, body image, and overall quality of life. Nurses play an important role in maintaining and restoring oral cavity health in their clients through nursing interventions and client education. Chart 54-1 lists ways for clients to maintain a healthy oral cavity.

STOMATITIS

■ OVERVIEW

Stomatitis is characterized by painful, single or multiple ulcerations of the oral mucosa that appear as inflammation and denudation of the oral mucosa, impairing the protective lining of the mouth. These ulcerations are commonly referred to as canker sores. Although the terms *stomatitis* and *mucositis* may be used interchangeably, stomatitis is contained in the oral cavity, and mucositis may be more generalized throughout the mucous membranes. The ulceration causes pain, and open areas predispose the individual to bleeding and infection. Although infection remains the most life-threatening complication of stomatitis, pain is the most common complaint (Eilers, 1997). Mild erythema (redness) may respond to topical treatments, whereas extensive stomatitis may require treatment with opioid analgesics.

Stomatitis is classified according to the cause of the inflammation. *Primary* stomatitis includes aphthous stomatitis, herpes simplex stomatitis, and traumatic ulcers. *Secondary* stomatitis generally results from infection by opportunistic viruses or bacteria, particularly in clients with immunosuppressive disorders.

■ Pathophysiology

The oral mucosa is a protective lining of stratified, squamous, and nonkeratinizing epithelium that extends from the mouth at the junction of the lips to the oropharynx (throat). Inflammatory processes induced by infectious agents, allergy, vitamin deficiency, systemic disease, or antineoplastic drugs cause injury to oral cavity membranes. Cells that are damaged by the inflammatory process slough off, leading to an ulcerated oral mucosa. The ulcerations formed are painful, and bleeding results secondary to erosion of oral mucous membranes (Eilers, 1997).

■ Etiology

Stomatitis can result from infection, allergy, vitamin deficiency, systemic disease, chemotherapy, or radiation. Infectious agents, such as bacteria and viruses, may have a role in the development of recurrent aphthous stomatitis. L-forms of streptococcus bacteria have been isolated from aphthous ulcers. Although viruses have not been successfully cultured from aphthous lesions, recurrent lesions have been associated with latent zoster or cytomegalovirus (CMV).

The implication that certain foods trigger allergic responses that result in the formation of aphthous ulcers remains controversial. Foods such as coffee, potatoes, cheese, nuts, citrus fruits, and gluten may be precipitating factors. In some cases, strict elimination diets have resulted in the improvement of ulcers. Deficiencies in vitamin B_{12}, folate, and iron associated with malnutrition can contribute to the formation of stomatitis.

Systemic diseases such as human immunodeficiency virus (HIV) infection and chronic renal failure can also predispose a person to stomatitis. Approximately 50% of first-degree relatives of individuals with aphthous ulcers also have the disease, suggesting a genetic link to stomatitis (Woo & Sonis, 1996). Treatment of disease states such as cancer can predispose an individual to the development of painful stomatitis or mucositis. Thirty-nine to fifty percent of clients undergoing chemotherapy or radiation to the head and neck for cancer re-

CLIENT EDUCATION GUIDE
Maintaining a Healthy Oral Cavity

- Perform a self-examination of your mouth every month; report any unusual finding.
- Be sure to eat a balanced diet.
- Brush and floss your teeth every day. Set a routine and keep to it.
- Manage your stress as much as possible; learn how to maintain your emotional health.
- Avoid contact with agents that may cause inflammation of the mouth, such as mouthwashes that contain alcohol.
- If possible, avoid medications that may cause inflammation of the mouth or reduce the flow of saliva.
- Be aware of any changes in the occlusion of your teeth, mouth pain, or swelling; seek medical attention promptly.
- See your dentist regularly; have problems attended to promptly.
- If you wear dentures, make sure they are in good repair and fit properly.

port experiencing stomatitis (Hyland, 1997). The severity of stomatitis is related to the type and dose of therapy, as well as to client-related factors, such as pretreatment oral health (Eilers, 1997). (See Chapter 25 for nursing care of the client undergoing radiation and chemotherapy.)

The symptoms of stomatitis range in severity from a dry, painful mouth to open ulcerations, predisposing the client to infection. Mouth ulcerations can alter nutritional status as a result of difficulty with food ingestion or swallowing. When severe, stomatitis and the edema that can accompany it have the potential to impact airway integrity.

Incidence/Prevalence

Aphthous stomatitis is the most common oral lesion treated by primary care providers. It has been found to affect more than 50% of the population and is especially common in North America (Peterson & Baughman, 1996). The incidence of stomatitis in clients undergoing cancer chemotherapy is approximately 40% (Beck, 1996).

> ### WOMEN'S HEALTH CONSIDERATIONS
> A hormonal influence has been suggested in relation to women and aphthous stomatitis. Women generally have a higher prevalence of the disorder, with an increased incidence of oral ulceration during the luteal phase of the menstrual cycle. A moderation or absence of lesions during pregnancy has been attributed to increased steroid levels (Peterson & Baughman, 1996).

Primary Stomatitis
APHTHOUS STOMATITIS

Aphthous stomatitis is a noninfectious inflammatory condition of the oral mucosa. Aphthous ulcers are categorized as minor, major, or herpetiform. Eighty percent of aphthous lesions are minor ulcers, measuring less than 0.4 inch (1 cm) in diameter and occurring in groups of up to five lesions. These lesions appear most commonly on the buccal mucosa, soft palate, oropharyngeal mucosa, and lateral and ventral areas of the tongue. The lesions appear as shallow, painful ulcerations covered by a yellow-gray pseudomembrane and exterior ery-

thematous ring. Major aphthous ulcers make up 7% to 20% of aphthous ulcers, are larger than 1 cm, persist for months, and may heal with scarring. Herpetiform ulcers make up 7% to 10% of aphthous ulcers, occur in groups of 10 or more, and are usually located in the posterior part of the mouth (Woo & Sonis, 1996).

HERPES SIMPLEX STOMATITIS

The herpes simplex virus (HSV) is responsible for the development of primary herpes simplex stomatitis, also called acute herpetic stomatitis. The uniformly sized vesicles occur most often on the tongue, palate, and buccal and labial mucosae. The vesicles rupture soon after appearing, leaving painful, ulcerated areas surrounded by erythematous margins. The lesions at this stage are similar to aphthous ulcers. The ulcerated areas heal in 10 to 14 days. The mucosal vesicles are generally accompanied by acute inflammation of the gingiva, occasionally with herpetic lesions. The tongue has a characteristic white coating, and the client complains of a foul breath. Primary HSV infection is characterized by symptoms of generalized infection, including malaise, fever, and lymphadenopathy.

HSV enters injured oral mucosal tissue, where it replicates in the cells of the dermis and epidermis, resulting in primary HSV infection. Although stomatitis caused by HSV can occur as either a primary or secondary (recurrent) infection, secondary infections are more common. Two types of HSV have been identified: HSV type 2, which causes genital lesions (discussed in Chapter 77), and HSV type 1, which is responsible for nongenital lesions.

HSV infection is extremely common. Primary herpetic stomatitis is usually contracted in childhood but may be seen in adults. Immunocompromised clients tend to experience more severe and extensive HSV infections.

VINCENT'S STOMATITIS

Vincent's stomatitis, or acute necrotizing stomatitis, is an acute bacterial infection of the gingiva characterized by erythema, ulceration, and necrosis of the gingival margins. The gingival papillae between the teeth appear worn away and raw. The gingivae often bleed spontaneously or from mild irritation, such as chewing. Clients complain of severe pain; foul breath; thick, ropy secretions; and increased salivation. Systemic clinical manifestations can include malaise, poor appetite, and occasionally, enlargement of cervical lymph nodes.

The disease has a sudden onset and is related to a decreased resistance of tissues to normal oral bacterial flora. Systemic etiologic factors that decrease tissue resistance include poor nutrition, leukemia, and severe infections such as pyelonephritis. Poor oral hygiene and extreme emotional stress have been suggested as contributing factors.

Necrotizing gingivitis occurs primarily in adults, and the incidence seems to increase with aging. Older adults have an increased susceptibility to infections because of decreased immunocompetence.

TRAUMATIC ULCERS

Oral trauma is thought to be the most common precipitating factor in the development of recurrent aphthous stomatitis

(Peterson & Baughman, 1996). Traumatic ulcers can develop at the site of an injury. Traumatic insults, such as injuries from dental procedures, cheek biting, and hot foods, can lead to ulceration. Such injuries can also allow the entry of bacteria, resulting in secondary infection.

Traumatic ulcers are commonly found in clients with malocclusion, ill-fitting dentures, or broken teeth and in those who habitually bite their oral mucosa. In addition, individuals with recurrent aphthous stomatitis are predisposed to developing additional ulcers at the site of a traumatic injury.

Secondary Stomatitis

LICHEN PLANUS

Lichen planus is an inflammatory mucocutaneous disease involving both the skin and the oral mucous membranes. The lesions may be active or in remission, with external lesions affecting the extremities and the genitalia. Symmetric white oral lesions of various patterns appear on the tongue and buccal and labial mucosae. Eighty percent of all lichen planus lesions are bilateral, appearing on the buccal mucosa (Burkhart, Burkes, & Burker, 1997). The remaining 20% are localized to the tongue or lips.

The etiology of the disease is unknown, but recent developments indicate that there may be a cell-mediated immune response involved in the progression of the lesions. Disease states such as diabetes and hypertension may invoke lichenoid reactions from the medications used to treat these conditions. Oral lichen planus may also be associated with hepatitis C infection (Bagan et al., 1998). Local irritants and trauma are contributing factors associated with the progression of lichenoid lesions. There has been conflicting evidence suggesting stress as a mediator of lichen planus. In addition, the chronic inflammatory nature of lichen planus may prove to be a risk factor for oral cancer.

Lichen planus affects 1% to 2% of the population, occurring more often in women than in men and occurring most often in clients ages 40 to 50 years (Burkhart, Burkes, & Burker, 1997). It occurs in all races, with variations in severity among the racial groups. Although the oral lesions themselves are often asymptomatic, an erosive form of the disorder can cause pain that interferes with speech and swallowing. The diagnosis of lichen planus is confirmed through tissue biopsy.

CANDIDIASIS (MONILIASIS)

In oral candidiasis, white plaquelike lesions appear on the tongue, palate, pharynx, and buccal mucosa (Figure 54-1). When these patches are wiped away, the underlying surface appears red and sore (Sheff, 1999). Clients rarely complain of actual pain but describe the lesions as dry or hot.

Candida albicans is part of the normal flora of the oral cavity. **Candidiasis,** also called moniliasis, is a fungal infection resulting from an overgrowth of this normal flora. With recurrent candidiasis, as with all secondary stomatitis, a causative systemic disorder should be sought. Antibiotic therapy destroys the normal flora that usually prevent fungal infections; thus candidiasis can occur in clients receiving long-term antibiotic therapy. Candidiasis of the oral cavity is common in clients undergoing immunosuppressive therapy (chemotherapy, radiation, steroid therapy, or antirejection medication). For example, chemotherapy affects the rapidly dividing cells of the oral mucosa, leading to ulcerations that have a propensity to become infected secondary to a decreased immune response. Candidiasis is also very common among HIV-infected individuals, becoming increasingly likely as CD4+ cell counts fall (Klaus & Grodesky, 1998).

> ### CONSIDERATIONS FOR OLDER ADULTS
> Older adults are especially at high risk for candidiasis because aging causes a decrease in immune function. The risk increases for clients who are diabetic, malnourished, or under emotional stress. Older adults who wear dentures may use soft denture liners that provide comfort but can also be colonized by *C. albicans,* contributing to denture stomatitis (Dixon, Breeding, & Faler, 1999).

▶ COLLABORATIVE MANAGEMENT

● Assessment

HISTORY

The nurse collects information concerning possible etiologic factors, such as recent infections, a history of stomatitis, nutritional compromise, oral hygiene habits, oral trauma, stress, or immunocompromise. A medication history should also be collected. The nurse records the course of the current outbreak and ascertains if episodes of stomatitis are recurrent. The client is asked if the lesions interfere with swallowing or eating.

PHYSICAL ASSESSMENT/CLINICAL MANIFESTATIONS

While examining the oral cavity, the nurse wears nonsterile gloves for protection against infection. Adequate lighting, including a flashlight or penlight, and a tongue blade facilitate the examination. The nurse assesses the oral cavity for lesions, coating, cracking, and fissures. Characteristics of the lesions are described in terms of location, size, shape, color, and drainage. Any odors that may be present are noted and described.

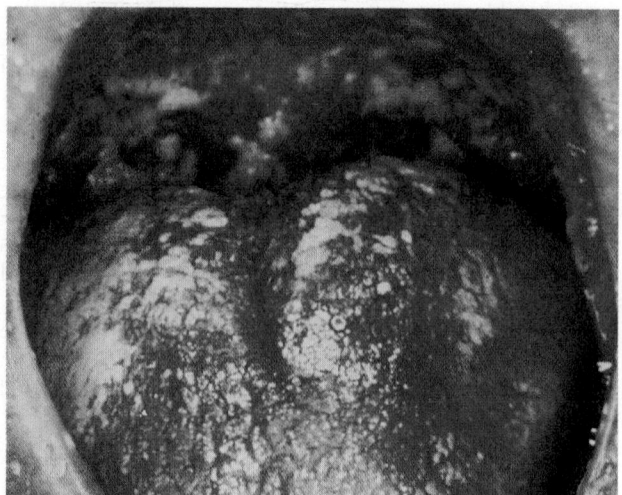

Figure 54-1 ● Oral candidiasis. (From Radford, J., & Thatcher, N. [1988]. The toxicity of cancer chemotherapy in adults. *Cancer Care, 5,* 4-7.)

If lesions are noted along the pharynx, and if the client reports dysphagia or pain on swallowing, the nurse should suspect that the lesions may extend farther down the esophagus. Additional diagnostic testing may be required.

The physical examination may also include examination of the cervical and submandibular lymph nodes for swelling. Any elevation in temperature is noted.

◼ LABORATORY ASSESSMENT

Laboratory tests are usually not needed. However, serum albumin, vitamin B$_{12}$, folate, and iron levels may be obtained if nutritional status appears to be compromised. A complete blood count may reveal the presence of infection, neutropenia, or anemia. A Tzank smear can assist in distinguishing between herpetic and aphthous ulcers. Fluid from herpetic vesicles in herpes simplex stomatitis may be obtained for viral culture. Bacterial culture of exudate from the oral mucosa validates Vincent's stomatitis or secondary infection. A potassium hydroxide slide preparation or a routine culture and Gram stain can help identify *Candida* organisms.

● Interventions

Interventions for stomatitis are aimed toward the promotion of oral health through scrupulous oral hygiene and careful food selection.

ORAL HYGIENE. The nurse or assistive nursing personnel uses a soft-bristled toothbrush or disposable foam swabs (toothettes) to stimulate gums and clean the oral cavity. The nurse encourages frequent rinsing of the mouth with any of the following: sodium bicarbonate solution, warm saline, or hydrogen peroxide solution. The client should avoid commercial mouthwashes because they have a high alcohol content, causing a burning sensation in irritated or ulcerated oral mucosa.

The nurse instructs the client to increase mouth care to every 2 hours and twice at night if the stomatitis is not controlled. Frequent gentle mouth care enhances debridement of ulcerated lesions and can prevent superinfections. Frequent oral care also promotes a general feeling of well-being. Chart 54-2 lists measures for special oral care.

DRUG THERAPY. Anti-infective agents, including antibiotics and antifungals, may be necessary for control of infection in the client with stomatitis. The nurse administers anti-infectives as ordered and provides instruction on how to take them. The health care provider prescribes systemic antibiotics severe recurrent or Vincent's stomatitis. Investigations have linked recurrent aphthous stomatitis to strains of L-streptococci. Tetracycline syrup 250 mg/10 mL four times a day for 10 days may be prescribed. The client rinses for 2 minutes and swallows the syrup, thus obtaining both topical and systemic therapy. Chlorhexidine, an oral rinse, can be beneficial in preventing infection, since it is active against numerous bacteria and fungi. However, chlorhexidine prepared in the United States is 9.6% alcohol and therefore may cause stinging and burning on administration. Chlorhexidine causes a brown discoloration of the teeth that can be removed with oxidizing agents and abrasives.

Antibiotics are of little value in viral or fungal stomatitis unless a secondary infection is present. Systemic antibiotics are ineffective for lichen planus and are not recommended.

A regimen of intravenous (IV) acyclovir (Zovirax) is usually prescribed for immunocompromised clients who contract herpes simplex stomatitis. Acyclovir is typically administered to clients with normal renal function at a dose of 5 mg/kg, infused at a constant rate over a 1-hour period every 8 hours for 7 days. Clients with competent immune systems may be given acyclovir in oral or topical form.

For clients with oral candidal infection, an antifungal agent is prescribed, such as nystatin (Mycostatin, Nadostine) oral suspension 600,000 units four times daily for 7 to 10 days. The nurse teaches the client to swish the solution around in the mouth before swallowing. Oral troches (lozenges) may also be effective. Clients who are taking inhaled steroids should be advised to use a spacer to decrease the amount of medication left in the mouth. In addition, the client should rinse the mouth with warm water after using inhalers, to rinse away any deposited drug (Shuster, 1998). Systemic steroids can be of benefit in long-standing lichen planus.

ANALGESICS. Interventions for clients with stomatitis should include pain control, because pain is consistently present during an outbreak. The nurse performs a comprehensive assessment of pain that includes the following: location, characteristics, onset and duration, frequency, quality, intensity, severity, and precipitating factors.

Topically applied agents or oral analgesics temporarily relieve severe oral pain (Table 54-1). Agents containing 20% benzocaine provide temporary pain relief and can be applied

---

CHART 54-2

BEST PRACTICE *for*
Care of Clients with Problems of the Oral Cavity

- Remove dentures if the client has severe stomatitis or oral pain.
- Encourage the client to perform oral hygiene, or provide it after each meal and as often as needed.
- Increase mouth care to every 2 hours or more often if stomatitis is not controlled.
- Use a soft toothbrush, toothette, or gauze for oral care.
- Encourage frequent rinsing of the mouth with hydrogen peroxide, warm saline, sodium bicarbonate (baking soda) solution, or a combination of these solutions.
- Teach the client to avoid commercial mouthwashes and lemon-glycerin swabs.
- Assist the client in selecting soft, bland, and nonacidic foods.
- Apply topical analgesics or anesthetics as ordered by the physician and monitor their effectiveness.

TABLE 54-1	DRUGS COMMONLY USED FOR ORAL PAIN RELIEF

ORAL AGENTS
- Lidocaine 2%, viscous
- Diphenhydramine elixir
- Opioids such as acetaminophen with codeine (codeine phosphate 12 mg, acetaminophen 120 mg/5 mL) and morphine sulfate

TOPICAL AGENTS
- Dyclonine (Dyclone) 0.5%
- Benzocaine 20%
- Lidocaine protective gel (Zilactin-L)

to the affected areas three to four times daily. Fifteen milliliters of 2% viscous lidocaine every 3 hours (maximum of 8 doses per day) can be used as a gargle or mouthwash.

The health care provider often prescribes topical swishes for herpes simplex stomatitis and lichen planus. These suspensions can be offered in frozen form; the numbing effects of the cold provide longer analgesia. Topical corticosteroids are indicated for aphthous ulcers, lichen planus, and the lesions of primary herpes simplex virus (HSV) infection. Triamcinolone cream is applied with the finger or a cotton-tipped applicator, or the corticosteroid can be injected directly into the lesion.

Occasionally, systemic approaches to pain relief need to be employed. For moderate to severe stomatitis, around-the-clock administration of combinations of opioid and nonopioid analgesics, such as acetaminophen and codeine, is recommended. If the pain is unrelieved, or if the stomatitis is severe, morphine may be used until healing occurs. Any time a client receives an intervention for pain, the nurse monitors the effectiveness of the pain control measures through an ongoing assessment of the pain experience.

TUMORS

OVERVIEW

Oral cavity tumors can be benign, premalignant, or malignant. Whether benign or malignant, tumors of the oral cavity impact many daily functions. Activities such as swallowing, chewing, and speaking can be affected. Pain accompanying the tumor can also impose limitations on daily activities and self-care. Oral cavity tumors affect body image, especially if treatment involves removal of the tongue or part of the mandible, or requires a tracheostomy.

Premalignant Lesions

LEUKOPLAKIA

Leukoplakia presents as slowly developing changes in the oral mucous membranes that are characterized by thickened, white, firmly attached patches. These patches appear slightly raised and sharply circumscribed. Leukoplakial lesions undergo malignant transformation in approximately 3% to 6% of cases (Olsen, 1999). Although leukoplakia can be found anywhere on the oral mucosa, lesions on the lips or tongue are more likely to progress to malignancy. Leukoplakia results from mechanical factors that cause long-term oral mucous membrane irritation, such as poorly fitting dentures, chronic cheek nibbling, or broken or poorly repaired teeth. In addition, oral hairy leukoplakia can be found in clients with HIV infection. The use of tobacco products has also been implicated in the development of leukoplakia, which is sometimes referred to as "smoker's patch." Oral leukoplakia can be confused with oral candidal infection. However, unlike candidal infection, leukoplakia cannot be removed by scraping.

Leukoplakia is the most common oral lesion among adults; it affects 3% of the population and accounts for 18% of all oral lesions (Shugars & Patton, 1997). Oral hairy leukoplakia is an early manifestation of HIV infection and is highly correlated with progression from HIV infection to acquired immunodeficiency syndrome (AIDS). Leukoplakia not associated with HIV infection is more often seen in people over age 40. Men have twice the incidence of leukoplakia that women have, but this ratio is changing because increasing numbers of women are smoking.

ERYTHROPLAKIA

Erythroplakia presents as a red, velvety mucosal lesion on the surface of the oral mucosa. There is a higher degree of malignant transformation in erythroplakia than in leukoplakia. As such, these lesions should be regarded with suspicion and analyzed by biopsy. Erythroplakia is most commonly found on the floor of the mouth, tongue, palate, and mandibular mucosa. Erythroplakia can be difficult to distinguish from inflammatory or immune reactions.

Malignant Tumors

SQUAMOUS CELL CARCINOMA

PATHOPHYSIOLOGY. More than 90% of oral cancers are squamous cell carcinomas that begin on the surface of the epithelium. Over a period of many years, premalignant (or dysplastic) changes begin. Cells begin to vary in size and shape; alterations in the thickness of the lining of the epithelium develop, resulting in atrophy. These tumors usually grow slowly, and the lesions may be large before the onset of symptoms unless ulceration is present. Mucosal erythroplasia is the earliest sign of oral carcinoma. Oral lesions that appear as red, raised, eroded areas are suspicious for carcinoma.

The American Joint Committee on Cancer has devised the TNM classification system for tumors of the lip and oral cavity (Table 54-2). Each lesion is defined by the following:

T—the size or degree of penetration of the tumor
N—the presence, size, number, and location of involved cervical lymph nodes
M—the presence of distant metastasis (spread)

ETIOLOGY. Squamous cell carcinoma is the most common oral malignancy. Squamous cell carcinomas can be found on the lips, tongue, buccal mucosa, and oropharynx. The major risk factors in the development of oral cancers are increasing age, tobacco use, and alcohol ingestion. Ninety-five percent of all oral cancers occur in people over 40 years of age. Tobacco use in any form (e.g., smoking or chewing tobacco) can increase the risk of cancer by 5% to 25%. The use of smokeless tobacco has nearly tripled in the last 20 years. This form of tobacco contains carcinogens and large quantities of nicotine, which can lead to nicotine addiction. Alcohol ingestion can potentiate the carcinogenic effects of tobacco.

An increased rate of oral carcinoma is found in individuals with certain occupations, such as textile workers, plumbers, and coal and metal workers. Additional factors, such as sun exposure, poor dietary habits, poor oral hygiene, and infection with the human papillomavirus (HPV), require further research.

Common signs and symptoms of oral carcinoma include unusual lumps or thickening of the buccal mucosa, or red or white patches appearing on the gums, tongue, or oral mucous membranes. Cancers of the lip are strongly associated with chronic exposure to the sun and often present as a sore that fails to heal. Soreness, pain, or a burning sensation may also be present. In later stages, the client may experience difficulty chewing or swallowing. Advanced cancers of the tongue can cause

TABLE 54-2 • TNM CLASSIFICATION FOR TUMORS OF THE LIP AND ORAL CAVITY

PRIMARY TUMOR (T)
- T_X Primary tumor cannot be assessed
- T_0 No evidence of primary tumor
- T_{is} Carcinoma in situ
- T_1 Tumor 2 cm or less in greatest dimension
- T_2 Tumor more than 2 cm but not more than 4 cm in greatest dimension
- T_3 Tumor more than 4 cm in greatest dimension
- T_4 (Lip) Tumor invades adjacent structures (e.g., through the cortical bone, the tongue, and the skin of the neck)
- T_4 (Oral cavity) Tumor invades adjacent structures (e.g., through the cortical bone, into the deep [extrinsic] muscle of the tongue, the maxillary sinus, and the skin)

LYMPH NODE (N)
- N_X Regional lymph nodes cannot be assessed
- N_0 No regional lymph node metastasis
- N_1 Metastasis in a single ipsilateral lymph node, 3 cm or less in greatest dimension
- N_2 Metastasis in a single ipsilateral lymph node, more than 3 cm but not more than 6 cm in greatest dimension; or multiple ipsilateral lymph nodes, none more than 6 cm in greatest dimension; or bilateral or contralateral lymph nodes, none more than 6 cm in greatest dimension
  - N_{2a} Metastasis in a single ipsilateral lymph node more than 3 cm but not more than 6 cm in greatest dimension
  - N_{2b} Metastasis in multiple ipsilateral lymph nodes, none more than 6 cm in greatest dimension
  - N_{2c} Metastasis in bilateral or contralateral lymph nodes, none more than 6 cm in greatest dimension
- N_3 Metastasis in a lymph node more than 6 cm in greatest dimension

DISTANT METASTASIS (M)
- M_X The presence of distant metastasis cannot be assessed
- M_0 No distant metastasis
- M_1 Distant metastasis

STAGE GROUPING

0	T_{is}	N_0	M_0
I	T_1	N_0	M_0
II	T_2	N_0	M_0
III	T_3	N_0	M_0
	T_1	N_1	M_0
	T_2	N_1	M_0
	T_3	N_1	M_0
IV	T_4	N_0	M_0
	T_4	N_1	M_0
	Any T	N_2	M_0
	Any T	N_3	M_0
	Any T	Any N	M_1

From American Joint Committee on Cancer. O.H. Beahrs, et al. (Eds.). (1998). *Manual for staging of cancer* (3rd ed.). Philadelphia: J.B. Lippincott.

pain that radiates to the ear. Cervical lymph nodes may become enlarged, hardened, and fixed secondary to metastatic invasion.

INCIDENCE/PREVALENCE. Carcinomas of the oral cavity account for approximately 6% of all cancers diagnosed each year in the United States. In 1999 in the United States, approximately 30,000 cases of oral cancer were diagnosed, and 8000 deaths were attributed to the disease (Greenlee et al., 2000). Worldwide, cancers of the mouth and pharynx account for 363,000 new cases and 200,000 deaths annually (Parkin, Pisani, & Ferlay, 1999).

CONSIDERATIONS FOR OLDER ADULTS
The incidence of oral cancer is expected to increase as the population of older adults increases. Carcinoma of the oral cavity is primarily a disease of older adults that is prevalent in the sixth and seventh decades of life.

WOMEN'S HEALTH CONSIDERATIONS
Along with an increase in tobacco use among women, there has been an increase in oral cancer rates among women. The estimated incidence for women in the United States is 6.4 per 100,000 (Parkin, Pisani, & Ferlay, 1999).

CULTURAL CONSIDERATIONS
African Americans have a higher rate of oral carcinoma than Caucasians (Shugars & Patton, 1997). The relative 5-year survival rate for Caucasians with cancer of the oral cavity or pharynx is 55%, compared with a relative 5-year survival rate of 32% for African Americans with oral cancer (National Cancer Institute, 1999). Higher mortality rates from oral cancer have been associated with limited access to health care.

■ BASAL CELL CARCINOMA

Basal cell carcinoma of the oral cavity occurs primarily on the lips. The lesion is asymptomatic and resembles a raised scab. With time, the lesion evolves into a characteristic ulcer with a raised pearly border. Basal cell carcinomas do not metastasize but can aggressively involve the skin of the face. The major etiologic factor in basal cell carcinoma is exposure to sunlight.

Basal cell carcinoma occurs as a result of the failure of basal cells to mature into keratinocytes. It is the second most common type of oral cancer but is much less common than squamous cell carcinoma.

CULTURAL CONSIDERATIONS
Clients who work outdoors or who sunbathe excessively, especially Caucasians with fair skin, are more likely to have basal cell carcinomas.

■ KAPOSI'S SARCOMA

Kaposi's sarcoma is a malignant lesion arising in blood vessels. Kaposi's sarcoma is usually painless and appears as a raised purple nodule or plaque. In the mouth the hard palate is the most common site of Kaposi's sarcoma, but it can also be found on the gums, tongue, or tonsils. It is most often associated with AIDS. (See Chapter 22 for a complete discussion of Kaposi's sarcoma.)

Activity Link

► COLLABORATIVE MANAGEMENT
● Assessment
■ HISTORY

A priority for nurses in the prevention and detection of oral cancers is the identification of high-risk groups. Individuals at high risk for developing oral cancer tend to use large amounts of alcohol and tobacco and are over 40 years of age. The nurse asks about occupation and exposure to known oral carcinogens or irritants, such as sunlight or other source of ultraviolet radiation. A family history of cancer and a history of previous oral cancer alert health care providers to be especially observant for signs of cancer.

The nurse assesses the client's routine oral hygiene regimen and use of dentures or oral appliances, which might add to discomfort or mechanically irritate the mucosa. The client should be asked about bleeding, which might indicate an ulcerative lesion. The nurse determines the status of the client's past and current appetite and nutritional state, including difficulty with chewing or swallowing. A continuing trend of weight loss may be related to metastasis, heavy alcohol intake, difficulty in eating or chewing, or an underlying disorder.

■ PHYSICAL ASSESSMENT/CLINICAL MANIFESTATIONS

An examination of the oral cavity requires adequate lighting for proper visualization. The nurse thoroughly inspects the oral cavity for any lesions, evidence of pain, or restriction of movement. Using a tongue blade, the nurse can visually examine all areas of the oral cavity. The nurse notes any alteration in speech attributable to tongue restriction. Following inspection, the advanced-practice nurse uses bimanual palpation of any visible nodules to determine size and fixation. The cervical lymph nodes should also be palpated (Figure 54-2).

■ PSYCHOSOCIAL ASSESSMENT

The functioning and appearance of the oral cavity are strongly linked with body image and quality of life. Therefore the nurse assesses the impact of oral lesions on the client's self-concept. In addition, the nurse assesses the client for any educational or cultural needs regarding instruction or therapy and evaluates the client's support system and past mechanisms of coping.

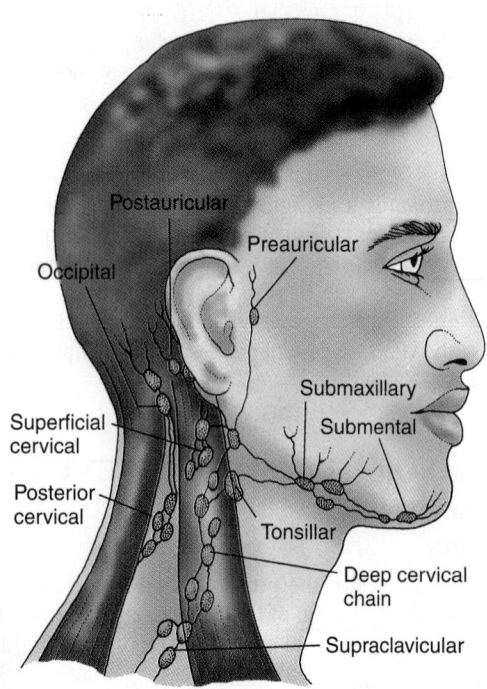

Figure 54-2 ● The lymph nodes of the cervical region.

Postauricular

Preauricular

Occipital

Superficial cervical

Posterior cervical

Submaxillary

Submental

Tonsillar

Deep cervical chain

Supraclavicular

■ RADIOGRAPHIC ASSESSMENT

The purpose of radiologic diagnostic tests for cancer of the oral cavity is to assess the extent and spread of the tumor. Computed tomography (CT) scans are helpful in determining the extent of the tumor and lymphatic or bone involvement.

■ OTHER DIAGNOSTIC ASSESSMENT

Biopsy is the definitive method for diagnosis of oral cancer; therefore the physician obtains a biopsy specimen of the oral tissue to assess for malignant or premalignant changes. Incisional biopsies allow for collection of normal and abnormal tissue. An intraoral biopsy can be done with the client under local anesthesia. In very small lesions, an excisional biopsy can permit complete tumor removal. Magnetic resonance imaging (MRI) is useful in detecting perineural involvement and in evaluating thickness in cancers of the tongue. Both CT and MRI can be used to determine metastatic spread to the liver or lungs if further staging of the disease is warranted.

An aqueous solution of toluidine blue 1% can be applied to oral lesions to determine if they are malignant. This preparation stains malignant lesions, leaving normal tissue unaffected. However, a lesion that is the result of an inflammatory process may also pick up the stain, leading to a false-positive result. Although a biopsy is still needed to confirm a cancer diagnosis, toluidine blue may be useful for screening high-risk individuals.

> ### CRITICAL THINKING CHALLENGE
> You are a nurse in a busy family practice clinic. A 67-year-old woman comes in for her annual physical examination. In the course of providing her recent health history, she tells you that she has developed several white patches on her tongue "that won't go away, no matter what I do."
> * What questions would be appropriate for the nurse to ask this client in gathering more of her health history?
> * What aspects of the oral cavity assessment should the nurse pay particular attention to?
>
> For suggested answer guidelines, go to SIMON http://www.wbsaunders.com/SIMON/Iggy/.

● Analysis

■ COMMON NURSING DIAGNOSES AND COLLABORATIVE PROBLEMS

The following are priority nursing diagnoses for clients with malignant tumors of the oral cavity:

1. **Risk for Ineffective Airway Clearance** related to obstruction by the tumor, edema, or secretions
2. **Impaired Oral Mucous Membrane** related to effects of the tumor

■ ADDITIONAL NURSING DIAGNOSES AND COLLABORATIVE PROBLEMS

In addition to the common nursing diagnoses, clients with tumors of the oral cavity may have one or more of the following:

* **Impaired Verbal Communication** related to the tumor or surgery
* **Disturbed Body Image** related to impaired oral mucous membrane, surgery, chemotherapy, or radiation therapy
* **Acute Pain** related to impaired oral mucous membrane
* **Risk for Infection** related to impaired oral mucous membrane

- Impaired Swallowing related to presence of the oral tumor, surgery, or radiation
- Imbalanced Nutrition: Less Than Body Requirements related to pain and/or edema

▶ Planning and Implementation

■ RISK FOR INEFFECTIVE AIRWAY CLEARANCE

NOC PLANNING: EXPECTED OUTCOMES. The client with a malignant tumor of the oral cavity is expected to maintain a patent airway as evidenced by effective coughing, increased air exchange, and the absence of aspiration.

INTERVENTIONS. Extensive tumor involvement and tenacious secretions can impede airway patency. Nursing measures for maintaining airway patency center on assessment for dyspnea, inability to cough effectively, or inability to swallow.

NONSURGICAL MANAGEMENT. The nurse assesses for difficulty breathing and/or decreased air exchange and dysphagia. Measures to increase air exchange, remove secretions, and prevent aspiration are instituted (Chart 54-3).

NIC AIRWAY MANAGEMENT. The nurse assesses for dyspnea resulting from the obstructive presence of the tumor or from excessive secretions. The nurse assesses the quality, rate, and depth of respirations and auscultates the lungs for decreased or absent ventilation, or for the presence of adventitious sounds. If oral secretions are excessive or thick, the nurse attempts to aid the client in expectorating secretions. To increase air exchange, the client is placed in a semi-Fowler's or high Fowler's position to maximize ventilation potential. Secretions can be mobilized by encouraging fluids to help liquefy secretions, by chest physiotherapy, and by measures to encourage effective coughing. If oral secretions remain problematic, oral suction equipment with a dental tip or a tonsil tip (Yankauer catheter) can be employed.

If edema is associated with oral cavity lesions, the client may receive steroids for reducing inflammation. Antibiotics may be ordered if infection is present, since infection can increase inflammation and edema in the lesion. A cool mist supplied by a face tent may assist with oxygen transport and control of edema.

NIC COUGH ENHANCEMENT. Measures that promote deep inhalation generate high intrathoracic pressure, which assists the client in producing an effective cough to mobilize secretions. The nurse assists the client to a sitting position with the head slightly flexed and the knees flexed. The nurse then instructs him or her to take several deep breaths, hold the breath for 2 seconds, and then cough two to three times in succession. He or she is instructed to follow coughing with several maximal inhalation breaths. The client can also be instructed to enhance coughing by inhaling deeply several times and coughing at the end of exhalation.

NIC ASPIRATION PRECAUTIONS. Aspiration precautions prevent or minimize the risk factors associated with aspiration. The nurse assesses the client's level of consciousness, gag reflex, and ability to swallow. To prevent aspiration, the client is placed upright at 90 degrees (high Fowler's position). As a precaution, suction equipment should be kept nearby.

Clients at risk of aspiration should be fed in small amounts; thickened liquids can be used to prevent gagging.

SURGICAL MANAGEMENT. The client with an oral lesion may require a tracheostomy preoperatively. This may be due to the extent of surgical excision required to remove the tumor, or it may be due to excessive edema. A tracheostomy re-establishes a patent airway and can be performed by the physician with the client under local or general anesthesia. The tracheostomy tube is usually left in place until edema resolves and the airway is patent. If the tumor is the major cause of the oral airway blockage, however, the tracheostomy may be maintained through the perioperative period until oral healing begins, and in some cases it may be permanent. After postoperative edema resolves, the client is decannulated (the tracheostomy tube is removed). (Refer to Chapter 28 for nursing care of the client with a tracheostomy.)

CHART 54-3

NIC INTERVENTION ACTIVITIES for The Client with Oral Cancer

Airway Management: *Facilitation of patency of air passages*
- Position the client to maximize ventilation potential.
- Remove secretions by encouraging coughing or suctioning.
- Instruct how to cough effectively.
- Auscultate breath sounds, noting areas of decreased or absent ventilation and presence of adventitious sounds.
- Administer humidified air or oxygen, as appropriate.
- Position to alleviate dyspnea.
- Monitor respiratory and oxygenation status, as appropriate.

Cough Enhancement: *Promotion of deep inhalation by the client with subsequent generation of high intrathoracic pressures and compression of underlying lung parenchyma for the forceful expulsion of air*
- Assist the client to a sitting position with the head slightly flexed, shoulders relaxed, and knees flexed.
- Encourage client to take several deep breaths.
- Encourage client to take a deep breath, hold it for 2 seconds, and cough two or three times in succession.
- Instruct client to inhale deeply, bend forward slightly, and perform three or four huffs (against an open glottis).
- Instruct client to inhale deeply several times, to exhale slowly, and to cough at the end of exhalation.
- Instruct client to follow coughing with several maximal inhalation breaths.
- Promote systemic fluid hydration, as appropriate.

Aspiration Precautions: *Prevention or minimization of risk factors in the client at risk for aspiration*
- Monitor level of consciousness, cough reflex, gag reflex, and swallowing ability.
- Monitor pulmonary status.
- Maintain an airway.
- Position upright 90 degrees or as far as possible.
- Feed in small amounts.
- Avoid liquids or use thickening agent.
- Offer foods or liquids that can be formed into a bolus before swallowing.
- Cut food into small pieces.
- Request medication in elixir form.
- Break or crush pills before administration.
- Keep head of bed elevated 30 to 45 minutes after eating.

NIC intervention activities selected from McCloskey, J.C., & Bulechek, G.M. (2000). *Nursing interventions classification (NIC)* (3rd ed.). St. Louis: Mosby. No part of this work is to be altered without prior written permission from the Publisher.

IMPAIRED ORAL MUCOUS MEMBRANE

PLANNING: EXPECTED OUTCOMES. The client with a malignant tumor of the oral cavity is expected to maintain or re-establish oral mucosal integrity.

INTERVENTIONS. Both the presence of tumors of the oral cavity and the effects of treatment of oral tumors pose threats to the integrity of the oral mucosa. Oral cavity lesions can be treated by surgical excision, by nonsurgical treatments such as radiation or chemotherapy, or by a combination of treatments (referred to as multimodal therapy), which is the most expensive treatment option (see the Cost of Care box below). Nursing interventions focus primarily on the restoration and maintenance oral health.

NONSURGICAL MANAGEMENT. The purpose of nonsurgical management is to promote tissue healing and to maintain and promote oral hygiene for the client with oral lesions.

ORAL CARE. The nurse works with the client to establish an oral hygiene routine. Ideally, oral hygiene is performed every 2 hours for ulcerated lesions or infection, or in the immediate postoperative period. Modifications might be needed because of oral discomfort, bleeding, or edema. Oral care with a soft-bristled toothbrush is preferred. In the event of a fall in the platelet count below 40,000/mm^3, the client should be switched to an ultrasoft "chemobrush." The use of toothettes or a disposable foam brush is discouraged because these products may not adequately control bacteremia-promoting plaque (Toth et al., 1995)(see the Evidence-Based Practice for Nursing box at right). Lubricant can be applied to moisten the lips and oral mucosa as needed.

Clients with ulcerative or bleeding lesions should avoid using commercial mouthwashes and lemon-glycerin swabs. Commercial mouthwashes contain alcohol, and lemon-glycerin swabs are acidic. These substances can cause a burning sensa-

tion and contribute to drying of the oral mucous membranes. The nurse encourages frequent rinsing of the mouth with sodium bicarbonate solution, warm saline, or hydrogen peroxide solution (see also Chart 54-2).

RADIATION THERAPY. Radiation therapy has been used alone, as well as in conjunction with surgery and chemotherapy, in the treatment of cancer of the oral cavity. The goal of radiation therapy is tumor eradication while preserving function and appearance. There are several ways to apply radiotherapy. In collaboration with the client, the physician chooses the best mode on the basis of the tumor site and staging.

Radiation therapy for oral cancers can be given by external beam or interstitial implantation. External beam radiation passes through the skin or mucous membrane to the tumor site. Typically, treatments are given as five daily treatments per week over a 6- to 9-week period. Special precautions are taken to minimize the dose of radiation to the brain or spinal cord. Another option is the implantation of radioactive substances (interstitial radiation therapy) to either boost the dosage or deliver a radiation dose close to the tumor bed. This form of implant therapy can be curative in early-stage lesions in the floor of the mouth or anterior tongue, or to add an ad-

---

EVIDENCE-BASED PRACTICE
FOR NURSING

Do foam swabs work as well as toothbrushes to remove dental plaque?

Pearson, L. (1996). A comparison of the ability of foam swabs and toothbrushes to remove dental plaque: Implications for nursing practice. *Journal of Advanced Nursing, 23,* 62-69.

The purpose of this study was to compare the effectiveness of a toothbrush and a foam swab in the removal of dental plaque over a 6-day period. Three experiments were conducted using the mouth of the author and a volunteer. A plaque scoring system was used to quantify the amount of plaque left on teeth adjacent to periodontal tissue. Plaque amounts were measured at the gum-tooth margin (gingival crevice plaque) and between teeth (approximal plaque).

At the end of 6 days, the ability of the toothbrush to remove plaque was noted to be superior to that of the foam swab; the toothbrush usually achieved complete removal of all visible plaque from the sites examined. The sites cleansed by the foam swabs revealed remaining plaque after using the "scrubbing" or "swabbing" technique outlined. When plaque was allowed to accumulate over a 6-day period, similar results were obtained. This study suggests that toothbrush use is more effective than foam swabs in removing plaque, but results could be impacted by user technique.

Critique. The very small sample size (2), as well as the use of the researcher as a study subject, may have permitted bias to be introduced into this study. It is also unclear who assigned the plaque scores to the study subjects. However, as nursing builds knowledge for evidence-based practice, the efficiency and utility of using these two mouth cleansing modalities need further examination.

Implications for Nursing. Nurses need to consider the aim of the intervention in selecting an instrument for mouth care. If the aim is to hydrate oral mucosa, a foam swab will deliver moisture to the tissues in an adequate fashion. Also, if damage to fragile oral mucosal tissue is a concern, a foam swab causes minimal damage. However, if removal of dental debris is the aim of mouth care, then the selection of a toothbrush appears to be more appropriate. This becomes important, since controlling plaque is a concern for those clients who may be immunocompromised (the overgrowth and invasion of organisms from plaque can be of concern).

COST OF CARE
IMPLICATIONS FOR NURSING

ORAL CAVITY PROBLEMS

Cost of Care
- The cost of medical-surgical care for clients with oral cancer in the United States is thought to be approximately $3.7 billion.
- The variables identified as being significantly associated with treatment costs are TNM stage, single-modality treatment versus multimodality treatment, and comorbidity grade.
- The majority of costs are incurred during the treatment phase.

Implications for Nursing
The majority of the costs associated with oral cavity cancer care are incurred during treatment, especially if treatment involves a combination of surgery, chemotherapy, and radiation. Measures to permit early identification and treatment of the disease at a stage where single-modality treatment can be used more effectively would yield substantial decreases in management costs. Client education about the risk factors for oral cancer plus rigorous assessment of those with high-risk profiles (e.g., heavy alcohol and tobacco use) would be cost-effective in reducing the incidence and permitting early diagnosis and treatment of the disease.

Data from Funk, G.F., et al. (1998). Cost-identification analysis in oral cavity cancer management. *Otolaryngology–Head and Neck Surgery, 118*(2), 211-220.

ditional boost of radiation to a tumor that received external beam radiation.

Interstitial radiation is used for smaller lesions that do not infiltrate surrounding tissues. The following can be radioactive materials:

* Seeds, which are permanently implanted into the tissue (usually for tumors unable to be completely excised, or in neck nodes)
* Needles or wires, which are extracted at the end of therapy
* Radiation catheters or holders, which are loaded with radioactive materials
* A "mold" of radioactive material placed directly over the lesion for a specific time

The dose of interstitial therapy is often difficult to calculate. With the exception of radioactive seeds, which have a low level of activity, clients receiving interstitial radiation are usually hospitalized for the duration of treatment. Radiation isolation precautions must be instituted while the materials are active or in place. A tracheostomy may be required with interstitial implants because of edema and increased oral secretions. (See Chapter 25 for nursing care of clients undergoing radiation therapy.)

CRITICAL THINKING CHALLENGE

The white patches on your client's tongue have been diagnosed as leukoplakia. In addition, a biopsy performed on a nodule located on the floor of the mouth was determined to be squamous cell carcinoma. The client is preparing to undergo surgical excision and adjunctive treatment with radiation.

* What should the nurse include in the preoperative teaching for this client?
* What complications from the treatment is this client at risk for?
* What measures should the nurse include in the oral hygiene care for this client?

For suggested answer guidelines, go to [SIMON] http://www.wbsaunders.com/SIMON/Iggy/.

CHEMOTHERAPY. The client may receive one or more chemotherapeutic agents (Table 54-3). The advantages of chemotherapy instead of, or as an adjunct to, surgery or radiation for cancer of the oral cavity continue to be evaluated.

Recent trials have been conducted on the use of two individual agents—mitomycin and cisplatin—to prevent local recurrence and improve survival. Response rates have varied from 0% to 30% (Vikram, 1998; Witt, 1998). The nurse instructs the client undergoing chemotherapy about the anticipated side effects of the medication, which vary with each agent. The nurse administers antiemetic medications as prescribed and provides other comfort measures as needed.

SURGICAL MANAGEMENT. The physician can often excise small, noninvasive lesions of the oral cavity in an ambu-

latory setting with local anesthesia. The surgical defect is usually small enough to be closed by sutures. These smaller lesions are also responsive to carbon dioxide laser therapy or *cryotherapy* (extreme cold application), which can be performed as an ambulatory care procedure in a surgical center (but may require general anesthesia).

Small oral cancers are equally responsive to radiation therapy and to surgery. More invasive lesions (stage III and IV) require more extensive surgical excision and result in a greater loss of function and disfigurement. Not all lesions can be excised by the peroral approach (through the mouth). The goal of surgical resection is the removal of the tumor with a surgical margin that is free of tumor involvement.

PREOPERATIVE CARE. Before excision of a lesion of the oral cavity, the nurse assesses and documents the client's level of understanding of the disease process, the rationale for the surgery, and the planned intervention. Information is reinforced as needed. The nurse identifies family members or other caregivers and includes them in health teaching.

For small, local excisions, postoperative restrictions include a liquid diet for a day, then soft foods. There are no activity limitations, and postoperative analgesics are prescribed.

The nurse instructs the client undergoing large surgical resections about the following:

* The placement of a temporary tracheostomy for approximately 10 days and the concomitant nursing care (oxygen therapy and suctioning)
* Temporary loss of speech due to the tracheostomy
* The need for vital signs to be taken frequently postoperatively
* The need to take nothing by mouth (remain on NPO status) for 10 to 14 days until intraoral suture lines are healed
* The need to have IV lines in place for medication delivery and hydration
* Postoperative medications and activity (out of bed on the first postoperative day)
* Any surgical drains

The nurse also assesses the client's ability to read and write. The client and nurse select the method of communication to use postoperatively with staff and family members (e.g., Magic Slate, picture board, or pad and pencil).

OPERATIVE PROCEDURES. Three factors influence the type of surgery performed for oral cancers: the size and location of the tumor, tumor invasion into the bone, and the presence of metastasis to neck lymph nodes (Olsen, 1999). Small tumors (2 cm or less) located near the mouth opening can be excised periorally (inside the mouth). Otherwise, an external approach may be used. The surgeon may approach the oral cavity from under the mandible or may split the lower lip and retract the lips and cheek for exposure. The mandible is occasionally split as well and pushed aside for oral access; it is wired at the end of the operation. The most extensive oral operations are composite resections, which combine partial or total **glossectomy** (tongue removal) and partial mandibulectomy. In the *commando (co-mandible) procedure,* the surgeon excises a segment of the mandible with the oral lesion, usually in conjunction with a radical neck dissection (see Chapter 29). If the anterior mandible is resected to treat tumor invasion in that area, the mandible is reconstructed after the

TABLE 54-3	COMMON CHEMOTHERAPEUTIC DRUGS USED IN CLIENTS WITH SQUAMOUS CELL CARCINOMA OF THE HEAD AND NECK
• Methotrexate	• Doxorubicin
• Bleomycin	• Vincristine
• Cisplatin (*cis*-platinum)	• 5-Fluorouracil
• Cyclophosphamide	• Hydroxyurea

resection to decrease speech and swallowing problems postoperatively and improve appearance. For clients undergoing a complete glossectomy, a prosthesis will be necessary to aid in swallowing and speech.

Metastasis to cervical lymph nodes usually indicates a poor prognosis for clients with cancer of the oral cavity. In clients with cervical node metastasis, a neck dissection may also be performed. A radical neck dissection involves the removal of submental; submandibular; upper, mid, and lower jugular; and posterior triangular levels of the cervical lymph nodes, along with cranial nerve XI, the internal jugular vein, and the sternocleidomastoid muscle. Modified and selective neck dissections may be done in individuals with minimal lymph node involvement.

POSTOPERATIVE CARE. Postoperative care of the client with cancer of the oral cavity focuses on airway management as a priority. The client will have a temporary tracheostomy placed, requiring intensive nursing care to promote airway clearance. In addition, care must be taken to protect the surgical incision site from mechanical damage and infection. Nursing interventions to relieve pain or discomfort and promote nutrition are also important.

Maintaining Airway Patency. After extensive excision or resection, the most important nursing intervention is maintaining airway patency. The client may not recall on awakening from anesthesia that a tracheostomy tube is in place and may initially panic because of the inability to speak. The nurse reminds the client why he or she cannot speak and provides reassurance that the vocal cords are intact (unless a total laryngectomy has been performed, then the loss of voice is permanent). The nurse provides the client with the predetermined method of communication.

Nursing interventions are aimed at keeping the temporary tracheostomy patent. Frequent suctioning, using sterile technique, may be required for excessive secretions. Humidified oxygen may be ordered to help liquefy secretions in the early postoperative phase. After the immediate postoperative phase, the client may be able to cough effectively enough to decrease the need for suctioning. After oral edema has decreased and the tracheostomy tube has been changed to a noncuffed type, the client can speak by plugging the stoma with the fingertip. The nurse and physician determine the appropriateness of instructing the client in this technique. (See Chapter 28 for care of the client with a tracheostomy.)

When the client has been determined to have an adequate airway through the areodigestive tract and can effectively clear secretions by coughing, the tracheostomy tube is removed. An airtight dressing is placed over the tracheostomy site, and the incision heals without the need for sutures. The client is instructed to press fingers over the dressing to prevent the incision from separating during coughing (Reese, 1996).

Clients who have undergone extensive resection may have slurred speech or difficulty in speaking. The nurse assesses the need for consultation with a speech/language pathologist.

Protecting the Operative Area. The surgical incision site requires careful attention to avoid infection. The nurse or assistive nursing personnel provides gentle mouth care for cleaning away thick secretions and stimulating the flow of saliva. The delivery of oral care depends on the nature and extent of the surgical procedure. Oral care should be provided every 4 hours in the early postoperative phase. The presence of unusual odors from the mouth can indicate infection. In the early postoperative phase, care must be taken to avoid disruption of the suture line during oral hygiene.

The nurse elevates the head of the bed to at least 30 degrees to assist in decreasing edema by gravity. If skin grafting was done, the nurse inspects the donor site (generally on the anterior thigh) during every nursing shift for bleeding or manifestations of infection. (See Chapter 29 for specific nursing care of the client with a radical neck dissection.)

Relieving Pain. To provide optimal pain relief in the postoperative period, the nurse relies on subjective and objective data to assess the need for analgesics and the effectiveness of the medications given. The goal of pain medication during this period is relief of pain while allowing the client to function at an optimal level. Clients who have undergone surgery for oral carcinomas describe their pain as throbbing or pounding. IV morphine is usually the initial postoperative pain medication given. Oral acetaminophen combined with codeine (Tylenol with Codeine) may be used for systemic relief of moderate pain.

Promoting Nutrition. Clients who have undergone extensive resections of the oral cavity remain on NPO status for 5 to 7 days or longer. This allows healing in the oral cavity before food contacts the incision. Nasogastric feeding or total parenteral nutrition is needed during this time (see Chapter 61). The tubes are usually inserted in the operating room.

When oral fluid intake is begun, the nurse assesses for and documents difficulty in swallowing, aspiration, or leakage of saliva or fluids from the suture line. Nursing care should also include the monitoring of weight and hydration. Nutritional supplementation may be used to improve the client's quality of life (see the Legal/Ethical Issues in Health Care box below). Clients experiencing weight loss or having difficulty maintaining hydration may be candidates for gastrostomy tube placement.

A speech/language pathologist is often consulted to assist with swallowing techniques. A swallowing impairment may be temporary or permanent. The client is encouraged to perform swallowing exercises.

Legal/Ethical Issues IN HEALTH CARE

NUTRITIONAL SUPPLEMENTATION IN CLIENTS UNDERGOING RADIATION TREATMENTS

Maintaining optimal nutritional status for individuals with oral carcinoma is a difficult task, considering the many aspects of digestion impacted by the disease and treatment. Radiation therapy can pose additional challenges to nutrition because of the decreased saliva flow and alterations in taste that can result. Not only does increasing evidence point to nutritional status as a predictor of overall survival, but the ability to eat and enjoy food is an important component of quality of life.

The purpose of the study by McCarthy and Weihofen (1999) was to describe the effect of nutritional supplements on the food intake of clients undergoing radiotherapy. Forty clients beginning external beam radiation therapy were given weekly dietary counseling. The daily food intake was recorded 3 days per week for 4 weeks. One half of the subjects were assigned to ingest a nutritional supplement between meals and at bedtime. Findings suggested that those who ingested the nutritional supplements significantly increased their total caloric and protein intake while not reducing their food-derived caloric and protein intake. Based on this study, the addition of nutritional supplements to the normal food intake for clients undergoing radiotherapy for the treatment of oral cancer may be a viable option in helping to maintain adequate nutrition.

From McCarthy, D. & Weihofen, D. (1999). The effect of nutritional supplements on food intake in patients undergoing radiotherapy. *Oncology Nursing Forum, 26*(5), 897-900.

● Community-Based Care

Continuing care for the client with an oral tumor depends on the severity of the tumor, the treatment for the tumor, and available support systems. Most clients are maintained at home during follow-up care. Ongoing nutritional management remains a vital part of the treatment plan. In addition, the short- and long-term effects of the treatment for cancers of the oral cavity must be monitored once the client is discharged home.

■ HOME CARE MANAGEMENT

If radiation therapy is part of the client's treatment plan, home care considerations include preparatory information and management strategies. Complications due to radiation to the head or neck can be acute or delayed. Acute effects include treatment-related mucositis, stomatitis, and alterations in taste. Long-term effects such as xerostomia (excessive mouth dryness) and dental decay require ongoing oral care, the use of saliva substitutes, and follow-up dental visits. Although ongoing dental care is important, the possible adverse effects that radiation has on the cellular elements of the bone make elective oral surgical procedures, such as tooth extraction, impossible in the area of the radiation. Fatigue, which can be either short or long term, is a common side effect of radiation and chemotherapy.

The client whose tracheostomy has been removed is often taking a soft diet by mouth before discharge. Occasionally, however, clients are discharged from the hospital while still requiring tracheostomy suction, oral suction, and nasogastric feedings. Suction equipment, nutritional supplies, and nursing care can be provided by home care companies. (See Chapter 61 for home care preparation for the client receiving home parenteral nutrition and Chapter 28 for home care preparation for the client with a tracheostomy.)

■ HEALTH TEACHING

The nurse instructs the client and family about medications, diet or feedings, any treatments (such as tracheostomy care, suture line care, and dressing changes), and early symptoms of infection.

Alterations in taste and dysphagia make maintaining adequate nutritional status a challenge. Alterations in taste occur when the taste buds are included in the radiation treatment field. Taste sensation begins to return several weeks after the completion of treatment. Changes in taste include aversions for meat, such as beef or pork, and metallic tastes in the mouth. Clients can be taught to add seasonings to foods, to use gravies or sauces to make foods more palatable, and to use high-protein foods such as cheeses, milk, eggs, puddings, and legumes in place of meat. Clients with dysphagia are instructed in swallowing exercises. Thickened liquids are recommended, since thin liquids, such as water, are difficult to control during swallowing. In collaboration with the dietitian, the nurse instructs the client and family on how to assess the nutritional intake of the client who is just beginning to eat. Liquid dietary supplements are usually recommended at this time. If bleeding is a problem, or if mucositis is present, a diet of soft foods that will not cause injury to the mucous membranes is preferred.

The nurse instructs the client and/or family members to inspect the oral cavity daily for areas of redness, indicating the onset of mucositis, or for lesions indicative of stomatitis. Meticulous oral hygiene should be continued in the postoperative phase, especially if adjuvant chemotherapy or radiation is planned or underway. The nurse reinforces the oral hygiene routine, putting particular emphasis on the need for frequent rinsing of the oral cavity to reduce the number of microorganisms and maintain hydration. The client should use a chemobrush, should rinse the chemobrush with hydrogen peroxide and water following each use, and should change chemobrushes weekly.

If the salivary glands were part of the radiation field, the client is instructed in the daily use of a fluoride gel to prevent dental caries. A 1% sodium fluoride gel is placed in a customized applicator that completely covers the tooth surface. This applicator is worn for 10 minutes daily. Saliva production is greatly reduced as a consequence of radiation. The resulting xerostomia results in the inability to eat dry foods. The nurse instructs the client in the use of saliva substitutes.

Skin reactions are also a common side effect of radiation. The nurse should instruct the client to avoid sun exposure, to avoid perfumed lotions or powders, and to cleanse the face or neck area with a gentle, nondeodorant soap.

To increase retention of the information, the client and the family demonstrate the skills they are taught. The nurse evaluates and documents their understanding of the treatments.

🐾 CONSIDERATIONS FOR OLDER ADULTS

For the older client with metastatic or invasive oral cancer, skilled home care or nursing home services are required for pain management, nutrition maintenance, and emotional support. Older adults often take subtherapeutic doses of analgesics for fear of becoming addicted. The home care nurse teaches the client about the need to promote comfort to improve nutrition and prevent depression. Chart 54-4 summarizes the focused nursing assessment for the older adult with oral cancer. (See Chapter 7 for further information on pain management in older adults.)

■ HEALTH CARE RESOURCES

Clients who have undergone composite resection often require community services, because they have both physical and psychosocial needs. Clients who have undergone surgical excision experience depression related to a change in body image. Excision of a portion of the mandible can leave a facial defect that may be difficult to hide. A social worker or other health care professional may be needed for client and family counseling. Clients who have undergone a total glossectomy may be able to speak with special training and the use of an intraoral prosthesis fashioned by a maxillofacial prosthodontist. The prosthesis is similar to dentures, with augmentation to approximate the oral articulating surfaces.

CHART 54-4

FOCUSED ASSESSMENT of
The Older Adult with Oral Cancer

- Assess the mouth and surrounding tissues for candidiasis, mucositis, pain, and loss of appetite and taste.
- Monitor the client's weight.
- Monitor nutritional and fluid intake.
- Assess for difficulty in eating or speech.
- Assess pain status and measures used to control pain.
- Monitor the client's response to medications.
- Identify psychosocial problems, such as depression, anxiety, and fear.

The nurse consults the social worker or case manager for assistance in obtaining special equipment or nutritional resources required by the client at home. The case manager assesses the financial needs of the client and makes referrals to government, community, and religious organizations as needed.

● Evaluation: Outcomes

NOC The nurse evaluates the care of the client with a malignant tumor of the oral cavity on the basis of the identified nursing diagnoses and collaborative problems. The expected outcomes include that the client:

- Maintains a patent oral airway through removal of oral secretions
- Maintains nutritional status by eating foods that are well tolerated and nutritious
- Communicates thoughts and feelings to family members, friends, and health care personnel
- Maintains the integrity of the oral mucous membrane

DISORDERS OF THE SALIVARY GLANDS

Acute Sialadenitis

■ OVERVIEW

Acute sialadenitis, the inflammation of a salivary gland, can be caused by infectious agents, irradiation, or immunologic disorders. Salivary gland inflammation can have a bacterial or viral etiology. Acute sialadenitis can be caused by infection with cytomegalovirus (CMV). The most common bacterial organisms are *Staphylococcus aureus*, *Staphylococcus pyogenes*, *Streptococcus pneumoniae*, and *Escherichia coli*. This disorder most commonly affects the parotid or submandibular gland in adults.

A decrease in the production of saliva (as in dehydrated or debilitated clients or in those who are on NPO status postoperatively for an extended time) usually precipitates acute sialadenitis. The bacteria or viruses enter the gland through the ductal opening in the oral cavity. Systemic medications, such as phenothiazines, chloramphenicol, and oxytetracycline, can also precipitate an episode of acute sialadenitis. Untreated infections of the salivary glands can evolve into abscesses, which can rupture and spread infection into the tissues of the neck and the mediastinum.

Clients who receive radiation for the treatment of cancers of the head and neck or thyroid may develop decreased salivary flow, predisposing them to acute or persistent sialadenitis. The effect of radiation on the salivary glands is rapid and dose related (Mandel & Mandel, 1999; McEwen & Sanchez, 1997). Immunologic disorders such as HIV infection can cause enlargement of the parotid gland that can be due to secondary infection. Sjögren's syndrome, an autoimmune disorder, is characterized by chronic salivary gland enlargement and inflammation (see Chapter 21).

► COLLABORATIVE MANAGEMENT

● Assessment

During the initial interview, the nurse assesses for any predisposing factors for sialadenitis, such as ionizing radiation to the head or neck area. The nurse asks about systemic illnesses such as HIV infection and collects a thorough medication history.

The presence of dehydration can be noted by assessing the oral cavity and the skin for turgor. Other assessment findings include pain and swelling of the face over the affected gland. Cranial nerve function is tested, since the branches of the facial nerve lie close to the salivary glands. Fever and general malaise also occur, and purulent drainage can often be massaged from the affected duct in the oral cavity (Chart 54-5).

● Interventions

Collaborative management includes the administration of IV fluids and measures such as the following to treat the underlying cause and increase the flow of saliva:

- Hydration
- Application of warm compresses
- Massage of the gland
- Use of a saliva substitute
- Use of **sialagogues** (substances that stimulate the flow of saliva)

Sialagogues include lemon slices and fruit- or citrus-flavored candy. Massage is accomplished by milking the edematous gland with the fingertips toward the ductal opening. Elevation of the head of the bed promotes gravity drainage of the edematous gland.

Acute sialadenitis is best prevented by adherence to routine oral hygiene. This practice prohibits infections from ascending to the salivary glands from the oral cavity.

Postirradiation Sialadenitis

The salivary glands are sensitive to ionizing radiation, such as from radiation therapy or radioactive iodine treatment of thyroid cancers. Exposure of the glands to radiation produces **xerostomia** (very dry mouth caused by severe reduction in the flow of saliva) within 24 hours. Radiation to the salivary glands can also produce pain and edema, which generally abate after several days.

Xerostomia may be temporary or permanent, depending on the dose of radiation and the percentage of total salivary gland tissue irradiated. Little can be done to relieve the client's dry mouth during the course of radiation therapy. Frequent sips of water and frequent mouth care, especially before meals, are the most effective interventions. After the course of radiation therapy has been completed, saliva substitutes may provide moisture for 2 to 4 hours at a time. Over-the-counter solutions are available, or solutions may be mixed with methylcellulose (Cologel), glycerin, and saline.

Salivary Gland Tumors

■ OVERVIEW

Tumors of the salivary glands are relatively rare; they constitute 5% of all oral tumors. Initially they present as slow-growing, painless masses (McEwen & Sanchez, 1997). Malignant tumors are characterized by more rapid growth than that of be-

---

CHART 54-5

KEY FEATURES of Sialadenitis

- Swelling on the sides of the face or under the tongue, which increases when the client eats
- Alteration in the quantity or appearance of saliva
- Pain, especially during eating
- Purulent drainage from the affected duct

nign tumors and are generally associated with pain. Involvement of the facial nerve, more common with malignant tumors, results in facial weakness or paralysis (partial or total) on the affected side. Needle aspiration biopsy and open biopsy are useful procedures in establishing a diagnosis.

▶ COLLABORATIVE MANAGEMENT

● Assessment

The nurse collects information concerning prior radiation exposure, since radiation to the head and neck areas is associated with the occurrence of salivary gland tumors. Salivary gland malignancies present as localized, firm masses. In advanced stages of salivary gland tumors, the nurse may note a large preauricular mass accompanied by facial nerve paralysis. Submandibular and minor salivary gland tumors may be tender or painful. Tumor invasion of the hypoglossal nerve causes impaired movement of the tongue, and a loss of sensation can follow. The nurse pays particular attention to assessment of the facial nerve because of its close proximity to the salivary glands. The nurse assesses the client's ability to:

- Wrinkle the brow
- Raise the eyebrows
- Squeeze the eyes shut
- Wrinkle the nose
- Pucker the lips
- Puff out the cheeks
- Grimace or smile

● Interventions

The treatment of choice for both benign and malignant tumors of the salivary glands is surgical excision. However, radiation therapy is often used for salivary gland cancers that are large, have recurred, show evidence of residual disease after excision, or are highly malignant.

Clients who have undergone **parotidectomy** (surgical removal of the parotid glands) or submandibular gland surgery are at risk for weakness or loss of function of the facial nerve because the nerve courses directly through the gland. Facial nerve repair with autogenous nerve grafting can be done at the time of surgery. The majority of studies support combining surgery with postoperative radiation for advanced disease.

ONLINE RESOURCES

For suggested readings and Internet resources, go to http://www.wbsaunders.com/SIMON/Iggy/.

SELECTED BIBLIOGRAPHY

Asterisk indicates a classic or definitive work on this subject.

Aubertin, M.A. (1997). Home care of the elderly oral cancer patient. *Home Healthcare Nurse, 15*(6), 381-390.

Bagan, J., et al. (1998). Preliminary investigation of the association of oral lichen planus and hepatitis C. *Oral Surgery, Oral Medicine, Oral Pathology, Oral Radiology, and Endodontics 85*(5), 532-535.

*Barnes, L., et al. (1996). Basaloid squamous cell carcinoma of the head and neck: Clinicopathological features and differential diagnosis. *Annals of Otology, Rhinology, and Laryngology, 105,* 75-82.

*Beck, S. (1996). Mucositis. In S. Groenwald et al. (Eds.), *Cancer symptom management* (pp. 308-323). Boston: Jones & Bartlett.

Burkhart, N.W., Burkes, E.J., & Burker, E.J. (1997). Meeting the educational needs of patients with oral lichen planus. *General Dentistry,* 126-131.

Dixon, D., Breeding, L., & Faler, T. (1999). Microwave disinfection of denture base materials colonized with *Candida albicans. Journal of Prosthetic Dentistry, 81*(2), 207-214.

*Dose, A. (1995). The symptom experience of mucositis, stomatitis, and xerostomia. *Seminars in Oncology Nursing, 11*(4), 248-255.

Eilers, J. (1997). Stomatitis as a side effect of cancer treatment. *Quality of Life: A Nursing Challenge, 5*(3), 68-74.

Freer, S.K. (2000). Use of an oral assessment tool to improve practice. *Professional Nurse, 15*(10), 635-639.

Greenlee, R., et al. (2000). Cancer statistics, 2000. *Ca: A Cancer Journal for Clinicians, 50*(1), 7-33.

Hyland, S. (1997). Assessing the oral cavity. In M. Frank-Stromborg & S. Olsen (Eds.), *Instruments for clinical health care research* (2nd ed.). Boston: Jones & Bartlett.

Klaus, B., & Grodesky, M. (1998). Common oral manifestations seen in patients with HIV/AIDS. *Nurse Practitioner, 23*(6), 134-139.

Mandel, S., & Mandel, R. (1999). Persistent sialadenitis after radioactive iodine therapy: Report of two cases. *Journal of Oral Maxillofacial Surgery, 57*(7), 738-741.

McCarthy, D., & Weihofen, D. (1999). The effect of nutritional supplements on food intake in patients undergoing radiotherapy. *Oncology Nursing Forum, 26*(5), 897-900.

McEwen, D., & Sanchez, M. (1997). A guide to salivary gland disorders. *AORN Journal, 65*(3), 554-566.

National Cancer Institute. (1999). *SEER cancer incidence public-use database CD-ROM, 1973-1999,* Bethesda, MD: Public Health Service, U.S. Department of Health and Human Services.

Olsen, M. (1999). Oral cavity cancer. In C. Miaskowski & P. Buchsel (Eds.), *Oncology nursing: Assessment and clinical care* (pp. 1177-1201). St. Louis: Mosby.

Parkin, D., Pisani, P., & Ferlay, J. (1999). Global cancer statistics. *CA: A Cancer Journal for Clinicians, 49*(1), 33-64.

*Pearson, L. (1996). A comparison of the ability of foam swabs and toothbrushes to remove dental plaque: Implications for nursing practice. *Journal of Advanced Nursing, 23,* 62-69.

*Peterson, M.J., & Baughman, R. (1996). Recurrent aphthous stomatitis: Primary care management. *Nurse Practitioner, 21*(5), 36-47.

*Ransier, A., et al. (1995). A combined analysis of a toothbrush, foam brush, and a chlorhexidine-soaked foam brush in maintaining oral hygiene. *Cancer Nursing, 18*(5), 393-396.

*Reese, J. (1996). Head and neck cancers. In R. McCorkle et al. (Eds.), *Cancer nursing: A comprehensive textbook* (2nd ed., pp. 773-795). Philadelphia: W.B. Saunders.

Sheff, B. (1999). Oral *Candida albicans. Nursing99, 29*(7), 25.

Shugars, D., & Patton, L. (1997). Detecting, diagnosing, and preventing oral cancer. *Nurse Practitioner, 22*(6), 105-129.

Shuster, J. (1998). Inhaled steroids and oral candidiasis. *Nursing98,* May, p.25.

*Toth, B., et al. (1995). Minimizing oral complications of cancer treatment. *Oncology, 9*(9), 851-858.

Vikram, B., (1998). Adjuvant therapy in head and neck cancer. *Ca: A Cancer Journal for Clinicians, 48*(4): 199-209.

Walton, J.C., Miller, J., & Tordecilla, L. (2001). Elder oral assessment and care. *MEDSURG Nursing, 10*(1), 37-44.

Witt, M.E. (1998). Radiation and chemotherapy as combined treatment for advanced head and neck cancer. *MEDSURG Nursing, 7*(3), 159-164.

*Woo, S., & Sonis, S. (1996). Recurrent aphthous ulcers: A review of diagnosis and management. *Journal of the American Dental Association, 127,* 1202-1211.

Interventions for Clients with Esophageal Problems

CONSTANCE VISOVSKY

Learning Objectives

After studying this chapter, you should be able to:

1. Explain the pathophysiology of gastroesophageal reflux disease (GERD).
2. Assess the client who is experiencing GERD.
3. Plan the nursing care for clients with GERD.
4. Develop a postoperative teaching plan for the client having a hiatal hernia repair.
5. Identify the differences in the incidence of esophageal cancer among cultural groups.
6. Describe the risk factors for esophageal cancer.
7. Analyze assessment data to determine common nursing diagnoses for the client with esophageal cancer.
8. Discuss the priorities for postoperative care of the client undergoing surgery for esophageal cancer.
9. Plan community-based care for clients diagnosed with esophageal cancer.

SIMON

Go to http://www.wbsaunders.com/SIMON/Iggy/ for self-assessment questions related to these Learning Objectives.

Esophageal disorders affect approximately 546,000 people in the United States. One third of the population experiences symptoms associated with the reflux of stomach acid into the esophagus. Impaired gastroesophageal motility resulting from achalasia or diverticula is responsible for 400,000 visits to health care providers annually (see the Cost of Care Box on p. 1193).

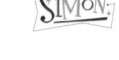
The esophagus is a hollow, distensible muscular tube located behind the trachea that acts primarily as a conduit for food from the mouth to the stomach. It passes through the diaphragm at the esophageal hiatus and extends to the gastroesophageal junction. The esophagus is susceptible to a variety of inflammatory, structural, motor, and neoplastic disorders. Collaborative management involves medical and surgical therapies in addition to diet and lifestyle modifications. Nurses have a significant role in assisting clients in making the lifestyle changes necessary for the successful prevention and management of esophageal disorders.

GASTROESOPHAGEAL REFLUX DISEASE

OVERVIEW

Esophageal reflux is defined as the backward flow of gastrointestinal contents into the esophagus. Reflux produces its characteristic symptoms by exposing the esophageal mucosa to the irritating effects of gastric and/or duodenal contents, resulting in inflammatory changes of the esophageal mucosa. A person with acute symptoms of inflammation is often described as having **reflux esophagitis,** a hallmark of gastroesophageal reflux disease (GERD). Reflux esophagitis is graded according to the extent and severity of the lesions.

Pathophysiology

The following physiologic factors are implicated in the development of GERD (Tucker & Schumann, 1999):

- An incompetent lower esophageal sphincter
- Irritation from the refluxate
- Abnormal esophageal clearance
- Delayed gastric emptying

The reflux of gastric contents into the esophagus is normally prevented by the presence of two high-pressure areas that remain relatively contracted in the resting phase. A 3-cm (1.2-inch) segment at the proximal end of the esophagus is called the upper esophageal sphincter (UES). Another 2- to 4-cm (0.8- to 1.6-inch) portion just proximal to the gastroesophageal junction is called the lower esophageal sphincter (LES). The function of the LES is supported by its anatomic placement in the abdomen, where the surrounding pressure is significantly higher than in the low-pressure thorax. Sphincter function is also supported by the acute angle (angle of His) that is formed as the esophagus enters the stomach. Esophageal reflux can occur when gastric volume or intra-abdominal pressure is elevated, when the sphincter tone of the LES is decreased, or when the LES undergoes inappropriate relaxation.

COST OF CARE
IMPLICATIONS FOR NURSING

ESOPHAGEAL PROBLEMS

Cost of Care
- Ambulatory care for clients with Barrett's esophagus costs approximately $103 per month, or $1241 per year.
- Clients with low-grade dysplasia (tissue changes) are three times as likely to have more than 3 endoscopies per year as compared to clients who do not have dysplasia.
- Endoscopies and clinic visits account for 31% and 5.9%, respectively, of the monthly medical costs.
- The medication costs per month for clients with Barrett's esophagus is $65.
- Proton-pump inhibitors account for 64.6% of the total medication cost.
- Medications account for more than 50% of the total cost of care.

Implications for Nursing
Prolonged gastrointestinal reflux leading to Barrett's esophagus or disease results in a relatively high cost of care in terms of the need for health care services. Clients require ongoing monitoring by endoscopy for dysplastic changes in the mucosa, long-term medication adherence to control reflux, and primary care provider visits. Nurses can play an integral role in the prevention of gastrointestinal reflux by educating their clients about the risk factors for developing reflux, strategies for managing reflux, and the necessity of making lifestyle adjustments that prevent esophageal damage.

Data from Eloubeidi, M., et al. (1999). A cost analysis of outpatient care for patients with Barrett's esophagus in a managed care setting. *The American Journal of Gastroenterology, 94*(8), 2033-2036.

An individual experiencing reflux may be asymptomatic and relatively unaware that reflux is occurring. However, the esophagus has only a limited resistance to the damaging effects of the acidic gastrointestinal (GI) contents. The pH of acid secreted by the stomach ranges from 1.5 to 2.0, whereas the pH of the distal esophagus is normally neutral (6.0 to 7.0). Repeated exposure of the esophageal mucosa to highly acid gastric secretions is associated with the development of erosive esophagitis.

Refluxed material is returned to the stomach by a combination of gravity, saliva, and peristalsis. The effectiveness of the clearance mechanism is very important. An inflamed esophagus cannot eliminate the refluxed material as quickly or efficiently as a healthy one, and therefore the duration of exposure increases with each reflux episode.

Hyperemia (increased blood flow) and erosion occur in the esophagus in response to the chronic inflammation. Gastric acid and pepsin are responsible for the tissue injury. Minor capillary bleeding often accompanies the erosion, but frank hemorrhage is rare. During the process of healing, the body may substitute a columnar epithelium (Barrett's epithelium) for the normal squamous cell epithelium of the lower esophagus. Although this new tissue is more resistant to acid and therefore supports esophageal healing, it is considered premalignant and is associated with an increased risk of cancer in 10% to 15% of clients with prolonged GERD (Sharma, 1999). The fibrosis and scarring that accompanies the healing process can produce esophageal stricture, resulting in a narrowing of the esophageal lumen. The stricture leads to progressive difficulty in swallowing. Uncontrolled esophageal reflux also creates a risk for other serious complications such as esophageal ulceration, hemorrhage, and aspiration pneu-

---

TABLE 55-1 • FACTORS CONTRIBUTING TO DECREASED LOWER ESOPHAGEAL SPHINCTER PRESSURE

- Fatty foods
- Caffeinated beverages, such as coffee, tea, and cola
- Chocolate
- Nicotine in cigarette smoke
- Calcium channel blockers
- Nitrates
- Peppermint, spearmint
- Alcohol
- Anticholinergic drugs
- High levels of estrogen and progesterone
- Nasogastric tube placement

---

monia. GERD has been implicated as one of the causes of adult-onset asthma, laryngitis, and dental deterioration.

Etiology

Current evidence suggests that GERD is a result of impaired LES function, which permits the reflux of gastric contents into the esophagus and the subsequent exposure of the esophageal mucosa to gastric contents from impaired esophageal clearance (Claussen, 1999). Currently, the role that hiatal hernia (see p. 1198) plays in the development of GERD is controversial, because each of these disorders often present independently of one another. Nighttime reflux tends to result in prolonged exposure of the esophagus to acid because recumbency tends to impair peristalsis and gravity clearance mechanisms.

Gastric distention caused by the ingestion of large meals or by conditions associated with delayed gastric emptying predispose the client to reflux. A number of individual factors, including certain foods and medications, have been identified as influencing the tone and contractility of the LES (Table 55-1). Clients who have a nasogastric tube often experience compromised esophageal sphincter function. The tube keeps the cardiac sphincter open and allows acidic contents from the stomach to enter the esophagus. Other factors that increase intra-abdominal and intragastric pressure (e.g., wearing tight belts, obesity, bending over, and ascites) overcome the gastroesophageal pressure gradient maintained by the LES and allow reflux to occur.

Incidence/Prevalence

The incidence of GERD is approximately 2% to 3% per year and affects 25% to 35% of the population. Ten percent of the population reports experiencing symptoms of reflux daily, and 44% report experiencing symptoms once a month (Scott & Gelhot, 1999). Gastroesophageal reflux disease (GERD) can occur at any age but is more common in people over 45 years of age. The incidence of GERD may be underestimated because many people with mild disease relate the symptoms to episodes of stress or dietary indiscretion.

CULTURAL CONSIDERATIONS
The prevalence of GERD is higher in females than in males and is found more often in Caucasians than in other ethnic groups. Severe esophagitis is more common in males than in females and is more prevalent in Caucasians than in African Americans.

► COLLABORATIVE MANAGEMENT
● Assessment
■ HISTORY

The nurse assesses the client for a history of heartburn or atypical chest pain associated with the reflux of gastrointestinal contents. The client is assessed for dysphagia (difficulty swallowing) or odynophagia (painful swallowing), either of which can indicate the development of a stricture. The nurse further investigates whether the client has a history of newly diagnosed asthma, morning hoarseness, or pneumonia, which are suggestive of severe reflux reaching the pharynx or mouth and/or pulmonary aspiration.

■ PHYSICAL ASSESSMENT/CLINICAL MANIFESTATIONS

The clinical manifestations of reflux may vary substantially in severity (Chart 55-1).

DYSPEPSIA. A diagnosis of GERD is made principally by a history of **dyspepsia** (also called pyrosis or heartburn), which is the characteristic symptom. Clients often describe this pain as a substernal or retrosternal burning sensation that tends to move up and down the chest in a wavelike fashion. If severe, the pain may radiate to the neck or jaw or may be referred to the back. The pain typically worsens when the client bends over, strains, or is in a recumbent position.

With severe GERD, the pain occurs after each meal and persists for 20 minutes to 2 hours. Clients usually experience prompt relief by ingesting fluids or antacids or by maintaining an upright posture. Some clients experience *atypical chest pain,* which mimics angina and needs to be carefully differentiated from cardiac disease.

REGURGITATION. **Regurgitation,** which is associated with neither belching nor nausea, is another common symptom. The client reports the occurrence of warm fluid traveling up the throat. If the fluid reaches the level of the pharynx, the client notes a sour or bitter taste in the mouth. This effortless regurgitation can even occur when the client is in an upright position. The danger of aspiration is increased if regurgitation occurs when the client is in a recumbent position.

If the client experiences regurgitation, the nurse carefully auscultates the chest for crackles, which is an indication of associated aspiration. The nurse assesses for coughing, hoarseness, or wheezing at night, which may be related to recumbent regurgitation. Assessment for bronchitis may be necessary in clients experiencing long-term regurgitation.

CHART 55-1

KEY FEATURES *of*
Gastroesophageal Reflux Disease

- Dyspepsia (heartburn or pyrosis)
- Regurgitation (may lead to aspiration or bronchitis)
- Coughing, hoarseness, or wheezing at night
- Water brash
- Dysphagia
- Odynophagia (painful swallowing)
- Chest pain
- Belching
- Flatulence

HYPERSALIVATION. A reflex salivary hypersecretion known as **water brash** occurs in response to reflux. Water brash must be carefully distinguished from regurgitation. The client reports a sensation of fluid in the throat, but unlike with regurgitation, there is no bitter or sour taste.

DYSPHAGIA AND ODYNOPHAGIA. Chronic GERD can involve **dysphagia** (difficulty in swallowing). Dysphagia may be the presenting symptom in 33% of clients with GERD. This symptom is usually fairly mild; it is not progressive and occurs with the first swallow of each meal. Dysphagia does not interfere with oral nutrition and does not produce weight loss. Careful assessment is required if a client reports progressive or persistent dysphagia, because this usually indicates the development of a stricture or cancer. The nurse assesses the following:
- The degree of dysphagia
- Whether dysphagia occurs with the ingestion of solids, liquids, or both
- Whether dysphagia is intermittent or occurs with each swallowing effort

Odynophagia (painful swallowing) is a possible symptom of GERD but is relatively rare in people with uncomplicated reflux disease. Severe and long-lasting chest pain may be present if spasms occurring in the esophagus cause the muscle to contract with excess force. The resulting pain can be agonizing and last for hours.

OTHER CLINICAL MANIFESTATIONS. Eructation (belching), flatulence (gas), or bloating after eating are other common complaints. Nausea and vomiting occur infrequently, and unplanned weight loss is rare.

■ RADIOGRAPHIC ASSESSMENT

No single test is considered to be a gold standard for diagnosing GERD. A barium swallow can be used to rule out complications associated with GERD or to evaluate dysphagia, but it is not sensitive enough to be diagnostic. The most accurate method of diagnosing gastroesophageal reflux disease (GERD) is 24-hour pH monitoring; this involves placing pH probes 2 inches (5 cm) above the lower esophageal sphincter (LES). A barium swallow with fluoroscopy then outlines the structure of the esophagus and its peristaltic patterns. Twenty-four hour ambulatory pH monitoring is widely used but is helpful only in evaluating acid reflux. Endoscopy is useful in diagnosing or evaluating reflux esophagitis or in monitoring complications such as Barrett's esophagus. During endoscopy, tissue samples can be obtained for biopsy, and strictures can be dilated (see Chapter 53).

■ OTHER DIAGNOSTIC ASSESSMENT

The health care provider orders esophageal manometry, or motility testing, when the diagnosis is uncertain. Water-filled catheters are inserted via the client's nose or mouth and are connected to transducers that record pressures from various sites in the esophagus as the catheters are withdrawn. Manometry quantifies the resting pressure of the LES and helps to evaluate sphincter competence, but when used alone it is not sensitive or specific enough to establish a diagnosis of GERD.

In Bernstein's test, an acidic solution is infused via a tube inserted into the distal esophagus. Clients with normal esophageal mucosa experience no symptoms when acid is infused, but clients with esophagitis experience immediate heartburn.

Scintigraphy involves preloading the stomach with a liquid radioisotope via the mouth or a tube. Scintillation counts are performed over the lower esophagus and are compared with counts obtained over the stomach. If a client is experiencing frequent reflux, the radioisotope will be refluxed back into the esophagus, which significantly elevates the scintillation counts over the lower esophageal region. Scintigraphy may be used in conjunction with pH monitoring.

● Interventions

Interventions begin with thorough teaching that GERD is a chronic condition that warrants ongoing management. This knowledge base is essential for a client's understanding of and adherence to the prescribed regimen of drugs, diet therapy, and lifestyle modifications.

NONSURGICAL MANAGEMENT. The goals of treatment for GERD are the relief of symptoms, treatment of esophagitis, and prevention of complications such as strictures or Barrett's esophagus. Although GERD can be controlled by diet therapy, education, lifestyle changes, and drug therapy, it is important to note that, even after the esophagitis is healed, 40% to 80% of clients relapse in 6 months after their medication is discontinued.

DIET THERAPY. Diet therapy is used to relieve symptoms in clients with relatively mild GERD. In collaboration with the dietitian, the nurse explores the client's basic meal patterns and food preferences. The nurse and dietitian work with both the client and the family to plan modifications that may decrease reflux symptoms. For adherence at home to be successful, it is essential that family members who do the shopping and cooking be included in this discussion.

In conjunction with the dietitian, the nurse counsels the client to limit or eliminate foods that decrease LES pressure. The client should also restrict spicy and acidic foods (e.g., orange juice, tomatoes) until esophageal healing can occur, because these foods irritate the inflamed tissue and cause heartburn (Goldsmith, 1998).

Because large meals increase the volume of and pressure in the stomach and delay gastric emptying, the nurse or dietitian instructs the client to eat four to six small meals each day rather than three large ones. Carbonated beverages should also be avoided because they increase pressure in the stomach. Clients are encouraged to avoid evening snacks and to eat no food for at least 3 hours before going to bed, because reflux episodes are most damaging at night. Clients may have the most difficulty adhering to the restriction of evening snacks. The nurse also advises the client to eat slowly and chew thoroughly to facilitate digestion and prevent eructation (belching). The client is encouraged to investigate which particular diet changes best reduce the frequency and severity of symptoms.

CLIENT EDUCATION. The nurse educates the client about the risk factors for the development of reflux, including contributing lifestyle factors. Lifestyle factors that can exacerbate the disease are reviewed, and the client is counseled on ways to eliminate them. The nurse also educates the client regarding the need for ongoing monitoring, particularly if the client has developed strictures, ulcerations, or Barrett's esophagus.

LIFESTYLE CHANGES. The control of GERD involves some lifestyle adjustments on the part of the client. For example, he or she is instructed to elevate the head of the bed by 8 to 12 inches for sleep to prevent nighttime reflux. In addition, he or she is instructed to sleep in the left lateral decubitus position to minimize the effects of nighttime episodes of reflux (see the Evidence-Based Practice for Nursing box below). Nighttime reflux is extremely common, and infrequent swallowing in combination with a recumbent position significantly impairs esophageal clearance. Although wooden blocks have traditionally been recommended to elevate the head of the bed, foam wedges may also achieve satisfactory results. The client or the client's spouse or partner may find elevation of the bed unacceptable at first. The nurse emphasizes the importance of this intervention and investigates all possible approaches for achieving compliance (Chart 55-2).

For clients with a history of smoking, the nurse explores the possibility and means of smoking cessation and makes the appropriate referrals. The nurse explains that smoking causes a prompt and significant drop in LES pressure and optimally should be stopped. The nurse also explores the client's normal pattern and amount of alcoholic beverage use. The client is taught about the effects of alcohol on LES sphincter pressure. The nurse can assist the client in finding appropriate alcohol cessation programs if needed.

EVIDENCE-BASED PRACTICE
FOR NURSING

What sleeping position would be most beneficial for clients with gastroesophageal reflux disease?

Khoury, R., et al. (1999). Influence of spontaneous sleep positions on nighttime recumbent reflux in patients with gastroesophageal reflux disease. *The American Journal of Gastroenterology, 94*(8), 2069-2073.

The purpose of this study was to investigate the influence of body position during sleep on recumbent reflux in 10 clients with gastroesophageal reflux disease. The 10 subjects (3 female, 7 male) were fed a standardized, high-fat dinner and bedtime snack. A single-channel pH probe was placed 5 cm above the lower esophageal sphincter (LES) in each client to measure the percentage of reflux episodes (pH <4) that occurred during four sleeping positions. A body position sensor taped to the client's sternum recorded spontaneous changes in posture during sleep.

The right lateral position was associated with the greatest percentage of time the pH remained under 4 and longer esophageal acid clearance when compared to the left, supine, and prone positions. The supine position resulted in a greater overall number of gastroesophageal reflux episodes that occurred within 1 minute of assuming this position. This study determined that the preferred sleeping position for clients with gastroesophageal reflux is the left lateral position.

Critique. Although the sample size was small, this was the first study to examine the effects of sleeping positions on recumbent reflux in clients with gastroesophageal reflux.

Implications for Nursing. Previous research supports the theory that body position influences gastroesophageal reflux. Nurses can incorporate information concerning sleeping position into their teaching plan for clients faced with damaging nighttime reflux. In addition to elevating the head of the bed, clients can be instructed to lie in the left lateral position for sleep to reduce the number of reflux episodes and the length of time the esophageal mucosa is exposed to acidic contents.

CHART 55-2

CLIENT EDUCATION GUIDE
Lifestyle Modifications to Control Reflux

- Eat four to six small meals a day.
- Limit or eliminate fatty foods, coffee, tea, cola, and chocolate.
- Reduce or eliminate from your diet any food or spice that causes pain.
- Limit or eliminate alcohol and tobacco.
- Do not snack in the evening, and take no food for 2 to 3 hours before you go to bed.
- Eat slowly, and chew your food thoroughly to reduce belching.
- Remain upright for 1 to 2 hours after meals, if possible.
- Elevate the head of your bed 8 to 12 inches using wooden blocks or a foam wedge. Never sleep flat in bed.
- If you are overweight, lose weight.
- Do not wear constrictive clothing.
- Avoid heavy lifting, straining, and working in a bent-over position.

If the client is obese, the nurse collaborates with the dietitian to examine approaches to weight reduction. Decreasing intra-abdominal pressure often reduces reflux symptoms.

Other lifestyle factors cause increased abdominal pressure, and the nurse explores these with the client. Wearing constrictive clothing, lifting heavy objects or straining, and working in a bent-over or stooped position should be avoided. The nurse emphasizes that these general adaptations are an essential and effective component of disease management and can produce prompt results in uncomplicated cases.

DRUG THERAPY. Some medications can cause reflux. Therefore the nurse, in conjunction with the primary health care provider, explores the possibility of eliminating from the client's regimen those medications implicated in reflux. Three principles guide drug therapy for gastroesophageal reflux: (1) to inhibit gastric acid secretion, (2) to accelerate gastric emptying, and (3) to protect the gastric mucosa (Chart 55-3).

Antacids. In uncomplicated cases of GERD, antacids are effective for occasional episodes of heartburn. Antacids act by elevating the pH level of the gastric contents, thereby deactivating pepsin. They are inadequate for the control of frequent symptoms because their duration of action is too short and their nighttime effectiveness is minimal.

Antacids containing aluminum hydroxide or magnesium hydroxide may be used. Maalox and Mylanta consist of a combination of these two agents, and clients often tolerate them better because they produce fewer side effects such as constipation and diarrhea. The nurse instructs the client to take the antacid 1 hour before and 2 to 3 hours after each meal. Some antacids are prepared as double-strength (DS) suspensions or tablets. The advantage of DS preparations is that the client can take a smaller amount of the drug. For example, 30 mL of regular Mylanta equals 15 mL of Mylanta-II (DS preparation).

Gaviscon, a combination of aluminum hydroxide and magnesium carbonate, is a commonly used and very effective medication for GERD. It forms a viscous foam that floats on top of the gastric contents and theoretically decreases the incidence of reflux. If reflux occurs, the foam enters the esophagus first and buffers the acid in the refluxed material. The nurse reminds the client to take this drug when food is in the stomach.

Histamine Receptor Antagonists. Histamine blockers, such as famotidine (Pepcid), ranitidine (Zantac), cimetidine (Tagamet), and nizatidine (Axid) are the main pharmacologic means of inhibiting gastric acid secretion. With histamine receptor antagonists available over the counter (OTC) and widely advertised for heartburn, many clients self-medicate before seeking professional assistance from their health care provider. When clients who have self-medicated with OTC preparations experience uncontrolled symptoms, the health care provider usually prescribes a *higher* dose of a histamine receptor antagonist.

Cimetidine (Tagamet) is not used as often as the longer-acting preparations. It has an inhibitory effect on the elimination of certain other medications, and therefore significant drug interactions can occur in clients taking warfarin, theophylline, phenytoin, nifedipine, or propranolol. Ranitidine and the other preparations are longer acting, and less frequent dosing is necessary. They also appear to produce fewer side effects and are safe for long-term administration. Although these drugs do not affect the occurrence of reflux directly, they do reduce gastric acid secretion, provide symptomatic improvement, and support healing of the inflamed esophageal tissue.

The proton pump inhibitors, such as omeprazole (Prilosec), lansoprazole (Prevacid), and rabeprazole (Aciphex), demonstrate effective, long-acting inhibition of gastric acid secretion. They are typically reserved for the treatment of severe GERD that is refractory to treatment with histamine blockers, and they play an important role in maintaining the remission of both GERD and Barrett's esophagus. These potent drugs can reduce gastric acid secretion by about 90% over a 24-hour period and can be given in a single daily dose. If once-a-day dosing fails to control symptoms, twice-a-day dosing is appropriate (Sharma, 1999). For example, omeprazole (Prilosec) is usually prescribed as a 20-mg oral dose once a day for 4 to 8 weeks. Complete healing of esophagitis is seen in 80% to 97% of clients (Tucker & Schumann, 1999). Proton pump inhibitors promote rapid tissue healing, but recurrence is common when the drug is stopped.

Other Drugs. Prokinetic drugs are used to accelerate gastric emptying and improve lower esophageal sphincter (LES) pressure and esophageal peristalsis. The health care provider may add bethanechol (Urecholine) or metoclopramide (Reglan) to the drug regimen for clients who experience severe and ongoing symptoms of reflux.

Bethanechol is a cholinergic drug; it increases the secretion of gastric acid and usually requires the simultaneous administration of a histamine receptor antagonist and antacids. Bethanechol is usually prescribed in 25-mg doses four times a day. The nurse teaches the client to take bethanechol 30 to 60 minutes before meals and warns the client about the typical side effects, which include abdominal cramping, diarrhea, increased salivation, and urinary urgency.

The primary action of metoclopramide is to increase the rate of gastric emptying. It does not affect gastric acid secretion or directly heal esophageal tissue. Its use is also associated with a high incidence of neurologic and psychotropic side effects such as fatigue, anxiety, ataxia, and hallucinations. Long-term use is not recommended.

SURGICAL MANAGEMENT. Antireflux surgery is usually indicated for otherwise healthy clients who have failed to respond to medical treatment or to demonstrate complications related to GERD or for whom the cost of long-term drug ther-

CHART 55-3

DRUG THERAPY *for* Gastroesophageal Reflux Disease (GERD)

Drug	Usual Dosage	Nursing Interventions	Rationale
Antacids, either aluminum or magnesium salts	30 mL PO between meals and as needed (PRN) throughout the day and at bedtime	Give 1 hr before meals, 2-3 hr after meals, and at bedtime. Give prn as instructed by physician. Observe the client for constipation or diarrhea. Suggest the use of combination mixtures or alternating use of aluminum and magnesium products.	Antacids neutralize acid and produce prompt relief of heartburn. Aluminum products produce constipation, and magnesium products induce diarrhea. Balancing their effects is important for client adherence.
Gaviscon, antacid plus alginic acid	1 tablet or 10-20 mL PO throughout the day and at bedtime	Give after meals and at bedtime.	Alginic acid forms a viscous foam that floats on top of the gastric contents, impeding reflux or buffering its effects when it occurs.
Histamine receptor antagonists		Instruct the client to take the drug with meals.	These drugs dramatically suppress gastric acid secretion and promote healing.
Cimetidine (Tagamet)	300 mg qid PO or 900-1200 mg PO at bedtime	Observe the client for side effects; fatigue, headache, and diarrhea are common. Instruct client about potential toxicity with some medications.	
Ranitidine (Zantac)	150 mg bid PO	Administer with meals and at bedtime.	Ranitidine and famotidine are more potent, longer-acting drugs, yet they produce fewer side effects.
Famotidine (Pepcid)	40 mg PO daily or 20 mg bid PO		
Nizatidine (Axid)	150 mg bid PO	Use cautiously and in reduced dosages in clients with renal disease. Observe for dysrhythmias. Do not mix with tomato-based, mixed-vegetable juices; apple juice is the preferred choice.	Clients need an adequate creatinine clearance to prevent drug toxicity. Dysrhythmias are common adverse effects of the drug. This drug may be less potent when mixed with tomato-based, mixed-vegetable juices.
Bethanechol (Urecholine)	25 mg qid PO	Instruct the client to take the drug 30-60 min before meals. Continue with antacids and histamine receptor antagonists as ordered. Observe the client for typical side effects: abdominal cramping, diarrhea, urinary urgency, and increased salivation. Counsel the client about the control of side effects.	This drug increases lower esophageal sphincter (LES) pressure and increases the rate of esophageal clearance. Bethanecol has cholinergic effects and increases the secretion of gastric acid. Typical associated cholinergic effects occur with the use of bethanechol.
Metoclopramide (Reglan)	10 mg tid or qid PO	Instruct the client to take the drug before meals. Teach the client to report any neurologic or psychotropic side effects, such as restlessness, anxiety, ataxia, or hallucinations.	This drug increases the rate of gastric emptying. Long-term drug use produces adverse effects in up to one third of clients.
Omeprazole (Prilosec, Losec✚)	20-30 mg PO daily	Instruct the client to take the drug before meals. Observe the client for typical side effects: abdominal cramping, diarrhea, headache.	Gastric acid suppression is greater than 90%. Action is prolonged, but gastrointestinal effects are severe in some clients.
Lansoprazole (Prevacid)	15 mg PO daily for gastroesophageal reflux disease (GERD) Up to 60 mg PO for gastrointestinal ulcers or Zollinger-Ellison syndrome	Instruct the client to take the drug before meals. For the client who has difficulty swallowing or has a nasogastric tube, open the capsule and mix granules in apple juice (or applesauce if not tube fed).	Same as above. The drug is safe to administer by opening (not crushing) the capsule.

apy is prohibitive. Various surgical procedures may be used. The three major surgical procedures are Nissen fundoplication, the Hill repair, and the Belsey repair (Figure 55-1).

In each of these procedures, the surgeon wraps and sutures the gastric fundus around the esophagus, which anchors the LES area below the diaphragm and reinforces the high-pressure area. For a more complete description of the three major procedures, see Operative Procedures (Hiatal Hernia), p. 1202.

The Client Care Plan on pp. 1199 and 1200 outlines the nursing care of clients undergoing esophageal surgery. Clients who have surgery are encouraged to continue following the basic antireflux regimen of antacids and diet therapy, because the rate of recurrence is significant.

Placement of the synthetic Angelchik prosthesis is also used for clients with severe reflux. This surgical procedure is associated with fewer long-term problems with achalasia (failure of the lower esophageal muscles and sphincter to relax properly). The surgeon performs a laparotomy and ties a C-shaped silicone prosthesis filled with gel around the distal esophagus (Figure 55-2). The prosthesis anchors the LES in the abdomen and reinforces sphincter pressure. Dysphagia is the primary complication of this procedure.

HIATAL HERNIA

■ OVERVIEW

The esophageal hiatus is the opening in the diaphragm through which the esophagus passes from the thorax to the abdomen. **Hiatal hernias,** also called diaphragmatic hernias, involve the protrusion of the stomach through the esophageal hiatus of the diaphragm into the thorax. Clients with hiatal hernias may be completely asymptomatic or may experience daily symptoms similar to those of clients with GERD.

■ Pathophysiology

The two major types of hiatal hernias are sliding hernias and paraesophageal (rolling) hernias.

■ SLIDING HERNIA

Sliding hernias are the most common type of hernia and account for 90% of the total number of hiatal hernias. The esophagogastric junction and a portion of the fundus of the stomach slide upward through the esophageal hiatus into the thorax (Figure 55-3). The hernia generally moves freely and slides into and out of the thorax during changes in position or intra-abdominal pressure. Although volvulus (twisting) and obstruction do occur rarely, the major concern in a client with a sliding hernia is the development of esophageal reflux and its complications. The development of reflux appears to be related to chronic exposure of the lower esophageal sphincter (LES) to the low pressure of the thorax, which significantly reduces the effectiveness of the LES. Symptoms associated with LES pressure are worsened by positions that favor reflux, such as bending or lying supine.

■ ROLLING HERNIA

With paraesophageal hernias, the gastroesophageal junction remains in its normal intra-abdominal location, but the fundus

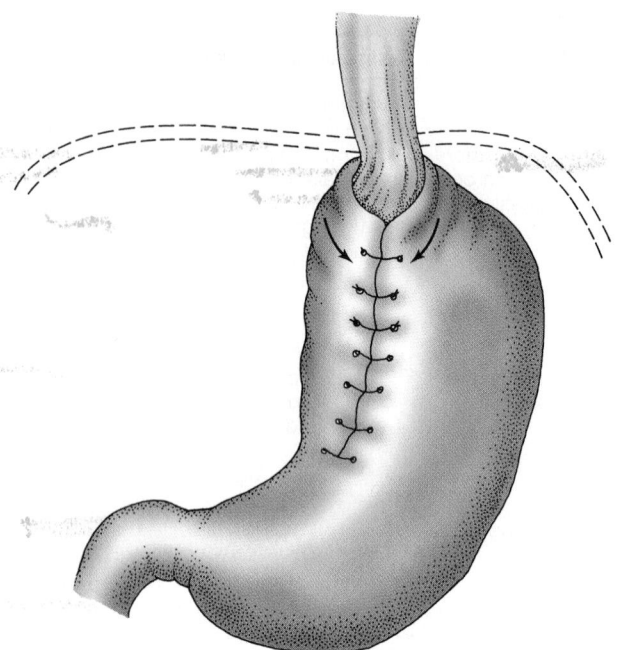

Figure 55-1 ● Nissen fundoplication for gastroesophageal reflux disease or hiatal hernia repair.

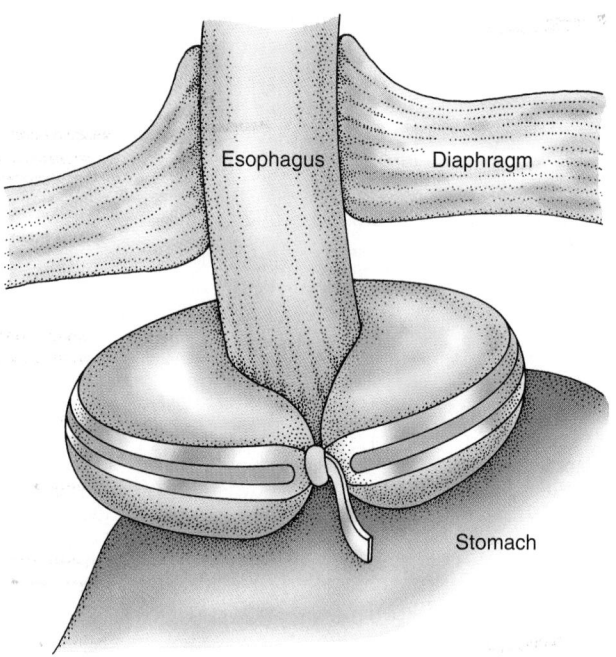

Figure 55-2 ● Placement of the Angelchik antireflux prosthesis.

(and possibly portions of the stomach's greater curvature) roll through the esophageal hiatus and into the thorax beside the esophagus (see Figure 55-3). The herniated portion of the stomach may be small or quite large; in rare cases, the stomach completely inverts into the thorax. Reflux is rarely a concern because the LES remains anchored below the diaphragm, but the risks of volvulus, obstruction, and strangulation are high. The development of iron deficiency anemia is common, because slow bleeding secondary to venous obstruction causes the gastric mucosa

NURSING DIAGNOSIS NO. 1 • Risk for Infection related to surgical incision

Expected Outcomes	Nursing Interventions	Rationale
The client will manifest no signs or symptoms of infection.	Do not reposition or replace the nasogastric tube. Do not perform endotracheal suctioning on a client with esophageal anastomosis or repair.	Moving the tube can cause trauma, which could puncture or irritate the incision; trauma to the area might open a potential route of infection.
	Encourage the client to suction or expectorate oral secretions rather than swallow them.	Clients are kept on nothing by mouth (NPO) status to avoid active peristalsis.
	Assess the cutaneous suture line for redness, drainage, and other signs of infection. Observe the dressing for bleeding; document and report any findings to the physician.	Monitor the client to detect complications and early signs of infection as soon as possible.
	Clean sutures once each shift with half-strength peroxide; dry the area and apply a small amount of antibacterial ointment.	Cleaning removes crusts and secretions, which could be an ideal media for bacterial growth.
	Monitor vital signs per the physician's orders. **D**	Monitoring provides early detection of and intervention for hemorrhage or infection.
	Document and report any significant changes to the physician.	

NURSING DIAGNOSIS NO. 2 • Risk for Imbalanced Nutrition: Less than Body Requirements related to NPO status and surgical disruption of the esophagus

The client will maintain adequate nutritional intake by nasogastric tube until oral feedings are begun.	Remind the client of NPO status when he or she is alert. **D**	Older clients may demonstrate memory deficit; clients are often on NPO status until the intraoral incision is healed.
	Monitor IV hydration while the client is on NPO status and before tube feedings are begun; monitor and record intake and output every shift.	Monitor hydration status for overload or retention; older clients are often susceptible to overload of fluids.
	Assess and document bowel sounds every shift until tube feedings are well tolerated.	Establish a baseline for bowel sounds; the return of bowel sounds postoperatively is often an indication to begin tube feedings.
	Measure and record the client's weight daily. **D**	Weight gives information on fluid status.
	Maintain proper functioning of the nasogastric tube; while it is attached to suction, measure and record drainage every shift. When tube feedings are begun, flush the tube carefully with water after each feeding or medication administration.	Monitor and maintain patency to permit drainage and to allow a route for the administration of medications and nutrition.
	Elevate the head of the bed 30 degrees at rest and 90 degrees for feeding and for ½ hr after feeding.	Raising the head helps prevent reflux; the incidence of reflux is greatest during and ½ hr after tube feedings.
	Provide the client with written and oral instructions regarding tube feedings.	Written and oral instructions provide the client with resources when the nurse is not available.
	Include the family/significant other in all teaching.	Including loved ones ensures support for the client to perform the procedures.
	Have the client give a return demonstration of the procedure.	A return demonstration aids in retention of the learned procedure and provides a means of evaluation for the nurse.
	When oral fluids are begun, assess and document swallowing difficulties, aspiration, or leakage, including signs of increased pulse rate, increased temperature, increased respiratory rate, subcutaneous emphysema, or a change in chest tube drainage indicating contamination from the gastrointestinal tract.	Clients occasionally have difficulty swallowing after esophageal surgery; assessment provides documentation of a real or perceived difficulty. The nurse observes carefully for signs of leakage from the esophageal anastomosis site or from a perforation.
	If the client is experiencing difficulty in swallowing, consult a speech-language pathologist for assessment or assistance in swallowing.	Speech-language pathologists are often experts at evaluating swallowing disorders; providing the client with techniques of head positioning, breath holding, or oral exercises can help overcome minor swallowing difficulties.
	Collaborate with the dietitian as appropriate.	A change in food consistency often eases swallowing difficulties.
	Observe the client for any epigastric burning, retrosternal or back pain, or pain radiating to the chin or shoulder indicative of esophageal reflux; document any findings.	Esophageal reflux, once documented, can be treated by positioning the client or dietary changes; analgesics may be required before mealtimes.

D Indicates tasks that can be delegated to assistive nursing personnel.

Continued

𝒞LIENT 𝒞ARE 𝒫LAN • THE CLIENT UNDERGOING TRADITIONAL OPEN ESOPHAGEAL SURGERY—cont'd

NURSING DIAGNOSIS NO. 3 • Acute Pain related to incision; Chronic Pain related to reflux

Expected Outcomes	Nursing Interventions	Rationale
The client will verbalize control of pain, facilitating adequate nutritional intake and participation in activities of daily living.	Assess and document the level of pain, relying on subjective and objective symptoms of pain and pain relief. Assess and document the relief obtained from the analgesic regimen.	Clients are often unwilling to demonstrate evidence of pain and often are unwilling to use analgesics, particularly opioids, as often as prescribed.
	Assess the client for pain related to esophageal reflux or perforation: epigastric burning; pain radiating to the shoulder, chin, or back; change in vital signs; change in character of chest tube drainage (if present); subcutaneous emphysema. Document and report all findings to the physician.	Early detection of esophageal perforation is imperative to begin effective treatment; documentation of reflux communicates to other health care workers the need to prevent reflux aspiration.
	Instruct the client to keep the head of the bed raised 30 degrees at all times and 90 degrees at meals and for ½ hr after meals. **D**	Raising the head of the bed not only reduces edema by facilitating gravity drainage but also facilitates food passage and prevents esophageal reflux.
	Explore dietary modifications with the client to alleviate discomfort related to reflux.	Smaller, more frequent meals with a change in food consistency can reduce the discomfort associated with reflux.
	Explore various positioning changes to facilitate food passage and alleviate symptoms of reflux.	Varying the positions assumed while eating and after eating can reduce the discomfort associated with reflux or dysphagia.
	Instruct the client to use analgesic medication ½ hr before meals, chest physiotherapy, and other treatments as needed.	Ensuring a peak analgesic effect during activities that the client reports as being most uncomfortable can increase compliance with those activities and efforts to obtain adequate nutritional intake.
	Instruct the client and family/significant other about the timing, side effects, and restrictions of the prescribed medications; provide written and oral instructions.	Written and oral instructions are given because the client may have memory loss.
	Instruct the client to monitor his or her own comfort.	The client gains a feeling of control concerning discomfort.

D Indicates tasks that can be delegated to assistive nursing personnel.

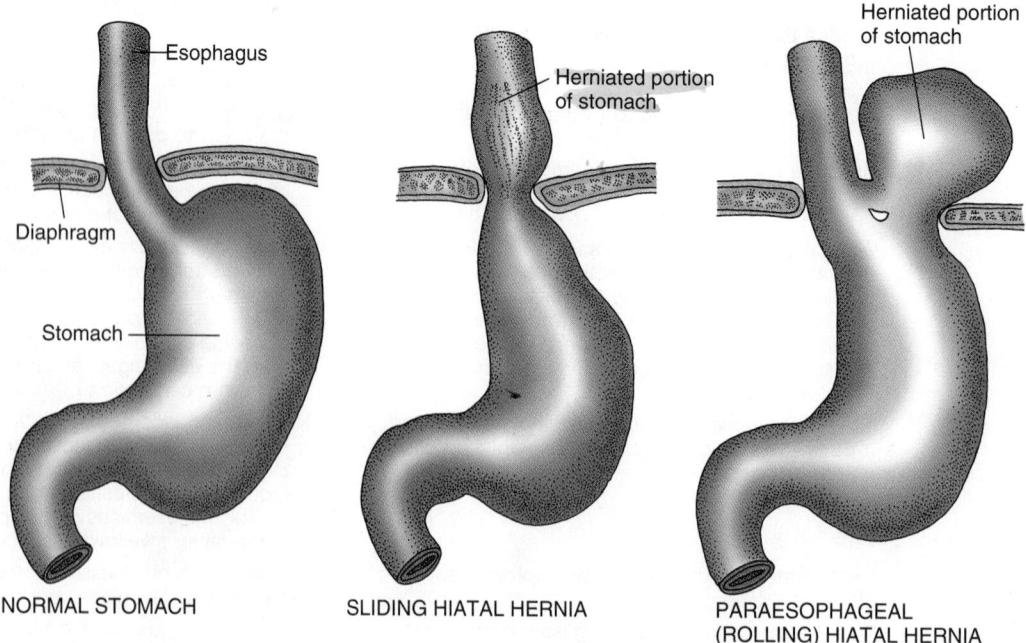

NORMAL STOMACH SLIDING HIATAL HERNIA PARAESOPHAGEAL (ROLLING) HIATAL HERNIA

Figure 55-3 ● A comparison of the normal stomach and sliding and paraesophageal (rolling) hiatal hernias.

to become engorged and ooze. Significant bleeding or hemorrhage is rare.

Etiology

Sliding hiatal hernias are believed to develop from muscle weakening in the esophageal hiatus, which loosens the esophageal supports and permits the lower portion of the esophagus to rise into the thorax. Congenital weaknesses, trauma, obesity, or surgery may also play a significant role. The development of the hernia is the result of the combined effects of weakened support structures and prolonged increases in abdominal pressure.

Muscle weakening does not appear to cause paraesophageal hernias. Instead, it is theorized that the stomach is not properly anchored below the diaphragm, and the hernia results from an anatomic defect rather than a structural weakness. Paraesophageal hernias can also be caused by previous esophageal surgeries, including sliding hernia repair.

Incidence/Prevalence

Hiatal hernia is one of the more common disorders that affect the upper gastrointestinal tract, and it affects women more often than men. Hiatal hernias have been reported in up to 20% of adults (Crawford, 1999).

CONSIDERATIONS FOR OLDER ADULTS
The incidence of sliding hiatal hernias increases with age in both genders and reaches a prevalence of approximately 60% in the sixth decade of life. As many as 80% of clients with hiatal hernias are asymptomatic or experience only mild, transient symptoms associated with reflux.

► COLLABORATIVE MANAGEMENT
Assessment

The nurse carefully assesses for heartburn, regurgitation, pain, dysphagia, and belching. An assessment of the client's general physical appearance and nutritional status is also included. The nurse notes the location, onset, duration, quality, and aggravating and alleviating factors associated with the presence of pain. The primary symptoms of sliding hiatal hernias are associated with reflux. The nurse auscultates the thorax and lungs, as pulmonary symptoms similar to asthma may be triggered by episodes of aspiration, particularly at night. A detailed history is crucial in attempting to differentiate angina from noncardiac chest pain due to gastroesophageal reflux. Symptoms resulting from hiatal hernia typically worsen after a meal or when the client is in a recumbent position (Chart 55-4).

In clients with paraesophageal (rolling) hernias, the nurse assesses for symptoms related to the stretching or displacement of thoracic contents by the hernia. Clients may report a feeling of fullness after eating and may even experience breathlessness or a feeling of suffocation if the hernia interferes with breathing. Some clients experience chest pain associated with reflux that mimics angina.

The barium swallow study with fluoroscopy is the most specific diagnostic test for identifying hiatal hernia. Paraesophageal hernias are usually clearly visible, and sliding hernias can often be observed as the client is moved through a series of positions that increase intra-abdominal pressure.

CHART 55-4

KEY FEATURES *of*
Hernias

Sliding Hiatal Hernias
- Heartburn
- Regurgitation
- Chest pain
- Dysphagia
- Belching

Paraesophageal Hernias
- Feeling of fullness after eating
- Breathlessness after eating
- Feeling of suffocation
- Chest pain that mimics angina
- Worsening of manifestations in a recumbent position

Clients with sliding hernias usually experience symptoms of reflux. Therefore any or all of the diagnostic tests used for gastroesophageal reflux disease (GERD) may be used to fully evaluate the extent of reflux and the degree of esophageal damage (see Other Diagnostic Assessment [GERD], p. 1194).

Interventions

Clients with hiatal hernias may be managed either medically or surgically. The health care provider's choice of management is based on the severity of the client's symptoms and the risk of serious complications. Sliding hiatal hernias are most commonly treated medically. Large paraesophageal hernias can become strangulated or obstructed; therefore early surgical repair is encouraged.

NONSURGICAL MANAGEMENT. The interventions for clients with hiatal hernia closely follow those outlined for clients with GERD and include drug therapy, diet therapy, lifestyle modifications, and client education. The health care provider typically prescribes antacids and histamine receptor antagonists, such as ranitidine (Zantac), in an attempt to control reflux and its symptoms.

Diet therapy is also an integral part of the conservative management of hiatal hernia and follows the guidelines discussed earlier for GERD, p. 1195. The client is encouraged to avoid eating in the late evening and to avoid foods associated with reflux. In collaboration with the dietitian, the nurse works with the client to modify the diet to reduce body weight (if appropriate), because obesity increases intra-abdominal pressure and worsens both the hernia and the symptoms of reflux.

The nurse carefully explains the underlying condition to increase the client's understanding of the disorder and increase adherence to the treatment regimen. Teaching about positioning, as described earlier for GERD (p. 1195) is also extremely important. It is essential that clients:

- Sleep at night with the head of the bed elevated 8 to 12 inches
- Remain upright for several hours after eating
- Avoid straining or excessive vigorous exercise
- Refrain from wearing clothing that is tight or constrictive around the abdomen

SURGICAL MANAGEMENT. The physician usually schedules surgery when the risk of complications is high or when damage from chronic reflux becomes severe.

PREOPERATIVE CARE. If the surgery is not urgent, the surgeon encourages clients who are overweight to lose weight before surgery. Clients are advised to quit or significantly reduce smoking. As part of preoperative teaching, the nurse reinforces the surgeon's instructions and prepares the client for the postoperative course.

Before developing the teaching plan, the nurse must know which surgical approach is planned. For the thoracic surgical approach, for example, the client is taught about chest tubes. The nurse also informs the client that a nasogastric tube will be inserted during surgery and will remain in place for several days. Oral intake is started gradually with clear liquids after peristalsis is re-established, or to stimulate peristalsis. The nurse also instructs the client about techniques for effective deep breathing and use of the incentive spirometer. These measures are essential to prevent postoperative respiratory complications. The high incision makes deep breathing extremely painful for the client. The nurse educates the client concerning the aspects of postoperative pain and assures the client that adequate postoperative analgesia will be administered.

OPERATIVE PROCEDURES. Although several hiatal hernia repair procedures are in use, each involves reinforcement of the lower esophageal sphincter (LES) through some degree of fundoplication. The surgeon wraps a portion of the stomach fundus around the distal esophagus to anchor it and reinforce the LES. The eventual recurrence for either type of hernia following surgical repair is 10% to 15% over 5 years (Ferguson, 1997).

The **Nissen repair** is the most commonly used procedure (see Figure 55-1) for hiatal hernia repair. An abdominal approach is usually chosen. The surgeon wraps the fundus a full 360 degrees around the lower esophagus. The sphincter reinforcement is tight and usually controls reflux effectively. Laparoscopic Nissen fundoplication (LNF) is a relatively new surgical technique that involves the creation of an antireflux valve or fundoplication laparoscopically through 5 ½-inch incisions in the abdomen. The fundus is then wrapped 360 degrees around the LES to strengthen it (Vaca et al., 1998).

In the Hill repair, an abdominal approach is also used, but the fundoplication is wrapped 180 degrees around the esophagus. The angle of His is restructured to accentuate the angle at which the esophagus enters the stomach. The Belsey repair usually involves a 280-degree esophageal wrap and uses a thoracic approach.

Surgeons do not agree about which surgical repair is most appropriate or effective, because each procedure has unique advantages and disadvantages. For example, the laparoscopic Nissen fundoplication is associated with all the risks of a major surgery; pneumonia, myocardial infarction, wound infection, and bleeding (Vaca et al., 1998).

POSTOPERATIVE CARE. Postoperative care following hiatal hernia repair closely follows that required after any esophageal surgery (see the Client Care Plan on pp. 1199 and 1200). The nurse carefully assesses for complications of fundoplication surgery and reports their occurrence to the physician (Chart 55-5).

Respiratory Care. The primary focus of postoperative care is the prevention of respiratory complications. The nurse or assistive nursing personnel elevates the head of the client's bed at least 30 degrees to lower the diaphragm and facilitate

---

CHART 55-5

BEST PRACTICE *for*
Assessment of Postoperative Complications Related to Fundoplication Procedures

COMPLICATION	ASSESSMENT FINDINGS
Temporary dysphagia	The client has difficulty swallowing when oral feeding begins.
Gas bloat syndrome	The client has difficulty belching to relieve distention.
Atelectasis, pneumonia	The client experiences dyspnea, chest pain, and/or fever.
Obstructed nasogastric tube	The client experiences nausea, vomiting, and/or abdominal distention. The nasogastric tube does not drain.

---

lung expansion. The client is assisted out of bed and is ambulated as soon as possible. The incision must be supported during coughing to reduce pain and to prevent excessive strain on the suture line, especially with obese clients.

Incentive spirometry and deep breathing are routinely used after surgery to maintain patency of the airways. Adequate analgesia is essential for client compliance and should be administered as needed. Clients with a smoking history or chronic airway limitation (chronic obstructive pulmonary disease, asthma) require more aggressive respiratory management by the respiratory therapist to prevent atelectasis and pneumonia. Clients with large hiatal hernias are at high risk for developing respiratory complications.

Nasogastric Tube Management. Postoperative management also involves the care of the nasogastric (NG) tube. Inserting a large-diameter NG tube during surgery prevents the fundoplication wrap from becoming too tight around the esophagus. The nasogastric drainage is initially dark brown with old blood but should become normal yellowish green within the first 8 hours after surgery. The nurse checks every 4 to 8 hours for proper placement of the tube in the stomach. The NG tube should be properly anchored so it cannot be displaced, because it cannot be safely reinserted without risking perforation of the incision.

Frequent assessment of the patency of the tube is essential to keep the stomach decompressed; this prevents retching or vomiting, which can strain or rupture the stomach sutures. Because the tube is irritating, the nurse or assistive nursing personnel provides frequent oral hygiene. The nurse also assesses the client's hydration status regularly, including accurate measures of intake and output. Adequate fluid replacement helps to thin respiratory secretions.

Nutritional Care. The client may begin oral intake with clear fluids after peristalsis is re-established or in an effort to stimulate peristalsis. Some surgeons create a temporary gastrostomy for feeding to allow for undisturbed healing of the repair. The client gradually progresses to a near-normal diet during the first 6 weeks. A few foods, such as caffeinated or carbonated beverages and alcohol, are either restricted or eliminated. The food storage area of the stomach is reduced by the surgery, and meals need to be both smaller and more frequent.

The nurse carefully supervises the first oral feedings, because temporary dysphagia is common. Persistent dysphagia usually indicates that the fundoplication is too tight, and dilation may be required.

Another common complication of fundoplication surgery is the gas bloat syndrome, in which clients are unable to voluntarily eructate (belch). The syndrome is usually temporary but may persist. The nurse teaches the client to avoid drinking carbonated beverages, eating gas-producing foods (especially high-fat foods), chewing gum, and drinking with a straw.

Many clients acquire the habit of aerophagia (air swallowing) from attempting to reverse or clear acid reflux. The nurse teaches these clients to consciously relax before and after meals, eat and drink slowly, and chew all food thoroughly.

Air in the stomach that cannot be removed by belching can be extremely uncomfortable. Frequent position changes and ambulation are effective interventions for eliminating air from the gastrointestinal tract.

● Community-Based Care

Clients undergoing one of the three major surgical repairs require activity restrictions during the 4- to 6-week postoperative recovery period. For laparoscopic surgery, activity is typically restricted for a shorter time, and the client can return to his or her usual lifestyle more quickly. For long-term management, the nurse teaches the client and family about appropriate diet modifications, but the use of stool softeners or bulk laxatives is recommended for the first postoperative weeks until healing is complete. The nurse instructs the client to avoid straining and prevent constipation.

The client is taught to inspect the healing incision daily and to notify the physician or health care provider if swelling, redness, tenderness, discharge, or fever occurs. The nurse advises the client to avoid contact with people with respiratory infections and to contact the physician if symptoms of a cold or influenza develop. Persistent coughing can cause the incision or the fundoplication to dehisce. The client is also advised to avoid smoking.

The nurse and dietitian educate the entire family or significant other about diet. Full support is essential for the client to successfully modify the size and timing of meals. Relatively few ongoing diet restrictions are needed, but overeating or eating the wrong types of foods can produce discomfort if the client cannot belch. The client avoids foods that produce discomfort, and the nurse encourages cautious experimentation with new foods. The nurse instructs the client to report the recurrence of reflux symptoms to the health care provider.

Although severe surgical complications are relatively rare, conditions such as gas bloat syndrome and dysphagia are common and may persist. The nurse helps the client prepare for these problems and for the potential that reflux may not be completely controlled or may occur again. Although surgery controls the condition, a cure is rare, and lifestyle modifications need to be ongoing.

ACHALASIA

▌ OVERVIEW

Achalasia is an esophageal motility disorder in which the lower esophageal sphincter (LES) fails to relax properly with swallowing and in which the normal peristalsis of the esophagus is replaced with abnormal contractions. It is characterized by chronic and progressive dysphagia. Regurgitation of ingested food may also occur, especially at night, resulting in

aspiration. If left untreated, progressive dysphagia can result in weight loss. Chest pain is experienced by one third of clients with the disorder.

Achalasia is thought to result from esophageal denervation (loss of nerve impulse passage). The exact cause of denervation is unknown. A genetic basis to the disorder has been proposed as suggested by occasional familial clustering and phenotype (observable characteristics) association.

Over time, peristaltic failure plus spasm can produce a massively dilated esophagus, which further slows food passage. Achalasia is an uncommon disorder that usually manifests itself in young adulthood. Both genders appear to be equally affected. Approximately 5% to 10% of individuals with this disorder develop esophageal squamous cell carcinoma (Crawford, 1999). Complications of achalasia also include esophageal candidiasis, lower esophageal diverticula, airway obstruction, and aspiration pneumonia.

➤ COLLABORATIVE MANAGEMENT
▌ Assessment

The nurse assesses for the primary symptoms of achalasia, such as dysphagia and regurgitation of solids, liquids, or both. The client is asked about the presence of chest pain associated with these symptoms.

Achalasia is often a chronic condition. The symptoms worsen over time, which poses an increased threat to health and functioning as the disorder progresses. The nurse questions the client about factors that aggravate the symptoms (e.g., body position or diet changes) as well as medications or home treatments that relieve the symptoms. The client is asked about a history of previous esophageal surgery or trauma, which compound the progressive dysphagia. Respiratory history and current respiratory-associated symptoms are particularly important with regard to their direct relationship to reflux, regurgitation, and aspiration.

To determine the effect of the esophageal symptoms, the nurse obtains a nutritional history, including dietary habits, food tolerances, and weight loss. The nurse also notes the presence of halitosis (foul mouth odor), which can be caused by the regurgitation of previously ingested food. The nurse auscultates the lungs for adventitious sounds secondary to pulmonary aspiration of retained saliva and food. The nurse or assistive nursing personnel weighs the client and compares this weight with the client's usual weight.

A chest x-ray study reveals a distorted and dilated tubular esophagus, the absence of a gastric air bubble and, occasionally, a tubular mediastinal mass next to the aorta. A barium swallow reveals esophageal dilation with a persistent beaklike narrowing at the terminal esophagus—the hallmark of a nonrelaxing LES. Esophageal manometry typically reveals an elevated resting LES pressure and incomplete sphincter relaxation when the client swallows. Endoscopy is used to evaluate the appearance of the esophageal mucosa, especially for changes associated with cancer or the presence of candida.

● Interventions

The symptoms associated with achalasia can be treated with a variety of approaches. A combination of dietary measures, pharmacologic agents, esophageal dilation and surgery are used.

DRUG AND DIET THERAPY. Mild cases of achalasia can be managed with calcium channel blockers or nitrates to reduce LES pressure. Drug therapy is given for symptom relief and is not recommended as an alternative to more definitive therapy.

The nurse advises the client to experiment with changes in diet because they can often ease the pressure and reflux associated with achalasia. The nurse discusses with the client any food habits he or she has noted that aggravate or relieve the symptoms. Semisoft foods are often better tolerated, as are warm foods and liquids. Eating four to six smaller meals rather than three large meals during the day facilitates the passage of food. The nurse collaborates with the dietitian for additional suggestions about diet changes and nutritional balance.

Nocturnal reflux of foods and liquids from the dilated esophagus into the hypopharynx and oral cavity often can be prevented if the client sleeps with the head of the bed elevated or in a semisitting position. The nurse also advises the client to experiment with various changes in position while eating, because such changes can reduce pressure sensations during meals. Some clients benefit from arching the back while swallowing. The nurse cautions the client to avoid wearing restrictive clothing, which can increase esophageal pressure and regurgitation.

ESOPHAGEAL DILATION. More severe cases of achalasia require dilation of the LES. The traditional treatment involves the passage of progressively larger sizes of esophageal bougies (dilators). Balloon dilation of the esophagus (using polyurethane balloons on a catheter) is considered the most effective treatment for achalasia. The procedure is performed on an ambulatory care basis. Typically, pneumatic dilators are positioned across the esophageal junction with fluoroscopy and local anesthesia. The balloon, which is filled with air or water, is inflated to a predetermined level for 30 to 60 seconds (Figure 55-4). This method lowers the basal LES pressure by tearing the esophageal sphincter muscle fibers.

After the procedure, the nurse monitors the client for bleeding and signs of perforation, such as chest and shoulder pain, elevated temperature, subcutaneous emphysema (air under the skin), or hemoptysis (coughing up blood). The client is taught to expectorate rather than swallow any secretions that may be produced. The client is also instructed to take nothing by mouth (NPO) for 1 hour and is instructed to limit dietary intake to liquids for 24 hours. The procedure may be repeated in 2 to 3 months if needed. Most clients report improvement in swallowing.

ESOPHAGOMYOTOMY. Surgical procedures for clients with achalasia are aimed at facilitating the passage of food. **Esophagomyotomy,** in which the LES is incised, has been used successfully for decades. Both thoracic and abdominal approaches can be used. An antireflux wrap (**fundoplication**) may or may not be part of the procedure.

Esophagomyotomy is a more complex surgical treatment for achalasia. General anesthesia is required, and the client is hospitalized for several days. A thoracotomy approach permits exposure of the esophagus. The surgeon cuts muscle fibers around the LES to open the sphincter and thereby provide less obstruction to food passage.

For long-term refractory achalasia, the surgeon may attempt excision of the affected portion of the esophagus, with

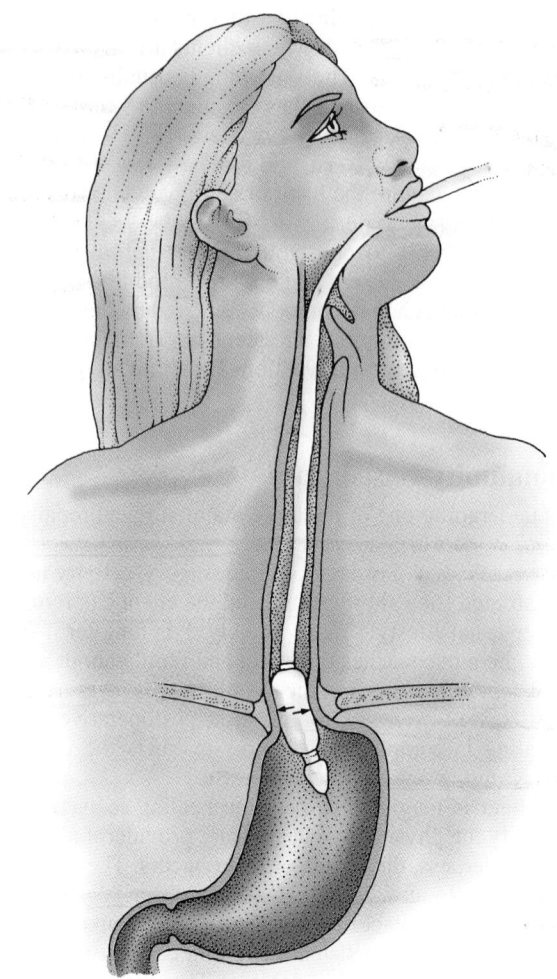

Figure 55-4 ● Balloon (pneumatic) dilation of the lower esophagus.

or without replacement by a segment of colon or jejunum (partial esophagectomy).

Postoperative care for clients undergoing esophagomyotomy or esophagectomy includes managing chest tubes and drains, assessing healing of the thoracotomy or abdominal incision, pain control, and managing nasogastric feedings. (See Chapter 19 for general postoperative care and Chapter 30 for care of the client with a thoracotomy.)

ESOPHAGEAL TUMORS

OVERVIEW

Tumors occurring in the esophagus can be benign or malignant. Benign tumors, usually in the form of leiomyomas, are extremely uncommon and are usually asymptomatic. No specific treatment is required unless they produce symptoms, and then they are generally removed.

Worldwide, esophageal cancer is the third most common gastrointestinal (GI) cancer and the eighth most common cancer (Parkin, Pisani, & Ferlay, 1999). A relatively uncommon cancer in the United States, it represents about 6% of all cancers of the GI tract, and mortality from the disease remains very high (Landis et al., 1999).

Pathophysiology

Most malignant esophageal tumors arise from the epithelium. Fifteen percent of all esophageal cancers are located in the upper esophagus and are primarily squamous cell in origin. Thirty-five percent of tumors appear in the mid-thoracic region and can be either squamous cell or adenocarcinomas. The lower esophagus is the site of approximately 50% of all esophageal cancers, primarily adenocarcinomas. The local and regional lymphatic spread of the disease differs according to the site of the original tumor. It has been proposed that esophageal cancers result from mutations in suppressor genes and proto-oncogenes (see Chapter 24 for a more complete discussion).

Esophageal tumors exhibit rapid local growth because there is no serosal layer to limit their extension. Because the esophageal mucosa is richly supplied with lymphatics, there is early spread of tumors to lymph nodes. Esophageal tumors can protrude into the esophageal lumen and either take on a flattened and infiltrative form to cause thickening of the lumen or manifest as a necrotic ulceration that invades deeply into surrounding tissue. In rare cases the lesion may be confined to the epithelial layer (in situ). In the majority of cases, the tumor is relatively large and well established on diagnosis.

Etiology

In the United States, the two primary risk factors associated with the development of squamous cell carcinoma of the esophagus are tobacco use and alcohol ingestion. The compounds in tobacco smoke may be responsible for the genetic mutations seen in one half of esophageal tumors. A smoker has two to six times the risk of eventually developing esophageal cancer than does a nonsmoker. Some alcoholic beverages contain potent carcinogens that may be responsible for the development of esophageal tumors. Smoking and alcohol ingestion act synergistically in the development of esophageal cancer.

Long-term exposure to gastric contents, such as that caused by gastroesophageal reflux disease (GERD), also plays a role in esophageal cancer development. Exposure to acid and pepsin leads to the replacement of normal distal squamous mucosa with columnar epithelium as a response to tissue injury, causing Barrett's disease or esophagus. This tissue undergoes dysplasia and, ultimately, malignant transformation.

In other parts of the world where esophageal cancer is common, the incidence of squamous cell carcinoma appears to be linked to high levels of nitrosamines (which are found in pickled and fermented foods) and foods high in nitrate. Diets that are chronically deficient in fresh fruits and vegetables have been implicated in the development of squamous cell carcinoma.

Certain genetic factors may have a role in the development of esophageal cancer. Overexpression and/or mutations of the p53 tumor suppressor gene have been found in esophageal cancer. In addition, the presence of the p53 gene may be an indication of advanced disease. Tumor cells with a mutated p53 gene have demonstrated resistance to chemotherapy.

Incidence/Prevalence

In the United States, cancer of the esophagus accounts for fewer than 1% of all newly diagnosed cancers and 6% of all tumors involving the gastrointestinal tract. In 1999 there was an estimated 316,000 new cases of esophageal cancer and 286,000 deaths worldwide (Parkin, Pisani, & Ferley, 1999). Although squamous cell cancer accounts for most cases, the rate of adenocarcinoma of the esophagus is also rapidly increasing. It is usually found at the gastroesophageal junction and the distal portion of the esophagus. The greatest incidence of adenocarcinoma can be found in Caucasian males of middle to upper socioeconomic status (Quinn & Reedy, 1999).

Esophageal cancer is extremely virulent and has a 5-year survival rate of less than 5%.

> **CULTURAL CONSIDERATIONS**
>
> Over the past several decades there have been statistically significant annual increases in the incidence of squamous cell cancer of the esophagus in the United States, particularly in African Americans. Mortality rates for esophageal cancer are now second only to those for cancer of the lung.
>
> The incidence of esophageal cancer is extremely high in areas of northwest China, the Caspian Sea (around Russia and Iran), Japan, and the Transkei region of southern Africa. In these groups, the disease is found primarily in the upper to middle esophageal area. Residents of some provinces in China have a 30% to 40% probability of dying from esophageal cancer. The causes of these extreme variations are being researched but have not been satisfactorily explained.

▶ COLLABORATIVE MANAGEMENT

● Assessment

■ HISTORY

The nurse assesses the client's racial and cultural background, age, sex, and any pertinent history of alcohol consumption, tobacco use, dietary habits, and other esophageal problems (e.g., dysphagia, stricture, or reflux). In collaboration with the dietitian, the nurse also collects a nutrition history, including the ingestion of pickled foods, changes in appetite, changes in taste, or a decline in weight. The degree of weight loss over time is also an important consideration.

Cancer of the esophagus is a silent tumor in its early stages, with few signs to identify on assessment. By the time the tumor causes symptoms, it usually has spread rather extensively.

■ PHYSICAL ASSESSMENT/CLINICAL MANIFESTATIONS

The primary clinical manifestations of esophageal cancer are dysphagia (most common) and weight loss (Brooks-Brunn, 2000). The nurse carefully assesses the degree and severity of dysphagia. Tumor-induced dysphagia is both persistent and progressive. It is initially associated with swallowing solids, particularly meat, and then progresses rapidly over a period of weeks or months to difficulty in swallowing soft foods and liquids. Late in the disease, even saliva can induce choking. Clients usually report a sensation that food is sticking in the throat or in the substernal area. Careful assessment of the dysphagia is an important part of the diagnosis because the dysphagia associated with other esophageal disorders is not usually continuous. Dysphagia does not usually appear until at least 60% of the esophageal diameter is narrowed by the tumor.

Odynophagia (painful swallowing) is present in most clients and is reported as a steady, dull, substernal pain that may radiate. The presence of severe or persistent pain often indicates tumor invasion of the mediastinal structures. The nurse also assesses for the occurrence of regurgitation, vomiting, foul breath, and chronic hiccups, which often accompany advanced disease. In most clients, pulmonary complications develop at some point, and the nurse assesses for the presence of chronic cough, increased secretions, and a history of recent infections.

Tumors in the upper esophagus may involve the larynx and thus cause hoarseness. Chart 55-6 summarizes the clinical manifestations of esophageal tumors.

■ PSYCHOSOCIAL ASSESSMENT

The symptoms and diagnosis of esophageal cancer can affect a client in profound ways. The disease produces significant daily symptoms, requires major modifications in basic eating patterns, and is terminal. The fear of choking can transform normal mealtimes into frightening experiences that the client may wish to avoid. The nurse carefully assesses the client's response to the diagnosis and prognosis and explores his or her coping strengths and resources. The impact of the disease on the usual pattern of activities is also assessed. The nurse also assesses the availability of support systems and the potential financial impact of the disease and its treatment.

■ RADIOGRAPHIC ASSESSMENT

To arrive at a diagnosis of esophageal cancer, the physician first uses a barium swallow study with fluoroscopy. The tumor margins of large masses can often be outlined during this test. A definitive diagnosis of cancer necessitates histologic evidence by means of a tissue biopsy.

■ OTHER DIAGNOSTIC ASSESSMENT

The definitive diagnosis of esophageal cancer is made by esophagogastroduodenoscopy (EGD) with biopsies of the esophagus and tumor. The physician performs an endoscopic examination to inspect the esophagus and to obtain specimens for cytologic studies and staging. Multiple tissue samples may be required when the suspected tumor is in the distal esophagus, because clear tissue samples are difficult to obtain.

A complete staging workup is performed to determine the extent of the disease. A computed tomography (CT) scan assists in identifying metastatic disease that can be present in the chest or abdomen. Positron emission tomography (PET) is a newer technology that may identify metastatic disease with more accuracy than a CT scan. Metastasis can also be diagnosed by bone and brain scans or exploratory laparoscopy. An endoscopic ultrasound (EUS) is a staging technique that can help determine the size and depth of tumor invasion. (These tests are described elsewhere in this text.)

> **CRITICAL THINKING CHALLENGE**
>
> You are gathering the initial history on a 65-year-old female Asian client admitted with dysphagia and a recent weight loss of 20 pounds over 3 months. The client states she used to smoke 2 packs of cigarettes per day for 30 years but quit 15 years ago. The client also admits to a 5-year history of gastrointestinal reflux, especially after eating in the late evening.
> * What lifestyle and cultural factors place this client at risk for esophageal cancer?
> * What specific questions would you ask concerning her swallowing difficulties?
> * What additional clinical manifestations should you inquire about?

For suggested answer guidelines, go to SIMON http://www.wbsaunders.com/SIMON/Iggy/.

▶ Analysis

■ COMMON NURSING DIAGNOSES AND COLLABORATIVE PROBLEMS

The priority nursing diagnosis for clients with cancer of the esophagus is Imbalanced Nutrition: Less than Body Requirements related to impaired swallowing.

■ ADDITIONAL NURSING DIAGNOSES AND COLLABORATIVE PROBLEMS

In addition to the common nursing diagnosis, the client with esophageal cancer may develop any of the following due to the impact of the disease and/or treatment:

* Risk for Aspiration related to impaired swallowing secondary to esophageal strictures
* Impaired Swallowing related to obstruction by the tumor or the effects of radiotherapy
* Acute Pain or Chronic Pain related to the pressure of the tumor mass in the esophagus or mediastinum
* Ineffective Coping and Compromised Family Coping related to the effects of the disease and to the terminal prognosis
* Anticipatory Grieving related to declining physical status and terminal prognosis
* Spiritual Distress related to impending death

The additional collaborative problem is Potential for Metastasis due to the close proximity of the esophagus to other body structures.

▶ Planning and Implementation

■ IMBALANCED NUTRITION: LESS THAN BODY REQUIREMENTS

NOC PLANNING: EXPECTED OUTCOMES. The major concern for a client with esophageal cancer is weight loss secondary to dysphagia. Therefore the client is expected to ingest

---

CHART 55-6
KEY FEATURES *of* **Esophageal Tumors**
• Persistent and progressive dysphagia (most common feature)
• Feeling of food sticking in the throat
• Odynophagia (painful swallowing)
• Severe, persistent chest or abdominal pain or discomfort
• Regurgitation
• Chronic cough with increasing secretions
• Hoarseness
• Anorexia
• Nausea and vomiting
• Weight loss (often >20 pounds)
• Changes in bowel habits (diarrhea, constipation, bleeding)

a sufficient quantity of balanced nutrients to meet the body's needs and to maintain a stable weight.

INTERVENTIONS. Interventions to maintain or improve the nutritional status of the client must focus on treatments to remove or shrink the obstructive tumor and on ameliorating the effects of treatment that can impact nutritional status.

Treatment options for cancer of the esophagus that can assist in both disease and nutrition management include the following:

- Nutritional support
- Radiotherapy
- Photodynamic therapy
- Dilation of strictures
- Prosthesis insertion
- Chemotherapy
- Surgical removal of the tumor

Much has been done over the last decade to try to improve the outcome for clients diagnosed with esophageal cancer. The typical treatment plan uses a combination of the above approaches. The current trend includes chemotherapy with or without surgery in an effort to improve the odds of obtaining a cure. Clients with cancer of the esophagus can experience many problems, and relieving symptoms becomes an essential consideration.

NIC NUTRITION THERAPY. The purpose of nutrition therapy is the administration of food and fluids to support the metabolic processes of a client who is malnourished or at high risk for becoming malnourished. A thorough nutritional assessment provides members of the health care team with baseline information concerning the client's nutritional status. The dietitian determines the caloric needs of the client to meet nutritional requirements. The nurse or assistive nursing personnel weighs the client daily. Careful positioning is essential for a client who is experiencing frequent regurgitation or who has prosthetic tubes to keep the esophagus patent. The nurse teaches the client to remain upright for several hours after meals and to avoid lying completely flat. The head of the bed is always elevated 30 degrees or more to prevent reflux.

Semisoft foods and thickened liquids are preferred because they are easier to swallow. Caloric intake and the amount of fluids ingested are monitored daily to monitor progress toward nutritional goals. In addition, liquid nutritional supplements can be used between feedings to increase caloric intake. Ongoing efforts are made to preserve the ability to swallow, but feeding tubes may be needed temporarily when dysphagia is severe. In clients with complete obstruction or life-threatening fistula formation, it may be necessary to create a gastrostomy or jejunostomy. The nurse monitors laboratory and clinical indicators of nutritional status. The client may also benefit from diet teaching and planning.

NIC SWALLOWING THERAPY. The nurse consults with the speech-language pathologist to assist with oral exercises to improve swallowing. A lollipop given to the client to suck on can enhance tongue strength. The client is instructed to reach for food particles on the lips or chin using the tongue. In preparation for swallowing, the nurse assists the client to position the head in forward flexion (chin tuck). The client is instructed to place food at the back of the mouth. The nurse

monitors for the sealing of lips and for tongue movements while eating and also checks for pocketing of food after swallowing. It is important the nurse monitor for signs of aspiration. Family members and/or caregivers are taught how to feed the client, monitor for aspiration, and institute appropriate measures should choking occur. Chart 55-7 provides a summary of NIC interventions.

NONSURGICAL MANAGEMENT. Treatment decisions are based on the location and size of the tumor, the presence of metastasis, the client's concurrent health status, and the client's ability to withstand radical surgery.

The focus of nonsurgical treatment is palliative care. The outcomes of palliative care are the relief of symptoms and improved duration of survival. A combination of chemotherapy, radiation, pain control, and nutritional support measures can be used. The physician selects nonsurgical management when a client is either unable or unwilling to undergo extensive surgery.

RADIATION THERAPY. Radiation therapy to manage esophageal cancer is only moderately effective and can be used alone or in combination with other modalities. Used alone, radiation has been effective in the palliation of advanced esophageal cancer, with improvement in symptoms in 50% to 76% of cases (Behrend, 1999). Radiation therapy is contraindicated for clients with tracheoesophageal fistula,

---

CHART 55-7

NIC INTERVENTION ACTIVITIES *for*
The Client with Esophageal Problems

Nutrition Therapy: *Administration of food and fluids to support metabolic processes of a client who is malnourished or at high risk for becoming malnourished*
- Determine—in collaboration with the dietitian, as appropriate—number of calories and type of nutrients needed to meet nutrition requirements.
- Assist the client to a sitting position before eating or feeding.
- Encourage the client to select semisoft food, if lack of saliva hinders swallowing.
- Select malts, shakes, and ice cream to supplement nutrition
- Monitor food/fluid ingested and calculate daily caloric intake, as appropriate
- Determine need for nasogastric tube feedings

Swallowing Therapy: *Facilitating swallowing and preventing complications of impaired swallowing*
- Collaborate with speech therapist to instruct client/family about swallowing exercise regimen.
- Explain the rationale of the swallowing regimen to client/family.
- Provide a lollipop for client to suck on to enhance tongue strength, if appropriate.
- Assist client to position head in forward flexion in preparation for swallowing ("chin tuck").
- Assist client to place food at back of mouth and on unaffected side.
- Monitor for signs and symptoms of aspiration.
- Instruct family/caregiver how to position, feed, and monitor client.
- Instruct client/caregiver on emergency measures for choking.

NIC intervention activities selected from McCloskey, J.C., & Bulechek, G.M. (Eds.). (2000). *Nursing interventions classification (NIC)* (3rd ed.). St. Louis: Mosby. No part of this work is to be altered without prior written permission from the Publisher.

mediastinitis, mediastinal hemorrhage, or infiltration of the cancer to the trachea or bronchus (Gregoire & Fitzpatrick, 1998). Radiation reduces tumor size and offers clients consistent short-term relief. Although higher doses of radiation demonstrate better results, esophageal stricture or stenosis can result in 30% to 50% of clients requiring esophageal dilation. Normal esophageal tissue is very sensitive to the effects of radiation. The treatment is typically administered in twenty episodes over 4 weeks.

In the first weeks of treatment, radiation produces edema and epithelial desquamation, which often create acute esophagitis and odynophagia (painful swallowing). Profound anorexia, nausea, and vomiting may also result. Symptoms persist until treatment is completed. The nurse assesses the client frequently to determine the incidence and severity of symptoms. Systemic analgesics are often required to control discomfort, and the nurse administers topical lidocaine (Viscous Xylocaine) before each attempt at oral feeding.

The nurse works with the client to modify the diet to meet nutritional needs and maintain comfort. Small, frequent, soft or semiliquid meals are offered. Sweet, light foods are often tolerated best, and protein powder may be used to supplement the nutritional content of the diet. The nurse maintains accurate records of calorie counts, intake and output, and daily weights and also assesses skin turgor and mucous membranes regularly. In collaboration with the physician and dietitian, the nurse assesses the need for enteral nutrition if oral intake is insufficient.

For clients receiving radiation therapy, frequent gentle mouth care is important. Clients are at risk for monilial esophagitis, and the nurse is alert to any abrupt worsening of symptoms. Chapter 25 describes additional nursing interventions for the client undergoing radiation therapy.

PHOTODYNAMIC THERAPY. Photodynamic therapy (PDT) was originally used for the treatment of skin cancer. In 1995 it was approved for use as a palliative treatment for individuals with advanced esophageal cancer, who are not candidates for surgery. The client is injected with porfimer sodium (Sanofi Pharmaceuticals, New York), a light-sensitive drug that acts to amass cancer cells. Two days after the injection, a fiberoptic probe with a light at the tip is threaded into the esophagus. The light activates the Photofrin, destroying only cancer cells. PDT is far less invasive than surgery and is performed on an ambulatory care basis under conscious sedation.

The side effects of Photofrin are rare but include nausea, fever, and constipation. After the procedure, the client is given written guidelines concerning photosensitivity measures. The client is instructed to avoid exposure to sunlight for 1 month. Sunglasses and protective clothing that covers all exposed body areas are essential. The client may experience chest pain secondary to tissue damage and will require pain relief with opioids for a short time. The client is instructed to follow a clear liquid diet for 3 to 5 days after the procedure and advance to full liquids as tolerated (Durkin, 1999).

ESOPHAGEAL DILATION. Esophageal dilation may be performed as necessary throughout the course of the disease to achieve temporary but immediate relief of dysphagia. Esophageal dilation can be performed on an ambulatory care basis. The physician uses dilators to tear soft tissue, widening the esophageal lumen. In most cases, malignant tumors may

be dilated safely, but perforation remains a significant risk. Bacteremia can also occur. To reduce the risk of endocarditis, the American Heart Association recommends prophylaxis with antibiotics (Behrend, 1999). The treatment is repeated as often as needed to preserve the client's ability to swallow (see p. 1204).

PROSTHESIS INSERTION. The physician may insert a semirigid prosthesis to bypass disabling dysphagia and to prevent aspiration in clients who have advanced disease or tracheoesophageal (TE) or esophagobronchial (EB) fistulas. Prosthesis insertion can maintain an open esophagus and preserve the client's ability to receive oral nourishment and thus palliate the symptoms related to obstruction. The procedure is not without risk, and acute complication rates have been reported to occur in 16% to 18% of clients (Raltz & Kozarek, 1999). The prosthesis can become dislodged, migrate, or perforate the esophagus as tumor bulk increases.

The nurse's primary care emphasis is the prevention of aspiration. The prosthesis interrupts the function of the lower esophageal sphincter (LES) and permits the free reflux of gastric contents. The nurse supervises the client closely, offers small oral feedings, and ensures that the client does not lie flat in bed.

CHEMOTHERAPY. The use of chemotherapy in the treatment of esophageal cancer has been only moderately effective. The two chemotherapeutic agents used to treat squamous cell carcinoma are 5-fluorouracil (5-FU) and cisplatin. Currently, there is no standard treatment for adenocarcinoma of the esophagus. Chemotherapy can be given before surgery to decrease tumor size, thereby facilitating surgical resection (Quinn & Reedy, 1999). Chemotherapy appears to be more effective when given in combination with radiation. Cisplatin and 5-FU make the tumor cells more sensitive to the effects of radiation. Chemotherapy can be administered concurrently with radiotherapy before surgery. This treatment is thought to provide the client with the best chance of cure.

CRITICAL THINKING CHALLENGE

Your client has been diagnosed with esophageal cancer and is undergoing preoperative radiation for tumor reduction before surgical resection.

- What possible complications related to this treatment should the nurse assess for?
- What nursing interventions could be instituted to assist the client in maintaining adequate nutritional intake?
- What should the nurse include in the teaching plan for this client?

For suggested answer guidelines, go to SIMON http://www.wbsaunders.com/SIMON/Iggy/.

SURGICAL MANAGEMENT. Radical surgery represents the only definitive treatment for esophageal cancer and is the preferred treatment for clients with no evidence of advanced disease. The goals of surgical resection vary from palliation to cure. Esophagectomy is an extensive surgical procedure and is associated with significant morbidity and mortality. Mortality from the surgical procedure ranges from 10% to 20%. Complications from surgery (e.g., fistula formation, abscess, and respiratory complications) occur in 20% to 50% of individuals (Behrend, 1999; Mayer, 1998).

PREOPERATIVE CARE. Preoperative preparation for clients undergoing esophagectomy or esophagogastrostomy can be quite extensive. Clients are advised to stop smoking 2 to 4 weeks before surgery to enhance their pulmonary functioning. Client preparation for surgery may include 5 days to 2 to 3 weeks of nutritional support in an effort to improve their nutritional status and decrease postoperative morbidity. Ideally, this supplementation is given orally, but most clients usually require tube feeding or parenteral nutrition. The role of parenteral nutritional support in these clients remains controversial (Sikora et al., 1998). The nurse carefully monitors the client's weight, intake and output, and fluid and electrolyte balance. A preoperative dental evaluation may be required to remove pre-existing dental caries. Meticulous oral care is performed four times daily to decrease the risk of postoperative infection.

Preoperative nursing care also focuses on teaching and on psychologic support. The nurse ensures that the client is knowledgeable about the surgery and its outcomes. The physician's instructions are clarified and reinforced as needed. The nurse explains the following:

- The number and sites of all incisions and drains
- The placement of a jejunostomy tube for initial enteral feedings
- The need for chest tubes if the pleural space is entered
- The purpose of the nasogastric tube
- The need for intravenous (IV) infusion

The client visits the critical care unit, if possible, and initiates contacts with unit staff.

The nurse instructs the client about routines for turning, coughing, deep breathing, and chest physiotherapy. The crucial nature of postoperative respiratory care is emphasized. The nurse addresses the probable need for ventilator support, because respiratory management is a major focus of postoperative care. If colon interposition is planned, the client also undergoes a complete bowel preparation with laxatives and enemas before surgery.

The client facing a serious illness and extensive surgery can be expected to display feelings of grief and anxiety. The nurse encourages the client to talk about personal feelings and fears and involves the family or significant others in all preoperative teaching and discussions. A primary nurse or case manager can be extremely helpful in providing continuity of care and support to the entire family.

OPERATIVE PROCEDURES. A subtotal or total *esophagectomy* is usually required because tumors are often quite large and involve distant lymph nodes. Several procedures have been used, but the preferred surgical procedure is an **esophagogastrostomy.** The diseased portion of the esophagus is removed, and the cervical portion is anastomosed (connected) to the stomach. The cervical portion of the stomach is then brought up into the thorax through the esophageal hiatus (Figure 55-5). A vagotomy is also usually performed with this type of resection, resulting in hypertonicity of the pylorus. A pyloromyotomy is created to prevent gastric motility disturbances. Lastly, a jejunostomy tube is placed for postoperative enteral feeding.

For a client with early stage tumors of the lower third of the esophagus, a transhiatal esophagectomy is the preferred surgical approach. The surgery is performed through an upper midline cervical incision. With this approach there is no entry into the pleural space, thereby minimizing respiratory complications.

For a client with tumors in the upper esophagus, radical neck dissection and laryngectomy may also be required because of the spread of disease to the larynx. The surgeon may perform a colon interposition when the tumor involves the stomach or the stomach is otherwise unsuitable for anastomosis. A section of right or left colon is removed and brought up into the thorax to substitute for the esophagus (see Figure 55-5).

These surgical procedures pose cardiovascular risks for the client. Intraoperative hypotension can result from pressure on the posterior heart. Decreased lymphatic pulmonary clearance can predispose the client to pulmonary edema when mediastinal lymph nodes and lymphatics are resected. The stress placed on the heart by extensive surgery can increase the risk of myocardial ischemia and dysrhythmias, especially if the client has underlying coronary disease.

The client with compromised nutritional status or prior radiation or chemotherapy is predisposed to an increased risk of infection. For clients who undergo more radical surgical procedures, there is a serious risk of leakage at the anastomosis site. This situation is especially true with colon interpositions because several anastomosis sites are vulnerable to the effects of tension, poor blood supply, and delayed healing. Mediastinitis resulting from an anastomotic leak can lead to fatal sepsis.

POSTOPERATIVE CARE. The client requires meticulous postoperative care and is at risk for multiple serious complications. The Client Care Plan on pp. 1199 and 1200 outlines client interventions for esophageal surgery.

Respiratory Care. Respiratory care is the *highest* postoperative priority, and the client is usually intubated and mechanically ventilated for at least the first 24 hours. Postoperative pulmonary complications include atelectasis and pneumonia. The risk of postoperative pulmonary complications is increased in the client who has received preoperative radiation. Once the client is extubated, the nurse begins deep breathing, turning, and coughing routines. Chest physiotherapy is initiated as ordered, usually every 2 to 4 hours. The nurse assesses the client for decreased breath sounds and shortness of breath every 1 to 2 hours. Incisional support and adequate analgesia are essential for effective coughing and should be administered regularly if the client's vital signs remain stable. The nurse keeps the client in a semi-Fowler's or high Fowler's position to support ventilation and prevent reflux. The physician prescribes prophylactic antibiotics and supplemental oxygen; blood gases are ordered regularly. The nurse ensures the patency of the water seal drainage system for chest tubes and monitors for changes in the volume or color of the drainage.

Cardiovascular Care. Hypotension can occur secondary to pressure placed on the posterior heart and may respond well to vigorous IV fluid administration. The nurse also monitors for signs and symptoms of fluid volume overload, particularly in clients who have undergone lymph node dissection. The nurse assesses for edema, crackles in the lungs, and increased jugular venous pressure. In the immediate postoperative phase, the client may be admitted to the intensive care unit. Critical care nurses assess hemodynamic parameters such as cardiac output, cardiac index, and systemic vascular resistance every 2 hours to monitor for myocardial ischemia.

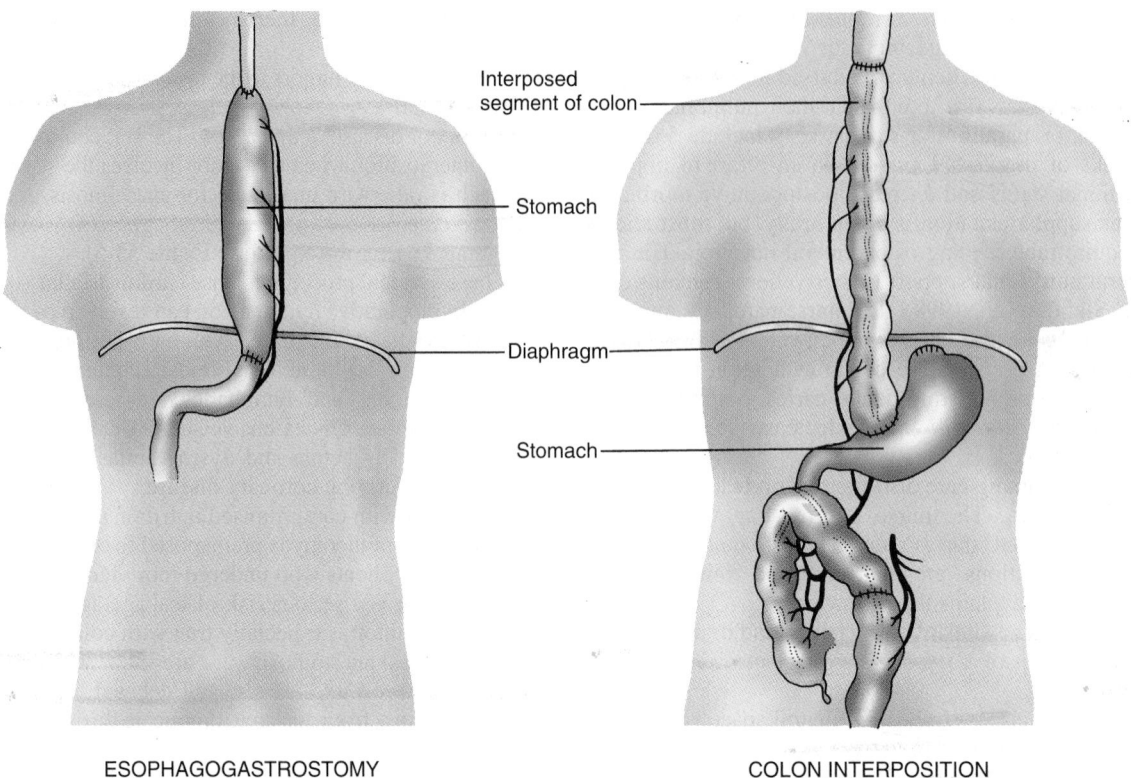

ESOPHAGOGASTROSTOMY   COLON INTERPOSITION

Figure 55-5 ● Surgical approaches to the treatment of esophageal cancer.

Atrial fibrillation is a dysrhythmia that results from irritation of the vagus nerve during surgery. Management of atrial fibrillation can include digitalization, beta blockers, or cardioversion. (See Chapter 34 for more information on atrial fibrillation.)

Wound Management. Wound management is another significant postoperative concern because the client typically has multiple incisions and drains. The nurse provides incisional support during turning and coughing to prevent dehiscence. Wound infection usually occurs 4 to 5 days after surgery. Postoperative leakage from the site of anastomosis is a dreaded complication that can appear 2 to 10 days after surgery. If an anastomic leak occurs, all oral intake is discontinued and is not resumed until the leak has healed. Nutrition may be given through the jejunostomy tube during the healing process. The nurse carefully assesses for fever, fluid accumulation, general signs of inflammation, and symptoms of early shock (e.g., tachycardia, tachypnea) and reports these findings to the health care provider immediately.

Nasogastric Tube Management. A nasogastric (NG) tube is placed intraoperatively to decompress the suture line. The nurse monitors the NG tube for patency and carefully secures the tube to prevent dislodgment, which can disrupt the sutures at the anastomosis. The nurse *does not* independently irrigate or reposition the NG tube in clients who have undergone esophageal surgery. The initial nasogastric drainage is bloody but should change to a greenish yellow color by the end of the first postoperative day. The continued presence of blood may indicate bleeding at the suture line. The nurse provides oral hygiene every 2 to 4 hours while the tube is in place (Chart 55-8).

CHART 55-8

BEST PRACTICE *for*
Managing the Client with a Nasogastric Tube After Esophageal Surgery

- Check for tube placement every 4 to 8 hours.
- Ensure that the tube is patent (open) and draining; drainage should turn from bloody to yellowish green by the end of the first postoperative day.
- Secure the tube well to prevent dislodgment.
- Do not irrigate or reposition the tube without a physician's order.
- Provide meticulous oral and nasal hygiene every 2 to 4 hours.
- Keep the head of the bed elevated to at least 30 degrees.
- When the client is permitted to have a small amount of water, place the client in an upright position and observe for dysphagia (difficulty swallowing).
- Observe for leakage from the anastomosis site, as indicated by fever, fluid accumulation, and manifestations of early shock (tachycardia, tachypnea, altered mental status).

Nutritional Care. The nutritional management of the client who has undergone an esophageal surgery is an early postoperative concern. On the second postoperative day, initial feedings begin through the jejunostomy tube. The feedings are slowly increased over the next several days. Feeding by this method can be discontinued once the client is taking adequate oral nutrition. However, some clients may require jejunostomy feedings for approximately 1 month if small amounts of aspiration are detected.

Before beginning oral feedings, a cine-esophagram study is performed to detect the presence of anastomotic leaks, strictures, or signs of aspiration. If no leaks are detected, an esophageal diet is begun, starting with liquids. If liquids are well tolerated, the client's diet is advanced to include semi-solid foods and then solid foods. The nurse supervises the client during all initial swallowing efforts and ensures that he or she is in an upright position. The food storage area of the stomach has been radically decreased, and gravity is the client's only real defense against reflux. The nurse continues to assess for signs of leakage.

The client is instructed to consume 6 to 8 meals per day and to ingest fluids between, rather than with, meals to prevent diarrhea. Diarrhea can occur 20 minutes to 2 hours after eating and can be symptomatically managed with loperamide before meals. The diarrhea is thought to be the result of **vagotomy syndrome,** which develops as a result of the interruption of vagal fibers to the abdominal viscera during surgery. This syndrome is diminished by pyloroplasty.

◎ CRITICAL THINKING CHALLENGE

Your client has completed a course of preoperative radiation therapy, and has undergone an esophagogastrostomy as part of her esophageal cancer treatment.

- What postoperative complications should you assess for and why?
- What nursing interventions would be most appropriate for preventing postoperative complications?

For suggested answer guidelines, go to 〔SIMON〕 http://www.wbsaunders.com/SIMON/Iggy/.

● Community-Based Care

Clients with esophageal cancer have many challenges to face once they are discharged home. The combination treatment regimens cause long-lasting side effects, such as fatigue and weakness. These complex treatments also require the client to be knowledgeable about symptom management and to know when to report issues of concern to the health care provider. (See Chapter 25 for care of the client undergoing radiation therapy and chemotherapy.)

▪ HOME CARE MANAGEMENT

The care given in the hospital is continued after discharge to the community. Ongoing respiratory care is a priority, and family members are instructed to assist with ambulation, splinting incisions, and use of the incentive spirometer. The nurse teaches the family to protect the client from infection and to contact the physician immediately if signs of respiratory infection develop. The client is encouraged to be as active as possible and to avoid excessive bedrest and its complications at all costs.

▪ HEALTH TEACHING

Wound healing is also an ongoing concern. The nurse teaches the client and family to inspect the incisions daily for redness, tenderness, swelling, odor, and discharge. The client and family are instructed to report a temperature greater than 101° F (38.3° C).

The nurse prepares written instructions about the signs of anastomosis leakage and the importance of reporting them to

---

𝓛EGAL/𝓔THICAL 𝓘SSUES IN HEALTH CARE

WITHHOLDING FOOD AND FLUIDS

Providing nutrition and hydration by means of IV catheters or gastric intubation raises many issues. Societal norms surround the provision of food and fluids to individuals who are deemed vulnerable, and this act is viewed differently than complex medical interventions. In addition, there is concern that withholding food and fluids may cause discomfort or suffering. Although there is agreement that ethical principles should be used to guide decision making in the provision or withdrawal of food and fluids, there is evidence to suggest that there are few potential benefits to providing nutrition to those with terminal or protracted illnesses.

Although there are no easy answers to this dilemma, a guide to decision making is suggested. The first consideration should be the previous wishes and evidence of current sensation of the individual involved. Second, the benefits and burdens of nutrition and hydration need to be evaluated in terms of long- and short-term goals. Finally, the interests of all parties involved should be represented. Clinicians should focus on reaching a consensus by incorporating an existing knowledge of feeding and hydration with consideration based on the wishes of the individual. The views of all stakeholders, and the given benefits and burdens of each case should also weigh in the decision.

From Daly, B. (2000) The special challenges of withholding food and fluids. *Gerontological Nursing, 26*(9), 25-31.

---

the physician or other health care provider immediately. The client and family members are instructed to report the presence of fever and a swollen, painful neck incision, which indicates a cervical anastomotic leak (Gregoire & Fitzpatrick, 1998).

Nutritional support also remains a concern. The nurse encourages the client to continue increasing oral feedings as tolerated. The client is reminded to eat a high-calorie, high-protein diet that contains soft and easily swallowed foods. Meals should be small and frequent, and nutritionally empty foods are avoided. Eggnogs and milkshakes may be easily prepared and enriched to supplement meals. The client needs to learn what foods can be tolerated and needs to adjust his or her eating pattern to ingest food more slowly than before. Individuals who have undergone esophageal resection can lose up to 10% of their body weight. The client is taught to monitor his or her weight at home and to report a weight loss of 5 pounds or more. If sufficient oral intake is not possible, the family may need instruction about tube feedings or parenteral nutrition at home. (See the Legal/Ethical Issues in Health Care box above.)

The nurse emphasizes the importance of keeping the client upright after meals and elevating the head of the bed on blocks. Families are counseled that dysphagia or odynophagia may recur because of stricture, reflux, or cancer recurrence. These symptoms should be promptly reported to the health care provider.

Despite radical surgery, the client with cancer of the esophagus still has a terminal illness and a relatively short life expectancy. Emphasis is placed on maximizing quality of life. Realistic planning is important as the client's condition eventually worsens, and the client and family are assisted to plan for the future together. The nurse assists family members in exploring formal and informal sources of support. When needed, the nurse helps the family or significant others arrange for hospice care.

■ HEALTH CARE RESOURCES

The nurse initiates referrals to community or home care organizations to assist the family in providing the needed home care. The client may need transportation to the radiation treatment center 5 times per week for up to 6 weeks. Oncology nursing care may be needed to monitor and evaluate the client who is receiving chemotherapy at home through venous access devices or portable infusion pumps. In addition, the nurse informs the family about the services available through the American Cancer Society. The nurse may also acquaint the family with area hospice services for future planning.

● Evaluation: Outcomes

NOC The nurse evaluates the care of the client with esophageal cancer on the basis of the identified nursing diagnoses and collaborative problems. The expected outcomes are that the client:

- Maintains hemodynamic stability free of cardiovascular complications
- Maintains a patent airway free of respiratory complications
- Is free of infection
- Is able to consume adequate nutrition and maintain a stable weight
- Is able to swallow comfortably
- States that pain is controlled through pharmacologic and nonpharmacologic pain control measures
- Successfully adapts to the stresses surrounding the diagnosis and treatment with meaningful support from family or significant others

DIVERTICULA

■ OVERVIEW

Diverticula are sacs resulting from the herniation of esophageal mucosa and submucosa into surrounding tissue. Clients complain of dysphagia, regurgitation, nocturnal cough, and halitosis (bad breath).

Diverticula may develop anywhere along the length of the esophagus. No environmental risk factors are known to be involved in the development of esophageal diverticula. The incomplete or late opening of the cricopharyngeal muscle during swallowing leads to high pressures in the hypopharynx and leads to *Zenker's diverticulum,* the most common form. Zenker's diverticulum occurs most often in older adults. Clients with esophageal diverticula can be at risk for esophageal perforation because the mucosa is without the protection of the normal esophageal muscle layer.

► COLLABORATIVE MANAGEMENT

The diagnosis of esophageal diverticula is made by x-ray examination and barium swallow. Endoscopy must be performed with strict care in these clients, because perforation can occur.

Diet therapy and positioning are the major interventions for controlling symptoms related to diverticula. The dietitian as-

sists the client in exploring variations in the size and frequency of meals and in food texture and consistency. Semisoft foods and smaller meals are often best tolerated and may reduce or relieve the symptoms of pressure and reflux. Individual food tolerances and intolerances are explored with the client.

As with other forms of reflux, nocturnal problems associated with diverticula are best managed by sleeping with the head of the bed elevated and avoiding the recumbent position for at least 2 hours after eating. The client is also counseled to avoid vigorous exercise after meals. The nurse advises the client to avoid restrictive clothing and frequent stooping or bending.

Surgical management is aimed at excising the diverticula and reapproximating the mucosa. Most physicians use the cervical surgical approach above the clavicle. Postoperatively, the client takes nothing by mouth for several days to promote healing and receives IV fluids for hydration, tube feedings, and then oral fluid and food. The nurse provides pain relief measures and monitors for complications such as bleeding or perforation. A nasogastric (NG) tube is placed during surgery for decompression and is *not* irrigated or repositioned unless specifically ordered by the surgeon. This tube may be used later for feeding.

Community-based care includes teaching the client and family about the following:

- Tube feeding and resuming an oral diet
- Positioning guidelines to prevent reflux
- Warning signs of complications

Community resources are usually not needed for uncomplicated cases.

TRAUMA

■ OVERVIEW

Trauma to the esophagus can result from blunt injuries, chemical burns, surgery or endoscopy, or the stress of protracted severe vomiting (Table 55-2). Trauma may affect the esophagus directly, impairing swallowing and nutrition, or it may create problems and complications in related structures such as the lungs or mediastinum. The incidence of most forms of esophageal trauma is low in adults.

When excessive force is exerted on the esophageal mucosa, it may perforate or rupture, allowing the caustic acid secretions to enter the mediastinal cavity. These tears are associated with a high mortality rate related to shock, respiratory impairment, or sepsis.

Chemical injury is usually a result of the accidental or intentional ingestion of caustic substances. The oral cavity is also usually damaged, and the damage is rapid and severe. Acid burns tend to affect the superficial layers of the esophagus, whereas alkaline substances cause deeper penetrating injuries.

TABLE 55-2 ● CAUSES OF ESOPHAGEAL PERFORATION
• Straining
• Seizures
• Trauma
• Foreign objects
• Instruments or tubes
• Chemical injury
• Complications of esophageal surgery
• Ulcers

Strong alkalis can cause full perforation of the esophagus within 1 minute. Additional problems may include aspiration pneumonia and hemorrhage. Strictures may develop as scar tissue forms. Table 55-3 lists caustic substances commonly found in the home.

► COLLABORATIVE MANAGEMENT

Most clients with esophageal trauma are initially evaluated and treated in the emergency department. Assessment focuses on the nature of the injury and the circumstances surrounding it. The nurse assesses for the presence of an airway, chest pain, dysphagia, vomiting, and bleeding.

If the risk of extending the damage is not excessive, the physician may order an x-ray or endoscopic study to evaluate tears or perforation. A computed tomography (CT) scan of the chest reveals the presence of mediastinal air.

After the injury, the client is allowed nothing by mouth to prevent further leakage of esophageal secretions. Esophageal and gastric suction is used for drainage and to rest the esophagus. Esophageal rest is maintained for at least 10 days after injury to allow for initial healing of the mucosa. The physician orders total parenteral nutrition (TPN) to provide calories and protein for wound healing while the client is not eating.

To prevent sepsis, the physician prescribes broad-spectrum antibiotics. High-dose corticosteroids may be administered to suppress inflammation and prevent strictures. The physician may prescribe opioid and nonopioid analgesics for pain management. When caustic burns involve the oral cavity, topical agents, such as 50/50 diphenhydramine hydrochloride (Benadryl) and kaolin with pectin (Ka-Pectolin) or topical lidocaine (Viscous Xylocaine), may be used for topical analgesia and local anti-inflammatory action.

If nonsurgical management is not effective in healing traumatized esophageal tissue, the client may need surgery to remove the damaged tissue. The client with severe injuries may require resection of part of the esophagus with a gastric pull-through and repositioning or replacement by a bowel segment. (See Surgical Management [Esophageal Tumors], pp. 1208 and 1209.)

ONLINE RESOURCES

For suggested readings and Internet resources, go to http://www.wbsaunders.com/SIMON/Iggy/.

SELECTED BIBLIOGRAPHY

Behrend, S.W. (1999). Esophageal cancer. In Miaskowski, C. & Buchsel, P. (Eds.), *Oncology nursing: Assessment and clinical care* (pp. 889-917). St. Louis: Mosby.

Brooks-Brunn, J.A. (2000). Esophageal cancer: An overview. *MEDSURG Nursing, 9*(5), 248-254.

Cameron, A. (1999). Barrett's esophagus: Prevalence and size of hiatal hernia. *The American Journal of Gastroenterology, 94*(8), 2054-2059.

Claussen, J. (1999). Gastroesophageal reflux disease: A rational approach to management. *Clinician Reviews, 9*(6), 69-82.

Crawford, J. (1999). The gastrointestinal tract. In R.S. Cotran et al. (Eds.), *Robbins pathologic basis of disease* (6th ed., pp. 775-787). Philadelphia: W.B. Saunders.

Daly, B. (2000). The special challenges of withholding artificial nutrition and hydration. *Journal of Gerontological Nursing, 26*(9), 25-31.

Durkin, S. (1999). Photodynamic therapy: A cancer treatment for the 21st century. *Gastroenterology Nursing, 22*(3), 115-120.

Eloubeidi, M., et al. (1999). A cost analysis of outpatient care for patients with Barrett's esophagus in a managed care setting. *The American Journal of Gastroenterology, 94*(8), 2033-2036.

Fackeer, W.K., & Richter, J.E., (2000). Refractory GERD: What next? *Consultant,* May, pp. 973-983.

Ferguson, M.K. (1997). Pitfalls and complications of antireflux surgery: Nissen and Collis-Nissen techniques. In Fell & Bains (Eds.), *Chest surgery clinics of North America* (pp. 489-509). Philadelphia: W.B. Saunders.

Goldsmith, C. (1998). Gastroesophageal reflux disease. *American Journal of Nursing, 98*(9), 44-45.

Gregoire, A.S., & Fitzpatrick, E. (1998). Esophageal cancer: Multisystem nursing management. *Dimensions of Critical Care Nursing, 17*(1), 28-36.

Kessenich, C. (1999). Differential diagnosis of chest pain: A case report. *Gastroenterology Nursing, 22*(1), 10-13.

Khoury, R., et al. (1999). Influence of spontaneous sleep positions on nighttime recumbent reflux in patients with gastroesophageal reflux disease. *The American Journal of Gastroenterology, 94*(8), 2069-2073.

Landis, S.H., et al. (1999). Cancer statistics 1999. *CA: A Cancer Journal for Clinicians, 49*(1), 8-31.

Mayer, R. (1998). Gastrointestinal tract cancer. In A.S. Fauci, E. Braunwald, & K.J. Isselbacher (Eds.), *Harrison's principles of internal medicine* (14th ed., pp. 568-577). New York: McGraw-Hill.

O'Connor, J., Falk, G., & Richter, J. (1999). The incidence of adenocarcinoma and dysplasia in Barrett's esophagus. *The American Journal of Gastroenterology, 94*(8), 2037-2042.

TABLE 55-3	ACTIVE INGREDIENTS OF COMMON HOUSEHOLD CORROSIVES	
Types	**Corrosive**	**Active Ingredient**
Acids		
Liquid	Mister Plumber	Sulfuric acid 8.5%
	Lysol Toilet Bowl Cleaner	Hydrochloric acid
	Sno-Bol Toilet Bowl Cleaner	Hydrochloric acid 15%
Granular	ZUD Rust and Stain Remover	Oxalic acid
	Sani-Flush Toilet Bowl Cleaner	Sodium bisulfite 75%
	Vanish Toilet Bowl Cleaner	Sodium acid sulfate 62%
Alkalis	Liquid Drāno	Sodium hydroxide 9.5%
	Crystal Drāno	Sodium hydroxide 80%
	Liquid Plumr	Sodium hypochlorite and hydroxide 8%
	Easy-Off Liquid Oven Cleaner	Sodium hydroxide
	Mr. Muscle Oven Cleaner	Sodium hydroxide
	Industrial/ Professional Drāno	Sodium hydroxide 32%
	Ammonia	Ammonium hydroxide
Bleaches	Clorox Peroxide	
Thermal agents	Dry ice Hot water	
Detergents	Cascade (dish)	Sodium tripolyphosphate
	Amway (dish)	Sodium tripolyphosphate

Parkin, D.M., Pisani, P., & Ferlay, J. (1999). Global cancer statistics. *CA: A Cancer Journal for Clinicians, 49*(1), 33-64.

Quinn, K., & Reedy, A. (1999). Esophageal cancer: Therapeutic approaches and nursing care. *Seminars in Oncology Nursing, 15*(1), 17-25.

Raltz, S., & Kozarek, R. (1999). Do age, gender, or tumor location affect outcomes when using metallic stents in the palliative treatment of esophageal carcinoma? *Gastroenterology Nursing, 22*(6), 249-253.

Scott, M., & Gelhot, A.R. (1999). Gastroesophageal reflux disease: Diagnosis and management. *American Family Physician, 59*(5), 1161-1169.

Sharma, P. (1999). Barrett's esophagus: Put guidelines into practice. *Patient Care for the Nurse Practitioner, 2*(9), 23-26.

Sikora, S., et al. (1998). Role of nutrition support during induction chemoradiation therapy in esophageal cancer. *Journal of Parenteral and Enteral Nutrition, 22*(1), 18-21.

Tucker, K., & Schumann, L. (1999). Gastroesophageal reflux disease. *The Clinical Advisor,* April, pp. 52-58.

Vaca, K., et al. (1998). The role of laparoscopic Nissen fundoplication in gastroesophageal reflux disease. *MEDSURG Nursing, 7*(6), 364-370.

Interventions for Clients with Stomach Disorders

CONSTANCE VISOVSKY

Learning Objectives

After studying this chapter, you should be able to:

1. Compare etiologies and assessment findings of acute and chronic gastritis.
2. Describe the key components of collaborative management for clients with gastritis.
3. Compare and contrast assessment findings associated with gastric and duodenal ulcers.
4. Identify the most common medical complications that can result from peptic ulcer disease (PUD).
5. Analyze assessment data to determine common nursing diagnoses associated with PUD.
6. Develop a teaching plan related to drug therapy for clients experiencing PUD.
7. Prioritize interventions for clients with upper gastrointestinal bleeding.
8. Plan preoperative and postoperative care for the client undergoing gastric surgery.
9. Develop a community-based plan of care for clients who have undergone gastric surgery.
10. Evaluate outcomes for clients with PUD.
11. Explain Zollinger-Ellison syndrome and its associated clinical manifestations.
12. Analyze risk factors for gastric carcinoma, including cultural considerations.
13. Plan postoperative care for clients who have undergone surgery for gastric cancer.
14. Discuss the psychologic and emotional concerns of clients with gastric cancer.

Go to http://www.wbsaunders.com/SIMON/Iggy/ for self-assessment questions related to these Learning Objectives.

Although only a few diseases affect the stomach, they can be very serious and in some cases life threatening. The most common disorders include gastritis, peptic ulcer disease, Zollinger-Ellison syndrome, and gastric carcinoma (cancer).

GASTRITIS

■ OVERVIEW

Gastritis is defined as inflammation of the gastric mucosa (stomach lining). It can be diffuse or localized and can be classified according to cause, cellular changes, or distribution of the lesions. Gastritis can be designated as erosive (acute gastritis, stress ulcers) or nonerosive (chronic gastritis). Although the mucosal changes accompanying acute gastritis typically resolve after several months, this is not true for chronic gastritis.

■ Pathophysiology

Prostaglandins provide a protective mucosal barrier that prevents the stomach from digesting itself by a process called acid autodigestion. If there is a break in the protective barrier, mucosal injury occurs. The resulting injury is compounded by histamine release and vagal nerve stimulation. Hydrochloric acid can then diffuse back into the mucosa and injure small vessels. This back-diffusion results in edema, hemorrhage, and erosion of the stomach's lining. The pathologic changes of gastritis include vascular congestion, edema, acute inflammatory cell infiltration, and degenerative changes in the superficial epithelium of the stomach lining.

The early pathologic manifestation of gastritis is a thickened, reddened mucous membrane with prominent rugae, or folds. As the disease progresses, the walls and lining of the stomach thin and atrophy. With progressive gastric atrophy from chronic mucosal injury, the function of the parietal (acid-secreting) cells decreases and the source of intrinsic factor is lost. The intrinsic factor is critical for absorption of vitamin B_{12}. When body stores of vitamin B_{12} are eventually depleted, pernicious anemia results. The amount and concentration of acid in stomach secretions gradually decrease until the secretions consist of only mucus and water.

Chronic gastritis is associated with an increased risk of gastric cancer as the persistent inflammation extends deep into the mucosa, causing destruction of the gastric glands and cellular changes. Hemorrhage may occur after an episode of acute gastritis or with ulceration caused by chronic gastritis.

ACUTE GASTRITIS

Inflammation of the gastric mucosa or submucosa after exposure to local irritants can result in acute gastritis. Various degrees of mucosal necrosis and inflammatory reaction occur in acute disease. The diagnosis cannot be based solely on clinical symptoms without an endoscopic examination. Complete regeneration and healing usually occur within a few days. If the stomach muscle is not involved, complete recovery usually occurs with no residual evidence of gastric inflammatory reaction.

CHRONIC GASTRITIS

Chronic gastritis appears as a patchy, diffuse (spread out) inflammation of the mucosal lining of the stomach. Chronic gastritis usually heals without scarring, but it can progress to hemorrhage and the formation of an ulcer.

Chronic gastritis may be categorized as type A, type B, or atrophic. Type A (nonerosive) chronic gastritis refers to an inflammation of the glands, as well as the fundus and body of the stomach. Type B chronic gastritis usually affects the glands of the antrum but may involve the entire stomach. In atrophic chronic gastritis, diffuse inflammation and destruction of deeply located glands accompany the condition. Chronic atrophic gastritis affects all layers of the stomach, thus decreasing the number of cells. The muscle becomes thickened, and inflammation is present. Chronic atrophic gastritis is characterized by total loss of fundal glands, minimal inflammation, thinning of the gastric mucosa, and intestinal metaplasia (abnormal tissue development).

Etiology

ACUTE GASTRITIS

The onset of infection with *Helicobacter pylori* can result in acute gastritis. *H. pylori* is a gram-negative, spiral-shaped organism that penetrates the mucosal gel layer of the gastric epithelium. Although it is uncommon, other forms of bacterial gastritis from organisms such as staphylococci, streptococci, *Escherichia coli,* or salmonella can cause life-threatening consequences such as sepsis and extensive tissue necrosis (Friedman & Peterson, 1998). Other infectious causes of acute gastritis can be found in clients with immunosuppressive disorders. In clients with acquired immunodeficiency syndrome (AIDS), for example, gastric erosions can be found with herpes simplex viral infection and disseminated cytomegalovirus (CMV) infection.

Nonsteroidal anti-inflammatory drug (NSAID) use poses a risk for the development of acute gastritis. Gastritis occurs in 5% to 25% of NSAID users, but the exact mechanism of the role of NSAIDs in the development of gastritis is not well understood. Other drugs, including alcohol, cytotoxic agents, caffeine, and corticosteroids, have also been implicated; however, scientific evidence is lacking. Acute gastritis is also caused by local irritation from radiation therapy and accidental or intentional ingestion of corrosive substances, including acids or alkalis (such as lye and drain cleaners [Mister Plumber, Drano]). In the client who is allowed nothing by mouth (NPO), gastritis may result from lack of stimulation of normal secretions. Acute stress-induced gastritis, characterized by multiple shallow erosions of the proximal stomach, may be present in 80% to 100% of critically ill clients.

CHRONIC GASTRITIS

Type A gastritis has been associated with the presence of antibodies to parietal cells and intrinsic factor; therefore an autoimmune pathogenesis for this type of gastritis has been proposed. Parietal cell antibodies have been found in 90% of clients with pernicious anemia and in more than one half of individuals with type A gastritis. A genetic link to this disease, with an autosomal dominant pattern of inheritance, has been noted in the relatives of clients with pernicious anemia (Centanni et al., 1999).

The most common form of the disease is type B gastritis, caused by *H. pylori* infection. There is a direct correlation between the number of organisms and the degree of cellular abnormality present. Although serum antibodies have been isolated in some clients, it is believed that these antibodies are not representative of an autoimmune process but are the result of prolonged inflammation. Fifty percent of clients who have gastric ulcers have associated chronic gastritis.

Chronic local irritation and toxic effects caused by alcohol ingestion, radiation therapy, and smoking have been implicated in the development of chronic gastritis. Surgical procedures that involve the pyloric sphincter, such as the Billroth II procedure, can lead to gastritis by causing reflux of alkaline secretions into the stomach. Other systemic disorders such as Crohn's disease, graft-versus-host disease, and uremia can also precipitate the development of chronic gastritis.

CHRONIC ATROPHIC GASTRITIS. Atrophic gastritis is a type of chronic gastritis that is seen most often in older adults. It can occur after exposure to toxic substances in the workplace (e.g., benzene, lead, and nickel) or *H. pylori* infection, or it can be related to autoimmune factors.

Although atrophic gastritis is often present in people with gastric cancer, it is not always considered a precancerous lesion. Gastric carcinoma develops in fewer than 10% of clients who have atrophic gastritis. Chart 56-1 lists guidelines for preventing gastritis.

Incidence/Prevalence

Approximately 2.7 million people in the United States have been diagnosed with gastritis. The incidence of gastritis is higher in men than in women; however, it has been suggested that more women have chronic atrophic gastritis. Acute and

---

CHART 56-1

CLIENT EDUCATION GUIDE
Gastritis Prevention

- Avoid drinking excessive amounts of alcoholic beverages.
- Use caution in taking large doses of aspirin, nonsteroidal anti-inflammatory drugs (such as ibuprofen), and corticosteroids. Prolonged use of small doses of corticosteroids may also cause gastritis.
- Avoid excessive intake of caffeine-containing beverages.
- Avoid eating contaminated foods or drinking contaminated water.
- Stop smoking.
- Protect yourself against exposure to toxic substances in the workplace, such as lead and nickel.
- Seek medical treatment if you are experiencing symptoms of esophageal reflux (see Chapter 55).

chronic forms of the disease are more prevalent in heavy smokers and persons who abuse alcohol. The incidence of chronic gastritis increases with age.

▶ COLLABORATIVE MANAGEMENT

● Assessment

■ PHYSICAL ASSESSMENT/CLINICAL MANIFESTATIONS

Physical assessment findings may include abdominal tenderness and bloating, **hematemesis** (vomiting blood), or **melena** (traces of blood in the stool). In stress-induced gastritis, symptoms of intravascular volume depletion and shock may be present.

ACUTE GASTRITIS. Symptoms of acute gastritis can range from mild to severe. Epigastric discomfort, anorexia, cramping, nausea, and vomiting may be present. In some cases, gastric hemorrhage is the presenting symptom (Chart 56-2). The symptoms last only a few hours or days and vary with the cause. Aspirin-related gastritis may result in dyspepsia (heartburn). Gastritis from alcohol abuse may cause vomiting and hematemesis. Gastritis or food poisoning caused by endotoxins, such as staphylococcal endotoxin, has an abrupt onset; severe nausea and vomiting often occur within 5 hours of ingestion of the contaminated food.

CHRONIC GASTRITIS. Chronic gastritis causes few symptoms. Clients may complain of nausea, vomiting, or upper abdominal discomfort. Periodic epigastric pain may simulate ulcer-like distress, which is relieved on ingestion of food. Some clients may have anorexia, and pain may be exacerbated by eating fatty or spicy foods (see Chart 56-2).

■ DIAGNOSTIC ASSESSMENT

Esophagogastroduodenoscopy (EGD) via an endoscope with biopsy is the gold standard for diagnosing gastritis, as well as detecting the presence of *H. pylori*. The health care provider uses biopsy to establish a definitive diagnosis of the type of gastritis. If lesions are patchy and diffuse, biopsy of several suspicious areas may be necessary to avoid misdiagnosis. A cytologic examination of the biopsy specimen is performed to confirm or rule out gastric cancer.

CHART 56-2
KEY FEATURES *of*
Gastritis

Acute Gastritis
- Rapid onset of epigastric pain or discomfort
- Nausea and vomiting
- Hematemesis (vomiting blood)
- Gastric hemorrhage
- Dyspepsia (heartburn)
- Anorexia

Chronic Gastritis
- Vague complaint of epigastric pain that is relieved by food
- Anorexia
- Nausea or vomiting
- Intolerance of fatty and spicy foods
- Pernicious anemia

● Interventions

Clients with gastritis are not often seen in the acute care setting unless they have an exacerbation of acute or chronic gastritis that results in fluid and electrolyte imbalance or bleeding. Management is directed toward supportive care for relieving the symptoms and removing the cause of discomfort.

Acute gastritis is treated symptomatically and supportively because the healing process is spontaneous, usually occurring within a few days. When the cause is removed, pain and discomfort usually subside. If hemorrhage is severe, a blood transfusion may be necessary. Fluid replacement is indicated in clients with severe fluid loss. Surgery, such as partial gastrectomy, pyloroplasty, and/or vagotomy, may be indicated for clients with major bleeding or ulceration. Treatment of chronic gastritis varies with the cause. General treatment goals include the eradication of causative agents, treatment of any underlying disease (e.g., uremia, Crohn's disease), and avoidance of toxic substances (e.g., alcohol, tobacco, nonsteroidal anti-inflammatory drugs [NSAIDs]).

NONSURGICAL MANAGEMENT. The identification and elimination of the causative factors, such as eradication of *H. pylori* infection, is the primary treatment modality. Drugs and diet therapy are also used in the treatment of gastritis.

DRUG THERAPY. In the acute phase, the nurse directs actions toward relief of pain and discomfort. The health care provider may order medications that block and buffer gastric acid secretions to relieve pain.

H$_2$-receptor antagonists are commonly used to block gastric secretions. These agents include ranitidine (Zantac), famotidine (Pepcid), and nizatidine (Axid). Sucralfate (Carafate, Sulcrate✦), a mucosal barrier fortifier, may also be prescribed. Antacids used as buffering agents include aluminum hydroxide combined with magnesium hydroxide (Maalox) and aluminum hydroxide combined with simethicone and magnesium hydroxide (Mylanta) (Chart 56-3). The nurse monitors for symptom relief and side effects of these medications and notifies the health care provider of any untoward effects or worsening of gastric distress.

Clients with chronic gastritis may require vitamin B$_{12}$ for prevention or treatment of pernicious anemia. If *H. pylori* is found in biopsy specimens, the health care provider may treat the infection and reverse or prevent impairment of mucosal defenses. A common drug regimen for *H. pylori* infection is bismuth subsalicylates (Pepto-Bismol), metronidazole (Flagyl, Novonidazol✦), and tetracycline or ampicillin (Amcill, Ampicin✦).

The nurse, health care provider, or pharmacist instructs clients about the medications associated with gastric irritation. These medications include chemotherapeutic agents, corticosteroids, erythromycin (E-Mycin, Erythromid✦), and NSAIDs, such as aspirin, indomethacin (Indocin, Novomethacin✦) and ibuprofen (Motrin, Advil, Amersol✦, Novo-Profen✦).

The health care provider may change the dose, frequency, or type of medication if symptoms of gastric irritation appear or persist. The nurse instructs clients to avoid stomach-irritating over-the-counter (OTC) medications, such as aspirin and ibuprofen.

DIET THERAPY. The nurse or dietitian instructs the client with gastric disease to limit intake of any foods and spices

CHART 56-3

DRUG THERAPY *for* Peptic Ulcer Disease

Drug	Usual Dosage	Nursing Interventions	Rationale
ANTACIDS			
Magnesium hydroxide with aluminum hydroxide (Maalox, Mylanta)	50-80 mEq 1 hr + 3 hr pc (after meals) + hs (at bedtime)	Give 2 hr after meals and at bedtime.	Hydrogen ion load is high after ingestion of foods.
		Use liquid rather than tablets.	Suspensions are more effective than chewable tablets.
		Do not give other drugs within 1-2 hr of antacids.	Antacids interfere with absorption of other drugs.
		Assess the client for a history of renal disease.	Hypermagnesemia may result.
		Assess the client for a history of congestive heart failure.	These antacids have a high sodium content.
		Observe the client for the side effect of diarrhea.	Magnesium often causes diarrhea.
Aluminum hydroxide (Amphojel)	50-80 mEq 1 hr + 3 hr pc + hs	Give 1 hr after meals and at bedtime.	Hydrogen ion load is high after ingestion of food.
		Use liquid rather than tablets if palatable.	Suspensions are more effective than chewable tablets.
		Do not give other drugs within 1-2 hr of antacids.	Antacids interfere with absorption of other drugs.
		Observe the client for the side effect of constipation. If constipation occurs, consider alternating with magnesium antacid.	Aluminum causes constipation, and magnesium has a laxative effect.
		Use for clients with renal failure.	Aluminum binds with phosphates in the gastrointestinal (GI) tract.
H₂ ANTAGONISTS			
Ranitidine (Zantac)	150 mg bid or 300 mg hs PO; 50 mg q6h IV or 8 mg/hr IV (continuous)	Give single dose at bedtime.	Bedtime administration suppresses nocturnal acid production.
Famotidine (Pepcid)	40 mg once daily or in two divided doses PO; 20 mg q12h IV	Give single dose at bedtime.	Bedtime administration suppresses nocturnal acid production. Compliance may improve with less frequent administration.
Nizatidine (Axid)	150 mg bid or 300 mg hs PO	Give single dose at bedtime.	Bedtime administration suppresses nocturnal acid production. Compliance may improve with less frequent administration.
Sucralfate (Carafate, Sulcrate❋)	1 g qid or 2 g bid PO	Give 1 hr before and 2 hr after meals, and at bedtime.	Food may interfere with drug's adherence to mucosa.
		Do not give within 30 min of giving antacids or other drugs.	Antacids may interfere with effect.

that cause distress. Tea, coffee, cola, chocolate, mustard, paprika, cloves, pepper, and hot spices may increase discomfort. Alcohol and tobacco should also be avoided.

After the client has an acute episode of gastritis, the nurse helps him or her to identify foods that aggravate discomfort. New foods should be introduced one at a time. Avoidance of substances that cause symptoms is important. Most clients seem to progress better with a soft, bland diet and smaller, more frequent meals.

STRESS REDUCTION. The nurse may assist the client with various techniques that reduce stress and discomfort, such as progressive relaxation, cutaneous stimulation, guided imagery, and distraction. (See Chapter 4 for a discussion of these therapies.)

SURGICAL MANAGEMENT. Partial gastrectomy, pyloroplasty, vagotomy, or even total gastrectomy may be indicated for clients who have major bleeding caused by severe erosive gastritis. Such surgery is necessary only if more conservative measures have not controlled the bleeding. Surgical interventions are discussed under Surgical Management (Peptic Ulcer Disease), p. 1228.

PEPTIC ULCER DISEASE

■ OVERVIEW

A **peptic ulcer** is a mucosal lesion of the stomach or duodenum. The term *peptic ulcer* is used to describe both gastric and duodenal ulcers. **Peptic ulcer disease (PUD)** results

CHART 56-3

DRUG THERAPY *for* Peptic Ulcer Disease—cont'd

Drug	Usual Dosage	Nursing Interventions	Rationale
ANTISECRETORY AGENTS			
Omeprazole (Prilosec, Losec✤)	20 mg bid or 40 mg hs PO	Have the client take capsule whole; do not crush.	Delayed-release capsules allow absorption after granules leave the stomach.
		Give single dose at bedtime for ulcer disease.	Bedtime administration suppresses nocturnal acid production.
Lansoprazole (Prevacid)	15 or 30 mg hs PO	Give single dose at bedtime for ulcer disease; do not crush.	Bedtime administration suppresses nocturnal acid production.
Rabeprazole (AcipHex)	20 mg once daily PO	Take following the morning meal.	Drug promotes healing and symptom relief of duodenal ulcers.
		Do not crush capsule.	Drug is a sustained-release capsule.
PROSTAGLANDIN ANALOGS			
Misoprostol (Cytotec)	200 μg qid PO	Take with food.	Drug protects against nonsteroidal anti-inflammatory drug (NSAID)–induced ulcers.
		Avoid magnesium-containing antacids.	Both misoprostol and magnesium-containing antacids can cause diarrhea.
ANTIMICROBIALS			
Clarithromycin (Biaxin)	500 mg tid PO	Antimicrobials should be given as part of therapy to eradicate *Helicobacter pylori* infection.	*H. pylori* is a gram-negative bacterium implicated in the development of peptic ulcer disease (PUD).
Amoxicillin (Amoxil)	1 g bid PO	The selection of the specific drug depends on its effectiveness, side effects, and drug interactions.	
Tetracycline	500 mg qid PO		
Metronidazole (Flagyl)	250 mg tid and hs PO		

when gastric mucosal defenses become impaired and no longer protect the epithelium from the effects of acid and pepsin (Figure 56-1).

Pathophysiology

GASTRIC ULCERS

Acid, pepsin, and *Helicobacter pylori* infection play an important role in the development of gastric ulcers. The gastric mucosal barrier overlies the epithelium. The secretion of mucus and bicarbonate provides a first line of defense in maintaining a near-normal pH on the gastric epithelium and protects the mucosal barrier against acid. Gastromucosal prostaglandins increase the barrier's resistance to ulceration. The integrity of the barrier is enhanced by the rich blood supply of the mucosa of the stomach and duodenum.

When a break in the mucosal barrier occurs, hydrochloric acid injures the epithelium. Gastric ulcers may then result from back-diffusion of acid or dysfunction of the pyloric sphincter (see Figure 56-1). Without normal functioning and competence of the pyloric sphincter, bile refluxes into the stomach. This reflux of bile acids may break the integrity of the mucosal barrier and produce hydrogen ion back-diffusion, which leads to mucosal inflammation. Toxic agents

and bile then destroy the lipid plasma membrane of the gastric mucosa.

Gastric emptying is often delayed in clients with gastric ulceration; this causes regurgitation of duodenal contents, which compounds the gastric mucosal injury. A decreased blood flow to the gastric mucosa may also alter the defense barrier and thereby allow ulceration to occur. Characteristically, gastric ulcers are deep and penetrating, and they usually occur on the lesser curvature of the stomach, near the pylorus (Figure 56-2).

DUODENAL ULCERS

Ninety-five percent of duodenal ulcers occur in the first portion of the duodenum. Duodenal ulcers present as deep, sharply demarcated lesions that penetrate through the mucosa and submucosa into the muscularis propria (muscle layer). The floor of the ulcer consists of a necrotic area residing on granulation tissue and surrounded by areas of fibrosis.

The characteristic feature of a duodenal ulcer is high gastric acid secretion, although a wide range of secretory levels is found. In clients with duodenal ulcers, pH levels are low in the duodenum for long periods. Protein-rich meals, calcium, and vagal excitation stimulate acid secretion. Combined with

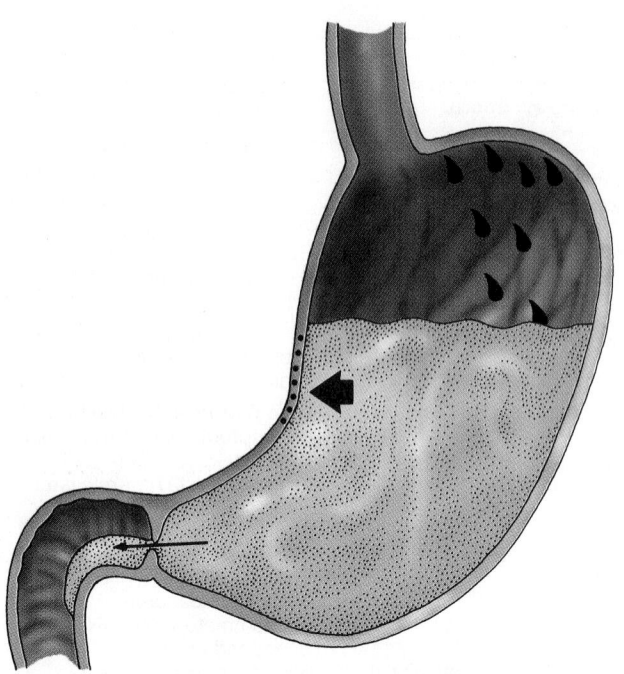

Conditions favoring the development of **gastric ulcers** are normal gastric acid secretion and delayed stomach emptying with *increased diffusion of gastric acid back into the stomach tissues*.

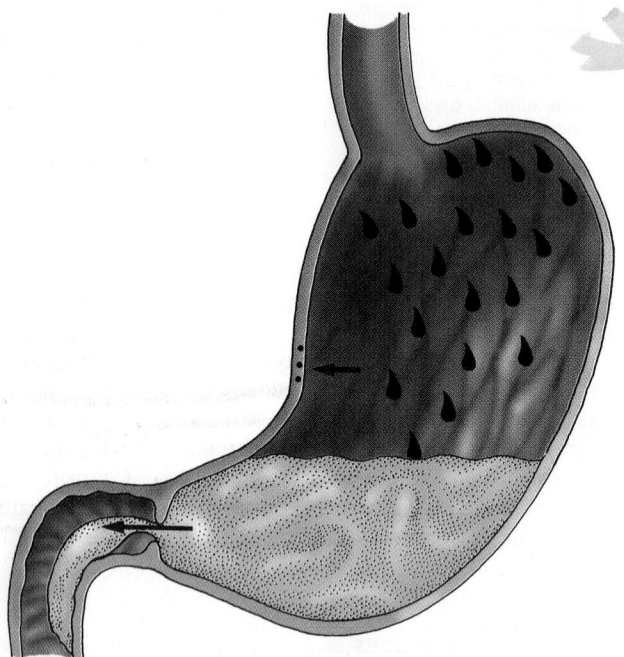

Conditions favoring the development of **duodenal ulcers** are normal diffusion of acid back into stomach tissues with *increased secretion of gastric acid* and *increased stomach emptying*.

Figure 56-1 ● The pathophysiology of peptic ulcer.

hypersecretion, a rapid emptying of food from the stomach reduces the buffering effect of food and delivers a large acid bolus to the duodenum (see Figure 56-1). Inhibitory secretory mechanisms and pancreatic secretion may be insufficient to control the acid load.

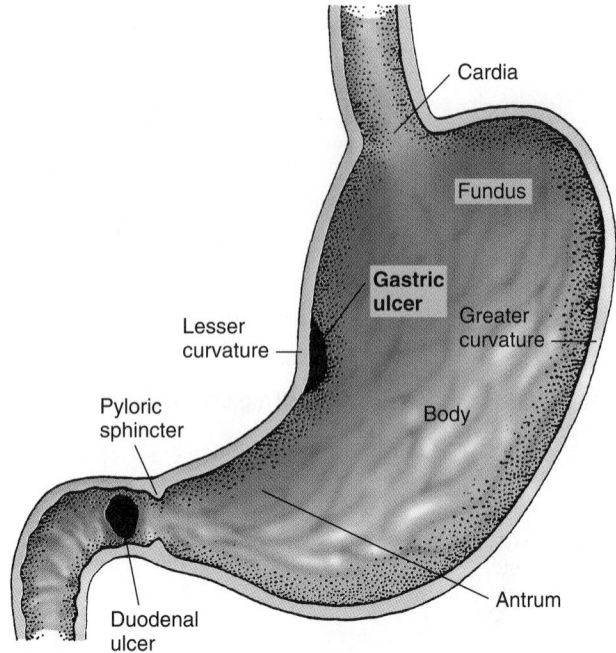

Figure 56-2 ● The most common sites for peptic ulcers.

Up to 95% to 100% of clients with duodenal ulcer disease have confirmed *H. pylori* infection (Friedman & Peterson, 1998). *H. pylori* produces substances that damage the gastric mucosa. Urease produced by *H. pylori* catalyzes the hydrolysis of urea to ammonia. Hydrogen ions are then released in response to the presence of ammonia and contribute further to gastric mucosal damage.

STRESS ULCERS

Stress ulcers are acute gastric mucosal lesions occurring after an acute medical crisis or trauma. Stress ulcers have been associated with head injury, burns, respiratory failure, shock, and sepsis. Bleeding caused by gastric erosion is the principal manifestation of acute stress ulcers.

Multifocal lesions associated with stress ulcers occur in the proximal portion of the stomach and duodenum. These lesions begin as focal areas of ischemia and evolve into erosions and ulcerations that may progress to massive hemorrhage. Little is known of the exact etiology of stress ulcers; however, in the presence of elevated levels of hydrochloric acid, ischemic areas can progress to erosive gastritis and subsequent ulcerations.

COMPLICATIONS OF ULCERS

The most common complications of PUD are hemorrhage, perforation, pyloric obstruction, and intractable disease.

HEMORRHAGE. Hemorrhage occurs in approximately 15% to 25% of clients with PUD and is the most serious complication (Figure 56-3). It tends to occur more often in clients with gastric ulcers and in older adults. Of those with an initial bleed, 40% experience a recurrence of bleeding if underlying infection with *H. pylori* remains untreated or if therapy does not include an H₂ antagonist. With massive bleeding, the client

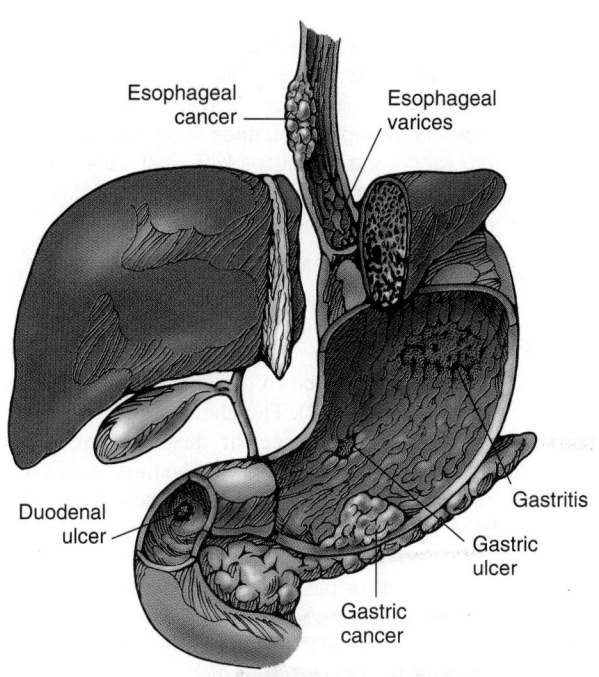

Figure 56-3 ● Common causes of upper gastrointestinal bleeding.

vomits bright red or coffee-ground blood (hematemesis). Hematemesis usually indicates bleeding at or above the duodenojejunal junction (upper gastrointestinal [GI] bleeding).

Minimal bleeding from ulcers is manifested by occult blood in a tarry stool (melena). Melena may occur in clients with gastric ulcers but is more common in those with duodenal ulcers. Gastric acid digestion of blood typically results in a granular dark vomitus (coffee-ground appearance); the digestion of blood within the duodenum and small intestine may result in a black stool.

PERFORATION. Perforation into the peritoneal cavity occurs in approximately 2% to 3% of clients with duodenal ulceration. Simultaneous hemorrhage accompanies perforation in 10% of clients and carries a 6% to 7% mortality rate (Blackington, 1999). In clients with perforation, the gastroduodenal contents (acid peptic juice, bile, and pancreatic juice) empty through the anterior wall of the stomach or duodenum into the peritoneal cavity. Sudden, sharp pain begins in the mid-epigastric region and spreads over the entire abdomen. The amount of pain correlates with the amount and type of GI contents spilled. The characteristic pain causes the client to be apprehensive. The abdomen is tender, rigid, and boardlike, and the client assumes the knee-chest position in an attempt to decrease the tension on the abdominal muscles. The client may become desperately ill within hours. Chemical peritonitis soon occurs; bacterial septicemia and hypovolemic shock follow. Peristalsis diminishes, and paralytic ileus develops. Peptic ulcer perforation is considered a surgical emergency.

PYLORIC OBSTRUCTION. Pyloric obstruction occurs in 2% to 4% of clients and is manifested by vomiting caused by stasis and gastric dilation. Obstruction occurs at the pylorus (the gastric outlet) and is caused by scarring, edema, inflammation, or a combination of these factors.

Symptoms of gastric outlet obstruction include abdominal bloating, nausea, and vomiting. When vomiting persists, the client may experience hypochloremic (metabolic) alkalosis from loss of large quantities of acid gastric juice (hydrogen and chloride ions) in the vomitus. Hypokalemia may also result from the vomiting or metabolic alkalosis. The health care provider typically hospitalizes the client so he or she may receive intravenous (IV) fluid and electrolyte replacement.

INTRACTABLE DISEASE. One third of all clients with ulcers have a single episode with no recurrence. Intractability may develop from complications of ulcers, excessive stressors in the client's life, or an inability to adhere to long-term therapy. The client no longer responds to conservative management, or recurrences of symptoms interfere with activities of daily living (ADLs). In general, the client continues to have recurrent pain and discomfort despite treatment. Clients who fail to respond to traditional treatments or who have a relapse following discontinuation of therapy should be referred to a gastroenterologist.

▌Etiology

Peptic ulcer development is primarily associated with nonsteroidal anti-inflammatory drug (NSAID) use and bacterial infection with *H. pylori*. NSAIDs (such as aspirin or ibuprofen) break down the mucosal barrier and disrupt the mucosal protection mediated systemically by cyclooxygenase (COX) inhibition. In addition, NSAIDs cause the depletion of endogenous prostaglandins, resulting in local gastric mucosal injury. The risk of developing PUD is 5 to 20 times higher in individuals who use NSAIDs than in the general population (Graham et al., 1999c). GI complications from NSAID use can occur at any time, even after long-term uncomplicated use. NSAID-related ulcers are difficult to treat, even with long-term therapy, since these ulcers have a high rate of recurrence.

Certain drugs may contribute to gastroduodenal ulceration by altering gastric secretion, producing localized damage to mucosa and interfering with the healing process. Theophylline (Theo-Dur) and caffeine stimulate hydrochloric acid production. Caffeine may contribute to vascular stasis and mucosal anoxia. The use of corticosteroids is also associated with an increased incidence of peptic ulceration.

H. pylori infection is transmitted from person to person, but exactly how this transmission takes place remains unknown. In one study, *H. pylori* was successfully cultivated from vomitus and occasionally from stool and saliva, indicating that the organism may be transmissible during GI tract illness, particularly if the person is vomiting (see the Evidence-Based Practice for Nursing box on p. 1222).

▌Incidence/Prevalence

In the United States, there are 450,000 new cases of PUD diagnosed each year, and a total of 4 million people see a health care provider for health issues related to peptic ulcers. The prevalence of peptic ulcers has risen from a rate of 19.9 per 1000 persons to a rate of 23 per 1000 (Astarita, 1999). The prevalence of duodenal ulcers ranges from 6% to 15%, and they occur with equal frequency in men and women. Sixty percent of duodenal ulcers recur within 1 year, and 90% recur

EVIDENCE-BASED PRACTICE FOR NURSING

Fecal and oral shedding of *Helicobacter pylori* from healthy infected adults

Parsonnet, J., Shmuely, H. & Haggerty, T. (1999). Fecal and oral shedding of *Helicobacter pylori* from healthy adults. *Journal of the American Medical Association, 282*(23), 2240-2245.

The purpose of this study was to determine how humans shed the organism *Helicobacter pylori* into the environment. A controlled clinical experiment involving healthy volunteers recruited through advertisement was conducted from February through December 1998. All subjects meeting eligibility criteria underwent serum immunoglobulin G (IgG) and 13C breath testing for *H. pylori* infection. A total of 16 asymptomatic *H. pylori*–infected adults and 10 uninfected adults participated in the study.

The *H. pylori*–infected subjects were given a cathartic (sodium phosphate) and an emetic (ipecac). One uninfected control subject also underwent the emesis portion of the experiment. Stool samples were collected during the 8 hours following cathartic administration. Following an overnight fast, subjects were administered 5 mL of ipecac followed by 480 mL of water. A saliva sample was obtained before and following emesis. Air samples were tested throughout the emesis period by using agar plates with a Fluoropore filter covering half of the plate's diameter. A new plate was replaced every 30 minutes. Ten subjects had a second air sampler placed 1.2 m away to determine the radius of bacterial aerosolization. The 10 uninfected subjects provided normal stool and saliva samples.

All vomitus samples from infected subjects grew *H. pylori*, often in high quantities. Air samples taken during vomiting episodes grew *H. pylori* in 37.5% of infected subjects. Saliva tested before and after vomiting grew small quantities of *H. pylori*. Only 22 (21.8%) of 101 stools from infected subjects grew the organism, and no stools or other samples from uninfected subjects contained *H. pylori*.

Critique. Although the sample in this case control study is relatively small, this study provides intriguing evidence of the presence and possible routes of transmission of *H. pylori*.

Implications for Nursing. Since *H. pylori* can be cultured from both vomitus and stools of healthy *H. pylori*–infected individuals, there may be implications for modifications in nursing practice and client education. Since much of the culture grew from vomitus, episodes of emesis could be a mechanism for the spread of *H. pylori* into the environment by means of gastric-oral transmission. Organisms are also dispersed into the air during periods of emesis. *H. pylori* was also cultured from saliva of infected individuals, inferring an oral-oral transmission. Since transmission of *H. pylori* has been demonstrated to occur under conditions that induce vomiting, further research is needed to determine the extent of nursing interventions necessary during episodes of gastrointestinal illness to prevent spread of the organism. Furthermore, as more is learned about *H. pylori* transmission, client education initiatives to prevent spread within households may also be necessary.

within 2 years. The incidence of gastric ulcers is not really known, since some afflicted individuals are asymptomatic (Friedman & Peterson, 1998).

CONSIDERATIONS FOR OLDER ADULTS

Both duodenal and gastric ulcers occur more often following the sixth decade of life. Older adults tend to use over-the-counter (OTC) remedies, often delaying appropriate treatment for symptoms of PUD. In addition, they often suffer from one or more chronic illnesses that require the use of medications that can precipitate or worsen PUD. There is also evidence that older adults may be at increased risk for complications and death following acute peptic ulcer bleeding.

CULTURAL CONSIDERATIONS

Rates of *H. pylori* infection are reportedly higher in African Americans and Hispanics. *H. pylori* infection is also more common in developing countries and among those living in overcrowded living conditions with poor sanitation and water supplies (Blackington, 1999).

▶ COLLABORATIVE MANAGEMENT

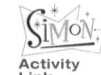

▶ Assessment

■ HISTORY

The nurse collects data related to the causes and risk factors for peptic ulcer disease (PUD). The client is questioned about dietary factors that can influence the development of PUD, such as alcohol intake and tobacco use. The nurse notes if certain foods, such as tomatoes, or caffeinated beverages precipitate or worsen symptoms. Information regarding actual or perceived daily stressors is also elicited.

A history of current or past medical conditions focuses on gastrointestinal (GI) tract problems, particularly any history of diagnosis or treatment for *H. pylori* infection. A complete evaluation of all prescription and OTC medications is obtained. The nurse specifically inquires if the client is taking corticosteroids, aspirin, or other nonsteroidal anti-inflammatory drugs (NSAIDs). The nurse also asks whether the client has ever undergone radiation treatments.

A history of GI upset, pain and its relationship to eating and sleep patterns, and actions taken to relieve pain is also important. The nurse inquires about any changes in the character of the pain, since this may signal the development of complications. For example, if pain that was once intermittent and relieved by food and antacids becomes constant and radiates to the back or upper quadrant, this may indicate impending ulcer perforation. It is important to note that many individuals with active duodenal or gastric ulcers report having no ulcer symptoms.

■ PHYSICAL ASSESSMENT/CLINICAL MANIFESTATIONS

Physical assessment findings may reveal epigastric tenderness, usually located at the midline between the umbilicus and the xiphoid process. If perforation into the peritoneal cavity is present, the client will exhibit a rigid, boardlike abdomen accompanied by rebound tenderness. Initially, auscultation of the abdomen may reveal hyperactive bowel sounds, but these may diminish with progression of the disorder.

Dyspepsia (indigestion), which is defined as discomfort centered around the epigastrium or upper abdomen, is the most commonly reported symptom associated with PUD. This pain or discomfort is described as sharp, burning, or gnawing. Some clients may perceive discomfort as a sensation of abdominal pressure or of fullness or hunger. Pain is less often the initial complaint in the older client. In this age-group, melena is often the presenting sign.

Gastric ulcer pain often occurs in the upper epigastrium with localization to the left of the midline and may be accentuated by food. *Duodenal* ulcer pain is usually located to the right of the epigastrium (Table 56-1). The pain associated with a duodenal ulcer occurs 90 minutes to 3 hours after eating and often awakens the client at night. Pain may also be exacerbated by certain foods (such as tomatoes, hot spices, fried

TABLE 56-1 • DIFFERENTIAL FEATURES OF GASTRIC AND DUODENAL ULCERS

Feature	Gastric Ulcer	Duodenal Ulcer
Age	Usually 50 yr or older	Usually 40-50 yr
Gender	Male/female ratio of 1.1:1	Equal male/female ratio
Blood group	No differentiation	Most often type O
General nourishment	May be malnourished	Usually well nourished
Stomach acid production	Normal secretion or hyposecretion	Hypersecretion
Occurrence	Mucosa exposed to acid-pepsin secretion	Mucosa exposed to acid-pepsin secretion
Clinical course	Healing and recurrence	Healing and recurrence
Pain	Occurs $1/2$-1 hr after a meal; at night: rarely	Occurs 90 min-3 hr after a meal; at night: often awakens client between 1 and 2 AM
	Accentuated by ingestion of food	Relieved by ingestion of food
Response to treatment	Healing with appropriate therapy	Healing with appropriate therapy
Hemorrhage	Hematemesis more common than melena	Melena more common than hematemesis
Malignant change	Perhaps in less than 10%	Rare
Recurrence	Tends to heal and recurs often in the same location	60% recur within 1 yr; 90% recur within 2 yr
Surrounding mucosa	Atrophic gastritis	No gastritis

foods, onions, alcohol, or caffeine drinks) and certain medications (such as aspirin, NSAIDs, or corticosteroids).

Vomiting may be a symptom accompanying ulcer disease, most commonly in conjunction with pyloric sphincter dysfunction. It results from gastric stasis associated with pyloric obstruction. Appetite is generally maintained in clients with a peptic ulcer unless pyloric obstruction is present.

To assess for fluid volume deficit, which can occur secondary to bleeding, the nurse takes orthostatic vital signs of all clients suspected of PUD. Orthostatic changes are characterized by a decrease of more than 20 mm Hg in systolic blood pressure, a decrease of 10 mm Hg in diastolic blood pressure, and/or an increase in pulse when the client rises from a lying to an erect (sitting or, if possible, standing) position. The nurse also assesses for dizziness, especially when the client is upright, since this is another symptom of fluid volume deficit.

> ⊙ **CRITICAL THINKING CHALLENGE**
>
> A client with a long-standing history of rheumatoid arthritis comes to the clinic where you work with complaints of vague, episodic epigastric abdominal discomfort over the last month.
> • During the initial interview, what pertinent questions should you ask regarding this client's symptoms?
> • How might the treatment for arthritis relate to the client's symptoms?
> • What might you expect to find when assessing this client?
>
> For suggested answer guidelines, go to 〔SIMON〕 http://www.wbsaunders.com/SIMON/Iggy/.

■ PSYCHOSOCIAL ASSESSMENT

The nurse assesses the impact of ulcer disease on the client's lifestyle, occupation, family, and social and leisure activities. Questions about lifestyle, occupation, and leisure can yield important information. The nurse evaluates the impact that lifestyle changes will have on the client. This assessment determines the client's ability to comply with the prescribed treatment regimen and to obtain the needed social support to alter his or her lifestyle.

■ LABORATORY ASSESSMENT

Hemoglobin and hematocrit values may be low, indicating bleeding. The stool specimen may be positive for occult blood if bleeding is present.

■ RADIOGRAPHIC ASSESSMENT

A barium examination of the GI tract can be used to establish a duodenal ulcer. A duodenal ulcer appears as a discrete crater in the duodenal bulb. This is often the initial test for a client who does not have severe symptoms. If perforation is suspected, the health care provider usually first orders a flat-plate film of the abdomen to identify the presence of free air.

■ OTHER DIAGNOSTIC ASSESSMENT

The major diagnostic test for PUD is esophagogastroduodenoscopy (EGD), which is the most accurate means of establishing a diagnosis. Visualization of the ulcer crater by EGD allows the health care provider to take specimens for *H. pylori* testing and for biopsy and cytologic studies for ruling out gastric cancer (see the Legal/Ethical Issues in Health Care box on p. 1224). EGD may be repeated at 4- to 6-week intervals while the health care provider evaluates the progress of healing in response to therapy.

Urea breath testing has been employed to detect *H. pylori* when endoscopy is not clinically indicated. To perform this test, the client must be on NPO status after midnight on the night before the test. The client drinks a carbon-enriched urea solution. The presence of *H. pylori* will cause the bacteria to break down the solution and release carbon dioxide, which the client inhales in a collection container for analysis. The carbon dioxide excreted in the breath is then measured and compared with a baseline measurement to determine the presence of *H. pylori*. In addition to its noninvasive nature, this test assesses the entire stomach and may prove especially helpful after the client has been treated to determine if treatment was successful (Blackington, 1999).

A second noninvasive test for *H. pylori* involves IgG serologic testing. Infection with *H. pylori* causes immunoglobulin

QUALITY OF CARE FOR MEDICARE CLIENTS WITH PEPTIC ULCER DISEASE

Economic constraints on the health care system have resulted in efforts to provide cost-effective, high-quality care. In an effort to improve the quality of care delivered to Medicare beneficiaries with peptic ulcer disease (PUD), a chart review of 2644 Medicare beneficiaries was conducted to measure compliance with National Institute of Health (NIH) guidelines for the detection and treatment of *Helicobacter pylori* in PUD.

In this particular study, only 57% of hospitalized Medicare recipients with PUD were tested for *H. pylori*. In addition, only 74% of clients with known *H. pylori* infection were treated with appropriate antimicrobial therapy. Medical record review also noted that 74% of clients were screened for nonsteroidal anti-inflammatory drug (NSAID) use. Only 24% had documented counseling regarding the risks associated with NSAID use, and only 2% had documented education of the ulcer-associated risks of NSAID use.

Although limited documented education may be in part to blame for the poor quality of care regarding *H. pylori*–related ulcers, NIH clinical practice guidelines for the diagnosis and treatment of peptic ulcer disease are clearly underutilized. Quality improvement initiatives are needed to improve the care delivered to Medicare beneficiaries with PUD. *H. pylori* screening and treatment guidelines need to be enforced to ensure that appropriate treatment is received, especially by older adults.

Data from Offman, J., et al. (2000). The quality of care for Medicare patients with peptic ulcer disease. *American Journal of Gastroenterology* 95(1), 106-113.

antibodies to form. Although antibody assays have a high sensitivity and specificity (>95%) for detecting *H. pylori,* antibody assays cannot be used to document eradication of the organism, since antibody levels can remain elevated despite successful treatment.

A complete medication history needs to be obtained before diagnostic testing is done for *H. pylori*. False-negative results could be obtained if the client has received antibiotic treatment, used a bismuth preparation (Pepto-Bismol), or used a proton-pump inhibitor within the 4-week period before testing for *H. pylori*. Other medications, such as misoprostol, sucralfate, or an H_2 blocker administered within the week before the test may also yield a false-negative result. Use of over-the-counter medications (OTC), such as Pepcid AC, Tagamet, and Zantac, can also affect test results.

▶ Analysis

■ COMMON NURSING DIAGNOSES AND COLLABORATIVE PROBLEMS

The following are priority nursing diagnoses for clients with peptic ulcer disease (PUD):

1. Acute Pain or Chronic Pain related to gastric and/or duodenal mucosal injury
2. Risk for Deficient Fluid Volume related to hemorrhage or vomiting

■ ADDITIONAL NURSING DIAGNOSES AND COLLABORATIVE PROBLEMS

In addition to the common nursing diagnoses, clients with PUD may have one or more of the following:

- Ineffective Therapeutic Regimen Management related to long-term treatment and lifestyle changes
- Ineffective Coping related to intractable progressive disease
- Imbalanced Nutrition: Less Than Body Requirements related to anorexia, nausea, or diet constraints
- Disturbed Sleep Pattern related to discomfort
- Risk for Falls related to orthostatic hypotension
- A collaborative problem that could occur is Potential for Metabolic Alkalosis.

▶ Planning and Implementation

■ ACUTE PAIN; CHRONIC PAIN

NOC **PLANNING: EXPECTED OUTCOMES.** PUD causes significant discomfort that impacts many aspects of daily living. The client with PUD is expected to experience reduction or alleviation of pain as indicated by self-report.

INTERVENTIONS. Interventions to manage pain related to PUD are accomplished with specific ulcer therapy and dietary modifications. One of the primary purposes for employing drug therapy in the management of PUD is to reduce or eliminate pain. Analgesics are not the mainstay of pain relief for PUD. Instead, the ulcer drug regimen itself promotes relief of pain by eradicating *H. pylori* infection and promoting healing of gastric mucosa.

The nurse performs a comprehensive pain assessment that includes the following aspects of pain:

- Location
- Characteristics
- Onset/duration
- Frequency
- Quality
- Severity
- Precipitating and alleviating factors

Any changes in the characteristics or location of peptic ulcer pain are carefully assessed, since such changes often accompany the development of complications. The nurse teaches the client to eliminate factors (such as spicy foods) that can precipitate or increase pain from ulcer disease.

Measures to promote adequate rest and sleep may be necessary, since ulcer pain can cause the client to awaken. The nurse assists the client in achieving compliance with the medication regimen, since adherence to the drug regimen will promote relief of pain and discomfort. The client's satisfaction with the level of pain relief achieved is monitored.

DRUG THERAPY. The primary goals of drug therapy in the treatment of PUD are (1) to provide pain relief, (2) to eradicate *H. pylori* infection, (3) to heal ulcerations, and (4) to prevent recurrence (see Chart 56-3). Several different regimens can be used to achieve these goals. In selecting a therapeutic drug regimen, the health care provider must consider the efficacy of the treatment, the anticipated side effects, the ability of the client to comply with the regimen, and the cost of the treatment (Astarita, 1999).

Although numerous drugs have been evaluated for the treatment of *H. pylori* infection, no single agent has been used successfully against the organism. Current practice involves using a combination of agents to achieve treatment goals. The most successful regimen used is a triple therapy consisting of a bismuth compound, metronidazole, and either amoxicillin or tetracycline. Triple therapy is supple-

COST OF CARE
IMPLICATIONS FOR NURSING

PEPTIC ULCER DISEASE

Cost of Care

- The cost of selected 2-week regimens for the treatment of *Helicobacter pylori*–associated peptic ulcer disease (PUD) ranges from $75 to $215, depending on the extent and combination of drugs used.
- Treatment of *H. pylori*–associated PUD decreases the need for hospitalization secondary to bleeding episodes. This reduces the economic burden to the health care system.
- The direct and indirect costs of diagnosis and treatment account for $5 billion to $6 billion annually.
- Treatment of *H. pylori*–related PUD provides substantial savings in terms of direct costs (e.g., medications, office visits) and indirect costs (lost workdays due to the illness).

Implications for Nursing

The treatment of *H. pylori*–associated PUD reduces recurrence from 80% to less than 10% in 1 year. However, in clinical practice, appropriate antimicrobial therapy is underutilized. Nurses need to understand the pathogenesis of PUD in order to advocate for appropriate treatment for their clients. In addition, nurses need to educate their clients concerning the role of *H. pylori* infection in ulcer disease in order to assist them in effective management of this disorder.

Data from Lane, L., & Fendrick, A.M. (1998). *Helicobacter pylori* and peptic ulcer disease. *Postgraduate Medicine, 103*(3), 231-243; and Graham, D., et al. (1999). Recognizing peptic ulcer disease: Keys to clinical and laboratory diagnosis. *Postgraduate Medicine, 105*(3), 113-128.

CHART 56-4

NURSING FOCUS *on the* **OLDER ADULT**
Giving Ulcer Medications Safely

- Assess the client's complete drug regimen. Older adults are more susceptible to adverse side effects from multiple drugs.
- Monitor the client carefully for signs of adverse effects.
- Keep dosage schedules simple when a client is at home.
- Assess the client's understanding of instructions related to medications. Provide a written list and instructions for each medication.

---

mented by the addition of an H_2-receptor antagonist to facilitate ulcer healing and prevent recurrence (see the Cost of Care box above). Although this regimen is the most effective and least expensive, adherence to the regimen is difficult for most clients. A client must consume medications four times daily, and adverse effects occur in 20% to 30% of individuals, especially older adults (Chart 56-4). Recently, some strains of *H. pylori* have begun to demonstrate metronidazole resistance, raising concerns about long-term treatment with this regimen.

HYPOSECRETORY DRUGS. Hyposecretory drugs produce a reduction in gastric acid secretions. These drugs include antisecretory agents, H_2-receptor antagonists, and prostaglandin analogs (see Chart 56-3).

ANTISECRETORY AGENTS. Omeprazole (Prilosec), lansoprazole (Prevacid), and the newest proton pump inhibitor, rabeprazole (Aciphex) suppress the H^+,K^+-ATPase enzyme system of gastric acid production. These medications are available as sustained-release tablets; therefore they must not be crushed before administration.

H_2-RECEPTOR ANTAGONISTS. Drugs that block histamine-stimulated gastric secretions are effective in the management of ulcer disease. These medications may be used for indigestion and heartburn, and lower-dose forms are available in over-the-counter (OTC) products. H_2-receptor antagonists block the action of the H_2 receptors of the parietal cells, thus inhibiting gastric acid secretion. The most common drugs are ranitidine (Zantac), famotidine (Pepcid), and nizatidine (Axid). These drugs are typically administered in a single dose at bedtime and are used for 4 to 6 weeks in combination with triple therapy.

PROSTAGLANDIN ANALOGS. Prostaglandins are naturally abundant in the gastrointestinal (GI) tract and have been shown to be effective in clinical trials in the treatment of duodenal ulcers. Prostaglandin analogs reduce gastric acid secretion and enhance gastric mucosal resistance to tissue injury. Misoprostol (Cytotec), the most commonly used drug in this category, *prevents* NSAID-induced ulcers. Some NSAIDs are being manufactured in combination with misoprostol. A significant adverse effect of this drug is uterine contraction; therefore its use is contraindicated in pregnant women.

ANTACIDS. Antacids buffer gastric acid and prevent the formation of pepsin. Antacids have demonstrated effectiveness in accelerating the healing of duodenal ulcers. Liquid suspensions are the most therapeutic form, but tablets may be more convenient and enhance compliance. The most widely used preparations are mixtures of aluminum hydroxide and magnesium hydroxide, since this combination overcomes the unpleasant GI side effects of either of these preparations when used alone. Mylanta and Maalox are examples of this type of combination antacid formulation. The aluminum and magnesium hydroxide combination products neutralize well at small doses. Aluminum and magnesium-based products must also be administered cautiously to those with renal impairment, since these substances cannot be eliminated adequately by the kidneys and are consequently retained in excessive amounts in the body.

The nurse instructs the client that to achieve a therapeutic effect, sufficient antacid must be ingested to neutralize the hourly production of acid. For optimal effect, antacids are given about 2 hours after meals to reduce the hydrogen ion load in the duodenum. Antacids may be effective from 30 minutes to 3 hours after ingestion. Antacids taken with an empty stomach are quickly evacuated; thus the neutralizing effect is reduced. Calcium carbonate (Tums) is a potent antacid, but it triggers gastrin release, causing a rebound acid secretion. Therefore its use in acid inhibition is not recommended.

Antacids can interact with certain drugs, such as phenytoin (Dilantin), tetracycline, and ketoconazole, and interfere with their effectiveness. The nurse determines what other drugs the client is using before recommending a specific antacid. Medications are administered 1 to 2 hours before or after the antacid. The nurse informs the client that flavored antacids, especially wintergreen, should be avoided. The flavoring increases the emptying time of the stomach; thus the desired effect of the antacid is negated.

The nurse teaches the client with past or present heart failure to avoid antacids containing a high sodium content, such as aluminum hydroxide, magnesium hydroxide, sodium bicarbonate, and simethicone combination products (Gelusil and Mylanta). Magaldrate (Riopan) has the lowest sodium concentration.

MUCOSAL BARRIER FORTIFIERS. Sucralfate (Carafate) is sulfonated disaccharide that forms complexes with proteins at the base of a peptic ulcer. This protective coat prevents further digestive action of both acid and pepsin.

Sucralfate does not inhibit acid secretion. Rather, it binds bile acids and pepsins, reducing injury from these substances. Sucralfate may be used in conjunction with H_2-receptor antagonists and antacids but should not be administered within 1 hour of the antacid. Sucralfate is given on an empty stomach 1 hour before each meal and at bedtime. The main side effect of this drug is constipation.

DIET THERAPY. The value of diet in the management of ulcer disease is highly controversial. There is no evidence that dietary restriction reduces gastric acid secretion or promotes tissue healing, although a bland diet may assist in relieving symptoms. Food itself acts as an antacid by neutralizing gastric acid for 30 to 60 minutes. An increased rate of gastric acid secretion, called rebound, may follow. If diet therapy is used, it may be directed toward neutralizing acid and reducing hypermotility, which may alleviate symptoms.

The nurse instructs the client to avoid substances that increase gastric acid secretion. This includes caffeine-containing beverages (coffee, tea, and cola). Both caffeinated and decaffeinated coffees should be avoided, since coffee contains peptides that stimulate gastrin release.

In collaboration, the nurse and dietitian teach the client to exclude any foods that cause discomfort. A bland, nonirritating diet is recommended during the acute symptomatic phase. Bedtime snacks are avoided because they may stimulate gastric acid secretion. Eating six smaller daily meals may help, but this regimen is no longer a regular part of therapy. There is no evidence to support the theory that eating six daily meals promotes healing of the ulcer, and this practice actually stimulates gastric acid secretion. Clients should avoid alcohol and tobacco because of their stimulatory effects on gastric acid secretion.

■ **RISK FOR DEFICIENT FLUID VOLUME**

PLANNING: EXPECTED OUTCOMES. Fluid volume loss secondary to the development of complications is a risk associated with PUD. Blood loss due to hemorrhage can carry significant morbidity and mortality. Fluid volume loss secondary to vomiting can lead to dehydration and electrolyte imbalances. The client with peptic ulcer disease (PUD) is expected to benefit from prevention or early detection of disease complications.

INTERVENTIONS. Monitoring and early recognition of complications are critical to the successful management of PUD. Interventions aimed at managing complications associated with PUD include prevention and/or management of bleeding, perforation, and gastric outlet obstruction. In some cases, surgical treatment of complications becomes necessary.

HYPOVOLEMIA MANAGEMENT. The purpose of managing hypovolemia is to expand intravascular fluid in a client who is volume depleted. The nurse or assistive nursing personnel monitors vital signs and observes for fluid loss from bleeding or vomiting. The nurse carefully monitors the client's fluid status, including intake and output. Fluid re-

placement in older adults should be closely monitored to prevent fluid overload. An infusion pump is used to ensure accurate delivery of the desired volume. Serum electrolytes are also monitored, since depletions from vomiting or nasogastric suctioning must be replaced. The nurse should ensure that two large-bore peripheral IV catheters are inserted so that both fluids and blood lost to vomiting or hemorrhage can be replaced. Volume replacement with isotonic crystalloid solutions (0.9 normal saline solution, or lactated Ringer's solution) should be started immediately, since adequate fluid volume replacement is essential. The health care provider may order blood products, such as packed red blood cells, to expand volume and correct abnormalities in the complete blood count (CBC). For clients with active bleeding, fresh frozen plasma may be given if the prothrombin time is 1.5 times higher than the midrange control value. To prevent injury from falls secondary to orthostatic hypotension, the client is assisted with ambulation.

BLEEDING REDUCTION: GASTROINTESTINAL. The purpose of interventions to reduce bleeding is to limit the amount of blood loss from the upper and lower gastrointestinal (GI) tract resulting from complications related to PUD. The nurse monitors the client for signs and symptoms indicating GI bleeding. All excretions are observed for the presence of frank or occult bleeding. With GI bleeding, the presence of frank blood or coffee-ground vomitus may be observed. Stools can contain frank blood or appear black and tarry. Occult blood loss may be detected by stool examination and may be accompanied by progressive iron deficiency anemia.

The nurse monitors the client's hematocrit, hemoglobin, and coagulation studies for changes from the baseline measurements. The nurse or assistive nursing personnel monitors vital signs. With mild bleeding (less than 500 mL), slight feelings of weakness and mild perspiration may be present. When blood loss exceeds 1 L/24 hr, signs and symptoms of shock may be manifested, such as hypotension, chills, palpitations, diaphoresis, and a weak, thready pulse. (See Chapter 38 for the treatment of shock.)

The nurse immediately notifies the health care provider of major bleeding. Transfusion therapy may be required to replace blood loss. (See Chapter 40 for nursing interventions for clients undergoing blood transfusion.) The health care provider may order H_2 blockers to avoid extremes in gastric pH levels. If appropriate and as ordered, the nurse inserts a nasogastric (NG) tube, monitors secretions, and performs nasogastric lavage to decompress the stomach and alleviate bleeding. In addition, the client and family are instructed to avoid the use of anti-inflammatory medications that can precipitate or worsen GI bleeding.

NIC interventions are summarized in Chart 56-5.

NONSURGICAL MANAGEMENT. Because prevention or early detection of complications is critical in obtaining a satisfactory outcome, the nurse monitors the client carefully and immediately reports changes to the health care provider. The type of nonsurgical intervention selected will depend on the type and severity of the complication.

The goals of therapeutic interventions for bleeding secondary to PUD are as follows:
- Cessation of the acute bleeding episode
- Prevention of rebleeding

CHART 56-5

NIC INTERVENTION ACTIVITIES for
The Client with Stomach Disorders

Hypovolemia Management: *The expansion of intravascular fluid volume in a client who is volume depleted*
- Monitor vital signs, as appropriate.
- Monitor fluid status, including intake and output, as appropriate.
- Monitor for fluid loss (e.g., bleeding, vomiting, diarrhea, perspiration, and tachypnea).
- Arrange availability of blood products for transfusion, if necessary.
- Administer blood products (e.g., platelets and fresh frozen plasma), as appropriate.
- Monitor for blood reaction, if appropriate.

Bleeding Reduction: Gastrointestinal: *The limitation of the amount of blood loss from the upper and lower gastrointestinal tract and related complications*
- Monitor for signs and symptoms of persistent bleeding (e.g., check all secretions for frank or occult blood).
- Hematest all excretions and observe for blood loss in emesis, sputum, feces, urine, nasogastric drainage, and wound drainage, as appropriate.
- Document color, amount, and character of stools.
- Monitor coagulation studies and complete blood count (CBC) with WBC differential.
- Insert nasogastric tube to suction and monitor secretions, if appropriate
- Perform nasogastric lavage, as appropriate.
- Avoid extremes in gastric pH level by administration of appropriate medication (e.g., antacids or histamine-2 blocking agent).
- Instruct the client and/or family on the need for blood replacement, as appropriate.
- Instruct the client and/or family to avoid the use of anti-inflammatory medications (e.g., aspirin and ibuprofen).

NIC intervention activities selected from McCloskey, J.C., & Bulechek, G.M. (2000). *Nursing interventions classification (NIC)* (3rd ed.). St. Louis: Mosby. No part of this work is to be altered without prior written permission from the Publisher.
WBC, White blood cell.

A combination of several different therapeutic interventions, including endoscopic therapy, acid suppression, NG tube placement, and saline lavage, can be used to control acute bleeding and prevent rebleeding. Therapeutic trials have been conducted to determine the optimal treatment for bleeding due to peptic ulcers. Endoscopic therapy and suppression of gastric acid are the primary therapies used to control active bleeding caused by PUD. H_2-receptor antagonists, proton pump inhibitors, and antacids are the primary medications used to treat this bleeding.

ENDOSCOPIC THERAPY. Endoscopic therapy via an esophagogastroduodenoscopy (EGD) can assist in achieving homeostasis during an acute bleeding episode. The three primary methods of endoscopic therapy are (1) thermal contact using a heater probe or multi-electrocoagulation, (2) injection of the bleeding site with diluted epinephrine or a sclerosing agent (alcohol), and (3) laser therapy. All three methods are effective in achieving blood clot formation. Thermal contact and injection are most commonly used. Laser therapy is costly and therefore is used less often. Endoscopic therapy is most beneficial for clients with active bleeding; however, persistent or re-bleeding despite endoscopic therapy continues to be problematic. No consensus has been reached on the appropriate management of re-bleeding.

ACID SUPPRESSION. Aggressive acid suppression is used to prevent re-bleeding. When acute bleeding is stopped and clot formation has taken place within the ulcer crater, the clot remains in contact with gastric contents. Acid-suppressive agents are used to stabilize the clot by raising the pH level of gastric contents. Several drugs are used to achieve acid suppression in clients with a bleeding episode. H_2-receptor antagonists prevent acid from being produced by parietal cells. Proton pump inhibitors prevent the transport of acid across the parietal cell membrane, whereas antacids buffer acid produced in the stomach.

NASOGASTRIC TUBE PLACEMENT. Upper GI bleeding may require the health care provider or nurse to insert a nasogastric (NG) tube to:
- Ascertain the presence or absence of blood in the stomach
- Assess the rate of bleeding
- Prevent gastric dilation
- Administer saline lavage

Nasogastric aspiration is an important part of diagnostic and prognostic evaluation of the client. The presence of red blood in emesis, nasogastric aspirate, or stools is correlated with a poor outcome (Terdiman, 1998).

Once the NG tube is placed, confirmation of proper positioning of the tube is determined by x-ray examination. The nurse irrigates the NG tube to maintain its patency and prevent obstruction with clotted blood.

SALINE LAVAGE. Saline lavage requires the insertion of a large-bore NG tube with instillation of saline in volumes of 50 to 200 mL. The saline and blood are repeatedly withdrawn until returns are clear or light pink and without clots. For protection against exposure to blood, practitioners may use the following procedure with a closed system for irrigation and suction. A Y-connector is attached to the NG tube, and an IV bag of normal saline is attached to tubing at one end of the Y-connector. The opposite connector is attached to tubing connected to wall suction. After the stomach is initially drained by suctioning, the tubing attached to the wall suction is clamped off, and up to 200 mL of normal saline is allowed to drain into the client through the NG tube. After the saline is instilled, the tube connecting the saline to the NG tube is clamped off, and the clamp to suction is released. The nurse instructs the client to lie on the left side during this procedure to limit the flow of saline out of the stomach and prevent aspiration.

NONSURGICAL MANAGEMENT OF PERFORATION. To prevent peritonitis from GI contents that have entered the peritoneum, perforation is managed by the immediate replacement of fluid, blood, and electrolytes and the administration of antibiotics. The nurse maintains nasogastric suction to drain gastric secretions and thus prevent further peritoneal spillage. The client remains on NPO status, and the nurse carefully monitors intake and output. The nurse or assistive nursing personnel checks vital signs at least hourly and monitors the client for clinical manifestations of septic shock, such as fever, pain, tachycardia, lethargy, or anxiety.

NONSURGICAL MANAGEMENT OF PYLORIC OBSTRUCTION. Pyloric obstruction is caused by edema, spasm, or scar tissue. Symptoms of obstruction related to difficulty in emptying the stomach include feelings of fullness, distention, or nausea after eating, as well as vomiting of copious amounts of undigested food.

Treatment of obstruction is directed toward restoration of fluid and electrolyte balance and decompression of the dilated stomach. Obstruction related to edema and spasm generally responds to medical therapy. First, the stomach must be decompressed with nasogastric suction; next, interventions are directed at correcting metabolic alkalosis and dehydration. The NG tube is clamped after about 72 hours, and the client is checked for retention of gastric contents. If the amount retained is not more than 350 mL in 30 minutes, the health care provider may allow oral fluids. In some cases, surgical intervention may be required.

CRITICAL THINKING CHALLENGE

Your client has been diagnosed with a nonsteroidal anti-inflammatory drug (NSAID)–induced duodenal ulcer, and the presence of *H. pylori* infection has been confirmed.

- What complications of peptic ulcer disease (PUD) is this client most at risk for?
- What dietary instructions should you give to this client?
- What should you teach this client about the medical treatment for PUD?

For suggested answer guidelines, go to SIMON http://www.wbsaunders.com/SIMON/Iggy/.

SURGICAL MANAGEMENT. New guidelines for the treatment of PUD that include *H. pylori* eradication and the development of nonsurgical means of controlling bleeding have led to a decline in the need for surgical intervention. In PUD, surgical intervention is used to:

- Reduce the acid-secreting ability of the stomach
- Treat clients who do not respond to medical therapy
- Treat a surgical emergency that develops as a complication of PUD

PREOPERATIVE CARE. Before surgery, an NG tube is inserted and connected to suction to remove secretions and empty the stomach. This allows surgery to take place without contamination of the peritoneal cavity by gastric secretions. Chart 56-6 describes the procedure for inserting the NG tube and nursing care associated with NG tube maintenance. The NG tube remains in place postoperatively to prevent the accumulation of secretions, which may lead to vomiting or gastrointestinal (GI) distention and pressure on the suture line.

Other preoperative nursing measures for the client undergoing gastric surgery are the same as those for any client undergoing abdominal surgery and general anesthesia (see Chapter 17).

CHART 56-6

BEST PRACTICE for Nasogastric Tubes

1. Inform the client about the procedure and its potential discomfort.
2. Seat the client with pillows behind the shoulders.
3. Lubricate the tube with a water-soluble lubricant.
4. Measure the length of the tube to be passed.
   a. Measure from the bridge of the nose to the earlobe to the xiphoid process.
   b. Indicate this length with a piece of tape on the tube.

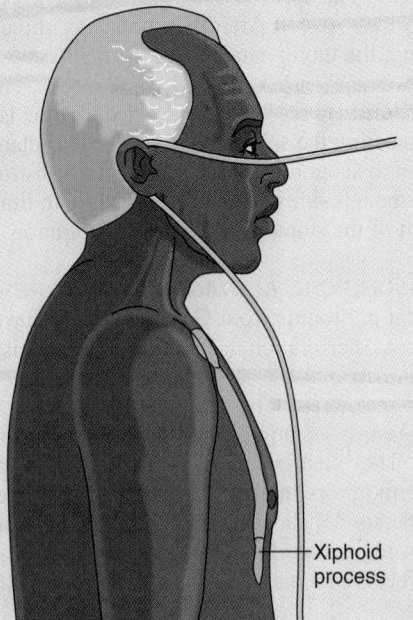

Xiphoid process

5. Determine which nostril is more patent.
6. Encourage the client to swallow or drink water if the level of consciousness and treatment plan permit.

7. Insert the tube.
   a. Pass the tube gently into the nasopharynx. Ask the client to swallow repeatedly while the tube is advanced.
   b. If resistance is met, rotate the tube slowly, aiming downward and toward the closer ear.
   c. In the intubated or semiconscious client, flex the client's head toward the chest while passing the tube.
8. Withdraw the tube immediately if any change is noted in the client's respiratory status.
9. Test for tube placement by using one or more of the following techniques:
   a. Obtain a sample of the gastric contents by aspirating with a 50-mL catheter-tipped syringe.
   b. Test the pH of the gastric contents (should be between 1 and 3.5).
   c. Obtain an order for an x-ray study to confirm placement.
10. Connect the tube to suction at low pressure.
    a. The Levin tube is connected to intermittent low suction.
    b. The Salem sump or Anderson tube is connected to continuous low suction.
11. Secure the tube to the client's nose with adhesive tape and to the client's gown.
    a. Tie a slipknot around the tube with a rubber band.
    b. Pin a rubber band to the client's gown.
12. Check the client's intake and output every 4 hr or more often, as indicated.
13. Observe the client for nausea, vomiting, abdominal fullness, or distention.
14. If irrigation is indicated, use only a normal saline solution.
15. Observe the client for alterations in fluid and electrolyte balance.
16. If indicated, instruct the client about movement that will not dislodge the tube and cause nasal irritation.
17. Remove the adhesive tape securing the tube to the nose daily and prn to clean skin; reapply tape.

OPERATIVE PROCEDURES. There is no definitive single procedure for PUD. The most commonly performed surgical procedures are gastroenterostomy, vagotomy and pyloroplasty.

Gastroenterostomy. A simple **gastroenterostomy** permits neutralization of gastric acid by regurgitation of alkaline duodenal contents into the stomach. The surgeon creates a passage between the body of the stomach and the small bowel, often the jejunum (Figure 56-4). The benefit may be offset by interference with acid inhibition of gastrin release, which results in a net increase in acid secretion.

If the gastroenterostomy drains the stomach, it reduces motor activity in the pyloroduodenal area. Drainage of the gastric contents diverts acid from the ulcerated area and facilitates healing. However, the secretory capacity of the parietal cell mass of the stomach has not been reduced, and the gastrin mechanism continues to function. For this reason, a vagotomy is usually combined with gastroenterostomy for reduction of the vagal influences.

Vagotomy. Three types of **vagotomy** have been used in the treatment of duodenal ulcers: truncal vagotomy, selective vagotomy, and proximal gastric vagotomy (Figure 56-5). Vagotomy eliminates the acid-secreting stimulus to gastric cells and decreases the responsiveness of parietal cells. In a truncal vagotomy, the vagal trunks are transected and the antrum is removed. The remaining stomach is anastomosed to the proximal duodenum (Billroth I) or to a loop of jejunum (Billroth II) (Figures 56-6 and 56-7).

With selective vagotomy, only the branches of the vagus nerve that supply the stomach are transected; the remaining abdominal viscera still has intact vagal innervation. Selective vagotomy results in a more complete response, reduced ulcer recurrence, and fewer postoperative complications.

Proximal gastric vagotomy interrupts the nerve supply to only the acid-secreting portion of the stomach; it spares the branches of the vagus nerve that innervate the antrum, making pyloroplasty unnecessary.

Pyloroplasty. The surgeon often performs **pyloroplasty** in conjunction with a vagotomy to widen the exit of the pylorus. This facilitates emptying of stomach contents. The most common procedure is the Heineke-Mikulicz pyloroplasty (Figure 56-8). In this procedure the surgeon enlarges the pyloric stricture by incising the pylorus longitudinally and sutures the incision transversely.

POSTOPERATIVE CARE. The postoperative care is similar for all of the surgical procedures (see the Client Care Plan on p. 1231). The nurse provides the usual postoperative care for clients who have had general anesthesia (see Chapter 19).

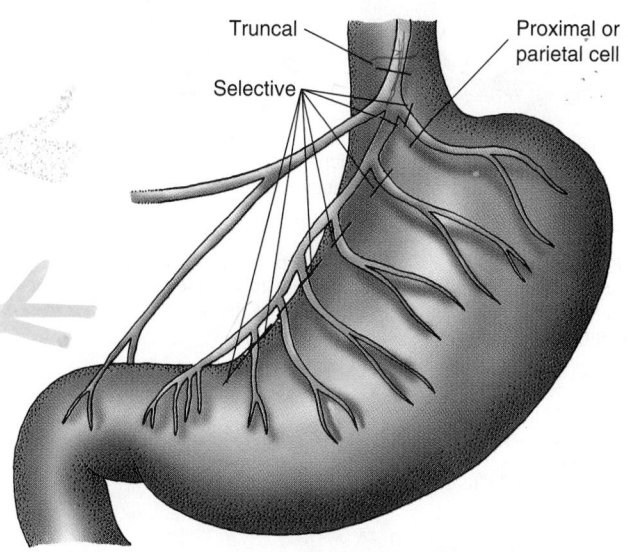

Figure 56-5   ●   The types of vagotomies.

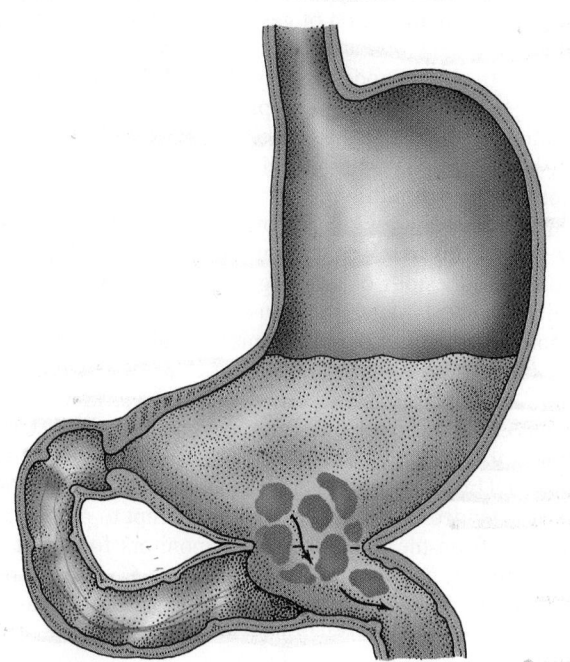

Figure 56-4   ●   Gastroenterostomy (the creation of a passage between the body of the stomach and the jejunum).

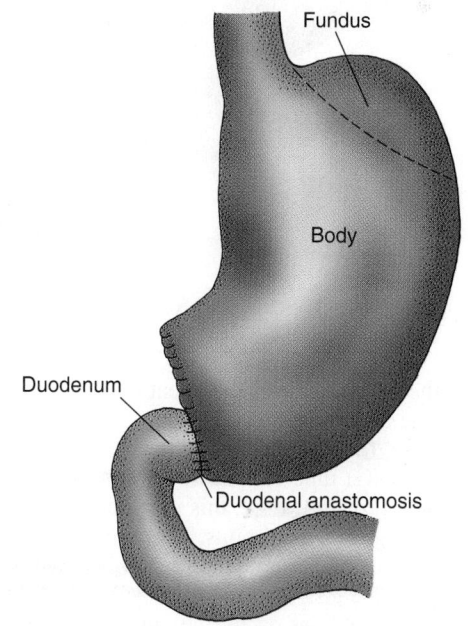

Figure 56-6   ●   The Billroth I procedure (gastroduodenostomy). The distal portion of the stomach is removed, and the remainder is anastomosed to the duodenum. The shading shows the portion removed.

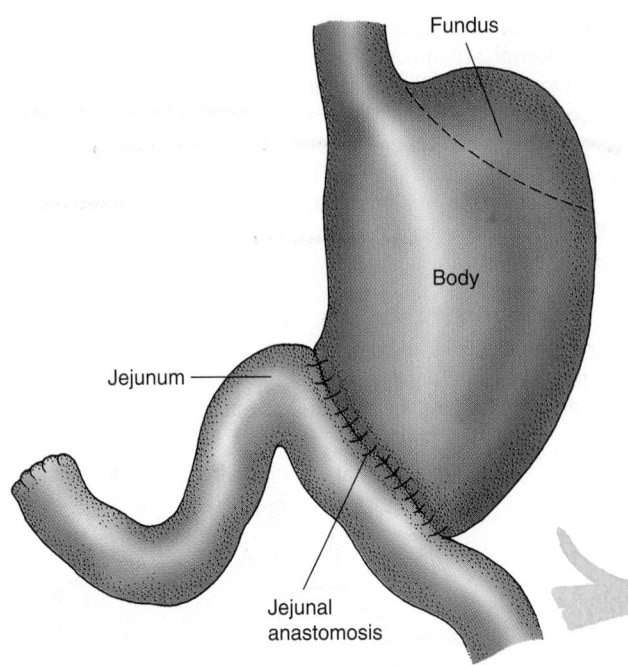

Figure 56-7 ● The Billroth II procedure (gastrojejunostomy). The lower portion of the stomach is removed, and the remainder is anastomosed to the jejunum. The shading shows the portion removed. A remaining duodenal stump is closed.

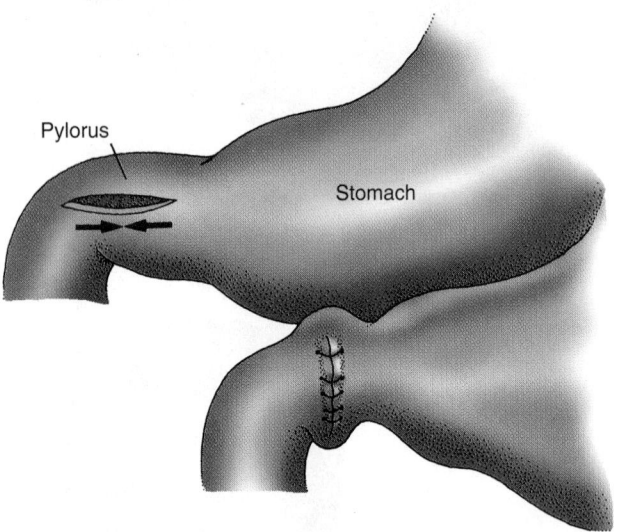

Figure 56-8 ● The Heineke-Mikulicz pyloroplasty.

In addition, the nurse monitors the client for the development of postoperative complications.

Nasogastric Tube Management. The nurse monitors the nasogastric (NG) tube for patency and carefully secures the tube to prevent dislodgment; this is critical for preventing the retention of gastric secretions. The nurse monitors the client to make sure that no more than a scant amount of blood drains from the tube and that abdominal distention does not develop. If these problems occur, the nurse reports them immediately to the surgeon. Irrigation or repositioning of the NG tube is not done after gastric surgery unless specifically ordered by the surgeon.

Monitoring for Postoperative Complications. The nurse observes the client carefully for possible complications and reports them immediately to the health care provider. In the immediate postoperative period, many complications may occur. Table 56-2 summarizes surgical procedures and potential complications.

A disruption in the patency of the NG tube can result in *acute gastric dilation* postoperatively; this is manifested by epigastric pain and a feeling of fullness, hiccups, tachycardia, and hypotension. Irrigation or replacement of the NG tube by order of the surgeon can relieve these symptoms.

Dumping syndrome is a term that refers to a constellation of vasomotor symptoms after eating, especially following a Billroth II procedure. This syndrome is believed to occur as a result of the rapid emptying of gastric contents into the small intestine, which shifts fluid into the gut, causing abdominal distension. The nurse observes for *early* manifestations of this syndrome, which typically occurs within 30 minutes of eating. Symptoms include vertigo, tachycardia, syncope, sweating, pallor, palpitations, and the desire to lie down.

Late dumping syndrome, which occurs 90 minutes to 3 hours after eating, is caused by a release of an excessive amount of insulin. The insulin release follows a rapid rise in the blood glucose level that results from the rapid entry of high-carbohydrate food into the jejunum. The nurse observes for intestinal manifestations, including dizziness, lightheadedness, palpitations, diaphoresis, and confusion.

Dumping syndrome is managed by dietary measures that include decreasing the amount of food taken at one time and eliminating liquids ingested with meals. In collaboration with the dietitian, the nurse instructs the client to consume a high-protein, high-fat, low-carbohydrate diet (Table 56-3). Pectin administered in the form of a dry powder may *prevent* the syndrome. A somatostatin analog, octreotide, may be ordered in severe cases.

Alkaline *reflux gastropathy,* also known as *bile reflux gastropathy,* is a complication of gastric surgery in which the pylorus is bypassed or removed (e.g., pyloroplasty, gastric resection with gastroduodenostomy [Billroth I procedure], and gastrojejunostomy [Billroth II procedure]). Endoscopic examination reveals regurgitated bile in the stomach and mucosal hyperemia. Symptoms include early satiety, abdominal discomfort, and vomiting.

Delayed gastric emptying is often present after gastric surgery and usually resolves within 1 week. Edema at the anastomosis or adhesions obstructing the distal loop may be mechanical causes. Metabolic causes (such as hypokalemia, hypoproteinemia, or hyponatremia) should be considered. The edema is resolved with nasogastric suction, maintenance of fluid and electrolyte balance, and proper nutrition.

Afferent loop syndrome may occur when the duodenal loop is partially obstructed after a Billroth II resection. Pancreatic and biliary secretions fill the intestinal loop, which becomes distended. Painful contractions attempt to propel these secretions from the loop. The nurse monitors for clients reporting abdominal bloating and pain 20 to 60 minutes after eating, often followed by nausea and vomiting. Treatment consists of surgical correction of the incomplete loop obstruction.

Recurrent ulceration occurs in approximately 5% of clients who have undergone gastric surgery for PUD. Recurrent ulcers can be due to incomplete vagotomy or persistent *H. pylori* in-

CLIENT CARE PLAN • THE CLIENT RECOVERING FROM GASTRIC SURGERY

NURSING DIAGNOSIS NO. 1 • Acute Pain or Chronic Pain related to gastric or mucosal injury or gastric surgery

Expected Outcomes	Nursing Interventions	Rationale
The client is expected to experience reduced pain as evidenced by verbalization of pain reduction or alleviation.	Teach the client what to expect regarding the postoperative pain experience. Explain possible effects of fatigue and anxiety. Instill a sense of control of the situation in relation to the temporary nature of the problem.	These interventions reduce the client's anxiety level and fatigue. Increased anxiety and fatigue ultimately intensify the pain experience by reducing the body's or mind's adaptive capacity to deal with uncomfortable stimuli or situations.
	Assess the client's sleep patterns and the influence of pain on sleep. **D**	Sleep disturbances are common with ulcer disease, and pain may exacerbate this problem.
	Encourage rest and provide an opportunity for rest during the day. **D**	Fatigue can intensify the pain experience.
	Administer appropriate analgesics as ordered for postoperative pain. Administer antiulcer therapy as ordered.	Analgesics are used in conjunction with comfort measures to reduce or alleviate postoperative pain. Pain control secondary to gastric mucosal injury is treated with agents to decrease gastric acid secretion, promote healing, and eradicate *H. pylori* infection.
	Teach nonpharmacologic techniques used in conjunction with medications to promote comfort, such as relaxation, cutaneous stimulation, and massage.	Nonpharmacologic pain relief measures provide an additional means of managing pain and discomfort.
	Encourage positioning to improve chest expansion (i.e., semi-Fowler's position or reclining). Demonstrate techniques to splint the incision during coughing. **D**	Proper positioning and incision splinting can lessen pain associated with movement and encourage deep breathing and coughing to prevent postoperative respiratory problems.
	Avoid, or use with caution, drugs that decrease mucosal resistance (aspirin, nonsteroidal anti-inflammatory drugs [NSAIDs], steroids) or drugs that alter gastric acid production. Discourage the use of stimulants (e.g., caffeine and nicotine) or spices (e.g., mustard, paprika, pepper, and Tabasco sauce) that are known to cause pain or discomfort.	Identification of factors that can exacerbate pain or discomfort can assist the client in eliminating individualized pain triggers. Certain substances are known gastric irritants and should be avoided.
	Eliminate the use of alcohol. Avoid the concurrent use of alcohol and aspirin.	Alcohol irritates the mucosal lining and may provoke gastritis. Alcohol and aspirin together greatly irritate the mucosal lining.
	Identify increases in pain or changes in pain characteristics. Instruct the client to report signs of complications, a feeling of fullness, weakness, or hematemesis.	Increasing pain or discomfort may indicate the development of complications.
	Gradually increase food until the client is able to eat three to six meals a day. **D**	Return of function of the stomach and intestines is evaluated postoperatively.
	If discomfort recurs, decrease the size of meals and the amount of fluids. **D**	Small enteral feedings are better tolerated than three large meals per day. Fluids should be offered between meals.

NURSING DIAGNOSIS NO. 2 • Risk for Deficient Fluid Volume related to vomiting, hemorrhage, or perforation

The client is expected to maintain vascular, cellular, and intracellular perfusion as evidenced by: • Intact mental status • Stable blood pressure • Warm, dry skin • Urine output of at least 30 mL/hr	Assess for nausea, vomiting, tarry stools, occult or frank blood in stools, thirst, diaphoresis, pain, tachycardia, and hypotension.	Assessment detects fluid volume deficit and evaluates its severity.
	Assess urine output and hemoglobin and hematocrit values.	Early detection of hypovolemia secondary to fluid volume depletion or hemorrhage can prevent excessive losses.
	Monitor client's fluid status, including intake and output. **D** Replace fluids and administer blood products as ordered by the health care provider.	If fluid volume deficit occurs, these same interventions assess the effectiveness of treatment.

D Indicates tasks that can be delegated to assistive nursing personnel.

TABLE 56-2 • SURGICAL MANAGEMENT OF PEPTIC ULCER DISEASE AND POTENTIAL COMPLICATIONS OF PEPTIC ULCER DISEASE

Surgery	Description	Possible Adverse Effects
Vagotomy Truncal (total abdominal vagotomy)	Cuts the vagus nerve at the esophageal level; severs both anterior and posterior trunks; destroys vagal and abdominal innervation; destroys gastrointestinal (GI) motility	Gastric emptying is inhibited; pyloroplasty or antrectomy must be performed to prevent gastric stasis. Some clients experience a feeling of fullness after eating (33%), dumping syndrome (10%), or diarrhea (10%).
Selective	Cuts the vagus nerve to the stomach, but other abdominal innervation remains; acid production stops	Gastric emptying is inhibited; pyloroplasty or antrectomy must be performed to prevent gastric stasis.
Proximal, or parietal cell (can be done without pyloroplasty or antrectomy)	Cuts the parietal branches of the vagus nerve; alters innervation to acid-producing cells but does not alter GI motility	Few negative consequences because innervation of the antrum and the pyloric sphincter remains.
Vagotomy with antrectomy	Cuts the vagus nerve and removes the antrum (lower half) of the stomach; removes the source of gastrin secretion	Some clients may have a feeling of fullness after eating, dumping syndrome, diarrhea, anemia, malabsorption, or recurrent ulceration.
Pyloroplasty	Enlarges the pylorus by surgically enlarging the pyloric sphincter	The stomach may empty too rapidly; alkaline reflux gastropathy can occur.
Vagotomy and pyloroplasty	Cuts the right and left branches of the vagus nerve; widens the existing pyloric sphincter to prevent stasis and to enhance emptying of the stomach	The stomach may empty too rapidly; alkaline reflux gastropathy can occur.
Subtotal gastrectomy Billroth I (gastroduodenostomy after resection) hemigastrectomy	Removes the distal one third to one half of the stomach and anastomoses with the duodenum; removes the antral portion of the stomach and the pylorus	Dumping syndrome, anemia, malabsorption, weight loss, or alkaline reflux may occur.
Billroth II (gastrojejunostomy after resection)	Removes the distal segment of the stomach and antrum and anastomoses with the jejunum; retains the duodenum; secretions of the liver and pancreas flow to the jejunum; preferred procedure	Afferent loop syndrome, malabsorption-related weight loss, vitamin B_{12} deficiency, alkaline reflux, or dumping syndrome may occur.
Total gastrectomy (esophagojejunostomy)	Removes the stomach from the level of the lower esophageal sphincter to the duodenum and anastomoses the duodenum to the esophagus	Gastric function is altered. Dumping syndrome and anemia may occur.

fection. Recurrence is most common following vagotomy with antrectomy, and ulcerations tend to occur at the site of anastomosis (stomal or marginal ulcer) or immediately distal in the small intestine. Abdominal pain, usually located in the epigastrium, is the most commonly reported symptom of recurrent peptic ulcer. The health care provider may order H_2-receptor antagonists and proton pump inhibitors to assist with the healing process. The eradication of *H. pylori* in the case of recurrent stomal ulcerations is controversial.

NUTRITIONAL MANAGEMENT. Several problems related to nutrition develop as a result of partial removal of the stomach, including deficiencies of vitamin B_{12}, folic acid, and iron; impaired calcium metabolism; and reduced absorption of calcium and vitamin D. These problems are caused by a shortage of intrinsic factor. The shortage results from the resection and from inadequate absorption because of rapid entry of food into the bowel. In the absence of intrinsic factor, clinical manifestations of pernicious anemia occur. The nurse should assess for the development of atrophic glossitis secondary to vitamin B_{12} deficiency. In atrophic glossitis, the tongue takes on a shiny and "beefy" appearance. The client may also have signs of anemia secondary to folic acid and iron deficiency. The nurse monitors the complete blood count (CBC) for signs of megaloblastic anemia and leukopenia. These manifestations are corrected by the administration of vitamin B_{12}. The health care provider may also prescribe folic acid or iron preparations.

● Community-Based Care

Clients may be discharged from the hospital as long as there is no evidence of ongoing bleeding, orthostatic changes, or cardiopulmonary distress or compromise. Clients discharged following treatment for peptic ulcer disease (PUD) and/or complications secondary to the disease must face several challenges in order to manage the disease successfully. Long-term adherence to medication regimens requires the client to take many oral medications on a daily basis. Permanent lifestyle alterations in dietary habits must also be made. Clients must be knowledgeable about complications related to PUD and know when to report symptoms to the health care provider.

■ HOME CARE MANAGEMENT

Clients are discharged to the home, subacute unit, or skilled nursing facility to continue recuperation. Clients who have undergone surgery or have had complications, such as hemor-

TABLE 56-3 • DIET FOR DUMPING SYNDROME

Food Group	Foods Allowed or Encouraged	Foods to Use with Caution	Foods That Must Be Excluded
Soups		Fluids 1 hr before and after meals	Spicy soups
Meat and meat substitutes	8 oz or more per day: fish poultry, beef, pork, veal, lamb, eggs, cheese, and peanut butter		Spicy meats or meat substitutes
Potato and substitutes	Potato, rice, pasta, starchy vegetables	Foods made with milk	Highly spiced potatoes or substitutes
Bread and cereal	White bread, rolls, muffins, crackers, and cereals	Whole-grain bread, rolls, crackers, and cereals	Breads with frosting or jelly, sweet rolls, and coffee cake
Vegetables	Two or more cooked vegetables	Gas-producing vegetables, such as cabbage, onions, broccoli, or raw vegetables	
Fruits	Limit three per day: unsweetened cooked or canned fruits	Unsweetened juice or fruit drinks 30-45 min after meals; fresh fruit	Sweetened fruit or juice
Beverages	Dietetic drinks	Limit to 1 hr after meals; caffeine-containing beverages, such as coffee, tea, and cola; if tolerated, diet carbonated beverages	Milk shakes, malts, and other sweet drinks; regular carbonated beverages and alcohol
Fats	Margarine, oils, shortening, butter, bacon, and salad dressings	Mayonnaise	Any fats with milk products
Desserts	Fruit (see Fruits)	Sugar-free gelatin, pudding, and custard	All sweets, cakes, pies, cookies, candy, ice cream, and sherbet
Seasonings and miscellaneous	Diet jelly, diet syrups, sugar substitutes	Excessive amounts of salt	Excessive amounts of spices, sugar, jelly, honey, syrup, or molasses

GENERAL PRINCIPLES
- Five to six small meals daily
- Relatively high fat and protein content
- Low roughage
- Relatively low carbohydrate content
- No milk, sweets, or sugars
- Liquid between meals *only*

rhage, may require visits from a home care nurse to assess clinical progress.

■ HEALTH TEACHING

The primary focus of home care preparation is client teaching regarding risk factors for the recurrence of PUD; clients are also taught to recognize and report the development of complications related to the disease process or surgical intervention.

The nurse instructs the client and family or significant others about factors related to the development of an ulcer. A risk assessment assists in identifying gastric irritants and lifestyle stressors that may be contributory to ulcer formation. Strategies for lifestyle changes are developed together with the client. The nurse teaches about symptoms that should be brought to the attention of the health care provider after discharge from the hospital, such as abdominal pain; nausea and vomiting; black, tarry stools; and weakness or dizziness. To demonstrate understanding, the client describes the symptoms back to the nurse.

The nurse also teaches the client about diets to be used for avoiding postprandial distention or dumping syndrome. For postsurgical clients, especially those who have undergone partial stomach removal, a smaller meal may be required. In collaboration with the dietitian, the nurse instructs the client to:

- Eat small, frequent meals
- Avoid drinking liquids with meals
- Abstain from foods that contribute to discomfort
- Eliminate caffeine and alcohol consumption
- Begin a smoking cessation program
- Receive B_{12} injections, as appropriate

The client is also taught to avoid any over-the-counter (OTC) product containing aspirin or ibuprofen. The nurse emphasizes the importance of adhering to the treatment regimen. Long-term medication compliance is critical for eradicating *H. pylori* infection and achieving healing of the ulcer. The importance of keeping all follow-up appointments is also emphasized, since early detection of recurrence or the development of complications is desirable.

The nurse helps the client to identify situations that cause stress, describe feelings during stressful situations, and develop a plan for coping with stressors (Chart 56-7). The nurse encourages the client to learn and use relaxation techniques, such as exercise, biofeedback, humor, and imagery (see Chapter 4). Psychotherapy may be indicated to help some clients cope with excessive anxiety or stress. Ulcer disease is difficult to eradicate, so it is essential for the client and family to understand how modifying living, working, and eating habits minimizes the risk of ulcer recurrence.

■ HEALTH CARE RESOURCES

Following discharge, home care nursing visits may be indicated if clients and family members or significant others require instruction or assistance with follow-up care, such as dressing changes, monitoring of potential complications, and continued nutritional problems.

● Evaluation: Outcomes

NOC The nurse evaluates the care of the client with peptic ulcer disease (PUD) on the basis of the identified nursing diagnoses and collaborative problems. The expected outcomes are that the client:

- Maintains hemodynamic stability, free of disease or surgical complications
- States that pain is reduced or alleviated by prescribed interventions
- Identifies potential causes and risks of disease recurrence
- Avoids the intake of irritating foods and beverages
- Avoids smoking
- Avoids over-the-counter medications containing aspirin or ibuprofen
- Identifies early symptoms of recurrence or complications
- Identifies and copes successfully with stressful situations
- Adheres to long-term medication regimen and appropriate follow-up with the health care provider

---

CHART 56-7

FOCUSED ASSESSMENT *of*
Ambulatory Care with Ulcer Disease

Assess gastrointestinal and cardiovascular status, including:
- Vital signs, including orthostatic vital signs
- Skin color
- Presence of abdominal pain (location, severity, character, duration, precipitating factors, and relief measures)
- Character, color, and consistency of stools
- Changes in bowel elimination pattern
- Hemoglobin and hematocrit
- Bowel sounds; palpate for areas of tenderness

Assess nutritional status, including:
- Dietary patterns and habits
- Intake of caffeine and alcohol
- Relationship of food to symptoms

Assess medication history.
- Use of steroids
- Use of nonsteroidal anti-inflammatory drugs (NSAIDs)
- Use of over-the-counter medications

Assess client's coping style
- Recent stressors
- Past coping style

Assess client's understanding of illness and ability to comply with therapeutic regimen.
- Symptoms to report to health care provider
- Expected and side effects of medications
- Food and drug interactions
- Need for smoking cessation

ZOLLINGER-ELLISON SYNDROME

■ OVERVIEW

Zollinger-Ellison syndrome (ZES) is manifested by upper gastrointestinal (GI) tract ulceration, increased gastric acid secretion, and the presence of a non–beta cell islet tumor of the pancreas, called a gastrinoma. Affected individuals may have more than one gastrinoma. Approximately two thirds of gastrinomas are malignant. Recent developments indicate that a benign but aggressive form of the disease may exist (Yu et al., 1999). Although most gastrinomas grow slowly, a small portion of them develop rapidly and metastasize widely. Metastasis occurs mainly in the liver and regional lymph nodes. Gastrinoma remains a relatively uncommon disease, with an incidence of 1 to 3 new cases per year per million people.

In 20% to 60% of clients with ZES, the gastrinoma results from an autosomal dominant disorder called multiple endocrine neoplasia type 1 (MEN-1) syndrome. Gastrinomas contain multiple hormones, but adrenocorticotropic hormone (ACTH) is most commonly found. As a result, Cushing's syndrome with increased ACTH levels is reported in approximately 8% of clients with ZES.

In the early course of the disease, symptoms resemble those of peptic ulcer disease (PUD). However, these symptoms tend to progress, and they respond poorly to traditional ulcer therapy. Diarrhea may be a manifestation of this disorder, occurring in 40% of clients. The diarrhea may be associated with large amounts of hydrochloric acid secreted into the proximal duodenum. **Steatorrhea** (an excessive amount of fat in the feces) results from the inactivation of pancreatic lipase secondary to the large concentrations of acid and decreased amounts of bile acids.

► COLLABORATIVE MANAGEMENT

● Assessment

Radiographic and endoscopic findings for ZES are similar to those for PUD. However, infection with *Helicobacter pylori* is usually absent. The diagnosis is usually made by radioimmunoassay studies that reveal increased serum gastrin levels in conjunction with the clinical features of the disease.

● Interventions

The aim of therapy is to suppress acid secretion in order to control the client's symptoms. The H^+,K^+-ATPase inhibitors, such as lansoprazole and omeprazole (given as 60 mg/day in a single dose) are the drugs of choice to reduce gastric acid secretion and heal ulcers in clients with ZES. However, long-term treatment with these drugs can lead to significant decreases in vitamin B_{12} levels (Termanini et al., 1998). High doses of H_2-receptor antagonists, such as ranitidine (Zantac), are also effective in reducing gastric acid and providing symptom relief.

If medical therapy fails, the health care provider may choose to perform a vagotomy and pyloroplasty to supplement pharmacologic means of controlling hypersecretion. A total gastrectomy is the surgical approach of choice for this disorder if vagotomy, pyloroplasty, and medical therapy are inadequate. (See the earlier discussion of these surgeries under Surgical Management [Peptic Ulcer Disease], p. 1228.)

The consequences of the malignant properties of the tumor are now being more widely recognized, and complete surgical resection of the tumor appears to be the optimal treatment. Clients with aggressive disease can also be treated with chemotherapeutic agents such as 5-fluorouracil and doxorubicin to reduce the tumor and control symptoms.

GASTRIC CARCINOMA

■ OVERVIEW

Gastric carcinoma refers to malignant neoplasms in the stomach. Adenocarcinomas account for 85% to 95% of all gastric cancers (Mayer, 1998, O'Connor, 1999). The remaining 15% are due to non-Hodgkin's lymphoma and leiomyosarcomas. In the United States, 30% of gastric cancers are in the distal stomach, 20% are in the midsection of the stomach, and 37% arise in the proximal third of the stomach. The remaining cases of gastric carcinoma involve the entire stomach. The onset is insidious, and the disease is often advanced when detected.

■ Pathophysiology

Gastric adenocarcinoma can be characterized as *intestinal* or *diffuse.* Intestinal adenocarcinomas result from atrophic gastritis or intestinal metaplasia, both of which are considered precancerous conditions. The diffuse form of the disease is found primarily in areas where gastric cancer is endemic. Early, superficial gastric cancers produce no notable symptoms. On microscopic examination, the cells resemble intestinal metaplasia (abnormal tissue development).

Gastric cancers spread by direct extension through the gastric wall and into regional lymphatics. The intramural lymphatics readily allow horizontal spread within the gastric wall. Extramural lymphatics carry tumor deposits to lymph nodes in more than 50% of operable cases. Direct invasion of and adherence to adjacent organs (e.g., the liver, pancreas, and transverse colon) may also result. Hematogenous spread via the portal vein to the liver and via the systemic circulation to the lungs and bones is the most common mode of metastasis. Peritoneal seeding of cancer cells from the involved gastric serosa to the omentum, peritoneum, ovary, and pelvic cul-de-sac can also occur.

In people with advanced gastric cancer, there is invasion of the muscularis (stomach muscle) or beyond. These lesions are not amenable to curative resection. Most clients in the United States have advanced (stage III or stage IV) disease when diagnosed. The 5-year survival rate following surgical resection is 20% to 25% for tumors located in the distal stomach, 10% for proximal tumors, and 5% when the entire stomach is involved (Hawkins, 1999).

■ Etiology

Recent evidence has provided a strong link between infection with *H. pylori* and the subsequent development of gastric cancer. Metabolic products produced by the organism transform the gastric mucosa while producing a state of chronic inflammation. Such chronic inflammatory states can induce cancer by increasing cell proliferation and free radical formation.

Clients with pernicious anemia, gastric polyps, chronic atrophic gastritis, and achlorhydria (absence of secretion of hydrochloric acid) are two to three times more likely to develop gastric cancer.

Gastric cancer seems to be positively correlated with the ingestion of pickled foods, salted fish, salted meat, and nitrates from processed foods, as well as a high consumption of salt. The ingestion of these foods over a long period of time can lead to atrophic gastritis, a precancerous condition.

The role of cigarette smoking and alcohol consumption in the development of gastric carcinoma is controversial, although some studies support the conclusion that smokers are 1.5 to 3 times more likely to develop gastric cancer as compared with nonsmokers (O'Connor, 1999).

Genetic factors may play a role in the development of gastric cancer; an increased incidence of the disease has been noted among direct relatives of clients with gastric cancer. First-degree relatives of individuals with gastric cancer are two to three times more likely to develop the disease themselves. In addition, individuals with type A blood appear to have a slight risk of gastric cancer.

Gastric surgery, especially a Billroth II procedure, seems to increase the risk for gastric cancer because of the eventual development of atrophic gastritis, which results in changes to the mucosa. Clients with Barrett's esophagus have an increased risk of adenocarcinoma of the gastric cardia.

■ Incidence/Prevalence

Although the incidence of gastric cancer is decreasing in the United States, it is the fourteenth most common cause of all cancer-related deaths, and it is one of the top five causes of cancer-related deaths for minority populations (O'Connor, 1999). Men appear to have a greater incidence of developing the disease than women, and the average age of onset is from 50 to 70 years of age.

> #### CULTURAL CONSIDERATIONS
> Japan, Chile, and Costa Rica have the highest incidence of gastric cancer. In some Nordic countries, such as Scandinavia, an increased incidence and prevalence of the disease has been noted over the last several decades. Native Americans, African Americans, and Hispanics are two times as likely to develop gastric cancer as compared with Caucasians (O'Connor, 1999).

► COLLABORATIVE MANAGEMENT
● Assessment
■ HISTORY

The nurse questions the client regarding the known risk factors for the development of gastric cancer. The nurse elicits information regarding preferred foods, especially pickled, salted, or smoked foods. Information regarding tobacco use and alcohol ingestion is also gathered. The nurse inquires if the client has ever been diagnosed or treated for *H. pylori* infection, gastritis, or pernicious anemia. The nurse notes if the client has a history of gastric surgery or polyps. The nurse also inquires if any of the client's immediate relatives have been diagnosed with gastric cancer. If known, the nurse makes a notation of the client's blood type.

PHYSICAL ASSESSMENT/CLINICAL MANIFESTATIONS

Although clients with *early* gastric cancer may be asymptomatic, indigestion (heartburn) and abdominal discomfort are the *most* common symptoms (Chart 56-8). These symptoms are often ignored, however, or a change in diet or use of antacids relieves them. As the tumor grows, these symptoms become more severe and do not respond to diet changes or antacids. Epigastric, back, or retrosternal pain is also an early symptom that may go unrecognized. Two thirds of clients will complain of epigastric pain following eating. This pain is described as a vague feeling of fullness or discomfort (Hawkins, 1999).

In *advanced* gastric carcinoma, progressive weight loss, nausea, and vomiting can occur. Vomiting represents pronounced dilation, thickening of the stomach wall, or pyloric obstruction. Obstructive symptoms appear earlier with tumors located near the pylorus than with fundic lesions. Clients with advanced disease may have weakness, fatigue, and anemia.

Physical assessment findings in advanced disease may be absent, or a palpable epigastric mass may suggest hepatomegaly from metastatic disease. Hard, enlarged lymph nodes in the left supraclavicular chain, left axilla, or umbilicus may be the result of metastasis from gastric cancer. Masses on the right suggest metastasis in the perigastric lymph nodes or liver. Signs of distant metastasis include the following:

- Virchow's (sentinel or signal) nodes (enlarged supraclavicular lymph nodes, especially on the left)
- Blumer's shelf, resulting from peritoneal seeding that produces a firm mass palpable on rectal or vaginal examination
- "Sister Mary Joseph nodes" (subcutaneous periumbilical deposits)
- Krukenberg's tumor (metastatic ovarian nodules)

LABORATORY ASSESSMENT

In clients with advanced disease, anemia is evidenced by low hematocrit and hemoglobin values. Clients may have macrocytic or microcytic anemia associated with decreased iron or

vitamin B_{12} absorption. The stool may be positive for occult blood.

Hypoalbuminemia and abnormal results of liver tests (such as bilirubin and alkaline phosphatase) occur with advanced disease and with hepatic metastasis. The level of carcinoembryonic antigen (CEA) is elevated in *advanced* cancer of the stomach.

RADIOGRAPHIC ASSESSMENT

A double-contrast upper gastrointestinal (GI) series is usually the first diagnostic test. The use of a double-contrast medium assists in the detection of small lesions. A polypoid mass, ulcer crater, or thickened fibrotic gastric wall may suggest gastric cancer.

A computed tomography (CT) scan is used to evaluate gastric malignancies. CT scans of the chest, abdomen, and pelvis are used in determining the extent of the disease.

OTHER DIAGNOSTIC ASSESSMENT

The health care provider uses esophagogastroduodenoscopy (EGD) for definitive diagnosis of gastric cancer. The lesion can be visualized directly, and biopsies of all visible lesions can be obtained to determine the presence of cancer cells. During the endoscopy, an endoscopic ultrasound (EUS) of the gastric mucosa can also be performed. This technology allows the health care provider to evaluate the depth of the tumor and the presence of lymph node involvement that permits more accurate staging of the disease.

▶ Interventions

Management of gastric cancer includes drug therapy, radiation, and/or surgery.

NONSURGICAL MANAGEMENT. The treatment of gastric cancer is highly dependent on the stage of the disease. Surgical resection of the tumor is usually combined with chemotherapy and/or radiation. Radiation and chemotherapy commonly prolong survival of clients with advanced gastric disease.

DRUG THERAPY. The role of chemotherapy in gastric cancer remains uncertain. No specific chemotherapeutic protocol has had a positive effect on survival. Chemotherapy with single agents such as fluorouracil (5-FU), doxorubicin, mitomycin-C, cisplatin, and etoposide have been used, but the use of a combination of agents appears to have superior results. Bone marrow suppression, nausea, and vomiting are common side effects. Chapter 25 discusses chemotherapy in detail.

RADIATION THERAPY. Although gastric cancers are somewhat sensitive to the effects of radiation, the use of this treatment is limited, since the disease is often widely disseminated to other abdominal organs on diagnosis. Organs such as the liver and kidneys, as well as the spinal cord, have limits as to the amount of radiation they can endure. Postoperative radiation has not significantly increased survival. Intraoperative radiotherapy (IORT) is available at only a few institutions in the United States, since special operative suites, equipment, and personnel are required.

CHART 56-8

KEY FEATURES *of*
Early Versus Advanced Gastric Cancer

Early Gastric Cancer
- Indigestion
- Abdominal discomfort initially relieved with antacids
- Feeling of fullness
- Epigastric, back, or retrosternal pain
(NOTE: Many clients with early gastric cancer have no clinical manifestations.)

Advanced Gastric Cancer
- Nausea and vomiting
- Obstructive symptoms
- Iron deficiency anemia
- Palpable epigastric mass
- Enlarged lymph nodes
- Weakness and fatigue
- Progressive weight loss
- Signs of distant metastasis
  Virchow's nodes
  Blumer's shelf
  "Sister Mary Joseph nodes"
  Krukenberg's tumor

The most common side effects experienced by clients undergoing radiation include impaired skin integrity, fatigue, and anorexia. Nausea, vomiting, and diarrhea may occur approximately 1 week after treatment is initiated and diminish a month or more after treatment ends. (See Chapter 25 for more information on radiation therapy.) The most common potential problems of IORT are hemorrhage and fistula development.

SURGICAL MANAGEMENT. Surgical resection is the preferred method for treating gastric cancer. The primary surgical procedures for the treatment of gastric cancer are total gastrectomy and subtotal gastrectomy. In early stages, surgery plus adjuvant chemotherapy or radiation may be curative. Most clients with advanced disease are candidates for palliative surgical treatment. Metastasis in the supraclavicular lymph nodes (Virchow's nodes), inguinal lymph nodes, liver, umbilicus, or perirectal wall indicates that the opportunity for cure by resection has been lost. Palliative resection may significantly improve the quality of life for a client suffering from obstruction, hemorrhage, or pain.

PREOPERATIVE CARE. The health care provider gives the client and family an explanation of the disease and the available treatment options (potentially curative or palliative). The nurse reinforces and clarifies the information given. Preoperative care is similar to that provided for the client undergoing general anesthesia and abdominal surgery (see Chapter 17).

OPERATIVE PROCEDURES. When the tumor is located in the mid or distal (lower) portions of the stomach, a subtotal gastrectomy is typically performed. The surgeon uses a Billroth I or Billroth II procedure (discussed earlier under Operative Procedures [Peptic Ulcer Disease], p. 1229). The omentum, spleen, and relevant nodes are also removed.

For the client with a resectable growth in the upper third of the stomach, a total gastrectomy is performed (Figure 56-9). In this procedure the surgeon removes the entire stomach along with en bloc removal of the lymph nodes and omentum. The surgeon sutures the esophagus to the duodenum or jejunum to re-establish continuity of the GI tract. More radical surgery involving removal of the spleen and distal pancreas is controversial. The overall mortality rate for clients undergoing total gastrectomy surgery is 10% to 15% (Hawkins, 1999). For clients with advanced disease, total gastrectomy is performed only when gastric bleeding or obstruction is present.

Clients with tumors at the gastric outlet who are not candidates for subtotal or total gastrectomy may undergo gastroenterostomy for palliation. The surgeon creates a passage between the body of the stomach and the small bowel, often the duodenum (see Figure 56-4).

POSTOPERATIVE CARE. Clients require the standard postoperative care that is given to those who have had general anesthesia (see Chapter 19). Complications after gastric surgery may include the following:
- Pneumonia
- Anastomotic leak
- Hemorrhage
- Reflux aspiration
- Sepsis
- Reflux (acute) gastritis (discussed earlier under Acute Gastritis, p. 1216)

- Paralytic ileus
- Bowel obstruction
- Wound infection
- Dumping syndrome (discussed earlier under Monitoring for Postoperative Complications [Peptic Ulcer Disease], p. 1230).

The nurse monitors the client for the development of postoperative complications. The nurse auscultates the lungs for adventitious sounds and monitors for the return of bowel sounds. Monitoring vital signs is performed as appropriate to detect signs of infection or bleeding. Aggressive pulmonary exercises and early ambulation can help prevent respiratory complications and deep vein thrombosis. The nurse also inspects the operative site every 8 hours for the presence of redness, swelling, or drainage, which indicates wound infection. The nurse also ensures proper positioning of the client to prevent aspiration from reflux.

Since weight loss is problematic for clients with gastric cancer, nutrition therapy is a vital aspect of preoperative and postoperative management. Preoperatively, compression by the tumor can impede adequate nutritional intake. To correct malnutrition before surgery, the health care provider may prescribe supplements to the diet and/or total parenteral nutrition (TPN). Vitamin, mineral, iron, and protein supplements are essential for correction of nutritional deficits.

Postoperatively, the client's inability to ingest normal-size meals, along with poor nutrient absorption due to decreased stomach size, can prevent the client from taking in adequate nutrition. Therefore the surgeon may place an enteral feeding tube during surgery for continued nutritional support. When feasible, oral intake should begin with fluids and progress to solids as tolerated. For clients who have undergone gastric surgery, regurgitation may result from overeating or from eating too quickly.

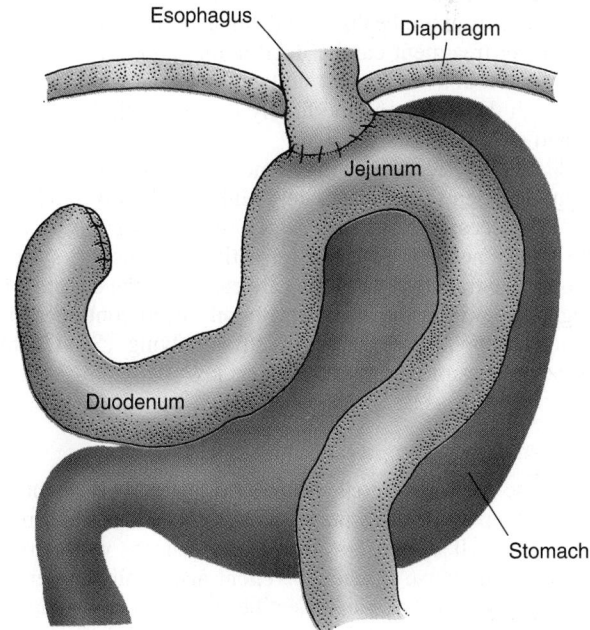

Figure 56-9 ● Total gastrectomy, with anastomosis of the esophagus to the jejunum (esophagojejunostomy), is the principal medical intervention for extensive gastric cancer.

After oral feedings are restarted, the nurse observes the client for signs and symptoms of dumping syndrome and teaches the manifestations and management of this syndrome. The client is advised to eat six small meals per day and to consume a diet high in protein and fat but low in carbohydrate-rich foods (see Table 56-3). Liquids should not be taken with meals. Milk and dairy products are usually eliminated because many clients are lactose-intolerant and have symptoms after the ingestion of milk-containing products.

In collaboration with the dietitian, the nurse guides the client and family in providing the most nutrients and calories. Counseling about methods of preparation and types of foods that increase caloric and protein intake is essential. The nurse maintains intake, output, and calorie counts on a daily basis and records weights at least weekly. Anemia, as well as vitamin B_{12} and folate deficiency, can result following gastrectomy. Oral folate and iron replacement and vitamin B_{12} injections can help correct these deficiencies.

● Community-Based Care

Clients who have undergone total gastrectomy and those who are debilitated with advanced gastric cancer are discharged to home with maximal assistance or to a subacute unit or skilled nursing facility. Clients who have undergone subtotal gastrectomy and are not debilitated may be discharged to home with partial assistance for activities of daily living (ADLs). Recurrence of the cancer is common, and clients will need regular follow-up examinations and radiographic assessments. A case manager may be assigned to ensure continuity of care and thorough follow-up with diagnostic testing.

■ HOME CARE MANAGEMENT

Gastric cancer is considered a life-threatening illness; therefore the client and family members require physical and emotional care from the health care team. The side effects of gastric cancer treatment can be debilitating, and clients need to learn symptom management strategies. Hospice programs can help both the client and the family to cope with these physical and emotional needs.

Clients may fear returning home because of their inability to care for themselves adequately. Enlisting family and health care resources for the client may ease some of this anxiety. The family needs adequate information and support systems to make the transition to home care easier for the client. If the prognosis is poor, the client and family need continued professional support to cope with death and dying. (See Chapter 9 for a discussion of end-of-life care.)

■ HEALTH TEACHING

The nurse instructs the client and family members about any continuing postoperative needs, adjuvant treatment, and nutrition therapy. If clients are discharged to home with surgical dressings, the nurse teaches the client and family to perform dressing changes. The nurse identifies the signs and symptoms of incisional infection (e.g., fever, redness, and drainage) that are to be reported.

Clients who will be receiving radiation therapy or chemotherapy require instructions related to the side effects of these treatments. Nausea and vomiting are common side effects of chemotherapy, and instruction in the use of prescribed antiemetics may be needed. (See Chapter 25 for education for clients receiving chemotherapy or radiation therapy.)

The nurse, in conjunction with the dietitian, educates the client and family concerning the type and quantity of foods that will provide optimal nutritional value. Interventions to minimize dumping syndrome are also emphasized (see Table 56-3).

■ HEALTH CARE RESOURCES

A home care referral provides ongoing assessment, assistance, and encouragement to the client and family or significant others at home. A home care nurse can help with physical care procedures and can also provide valuable psychologic support. Additional referrals to a dietitian, professional counselor, or clergy may be necessary. Referral to a hospice agency can be of great assistance. Hospice care may be delivered in the home or in an institutional setting. Appropriate support groups (such as I Can Cope, provided by the American Cancer Society) can be a major resource.

ONLINE RESOURCES

For suggested readings and Internet resources, go to http://www.wbsaunders.com/SIMON/Iggy/.

SELECTED BIBLIOGRAPHY

Aronson, B. (1998). Update on peptic ulcer drugs. *American Journal of Nursing, 98*(1), 41-46.

Astarita, T. (1999). Update on peptic ulcer disease management. *Patient Care for the Nurse Practitioner, 2*(12), 39-51.

Blackington, E. (1999). The gastric demon. *ADVANCE for Nurse Practitioners, 7*(8), 37-44.

Centanni, M., et al. (1999). Atrophic body gastritis in patients with autoimmune thyroid disease: An underdiagnosed association. *Archives of Internal Medicine, 159*(15), 1726-1730.

Cromwell, D., et al. (1999). Can restrictions on reimbursement for antiulcer drugs decrease Medicaid pharmacy costs without increasing hospitalizations? *Health Services Research, 33*(6), 1593-1608.

Curtas, S. (1999). Diagnosing gastrointestinal malignancies. *Seminars in Oncology Nursing, 15*(1), 10-16.

Friedman, L., & Peterson, W. (1998). Peptic ulcer and related disorders. In A.S. Fauci, E. Braunwald, & K.J. Isselbacher (Eds.), *Harrison's principles of internal medicine* (14th ed., pp. 1596-1616). New York: McGraw-Hill.

Graham, D., et al. (1999a). Practical advice on eradicating *Helicobacter pylori* infection. *Postgraduate Medicine, 105*(3), 137-148.

Graham, D., et al. (1999b). Recognizing peptic ulcer disease: Keys to clinical and laboratory diagnosis. *Postgraduate Medicine, 105*(3), 113-128.

Graham, D., et al. (1999c). Scope and consequences of peptic ulcer disease: How important is asymptomatic *Helicobacter pylori* infection? *Postgraduate Medicine, 105*(3), 100-108.

Hawkins, B. (1999). Stomach cancer. In C. Miaskowski & P. Buchsel (Eds.), *Oncology nursing: Assessment and clinical care* (pp. 1015-1030). St. Louis: Mosby.

Heslin, J.M. (1997). Peptic ulcer disease. *Nursing97, 27*(1), 34-40.

Lane, L., & Fendrick, A.M. (1998). *Helicobacter pylori* and peptic ulcer disease. *Postgraduate Medicine, 103*(3), 231-243.

Levy, R., & Feld, A. (1999). Increasing patient adherence to gastroenterology treatment and prevention regimens. *American Journal of Gastroenterology, 94*(7), 1734-1742.

Marshall, J., Collins, S., & Gafni, A. (2000). Prediction of resource utilization and case cost for acute nonvariceal upper gastrointestinal hemorrhage at a Canadian community hospital. *American Journal of Gastroenterology, 94*(7), 1841-1846.

Mayer, R. (1998). Gastrointestinal tract cancer. In A.S. Fauci, E. Braunwald, & K.J. Isselbacher (Eds.), *Harrison's principles of internal medicine (*14th ed., pp. 568-578). New York: McGraw-Hill.

Navuluri, R., & Yue, S. (1999). Understanding peptic ulcer disease pharmacotherapeutics. *Nurse Practitioner, 24*(3), 128-132.

Norton, J.A., Fraker, D.L., & Alexander, H.R. (1999). Surgery to cure Zollinger-Ellison syndrome. *New England Journal of Medicine, 341*(9), 635-644.

O'Connor, K. (1999). Gastric cancer. *Seminars in Oncology Nursing, 15*(1), 26-35.

Offman, J., et al. (2000). The quality of care for Medicare patients with peptic ulcer disease. *American Journal of Gastroenterology 95*(1), 106-113.

Parkman, H., MacMillan Rodney, W., & Rogers, H. (2001). Empiric therapy for nonulcer dyspepsia. *Patient Care for the Nurse Practitioner, 3*(1), 23-24.

Parsonnet, J., Shmuely, H., & Haggerty, T. (1999). Fecal and oral shedding of *Helicobacter pylori* from healthy adults. *Journal of the American Medical Association, 282*(23), 2240-2245.

Ridenour, K. (1998). Medication history and *Helicobacter pylori* testing. *Gastroenterology Nursing, 21*(1), 24-25.

Saddler, D. (1999). Education for the gastroenterology cancer patient. *Gastroenterology Nursing, 22*(3), 121-126.

Schwartz, R., Karpeh, M., & Brennan, M. (1999). In J.M. Daly, T.P.J. Hennessy, & J.V. Reynolds (Eds.), *Management of upper gastrointestinal cancer* (pp. 83-101). Philadelphia: W.B. Saunders.

Terdiman, J. (1998). Update on upper gastrointestinal bleeding: Basing treatment decisions on patient's risk level. *Postgraduate Medicine, 103*(6), 43-63.

Termanini, B., et al. (1998). Effect of long-term gastric acid suppressive therapy on serum vitamin B_{12} levels in patients with Zollinger-Ellison syndrome. *American Journal of Medicine, 104*(5), 422-430.

Weber, H.C., et al. (1997). Studies on the interrelation between Zollinger-Ellison syndrome, *Helicobacter pylori,* and proton pump inhibitor therapy. *Gastroenterology, 112*(1), 84-91.

Yu, F., et al. (1999). Prospective study of the clinical course, prognostic factors, causes of death and survival in patients with long-standing Zollinger Ellison syndrome. *Journal of Clinical Oncology, 17*(2), 615-630.

Interventions for Clients with Noninflammatory Intestinal Disorders

CONSTANCE VISOVSKY

Learning Objectives

After studying this chapter, you should be able to:

1. Explain the risk factors for irritable bowel syndrome (IBS) and cancer of the colon.
2. Develop a teaching-learning plan for clients with IBS.
3. Differentiate the most common types of hernias.
4. Develop a plan of care for a client undergoing a hernia repair.
5. Interpret diagnostic assessments for clients with colorectal cancer.
6. Discuss the psychosocial aspects associated with colorectal cancer and related surgeries.
7. Explain the role of the nurse in managing the client with colorectal cancer.
8. Develop a perioperative plan of care for a client undergoing a colon resection and colostomy.
9. Construct a community-based teaching-learning plan for clients requiring colostomy care.
10. Identify community-based resources for clients with colorectal cancer.
11. Analyze the differences between small-bowel and large-bowel obstructions.
12. Describe assessment findings associated with mechanical and nonmechanical obstructions.
13. Explain the role of the nurse when caring for clients with nasogastric tubes.
14. Develop a plan of care for a client experiencing intestinal obstruction.
15. Prioritize nursing care for the client with abdominal trauma.

SiMON

Go to http://www.wbsaunders.com/SIMON/Iggy/ for self-assessment questions related to these Learning Objectives.

The most common presenting symptoms associated with noninflammatory intestinal disorders include alterations in bowel patterns, abdominal pain, and rectal bleeding (Figure 57-1). Symptoms of this type require investigation, since they can be associated with serious illnesses, such as intestinal obstruction or colorectal cancer.

IRRITABLE BOWEL SYNDROME

OVERVIEW

Irritable bowel syndrome (IBS) is the most common digestive disorder seen in clinical practice. IBS is a functional gastrointestinal (GI) disorder, characterized by the presence of chronic or recurrent diarrhea, constipation, and/or abdominal pain and bloating (Alderman, 1999). IBS is estimated to occur in 10% to 22% of the population of the United States. It is believed to be due to impairment in the motor or sensory function of the GI tract. Motility changes result in changes in the normal bowel elimination pattern to a pattern of diarrhea, constipation, or alternating diarrhea and constipation. Symptoms of IBS typically begin to appear in young adulthood. The exact cause is unknown, since no structural or infectious etiology has been identified. Physical factors, such as diverticular disease, ingestion of coffee or other gastric stimulants, or lactose intolerance may contribute to IBS. IBS follows a pattern of intermittent remissions and exacerbations.

The diagnosis of IBS is made by careful history taking, documenting the presence of characteristic symptoms; laboratory tests; and any other diagnostic tests to exclude a more serious condition. There are no specific biomarkers for IBS, but characteristic symptoms known collectively as the Manning criteria are typically present in clients with IBS. The Manning criteria include abdominal pain relieved by defecation or associated with changes in stool frequency or consistency, abdominal distention, the sensation of incomplete evacuation of stool, and the presence of mucus with stool passage. Bowel function changes progressively and eventually forms the characteristic pattern.

Recent studies have demonstrated that clients with IBS experience alteration in rectal visceral sensation. Balloon distention in the rectum or sigmoid colon resulted in abdominal

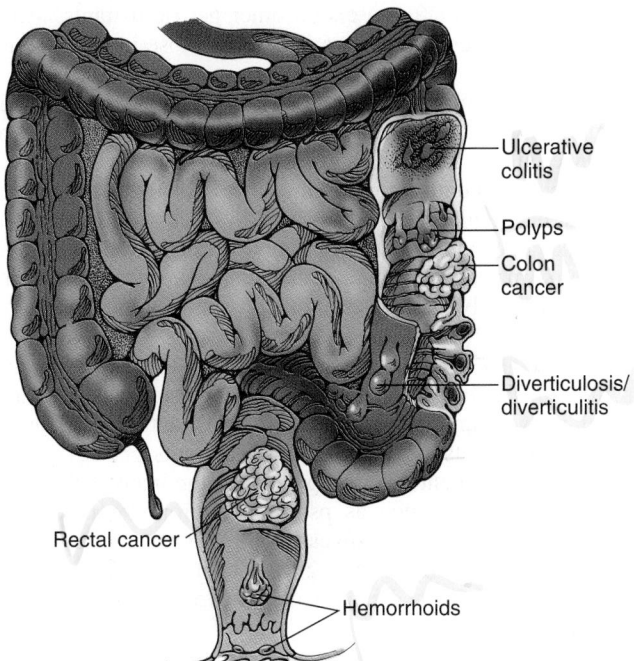

Ulcerative colitis

Polyps

Colon cancer

Diverticulosis/ diverticulitis

Rectal cancer

Hemorrhoids

Figure 57-1 ● Common causes of lower gastrointestinal bleeding.

pain at levels higher in clients with IBS than in those without IBS (Schmulson et al., 2000).

The course of the illness is generally specific to the client, and most clients can identify factors that precipitate exacerbations, such as diet, stress, or anxiety. There are no changes in the bowel mucosa and therefore no serious health consequences. However, the irregular bowel patterns and associated cramps often wreak havoc on the person's lifestyle. Psychosocial factors have been thought to play a significant role in IBS. However, the evidence is often contradictory (Carlson, 1998). Food intolerance may be associated with IBS. Dairy products and grains can contribute to bloating, flatulence, and distention. In one study, individuals who reported intolerances to multiple foods were more likely to report IBS (Locke et al., 2000). Finally, IBS symptoms have also been associated with analgesic use (see the Evidence-Based Practice for Nursing box at right).

> ### WOMEN'S HEALTH CONSIDERATIONS
> The prevalence of IBS in women is 2:1 as compared with men. Furthermore, several studies indicate that there may be a link between a history of physical, sexual, or emotional abuse and the subsequent development of IBS in women (Toner & Akman, 2000).

► COLLABORATIVE MANAGEMENT
● Assessment

The client is asked about a history of abdominal pain, changes in the bowel pattern or consistency of stools, and the passage of mucus. The nurse collects information on all medications the client is taking, since many medications cause GI symptoms similar to those of IBS. A careful dietary history, including the use of caffeinated beverages or beverages sweet-

ened with sorbitol or fructose, which can cause bloating or diarrhea, should be elicited.

A flare-up consisting of worsening cramps, abdominal pain, and diarrhea or constipation usually brings the client to the health care provider. The most common symptom of IBS is pain in the left lower quadrant of the abdomen. The client reports increased pain after eating and relief after a bowel movement. Nausea may be associated with mealtime and defecation. The crampy abdominal patterns are accompanied by constipation or diarrhea. The constipated stools are small and hard and are generally followed by several softer stools. The diarrheal stools are soft and watery, and mucus is often present in the stools. Clients with IBS often complain of belching, gas, anorexia, and bloating.

The client generally appears well, with a stable weight, and nutritional and fluid levels are within normal ranges. The nurse inspects and auscultates the abdomen. Bowel sounds are generally within normal range and may be somewhat quiet with constipation. On percussion of the abdomen, tympanic sounds may be heard over loops of filled bowel. On palpation, there may be diffuse (widespread) tenderness, which is generally worse if the sigmoid colon is palpable. The rectal examination may reveal hard or soft stool.

Routine laboratory work (including a complete blood count [CBC], serologic tests, serum albumin, erythrocyte sedimentation rate, and stools for occult blood) is normal in IBS. The health care provider typically orders a barium enema examination for clients suspected of having IBS. Colonic spasm is often noted during the procedure; however, this finding is not diagnostic. In the absence of other diagnostic findings, colonic spasm supports the diagnosis (Figure 57-2).

The evaluation of IBS is not complete without flexible sigmoidoscopy in adults younger than 40 years of age or colonoscopy in adults older than 40 years of age. A colonoscopy often demonstrates intense spastic contractions, which often stimulate painful sensations. Otherwise, the bowel mucosa appears continuous, smooth, and pink.

▶ Interventions

The client with IBS is most often cared for on an ambulatory basis. Interventions are directed at education, dietary modification, drug therapy, and stress management.

CLIENT EDUCATION. The nurse educates the client regarding the chronic nature of the disorder. Education is also directed at identifying food intolerances and needed dietary modifications. Information regarding what constitutes normal bowel function and laxative abuse is provided. The client must be alert to the urge to defecate and evacuate promptly to avoid straining and should plan to allow time and privacy in the bathroom.

DIET THERAPY. The initial treatment of IBS focuses on dietary modifications. The nurse assists the client in identifying and eliminating offending or upsetting foods. He or she is advised to limit caffeine and to avoid alcohol, beverages that

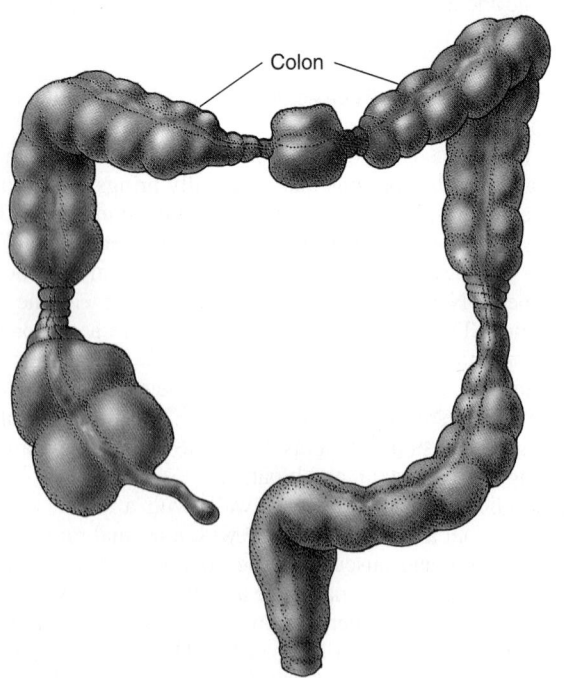

Figure 57-2 ● Spastic contractions of the colon as they occur with irritable bowel syndrome.

Colon

contain sorbitol or fructose, and other gastric irritants. Milk and milk products are to be avoided if lactose intolerance is suspected.

Fiber supplements are usually recommended whatever the predominant symptom may be. Dietary fiber and bulk help produce bulky, soft stools and establish regular bowel habits. The client should ingest approximately 30 to 40 g of fiber each day. Eating regular meals, drinking 8 to 10 cups of liquid each day, and chewing food slowly promote normal bowel function. The nurse may need to collaborate with the dietitian to help the client and family or significant others with meal planning.

DRUG THERAPY. Drug therapy is directed at the major symptom. The health care provider may prescribe bulk-forming laxatives, antidiarrheal agents, $5HT_3$ antagonists, anticholinergic agents, or tricyclic antidepressants.

For the treatment of constipation-predominant IBS, bulk-forming laxatives, such as psyllium hydrophilic mucilloid (Metamucil) or calcium polycarbophil (Mitrolan), are generally taken at mealtimes with a glass of water. The hydrophilic properties of these medications help prevent dry, hard, or liquid stools.

Diarrhea-predominant IBS is typically treated with antidiarrheal agents, such as diphenoxylate hydrochloride with atropine sulfate (Lomotil) or loperamide (Imodium) (Chart 57-1).

For IBS where pain is the predominant symptom, anticholinergics or antispasmodics, such as dicyclomine hydrochloride (Bentyl) and propantheline bromide (Pro-Banthine), help relieve abdominal cramping and intestinal spasm. Tricyclic antidepressants have also been successfully used in this form of IBS. It is unclear whether their effectiveness is due to the antidepressant or anticholinergic effects of the drugs. If clients experience postprandial discomfort (discomfort after eating), they should take these medications 30 to 45 minutes before mealtime.

STRESS MANAGEMENT. Stress management is based on the client's current and ongoing stressors and available resources. After the nurse completes a detailed psychosocial assessment, the nurse and the client set expected outcomes and plan appropriate interventions. Relaxation techniques can help the client learn skills for managing the illness. Understanding the illness empowers the client to take certain actions (e.g., diet modification and exercise) that can significantly affect the course of the illness.

If the client is in a stressful work or family situation, personal counseling may be helpful. The nurse may need to make appropriate referrals or assist in making appointments. The opportunity to discuss problems and attempt creative problem solving is often helpful. The nurse teaches the client that regular exercise is important for managing stress and promoting regular bowel elimination.

HERNIATION

■ OVERVIEW

A **hernia** is a weakness in the abdominal muscle wall through which a segment of the bowel or other abdominal structure protrudes. Hernias can also penetrate through any other defect in the abdominal wall, through the diaphragm, or through other structures in the abdominal cavity.

Defects in the muscle wall result from weakened collagen or widened spaces at the inguinal ligament. These muscle weaknesses can be inherited or acquired as part of the aging process. Increases in intra-abdominal pressure as a result of pregnancy, obesity, abdominal distention, ascites, heavy lifting, or coughing can contribute to their occurrence.

The most common types of abdominal hernias (Figure 57-3) are indirect, direct, femoral, umbilical, and incisional. An *indirect* inguinal hernia is a sac formed from the peritoneum that contains a portion of the intestine or omentum. The hernia pushes downward at an angle into the inguinal canal. In males, indirect inguinal hernias can become large and often descend into the scrotum. *Direct* inguinal hernias, in contrast, pass through a weak point in the abdominal wall.

Femoral hernias protrude through the femoral ring. A plug of fat in the femoral canal enlarges and eventually pulls the peritoneum and often the urinary bladder into the sac. *Umbilical* hernias are congenital or acquired. Congenital umbilical hernias appear in infancy. Acquired umbilical hernias directly result from increased intra-abdominal pressure. They are most commonly seen in obese individuals.

Incisional, or ventral, hernias occur at the site of a previous surgical incision. These hernias result from inadequate healing of the incision, which is most often caused by postoperative wound infections, inadequate nutrition, and obesity.

Hernias may also be classified as **reducible,** irreducible (incarcerated), or strangulated. A hernia is reducible when the contents of the hernial sac can be placed back into the abdominal cavity by gentle pressure. An **irreducible** (incarcerated) hernia cannot be reduced or placed back into the abdominal cavity. Any hernia that is not reducible requires immediate surgical evaluation.

A hernia is **strangulated** when the blood supply to the herniated segment of the bowel is cut off by pressure from the hernial ring (the band of muscle around the hernia). If a hernia is strangulated, there is ischemia and obstruction of the bowel loop. This can lead to necrosis of the bowel and possibly bowel perforation. Signs of strangulation are abdominal distention, nausea, vomiting, pain, fever, and tachycardia.

The most important elements in the development of a hernia are congenital or acquired muscle weakness and increased intra-abdominal pressure. The most significant factors contributing to increased intra-abdominal pressure are obesity, pregnancy, and lifting of heavy objects.

Indirect inguinal hernias, the most common type, are most frequent in men because they follow the tract that develops when the testes descend into the scrotum before birth. Direct

CHART 57-1

DRUG THERAPY *for* the Treatment of Diarrhea-Predominant Irritable Bowel Syndrome

Drug	Usual Dosage	Nursing Interventions	Rationale
Diphenoxylate hydrochloride and atropine sulfate (Lomotil)	1 tablet 6 times/day; no more than 6 tablets in 24 hr	Assess for abdominal distention, pain, and fever.	These symptoms may indicate a bacterial organism in the gastrointestinal (GI) tract. Diarrhea should not be suppressed in the presence of GI infection.
		Assess for sedation, dry mouth, urinary retention, and rash.	These are common side effects.
Loperamide (Imodium)	2 mg after each loose stool; maximum of 16 mg/day	Assess for abdominal distention, pain, and fever.	These symptoms may indicate a bacterial organism in the GI tract. Diarrhea should not be suppressed if GI infection is present.

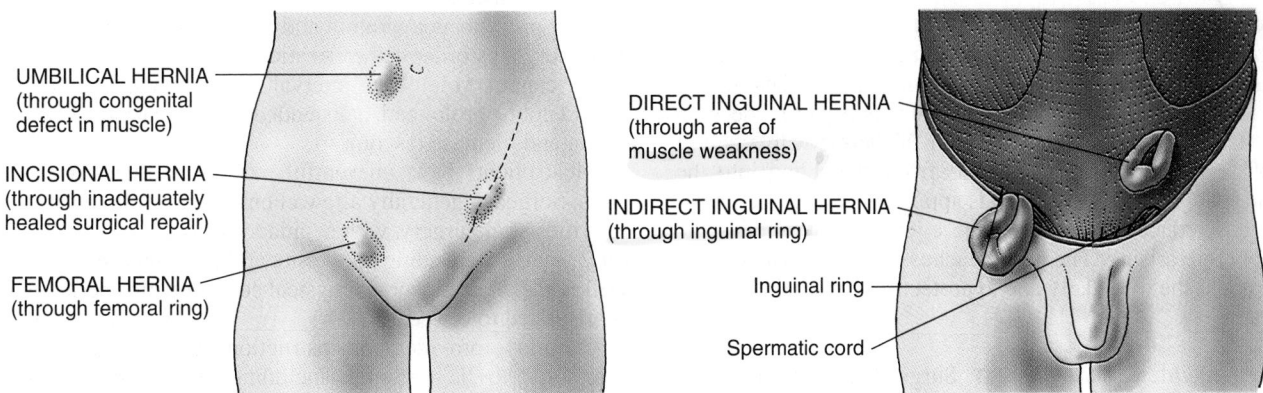

UMBILICAL HERNIA (through congenital defect in muscle)

INCISIONAL HERNIA (through inadequately healed surgical repair)

FEMORAL HERNIA (through femoral ring)

DIRECT INGUINAL HERNIA (through area of muscle weakness)

INDIRECT INGUINAL HERNIA (through inguinal ring)

Inguinal ring

Spermatic cord

Figure 57-3 ● The types of abdominal hernia.

hernias occur more often in older adults. Femoral and adult umbilical hernias are most common in obese or pregnant women. Incisional hernias can occur in people who have undergone abdominal surgery.

> ### CONSIDERATIONS FOR OLDER ADULTS
> The older adult with a strangulated hernia may not complain of pain but instead may present with nausea and vomiting. The nurse must carefully evaluate the client complaining of any of these symptoms, since they may require immediate medical and eventually surgical intervention.

► COLLABORATIVE MANAGEMENT

◗ Assessment

The client with a hernia typically comes to the health care provider's office or the emergency department with a complaint of a "lump" or protrusion felt at the involved site. The development of the hernia may be associated with straining or lifting.

To perform an abdominal assessment, the nurse inspects the abdomen when the client is lying and again when he or she is standing. If the hernia is reducible, it may disappear when the client is lying flat. The examiner asks the client to strain or perform the Valsalva maneuver and observes for bulging. The abdomen is auscultated for active bowel sounds. Absent bowel sounds may indicate obstruction and strangulation.

To palpate the hernia, the health care provider gently examines the ring and its contents by inserting a finger in the ring and noting any changes when the client coughs. The nurse never forces the hernia to reduce; that maneuver could cause strangulated intestine to rupture.

If a male client suspects a hernia in his groin, the health care provider has him stand for the examination. Using the right hand for the client's right side and the left hand for the client's left side, the health care provider invaginates the loose scrotal skin with the index finger, following the spermatic cord upward to the external inguinal cord. At this point, the client is asked to cough, and the health care provider notes any palpable herniation.

◗ Interventions

The type of treatment selected will depend on client factors, as well as the type of hernia.

NONSURGICAL MANAGEMENT. If the client is not a surgical candidate and the hernia is incarcerated, no attempt should be made to reduce the hernia. Instead, the health care provider may prescribe a truss. A truss is a pad made with firm material; it is held in place over the hernia with a belt to help keep the abdominal contents from protruding into the hernial sac. If a truss is used, it is applied only after the physician has reduced the hernia. The client usually applies the truss before arising. The nurse teaches the client to assess the skin under the truss daily and to protect it with a light layer of powder.

SURGICAL MANAGEMENT. Surgical repair of a hernia is the treatment of choice. Surgery is often performed on an ambulatory care basis for adult clients who have no pre-existing health conditions that would complicate the operative course. In same-day surgery centers, anesthesia may be local, regional, or general, and the surgery may be laparoscopic. More extensive surgery, such as a bowel resection or temporary colostomy, may be necessary if strangulation results in a gangrenous section of bowel. Clients undergoing extensive surgery are hospitalized for a longer period of time.

Herniorrhaphy is the surgery of choice for hernia repair. Hernioplasty is performed less often but can be performed in conjunction with a herniorrhaphy.

PREOPERATIVE CARE. The nurse prepares the client for surgery (see Chapter 17). He or she may be instructed to have one or two enemas the night before or the morning of surgery, depending on the surgeon's preference. If outpatient surgery is planned, the nurse assists the client in making appropriate arrangements for travel to home and for home care.

OPERATIVE PROCEDURES. During a **herniorrhaphy,** the surgeon makes an abdominal incision and places the contents of the hernial sac back into the abdominal cavity before closing the opening. When a **hernioplasty** is performed, the surgeon reinforces the weakened muscle wall with mesh, fascia, or wire. The surgeon may opt to perform the surgery through a laparoscope instead of using the open surgical method.

POSTOPERATIVE CARE. Postoperative care of the client is the same as that described in Chapter 19, except that clients who have undergone surgery for hernias are told to avoid coughing. To promote lung expansion, the nurse encourages deep breathing and frequent turning. With repair of an indirect inguinal hernia, the physician often orders a scrotal support and ice bags to be applied to the scrotum to prevent swelling, which often contributes to pain. Elevation of the scrotum with a soft pillow helps prevent and control swelling. The nurse encourages early ambulation on the day of surgery if it is not contraindicated by scrotal swelling or pre-existing conditions. Ambulation helps promote comfort and a feeling of well-being and decreases the risk of postoperative complications.

In the immediate postoperative period, the client may experience difficulty voiding. The nurse allows the male client to stand to allow a more natural position for gravity to facilitate voiding and bladder emptying. Techniques to stimulate voiding, such as allowing water to run, may also be used. Careful monitoring of intake and output alerts the nurse to voiding problems early. The nurse carefully palpates the abdomen for distention. A fluid intake of at least 1500 to 2500 mL/day prevents dehydration and maintains urinary function. Most surgeons order catheterization every 6 to 8 hours if the client cannot void. The interval between catheterizations should not be prolonged; a distended bladder can stress the incision and increase discomfort.

Most clients have uneventful recoveries after hernia repairs. Surgeons generally allow clients to return to their usual activities after surgery, with avoidance of straining and lifting for 2 weeks. Depending on the site and the extent of repair, as well as the client's general physical condition, this period may be extended to 6 weeks.

The nurse provides oral instructions and a written list of symptoms to be reported, including fever, chills, wound drainage, redness or separation of the incision, and increasing incisional pain.

The client is also instructed to keep the wound dry and clean and to replace the sterile dressing daily if indicated. Showering is permitted if allowed by the surgeon.

COLORECTAL CANCER

■ OVERVIEW

Cancer of the colon and rectum is the third most common cancer in the United States and occurs equally in men and women. Cancer of the colon ranks third in estimates for cancer deaths in the United States (Greenlee et al., 2000). Colorectal cancer can occur at any age but is most prevalent in individuals over the age of 50. Although the death rate from large-bowel cancer may be decreasing slightly, this disease is lethal in a significant number of cases because it is often not detected until an advanced stage, when metastasis has occurred.

■ Pathophysiology

Ninety-five percent of colorectal cancers are adenocarcinomas. Adenocarcinomas are tumors that arise from the glandular epithelial tissue of the colon. Colorectal cancer develops as a multistep process, resulting in a number of molecular changes, such as loss of key tumor suppressor genes and activation of certain oncogenes that alter colonic mucosa cell division. The increased proliferation of the colonic mucosa forms polyps that can be transformed into malignant tumors. The majority of colorectal cancers are believed to arise from adenomatous polyps that present as a visible protrusion from the mucosal surface of the bowel.

Tumors occur in different areas of the colon, with 70% occurring on the right side of the proximal colon. The percentages in Figure 57-4 indicate an increased incidence of cancer in the proximal sections of the large intestine in the last 20 years.

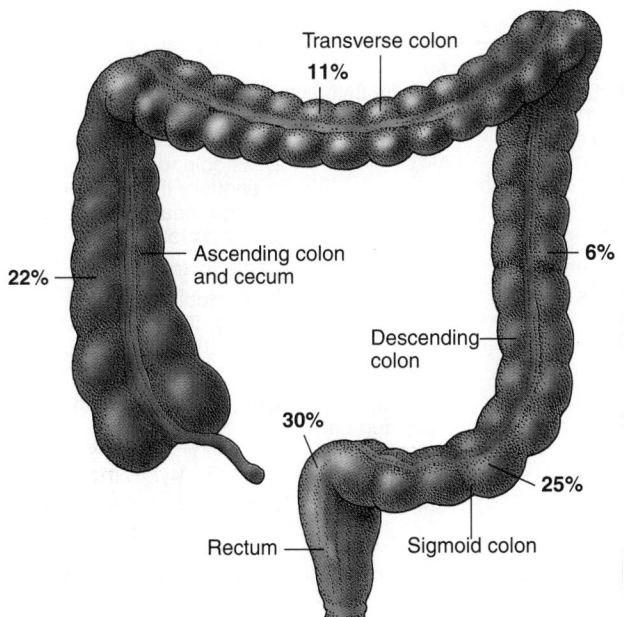

Transverse colon
11%

Ascending colon and cecum

22%

6%

Descending colon

30%

25%

Rectum   Sigmoid colon

Figure 57-4 ● The incidence of cancer in relation to colorectal anatomy.

Colorectal cancer can metastasize by means of direct extension or by spreading through the blood or lymph. The tumor may spread locally into the four layers of the bowel wall and into neighboring organs. The tumor may enlarge into the lumen of the bowel or spread through the lymphatics or the circulatory system. The circulatory system is entered directly from the primary tumor through blood vessels in the bowel or via the lymphatics. The liver is the most frequent site of metastasis from circulatory spread. Of clients with colorectal cancer, 15% to 30% will develop metastasis to the liver in spite of surgical resection of the tumor. Metastasis to the lungs, brain, bones, and adrenal glands may also be found. Colon tumors can also spread by peritoneal seeding during surgical resection of the tumor. Seeding occurs when a tumor is excised and cancer cells break off from the tumor into the peritoneal cavity.

Complications related to the increasing growth of the tumor locally or through metastatic spread include bowel obstruction or perforation with resultant peritonitis, abscess formation, and fistula formation to the urinary bladder or the vagina. The tumor may invade neighboring blood vessels and cause frank bleeding. A tumor growing into the bowel lumen can gradually obstruct the intestine and eventually block it completely. Tumor extending beyond the bowel wall may place pressure on neighboring organs (uterus, urinary bladder, and ureters) and cause symptoms that mask those of the cancer. Twenty percent of clients diagnosed with colorectal cancer are diagnosed at the time of an emergency hospitalization for bowel obstruction or other life-threatening complication (Hardcastle, 1997).

■ Etiology

Risk factors for the development of colorectal cancer include genetic predisposition, personal and dietary factors, and inflammatory bowel disease.

■ GENETIC PREDISPOSITION

Individuals with a first-degree relative diagnosed with colorectal cancer have a threefold to fourfold risk of developing the disease. An autosomal dominant inherited genetic disorder known as familial adenomatous polyposis (FAP) accounts for 1% of colorectal cancers. In these individuals, thousands of adenomatous polyps develop over the course of 10 to 15 years and have a 100% chance of becoming malignant. By the age of 20, most individuals require surgical intervention to prevent cancer. Hereditary nonpolyposis colorectal cancer (HNPCC) is another autosomal dominant disorder and accounts for 10% of all colorectal cancers. This disorder is characterized by the development of colorectal cancer at an average age of 45 years (Cavalieri & Franklin, 1998; Saddler & Ellis, 1999). Clients with this type of genetic disorder may also have a higher incidence of endometrial, ovarian, and ureteral cancers.

■ PERSONAL FACTORS

Approximately 75% of all colorectal cancers have no known predisposing cause. Age is considered a risk factor in the development of colorectal cancer, since 95% of cases are diagnosed in persons over 50 years of age. Individuals who have been diagnosed and treated for colorectal cancers have an increased risk of developing a second primary colorectal cancer, often at the site of the surgical anastomosis. Individuals with adenomatous polyps are at an increased risk of developing colorectal cancer. Such individuals need regular follow-up with colonoscopy to visualize and remove polyps.

DIETARY FACTORS

It is theorized that decreased bowel transit time and certain foods containing chemical mutagens may place individuals at risk for colorectal cancer (Table 57-1). These foods also aid in decreasing bowel transit time, which would increase the time that the bowel is exposed to carcinogens (cancer-causing substances). A high-fat diet, particularly animal fat from red meats, increases bile acid secretion and anaerobic bacteria, which are thought to be carcinogenic within the bowel. Fried and broiled meats and fish are also thought to contain chemical mutagens that are carcinogenic. Diets with large amounts of refined carbohydrates that lack fiber decrease bowel transit time.

INFLAMMATORY BOWEL DISEASE

Inflammatory bowel diseases, such as ulcerative colitis and Crohn's disease, pose an increased risk of colorectal cancer, especially if the disease has had a long, severe course.

Incidence/Prevalence

Americans have a 6% lifetime risk of developing colorectal cancer. Approximately 130,000 people in the United States were diagnosed with colorectal cancer in 1999, with an estimated 55,000 deaths (Landis et al., 1999). Most clients with colorectal cancer are older than 50 years of age; only 2% to 6% are younger than 40 years of age. The peak incidence of colorectal cancer occurs in the sixth decade of life. The overall incidence of colorectal cancer is equivalent in men and women, with cancer of the rectum being more common in men. Anal cancers account for approximately 4% of colorectal cancers.

> 〰 **CULTURAL CONSIDERATIONS**
> Both male and female African Americans have an increased frequency of colorectal cancer in advanced stages at the time of diagnosis, and consequently an increase in death rates from colorectal cancer, as opposed to male and female Caucasian Americans (Saddler & Ellis, 1999). The incidence of colorectal cancer is higher in industrialized regions of the world, with the highest rates found in North America and Australia.

TABLE 57-1 • FOODS THAT AFFECT A PERSON'S RISK FOR COLORECTAL CANCER

FOODS TO AVOID
- Red meat
- Animal fat
- Fatty foods
- Fried or broiled meats and fish
- Refined carbohydrates (e.g., concentrated sweets)

FOODS TO CONSUME
- Fruits and vegetables, especially cruciferous vegetables from the cabbage family (e.g., broccoli, cabbage, cauliflower, brussels sprouts)
- Whole-grain products
- Adequate fluids, especially water

► COLLABORATIVE MANAGEMENT
● Assessment

HISTORY

In taking a history from a client with colorectal cancer, the nurse obtains the client's diet history and asks about major risk factors, such as a personal history of breast, ovarian, or endometrial cancer; ulcerative colitis; Crohn's disease; familial polyposis; or adenomas; or a family history of colorectal cancer. The nurse also assesses the client's participation in age-specific screening guidelines for colorectal cancer (Chart 57-2).

The nurse also asks about changes in bowel habits, such as diarrhea or constipation, with or without blood in the stool. The client may also report fatigue (related to anemias), abdominal fullness, pain, or weight loss, which, unfortunately, are signs of advanced disease.

PHYSICAL ASSESSMENT/CLINICAL MANIFESTATIONS

The signs of colorectal cancer depend on the location of the tumor. However, the most common signs are rectal bleeding, anemia, and a change in the stool. Stools may contain microscopic amounts of blood that are not noticeably visible, or the client may have mahogany-colored or bright red stools. Gross blood is not usually detected with tumors of the right side of the colon but is common (but not massive) with tumors of the left side of the colon and the rectum.

Tumors arising in the transverse and descending colon result in symptoms of obstruction as growth of the tumor impedes the passage of stool. The client may complain of "gas pains," cramping, or incomplete evacuation. Tumors arising in the rectosigmoid colon are associated with hematochezia (the passage of red blood via the rectum), straining to pass stools, and narrowing of stools. Clients may complain of dull

---

CHART 57-2

BEST PRACTICE for
Screening Guidelines for Colorectal Cancer

AGE	FAMILY HISTORY	DIAGNOSTIC EXAMINATIONS
10	FAP	DRE, colonoscopy; repeat annually if polyps present; repeat in 3 yr if no polyps found
Late teens	HNPCC	Same as for FAP
25	None	DRE, stool guaiac, colonoscopy; if negative, repeat in 3-5 yr; otherwise, repeat in 1 yr to monitor
40	One or more first-degree relatives	DRE, stool guaiac, colonoscopy; if negative, repeat in 3-5 yr; otherwise, repeat in 1 yr to monitor
50	None	DRE, stool guaiac, colonoscopy; if negative, repeat in 3-5 yr; otherwise repeat in 1 yr to monitor

Data from Jessup, J., et al. (1997). Diagnosing colorectal carcinoma: Clinical and molecular approaches. *CA: A Cancer Journal for Clinicians, 47*(2), 70-92.
DRE, Digital rectal examination; *FAP,* familial adenomatous polyposis; *HNPCC,* hereditary nonpolyposis colorectal cancer.

pain. Right-sided tumors can grow quite large without disrupting bowel patterns or appearance, since the stool consistency is more liquid in this part of the colon. These tumors ulcerate and bleed intermittently, so stools can contain dark or mahogany-colored blood. A mass may be palpated in the lower right quadrant, and the client often has anemia secondary to blood loss.

Examination of the abdomen begins with assessment for obvious distention or masses. Visible peristaltic waves accompanied by high-pitched or tingling bowel sounds may indicate a partial bowel obstruction from the tumor. Total absence of bowel sounds after listening for 5 full minutes indicates a complete bowel obstruction. Palpation and percussion are performed to evaluate the liver and spleen for enlargement and to evaluate for masses along the colon. The health care provider may perform a digital rectal examination to palpate the rectum and lower sigmoid colon for masses.

PSYCHOSOCIAL ASSESSMENT

The psychologic consequences associated with a diagnosis of colorectal cancer are many. Clients must cope with a diagnosis that inspires fear and anxiety about treatment, pain, possible disfigurement, and a shortened life span. In addition, if the cancer is believed to have a genetic origin, there is anxiety concerning implications for the client's immediate family members. Possible loss of health insurance and excessive costs of genetic testing are also sources of fear and anxiety.

LABORATORY ASSESSMENT

COMPLETE BLOOD COUNT AND BLOOD CHEMISTRIES. Hemoglobin and hematocrit values are usually decreased as a result of the intermittent bleeding associated with the tumor. Colorectal cancer that has metastasized to the liver will cause liver function tests to be elevated.

FECAL OCCULT BLOOD TESTS. A positive test result for occult blood in the stool (**fecal occult blood test [FOBT]**) confirms bleeding in the gastrointestinal (GI) tract. False-positive reactions can be caused by a number of foods and medications. The client avoids meat, peroxidase-containing foods (horseradish and beets), aspirin, and vitamin C for 48 hours before giving a stool specimen. The nurse assesses whether the client is taking anti-inflammatory drugs (such as ibuprofen, corticosteroids, or salicylates). These medications may be discontinued for a period before the test to reduce the risk of a false-positive result (Held-Warmkessel, 1998). Two separate stool samples should be tested on 3 consecutive days. Negative results do not completely rule out the possibility of colorectal cancer.

ONCOFETAL ANTIGEN TESTING. Carcinoembryonic antigen (CEA) may be elevated in 70% of people with colorectal cancer. There is no relationship between the CEA level and the cancer stage. CEA is not specifically associated with the colorectal cancer, and it may be elevated in the presence of other benign or malignant diseases and in smokers. CEA is often used to monitor the effectiveness of treatment and identify disease recurrence.

RADIOGRAPHIC ASSESSMENT

BARIUM ENEMA. A double-contrast barium enema (air and barium are instilled into the colon) provides better visualization of polyps and small lesions than barium alone. This test may demonstrate an occlusion in the bowel, where the tumor is decreasing the size of the lumen.

COMPUTED TOMOGRAPHY. Computed tomography (CT) of the abdomen, pelvis, lungs, or liver helps confirm the existence of a mass and the extent of disease.

CHEST X-RAY STUDY. A chest x-ray study and liver scan may locate distant sites of metastasis.

> ### CRITICAL THINKING CHALLENGE
> You are gathering the initial history for a 44-year-old woman admitted to your unit with intermittent rectal bleeding over the last 3 months. The client states that her maternal uncle died of colorectal cancer at the age of 52.
> - What personal factors place this client at risk for colorectal cancer?
> - What specific questions would you ask concerning the rectal bleeding she reports?
> - What abnormalities in laboratory values would you suspect?
>
> For suggested answer guidelines, go to SIMON http://www.wbsaunders.com/SIMON/Iggy/.

OTHER DIAGNOSTIC ASSESSMENT

SIGMOIDOSCOPY. A sigmoidoscopy provides visualization of the lower colon using a fiberoptic scope. Polyps can be visualized, and samples can be taken for biopsy.

COLONOSCOPY. A colonoscopy provides visualization of the entire large bowel from the rectum to the ileocecal valve. As with sigmoidoscopy, polyps can be visualized and removed, and tissue samples can be taken for biopsy. Colonoscopy is the definitive test for the diagnosis of colorectal cancer.

LIVER SCAN. A liver scan may locate distant sites of metastasis.

◆ Analysis

COMMON NURSING DIAGNOSES AND COLLABORATIVE PROBLEMS

The priority nursing diagnosis for clients with colorectal cancer is Anticipatory Grieving related to the diagnosis of a potentially terminal illness, a disturbance in body image, and the possible loss of fecal continence. The priority collaborative problem is Potential for Metastasis.

ADDITIONAL NURSING DIAGNOSES AND COLLABORATIVE PROBLEMS

In addition to the common nursing diagnoses and collaborative problems, clients with colorectal cancer may develop one or more of the following:
- Acute Pain or Chronic Pain related to tumor obstruction of the intestine, with possible pressure on other organs
- Disturbed Body Image related to the creation of a stoma or fear of incontinence

- Compromised Family Coping related to alteration in roles, lifestyle changes, and fear of the client's death
- Imbalanced Nutrition: Less Than Body Requirements related to the diagnostic workup
- Fear related to the disease process
- Powerlessness related to the presence of a life-threatening illness and its treatment

▶ Planning and Implementation

■ ANTICIPATORY GRIEVING

NOC PLANNING: EXPECTED OUTCOMES. A client faced with a diagnosis of colorectal cancer experiences feelings and anxieties that can tax his or her ability to cope with present and future issues related to the disease and treatment. The client with colorectal cancer is expected to identify, develop, and use effective coping methods in dealing with the perceived changes and losses experienced.

INTERVENTIONS. The client and family are faced with a possible loss of or alteration in body functions. Medical and surgical interventions for the treatment of colorectal cancer may result in cure, disease control, or palliation. Interventions are designed to assist the client in formulating effective strategies for expressing feelings of grief and developing coping skills.

The nurse observes and identifies the following:
- The client's and family's current methods of coping
- Effective sources of support used in past crises
- The client's and family's present perceptions of the health problem
- Signs of anticipatory grief, such as crying, anger, and withdrawal from usual relationships

The nurse encourages the client to verbalize feelings about the diagnosis, treatment, and anticipated alteration in body functions if a colostomy is planned (see later discussion of the operative procedure under Surgical Management, p. 1249). Sadness, anger, feelings of loss, and depression are normal responses to this change in body functions.

If a colostomy is planned, the nurse teaches the client what to expect about the appearance and care of the colostomy. Postoperatively, the client is encouraged to look at and touch the stoma. When the client is physically able, the nurse asks him or her to participate in colostomy care. Participation helps to restore the client's sense of control over his or her lifestyle and thus facilitates improved self-esteem.

NIC GRIEF WORK FACILITATION. The purpose of grief work is to assist the client with the resolution of a significant loss. The nurse assists in identifying the nature of and reaction to the loss. Encouraging the client to verbalize feelings and identify fears helps to move him or her through the appropriate phases of the grief process. The nurse establishes a trusting, ongoing relationship with the client and provides support through the personal grieving stages.

The nurse, in collaboration with the psychologist when appropriate, assists the client in identifying personal coping strategies. The client is encouraged to implement cultural, religious, and social customs associated with the loss and to identify sources of community support available to the client and family. Modifications in lifestyle can be anticipated in clients with a diagnosis of colorectal cancer. The nurse assists

in identifying the necessary modifications in lifestyle that may be necessary. The chaplain, social worker, and/or family assists in discussions and decisions concerning treatment, the prognosis, and end-of-life decisions, as appropriate.

NIC GENETIC COUNSELING. Genetic counseling entails the use of an interactive helping process focusing on the prevention of a genetic disorder or on the ability to cope with a family member who has a genetically based disorder. The nurse may be asked to provide a referral to a genetics center by clients who are believed to have familial colorectal cancers. Specially trained nurses can discuss the purposes and goals of genetic testing. Privacy and confidentiality need to be ensured. A review of the family history may provide important information concerning the pattern of colorectal cancer inheritance. To make an informed decision, the client and family need information about the advantages, risks, and costs of appropriate genetic tests. The nurse will need to carefully monitor the client's response on learning of his or her genetic risk factors.

NIC interventions are summarized in Chart 57-3.

■ POTENTIAL FOR METASTASIS

PLANNING: EXPECTED OUTCOMES. The client with colorectal cancer is expected to not have the cancer spread to vital organs; thus the client's life expectancy will be increased and the quality of life will be improved.

INTERVENTIONS. Although surgical resection is the primary means used to control the disease, several adjuvant

---

CHART 57-3

NIC INTERVENTION ACTIVITIES for The Client with Noninflammatory Intestinal Disorders

Grief Work Facilitation: *Assistance with the resolution of a significant loss*
- Assist the client to identify the nature of the attachment to the lost object or person.
- Assist the patient to identify the initial reaction to the loss.
- Encourage expression of feelings about the loss.
- Instruct in phases of the grieving process, as appropriate.
- Support progression through personal grieving stages.
- Include significant others in discussions and decisions, as appropriate.
- Assist to identify personal coping strategies.
- Encourage client to implement cultural, religious, and social customs associated with the loss.
- Identify sources of community support.
- Assist in identifying modifications needed in lifestyle.

Genetic Counseling: *Use of an interactive helping process focusing on assisting an individual, family, or group, manifesting or at risk for developing or transmitting a birth defect or genetic condition, to cope.*
- Provide privacy and ensure confidentiality.
- Discuss the client's purpose, goals, and agenda for the genetic counseling session.
- Discuss the advantages, risks, and costs of genetic tests.
- Monitor response when patient learns about own genetic risk factors.
- Provide referral to genetic health care specialists, as necessary.

NIC intervention activities selected from McCloskey, J.C., & Bulechek, G.M. (2000). *Nursing interventions classification (NIC)* (3rd ed.). St. Louis: Mosby. No part of this work is to be altered without prior written permission from the Publisher.

therapies are employed as well. Adjuvant therapies are administered before or after surgery to affect a cure and to prevent recurrence.

NONSURGICAL MANAGEMENT. The type of therapy used is based on the pathologic staging of the disease. Dukes' staging classification is most often used. This method classifies colorectal tumors by designating them as either A, B, C, or D according to the depth of invasion into the mucosa and distant spread.

Dukes' stage A indicates that the tumor has penetrated into, but not through, the bowel wall. Stage B indicates that the tumor has penetrated through the bowel wall. Stage C indicates that the tumor has penetrated through the bowel wall and that there is lymph node involvement. Stage D indicates that the tumor has metastasized to any of a number of distant sites.

RADIATION THERAPY. The administration of preoperative radiation therapy has not improved overall survival from colorectal cancer but has been effective in providing local or regional control of the disease. Postoperative radiation has not demonstrated any consistent improvement in survival or recurrence. As a palliative measure, radiation therapy may be used to control pain, hemorrhage, bowel obstruction, or metastasis to the lung in advanced disease. Unlike the case with colorectal cancer, radiation therapy is almost always a part of the treatment plan for rectal cancer. The nurse explains the radiation therapy procedure to the client and family and monitors for possible side effects (e.g., diarrhea and fatigue). (See Chapter 25 for care of clients undergoing radiation therapy.)

CHEMOTHERAPY. Adjuvant chemotherapy after primary surgery is recommended for clients with stage II (Dukes' stage B_2) or stage III (Dukes' stage C) disease to improve survival. The drug of choice is intravenous (IV) 5-fluorouracil (5-FU) with or without levamisole or leucovorin. The side effects of 5-FU and levamisole or leucovorin are diarrhea, mucositis, and skin effects. Oxaliplatin is a relatively new platinum analog chemotherapeutic agent. It has been used with 5-FU and levamisole or leucovorin with good results in clients with metastatic disease. The dose-limiting toxicity for this agent is peripheral sensory neuropathy.

In 1997 irinotecan (Camptosar) was approved as second-line treatment for metastatic disease if disease has recurred or progressed after treatment with 5-FU. With this drug, myelosuppression (bone marrow suppression) and diarrhea are the most frequent dose-limiting toxicities. Current clinical trials using a 17-1A monoclonal antibody and a colorectal tumor vaccine are in progress. In addition, new oral agents consisting of a fluorinated pyrimidine and leucovorin are being tested. Intrahepatic arterial chemotherapy, often with 5-FU, may be administered to clients with liver metastasis.

SURGICAL MANAGEMENT. Surgical removal of the tumor with margins free of disease is the best method of ensuring removal of colorectal cancer. The size of the tumor, its location, the extent of metastasis, the integrity of the bowel, and the condition of the client determine which surgical procedure is performed for colorectal cancer (Table 57-2). Because the majority of colorectal cancers are diagnosed when the cancer has extended beyond the tumor, the three most common surgeries

performed are *hemicolectomy* (resection of the tumor and regional lymph nodes) with reanastomosis, *colon resection* with *colostomy (temporary or permanent),* and *abdominoperineal resection* (Saddler & Ellis, 1999).

Small tumors indicate an early stage of cancer and are well differentiated without evidence of vascular or lymphatic invasion. They can be removed with clean margins and may be treated with local excision and close follow-up. A transanal approach without an abdominal incision is the technique most commonly used; this approach decreases the risk for postoperative complications and shortens the hospital stay. Only 5% of clients with colorectal cancer, however, meet the criteria of early-stage cancer. Currently, clinical trials are being conducted to evaluate the use of laparoscopic techniques in the treatment of colorectal cancer.

HEMICOLECTOMY AND COLON RESECTION. A **hemicolectomy** involves excision of the involved area of the colon, leaving an area of clean margins. If the integrity of the intestine is optimal (e.g., without inflammation, as with bowel obstruction or perforation), and if the rectal sphincter can be left intact, reanastomosis can usually be accomplished and an ostomy can be avoided. If healing of a reanastomosed bowel is thought to be in jeopardy, a temporary or permanent colostomy will be performed. A **colostomy** is the surgical creation of an opening of the colon onto the surface of the abdomen.

Preoperative Care. The nurse helps the client to prepare for colon resection by reinforcing the physician's explanation of the planned surgical procedure. The client is told as accurately as possible what anatomic and physiologic changes will occur with surgery. The location and number of incision sites and drains are also discussed.

Before evaluating the tumor and colon during surgery, the physician may not be able to determine whether a colostomy will be necessary. If this is the case, the physician informs the client that a colostomy is a possibility. If the surgeon informs

---

TABLE 57-2 • SURGICAL PROCEDURES FOR COLORECTAL CANCERS IN VARIOUS LOCATIONS

RIGHT-SIDED COLON TUMORS
- Right hemicolectomy for smaller lesions
- Right ascending colostomy or ileostomy for large, widespread lesions
- Cecostomy (opening into the cecum with intubation to decompress the bowel)

LEFT-SIDED COLON TUMORS
- Left hemicolectomy for smaller lesions
- Left descending colostomy for larger lesions (e.g., the Hartmann procedure)

SIGMOID COLON TUMORS
- Sigmoid colectomy for smaller lesions
- Sigmoid colostomy for larger lesions (e.g., the Hartmann procedure)
- Abdominoperineal resection for large, low sigmoid tumors (near the anus) with colostomy (the rectum and the anus are completely removed, leaving a perineal wound)

RECTAL TUMORS
- Resection with anastomosis or pull-through procedure (preserves anal sphincter and normal elimination pattern)
- Colon resection with permanent colostomy
- Abdominoperineal resection with colostomy

the client that a colostomy is inevitable, the nurse consults an enterostomal therapist (ET) to advise on optimal placement of the ostomy and instructs the client about the rationale and general principles of ostomy care. An ET is a registered nurse who has completed specialized training and is certified in ostomy nursing care. Some are also certified in wound and incontinence care.

The client who requires low rectal surgery is faced with the risk of postoperative sexual dysfunction and urinary incontinence as a result of nerve damage during surgery. The physician discusses the risk for these problems with the client before surgery and allows him or her to verbalize concerns and questions related to this risk. The nurse reinforces teaching about abdominal surgery performed with the client under general anesthesia and reviews the routines for turning and deep breathing (see Chapter 17).

If the bowel is not obstructed or perforated, elective surgery is planned. The client receives a thorough cleaning of the bowel, or "bowel prep," to minimize bacterial growth and prevent complications. In preparation for the bowel prep, the client is usually instructed to restrict the diet to clear liquids for 1 to 2 days before surgery. Mechanical cleaning is accomplished with laxatives and enemas or with "whole-gut lavage." For whole-gut lavage, the client usually ingests large quantities of a sodium sulfate and polyethylene glycol solution (e.g., GoLYTELY). This solution overwhelms the absorptive capacity of the small bowel and clears feces from the colon.

To reduce the risk of infection, the surgeon may prescribe oral or IV antibiotics to be given the day before surgery (Held-Warmkessel, 1998). Before surgery, a nasogastric (NG) tube is placed for decompression of the stomach following surgery. A peripheral IV line is also placed for fluid and electrolyte replacement while the client is taking nothing by mouth (NPO).

The client with colorectal cancer faces a serious illness with long-term consequences of the disease and treatment. A case manager can be very helpful in identifying client and family needs, as well as continuity of care and support.

Operative Procedure. The surgeon makes an incision in the abdomen and explores the abdominal cavity to determine if the tumor can be removed. The portion of the colon with the tumor is excised, and the two open ends of the bowel are irrigated before **anastomosis** (reattachment) of the colon. If an anastomosis is not feasible because of the location of the tumor or the bowel is inflamed, a colostomy is created.

A colostomy may be created in the ascending, transverse, descending, or sigmoid colon (Figure 57-5). One of three basic techniques is used to construct a colostomy. A loop **stoma** (surgical opening) is made by bringing a loop of colon to the skin surface, severing and everting the anterior wall, and suturing it to the abdominal wall. Loop colostomies are usually performed in the transverse colon and are usually temporary (Bradley & Pupiales, 1997). An external rod is used to support the loop until the intestinal tissue adheres to the abdominal wall. Care must be taken to avoid displacing the rod, especially during appliance changes.

An end stoma is often constructed, most often in the descending or sigmoid colon, when a colostomy is intended to

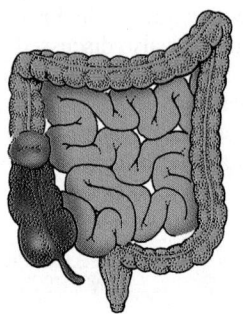

The **ascending colostomy** is done for right-sided tumors.

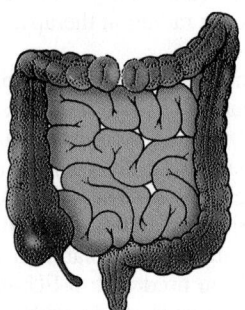

The **transverse (double-barreled) colostomy** is often used in such emergencies as intestinal obstruction or perforation because it can be created quickly. There are two stomas. The proximal one, closest to the small intestine, drains feces. The distal stoma drains mucus.

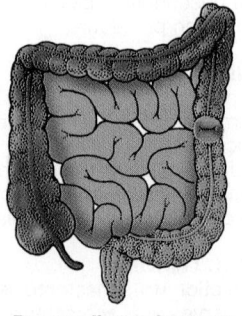

Descending colostomy

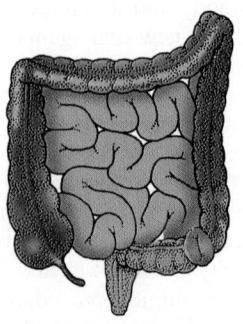

Sigmoid colostomy

Figure 57-5 ● Different locations of colostomies in the colon.

be permanent. It may also be done in conjunction with a Hartmann procedure, when the surgeon oversews the distal stump of the colon and places it in the abdominal cavity, preserving it for future reattachment. An end stoma is constructed by severing the end of the proximal portion of the bowel and bringing it out through the abdominal wall.

The least common colostomy is the double-barrel stoma, which is created by dividing the bowel and bringing both the proximal and distal portions to the abdominal surface to create two stomas. The proximal stoma (closest to the client's head) is the functioning stoma and eliminates stool; the distal stoma (farthest from the head) is considered nonfunctioning, although it may secrete some mucus. The distal stoma is sometimes referred to as a mucous fistula.

Postoperative Care. Clients who have undergone a colon resection without a colostomy receive care similar to that of clients undergoing any abdominal surgery (see Chapter 19).

Colostomy Management. The client who has a colostomy created may return from surgery with an ostomy pouch system in place. If there is no pouch system in place, a petrolatum gauze dressing is usually placed over the stoma to keep it moist, and this is covered with a dry, sterile dressing. In collaboration with the enterostomal therapist (ET), the nurse places a pouch system as soon as possible. The colostomy pouch system allows more convenient and acceptable collection of stool than a dressing does.

The nurse assesses the color and integrity of the stoma. A healthy stoma should be reddish pink and moist and will protrude about ¾ inch (2 cm) from the abdominal wall. A small amount of bleeding at the stoma is common.

The nurse reports any of the following problems related to the colostomy to the surgeon:

- Signs of ischemia and necrosis (dark red, purplish, or black color; dry, firm, or flaccid)
- Unusual bleeding
- Mucocutaneous separation (breakdown of the suture line securing the stoma to the abdominal wall)

The nurse also assesses the condition of the peristomal skin and frequently checks the pouch system for proper fit and signs of leakage. The peristomal skin should be intact, smooth, and without redness or excoriation.

The colostomy should start functioning 2 to 4 days postoperatively. When the colostomy begins to function, the pouch may need to be emptied frequently because of excess gas collection. It should be emptied when it is one-third to one-half full of stool. Stool is liquid immediately postoperatively but becomes more solid, depending on where in the colon the stoma was placed. For example, the stool from a colostomy in the ascending colon is liquid, the stool from a colostomy in the transverse colon is pasty, and the stool from a colostomy in the descending colon is more solid (similar to usual stool expelled from the rectum).

ABDOMINOPERINEAL RESECTION. When rectal tumors are present, the rectum and rectal support structure may need to be removed. An abdominoperineal resection usually requires a permanent colostomy for evacuation. However, with improvements in surgical techniques, more clients can undergo a colon resection with the rectal sphincter left intact; thus the need for a colostomy is avoided.

Preoperative Care. The preoperative care for the client undergoing an abdominoperineal resection is similar to that provided for the client undergoing a colon resection.

Operative Procedure. The surgeon removes the distal sigmoid colon, the rectosigmoid colon, the rectum, and the anus through combined abdominal and perineal incisions. A permanent end-sigmoid colostomy is created.

Postoperative Care. Postoperative care after an abdominoperineal resection is similar to that given after a colon resection with the creation of a sigmoid colostomy. The nurse collaborates with the ET to provide colostomy care and client and family education. In addition, the nurse monitors for postoperative complications, including pneumonia, dehydration, anastomotic leakage, and wound infection.

Wound Management. The perineal wound is generally surgically closed, and two bulb suction drains, such as Jackson-Pratt drains, are placed in the wound or through stab wounds near the wound. The drains help prevent drainage from collecting within the wound and are usually left in place for several days, depending on the character and amount of drainage.

Monitoring drainage from the perineal wound and cavity is important because of the possibility of infection and abscess formation. Serosanguineous drainage from the perineal wound may be observed for 1 to 2 months after surgery. Complete healing of the perineal wound may take 6 to 8 months. This wound can be a greater source of discomfort than the abdominal incision and ostomy, and more care may be required. The client may experience phantom rectal sensations because sympathetic innervation for rectal control has not been interrupted. Rectal pain and itching may occasionally occur after healing; however, there is no known physiologic explanation for these sensations. Interventions may include use of antipruritic medications, such as benzocaine, and sitz baths. The nurse continually assesses for signs of infection, abscess, or other complications and implements methods for promoting wound drainage and comfort (Chart 57-4).

Colostomy Management. The care of the permanent colostomy created as a result of the abdominal-perineal re-

---

CHART 57-4

BEST PRACTICE *for*
Perineal Wound Care

Wound Care
- Place an absorbent dressing (Kerlix or abdominal pad) over the wound.
- Instruct the client that he or she may:
    Use a feminine napkin as a dressing
    Wear jockey-type shorts rather than boxers

Comfort Measures
- If ordered, soak the wound area in a sitz bath for 10 to 20 minutes three or four times per day.
- Administer pain medication as ordered and assess its effectiveness.
- Instruct the client about permissible activities. The client should:
    Assume a side-lying position in bed; avoid sitting for long periods
    Use foam pads or a soft pillow to sit on whenever in a sitting position
    Avoid the use of air rings or rubber doughnut devices

Prevention of Complications
- Maintain fluid and electrolyte balance by monitoring intake and output and by monitoring output from the perineal wound.
- Observe suture line integrity and monitor wound drains; watch for erythema, edema, bleeding, purulent drainage, unusual odor, and excessive or constant pain.

section is similar to that of a hemicolectomy with a colostomy (see Surgical Management, p. 1249).

CRITICAL THINKING CHALLENGE

Your client is about to undergo a colon resection with the creation of a temporary colostomy for colorectal cancer.
- What preoperative teaching should be included for this client?
- What physical parameters should you assess the stoma for in the early postoperative period?
- What postoperative complications should you monitor for?

For suggested answer guidelines, go to SIMON http://www.wbsaunders.com/SIMON/Iggy/.

Community-Based Care

Clients undergoing an uncomplicated colon resection are typically hospitalized for 5 to 7 days. Discharge planning with the assistance of a discharge planner or case manager assists clients and their families in coping with the immediate postoperative phase of recovery. Following hospitalization for surgery, the client with colorectal cancer is usually managed at home. Radiation therapy or chemotherapy is typically done on an ambulatory (outpatient) basis. For the client with advanced cancer, hospice care is an option (see Chapter 9).

HOME CARE MANAGEMENT

The nurse assesses all clients for their ability to perform incision care and activities of daily living (ADLs) within limitations. For clients requiring assistance with these activities, home care visits by nurses or assistive nursing personnel can be provided.

For the client who has undergone a colostomy, the nurse or case manager reviews the home situation to aid the client in arranging for care. Ostomy products should be kept in an area (preferably the bathroom) where the temperature is neither hot nor cold (skin barriers may become stiff or melt in extreme temperatures) to ensure proper functioning. The enterostomal therapist (ET) may serve as a consultant after the client is discharged home to ensure continuity of care.

No changes are needed in sleeping accommodations. A rubber covering may initially be placed over the bed mattress if clients feel insecure about the pouch system. The client may consume his or her usual diet on discharge.

HEALTH TEACHING

Before discharge, clients are instructed to avoid lifting heavy objects or straining on defecation to prevent tension on the anastomosis site. The client is advised to avoid driving for 4 to 6 weeks while the incision heals. A stool softener may be prescribed to keep stools at a soft consistency for ease of passage. Clients are instructed to note the frequency, amount, and character of the stools. In addition to this information, the nurse teaches all clients with colon resections to watch for and report clinical manifestations of intestinal obstruction and perforation (e.g., cramping, abdominal pain, nausea, and vomiting). A normal diet may be resumed; however, the client is advised to avoid gas-producing foods and carbonated beverages. Four to six weeks may be required to establish the effects of certain foods on bowel patterns.

COLOSTOMY CARE. Rehabilitation after ostomy surgery requires that clients and family members learn the principles of colostomy care and the psychomotor skills needed to facilitate this care. Providing information is important, but the nurse must also allow adequate opportunity for clients to learn the psychomotor skills involved in ostomy care before discharge. Sufficient practice time is planned for clients and family or significant others so that they can handle, assemble, and apply all ostomy equipment. The nurse teaches clients and family or other caregiver about the following:

- The normal appearance of the stoma
- Signs and symptoms of complications
- Measurement of the stoma
- The choice, use, care, and application of the appropriate appliance to cover the stoma
- Measures to protect the skin adjacent to the stoma
- Dietary measures to control gas and odor
- Resumption of normal activities, including work, travel, and sexual intercourse

The appropriate pouch system must be selected and fitted to the stoma. Clients with flat, firm abdomens may use either flexible (bordered with paper tape) or nonflexible (full skin barrier wafer) pouch systems. A firm abdomen with lateral creases or folds requires a flexible system. Clients with deep creases, flabby abdomens, a retracted stoma, or a stoma that is flush or concave to the abdominal surface benefit from a convex appliance with a stoma belt (Bradley & Pupiales, 1997). This type of system presses into the skin around the stoma, causing the stoma to protrude. This protrusion helps tighten the skin and prevents leaks around the stoma opening onto the peristomal skin.

Measurement of the stoma is necessary to determine the correct size of the stomal opening on the appliance. The opening should be large enough not only to cover the peristomal skin but also to avoid stomal trauma. The stoma will shrink within 6 to 8 weeks of surgery; therefore it needs to be measured at least once weekly during this time and as needed if the client gains or loses weight. The client and family caregiver should be taught to trace the pattern of the stomal area on the wafer portion of the appliance and to cut an opening about $\frac{1}{8}$ to $\frac{1}{16}$ inch larger than the stomal pattern to ensure that stomal tissue will not be constricted (Catanzaro & Serembus, 1998).

Skin preparation may include clipping peristomal hair or shaving the area to achieve a smooth surface, prevent unnecessary discomfort when the wafer is removed, and minimize the risk of infected hair follicles. The client is advised to avoid using moisturizing soaps to clean the area because the lubricants can interfere with adhesion of the appliance. The client and family caregiver are taught to apply a skin sealant and allow it dry before application of the appliance (colostomy bag) to facilitate less painful removal of the tape or adhesive. If peristomal skin becomes raw, the client or caregiver checks to see whether the sealant contains alcohol and, if so, reconsiders using it to avoid causing a burning sensation to the skin. Stoma powder or paste, or a combination, may also be used for erythematous peristomal skin. The paste is also used to fill in crevices and creases to create a flat surface for the faceplate of the colostomy bag. If the client develops a fungal rash, an antifungal cream or powder is used, as ordered.

Control of gas and odor from the colostomy is often a significant goal for clients with new ostomies. Although a leaking or inadequately closed pouch is the usual cause of odor, flatus can also contribute to the odor. The nurse teaches the client and family caregiver that although there are generally no forbidden foods for ostomates, certain foods and habits can cause flatus or contribute to odor when the pouch is open. Broccoli, brussels sprouts, cabbage, cauliflower, cucumbers, mushrooms, and peas often cause flatus, as does chewing gum, smoking, drinking beer, and skipping meals. Crackers, toast, and yogurt can help prevent gas. Asparagus, broccoli, cabbage, turnips, eggs, fish, and garlic contribute to odor when the pouch is open. Buttermilk, cranberry juice, parsley, and yogurt will help prevent odor; charcoal filters, pouch deodorizers, or placement of a breath mint in the pouch will eliminate odors. The client should be cautioned not to put aspirin tablets in the pouch because they may cause ulceration of the stoma (Table 57-3).

The client with a sigmoid colostomy may benefit from colostomy irrigation to regulate elimination. However, most clients with a sigmoid colostomy can become regulated through diet. An irrigation is similar to an enema but is administered through the stoma rather than the rectum.

In addition to instructing the client about the clinical manifestations of obstruction and perforation, the nurse also advises the client with a colostomy to report any fever or sudden onset of pain or swelling around the stoma. Other assessments performed by the home care nurse are listed in Chart 57-5.

PSYCHOSOCIAL PREPARATION. The diagnosis of cancer can be emotionally immobilizing for the client and family or significant others, but treatment may be welcomed because it may provide hope for control of the disease. The nurse explores the client's reactions to the illness and perceptions of planned interventions.

The client's reaction to ostomy surgery, which may include disfigurement, may involve the following:
- Fear of not being accepted by others
- Feelings of grief related to disturbance in body image
- Concerns about sexuality

The nurse allows the client to verbalize his or her feelings. By teaching how to physically manage the ostomy, the nurse can help the client begin to restore self-esteem and improve body image. Inclusion of family and significant others in the rehabilitation process may help maintain relationships and raise the client's self-esteem. Anticipatory instruction includes information on leakage accidents, odor control measures, and adjustments to resuming normal sexual relationships.

■ HEALTH CARE RESOURCES

Several resources are available to complement nursing care, maintain continuity of care in the home environment, and provide for client needs that the nurse is not able to meet. The nurse makes a referral to the case manager or social worker, who can provide further emotional counseling to the client and family or significant others, aid in managing the financial concerns that the client and family may have, or arrange home care or extended care (e.g., in a nursing home, group home, or hospice) as needed.

The nurse makes a referral to the enterostomal therapist (ET) to aid in preoperative stoma teaching, evaluate and mark the stoma site, and provide consultation for problems in care. The enterostomal therapist (ET) may also conduct an ambulatory care clinic for ongoing client needs.

Information about the United Ostomy Association, a self-help group of people who have ostomies, is provided. Literature, such as the organization's publication *(Ostomy Quarterly),* and information about a local chapter are given to the client. This organization conducts a visitor program that sends specially trained visitors (who have an ostomy) to talk with clients. After obtaining the client's consent, the nurse makes a referral to the visitor program so that the visitor can see the client both preoperatively and postoperatively. A physician's consent for visitation is generally necessary.

The local division or unit of the American Cancer Society (ACS) can help provide necessary medical equipment and supplies, home care services, travel accommodations, and other resources for the client who is undergoing cancer treatment or ostomy surgery. The nurse informs the client and family of the programs available through the local division or unit.

Because of short hospital stays, clients with new ostomies receive most of their instruction on colostomy care from nurses working for home care agencies. This resource also facilitates provision for physical care needs, medication management, and emotional support for clients with or without colostomies. If the client has advanced colorectal cancer, a referral for hospice services in the home, nursing home, or other long-term care setting may be appropriate. The home care nurse informs the client and family about what ostomy supplies are needed and where they can be purchased. Price and location are considered before recommendations are made.

● Evaluation: Outcomes

NOC The nurse evaluates the care of the client with colorectal cancer on the basis of the identified nursing diagnoses and collaborative problems. The expected outcomes are that the client:
- Maintains hemodynamic stability following surgery
- Is free of infection and postoperative complications
- Demonstrates appropriate incision care and, if applicable, appropriate colostomy care with minimal assistance
- Acquires or maintains effective coping patterns throughout the diagnosis, treatment, and rehabilitative phases of recovery

INTESTINAL OBSTRUCTION

■ OVERVIEW

Intestinal obstruction is defined as "a partial or complete obstruction of the small or large bowel that impedes the natural progression of digestive processing" (Shelton, 1999, p. 478). Intestinal obstruction is a common and serious disorder caused by a variety of conditions and is associated with significant morbidity. Bowel obstruction accounts for up to 20% of emergency admissions to a surgical service. It can occur anywhere in the intestinal tract, although the ileum in the small intestine (the narrowest part of the intestinal tract) is the most common site. The nurse assesses for clinical manifestations of obstruction in all clients with gastrointestinal (GI) disorders, since obstruction occurs fairly often and is associated with a variety of conditions.

■ Pathophysiology

Intestinal obstructions can be partial or complete and are classified as mechanical or nonmechanical. In **mechanical ob-**

TABLE 57-3 • SOLUTIONS TO SPECIAL PROBLEMS IN OSTOMY USE

Problems	Solutions
ODOR	
Foods	
Dairy products (boiled milk, eggs, and some cheese), fish, onion, garlic, coffee, alcohol, nuts, prunes, beans, cabbage, cucumbers, asparagus, radishes, broccoli, turnips, peas, highly seasoned foods	Spinach, cranberry juice, yogurt, buttermilk, dark green vegetables (parsley is particularly helpful), increased vitamin C in food or vitamin preparations
Drugs	*Oral Medications*
Antibiotics, vitamins, iron	Chlorophyll tablets (Derifil) for fecal odors (absorb gas) Charcoal tablets Bismuth bicarbonate (0.6 g tid with meals) Bismuth subgallate (Devrom or Biscaps) 1 or 2 tablets with meals and 1 tablet at bedtime
	Pouch Preparations Odor-proof pouch or pouch with odor-control mechanism Manufactured preparations (place small amounts in pouch): Banish II or Superbanish (United), Odor-Guard (Marlan), Ostobon (Pettibone Labs), activated charcoal, ostomy deodorant (Sween), Nilodor, Devko tablets (Parthenon), D-Odor, M-9 (Mason Lab) Sodium bicarbonate solution (soaked cotton balls in pouch) Vanilla, peppermint, lemon, or almond extracts (put 10 drops into pouch or soak cotton balls) Favorite spice, cloves, or cinnamon (place ¼ tsp in pouch) Mouthwash (e.g., Cēpacol, Listerine) (several drops in pouch or soaked cotton balls in pouch)
	Cleaning Reusable Pouches Wisk and water (1:1 solution) Baking soda and water (1:1 solution) Household white vinegar and water (1:1 solution) Manufactured products: Uri-Kleen, Uni-Wash (United), Peri-Wash (Sween), Skin Care cleaner (Bard) Baking soda (after drying the pouch, powder inside with baking soda)
FLATULENCE	
Activities	
Eating fast and talking at same time, gum chewing, smoking, snoring, skipping meals, emotional upset	Avoid these activities; eat solids before taking liquids
Foods	*Pouch Adaptation*
Mushrooms, onions, beans, cabbage, brussels sprouts, spinach, cheese, eggs, beer, carbonated beverages, fish, highly seasoned foods, some fruit drinks, corn, pork, peas, coffee, high-fat foods	Use pouches with gas or odor filters
SKIN IRRITATION	
Allergy	
Erythema, erosion, edema, weeping, bleeding, itching, burning, stinging, irritation the same shape as the allergic material	Creams: Sween cream, Unicare cream, or Hollister Skin Conditioning Cream (use small amount and rub in; tapes will adhere when dry)
Chemical Exposure	Powders (karaya gum, Stomahesive, cornstarch) used with skin gel (Skin Prep, Skin Gel)
Stool, urine, glues, solvents, soaps, detergents, proteolytic digestive enzymes	Antacids: aluminum hydroxide (Amphojel, Maalox) used with skin sealant (Skin Prep, Skin Gel)
Epidermal Hyperplasia	Skin sealant alone (for slightly reddened skin)
Increased formation of epidermal cells causing a generalized thickening of the outer layer of the skin	Skin barriers: one application left on for 24 hr or longer may clear irritations quickly Pastes (Hollister Premium, Stomahesive) used to fill in creases and spaces
Mechanical Trauma	Hair dryer on cool setting to decrease moisture
Pressure, friction, or stripping of the skin (e.g., adhesives, tape, belts)	Do not patch or tape leaks; correct the leakage problem immediately
Infection	*For Candidiasis*
Candida albicans infection indicated by pustular, reddened, weepy, white spots	Use nystatin (Mycostatin) powder; cover with skin sealant (Skin Prep or Skin Gel)
Radiation Therapy	
Erythema, weeping	Use drying agent (e.g., acroflavin) Place skin barrier (Stomahesive) over site

FOCUSED ASSESSMENT *of*
The Home Care Client with a Colostomy

Assess gastrointestinal status, including:
- Dietary and fluid intake and habits
- Presence or absence of nausea and vomiting
- Weight gain or loss
- Bowel elimination pattern and characteristics and amount of effluent (stool)
- Bowel sounds

Assess condition of stoma, including:
- Location, size, protrusion, color, and integrity
- Signs of ischemia, such as dull coloring or dark or purplish bruising

Assess periostomal skin for:
- Presence or absence of excoriated skin, leakage underneath drainage system
- Fit of appliance and effectiveness of skin barrier and appliance

Assess client's and family's coping skills, including:
- Self-care abilities in the home
- Acknowledgment of changes in body image and function
- Sense of loss

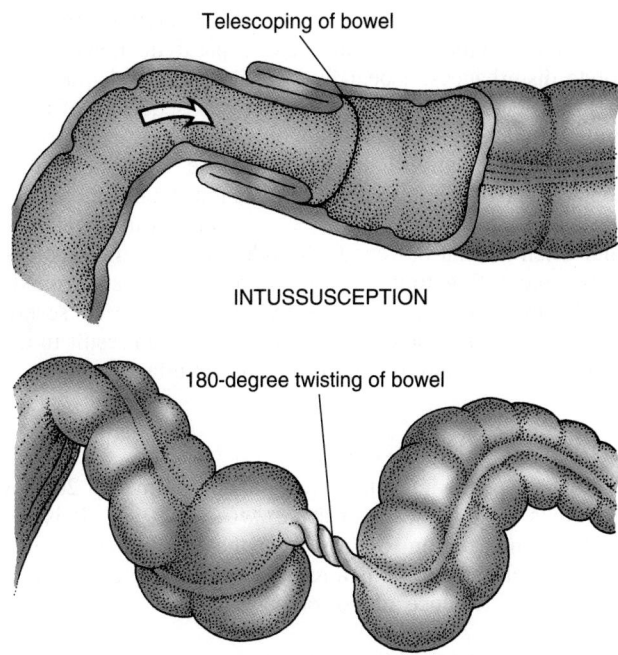

INTUSSUSCEPTION

VOLVULUS

Figure 57-6 ● Two types of mechanical obstruction.

struction, the bowel is physically obstructed by disorders outside the intestine (e.g., adhesions or hernias) or by blockages in the lumen of the intestine (e.g., tumors, inflammation, strictures, or fecal impactions). **Nonmechanical obstruction** (also known as paralytic ileus or adynamic ileus because it is a result of neuromuscular disturbance) does not involve a physical obstruction in or outside the intestine. Instead, peristalsis is decreased or absent, resulting in a slowing of the movement or a backup of intestinal contents.

Intestinal contents are composed of ingested fluid and saliva; gastric, pancreatic, and biliary secretions; and swallowed air. In both mechanical and nonmechanical obstructions, the intestinal contents accumulate at and above the area of obstruction. Intestinal distention results from the intestine's inability to absorb the contents and mobilize them down the intestinal tract. To compensate for the lag, peristalsis increases in an effort to move the intestinal contents forward. The increase in peristalsis stimulates more secretions, which leads to additional distention. This causes edema of the bowel with increased capillary permeability. Plasma leaking into the peritoneal cavity and fluid trapped in the intestinal lumen markedly decrease the absorption of fluid and electrolytes into the vascular space. Reduced circulatory blood volume and electrolyte imbalances typically occur. Hypovolemia ranges from mild to extreme (hypovolemic shock).

Specific fluid and electrolyte problems result, depending on the part of the intestine that is blocked. An obstruction high in the small intestine causes a loss of gastric hydrochloride, which can lead to *metabolic alkalosis.* Obstruction below the duodenum but above the large bowel results in loss of both acids and bases, so that acid-base imbalance is usually not compromised. Obstruction at the end of the small intestine and lower in the intestinal tract causes loss of alkaline fluids, which can lead to *metabolic acidosis.*

If the resultant hypovolemia is severe, renal insufficiency or even death can occur. Bacterial peritonitis with or without actual perforation can also result. Bacteria in the intestinal contents lie stagnant in the obstructed intestine. This is not a problem unless the blood flow to the intestine is compro-

mised. However, with so-called closed-loop obstruction (blockage in two different areas) or a **strangulated obstruction** (obstruction with compromised blood flow), the risk for peritonitis is greatly increased. Bacteria without blood supply can form an endotoxin, and release of the endotoxin into the peritoneal or systemic circulation results in septic shock. With a strangulated obstruction, major blood loss into the intestine and the peritoneum can result. Current mortality rates for bowel obstruction range from 3.5% to 6% but may be as high as 14% in older adults.

Etiology

Mechanical obstruction can result from adhesions, tumors, hernias, fecal impactions, strictures due to Crohn's disease or radiation, intussusception (telescoping of a segment of the intestine within itself), volvulus (twisting of the intestine), fibrosis due to disorders such as endometriosis, and vascular disorders (e.g., emboli and arteriosclerotic narrowing of mesenteric vessels) (Figure 57-6). In individuals age 65 or older, diverticulitis and tumors are the most common causes of obstruction.

Regardless of age, adhesions are the most common cause of mechanical obstruction, accounting for 45% to 60% of cases. Adhesions are bands of granulation and scar tissue that develop as a result of an inflammatory response, encircling the intestine and constricting its lumen.

Paralytic, or **adynamic, ileus** is a nonmechanical obstruction caused by physiologic, neurogenic, or chemical imbalances associated with decreased peristalsis from trauma or the effect of a toxin on autonomic intestinal control. Adynamic ileus occurs to some degree following abdominal surgery or trauma. Paralytic ileus can be caused by handling of the intestines during abdominal surgery; intestinal function is lost for a few hours to several days.

Thoracic diseases such as myocardial infarction, rib fracture, and pneumonia can also cause paralytic ileus. Electrolyte disturbances, especially hypokalemia, predispose the client to ileus. Paralytic ileus can be a consequence of peritonitis, since leakage of colonic contents causes severe irritation and triggers an inflammatory response. Vascular insufficiency to the bowel, also referred to as intestinal ischemia, is a potential cause of adynamic ileus. Vascular insufficiency results when arterial or venous thrombosis or an embolus decreases blood flow to the mesenteric blood vessels surrounding the intestines, as in congestive heart failure or severe shock. Severe insufficiency of blood supply can result in infarction of surrounding organs (e.g., bowel infarction).

Incidence/Prevalence

Obstruction of the intestines occurs in approximately 20% of all clients who are seen for acute abdominal pain. It is the most common reason for surgery of the small intestine. Because bowel obstruction is a result of other disorders, statistics on the incidence of bowel obstruction are not readily available.

Obstruction of the intestines occurs in all age-groups, but the incidence differs with age. In adults, 75% of all obstructions occur in the small intestine and 15% occur in the large intestine. In order of occurrence, adhesions, hernias, and tumors are the most common causes of small-bowel obstruction; cancer of the colon, diverticulitis, and volvulus cause most large-bowel obstructions in adults.

> ### CONSIDERATIONS FOR OLDER ADULTS
> The physiologic changes associated with aging, such as decreased peristalsis and decreased mobility, contribute to fecal impactions in older adults. Fecal impactions can lead to partial or complete bowel obstruction.

➤ COLLABORATIVE MANAGEMENT

● Assessment

HISTORY

The nurse collects information concerning the following:
- Past or recent abdominal surgery
- Radiation therapy
- History of inflammatory bowel disease
- Gallstones
- Hernias
- Trauma
- Peritonitis
- Cancer

The client is asked about recent occurrence of nausea or vomiting. The nurse also asks about the passage of flatus and the time, character, and consistency of the last bowel movement. Singultus (hiccups) is common with all types of intestinal obstruction.

The nurse assesses for a family history of colorectal cancer and asks the client about blood in the stool or a change in bowel pattern. The body temperature with obstruction is rarely higher than 100° F (37.8° C). A temperature higher than this, with or without guarding and tenderness, and a sustained elevation in pulse indicate a strangulated obstruction or peritonitis.

■ PHYSICAL ASSESSMENT/CLINICAL MANIFESTATIONS

MECHANICAL OBSTRUCTION. The client with mechanical obstruction in the small intestine often has mid-abdominal pain or cramping. The pain can be sporadic, and the client may feel comfortable between episodes. If strangulation is present, the pain becomes more localized and steady. Vomiting often accompanies obstruction and is more profuse with obstructions in the proximal small intestine. The vomitus may contain bile and mucus or be orange-brown and foul smelling as a result of bacterial overgrowth with low ileal obstruction. Obstipation (no passage of stool) and failure to pass flatus accompany complete obstruction. Diarrhea may be present in partial obstruction.

Mechanical colonic obstruction causes a milder, more intermittent colicky abdominal pain than is seen with small-bowel obstruction. Lower abdominal distention may be present, as well as obstipation, or ribbon-like stools if obstruction is partial. Alterations in bowel patterns and blood in the stools accompany the obstruction if colorectal cancer or diverticulitis is the cause.

On examination of the abdomen, the nurse may observe abdominal distention, which is common in all forms of intestinal obstruction. Peristaltic waves may also be visible. The nurse auscultates for proximal high-pitched bowel sounds (**borborygmi**), which are associated with cramping early in the obstructive process as the intestine tries to push the mechanical obstruction forward. In later stages of mechanical obstruction, the bowel sounds are absent, especially distal to the obstruction. Abdominal tenderness and rigidity are usually minimal. The presence of a tense, fluid-filled bowel loop mimicking a palpable abdominal mass may signal a closed-loop, strangulating small-bowel obstruction.

NONMECHANICAL OBSTRUCTION. In most types of nonmechanical obstruction (paralytic, or adynamic, ileus), the pain is described as a constant, diffuse discomfort. Colicky cramping is not characteristic of this type of obstruction. Pain associated with obstruction attributable to vascular insufficiency or infarction is usually severe and constant. On inspection, abdominal distention is typically present. On aus-

CHART 57-6

KEY FEATURES of
Small-Bowel and Large-Bowel Obstructions

Small-Bowel Obstructions	Large-Bowel Obstructions
Abdominal discomfort/pain, possibly accompanied by visible peristaltic waves in upper and mid abdomen	Intermittent lower abdominal cramping
Upper or epigastric abdominal distention	Lower abdominal distention
Nausea and early, profuse vomiting	Minimal or no vomiting (may contain fecal material)
Obstipation	Obstipation or ribbon-like stools
Severe fluid and electrolyte imbalances	No major fluid and electrolyte imbalances
Metabolic alkalosis	Metabolic acidosis

cultation of the abdomen, the nurse notes decreased bowel sounds in early obstruction and absent bowel sounds in later stages. Vomiting of gastric contents and bile is frequent, but the vomitus rarely has a foul odor and is rarely profuse. Obstipation may or may not be present. Chart 57-6 compares small-bowel and large-bowel obstructions.

LABORATORY ASSESSMENT

There is no definitive laboratory test to confirm a diagnosis of mechanical or nonmechanical obstruction. White blood cell (WBC) counts may be normal unless there is a strangulated obstruction, in which case there may be leukocytosis (increased WBCs). Hemoglobin, hematocrit, creatinine, and blood urea nitrogen (BUN) values are often elevated, indicating dehydration. Serum sodium, chloride, and potassium concentrations are reduced because of loss of fluid and electrolytes. Elevations in serum amylase levels may be found with strangulating obstructions, which can damage the pancreas.

High obstruction in the small intestine is likely to show an elevated serum venous carbon dioxide concentration and other values indicative of metabolic alkalosis. Obstruction in the large intestine is likely to show a low serum venous carbon dioxide concentration and other values suggestive of metabolic acidosis.

RADIOGRAPHIC ASSESSMENT

The health care provider obtains flat-plate and upright abdominal x-ray films as soon as an obstruction is suspected. Distention of loops of intestine with fluid and gas in the small intestine, in conjunction with the absence of gas in the colon, indicates an obstruction in the small intestine. However, x-ray findings are often normal when a strangulated obstruction actually exists in the small intestine. Therefore obstruction cannot be ruled out on the basis of x-ray findings.

Obstruction of the large intestine often shows gas distention of the colon on abdominal x-ray studies. A finding of free air under the diaphragm on abdominal x-ray examination indicates a perforated intestine.

OTHER DIAGNOSTIC ASSESSMENT

The diagnostic examination chosen depends on the suspected location of the obstruction. The physician may perform endoscopy (sigmoidoscopy or colonoscopy) or a barium enema study to determine the cause of the obstruction, except in cases where perforation is suspected. A computed tomography (CT) scan is useful in uncovering the cause and location of the obstruction and may be the diagnostic tool of choice when symptoms are severe (see the Cost of Care Box at right).

• Interventions

Interventions are aimed at uncovering the cause and relieving the obstruction. Intestinal obstructions can be relieved by nonsurgical or surgical means. If the obstruction is partial and there is no evidence of strangulation, nonsurgical management is the treatment of choice. Decompression of the intestinal tract is initiated along with fluid and electrolyte replacement.

NONSURGICAL MANAGEMENT. Paralytic ileus responds well to nonsurgical methods of relieving obstruction.

Nonsurgical approaches are also preferred in the treatment of clients with terminal disease associated with bowel obstruction. In addition to being on NPO status, clients with intestinal obstruction typically have a nasogastric or, more rarely, nasointestinal tube inserted. These tubes provide decompression of the bowel by draining fluid and air and are attached to suction; the type of suction depends on the type of tube inserted.

NASOINTESTINAL TUBES. The physician *occasionally* inserts nasointestinal (NI) tubes (such as the Miller-Abbott, Cantor, and Harris tubes) for obstruction of the small intestine. These longer tubes extend into the small intestine. Mercury-filled balloons at the end of a lumen act as a bolus of food, stimulating peristalsis and advancing down the intestinal tract. The Cantor and Harris tubes are single-lumen tubes with mercury-filled balloons at the tips and suction ports within the same lumen, proximal to the tip. The Miller-Abbott tube has two separate lumens for mercury and drainage.

The nurse assists with progression of the tube by helping the client change position every 2 hours and, if ordered, by advancing the tube 3 to 4 inches at specified times. These tubes are never taped to the nose until they reach a specified position in the intestine. As the tube is being inserted and advanced, it drains by gravity. The nurse monitors the drainage; if drainage stops, the nurse obtains a physician's order to inject 10 mL of air. The nurse does not irrigate the NI tube with fluid without an order by the health care provider. If ordered, the nurse attaches low intermittent suction to the suction lumen when the tube has stopped advancing.

COST OF CARE
IMPLICATIONS FOR NURSING

INTESTINAL OBSTRUCTION

Cost of Care
- The cost of plain abdominal films in the diagnosis of intestinal obstruction is approximately $200 to $300 and provides an overall accuracy of 57%.
- A barium swallow or enema can cost $300 to $500, with an overall accuracy of 78%.
- Computed tomography (CT) can cost $500 to $800. The overall accuracy of CT in diagnosing intestinal obstruction ranges from 91% to 97%.
- The use of ultrasound in the diagnosis of intestinal obstruction is gaining popularity. The cost of this procedure is $300 to $600, with an overall accuracy of 81% to 96%.
- Laparoscopy is indicated to evaluate the need for laparotomy. The cost of this procedure can range from $1000 to $2000, with an overall accuracy of 94%.

Implications for Nursing
There are a variety of diagnostic tests that can be used in confirming the diagnosis of intestinal obstruction. Excessive costs to the health care system occur when an inappropriate diagnostic test is chosen, or if because of inadequate preparation, the examination needs to be repeated. Advanced-practice nurses require a working knowledge of diagnostic testing in order to ensure that their clients undergo the appropriate examination. Nurses responsible for preparing clients to undergo diagnostic procedures should ensure that proper preparation for the examination has been carried out (e.g., bowel prep, maintaining NPO status) to avoid inaccurate or incomplete results requiring the client to undergo additional testing that could add to the client burden and health care costs.

Data from Shelton, B. (1999). Intestinal obstruction. *AACN Clinical Issues: Advanced Practice in Acute and Critical Care, 10*(4), 478-491.

Most health care providers avoid the use of NI tubes because insertion of the mercury-filled lumen is often difficult; the time it takes to insert the tube also delays treatment. Insertion of this tube can be uncomfortable for clients.

NASOGASTRIC TUBES. Most clients with an obstruction have at least a **nasogastric (NG) tube** in place unless the obstruction is mild. Salem sump and Anderson tubes are examples of NG tubes that sit distally in the stomach and are attached to *low continuous* suction. Levin tubes are connected to *low intermittent* suction.

At least every 4 hours, the nurse assesses the client with an NG tube for proper placement of the tube, tube patency, and output. The nasal skin is also monitored daily for integrity. The nurse assesses for peristalsis by auscultating for bowel sounds with the suction disconnected (suction will mask peristaltic sounds).

The nurse questions the client regarding the passage of flatus and records the passage, amount, and character of bowel movements daily. Abdominal girth is measured at the same point each day. The client is also assessed for nausea and asked to report this manifestation.

NG tubes must be monitored for proper functioning. Occasionally, NG tubes move out of optimal drainage position or become plugged. In this case, the nurse notes a decrease in gastric output or stasis of the tube's contents. The client is assessed for nausea, vomiting, increased abdominal distention, and placement of the tube. If the NG tube is repositioned or replaced, confirmation of proper placement is obtained by x-ray examination before use. After appropriate placement is established, the contents are aspirated and the tube is irrigated with 30 mL of normal saline every 4 hours or as needed to maintain patency.

OTHER NONSURGICAL TECHNIQUES. Most types of nonmechanical obstruction respond to nasogastric decompression in conjunction with medical treatment of the primary disorder. Incomplete mechanical obstruction can sometimes be successfully treated without surgery. Obstruction caused by fecal impaction usually resolves after disimpaction and enema administration. Intussusception may respond to hydrostatic pressure changes during a barium enema.

FLUID AND ELECTROLYTE REPLACEMENT. IV fluid replacement and maintenance are indicated for all clients with intestinal obstruction, since the client is on NPO status and fluid and electrolyte loss (particularly potassium) through vomiting and nasogastric suction is great. On the basis of serum electrolytes and blood urea nitrogen (BUN) levels, the health care provider orders aggressive fluid replacement with 2 to 4 L of normal saline or lactated Ringer's solution with potassium added. Care must be taken with clients who are prone to fluid overload (e.g., the client with a history of congestive heart failure). The nurse carefully monitors lung sounds, weight, and intake and output parameters. Blood replacement may be indicated in strangulated obstruction because of blood loss into the bowel or peritoneal cavity.

The nurse or assistive nursing personnel monitors the client's vital signs and other measures of fluid status (e.g., urine output, skin turgor, and mucous membranes). Edema from third spacing is assessed because fluid is lost, mostly from the vascular space, into surrounding spaces (e.g., the

peritoneal cavity). In collaboration with the dietitian, the physician may order total parenteral nutrition (TPN) to improve the nutritional status of the client, especially if he or she has had chronic nutritional problems and has been on NPO status for an extended period. Chapter 61 discusses the nursing care of clients receiving TPN.

Because of fluid losses, the client with intestinal obstruction is characteristically thirsty. The nurse provides frequent mouth care to help maintain moist mucous membranes. Lemon-glycerin swabs are avoided because they can increase mouth dryness. A small amount of ice chips may be allowed if the client is not having surgery; however, the health care provider should be consulted first. Ice chips can provide more free water than electrolytes; thus potassium and hydrochloric acid are washed out of the NG tube. The nurse monitors intake and output carefully to avoid electrolyte imbalance and false interpretation of gastric output measurements.

PAIN MANAGEMENT. The abdominal distention commonly noted with intestinal obstruction can cause a great deal of discomfort, especially when distention is severe. The colicky, crampy pain that comes and goes with mechanical obstruction and the nausea, vomiting, dry mucous membranes, and thirst contribute to the client's discomfort. The nurse continually assesses the character and location of the pain and immediately reports any pain that significantly increases or changes from a colicky, intermittent type to a constant discomfort. Such changes can indicate perforation of the intestine or peritonitis.

Opioid analgesics are normally withheld in the diagnostic period so that clinical manifestations of perforation or peritonitis are not masked. The nurse explains to the client and family the rationale for not giving analgesics. In addition, if analgesics such as morphine or meperidine are given, they slow intestinal motility and can cause vomiting. The nurse must be alert to this side effect, because nausea and vomiting are also signs of NG tube obstruction or worsening bowel obstruction.

The nurse helps the client obtain a position of comfort with frequent position changes to promote increased peristalsis. A semi-Fowler's position helps alleviate the pressure of abdominal distention on the chest. Not only is this a good comfort technique, but it also facilitates adequate thoracic excursion and normal breathing patterns.

Discomfort is generally less with nonmechanical obstruction than with mechanical obstruction. With both types of obstruction, discomfort is aggravated by ingestion of food or fluids.

DRUG THERAPY. If strangulation is thought to be likely, the health care provider prescribes IV broad-spectrum antibiotics. In addition, in cases of partial obstruction or paralytic ileus, medications that enhance gastric motility, such as octreotide acetate (Sandostatin), may be used.

SURGICAL MANAGEMENT. In all cases of complete mechanical obstruction and in many cases of incomplete mechanical obstruction, surgical intervention is necessary to relieve the obstruction. A strangulated obstruction is inevitably complete, and surgical intervention is always required. An **exploratory laparotomy** (a surgical opening of the abdominal cavity to investigate the cause of the obstruction) is initially performed for most clients with obstruction. More specific surgical procedures depend on the cause of the obstruction.

PREOPERATIVE CARE. The nurse provides preoperative teaching as discussed in Chapter 17. If time permits, all clients who require surgery for obstruction undergo nasogastric intubation and suction before surgery. However, in cases of complete obstruction, surgery should proceed without delay.

OPERATIVE PROCEDURES. The surgeon enters the abdominal cavity and explores for obstruction. If adhesions are found to be the cause of the obstruction, the adhesions are lysed (cut and released). Obstruction caused by a tumor or diverticulitis requires a colon resection with primary anastomosis or a temporary or permanent colostomy. If obstruction is caused by intestinal infarction, an embolectomy, thrombectomy, or colon resection (partial removal) may be necessary, particularly if the intestine is gangrenous.

POSTOPERATIVE CARE. Postoperative care for the client undergoing an exploratory laparotomy with lysis of adhesions, colon resection, thrombectomy, or embolectomy is similar to that described in Chapter 19. All clients have an NG tube in place until peristalsis (as characterized by the return of bowel sounds) resumes. The NG tube is removed slowly by first discontinuing suction and then clamping the tube for a scheduled amount of time. Residual drainage is checked at each stage to assess peristalsis without decompression before removing the NG tube entirely.

● Community-Based Care

All clients with intestinal obstruction are hospitalized for monitoring and treatment. The length of stay varies according to the type of obstruction, the treatment, and the presence of complications. Clients who have complicated obstruction, such as strangulation or incarceration, are at greater risk for peritonitis, sepsis, and shock. The hospital stay may be up to several weeks, depending on the severity of complications.

Clients with nonmechanical (adynamic) intestinal obstruction are less likely to require a lengthy hospitalization because of the obstruction alone. Adynamic obstruction generally responds to NG intubation and suction within a few days.

■ HOME CARE MANAGEMENT

For the client who has had an intestinal obstruction, preparation for home care depends on the cause of the obstruction and the treatment required. Clients who have resolution of obstruction without surgical intervention are assessed for their knowledge of strategies to avoid recurrent obstruction. For example, if fecal impaction was the cause of the obstruction, the nurse assesses the client's ability to carry out a bowel regimen independently. For clients who have undergone surgery, the nurse evaluates their ability to function at home with the added tasks of incision care and possibly colostomy care.

■ HEALTH TEACHING

The nurse instructs the client to report any abdominal pain or distention, nausea, or vomiting, with or without constipation, since these symptoms might indicate recurrent obstruction.

The client should be reassured, however, that recurrent paralytic ileus is not usually a problem. The client who has had mechanical obstruction as a result of fecal impaction (often the older adult) needs to have a structured bowel regimen to prevent recurrence (Chart 57-7). The nurse instructs this client to adhere to high-fiber diets, to exercise, and to drink at least 24 ounces of water daily, unless contraindicated. The physician may also order bulk-forming laxatives to help maintain a consistent elimination pattern.

The nurse teaches the client who has had surgery about incision care, drug therapy, and activity limitations. Drug therapy consists of an oral opioid analgesic, such as oxycodone hydrochloride with acetaminophen (Tylox, Percocet, Endocet✤), to be taken as needed for incisional discomfort. As with any opioid therapy, a stool softener is added to the medication regimen to prevent constipation and possible recurrent obstruction.

With resolution of obstruction, educational efforts by the nurse are aimed at prevention of obstruction by examining the cause of the obstruction and how to prevent recurrence. The nurse also reinforces important signs and symptoms to report to the health care provider. The client who had curative treatment of the underlying cause most likely requires less support than the client who underwent treatment of obstruction related to a serious disease that will require further treatment. The client is encouraged to express fears and concerns about the future. The nurse assesses the client's understanding and needs with regard to treatment plans.

■ HEALTH CARE RESOURCES

The need for follow-up appointments depends on the cause of the obstruction and the treatment required. If the client is at risk for fecal impaction, the nurse can arrange for a home care nurse to assess the gastrointestinal (GI) function and dietary habits of the client on an ongoing basis. Arrangements should also be made for the services of a home care nurse if the client needs help with incision or colostomy care. Medicare guidelines or insurance precertification requirements must be met before approval is given for home care visits. The discharge planner or case manager assist in setting up home care follow-up.

CHART 57-7

NURSING FOCUS *on the* **OLDER ADULT**
Fecal Impaction

- Teach the client to eat high-fiber foods, including plenty of raw fruits and vegetables and whole-grain products.
- Encourage the client to drink adequate amounts of fluids, especially water.
- Do not routinely administer a laxative; teach the client that laxative abuse decreases abdominal muscle tone and contributes to an atonic colon.
- Encourage the client to exercise regularly, if possible. Walking every day is an excellent exercise for promoting intestinal motility.
- Use natural foods to stimulate peristalsis, such as warm beverages and prune juice.
- Take bulk-forming products, such as Metamucil, to provide fiber.
- Check the client's stool for amount and frequency; oozing of soft or diarrheal stool often indicates a fecal impaction.
- Have the client sit on a toilet or bedside commode, rather than on a bedpan, for elimination.

ABDOMINAL TRAUMA

OVERVIEW

Abdominal trauma is defined as injury to the structures located between the diaphragm and the pelvis, which occurs when the abdomen is subjected to blunt or penetrating forces. Organs injured may include the large or small bowel, liver, spleen, duodenum, pancreas, kidneys, and urinary bladder.

At least one half of all blunt abdominal trauma occurs from motor vehicle accidents (MVAs) (Sommers & Johnson, 1997). Other causes of blunt trauma include falls, aggravated assaults, and contact sports. *Penetrating abdominal trauma* is caused by gunshot wounds, stabbing, or impalement with an object. The liver is the most commonly injured organ in blunt and penetrating trauma. The spleen is the most commonly injured organ in blunt abdominal trauma. The small intestine is the third most commonly injured organ in abdominal trauma; 80% of injuries are caused by gunshot wounds (GSWs).

> ### CULTURAL CONSIDERATIONS
>
> MVAs are three times more common in males than in females in the 15- to 24-year age-group. In the 15- to 34-year age-group, European Americans (Caucasians) have a death rate from MVAs that is 40% higher than that of African Americans (Sommers & Johnson, 1997). Penetrating injuries from GSWs and stab wounds are more common in preteen and young adults than in older adults and are more common in African Americans than in European Americans.

► COLLABORATIVE MANAGEMENT

● Assessment

In the emergency phase of treatment, health care providers focus on the risks of hemorrhage, shock, and peritonitis. Mental status and skin perfusion are *priority* nursing assessments, with skin perfusion being the most reliable clinical guide in assessing hypovolemic shock:

- In a person with mild shock, the skin is pale, cool, and moist.
- With moderate shock, diaphoresis is more marked and urine output ceases.
- With severe shock, changes in mental status are manifested by agitation, disorientation, and recent memory loss.

The nurse assesses for abdominal trauma by asking the client about the presence, location, and quality of pain. The abdomen, flanks, back, genitalia, and rectum are inspected for contusions, abrasions, lacerations, ecchymosis, penetrating injuries, and symmetry. All of the client's clothes must be removed. If pneumatic garments such as antishock trousers are in place, they are usually not removed unless aggressive fluid replacement has been given to the client, a surgical team is available to immediately intervene, and the attending physician orders it to be done. After pneumatic garments are removed, uncontrolled hemorrhage can occur. Antishock trousers have a constrictive effect on hemorrhage in the trunk and facilitate circulatory return to the heart. However, they can cause compartment syndrome to the lower extremities; consequently, their use is controversial.

Inspection of the abdomen may reveal distention. To perform an adequate inspection, the nurse turns the client while maintaining spinal immobilization. Ecchymosis may signify internal bleeding. Ecchymosis present in the distribution of a lap seat belt should be reported to the health care provider immediately, since investigation for occult injury to the bowel is necessary. Ecchymosis around the umbilicus is known as **Cullen's sign,** and ecchymosis on either flank (known as **Turner's sign**) may indicate retroperitoneal bleeding into the abdominal wall.

The nurse auscultates the abdomen for bowel sounds. Absent or diminished bowel sounds may be caused by the presence of blood, bacteria, or a chemical irritant in the abdominal cavity. The nurse also auscultates for bruits in the abdomen, which indicate renal artery injury.

During percussion, an abnormal sign associated with abdominal trauma is resonance over the right flank with the client lying on the left side. This is known as **Ballance's sign** and is found with a ruptured spleen. Resonance over the normally dull liver is due to free air, which is pathologic. Palpation for lower rib fractures should increase suspicion of liver or spleen injuries. Injury to the spleen is present in 20% of individuals with left lower rib fractures. Liver injury is present in 10% of individuals with right lower rib fractures. The presence of **Kehr's sign,** left shoulder pain resulting from diaphragmatic irritation, may be present in splenic injury.

Dullness over hollow organs that normally contain gas, such as the stomach and the large and small intestines, may indicate blood or fluid. Light abdominal palpation identifies areas of tenderness, rebound tenderness, guarding, rigidity, and spasm. If the nurse palpates a mass, it may be blood or a fluid collection.

The client without obvious significant bleeding or definite signs of peritoneal irritation undergoes abdominal radiography, diagnostic peritoneal lavage (DPL), and computed tomography (CT). For peritoneal lavage, the physician inserts a large-bore catheter into the abdomen and allows fluid to enter the abdominal cavity. If the return drainage from the abdomen is pink or grossly bloody, the health care team prepares the client for surgery. Abdominal ultrasound has recently been used successfully in diagnosing blunt abdominal trauma and may replace CT and DPL for diagnosis (Levins, 2000). Clients with hemodynamic instability or peritonitis are candidates for immediate laparotomy.

● Interventions

Nonsurgical and surgical interventions are aimed at preserving or restoring hemodynamic stability, preventing or decreasing blood loss, and preventing complications.

NONSURGICAL MANAGEMENT. Nursing interventions include placement of at least two large-bore IV catheters in the upper extremities. IV catheters are not used in the lower extremities; if the vasculature has been injured, fluid can pool in the abdomen. The health care provider may insert a central venous catheter to assist with rapid fluid volume infusion. IV fluid consists of a balanced saline solution, crystalloids, and possibly blood.

The following physiologic parameters are monitored:

- Arterial blood gases
- Complete blood count (CBC)
- Serum electrolyte, glucose and amylase, and blood urea nitrogen (BUN) determinations
- Liver function tests
- Clotting studies

Measuring arterial blood gases may be of assistance in determining the severity of shock. Hemoglobin and hematocrit values do not initially reflect true blood loss; values can be skewed because of hemoconcentration from volume loss or the dilutional effects of IV fluids. Serial hemoglobin and hematocrit measurements may be more accurate in determining true blood loss. An elevated white blood cell (WBC) count may indicate a ruptured spleen or intestinal injury. Elevated levels of serum transaminases may indicate liver injury. Elevation of serum amylase activity may signal injury to the pancreas or the bowel. All laboratory work is compiled so that values can be compared and subtle changes noted.

Continuous cardiac monitoring is begun in the emergency department. The nurse inserts an indwelling urinary (Foley) catheter unless there is blood at the urinary meatus. Initially and hourly thereafter, the nurse evaluates urine output for bleeding and specific gravity. Laboratory tests indicate the amount of blood and protein in the urine. If there is an open abdominal wound or evisceration, the nurse covers it with a sterile dry dressing unless the physician orders otherwise. Unless it is contraindicated, as in the case of a concomitant skull fracture, the physician or nurse inserts a nasogastric (NG) tube, which is kept in place to identify bleeding and to minimize the risk of vomiting and aspiration. Antibiotics are administered as ordered to reduce the risk of peritonitis.

If the client with known abdominal trauma has no definite clinical manifestations of active bleeding or abdominal injury, he or she is admitted to the hospital for observation. Blunt trauma can cause active, but often not obvious, damage. The nurse assesses for abdominal or referred pain and nausea. Every 15 to 30 minutes in the early postinjury period and then hourly, the nurse evaluates the client's:

- Mental status
- Vital signs
- Clinical findings, such as vomiting, guarding, rigidity, or rebound tenderness
- Skin temperature
- Bowel sounds
- Urine output

The nurse reports any change immediately to the health care provider. It is more important for the nurse to recognize the high risk of an active abdominal injury and assess for general signs of abdominal injury (e.g., hemorrhage and peritonitis) than to identify the exact nature of the abdominal injury. Analgesics for pain are not prescribed at this time so that clinical manifestations are not masked or overlooked. The nurse explains the rationale for withholding analgesics to the client and family or significant others.

SURGICAL MANAGEMENT. For the client with severe abdominal trauma, the surgeon performs an exploratory laparotomy and repairs abdominal injuries immediately if there are definite signs of peritoneal irritation. These signs include rebound tenderness, significant blood loss, evisceration, or a gunshot wound (GSW) with possible peritoneal involvement.

Most stab wounds require exploratory laparotomy, but as many as 25% are superficial and do not involve the peritoneum. Using local anesthesia, the surgeon explores and cleans superficial stab wounds; the client does not require an exploratory laparotomy.

Before discharge from the hospital, the client who has experienced abdominal trauma is taught the signs and symptoms of abdominal bleeding whether or not surgery has been performed. The nurse instructs the client to report abdominal

pain, nausea, vomiting, bloody or black stools, fever, weakness, and dizziness.

Hemorrhage can occasionally occur weeks after blunt abdominal trauma, despite medical evaluation. For the client who undergoes surgery or exploration of wounds, the nurse provides instructions on wound care before discharge from the hospital.

POLYPS

▌OVERVIEW

Polyps in the intestinal tract are small growths covered with mucosa and attached to the surface of the intestine. Although most are benign, polyps are significant in that some have the potential to become malignant.

Polyps are identified by their tissue type. The presence of adenomas always necessitates medical consultation because of their malignant potential. Although only 2% to 5% of adenomas progress to cancer, almost all colorectal cancers develop from an adenoma (Markowitz & Winawer, 1997). Adenomas are further classified as villous or tubular. Of these, villous adenomas pose a greater cancer risk.

Familial adenomatous polyposis (FAP) and hereditary nonpolyposis colorectal cancer (HNPCC) are inherited syndromes characterized by progressive development of colorectal adenomas. Unless these syndromes are treated, colorectal cancer inevitably occurs by the fourth to fifth decade of life (Markowitz & Winawer, 1997).

Other types of polyps include hyperplastic and hamartomatous polyps. Hyperplastic polyps, which include mucosal and inflammatory varieties, are entirely benign with no malignant potential. Hamartomatous polyps include juvenile and Peutz-Jeghers syndrome polyps. Although both types are generally benign, rare reports of malignant changes have been reported in juvenile polyps.

In addition to being classified by their tissue type, polyps are described according to their appearance (Figure 57-7). Pedunculated polyps are stalklike; a thin stem attaches them to the intestinal wall. They become elongated as peristalsis pulls them into the lumen of the intestine. Polyps attached to the intestinal walls by a broad base are described as sessile. A malignant polyp may be pedunculated or sessile.

▶ COLLABORATIVE MANAGEMENT

Polyps are usually asymptomatic and are discovered during routine diagnostic testing, including tests for blood in the stool. However, they can cause gross rectal bleeding, intestinal

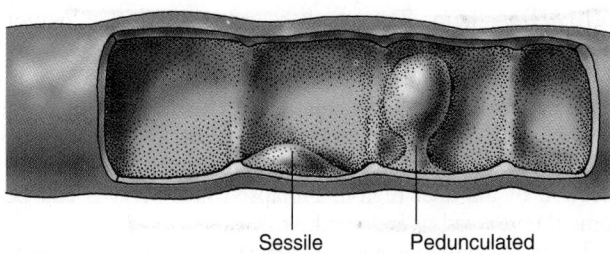

Sessile   Pedunculated

Figure 57-7 ● Pedunculated and sessile polyps. Pedunculated polyps, such as tubular adenomas, are stalklike. Sessile polyps, such as villous adenomas, are broad based.

obstruction, or intussusception (telescoping of the bowel). Diagnostic studies involve a barium enema examination and proctosigmoidoscopy or colonoscopy for ruling out cancer. Biopsy specimens of polyps can be obtained, or the entire polyp can be removed (polypectomy) with the use of an electrocautery snare that fits through the sigmoidoscope or colonoscope. This often eliminates the need for abdominal surgery to remove a suspicious or definitely malignant polyp. The client with FAP often requires a total colectomy (colon removal) to prevent the development of cancer.

Nursing care focuses on client education. The nurse instructs the client about the following:

* The nature of the polyp
* Clinical manifestations to report to the health care provider
* The need for regular, routine monitoring

The client with a known benign polyp that does not need to be removed has frequent sigmoidoscopic or colonoscopic examinations to monitor for any growth or change in the polyp or for an increase in the number of polyps. If the client has undergone a polypectomy, follow-up sigmoidoscopic or colonoscopic examinations are needed, because there is an increased risk of multiple polyps in the client who has had at least one polyp.

Nursing care of the client who has undergone a polypectomy of the colorectal area includes monitoring for abdominal distention and pain, rectal bleeding, mucopurulent rectal drainage, and fever.

A small amount of blood might appear in the stool after a polypectomy, but this should be temporary. Nursing care of the client who has undergone a total colectomy is described in Chapter 58 under Crohn's Disease.

HEMORRHOIDS

■ OVERVIEW

Hemorrhoids are unnaturally swollen or distended veins in the anorectal region. Hemorrhoids are common and not significant unless they cause pain or bleeding. The veins involved in the development of hemorrhoids are part of the normal structure in the anal region. With limited distention, the veins function as a valve overlying the anal sphincter that assists in continence. Increased intra-abdominal pressure causes elevated systemic and portal venous pressure, which is transmitted to the anorectal veins. Arterioles in the anorectal region shunt blood directly to the distended anorectal veins, which increases the pressure. With repeated elevations in pressure from increased intra-abdominal pressure and engorgement from arteriolar shunting of blood, the distended veins eventually separate from the smooth muscle surrounding them. The result is prolapse of the hemorrhoidal vessels.

Hemorrhoids can be internal or external (Figure 57-8). Internal hemorrhoids, which cannot be seen on inspection of the perineal area, lie above the anal sphincter. External hemorrhoids lie below the anal sphincter and can be seen on inspection of the anal region. Prolapsed hemorrhoids can become thrombosed or inflamed, or they can bleed.

The most common causes of repeated increased abdominal pressure resulting in hemorrhoids are straining at stool, pregnancy, portal hypertension, and colorectal cancer.

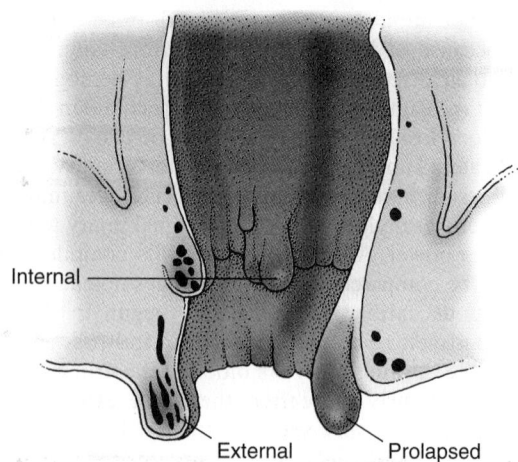

Figure 57-8 ● Internal, external, and prolapsed hemorrhoids. Internal hemorrhoids lie above the anal sphincter and cannot be seen on inspection of the anal area. External hemorrhoids lie below the anal sphincter and can be seen on inspection of the anal region. Hemorrhoids that enlarge, fall down, and protrude through the anus are called prolapsed hemorrhoids.

► COLLABORATIVE MANAGEMENT

▶ Assessment

The most common symptoms of hemorrhoids are bleeding and prolapse. Blood is characteristically bright red and is present on toilet tissue or outside the stool. Pain is a common symptom and is often associated with thrombosis, especially if thrombosis occurs suddenly. Other symptoms include itching and a mucous discharge. Diagnosis is made by inspection, digital examination, proctoscopy, or proctoscopic ultrasonography.

▶ Interventions

Interventions are typically conservative and are aimed at reducing symptoms with a minimum of discomfort, cost, and time lost from usual activities.

NONSURGICAL MANAGEMENT. Local treatment and diet therapy are initiated when symptoms begin. Cold packs applied to the anorectal region for a few minutes at a time beginning with the onset of pain and hot sitz baths three or four times a day are often enough to relieve discomfort, even if the hemorrhoids are thrombosed.

Witch hazel soaks (e.g., Tucks) are also effective for pain. Topical anesthetics, such as lidocaine (Xylocaine), are useful for severe pain. Dibucaine (Nupercainal) ointment, an over-the-counter remedy, may be applied for mild to moderate pain. This ointment should be used only temporarily, however, because it can mask worsening symptoms and delay diagnosis of a severe disorder. If itching or inflammation is present, the health care provider prescribes a steroid preparation, such as hydrocortisone. Cleansing the anal area with moistened cleansing tissues rather than standard toilet tissue helps to avoid irritation. The anal area should be cleansed gently by dabbing, rather than by wiping.

Diets high in fiber and fluids are recommended to promote regular bowel movements without straining. Stool softeners, such as docusate sodium (Colace), can be used temporarily. Irritating laxatives are avoided, as well as foods and beverages that can make hemorrhoids worse. Spicy foods, nuts, coffee, and alcohol can be irritating. Clients are encouraged to avoid sitting for long periods of time. The health care provider may prescribe oral analgesics for pain if the hemorrhoids are thrombosed.

Conservative treatment should alleviate symptoms in 3 to 5 days. If symptoms continue or recur frequently, the client may require surgical intervention.

SURGICAL MANAGEMENT. The surgeon can perform several procedures for symptomatic hemorrhoids. The type of surgery depends on the degree of prolapse, whether there is thrombosis, and the overall condition of the client. Surgical methods include sclerotherapy, elastic band ligation, cryosurgery, and hemorrhoidectomy.

In **sclerotherapy,** the surgeon injects a sclerosing agent into the tissues around the hemorrhoids to obliterate the vessels. Sclerotherapy can be done on an outpatient basis without long-term pain. However, it can be done only for low-grade hemorrhoids.

Elastic band ligation is considered a better method because of its success rate. One or two rubber bands are put on at one ambulatory care visit, and repeated visits may be needed for ligation of all hemorrhoids. Local pain after ligation does occur, and hemorrhage may also occur.

Cryosurgery, which can be done on an ambulatory care basis, involves freezing the hemorrhoid with a probe to cause necrosis. Because of its many disadvantages (e.g., profuse and foul drainage lasting up to 6 weeks; hemorrhage; large, painful skin tags; and incomplete destruction), cryosurgery is no longer a widely accepted method.

Hemorrhoidectomy, the standard treatment, can now be performed in an ambulatory care/same-day surgical setting. Approximately 10% of clients with symptomatic hemorrhoids undergo hemorrhoidectomies. The most common problem following a hemorrhoidectomy is pain, which is severe for 1 to 2 days after surgery. Urinary retention can also occur because of rectal spasms and anorectal tenderness. Hemorrhage, which may be internal and not visible or external, is a rare but potential complication.

The nurse teaches clients with hemorrhoids about the need for adhering to high-fiber, high-fluid diets to promote regular bowel patterns. The nurse advises clients to avoid stimulant laxatives, which are habit forming.

For clients who undergo any type of surgical intervention, the nurse monitors for hemorrhage and pain postoperatively. These clients, in particular, require ongoing interventions for pain because of its severity. Appropriate nursing interventions include the following:

- Assisting clients to a side-lying position
- Keeping fresh ice packs over the dressing until the packing is removed
- Use of moist heat (as in sitz baths) three or four times a day after the first 12 hours postoperatively

Vasodilation from the sitz bath redirects blood to the rectal area, which might cause the client to feel faint. The nurse may place an ice bag on the client's head during the sitz bath to prevent feelings of faintness. A flotation pad can be used under the buttocks for sitting.

The first postoperative bowel movement may be very painful. The physician usually prescribes stool softeners, such as docusate sodium, to begin on the first postoperative day.

Opioid analgesics are administered before the client attempts to defecate, and the caregiver should stay nearby during the first defecation. All clients who have undergone a hemorrhoidectomy are monitored for urinary retention.

MALABSORPTION SYNDROME

OVERVIEW

Malabsorption is a syndrome associated with a variety of disorders and intestinal surgical procedures. Malabsorption interferes with the ability to absorb nutrients and is a result of a generalized flattening of the mucosa of the small intestine. With various disorders, physiologic mechanisms limit absorption of nutrients because of one or more of the following abnormalities:

- Bile salt deficiencies
- Enzyme deficiencies
- Presence of bacteria
- Disruption of the mucosal lining of the small intestine
- Altered lymphatic and vascular circulation
- Decrease in the gastric or intestinal surface area

The nutrient involved in malabsorption depends on the type and location of the abnormality in the intestinal tract.

Deficiencies of bile salts can lead to malabsorption of fats and fat-soluble vitamins. Bile salt deficiencies can result from decreased synthesis of bile in the liver, bile obstruction, or alteration of bile salt absorption in the small intestine.

Enzymes normally found in the intestine split disaccharides (complex sugars) to monosaccharides (simple sugars). Examples of these enzymes are lactase, sucrase, maltase, and isomaltase. Lactase deficiency is the most common disaccharide enzyme deficiency. Without sufficient amounts of this enzyme, the body is not able to break down lactose. Lactase deficiency can be due to genetic transmission, injury to intestinal mucosa from viral hepatitis, bacterial proliferation in the intestine, or sprue. Deficiencies of the other disaccharide enzymes are rare.

Pancreatic enzymes are also necessary for absorption of vitamin B_{12}. With destruction or obstruction of the pancreas or insufficient pancreatic stimulation, these nutrients are malabsorbed. Chronic pancreatitis, pancreatic carcinoma, resection of the pancreas, and cystic fibrosis can cause these malabsorption problems.

Loops of bowel can accumulate intestinal contents, resulting in bacterial overgrowth, when there is a decrease in peristalsis. Bacteria at these sites break down bile salts, and fewer salts are available for fat absorption. These bacteria can also ingest vitamin B_{12}, which contributes to vitamin B_{12} deficiency. This phenomenon can occur after a gastrectomy or with progressive systemic sclerosis and diabetic enteropathy.

Disruption of the mucosal lining of the intestine is responsible for the malabsorption that occurs with celiac (nontropical) sprue, tropical sprue, Crohn's disease, and ulcerative colitis.

In celiac (nontropical) sprue, the absorptive surface area in the small intestine is lost; there is malabsorption of most nutrients. Celiac sprue is thought to be due to a genetic immune hypersensitivity response to gluten or its breakdown products or to result from the accumulation of gluten in the diet with peptidase deficiency.

Tropical sprue is caused by an infectious agent that has not been identified but is thought to be bacterial. Mucosal changes occur in a more widespread manner than in celiac sprue. However, the changes are not as severe as in celiac sprue. Tropical sprue results in malabsorption of fat, folic acid, and vitamin B_{12} in later stages of the disease.

The inflammation in Crohn's disease interferes with the surface of cells absorbing bile salts and therefore leads to fat malabsorption. In ulcerative colitis, protein loss may occur.

Obstruction to lymphatic flow in the intestine can lead to loss of plasma proteins along with loss of minerals (such as iron, copper, and calcium), vitamin B_{12}, folic acid, and lipids. Lymphatic obstruction can be caused by many conditions. Certain cancers, such as lymphoma, inflammatory states, radiation enteritis, Crohn's disease, Whipple's disease, congestive heart failure, and constrictive pericarditis, are causes of lymphatic obstruction.

Interference with blood flow to the intestinal mucosa, which occurs in celiac and superior mesenteric artery disease, results in malabsorption. With intestinal surgery, there is loss of the surface area needed to facilitate absorption. Resection of the ileum results in vitamin B_{12}, bile salt, and other nutrient deficiencies. Gastric surgery is one of the most common causes of malabsorption and maldigestion. Other conditions associated with maldigestion and malabsorption include small-bowel ischemia and radiation enteritis.

➤ COLLABORATIVE MANAGEMENT

● Assessment

Diarrhea is the classic symptom of malabsorption. It occurs secondary to unabsorbed nutrients, which add to the bulk of the stool, and unabsorbed fat. Steatorrhea (greater than normal amounts of fat in the feces) is a common sign. Steatorrhea is a result of bile salt deconjugation, nonabsorbed fats, or bacteria in the intestine. Not all clients with malabsorption will have diarrhea; instead, many clients manifest an increased stool mass. Other clinical manifestations include the following:

* Weight loss
* Bloating and flatus (carbohydrate malabsorption)
* Decreased libido
* Easy bruising (purpura)
* Anemia (with iron and folic acid or vitamin B_{12} deficiencies)
* Bone pain (with calcium and vitamin D deficiencies)
* Edema (caused by hypoproteinemia)

Laboratory studies reveal a decrease in mean corpuscular volume (MCV), mean corpuscular hemoglobin (MCH), and mean corpuscular hemoglobin concentration (MCHC). These decreases indicate hypochromic microcytic anemia resulting from iron deficiency. Increased MCV and variable MCH and MCHC values indicate macrocytic anemia resulting from vitamin B_{12} and folic acid deficiencies. Serum iron levels are low in protein malabsorption because of insufficient gastric acid for use of iron. Serum cholesterol levels may be low from decreased absorption and digestion of fat. Low serum calcium levels may indicate malabsorption of vitamin D and amino acids. Low levels of serum vitamin A (retinol) and carotene, its precursor, indicate a bile salt deficiency and malabsorption of fat. Serum albumin and total protein levels are low if protein loss occurs. A quantitative fecal fat analysis is elevated in either malabsorption or maldigestion.

A lactose tolerance test result that shows less than a 20% rise in the blood glucose level over the fasting blood glucose level indicates lactose intolerance. A monosaccharide test validates or rules out lactase deficiency. The xylose absorption test can reveal low urine and serum D-xylose levels if malabsorption in the small intestine is present, a common finding in celiac sprue. An abnormal D-xylose test can indicate bacterial overgrowth in the small intestine.

The Schilling test measures urinary excretion of vitamin B_{12} for diagnosis of pernicious anemia and a variety of other malabsorption syndromes. The bile acid breath test assesses the absorption of bile salt. If the client has bacterial overgrowth, the bile salts will become deconjugated, and the carbon dioxide level in the breath will peak earlier than expected.

Biopsy of the small intestine is performed via an oral endoscopic procedure for diagnosis of tropical sprue or celiac sprue. Ultrasonography is used to diagnose pancreatic tumors and tumors in the small intestine that are causing malabsorption. X-ray studies of the gastrointestinal (GI) tract reveal pancreatic calcifications, tumors, or other abnormalities that cause malabsorption. Barium enema examination shows mucosal changes representative of celiac sprue or other abnormalities.

● Interventions

Interventions for most malabsorption syndromes focus on avoidance of dietary substances that aggravate malabsorption and supplementation of nutrients. Surgical or nonsurgical management of the primary disease may be indicated. Drug therapy may also improve or resolve malabsorption.

Dietary management includes a low-fat diet for clients who have gallbladder disease, severe steatorrhea, cystic fibrosis, and progressive systemic sclerosis. A low-fat diet may or may not be indicated for pancreatic insufficiency, because this disorder improves with enzyme replacement. Some clinicians believe that limitation of fat intake is not necessary with enzyme replacement. Dietary intake of fat is actually beneficial to the client because it has a high amount of calories. After a total gastrectomy, a high-protein, high-calorie diet and small, frequent meals are recommended. Lactose-free or lactose-restricted diets are available for clients with lactase deficiency, and gluten-free diets are available for clients with celiac sprue.

The physician orders nutritional supplements according to the specific deficiency. Common supplements include the following:

* Water-soluble vitamins, such as folic acid, vitamin B_{12}, and vitamin B complex
* Fat-soluble vitamins, such as vitamin A, vitamin D, and vitamin K
* Minerals, such as calcium, iron, and magnesium
* Pancreatic enzymes, such as pancrelipase (Pancrease, Viokase)

Antibiotics are used to treat tropical sprue, Whipple's disease, and other disorders involving bacterial overgrowth. Tropical sprue is treated with trimethoprim/sulfamethoxazole (Bactrim, Septra). Bacterial overgrowth can be caused by a variety of disorders but is often treated with tetracycline and metronidazole (Flagyl, Novonidazol❧). Steroids are sometimes given in celiac disease to decrease inflammation.

Drug therapy is used to control the clinical manifestations of malabsorption. Antidiarrheal agents, such as diphenoxylate hydrochloride and atropine sulfate (Lomotil) or kaolin with pectin (Kaopectate, Kao-Con), are often used to control diar-

CHART 57-8

BEST PRACTICE *for*
Special Skin Care for Clients with Chronic Diarrhea

- Use medicated wipes or premoistened disposable wipes rather than toilet tissue to clean the perineal area.
- Clean the perineal area well with mild soap and warm water after each stool; rinse soap from the area well.
- If the physician allows, provide a sitz bath several times a day.
- Apply a thin coat of vitamin A & D ointment or other medicated protective covering, such as aloe products, after each stool.
- Keep the client off the affected buttock area.
- For open areas, cover with thin DuoDerm or Tegaderm occlusive dressing to promote rapid healing.
- Observe for fungal or yeast infections, which appear as dark red rashes. Obtain an order for medication if this problem occurs.

rhea and steatorrhea (see Chart 57-1). Anticholinergics, such as dicyclomine hydrochloride (Bentyl, Bentylol), are often given before meals to inhibit gastric motility. IV fluids may be necessary to replenish fluid losses associated with diarrhea.

The nurse provides special measures to protect the skin when diarrhea occurs (Chart 57-8). The nurse conducts an ongoing assessment for clinical manifestations of malabsorption and relates these to activities and dietary intake. For example, clients with steatorrhea are monitored for fluid and electrolyte imbalances and are encouraged to ingest electrolyte-rich liquids liberally. The nurse teaches clients the rationale for dietary, drug, and surgical management of nutritional deficiencies and evaluates interventions on the basis of changes in or resolution of clinical manifestations.

ONLINE RESOURCES

For suggested readings and Internet resources, go to http://www.wbsaunders.com/SIMON/Iggy/.

SELECTED BIBLIOGRAPHY

Alderman, J. (1999). Managing irritable bowel syndrome. *ADVANCE for Nurse Practitioners, 7*(1), 40-46.

American Cancer Society. (1997). Colorectal cancer. *CA: A Cancer Journal for Clinicians, 47*(2), 66-128.

Beackington, E. (2000). Irritable bowel syndrome: An update on treatment options. *Advance for Nurse Practitioners,* October, pp. 32-36.

Bonci, L., et al. (1998). Is malabsorption causing your patient's GI symptoms? *Patient Care,* March, pp. 93-116.

Bradley, M., & Pupiales, M. (1997). Essential elements of ostomy care. *American Journal of Nursing, 97*(7), 38-46.

Cantanzaro, J., & Serembus, J. (1998). High tech wound and ostomy care in the home setting. *Critical Care Nursing Clinics of North America, 10*(3), 327-338.

Carlson, E. (1998). Irritable bowel syndrome. *Nurse Practitioner, 23*(1), 82-93.

Cavalieri, J., & Franklin, B. (1998). Hereditary nonpolyposis colon cancer. *American Journal of Nursing, 98*(10), 42-43.

Clevenger, F., & Tepas, J. (1997). Perioperative management of patients with major trauma injuries. *AORN Journal, 65*(3), 583-594.

Greenlee, R., et al. (2000). Cancer statistics 2000. *CA: A Cancer Journal for Clinicians, 50*(1), 16.

Hardcastle, J.D. (1997). Colorectal cancer. *CA: A Cancer Journal for Clinicians, 47*(2), 66-68.

Harris, H., et al. (1999). Leukocytosis and free fluid are important indicators of isolated intestinal injury after blunt trauma. *Journal of Trauma, Injury, Infection, and Critical Care, 46*(4), 656-659.

Held-Warmkessel, J. (1998). Colon cancer: Prevention and detection strategies. *ADVANCE for Nurse Practitioners, 6*(7), 42-45.

Jenks, J.M., Morin, K.H., & Tomaselli, N. (1997). The influence of ostomy surgery on body image in patients with cancer. *Applied Nursing Research, 10*(4), 174-180.

Jeppesen, P., et al. (1997). Essential fatty acid deficiency in patients with severe fat malabsorption. *American Journal of Clinical Nutrition, 65,* 837-843.

Jessup, J.M., et al. (1997). Diagnosing colorectal carcinoma: Clinical and molecular approaches. *CA: A Cancer Journal for Clinicians, 47*(2), 70-92.

Koloski, N., Talley, N., & Boyce, P. (2000). The impact of functional gastrointestinal disorders on quality of life. *American Journal of Gastroenterology, 95*(1), 67-71.

Korsten, M., & Abittan, C. (1999). Obstipation and lower abdominal pain. *Clinical Advisor, 2*(6), 68-70.

Landis, S.H., et al. (1999). Cancer statistics, 1999. *Ca: A Cancer Journal for Clinicians, 49*(1), 8-32.

Lerman, C., et al. (1999). Genetic testing in families with hereditary nonpolyposis colon cancer. *Journal of the American Medical Association, 281*(17), 1618-1622.

Levins, T.T. (2000). Using ultrasound to assess blunt abdominal trauma. *Nursing2000, 30*(5), 32cc14-32cc15.

Locke, G.R., et al. (2000). Risk factors for irritable bowel syndrome: Role of analgesics and food sensitivities. *American Journal of Gastroenterology, 95*(1), 157-164.

Markowitz, A.J., & Winawer, S.J. (1997). Management of colorectal polyps. *CA: A Cancer Journal for Clinicians, 47*(2), 93-112.

O'Brien, B. (1999). Coming of age with an ostomy. *American Journal of Nursing, 99*(8), 71-74.

Pharmacia & Upjohn Company. (1997). Data on file. Kalamazoo, MI: Author.

Pontieri-Lewis, V. (2000). Colorectal cancer: Prevention and screening. *MEDSURG Nursing, 9*(1), 9-13.

Saddler, D., & Ellis, C. (1999). Colorectal cancer. *Seminars in Oncology Nursing, 15*(1), 58-69.

Schmulson, M., et al. (2000). Correlation of symptom criteria with perception thresholds during rectosigmoid distension in irritable bowel syndrome patients. *American Journal of Gastroenterology, 95*(1), 152-155.

Shelton, B. (1999). Intestinal obstruction. *AACN Clinical Issues: Advanced Practice in Acute and Critical Care, 10*(4), 478-491.

Sommers, M.S., & Johnson, S.A. (1997). *Davis's manual of nursing therapeutics for diseases and disorders.* Philadelphia: F.A. Davis.

Toner, B., & Akman, D. (2000). Gender role and irritable bowel syndrome: Literature review and hypothesis. *American Journal of Gastroenterology, 95*(1), 11-16.

Town, J. (1997). Bringing acute abdomen into focus. *Nursing97, 27*(5), 52-57.

Weber, T., et al. (1999). Novel hMLH1 and hMSH2 germline mutations in African-Americans with colorectal cancer. *Journal of the American Medical Association, 281*(24), 2316-2320.

Yoshii, H., et al. (1998). Usefulness and limitations of ultrasonography in the initial evaluation of blunt abdominal trauma. *Journal of Trauma, Injury, Infection and Critical Care, 45*(1), 45-51.

58

Interventions for Clients with Inflammatory Intestinal Disorders

CONSTANCE VISOVSKY

Learning Objectives

After studying this chapter, you should be able to:

1. Compare and contrast the typical physical assessment findings associated with appendicitis and peritonitis.
2. Prioritize nursing care for the client who has peritonitis.
3. Discuss the common causes of gastroenteritis.
4. Compare and contrast the pathophysiology and clinical manifestations of ulcerative colitis and Crohn's disease.
5. Analyze priority nursing diagnoses and collaborative problems for clients with chronic inflammatory bowel disease (IBD).
6. Explain the purpose of and nursing implications related to drug therapy for clients with IBD.
7. Formulate a postoperative plan of care for a client undergoing a colon resection/colectomy and colostomy or ileostomy.
8. Develop a teaching plan for a client needing community-based care for a new ostomy.
9. Identify expected outcomes for clients with chronic IBD.
10. Explain the role of diet therapy in managing the client with diverticular disease.
11. Describe the comfort measures that the nurse can use for the client with an anal abscess, fissure, or fistula.
12. Discuss ways that helminthic infestation, parasitic infection, and food poisoning can be prevented.

Go to http://www.wbsaunders.com/SIMON/Iggy/ for self-assessment questions related to these Learning Objectives.

Inflammatory bowel disease (IBD) is a condition of the small and/or large intestine involving inflammation that can be acute or chronic in duration. Chronic forms of IBD are characterized by periods of exacerbation and remission. Inflammatory and infectious intestinal disorders are often difficult to differentiate, since many of the characteristics of infectious processes mimic those of more chronic conditions. The nurse's involvement in assessing and managing intestinal disorders is essential to early diagnosis and successful treatment.

ACUTE INFLAMMATORY BOWEL DISORDERS

Appendicitis, peritonitis, and gastroenteritis are the most common acute inflammatory bowel problems. These disorders are potentially life threatening, and can have major systemic complications if not treated promptly.

Appendicitis

■ OVERVIEW

Appendicitis is acute inflammation of the vermiform appendix—the blind pouch attached to the cecum of the colon that is usually located in the right iliac region, just below the ileocecal valve. The appendix has no known function. As part of the cecum, it fills with food and empties on a regular basis. Inflammation of the appendix can occur when the lumen (opening) of the appendix is obstructed. Inflammation leads to infection as bacteria invade the wall of the appendix.

When the lumen is blocked, the mucosa continues to secrete fluid until the pressure within the lumen exceeds venous pressure. Blood flow to the appendix is restricted, and infection causes more swelling, which further impedes blood flow. Gangrene from hypoxia or perforation can occur within 24 to 36 hours. If this process occurs slowly, adjacent organs may wall off the area, and a localized abscess develops. If the infectious process occurs rapidly, peritonitis (inflammation of the peritoneum) may result. All complications of peritonitis are serious. Acute appendicitis is the most common cause of acute inflammation in the right lower quadrant. Consequently, it is one of the most common indications for emergency abdominal surgery.

When obstruction is present, calculi composed of fecal material (fecaliths), calcium phosphate–rich mucus, and inorganic salts may be the most common cause of the initial obstruction. Other causes of obstruction include tumors, viral infections, and worms. However, recent evidence points to ulceration of the mucosa as the primary cause of appendicitis (Silen, 1998). Infection by viral or fungal pathogens has been suggested as the cause of ulceration. Although appendicitis affects a person at any age, the peak incidence is between the ages of 20 and 30 years. Appendicitis affects men and women equally, except before 25 years of age, when males are affected more often than females at a 3:2 ratio (Silen, 1998).

It is thought that chronic infection of the appendix can occur, but this is not usually the cause of abdominal pain that lasts for weeks or months. Recurrent acute appendicitis does sometimes occur, often with complete remission of inflammation between acute attacks. In rare instances, acute appendicitis may be the first manifestation of Crohn's disease.

✺ CONSIDERATIONS FOR OLDER ADULTS

Appendicitis is relatively rare at extremes in age; however, perforation is more common in older people, causing a higher mortality rate. The diagnosis of appendicitis is difficult to establish in older adults, as symptoms of pain and tenderness are not as pronounced in this age-group. As a result, 30% of older clients with appendicitis develop perforation due to a delay in diagnosis. The development of peritonitis is associated with a 15% mortality rate in older adults (Silen, 1998).

► COLLABORATIVE MANAGEMENT
◗ Assessment

The history obtained from the client outlining the sequence of events provides the most important assessment of appendicitis. The most common symptom is abdominal pain, which results from contractions of the appendix or distention of its lumen. With *classic* appendicitis, abdominal pain in the epigastric or periumbilical area is the initial symptom. Pain may not be localized, however, and can exist anywhere in the abdomen or flanks. The pain at this time is described as mild or cramping. Nausea and vomiting follow in 50% to 60% of cases. As the inflammation spreads to the peritoneal surface, the pain becomes more steady and severe and the location shifts to the right lower quadrant. Abdominal pain that increases with cough or movement and is relieved by flexion of the right hip or the knees suggests a perforated appendix with peritonitis. Anorexia is a frequent finding associated with acute appendicitis.

Abdominal tenderness on palpation is the most common, important, and reliable symptom. In later stages of inflammation, tenderness becomes more localized and is noted with palpation of the right lower quadrant. This area is referred to as **McBurney's point;** it is located midway between the anterior iliac crest and the umbilicus in the right lower quadrant

(Figure 58-1). The nurse may feel tenseness of the muscles (muscle rigidity) over the tender area. Rigidity over the whole abdomen, accompanied by tense positioning and guarding, indicates a perforated appendix with peritonitis. Perforation rarely occurs within 24 hours of the onset of symptoms, but the incidence of peritonitis rises to as high as 80% after 48 hours. Rebound tenderness is a term used to describe a sensation of severe pain that occurs after deep pressure is applied and released. This maneuver involves pressing a finger into the abdomen at a point away from the pain and is performed by the physician or advanced-practice nurse.

The client's temperature is usually normal or slightly elevated at 99° to 100.5° F (37.2° to 38° C). A temperature of 101° F (38.2° C) or higher suggests the presence of peritonitis. As the temperature rises, a corresponding rise in pulse rate will be noted.

Because the clinical manifestations associated with many other medical conditions are similar to those of acute appendicitis, arriving at a diagnosis is often difficult. It is important for the nurse to determine the sequence of symptoms. For example, nausea and vomiting that precede abdominal pain often indicate gastroenteritis.

Clinical manifestations that do not follow the classic pattern can occur as a result of variations in the anatomic location of the appendix. The appendix can be located deep in the pelvis, in the right upper quadrant, or even in the left lower quadrant.

Laboratory findings do not establish the diagnosis, but there is often a moderate elevation of the white blood cell (WBC) count (leukocytosis) to 10,000 to 18,000/mm^3 with a "shift to the left" (an increased number of immature WBCs). A WBC elevation greater than 20,000/mm^3 may indicate a perforated appendix. An ultrasound study may show the presence of an enlarged appendix. If symptoms are recurrent or prolonged, a barium enema or computed tomography (CT) scan may reveal the presence of a fecalith.

◗ Interventions

All clients with suspected or confirmed appendicitis are hospitalized and examined by a surgeon. If the diagnosis is questionable, the health care team observes the client before surgical exploration.

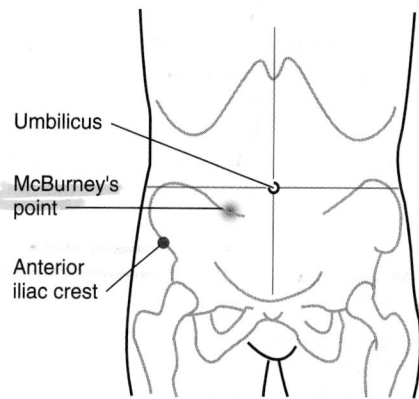

Umbilicus

McBurney's point

Anterior iliac crest

Figure 58-1 ◗ McBurney's point is located midway between the anterior iliac crest and the umbilicus in the right lower quadrant. This is the classic area for localized tenderness during the later stages of appendicitis.

NONSURGICAL MANAGEMENT. After admission to the hospital, the physician keeps the client with suspected or known appendicitis on nothing by mouth (NPO) status to prepare for the possibility of emergency surgery and to avoid aggravating the inflammatory process. The nurse administers intravenous (IV) fluids, as ordered, to prevent fluid and electrolyte imbalance and to replenish fluid volume. If the semi-Fowler's position can be tolerated, the nurse advises the client to maintain this position so that abdominal drainage, if any, can be contained in the lower abdomen.

Once the diagnosis of appendicitis is confirmed, the surgeon schedules surgery. The nurse may administer opioid analgesics, as ordered, while the client is being prepared for surgery. The client with suspected appendicitis should not receive laxatives or enemas, which can cause perforation of the appendix. Heat should never be applied to the abdomen because this may increase circulation to the appendix and result in increased inflammation and perforation.

SURGICAL MANAGEMENT. Surgery is required as soon as possible. If the diagnosis is not definitive but the client is at high risk for complications from suspected appendicitis, the surgeon may perform an exploratory laparotomy to rule out appendicitis.

PREOPERATIVE CARE. Preoperative teaching is often limited because the client is in pain or may be transferred to the operating suite for emergency surgery. The nurse prepares the client for general anesthesia and surgery (see Chapter 17).

OPERATIVE PROCEDURES. An **appendectomy** is the removal of the inflamed appendix. In a *traditional,* uncomplicated appendectomy, the surgeon removes the appendix through an incision approximately 3 inches (7.5 cm) long in the right lower quadrant. The incision is larger if the appendix is in an atypical position or if peritonitis is present.

An appendectomy is often done via **laparoscopy.** The surgeon makes several small incisions through which an endoscope is inserted. A cutting instrument is threaded through the endoscope, and the appendix is removed.

POSTOPERATIVE CARE. Postoperative care of the client who has undergone an appendectomy includes the care required for any client who has received general anesthesia (see Chapter 19). For clients who have undergone a traditional appendectomy, the incision is located over McBurney's point if the appendix was in the typical location. The incision may be as long as the length of the abdomen, depending on the area explored in surgery and the location of the appendix. Drains may have been inserted during the procedure if an abscess was present or if the appendix perforated. The drains are left in place for several days.

If peritonitis was present, a nasogastric (NG) tube is placed to decompress the stomach and prevent abdominal distention. IV antibiotics are typically prescribed if peritonitis or abscess is present. Opioid analgesics are administered for pain as needed. The client is typically out of bed on the evening of surgery or the first postoperative day. The client who has had an uncomplicated appendectomy via laparoscopy may stay overnight or may be discharged on the day of surgery. In this case, no NG tubes or drains are needed.

The client who has undergone an uncomplicated appendectomy usually recovers rapidly. After a traditional surgical procedure, he or she can resume normal activity in 2 to 4 weeks. If surgery has been complicated by perforation or peritonitis, he or she is hospitalized for 5 to 7 days or longer.

If the client is discharged to a home setting, the nurse assesses his or her ability to function with the added tasks of incision care, drug therapy, and some activity restrictions. The nurse assesses the home environment and the need for support to meet physical needs.

Peritonitis

OVERVIEW

Peritonitis is an acute inflammation of the endothelial lining of the abdominal cavity, or peritoneum. Peritonitis can be classified as primary or secondary, localized or generalized. Peritonitis is a life-threatening illness and is associated with several abdominal disorders.

Pathophysiology

PATHOLOGIC CHANGES

Normally, the peritoneal cavity contains approximately 50 mL of sterile fluid (transudate), which serves to prevent friction in the abdominal cavity during peristalsis (Hirsch & Caswell, 1999). When the peritoneal cavity is contaminated by bacteria, the body initially produces an inflammatory reaction that walls off a localized area to fight the infection. This local reaction involves vascular dilation and increased capillary permeability, allowing for transport of leukocytes and subsequent phagocytosis of the offending organisms. If this walling off process fails, the inflammation spreads and contamination becomes massive, resulting in diffuse peritonitis.

COMPLICATIONS

Vascular dilation continues, along with hyperemia (increased blood flow) and a fluid shift. The body responds to the infectious process by shunting extra blood to the area of inflammation. Fluid is shifted from the extracellular fluid (ECF) compartment into the peritoneal cavity, connective tissues, and gastrointestinal (GI) tract ("third spacing"). This shift of fluid out of the vascular space can result in a significant decrease in circulatory volume. The rate of decreasing circulatory volume is proportional to the degree of peritoneal involvement. Severely decreased circulatory volume can result in insufficient perfusion of the kidneys, leading to renal failure with electrolyte imbalance.

Peristalsis slows or stops in response to severe peritoneal infection, and the lumen of the bowel becomes distended with gas and fluid. Fluid that normally flows to the small bowel and the colon for reabsorption accumulates in the intestine in volumes of 7 to 8 L daily. The toxins or bacteria responsible for the peritonitis can also enter the bloodstream from the peritoneal area, leading to bacteremia or septicemia (bacterial invasion of the blood).

Respiratory problems can occur as a result of increased abdominal pressure against the diaphragm from intestinal distention and fluid shifts to the peritoneal cavity. Pain can interfere with ventilatory efforts when the client has an increased oxygen demand because of the infectious process.

TYPES OF PERITONITIS

Primary peritonitis is an acute bacterial infection that develops as a result of contamination of the peritoneum through the vascular system. Tuberculous peritonitis that arises from a tuberculin infection originating elsewhere in the body is a type of primary peritonitis. Clients with alcoholic cirrhosis and ascites, in the absence of a perforated organ, often manifest peritonitis, which may be due to leakage of bacteria through the wall of the intestine.

Secondary peritonitis is usually caused by bacterial invasion as a result of an acute abdominal disorder. Secondary peritonitis can develop as a result of a gangrenous bowel, perforation of the viscera by blunt or penetrating trauma, or bile leakage.

Etiology

Peritonitis is caused by contamination of the peritoneal cavity by bacteria or chemicals. Bacteria gain entry into the peritoneum by perforation or from an external penetrating wound. The most common causes of bacterial peritonitis are appendicitis and perforations associated with peptic ulcer disease, diverticulitis, a gangrenous gallbladder, or bowel obstruction. Bacterial invasion can also occur from an ascending infection through the reproductive tract, as in salpingitis or a septic abortion. Other causes of peritonitis include perforating tumors, ulcerative colitis, foreign bodies (from trauma), leakage or contamination during a surgical procedure, and infection by skin pathogens in clients undergoing continuous ambulatory peritoneal dialysis (CAPD). Bacteria responsible for peritonitis include *Escherichia coli, Streptococcus, Staphylococcus, Pneumococcus,* and *Gonococcus.* Chemical peritonitis arises from leakage of bile, pancreatic enzymes, and gastric acid.

Incidence/Prevalence

Primary peritonitis accounts for only a small percentage of the cases of peritonitis. The incidence of secondary peritonitis is difficult to determine because data usually relate to the underlying cause, such as appendicitis or peptic ulcer.

➤ COLLABORATIVE MANAGEMENT
● Assessment

HISTORY

The nurse questions the client regarding a history of abdominal pain and determines if the pain is localized or generalized. The nurse also asks about a history of a low-grade fever or recent spikes in temperature.

PHYSICAL ASSESSMENT/CLINICAL MANIFESTATIONS

Physical findings of peritonitis (Chart 58-1) depend on several factors: the stage of the disease, the ability of the body to localize the process by walling off the infection, and whether the inflammation has progressed to generalized peritonitis. The client typically appears acutely ill, lying still, possibly with the knees flexed. Movement is guarded, and the client may report and show signs of pain (e.g., facial grimacing) with coughing or movement of any type. During inspection, the nurse may observe progressive abdominal distention if the inflammation markedly reduces intestinal motility. The nurse may auscultate for bowel sounds, but these usually disappear with progression of the inflammation.

The cardinal signs of peritonitis are abdominal pain and tenderness. In the client with localized peritonitis, the abdomen is tender on palpation in a well-defined area of the abdomen with rebound tenderness in this area. With generalized peritonitis, tenderness is widespread. Abdominal wall rigidity is a common finding. The client may have a high fever because of the infectious process, with tachycardia occurring in response to the fever. The nurse assesses whether the client has dry mucous membranes with poor tissue turgor and a low urine output. A low urine output occurs because fluid accumulates in the peritoneal cavity, the GI tract, and connective tissues, resulting in a fluid deficit in the vascular space. Nausea and vomiting may also be present. Hiccups may occur as a result of diaphragmatic irritation. Depending on the severity of the peritonitis, the nurse may find that the client has a compromised respiratory status.

DIAGNOSTIC ASSESSMENT

White blood cell (WBC) counts are commonly elevated to 20,000/mm^3 with a high neutrophil count. A series of blood culture studies may be done to determine whether septicemia has occurred and to identify the causative organism to enable appropriate therapy.

The health care provider orders laboratory tests to assess fluid and electrolyte balance and renal status, including the following:
- Electrolytes
- Blood urea nitrogen (BUN)
- Creatinine
- Hemoglobin
- Hematocrit

Arterial blood gas values are obtained to assess respiratory function and acid-base balance.

CHART 58-1

KEY FEATURES *of*
Peritonitis

- Abdominal pain (localized, poorly localized, or referred to the shoulder or thorax)
- Rigid, boardlike abdomen
- Distended abdomen
- Nausea, anorexia, vomiting
- Diminishing bowel sounds
- Inability to pass flatus or feces
- Rebound tenderness in the abdomen
- High fever
- Tachycardia
- Dehydration from high fever (poor skin turgor)
- Decreased urine output
- Hiccups
- Possible compromise in respiratory status

Abdominal x-ray films are obtained to assess for free air or fluid in the abdominal cavity, which indicates perforation. The x-ray films may also show dilation, edema, and inflammation of the small and large intestines.

The physician may perform a diagnostic peritoneal lavage by instilling 1 L of fluid through a peritoneal dialysis catheter. Lavage fluid positive for peritonitis is characterized by the following: more than 500 WBCs/mL^3 of fluid, more than 50,000 red blood cells (RBCs)/mL, or the presence of bacteria on a Gram stain. Bile-stained green fluid may indicate a ruptured gallbladder or perforated intestine, which can lead to chemical peritonitis.

Interventions

All clients with peritonitis are hospitalized because of the severe nature of the illness. If complications are extensive, the client may be admitted to a critical care unit. Nursing interventions focus on the early identification of complications.

NONSURGICAL MANAGEMENT. The physician prescribes IV fluids and broad-spectrum antibiotics immediately after establishing the diagnosis of peritonitis. IV fluids are necessary to replace fluids collected in the peritoneum and bowel. Daily weight and intake and output are monitored to assess fluid status. A nasogastric (NG) tube is inserted to decompress the stomach and the intestine, and the client is on NPO status. The nurse administers oxygen, as ordered, according to the client's respiratory status. The health care provider will most likely institute pain management with IV analgesics, such as morphine sulfate administered via a patient-controlled analgesia (PCA) pump. Even with nonsurgical management of peritonitis, the nurse can expect the health care provider to order a surgical consultation in the event that surgery becomes necessary.

SURGICAL MANAGEMENT. Abdominal surgery is the optimal treatment for identifying and repairing the cause of the peritonitis. If the client is so critically ill that surgery would be life threatening, it may be delayed. Surgery focuses on controlling the contamination, removing foreign material from the peritoneal cavity, and draining collected fluid.

The surgeon performs an **exploratory laparotomy** to remove or repair the inflamed or perforated organ. The abdominal cavity is opened surgically and explored for inflamed and perforated organs or other abnormalities.

PREOPERATIVE CARE. The preoperative care for the client undergoing an exploratory laparotomy is similar to that described in Chapter 17 for the client receiving general anesthesia.

OPERATIVE PROCEDURES. For an exploratory laparotomy, the surgeon makes an incision through the abdominal wall and explores the abdominal cavity. Part or all of a perforated or inflamed organ may be removed, depending on that organ's function. For example, an appendectomy is performed for an inflamed appendix; a colon resection, with or without a colostomy, is indicated for a perforated diverticulum or perforated colon secondary to a tumor. Before the abdominal cavity is closed, the surgeon irrigates the peritoneum with antibiotic solutions. Two to four catheters may also be inserted to drain the cavity and provide a route for irrigation postoperatively.

POSTOPERATIVE CARE. Postoperative care is similar to that for other clients undergoing surgery (see Chapter 19). Clients with peritonitis may have actual or potential multisystem complications. Therefore the nurse initially monitors level of consciousness, vital signs, respiratory status (respiratory rate and breath sounds), and fluid and electrolyte status (intake and output and laboratory values) at least hourly.

Positioning. The nurse maintains the client in a semi-Fowler's position to promote drainage of peritoneal contents in the inferior region of the abdominal cavity. This position also facilitates adequate respiratory excursion in that the diaphragm and abdominal contents are impinging on respiratory muscles.

Wound Care. The client is likely to have multiple incisions and drains. Because contamination at the time of surgery impedes healing of an incision with edges well approximated (by first intention), incisions are allowed to heal by second or third intention. These incisions necessitate meticulous care involving manual irrigation or packing, as ordered by the surgeon. If the surgeon orders peritoneal irrigation through a drain, the nurse maintains sterile technique during manual irrigation, usually by using a catheter-tipped syringe. The nurse determines that the client is not retaining irrigant by ensuring the absence of abdominal distention or pain and by monitoring irrigant intake and output.

As a result of the loss of fluids from the extracellular space to the peritoneal cavity, IV fluid replacement and maintenance are indicated for all clients with peritonitis. Fluid volume deficit also occurs as a result of nasogastric suctioning and NPO status. Normal saline or a balanced saline solution with potassium is administered intravenously according to electrolyte, BUN, and serum creatinine values. To assess fluid volume, the nurse monitors the client's vital signs, urine output, skin turgor, integrity of mucous membranes, and most important, weight. The nurse also assesses for edema from third spacing.

> ### CONSIDERATIONS FOR OLDER ADULTS
> The older adult often does not have characteristic signs and symptoms of dehydration. A change in mental status may be an early sign of fluid deficit. The nurse assesses skin turgor on an older client using the skin over the forehead or sternum. The nurse provides frequent mouth care to help maintain moist mucous membranes. The use of lemon-glycerin swabs is avoided because they can increase dryness.

Community-Based Care

The length of hospitalization depends on the extent and severity of the infectious process. Clients who have a localized abscess drained and who respond to antibiotics and IV fluids without respiratory, renal, or cardiac complications are discharged in about a week. Clients who experience complications of peritonitis, along with sepsis or shock, may require mechanical ventilation or hemodialysis, with hospital stays lasting for several weeks. Discharge planning varies with the degree of involvement of all body systems. Some clients may be transferred to a subacute unit to complete their antibiotic therapy and recovery.

If the client is being discharged to home, the nurse assesses his or her ability to function at home with the added task of incision care and a diminished activity tolerance. The nurse provides the client with written and oral instructions to report the following:

- Unusual or foul-smelling drainage
- Swelling, redness, or warmth or bleeding from the incision site
- A temperature higher than 101° F (38.2° C)
- The presence of abdominal pain

The nurse also instructs the client in proper handwashing and dressing change techniques, which include directions to dress wounds separately to avoid cross-contamination.

The physician prescribes an oral opioid analgesic and possibly an antibiotic. The nurse reviews information about these medications with the client and caregiver. For clients taking opioid analgesics for any length of time, a stool softener should be prescribed.

The nurse also explains diet and activity limitations. Diet depends on the type of surgery performed and the client's specific food tolerances at the time of discharge. All clients are told to refrain from any lifting for *at least* 6 weeks. Other activity limitations are made on an individual basis with the physician's recommendation.

Peritonitis is a life-threatening and consequently frightening illness. Incisional care can be demanding, and activity intolerance can be overwhelming. If complications have resolved, the nurse reassures clients that they can realistically expect to resume their previous lifestyle. Convalescence is often longer than that required for other types of surgery, however, because of the multisystemic involvement.

Clients with an incision healing by second or third intention may require dressings, solution, and catheter-tipped syringes to irrigate the wound. The nurse may arrange for a home care nurse to assess, irrigate, or pack the wound and change the dressing as needed. If a client needs assistance with activities of daily living, a home care aide or temporary placement in a skilled care facility may be indicated. The case manager collaborates with the health care team to determine the most appropriate setting for community-based care.

Gastroenteritis

OVERVIEW

Acute diarrheal illnesses cause significant morbidity among young children and adults, especially in less-developed nations of the world. **Gastroenteritis** is an increase in the frequency and water content of stools and/or vomiting as a result of inflammation of the mucous membranes of the stomach and intestinal tract. Gastroenteritis primarily affects the small bowel and can be of either viral or bacterial origin. Both forms have similar manifestations and are considered self-limiting in their course unless complications occur. All organisms that are implicated in gastroenteritis cause diarrhea; however, the organisms discussed in this section have distinguishing characteristics.

Authors disagree on classification of the infectious diseases described as gastroenteritis. Some investigators include shigellosis when discussing gastroenteritis; others consider shigellosis separately as a dysentery type of illness. Dysenteries affect the *large* bowel; gastroenteritis affects the *small* bowel. Other authors classify infectious disease of the intestine as bacterial, viral, or parasitic, without using the term *gastroenteritis.*

Food poisoning is sometimes described in conjunction with gastroenteritis, with specific reference to the organism causing the food poisoning. Gastroenteritis, however, differs from food poisoning with regard to transmission in the body, incubation time, and effect on immunity.

The following discussion of gastroenteritis includes the viral forms (epidemic viral, rotavirus) and the bacterial forms (*Campylobacter, Escherichia coli,* and shigellosis) (Table 58-1). Organisms associated with food poisoning and parasitic infections are discussed under Food Poisoning, p. 1295.

Pathophysiology/Etiology

Infection with viral and bacterial organisms can produce gastrointestinal (GI) illnesses in which watery diarrhea is the primary feature. These disorders can be caused by noninflammatory, inflammatory, or penetrating mechanisms. The infecting organism (e.g., enterotoxigenic *E. coli*) can release enterotoxin

TABLE 58-1 • COMMON TYPES OF GASTROENTERITIS AND THEIR CHARACTERISTICS	
Type	**Characteristics**
VIRAL GASTROENTERITIS	
Epidemic viral	Caused by many parvovirus-type organisms Transmitted by the fecal-oral route in food and water Incubation period 10-51 hr Communicable during acute illness
Rotarvirus and Norwalk virus	Transmitted by the fecal-oral route and possibly the respiratory route Incubation in 48 hr Rotavirus is most common in infants and young children Norwalk virus affects young children and adults
BACTERIAL GASTROENTERITIS	
Campylobacter enteritis	Transmitted by the fecal-oral route or by contact with infected animals or infants Incubation period 1-10 days Communicable for 2-7 weeks
Escherichia coli diarrhea	Transmitted by fecally contaminated food, water, or fomites
Shigellosis	Transmitted by direct and indirect fecal-oral routes Incubation period 1-7 days Communicable during the acute illness to 4 weeks after the illness Humans possibly carriers for months

(a noninflammatory toxic substance specific to the intestinal mucosa), which results in diarrhea. The organism (e.g., *Shigella* or *Campylobacter*) can also attach itself to mucosal epithelium without penetrating it. Cells of the intestinal villi are then destroyed, and malabsorption results. Infections that are mediated by bacterial toxins cause the absorptive capacity of the distal small bowel and proximal colon to be overcome, resulting in diarrhea. Finally, the organism (e.g., rotavirus) can penetrate the intestine, causing cellular destruction, necrosis, and a potential for ulceration. Diarrhea occurs often with white blood cells (WBCs) or red blood cells (RBCs) present in the stool.

All of these situations result in *increased* GI motility, with fluids and electrolytes being secreted into the intestine at rapid rates. Invading organisms have increased capabilities of attaching to the intestinal mucosa if the normal intestinal flora is altered. This can occur in clients who are receiving antibiotics, are malnourished, or are debilitated. Two groups of viruses, the rotaviruses and Norwalk virus, as well as bacterial pathogens, are primary etiologic agents involved in the development of gastroenteritis.

TYPES OF GASTROENTERITIS

VIRAL GASTROENTERITIS. Many types of rotaviruses cause rotavirus gastroenteritis. The reservoir of these viruses is in humans. The viruses are transmitted via the fecal-oral route and possibly via the respiratory tract. Incubation is 48 hours. The period of communicability is during the acute stage and shortly after. Rotavirus infection is generally limited to infants and young children; by age 2 years, most children have acquired antibodies against most types of these viruses.

Norwalk virus infection can occur year-round and affects adults and children alike. This virus is spread by the oral-fecal route and is responsible for one third of all epidemics of viral gastroenteritis in developed countries. The virus is also a common cause of waterborne epidemics of gastroenteritis.

BACTERIAL GASTROENTERITIS. There are three general types of bacterial gastroenteritis:

* *E. coli* diarrhea ("traveler's diarrhea")
* *Campylobacter enteritis* ("traveler's diarrhea")
* *Shigellosis* (bacillary dysentery)

E. coli is the most common organism implicated in traveler's diarrhea. The reservoirs of *E. coli* are humans, who are often asymptomatic. The organism is transmitted through fecally contaminated food, water, or fomites (any other substance that transmits infection).

The etiologic feature of *Campylobacter* enteritis is the bacterium *Campylobacter jejuni;* reservoirs are domestic or wild animals and birds. *C. jejuni* is transmitted through the fecal-oral route by ingestion of water or food contaminated with feces or by direct contact with infected animals or infants. Incubation ranges from 1 to 10 days. The organism is communicable for several days to weeks throughout the course of the infection (usually 2 to 7 weeks).

Shigellosis is caused by infection with *Shigella* bacteria. Direct or indirect fecal-oral transmission can occur from an infected person or carrier. The incubation period before the illness is 1 to 7 days. The illness can be communicated during the acute phase and for up to 4 weeks after the onset of the illness. A person may be a carrier of this illness for months after the acute illness.

Incidence/Prevalence

Acute GI illnesses are the second most common disease worldwide. Acute diarrheal illnesses are the most common cause of morbidity and mortality among children and older adults in Asia, Africa, and Latin America. Gastroenteritis often occurs in epidemic outbreaks among groups of people.

Campylobacter enteritis occurs worldwide, commonly in epidemic outbreaks. Its incidence is highest during warm months. Diarrhea caused by *E. coli* also occurs worldwide, commonly in epidemics. The highest incidence is in areas of poor sanitation during warm months. Shigellosis occurs worldwide in every age-group but is most frequent in children under the age of 10 years. Children and older adults are more susceptible to *Shigella* because of their immature or depressed immune systems. Outbreaks of shigellosis are common in areas with crowded living conditions.

➤ COLLABORATIVE MANAGEMENT

● Assessment

The history elicited from the client can provide information related to the potential cause of the illness. The nurse questions the client regarding a recent history of travel, especially to tropical regions of Asia, Africa, or Central or South America. Traveler's diarrhea can begin 3 days to 2 weeks following the client's arrival.

The client who has gastroenteritis usually appears ill. Nausea and vomiting can occur with all types of gastroenteritis but are usually limited to the first 1 or 2 days of the illness. All clients with gastroenteritis classically have diarrhea, which varies in consistency and amount with the causative organism.

In clients with epidemic viral gastroenteritis, myalgia (muscle aches), headache, and malaise are often reported. The nurse notes slight abdominal distention. The nurse auscultates hyperactive bowel sounds and finds diffuse tenderness on palpation. However, there should be *no* rebound tenderness, which might indicate peritonitis. Depending on the amount of fluids lost through diarrhea and vomiting, the client may have varying degrees of dehydration manifested by the following:

* Poor skin turgor
* Dry mucous membranes
* Orthostatic blood pressure changes
* Hypotension
* Oliguria

In some cases, dehydration may be severe, and shock may occur if diarrhea is prolonged. Dehydration occurs rapidly in older adults.

Diarrhea associated with epidemic viral gastroenteritis is typically limited to 24 to 48 hours. In rotavirus gastroenteritis, there is an elevated temperature and watery diarrhea lasting 2 to 6 days. Mucus may be present in the stools of individuals infected with rotavirus. Infection with the Norwalk virus is characterized by the rapid onset of nausea, abdominal cramps, vomiting, and diarrhea. The illness is usually mild, lasting 24 to 48 hours (Greenberg, 1998). *Campylobacter* enteritis is a more severe disease with foul-smelling stools that contain blood and that can number 20 to 30 per day for up to

7 days. *E. coli* gastroenteritis may or may not involve blood or mucus in the stool; diarrhea can last for up to 10 days. *Shigella* causes stools containing blood and mucus, which can continue for up to 5 days.

As part of the laboratory assessment, Gram stain of stool is usually done before culture. Many white blood cells (WBCs) on Gram stain suggest shigellosis. The presence of WBCs and red blood cells (RBCs) in the stool indicates *Campylobacter* gastroenteritis.

A stool culture that is positive for enterotoxigenic *E. coli* is diagnostic of *E. coli* diarrhea. Culture of stool that is positive for *Shigella* when there are pus cells or WBCs present in the stool is diagnostic of shigellosis.

Sophisticated electron microscopy and immunoassay procedures can identify epidemic viral gastroenteritis or rotavirus gastroenteritis; however, such examinations are rarely done because they are expensive and tedious to perform.

● Interventions

For clients with most types of gastroenteritis, supportive treatment is instituted. Therapy is focused on fluid replacement, and the amount and route of fluid administration are determined by fluid status.

FLUID REPLACEMENT. For mild cases of gastroenteritis, the client is treated on an ambulatory care basis or in the nursing home if he or she is a resident there. If the fluid volume is severely depleted, the client is admitted to the hospital for administration of IV fluids. For older clients at home or in a long-term care setting, oral rehydration therapy (ORT) with commercially prepared rehydration products, such as Resol, may prevent hospitalization.

The nurse obtains weight, orthostatic blood pressure, and other vital sign measurements at the time of admission. Hypotonic IV fluids, such as half-strength normal saline (0.45% sodium chloride), are infused as ordered. The nurse monitors the client's vital signs, intake and output, and weight. A rapid gain or loss of 1 kg (2.2 pounds) of body weight is equivalent to the gain or loss of 1 L of fluid. Standard precautions are consistently observed when handling vomitus and stool.

The health care provider may order a potassium supplement to be added to IV fluids if the serum potassium level is low. To help assess renal function and prevent hyperkalemia, the nurse verifies that the client is voiding before and during potassium replacement. The client is advised to rest in bed, especially during periods of nausea or vomiting.

Depending on the type of gastroenteritis, the local health department may need to be notified. It is mandatory that every case of shigellosis be reported. In some endemic areas, *Campylobacter* enteritis needs to be reported on a case-by-case basis. Other types of gastroenteritis must be reported only if they occur in epidemic proportions. The nurse or case manager investigates state and local health department guidelines for reporting requirements.

DIET THERAPY. Diet therapy is the same for the client who remains at home as for the client in the hospital. If the client is not actively vomiting, the nurse recommends small volumes of clear liquids with electrolytes (e.g., Gatorade) for 24 hours. The frequency and amount of oral intake can be increased if nausea and vomiting are *not* present. If nausea and vomiting continue, the nurse withholds food and fluids until these symptoms subside. The nurse advises the client *not* to drink water, because it does not contain any electrolytes to replace those lost. After 24 hours, the diet for all clients can be advanced to include saltine crackers, toast, and jelly. When the client can tolerate this diet, bland foods (e.g., nonfat soup, custard, yogurt, cottage cheese, mashed or baked potatoes, and cooked vegetables) may be added. Caffeine is avoided, since it can increase intestinal motility. The client may progress to a regular diet as tolerated.

DRUG THERAPY. Drugs that suppress intestinal motility, such as anticholinergics and antiemetics, are *not* routinely given for bacterial or viral gastroenteritis. Use of these drugs can prevent the infecting organisms from being eliminated from the body. If the health care provider determines that antiperistaltic agents are necessary, an initial dose of loperamide 4 mg may be administered orally, followed by 2 mg after each loose stool, up to 16 mg/day. Bismuth subsalicylate (Pepto-Bismol) 30 mL or 2 tablets every 30 minutes for a maximum of 8 doses may be given to reduce the watery volume of the stool.

Treatment with antibiotics may be warranted if the gastroenteritis is due to bacterial infection with fever and severe diarrhea. The health care provider may order norfloxacin (Chibroxin, Noroxin) 400 mg twice a day PO or ciprofloxacin (Cipro) 500 mg twice a day PO for 3 days. If the gastroenteritis is due to shigellosis, anti-infective agents, such as trimethoprim/sulfamethoxazole (Septra, Bactrim), are administered.

For relatively short-term diarrhea of 24 to 48 hours' duration, the diagnosis is based primarily on the client's history and clinical manifestations without validation by a stool examination. When diarrhea is severe or persists for long periods, the stool is examined in an effort to determine the causative organism and to begin specific treatment. It should be determined if the diarrhea is caused by *Salmonella* or parasites, because these organisms respond to specific medications (see Parasitic Infection, p. 1292). Diarrhea that continues longer than 10 days is probably *not* due to gastroenteritis, and a thorough investigation for the cause is warranted.

SKIN CARE. Frequent stools that are rich in electrolytes and enzymes, as well as frequent wiping and washing of the anal region, can irritate the skin. The nurse teaches the client to avoid toilet paper and harsh soaps. Ideally, the client can gently clean the area with warm water or absorbent cotton, followed by thorough drying with absorbent cotton. Cream, oil, or gel can be applied to a damp, warm washcloth to remove excrement adhering to excoriated skin. Hydrocortisone cream or protective barrier cream should be applied to the skin between stools. Witch hazel compresses (e.g., Tucks) and sitz baths for 10 minutes, two to three times daily, can also relieve discomfort.

If leakage of stool is a problem, the client can put absorbent cotton next to the anal orifice and keep it in place with snug underwear. For clients who are incontinent, the nurse keeps the perineal and buttock areas clean and dry. The use of incontinent pads instead of briefs allows air to circulate to the skin and prevents irritation.

HEALTH TEACHING. During the acute phase of the illness, the nurse teaches about the importance of fluid replacement measures. The nurse teaches the client to follow the diet described earlier under Diet Therapy, p. 1273, and about any necessary medications. The nurse also teaches the client and family about the importance of minimizing the risk of transmission of gastroenteritis. Clients are advised to:

- Wash their hands meticulously with an antibacterial soap, especially after bowel movements, and maintain good personal hygiene
- Restrict the use of glasses, dishes, eating utensils, and tubes of toothpaste to themselves only
- Maintain clean bathroom facilities to avoid exposure to stool
- Inform the health care provider if symptoms persist beyond 3 days

Clients adhere to these precautions for up to 7 weeks after the illness or up to several months if *Shigella* was the offending organism. If the client is employed as a food handler, the public health department should be consulted for recommendations about the return to work (Chart 58-2).

CHRONIC INFLAMMATORY BOWEL DISEASE

Chronic inflammatory bowel disease (chronic IBD) refers to several inflammatory disorders of the gastrointestinal (GI) tract with no known etiology. Chronic IBDs may be divided into two major groups: ulcerative colitis and Crohn's disease (Table 58-2).

Ulcerative Colitis

OVERVIEW

Ulcerative colitis is a chronic inflammatory process affecting the mucosal lining of the colon or rectum. This chronic inflammatory process can result in loose stools containing blood and mucus, poor absorption of vital nutrients, and

---

CHART 58-2

CLIENT EDUCATION GUIDE
Measures to Prevent the Transmission of Gastroenteritis

- Wash your hands meticulously with an antibacterial soap, especially after having a bowel movement.
- Do not share your dishes, glasses, or toothpaste.
- Keep the commode clean to prevent exposure to your stool.
- Do not prepare or handle food that will be consumed by others.

---

thickening of the colon wall. Over time, the client experiences episodes of abdominal discomfort and extraintestinal manifestations of the disease that cause disruption of lifestyle. The affected client may have only minor periodic health problems, necessitating only ambulatory care, or serious problems, such as malnutrition and physical debilitation, requiring multiple hospitalizations.

Pathophysiology

Ulcerative colitis is characterized by diffuse inflammation of the intestinal mucosa; the result is a loss of surface epithelium with ulceration and possibly abscess formation. Generally, the disease begins in the rectum and proceeds in a uniform, continuous manner proximally toward the cecum. The inflammatory process progresses to epithelial cell damage and loss, leaving areas of ulceration. The colon appears ulcerated, reddened, and hemorrhagic. Ulcerative colitis is characterized by periods of remission and exacerbation.

Clients with *acute* ulcerative colitis may have vascular congestion, hemorrhage, edema, and ulceration of the bowel mucosa. As the disease course progresses, *chronic* changes in the colon occur. Fibrosis and retraction of the bowel result in muscle hypertrophy, deposition of fat and fibrous tissue, and a narrower and shorter colon. With long-term disease, dysplastic changes to the surface epithelium occur. These changes are associated with an increased risk of colon cancer.

Complications of ulcerative colitis include the following:

- Intestinal perforation with resultant peritonitis and fistula formation
- **Toxic megacolon**
- Hemorrhage
- Increased risk of colon cancer
- Abscess formation
- Malabsorption
- Bowel obstruction
- Extraintestinal clinical manifestations, such as arthritis

Table 58-3 describes these common complications.

Etiology

The exact cause of ulcerative colitis is unknown. A genetic basis of the disease has been proposed because of the increased incidence seen in families, certain ethnic groups, and twins. Immunologic theories, including autoimmune dysfunction, have been explored because of the extraintestinal manifestations of the disease. One hypothesis suggests that

---

TABLE 58-2 • DIFFERENTIAL FEATURES OF ULCERATIVE COLITIS AND CROHN'S DISEASE

Feature	Ulcerative Colitis	Crohn's Disease
Location	Begins in the rectum and proceeds in a continuous manner toward the cecum	Most often in the terminal ileum, with patchy involvement through all layers of the bowel
Etiology	Unknown	Unknown
Peak incidence at age	15-25 yr and 55-65 yr	15-40 yr
Stools	10-20 liquid, bloody stools per day	5-6 soft, loose stools per day, rarely bloody
Complications	Hemorrhage Perforation Fistulas Nutritional deficiencies	Fistulas Nutritional deficiencies

IBD results from an abnormal response to normal flora present in the intestines; another possibility is that there may be a defect in intestinal permeability that permits antigens to leak through the mucosa, stimulating an inflammatory response. Psychologic factors have also been implicated, since stress often results in a flare-up of the disease. However, there is little evidence to relate psychologic factors to the cause of the disease.

Incidence/Prevalence

There is a higher geographic distribution of the disease in northern Europe and North America. The annual incidence of ulcerative colitis is approximately 2 to 10 new cases per 100,000 persons. The prevalence is 40 to 100 cases per 100,000 people in the United States. There is a tenfold risk of the disease if an individual has a first-degree relative with the disease.

Peak incidence is between the ages of 15 and 25 years, with another peak occurring between ages of 55 and 65 years. Females are more often affected than men. Jewish Caucasians of European or Ashkenazic origin are at highest risk compared with other Caucasian groups (Rubin, 1998).

> ### CULTURAL CONSIDERATIONS
> Ulcerative colitis is four to five times more common among people of Jewish origin and commonly affects Caucasians in developed Western society. It is seen more often in individuals of Jewish European or Ashkenazic origin, but not in those of Sephardic origin. Although the disease is more common in Caucasians, the incidence in African Americans is increasing.

TABLE 58-3 • COMPLICATIONS OF ULCERATIVE COLITIS AND CROHN'S DISEASE

Complication	Description
Hemorrhage/ perforation	Lower gastrointestinal bleeding results from erosion of the bowel wall.
Abscess formation	Localized pockets of infection develop in the ulcerated bowel lining.
Toxic megacolon	Paralysis of the colon causes dilation and subsequent bowel obstruction.
Malabsorption	Essential nutrients cannot be absorbed through the diseased intestinal wall, causing anemia and malnutrition (most common in Crohn's disease).
Bowel obstruction	Obstruction results from toxic megacolon or cancer.
Fistulas	Fistulas can occur anywhere, but usually track between the bowel and bladder. Pyuria and fecaluria result.
Colorectal cancer	Clients with ulcerative colitis for 7-10 yr or longer have a high risk for colorectal cancer. This complication accounts for about one third of all deaths related to ulcerative colitis.
Extraintestinal complications	Complications include arthritis, hepatic and biliary disease (especially cholelithiasis), oral and skin lesions, and ocular disorders, such as iritis. The cause is unknown.

➤ COLLABORATIVE MANAGEMENT
● Assessment

▮ HISTORY

The nurse collects data on any family history of inflammatory bowel disease (IBD) and previous and current therapy for the illness, as well as dates and types of surgery. Obtaining a diet history is essential. The history should include the client's usual dietary patterns and the relationship of elimination patterns to intolerance of milk and milk products and greasy, fried, spicy, or hot foods. A history of weight loss may be seen in clients with severe disease.

The nurse asks about the symptoms of acute ulcerative colitis, which often include abdominal pain, cramping, urgency, and diarrhea with up to 10 to 20 liquid, bloody stools per day, as well as anorexia and fatigue. The client is questioned regarding his or her usual bowel elimination pattern; the color, consistency, and character of stools; and the presence or absence of blood in all stools. The nurse notes the relationship between the occurrence of diarrhea and the timing of meals, pain, emotional distress, and activity. The client is questioned regarding extraintestinal symptoms such as arthritis, mouth sores, vision problems, and skin disorders.

▮ PHYSICAL ASSESSMENT/CLINICAL MANIFESTATIONS

The client with ulcerative colitis may have symptoms that vary with the acuteness of onset and with complications of the disease process. The client may complain of abdominal pain, bloody diarrhea, and **tenesmus** (uncontrollable straining). Vital signs are usually within normal limits in mild disease. In more severe cases, the client may have a low-grade fever (99° to 100° F [37.2° to 37.8° C]). The physical assessment findings are typically nonspecific, and in milder cases the physical examination may be normal.

The nurse may note some mild abdominal distention along the colon. Palpation may reveal areas of increased or localized tenderness. Rebound tenderness may suggest peritonitis. The nurse may note localized areas of abdominal pain or cramping over areas of diseased bowel. The client may be febrile and tachycardic, indicating possible complications, such as peritonitis, dehydration, and bowel perforation.

▮ PSYCHOSOCIAL ASSESSMENT

The intestinal and extraintestinal symptoms associated with ulcerative colitis can be taxing. The nurse evaluates the client's understanding of the illness and its impact on his or her lifestyle. The client is encouraged and supported while the following are explored:
- The relationship of life events to disease exacerbations
- Stress factors that produce symptoms
- Family and social support systems
- Concerns regarding the possible genetic basis and associated cancer risks of the disease

Many clients are very apprehensive regarding the frequency of stools and the presence of blood. The uncontrollability of the disease symptoms, particularly diarrhea, can be disruptive and stress producing. More severe illness may limit the client's activities outside the home. As a result of the excessive diarrhea, the client may become dependent on the proximity of a bathroom. Eating may be associated with pain and cramping, as well as an increased frequency of stools. Mealtimes may become unpleasant experiences. Frequent visits to health care providers and vigilant monitoring of the colonic mucosa for dysplastic (irregular) changes can be anxiety provoking.

LABORATORY ASSESSMENT

As a result of chronic blood loss, hematocrit and hemoglobin levels may be low, reflecting anemia and a chronic disease state. An increased white blood cell (WBC) count and elevated erythrocyte sedimentation rate (ESR) are consistent with inflammatory disease. Sodium, potassium, and chloride concentrations may be depleted secondary to frequent diarrheal stools and malabsorption resulting from the diseased bowel. Hypoalbuminemia is found in clients with extensive disease.

Viral and bacterial dysenteries can cause symptoms similar to those of ulcerative colitis. Before an invasive diagnostic workup, the stools are examined for occult blood, ova (eggs), and parasites, and specimens for culture are obtained. Other problems must be ruled out before a definitive diagnosis of ulcerative colitis is made.

RADIOGRAPHIC ASSESSMENT

Barium enemas with air contrast demonstrate differences between Crohn's disease and ulcerative colitis and identify complications, mucosal patterns, and the distribution and depth of disease involvement. In early disease, the barium enema will show incomplete filling as a result of inflammation and fine ulcerations along the bowel contour. These ulcerations appear deeper in more advanced disease.

OTHER DIAGNOSTIC ASSESSMENT

The sigmoidoscopic examination is probably the most definitive diagnostic procedure for ulcerative colitis. The physician can directly visualize the sigmoid and transverse colon. Common findings include an edematous, friable bowel mucosa with a loss of vascular pattern and frequent ulcerations. Biopsy specimens can also be taken to determine if inflammation or dysplastic changes are present.

CRITICAL THINKING CHALLENGE

A 65-year-old female client is admitted to your unit with a 10-year history of mild to moderate ulcerative colitis. Recently she has noted an increasing amount of abdominal pain and cramping following meals. She has also experienced an increase in stools from 1 to 3 per day to 8 to 12 per day. She reports that the stools contain blood and mucus. Her vital signs are normal except for a slight increase in temperature to 100° F (37.8° C).

- What additional information in the history should you elicit from the client?
- What actions should you take considering this client's increase in temperature and gastrointestinal (GI) symptoms?
- What long-term consequences of the disease is this client most at risk for?

For suggested answer guidelines, go to SIMON http://www.wbsaunders.com/SIMON/Iggy/.

● Analysis

COMMON NURSING DIAGNOSES AND COLLABORATIVE PROBLEMS

The following are common nursing diagnoses for clients with ulcerative colitis:

1. Diarrhea related to inflammation of the bowel mucosa
2. Acute and Chronic Pain related to inflammation and ulceration of the bowel mucosa and accompanying skin irritation

The most common collaborative problem is Potential for Gastrointestinal Bleeding.

ADDITIONAL NURSING DIAGNOSES AND COLLABORATIVE PROBLEMS

In addition to the common nursing diagnoses and collaborative problems, clients with ulcerative colitis may have one or more of the following:

- Imbalanced Nutrition: Less Than Body Requirements related to diarrhea and malabsorption
- Disturbed Body Image related to increased bowel elimination or surgical intervention
- Activity Intolerance related to fatigue and anemia
- Ineffective Coping related to chronic physical illness and repeated hospitalizations
- Risk for Deficient Fluid Volume related to diarrhea
- Impaired Oral Mucous Membrane related to extraintestinal oral disease
- Anxiety related to increased risk of colon cancer and lifestyle interruptions

● Planning and Implementation

DIARRHEA

NOC **PLANNING: EXPECTED OUTCOMES.** A major concern for a client with ulcerative colitis is the occurrence of frequent, bloody diarrhea. The client with ulcerative colitis is expected to experience decreased diarrhea through measures to reduce the inflammation of the intestinal lining.

INTERVENTIONS. Many measures are used to relieve symptoms and to reduce intestinal motility, decrease inflammation, and promote intestinal healing. Medical management of ulcerative colitis is the preferred and initial treatment option.

NONSURGICAL MANAGEMENT. Nonsurgical management includes drug and diet therapy. The provision of physical and emotional rest are also important considerations.

NIC **DIARRHEA MANAGEMENT.** The purpose of diarrhea management (Chart 58-3) is the prevention and alleviation of diarrhea. It is important to instruct the client with exacerbations of diarrhea to record the color, volume, frequency, and consistency of stools to determine the severity of the problem. The nurse, in collaboration with the dietitian, assists in identifying factors that may cause or contribute to diarrhea.

The nurse monitors the skin in the perianal area for irritation and ulceration due to loose, frequent stools. Stool cultures may be sent if diarrhea continues. The client and family members are instructed in the appropriate use of antidiarrheal medications. The nurse or assistive nursing personnel weighs the client regularly. In severe exacerbations of the disease, the

CHART 58-3

NIC INTERVENTION ACTIVITIES *for*
The Client with Inflammatory Bowel Disease

Diarrhea Management: *Management and alleviation of diarrhea*
- Instruct client/family members to record color, volume, frequency, and consistency of stools.
- Identify factors (e.g., medications, bacteria, tube feedings) that may cause or contribute to diarrhea.
- Teach the client to eliminate gas-forming and spicy foods from diet.
- Suggest trial elimination of foods containing lactose.
- Instruct in low-fiber, high-protein, high-calorie diet, as appropriate.
- Teach client appropriate use of antidiarrheal medications.
- Monitor the skin in perianal area for irritation and ulceration.
- Weigh the client regularly.
- Perform actions to rest the bowel (NPO liquid diet).

Pain Management: *Alleviation of pain or a reduction in pain to a level of comfort that is acceptable to the client*
- Perform a comprehensive pain assessment to include location, characteristics, onset/duration, frequency, quality, intensity or severity of pain, and precipitating factors.
- Evaluate, with the client and the health care team, the effectiveness of past pain control measures that have been used.
- Reduce or eliminate factors that can precipitate or increase the pain experience (e.g., fear, fatigue, monotony, and lack of knowledge).
- Teach the use of nonpharmacologic measures (e.g., biofeedback, TENS, hypnosis, relaxation, guided imagery, music therapy, distraction, activity therapy, acupressure, hot/cold application, and massage) before, after and, if possible, during painful activities; before pain occurs or increases; and along with other pain relief measures.

NIC intervention activities selected from McCloskey, J.C., & Bulechek, G.M. (2000). *Nursing interventions classification (NIC)* (3rd ed.). St. Louis: Mosby. No part of this work is to be altered without prior written permission from the Publisher.
TENS, Transcutaneous electrical nerve stimulation.

nurse, in collaboration with the health care provider, performs actions to rest the bowel.

DRUG THERAPY. The health care provider prescribes a combination of drugs, including salicylate compounds, corticosteroids, immunosuppressants, and antidiarrheals.

Salicylate Compounds. Sulfasalazine (Azulfidine, PMS-Sulfasalazine✤) is one of the primary treatments for ulcerative colitis. It is thought to act by inhibiting prostaglandin synthesis. These compounds may be administered orally or rectally to reduce inflammation. Sulfasalazine is used to prevent recurrences of the disease, as well as to treat acute exacerbations of mild to moderate severity (Glickman, 1998). The usual dose of sulfasalazine is 2 to 4 g/day. The nurse teaches the client to take the drug with a full glass of water and to increase fluids throughout the day. The drug should be taken after meals to prevent GI discomfort. Blood dyscrasias, such as leukopenia and anemia, may occur.

Oral mesalamine (Asacol, Pentasa, Salofalk✤) is used for its anti-inflammatory effect in the acute phase of the illness. The recommended dose of Asacol is 800 mg three times a day or Pentasa 4 g daily in divided doses. Tablets should not be crushed, broken, or chewed. The drug is also available for rectal administration.

Olsalazine (Dipentum) 1 g daily is a salicylate used for maintenance therapy. Side effects of oral mesalamine include occasional flare-ups of colitis.

Clients with mild to moderate colitis of the distal bowel may be treated with mesalamine suppositories given two or three times daily or with retention enemas (Rowasa enema) given once daily at bedtime.

Corticosteroids. Oral or IV corticosteroid therapy may be prescribed during exacerbations of the disease. Prednisone (Deltasone, Winpred) 40 to 65 mg daily is usually given orally. For a severely ill client, prednisolone (Delta-Cortef) 45 to 60 mg daily may be given intravenously. Once clinical improvement has been established, the corticosteroids are tapered over a 2- to 3-month period following discharge because of the long-term adverse effects that commonly occur with steroid therapy. Examples include hyperglycemia (increased blood glucose), osteoporosis, peptic ulcer disease, and increased risk for infection. For clients with rectal symptoms, topical steroids in the form of small-retention enemas may be prescribed. Hydrocortisone rectal foam (Cortifoam) is ordered one to two times daily for 2 to 3 weeks, then every other day. Hydrocortisone enemas (Cortenema) are given at bedtime for 21 days, then tapered and discontinued.

Immunosuppressive Drugs. As single agents, immunosuppressive drugs are not effective in the treatment of ulcerative colitis. However, when given in combination with steroids, they may help to reduce the amount of steroids necessary to obtain a response. Cyclosporine given at 4 mg/kg/day can be beneficial in severely ill clients who might otherwise require a colectomy. Oral mercaptopurine (Purinethol) may be given at a dose of 1.5 to 2.5 mg/kg/day. The nurse observes for side effects of this medication, which include thrombocytopenia (decreased platelets), leukopenia (decreased white blood cells [WBCs]), anemia, renal failure, infection, headache, GI ulceration, stomatitis (oral cavity inflammation), and hepatotoxicity. Therefore it is important to monitor blood counts and note signs of infection.

Antidiarrheal Drugs. To provide symptomatic management of diarrhea, antidiarrheal drugs may be ordered. These drugs are given very cautiously, however, since they can precipitate colonic dilation and toxic megacolon. Common antidiarrheal drugs include diphenoxylate hydrochloride and atropine sulfate (Lomotil) and loperamide (Imodium).

DIET THERAPY. The severity of the client's ulcerative colitis determines the type of diet required. Clients may begin with one form of diet therapy and progress to a more advanced diet as symptoms diminish, with the goal of preventing hyperactive bowel activity.

Clients with severe symptoms are kept on NPO status to ensure bowel rest. The physician often orders total parenteral nutrition (TPN) for these clients (see Chapter 61). Clients with slightly less severe symptoms may be given elemental formulas, such as Vivonex or Ensure, which are absorbed in the upper bowel, thus minimizing bowel stimulation. Clients with significant but less severe symptoms may be restricted to a low-fiber (low-residue) diet. Clients following a low-fiber diet should avoid foods such as whole-wheat grains, nuts, and fresh fruits or fresh vegetables (Table 58-4). There is controversy whether fiber needs to be restricted during the chronic phase of the illness. If fiber intake does not induce symptoms, the intake of fiber need not be limited. However, because the role of diet in inflammatory bowel disease (IBD) is not well defined, and because individual tolerance to foods vary, clients with controlled symptoms may only need to limit or omit those foods that cause them discomfort or diarrhea.

Typically, lactose-containing foods are poorly tolerated and should be reduced or eliminated. All clients should be cautioned that caffeinated beverages, pepper, alcohol, and smoking are common GI stimulants that could cause discomfort.

REST. At the onset of treatment, activity is generally restricted because rest can reduce intestinal activity, provide comfort, and promote healing. The nurse ensures that the client has easy access to a bedpan, commode, or bathroom in case of urgency or tenesmus.

> **CRITICAL THINKING CHALLENGE**
> Your older client with ulcerative colitis has developed mouth ulcers and is complaining of stiffness in her joints. Her abdominal pain and diarrhea have improved with aggressive treatment, including immunosuppressives.
> - What relationship does the client's mouth sores and joint pain have to her disease process?
> - What possible complications of immunosuppressive therapy should you be alert for?
> - What laboratory values would be most important for you to monitor for in this client?
>
> For suggested answer guidelines, go to SIMON http://www.wbsaunders.com/SIMON/Iggy/.

TABLE 58-4 • GUIDELINES FOR A LOW-FIBER DIET

Foods Allowed	Foods Not Allowed
BEVERAGES Only 2 glasses of milk, if allowed, boiled or evaporated; strained fruit juices, coffee, tea, and carbonated beverages	Alcohol
EGGS Prepared in any manner, except fried	Fried
CHEESE Cottage, cream, milk, American, and Tillamook (use in small amounts)	Highly flavored
MEATS OR POULTRY Roasted, baked, or broiled tender beef, lamb, liver, veal, fish, chicken, or turkey	Tough meats, pork; fried or highly spiced meats
SOUPS Bouillon, broth, and strained cream soups from foods allowed	Any others
FATS Butter, margarine, oils, 30 mL (1 oz) of cream daily	None
VEGETABLES Canned or cooked vegetables, such as asparagus, beets, carrots, peas, potatoes, pumpkin, squash, spinach, and young string beans; tomato juice	Raw or whole cooked vegetables (e.g., potato with skin)
FRUITS Strained fruit juices; cooked or canned apples, apricots, Royal Ann cherries, peaches, pears, dried fruit purée, and ripe banana and avocado; all of the above *without skins or seeds*	All other raw or cooked fruits
BREAD AND CRACKERS Refined bread, toast, rolls, and crackers	Pancakes, waffles, and whole-grain bread or rolls
CEREALS Cooked cereal, such as Cream of Wheat, Malt-O Meal, strained oatmeal, cornmeal, cornflakes, puffed rice, Rice Krispies, and puffed wheat	Whole-grain cereals; other prepared cereals
POTATOES/RICE/PASTA White rice, macaroni, noodles, and spaghetti	Fried potato, potato chips, and brown rice
DESSERTS Gelatin desserts, tapioca, angel food or sponge cake, plain custards, water ice or ice cream without fruit or nuts, and rennet or simple puddings	Rich pastries, pies, and anything with nuts or dried fruit
SWEETS Sugar, jelly, honey, syrups, gumdrops, hard candy, plain creams, milk chocolate	Other candy; jam, marmalade
MISCELLANEOUS FOODS Cream sauce and plain gravy	Nuts, olives, popcorn, rich gravies, pepper, spices, and vinegar

Modified from Williams, S. R. (1998). *Nutrition and diet therapy* (8th ed.). St. Louis: Mosby.

SURGICAL MANAGEMENT. Approximately 20% to 25% of individuals with ulcerative colitis require a colectomy (Glickman, 1998). Indications for surgery include bowel perforation, toxic megacolon, hemorrhage, colon cancer, and conventional treatment failure. The surgeon may choose one of several surgical procedures to alleviate these problems.

TOTAL PROCTOCOLECTOMY WITH A PERMANENT ILEOSTOMY.
Total proctocolectomy (or colectomy) with a permanent ileostomy has traditionally been the standard surgical procedure for clients undergoing a colectomy.

Preoperative Care. When an ileostomy is indicated, the nurse provides extensive explanations to the client and family or significant other. Preoperative teaching includes aspects that relate to abdominal surgery (see Chapter 17) and those that relate to ileostomy. The surgeon consults with the enterostomal therapist (ET) preoperatively for recommendations on the location of the ostomy (stoma). (An ET is a nurse specializing and certified in skin and ostomy care.) A visit from an ostomate (a client with an ostomy) may be appropriate before surgery if the client agrees to this. The surgeon orders oral or parenteral antibiotics, such as neomycin sulfate (Mycifradin, Neo-fradin), as a bowel antiseptic. Mechanical cleansing of the bowel with enemas or laxatives may also be required.

Operative Procedure. During a total proctocolectomy with a traditional permanent ileostomy, the colon, rectum, and anus are removed, followed by closure of the anus. The surgeon brings the end of the terminal ileum out through the abdominal wall and forms a stoma, or ostomy. The stoma is usually placed in the right lower quadrant of the abdomen, below the belt line (Figure 58-2). The surgeon makes a perineal incision to remove the rectum and supporting tissues.

Postoperative Care. Initially after surgery, the output from the ileostomy is a loose, dark green liquid that may contain some blood. Over time, a process called ileostomy adaptation occurs. The small intestine begins to absorb increased amounts of sodium and water (a former function of the large intestine, which was removed by surgery). Stool volume decreases, becomes thicker (pastelike), and turns yellow-green or yellow-brown. The effluent (fluid material) usually has little odor or a sweet odor. Any foul or unpleasant odor may be a symptom of some underlying problem (e.g., blockage or infection).

Depending on the frequency and irritation of stool drainage, the client must wear a pouch system at all times. Disposable systems are most often used.

Prevention of skin problems (irritation, excoriation, ulceration) is critical for the client with an ileostomy. The output from the small intestine is rich in proteolytic enzymes and bile salts, which can quickly irritate and injure the skin. A pouch system that has some type of skin barrier (gelatin or pectin) provides sufficient protection for most clients. Other products are also available.

Most clients undergoing surgical intervention for ulcerative colitis have lived with chronic illness for some time. They may view surgery positively as a relief from the multiple problems caused by the disease. Initially, however, they may not perceive life with an ileostomy as a positive alternative.

Total proctocolectomy with a permanent ileostomy results in an alteration in appearance and body function. The goals for a client undergoing this procedure are to become proficient in self-care, to adapt his or her lifestyle to include care of an ostomy, and to successfully resume presurgery activities.

TOTAL COLECTOMY WITH A CONTINENT ILEOSTOMY.
As an alternative to the traditional ileostomy with an external pouch, the surgeon may create an internal system—a Kock's ileostomy or ileal reservoir. This procedure is sometimes referred to as a continent ileostomy. The surgeon constructs an intra-abdominal pouch or reservoir from the terminal ileum (Figure 58-3), where stool is stored in the pouch until it is drained by the client using a soft rubber catheter. The care of a Kock's ileostomy involves the connection of the pouch to the stoma, which is constructed with a nipple-like valve made from an intussuscepted portion of the ileum. The stoma is flush with the skin.

The nursing care of the client undergoing this procedure is similar to the care of the client undergoing a proctocolectomy with a permanent ileostomy (see the previous section). Immediately postoperatively, an indwelling Foley catheter is placed in the pouch, which is connected to low intermittent suction and irrigated as ordered.

The nurse monitors the character and quality of effluent (drainage). Approximately 2 weeks after surgery, the nurse teaches the client to drain the stoma. Initially, the pouch holds only 50 to 75 mL; over time, the pouch capacity reaches 500 to 700 mL. When the pouch needs to be emptied, the client experiences a sensation of fullness. The client drains the pouch several times a day and wears a small dressing over the stoma to keep it moist and to protect clothing from the moist stoma. This procedure has several advantages. The client does not need to wear an external pouch for collection of stool and experiences minimal skin problems. Unfortunately, the need

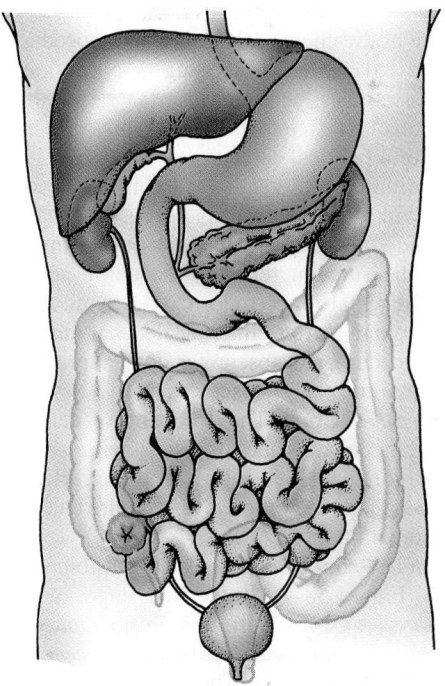

Figure 58-2 ● Total proctocolectomy with a permanent ileostomy. This involved removal of the colon, the rectum, and the anus with closure of the anus. Note the missing colon, rectum, and anus with the resultant stoma in the right lower quadrant.

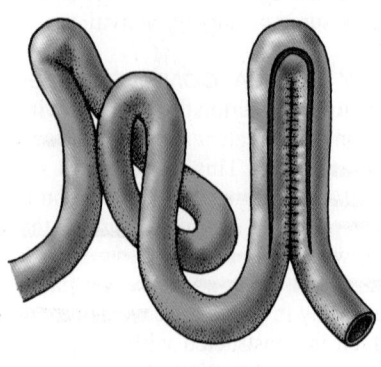
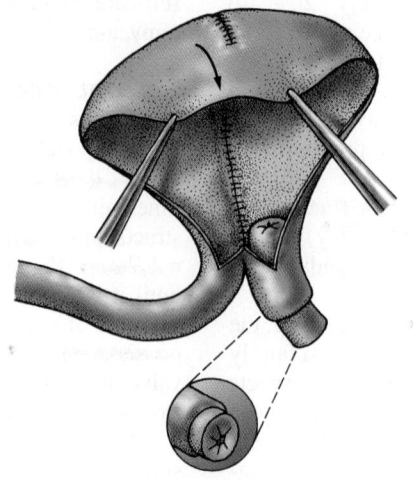
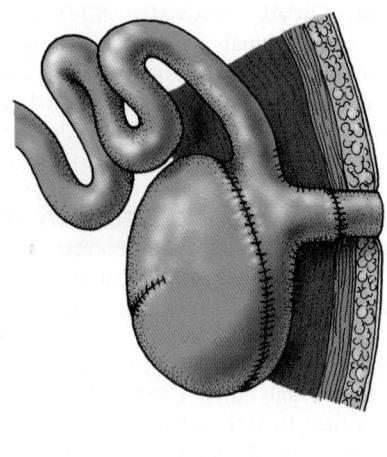
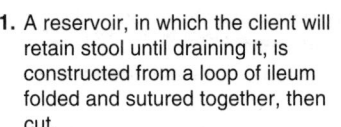

1. A reservoir, in which the client will retain stool until draining it, is constructed from a loop of ileum folded and sutured together, then cut.

2. A portion of the ileum is intussuscepted to form a nipple valve, and the upper part of the stitched and cut ileum is pulled down and sutured to form a pouch.

3. The nipple valve, which shuts tight against pressure from a filled pouch, is pulled through the stoma and sutured flush with the abdomen.

Figure 58-3 ● The creation of a Kock's (continent) ileostomy.

for frequent revisions and problems with leakage have made this procedure less desirable.

TOTAL COLECTOMY WITH ILEOANAL ANASTOMOSIS; ILEOANAL RESERVOIR.

During a total colectomy with ileoanal anastomosis, the surgeon removes the colon and the rectum and sutures the ileum into the anal canal. Usually continence is excellent following this procedure, but up to 20% of clients will have some nocturnal leakage of stool. The nursing care of the client undergoing this procedure is similar to the care of clients undergoing a colectomy. With an ileoanal anastomosis, perineal irritation is a common occurrence as a result of frequent, loose stools. The nurse should provide careful perineal care.

The creation of an ileoanal reservoir has become popular for clients with ulcerative colitis because it spares the rectal sphincter and eliminates the need for an ostomy. During this procedure, the surgeon removes the colon and sutures the ileum into the rectal stump to form a reservoir. If residual rectal mucosa remains after either an ileoanal anastomosis or a reservoir procedure, proctoscopy is done at predetermined intervals to monitor for dysplasia.

Preoperative Care. The preoperative care for a client undergoing an ileoanal anastomosis is similar to that for a client undergoing an ileostomy. However, clients will not have an ostomy and therefore do not require consultation with an enterostomal therapist (ET).

Operative Procedure. Ileoanal anastomosis occurs in two stages (Figure 58-4). In the first stage, the surgeon excises the rectal mucosa, performs an abdominal colectomy, constructs the reservoir or pouch to the anal canal, and creates a temporary loop ileostomy. The loop ileostomy is necessary to allow adequate healing of the internal pouch and all anastomosis sites and to allow for an increase in the capacity of the internal reservoir through fluid instillations. After 3 to 4 months the client returns to have the loop ileostomy closed.

Stool formation resembles that in clients who have undergone a traditional ileostomy.

Postoperative Care. The nurse provides the usual postoperative interventions for clients who have undergone abdominal surgery. All clients requiring surgical intervention for ulcerative colitis have an abdominal incision. Initially, most clients are maintained on NPO status and a nasogastric (NG) tube is used for suction.

■ ACUTE PAIN; CHRONIC PAIN

NOC PLANNING: EXPECTED OUTCOMES. The client with ulcerative colitis is expected to experience relief from painful abdominal cramping and skin irritation as indicated by self-report.

INTERVENTIONS. Pain control may be accomplished through pharmacologic and nonpharmacologic measures. The client's symptoms can cause physical discomfort, which can also contribute to emotional discomfort. The use of a variety of symptom-reducing interventions and supportive measures can provide increased comfort.

NIC PAIN MANAGEMENT. The purpose of pain management is the alleviation of pain or a reduction in pain to a level of comfort that is acceptable to the client (see Chart 58-3). The client with ulcerative colitis experiences abdominal pain and cramping, particularly with exacerbations of the disease. Increases in pain may also signal the development of complications such as peritonitis. Frequent bowel movements can cause skin irritation and increase the client's discomfort. The nurse performs a comprehensive pain assessment. With the client and the health care team, the nurse evaluates the effectiveness of past pain control measures used.

The nurse assists the client in reducing or eliminating factors that can precipitate or increase the pain experience. An-

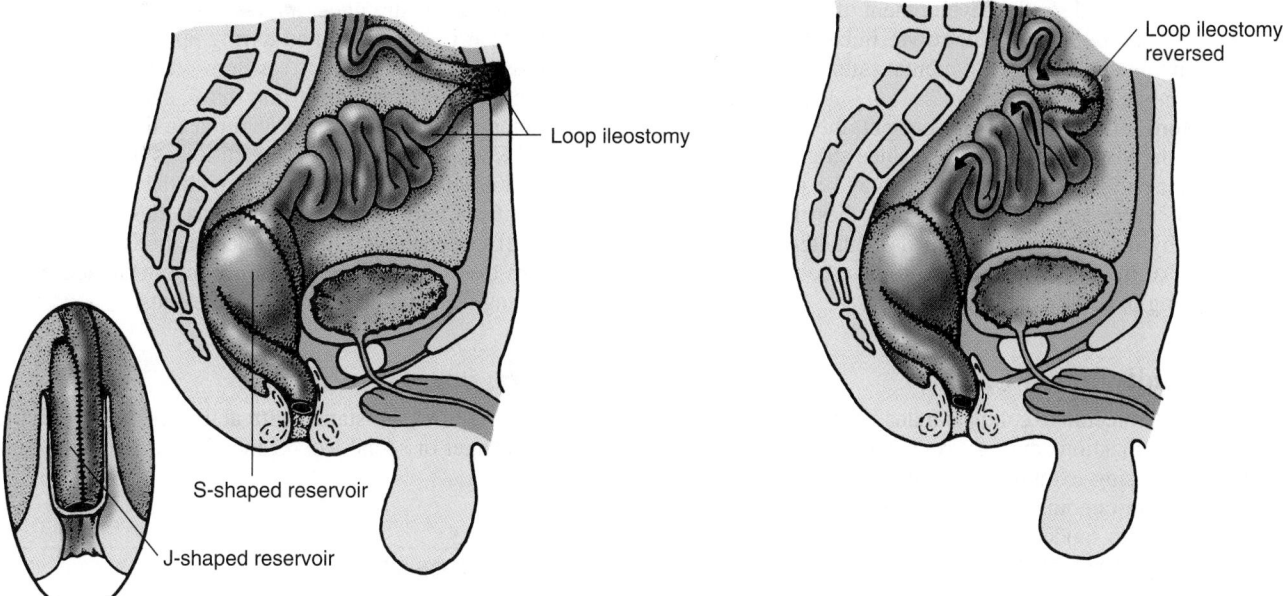

Stage 1.
After removal of the colon, a temporary loop ileostomy is created and an ileoanal reservoir is formed. The reservoir is created in an S-shaped reservoir (using three loops of ileum) or a J-shaped reservoir (suturing a portion of ileum to the rectal cuff, with an upward loop).

Stage 2.
After the reservoir has had time to heal–usually several months–the temporary loop ileostomy is reversed, and stool is allowed to drain into the reservoir.

Figure 58-4   ●   The creation of an ileoanal reservoir.

tidiarrheal medications may be prescribed to control diarrhea but must be used cautiously, since they can precipitate toxic megacolon. The client may benefit from diet teaching and meal planning as a means of decreasing abdominal discomfort related to cramping and bloating. Excoriated skin can contribute to pain and discomfort. Scrupulous skin care prevents painful excoriation of the skin. The nurse can also teach the client to use nonpharmacologic measures (e.g., biofeedback, music therapy, guided imagery) as a means of pain modification.

DRUG THERAPY. Antidiarrheal medications are used to control diarrhea and thereby reduce the resulting discomfort. These must be used with caution, since toxic megacolon can develop. The physician may prescribe anticholinergics, such as propantheline bromide (Pro-Banthine), before meals to provide relief from the pain and cramping that may occur with diarrhea. Opioids are used sparingly and cautiously, since these drugs can mask symptoms of life-threatening complications.

DIET THERAPY. Dietary measures help to control symptoms and thereby promote relief from discomfort. The nurse assesses the client's needs for diet teaching and evaluates the effects of implemented dietary measures on an ongoing basis.

PERINEAL SKIN CARE. Perineal skin can be irritated by frequent contact with loose stools and frequent cleaning. This irritation can be a major contributor to the client's discomfort. The nurse explains special measures for skin care. For example, cleaning the perineal area with mild soap and warm water after each bowel movement keeps the skin free of any stool.

Frequent sitz baths may be helpful, particularly after a bowel movement. The application of a thin coat of mineral oil, petroleum jelly, vitamin A and D ointment, aloe creams, or medicated foam applications may provide relief. Use of medicated wipes with witch hazel (e.g., Tucks) is soothing if the rectal area is tender or sensitive from the use of toilet tissue.

Various manufacturers of ostomies (e.g., Hollister and Convatec) produce a three-product system for skin care that may help prevent and heal perineal skin irritation, thus relieving discomfort. Such systems include a skin-cleaning solution, a moisturizing and healing cream, and a petroleum jelly–like ointment that prevents contact of moisture and stool with the skin.

■ POTENTIAL FOR GASTROINTESTINAL BLEEDING

PLANNING: EXPECTED OUTCOMES. The client with ulcerative colitis is expected to experience a reduction in or cessation of the gastrointestinal (GI) bleeding that accompanies chronic ulcerative colitis. The client is also expected to remain free of complications of the disease that can cause bleeding, such as perforation.

INTERVENTIONS. The nurse's primary responsibility is to monitor the client closely for signs and symptoms of GI bleeding resulting from acute disease or complications. All stools are monitored for blood, using both gross and occult examination. The nurse monitors the client's hematocrit, hemoglobin, and electrolyte values for abnormalities. The nurse or assistive nursing personnel monitors the client's vital signs.

The client is observed for the development of fever, tachycardia, fluid volume depletion, electrolyte imbalances, and severe abdominal pain. Changes in mental status may be noted, especially among older adults.

If symptoms of GI bleeding are present, the nurse notifies the health care provider immediately, since surgical intervention may be necessary. Blood products may be necessary for clients with severe anemia. The nurse readies the client for transfusion by inserting a large-bore IV catheter for the administration of blood. Chapter 56 describes the management of GI bleeding in detail.

Community-Based Care

The client with ulcerative colitis is managed at home but may require hospitalization during exacerbations. In addition, clients experiencing extraintestinal manifestations of the disease will require ongoing management of joint or skin problems. Clients with moderate to severe ulcerative colitis have more acute exacerbations than those with milder forms of the disease. Such clients may benefit from case manager services to coordinate and facilitate quality care in a cost-effective way.

HOME CARE MANAGEMENT

For clients with ulcerative colitis, home care management focuses on managing symptoms and monitoring for complications. The nurse instructs the client in measures to reduce or control abdominal pain, cramping, and diarrhea. The nurse also instructs the client and family members regarding symptoms that should be reported immediately to the health care provider. For clients returning home or transferring to nursing home or subacute care following surgery, ongoing respiratory care, incision care, ostomy care, and pain management are additional concerns.

HEALTH TEACHING

The nurse educates the client about the nature of ulcerative colitis with regard to its acute episodes, remissions, and symptom management. The nurse emphasizes that even though the cause is unknown, relapses can be resolved with proper health care.

The nurse teaches the client dietary measures to reduce bloating and cramping. The client needs to learn what foods are best tolerated and adjust his or her diet accordingly. The nurse teaches about prescribed medications and medication side effects to remain alert for. Clients taking immunosuppressive drugs should be taught to report signs of infection, such as sore throat, to the health care provider. The nurse prepares written instructions for the client and family members about the signs of colonic dilation and perforation and reiterates the importance of notifying the health care provider if these signs occur.

If the client has undergone a surgical diversion to manage colon effluent, the nurse or enterostomal therapist (ET) explains and demonstrates the required care. The client is encouraged to demonstrate self-care of the ileostomy. The nurse also teaches clients with an ileostomy to include adequate amounts of salt and water in their diets because the ileostomy promotes the loss of these elements. They are taught to be cautious in situations that promote profuse sweating or fluid loss, such as during strenuous physical activities, when environmental heat is excessive, and during episodes of diarrhea and vomiting. Chart 58-4 describes ileostomy care in detail.

A client with an ileostomy may have multiple concerns about management at home and about sexual and social adjustments. Considering possible sexual issues helps the client to identify and discuss these concerns with the sexual partner. Social situations may precipitate some anxieties related to decreased self-esteem and a disturbance in body image. The nurse helps the client explore possible concerns in addressing and resolving these potentially stressful events.

HEALTH CARE RESOURCES

If the client requires assistance with activities of daily living, the case manager or social worker may help arrange the serv-

---

CHART 58-4

CLIENT EDUCATION GUIDE
Ileostomy Care

Pouch Care
- Empty your pouch when it is one-third to one-half full.
- Change the pouch during inactive times, such as before meals, before retiring at night, on waking in the morning, and 2 to 4 hours after eating.
- Change the entire pouch system every 3 to 7 days.

Skin Protection
- Use a pectin-based skin barrier (not karaya gum) to protect your skin from contact with contents from the ostomy.
- Use skin care products, such as skin sealants and ostomy skin creams, if your skin continues to come into contact with ostomy contents.
- Watch your skin for any irritation or redness.

Diet
- Chew food thoroughly.
- Be cautious of high-fiber and high-cellulose foods. You may need to eliminate these from the diet if they cause severe problems (diarrhea, constipation, or blockage). Examples include popcorn, peanuts, coconut, Chinese vegetables, string beans, tough-fiber meats, shrimp and lobster, rice, bran, and skinned vegetables (tomatoes, corn, and peas).

Medications
- Avoid taking enteric-coated and capsule medications.
- Inform any health care provider who is prescribing medications for you that you have an ostomy. Before having prescriptions filled, inform your pharmacist that you have an ostomy.
- Do not take any laxatives or enemas. You should usually have loose stool and should contact a physician if no stool has passed in 6 to 12 hours.

Symptoms to Watch for
- Report any drastic increase or decrease in drainage to your health care provider.
- If stomal swelling, abdominal cramping, or distention occurs, or if ileostomy contents stop draining, do the following:
  - Remove the pouch with faceplate.
  - Lie down, assuming a knee-chest position.
  - Begin abdominal massage.
  - Apply moist towels to the abdomen.
  - Drink hot tea.
  - If none of these maneuvers is effective in resuming ileostomy flow, or if abdominal pain is severe, call your health care provider right away.

ices of a home care aide. If the client is discharged from the hospital with an ileostomy, the case manager makes a referral to a home care agency. A home care nurse can provide assessment and guidance in integrating ostomy care into the client's lifestyle and possibly provide wound care, including the monitoring of wound healing (Chart 58-5). The client needs to know where to purchase ostomy supplies, along with the name, size, and manufacturer's order number. The ET or case manager contacts local and regional supply companies for prices and availability of supplies.

The nurse or ET can identify the local ostomy support group by contacting the United Ostomy Association. A support group or the Crohn's and Colitis Foundation of America may be of assistance in obtaining supplies, as well as providing education for ostomates. The nurse also informs the client and family or significant others of available ostomy outpatient clinics and ETs. If the client agrees, a visit from an ostomate can be initiated or continued on an outpatient basis.

● Evaluation: Outcomes

NOC The nurse evaluates the care of the client with ulcerative colitis on the basis of the identified nursing diagnoses and collaborative problems. Expected outcomes may include that the client will:

- Be free of diarrhea, rectal bleeding, and cramping
- Maintain adequate hydration
- Understand the factors that can influence exacerbations of the disease
- Maintain ideal body weight
- Understand and adhere to the prescribed drug regimen
- Remain free of complications of the disease
- Identify and seek care for extraintestinal manifestations of the disease

In addition, the client with an ileostomy can be expected to:

- Engage in self-care of the ileostomy
- Maintain peristomal skin integrity
- Demonstrate behaviors that integrate ostomy care into his or her lifestyle
- Verbalize signs and symptoms of stoma complications

Crohn's Disease

▌ OVERVIEW

Crohn's disease, also known as *regional enteritis* or *granulomatous colitis,* is a chronic inflammatory bowel disease (IBD) that can affect any part of the gastrointestinal (GI) tract, from the mouth to the anus. Approximately one million people in the United States have the disease (Klonowski & Masoodi, 1999). The peak incidence is between 15 and 40 years of age. The cause of Crohn's disease is uncertain; however, infectious, genetic, and immune etiologies have been proposed.

Mycobacterium paratuberculosis has been proposed as an environmental stimulus that could be implicated in the development of Crohn's disease, since granulomas similar to those seen in individuals with pulmonary tuberculosis have been found on biopsy of the intestines of people with the disease. A genetic predisposition to the disease has also been proposed, since the disease tends to cluster in families and appears equally in identical twins. However, the most widely accepted cause is believed to be a defect in the immunoregulation of in-

flammation in the presence of bacteria or viruses in the intestinal tract, along with a genetic predisposition for the disease (Norton, 1998).

Chronic, nonspecific inflammation of the entire intestinal tract characterizes the disease, with the terminal ileum being the site most often affected. Eventually, deep fissures and ulcerations develop and often extend through all bowel layers, predisposing the individual to the development of bowel fistulas. The result is severe diarrhea and malabsorption of vital nutrients. Chronic pathologic changes include thickening of the bowel wall, resulting in narrowing of the bowel lumen and strictures. In advanced disease, the bowel mucosa demonstrates nodular swelling (granulomas) intermingled with deep ulcerations.

The complications associated with Crohn's disease are similar to those of ulcerative colitis. As shown in Table 58-3, hemorrhage is more common in ulcerative colitis but can occur in Crohn's disease as well (see the Evidence-Based Practice for Nursing box on p. 1284). Severe malabsorption by the small intestine is more common in clients with Crohn's disease. Cancer of the small bowel and colon may develop in the client with Crohn's disease but usually occurs after the disease has been present for 15 to 20 years. Fistula formation is a common complication of Crohn's disease. Fistulas can occur between segments of the intestine or present as cutaneous fistulas or perirectal abscesses. Fistulas can also extend from the bowel to other organs and body cavities, such as the bladder or vagina (Figure 58-5). Twenty to thirty percent of individuals with the disease will develop intestinal obstruction. Initially, obstruction results from inflammation and edema. Over time, fibrosis develops and obstruction results secondary to a narrowing of the bowel (Glickman, 1998).

CHART 58-5

FOCUSED ASSESSMENT *of*
Home Care of Clients with Inflammatory Bowel Disease

Assess gastrointestinal function and nutritional status, including:
- Abdominal cramping or pain
- Bowel elimination pattern; specifically frequency, characteristics and amount of stools, presence or absence of blood in stools
- Dietary and fluid intake and habits (include relationship of specific foods to cramping and stools)
- Weight gain or loss
- Signs and symptoms of dehydration
- Presence or absence of fever, rectal tenesmus, or urgency
- Bowel sounds
- Condition of perianal skin, including presence or absence of perianal fistula or abscess

Assess client's and family's coping skills, including:
- Current and ongoing stress level and coping style
- Availability of support system

Assess home environment, including:
- Adequacy and availability of bathroom facilities
- Opportunity for rest and relaxation

Assess ability to manage therapeutic regimen, including:
- Knowledge of medications
- Signs and symptoms to report
- Dietary management
- Availability of community resources
- Importance of follow-up care

EVIDENCE-BASED PRACTICE
FOR NURSING

What are the characteristics of clients with acute lower gastrointestinal bleeding related to Crohn's disease?

Belaiche, J., et al. (1999). Acute lower gastrointestinal bleeding in Crohn's disease: Characteristics of a unique series of 34 patients. *American Journal of Gastroenterology, 94*(8), 2177-2181.

The purpose of this study was to assess the characteristics of clients with lower gastrointestinal (GI) bleeding related to Crohn's disease. In this study, 34 clients presenting to the hospital with lower GI bleeding were identified and data concerning the following characteristics were analyzed: client characteristics, blood transfusion requirements, site of bleeding, treatment, and follow-up.

In eight clients, the first manifestation of Crohn's disease was an episode of severe bleeding. Clients received 1 to 5 units of blood. The hemorrhage was found to be more frequent in clients with colonic disease than in those with disease confined to the small bowel. In 95% of cases, bleeding was caused by an area of ulceration, usually found in the sigmoid colon. Treatment consisted of blood transfusions and supportive measures such as corticosteroids, immunosuppressants, or endoscopy to identify the lesion and to apply either laser coagulation or adrenaline to stop bleeding from the lesion. Treatment was successful in 80% of clients with a first-time bleed. Bleeding was not significantly associated with steroid therapy in this study. In follow-up, 12 clients experienced recurrent bleeding episodes.

Critique. The relatively small sample size and convenience sampling method limits the generalizability of the findings. The definition and severity of GI bleeding may vary across the several medical centers used for subject recruitment, although the authors attempted to standardize this by recruiting subjects who received 2 or more units of blood.

Implications for Nursing. Although the results of the study cannot be generalized to all clients with Crohn's disease, new data about the presentation of the disease and its course were presented. The characteristics of hemorrhagic forms of Crohn's disease are not well described in the literature. This study can serve to make nurses more aware of bleeding as a complication more often associated with the disease than was previously thought. Nurses who care for individuals with disease in the colon can monitor their clients more closely for GI bleeding. Also, the study finding that more conservative treatments were successful in treating 80% of first-time hemorrhages can be shared with clients. Finally, although steroids were not associated with the development of bleeding in this study, other medications can increase the risk of GI bleeding. Clients need to be taught to avoid nonsteroidal anti-inflammatory drugs or aspirin-containing products while taking steroids, since the risk of bleeding increases. In addition, concomitant warfarin treatment may also increase the risk of bleeding.

CULTURAL CONSIDERATIONS

Crohn's disease is more common among people of Jewish descent, Caucasians of Western cultures, and those of middle European origin. The incidence of Crohn's disease is 20% greater in women than in men.

► COLLABORATIVE MANAGEMENT

● Assessment

■ HISTORY

A detailed history will assist in uncovering signs and symptoms specific to Crohn's disease. A history of fever, abdominal pain, and loose stools is commonly seen in a client with Crohn's disease. He or she is asked about recent unintentional loss of weight. The nurse should ask about the frequency, consistency, and presence of blood in the stool. The nurse also ascertains if the client has any first-degree relatives with the disease.

■ PHYSICAL ASSESSMENT/CLINICAL MANIFESTATIONS

The nurse performs a thorough abdominal examination, assesses for clinical manifestations of the disease, and evaluates the client's nutritional and hydration status. When performing an abdominal assessment, the nurse often notes findings that are consistent with those in acute appendicitis (e.g., tenderness, guarded movement, and a palpable mass in the right lower quadrant).

On inspection of the abdomen, the nurse assesses for distention, masses, or visible peristalsis. Inspection of the perianal area may reveal ulcerations or fissures. During auscultation, bowel sounds may be decreased or absent in the client with severe inflammation or obstruction. An increase in high-pitched or rushing sounds may be present over areas of narrowed bowel loops. Muscle guarding, masses, rigidity, or tenderness may be noted on palpation.

The clinical presentation of Crohn's disease can vary greatly from client to client. Depending on the parts of the bowel involved, the nurse may identify several clinical manifestations. Most clients report diarrhea, abdominal pain, and low-grade fever. Fever is also commonly present with complications such as fistulas and severe inflammation. If the disease occurs only in the ileum, diarrhea occurs five or six times per day, often with a soft, loose stool. Steatorrhea (fatty diarrheal stools) is common. The stool may contain bright red blood, but this is a rare finding.

Abdominal pain from the inflammatory process is usually constant and is located in the right lower quadrant. Clients also experience periumbilical pain before and after bowel movements. If the lower colon is diseased, pain is often experienced in both lower abdominal quadrants.

Weight loss is experienced by approximately 80% of individuals with Crohn's disease. Clients often experience nutritional problems as a result of increased catabolism secondary to chronic inflammation, anorexia, malabsorption, or self-imposed dietary restrictions. The result is fluid and electrolyte imbalances, as well as protein, iron, vitamin, and mineral deficiencies.

The marked inflammatory bowel changes decrease the small bowel's ability to absorb nutrients, which may be worsened by surgery and fistulas. The nurse is acutely aware of how important it is to detect clinical manifestations of peritonitis, bowel obstruction, and nutritional and fluid imbalances. The early detection of a change in the client's status helps to minimize these life-threatening complications.

■ PSYCHOSOCIAL ASSESSMENT

The client experiencing Crohn's disease needs a complete psychosocial assessment. The chronicity of the problem and the troublesome complications can greatly affect clients and their families. The assessment should be ongoing and should continuously reflect the client's status, as well as the family's.

■ DIAGNOSTIC ASSESSMENT

The health care provider may order a number of laboratory studies for clients with Crohn's disease; however, no disease-specific tests are available to confirm the diagnosis. The re-

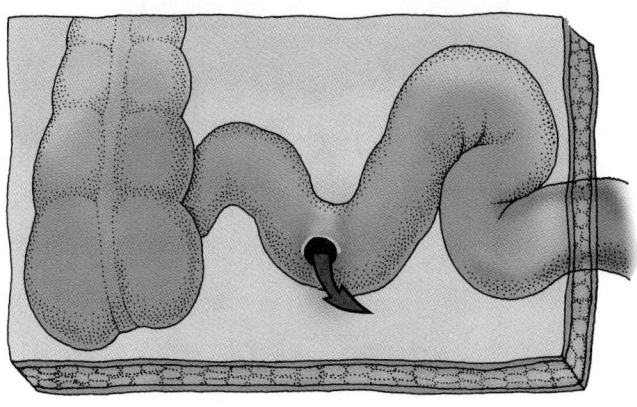

External enterocutaneous
(between skin and intestine)

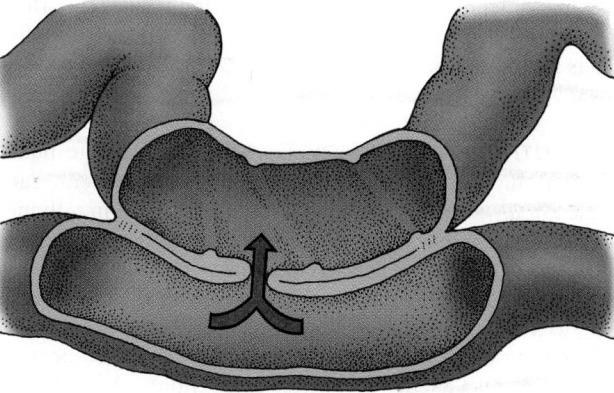

Enteroenteric
(between intestine and intestine)

Figure 58-5 ● The types of fistulas that are complications of Crohn's disease.

sults of laboratory tests often indicate the extent and severity of inflammation associated with the disease.

If bleeding is present, the client may experience anemia. The nurse may note decreased hemoglobin and hematocrit values as a result of slow blood loss. Serum levels of folic acid and cobalamin (vitamin B_{12} group) are generally low because of malabsorption, further contributing to anemia. Amino acid malabsorption may result in decreased albumin levels. An elevated erythrocyte sedimentation rate (ESR) is consistent with the presence of inflammation. White blood cells (WBCs) in the urine may indicate infection (pyuria), which may be caused by ureteral obstruction or an enterovesical (bowel to bladder) fistula. If significant diarrhea is present, the client will experience electrolyte losses, particularly potassium and magnesium.

The results of the contrast barium enema and upper gastrointestinal (GI) series often provide more specific diagnostic information. X-ray studies show narrowing, ulcerations, strictures, and fistulas consistent with Crohn's disease. In the acute illness, these tests are often deferred until the risk of perforation lessens.

Depending on which areas of the bowel are diseased, the sigmoidoscopic examination may not be diagnostic. If the rectosigmoid colon is involved, the physician may see ulcerations and inflamed mucosa, areas of fissure, fistula, and abscess formation of the perianal and perirectal areas.

Colonoscopy is used when other tests, especially the barium enema examination, have not led to a specific diagnosis.

● Interventions

Treatment of Crohn's disease is similar to that described earlier under Nonsurgical Management (Ulcerative Colitis), p. 1276.

NONSURGICAL MANAGEMENT. Specific interventions vary with the severity of disease and complications present.

DRUG THERAPY. The drugs used to manage Crohn's disease are similar to those used in the treatment of ulcerative colitis (see Drug Therapy [Ulcerative Colitis], p. 1277). Sulfasalazine (Asulfidine, PMS-Sulfasalazine♣) 1.5 to 2 g twice a day PO has been shown to be effective in treating exacerbations of Crohn's disease. Although glucocorticoids can be effective, sepsis can result from abscesses or fistulas that may

be present. These medications mask the symptoms of infection; therefore they must be used with caution and require vigilant monitoring by the nurse for signs of infection.

Metronidazole (Flagyl, Novonidazol♣) 250 to 500 mg three times a day PO has been helpful in clients with fistulas. Immunosuppressive therapy has been effective in clients with refractory disease or fistulas. Azathioprine (Imuran), an immunosuppressive agent, 50 mg/day for 12 months may be instituted. After that time the health care provider may attempt to withdraw the drug, but long-term therapy may be needed in some cases.

Since a defect in immunoregulation of inflammation may be implicated in the development of Crohn's disease, neutralization of a cytokine (specifically, tumor necrosis factor) may prove useful in decreasing bowel inflammation. A relatively new drug, infliximab (Remicade) a chimeric monoclonal antibody form of antitumor necrosis factor alpha, has been approved for use. The usual dose of 5 mg/kg has demonstrated efficacy in the treatment of active Crohn's disease and fistulas. Further investigation is needed to determine the long-term safety and efficacy of the drug (Mikula, 1999).

NUTRITIONAL MANAGEMENT. Long-standing nutritional deficits can have severe consequences for the client with Crohn's disease. Malnutrition can result in poor fistula and wound healing, loss of lean muscle mass, decreased immune system response, and increased morbidity and mortality. With severe exacerbations of the disease, the health care provider may order hospitalization to provide bowel rest and nutritional enhancement with total parenteral nutrition (TPN). For less severe exacerbations, the health care provider may prescribe an elemental diet using products such as Vivonex to induce remission. Elemental diets are absorbed in the jejunum and therefore permit rest of the distal small intestine and colon. Once remission is achieved, the health care provider will usually prescribe a low-residue diet. Nutritional supplements, such as Ensure or Sustacal, can be added to provide nutrients and added calories.

COMPLICATION MANAGEMENT. **Fistulas** (abnormal tract from intestine to skin or intestine to intestine) are common occurrences with acute exacerbations of Crohn's disease. Clients with fistulas often experience complications, such as systemic infections, skin problems, malnutrition, and fluid and electrolyte imbalances. Treatment of the client with a fistula is multidimensional and includes nutrition and electrolyte therapy, skin care, and prevention of infection.

ELECTROLYTE THERAPY. Establishing adequate nutrition and fluid and electrolyte balance takes priority in the care of the client with a fistula. GI secretions are high in volume, electrolytes, and enzymes. The client is at high risk for malnutrition, dehydration, and hypokalemia. The nurse assesses for these complications and collaborates with the health care team to manage them.

The physician orders fluids and electrolyte replacement by oral liquids and nutrients, as well as IV fluids. An antidiarrheal agent, such as diphenoxylate hydrochloride or atropine sulfate (Lomotil), may be prescribed to decrease fluid loss from diarrhea, but these drugs are not commonly used and must be given with caution.

When a fistula begins to develop, the client's nutritional status is usually compromised. After the fistula has developed, nutritional status worsens. The client requires at least 3000 calories/day to promote healing of the fistula. If the client cannot take adequate oral fluids and nutrients, the physician may order TPN. In collaboration with the dietitian, the nurse:

* Carefully monitors the client's tolerance to diet
* Assists the client in selecting high-calorie, high-protein, high-vitamin, low-fiber meals
* Offers enteral supplements, such as Ensure and Vivonex
* Records food intake for accurate calorie counts

SKIN CARE. Proteolytic enzymes and bile contribute to the problem of skin irritation and excoriation. Skin irritation needs to be prevented; this is usually accomplished through the use of skin barriers, application of pouches, and insertion of drains (Figure 58-6). By applying a pouch to the draining fistula, the nurse prevents skin irritation and can measure the effluent (drainage).

In one approach to drainage management, the nurse covers the area surrounding the fistula with barriers, such as Stomahesive or DuoDerm, and then applies a wound drainage system over the fistula, securing it to the protective dressing. The skin adjacent to the fistula is cleaned with normal saline solution and gently patted dry.

The nurse collaborates with the enterostomal therapist (ET) to provide wound management. Wound drainage must *never* be allowed to be in direct contact with skin without prompt cleaning, because intestinal fluid enzymes are caustic.

PREVENTION OF INFECTION. Clients with fistulas are at extremely high risk for intra-abdominal abscesses and sepsis. Intra-abdominal fistulas are treated with careful nursing interventions, containment of wound drainage, and antibiotic therapy. The nurse observes for subtle signs of infection or sepsis, such as fever, abdominal pain, or change in mental status.

SURGICAL MANAGEMENT. Surgery to remove diseased portions of intestine is controversial for clients with Crohn's disease because risk for recurrence is considerable. However, those who continue to have symptoms after long-term medical treatment and those with complications such as fistulas may undergo a small-bowel resection and anastomosis with or without a colon resection to improve quality of life (see the Legal/Ethical Issues in Health Care box on p. 1287).

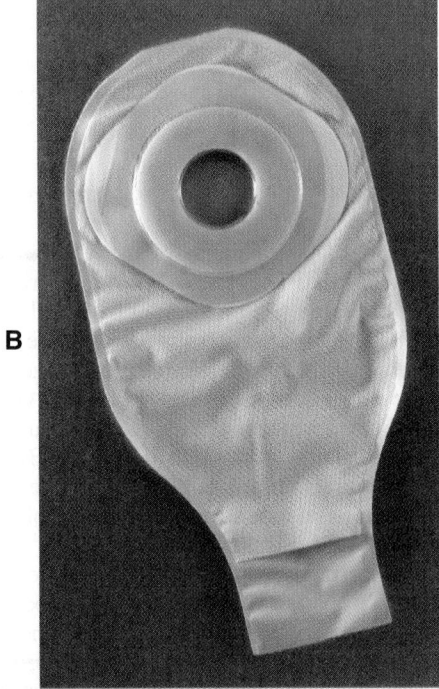

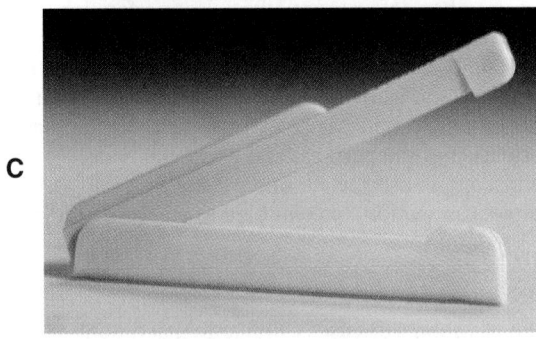

Figure 58-6 ● Skin barriers, such as wafers **(A),** are cut to fit ⅛ inch around fistula. A drainable pouch **(B)** is applied over the wafer and clamped **(C)** until the pouch is to be emptied. Effluent should drain into the bag and not contact the skin. (Courtesy ConvaTec, A Bristol-Myers Squibb Company, Skillman, NJ.)

Stricturoplasty may be performed for bowel strictures related to Crohn's disease. This procedure, which involves incising along the length of the stricture and suturing the incised area on the horizontal plane, allows for an increase in the bowel diameter. Preoperative and postoperative care for each

LEGAL/ETHICAL ISSUES IN HEALTH CARE

THE IMPACT OF SURGERY FOR CROHN'S DISEASE ON HEALTH-RELATED QUALITY OF LIFE

When clients are questioned regarding their concerns relative to the disease process, surgery appears to be one of their greatest worries, particularly if the surgery will require them to have an ostomy. This study examined whether surgical treatment of Crohn's disease modified health-related quality of life (QOL) as compared with inactive Crohn's disease, active disease, or healthy controls.

Clients with active Crohn's disease reported the lowest health-related QOL. The most important factor in determining health-related QOL is the severity of the disease and accompanying symptoms. It is apparent that the severe symptoms accompanying active disease seriously impair perceived QOL. QOL improves during disease remission, regardless of whether the remission was achieved by medical or surgical means. To improve QOL, it is more important to achieve remission, regardless of the approach used.

Data from Casellas, F., et al. (2000). Impact of surgery for Crohn's disease on health-related quality of life. *American Journal of Gastroenterology, 95*(1), 177-181.

of these surgical procedures is similar to care for clients undergoing other types of abdominal surgery.

Community-Based Care

The discharge care plan for the client with Crohn's disease is similar to that for the client with ulcerative colitis (see Community-Based Care [Ulcerative Colitis], p. 1282). The nurse or case manager helps the client with a draining fistula plan for care of the fistula at home.

HOME CARE MANAGEMENT

The interventions begun in the hospital to manage the disease need to be carried out to some extent in the home. Measures to control the disease and related symptoms and manage nutrition need to be reinforced. Supplies for wound and/or fistula care may be required. The client's home should be arranged so that the client has easy access to the bathroom, as well as privacy to perform fistula care. To ensure adequate nutrition, the client should have easy access to a well-supplied kitchen of readily prepared foods.

HEALTH TEACHING

The teaching plan for the client with Crohn's disease is similar to that for the client with ulcerative colitis. He or she is taught the usual course of the disease, symptoms of complications, and when to notify the health care provider. Medication teaching, including purpose, dose, and side effects, is incorporated into the teaching plan. The nurse, in collaboration with the dietitian, teaches the client to follow a low-residue, high-calorie diet and to avoid foods that cause discomfort.

The nurse teaches the client to provide for rest periods, especially during exacerbations of the disease. If stress appears to increase symptoms of the disease, the nurse may teach the client stress management techniques or recommend counseling. For long-term follow-up, the client is educated regarding the increased risk of bowel cancer and the advisability of having a colonoscopy yearly as a means of early detection of changes in the mucosa (Hirsch & Caswell, 1999).

If a client has developed a fistula, the nurse explains and demonstrates fistula care. The client needs opportunities to practice the care in the hospital. Ideally, the client should be independent in fistula care before leaving the hospital. However, because of the perirectal or vaginal location of the fistula or an obese abdomen, the client may need assistance in this care. If this is the case, a family member or a caregiver must learn and practice the care, or the nurse or case manager can arrange for home care services.

HEALTH CARE RESOURCES

The client discharged to home following resection and anastomosis may require visits from a home care nurse to assess the surgical wound and monitor for complications. The nurse assesses the client's and family's ability to monitor the progress of fistula healing and to watch for signs and symptoms of infection and sepsis. Home care nursing visits may also be appropriate for this purpose. A home care aide might be considered for clients who cannot meet their nutritional needs, who need help with meal preparation, and who need help in purchasing groceries.

If the client needs equipment for fistula care, such as skin barriers and wound drainage bags, the nurse or case manager contacts medical supply companies or local pharmacies to ascertain their availability and price (see the Cost of Care box above). A support group sponsored by the United Ostomy Association or a local hospital in the community may also be available to assist the client and family with physical, as well as psychosocial, needs.

COST OF CARE
IMPLICATIONS FOR NURSING

INFLAMMATORY BOWEL DISEASE

Cost of Care
- The average cost of hospitalization for Crohn's disease is $12,528 excluding physician's fees.
- The mean cost per admission for all cases of ulcerative colitis is $3726.
- Surgical treatment for Crohn's disease accounts for 49.8% of all admissions and accounts for 60% to 55% of all costs.
- Clients treated surgically for Crohn's disease had more costly hospitalizations than those treated medically.
- Total parenteral nutrition accounts for 63% of all pharmacy costs when clients are admitted for exacerbations of Crohn's disease.
- Admissions for Crohn's disease that include surgical interventions are the most costly.

Implications for Nursing
Chronic diseases such as Crohn's disease are characterized by periods of remission and exacerbation. Vigilant monitoring of the client's status by home care nurses could significantly reduce costs by identifying complications so that treatment is initiated in the early phases. Nurses play an important role in the education of their clients and families. Teaching initiatives that assist clients with symptom management and recognition of complications could possibly avoid more costly hospital admissions and subsequent invasive treatments. Therapies that decrease the number of surgical hospitalizations should reduce the cost of inpatient care associated with Crohn's disease.

Data from Cohen, R., et al. (2000). The cost of hospitalization for Crohn's disease. *American Journal of Gastroenterology, 95*(2), 524-530.

Diverticular Disease

■ OVERVIEW

Diverticula are congenital or acquired pouchlike herniations of the mucosa through the muscular wall of the small intestine or colon. **Diverticulosis** is the presence of many abnormal pouchlike herniations (diverticula) in the wall of the intestine. **Diverticulitis** is the term used to describe an inflammation of one or more diverticula.

■ Pathophysiology

Diverticula can occur in any part of the small or large intestine, but they occur most commonly in the sigmoid colon (Figure 58-7). The musculature of the colon hypertrophies, thickens, and becomes rigid, and herniation of the mucosa and submucosa through the colon wall is seen. Diverticula seem to occur at points of weakness in the intestinal wall, often at areas where blood vessels interrupt muscular continuity. The muscle weakness develops as part of the aging process.

In and of themselves, diverticula cause few problems. If undigested food or bacteria become trapped in a diverticulum, however, blood supply to that area diminishes and bacteria invade the diverticulum. Diverticulitis results when the diverticulum perforates and a local abscess forms. The perforated diverticulum can also progress to an intra-abdominal perforation with generalized peritonitis.

Bleeding from diverticula can range from minor, localized bleeding to massive hemorrhage. Minor bleeding is often due to localized inflammation in areas of vascular granulation tissue at the base of the diverticulum. Hemorrhage can result when a blood vessel is eroded within a diverticulum. Inflammation secondary to recurrent diverticulitis can lead to narrowing of the bowel lumen, which may result in obstruction.

Inflammation can also result in fistulas to other organs, such as the bladder and the vagina.

Diets with small amounts of fiber have been implicated in the development of diverticula in that they cause less bulky stool and possibly constipation. For diverticulosis and diverticulitis to occur, there must be an increase in intraluminal pressure and muscle contractions to move fecal material through the colon.

The etiologic factor in diverticulitis may be retained undigested food in diverticula, which compromises the blood supply to that area and facilitates bacterial invasion of the sac.

■ Incidence/Prevalence

The incidence of diverticulosis is difficult to determine, but it is estimated that millions of people are affected. Diverticular disease affects one third of adults over age 60 years. Although diverticulosis is common, only 1 out of 5 people with this disease displays symptoms. Diverticular disease occurs more often in men than in women (Isselbacher & Epstein, 1998).

> **⚘ CONSIDERATIONS FOR OLDER ADULTS**
> The incidence of diverticula increases with age. There is a reported incidence of 20% to 50% in Western populations over the age of 50 (Isselbacher & Epstein, 1998).

➤ COLLABORATIVE MANAGEMENT

● Assessment

■ HISTORY

Clients with diverticulosis are usually asymptomatic, and unless pain and/or bleeding develops, the condition may go undiagnosed or be found incidentally on routine colonoscopy. Occasionally, diverticulosis causes symptoms. For clients

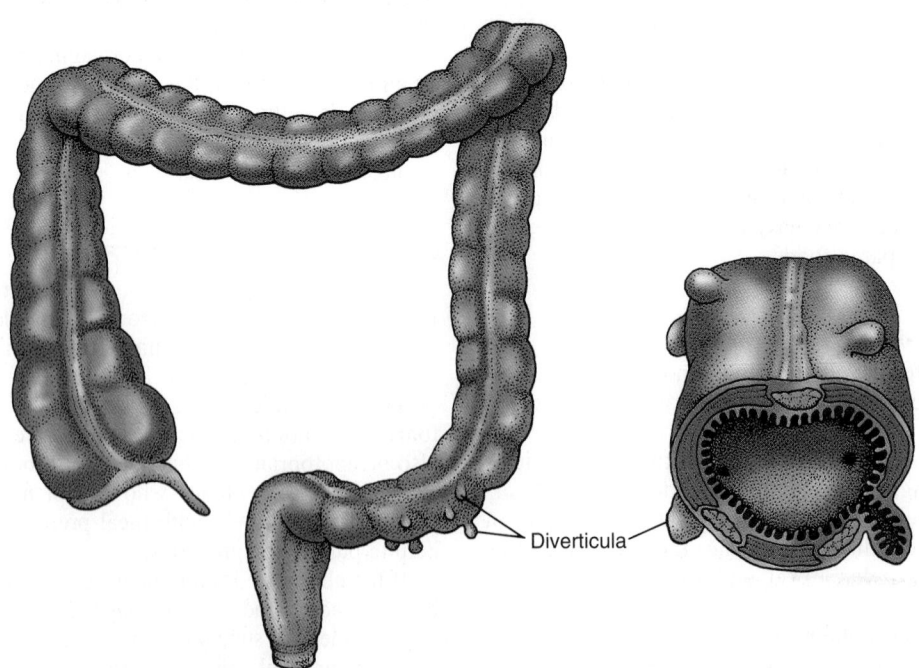

Diverticula

Figure 58-7 ● Several abnormal outpouchings, or herniations, in the wall of the intestine, which are diverticula. These can occur anywhere in the small or large intestine but are found most often in the sigmoid as shown in this figure. Diverticulitis is the inflammation of a diverticulum that occurs when undigested food or bacteria become trapped in the diverticulum.

with uncomplicated diverticulosis, the nurse asks about a history of intermittent pain in the left lower quadrant and a history of constipation. If diverticulitis is suspected, the client is asked about a history of fever and abdominal pain. The nurse inquires about recent bowel elimination patterns, since constipation may develop as a result of intestinal inflammation. The client is also questioned about the presence of bleeding from the rectum.

PHYSICAL ASSESSMENT/CLINICAL MANIFESTATIONS

On physical examination of the client with uncomplicated diverticulosis, no clinical manifestations of the disorder may be present. Occasionally the nurse may elicit tenderness on abdominal palpation.

The client with diverticulitis has abdominal pain, most often localized to the left lower quadrant. The pain may be intermittent at first but becomes progressively steady. Occasionally pain may be suprapubic or may occur on one side. Abdominal pain is generalized if peritonitis has occurred. The client's temperature is elevated, ranging from a low-grade fever to 101° F (38.2° C), and may be accompanied by chills. The nurse may note the presence of tachycardia secondary to fever. Nausea and vomiting are also commonly present.

On examination of the abdomen, the nurse may observe distention. Tenderness on palpation may be noted over the area involved (usually the left lower quadrant). The colon may be palpable. If localized peritoneal irritation is present, localized muscle spasm, guarded movement, and rebound tenderness are usually present. If generalized peritonitis is present, abdominal muscle spasm, guarding, and rebound tenderness are more diffuse.

If the perforated diverticulum is close to the rectum, the health care provider may palpate a tender mass during the rectal examination. Blood pressure checks may show orthostatic changes. If bleeding is massive, the client may have hypotension and dehydration that result in shock. If generalized peritonitis has occurred, sepsis and manifestations of hypotension and septic or hypovolemic shock can occur.

DIAGNOSTIC ASSESSMENT

For the client with uncomplicated diverticulosis, laboratory studies are not indicated. The client with diverticulitis, however, has an elevated white blood cell (WBC) count. Decreased hematocrit and hemoglobin values are noted if chronic or severe bleeding is present. In stool tests for occult blood, results are positive in 20% of clients (also called a positive guaiac). Urinalysis may show a few red blood cells (RBCs) if the left ureter is in proximity to a perforated diverticulum.

X-ray studies of the intestinal tract with barium contrast show diverticula. An upper gastrointestinal (GI) series shows diverticula of the small intestine, and barium enema examination shows diverticula of the large intestine. X-ray studies are not indicated in clients with uncomplicated diverticulosis, because symptoms are usually minimal or nonexistent.

The client with diverticulitis usually does *not* undergo a barium enema examination in the acute phase of the illness because of the risk of rupture of the inflamed diverticulum. A barium enema examination may be completed after the client has been treated with antibiotics and the inflammation has resolved. A flat-plate film of the abdomen may reveal free air

and fluid in the left lower quadrant, suggesting an abscess or free air under the diaphragm, indicating perforation. The health care provider may also order a computed tomography (CT) scan to diagnose an abscess or thickening of the bowel related to diverticulitis.

Ultrasonography, a noninvasive test, may reveal bowel thickening or an abscess. The physician may perform a sigmoidoscopy or colonoscopy *after the acute phase* of the illness, usually to rule out the presence of a tumor in the large intestine, particularly if the client has rectal bleeding. If the sigmoidoscope or colonoscope enters a diverticulum, however, the chances of perforating the diverticulum are high.

Interventions

Clients may be treated on an ambulatory care basis when symptoms are mild, with a temperature lower than 101° F (38.2° C) and a WBC count ranging from 13,000 to 15,000/mm³. The client who is an outpatient should be monitored for any prolonged or increased fever, abdominal pain, or blood in the stool.

Clients with moderate to severe diverticulitis require hospitalization. Clinical manifestations that suggest the need for admission are a temperature higher than 101° F (38.2° C), persistent abdominal pain for more than 3 days, or evidence of lower GI bleeding.

NONSURGICAL MANAGEMENT. For the client with diverticulitis, a combination of drug and diet therapy with rest to decrease inflammation and improve tissue perfusion is indicated. This plan is preferred for older adults and others with mild to moderate disease (Chart 58-6).

DRUG THERAPY. For clients with mild diverticulitis, the health care provider prescribes broad-spectrum antibiotics, such as metronidazole (Flagyl) plus trimethoprim/sulfamethoxazole (Bactrim, Septra) or ciprofloxacin (Cipro). A mild analgesic may be given for pain.

The health care provider admits clients with more severe pain to the hospital and orders IV fluids to correct dehydration, as well as IV antibiotics such as cefoxitin plus metro-

---

CHART 58-6

NURSING FOCUS *on the* **OLDER ADULT**
Diverticulitis

- Provide antibiotics, analgesics, and anticholinergics as ordered. Observe older clients carefully for side effects of these drugs, especially confusion (or increased confusion), urinary retention or failure, and orthostatic hypotension.
- Do not give laxatives or enemas. Teach the client and the family about the importance of avoiding these measures.
- Encourage the client to rest and to avoid activities that may increase intra-abdominal pressure, such as straining and bending.
- While diverticulitis is active, provide a *low*-fiber diet (see Table 58-4). When the inflammation resolves, provide a *high*-fiber diet. Teach the client and family about these diets and when they are appropriate.
- Because older clients do not always experience the typical pain or fever expected, observe carefully for signs of active disease.
- Perform frequent abdominal assessments to determine distention and tenderness on palpation.
- Check stools for occult or frank bleeding.

nidazole. Anticholinergics, such as propantheline bromide (Pro-Banthine), may reduce intestinal hypermotility. For clients with moderate to severe diverticulitis, an opioid analgesic, such as meperidine hydrochloride (Demerol) or morphine sulfate, can alleviate pain.

Laxatives are avoided because they increase intestinal motility. Enemas are avoided because they increase intraluminal pressure. The nurse assesses the client for clinical manifestations of fluid and electrolyte imbalance on an ongoing basis.

REST. The nurse instructs the client to remain in bed during the acute phase of illness. He or she is advised to refrain from lifting, straining, coughing, or bending to avoid an increase in intra-abdominal pressure, which can result in perforation of the diverticulum.

DIET THERAPY. During the acute phase of the illness, the client's diet is restricted to clear liquids. Clients who have more severe symptoms are admitted to the hospital and are kept on NPO status. A nasogastric (NG) tube is inserted if nausea, vomiting, or abdominal distention is severe. The nurse administers IV fluids, as ordered, for hydration. In collaboration with the dietitian, the client increases dietary intake slowly as symptoms subside. When inflammation has resolved and bowel function returns to normal, a fiber-containing diet is introduced gradually. If active diverticulitis recurs, fiber intake is stopped for the acute phase of the illness.

SURGICAL MANAGEMENT. The client with diverticulitis may need to undergo surgery for any of the following conditions:
- Rupture of the diverticulum with subsequent peritonitis
- Pelvic abscess
- Bowel obstruction
- Fistula
- Persistent fever or pain after 4 days of medical treatment
- Uncontrolled bleeding

The surgeon performs emergency surgery if peritonitis, bowel obstruction, or pelvic abscess is present. Colon resection, with or without a colostomy, is the most common surgical procedure for clients with diverticular disease.

PREOPERATIVE CARE. Preparation of the client for surgery depends on the severity of the condition. The surgery might be performed on an emergency basis, or it might be done with a few weeks' notice. The surgeon informs the client whether a temporary or permanent colostomy might be required.

If the client is *not* in the acute stage of diverticulitis, a thorough bowel preparation *may* be given, consisting of enemas and laxatives daily for 2 to 3 days before surgery. Because of the risk of perforation, however, the surgeon may forgo an aggressive bowel preparation. If the client has an acutely inflamed diverticulum or persistent fever and abdominal pain, the bowel preparation is most likely withheld.

The client who is to undergo emergency surgery or who has not responded to medical intervention is maintained on NPO status with an NG tube in place. He or she receives IV fluids with appropriate electrolyte replacements.

For clients without acute inflammation, a well-structured preoperative diet is ordered. The client usually has a low-fiber diet for 4 to 5 days, followed by a full-liquid diet for 2 days, then a clear-liquid diet the evening before surgery.

Preoperative teaching may include information about the possible need for a colostomy. If a colostomy is a possible outcome, the enterostomal therapist (ET) or office nurse describes its function and purpose. The nurse need not discuss colostomy care in detail unless the client wishes this information at this time.

OPERATIVE PROCEDURES. In a resection of the colon, the surgeon excises the portion that is inflamed or diseased and, if possible, creates an anastomosis of the colon to restore patency. Inflammation and infection, however, may preclude the feasibility of an anastomosis. If this is the case, the surgeon may perform a colostomy. Select clients may be candidates for colostomy closure and anastomosis after the bowel has been allowed to rest for 3 to 6 months.

POSTOPERATIVE CARE. The immediate physical care for clients undergoing a colon resection for diverticulitis is the same as that for clients undergoing abdominal surgery (see Chapter 19).

Wound Care. The client has a drain in place at the abdominal incision site for 2 to 3 days. If a colostomy has been performed, the stoma may be covered with petroleum gauze dressing because the colostomy does not drain for approximately 2 days, or a colostomy bag may be placed over the stoma. If the stoma is visible, the nurse monitors its color and integrity. The stoma should be pinkish to cherry red without retraction or prolapse into the abdomen.

Diet Therapy. The client is maintained on NPO status with an NG tube in place for 2 to 3 days after a colon resection with or without a colostomy. When peristalsis returns, the nurse removes the NG tube, according to the health care provider's order, and introduces clear liquids *slowly. Gradually,* the diet is advanced to solids, depending on the return of peristalsis and bowel function.

If the client has had a colostomy created, it should begin functioning in 2 to 4 days. Most clients who undergo surgery and colostomy formation for diverticulitis have a sigmoid colostomy because the sigmoid colon is the most common site of diverticulitis. Drainage from a sigmoid colostomy initially consists of loose stool, but eventually the stool becomes formed. A tight seal around the stoma is essential to avoid contact of feces with the skin. Colostomy care is detailed in Chapter 57.

Emotional Support. If a colostomy has been performed, the nurse gives the client an opportunity to express feelings about the ostomy. The nurse discusses these feelings with the client, acknowledging that anger and depression are normal responses. When the client is physically able, the nurse encourages him or her to look at the stoma and touch the apparatus.

⦿ Community-Based Care

The length of hospitalization for clients with diverticulitis ranges from 4 to 10 days, depending on the response to medical treatment and the need for surgery. Discharge plans vary according to the treatment.

▪ HOME CARE MANAGEMENT

For the client with diverticulitis who has responded to medical treatment, home care focuses on proper diet. The nurse assesses the client's ability to obtain and prepare the recommended high-fiber foods. The client who has required surgical intervention has the added responsibilities of incision care and possibly colostomy care, with some temporary limitations placed on activities.

■ HEALTH TEACHING

DIET THERAPY. All clients with diverticular disease require education regarding a high-fiber diet. For clients with diverticulosis, an increase in dietary fiber can regulate bowel function and bring about partial relief of symptoms. The nurse and dietitian encourage the client with diverticulosis to eat a diet high in cellulose and hemicellulose types of fiber. These substances can be found in wheat bran, whole-grain breads, and cereals. The client should ingest at least 25 to 35 g of fiber per day. This requirement can be derived from four slices of 100% whole-wheat bread and a 3-ounce serving of all-bran cereal. The nurse also teaches the client to eat fresh fruits and vegetables with high-fiber content to add bulk to stools.

The client who is not accustomed to eating high-fiber foods should add them to the diet gradually to avoid flatulence and abdominal cramping. If the client cannot tolerate the recommended fiber requirement, a bulk-forming laxative, such as psyllium hydrophilic mucilloid (Metamucil), can be taken to increase fecal size and consistency. An adequate intake of fluids will help to prevent the bloating that may accompany a high-fiber diet. The client should also avoid alcohol because it irritates the bowel. Clients are instructed to avoid foods containing seeds or indigestible material that may block a diverticulum, such as nuts, corn, popcorn, cucumbers, tomatoes, figs, strawberries, and caraway seeds. In collaboration with the dietitian, the nurse teaches the client that dietary fat intake should not exceed 30% of the total daily caloric intake.

Clients should *avoid all fiber* when they have symptoms of *diverticulitis* because high-fiber foods are irritating. As diverticulitis resolves, fiber can gradually be added until progression to a high-fiber diet is once again obtained. The client who has undergone surgery is usually taking solid food by the time of discharge from the hospital.

The nurse explains the usual disease course and factors that can exacerbate the disease to the client. Follow-up with the health care provider approximately 1 month following resolution of symptoms is recommended, and a repeat flexible sigmoidoscopy or barium enema may be preformed at that time.

SURGICAL FOLLOW-UP. Clients who have had abdominal surgery need oral and written instructions on incision care and the signs and symptoms to report to the health care provider. These are similar to the instructions given to clients after other types of abdominal surgery. The nurse provides instructions on colostomy care for clients who have a temporary or permanent colostomy.

GENERAL INSTRUCTIONS. The nurse instructs clients *with any type of diverticular disease,* orally and in writing, about signs and symptoms of acute diverticulitis, including fever, abdominal pain, and bloody, mahogany, or tarry stools. The client should be advised to avoid the use of laxatives (other than bulk-forming types) and enemas. All clients can also benefit from avoiding the activities that increase intra-abdominal pressure, such as straining at stool, bending, or lifting heavy objects.

The nurse reassures clients with diverticulosis that this disorder need not cause problems if a proper diet is followed. The client is informed that this illness does not commonly recur and that with proper diet and elimination patterns, recurring episodes and potential complications can be avoided.

The client with a colostomy has special needs with regard to the alteration in body image and loss of body function. The nurse encourages the client to verbalize concerns about body image.

Clients who have undergone surgery may need assistance with incision and colostomy care. The nurse or case manager arranges for a home care nurse to assess wound healing and proper functioning of the ostomy and the appliance. If the client is interested, the nurse can arrange for a visit from an ostomy volunteer or an enterostomal therapist (ET). For information about other ostomy resources, the nurse or the client can contact the United Ostomy Association.

ANORECTAL ABSCESS

■ OVERVIEW

Anorectal abscesses most often result from obstruction of the ducts of glands in the anorectal region by feces, foreign bodies, or trauma. Stasis of obstructing contents occurs and causes infection that spreads into adjacent tissue. Most abscesses begin as cryptitis (a pocket of infection in an anal crypt).

The client may experience diarrhea or rectal pain as the first symptom. There may be no clinical manifestations at the time of the first physical assessment, but local swelling, erythema, and tenderness on palpation are apparent within a few days after the onset of pain. If the abscess becomes chronic, discharge, bleeding, and pruritus (itching) may exist. Fever occurs if larger abscesses are present.

► COLLABORATIVE MANAGEMENT

Anorectal abscesses are managed by surgical incision and drainage. The physician can often incise simple perianal and ischiorectal abscesses using a local anesthetic. For clients with more extensive abscesses, a regional or general anesthetic may be needed. Systemic antibiotics are given only for clients who are immunocompromised, are diabetic, have valvular disease or a prosthetic valve, or have extensive subcutaneous fat. Incision and drainage in these clients is performed after antibiotic therapy.

Nursing interventions are focused on helping the client to maintain comfort and optimal perineal hygiene (Chart 58-7). The nurse encourages the use of sitz baths, analgesics, bulk-producing agents, and stool softeners during the perioperative period until healing occurs. The nurse also emphasizes the importance of ongoing perineal hygiene after all bowel movements and the maintenance of a regular bowel pattern with a high-fiber diet.

ANAL FISSURE

■ OVERVIEW

An anal fissure is a superficial erosion of the anal canal. Fissures can be primary or secondary, acute or chronic. *Primary* fissures are idiopathic with no known cause. *Secondary* fis-

CHART 58-7

BEST PRACTICE *for*
Promoting Perineal Comfort

- Keep the perineal area clean with mild soap.
- Pat the perineal area dry instead of rubbing it.
- Provide warm sitz baths or apply warm compresses to the area.
- If the area is acutely inflamed, apply cold packs.
- Provide a chair cushion or a soft, inflatable ring for the seated client. For the older or debilitated client, monitor the skin carefully to prevent pressure sores.
- Use absorbent pads for drainage, if any, and change them often.
- Use premoistened wipes for cleaning the perineal area after a bowel movement.
- Use witch hazel wipes (e.g., Tucks) to relieve pain.
- Give bulk-forming agents, such as psyllium mucilloid (Metamucil), as ordered, to reduce pain associated with defecation.
- Apply a topical anesthetic cream to the perineal area, as ordered.
- Give oral analgesics, as prescribed, for pain relief.
- Do not administer enemas or give potent laxatives.

sures are associated with another disorder (e.g., Crohn's disease, tuberculosis, or leukemia) or with trauma (e.g., from a foreign body, childbirth, or perirectal surgery). Constipated stool, diarrhea, or spasm of the anal sphincter is another possible cause.

► COLLABORATIVE MANAGEMENT

An acute anal fissure is superficial and resolves spontaneously or heals quickly with conservative treatment. Chronic fissures recur, and surgical treatment may be needed. Pain during and after defecation and bleeding noted outside the stool are the most common symptoms. Other clinical manifestations associated with chronic fissures are pruritus, urinary frequency or retention, dysuria, and dyspareunia (painful intercourse).

The health care provider makes the diagnosis by inspecting and stretching the perianal skin. If the client is having pain at the time of the examination, diagnostic testing is usually limited to inspection. If the client is not in severe pain, a digital examination and possibly a sigmoidoscopy are performed. When painless or multiple fissures are present, the physician may perform a barium enema and sigmoidoscopy to rule out an associated inflammatory bowel disorder.

Management of an acute fissure is nonsurgical, with interventions aimed at local, symptomatic pain relief and softening of stools to reduce trauma to the area. Warm sitz baths and analgesia are recommended along with the use of bulk-producing agents, such as psyllium hydrophilic mucilloid (Metamucil), which help minimize pain associated with defecation. If fissures do not respond to medical management within several days to weeks, surgical excision of the fissure with a local anesthetic may be necessary.

The nurse explains the appropriate pain control measures to the client. When nonsurgical management is initiated, the nurse instructs clients to notify the health care provider if pain is not relieved within a few days. The nurse instructs the client who undergoes surgery to continue with the same pain management and bowel regimen, including sitz baths, analgesics, and bulk-

forming agents. He or she is reminded to report any drainage or bleeding from the rectum to the health care provider.

ANAL FISTULA

■ OVERVIEW

An anal fistula, or *fistula in ano,* is an abnormal tract leading from the anal canal to the perianal skin. Most anal fistulas result from anorectal abscesses, which are caused by obstruction of anal glands (see Anorectal Abscess, p. 1291). Fistulas can also be associated with tuberculosis, Crohn's disease, or cancer.

► COLLABORATIVE MANAGEMENT

The client with an anal fistula has pruritus (itching), purulent discharge, and tenderness or pain that is worsened by bowel movements. The physician uses a proctoscope to identify the source of symptoms and to locate the fistula. Because fistulas do not heal spontaneously, surgery is necessary. To perform a fistulotomy, the surgeon incises the tissue overlying the tract and performs curettage (scraping) of the base. The incision site heals by secondary intention. In a client with a high fistula, a special surgical technique is necessary because important sphincters are often affected. Postoperatively, the nurse instructs the client about sitz baths, analgesics, and the use of bulk-producing agents or stool softeners to minimize pain.

PARASITIC INFECTION

■ OVERVIEW

Parasites can enter and invade the gastrointestinal (GI) tract and cause infections leading to varying degrees of illness. Parasites commonly enter through the mouth by means of fecal-oral transmission from the following:

- Contaminated food or water
- Oral-anal sexual practices
- Contact with feces from a contaminated person

Common parasites that cause infection in humans are *Entamoeba histolytica,* which causes amebiasis (amebic dysentery), *Giardia lamblia,* which causes giardiasis, and *Cryptosporidium.*

■ Infection with *Entamoeba histolytica*

Humans are the only known hosts for *E. histolytica* (also known as amebiasis). This organism occurs in cysts and trophozoites (sporozoan parasites). Trophozoites die rapidly after they leave the body in stool. Cysts, however, can remain viable in the right type of environment for weeks or months. Humans who eliminate cysts are infectious. Flies have been found to be vectors for transmission of the cysts, and transmission is increased in areas that use human excrement for fertilizer. Transmission occurs by the fecal-oral route.

Amebiasis occurs worldwide, but it is most prevalent and most severe in tropical areas. Prevalence rates are as high as 40% in areas with poor sanitation, crowding, and poor nutrition. Amebiasis causes 40,000 to 100,000 deaths annually worldwide. The disease causes less severe symptoms and often goes undiagnosed in temperate climates. The organism may occur in 2% to 5% of some populations in the United States.

E. histolytica either feeds on bacteria in the intestine or invades and ulcerates the mucosa of the large intestine. The parasite can be limited to the GI tract (intestinal amebiasis), or it can extend outside the intestines (extraintestinal amebiasis). People can have intestinal amebiasis without having any symptoms, or symptoms can range from mild to severe.

Infection with *Giardia lamblia*

G. lamblia is a protozoal parasite that causes superficial invasion, destruction, and inflammation of the mucosa in the small intestine. Like *E. histolytica*, *G. lamblia* has a trophozoite and cyst form, and cysts can transmit the organism. Humans are hosts to this organism, but beavers and dogs may be reservoirs for infection. *G. lamblia* is transmitted by the fecal-oral route. Giardiasis is a well-recognized problem in travelers, campers, male homosexuals, and immunosuppressed people.

Modes of transmission are similar to those for amebiasis; in the United States, however, giardiasis is much more prevalent and is the most common parasitic infection. Giardiasis affects only the intestinal system, causing acute diarrhea, chronic diarrhea, or malabsorption syndrome. The acute phase usually is self-limiting, lasting days or weeks. The chronic phase can last for years. Diarrhea is usually mild in both forms, but it can be severe. As stools increase in frequency, they become more watery, greasy, frothy, and malodorous with mucus. Weight loss and weakness are also common. Malabsorption can occur with diarrhea that continues for longer than 3 weeks. Manifestations result from malabsorption of fat, protein, vitamin B$_{12}$, and lactase deficiency.

Infection with *Cryptosporidium*

Cryptosporidium is another parasitic infestation transmitted by the fecal-oral route that is manifested by diarrhea. This infection commonly occurs in immunosuppressed clients, particularly those with human immunodeficiency virus (HIV). (See Chapter 22 for a discussion of HIV infection.)

► COLLABORATIVE MANAGEMENT

● Assessment

A thorough history can provide information about potential sources of exposure to parasitic infection. A history of travel to parts of the world where such infections are prevalent increases suspicion for infection with parasites. GI symptoms related to travel may be delayed as long as 1 to 2 weeks following the return home. A diet history is especially helpful if several people become ill. Common water supplies may be infected with *Giardia* or *Cryptosporidium*. Trichinosis should be considered if the client has ingested pork products.

Mild to moderate *E. histolytica* infestation causes clinical manifestations, including the daily passage of several strongly odoriferous stools, possibly with mucus but without blood, accompanied by abdominal cramping, flatulence, fatigue, and weight loss.

Clients experience characteristic remissions and recurrences. Severe amebic dysentery is manifested by frequent, more liquid, and odoriferous stools with mucus *and* blood. Fever up to 105° F (40° C), tenesmus (ineffectual and painful straining to defecate), generalized abdominal tenderness, and vomiting can also occur. The ulcerations characteristic of invading amebiasis that occur in the colon can cause pain, bleeding, and obstruction. Ulcerations can also be localized in the rectum, resulting in formed stool with blood. Complications are rare but include appendicitis and bowel perforation.

Extraintestinal amebiasis can occur without symptoms of intestinal infection. The most common form is amebic liver abscess, which causes symptoms of fever, pain, and an enlarged liver. The abscess can rupture, and death can result if the infection is not treated and complications occur.

The diagnosis of amebiasis is made by examination of stool for parasites. Because *E. histolytica* is difficult to detect, serial stool examinations are needed if the disease is suspected. The use of sigmoidoscopy may detect ulcerations in the rectum or colon. Exudate obtained during sigmoidoscopic examination is studied for the parasite. The white blood cell (WBC) count can be as high as 20,000/mm^3 when severe dysentery is present.

The diagnosis of giardiasis is also confirmed by stool examination for parasites. Because organisms may not be detected for at least 1 week after symptoms appear, multiple stool samples should be examined. Duodenal aspirate can also be examined for the parasite.

Infection with *Cryptosporidium* is usually self-limiting in individuals who are not immunocompromised. Drug therapy for clients with immunosuppression may consist of paromomycin 500 to 750 mg four times daily.

● Interventions

INTERVENTIONS FOR AMEBIASIS. Treatment for all types of amebiasis mandate the use of amebicide drugs. The physician commonly prescribes metronidazole (Flagyl, Novonidazol✦) and diloxanide furoate (Entamide), or diloxanide furoate and tetracycline hydrochloride (Sumycin) followed by chloroquine. Clients with severe dysentery require IV fluids for replacement and maintenance of fluid volume and possibly opiates, such as diphenoxylate hydrochloride and atropine sulfate (Lomotil), to control bowel motility. Clients with extraintestinal amebiasis or severe dehydration are hospitalized. Clients with asymptomatic, mild, or moderate disease are treated as outpatients with drug therapy. For all clients, at least three stools are examined for parasites at 2- to 3-day intervals, starting 2 to 4 weeks after drug therapy has been completed.

INTERVENTIONS FOR GIARDIASIS. Treatment for giardiasis is drug therapy. Metronidazole is the drug of choice, and the usual dose is 250 mg three times a day PO for 5 days. Tinidazole (Fasigyn) can be used as an alternative. Stools are examined 2 weeks after treatment is begun to assess for eradication.

The nurse explains modes of transmission and means to avoid the spread of infection and recurrent contact with parasitic organisms. Clients are taught that they can transmit the infection to others until amebicides effectively kill the parasites. The nurse instructs clients to:

- Avoid contact with stool
- Keep toilet areas clean
- Wash their hands meticulously with an antimicrobial soap after bowel movements
- Maintain personal hygiene
- Avoid stool from dogs and beavers

The client is also advised to avoid sexual practices that allow rectal contact until drug therapy is completed. The nurse informs the client that all household and sexual contacts should undergo stool examinations for parasites. If the water supply is suspected as the source, a sample is obtained and sent for analysis. Multiple infections are common in households, often as a result of contaminated water supplies. Well water and water from areas with inadequate or no filtration equipment can be sources of contamination.

HELMINTHIC INFESTATION

Helminths are wormlike animals; they are often parasitic and capable of causing infectious disease in humans. There are many species of helminths, which, for purposes of classification, are divided into three general categories:

- Roundworms (nematodes)
- Flukes (trematodes)
- Tapeworms (cestodes)

Helminths can cause various degrees of gastrointestinal (GI) symptoms in humans. Most often, they enter the human body through the skin or via the oral route with ingestion of food, water, or other substances contaminated with worms. Some helminths gain access to the human body via insects, such as flies and mosquitoes. Helminths that are typically transmitted via insects are limited to tropical areas, however, and are not discussed here. Flukes (trematodes), which are passed to humans via snail-contaminated water, are also limited to tropical and subtropical areas outside the United States and are not discussed here.

Roundworms

Roundworms are commonly the cause of helminthic infections in the United States and worldwide. These infections include enterobiasis, trichinosis, and hookworm.

Enterobiasis

Enterobiasis ("pinworm infection") is caused by *Enterobius vermicularis* and is the most common helminthic infection in the United States. It is transmitted by oral ingestion of contaminated food, drink, or fomites. The most common clinical manifestations of infection include nocturnal perianal pruritus, vaginitis, insomnia, and restlessness.

The client may have vague GI symptoms, such as abdominal pain, nausea, vomiting, and diarrhea. However, many infected clients have no symptoms. Diagnosis is made when eggs of the helminth are found on the perianal skin or on cellulose tape that has been applied to the perianal skin.

Treatment of enterobiasis includes meticulous handwashing techniques after defecation and before meals to prevent spread of the worms to others. Drug therapy is indicated for all clients with symptoms and in some clients who are infected but are not symptomatic. Household cohabitants of an infected client may be treated with drug therapy even if they are asymptomatic. Pyrantel pamoate (Antiminth, Combantrin✤) or mebendazole (Vermox, Nemasol✤) is given orally in one dose, which is repeated at 2 and 4 weeks.

Infection with pinworms is curable and is not usually associated with complications; however, recurrences are common.

Trichinosis

Trichinosis is another helminthic disease caused by roundworms. The incidence in the United States is 50 to 100 cases annually, but many mild or asymptomatic cases are not diagnosed, since the person is usually asymptomatic. *Trichinella spiralis*, which lives in the intestine of humans, pigs, bears, and rats, causes trichinosis. The organism is usually transmitted to people who ingest undercooked pork or pork products. Ingestion of other meats, such as ground beef, can also promote transmission if a meat grinder has been used for both beef and pork. Following ingestion, the larvae, encased in cysts, are released by the digestive action of acid and pepsin. Incubation is 12 hours to 28 days after ingestion. Clinical manifestations range from none to severe; death rarely results.

During the first week following infection, diarrhea results from the invasion of the gut by large numbers of the parasite. Abdominal pain, nausea, and vomiting may follow. During the second week, the larvae begin to invade the muscle, instigating a hypersensitivity reaction characterized by fever, periorbital and facial edema, and subconjunctival hemorrhage. Occasionally a rash or dyspnea develops. Two to three weeks after infection, symptoms of myositis, myalgia, and muscle weakness develop, particularly in the lower back, neck, jaw, biceps, and extraocular muscles. Vague muscle pain and malaise characterize the convalescence phase, which can last for several months.

A diagnosis of trichinosis is confirmed by a history of ingestion of raw or undercooked meat. White blood cell (WBC) and eosinophil counts are elevated for 2 weeks after meat is ingested. Biopsy of skeletal muscle shows larvae of the *Trichinella* organism. Worms are rarely seen in feces.

During the first week after infection, the client is treated with oral mebendazole. During the stage of muscle invasion, he or she must be hospitalized to receive high doses of corticosteroids.

Hookworms

Hookworms are also roundworms. They differ from pinworms and *Trichinella* in that they initially enter the human body through the skin. Hookworm disease is caused by either *Ancylostoma duodenale* or *Necator americanus*.

Hookworms infect a quarter of the world's population, but the disease is rare in areas outside the tropics or in areas with little rain. Worms are infective outside the body in warm, moist soil for up to 1 week. Transmission occurs when larvae penetrate through the skin. The organism can migrate to pulmonary capillaries via the bloodstream and enter alveoli. Cilia carry the organisms up the respiratory tree to the pharynx and the mouth, where they are swallowed and enter the GI tract. Hookworms probably also enter the GI tract when a person ingests contaminated food.

Early symptoms of hookworm disease include a pruritic, erythematous, raised vesicular inflammation of the skin. Infection in the GI tract may produce no symptoms, or it may cause anorexia, diarrhea, or mild abdominal and epigastric discomfort. Bleeding and anemia may occur when worms suck blood at sites of attachment in the GI tract. If blood loss is severe, the client may have symptoms of iron deficiency anemia, such as pallor, hair thinning, deformed nails, pica, and shortness of breath.

Diagnosis of hookworm infection is based on the presence of ova (eggs) in the feces. Occult blood is often present in the stool. There may be a low hemoglobin concentration and hematocrit value or a low serum iron level and high iron-binding capacity, indicating hypochromic microcytic anemia. The WBC counts and eosinophil counts are elevated.

All clients with symptoms receive iron therapy and a diet high in protein and vitamins for at least 3 months after anemia is corrected. Pyrantel pamoate (Antiminth) or mebendazole (Vermox) is given for a complete recovery. Severe hookworm disease can cause malabsorption and protein loss, necessitating nutritional support in addition to other treatments.

Tapeworms

Five types of tapeworms (cestodes) may infect humans: tapeworms found in cattle, fish, dogs pigs, and rodents. Tapeworm infections generally cause either no symptoms or only occasional GI upset, such as nausea, diarrhea, or abdominal pain.

Transmission of tapeworms occurs when a person ingests undercooked beef, raw fish, or other contaminated food or water or accidentally swallows infected lice or fleas from dogs. People can also accidentally ingest arthropods, such as cockroaches, in stored foods or cereals.

The diagnosis of tapeworm infestation is made by laboratory examination of eggs found in the stool (test of stool for ova and parasites). Clients are treated with medications for this type of infection.

• • •

When caring for clients with helminths, the nurse follows standard precautions or body substance precautions when in contact with any stool. All clients are taught to wash their hands after defecating and before eating. They should avoid ingesting undercooked beef, fish, or pork, as well as drinking water that may be contaminated. After petting dogs, clients should take care to keep their mouth closed and wash their hands. All stored foods should be kept tightly closed to avoid contamination by cockroaches and other insects.

FOOD POISONING

Foodborne illnesses are a common problem, with 6.5 cases occurring in the United States every year (Van Benden et al., 1999). Food poisoning has been linked to as many as 9000 deaths per year in the United States (Shewmake & Dillon, 1998). Food poisoning results when a person ingests infectious organisms in food. Unlike gastroenteritis, food poisoning is not directly communicable from person to person, and incubation periods are shorter. Like gastroenteritis, it causes diarrhea, nausea, and vomiting. The nurse can differentiate food poisoning from gastroenteritis by obtaining a thorough history of common food intake in clients who have common symptoms of acute diarrhea, nausea, and vomiting.

The common types of food poisoning are caused by pathogens and include the following (Table 58-5):

- Gram-negative Salmonella
- *Staphylococcal aureus*
- *Escherichia coli*
- Botulism

TABLE 58-5 • COMMON TYPES OF FOOD POISONING
STAPHYLOCOCCAL INFECTION   • Caused by contaminated meats and dairy products   • Can be transmitted by human carriers   • Causes abrupt onset of vomiting and diarrhea without fever
***ESCHERICHIA COLI* INFECTION**   • Caused by meat contaminated with animal feces   • Causes abrupt vomiting, diarrhea, abdominal cramping, and fever
BOTULISM   • Commonly associated with improperly canned foods, especially fruits and vegetables   • Nausea, vomiting, diarrhea, and weakness progressing to paralysis   • Diplopia, dysphagia, and dysarthria
SALMONELLOSIS   • Caused by contaminated food or drink but can be transmitted by the fecal-oral route   • Fever, nausea, vomiting, abdominal cramping, and diarrhea lasting for 3 to 5 days

All cases of botulism and salmonellosis need to be reported to the local health department. Cases of staphylococcal and *E. coli* food poisoning are reported if epidemic outbreaks occur.

Salmonellosis

Salmonellosis is a bacterial infection caused by the *Salmonella* organism. It can be transmitted by the "five Fs": flies, fingers, food, feces, and fomites.

Incubation is 8 to 48 hours after the person has ingested the contaminated food or liquid. Symptoms usually last for 3 to 5 days and include fever with or without chills, nausea, vomiting, cramping abdominal pain, and diarrhea, which may be bloody.

Salmonellosis is usually self-limiting, but bacteremia with localization in joints or bone may occur. The definitive diagnosis is made by stool culture. Treatment is symptomatic, and drug therapy is not usually indicated unless bacteremia occurs; in that case, the physician prescribes antibiotics.

Clients may be carriers of the bacterium for up to 1 year. The nurse instructs all clients with *Salmonella* gastroenteritis and their contacts to wash their hands before meals and after defecating to avoid transmission of the organism. The treatment for *Salmonella* infection is controversial, since antibiotics tend not to shorten the illness. In some studies, quinolones have been shown to be effective, but these are usually reserved for individuals with severe manifestations of the illness.

Staphylococcal Infection

Staphylococcus is associated with 25% of reported food poisoning outbreaks. *Staphylococcus* is found in meats and dairy products and can be transmitted by carriers of the organism. For staphylococcal food poisoning to occur, there must be contamination of food and a period of time (hours) during which the organisms multiply. This can take place during the slow cooling of food after it is cooked.

Symptoms of staphylococcal food poisoning include an abrupt onset of vomiting, abdominal cramping, and diarrhea. The person usually has symptoms 2 to 4 hours after ingesting the contaminated food. There is no fever, but the client is weak.

A diagnosis can be made when stool culture yields 100,000 enterotoxin-producing staphylococci; however, symptoms rarely last more than 24 hours, and people do not always seek medical attention. Antimicrobial drug therapy is not usually indicated unless an agent produces progressive systemic involvement. Parenteral fluids may be necessary if fluid volume is grossly depleted.

Escherichia coli Infection

E. coli is not usually associated with food poisoning. Since 1992, however, there have been several outbreaks of *E. coli* food poisoning in the United States. Enterohemorrhagic strains of *E. coli* produce cytotoxins that cause outbreaks of hemorrhagic colitis and hemolytic-uremic syndrome. Treatment of the client with *E. coli* food poisoning includes IV fluids and antibiotic therapy.

Botulism

Botulism is a paralytic disease resulting from ingestion of a toxin in food contaminated with *Clostridium botulinum*. Botulism is most commonly associated with home-canned foods, particularly vegetables, fruits, condiments, and less commonly, meat and fish. It can be associated with commercially prepared products and with products not adequately heated to destroy toxins before they are eaten.

Incubation is usually 18 to 36 hours. After this time, symptoms occur; illness may be mild or severe, with paralysis, respiratory failure, and death. Initial symptoms include diplopia, dysphagia, and dysarthria.

Weakness can progress rapidly from the neck to the arms, thorax, and legs. Paralytic ileus, severe constipation, and urinary retention can also occur. Nausea, vomiting, and abdominal pain may occur before or after the onset of paralysis.

The diagnosis is made on the basis of the client's history and a stool culture of *C. botulinum*. The serum may be positive for toxins.

Treatment with trivalent botulism antitoxin (ABE) is given as soon as the diagnosis is made if the client is not hypersensitive to it. The physician may lavage the stomach to stop absorption of toxin. All clients are hospitalized to observe for and treat respiratory paralysis. Nothing is given orally until swallowing and respiratory difficulties pass. The physician orders IV fluids as needed. If respiratory paralysis occurs, tracheostomy and mechanical ventilation are implemented. If ventilation can be maintained, the client can survive with no neurologic deficits after the illness.

To prevent botulism, the nurse teaches clients the importance of discarding cans of food that are punctured or swollen or that have defective seals. Containers for home-canned foods must be sterilized by boiling for 20 minutes to destroy *C. botulinum* spores before canning.

ONLINE RESOURCES

For suggested readings and Internet resources, go to http://www.wbsaunders.com/SIMON/Iggy/.

SELECTED BIBLIOGRAPHY

Belaiche, J., et al. (1999). Acute lower gastrointestinal bleeding in Crohn's disease: Characteristics of a unique series of 34 patients. *American Journal of Gastroenterology, 94*(8), 2177-2181.

Bernstein, C., et al. (2000). Direct hospital costs for patients with inflammatory bowel disease in a Canadian tertiary care university hospital. *American Journal of Gastroenterology, 95*(3), 677-683.

Borwell, B. (1997). The psychosexual needs of stoma patients. *Professional Nurse, 12*(4), 250-255.

Butterton, J., & Calderwood, S. (1998). Acute infectious diarrheal diseases and bacterial food poisoning. In A.S. Fauci, E. Braunwald, & K.J. Isselbacher (Eds.), *Harrison's principles of internal medicine* (14th ed., pp. 796-801). New York: McGraw-Hill.

Casellas, F., et al. (2000). Impact of surgery for Crohn's disease on health-related quality of life. *American Journal of Gastroenterology, 95*(1), 177-181.

Cohen, R., et al. (2000). The cost of hospitalization for Crohn's disease. *American Journal of Gastroenterology, 95*(2), 524-530.

Delco, F., & Sonnenberg, A. (1999). Commonalities in the time trends of Crohn's disease and ulcerative colitis. *American Journal of Gastroenterology, 94*(8), 2172-2176.

Eckes, L.M., & Norton, B.A. (1997). Ulcerative colitis: From medical management to ileal pouch anal anastomosis—A patient's perspective. *Gastroenterology Nursing, 20*(3), 91-100.

Glickman, R. (1998). Inflammatory bowel disease: Ulcerative colitis and Crohn's disease. In A.S. Fauci, E. Braunwald, & K.J. Isselbacher (Eds.), *Harrison's principles of internal medicine* (14th ed., pp. 1633-1645). New York: McGraw-Hill.

Greenberg, H. (1998). Viral gastroenteritis. In A.S. Fauci, E. Braunwald, & K.J. Isselbacher (Eds.), *Harrison's principles of internal medicine* (14th ed., pp. 1116-1118). New York: McGraw-Hill.

Hirsch, C., & Caswell, D. (1999). Gastrointestinal disorders. In American Association of Critical-Care Nurses—A. Gawlinski & D. Hamwi (Eds.), *Acute care nurse practitioner clinical curriculum and certification review* (pp. 618-722). Philadelphia: W.B. Saunders.

Isselbacher, K., & Epstein, A. (1998). Diverticular, vascular, and other disorders of the intestine and peritoneum. In A.S. Fauci, E. Braunwald, & K.J. Isselbacher (Eds.), *Harrison's principles of internal medicine* (14th ed., pp. 1648-1656). New York: McGraw-Hill.

Klonowski, E., & Masoodi, J. (1999). The patient with Crohn's disease. *RN, 62*(3), 32-37.

Lynn, R., & Friedman, L. (1998). Irritable bowel syndrome. In A.S. Fauci, E. Braunwald, & K.J. Isselbacher (Eds.), *Harrison's principles of internal medicine* (14th ed., pp. 1646-1648). New York: McGraw-Hill.

Martin, F. (1997). Ulcerative colitis. *American Journal of Nursing 97*(8), 38-39.

Mikula, C. (1999). Anti-TNF alpha: New therapy for Crohn's disease. *Gastroenterology Nursing, 22*(6), 245-248.

Mishkin, S. (1997). Dairy sensitivity, lactose malabsorption, and elimination diets in inflammatory bowel disease. *American Journal of Clinical Nutrition, 65*(2), 564-567.

Moore, S., et al. (1998). Nurse perceptions of ostomy patients and their ostomy care competence. *Home Care Provider, 3*(4), 214-220.

Northouse, L.L., et al. (1999). The concerns of patients and spouses after the diagnosis of colon cancer: A qualitative analysis. *Journal of Wound, Ostomy, and Incontinence Nursing, 26*(1), 8-17.

Norton, B. (1998). Crohn's disease: A review of medical, surgical and nutritional management. *ADVANCE for Nurse Practitioners, 6*(9), 42-50.

Olmstead, J. (1998). Evaluation and management of the patient with ulcerative colitis. *Gastroenterology Nursing, 21*(4), 176-180.

Rayhorn, N. (1999). Understanding inflammatory bowel disease. *Nursing99, 29*(12), 57-61.

Rubin, D. (1998). Small and large bowel dysfunction. In Jameson, J.L. (Ed.), *Principles of molecular medicine.* New Jersey: Humana Press.

Shewmake, R., & Dillon, B. (1998). Food poisoning. *Postgraduate Medicine, 103*(6), 125-131.

Silen, W. (1998). Acute appendicitis. In A.S. Fauci et al. (Eds.), *Harrison's principles of internal medicine* (14th ed., pp. 1658-1660). New York: McGraw-Hill.

Van Benden, C., et al. (1999). Multiple outbreak of Salmonella enterica serotype Newport infections due to contaminated alfalfa sprouts. *Journal of the American Medical Association, 281*(2), 158-162.

Worley, J. (1999). Diagnosis and management of inflammatory bowel disease. *Journal of the American Academy of Nurse Practitioners, 11*(1), 23-31.

Interventions for Clients with Liver Problems

JANICE TAZBIR

Learning Objectives

After studying this chapter, you should be able to:

1. Describe the pathophysiology and complications associated with cirrhosis of the liver.
2. Interpret laboratory test findings commonly seen in clients with cirrhosis.
3. Analyze assessment data from clients with cirrhosis to determine priority nursing diagnoses and collaborative problems.
4. Formulate a collaborative plan of care for the client with severe late-stage cirrhosis.
5. Identify emergency interventions for the client with bleeding esophageal varices.
6. Evaluate care for clients with cirrhosis.
7. Develop a community-based teaching plan for the client with cirrhosis of the liver.
8. Compare and contrast the transmission of hepatitis A, B, and C viral infections.
9. Explain ways in which each type of hepatitis can be prevented.
10. Discuss the primary concerns about the increasing incidence of hepatitis C in the United States.
11. Identify treatment options for clients with cancer of the liver.
12. Describe the typical complications that result from liver transplantation.

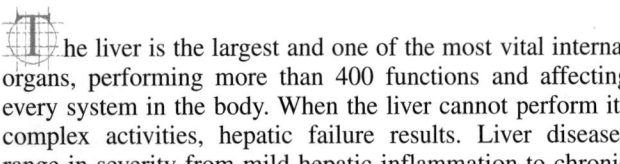

Go to http://www.wbsaunders.com/SIMON/Iggy/ for self-assessment questions related to these Learning Objectives.

The liver is the largest and one of the most vital internal organs, performing more than 400 functions and affecting every system in the body. When the liver cannot perform its complex activities, hepatic failure results. Liver diseases range in severity from mild hepatic inflammation to chronic end-stage cirrhosis.

CIRRHOSIS

OVERVIEW

Cirrhosis is a chronic, progressive liver condition. It usually develops insidiously and has a prolonged, destructive course. As an end-stage process, it is essentially an irreversible reaction to hepatic inflammation and necrosis.

Pathophysiology

Cirrhosis is characterized by diffuse fibrotic bands of connective tissue that distort the liver's normal architecture. Extensive degeneration and destruction of hepatocytes (hepatic [liver] cells) occur. In attempts to regenerate with new nodule formation, a disorganized lobular pattern develops. Flow alterations in the vascular system and lymphatic bile duct channels result from compression caused by the proliferation of fibrous tissue.

TYPES OF CIRRHOSIS

There are four major types of cirrhosis (Table 59-1):
1. Laënnec's, or alcoholic cirrhosis
2. Postnecrotic cirrhosis
3. Biliary cirrhosis
4. Cardiac cirrhosis

LAËNNEC'S CIRRHOSIS. Laënnec's cirrhosis, or alcoholic cirrhosis, is also called nutritional, or portal, cirrhosis. Alcohol has a direct toxic effect on the liver cells (hepatocytes) and causes liver inflammation (alcoholic hepatitis), which usually precedes the onset of alcoholic cirrhosis. Metabolic changes in the liver that are induced by alcohol lead to fatty infiltration of the hepatocytes and scarring between the lobules. The liver becomes enlarged, with cellular degeneration and infiltration by fat, leukocytes, and lymphocytes (white blood cells). As the inflammatory process decreases, the destructive phase increases. Early scar formation is caused by fibroblast infiltration and collagen formation. Damage to the hepatic parenchyma progresses as a result of malnutrition and repeated exposure to the hepatotoxin (alcohol). If alcohol is withheld, the fatty infiltration is reversible. If alcohol abuse continues, widespread scar tissue formation and fibrosis infiltrate the liver as a result of cellular necrosis.

TABLE 59-1 • MAJOR TYPES OF CIRRHOSIS OF THE LIVER

LAËNNEC'S CIRRHOSIS
- Most common type
- Caused by long-term use of alcohol
- Liver becomes enlarged, firm, and hard in early disease, and smaller and nodular in end-stage disease

POSTNECROTIC CIRRHOSIS
- Caused by massive hepatic cell necrosis, usually from acute viral hepatitis or exposure to certain hepatotoxins, such as industrial chemicals

BILIARY CIRRHOSIS
- Caused by chronic biliary obstruction, bile stasis, and inflammation
- Liver becomes fibrotic; hepatic cells are destroyed

CARDIAC CIRRHOSIS
- Caused by severe or chronic heart failure (also called vascular cirrhosis).
- Liver becomes enlarged and congested with venous blood, resulting in cell necrosis from anoxia

In early cirrhosis, the liver capsule is enlarged, firm, and hard. The regenerated nodules give the capsule a hobnailed, or bumpy, appearance. As the pathologic process of cirrhosis progresses, the liver shrinks in size. The capsule is covered with fine nodules surrounded by gray connective tissue.

POSTNECROTIC CIRRHOSIS. Postnecrotic cirrhosis occurs after massive liver cell necrosis. Broad bands of scar tissue cause the destruction of liver lobules and entire lobes. The liver enlarges and then becomes shrunken with large nodules, representing macronodular structural changes throughout the organ. Postnecrotic cirrhosis occurs most often as a complication of acute viral hepatitis or after exposure to industrial or chemical hepatotoxins (e.g., carbon tetrachloride). This type of cirrhosis is suspected in clients who exhibit signs of chronic liver disease and do not have a history of excessive alcohol intake.

BILIARY CIRRHOSIS. Biliary cirrhosis develops as a result of chronic biliary obstruction, bile stasis, inflammation, or diffuse hepatic fibrosis. *Primary* biliary cirrhosis results from intrahepatic bile stasis. *Secondary* biliary cirrhosis is caused by obstruction of the hepatic or common bile ducts, which produces bile stasis in the liver. The accumulation of excessive hepatic bile leads to progressive fibrosis, hepatocellular destruction, and regenerated nodules. Severe obstructive jaundice is a key clinical manifestation in both types of biliary cirrhosis.

CARDIAC CIRRHOSIS. Cardiac cirrhosis, or vascular cirrhosis, is associated with severe right-sided heart failure. It develops in clients with long-standing heart failure after cor pulmonale, constrictive pericarditis, and valvular insufficiency (see Chapter 35). The liver becomes enlarged, is congested with venous blood, and appears edematous and dark in color. The liver serves as a reservoir for large amounts of venous blood that the failing heart cannot pump back into the systemic circulation. The increase in hepatic volume and pressure causes severe venous congestion. The liver becomes anoxic, which results in hepatic cell necrosis and fibrosis.

■ COMPLICATIONS OF CIRRHOSIS

Common problems and complications associated with hepatic cirrhosis depend on the amount of damage sustained by the liver. The loss of hepatic function contributes to the development of metabolic abnormalities. Hepatic cell degeneration may lead to the following:
- Portal hypertension
- Ascites (accumulation of abdominal fluid)
- Bleeding esophageal varices
- Coagulation defects
- Jaundice
- Portal-systemic encephalopathy (PSE) with hepatic coma
- Hepatorenal syndrome

PORTAL HYPERTENSION. Portal hypertension, a persistent increase in pressure within the portal vein, is a major complication of cirrhosis. It results from increased resistance to or obstruction of the flow of blood through the portal vein and its tributaries. The blood meets resistance to flow and seeks collateral venous channels around the high-pressure area.

Blood flow backs into the spleen, causing splenomegaly. Veins in the esophagus, stomach, intestines, abdomen, and rectum become dilated. Portal hypertension can result in ascites, esophageal varices, prominent abdominal veins (caput medusae), and hemorrhoids.

ASCITES. Ascites is the accumulation of free fluid containing almost pure plasma within the peritoneal cavity. Increased hydrostatic pressure from portal hypertension causes plasma to leak into the peritoneal cavity. The accumulation of plasma protein, primarily albumin, in the peritoneal fluid reduces the amount of circulating plasma protein in the blood. When this decrease is combined with the inability of the liver to synthesize albumin because of impaired hepatocyte functioning, the effective serum colloid osmotic pressure is decreased in the circulatory system.

Increased hepatic lymph formation also contributes to ascites formation. The lymphatic system is unable to channel the increased amounts of lymph, and weeping of liver plasma ("liver sweat") occurs as a result. The decrease of effective intravascular circulation from massive ascites may cause renal vasoconstriction, triggering the renin-angiotensin system. This results in sodium and water retention, which increases hydrostatic pressure and lymph formation, and the vicious circle of ascites formation continues.

BLEEDING ESOPHAGEAL VARICES. As the blood backs up away from the liver, it enters the esophageal and gastric vessels that carry it into the systemic circulation. **Bleeding esophageal varices** occur when these fragile, thin-walled esophageal veins become distended or irritated and rupture. Variceal bleeding may be caused by the following:
- Any chemical irritant, such as alcohol, medications, and refluxed gastric acid
- Mechanical trauma from abrasions by poorly chewed food, vomiting, or nasogastric (NG) tube insertion
- Increased pressure in the esophagus caused by vigorous physical exercise, coughing, or retching and vomiting

Varices occur most often in the distal end of the esophagus but are also noted in the proximal esophagus and stomach. Gastric ulceration or erosion also puts the client at risk for hemorrhage from the stomach. Endoscopy, if possible, can differentiate between gastrointestinal and esophageal bleeding.

The client with bleeding esophageal varices loses large volumes of blood from hematemesis and may go into shock from hypovolemia. This condition is a medical emergency and needs immediate medical intervention (see Potential for Hemorrhage, p. 1308).

COAGULATION DEFECTS. With cirrhosis, there is a decrease in the synthesis of bile fats in the liver; this prevents the absorption of fat-soluble vitamins (e.g., vitamin K). Without vitamin K, clotting factors II, VII, IX, and X are not produced in sufficient quantities, and the client is susceptible to bleeding and easy bruising. Therefore when a client has bleeding esophageal varices, the blood does not clot and hemorrhage occurs.

CRITICAL THINKING CHALLENGE

You are the nurse for a client with Laënnec's cirrhosis. You go into the client's room and find the client in the bathroom vomiting what appears to be hematemesis (blood in the vomitus).

- What actions will you take?
- In what order of priority should you implement these interventions?
- How can you differentiate if this is a gastrointestinal bleed or an esophageal bleed?

For suggested answer guidelines, go to SIMON http://www.wbsaunders.com/SIMON/Iggy/.

JAUNDICE. **Jaundice** in clients with hepatic cirrhosis is caused by one of two mechanisms (Table 59-2): hepatocellular disease or intrahepatic obstruction. Hepatocellular jaundice develops because the liver cannot metabolize bilirubin. The liver's normal uptake of bilirubin from the blood is thus impaired. This decreased excretion results in excessive circulating bilirubin levels. Intrahepatic obstructive jaundice results from edema, fibrosis, or scarring of the hepatic bile channels and bile ducts, which interferes with normal bile and bilirubin excretion.

PORTAL-SYSTEMIC ENCEPHALOPATHY. **Portal-systemic encephalopathy (PSE)** is also known as **hepatic encephalopathy** and **hepatic coma** in the later stages. It is a clinical disorder seen in end-stage hepatic failure and cirrhosis. PSE is manifested by neurologic symptoms and is characterized by an altered level of consciousness, impaired thinking processes, and neuromuscular disturbances.

PSE may develop insidiously in clients with chronic liver disease and go undetected until the late stages. Symptoms develop rapidly in acute liver dysfunction. Four stages of development have been identified: prodromal, impending, stuporous, and comatose (Table 59-3). The client's symptoms may gradually progress to coma or fluctuate among the four stages.

The exact mechanisms of PSE have not been identified. The most probable cause is impaired ammonia metabolism. Most of the ammonia in the body is found in the gastrointestinal (GI) tract. Protein provided by the diet is transported to the liver by the portal vein. The liver breaks down protein by a series of enzymatic reactions. Protein is initially broken

down into glutamine (a nontoxic substance) and ammonia. Ammonia is further broken down into urea. Urea diffuses into the body fluids and is eventually excreted in the urine by the kidneys.

Some ammonia is normally formed in the GI tract by the action of intestinal bacteria on protein products. Gastric juices are also a source of ammonia, and peripheral tissue metabolism produces some ammonia. The kidney may be a source of endogenous ammonia if hypokalemia is present.

TABLE 59-2 • LABORATORY DIAGNOSTIC DIFFERENTIATION OF JAUNDICE			
Test	**Hepatocellular Jaundice**	**Obstructive Jaundice**	**Hemolytic Jaundice**
Serum bilirubin			
Indirect (unconjugated)	Increased	Slightly increased	Increased
Direct (conjugated)	Increased	Moderately increased	Normal
Urine bilirubin	Increased	Increased	None
Urobilinogen			
Stool	Normal to decreased	None	Increased
Urine	Normal to increased	None	Increased

TABLE 59-3 • STAGES OF PORTAL-SYSTEMIC ENCEPHALOPATHY

STAGE I: PRODROMAL
- Subtle manifestations that may not be recognized immediately
- Personality changes
- Behavior changes (agitation, belligerence)
- Emotional lability (euphoria, depression)
- Impaired thinking
- Inability to concentrate
- Fatigue, drowsiness
- Slurred or slowed speech
- Sleep pattern disturbances

STAGE II: IMPENDING
- Continuing mental changes
- Mental confusion
- Disorientation to time, place, or person
- Asterixis (see Figure 59-3)

STAGE III: STUPOROUS
- Progressive deterioration
- Marked mental confusion
- Stuporous, drowsy, but arousable
- Abnormal electroencephalogram tracing
- Muscle twitching
- Hyperreflexia
- Asterixis

STAGE IV: COMATOSE
- Unresponsiveness, leading to death in 85% of clients progressing to this stage
- Unarousable, obtunded
- Response to painful stimulus
- No asterixis
- Positive Babinski's sign
- Muscle rigidity
- Fetor hepaticus (characteristic liver breath—musty, sweet odor)
- Seizures

If the liver is incapable of adequate protein degradation and cannot convert ammonia to urea, an excessive amount of circulating ammonia develops. Elevated ammonia levels are toxic to central nervous system tissue (glial and nerve cells), interfering with normal cerebral metabolism and function.

Factors that may precipitate PSE include the following:
- High-protein diet
- Infections
- Hypovolemia (deficient fluid volume)
- Hypokalemia (deficient serum potassium)
- Constipation
- GI bleeding (causes a large protein load in the intestines)
- Drugs (e.g., hypnotics, opioids, sedatives, analgesics, diuretics)

PSE may also occur after paracentesis or shunting procedures. The prognosis for a client with PSE depends on the severity of the underlying cause, the precipitating factors, and the degree of liver dysfunction.

HEPATORENAL SYNDROME. The development of **hepatorenal syndrome** indicates a poor prognosis for the client with hepatic failure. It is one of the primary causes of death in end-stage cirrhosis. Progressive oliguric renal failure associated with hepatic failure results in functional impairment of kidneys with normal anatomic and morphologic features. This syndrome is manifested by the following:
- A sudden decrease in urinary flow
- Elevated blood urea nitrogen and creatinine levels, with abnormally decreased urine sodium excretion
- Increased urine osmolarity

Hepatorenal syndrome often occurs after clinical deterioration from GI bleeding or the onset of PSE. Drugs such as indomethacin (Indocin) and possibly acetaminophen (Tylenol, Exdol✿) and aspirin (acetylsalicylic acid [ASA]) may precipitate renal failure when administered to the client with cirrhosis. Hepatorenal syndrome is generally accompanied by elevated serum ammonia levels with an increase in jaundice and serum bilirubin levels. The kidneys cannot excrete these products in the urine. Hepatorenal syndrome may also complicate other liver diseases, including acute hepatitis and hepatic malignancy.

Etiology

The exact factors contributing to cirrhosis have not been clearly defined. There is a genetic component, with a familial tendency to develop cirrhosis and a familial hypersensitivity to alcohol in some people. Many alcoholics do not experience cirrhosis, whereas others have cirrhosis even when adequate nutrition is maintained.

The cause of cirrhosis varies with the type. Chronic infection with the hepatitis B virus is the number-one cause of cirrhosis in the world (Rollier et al., 1999). Laënnec's (alcoholic) cirrhosis results from the hepatotoxic effect of alcohol. Poor nutritional intake compounds the problem of a malnourished liver in most adults. Postnecrotic cirrhosis usually occurs after acute viral hepatitis, which may result from blood transfusions. It is seen after exposure to industrial or chemical hepatotoxins (e.g., carbon tetrachloride, arsenic, and phosphorus). Biliary cirrhosis results from chronic biliary obstruction and inflammation. Cardiac cirrhosis is associated with prolonged hepatic venous congestion. Cirrhosis often develops as an idiopathic process.

Incidence/Prevalence

Cirrhosis may develop at any age. Cirrhosis and chronic liver disease was the tenth leading cause of death in 1997, accounting for 25,175 deaths (Centers for Disease Control and Prevention [CDC], 1999). Of all cases of cirrhosis, 10% to 30% are postnecrotic and 5% to 10% are primary biliary. Laënnec's cirrhosis is the most common type of cirrhosis in industrialized countries. Most cases of cirrhosis could be prevented by eliminating alcohol intake. The death rate for cirrhosis in men is two times the rate for females, regardless race or ethnicity (National Institutes of Health [NIH], 1999).

> ### CULTURAL CONSIDERATIONS
> In the United States, mortality from cirrhosis is higher in African Americans and Hispanics (CDC, 1999). The cause is unknown.

► COLLABORATIVE MANAGEMENT

● Assessment

HISTORY

The nurse obtains historical data from clients with suspected cirrhosis, including age, sex, race, history of or present substance use, and employment history, especially exposure to harmful chemical toxins. The nurse determines whether there is a history of alcoholism in the family. The client is asked to describe his or her alcohol intake, including the amount consumed during a given period of time. The nurse also asks the client about previous medical conditions, such as acute viral hepatitis, biliary tract disorders, viral infections, blood transfusions, and a history of heart failure or respiratory disorders.

PHYSICAL ASSESSMENT/CLINICAL MANIFESTATIONS

Because cirrhosis has an insidious onset, many of the early signs and symptoms are vague and nonspecific. The client may report the following:
- Generalized weakness
- Weight loss
- GI symptoms (loss of appetite, early morning nausea and vomiting, dyspepsia, flatulence, and changes in bowel habits, with constipation and bouts of diarrhea)
- Abdominal pain and liver tenderness (both of which are often ignored by the client)

Hepatic function abnormalities are often detected when a physical examination or laboratory tests are completed for an unrelated illness or problem. The development of late signs of advanced cirrhosis may cause the client to seek medical treatment. GI bleeding, jaundice, ascites, and spontaneous bruising indicate deteriorating hepatic function and represent complications of cirrhosis.

The nurse thoroughly assesses the client with liver dysfunction or hepatic failure, because it affects every body system (Figure 59-1). The clinical picture and course vary from client to client depending on the severity of hepatic failure. An inspection may reveal the following:
- Obvious yellowing of the skin (jaundice) and the sclerae (icterus)
- Dry skin

NEUROLOGIC FINDINGS
Asterixis
Paresthesias of feet
Peripheral nerve degeneration
Portal-systemic encephalopathy
Reversal of sleep-wake pattern
Sensory disturbances

GASTROINTESTINAL (GI)
FINDINGS
Abdominal pain
Anorexia
Ascites
Clay-colored stools
Diarrhea
Esophageal varices
Fetor hepaticus
Gallstones
Gastritis
Gastrointestinal bleeding
Hemorrhoidal varices
Hepatomegaly
Hiatal hernia
Hypersplenism
Malnutrition
Nausea
Small nodular liver
Vomiting

RENAL FINDINGS
Hepatorenal syndrome
Increased urine bilirubin

ENDOCRINE FINDINGS
Increased aldosterone
Increased antidiuretic hormone
Increased circulating estrogens
Increased glucocorticoids
Gynecomastia

IMMUNE SYSTEM DISTURBANCES
Increased susceptibility to infection
Leukopenia

CARDIOVASCULAR FINDINGS
Cardiac dysrhythmias
Development of collateral circulation
Fatigue
Hyperkinetic circulation
Peripheral edema
Portal hypertension
Spider angiomas

PULMONARY FINDINGS
Dyspnea
Hydrothorax
Hyperventilation
Hypoxemia

HEMATOLOGIC FINDINGS
Anemia
Disseminated intravascular
    coagulation
Impaired coagulation
Splenomegaly
Thrombocytopenia

DERMATOLOGIC FINDINGS
Axillary and pubic hair changes
Caput medusae
Ecchymosis
Increased skin pigmentation
Jaundice
Palmar erythema
Pruritus
Spider angiomas

FLUID AND ELECTROLYTE
DISTURBANCES
Ascites
Decreased effective blood volume
Dilutional hyponatremia or
    hypernatremia
Hypocalcemia
Hypokalemia
Peripheral edema
Water retention

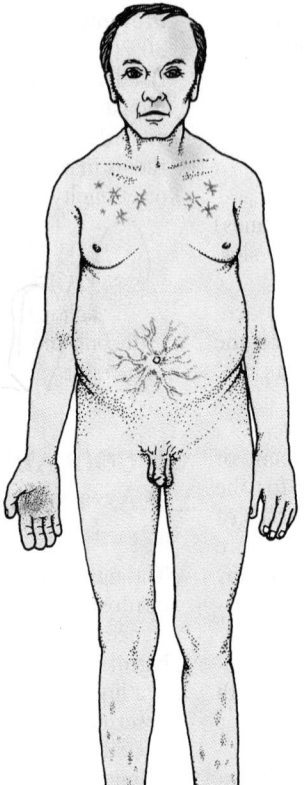

Figure 59-1 ● The clinical picture of a client with liver dysfunction. Signs and symptoms vary according to the progression of the disease. Early signs and symptoms are noted in color.

- Rashes
- Purpuric lesions, such as petechiae (round, pinpoint, red-purple lesions) or ecchymosis (large purple, blue, or yellow bruises)
- Warm and bright red palms of the hands (palmar erythema)
- Vascular lesions with a red center and radiating branches, known as "spider angiomas" (telangiectasias, spider nevi, or vascular spiders), on the nose, cheeks, upper thorax, and shoulders
- Peripheral dependent edema of the extremities and sacrum

ABDOMINAL ASSESSMENT. The nurse may readily detect *massive* ascites as a distended abdomen with bulging flanks. The umbilicus may protrude, and dilated abdominal veins (caput medusae) may radiate from the umbilicus. Ascites can cause physical problems; for example, orthopnea and dyspnea from increased abdominal distention can interfere with lung expansion. The client may have difficulty maintaining an erect body posture, and problems with balance may affect walking. The nurse inspects and palpates for the presence of inguinal or umbilical hernias, which are likely to develop in clients with ascites because of increased intra-abdominal pressure.

Minimal ascites is often more difficult to detect. Advanced assessment techniques, such as the percussion test for shifting dullness and the presence of a fluid wave, may be performed by the health care provider.

When performing an assessment of the abdomen, the nurse keeps in mind that hepatomegaly occurs in 60% of all cases of early cirrhosis. The advanced practice nurse or other health care provider palpates the right upper quadrant for **hepatomegaly** (enlarged liver) below the costal (rib cage) border. The presence of hepatomegaly may be determined by percussing for dullness over the enlarged liver.

The nurse measures the client's abdominal girth to evaluate the progression of ascites (Figure 59-2). To measure abdominal girth, the client lies flat while the nurse pulls a tape measure around the largest diameter of the abdomen. The girth is measured at the end of exhalation. The abdominal skin

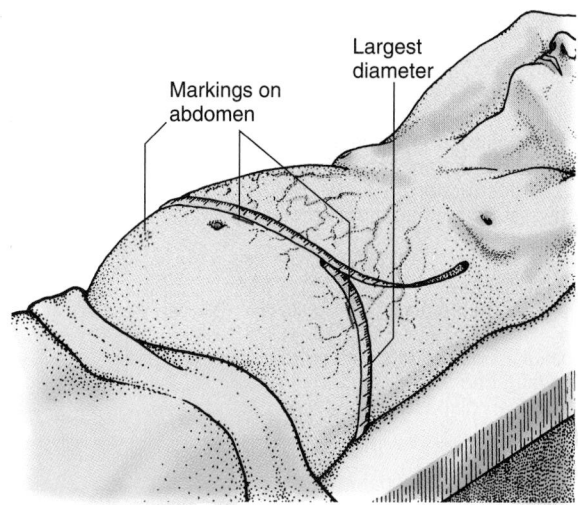

Figure 59-2 ● How to measure abdominal girth. With the client supine, the nurse brings the tape measure around the client and takes a measurement at the level of the umbilicus. Before removing the tape, the nurse marks the client's abdomen along the sides of the tape on the client's flanks (sides) and midline to ensure that later measurements are taken in the same place.

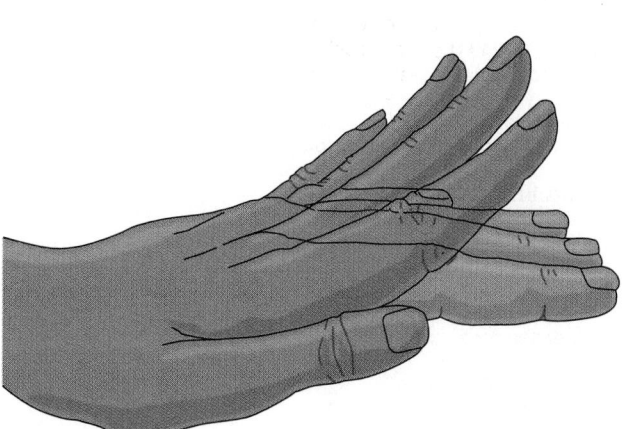

Figure 59-3 ● To elicit asterixis (flapping tremor), have the client extend the arm, dorsiflex the wrist, and extend the fingers. Observe for rapid, nonrhythmic extensions and flexions.

and flanks should be marked to ensure the same tape measure placement on subsequent readings.

OTHER PHYSICAL ASSESSMENT. The nurse assesses nasogastric (NG) tube drainage (if present), vomitus, and stool for the presence of blood. This may be indicated by frank blood in the excrement or by a positive result of an *o*-toluidine test for occult blood content (Hema-Check, Hematest). Gastritis, stomach ulceration, or oozing esophageal varices may be responsible for the presence of blood (**melena).**

The nurse may note fetor hepaticus, which is the distinctive breath odor of chronic liver disease and portal-systemic encephalopathy (PSE). It is characterized by a fruity or musty odor. Fetor hepaticus results from the inability of the damaged liver to metabolize and detoxify mercaptan, which is produced by bacterial degradation of methionine, a sulfurous amino acid.

Amenorrhea may occur in women, and men may exhibit testicular atrophy, **gynecomastia** (enlarged breasts), and impotence as a result of inactive hormones. Clients with problems of the hematologic system caused by hepatic failure may have bruising, **petechiae** (small, purplish hemorrhagic spots on the skin), and an enlarged spleen.

The nurse continually assesses the client's neurologic functioning. Subtle changes in mentation and personality often progress to coma, a late complication of PSE. The nurse also assesses for **asterixis** (liver flap or flapping tremor), a coarse tremor characterized by rapid, nonrhythmic extensions and flexions in the wrists and fingers. Asterixis also appears in the ankles, corners of the mouth, eyelids, and tongue. Figure 59-3 illustrates the technique used to elicit asterixis during physical assessment.

■ PSYCHOSOCIAL ASSESSMENT

The client with hepatic cirrhosis may undergo subtle or obvious personality, cognitive, and behavior changes, such as ag-

itation and belligerence. He or she may experience sleep pattern disturbances or may exhibit signs of emotional lability, euphoria, or depression. The nurse performs a psychosocial assessment to identify needs and help guide client care. For reasons unknown, individuals living in poorer, inner city communities experience a disproportionate percentage of liver disease (Frieden et al., 1999)

Repeated hospitalizations are common for clients with alcohol-induced cirrhosis who do not adhere to treatment plans. The nurse assesses the impact of the hospitalizations on the client's lifestyle and self-esteem. Social workers assess the client's financial capabilities to help determine whether assistance is needed.

■ LABORATORY ASSESSMENT

Characteristic abnormalities are common in laboratory studies of clients with liver disease (Table 59-4). Serum levels of aspartate aminotransferase (AST), alanine aminotransferase (ALT), and lactate dehydrogenase (LDH) are elevated because these enzymes are released into the blood with the destruction of hepatic cells. Alkaline phosphatase levels are sensitive to mild extrahepatic or intrahepatic biliary obstruction and therefore increase in clients with cirrhosis.

Total serum bilirubin levels also rise. Indirect bilirubin levels rise in clients with cirrhosis because of the inability of the failing liver to conjugate bilirubin. Therefore bilirubin is present in the urine (urobilinogen) in increased amounts. Fecal urobilinogen concentration is decreased in clients with biliary tract obstruction, which occurs in biliary cirrhosis. These clients exhibit light- or clay-colored stools.

Total serum protein and albumin levels are decreased in clients with severe or chronic liver disease as a result of decreased synthesis by the liver. Serum levels of globulins (alpha, beta, and gamma) are elevated because of their increased synthesis by the reticuloendothelial system of the liver, which indicates an immune response to hepatic disease.

Prothrombin time (PT) is prolonged because the liver decreases the synthesis of prothrombin, reflecting hepatocellular

TABLE 59-4 • ASSESSMENT OF ABNORMAL LABORATORY FINDINGS IN LIVER DISEASE

Abnormal Finding	Significance
SERUM ENZYMES	
Elevated serum aspartate aminotransferase (AST)	Hepatic cell destruction, hepatitis (most specific indicator)
Elevated serum alanine aminotransferase (ALT)	Hepatic cell destruction, hepatitis
Elevated lactate dehydrogenase (LDH)	Hepatic cell destruction
Elevated serum alkaline phosphatase	Obstructive jaundice, hepatic metastasis
BILIRUBIN	
Elevated serum total bilirubin	Hepatic cell disease
Elevated serum direct conjugated bilirubin	Hepatitis, liver metastasis
Elevated serum indirect unconjugated bilirubin	Cirrhosis
Elevated urine bilirubin	Hepatocellular obstruction, viral or toxic liver disease
Elevated urine urobilinogen	Hepatic dysfunction
Decreased fecal urobilinogen	Obstructive liver disease
SERUM PROTEINS	
Increased serum total protein	Acute liver disease
Decreased serum total protein	Chronic liver disease
Decreased serum albumin	Severe liver disease
Elevated serum globulin	Immune response to liver disease
OTHER TESTS	
Elevated serum ammonia	Advanced liver disease or portal-systemic encephalopathy (PSE)
Prolonged prothrombin time (PT) or INR	Hepatic cell damage and synthesis of prothrombin

INR, International Normalized Ratio.

or obstructive biliary tract disease. Anemia may be reflected by an altered complete blood count (CBC), with decreased hemoglobin and hematocrit values. The white blood cell (WBC) count may also be decreased. Increased toxins in the blood lead to premature cell death. Ammonia levels are elevated in the presence of advanced liver disease and PSE because the conversion of ammonia to urea for excretion is decreased.

■ RADIOGRAPHIC ASSESSMENT

Abdominal x-ray studies may reveal an enlarged liver, gas or cysts within the liver and biliary tract, calcification of the liver, and massive ascites.

The upper gastrointestinal (GI) radiographic series is an examination of the esophagus, stomach, and small bowel. It may show the presence of esophageal varices or gastric or duodenal ulceration, all of which complicate the care of a client with cirrhosis.

The physician may order angiographic studies to identify actual arterial bleeding sites within the stomach. A computed tomography (CT) scan is helpful in detecting minimal ascites and provides information about the volume and character of fluid collections.

■ OTHER DIAGNOSTIC ASSESSMENT

The physician may perform an esophagogastroduodenoscopy (EGD) to directly visualize the upper GI tract and to detect the presence of bleeding or oozing esophageal varices, stomach irritation and ulceration, or duodenal ulceration and bleeding. Injection sclerotherapy may be performed as a palliative measure during the endoscopic procedure to halt variceal bleeding (see Potential for Hemorrhage, p. 1308).

Radioisotope liver scans show abnormal hepatic thickening and identify liver masses. The physician may use liver biopsy as the definitive test for cirrhosis. A hepatic tissue biopsy reveals destruction and fibrosis of the hepatic cells, which is indicative of the disease.

■ Analysis

■ COMMON NURSING DIAGNOSES AND COLLABORATIVE PROBLEMS

The most common nursing diagnosis for clients with cirrhosis is Excess Fluid Volume related to portal hypertension (causing ascites) and decreased serum colloid osmotic pressure.

The following are the primary collaborative problems for clients with cirrhosis:
1. Potential for Hemorrhage
2. Potential for Portal-Systemic Encephalopathy (PSE)

■ ADDITIONAL NURSING DIAGNOSES AND COLLABORATIVE PROBLEMS

In addition to the common nursing diagnoses and collaborative problems, clients with cirrhosis may have one or more of the following:
- Imbalanced Nutrition: Less than Body Requirements related to anorexia, nausea, and faulty absorption, metabolism, and storage of nutrients and vitamins
- Ineffective Breathing Pattern related to ascites and decreased diaphragmatic excursion and pressure on the diaphragm from ascites
- Impaired Comfort related to abdominal pressure
- Risk for Infection related to a decreased number of white blood cells
- Risk for Impaired Skin Integrity related to pruritus secondary to jaundice, edema, and ascites
- Ineffective Coping related to a chronic and potentially fatal disease process
- Sexual Dysfunction related to altered hormonal function and decreased libido

- Disturbed Body Image related to distended abdomen and skin lesions

Additional collaborative problems include the following:
- Potential for Drug Toxicity
- Potential for Hypokalemia

▶ Planning and Implementation

▥ EXCESS FLUID VOLUME

NOC **PLANNING: EXPECTED OUTCOMES.** The client with cirrhosis is expected to experience a decrease in extravascular and intra-abdominal fluid as indicated by (1) a decrease or absence of ascites, (2) serum electrolytes within normal limits (WNL), and (3) blood pressure in expected range (IER).

INTERVENTIONS. Fluid accumulations are minimal during the early stages of ascites, and therefore interventions are aimed at preventing the accumulation of additional fluid and mobilizing the existing fluid collection. Nonsurgical treatment measures usually control ascites. If respiratory or abdominal functioning is compromised, surgical measures may be necessary. (See the Concept Map for chronic liver failure on p. 1306.)

NONSURGICAL MANAGEMENT. Supportive measures to control abdominal ascites include diet therapy, drugs, paracentesis, and comfort measures. The nurse also carefully monitors fluid and electrolyte status.

DIET THERAPY. The health care provider usually places the client with abdominal ascites on a low sodium diet as an initial means of controlling fluid accumulation in the abdominal cavity. The amount of daily sodium intake restriction typically varies from 500 mg to 2 g. In collaboration with the dietitian, the nurse explains the purpose of the diet and advises the client to eliminate table salt and salty foods. (See Chapter 13 for a list of high-sodium foods.) The absence of salt in low-sodium diets is distasteful to most people, so the dietitian suggests alternative flavoring additives such as lemon, vinegar, parsley, oregano, and pepper.

The health care provider may limit the client's fluid intake if serum sodium levels fall. The kidneys retain sodium, and dilutional hyponatremia results, primarily from excessive fluid volume. Intravenous (IV) and oral fluids are restricted to 1000 to 1500 mL/day in an effort to reverse the fluid overload and raise the serum sodium level. The nurse calculates the permitted amount of oral fluids on the basis of the ordered IV intake.

In general, clients with cirrhosis are malnourished and have multiple dietary deficiencies. Vitamin supplements, such as thiamine, folate, and multivitamin preparations, are typically added to the IV fluids because of the inability of the liver to store vitamins. Oral vitamins are given when IV fluid administration is discontinued.

DRUG THERAPY. The health care provider usually orders a diuretic to reduce fluid accumulation and to prevent cardiac and respiratory impairment.

The nurse monitors the effect of diuretic therapy by assessing intake and output, weighing the client daily, measuring abdominal girth, and monitoring electrolyte levels. Serious electrolyte imbalances, such as hypokalemia (decreased

potassium) and hyponatremia (decreased sodium), may accompany diuretic therapy. (See Chapter 13 for discussion of electrolyte imbalances.) Depending on the diuretic selected, the provider may order an oral or IV potassium supplement.

Clients with cirrhosis often require antacid therapy for GI symptoms. Because most antacids are high in sodium, the physician prescribes a low-sodium antacid such as magaldrate (Riopan).

PARACENTESIS. Abdominal **paracentesis** may be indicated if dietary restrictions and drug administration fail to control ascites (Chart 59-1). The procedure is performed at the bedside. The physician inserts a trocar catheter into the abdomen to remove and drain ascitic fluid from the peritoneal cavity.

Once a primary treatment modality for ascites, paracentesis is more commonly used as a diagnostic tool to examine ascitic fluid. It is also used as a palliative measure to relieve abdominal pressure, because ascites may cause severe respiratory and abdominal distress. To relieve acute symptoms, the physician slowly drains the ascitic fluid (usually 1 to 3 L). Hypovolemia with a fluid volume deficit may occur with rapid fluid removal, because these clients have adjusted to the excessive fluid volume in the abdomen. Rapid, drastic removal of ascitic fluid leads to decreased abdominal pressure, which may contribute to vasodilation and shock. The nurse observes for impending signs of shock from fluid shifts during and immediately after the procedure.

Repeated paracentesis procedures are contraindicated because of the increased incidence of protein depletion, hypovolemia, and electrolyte imbalances (hypokalemic alkalosis), which can contribute to the development of portal-systemic encephalopathy in the client with cirrhosis.

COMFORT MEASURES. Excessive ascitic fluid volume in the abdomen may cause the client to experience respiratory difficulty. Dyspnea may develop as a result of increased intra-abdominal pressure, which limits thoracic expansion and diaphragmatic excursion. The nurse or assistive nursing personnel elevates the head of the bed to at least 30 degrees or as high as the client wishes in an effort to minimize shortness of breath. The client is encouraged to sit in a chair. This upright position, with his or her feet elevated to discourage dependent ankle edema, often relieves dyspnea.

To weigh the client, the nurse or assistive nursing personnel uses a standard upright bedside scale (if the client can stand). Weighing on a bed scale necessitates that the client lie flat; this supine position can cause the client to feel increasingly short of breath and can increase anxiety.

NIC *FLUID/ELECTROLYTE MANAGEMENT.* The nurse monitors the client for fluid and electrolyte imbalances as a result of the disease or treatment. Laboratory tests, such as blood urea nitrogen (BUN), serum protein, hematocrit, and electrolytes help to determine fluid and electrolyte status. Nursing activities are listed in Chart 59-2.

SURGICAL MANAGEMENT. When medical management fails to control ascites, the physician may choose surgical intervention to divert ascites into the venous system by creating a shunt. However, the shunt has limited use as an effective treatment for ascites. Clients with ascites are poor sur-

Concept Map: Chronic Liver Failure

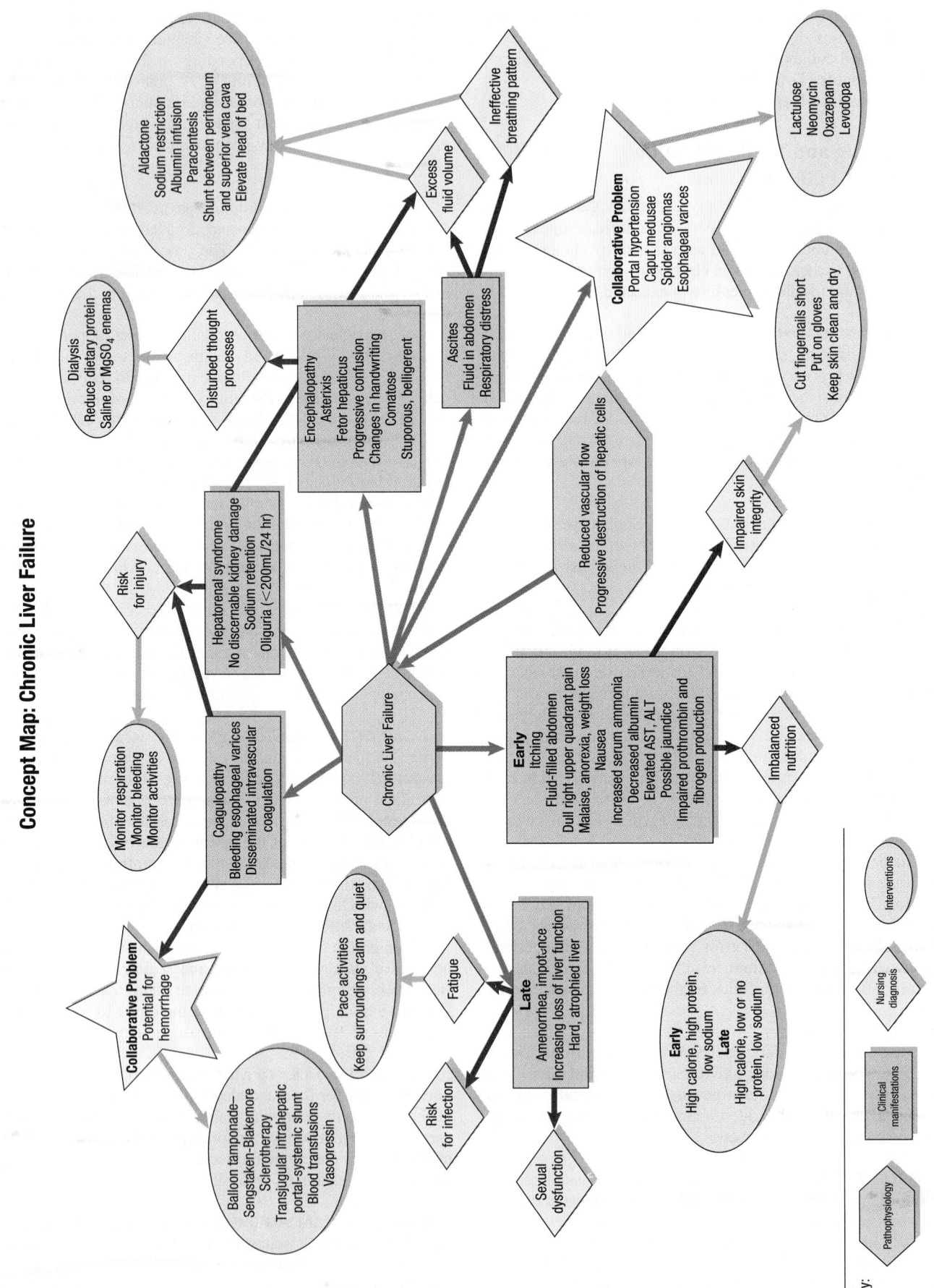

Key:

Interventions

Nursing diagnosis

Clinical manifestations

Pathophysiology

CHART 59-1

BEST PRACTICE *for*
Care of the Client Having a Paracentesis

- Explain the procedure, and answer the client's questions.
- Obtain vital signs, measure the client's abdominal girth, and weigh the client.
- Ask the client to void completely or drain the Foley catheter.
- Position the client. Assist him or her to sit in an upright position at the side of the bed with the feet propped on a stool. Support the client to maintain this position during the procedure.
- Monitor vital signs every 15 minutes during the procedure.
- Measure the drainage and record on the intake and output record.
- Describe the collected fluid (e.g., clear, straw-colored, hazy, or cloudy). Send specimens for laboratory analysis.
- After the physician removes the trocar catheter, apply a dressing to the puncture site. Assess for fluid leakage.
- Position the client in bed and maintain bedrest until vital signs are stable and return to baseline.

CHART 59-2

NIC INTERVENTION ACTIVITIES *for*
The Client with Cirrhosis

Fluid/Electrolyte Management: *Regulation and prevention of complications from altered fluid and/or electrolyte levels*
- Obtain laboratory specimens for monitoring of altered fluid and electrolyte levels (i.e. hematocrit, BUN, protein, sodium and potassium levels) as appropriate.
- Keep an accurate record of intake and output.
- Weigh daily and monitor trends.
- Monitor for signs and symptoms of fluid retention.
- Monitor vital signs, as appropriate.
- Administer prescribed supplemental electrolytes, as appropriate.

Bleeding Precautions: *Reduction of stimuli that may induce bleeding or hemorrhage in at-risk clients*
- Monitor the client closely for hemorrhage.
- Monitor for signs and symptoms of persistent bleeding (e.g., check all secretions for frank or occult blood)
- Monitor coagulation studies, including prothrombin time (PT), partial prothrombin time (PTT), fibrinogen, fibrin degradation/split products, and platelet counts, as appropriate
- Monitor orthostatic vital signs, including blood pressure.
- Use electric razor, instead of straight-edge, for shaving
- Use soft toothbrush or toothettes for oral care.
- Avoid injections (IV, IM, or SQ), as appropriate.
- Protect the client from trauma, which may cause bleeding.

Neurologic Monitoring: *Collection and analysis of client data to prevent or minimize neurologic complications*
- Monitor level of consciousness.
- Monitor level of orientation.
- Monitor recent memory, attention span, past memory, mood, affect, and behaviors.
- Monitor vital signs: temperature, blood pressure, pulse, and respirations.

NIC intervention activities selected from McCloskey, J.C., & Bulechek, G.M. (Eds.). (2000). *Nursing interventions classification (NIC)* (3rd ed.) St. Louis: Mosby. No part of this work is to be altered without prior written permission from the Publisher. *BUN,* Blood urea nitrogen.

gical risks because of their susceptibility to infection, as evidenced by the following:

- A decreased WBC count
- Disseminated intravascular coagulation (DIC)
- Bleeding esophageal varices
- Anesthesia reactions

Mortality in these clients having shunt procedures can be as great as 11% perioperatively; complication rates are approximately 30% (Ziser et al., 1999).

PREOPERATIVE CARE. Because the client with cirrhosis has many underlying medical problems, an optimal physical state is desired before surgery is performed. Electrolyte imbalances are corrected, and abnormal coagulation is treated with the administration of fresh frozen plasma and vitamin K. Packed red blood cells are made available for transfusion, because these clients have bleeding tendencies.

OPERATIVE PROCEDURES. One of several types of shunts may be created, such as the peritoneovenous and Denver shunts.

Peritoneovenous Shunt. A peritoneovenous shunt, also known as a peritoneojugular or LeVeen shunt (Figure 59-4), drains ascites through a one-way valve into a silicone rubber tube that terminates in the superior vena cava. A pressure gradient develops between the peritoneal cavity and the vena cava, facilitating the flow of ascitic fluid through the valve into the venous system. During inspiration, the diaphragm descends, which increases peritoneal fluid (ascites) pressure; pressure in the superior vena cava also increases, which creates the needed gradient. A pressure difference of greater than 3 cm H_2O is necessary to open the valve. The valve closes when the pressure is decreased.

After the shunt has been inserted, the client is expected to lose weight, show a decrease in abdominal girth, have increased urinary output, and exhibit an increased renal excretion of sodium. These clinical improvements result from restored adequate peripheral circulation.

Denver Shunt. The Denver shunt has a subcutaneous pump that can be manually compressed. It is often preferred for clients whose ascites contains large particles (common in neoplastic ascites). These particles can cause the flow to be-

come sluggish and result in a clotted shunt. Compressing the pump of the Denver shunt helps to irrigate the tubing to maintain patency.

POSTOPERATIVE CARE. The nurse provides the usual postoperative care for a client undergoing abdominal surgery (see Chapter 19). The nurse remains aware that the ascitic fluid is routed into the venous system, resulting in vascular volume expansion and hemodilution. The vital signs are monitored carefully; an increase in blood pressure reflects an increase in vascular volume. If the client has a central venous or pulmonary artery catheter in place, the nurse determines whether pressure is elevated. Breath sounds are auscultated for the presence of crackles, which indicates excessive lung fluid. A diuretic, such as furosemide (Lasix), is usually ordered to rid the body of excessive fluid.

The nurse notes any abnormal results of coagulation studies (prothrombin time [PT] and partial thromboplastin time [PTT]). Reabsorption of clotting factors in ascitic fluid may further inhibit an already altered clotting mechanism and lead to DIC and bleeding abnormalities.

The nurse or assistive nursing personnel measures the client's weight, abdominal girth, and urinary output each shift to determine the effectiveness of the shunting procedure.

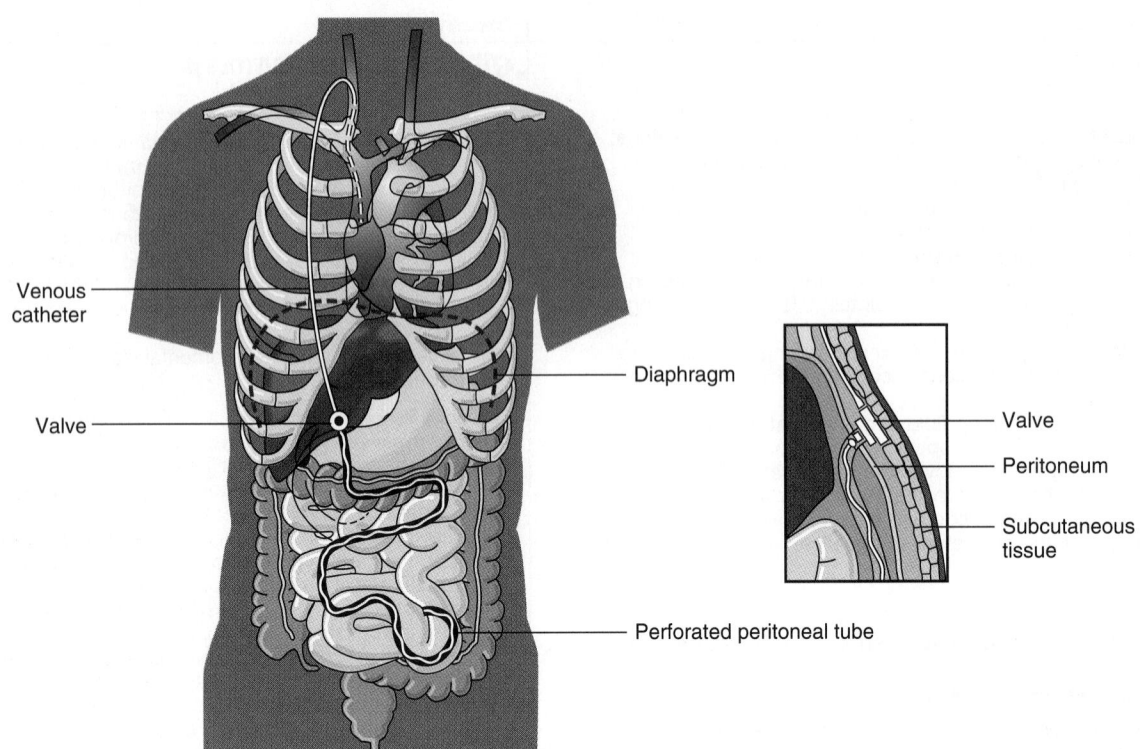

Figure 59-4 ● Peritoneovenous (LeVeen) shunting for treatment of ascites.

■ POTENTIAL FOR HEMORRHAGE

PLANNING: EXPECTED OUTCOMES. If the client experiences hemorrhage, it is expected to be controlled through medical and nursing interventions.

INTERVENTIONS. During the acute phase of bleeding, early interventions are based on identifying the source of bleeding and initiating treatment to halt it. Because massive esophageal bleeding can cause rapid blood loss, emergency interventions are initiated. If the client is a known alcoholic with a history of variceal bleeding, measures to treat the esophageal varices are initiated and therefore valuable time is not wasted looking for another source of bleeding.

NONSURGICAL MANAGEMENT. The health care team intervenes quickly to control bleeding by providing gastric intubation, balloon tamponade, drug therapy, replacement of blood products, injection sclerotherapy, or transjugular intrahepatic portal-systemic shunt (TIPS). The client is managed in the critical care unit. After the acute bleeding episode has been controlled, the client may require surgical intervention to decrease portal hypertension, thereby decreasing the risk of further variceal bleeding.

GASTRIC INTUBATION. Early in the hospitalization, the client's reports of hematemesis should be investigated. The physician usually inserts an 18-gauge Salem sump tube and lavages the stomach until the fluid returned is clear. The introduction of saline or water lavage may be used to achieve vasoconstriction of the bleeding gastric ulceration or varices. The physician may add norepinephrine (Levophed) to the solution to produce further constriction.

If endoscopy identifies the bleeding site as a gastric ulcer, the physician initiates medical treatment with drug therapy (antacids and histamine receptor antagonists) and blood product replacement. If bleeding continues from the ulcer, surgical intervention is necessary.

ESOPHAGOGASTRIC BALLOON TAMPONADE. If the physician suspects that hematemesis has occurred because of bleeding esophageal varices, he or she inserts an esophagogastric tamponade tube. Bleeding varices are a medical emergency and necessitate immediate intervention. The primary nursing intervention is maintaining a patent airway. Vomiting and the accumulation of blood in the oropharynx may result in aspiration, occlusion of the airway, and respiratory compromise. The nurse attempts to keep the client's oropharynx clear by suctioning secretions, turning the client's head, and keeping the head of the bed elevated during vomiting episodes to prevent aspiration.

Types of Esophagogastric Tubes. The classic method of treating bleeding esophageal varices is by compressing the bleeding vessels with an esophagogastric tube, such as the Sengstaken-Blakemore tube (Blakemore tube), which has two balloons. This type of tube is also referred to as a **tamponade tube.** When inflated, the large esophageal balloon compresses the esophagus. The smaller gastric balloon helps anchor the tube and exerts pressure against bleeding varices in the distal esophagus and the cardia of the stomach. A third lumen terminates in the stomach and is connected to suction, allowing the aspiration of gastric contents and blood. A Salem sump tube is used in conjunction with the Sengstaken-Blakemore tube and is placed in the proximal esophagus to enable clearing of collected esophageal secretions, saliva, and blood.

Insertion of an Esophagogastric Tube. Before the physician inserts the tube, the nurse inspects it and inflates and deflates the balloons to check for integrity and leaks. Each lumen is identified and labeled to prevent errors in adding or removing pressure and air volume.

The physician usually anesthetizes the client's nose and oropharynx, introduces the tube through the nares, and gently inserts it into the stomach. After tube placement is verified, the stomach is aspirated and irrigated. The gastric balloon is inflated with up to 300 mL of air. The nurse assists the physician in securing the tube and applying traction, which provides additional tamponading pressure. This is accomplished by taping the tube to the face guard of a football helmet or by securing it to an overbed traction apparatus and applying a 1-pound (0.45-kg) traction weight.

Care of the Client with an Esophagogastric Tube. Inflation of the esophageal balloon is measured with a sphygmomanometer. Pressure should be maintained between 20 and 25 mm Hg. The nurse periodically checks the balloon pressures and volumes to prevent loss of pressure (with further bleeding or erosion) or rupture of the esophagus caused by overinflation (Chart 59-3). The esophagogastric balloon is usually removed after 48 hours. The nurse attaches the esophageal and gastric drainage lumina to low intermittent suction and monitors the amount and type of drainage.

Placement of the tamponade tube should halt variceal bleeding. After bleeding is controlled, the traction is released, and esophageal pressure is gradually decreased. The gastric balloon is deflated, and the tube is removed. Another tube should be kept at the bedside for potential reinsertion if bleeding recurs.

The nurse and assistive nursing personnel should be alert for sudden respiratory compromise with acute distress caused by airway obstruction from upward displacement of the esophageal balloon. A pair of scissors is *always* kept at the bedside. If the tube becomes dislodged, the nurse cuts both balloon ports to rapidly deflate the balloon and quickly removes the tube.

BLOOD TRANSFUSIONS. Massive hemorrhage necessitates replacement by blood products. Blood is drawn to identify the client's blood type. Until the blood is available, the nurse administers large crystalloid (IV fluids) or colloid (plasma) volumes, as ordered, into large-bore IV access routes to maintain blood pressure.

The nurse administers packed red blood cells and fresh frozen plasma (per physician order and agency policy) to replace blood volume and clotting factors. The physician and the nurse monitor trends in hemoglobin and hematocrit levels, and additional blood products are transfused as indicated.

DRUG THERAPY. To prevent the incidence of esophageal hemorrhage, the client may be placed on propranolol (Inderal, Apo-Propranolol♣) therapy. By decreasing heart rate and systemic blood pressure, the chance of bleeding may be reduced.

In a client who is actively bleeding, the physician may use a vasoconstrictor (e.g., vasopressin [Pitressin]), to temporarily control hemorrhage by lowering pressure within the portal blood flow system. This drug causes contraction of smooth muscle in the vascular bed. By constricting preportal splanchnic arterioles, blood flow is decreased to the abdominal organs, which reduces portal pressure and portal blood flow.

Vasopressin is administered by infusion pump intravenously or through a catheter placed in the superior mesen-

---

CHART 59-3

BEST PRACTICE *for*
Care of Clients with Esophageal Tamponade Tubes

- Assist the physician with tube placement. Before the gastric balloon is inflated, make sure that a chest x-ray film is obtained and is available *immediately* on tube insertion.
- Elevate the head of the bed when the tube is in place.
- Clearly label all lumina of the tamponade tube.
- Keep a pair of scissors at the bedside. Cut the tube and remove it immediately if signs of respiratory distress or airway obstruction occur.
- Apply gentle tension to the tube by securing it to the face guard of a football helmet or by applying an overhead traction setup with a 1-pound (0.45-kg) traction weight.
- Apply a cut gauze sponge around the tube under the client's nose.
- Insert a drainage tube into the esophagus, above the inflated balloon, if the tamponade tube does not have an esophageal drainage port. If an esophageal drainage port is available, maintain drain patency.
- Provide the client with frequent mouth care.
- Restrain the client's hands loosely *if necessary* to prevent dislodgement of the tube.
- Maintain the specified balloon pressures and volumes. (Esophageal balloon pressure is measured in millimeters of mercury; gastric balloon volume is measured in milliliters or cubic centimeters.) Release the pressure at specified intervals. (The client may experience substernal pressure when the esophageal balloon is inflated. This is an expected feeling.)
- Assess the client's sudden report of back and upper abdominal pain. Monitor vital signs for a drop in blood pressure and an increase in the heart rate. Report these signs immediately.

---

teric artery. The IV route is indicated initially because it allows easy, rapid access. The insertion of a superior mesenteric artery catheter is an invasive procedure performed by the physician or radiologist through fluoroscopy. Both infusion methods have demonstrated effective short-term control of variceal bleeding, but recurrent hemorrhage is common. An initial bolus dose of 20 to 40 units of vasopressin in 100 to 200 mL of 5% dextrose in water (D_5W) is typically given, followed by a continuous infusion of 200 units in 500 mL of D_5W at 0.2 to 0.4 units/min.

The nurse closely monitors the pulse, blood pressure, and intake and output ratio of the client receiving vasopressin. The occurrence of abdominal cramping, chest pain, and cardiac dysrhythmias is noted and reported immediately to the health care provider. Vasopressin may precipitate acute angina or myocardial infarction in clients with coronary artery disease. The nurse immediately reports any abnormal assessment findings to the physician. Concurrent IV administration of nitroglycerin, a vasodilator, may help prevent vasoconstriction of the coronary arteries during vasopressin therapy.

INJECTION SCLEROTHERAPY. The use of endoscopic injection sclerotherapy in clients with bleeding esophageal varices is a treatment reserved for clients who have repeated hemorrhagic episodes despite conservative medical management. Before the endoscopy, the nurse obtains baseline vital signs values. The physician usually administers the first dose of sedative, usually diazepam (Valium) or midazolam hydrochloride (Versed). The physician sprays the client's throat with a topical anesthetic, such as benzocaine (Cetacaine).

Injection sclerotherapy is performed in conjunction with esophagogastroduodenoscopy. During the endoscopic examination, the physician introduces a sclerosing agent, or sclerosant, through a flexible injector (Figure 59-5).

Bleeding from the varices should stop within 2 to 5 minutes. If it continues, the physician makes a second injection attempt below the bleeding site. Prophylactic injection sclerotherapy may be performed on other distended, nonbleeding varices. Because the procedure is usually done during an acute bleeding episode, the nurse or assistive nursing personnel closely monitors the client's vital signs during this hour-long procedure, which is done at the bedside or in an endoscopy clinic.

The client may report noncardiac chest discomfort for 24 to 72 hours after the injection; this discomfort is relieved by analgesia. The nurse assesses the complaint of chest pain and administers pain medication. Esophageal perforation and ulceration are other complications of injection sclerotherapy and cause severe chest pain. The nurse immediately reports acute changes to the physician.

Because aspiration may occur and cause pneumonia and pleural effusion, the nurse assesses lung sounds for decreased aeration and adventitious sounds. After injection sclerotherapy, caution is necessary when nasogastric (NG) tubes are used and inserted. Some physicians prefer not to reinsert NG tubes to decrease the risk of injury to the sclerosed esophagus.

ENDOSCOPIC LIGATION.
Endoscopic variceal ligation uses bands to ligate the bleeding varices and can be used to prevent esophageal varices from bleeding. This procedure is similar to sclerotherapy except that the varices are ligated with bands instead of injected. This procedure is thought to be safer and more cost-effective than propranolol therapy in preventing esophageal varices from bleeding (Sarin et al., 1999).

TRANSJUGULAR INTRAHEPATIC PORTAL-SYSTEMIC SHUNT.
Insertion of a **transjugular intrahepatic portal-systemic shunt (TIPS)** is a nonsurgical procedure performed in the radiology department in a special procedures room or an interventional radiology suite. This procedure is usually reserved for clients who have not responded to any other nonsurgical management. With the client under IV conscious sedation, the physician passes a shunt through a catheter and implants it between the portal vein and the hepatic vein. This technique reduces portal venous pressures and therefore controls bleeding.

Before the procedure, the physician obtains informed consent from the client. The client should know that the procedure is painful even though droperidol (Inapsine), meperidine hydrochloride (Demerol), or midazolam hydrochloride (Versed) is given in high doses for IV conscious sedation. Complications may include stenosis and thrombosis. After TIPS, the client can usually go home within 2 to 4 days.

SURGICAL MANAGEMENT. Portal-systemic shunts are considered a last-resort intervention for clients with portal hypertension and esophageal varices. The high mortality rate associated with shunting procedures occurs because clients with end-stage liver disease have coagulation abnormalities, are susceptible to infection, tolerate anesthesia poorly, and have ascites. In recent years, liver transplantation has also been commonly performed for end-stage cirrhosis (see Liver Transplantation, p. 1324).

Surgical bypass shunting procedures decrease portal hypertension by diverting a portion of the portal vein blood flow from the liver. The goal is to decrease the incidence of variceal bleeding while maintaining sufficient blood flow to the liver, thereby preserving hepatocellular function.

PREOPERATIVE CARE. The client with hepatic cirrhosis has multiple underlying problems. The client with esophageal bleeding must be transfused before surgery with packed red blood cells and fresh frozen plasma to correct clotting deficiencies.

OPERATIVE PROCEDURES. The shunting procedures most commonly used are the portacaval and splenorenal shunts (Figure 59-6).

The portacaval shunt diverts the portal venous blood flow into the inferior vena cava to decrease portal pressure. The portal vein is anastomosed to the inferior vena cava. Splenorenal shunting involves splenectomy with anastomosis of the splenic vein and left renal vein. There are several variations of these procedures. With the *mesocaval* shunt, the superior mesenteric vein is anastomosed to the inferior vena cava.

Portal-systemic decompression shunting procedures are not as common as they once were because of complications such as bleeding, portal-systemic encephalopathy (PSE), shunt thrombosis, and infection, as well as the increase in number of liver transplants. A shunt may decrease the occurrence of variceal bleeding, but survival time is usually not prolonged.

POSTOPERATIVE CARE. The client is usually admitted to the critical care unit immediately after surgery. The extent of care needed depends on the client's preoperative health status, extent of hepatic disease, and magnitude of the procedure.

The nurse provides constant observation and careful monitoring, including a frequent assessment of vital signs, central venous pressure, and pulmonary artery pressure (if indicated), as well as an hourly intake and urinary output measurements. In collaboration with the physician and the respiratory therapist, the nurse monitors respiratory status if the client is intubated, protects the client's artificial airway (endotracheal tube), and checks the ventilator for correct settings. The usual postoperative care measures to prevent atelectasis and pneumonia are instituted.

Although the intubated client has an increased need for sedatives, the nurse exercises discretion in providing opioid anal-

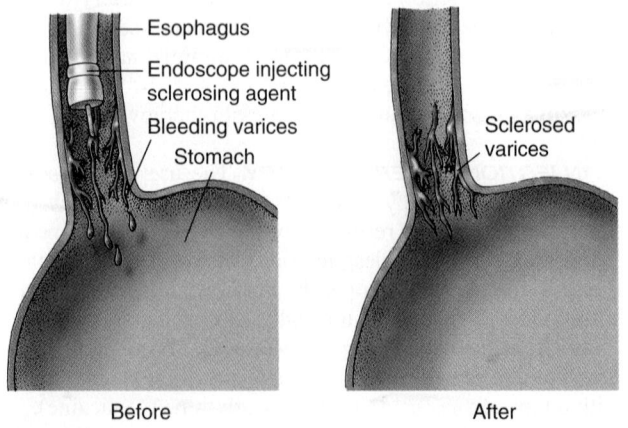

Esophagus
Endoscope injecting sclerosing agent
Bleeding varices
Stomach
Sclerosed varices

Before   After

Figure 59-5 ● Injection sclerotherapy.

gesics for pain relief and sedation during the postoperative period. These drugs are contraindicated in clients with chronic hepatic failure, because most drugs are metabolized in the liver.

After these shunting procedures, clients are susceptible to oliguria. They are often hypovolemic as a result of the following:

- Uncompensated blood loss
- Excessive fluid loss from prolonged exposure of the peritoneal space during surgery, resulting in fluid evaporation
- The recurrence of ascites
- Preoperative fluid restriction
- Diuretic therapy

The nurse administers the ordered fluid volume and assesses the effects of the volume by monitoring for increased blood pressure, decreased heart rate, and increased urinary output. Excessive increases in the central venous pressure or pulmonary artery pressure after fluid challenge are reported. Volume replacement may be given as fresh frozen plasma (to correct postoperative coagulopathy), IV solution boluses, and packed red blood cells.

Recurrent esophageal variceal bleeding after a portal-systemic shunt is not uncommon and may indicate the return of elevated portal pressures caused by a thrombosed (clotted) shunt. A rapid reaccumulation of abdominal fluid may also suggest a failed shunt or excessive sodium administration. The physician may need to reinstitute diuretic therapy. The nurse continues to measure the client's abdominal girth and reports sudden girth increases to the physician.

The nurse should be alert for the development of postshunt encephalopathy, because it is common in these clients (see care measures for portal-systemic encephalopathy [PSE] in the next section).

Clients requiring portal-systemic shunts have increased nutritional requirements and are often given total parenteral nutrition (TPN) to provide the needed calories, vitamins, and minerals. The nurse also administers albumin intravenously several times per day to replace the albumin lost in ascites. (See Chapter 61 for care associated with TPN administration.)

Bleeding Precautions. The nurse monitors the client closely for hemorrhage. Coagulation studies, including prothrombin time (PT), partial thromboplastin time (PTT), platelet count, and International Normalized Ratio (INR), are also monitored carefully. Chart 59-2 lists additional interventions for clients at risk for bleeding.

■ POTENTIAL FOR PORTAL-SYSTEMIC ENCEPHALOPATHY

PLANNING: EXPECTED OUTCOMES. It is expected that the nurse report and document findings for clients who exhibit signs of portal-systemic encephalopathy (PSE).

INTERVENTIONS. During the early stages of PSE in clients with hepatic cirrhosis, interventions are focused on decreasing ammonia formation in an effort to decrease progressive cerebral dysfunction. The diseased liver cannot convert ammonia to a less toxic form, and ammonia is carried by the circulatory system to the brain, where high levels of ammonia are toxic to normal cerebral function. The aim of PSE management is to halt this process.

Because ammonia is formed in the gastrointestinal (GI) tract by the action of bacteria on protein, nonsurgical treatment measures to decrease ammonia production include dietary limitations and drug therapy to reduce bacterial breakdown. The nurse collaborates with the dietitian and physician to plan and implement these treatment measures.

DIET THERAPY. The client with cirrhosis has increased nutritional requirements. The client needs high-carbohydrate, moderate-fat, and high-protein foods. The diet is often modified for clients who have elevated serum ammonia levels and exhibit the signs of PSE. The client's intake of dietary protein is typically limited in an effort to reduce the

NORMAL HEPATIC CIRCULATION   PORTACAVAL (END-TO-SIDE) SHUNT   SPLENORENAL (END-TO-SIDE) SHUNT

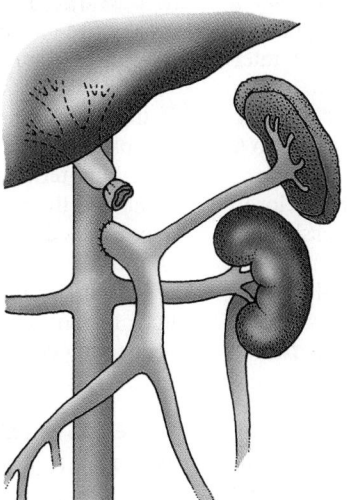
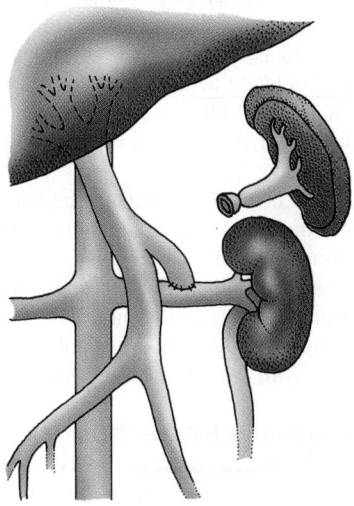

Portal vein
Spleen
Splenic vein
Left renal vein
Inferior vena cava

Figure 59-6 ● Surgical shunting diverts portal venous blood flow from the liver to decrease portal and esophageal pressure.

excessive breakdown of protein into ammonia by intestinal bacteria.

The diet for a client with PSE or elevated ammonia levels usually includes low-protein foods and simple carbohydrates, such as fruit juice. As the client's mental status deteriorates, proteins may be totally eliminated from the diet. When PSE fluctuates among the four stages, the nurse avoids giving foods high in protein content, such as meat, fish, poultry, eggs, and dairy products.

Clients with cirrhosis often experience GI bleeding, which results in the formation of increased amounts of ammonia as intestinal bacteria attempt to metabolize the blood cells. GI bleeding may precipitate hepatic coma (stage IV of PSE). These clients are maintained on nothing by mouth (NPO) status with a nasogastric (NG) tube or an esophageal tamponade tube, depending on the source of the bleeding. Nutritional maintenance with IV total parenteral nutrition is often necessary.

DRUG THERAPY. Several types of drugs can eliminate or reduce ammonia levels in the body.

LACTULOSE. The health care provider orders the administration of lactulose (Cephulac) to promote the excretion of ammonia in the stool. Lactulose, a disaccharide with high molecular weight, is a viscous, sticky, sweet-tasting liquid that the nurse administers either orally or by NG tube. When giving the drug orally, the nurse dilutes the lactulose with fruit juice to help the client tolerate the sweet taste. Lactulose retention enemas are often necessary when the client cannot tolerate oral administration or when liquids are contraindicated in the upper GI tract.

Lactulose creates an acidic environment in the bowel by keeping ammonia in its ionized state; this decreases the colon's pH from 7 to 5. This causes ammonia to leave the circulatory system and move into the colon, which reverses the normal passage of ammonia from the colon to the bloodstream. The acidic environment also discourages the growth of bacteria. Lactulose draws water into the bowel because of its high osmotic gradient, producing a laxative effect and facilitating the evacuation of ammonia from the bowel.

The desired effect of lactulose is two to three soft stools per day with an acidic fecal pH. During the acute phase of PSE, 20 to 30 g of lactulose is administered at 4-hour intervals until stools are achieved; the dosage is then decreased to three or four times per day. As a retention enema, 200 g of lactulose diluted in 1000 mL of water is administered at 4- to 6-hour intervals.

The nurse or assistive nursing personnel observes closely for watery diarrheal stools, which may signify excessive lactulose administration. The client may complain of intestinal bloating and cramping. The nurse also monitors daily for decreasing ammonia levels, which would reflect a positive effect of drug therapy, and for hypokalemia and dehydration, which can result from numerous stools.

NEOMYCIN SULFATE. Neomycin sulfate (Mycifradin Sulfate), a broad-spectrum antibiotic, is given to act as an intestinal antiseptic. It destroys the normal flora in the bowel, diminishing protein breakdown and decreasing the rate of ammonia production. Maintenance doses of neomycin are given orally but may also be administered as a retention enema.

Because constipation may lead to increased bacterial action on retained stool, with a resulting increase in ammonia

levels, stool softeners should be included in the long-term treatment plan. The administration of medications that are potentially toxic to the liver, such as opioid analgesics, sedatives, and barbiturates, must be restricted.

OTHER DRUGS. Because the client with PSE exhibits progressive neurologic changes and is often confused, combative, uncooperative, or belligerent, the nurse may need to give sedatives to prevent him or her from self-harm or harm of others. In such cases, the judicious use of drugs such as oxazepam (Serax) is warranted.

Levodopa (Dopar, Larodopa) has been used with some success in the treatment of chronic PSE. The use of levodopa (a precursor of dopamine and norepinephrine) is based on the theory that encephalopathy involves defective neurotransmitters. Deficient dopamine and norepinephrine are replaced by false transmitters—amine products from the breakdown of dietary protein. Synthetic levodopa provides the pathway for normal transmission.

NEUROLOGIC MONITORING. The nurse or assistive nursing personnel continually assesses for changes in level of consciousness and orientation (see Chart 59-2). An individualized neurologic assessment is developed for each client and includes the assessment of simple tasks such as name writing, bilateral handgrasping, and serial subtractions and additions.

The nurse also continually assesses for the presence of asterixis (liver flap) and fetor hepaticus (liver breath). These signs suggest worsening encephalopathy.

CRITICAL THINKING CHALLENGE

You are caring for a client in the prodromal stage of PSE.
- In planning care, which common medications are hepatotoxic and should be avoided?
- What type of dietary restrictions might be ordered?
- How will you maintain the client's safety?
- For what signs and symptoms indicating worsening PSE will you be observing?

For suggested answer guidelines, go to http://www.wbsaunders.com/SIMON/Iggy/.

● Community-Based Care

If the client with hepatic cirrhosis survives life-threatening complications, he or she is usually discharged to the home or to a long-term care facility after treatment measures have combated the acute medical problems. A home care referral may be needed if the client is discharged to the home. These chronically ill clients are often readmitted, and community-based care is aimed at preventing rehospitalization. The client may benefit from hospice care. A case manager is often needed to coordinate interdisciplinary care.

■ HEALTH TEACHING

The client is discharged to the home setting with an individualized teaching plan (Chart 59-4) that covers diet therapy, drug therapy, and alcohol abstinence.

DIET THERAPY. In collaboration with the dietitian, the nurse provides strict dietary instructions. Most clients need a diet high in calories, protein, and vitamins. Depending on the

CHART 59-4

CLIENT EDUCATION GUIDE
Cirrhosis

Diet Therapy
- Consume a diet high in calories, protein, and vitamins unless your health care provider has told you to avoid high-protein foods.
- If you have excessive fluid in the abdomen, follow the low-sodium diet prescribed for you.
- Eat small, frequent meals that are nutritionally well balanced.
- Include in your diet daily supplemental liquids (e.g., Ensure or Ensure Plus) and a multivitamin. Low-protein supplements are available if needed.

Drug Therapy
- Take the diuretics prescribed for you. If you experience weakness or cardiac irregularities, report these symptoms to your health care provider.
- Take the H_2-receptor antagonist prescribed for you to prevent gastrointestinal bleeding.
- Do *not* take any other medication unless specifically ordered by your health care provider.

Alcohol Abstinence
- Do not consume any alcohol.
- Seek support services for help.

presence or absence of ascites, the client may require a diet low in sodium. The dietitian plans meals and menus with the client's favorite foods and provides lists of foods high in calories, protein, and vitamins.

The client with portal-systemic encephalopathy (PSE) must avoid high-protein foods at home in an effort to decrease the incidence of progressive neurologic dysfunction. If the client's nutritional intake is decreased after discharge, multivitamin supplements and supplemental liquid feedings (e.g., Ensure) are usually needed.

DRUG THERAPY. The client is often discharged while receiving diuretics. The nurse provides written instructions and the health care provider's prescription for the diuretic. Written information about the signs and symptoms of potential electrolyte imbalances that may result from diuretic therapy (e.g., hypokalemia) is also essential. The client may need to take a potassium supplement.

If the client has had problems with bleeding from gastric ulcers, the provider prescribes antacids or an H_2-receptor antagonist agent, such as ranitidine hydrochloride (Zantac). The nurse provides written guidelines and administration schedules for all medications to be taken at home.

The nurse advises the client to avoid all over-the-counter medications and to consult the physician for follow-up medical care. The client is instructed to notify the physician immediately if any gastrointestinal (GI) bleeding is noted so that re-evaluation can be initiated quickly.

ALCOHOL ABSTINENCE. One of the most important aspects of ongoing care for the nurse to stress is the need for alcohol abstinence (see Chapter 8). Avoiding alcohol can do the following:
- Prevent further fibrosis of the liver from scarring
- Allow the liver to regenerate
- Prevent gastric and esophageal irritation
- Reduce the incidence of bleeding
- Prevent other life-threatening complications

HOME CARE MANAGEMENT

The nurse, case manager, client, and family or significant other should identify any physical adaptations needed to prepare the client's home for convalescence. The client's rest area should be close to a bathroom, because diuretic therapy increases the frequency of urination. If the client has difficulty reaching the toilet, additional equipment (e.g., urinals, bedpans, and bedside commodes) is necessary. Special, adult-sized incontinence pads or briefs may be helpful if the client has an altered mental status and has urinary incontinence.

Initial home activity may be limited for the client who has undergone surgical intervention. If the client experiences shortness of breath from massive ascites, elevating the head of the bed and maintaining the client in a semi-Fowler's to high Fowler's position may help alleviate respiratory distress. Alternatively, a reclining chair with a foot elevator may be used.

HEALTH CARE RESOURCES

The client with chronic cirrhosis may require a home care nurse to assess the client's tolerance of dietary restrictions. The home care nurse can also monitor the effectiveness of drug therapy or the surgical shunt in controlling ascites. Individual and group therapy sessions may be arranged to assist the client in dealing with alcohol abstinence. The nurse may refer the client and family to self-help groups, such as Alcoholics Anonymous and Al-Anon. The client may also desire spiritual support. Other possible resources include hospice and long-term care in a nursing home.

● Evaluation: Outcomes

NOC The nurse evaluates the care of the client with cirrhosis on the basis of the identified nursing diagnoses and collaborative problems. The expected outcomes include that the client will:
- Experience a decrease in or no ascites
- Have electrolytes within normal limits (WNL)
- Have blood pressure WNL
- Not experience hemorrhage, or be managed immediately if bleeding occurs
- Not experience PSE, or be managed immediately if PSE occurs
- Have the optimal quality of life possible

HEPATITIS

OVERVIEW

Hepatitis is the widespread inflammation of liver cells. *Viral* hepatitis is the most prevalent type and can be either acute or chronic. **Viral hepatitis** results from an infection caused by one of five major categories of viruses:
- Hepatitis A virus (HAV)
- Hepatitis B virus (HBV)
- Hepatitis C virus (HCV)
- Hepatitis D virus (HDV)
- Hepatitis E virus (HEV)

Hepatitis F and G have also been identified but are uncommon.

Liver injury with inflammation can also develop after exposure to a number of pharmacologic and chemical agents by inhalation, ingestion, or parenteral (IV) administration. *Toxic* and *drug-induced hepatitis* can result from exposure to hepatotoxins (e.g., industrial toxins, alcohol, and medications).

Hepatitis may also occur as a secondary infection during the course of infections with other viruses, such as Epstein-Barr, herpes simplex, varicella-zoster, and cytomegalovirus.

Clients usually recover from hepatitis but may have residual liver damage. Mortality from hepatitis is relatively low, but severe hepatitis may be fatal. With increasing numbers of people developing chronic hepatitis, the mortality is rising.

▮ Pathophysiology

After the liver has been exposed to causative agents (e.g., a virus), it becomes enlarged and congested with inflammatory cells, lymphocytes, and fluid, resulting in right upper quadrant pain and discomfort. As the disease process continues and progresses, the liver's normal lobular pattern becomes distorted as a result of widespread inflammation, necrosis, and hepatocellular regeneration. This distortion increases pressure within the portal circulation, interfering with the blood flow into the hepatic lobules. Edema of the liver's bile channels results in intrahepatic obstructive jaundice.

Specific data on the pathogenesis of hepatitis A, C, D, and E are limited. Clinical manifestations of acute HBV inflammation are determined by an immunologic response of the host (client). Immune complex–mediated tissue damage may contribute to the extrahepatic manifestations of acute hepatitis B. Clinical responses include an urticarial rash (hives) and arthritic joint pain.

There are three phases of hepatitis. The **preicteric** or prodromal phase begins with the infection and the start of signs and symptoms and generally lasts a week. The **icteric** phase starts with the onset of jaundice and lasts approximately 4 to 6 weeks. The **posticteric** or recovery phase of hepatitis is marked by active phagocytosis and enzyme activity; damaged hepatic cells are removed, allowing for regeneration of the cells. This phase may last up to 4 months. Unless serious complications develop, most clients recover normal hepatic function after a viral hepatic insult.

▮ CLASSIFICATION OF HEPATITIS AND ETIOLOGIES

VIRAL HEPATITIS. The five types of acute viral hepatitis vary by mode of transmission, manner of onset, and incubation periods (Table 59-5). These viruses are classified as enteral or parenteral in reference to the mechanism of transmission.

Enteral forms (hepatitis A and E) are transmitted by the fecal-oral route. Parenteral forms (hepatitis B, C, and D) are primarily transmitted via venous blood transfer or through intimate sexual contact. Vaccines to prevent hepatitis A and B are currently available.

HEPATITIS A. The causative agent of hepatitis A, hepatitis A virus (HAV), is a ribonucleic acid (RNA) virus of the enterovirus family. HAV is characterized by a mild course similar to that of a typical viral syndrome and often goes unrecognized. It is spread via the fecal-oral route by the oral ingestion of fecal contaminants. Sources of infection include contaminated water, shellfish caught in contaminated water, and food contaminated by food handlers infected with HAV. The virus may also be spread by oral-anal sexual activity. The incubation period of hepatitis A is usually 15 to 50 days. The disease is usually not life threatening. Individuals exposed to

the virus should be given immune globulin immediately and not later than 2 weeks after the exposure.

HEPATITIS B. Hepatitis B is caused by a double-shelled particle containing deoxyribonucleic acid (DNA) composed of a core antigen (HBcAg), a surface antigen (HBsAg), and an independent protein (HBeAg) that circulates in the blood.

The primary mode of transmission of hepatitis B virus (HBV) is via the skin and mucous membrane route by contamination with blood and serous fluid. Lower concentrations of HBV are also found in semen, vaginal fluid, and saliva. Although transmission can occur through bites, there are no documented cases of transmission through kissing. Hepatitis B may be spread through the following modes of transmission:

- Sexual contact with multiple partners (heterosexual and homosexual)
- Sharing needles
- Accidental needle sticks or injuries from sharp instruments in health care workers
- Blood transfusion
- Hemodialysis
- Acupuncture, tattooing, ear or body piercing
- Maternal-fetal route

The clinical course of hepatitis B may be varied. It may have an insidious onset with mild signs and symptoms, or it may result in serious complications such as fulminant hepatitis, chronic hepatitis, cirrhosis, and hepatocellular carcinoma, a rare but increasing problem in the United States. The incubation period is generally 45 to 180 days, but hepatitis B commonly develops 60 to 90 days after exposure. Chronic HBV infection develops in about 1% to 10% of adult clients with acute HBV infection (CDC, 1999).

HEPATITIS C. The causative virus of hepatitis C (HCV) is an enveloped, single-stranded RNA virus. It is transmitted by exposure of the skin and mucous membrane to blood and plasma; it is rarely transmitted sexually or from mother to fetus.

HCV is spread by contaminated items such as the following:

- Illicit IV drug needles (highest incidence)
- Tattoo, ear, or body piercing needles
- Razors, nail clippers, and scissors
- Toothbrushes and Water Piks
- Tampons or sanitary napkins
- Blood, blood products, or organ transplants received before 1992

Health care workers, such as nurses and phlebotomists, are also at risk for HCV infection following a needle stick injury with HCV-contaminated blood. HCV infection is also common in hemodialysis centers.

The incubation period for HCV is 21 to 140 days, with an average incubation period of 7 weeks. Approximately 85% of infected individuals develop chronic hepatitis (Hoofnagle, 1999). Approximately 2.7 million Americans are chronically infected with HCV, with 65% between 30 and 49 years of age (Alter, 1999). This suggests that the health care system may be burdened as infected individuals age and develop worsening liver damage (see the Cost of Care box on p. 1316).

Hepatitis C is a leading cause of cirrhosis and hepatocellular carcinoma worldwide. Approximately half of the liver transplants performed in the United States are for end-stage hepatitis C (Hepatitis Foundation International, 1999). Unfor-

TABLE 59-5 • DIFFERENTIAL FEATURES OF THE FIVE TYPES OF VIRAL HEPATITIS*

Hepatitis A	Hepatitis B	Hepatitis C	Hepatitis D	Hepatitis E
SYNONYMS				
Infectious hepatitis	Serum hepatitis	Post-transfusion hepatitis		Epidemic non-A, non-B hepatitis or enterically transmitted hepatitis
DIAGNOSIS OF ACUTE DISEASE				
Anti-HAV IgM in serum	HBsAg in serum	Anti-HCV in serum	Anti-HDV in serum	Anti-HEV in serum
INCUBATION PERIOD				
15-50 days	48-180 days	14-180 days	14-56 days	15-64 days
HIGH-RISK GROUPS				
More common in young children and institutional settings	All age-groups affected, especially drug addicts and health care personnel	All ages of drug users Persons with hemophilia	Drug addicts Persons with hepatitis B	Persons living in underdeveloped countries
SEASON				
Fall and early winter	All year	All year	All year	All year
TRANSMISSION				
Usually by oral-fecal route among persons living in close contact; ingestion of contaminated water or contaminated shellfish	Primarily blood; drug abuse, sexual contact, mother to child at birth	Primarily blood; drug abuse, sexual contact (rarely), mother to child at birth	Co-infects with hepatitis B; nonpercutaneous; close personal contact	Oral-fecal route; transmitted principally by contaminated water
CLINICAL FINDINGS				
Majority of type A infections (mild and anicteric); symptoms similar to those of influenza	Changes similar to those of hepatitis A	Changes similar to those of hepatitis A	Changes similar to those of hepatitis A, but symptoms often more severe than those in hepatitis A and hepatitis B	Resembles hepatitis A
	Fatigue, anorexia, low-grade fever, abdominal discomfort, arthralgias, rashes, enlarged and tender liver, light stools, dark urine, jaundice Elevated serum AST and ALT levels (early), hyperbilirubinemia, abnormal liver function test results	Tends to have more severe symptoms; sometimes necessitates hospitalization for extended periods	Often asymptomatic	
VIRUS IN FECES?				
Yes	Not infectious	Not identified	Not identified	Possible
VIRUS IN SERUM?				
Anti-HAV in serum during acute phase and incubation period is rare	HBsAg is in serum throughout the clinical course	Anti-HVC test is approximately 95% reliable; often takes up to 8 weeks to show antibody	Anti-HDV in serum	
NOSOCOMIAL PROBLEM?				
No	Yes	Yes	Yes	No
MORTALITY				
Less frequent	More frequent, chronic form can be fatal	More frequent, chronic form can be fatal	Increased	Unknown

Anti-HAV, antibody to HAV; IgM, immunoglobulin M; *HBsAg,* hepatitis B surface antigen; *anti-HCV,* antibodies to HCV; *anti-HDV,* antibodies to HDV; *anti-HEV,* antibodies to HEV; *AST,* aspartate aminotransferase; *ALT,* alanine aminotransferase; *HBIG,* hepatitis B immune globulin; *anti-HBs,* hepatitis B surface antibody; *anti-HBc,* hepatitis B core antibody; *anti-HBe,* hepatitis Be antibody.

Continued

TABLE 59-5 • DIFFERENTIAL FEATURES OF THE FIVE TYPES OF VIRAL HEPATITIS*—cont'd

Hepatitis A	Hepatitis B	Hepatitis C	Hepatitis D	Hepatitis E
INCIDENCE OF CHRONIC ACTIVE HEPATITIS AS A COMPLICATION				
Low	Approximately 15% will develop chronic form	Approximately 85% will develop chronic form	Yes	No
IMMUNE GLOBULIN (IG) (PROPHYLAXIS)				
IG	HBIG or IG	No		None; recommended IG
VACCINE				
Yes	Yes	No	Prevention of hepatitis B with vaccine prevents hepatitis D	No
ANTIBODY				
Anti-HAV	Anti-HBs, anti-HBc, anti-HBe	Anti-HCV	Anti-HDV	Anti-HEV

Anti-HAV, antibody to HAV; *IgM,* immunoglobulin M; *HBsAg,* hepatitis B surface antigen; *anti-HCV,* antibodies to HCV; *anti-HDV,* antibodies to HDV; *anti-HEV,* antibodies to HEV; *AST,* aspartate aminotransferase; *ALT,* alanine aminotransferase; *HBIG,* hepatitis B immune globulin; *anti-HBs,* hepatitis B surface antibody; *anti-HBc,* hepatitis B core antibody; *anti-HBe,* hepatitis Be antibody.

COST OF CARE
IMPLICATIONS FOR NURSING

HEPATITIS C

Cost of Care
- An estimated 3.9 million Americans, nearly 2% of the population, are chronically infected with hepatitis C.
- The cost of hepatitis C infections and related diseases is more than $600 million dollars per year.
- More than half of the liver transplants performed in the United States are for hepatitis C. The average first-year cost for a liver transplant exceeds $200,000.
- From the year 2010 through 2019, the projected cost in direct medical expenses is $10.7 billion, with 165,900 deaths due to chronic liver disease and 27,200 deaths due to hepatocellular carcinoma.

Implications for Nursing
Nurses are at high risk for getting hepatitis C and becoming part of these statistics. As these costs rise, health care will be impacted further from this disease. Nurses must strive to disseminate information about this disease to prevent others from obtaining it and to help reduce costs.

Data from Wong, J.B., et al. (2000). Estimating future hepatitis C morbidity, mortality, and costs in the United States. *American Journal of Public Health, 90*(10), 1562-1569.

LEGAL/ETHICAL ISSUES
IN HEALTH CARE

LIVER TRANSPLANTATION FOR CLIENTS WITH HEPATITIS C

More than half of the transplants performed in the United States are for clients with end-stage liver disease related to hepatitis B and hepatitis C. When these individuals receive a transplant, many "new livers" become reinfected with the hepatitis. As a result, another transplantation is required.

As of October 1999 more than 14,000 people are awaiting a transplant, and approximately 4500 transplants are performed each year. Is it ethical to provide transplants for individuals with hepatitis? Is it a lifesaving or life-prolonging procedure for these individuals? Is it an appropriate use of a scarce resource? Should the diagnosis come into consideration with transplantation, given that the clients often choose to participate in high-risk behaviors that make them susceptible to hepatitis C?

tunately, the newly transplanted liver often becomes reinfected with the virus (see the Legal/Ethical Issues box below, left).

HEPATITIS D. Hepatitis D (delta hepatitis, or HDV) is caused by a defective RNA virus that needs the helper function of HBV. HDV co-infects with HBV and needs its presence for viral replication. Hepatitis D can co-infect a client with HBV or can occur as a superinfection in a client with chronic HBV. Superinfection usually develops into chronic HDV. The incubation period is approximately 14 to 56 days. As with HBV, the disease is transmitted primarily by parenteral routes.

CULTURAL CONSIDERATIONS
In the United States, Canada, and northern Europe, hepatitis D (delta infection) is most prevalent in people exposed to blood and blood products (e.g., drug addicts and hemophiliacs).

The prevalence of hepatitis D usually corresponds to the prevalence of hepatitis B. Southern Italy, Africa, South America, and parts of Russia and Romania have a high prevalence, whereas northern Italy, Spain, Turkey, and Egypt have a moderate prevalence (CDC [Hepatitis Branch], 1997).

HEPATITIS E. The hepatitis E virus (HEV) was originally identified by its association with waterborne epidemics of hepatitis in the Indian subcontinent. Since then, it has occurred in epidemics in Asia, Africa, the Middle East, Mexico, and Central and South America. Many large outbreaks have occurred after heavy rains and flooding.

In the United States, hepatitis E has been found only in travelers returning from these endemic areas. The nonenveloped, single-stranded RNA virus is transmitted via the fecal-oral route, and the clinical course resembles that of hepatitis A. HEV has an incubation period of 15 to 64 days. There is no evidence at this time of a chronic form of HEV.

TOXIC AND DRUG-INDUCED (CHEMICAL) HEPATITIS. Two major types of toxic hepatitis have been recognized—direct toxic hepatitis and idiosyncratic toxic hepatitis.

DIRECT TOXIC HEPATITIS. Direct toxic hepatitis (DTH) results in necrosis and fatty infiltration of the liver. Agents causing toxic hepatitis are generally systemic poisons or are converted in the liver to toxic metabolites. People with repeated, regular exposure to an offending agent (e.g., alcohol [alcoholic hepatitis]) or with a dose-related toxicity range can have direct toxic hepatitis. For example, acetaminophen (Tylenol), a commonly used over-the-counter (OTC) analgesic, can cause severe hepatic necrosis when taken in large amounts, such as in suicide attempts or accidental ingestion by children.

Industrial toxins such as carbon tetrachloride, trichloroethylene, and yellow phosphorus also have a direct toxic effect on the liver.

IDIOSYNCRATIC TOXIC HEPATITIS. Idiosyncratic toxic hepatitis (ITH) results in morphologic changes to the liver that are similar to those found in viral hepatitis. In idiosyncratic drug reactions, the occurrence of hepatitis is unpredictable and uncommon. It may occur at any time during or shortly after exposure to the drug. Examples of agents that result in idiosyncratic toxic hepatitis are isoniazid (INH, Isotamine✦), an antituberculosis drug, and phenytoin (Dilantin), an anticonvulsant.

Treatment of toxic and drug-induced hepatitis is supportive. Transplantation may be considered if fulminating liver failure is present. Withdrawal of the suspected agent is indicated at the first sign of a reaction. Chemical exposure of the liver to drugs and toxins has resulted in the development of chronic active hepatitis and cirrhosis.

▣ COMPLICATIONS OF HEPATITIS

Failure of the liver cells to regenerate, with progression of the necrotic process, results in a severe and often fatal form of hepatitis known as **fulminant hepatitis.** This form of massive hepatic necrosis is rare.

Hepatitis is considered to be chronic when liver inflammation lasts longer than several months (usually defined as 6 months). **Chronic hepatitis** usually occurs as a result of hepatitis B or hepatitis C. Superimposed infection with hepatitis D (HDV) in clients with chronic HBV may also result in chronic hepatitis.

With **chronic active hepatitis (CAH),** liver damage is progressive and is characterized by hepatic necrosis, acute inflammation, and progressive fibrosis. The client may be asymptomatic for long periods of the hepatic disease process, or the continued fibrosis may lead to liver failure, cirrhosis, and death. Chronic active hepatitis may be manifested by the following:

- Persistent clinical symptoms and hepatomegaly
- The continual presence of HBsAg (hepatitis B surface antigen) or anti-HCV (HCV antibodies)
- Elevated, fluctuating serum levels of aspartate aminotransferase (AST), bilirubin, and alkaline phosphatase for 6 months or longer after the acute hepatitis episode

Liver biopsy is necessary to establish the diagnosis of chronic hepatitis.

In people with *chronic persistent* hepatitis and *chronic lobar* hepatitis, liver damage does not progress after the initial insult. These types of hepatitis result from infections with hepatitis B and C viruses. Most clients with chronic persistent hepatitis are asymptomatic, and physical findings are normal. Laboratory data may reveal a mild elevation of serum AST and alkaline phosphatase levels that may persist for up to 1 year. Routine screening of blood donors and the elimination

---

CHART 59-5

BEST PRACTICE *for*
Prevention of Viral Hepatitis in Health Care Workers

- Use standard precautions to prevent the transmission of disease between clients or between clients and health care staff (see Chapter 26).
- Eliminate needles and other sharps by substituting needleless systems. (Needle sticks are the major source of hepatitis B transmission in health care workers.)
- Take the hepatitis B vaccine (Hepatovax-B, Recombivax HB), which is given in a series of three injections. This vaccine also prevents hepatitis D. (See Chapter 26 for more information on this requirement of the United States Occupational Safety and Health Administration [OSHA].)
- For postexposure prevention of hepatitis A or B, seek medical attention immediately for immunoglobulin (IG) administration.
- Report all cases of hepatitis to the local health department.

CHART 59-6

CLIENT EDUCATION GUIDE
Prevention of Viral Hepatitis

- Maintain adequate sanitation and personal hygiene. Wash your hands before eating and after using the toilet.
- Drink water treated by a water purification system.
- If traveling in underdeveloped or nonindustrialized countries, drink only bottled water. Avoid food washed or prepared with tapwater, such as raw vegetables, fruits, and soups.
- Use adequate sanitation practices to prevent the spread of the disease between family members.
- Do not share bed linens, towels, eating utensils, or drinking glasses.
- Do not share needles for injection, body piercing, or tattooing.
- Do not share razors, nail clippers, toothbrushes, or Water Piks.
- Use a condom during sexual intercourse.

---

of commercial blood sources have virtually eliminated the incidence of hepatitis B or C caused by blood transfusion. Case reporting to local health departments for all types of *viral* hepatitis is mandatory. Measures to prevent viral hepatitis for health care workers and others in contact with infected clients are listed in Charts 59-5 and 59-6.

▣ Etiology

In addition to the hepatitis A, B, C, D, and E viruses, other causes of hepatitis include the following:

- Drugs, chemicals, and toxins
- Blood transfusion reactions from exposure to the hepatitis virus
- Hyperthyroidism
- Ingestion of ethyl alcohol (ETOH), resulting in alcoholic hepatitis
- Wilson's disease (increased serum copper)
- Other viruses, such as Epstein-Barr, cytomegalovirus, and yellow fever

▣ Incidence/Prevalence

There are an estimated 125,000 to 200,000 infections of hepatitis A every year. Approximately one third of Americans have evidence of past infection, but many are not aware that they were infected (CDC, 1999).

Hepatitis B occurs primarily in young adults between 20 and 39 years of age. The incidence of hepatitis B is between 140,000 to 320,000 infections each year. There has been a decrease during the first half of the 1990s, most likely as a result of the hepatitis B vaccine. Approximately 10% of clients with hepatitis B develop chronic hepatitis.

The prevalence of hepatitis C is highest in individuals with high-risk drug behaviors, such as sharing needles. The incidence is approximately 36,000 new infections per year. It is estimated that 4 million of the U.S. population has been infected. The chronic form develops in approximately 85% of those infected.

► COLLABORATIVE MANAGEMENT
◖ Assessment
▥ HISTORY

If viral hepatitis is suspected, the nurse asks the client whether he or she has had known exposure to a person with hepatitis. The nurse determines whether the client has had recent blood transfusions or undergoes hemodialysis for renal failure. The client should be asked about the following:

* Sexual activities
* Social activities
* Injectable drug use
* Recent ear or body piercing and/or tattooing
* Close living accommodations, such as military barracks, correctional institutions, overcrowded apartments, long-term care facilities
* Receiving blood, blood products, or a transplant before 1992

The client's employment history is obtained. The nurse specifically asks about employment as a health care worker. The client is asked about recent travel to a foreign country or to an area with inadequate environmental sanitation. The client is also questioned about the ingestion of water from a possibly contaminated source or the recent ingestion of shellfish.

▥ PHYSICAL ASSESSMENT/CLINICAL MANIFESTATIONS

VIRAL HEPATITIS. The courses and clinical manifestations of all five types of viral hepatitis are somewhat similar (see Table 59-5). The nurse assesses the client's general subjective complaints, determining whether symptoms occurred acutely (hepatitis A and E) or insidiously (hepatitis B and C).

The client may verbalize feelings of fatigue and loss of appetite. The nurse explores further to assess whether the client is experiencing the following:

* Abdominal pain
* Arthralgia (joint pain)
* Myalgia (muscle pain)
* Diarrhea/constipation
* Fever
* Irritability
* Lethargy
* Malaise
* Nausea/vomiting

The nurse lightly palpates the right upper abdominal quadrant to assess for liver tenderness. The client may report right upper quadrant pain with jarring movements. The skin, scle-

rae, and mucous membranes are inspected for the presence of jaundice. The client may present for medical treatment only after jaundice appears, believing that other vague symptoms are related to an influenza-like syndrome.

Jaundice in hepatitis results from intrahepatic obstruction and is caused by edema of the liver's bile channels. Dark urine and clay-colored stools are often reported by the client. The nurse obtains a urine and stool specimen for visual inspection and laboratory analysis. The skin is inspected for the presence of rashes in clients with suspected hepatitis B and hepatitis C. Irregular patches of redness or urticaria (hives) may occur. The client often reports pruritus (itching) and may have skin abrasions from scratching.

The client with hepatitis A usually has a fever, and the temperature may range from 100° to 104° F (38° to 40° C). Fever may be low-grade or absent with hepatitis B and hepatitis C.

TOXIC AND DRUG-INDUCED HEPATITIS. The clinical picture in toxic and drug-induced hepatitis depends on the causative agent. Idiosyncratic reactions may result in clinical manifestations that are indistinguishable from those of viral hepatitis or may simulate extrahepatic bile duct obstruction symptoms such as severe jaundice, rash, arthralgia, and fever.

▥ PSYCHOSOCIAL ASSESSMENT

Viral hepatitis usually occurs as an acute illness. Its symptoms may be mild and abate rapidly or go undetected. Emotional problems for affected clients often center on their anger about being sick and being fatigued. General malaise, inactivity, and vague complaints contribute to depression and despondency. These clients worry about the long-term effects and complications.

Clients with viral hepatitis often feel guilty about having exposed others to the virus. Infectious diseases such as hepatitis continue to have a social stigma. The client may feel embarrassed by the isolation and hygiene precautions that are imposed in the hospital and continue to be necessary at home. This embarrassment may cause the client to limit social interactions. Self-imposed visitor restrictions may be instituted by the client out of fear of spreading the virus to family and friends.

Family members are sometimes afraid of contracting the disease and may distance themselves from the client. The nurse allows the client and family to verbalize these feelings and explores the reasons for these fears. Precautionary isolation measures evoke anxiety for the client and the family.

Clients are unable to return to work until the results of blood tests for serologic markers are negative. The loss of wages and the cost of hospitalization for a client without insurance coverage may produce great anxiety and financial burden for the client and the family.

> **⟲ CRITICAL THINKING CHALLENGE**
>
> You are the nurse caring for a 52-year old man recently diagnosed with chronic hepatitis C. He denies any high-risk behavior but admits to getting a tattoo in Vietnam. How will you reply to his following questions?
> * Could I have gotten this by a tattoo?
> * Could my wife and children have hepatitis?
> * How could I not have known I had hepatitis?
> * What is the cure?
>
> For suggested answer guidelines, go to ⟨SIMON⟩ http://www.wbsaunders.com/SIMON/Iggy/.

■ LABORATORY ASSESSMENT

The presence of hepatitis A, B, and C is usually indicated by acute elevations in levels of liver enzymes, indicating liver cellular damage, and by specific serologic markers.

SERUM LIVER ENZYMES. Levels of alanine aminotransferase (ALT) may be elevated to more than 1000 mU/mL and may rise to as high as 4000 mU/mL in severe cases of viral hepatitis. Aspartate aminotransferase (AST) levels may rise to 1000 to 2000 mU/mL. Alkaline phosphatase levels may be normal (30 to 90 IU/L) or mildly elevated. Serum total bilirubin levels are elevated to greater than 2.5 mg/dL and are consistent with the clinical appearance of jaundice. Elevated levels of bilirubin are also present in the urine.

SEROLOGIC MARKERS/ENZYME ASSAYS. The presence of *hepatitis A* is established when hepatitis A virus (HAV) antibodies (anti-HAV) are identified in the blood. Ongoing inflammation of the liver by HAV is evidenced by the presence of immunoglobulin M (IgM) antibodies, which persist in the blood for 4 to 6 weeks. Previous infection is indicated by the presence of immunoglobulin G (IgG) antibodies. These antibodies persist in the serum and provide permanent immunity to HAV.

The presence of the *hepatitis B* virus (HBV) is established if serologic testing confirms the presence of hepatitis B antigen-antibody systems in the blood. HBV is a double-shelled DNA virus consisting of an inner core and an outer shell. Antigens located on the surface (shell) of the virus (HBsAg) and IgM antibodies to hepatitis B core antigen (anti-HBc IgM) are the most significant serologic markers. The presence of these markers establishes the diagnosis of hepatitis B. The client is considered infectious as long as HBsAg is present in the blood. Persistence of this serologic marker after 6 months or longer indicates a carrier state or chronic hepatitis. HBsAg levels normally decline and disappear after the acute hepatitis B episode. The presence of antibodies to HBsAg (anti-HBs) in the blood indicates recovery and immunity to hepatitis B.

Enzyme-linked immunosorbent assay (ELISA) is the initial screening test for clients suspected of being infected with *hepatitis C* virus (HCV), and it is the most commonly used enzyme test for HCV antibodies (anti-HCV). False-positive results can occur in clients with normal ALT levels and no risk factors. In these cases, a more specific assay called the recombinant immunoblot assay (RIBA) is used. Because HCV can often be detected within 2 to 3 weeks of exposure, the virus may be measured directly using the reverse transcription polymerase chain reaction (RT-PCR) test.

The presence of *hepatitis D* virus (HDV) can be confirmed by the identification of intrahepatic delta antigen or, more often, by a rise in the hepatitis D virus antibodies (anti-HDV) titer.

Hepatitis E virus (HEV) testing is usually reserved for travelers in whom hepatitis is present, but the viruses cannot be detected. The presence of the hepatitis E antibodies (anti-HEV) is found in individuals infected with the virus.

■ OTHER DIAGNOSTIC ASSESSMENT

Chronic hepatitis is diagnosed by percutaneous liver biopsy. The biopsy distinguishes between chronic active and chronic persistent hepatitis. It is also the gold standard test for assessing the extent of injury and prognosis of HCV disease. The finding of fatty infiltrates in liver biopsy specimens and in-

flammation with neutrophils is consistent with Laënnec's (alcohol-induced) hepatitis.

▶ Interventions

The client with viral hepatitis can be mildly or acutely ill depending on the severity of the inflammation. Most clients are not hospitalized. The plan of care for all clients with viral hepatitis is based on measures to rest the liver, promote cellular regeneration, and prevent complications (see the Client Care Plan on pp. 1320 and 1321).

NONSURGICAL MANAGEMENT. During the acute stage of viral hepatitis, interventions are aimed at resting the inflamed liver to promote hepatic cell regeneration. Rest is an essential intervention to reduce the liver's metabolic demands and increase its blood supply. Treatment is generally supportive.

PHYSICAL REST. The nurse and assistive nursing personnel assess the client's response to activity and rest periods. Strict bedrest may be indicated during the early icteric phase of hepatitis. The client is usually tired and expresses feelings of general malaise. Complete bedrest is usually not required, but rest periods alternating with periods of activity are indicated and are often sufficient to promote hepatic healing.

The nurse individualizes the client's plan of care and changes it as needed to reflect the severity of symptoms, fatigue, and the results of liver function tests and enzyme determinations. The client and nursing staff should adhere to scheduled rest periods. Activities such as self-care and ambulating are gradually added to the activity schedule as tolerated.

PSYCHOLOGIC REST. Emotional and psychologic rest is essential for the client. Because bedrest and inactivity can produce anxiety, the nurse includes diversional activities in the plan of care. The nurse asks the hospitalized client's family to bring in small craft projects, reading materials (e.g., magazines, books, newspapers), or a portable radio. Staff and family members are encouraged to spend time in the client's room.

DIET THERAPY. A special diet is usually not required. The diet should be high in carbohydrates and calories with moderate amounts of fat and protein. Small, frequent meals are often preferable to three standard meals. The nurse asks the client about food preferences, because favorite foods are tolerated better than randomly selected foods. The nurse or assistive nursing personnel encourages the client to select foods that are appealing. High-calorie snacks may be needed.

The health care provider typically orders supplemental vitamins. If caloric intake is low, the nurse may need to provide supplemental commercial feedings, such as Ensure.

DRUG THERAPY. An antiemetic to relieve nausea, such as trimethobenzamide hydrochloride (Tigan) and dimenhydrinate (Dramamine), may be prescribed. Prochlorperazine maleate (Compazine), a phenothiazine, is avoided because of its potential hepatotoxic effects.

There are no drugs specific for hepatitis A management. Interferon, a biologic response modifier given by injection over several months, has been approved for the treatment of *hepatitis B*. However, interferon has a number of side effects that often are so severe the client cannot continue the therapy. Side effects include flu-like symptoms of headaches, fever,

CLIENT CARE PLAN • THE CLIENT WITH VIRAL HEPATITIS

NURSING DIAGNOSIS NO. 1 • Activity Intolerance related to decreased metabolic energy production secondary to liver dysfunction.

Expected Outcomes	Nursing Interventions	Rationale
The client will gradually increase activity to the level experienced before hepatitis occurred.	Provide several periods of rest during the day. **D** Organize care so the client is not fatigued. **D** Reinforce the need for bedrest in the immediate recovery period. **D** Gradually add activities to the client's daily schedule. For example, self-care activities are allowed before ambulation. **D**	Rest promotes healing of the liver; inflammation of hepatic cells decreases.
	Provide or encourage diversional activities on the basis of the client's interests, such as reading, watching television, or doing small crafts. **D** Encourage family members and significant others to visit the client for short periods. **D** Place frequently used items close within reach. **D**	Diversions such as visits and independent activities decrease anxiety, which can prevent rest. The nurse needs to caution against excessive visitation, because the client may become more fatigued.

NURSING DIAGNOSIS NO. 2 • Imbalanced Nutrition: Less than Body Requirements related to anorexia, nausea, and vomiting

The client will achieve an optimal intake of nutrients and calories to promote liver tissue healing.	Provide a diet high in carbohydrates and calories; in collaboration with the dietitian, provide moderate amounts of fat and protein. Provide small, frequent meals that are attractively presented.	A diet high in carbohydrates and calories provides energy. Protein is needed for hepatic cell regeneration. The appearance of a large meal can cause anorexia. Eating a large quantity of food can cause abdominal distention and nausea or vomiting.
	Obtain a diet history to determine food preferences. Encourage significant others to bring in foods, if permitted. Allow the client to select meals from the menu. **D** Offer high-calorie, high-protein snacks such as milkshakes. **D** Provide supplemental vitamins and liquid feedings, such as Ensure or Ensure Plus, as ordered. Avoid fried and fatty foods, which can increase nausea.	
	Administer antiemetic medication, such as trimethobenzamide hydrochloride (Tigan), as ordered. Administer acid suppression therapy as ordered.	Antiemetics and acid suppression therapy minimize gastric distress, which allows the client to consume adequate oral nutrition.
	Remove noxious odors or move unpleasant objects or substances away from the client. **D**	Noxious odors or substances, such as a full bedside commode, can contribute to nausea.

D indicates tasks that can be delegated to assistive nursing personnel.

INR, International Normalized Ratio.

fatigue, loss of appetite, nausea, and vomiting. Other side effects include hair loss, depression, and bone marrow suppression that decreases white blood cell and platelet production.

Two antiviral drugs have recently been used to treat acute HBV: ribavirin (Virazole, Rebetol) and lamivudine (Epivir). Lamivudine is also used after liver and heart transplantation. Both of these drugs can cause sudden, severe anemia and cardiac arrest.

Hepatitis C can be treated with interferon (usually alfa), ribavirin (Virazole, Rebetol), or the more effective combination of Rebetol and interferon alfa-2b, a recombinant called Rebetron. Long-term results are better with the combination drug, which is now considered the first-line drug for HCV (Dougherty & Dreher, 2001).

COMFORT MEASURES. Some foods and smells may stimulate nausea. If possible, the nurse or assistive nursing personnel removes the stimulus causing the nausea. In an effort to stimulate appetite, the nurse or assistive nursing personnel provides mouth care or instructs the client to perform mouth care before meals. The meal may be more palatable when the client is sitting up in a chair. The nurse empties bedpans, urinals, and bedside commodes promptly and provides an air freshener for the room if the client can tolerate it.

SURGICAL MANAGEMENT. Liver transplantation may be performed for clients with chronic hepatitis, especially for hepatitis C, but many become reinfected (see the later discussion of liver transplantation, p. 1324).

$\mathcal{C}$LIENT $\mathcal{C}$ARE $\mathcal{P}$LAN • THE CLIENT WITH VIRAL HEPATITIS—cont'd

NURSING DIAGNOSIS NO. 3 • Deficient Knowledge related to causes of hepatitis and modes of transmission

Expected Outcomes	Nursing Interventions	Rationale
The client will verbalize knowledge about the causes of hepatitis and the modes of transmission.	Assess client's knowledge about disease and modes of transmission, and educate as necessary.	A baseline for the client's level of knowledge must be obtained.
	Instruct the client with hepatitis B or C that a chronic form of the disease may develop and that he or she will need monitoring once discharged.	If the client does not realize the risk for a chronic form, he or she may continue risk behaviors and accidentally infect others.
	If it is identified that the client has a drug or alcohol problem, refer to appropriate persons.	Abstaining from risk behaviors will help reduce transmission.
	Instruct clients that they should not donate blood.	The blood would be wasted because it is contaminated.
	Teach clients to modify sexual practices as directed by health care providers.	Depending on sexual practices, all types of viral hepatitis may be transmitted sexually.
	Use direct, nonjudgmental questions to identify risk behaviors.	Clients may not understand why they are being questioned about sexual and drug behaviors.

NURSING DIAGNOSIS NO. 4 • Risk for Impaired Skin integrity related to pruritus secondary to hepatic dysfunction

The skin will remain intact.	Keep the client's skin hydrated with proper moisture. Avoid hot baths, and use emollients. **D**	Dry skin can lead to more pruritus and make the skin more at risk to breakdown.
	Keep client's fingernails short, and encourage using knuckles if client must scratch. **D**	Fingernails may scratch and tear the skin.
	Administer antihistamines as prescribed, closely observing for sedation.	Antihistamines may relieve pruritus but may cause excessive sedation.

NURSING DIAGNOSIS NO. 5 • Ineffective Protection related to increased risk of bleeding secondary to decreased vitamin K absorption and possible thrombocytopenia

The client is free from bleeding.	Monitor prothrombin time, INR, and platelet levels.	Increased levels for prothrombin time and INR and decreased platelet levels indicate that the client is at greater risk for bleeding.
	Observe for signs of overt and occult bleeding (e.g., bleeding gums, gastrointestinal bleeding, tarry stools). **D**	If any type of bleeding occurs, the health care provider must be notified immediately.
	Avoid intramuscular injections whenever possible; use small-gauge needles if injection is necessary.	Intramuscular injections may cause bleeding.
	Administer vitamin K as ordered.	Vitamin K helps decrease the chance for bleeding.
	Teach client to use a soft toothbrush and an electric razor.	Less harsh objects help minimize injury to the mucosa and face.

D indicates tasks that can be delegated to assistive nursing personnel.

INR, International Normalized Ratio.

▶● Community-Based Care

▥ HEALTH TEACHING

The nurse teaches the client and the family to observe measures to prevent infection transmission (see Chart 59-6). In addition, the nurse instructs the client with viral hepatitis to avoid alcohol and any nonprescription, over-the-counter medications, particularly acetaminophen (Tylenol, Exdol♥) and sedatives, for 3 to 12 months because of the hepatotoxic effects (Chart 59-7). Clients who develop chronic hepatitis should always avoid these products.

The client must determine patterns for rest on the basis of physical tolerance of increased activity. The nurse encourages the client to increase activity gradually to prevent fatigue. The client should eat small, frequent meals of high-carbohydrate and low-fat foods. In collaboration with the dietitian, the nurse provides diet teaching and menu planning. The nurse teaches the client to follow precautionary measures and avoid sexual activity until the results of hepatitis B surface antigen (HBsAg) tests are negative.

▥ HOME CARE MANAGEMENT

Home care management varies according to the type of hepatitis. A primary focus is preventing the spread of the infection. For hepatitis transmitted by the fecal-oral route, careful handwashing and sanitary disposal of feces are important. Standard precautions are used for hepatitis transmitted percutaneously and permucosally. Education is therefore very important.

HEALTH CARE RESOURCES

Clients with viral hepatitis and their families may contact the local health department for further information on infection control and prevention. Clients discharged home with limited activity tolerance or minimal family support may need the assistance of a home care aide in performing activities of daily living, particularly meal preparation.

FATTY LIVER

A fatty liver is caused by the accumulation of triglycerides and other fats in the hepatic cells. In severe cases, fat may constitute as much as 40% of the liver's weight and cause changes in liver function. Minimal, temporary fatty changes are usually reversible by eliminating the cause. The most common cause of fatty liver is chronic alcoholism. Other causes include the following:

- Malnutrition
- Diabetes mellitus
- Obesity
- Pregnancy
- Prolonged total parenteral nutrition (TPN)
- Exposure to large doses of drugs toxic to the liver

Fatty infiltration of the liver may result from faulty fat metabolism in the liver and the mobilization of fatty acids from adipose tissue.

Many clients with a fatty liver are asymptomatic. The most common and typical finding is hepatomegaly. Other symptoms include the following:

- Right upper abdominal pain
- Ascites
- Edema
- Jaundice
- Fever
- Signs of late cirrhosis, depending on the severity of the fat infiltration and the longevity of the occurrence

A liver biopsy confirms excessive fat in the liver. Interventions are aimed at removing the underlying cause of the infiltration and providing dietary restrictions.

HEPATIC ABSCESS

OVERVIEW

Although hepatic abscesses are uncommon, they carry a high mortality rate. Liver abscesses occur when the liver is invaded by bacteria or protozoa. These organisms destroy the liver tissue, producing a necrotic cavity filled with infective agents, liquefied liver cells and tissue, and leukocytes. The infectious necrotic tissue walls off the abscess from the healthy liver.

A *pyogenic* liver abscess occurs when bacteria invade the liver. Infecting organisms include *Escherichia coli* and *Klebsiella, Enterobacter, Salmonella, Staphylococcus,* and *Enterococcus* species. A pyogenic abscess is generally solitary and confined to the right lobe, but occasionally they are multiple in nature. The usual cause is acute cholangitis, which occurs as a complication of cholelithiasis. Pyogenic liver abscesses may also result from liver trauma, abdominal peritonitis, and sepsis, or an abscess can extend to the liver after pneumonia or bacterial endocarditis.

The protozoan *Entamoeba histolytica* causes an *amebic* hepatic abscess, which may occur after amebic dysentery. These abscesses usually occur in the form of a single abscess in the right hepatic lobe.

► COLLABORATIVE MANAGEMENT

Clients with hepatic abscesses are generally ill. On occasion, an abscess is not diagnosed until autopsy. In clients with a pyogenic liver abscess, the onset of symptoms is usually sudden. Amebic abscesses cause a more insidious onset of symptoms. Common complaints include the following:

- Right upper abdominal pain with a palpable, tender liver
- Anorexia
- Weight loss
- Nausea and vomiting
- Fever and chills
- Shoulder pain
- Dyspnea
- Pleural pain if the diaphragm is involved

A hepatic abscess is usually diagnosed by liver scan. Hepatic arteriography differentiates an abscess from a malignancy. Blood cultures assist in identifying the causative organism in pyogenic abscesses, and stool cultures may identify *E. histolytica*. With ultrasonographic guidance, a liver abscess may be aspirated percutaneously. Surgical drainage is indicated only for a single pyogenic abscess or for an amebic abscess that fails to respond to long-term antibiotic treatment.

LIVER TRAUMA

OVERVIEW

The liver is the most common organ to be injured in clients with penetrating trauma of the abdomen (e.g., gunshot wounds, stab wounds, and rib fractures) and is the second most commonly injured organ in clients who have blunt abdominal trauma. Liver damage or injury should be suspected whenever any upper abdominal or lower chest trauma is sustained. The liver is often injured by steering wheels in vehicular accidents. Common injuries to the liver include simple lacerations, multiple lacerations, avulsions (tears), and crush injuries.

The liver is a highly vascular organ and receives approximately 29% of the body's cardiac output. When hepatic trauma occurs, blood loss can be massive. The client may exhibit signs of hemorrhagic shock, such as the following:

- Hypotension
- Tachycardia
- Tachypnea
- Pallor
- Diaphoresis
- Cool, clammy skin
- Confusion

A decreased hematocrit may confirm suspected blood loss. Clinical manifestations include right upper quadrant pain with abdominal tenderness, distention, guarding, and rigidity. Abdominal pain exaggerated by deep breathing and referred to the right shoulder (Kehr's sign) may indicate diaphragmatic irritation (Chart 59-8).

► COLLABORATIVE MANAGEMENT

When hepatic and other abdominal organ trauma is suspected, the physician performs an emergency peritoneal lavage to confirm injury. If trauma is present, the lavage reveals gross blood or a high red blood cell count.

The physician then performs an exploratory laparotomy to identify and control the source and type of bleeding. Minor surgical interventions, such as suture placement, wound packing, decompression, or a combination of these procedures, are often performed to halt bleeding. Liver lobe resection is required in some extensive liver injuries.

Clients with hepatic trauma require the administration of multiple blood products, packed red blood cells, and fresh frozen plasma, as well as massive volume infusion to maintain adequate hydration. Postoperatively, the client with hepatic trauma is admitted to a critical care unit. The nurse monitors the client for persistent bleeding. Complete blood count and coagulation studies must be closely monitored for trends in changes.

CANCER OF THE LIVER

■ OVERVIEW

Primary hepatic cancer, or **hepatocellular carcinoma** (cancer originating in the liver), is one of the leading causes of death in the world. The incidence is higher in African-American males and is increasing in people age 40 to 60 years of age (El-Serag & Mason, 1999). Possible reasons for this trend include the increase in people with hepatitis B and hepatitis C infections, which often lead to cancer of the liver.

> ≋ **CULTURAL CONSIDERATIONS**
>
> Hepatocellular carcinoma (HCC) is rare in the United States but is one of the most common malignancies in other parts of the world (e.g., Africa). The geographic variation probably reflects the prevalence of chronic hepatitis B and chronic hepatitis C infection in other countries. Hepatitis B or C virus is thought to be the primary carcinogen in as many as 80% of clients with HCC worldwide. Men are affected three times more than women, and blacks worldwide are affected twice as often as Caucasians (El-Serag & Mason, 1999).

CHART 59-8

KEY FEATURES *of*
Liver Trauma

- Right upper quadrant pain with abdominal tenderness
- Abdominal distention and rigidity
- Guarding of the abdomen
- Increased abdominal pain exaggerated by deep breathing and referred to the right shoulder (Kehr's sign)
- Indicators of hemorrhage and hypovolemic shock:
  Tachycardia
  Tachypnea
  Pallor
  Diaphoresis
  Cool, clammy skin
  Confusion or other change in mental state

Carcinoma of the liver most often develops as a metastatic process. Because of the increased vascularity of the liver, the organ is a common site for metastasis from (1) primary cancers of the esophagus, stomach, colon, rectum, breasts, and lungs; or (2) a malignant melanoma.

Between 30% and 70% of clients with primary hepatic cancer also have cirrhosis, and the risk is 40 times greater in clients with cirrhosis. Men with cirrhosis are more likely than women to develop HCC. Increased testosterone and decreased estrogens may promote the development of HCC in men with cirrhosis (Tanaka et al., 2000).

Primary hepatic cancer has also been associated with trauma, nutritional deficiencies, and exposure to carcinogens and hepatotoxins, such as aflatoxin, thorium dioxide, *Senecio* alkaloids, and the fungus *Aspergillus*.

► COLLABORATIVE MANAGEMENT

Clients with liver metastasis initially complain of epigastric or right upper quadrant abdominal pain, fatigue, anorexia, and weight loss. Later they typically experience the same manifestations of HCC, such as jaundice, ascites, bleeding, and encephalopathy. A nuclear radioisotope liver scan detects metastasis in many cases, but ultrasonography with needle biopsy may be required to confirm the metastasis.

Liver cancer is usually fatal within 6 months of diagnosis. Surgical management may be indicated for clients with a single metastatic lesion confined to one liver lobe. Liver lobe resection for surgical excision of metastasis has been successful in achieving survival rates of up to 5 years.

Unfortunately, 75% of clients are not candidates for surgical excision because their tumors are unresectable. A newer procedure, cryosurgical ablation of the liver, has produced remissions that offer hope for long-term survival (Leininger, 1997). In this procedure, the surgeon makes a subcostal or midline abdominal incision and selects which tumors are appropriate for either resection or cryoablation. The cryotherapy probes circulate liquid nitrogen and freeze the tumors. Postoperatively, the client is admitted to the critical care unit for monitoring of complications, including hypothermia, renal failure, and bleeding.

Other standard treatments for liver cancer include high-dose chemotherapy, usually with fluorouracil (5-FU) and hepatic artery ligation to deprive the metastatic lesion of oxygen. Both treatments can be accomplished without systemic effect because of the unique portal vein circulation in the liver. Hepatic chemotherapy is administered by a surgically implanted infusion pump, which enables controlled infusion for up to 14 days at a time. (See Chapter 25 for a discussion of intra-arterial chemotherapy.) Transplantation may also be used to treat liver cancer.

LIVER TRANSPLANTATION

■ OVERVIEW

The first liver transplantation was performed in 1963, and in 1983 it was decided that liver transplantation no longer be considered experimental. In 1998, 4487 liver transplants were performed, and 1-year survival rates are now approximately 84% (United Network for Organ Sharing (UNOS), 1998). The client with end-stage liver disease who has not responded to conventional medical or surgical intervention is a potential candidate for liver transplantation. In the adult, diseases treated by liver transplantation include the following:

- Primary or secondary biliary cirrhosis
- Chronic active hepatitis with cirrhosis
- Hepatic metabolic diseases, such as protoporphyria and Wilson's disease
- Budd-Chiari syndrome (hepatic vein thrombosis)
- Primary sclerosing cholangitis
- Lannëac's cirrhosis, if the person has abstained from alcohol

Liver transplantation is not commonly performed for clients with malignant neoplasms. Because the tumor is likely to recur in immunosuppressed clients, the procedure remains controversial.

The client for potential transplantation undergoes extensive physiologic and psychologic assessment and evaluation by physicians and transplant coordinators to identify contraindications to the procedure.

Clients who are not considered candidates for transplantation are those with severe end-stage liver disease with life-threatening complications, such as the following:

- Repeated episodes of esophageal variceal bleeding
- Sepsis
- Severe cardiovascular instability with advanced cardiac disease
- Acquired immunodeficiency syndrome (AIDS)
- Diabetes mellitus
- Severe respiratory disease

Additional identified risk factors include the existence of the following:

- Portal vein thrombosis
- Advanced catabolic state
- Active alcoholism
- Age older than 60 years
- Primary and metastatic malignant disease
- A lack of knowledge and understanding of the procedure and necessary postoperative care measures
- A poor psychosocial support system
- Psychologic instability

Liver transplantation has become the most effective treatment for clients with an increasing number of acute and chronic liver diseases, although they are more common in children than in adults. Indications and contraindications continue to vary among transplantation centers and are continually revised as treatment options change and surgical techniques improve.

Donor livers are obtained primarily from head trauma victims and in the United States. They are distributed through a nationwide program, the United Network of Organ Sharing (UNOS). This system distributes donor livers on the basis of regional considerations and recipient acuity. A new program for living donors has also been established. Recipients with the highest level of acuity receive highest priority.

■ Acute Graft Rejection

The success of all transplantations has greatly improved since the introduction in 1980 of cyclosporine (cyclosporin A), an immunosuppressant drug. Cyclosporine has been the primary agent to prevent rejection of the donor organ graft, but azathioprine (Imuran) and prednisone (Deltasone) are also used. Most recipients receive a combination of cyclosporine, steroids, and azathioprine.

A newer immunosuppressant agent discovered in 1984, tacrolimus (FK 506), is more potent than cyclosporine. FK 506 has been shown to be effective as a form of rescue therapy for clients who continue to reject a liver graft. Mycophenolate mofetil (CellCept) is the one of the newest approved immunosuppressants for the treatment of rejection in liver transplants and for those who are unable to tolerate cyclosporin or FK 506.

A majority of clients still experience a rejection response after liver transplantation beginning 1 to 2 weeks after surgery. Clinical manifestations of acute rejection include tachycardia, fever, right upper quadrant or flank pain, decreased bile pigment and volume, and increasing jaundice. Laboratory findings include elevated serum bilirubin, alkaline phosphatase levels, and increased prothrombin time and aminotransferase levels.

Transplant rejection is treated with IV doses of methylprednisolone (Solu-Medrol). If this drug is not effective, antibodies to lymphocytes such as muromonab-CD3 (OKT3) may also be used. OKT3 is T-cell specific and is more potent, but it increases the client's risk of infection. Mycophenolate mofetil may also be used against rejection. As with all rejection treatments, the client is at a greater risk for infection. If none of these drugs is effective, a rapid deterioration of liver function occurs. Multisystem organ failure, including respiratory and renal involvement, develops along with diffuse coagulopathies and portal-systemic encephalopathy. The only alternative for treatment is emergency transplantation.

■ Infection

Infection is another potential threat to the transplanted graft and the client's survival. Immunosuppressant therapy, which must be used to prevent and treat organ rejection, significantly increases the client's susceptibility to and risk for infection. Other risk factors include the presence of multiple tubes and intravascular lines, immobility, and prolonged anesthesia.

The average liver transplant client acquires at least one bacterial infection and has a 40% to 50% chance of developing a viral or fungal infection. In the early post-transplantation period, common infections include pneumonia, wound infections, and urinary tract infections. Opportunistic infections usually develop after the first postoperative month and include cytomegalovirus, mycobacterial infections, and parasitic infections. Latent infections such as tuberculosis and herpes simplex are often reactivated.

Transplant complications cause clients to be very anxious. The nurse and other members of the health care team assure the client that these problems are common and usually successfully treated (see the Evidence-Based Practice for Nursing on box at right).

The physician prescribes broad-spectrum antibiotics for prophylaxis during and after surgery. The nurse obtains culture specimens from all lines and tubes and collects specimens for culture at predetermined time intervals as dictated by the agency's policy. If an infection is detected, the physician prescribes organism-specific anti-infective agents.

■ Other Complications

The biliary anastomosis is susceptible to breakdown, obstruction, and infection. If leakage occurs or if the site becomes necrotic or obstructed, an abscess can form or peritonitis, bacteremia, and cirrhosis may develop. Other potential complications include the following:

- Hemorrhage
- Hepatic artery thrombosis
- Fluid and electrolyte imbalances

EVIDENCE-BASED PRACTICE
FOR NURSING

How much anxiety is experienced by clients undergoing a liver transplant?

Chappell, S., & Case, P. (1997). Anxiety in liver transplant patients. *MEDSURG Nursing, 6*(2), 98-103.

The purpose of this study was to describe the anxiety of adult liver transplant recipients during their hospitalization. Speilberg's model of state and trait anxiety was the framework for the study. Speilberg's State Trait Anxiety Inventory (STAI) and a visual analog scale (VAS) were completed at the following stages: admission for transplantation, transfer to the nursing floor, first liver biopsy, first signs of infection, first signs of a rejection episode, immediately after the first teaching session with the transplant coordinator, and discharge from the hospital. The highest mean anxiety scores occurred at the first liver biopsy, the first episode of rejection, and the first infection.

Critique. Although the sample size for this study was small, the researchers aimed to explore the psychosocial aspects of this major surgery and life-changing event. Data from this study can help nurses better care for their clients by addressing both their psychosocial needs and their physical needs.

Implications for Nursing. Nurses should anticipate that clients will be extremely anxious during the first liver biopsy and during episodes of rejection or infection. Nurses caring for clients during these procedures and times should exercise additional support. Other people on the health care team, as well as the clients' families, should also be made aware that clients will experience anxiety at these times; they should be taught to be as supportive and understanding as possible.

TABLE 59-6 • ASSESSMENT AND PREVENTION OF COMMON POSTOPERATIVE COMPLICATIONS ASSOCIATED WITH LIVER TRANSPLANTATION

Assessment	Prevention
ACUTE GRAFT REJECTION Occurs from the fourth to tenth postoperative day Manifested by tachycardia, fever, right upper quadrant (RUQ) or flank pain, diminished bile drainage or change in bile color, or increased jaundice Laboratory changes include increased levels of serum bilirubin, transaminases, and alkaline phosphatase, as well as prolonged prothrombin time.	Prophylaxis with immunosuppressant agents, such as cyclosporine Early diagnosis to treat with more potent antirejection drugs, such as muromonab-CD3 (OKT3)
INFECTION Can occur at any time during recovery Frequent cultures of tubes, lines, and drainage Manifested by fever or excessive, foul-smelling drainage (urine, wound, or bile); other indicators depend on location and type of infection Early removal of invasive lines Good handwashing	Antibiotic prophylaxis Early diagnosis and treatment with organism-specific anti-infective agents
HEPATIC COMPLICATIONS (BILE LEAKAGE, ABSCESS FORMATION, HEPATIC THROMBOSIS) Manifested by decreased bile drainage, increased RUQ abdominal pain with distention and guarding, nausea or vomiting, increased jaundice, and clay-colored stools Laboratory changes include increased levels of serum bilirubin and transaminases	Keep T-tube in dependent position and secure to client; empty frequently, recording quality and quantity of drainage Report manifestations to physician immediately May necessitate surgical intervention
ACUTE RENAL FAILURE Caused by hypotension, antibiotics, cyclosporine, acute liver failure, or hypothermia Indicators of hypothermia include shivering, hyperventilation, increased cardiac output, vasoconstriction, and alkalemia Early indicators of renal failure include changes in urine output, increased BUN and creatinine levels, and electrolyte imbalance	Monitor all drug levels with nephrotoxic side effects Prevent hypotension Observe for early signs of renal failure and report them immediately to the physician

*BUN, Blood urea nitrogen

- Pulmonary atelectasis
- Acute renal failure
- Chronic graft rejection
- Psychologic maladjustment

► COLLABORATIVE MANAGEMENT

Care of the client undergoing liver transplantation requires an interdisciplinary team approach. Case managers are an important part of the team. After the client is identified as a candidate and a donor organ is procured, the actual liver transplantation surgical procedure usually takes 8 hours. The length of the procedure can vary greatly. The procedure involves five anastomoses between recipient and donor organs, including the following vascular anastomosis sites:

- Suprahepatic inferior vena cava
- Infrahepatic vena cava
- Portal vein
- Hepatic artery
- Biliary tract

The biliary anastomosis site varies depending on the client's extrahepatic biliary tract. Two common sites are end-to-end anastomosis between the donor and the recipient common bile duct and anastomosis between the donor common bile duct and the recipient jejunum.

In the immediate postoperative period, the client who has undergone liver transplantation is managed in the critical care unit and requires aggressive monitoring and care. The nurse assesses for signs and symptoms of complications of surgery and immediately reports their occurrence to the physician (Table 59-6).

The nurse monitors the client's temperature and reports temperatures greater than 100° F (38° C) and increased abdominal pain, distention, and rigidity, which are indicators of peritonitis. Nursing assessment also includes monitoring for a change in neurologic status that could indicate encephalopathy from a nonfunctioning liver. Signs of coagulopathy (e.g., continuous bloody oozing from a catheter, a drain, and incision sites; petechiae; or ecchymosis) are reported to the physician immediately because they can indicate impaired function of the transplanted liver.

ONLINE RESOURCES

For suggested readings and Internet resources, go to http://www. wbsaunders.com/SIMON/Iggy/.

SELECTED BIBLIOGRAPHY

Alter, M. (1999). *Epidemiology of hepatitis C.* NIH Consensus Development Conference on Management of Hepatitis C; http://gi.ucsf.edu/ALF/CC/CCMAlter.html.

Bockhold, K.M. (2000). Who's afraid of hepatitis C? *American Journal of Nursing, 100*(5), 26-31.

Centers for Disease Control and Prevention (Hepatitis Branch) (April 28, 1997). *Epidemiology and prevention of viral hepatitis A to E: An overview;* http://www.cdc.gov/ncidod/diseases/hepatitis/slideset/httoc.htm.

Centers for Disease Control and Prevention. (1999). *Hepatitis fact sheet;* http://www.cdc.gov/ncidod/diseases/hepatitis.htm.

Chappell, S., Case, P. (1997). Anxiety in liver transplant patients. *MEDSURG Nursing, 6*(2), 98-103.

Dougherty, A.S., & Dreher, H.M. (2001). Hepatitis C: Current treatment strategies for an emerging epidemic. *MEDSURG Nursing, 10*(1), 9-13.

El-Sarag, H., & Mason, A. (1999). Rising incidence of hepatocellular carcinoma in the United States. *New England Journal of Medicine, 340*(10), 745-750.

Frieden, T., et al. (1999). Chronic liver disease in central Harlem: The role of alcohol and viral hepatitis. *Hepatology, 29*(3), 883-888.

Groen, K.A. (1999). Primary and metastatic liver cancer. *Seminars in Oncology Nursing, 15*(1), 48-57.

Hepatitis Foundation International. (September 1999). *Hepatitis fact sheet;* http://hepfi.org/Hepinfo/FACT%201-99.htm.

Hoofnagle, J. (1999). Hepatitis C: *The clinical spectrum of disease.* NIH Consensus Development Conference on Management of Hepatitis C; http://www.hepnet.com/hepc/hoofnagl.html.

Leininger, S.M. (1997). Managing patients with cryosurgical ablation of the prostate and liver. *MEDSURG Nursing, 6*(6), 359-363, 386.

LoBiondo-Wood, G., et al. (1997). Impact of liver transplantation on quality of life: A longitudinal perspective. *Applied Nursing Research, 10*(1), 27-32.

National Institutes of Health (Hepatitis Branch). (September 1999). *Program and abstracts.* NIH Consensus Development Conference on Management of Hepatitis C; http://odp.od.nih.gov/consensus/cons/105/105_abstract.pdf.

Neuman, A., et al. (1998). Hepatitis C viral dynamics in vivo and the antiviral efficacy of interferon-alpha therapy. *Science, 282,* 103-107.

Rollier, C., et al. (1999). Protective and therapeutic effect of DNA-based immunization against Hepadnavirus large envelope protein. *Gastroentereology, 116*(3), 658-665.

Sarin, S., et al. (1999). Comparison of endoscopic ligation and propranolol for the primary prevention of variceal bleeding. *New England Journal of Medicine, 340,* 988-993.

Shovein, J.T., et al. (2000). Hepatitis A: How benign is it? *American Journal of Nursing, 100*(3), 43-47.

Starzl, T., et al. (1997). Liver transplantation. *Gastroenterology, 112*(1), 288-291.

Tanaka, K, et al. (2000). Serum testosterone: Estradiol ration and the development of hepatocellular carcinoma among male cirrhotic patients. *Cancer Research, 60*(18), 5106-5110.

United Network for Organ Sharing. (1998). *1998 Annual Report;* http://www.unos.org.

Wiley, T., et al. (1998). Impact of alcohol on the histological and clinical progression of hepatitis C infection. *Hepatology, 28*(3), 805-809.

Wong, J.B., et al. (2000). Estimating future hepatitis C morbidity, mortality, and costs in the United States. *American Journal of Public Health, 90*(10), 1562-1569.

Ziser, A., et al. (1999). Morbidity and mortality in cirrhotic patients undergoing anesthesia and surgery. *Anesthesiology, 90*(1),42-53.

Interventions for Clients with Problems of the Gallbladder and Pancreas

E. JEAN HAYES

Learning Objectives

After studying this chapter, you should be able to:

1. Identify the common causes of cholecystitis and cholelithiasis (gallbladder disease).
2. Explain the role of testing in diagnosis of gallbladder disease.
3. Compare postoperative care of clients undergoing a traditional cholecystectomy with that of clients undergoing a laparoscopic cholecystectomy.
4. Develop a community-based teaching plan for clients with gallbladder disease, including care of a T-tube.
5. Compare and contrast the pathophysiology of acute and chronic pancreatitis.
6. Interpret common assessment findings associated with acute pancreatitis and those associated with chronic pancreatitis.
7. Prioritize nursing care for clients with acute pancreatitis and clients with chronic pancreatitis.
8. Explain the use and adverse effects of drug therapy for clients with chronic pancreatitis.
9. Develop a postoperative plan of care for clients undergoing a Whipple procedure.
10. Construct a discharge plan for care of clients with pancreatic cancer in the community.
11. Discuss the psychosocial needs of the client with pancreatic cancer and associated nursing interventions.

Go to http://www.wbsaunders.com/SIMON/Iggy/ for self-assessment questions related to these Learning Objectives.

Disorders of the gallbladder and pancreas begin as single-organ processes, but the inflammatory response may extend to other organs if the primary disorder is not treated. This occurs because of the anatomic proximity of the liver, gallbladder, and pancreas and because the flow of bile from the liver through the biliary (gallbladder) ductal system may be impeded. Inflammation of the gallbladder, liver, or pancreas is caused by obstruction in the biliary system from gallstones, edema, stricture, or tumors. For example, gallstones impacted in the cystic duct cause cholecystitis; gallstones lodged in the ampulla of Vater impede the flow of bile and pancreatic secretions, which can result in pancreatitis.

BILIARY DISORDERS

Cholecystitis

■ OVERVIEW

The two most common problems that occur within the biliary tree are stone formation (cholelithiasis) and associated chronic inflammation (cholecystitis). Cholecystitis may occur as an acute or chronic inflammation of the gallbladder wall (Table 60-1). Chronic inflammation may be complicated by an acute attack if an obstruction is present.

■ Pathophysiology

■ ACUTE CHOLECYSTITIS

Acute **cholecystitis** (inflammation of the gallbladder) usually develops in association with **cholelithiasis** (gallstones). Either condition may occur singly, but they frequently occur together. Cholelithiasis is discussed in detail later in this chapter (p. 1333).

Acalculous **cholecystitis** (inflammation occurring in the absence of gallstones) is believed to be due to bacterial invasion via the lymphatic or vascular route. *Escherichia coli* is the most common causative bacterium found, but group D *Streptococcus, Salmonella,* and *Staphylococcus* may also be found.

Acute cholecystitis usually follows obstruction of the cystic duct by a stone, which evokes the inflammatory response. This response may be the result of a mechanical, chemical, or

TABLE 60-1 • COMPARISON OF ACUTE AND CHRONIC CHOLECYSTITIS

Acute Cholecystitis	Chronic Cholecystitis
Inflammation present	Inflammation followed by fibrosis
Most commonly occurs as a result of cholelithiasis (gallstones) but can occur from bacterial invasion or biliary spasm	Most commonly occurs as a result of cholelithiasis
Bile obstruction *not* common	Bile obstruction common; may result in cholangitis and pancreatitis
Jaundice *not* common	Jaundice very common

bacterial process (Greenberger & Isselbacher, 1998). When the gallbladder is inflamed, trapped bile is reabsorbed and acts as a chemical irritant to the gallbladder wall; that is, the bile has a toxic effect. The presence of bile, in combination with impaired circulation, edema, and distention of the gallbladder, causes ischemia of the gallbladder wall. The result is tissue sloughing with necrosis and gangrene. Perforation (rupture) of the gallbladder wall may occur. If the perforation is small and localized, an abscess may form. Peritonitis may result if the perforation is large.

In some cases, painful episodes of cholecystitis may be the result of organ or bile duct spasticity. The spasticity temporarily prevents the release of an adequate amount of bile for fat digestion.

■ CHRONIC CHOLECYSTITIS

Chronic cholecystitis results, possibly from repeated bouts of acute or subacute cholecystitis, when gallbladder muscle wall disease and inefficient emptying of bile by the gallbladder persist. Gallstones are almost always present. In chronic cholecystitis, the gallbladder becomes fibrotic and contracted, which results in decreased motility and deficient absorption.

Pancreatitis and **cholangitis** (inflammation of the common bile duct) can occur as complications of cholecystitis. Pancreatitis and cholangitis result from the backup of bile throughout the biliary tract. Bile obstruction leads to jaundice.

Jaundice (yellow discoloration of the skin and mucous membranes) and **icterus** (yellow discoloration of the sclerae) can occur in clients with acute cholecystitis but is most commonly seen in clients with chronic gallbladder inflammation. Impeded or obstructed bile flow caused by edema of the ducts or gallstones contributes to *extrahepatic obstructive* jaundice. Jaundice in cholecystitis may also be caused by direct liver involvement. Inflammation of the liver's bile channels or bile ducts may cause *intrahepatic* obstructive jaundice, resulting in an increase in circulating levels of bilirubin, the principal pigment of bile.

When the concentration of bilirubin in the blood increases to greater than 2.5 mg/dL, jaundice occurs (Pagana & Pagana, 1998). In a person with obstructive jaundice, the normal flow of bile into the duodenum is blocked, allowing excessive bile salts to accumulate in the skin. This accumulation of bile salts leads to pruritus (itching) or a burning sensation. The bile flow blockage also prevents bilirubin from reaching the large intestine, where it is converted to urobilinogen. Because urobilinogen accounts for the normal brown color of feces, clay-colored stools result. Water-soluble bilirubin is normally excreted by the kidneys in the urine. When an excess of circulating bilirubin occurs, the urine becomes dark and foamy because of the kidneys' effort to clear the bilirubin.

■ Etiology

The exact etiology of cholecystitis is unknown. In addition to the formation of gallbladder calculi, causes of acute cholecystitis include the following:

- Trauma
- Inadequate blood supply
- Prolonged anesthesia and surgery
- Adhesions
- Edema
- Neoplasms (tumors)
- Long-term fasting
- Prolonged dehydration
- Gallbladder trauma
- Prolonged immobility
- Excessive opioid use

Any condition that affects the regular filling or emptying of the gallbladder or causes "gallbladder shock" (a decrease in blood flow to the gallbladder) can result in acute cholecystitis. Cholecystitis has also been attributed to anatomic problems such as twisting or kinking of the gallbladder neck or cystic duct resulting in pancreatic enzyme reflux into the gallbladder.

■ Incidence/Prevalence

More than 20 million persons in the United States have gallbladder disease, which causes more than 800,000 hospitalizations each year (see the Cost of Care Box on p. 1329). Gallstones are very common in the United States, with approximately 20% of the population being affected. Native Americans, particularly the Pima Indians of Arizona, have an unusually high incidence of gallstones, with Mexican Americans and Caucasians following (Everhart et al., 1999; Price & Wilson, 1997). A high incidence of biliary tract disease and cholecystitis occurs in people with a sedentary lifestyle, a familial tendency to biliary disease, obesity, or diabetes mellitus.

> **WOMEN'S HEALTH CONSIDERATIONS**
> The incidence of gallbladder disease is higher in women, especially Caucasian women. By age 60 years, nearly one third of obese women develop biliary disease (Allen & Phillips, 1997).

► COLLABORATIVE MANAGEMENT
● Assessment
■ PHYSICAL ASSESSMENT/CLINICAL MANIFESTATIONS

Clients with acute cholecystitis frequently present with pain, although clinical manifestations vary in intensity and frequency (Chart 60-1).

The nurse or assistive nursing personnel obtains the client's height and weight and determines his or her sex, age, race, and ethnic group. The nurse asks about food preferences and determines whether excessive fat and cholesterol are included in the diet. The client is asked whether any foods are

COST OF CARE
IMPLICATIONS FOR NURSING

GALLBLADDER DISORDERS

Cost of Care

- Approximately 800,000 hospitalizations occur each year for gallstone disease at a cost exceeding $2 billion annually.
- The cost of medical care for the client with a biliary disorder varies according to the type of problem present and the medical/surgical management needed to resolve the problem.
- Obesity is a major contributing factor to the formation of gallstones, a major cause of cholecystitis.
- The health-related economic cost of obesity to U.S. business represents approximately 5% of the total medical costs.
- Surgical management of gallbladder disease, without complications, can cost from a low of approximately $4000 to a high of around $12,000. Complications will increase the cost expenditure.
- Laparoscopic cholecystectomy has reduced the length of stay and the cost of treatment of gallbladder disease.

Implications for Nursing

Because of the high cost of obesity, and the significance of obesity to gallbladder disorders, nurses need to become familiar with the management of obesity. The nurse will want to consult with a nutritionist or dietitian to develop a dietary plan for the client. The plan needs to allow the client to reduce weight in a slow, safe manner, since rapid weight loss is a causative factor in gallstone formation. Preventing the formation of gallstones will decrease the number of surgeries needed each year.

Nurses need to continue to be proficient in providing care for the client undergoing an outpatient laparoscopic procedure, including preoperative and postoperative teaching to prevent complications. The prevention of complications will reduce the cost factor by decreasing the number of days the client will need to stay in the hospital and lowering the number of interventions such as antibiotic therapy.

Data from Thompson, D., et al. (1998). Estimated economic costs of obesity to U.S. business, *American Journal of Health Promotion, 13*(2), 120-127; and Howard, D.E., & Fromm, H. (1999). Nonsurgical management of gallstone disease, *Gastroenterology Clinics of North America, 28*(1), 133-141.

---

not tolerated. The nurse asks whether any of the following gastrointestinal (GI) symptoms occur in relation to the intake of fatty food: flatulence, dyspepsia (indigestion), eructation (belching), anorexia, nausea, vomiting, and abdominal pain or discomfort.

The client is asked to describe the pain, including its intensity and duration, precipitating factors, and any measures that relieve it. The pain may be described as indigestion of varying intensity, ranging from a mild, persistent ache to a steady, constant pain in the right upper abdominal quadrant. The pain may radiate to the right shoulder or scapula. The abdominal pain of chronic cholecystitis may be vague and nonspecific. The usual pattern of more acute pain is episodic. Clients often refer to these episodes as "gallbladder attacks."

The nurse also asks the client to describe his or her daily activity or exercise routines to determine whether his or her lifestyle is sedentary. The client is questioned whether there is a family history of gallbladder disease, since there is a familial tendency for biliary tract diseases. If the client is female, the nurse also determines whether estrogen replacement therapy (ERT) is being taken, because this therapy may contribute to biliary disorders.

Because of gallbladder tenderness, it is difficult to use abdominal palpation and percussion in assessment of the client with acute cholecystitis. With right subcostal palpation, pain

CHART 60-1

KEY FEATURES *of*
Cholecystitis

- Episodic or vague abdominal pain or discomfort that can radiate to the right shoulder
- Pain triggered by a high-fat or high-volume meal
- Anorexia
- Nausea or vomiting
- Dyspepsia
- Eructation
- Flatulence
- Feeling of abdominal fullness
- Rebound tenderness (Blumberg's sign)
- Fever
- Jaundice, clay-colored stools, dark urine, steatorrhea (most common with chronic cholecystitis)

---

increases with deep inspiration (Murphy's sign). Guarding and rigidity, as well as rebound tenderness (Blumberg's sign), are reliable indicators of peritoneal irritation.

Assessment for rebound tenderness and deep palpation are reserved for physicians and advanced-practice nurses. To elicit rebound tenderness, the nurse pushes his or her fingers deeply and steadily into the client's abdomen, then quickly releases the pressure. Pain that results from the rebound of the palpated tissue indicates peritoneal inflammation. Deep palpation below the liver border in the right upper quadrant may reveal a sausage-shaped mass, representing the distended, inflamed gallbladder. Percussion over the posterior rib cage intensifies localized abdominal pain.

In *chronic* cholecystitis, clients may have insidious symptoms and may not seek medical treatment until late symptoms such as jaundice, clay-colored stools, and dark urine result from an obstructive process. Steatorrhea (fatty stools) occurs because fat absorption is decreased owing to the lack of bile. Bile is needed for the absorption of fats and fat-soluble vitamins in the intestine. As with any inflammatory process, the client may have an elevated temperature of 99° to 102° F (37° to 39° C), tachycardia, and dehydration from fever and vomiting.

■ DIAGNOSTIC ASSESSMENT

There are no laboratory tests specific for gallbladder disease. A differential diagnosis must rule out other diseases that may cause similar symptoms, such as peptic ulcer disease, gastroesophageal reflux disorder, and pancreatitis. Serum levels of alkaline phosphatase, aspartate aminotransferase (AST), and lactate dehydrogenase (LDH) may be elevated, indicating abnormalities in liver function. The direct (conjugated) and indirect (unconjugated) serum bilirubin levels are elevated if an obstructive process is present. An increased white blood cell (WBC) count with a left shift on the differential count indicates inflammation. If there is pancreatic involvement, serum and urine amylase levels are elevated.

Ultrasonography of the right upper quadrant is the best diagnostic test for cholecystitis and has largely replaced the older cholecystogram. It is safe, accurate, and painless. Acute cholecystitis is evidenced by edema of the gallbladder wall and pericholecystic fluid, both of which are determined by the ultrasound (Nahrwold, 1997). The health care provider may also order an upper GI radiographic series to rule out other causes of abdominal pain, such as gastritis and peptic ulcer disease. A cholecystogram may be ordered if other diagnostic tests are inconclusive.

A hepatobiliary scan with cholecystokinin using technetium ^{99m}Tc disofenin or mebrofenen can be performed to visualize the gallbladder and determine patency of the biliary system. The pretest fasting period for this scan can be as short as 4 hours, making it preferable to a diagnostic study that would require a longer fasting time. Visualization of the gallbladder excludes the diagnosis of acute cholecystitis with a high degree of certainty (Fischbach, 2000).

▶ Interventions

Nonsurgical treatment measures prescribed during the acute phase of cholecystitis are directed at resting the inflamed gallbladder in an effort to reduce the inflammatory process and relieve the pain. Because of the risk of sepsis and perforation, however, acute cholecystitis is generally managed surgically.

NONSURGICAL MANAGEMENT. Nonsurgical measures to relieve pain include diet and drug therapy. The physician, nurse, and dietitian often collaborate when implementing these interventions.

DIET THERAPY. For clients with acute cholecystitis, the health care provider may recommend withholding food and fluids or modifying the diet by avoiding high-fat or high-volume meals. These dietary measures decrease stimulation of the gallbladder and help prevent pain, nausea, and vomiting. For clients with severe nausea and vomiting, decompression of the stomach may be necessary. A nasogastric tube is inserted to empty the stomach contents. (The nurse's role in caring for a client with a nasogastric [NG] tube is described in Chapter 58.)

The nurse encourages the client with chronic cholecystitis to consume a low-fat diet to decrease stimulation of the gallbladder. Smaller, more frequent meals assist some clients in tolerating food better.

CRITICAL THINKING CHALLENGE

Your client with chronic cholecystitis tells you that she has been avoiding fried foods and eating a low-fat diet but is still having problems with pain and nausea after meals. You want to determine what she considers to be "low fat."

- Using a daily caloric intake of 1800 calories, determine how many grams of fat your client can consume to remain at a 20% total dietary fat intake.
- What questions might you ask her to evaluate whether she can determine the percentage of fat in a food item by reading the label?
- Who else might you involve in this client's care to assist with nutritional needs?

For suggested answer guidelines, go to SIMON http://www.wbsaunders.com/SIMON/Iggy/.

DRUG THERAPY. For clients in severe pain, the health care provider may order opioid analgesics, such as meperidine hydrochloride (Demerol), to relieve abdominal pain and spasm. Traditionally, morphine has not been given, because it can cause spasms of the sphincter of Oddi and increase pain. Meperidine, like all opioids, can increase smooth muscle tone in the biliary tract as well, causing biliary and pancreatic se-

cretions to decrease and bile duct pressure to increase. This can also result in spasms of the sphincter of Oddi (Pasero, 1998). Antispasmodic agents, such as anticholinergics (e.g., dicyclomine hydrochloride [Bentyl, Lomine✦]), may be used to relax the smooth muscles, preventing biliary contraction. Decreased muscle contraction minimizes secretions and assists in the reduction of pain. The health care provider usually prescribes antiemetics, such as trimethobenzamide hydrochloride (Tigan), to relieve nausea and vomiting.

SURGICAL MANAGEMENT. The usual surgical treatment of clients with acute and chronic cholecystitis is cholecystectomy, the removal of the gallbladder. Two operative procedures are available to the surgeon for performing a cholecystectomy: the traditional open approach and laparoscopic laser cholecystectomy.

TRADITIONAL CHOLECYSTECTOMY. Use of the traditional surgical approach has markedly declined during the past decade. The client undergoing this surgery is usually hospitalized for several days following the procedure.

Preoperative Care. The nurse provides the usual preoperative care in the operating suite on the day of surgery (see Chapter 17). The nurse reinforces teaching of aggressive measures to prevent respiratory complications. To minimize abdominal/incisional jarring during coughing, deep breathing, and turning, the nurse demonstrates splinting methods using a pillow or folded blanket. These clients, especially older adults and smokers, are also susceptible to postoperative atelectasis. The nurse instructs the client in the use of sustained maximal inspiration (SMI) devices, such as an incentive spirometer.

The importance of early mobilization in preventing complications is also emphasized. The nurse informs the client to expect to get out of bed the evening of surgery.

Operative Procedure. The surgeon not only removes the gallbladder through a right subcostal incision but also often explores the biliary ducts for the presence of stones. If the common bile duct is explored, the surgeon typically inserts a T-tube drain to ensure patency of the duct (Figure 60-1). Trauma to the common bile duct stimulates inflammation, which can impede bile flow and contribute to bile stasis. In addition, the surgeon usually inserts a drainage tube, such as a Jackson-Pratt (JP) drain. This drainage tube is positioned in the gallbladder bed to prevent fluid accumulation. The drainage is usually serosanguinous (serous fluid mixed with blood) and is bile stained in the first 24 hours postoperatively.

Postoperative Care. Postoperative incisional pain relief after a traditional cholecystectomy is usually achieved with meperidine hydrochloride (Demerol) using a patient-controlled analgesia (PCA) pump. The client participates in coughing and deep breathing exercises more readily when pain is minimized. Therefore the nurse plans for the coughing and deep breathing exercises to be performed when pain relief is optimal.

Antiemetics may be necessary for clients with episodes of postoperative nausea and vomiting. The nurse administers the antiemetic early, as ordered, to prevent retching associated with vomiting and thus decrease the incidence of pain related to muscle straining.

The nurse cares for the incision, the surgical drain, and the T-tube. The surgeon typically removes the surgical dressing and drain within 24 to 48 hours after surgery. The T-tube,

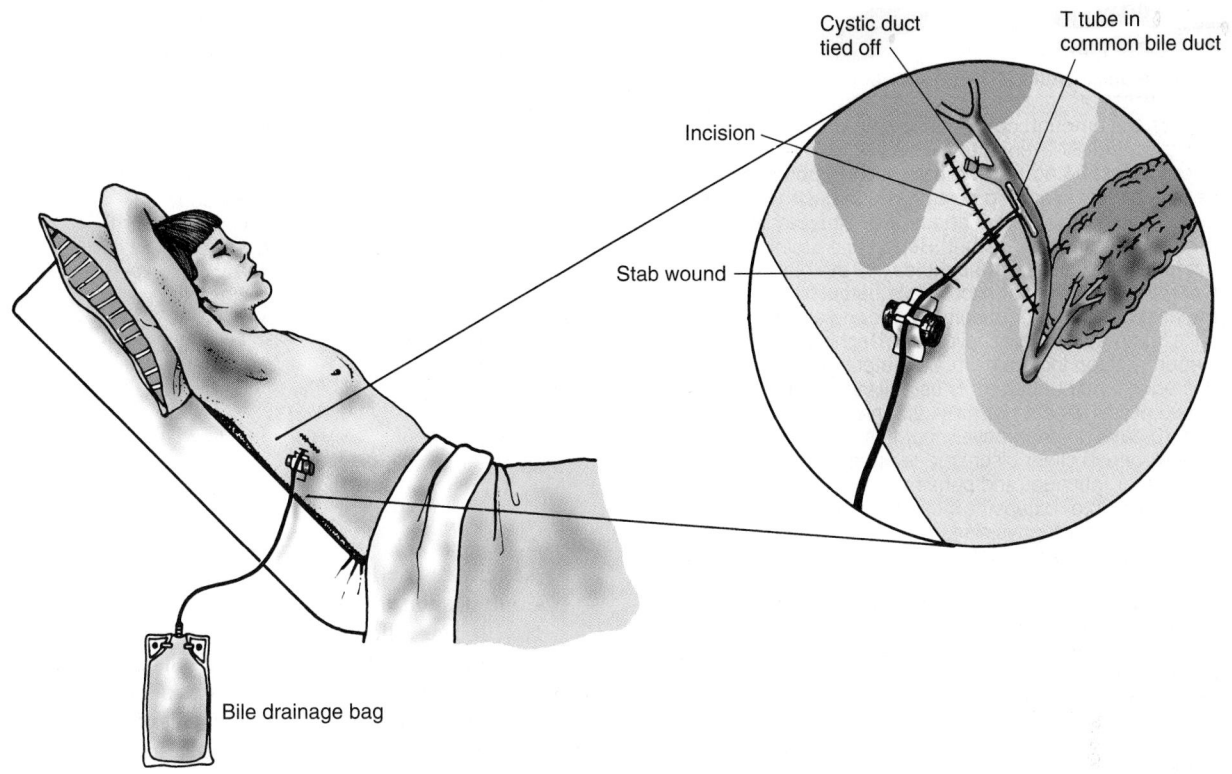

Figure 60-1 ● Placement of a T-tube.

however, may remain in place for 6 weeks or longer. Chart 60-2 highlights the important nursing care activities associated with the T-tube system.

The client usually receives nothing by mouth (NPO) for about 8 to 24 hours postoperatively. If gallbladder disease is severe, a nasogastric (NG) tube provides stomach decompression during this period. When peristalsis returns, the nurse removes the NG tube as ordered. The physician places the client on a clear liquid diet. The nurse gradually advances the diet from clear liquids to solid foods as tolerated. Within a day or two, the client resumes the ingestion of solid foods and is discharged to home.

The amount of fat allowed in the client's diet after a cholecystectomy depends on his or her tolerance of fat. In the early postoperative period, if bile flow is reduced, a low-fat diet may reduce discomfort and prevent nausea. For most clients, a special diet is not required. The nurse advises the client to eat nutritious meals and avoid excessive intake of fat. If the client is obese, the nurse recommends a weight reduction program. The nurse collaborates with the physician and the dietitian in planning the appropriate diet.

LAPAROSCOPIC CHOLECYSTECTOMY. Laparoscopic cholecystectomy, introduced in 1988, has quickly gained in popularity (see the Clinical Pathway on p. 1852). It is now considered the treatment of choice by many surgeons and is performed more often than the traditional open cholecystectomy. From studies involving 4000 clients undergoing a laparoscopic cholecystectomy, data show very positive results, including the following:

- Complications are very uncommon.
- Conversion to open cholecystectomy is about 5%.
- The death rate is very low (i.e., <0.1%).
- Bile duct injuries are rare.

These data indicate why the laparoscopic approach to gallbladder removal is now considered the "gold standard" (Greenberger & Isselbacher, 1998).

Preoperative Care. The laparoscopic procedure is commonly done on an ambulatory care basis in a same-day surgery suite. The surgeon explains the procedure; the nurse answers questions and reinforces the physician's instructions. There is no special preoperative preparation for the client. However, the physician typically orders the usual preoperative laboratory tests and requires the client to be on NPO status before the surgery. Chapter 17 describes general preoperative care for the client undergoing anesthesia.

Operative Procedure. The surgeon makes a 10-mm midline puncture at the umbilicus. The abdominal cavity is insufflated with 3 to 4 L of carbon dioxide. Gasless laparoscopic cholecystectomy using abdominal wall lifting devices is a more recent innovation. This technique results in improved pulmonary and cardiac function (Strasberg, 1999). A trocar catheter is inserted, through which a laparoscope is introduced. The laparoscope is attached to a video camera, and the abdominal organs are viewed on a monitor. The surgeon makes three small punctures through which to introduce laparoscopic forceps to manipulate the gallbladder. A laser is used to dissect the gallbladder away from the liver bed and to close off the cystic artery and the duct. The surgeon mobilizes the gallbladder, aspirates the bile and crushes any large stones, and then extracts the gallbladder through the umbilical port.

Postoperative Care. Removing the gallbladder with the laparoscopic technique reduces the risk of wound complications. Some clients have a problem with "free air pain" from

CHART 60-2

BEST PRACTICE *for*
Care of the Client with a T-Tube

- Assess the amount, color, consistency, and odor of drainage initially every 2 to 4 hours, then every 8 hours after the first 24 hours. In the immediate postoperative period, expect bloody drainage, which changes to green-brown bile. Bile output is about 400+ mL/day with a gradual decrease in amount. Report bile drainage amounts in excess of 1000 mL/day to the physician.
- Collect and administer excess bile output to the client by the nasogastric tube (uncommon), or give synthetic bile salts, such as dehydrocholic acid (Decholin).
- Report sudden increases in bile output after a normally decreasing output pattern is established. (The hospital-based nurse will not normally observe this, since it occurs 9 to 10 days postoperatively, but this information should be included in client discharge teaching.)
- Assess for foul odor and purulent drainage, which indicate infection or extensive inflammation. Report changes in drainage to the physician.
- Inspect the skin around the T-tube insertion site for signs of inflammation, including redness, swelling, and erythema, and observe for frank bile leakage. Keep the dressing dry. (Use the hospital's procedure and provide drain care and dressing change per protocol. The site is usually cleaned and the dressing changed daily.)
- Keep the drainage system below the level of the gallbladder. Maintain the client in the semi-Fowler's position.
- *Never* irrigate, aspirate, or clamp a T-tube without a physician's order.
- Assess the drainage system for pulling, kinking, or tangling of tubing, especially when the client is positioned toward the right side. Assist the client with early turning and ambulation. Drape and secure the section of the T-tube emerging from the stab wound over a small roll of gauze taped to the client's skin to help prevent its lumen from occluding as a result of pressure.
- When ordered by the physician, raise the drainage bag to the level of the abdomen (usually on the fourth or fifth postoperative day). Then assess the client for feelings of fullness, nausea, or pain.
- When the client is allowed to eat, clamp the T-tube for 1 to 2 hours (per physician's orders) before and after meals. Assess the client's response to determine tolerance of food.
- Observe stools for return of brown color 7 to 10 days postoperatively.

TABLE 60-2 • FOODS FOR CLIENTS WITH CHOLECYSTITIS OR CHOLELITHIASIS TO AVOID	
FOODS HIGH IN CHOLESTEROL	**GAS-FORMING VEGETABLES**
Dairy Products	• Cabbage
• Whole milk	• Onions
• Ice cream	• Broccoli
• Butter	• Cauliflower
• Cream	• Sauerkraut
• Cheese	• Radishes
	• Cucumbers
Other Foods	• Beans
• Fried, fatty foods	
• Rich pastries	
• Gravies	
• Nuts	
• Chocolate	
• Egg yolks	
• Avocado	

- Activity restrictions
- Complication recognition
- Health care follow-up

In postoperative teaching and discharge planning, the nurse should include a supportive spouse, family member, or significant other to provide reinforcement of information and to assist the client in adhering to the treatment plan.

Diet therapy for the client who has undergone a cholecystectomy is based on his or her tolerance of fats. The nurse or dietitian consults with the client to develop a nutrition program that includes nutritious, well-balanced meals that include the client's preferences, when possible. If the client has a poor tolerance of fats, a low-fat diet is developed and a list of foods to avoid is provided (Table 60-2). The dietitian may provide printed menu-planning guidelines. Some clients need to maintain a low-fat diet for 6 months or longer. They are advised to add fatty foods to the diet slowly and as tolerated.

If the client has problems tolerating three large meals a day, the nurse advises him or her to try smaller, more frequent meals. If the client is obese, a weight reduction diet is recommended and teaching is tailored to provide appropriate dietary guidelines.

Clients are leaving the hospital sooner after traditional open gallbladder surgery than in the past. Since a T-tube is usually left in place for several weeks, clients are sent home with the drainage systems intact. The nurse instructs the client and one or more family members to inspect the incision wound and the T-tube drainage site for signs and symptoms of inflammation. These signs and symptoms include redness, swelling, warmth, extreme tenderness, excessive drainage, and increased incisional pain. Any of these findings should be reported to the health care provider. The nurse provides oral and written instructions for drainage tube care (Chart 60-3).

The client with cholecystitis who either refuses or postpones surgery must be instructed on the signs of potential complications of chronic cholecystitis, including fever, recurrent abdominal pain, and jaundice. If these signs occur, the client should notify the health care provider for prompt medical care.

carbon dioxide retention in the abdomen. The nurse teaches about the importance of early ambulation to promote absorption of the carbon dioxide. Far less opioid analgesia is necessary after the laparoscopic procedure than following the open cholecystectomy procedure.

The client is usually discharged from the hospital or surgery center within 1 day. Following laparoscopic surgery, the client can return to usual activities, including work, much sooner than if an open cholecystectomy had been done. Most clients are able to resume usual activities within 1 to 3 weeks.

● Community-Based Care

▥ HEALTH TEACHING

With a cholecystectomy, discharge teaching for the client and the family may include the following:

- Pain management
- Diet therapy
- Wound, drain, and incision care

▥ HOME CARE MANAGEMENT

After a traditional cholecystectomy, clients usually need short-term assistance with procuring foods, preparing meals, performing dressing changes, and caring for the T-tube. Clients who have undergone traditional gallbladder surgery may also need transportation to follow-up appointments with the health care provider. The surgeon typically allows these clients to return to their usual activities 4 to 6 weeks after surgery.

■ HEALTH CARE RESOURCES

For clients at home with a T-tube or for those older adults who cannot manage self-care, a home care nurse may be needed to provide support and follow-up nursing care and teaching. The home care nurse assesses the client's adaptation to the treatment plan and evaluates wound healing and the integrity of the T-tube drainage system. The home care nurse also determines the need for further wound and skin care interventions and implements these interventions as needed.

Cholelithiasis
■ OVERVIEW

Cholelithiasis, the presence of one or more gallstones, is the most common disorder of the biliary tract. It is estimated that 16 to 20 million persons in the United States have gallstones, with approximately 1 million new cases developing each year (Greenberger & Isselbacher, 1998). Gallstones form when bile, stored in the gallbladder, hardens into stonelike material. In more than 90% of clients with cholecystitis, the cause of inflammation is bile stasis resulting from impaction of the cystic duct by gallstones. Chronic cholecystitis occurs when repeated episodes of cystic duct obstruction result in chronic inflammation.

■ Pathophysiology
■ PATHOLOGIC CHANGES

The exact pathophysiology of gallstone formation is not clearly understood, but abnormal metabolism of cholesterol and bile salts plays an important role in their formation. Contributing factors may include the following:

- Supersaturation of bile with cholesterol
- Excessive bile salt losses
- Decreased gallbladder-emptying rates
- Changes in bile concentration or bile stasis within the gallbladder

Gallstones may lie dormant within the gallbladder or may move to other areas of the biliary tree as the gallbladder empties and refills with bile. Stones may migrate and lodge within the gallbladder neck, cystic duct, or common bile duct, causing obstruction (Figure 60-2). Common bile duct stones are seen in 20% of clients age 65 years or older who undergo a cholecystectomy (Howard & Fromm, 1999). Gallstones interfere with or totally obstruct normal bile flow from the gallbladder to the duodenum, causing vascular congestion as a result of impeded venous return. Edema and congestion occur and contribute to the initial inflammatory process. When bile cannot flow from the gallbladder, the stasis of bile and local irritation from the gallstones lead to cholecystitis (see Acute Cholecystitis, p. 1327).

Cholangitis, usually associated with choledocholithiasis (common bile duct stones), involves infection of the bile ducts. *Ascending* cholangitis (inflammation of the biliary tree) occurs after bacterial invasion of the ducts. Bacterial invasion can lead to life-threatening *suppurative* cholangitis when symptoms are not recognized quickly and pus accumulates in the ductal system.

■ TYPES OF GALLSTONES

The gallbladder provides an excellent environment for the production of gallstones. In particular, the gallbladder only occasionally mixes its normally abundant mucus with its highly viscous, concentrated bile. The constant temperature within the gallbladder also contributes to stone formation by delaying bile emptying, causing biliary stasis.

Gallstones are composed of substances normally found in bile, such as cholesterol, bilirubin, bile salts, calcium, and various proteins. Stones are classified as either cholesterol stones or pigment stones.

Cholesterol stones form as a result of metabolic imbalances of cholesterol and bile salts. They are the most common type found in people in the United States, accounting for 90% of all gallstones, and generally originate from the gallbladder (Howard & Fromm, 1999).

■ Etiology

There appears to be a familial tendency in the development of cholelithiasis, but this may be related to familial dietary habits (excessive dietary cholesterol intake) and familial sedentary lifestyles. Gallstones are seen more frequently in obese clients, probably as a result of impaired fat metabolism or increased cholesterol. Cholesterol-lowering drugs, which lower cholesterol levels in the blood, actually increase the amount of cholesterol secreted in bile. Age is also a factor, with people over 60 years of age more likely to develop stones than

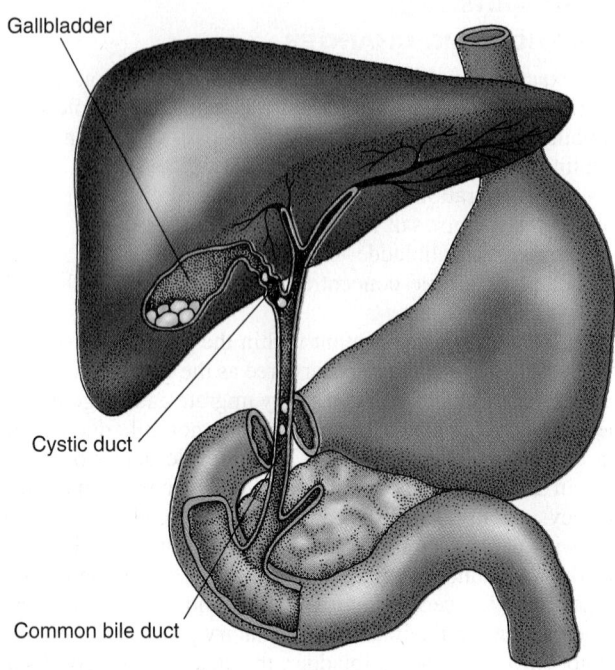

Gallbladder

Cystic duct

Common bile duct

Figure 60-2 ● Gallstones within the gallbladder and obstructing the common bile and cystic ducts.

younger people. Persons with type 1 diabetes are also at increased risk for the development of gallstones and cholecystitis because of the higher levels of fatty acids (triglycerides) they generally have.

Cholesterol is increased following rapid weight loss, when the liver excretes extra cholesterol into bile (National Institutes of Health [NIH], 1999). The ingestion of low-calorie or liquid protein diets also increases the susceptibility to gallstone development. These diets cause the liberation of cholesterol from tissues; the cholesterol is excreted as crystals in bile. Alcohol abuse may contribute to the formation of pigment stones, but alcohol in moderate amounts appears to reduce the formation of cholesterol stones (Howard & Fromm, 1999). Cholelithiasis is seen with hemolytic blood disorders, with bowel disease such as Crohn's disease, and after jejunoileal bypass surgery as a treatment of morbid obesity.

WOMEN'S HEALTH CONSIDERATIONS

Women who are between 20 and 60 years of age are twice as likely to develop gallstones as men. Obesity is a major risk factor for gallstone formation, especially in women (NIH, 1999). Pregnancy tends to worsen gallstone formation. Pregnancy, as well as drugs such as estrogen and birth control pills, especially the older oral contraceptives, alter hormone levels and delay muscular contraction of the gallbladder, causing a decreased rate of bile emptying. The incidence of gallstones is higher in women who have had multiple pregnancies. Combinations of causative factors increase the incidence of stone formation, especially in women. For example, an obese pregnant woman or an obese woman taking birth control pills may be at higher risk.

Incidence/Prevalence

Cholelithiasis is common and a major source of morbidity in the United States, accounting for 800,000 hospitalizations

each year for both men and women at a cost exceeding $2 billion annually (Howard & Fromm, 1999). Because gallstones are so prevalent, with up to 20 million persons having the disorder, several thousand deaths are attributed to them each year. This places gallstone disorder among the most common causes of death due to nonmalignant digestive disease (Everhart et al., 1999). The incidence of gallstone disease increases with age: 50% of women and 16% of men in their 70s and 80% of men and women in their 80s have the disorder (Howard & Fromm, 1999). Male clients who have cholelithiasis are usually 50 years of age or older. Two thirds of people with gallstones also experience chronic cholecystitis (Greenberger & Isselbacher, 1998).

CULTURAL CONSIDERATIONS

Gallstones are more prevalent among Native Americans and less prevalent among African Americans and Asians (Howard & Fromm, 1999). There is a lower prevalence of gallbladder disease among both non-Hispanic black men and women than among non-Hispanic whites. Age-standardized prevalence is similar for non-Hispanic white and Mexican-American men, with both having a higher prevalence than non-Hispanic black men. Among women, the age-adjusted prevalence is highest for Mexican Americans, followed by non-Hispanic whites and non-Hispanic blacks (Everhart et al., 1999).

▶ COLLABORATIVE MANAGEMENT
◗ Assessment

The same historical database may be obtained for clients with cholecystitis and clients with cholelithiasis (see Assessment [Cholecystitis], p. 1328).

◼ PHYSICAL ASSESSMENT/CLINICAL MANIFESTATIONS

The severity of pain and presentation of symptoms in the client with cholelithiasis depend on the following:
- Whether the stone is stationary or mobile
- The size and location of the stone
- The degree of obstruction
- The presence and extent of inflammation

Initially, the pain of cholelithiasis is usually a steady, mild ache located in the mid-epigastric area. It may increase in intensity and duration and may radiate to the right shoulder or back.

The severe pain of **biliary colic** is produced by obstruction of the cystic duct of the gallbladder. When a stone is moving through or is lodged within the duct, tissue spasm occurs in an effort to mobilize the stone through the small duct. This intense pain may be so severe that it is accompanied by tachycardia, pallor, diaphoresis, and prostration (extreme exhaustion).

Any of the clinical manifestations seen in acute or chronic cholecystitis may occur in cholelithiasis (see Chart 60-1). Clients with chronic cholecystitis and acute ductal obstruction may experience the excruciating pain of biliary colic as well. On inspection, the nurse may observe jaundice of the skin, the sclerae, the upper palate, and the oral mucous membranes. If gallstones occlude the common bile duct, prolonged severe inflammation and hepatic damage may also occur.

■ LABORATORY ASSESSMENT

There are no specific laboratory tests for cholelithiasis. As in cholecystitis, the serum alkaline phosphatase, lactate dehydrogenase, aspartate aminotransferase, and direct and indirect bilirubin levels may be elevated. Examination of a random stool specimen may reveal absent or low levels of urobilinogen in the feces, indicating an obstructive process. If pancreatic involvement accompanies gallstone impaction, serum and urine amylase levels are elevated.

■ RADIOGRAPHIC ASSESSMENT

Calcified gallstones are easily visualized on abdominal x-ray examination. An oral cholecystogram is diagnostic when the stones are radiopaque. The physician may order intravenous (IV) cholecystography (or cholangiography) for clients who are unable to absorb oral contrast agents.

Percutaneous transhepatic cholangiography is a fluoroscopic examination of the biliary ducts and may be used to diagnose obstructive jaundice and visualize stones located in the ducts. Another procedure that permits radiographic visualization of the common bile duct, pancreas, pancreatic ducts, and biliary tree is endoscopic retrograde cholangiopancreatography (ERCP). This procedure permits the gastroenterologist to precisely pinpoint the nature of a biliary obstruction (see Chapter 53).

■ OTHER DIAGNOSTIC ASSESSMENT

Ultrasound of the gallbladder is most commonly used procedure to determine the presence of stones within the biliary system. It is the test of choice to confirm the diagnosis of cholelithiasis and to distinguish between obstructive and nonobstructive jaundice. Ultrasound of the gallbladder is reported to be 95% accurate in detecting gallstones. The exception is a stone found in the common bile duct, which rarely visualizes on ultrasound (McCormick, 1999).

> **⟳ CRITICAL THINKING CHALLENGE**
>
> Your client is scheduled to have an ERCP performed in the morning. She asks you how this test can determine what is causing her jaundice and expresses concern about the safety of the procedure.
> * What answers will you give this client?
> * How does jaundice develop in the biliary tree?
> * What does an ERCP detect that other procedures might not?
> * What are the risks and benefits of an ERCP?
> * What postprocedure assessments and interventions will you need to provide for this client?
>
> For suggested answer guidelines, go to SIMON http://www.wbsaunders.com/SIMON/Iggy/.

● Interventions

The health care provider may institute supportive medical treatment for clients with cholelithiasis as an alternative to or before surgical removal of the gallbladder and gallstones.

NONSURGICAL MANAGEMENT. Two thirds of gallstones are asymptomatic, or silent (Howard & Fromm, 1999). Asymptomatic stones are usually managed conservatively with no medical or surgical intervention. Acute pain occurs when the gallstones partially or totally obstruct the cystic or

common bile duct. Measures aimed at resting the inflamed gallbladder are the same as those discussed earlier for cholecystitis, p. 1330. Symptomatic clients require treatment, and laparoscopic cholecystectomy is the accepted first-line therapy (Strasberg, 1999).

DIET THERAPY. In general, the client must adhere to a low-fat diet to prevent further pain of biliary colic. If gallstones are causing an obstruction of bile flow, the health care provider may order replacement of fat-soluble vitamins (such as vitamins A, D, E, and K) and the administration of bile salts to facilitate digestion and vitamin absorption. Food and fluids are withheld if nausea and vomiting occur.

DRUG THERAPY. Pain caused by acute obstruction with gallstones necessitates opioid analgesia with meperidine hydrochloride (Demerol). Older clients should not be given Demerol, since it can cause acute confusion and nausea (see Chapter 7). Morphine is usually not used, because it is thought to cause biliary spasm and constrict the sphincter of Oddi. Antispasmodic or anticholinergic drugs, such as dicyclomine hydrochloride (Bentyl, Lomine✤), may be given to relax smooth muscles and decrease ductal tone and spasm. The health care provider orders antiemetics to control nausea and vomiting.

Bile acid therapy has been effective in dissolving gallstones, depending on the type of stones. Chenodeoxycholic acid (CDCA; chenodiol; Chenix) and ursodeoxycholic acid (UDCA; ursodiol; Actigall) reduce cholesterol stones by unsaturating bile. They do this by decreasing coupling of cholesterol to bile acids during bile secretion. Adverse effects of chenodiol are lessened when it is used in conjunction with ursodiol. Ursodiol has also been shown to be effective in preventing gallstone formation after rapid weight loss (Howard & Fromm, 1997).

Chenodiol may be effective in dissolving small stones (less than 5 mm). This treatment is generally reserved for older adults who have mild or asymptomatic gallstone disease and those who are poor surgical risks. Unfortunately, it may take up to 2 years to dissolve gallstones, and compliance with taking medications over an extended length of time can be a problem. These drugs are expensive, and stones can recur if the client is not maintained on low drug dosages for even more prolonged periods. The nurse observes for and reports diarrhea, the common side effect of chenodiol therapy.

Ursodiol has been approved in the United States as an anticholelithic agent since 1988. This drug dissolves small (less than 20-mm) cholesterol gallstones. As is the case for chenodiol, ursodiol may take up to 1 year to dissolve the stone or stones. Moreover, in up to 50% of treated clients, the stones recur within 5 years. Therefore this treatment is best for clients who have mild or infrequent clinical manifestations, those who refuse surgery, or those who are poor surgical risks.

Obstructive jaundice in cholelithiasis is caused by impeded bile flow through the common bile duct as a result of gallstone obstruction. It may lead to excessive accumulation of bile salts in the skin. As a result, severe pruritus may occur. Cholestyramine resin (Questran) binds with bile acids in the intestine, forming an insoluble compound that is excreted in the feces. As a result, excessive bile salts are removed and itching is decreased. The nurse mixes the powder form of the drug with fruit juices or milk. It should be given before meals and at bedtime.

EXTRACORPOREAL SHOCK WAVE LITHOTRIPSY.

Extracorporeal shock wave lithotripsy is a noninvasive procedure that is used for ambulatory treatment of clients with gallstones in some settings. A machine–a lithotriptor–generates powerful shock waves to shatter the gallstones (Figure 60-3). Clients who are eligible for this procedure must have three or fewer cholesterol stones (measuring between 5 and 30 mm), have a functioning gallbladder, and have no history of liver or pancreatic disease. Clients who have pacemakers or who are pregnant are not candidates for lithotripsy.

During the hour-long procedure, up to 1500 shocks are repeated until the gallstone is completely fragmented. The minute particles are then able to travel through the biliary ductal system to be excreted via the intestines. Because some clients experience mild pain as gallbladder spasms occur in an effort to expel the tiny stone fragments, the physician may use IV conscious sedation with fentanyl citrate (Alfenta, Sublimaze) or midazolam hydrochloride (Versed).

Eating and drinking are permitted almost immediately after the procedure. The nurse informs the client that right upper quadrant discomfort after the procedure is not uncommon and usually resolves within 2 days. Acetaminophen (Tylenol, Exdol✚) often provides enough analgesia to relieve this pain.

PERCUTANEOUS TRANSHEPATIC BILIARY CATHETER INSERTION.

The physician may insert a percutaneous transhepatic biliary catheter under fluoroscopic guidance. This procedure decompresses obstructed extrahepatic ducts so that bile can flow (Figure 60-4). It is primarily used for inoperable hepatic, pancreatic, or bile duct carcinoma. It may be a nonsurgical alternative for the treatment of biliary obstruction caused by gallstones and hepatic dysfunction associated with obstructive jaundice and biliary sepsis in high-risk candidates. Nursing care associated with this treatment is outlined in Chart 60-4.

SURGICAL MANAGEMENT.

One of several procedures may be indicated in the surgical treatment of cholelithiasis (Table 60-3). **Cholecystotomy** (an opening into the gallbladder) may be an emergency procedure to remove gallstones. This procedure is often performed for older adults or critically ill clients with life-threatening multisystem problems who may not withstand a prolonged surgical procedure. If the stones are located in the common bile duct, a **choledocholithotomy** (an incision into the common bile duct to remove stones) is necessary. If the common bile duct is explored, the surgeon inserts a T-tube drain into the duct to ensure patency until edema subsides and to allow collection of excessive bile drainage.

A simple, traditional **cholecystectomy** or laparoscopic cholecystectomy is performed when stones are confined to the gallbladder. The common bile duct and adjacent ducts are explored for the presence of additional stones or stone fragments and crystals in this traditional surgical procedure (see Surgical Management [Cholecystitis], p. 1330).

After a cholecystectomy with T-tube placement, the surgeon may prescribe drugs to stimulate bile production and bile flow from the liver. Bile flow promotes the digestion and absorption of fat, fat-soluble vitamins, and cholesterol in the duodenum. Hydrocholeretic drugs, such as dehydrocholic acid (Decholin, Cholan), which are synthetic bile salts, increase the solubility of cholesterol. Increased solubility prevents the accumulation of cholesterol in bile, thereby decreasing the recurrence of biliary calculi and promoting drainage of (potentially infected) bile through the T-tube drainage system.

A postoperative T-tube cholangiogram can identify retained stones. Direct visualization of the biliary tract with an endoscope **(choledochoscopy)** enables the removal of calculi retained in the common bile duct. Choledochoscopy is performed through a T-tube or an incision into the common bile duct. An instrument with a small, basket-like attachment is used to snare the stone (Figure 60-5). If this method fails, a fiberoptic endoscope is introduced into the duodenum. An incision into the papillae (papillotomy) allows the stone to pass into the duodenum.

The preoperative and postoperative nursing care measures for the client undergoing gallbladder surgical procedures are

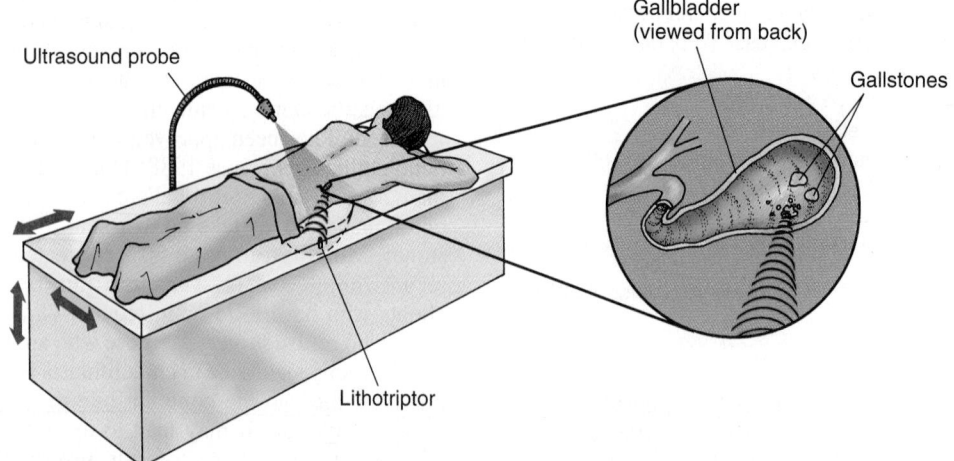

Figure 60-3 ● Biliary lithotripsy. With the assistance of a computer and an ultrasound monitor, the physician positions the client over a shock wave generator (lithotriptor) by means of a table that moves upward and downward, forward and backward, and from side to side. When the client is positioned properly, the physician fires the lithotriptor. Particles slough off the gallstones until they are completely fragmented, and the fragments pass through the biliary ductal system.

the same as those for cholecystectomy (see Surgical Management [Cholecystitis], p. 1330).

An additional therapeutic intervention, used in conjunction with or as an alternative to surgery, is endoscopic retrograde cholangiopancreatography (ERCP). This procedure allows the physician radiographic visualization of the common bile duct, gallbladder, pancreatic ducts, and biliary tree. Since about 10% of clients with gallstone disease also have common duct stones, this can be significant (Nahrwold, 1997). If gallstones are present in the bile ducts, the surgeon may use ERCP in removing them, either before or during gallbladder surgery.

Community-Based Care

Most often, the client with cholelithiasis has surgery and is discharged to home postoperatively (see Community-Based Care [Cholecystitis], p. 1332). The client may be discharged with a T-tube drainage system intact (see Chart 60-3) and will need instructions as to care of the tube.

The nurse provides information to the client and family about the potential for **postcholecystectomy syndrome,** in which the clinical manifestations of biliary tract disease occur following cholecystectomy in a small percentage of clients. Postcholecystectomy syndrome is caused by residual or recurring calculi, inflammation, or stricture of the common bile duct.

The nurse instructs the client to report symptoms of biliary tract disease, including jaundice of the skin or sclera, darkened urine, light-colored stools, pain, fever, or chills, to the physician or nurse practitioner.

Cancer of the Gallbladder

OVERVIEW

Primary cancer of the gallbladder is rare and is more common in women than in men (NIH, 1999). Adenocarcinoma and squamous cell carcinoma of the gallbladder account for the

majority of gallbladder cancers. They typically infiltrate the liver and ducts, as well as the gallbladder. These rare gallbladder carcinomas appear more frequently in clients with pre-existing chronic cholecystitis and cholelithiasis.

The diagnosis of gallbladder cancer is difficult. Early symptoms, when present, are insidious in onset and similar to those of chronic cholecystitis and cholelithiasis. Characteristic signs and symptoms include the following:

- Anorexia
- Weight loss

CHART 60-4

BEST PRACTICE *for*
The Client with a Transhepatic Biliary Catheter

- Change the catheter insertion site dressing daily, according to the hospital's policy. Recommended care includes cleaning the skin with hydrogen peroxide and applying antibiotic ointment and a small sterile dressing to the site.
- During the first several days after catheter insertion, unclamp the catheter and allow it to drain into an external drainage system (per physician's order).
- Using a three-way stopcock system located between the catheter and the drainage bag, irrigate the catheter twice daily with 5 to 20 mL of bacteriostatic (preservative-free) saline. Check the physician's orders for the amount of solution and the frequency of irrigation. Flush the tubing to the client and to the bag to ensure that the tubing is patent. (Occlude the stopcock with a sterile cap when the irrigation procedure is complete.)
- Instruct the client that he or she may experience discomfort during irrigation. Observe for abdominal cramping or excessive pain, and notify the physician if any occurs.
- If pain is severe and abdominal rigidity develops, notify the physician immediately.
- Assess the client for decreasing jaundice. Stools should change from clay color to normal brown, and urine should change from dark to straw color. Monitor serum bilirubin test results for decreasing levels.
- Assess the client for fever, chills, and hypotension, and report these findings to the physician.
- Inspect the catheter for the presence of blood, and notify the physician immediately if any occurs.
- Inspect the catheter for patency.
- The drainage bag should remain in a dependent position. Do not place the bag on the bed or above the level of the client.
- Affix the bag to the client's gown (not to the bed).
- Provide discharge instructions to the client or a family member, including:
  Dressing care
  Signs of catheter malfunction, infection, and dislodgment
  Outpatient and cholangiography appointments

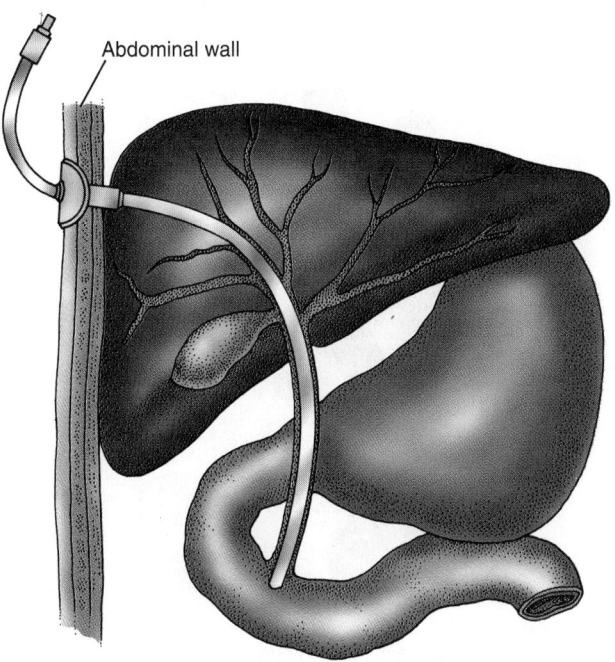

Figure 60-4 ● Transhepatic biliary catheterization.

Label: Abdominal wall

TABLE 60-3 · COMMON GALLBLADDER SURGICAL PROCEDURES

Surgical Procedure	Description
Traditional cholecystectomy	Removal of the gallbladder through a high (subcostal) abdominal incision
Laparoscopic laser cholecystectomy	Removal of the gallbladder by laser through a laparoscope
Cholecystotomy	Incision into the gallbladder to remove gallstones
Choledochotomy	Incision into the common bile duct
Choledocholithotomy	Incision into the common bile duct to remove gallstones

- Nausea
- Vomiting
- General malaise
- Jaundice
- Hepatosplenomegaly
- Chronic, progressively severe epigastric or right upper quadrant pain

A moderately tender, irregularly shaped mass may be palpated. Often, gallbladder carcinoma is discovered during other procedures for diagnosis of suspected cholecystitis or during cholecystectomy.

► COLLABORATIVE MANAGEMENT

The prognosis for the client with cancer of the gallbladder is poor. Three treatments are used: surgery, radiation therapy, and chemotherapy. Surgical intervention, when performed, is usually extensive. A bile drainage tube (transhepatic biliary catheter) may be inserted to relieve symptoms such as jaundice and itching (see Chart 60-4).

PANCREATIC DISORDERS
Acute Pancreatitis
▇ OVERVIEW

Acute pancreatitis is a serious and, at times, life-threatening inflammatory process of the pancreas. This inflammatory process is brought on by a premature activation of pancreatic enzymes that destroy ductal tissue and pancreatic cells, resulting in autodigestion and fibrosis of the pancreas. The pathologic changes occur in variable degrees. The severity of pancreatitis depends on the extent of inflammation and tissue destruction. Pancreatitis can range from mild involvement evidenced by edema and inflammation to necrotizing hemorrhagic pancreatitis (NHP). NHP affects approximately 20% of clients diagnosed with pancreatitis and is characterized by diffusely bleeding pancreatic tissue with fibrosis and tissue death.

▇ Pathophysiology

The pancreas is unusual in that it functions as both an exocrine gland and an endocrine gland. The primary endocrine disorder is diabetes and is discussed in Chapter 65. The exocrine function of the pancreas is responsible for secreting enzymes that assist in the breakdown of starches, proteins, and fats. These enzymes are normally secreted in the inactive form and become activated once they enter the intestine. Early activation (i.e., activation within the pancreas rather than the intestinal lumen) results in the inflammatory process of pancreatitis. Direct toxic injury to the pancreatic cells and the production and release of pancreatic enzymes (trypsin, elastase, phospholipase A, lipase, and kallikrein) result from the obstructive damage. Following pancreatic duct obstruction, increased pressure within the pancreas and the pancreatic ducts may contribute to ductal rupture, allowing spillage of trypsin and other enzymes into the pancreatic parenchymal tissue. In acute pancreatitis, four major pathophysiologic processes occur: lipolysis, proteolysis, necrosis of blood vessels, and inflammation.

▇ LIPOLYSIS

The hallmark of pancreatic necrosis is enzymatic fat necrosis of the endocrine and exocrine cells of the pancreas caused by the enzyme lipase. Fatty acids are released during this lipolytic process and combine with ionized calcium to form a soap-like product. The initial rapid lowering of serum calcium levels is not readily compensated for by the parathyroid gland. Because the body needs ionized calcium and cannot use bound calcium, hypocalcemia occurs.

▇ PROTEOLYSIS

The pathogenesis of pancreatitis involves **autodigestion** of the pancreatic parenchyma by the enzymes normally produced by the pancreas (Figure 60-6). Trypsin is the key element that activates all other proteolytic enzymes involved in autodigestion.

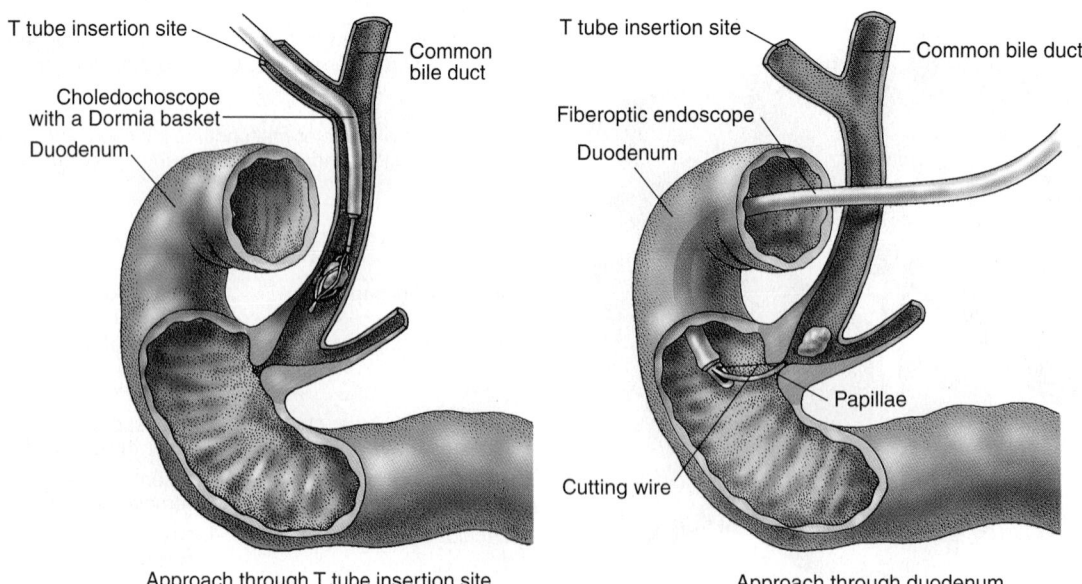

Approach through T tube insertion site

Approach through duodenum

Figure 60-5 ● Choledochoscopic removal of gallstones.

The agent that triggers the premature activation of trypsin to trypsinogen has not been identified and is being investigated. Proteolysis involves the splitting of proteins by hydrolysis of the peptide bonds, resulting in the formation of smaller polypeptides. Proteolytic activity may lead to thrombosis and gangrene of the pancreas. Pancreatic destruction may be localized and confined to one area or may involve the entire organ.

NECROSIS OF BLOOD VESSELS

Elastase is activated by trypsin and causes elastic fibers of the blood vessels and ducts to dissolve. The necrosis of blood vessels results in bleeding, ranging from minor bleeding to massive hemorrhage of pancreatic tissue. Another pancreatic enzyme, kallikrein, causes the release of vasoactive peptides, bradykinin, and a plasma kinin known as kallidin. These substances contribute to vasodilation and increased vascular permeability, further compounding the hemorrhagic process. This massive destruction of blood vessels by necrosis may lead to generalized hemorrhage with blood escaping into the retroperitoneal tissues. The client with hemorrhagic pancreatitis is critically ill, and extensive pancreatic destruction and shock may lead to death. The majority of deaths in clients with acute pancreatitis result from irreversible shock.

INFLAMMATION

The inflammatory stage occurs when leukocytes cluster around the hemorrhagic and necrotic areas of the pancreas. A second-ary bacterial process may lead to suppuration (pus formation) of the pancreatic parenchyma or the formation of an abscess (see later discussion under Pancreatic Abscess, p. 1348). Infected lesions that are mild may be absorbed. When infected lesions are severe, calcification and fibrosis occur. If the infected fluid becomes walled off by fibrous tissue, a pancreatic pseudocyst is formed (see Pancreatic Pseudocyst, p. 1349).

THEORIES OF ENZYME ACTIVATION

Several theories explain the triggering mechanisms leading to enzyme activation in acute pancreatitis. The *bile reflux* ("common channel") theory proposes that an obstruction of the common channel (the common bile duct and the main pancreatic duct channel) causes reflux of the bile into the pancreatic tissue, resulting in activation of the enzymes. Not all biliary tracts have this common channel. If the common channel is absent, the common bile and pancreatic ducts merge into the duodenum separately.

According to the *hypersecretion-obstruction* theory, the pancreatic duct ruptures and the resulting disruption or tearing of the cell membrane allows pancreatic secretions and enzymes to leak back into the parenchymal tissue.

The exact mechanism of *alcohol-induced* changes in pancreatitis is unclear. Alcohol appears to have a direct metabolic effect on the pancreas by stimulating hydrochloric acid and secretin production, which in turn stimulates exocrine functions of the pancreas. Alcohol also causes edema of the duodenum and the ampulla of Vater, obstructing the flow of pancreatic se-

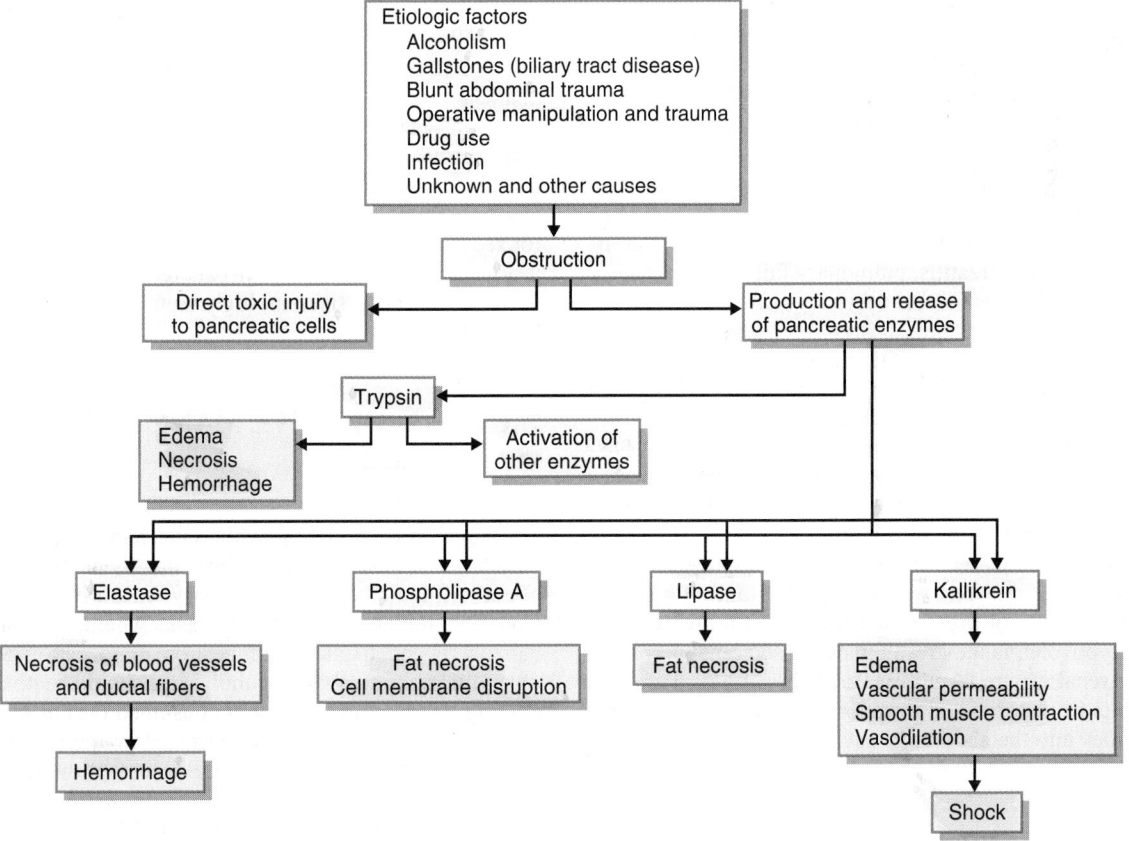

Figure 60-6 ⬤ The process of autodigestion in acute pancreatitis.

cretions. Alcohol may decrease the tone of the sphincter of Oddi and cause sphincter spasm and duodenal reflux.

According to the fourth theory, reflux of duodenal contents can occur from biliary tract disease, gallstones in the bile duct (causing the sphincter of Oddi to dilate), or a generalized loss of tone caused by alcohol ingestion. Duodenal contents can enter the pancreatic duct through the weakened sphincter, activating the pancreatic enzymes.

The generalized abdominal pain of acute pancreatitis is related to peritoneal irritation. Ductal release of digested proteins and lipids into the peripancreatic tissues, along with stretching of the pancreatic tissue, causes the seepage of these substances into the mesentery. The resultant peritonitis stimulates the sensory nerves, contributing to intense pain in the back and flanks.

■ COMPLICATIONS OF ACUTE PANCREATITIS

Acute pancreatitis may result in severe, life-threatening complications. Jaundice occurs from swelling of the head of the pancreas, which impedes bile flow through the common bile duct. The bile duct may also be compressed by calculi or a pancreatic pseudocyst. The resulting total bile flow obstruction causes severe jaundice. Transient hyperglycemia occurs as a result of the release of glucagon, as well as the decreased release of insulin due to damage to the pancreatic islet cells. Total destruction of the pancreas may occur, leading to type 1 diabetes.

Left lung pleural effusions frequently develop in the client with acute pancreatitis. Amylase effusions probably occur when exudate containing pancreatic enzymes passes from the peritoneal cavity into the pleural cavity via the transdiaphragmatic lymph channels. Atelectasis and pneumonia may also occur, especially in older clients.

Multisystem organ failure occurs as a sequela to necrotizing hemorrhagic pancreatitis (NHP). The client is at risk for acute respiratory distress syndrome (ARDS). This severe form of pulmonary edema is caused by disruption of the alveolar-capillary membrane and is a serious complication of acute pancreatitis. (See Chapter 32 for a discussion of ARDS.) In acute pancreatitis, pulmonary failure accounts for more than half of all deaths that occur in the first 7 days of the disease.

Coagulation defects are another major potential complication and may result in death. Complex physiologic changes in the pancreas cause the release of necrotic tissue and enzymes into the bloodstream, resulting in altered coagulation. Disseminated intravascular coagulation (DIC) involves hypercoagulation of the blood, with consumption of clotting factors and the development of microthrombi.

Shock in acute pancreatitis results from peripheral vasodilation from the released vasoactive substances and the retroperitoneal loss of protein-rich fluid from proteolytic digestion. Hypovolemia may result in decreased renal perfusion and acute renal failure (Ambrose & Dreher, 1996). Paralytic ileus results from peritoneal irritation and seepage of pancreatic enzymes into the abdominal cavity.

■ Etiology

In many cases, the cause of pancreatitis is not known. Many factors can produce injury to the pancreas. The most com-

monly cited factor is biliary tract disease, with gallstones accounting for 45% of the cases of obstructive pancreatitis. Excessive alcohol ingestion is the second leading cause of pancreatitis. Iatrogenic acute pancreatitis may occur as a result of trauma from surgical manipulation after biliary tract, pancreatic, gastric, and duodenal procedures, such as cholecystectomy, the Whipple procedure, and partial gastrectomy. The trauma may also originate as a complication of the diagnostic procedure endoscopic retrograde cholangiopancreatography (ERCP).

Other etiologic factors include the following:
- Trauma: external (blunt trauma) or operative
- Pancreatic obstruction: tumors, cysts, or abscesses; abnormal organ structure
- Metabolic disturbances: hyperlipidemia, hyperparathyroidism, or hypercalcemia
- Renal disturbances: failure or transplantation
- Familial, inherited conditions
- Penetrating gastric or duodenal ulcers, resulting in peritonitis
- Viral infections, such as coxsackievirus B infection
- Toxicities of drugs, including opiates, sulfonamides, thiazides, steroids, and oral contraceptives (The exact mechanism by which these and other drugs cause pancreatitis is unknown.)

■ Incidence/Prevalence

Steady, heavy alcohol intake for 5 to 10 years is likely to be the causative mechanism for pancreatitis in the middle-aged male population. Episodes of acute pancreatitis usually occur after excessive alcohol consumption. These attacks are especially common during holidays and vacations. Women are affected most often after cholelithiasis and biliary tract disturbances.

Death occurs in approximately 10% of clients with acute pancreatitis, but with early diagnosis and treatment, mortality can be reduced. Death occurs at a higher rate in older adults and in clients with postoperative pancreatitis. The prognosis for recovery is favorable for pancreatitis associated with biliary tract disease and poor if pancreatitis accompanies alcoholism. Mortality rises as high as 60% when necrosis and hemorrhage occur.

▶ COLLABORATIVE MANAGEMENT
Activity Link

● Assessment

■ HISTORY

The nurse asks the client with acute pancreatitis to indicate why he or she is seeking medical treatment. Most often, the client will indicate that the primary reason is to obtain relief from abdominal pain. The nurse asks whether the abdominal pain is related to alcohol ingestion or to eating a high-fat meal. Information about alcohol usage should be obtained, including the amount of alcohol consumed during what period of time (i.e., years of consumption, how much usually consumed over a particular period). Because of the familial connection, the client is questioned about a family history of alcoholism, pancreatitis, or biliary tract disease. The client is questioned concerning a personal history of any biliary tract problems, such as gallstones. The nurse further determines whether any abdominal surgical interventions, such as cholecystectomy, or diagnostic procedures, such as ERCP, have been performed recently.

The nurse assesses for the presence of other medical problems known to cause pancreatitis, including peptic ulcer disease, renal failure, vascular disorders, hyperparathyroidism, and hyperlipidemia. The client is also asked whether any recent viral infections have been experienced and to list all prescription and over-the-counter (OTC) drugs taken recently.

▥ PHYSICAL ASSESSMENT/CLINICAL MANIFESTATIONS

Diagnosis of pancreatitis is made on the basis of the clinical presentation combined with the results of diagnostic studies—both laboratory and radiologic. Clinical manifestations of acute pancreatitis vary widely and depend on the severity of the inflammation. Typically, a client is diagnosed after presenting with abdominal pain that localizes in the epigastrium; this is the most frequent symptom. The nurse obtains in-depth data about the pain. The client often states that the pain had a sudden onset, is located in the mid-epigastric area or the left upper quadrant, and radiates to the back, left flank, or left shoulder. The pain is described as intense and continuous, and it is worsened by lying in the supine position. Often the client finds relief by assuming the fetal position (with the knees drawn up to the chest and the spine flexed) or when sitting upright and bending forward. The client may report weight loss resulting from nausea and vomiting.

When performing an abdominal assessment, the nurse may find the following on inspection:

- Generalized jaundice
- Gray-blue discoloration of the abdomen and periumbilical area (**Cullen's sign**)
- Gray-blue discoloration of the flanks (**Turner's sign**), caused by pancreatic enzyme leakage to cutaneous tissue from the peritoneal cavity

The nurse listens for bowel sounds; absent or decreased bowel sounds usually indicate paralytic (adynamic) ileus. On light palpation, the nurse notes abdominal tenderness, rigidity, and guarding as a result of peritonitis. A palpable mass may be found if a pancreatic pseudocyst is present. Pancreatic ascites creates a dull sound on percussion.

The nurse or assistive nursing personnel takes and records vital signs frequently to assess for elevated temperature, tachycardia, and decreased blood pressure. The nurse uses these data to determine whether complications are occurring. Respiratory complications, such as left lung pleural effusions, atelectasis, and pneumonia, are common in clients with acute pancreatitis. The nurse auscultates the lung fields for adventitious sounds or decreased aeration and observes respirations for dyspnea or orthopnea.

Changes in vital signs may indicate the life-threatening complication of shock. Hypotension and tachycardia may result from pancreatic hemorrhage, excessive fluid volume shifting, or the toxic effects of abdominal sepsis from enzyme damage. The nurse also observes the client for changes in behavior and sensorium that may be related to alcohol withdrawal, hypoxia, or impending sepsis with shock (see Chapter 8).

▥ PSYCHOSOCIAL ASSESSMENT

Excessive alcohol intake, particularly in men, is the most frequent cause of acute pancreatitis. Thus the nurse tactfully explores the client's alcohol intake history. The nurse and the client should discuss the intake of alcohol and the reasons for overindulging. The nurse asks him or her when increased drinking episodes occur, in particular, whether binges occur during holidays, vacations, or weekends or revolve around particular activities, such as card playing or television viewing. The client is also questioned about any recent traumatic event that may have contributed to increased alcohol consumption, such as the death of a family member or a job loss.

▥ LABORATORY ASSESSMENT

Diagnostic laboratory abnormalities are found in clients with acute pancreatitis (Table 60-4). Elevated serum amylase and lipase levels provide the most reliable and direct evidence of pancreatitis and are considered the cardinal diagnostic signs. Serum amylase levels usually increase within 12 to 24 hours and remain elevated for 3 to 4 days. A level of serum amylase three times greater than normal is considered diagnostic (Greenberger, Toskes, & Isselbacher, 1998). Persistent elevations of amylase levels may be an indicator of pancreatic abscess or pseudocyst (Lillemoe & Yeo, 1998). Lipase is considered more specific in the diagnosis of acute pancreatitis, and serum levels remain elevated for up to 2 weeks. Because serum lipase levels stay elevated for such a long time, the physician may find this test useful in diagnosing clients who are not examined until several days after the initial onset of symptoms (Hoerner, 1998). Amylase levels in 24-hour urine collections are also elevated as a result of the inflammatory process and remain elevated for up to 2 weeks. However, testing the urine for amylase is no more sensitive than testing serum amylase, yet it costs more. Testing the urine is sometimes useful several days after the onset of symptoms, when serum amylase levels may be normal.

If pancreatitis is accompanied by biliary dysfunction (biliary pancreatitis), serum bilirubin and alkaline phosphatase

TABLE 60-4 ⦁ CAUSES OF LABORATORY DIAGNOSTIC ABNORMALITIES IN ACUTE PANCREATITIS	
Abnormal Finding	**Cause**
CARDINAL DIAGNOSTIC TESTS	
Increased *serum* amylase	Pancreatic cell injury
Elevated *serum* lipase	Pancreatic cell injury
Elevated *urine* amylase	Pancreatic cell injury
OTHER DIAGNOSTIC TESTS	
Elevated serum glucose	Pancreatic cell injury, resulting in impaired carbohydrate metabolism; decreased insulin release
Decreased serum calcium	Fatty acids combined with calcium; seen in fat necrosis
Elevated bilirubin	Hepatobiliary obstructive process
Elevated aspartate transaminase (AST)	Hepatobiliary involvement
Elevated white blood cell count	Inflammatory response

levels are usually elevated. A sensitive indicator of biliary obstruction in acute pancreatitis is serum alanine aminotransferase (ALT). A threefold or greater rise in concentration offers a 95% probability that the diagnosis of acute biliary pancreatitis is correct (Baillie, 1997). Elevated white blood cell (WBC) count and serum glucose levels are also common in acute pancreatitis (Ambrose & Dreher, 1996).

Decreased serum calcium and magnesium levels are seen with fat necrosis. Calcium levels may fall and remain decreased for 7 to 10 days. Calcium levels that consistently remain below 8 mg/dL are associated with a poor prognosis.

RADIOGRAPHIC ASSESSMENT

Computed tomography (CT) provides a reliable diagnosis of acute pancreatitis. This noninvasive technique may be used to rule out pancreatic pseudocyst or ductal calculi. A chest x-ray film may reveal elevation of the left side of the diaphragm or pleural effusion.

OTHER DIAGNOSTIC ASSESSMENT

In the client with severe pancreatitis, ultrasonography and magnetic resonance imaging (MRI) of the pancreas help confirm an initial clinical impression, assess for the degree of inflammatory resolution, and reveal common bile duct dilation from obstruction or gallstones. The MRI study provides information similar to that of a CT scan but is much more costly and offers no real advantage over the less expensive CT scan. Endoscopic retrograde cholangiopancreatography (ERCP) is the definitive test to locate and assist in removing gallstones, which can cause biliary pancreatitis.

Analysis

COMMON NURSING DIAGNOSES AND COLLABORATIVE PROBLEMS

The following are priority nursing diagnoses for clients with acute pancreatitis:

1. Acute Pain related to the effects of pancreatic inflammation and enzyme leakage
2. Imbalanced Nutrition: Less Than Body Requirements related to the effects of pancreatic dysfunction, nausea, vomiting, and anorexia

ADDITIONAL NURSING DIAGNOSES AND COLLABORATIVE PROBLEMS

In addition to the common nursing diagnoses, clients with acute pancreatitis may have one or more of the following:

- Deficient Fluid Volume related to pancreatic hemorrhage, fluid loss into the abdominal cavity, nausea and vomiting, and nasogastric suctioning
- Ineffective Breathing Pattern related to the complications of pleural effusion or acute respiratory distress syndrome (ARDS)
- Risk for Activity Intolerance related to debilitation
- Anxiety related to severe illness and a possibly chronic condition
- Disturbed Sleep Pattern related to pain
- Impaired Health Maintenance related to insufficient knowledge about the illness, its causative factors, and the treatment plan

The client with pancreatitis is also likely to have the following collaborative problems:

- Potential for Hyperglycemia
- Potential for Hemorrhage
- Potential for Fluid and Electrolyte Imbalances

Planning and Implementation

ACUTE PAIN

NOC PLANNING: EXPECTED OUTCOMES. The client with acute pancreatitis is expected to verbalize a decrease in or absence of abdominal pain, as evidenced by a pain scale measurement.

INTERVENTIONS. Abdominal pain is the prominent symptom of pancreatitis. The main focus of nursing care is aimed at reducing discomfort and pain by the use of interventions that decrease gastrointestinal (GI) tract activity, thus decreasing pancreatic stimulation. Pain assessment to measure the effectiveness of these interventions is a vital nursing activity (see Chapter 7).

NONSURGICAL MANAGEMENT. The health care team initially attempts to achieve pain relief with nonsurgical interventions, which include fasting, drug therapy, and comfort measures.

FASTING. In an effort to rest the pancreas and reduce pancreatic enzyme secretion, food and fluids are withheld in the acute period. The health care provider orders IV fluid administration to maintain hydration. IV replacement of calcium and magnesium may also be needed.

Nasogastric drainage and suction may be necessary to decrease gastric distention and to suppress pancreatic secretion. Gastric decompression prevents gastric digestive juices from flowing into the duodenum. Because paralytic (adynamic) ileus is a common complication of acute pancreatitis, prolonged nasogastric intubation may be necessary. The nurse assesses for the presence of bowel sounds before the nasogastric (NG) tube is removed.

NIC *ANALGESIC ADMINISTRATION* (Chart 60-5). Pain management for acute pancreatitis should begin with titration of opioids by means of patient-controlled analgesia (PCA). Meperidine hydrochloride (Demerol) is the traditional drug of choice for relieving abdominal pain associated with acute pancreatitis (Pasero, 1998). It has been thought that meperidine hydrochloride causes less incidence of spasm of the smooth musculature of the pancreatic ducts and the sphincter of Oddi than do other analgesics such as morphine. In mild pancreatitis, the pain usually subsides in 3 to 4 days; however, with severe acute pancreatitis, the abdominal pain and tenderness may persist for up to 2 weeks. The nurse individualizes dosages and intervals of medication administration, as ordered, according to the severity of the disease and the symptoms.

> **CRITICAL THINKING CHALLENGE**
> Your client with acute pancreatitis tells you that he is not getting much relief from the pain with the shots you are giving him every 4 hours.
> - What should you include in this client's comprehensive pain assessment?

CHART 60-5

NIC **INTERVENTION ACTIVITIES** *for*
The Client with Acute Pancreatitis

Analgesic Administration: *Use of pharmacologic agents to reduce or eliminate pain*
- Determine pain location, characteristics, quality, and severity before medicating client.
- Check medical order for drug, dose, and frequency of analgesic prescribed.
- Choose the appropriate analgesic or combination of analgesics when more than one is prescribed.
- Choose the IV route, rather than IM, for frequent pain medication injections, when possible.
- Attend to comfort needs and other activities that assist relaxation to facilitate response to analgesia.
- Administer analgesics around-the-clock to prevent peaks and troughs of analgesia, especially with severe pain.
- Administer adjuvant analgesics and/or medications when needed to potentiate analgesia.
- Consider use of continuous infusion, whether alone or in conjunction with bolus opioids, to maintain serum levels.
- Institute safety precautions for those receiving narcotic analgesics, as appropriate.
- Correct misconceptions/myths client or family members may hold regarding analgesics, particularly opioids (e.g., addiction and risks of overdose).
- Evaluate the effectiveness of analgesic at regular frequent intervals after each administration, but especially after the initial doses, also observing for any signs and symptoms of untoward effects (e.g., respiratory depression, nausea and vomiting, dry mouth, and constipation).
- Document response to analgesic and any untoward effects.
- Implement actions to decrease untoward effects of analgesics (e.g., constipation and gastric irritation).
- Collaborate with the health care provider if drug, dose, route of administration, or interval changes are indicated, making specific recommendations based on equianalgesic principles.

Pain Management: *Alleviation of pain or a reduction in pain to a level of comfort that is acceptable to the client*
- Perform a comprehensive assessment of pain to include location, characteristics, onset/duration, frequency, quality, intensity or severity of pain, and precipitating factors.
- Observe for nonverbal cues of discomfort, especially in those unable to communicate effectively.
- Ensure that client receives attentive analgesic care.
- Consider cultural influences on pain response.
- Determine the impact of the pain experience on quality of life (e.g., sleep, appetite, activity, cognition, mood, relationships, performance of job, and role responsibilities).
- Evaluate, with the client and the health care team, the effectiveness of past pain control measures that have been used.
- Control environmental factors that may influence the client's response to discomfort (e.g., room temperature, lighting, and noise).
- Reduce or eliminate factors that precipitate or increase the pain experience (e.g., fear, fatigue, monotony, and lack of knowledge).

- Consider the client's willingness to participate, ability to participate, preference, support of significant others for method, and contraindications when selecting a pain relief strategy.
- Select and implement a variety of measures (e.g., pharmacologic, nonpharmacologic, interpersonal) to facilitate pain relief, as appropriate).
- Provide the person optimal pain relief with prescribed analgesics.
- Implement the use of patient-controlled analgesia (PCA), if appropriate.
- Use pain control measures before pain becomes severe.
- Verify level of discomfort with client, note changes in the medical record, and inform other health professionals working with the client.
- Evaluate the effectiveness of the pain control measures used through ongoing assessment of the pain experience.
- Institute and modify pain control measures on the basis of the client's response.
- Promote adequate rest/sleep to facilitate pain relief.
- Notify the health care provider if measures are unsuccessful or if current complaint is a significant change from client's past experience of pain.
- Inform other health care professionals/family members of nonpharmacologic strategies being used by the client to encourage preventive approaches to pain management.
- Use a multidisciplinary approach to pain management, when appropriate.
- Consider referrals for client, family, and significant others to support groups and other resources, as appropriate.
- Provide accurate information to promote family's knowledge of and response to the pain experience.
- Incorporate the family in the pain relief modality, if possible.
- Monitor client satisfaction with pain management at specified intervals.

Patient-Controlled Analgesia (PCA) Assistance: *Facilitating client control of analgesic administration and regulation*
- Collaborate with health care providers, client, and family members in selecting the type of narcotic to be used.
- Ensure that the client is not allergic to the analgesic to be administered.
- Teach the client and family to monitor pain intensity, quality, and duration.
- Teach the client and family to monitor respiratory rate and blood pressure.
- Teach the client and family members how to use the PCA device.
- Teach the client and family members the action and side effects of pain-relieving agents.
- Document client's pain, amount and frequency of drug dosing, and response to pain treatment in a pain flow sheet.
- Recommend a bowel regimen to avoid constipation.
- Consult with clinical pain experts for a client who is having difficulty achieving pain control.

NIC intervention activities selected from McCloskey, J.C., & Bulechek, G.M. (2000). *Nursing interventions classification (NIC)* (3rd ed.). St. Louis: Mosby. No part of this work is to be altered without prior written permission from the Publisher.

- What medication is he probably receiving, and why?
- What actions should you take in regard to his statement about lack of adequate pain relief?
- What options does the health care team have for pain management?

For suggested answer guidelines, go to SIMON http://www.wbsaunders.com/SIMON/Iggy/.

DRUG THERAPY. Decreasing the release of secretin reduces pancreatic stimulation. Secretin is an intestinal hormone that stimulates the release of enzymes and bicarbonate from the pancreas when acidic chyme is present in the duodenum. Antacids administered orally or via an NG tube that is clamped for 20 minutes after administration neutralize gastric secretions. The health care provider orders histamine receptor antagonists, such as ranitidine hydrochloride (Zantac), to decrease hydrochloric acid production so that pancreatic enzymes are not activated by an acidic pH. These interventions are also useful in reducing the occurrence of GI erosion and bleeding. Anticholinergics, such as dicyclomine hydrochloride (Bentyl, Lomine✿), are indicated to decrease vagal stimulation, decrease GI motility, and inhibit pancreatic enzyme and bicarbonate volume and concentration. However, these drugs can cause unwanted side effects for older adults, such as dry mouth, urinary retention, constipation, and acute confusion.

An additional drug that the care provider might prescribe is somatostatin or its synthetic analog, octreotide. This is used in an attempt to decrease pancreatic activity, but the research is still inconclusive about the value of the therapy (Uhl et al., 1999).

COMFORT MEASURES. Helping the client to assume the fetal position (with the legs drawn up to the chest) may decrease the abdominal pain of pancreatitis.

If the client has an NG tube in place, the nurse provides frequent oral hygiene measures to keep mucous membranes moist and free of inflammation or crusting. Because of the drying effect of anticholinergic drugs and the absence of oral fluids, the mouth and oral cavity may be extremely dry, resulting in considerable discomfort.

Lowering the client's anxiety level may also substantially reduce pain. The nurse provides thorough explanations of procedures. The client is encouraged to express the emotions and responses he or she is experiencing. The nurse also provides reassurance and diversional activities, such as television, music, and reading material, and encourages visitors to direct attention away from the pain.

SURGICAL MANAGEMENT. Surgical intervention for acute pancreatitis is usually not indicated. However, complications of pancreatitis, such as pancreatic pseudocyst and abscess, may necessitate surgical drainage. If pancreatitis is caused by biliary tract obstruction, the physician may perform a laparotomy (abdominal exploration) for common bile duct exploration and the release of obstruction.

PREOPERATIVE CARE. In addition to general preoperative care measures, the client usually has an NG tube inserted and begins receiving IV fluids. The client is frequently in pain, a factor that inhibits the learning process, so the nurse provides preoperative teaching in a manner that takes the client's comfort level into account. Postoperative reminders may be needed to reinforce the preoperative learning. The nurse teaches the client to expect a pancreatic drainage tube and explains its care during the postoperative period. The nurse needs to be certain that the client knows how to promote respiratory function by turning, coughing, deep breathing, and splinting the incision, because the client with an NG tube is at increased risk for postoperative pulmonary complications.

OPERATIVE PROCEDURE. When an abscess or pseudocyst is incised and drained with the client under general anesthesia, drainage tubes are inserted, sutured in place, and connected to low suction (80 mm Hg or less) to prevent further tissue erosion.

POSTOPERATIVE CARE. Postoperatively, the nurse monitors drainage tubes for patency by assessing for kinks in the tubes and maintaining the ordered drain suction pressure and system integrity. The nurse records the output amount from the drain and describes the character of the drainage. A sump type of drain is usually inserted. The nurse ascertains that the drain is functioning, as indicated by a hissing noise from the sump lumen.

The nurse provides meticulous skin care and dressing changes. The client is monitored for the first signs of redness or skin irritation because pancreatic enzyme drainage is particularly excoriating to the skin. Skin barriers, such as a Stomahesive wafer around the drainage tube, are applied to repel drainage from the skin. The nurse continually assesses for further deterioration of the tissue. The nurse should also collaborate with an enterostomal therapist (ET) for measures to promote skin integrity, such as the use of individualized ostomy appliances and the application of topical ointments.

■ IMBALANCED NUTRITION: LESS THAN BODY REQUIREMENTS

NOC **PLANNING: EXPECTED OUTCOMES.** The client with acute pancreatitis is expected to have sufficient nutritional intake to maintain body weight and a decrease in pancreatic stimulation.

INTERVENTIONS. The client is maintained on NPO status in the early stages of pancreatitis. Clients who have severe pancreatitis and are unable to eat for 7 to 10 days should receive nutritional support in the form of total parenteral nutrition (TPN) (see Chapter 61) or total enteral nutrition (TEN) (see the Evidence-Based Practice for Nursing box on p. 1345). If TPN is used for nutritional support, the nurse assesses for glucose intolerance by monitoring for elevated blood glucose levels. This is extremely important in clients with pancreatitis because pancreatic dysfunction affects the release of insulin. Some clients require insulin administration during an acute episode of the disease. TEN has been shown to produce fewer episodes of glucose elevation and other complications associated with the use of TPN yet has been shown to be as effective in maintaining nutritional status (Scolapio et al., 1999).

When food is tolerated during the recovery phase, the health care provider generally orders small, frequent, moderate- to high-carbohydrate, high-protein, low-fat meals. Foods should be bland with little spice; caffeine-containing foods (tea, coffee, cola, and chocolate), as well as alcohol, should be avoided.

To boost caloric intake, commercial liquid nutritional preparations, such as Ensure and Isocal, supplement the diet. If caloric intake is less than desired, an NG tube may be required for additional nutrition via enteral feedings. The health care provider may also prescribe fat-soluble and other vitamin and mineral replacement supplements.

● Community-Based Care

■ HEALTH TEACHING

Education needs to be started early in the hospitalization period—as soon as the acute episodes of pain have subsided. The nurse assesses the client's and family members' or significant others' knowledge of the disease.

The goals of discharge planning and education are to avoid further episodes of pancreatitis and prevent progression to a chronic disease. The nurse instructs the client to abstain from

EVIDENCE-BASED PRACTICE FOR NURSING

What is the best method for ensuring optimal nutrition in clients with acute pancreatitis? Is early total enteral nutrition (TEN) or total parenteral nutrition (TPN) going to provide the client with mild acute pancreatitis the best nutrition?

McClave, S., et al. (1997). Comparison of the safety of early enteral vs parenteral nutrition in mild acute pancreatitis. *Journal of Parenteral and Enteral Nutrition, 21*(1), 14-20.

Acute pancreatitis creates a catabolic stress state that promotes, among other things, nutritional deterioration. Total parenteral nutrition (TPN) has been the standard of practice for providing exogenous nutrients while avoiding pancreatic stimulation. Based on evaluation of other studies conducted, the authors determined that more information was needed to determine if the widespread use of TPN was warranted. Clients admitted to the hospital with acute pancreatitis were prospectively randomized to receive either total enteral nutrition (TEN) (nasojejunal route) or TPN. There were no differences on admission in mean age, Ranson criteria, multiple organ failure score (MOF), or APACHE III score between the TEN and TPN groups. Both groups were studied, and the authors found that TEN was as safe and effective as TPN and had some advantages over TPN: less costly, more rapid resolution of the toxicity, and less stress-induced hyperglycemia.

Critique. Because of the small sample size of 32 (16 per group), the cost of nutrition was the only study end point to reach statistical significance. The study was performed in clients with mild acute pancreatitis, predominantly alcoholic related, so results may not be directly applied to persons with severe acute pancreatitis.

Implications for Nursing. The nurse caring for a client with acute pancreatitis needs to recognize the impact the illness has on the nutritional well-being of the individual. The traditional method of treatment includes avoiding pancreatic stimulation by having the client remain on NPO status (receiving nothing by mouth) and using alternative nutritional support. The nurse needs to familiarize himself or herself with the unique needs of the client with jejunal feeding. Traditional complications associated with TPN may also be decreased, such as fewer episodes of hyperglycemia and fewer nosocomial infections.

alcohol to prevent further pain attacks and extension of inflammation and pancreatic insufficiency. The client is told that if alcohol is consumed, pain will be experienced, and further autodigestion of the pancreas will lead to chronic pancreatitis and chronic pain.

The nurse also teaches the client to notify the health care provider after discharge to home if acute abdominal pain or biliary tract disease (as evidenced by jaundice, clay-colored stools, or darkened urine) occurs. These signs and symptoms are possible indicators of complications or disease progression.

■ HOME CARE MANAGEMENT

Home care preparation will need to be individualized for each client's circumstances. Some clients with acute pancreatitis may be severely weakened from their acute illness and need to confine activity to one floor, limiting stair climbing and other strenuous activities until they regain their strength.

■ HEALTH CARE RESOURCES

Clients with acute pancreatitis require visits by a home care nurse if the hospital course was complicated. In these cases, home care may be needed for wound care and assistance with

activities of daily living (ADLs). The client requires medical follow-up with the primary care physician or nurse practitioner for monitoring of the disease process. For clients with alcoholism, the nurse provides information about groups such as Alcoholics Anonymous (AA). Family members may attend support groups such as Al-Anon and Al-Ateen.

● Evaluation: Outcomes

NOC The nurse evaluates the care of the client with acute pancreatitis on the basis of the identified nursing diagnoses and collaborative problems. The expected outcomes include that the client will:

- Experience an alleviation of or reduction in abdominal pain, as indicated by self-report
- Maintain adequate nutritional intake with a decrease in pancreatic stimulation as evidenced by weight maintenance
- Not experience a recurrence of pancreatitis

Chronic Pancreatitis

■ OVERVIEW

Chronic pancreatitis is a progressive, destructive disease of the pancreas, characterized by remissions and exacerbations (recurrence). Inflammation and fibrosis of the tissue contribute to pancreatic insufficiency and diminished function of the organ. Chronic pancreatitis usually develops after repeated episodes of alcohol-induced acute pancreatitis. It may also be associated with chronic obstruction of the common bile duct. Chronic pancreatitis may develop in the absence of a known acute disorder. Relief of pain, prevention of recurrence of attacks, prevention of complications, and nutritional support are the principal interventions.

■ Pathophysiology

■ TYPES OF CHRONIC PANCREATITIS

Alcohol-induced chronic pancreatitis is also known as *chronic calcifying pancreatitis (CCP)*. Protein precipitates that plug the ducts and lead to ductal obstruction, atrophy, and dilation characterize CCP. As the protein plugging becomes diffuse, the epithelium of the ducts undergoes histologic changes, resulting in metaplasia (cell replacement) and ulceration. This inflammatory process causes fibrosis of the pancreatic tissue. Intraductal calcification and marked pancreatic parenchymal destruction develop in the late stages. Cystic sacs containing pancreatic secretions and enzymes form on the pancreas. The organ becomes hard and firm as a result of acinar cell atrophy and pancreatic insufficiency.

Chronic obstructive pancreatitis develops from inflammation, spasm, and obstruction of the sphincter of Oddi. Inflammatory and sclerotic lesions occur in the head of the pancreas and around the ducts, causing an obstruction and backflow of pancreatic secretions (see Complications of Acute Pancreatitis, p. 1340).

■ PATHOLOGIC CHANGES

Pancreatic insufficiency in chronic pancreatitis is characterized by the loss of exocrine function. Pancreatic exocrine secretion is divided into two components: aqueous bicarbonate and enzymes.

The aqueous component neutralizes the duodenal contents and pancreatic enzymes that are essential to normal digestion and absorption. Most clients with chronic pancreatitis have a decreased output of pancreatic secretion and bicarbonate. Pancreatic enzyme secretion must be reduced by more than 80% to produce steatorrhea resulting from severe malabsorption of fats. These characteristic stools are pale, bulky, and frothy and have an offensive odor. The action of colonic bacteria on unabsorbed lipids and proteins is responsible for the foul odor. On inspection of the stools, the fat content is visible. In severe chronic pancreatitis, stool fat output may exceed 40 g/day.

Fat malabsorption also contributes to weight loss and muscle wasting (a decrease in muscle mass) and leads to general debilitation of the client. Protein malabsorption results in a "starvation" edema of the feet, legs, and hands caused by decreased levels of circulating albumin.

The loss of pancreatic endocrine function is responsible for the development of frank diabetes mellitus in clients with chronic pancreatic insufficiency. (See Chapter 65 for a complete discussion of diabetes mellitus.)

The client with chronic pancreatitis may have pulmonary complications, such as pleuritic pain, pleural effusions, and pulmonary infiltrates. Pancreatic ascites may impede diaphragmatic excursion and decrease lung expansion, resulting in impaired ventilation. In the ill client with chronic pancreatitis, acute respiratory distress syndrome (ARDS) may develop.

▌ Etiology

The cause of chronic calcifying pancreatitis is persistent excessive alcohol intake that results in repeated episodes of acute pancreatitis. The most common cause of chronic obstructive pancreatitis is cholelithiasis and biliary tract disease, which results in persistent inflammation. Other etiologic factors include pancreatic pseudocyst, postoperative ductal scarring, and cancer of the pancreas or duodenum. All of these factors can produce obstruction of the pancreatic duct. Prolonged starvation and prolonged use of parenteral feedings for nutritional support can result in pancreatic atrophy, causing pancreatic insufficiency.

▌ Incidence/Prevalence

Approximately 75% of clients with chronic pancreatitis are alcoholics (Price & Wilson, 1997). Alcohol-induced pancreatitis is predominantly found in men, but the incidence in women is increasing. In women, chronic pancreatitis occurs more commonly among those with biliary tract disease (cholecystitis and cholelithiasis). The age at occurrence of chronic pancreatitis is variable but is usually between 45 and 60 years.

➤ COLLABORATIVE MANAGEMENT
◖ Assessment

Clinical manifestations of chronic pancreatitis differ from those of an acute inflammation, although, as with acute pancreatitis, abdominal pain is the major clinical manifestation (Chart 60-6). The client with chronic pancreatitis typically describes the pain as a continuous burning or gnawing dullness

---

CHART 60-6

KEY FEATURES *of*
Chronic Pancreatitis

- Intense abdominal pain (major clinical manifestation) that is continuous and burning or gnawing
- Abdominal tenderness
- Ascites
- Possible left upper quadrant mass (if pseudocyst or abscess is present)
- Respiratory compromise manifested by adventitious or diminished breath sounds, dyspnea, or orthopnea
- Steatorrhea; clay-colored stools
- Weight loss
- Jaundice
- Dark urine
- Polyuria, polydipsia, polyphagia (diabetes mellitus)

---

with periods of acute exacerbation. The pain is intense and relentless. The frequency of acute exacerbations may increase as the pancreatic fibrosis develops.

The nurse performs the same abdominal assessment as for clients with acute pancreatitis, but the findings may not be as significant. Abdominal tenderness is less intense. A mass may be palpated in the left upper quadrant, which is indicative of a pancreatic pseudocyst or abscess (see Pancreatic Pseudocyst, p. 1349). Massive pancreatic ascites may be present, producing dullness on abdominal percussion. Because respiratory complications can accompany the condition, the nurse auscultates the lung fields for adventitious sounds or decreased aeration and observes for dyspnea or orthopnea.

The client is asked to collect a random stool specimen, if able, or is asked to describe the stools. The nurse or assistive nursing personnel collects the stool specimen for diagnostic studies. The specimen may show the presence of steatorrhea (foul-smelling fatty stools that may increase in volume as pancreatic insufficiency progresses and lipase production decreases). The nurse observes the client's anal area for excoriation resulting from frequent defecation.

The client may also experience weight loss, muscle wasting, jaundice, dark urine, and the signs and symptoms of diabetes mellitus, such as polyuria, polydipsia, and polyphagia.

In chronic pancreatitis, significant laboratory findings include normal or moderately elevated serum amylase and lipase levels. Obstruction of the intrahepatic bile duct can cause elevated serum bilirubin and alkaline phosphatase levels. Transient elevations in serum glucose levels are common and can be detected by blood glucose monitoring, both fasting and nonfasting.

The only definitive diagnostic test for chronic pancreatitis is the identification of calcification of pancreatic tissue in a biopsy specimen. If direct evidence of chronic pancreatitis is needed, the health care provider may order a secretin test. This test is the most sensitive and specific for chronic pancreatitis, other than histology (Amann, DiMagno, & Rubin, 1997). Secretin is an intestinal hormone that stimulates hepatic and pancreatic secretion. In this test, the client swallows a double-lumen gastrointestinal (GI) tube. The tip should reach the duodenum, with the proximal lumen port located in the stomach. Gastric and duodenal contents are aspirated before and after IV administration of secretin. An abnormal volume of enzymes and bicarbonate in the GI contents may indicate chronic pancreatitis.

Abdominal ultrasonography is also a helpful diagnostic tool, especially to reveal pseudocysts. Endoscopic retrograde cholangiopancreatography (ERCP) may reveal ductal system abnormalities, such as calcification and strictures, or it may delineate the presence of pancreatic pseudocyst.

● Interventions

The focus of caring for the client with chronic pancreatitis is to manage pain, assist in maintaining a sufficient nutritional intake, and prevent recurrence.

NONSURGICAL MANAGEMENT. Nonsurgical interventions primarily include drug and diet therapy.

DRUG THERAPY. The major intervention for the pain of chronic pancreatitis is drug therapy. In addition, the nurse teaches the client to avoid ingesting irritating substances that can precipitate pain.

NIC *Analgesic Administration* (see Chart 60-5). The nurse medicates the client, as ordered, according to the assessment of the level and intensity of pain and evaluates the effectiveness of the drug intervention. Opioid analgesia with meperidine hydrochloride (Demerol) is most frequently used, but opioid dependency may become a problem. Nonopioid analgesics may be tried to relieve pain. (See Chapter 7 for other interventions for chronic pain.)

If drug dependency becomes a problem, behavior modification programs and drug and alcohol counseling will be necessary. The health care provider may need to admit these clients to drug and alcohol dependency programs.

Enzyme Replacement. Pancreatic enzymes (non–enteric-coated preparations) are essential dietary supplements (Chart 60-7). These are given with meals or snacks to aid in digestion and absorption of fat and protein. Drugs such as pancreatin (Donnazyme) and pancrelipase (Cotazym, Viokase, or Pancrease) are prescribed in capsule, tablet, or powder form and contain amylase, lipase, and protease. Cotazym also contains calcium carbonate to increase depleted calcium levels. The nurse mixes the powder form in applesauce or fruit juice to make it more palatable. Enzyme preparations should not be mixed with foods containing proteins, because the enzymatic action dissolves the food into a watery substance. The nurse advises the client to wipe his or her lips with a wet towel to prevent the skin irritation and breakdown that residual enzymes can cause.

The dosage of pancreatic enzymes depends on the severity of the malabsorption and maldigestion. The nurse records the number and consistency of stools per day to monitor the effectiveness of enzyme therapy. If pancreatic enzyme treatment is effective, the stools should become less frequent and less fatty.

Insulin Therapy. If the client has diabetes, the health care provider prescribes insulin or oral hypoglycemic agents for glucose control. Clients maintained on total parenteral nutrition (TPN) are particularly susceptible to labile glucose levels and may require regular insulin additives to the solution. The nurse closely monitors blood glucose levels so that hyperglycemia is controlled and insulin or diabetic shock is prevented. The use of glucometers allows frequent assessment of glucose levels during the critical insulin dosage adjustment period. The nurse, laboratory tech-

---

CHART 60-7

◗ **CLIENT EDUCATION GUIDE**
◗ **Enzyme Replacement for the Client with Chronic Pancreatitis**

- Give pancreatic enzymes with meals and snacks.
- Administer pancreatin after antacid or H_2 blockers; decreased pH inactivates drug.
- Tell the client to swallow the tablets without chewing to minimize oral irritation.
- Mix the powder form in applesauce or fruit juice.
- Do not mix enzyme preparations in protein-containing foods.
- Have the client wipe his or her lips after taking enzymes to avoid skin irritation.
- Do not crush enteric-coated preparations.
- Monitor serum uric acid levels (pancrelipase can cause an increase in uric acid levels).

---

nician, or assistive nursing personnel checks glucose levels every 2 to 4 hours.

Other Drugs. The health care provider may also prescribe histamine receptor antagonists, such as ranitidine hydrochloride (Zantac), to decrease gastric acid. Gastric acid destroys the lipase needed to break down fats. Controlling the acidity of the stomach with H_2 blockers or proton pump inhibitors or neutralizing stomach acid with oral sodium bicarbonate may enhance the effectiveness of the non–enteric-coated enzyme therapy. Subcutaneous octreotide (Sandostatin), a growth hormone similar to somatostatin, is ordered by some physicians if pain and diarrhea persist (Amann, DiMagno, & Rubin, 1997).

DIET THERAPY. Protein and fat malabsorption results in significant weight loss and decreased muscle mass in the client with chronic pancreatitis. Therefore the nutritional interventions for acute pancreatitis are also relevant for the chronic phase of pancreatitis. The client often limits food intake to avoid the recurrent pain, which is exacerbated by eating. For this reason, nutrition maintenance is often difficult to achieve, and clients are provided with TPN or total enteral nutrition (TEN), including vitamin and mineral replacement.

For long-term dietary management, the client needs an increased number of calories, up to 4000 to 6000 calories/day, to maintain weight. Foods high in carbohydrates and protein also assist in the healing process. Foods high in fat are avoided because they cause or increase diarrhea.

SURGICAL MANAGEMENT. Surgery is not a primary intervention for the treatment of chronic pancreatitis. However, it may be indicated for intractable abdominal pain, incapacitating relapses of pain, or complications such as abscesses and pseudocysts.

The underlying pathologic changes determine the procedure indicated. The surgeon incises and drains an abscess or pseudocyst. Cholecystectomy or choledochotomy (incision of the common bile duct) may be indicated if biliary tract disease is an underlying cause of pancreatitis. If the pancreatic duct sphincter is fibrotic, the surgeon performs a sphincterotomy (incision of the sphincter) to enlarge it.

In pancreaticojejunostomy, the pancreatic duct is opened and anastomosed to the jejunum to relieve obstruction. This procedure relieves pain and preserves pancreatic tissue and function. The preoperative and postoperative care is similar to that for clients undergoing the Whipple procedure (discussed under Surgical Management [Pancreatic Carcinoma], p. 1352). A partial pancreatectomy (resection of the pancreas) may be performed for clients with advanced pancreatitis or disabling pain. Vagotomy with gastric antrectomy is done to alter nerve stimulation and decrease pancreatic secretion. (See Chapter 56 for a discussion of nursing care.)

In a few cases, pancreas transplantation may be done. However, this procedure is performed most often for clients with severe, uncontrolled diabetes. Chapter 65 discusses pancreas transplantation.

● Community-Based Care

The care of the client with pancreatitis usually involves a case manager or discharge planner. A community-based case manager may continue to follow the client while he or she requires health care in the home or other community-based setting.

■ HEALTH TEACHING

Because there is no known cure for chronic pancreatitis, client and family education is aimed at preventing further acute exacerbations of this chronic disease, providing long-term care, and promoting health maintenance (Chart 60-8).

DIET THERAPY. The nurse instructs the client to avoid known precipitating factors, such as the ingestion of caffeinated beverages and alcohol. The dietitian elicits the participation of the family or significant other in diet planning and food preparation. Diet teaching focuses on eating bland, low-fat, frequent meals and avoiding rich, fatty foods. The nurse and dietitian stress the importance of dietary compliance and the need for increased nutritional intake to prevent acute exacerbations of this chronic illness. Written instructions on diet and pancreatic enzyme replacement therapy are essential.

The nurse instructs the client and family members or significant others on the importance of adhering to the pancreatic enzyme replacement treatment. The client must take the prescribed enzymes with meals and snacks to aid in the digestion of food and promote the absorption of fats and proteins. The nurse teaches the client to take the enzymes at the beginning of the meal and to report to the health care provider any increase in the occurrence of foul-smelling, frothy, fatty stools; abdominal distention; and cramping so that pancreatic enzyme replacement may be increased as needed. The client should report any skin excoriation or breakdown so that therapeutic interventions to promote skin integrity can be instituted.

CHART 60-8

CLIENT EDUCATION GUIDE
Prevention of Exacerbations of Chronic Pancreatitis

- Avoid things that make your symptoms worse, such as drinking caffeinated beverages.
- Avoid alcohol ingestion; refer to self-help group for assistance.
- Avoid nicotine.
- Eat bland, low-fat, high-protein, moderate-carbohydrate meals; avoid gastric stimulants, such as spices.
- Eat small meals and snacks high in calories.
- Take the pancreatic enzymes that have been prescribed for you with meals.
- Rest frequently; restrict your activity to one floor until you regain your strength.

SKIN CARE. The frequency of defecation (whether continent or incontinent) poses challenging skin care problems. The nurse instructs the client to keep his or her skin dry and free of the abrasive fatty stools, which are excoriating to the skin. The skin should be cleaned thoroughly after each stool and a soothing emollient, such as Sween, applied. To prevent breakdown and maintain skin integrity, a skin barrier may be needed. Many products on the market, such as zinc oxide cream, actively repel stool from the skin.

DRUG THERAPY. The client and family members must be able to state the desired effect of the prescribed drugs, the schedule for drug administration, and potential side effects. The nurse provides written guidelines as reinforcement.

If the client develops diabetes mellitus as a result of chronic pancreatitis from endocrine dysfunction, management of elevated glucose levels after discharge from the hospital may necessitate oral hypoglycemic agents or insulin injections. If this is the case, the client and the family require in-depth teaching concerning diabetes, its signs and symptoms, medical management, insulin administration, dietary management, urine and blood glucose monitoring, and general care information. (See Chapter 65 for a discussion of diabetes.)

■ HOME CARE MANAGEMENT

Client with chronic pancreatitis are usually discharged to home, but some may require care in a long-term care setting. If the client is discharged to home, the activity area should be limited to one floor until he or she regains strength and can increase activity. Toilet facilities must be easily accessible because of chronic steatorrhea and frequent defecation. If toilet facilities are not available in the immediate rest area, a bedpan or bedside commode is obtained for the home.

■ HEALTH CARE RESOURCES

Chronic illnesses are devastating for families. The high costs of medical insurance, medical treatment, and drug therapy cause serious financial problems. Often the client with chronic pancreatitis is unable or unwilling to work. Case management to coordinate care and manage resources should be instituted during hospitalization and continue throughout the course of the illness.

The client may require home visits by nurses and a dietitian, depending on the severity of the chronic health problems and home maintenance and support needs. The home care nurse assesses the client for pain management, compliance with dietary guidelines and alcohol abstinence, the effectiveness of pancreatic enzyme therapy, and psychosocial adaptation to a chronic illness.

The nurse or case manager refers the client to a counselor or a self-help group, such as Alcoholics Anonymous, if appropriate.

Pancreatic Abscess
■ OVERVIEW

Pancreatic abscesses are the most serious complication of pancreatitis. If untreated, they are always fatal. After surgery, the recurrence rate is higher than 30%. The abscesses form from collections of purulent liquefaction of the necrotic pancreas.

Pancreatic abscesses occur after severe acute pancreatitis, exacerbations of chronic pancreatitis, or biliary tract surgery. The development of either a single abscess or multiple abscesses results from extensive inflammatory necrosis of the pancreas that is readily invaded by infectious organisms such as *Escherichia coli, Klebsiella, Bacteroides, Staphylococcus,* and *Proteus.* They can erode through the retroperitoneum into the bowel mesentery, the mediastinum, the pleural space, or the pelvis.

► COLLABORATIVE MANAGEMENT

Clients with pancreatic abscesses often appear more seriously ill than clients with pseudocysts. Clinical manifestations are similar; however, the temperature in clients with abscesses may spike to as high as 104° F (40° C). Blood cultures are helpful in revealing the infective organism. Pleural effusions commonly accompany these abscesses. Ultrasonography and computed tomography (CT) cannot differentiate between pancreatic pseudocysts and abscesses.

Pancreatic abscesses that are not surgically drained carry 100% mortality. Drainage should be performed as soon as possible to prevent sepsis. Antibiotic treatment alone does not resolve the abscess. Mortality remains as high as 60%, even after surgical drainage. Many clients require multiple drainage procedures for recurrent abscesses.

> ### CRITICAL THINKING CHALLENGE
> Your client has indicated that he does not intend to alter his alcohol consumption after he is discharged; in fact, he plans to stop for a drink at his favorite bar on the way home after his release later today.
> * What is the connection between alcohol consumption and chronic pancreatitis?
> * What questions should you ask to determine if the client fully understands the connection between alcohol consumption and recurrence of pancreatitis?
> * What resources are available to him to assist with his alcohol problem?
> * What nursing diagnoses are appropriate for this client?

For suggested answer guidelines, go to [SIMON] http://www.wbsaunders.com/SIMON/Iggy/.

Pancreatic Pseudocyst
■ OVERVIEW

Pancreatic pseudocysts develop as a complication of acute or chronic pancreatitis. **Pseudocysts** occur in pancreatitis caused by alcoholism, biliary tract disease, or abdominal or surgical trauma. Pseudocysts develop in 10% to 20% of all people with pancreatitis, and mortality is reported at approximately 10%.

Pancreatic pseudocysts, or false cysts, are so named because, unlike true cysts, they do not have an epithelial lining. Pseudocysts are encapsulated saclike structures that form on or surround the pancreas. The pseudocyst wall is inflamed, vascular, and fibrotic. It may contain up to several liters of straw-colored or dark-brown viscous fluid, the enzymatic exudate of the pancreas.

► COLLABORATIVE MANAGEMENT

A pseudocyst can be palpated as an epigastric mass in approximately 50% of cases. The primary presenting symptom is epigastric pain radiating to the back. Other common clinical manifestations include abdominal fullness, nausea, vomiting, and jaundice.

Pseudocysts are diagnosed, and their growth and resolution monitored, by serial abdominal ultrasonographic examination or CT.

Complications of pseudocyst formation include the following:
* Hemorrhage
* Infection
* Obstruction of the bowel, biliary tract, or splenic vein
* Abscess
* Fistula formation
* Pancreatic ascites

Pseudocysts may spontaneously resolve, or they may rupture and produce hemorrhage. Surgical intervention is necessary if the pseudocyst does not resolve within 6 weeks or if complications develop. To accomplish internal drainage, the surgeon creates an opening (ostomy) between the pseudocyst and the stomach (cystogastrostomy), the jejunum (cystojejunostomy), or the duodenum (cystoduodenostomy). To provide external drainage, the surgeon inserts a sump drainage tube to remove pancreatic secretions and exudate. Pseudocysts recur in almost 10% of cases. Pancreatic fistulas are common after surgery, and skin breakdown from corrosive pancreatic enzymes presents a major nursing care challenge (see earlier discussion under Postoperative Care [Acute Pancreatitis], p. 1344).

Pancreatic Carcinoma
■ OVERVIEW

Cancer of the pancreas is one of the leading causes of cancer-related mortality, accounting for 2% to 3% of the new cancer cases each year and for high costs of care (see the Cost of Care Box on p. 1350) (Sauter & Coleman, 1999).

■ Pathophysiology

Pancreatic tumors usually originate from epithelial cells of the pancreatic ductal system. If the tumor is discovered in the early stages, the tumor cells may be localized within the glandular organ; however, this is highly unlikely. Most often, the tumor is discovered in the late stages of development and may be a well-defined mass or is diffusely spread throughout the pancreas.

The tumor may be a primary cancer, or it may result from metastasis from cancers of the lung, breast, thyroid, or kidney or from skin melanoma. Primary pancreatic tumors are generally adenocarcinomas and grow in well-differentiated glandular patterns. Pancreatic adenocarcinoma grows rapidly and spreads to surrounding organs (stomach, duodenum, gallbladder, and intestine) by direct extension and invasion of lymphatic and vascular systems. This highly metastatic lesion may eventually invade the lung, peritoneum, liver, spleen, and lymph nodes.

Clinical manifestations depend on the site of origin or metastasis. The head of the pancreas is the most common site of pancreatic carcinoma. Pancreatic tumors are usually small lesions with poorly defined margins. Jaundice results from tumor compression and obstruction of the common bile duct and from gallbladder dilation, causing the organ to enlarge.

Carcinomas of the body and tail of the pancreas are usually large and invade the entire tail and body. These tumors may

COST OF CARE
IMPLICATIONS FOR NURSING

PANCREATIC CANCER

Cost of Care
- Pancreatic cancer ranks eleventh in incidence and fifth in cancer deaths.
- Total annual costs are $4.9 billion (men: $3.0 billion; women: $1.9 billion).
- Total direct costs are $881.3 million.
  - Seventy-one percent of total direct costs ($627.1 million/ $881.3 million) are for those over 65 years of age.
  - Total hospital costs are 77% ($679.5 million/$881.3 million) of total direct costs.
- Total indirect costs are $4 billion.
  - Sixty-three percent of total indirect costs ($2518.43 million/$4018 million) are for those ages 45 to 64 years.
  - Mortality costs are $3.7 billion—93% ($3739 million/$4018 million) of indirect costs.

Implications for Nursing
Pancreatic cancer has a very low 5-year survival rate, with fewer than 20% of those diagnosed with the disease living longer than 1 year after diagnosis.

Because of the cost of pancreatic cancer, it is important that nurses recognize the role they might play in the disease process. This role might include education about the risk factors and prevention, the signs and symptoms, and the treatment of this cancer.

Currently there is no known diagnostic test to predict the individual's susceptibility to this type of cancer, nor is the exact cause of the cancer known.

Nurses need to identify who might be at higher risk to develop pancreatic cancer: some possible links have been shown with alcohol and caffeine consumption and with a diet high in fat and protein. Smoking is known to be the single most significant risk factor for the development of pancreatic cancer. These actual and potential risk factors are modifiable.

Data from Wilson, L., & Lightwood, J. (1999). Pancreatic cancer: Total costs and utilization of health services, *Journal of Surgical Oncology, 71*(3), 171-181; and Sauter, P.L., & Coleman, J. (1999). Pancreatic cancer: A continuum of care. *Seminars in Oncology Nursing, 15*(1), 36-47.

be palpable abdominal masses, especially in the thin client. Through metastatic spread via the splenic vein, metastasis to the liver may cause hepatomegaly (enlargement of the liver up to two to three times its normal size). Carcinomas of the body and tail spread more extensively than do pancreatic head carcinomas, with invasion of the retroperitoneum, vertebral column, spleen, adrenal glands, colon, or stomach. Regardless of where it originates, pancreatic cancer spreads rapidly through the lymphatic and venous systems to other organs.

Thrombophlebitis is a common complication of pancreatic carcinoma. It is attributed to an increase in the levels of thromboplastic factors in the blood. Necrotic products of the pancreatic tumor are believed to have thromboplastic properties, resulting in the blood's hypercoagulable state. Thrombophlebitis is due to the client's confinement to bed and extensive surgical manipulation.

Etiology

The exact cause of pancreatic carcinoma is unknown. The single most prevalent risk factor for pancreatic cancer is smoking. A diet high in protein and fat, and high coffee or alcohol consumption have also been investigated for possible linkage to the disease, but current studies do not show a substantial direct association (Sauter & Coleman, 1999). Research does

support the theory that there might be a genetic link in the development of pancreatic cancer (McEwen et al., 1996).

Incidence/Prevalence

Approximately 28,000 people develop pancreatic cancer each year, and an equal number of people die from the disease each year. Fewer than 20% of persons diagnosed with pancreatic cancer survive longer than 1 year after diagnosis (Sauter & Coleman, 1999).

CONSIDERATIONS FOR OLDER ADULTS
The incidence of pancreatic cancer increases with age. The highest rates of incidence are in people between 60 and 70 years of age, and pancreatic cancer rarely develops before the age of 50. The disease appears to be somewhat more common in men than in women, but the difference is slight (Mayer, 1999; Sauter & Coleman, 1999).

CULTURAL CONSIDERATIONS
Cancer of the pancreas occurs in developed countries. A slightly higher incidence among African Americans has been reported (Sauter & Coleman, 1999).

► COLLABORATIVE MANAGEMENT
● Assessment

Pancreatic cancer often presents in an insidious manner. The presenting symptoms depend somewhat on the location of the tumor. The first clue to the presence of pancreatic carcinoma may be the appearance of jaundice, which is a late sign (Chart 60-9). Jaundice appears as the initial sign in two thirds of all cases because the gallbladder and liver are commonly involved. As the tumor spreads, the green-gold skin color associated with obstructive jaundice progressively worsens. On noting the jaundice, the nurse asks the client whether the color of the stool and urine has changed. As a result of the obstructive process, the stool is clay colored and the urine is dark and frothy. The nurse inspects the skin for dryness and scratch marks, indicating pruritus from jaundice. The nurse also assesses the sclerae for icterus and the mucous membranes for signs of jaundice.

By the time jaundice appears, the pancreatic carcinoma is usually in an advanced stage. The nurse may be able to palpate the enlarged gallbladder and liver. In advanced cases of pancreatic carcinoma, the tumor may be palpated as a firm, fixed mass in the left upper abdominal quadrant or epigastric region.

The most common complaint, often misinterpreted by even the client, is fatigue. This fatigue is described as a diminished energy level and an increased need for rest disproportionate to the level of activity. The client notices an inability to perform usual physical or intellectual activities (Sauter & Coleman, 1999).

The nurse questions the client about abdominal pain, which may be described as a vague, constant dullness in the upper abdomen and nonspecific in nature. Pain, a common early complaint in clients with pancreatic carcinoma, is also present in the advanced stages of the disease. Pain may be related to eating or activity.

CHART 60-9
KEY FEATURES *of* **Presenting Signs and Symptoms of Pancreatic Carcinoma**

- Jaundice (lesions of pancreatic head only)
- Clay-colored stools
- Dark urine
- Abdominal pain: usually vague, dull, or nonspecific
- Weight loss
- Anorexia
- Nausea or vomiting
- Glucose intolerance
- Splenomegaly
- Flatulence
- Gastrointestinal bleeding
- Ascites
- Leg or calf pain (from thrombophlebitis)
- Weakness

In addition, the nurse asks the client whether he or she is experiencing pain in other areas of the body. Referred back pain may be caused by pressure on the nerve plexus. Some clients have leg or calf pain with swelling and redness as a result of thrombophlebitis, a complication of pancreatic carcinoma.

The nurse or assistive nursing personnel weighs the client and determines the extent of weight loss and whether it has occurred rapidly. The client is questioned about food intake and intolerances. Anorexia accompanied by early satiety, nausea, flatulence, and vomiting is common. Gastrointestinal (GI) bleeding may develop from esophageal or gastric varices caused by the tumor pressing on the portal vein. A new diagnosis of diabetes is found in some clients.

The nurse performs a general abdominal assessment. In particular, the nurse percusses the abdomen for dullness, which may indicate the presence of ascites. Pancreatic ascites occurs in the advanced stages of the disease process.

There are no specific blood tests to diagnose pancreatic carcinoma. Serum amylase and lipase levels, as well as alkaline phosphatase and bilirubin levels, are elevated. The degree of elevation depends on the acuteness or chronicity of the pancreatic and biliary damage. Elevated carcinoembryonic antigen (CEA) levels occur in 80% to 90% of clients with pancreatic carcinoma. This test may provide early information about the presence of tumor cells. CA 19-9, another tumor marker, has been found to be the most useful serologic test for monitoring a proven diagnosis and for continuing surveillance of the cancer for potential spread or recurrence (Sauter & Coleman, 1999).

Computed tomography (CT) can confirm the presence of a tumor and can differentiate the tumor from a cyst. Biopsy of pancreatic tissue by needle aspiration reveals malignant cells. Ultrasonographic examinations do not distinguish pancreatic carcinoma from other pancreatic disorders. Endoscopic retrograde cholangiopancreatography (ERCP) visualization and cytologic study of aspirate provide the most definitive diagnostic data. An alternative to ERCP is a percutaneous transhepatic biliary cholangiogram with placement of a percutaneous transhepatic biliary drain (PTBD). This drain decompresses the blocked biliary system by draining bile, either internally or externally (Sauter & Coleman, 1999). Aspiration of pancreatic ascitic fluid by abdominal paracentesis may reveal malignant cells and elevated amylase levels. When the secretin test is performed (see Assessment [Chronic Pancreatitis], p. 1346), duodenal or gastric aspirate may reveal malignant cells.

EVIDENCE-BASED PRACTICE
FOR NURSING

Improving the quality of life for clients with pancreatic cancer: A cooperative team approach by a diverse group of health care providers can improve the life experiences of persons with pancreatic cancer

Sauter, P.K., & Coleman, J. (1999). Pancreatic cancer: A continuum of care. *Seminars in Oncology Nursing, 15*(1), 36-47.

A diagnosis of pancreatic cancer leads a person to consider both quality and quantity of life, since cancer of the pancreas is a disease with a poor prognosis. Many physical symptoms are associated with advanced disease—symptoms that are sometimes feared more that the cancer itself. Fewer than 20% of clients diagnosed with pancreatic cancer live longer than 1 year after diagnosis, and only 3% survive for 5 years. The authors' objectives were to provide information about the etiology, manifestations, treatment, and symptom management of pancreatic cancer. To this end, information was gathered from textbooks, research studies, and review articles. The course of the disease was tracked, from diagnosis to medical management, with appropriate nursing interventions identified for all aspects of care. It was recommended that the nurse place emphasis on empowering the client and caregivers in the management of the disease, when possible.

Critique. Although the authors presented detailed information on the medical management of the disease, they did not provide the same detailed information on ways to involve or empower the client. An excellent research suggestion was given: develop an accurate marker for pancreatic cancer that can be easily detected in a screening test for persons at risk for the disease. Research needs to make progress in the identification of a genetic marker to identify familial links to pancreatic cancer.

Implications for Nursing. Providing care for the client with pancreatic cancer presents many nursing challenges. The nurse needs to understand the disease progression and its multiple treatments in order to provide knowledgeable care to the client. Caring for the client with pancreatic cancer needs to be rendered in a manner that empowers both the client and the caregivers. To accomplish this, the nurse needs to become an integral part of the health care team, which can address treatment, symptom management, and meeting the psychologic, social, and spiritual needs of the client and family as the disease progresses.

Interventions

Management of the client with pancreatic carcinoma is geared toward preventing tumor spread and decreasing pain. These measures are not curative, only palliative (see the Evidence-Based Practice for Nursing box above). The cancers are often multifocal and recur despite treatment.

NONSURGICAL MANAGEMENT. As in other types of cancer, chemotherapy or radiation is used to relieve pain. (See Chapter 25 for nursing interventions associated with these treatment modalities.)

DRUG THERAPY. In an effort to keep the pain under control, the nurse medicates the client, as ordered, with opioid analgesics (usually morphine) and provides comfort measures before the pain escalates and reaches a peak. Because of the poor prognosis, drug dependency is not a consideration. High doses of opioid analgesics may be needed for the intense abdominal and back pain that occurs in the late stages of the disease.

Chemotherapeutic interventions for pancreatic carcinoma have had limited success. Combining agents such as fluorouracil (5-fluorouracil [5-FU]) and carmustine (BCNU) has been more successful than single-agent chemotherapy. 5-FU is an antimetabolite that interferes with deoxyribonucleic acid (DNA) synthesis in rapidly dividing cells. Two other drugs prescribed are mitomycin (Mutamycin), an antitumor antibiotic that inhibits synthesis of ribonucleic acid (RNA), and streptozocin (Zanosar), a nitrosourea that interferes with the replication of DNA. The nurse provides the client with symptomatic relief and comfort measures for the adverse effects of chemotherapeutic agents, such as nausea and vomiting. Gemcitabine, a new cytotoxic agent, is now standard therapy for the treatment of clients whose cancer is nonresectable or whose cancer has metastasized. The major benefit to the client is pain management, with shrinkage of tumor size and prolonged survival a secondary benefit (Sauter & Coleman, 1999).

RADIATION THERAPY. Intensive external beam radiation therapy to the pancreas may offer pain relief by shrinking tumor cells, alleviating obstruction, and improving food absorption; it does not improve survival rates. Implantation of radioactive iodine (^{125}I) seeds, in combination with systemic or intra-arterial administration of floxuridine (FUDR), has also been used. The client may experience discomfort during and after the radiation treatments. Supportive nursing interventions for the relief of symptoms are indicated.

SURGICAL MANAGEMENT. Complete surgical resection of the pancreatic tumor offers the individual with pancreatic cancer the only effective treatment, but the surgery is only possible in a small percentage of cases. The mean survival rate for clients with nonresectable pancreatic cancer is 6 months after diagnosis (Mayer, 1999). Clients with tumors confined to the head of the pancreas are candidates for curative resection. Clients with tumors of the body and tail generally are not candidates for surgery, because in most cases their tumors have spread to other organs. The surgeon may perform either a total pancreatectomy or the Whipple procedure (pancreaticoduodenectomy).

PREOPERATIVE CARE. The client with pancreatic carcinoma is a poor surgical risk because of malnutrition and debilitation. A nasogastric (NG) tube for decompression is inserted, and the administration of IV fluids or total parenteral nutrition (TPN) is typically started before surgery.

The client experiences anorexia with early satiety and often experiences nausea and vomiting, making the oral intake of nutrition difficult to maintain. Management is geared toward providing optimal nutrition preoperatively and postoperatively.

Tube Feedings. As long as intestinal function is adequate, the client may be maintained nutritionally with enteral tube feedings. When tube feedings are tolerated, a small-lumen silicone feeding tube, such as a Dobbhoff tube, is inserted to avoid the complications of larger-lumen tubes, such as sinusitis and nasal irritation. Commercially prepared products chosen by the health care provider or dietitian provide specific nutrients. Feedings are given by bolus or continuous infusion, depending on the client's tolerance and residual volumes.

Often, in the late stages of pancreatic carcinoma or during the Whipple procedure, the physician inserts a small catheter into the jejunum (jejunostomy) so that enteral feedings may be given. This feeding method is preferred to prevent reflux and to facilitate absorption. Feedings are initiated in low concentrations and volumes and are gradually increased as tolerated. The nurse delivers feedings by means of a tube-feeding pump to maintain a constant volume and assesses for diarrhea frequency as a means of measuring tolerance (see Chapter 61).

Total Parenteral Nutrition. For optimal nutrition, hyperalimentation by TPN may be necessary in addition to tube feedings or as a single measure to provide nutrition. When central venous access is required, a Hickman catheter or other type of catheter may be necessary. Meticulous IV line care is an important nursing measure to prevent catheter sepsis. Sterile dressing changes and site observation are extremely important (see Chapter 14). The nurse also performs finger sticks to obtain blood for glucose measurements. These measurements help to monitor the client's pancreatic function and tolerance of dextrose in the solution. Additional nursing care measures for the client receiving TPN are given in Chapter 61.

OPERATIVE PROCEDURES. The Whipple procedure (radical pancreaticoduodenectomy) involves extensive surgical manipulation and is used to treat cancer of the head of the pancreas. The procedure entails removal of the proximal head of the pancreas, the duodenum, a portion of the jejunum, the stomach (partial or total gastrectomy), and the gallbladder, with anastomosis of the pancreatic duct (pancreaticojejunostomy), the common bile duct (choledochojejunostomy), and the stomach (gastrojejunostomy) to the jejunum (Figure 60-7). In addition, the surgeon may remove the spleen (splenectomy).

As a palliative measure to relieve biliary obstruction in the likelihood of extensive tumor invasion, a cholecystojejunostomy may be done as a bypass procedure.

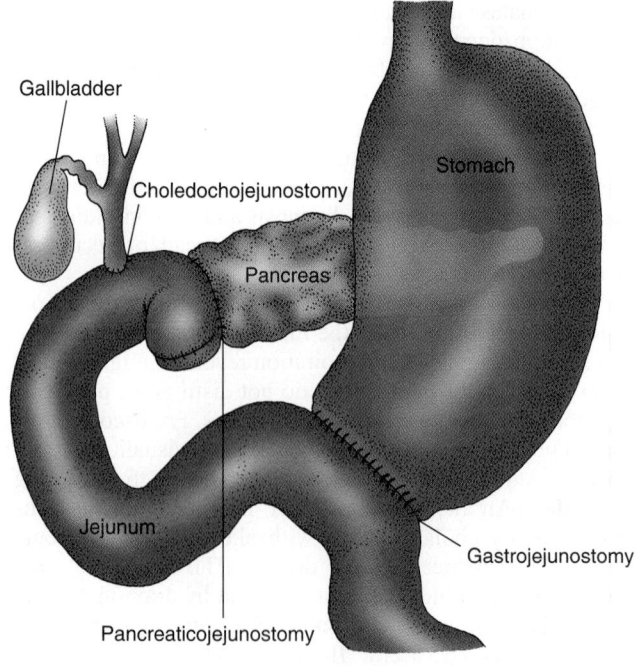

Figure 60-7 ● The three anastomoses that constitute the Whipple procedure: choledochojejunostomy, pancreaticojejunostomy, and gastrojejunostomy.

POSTOPERATIVE CARE. In addition to routine postoperative care measures, the client who has undergone a radical pancreaticoduodenectomy requires intensive nursing care and is usually admitted to a surgical critical care unit. The nurse assesses for potential complications of the Whipple procedure (Table 60-5).

Gastrointestinal Drainage Monitoring. The monitoring of gastrointestinal (GI) drainage and NG tube patency is an important aspect of postoperative nursing care. Drainage tubes are strategically placed during surgery to remove drainage and secretions from the area and to prevent stress on the anastomosis sites. The nurse assesses the tubes and drainage devices for undue stress or kinking and maintains the drainage tubes in a dependent position. The suction pressure gauge is checked frequently to maintain the desired suction level. Most often, Salem sump tubes are used and connected to low continuous suction (80 mm Hg or less) to maintain drain patency.

The nurse monitors the drainage for color, consistency, and amount. The drainage should be serosanguineous; the appearance of clear, colorless, bile-tinged drainage or frank blood with an increase in output may indicate disruption or leakage of an anastomosis site. Most of the disruptions of the anastomosis site occur within a week to 10 days after surgery. Hemorrhage can occur as an early or late complication.

If the NG tube is obstructed, the nurse instills air first. If this method does not keep the drainage lumen open, irrigation with 10 to 20 mL of normal saline is gently performed. If the problem continues, the nurse may need to notify the physician for additional interventions.

The development of a fistula (an abnormal passageway) is the most common and most serious postoperative complication. Biliary, pancreatic, or gastric fistulas result from partial or total breakdown of an anastomosis site. The secretions that drain from the fistula contain bile, pancreatic enzymes, or gastric secretions, depending on which anastomosis site is ruptured. These secretions, particularly pancreatic fluid, are corrosive and irritating to the skin, and internal leakage causes a chemical peritonitis. Peritonitis (inflammation and infection of the peritoneum) necessitates treatment with multiple antibiotics.

Positioning. The nurse places the client in the semi-Fowler's position to reduce stress on the suture line and anastomosis site, as well as to optimize lung expansion. Stress on the gastric suture line can be minimized by maintaining NG tube drainage at a low suction level to keep the remaining stomach (if a partial gastrectomy is done) or the jejunum (if a total gastrectomy is done) free of excessive fluid buildup and pressure. The NG tube is also used to reduce stimulation of the remaining pancreatic tissue.

Assessment of Fluids and Electrolytes. Because the Whipple procedure is extensive and can take 6 to 10 hours to complete, maintaining fluid and electrolyte balance can be difficult. Clients tend to experience significant intraoperative blood loss and postoperative bleeding. The intestine is exposed to air for long periods, and evaporation of fluid occurs. Significant losses of fluid and electrolytes occur from NG and other drainage tubes. In addition, these clients are usually malnourished and have low serum levels of protein and albumin, which maintain colloid osmotic pressure within the circulating system. Reduction in the serum osmotic pressure makes the client susceptible to third spacing of body fluids, with fluid moving from the intravascular to the interstitial space, resulting in shock.

For these reasons, the nurse closely monitors vital signs for decreased blood pressure and increased heart rate, decreased vascular pressures with a central venous line or pulmonary artery catheter (Swan-Ganz catheter), and decreased urine output to detect early signs of hypovolemia and prevent shock. The nurse is also alert for pitting edema of the extremities, dependent edema in the sacrum and back, and an intake that far exceeds output. Nutritional repletion via hyperalimentation and the administration of albumin promote the shift of fluid from the interstitial space back into the intravascular space.

Maintenance of ordered IV fluid volume replacement is important. The nurse monitors hemoglobin and hematocrit values to assess for blood loss and the need for blood transfusions. Electrolyte values are reviewed for decreased serum levels of sodium, potassium, chloride, and calcium. IV fluid concentrations must be altered to correct these electrolyte imbalances. The physician orders replacement of electrolytes as needed.

TABLE 60-5 • POTENTIAL COMPLICATIONS OF THE WHIPPLE PROCEDURE

CARDIOVASCULAR COMPLICATIONS
- Hemorrhage at anastomosis sites with hypovolemia
- Myocardial infarction
- Heart failure
- Thrombophlebitis

PULMONARY COMPLICATIONS
- Atelectasis
- Pneumonia
- Pulmonary embolism
- Acute respiratory distress syndrome
- Pulmonary edema

GASTROINTESTINAL COMPLICATIONS
- Adynamic (paralytic) ileus
- Gastric retention
- Gastric ulceration
- Bowel obstruction from peritonitis
- Pancreatitis
- Hepatic failure
- Thrombosis to mesentery

WOUND COMPLICATIONS
- Infection
- Dehiscence
- Fistulas: pancreatic, gastric, and biliary

METABOLIC COMPLICATIONS
- Unstable diabetes mellitus
- Renal failure

> **CRITICAL THINKING CHALLENGE**
>
> Your client had a Whipple procedure performed 3 days ago, and he has come to your unit from the surgical intensive care unit. He still has an NG tube to low suction and a wound drain in place.
> - What physical assessments need to be made initially on placement in your care unit?
> - Which postoperative complications would you assess the client for at this point?
> - What changes in nasogastric output might signify a complication? What should the normal output look like?
>
> For suggested answer guidelines, go to SIMON http://www.wbsaunders.com/SIMON/Iggy/.

Glucose Monitoring. Immediately after the Whipple procedure, the client may have transient hyperglycemia or hypoglycemia as a result of stress and surgical manipulation of the pancreas. Most of the endocrine cells (islets of Langerhans, responsible for insulin and glucose secretion) are located in the body and tail of the pancreas. In most clients, up to half of the gland remains, and diabetes does not develop; however, a large number of clients are diabetic before surgery. The nurse monitors glucose levels frequently during the early postoperative period and administers insulin injections, as prescribed.

▶ Community-Based Care

The client with pancreatic cancer is usually followed by a case manager, both in the hospital and in the home or other community-based setting. The role of the case manager is to ensure that the client receives cost-effective treatment and that his or her biopsychosocial needs are met.

▦ HEALTH TEACHING

When the client is discharged to home, many of the care measures are palliative and aimed at providing relief of symptoms such as pain. Care measures and teaching information are similar to those for clients with chronic pancreatitis.

In many cases, the diagnosis of pancreatic cancer is made a few months before death occurs. The client needs time to adjust to the diagnosis, which is usually made too late for cure or prolonged survival. The nurse helps the client identify what needs to be done to prepare for death. For example, the client may want to write a will or see family members and friends whom he or she has not seen recently. The client needs to make specific requests for the funeral or memorial service known to family members or significant others. These actions help the client prepare for death in a dignified manner. Chapter 9 discusses anticipatory grieving and preparation for death in detail.

▦ HOME CARE MANAGEMENT

The stage of progression of pancreatic carcinoma and available home care resources dictate whether the client can be discharged to home or whether additional care is needed in a skilled nursing facility or hospice. Home care preparations depend on the client's physical and activity limitations and should be tailored to his or her needs. The nurse needs to coordinate care with the client and whoever will be used as the care provider after discharge from the hospital—home care provider, hospice care provider, or extended care provider.

The client and family need emotional support to deal with issues related to this illness. The nurse assists family members in ascertaining realistically and objectively the amount of physical care required for the client. The family members must be told that their own physical and emotional health is at risk during this stressful period and that supportive counseling is indicated. If the family does not have a religious affiliation or a spiritual leader (e.g., a minister or a rabbi) to provide support, the nurse suggests alternative counseling options. It is appropriate for the nurse to make the initial contact or appointment according to the client's or family's wishes.

▦ HEALTH CARE RESOURCES

Regular home care nursing and assistive nursing personnel visits are scheduled to assist the client and family by providing physical, psychologic, and supportive care. The nurse supplies information about local hospice care (see Chapter 9) and cancer support groups.

ONLINE RESOURCES

For suggested readings and Internet resources, go to http://www. wbsaunders.com/SIMON/Iggy/.

SELECTED BIBLIOGRAPHY

Asterisk indicates a classic or definitive work on this subject.

Allen, K.M., & Phillips, J.M. (1997). *Women's health across the lifespan: A comprehensive perspective.* Philadelphia: J.B. Lippincott.

Amann, S.T., DiMagno, E., & Rubin, W. (1997). Pancreatitis: Diagnostic and therapeutic interventions. *Patient Care, 31*(11), 200-202, 205-212, 215-216.

*Ambrose, M.S., & Dreher, H.M. (1996). Pancreatitis: Managing a flare-up. *Nursing, 26*(4), 33-39.

American Cancer Society. (2000). *Cancer facts and figures—2000.* Report No. 00-300M-No.5008.00 Atlanta: Author.

*Bagg, A. (1988). Whipple's procedure: Nursing guidelines. *Critical Care Nurse 8*(5), 34-45.

Baillie, J. (1997). Treatment of acute biliary pancreatitis. *New England Journal of Medicine, 336*(4), 286-287.

Banks, P. (1997). Practice guidelines in acute pancreatitis. *American Journal of Gastroenterology, 92*(3), 377-386.

Barton-Burke, M. (1999). Gemcitabine: A pharmacologic and clinical overview. *Cancer Nursing, 22*(2), 176-183.

*Carson, C., Seidel, S., & Bushmiaer, M. (1996). Recovery from laparoscopic cholecystectomy procedures. *AORN Journal, 63*(6), 1099-1113.

*Conner, M., & Deane, D. (1995). Patterns of patient controlled analgesia and intramuscular analgesia. *Applied Nursing Research, 8*(2), 67-72.

Cooper, A.D. (1999). Bile salts: Metabolic, pathologic, and therapeutic considerations. *Gastroenterology Clinics of North America, 28*(1), xi, 1-245.

Coyne, P.J. (1998a). Pain control: Assessing and treating the pain of pancreatitis. *American Journal of Nursing, 98*(11), 14, 16.

Coyne, P.J. (1998b.) *Pancreatitis.* In M. McCaffery & C. Passero. (Eds.), *Pain: Clinical manual* (2nd ed.). St. Louis: Mosby.

Everhart, J.E., et al. (1999). Prevalence and ethnic differences in gallbladder disease in the United States. *Gastroenterology, 177*(3), 632-639.

*Fain, J.A., & Amato-Vealey, E. (1988). Acute pancreatitis: A gastrointestinal emergency. *Critical Care Nurse, 8*(6), 47-63.

Fischbach, F. (2000). *A manual of laboratory and diagnostic tests* (6th ed.). Philadelphia: J.B. Lippincott.

Greenberger, N., Isselbacher, K. (1998). Diseases of the gallbladder and bile ducts. In A.S. Fauci, C. Braunwald, & K.J. Isselbacher (Eds.), *Harrison's principles of internal medicine* (14th ed., p. 1504). New York: McGraw-Hill.

Greenberger, N., Toskes, P.P., & Isselbacher, K.J. (1998). Acute and chronic pancreatitis. In A.S. Fauci, C. Braunwald, & K.J. Isselbacher (Eds.), *Harrison's principles of internal medicine* (14th ed., pp. 1741-1752). New York: McGraw-Hill.

Held-Warmkessel, J., Volpe, H., & Waldman, A.R. (1998). Symptom management for patients with pancreatic cancer. *Clinical Journal of Oncology Nursing, 2*(4), 135-139.

Hoerner, M. (1998). Continuing education forum: Diagnosis and management of acute pancreatitis. *Journal of the American Academy of Nurse Practitioners, 10*(10), 471-477.

Howard, D.E., & Fromm, H. (1999). Nonsurgical management of gallstone Disease. *Gastroenterology Clinics of North America, 28*(1), 133-144.

Izbicki, J.R., et al. (1999). Surgical treatment of chronic pancreatitis and quality of life after operation. *Surgical Clinics of North America, 79*(4), 913-944.

Katz, J. (1997). Back to basics: Providing effective patient teaching. *American Journal of Nursing, 97*(5), 33-36.

*Kowdley, K. (1996). Update on therapy for hepatobiliary diseases. *Nurse Practitioner, 21*(7), 78-88.

Krumberger, J. (1999). Ask the experts: What is the most current recommendation for analgesic agents and pain management in patients with pancreatitis and other obstructive gastrointestinal disorders? *Critical Care Nurse, 19*(2), 110-111.

Levin, B. (1999). Gallbladder carcinoma. *Annals of Oncology, 10* (Suppl. 4), 129-130.

Lillemoe, K. (1998). Palliative therapy for pancreatic cancer. *Surgical Oncology Clinics of North America, 7*(1), 199-216.

Lillemoe, K., & Yeo, C. (1998). Management of the complications of pancreatitis. *Current problems in Surgery, 35,* 3-98.

Mayer, R. (1999). *Pancreatic cancer;* http://www.harrisononline.com.

McClave, S.A., et al. (1997). Comparison of the safety of early enteral vs parenteral nutrition in mild acute pancreatitis. *Journal of Parenteral and Enteral Nutrition, 21*(1), 14-20.

McCormick, M.E. (1999). Endoscopic retrograde cholangiopancreatography. *American Journal of Nursing, 99*(2), 24HH-JJ.

*McEwen, D., et al. (1996). Managing patients with pancreatic cancer. *AORN Journal, 64*(5), 716-734.

*McGrath, P., Sloan, D., & Kenady, D. (1996). Surgical management of pancreatic carcinoma. *Seminars in Oncology, 23*(2), 200-212.

Meissner, J.E. (1997). Disease review: Caring for patients with pancreatitis. *Nursing, 27*(10), 50-51.

Nahrwold, D.L. (1997). Gallstone disease: Update on diagnostic and therapeutic options. *Consultant, 37*(8), 2049-2052, 2057-2058.

National Institutes of Health. (1999). Gallstones; http://www.niddk.nih.gov/health/digest/pubs/gallstns/gallstns.htm.

Norton, I.D., & Petersen, B.T. (1999). Interventional treatment of acute and chronic pancreatitis: Endoscopic procedures. *Surgical Clinics of North America, 79*(4), 895-911, xii.

Nowazek, V. (1996). Nursing management of the patient with acute pancreatitis. In S.D. Ruppert, J.G. Kernicki, & J.T. Dolan (Eds.), *Dolan's critical care nursing* (2nd ed., pp. 832-847). Philadelphia: F.A. Davis.

Pagana, K.D., & Pagana, T.J. (1998). *Mosby's manual of diagnostic and laboratory tests,* St. Louis: Mosby.

Pasero, C. (1998). Assessing and treating the pain of pancreatitis. *American Journal of Nursing, 98*(11), 14, 16.

Peterson, A. (1997). Analgesics. *RN, 60*(4), 45-50.

*Pinto, K. (1996). Acalculous cholecystitis: A case report. *Nurse Practitioner, 21*(10), 120-122.

Price, S.A., & Wilson, L. (1997). *Pathophysiology: Clinical concepts of disease processes* (5th ed., pp. 376-383, 396-400). St. Louis: Mosby.

Runzi, M., & Layer, P. (1999). Nonsurgical management of acute pancreatitis: Use of antibiotics. *Surgical Clinics of North America, 79*(4), 759-765, xii.

Rutecki, G.W., & Whittier, F.C. (1998). Decision points in hypocalcemia: Is emergent therapy required? Complications may include tetany, seizures, and arrhythmias. *Journal of Critical Illness, 13*(2), 84-86, 89-90.

Sauter, P.K., & Coleman, J. (1999). Pancreatic cancer: A continuum of care. *Seminars in Oncology Nursing, 15*(1), 36-47.

Scolapio, J.S., Mahli-Chowla, N., & Ukleja, A. (1999). Nutrition supplementation in patients with acute and chronic pancreatitis. *Gastroenterology Clinics of North America, 28*(3), 695-707.

Simon, J.A. & Hudes, E.S. (1998). Serum ascorbic acid and other correlates of gallbladder disease among U.S. adults. *American Journal of Public Health, 88*(8), 1208-1212.

Simpson, J.P., Savarise, M.T., & Moore, J. (1999). Outpatient laparoscopic cholecystectomy: What predicts the need for admission? *American Surgeon, 65*(6), 525-528.

Snow, L.L., et al. (1999). Management of bile duct stones in 1527 patients undergoing laparoscopic cholecystectomy. *American Surgeon, 65*(6), 530-545.

*Steer, M.L., Waxman, I., & Freedman, S. (1995). Chronic pancreatitis. *New England Journal of Medicine, 332*(22), 1482-1490.

Strasberg, S. (1999). Laparoscopic biliary surgery. *Gastroenterology Clinics of North America, 28*(1), 117-130.

Thompson, D., et al. (1998). Estimated economic costs of obesity to U.S. business. *American Journal of Health Promotion, 13*(2), 120-127.

*Tierney, L.M., McPhee, S.J., & Papadakis, M.A. (1996). *Current medical diagnosis and treatment* (35th ed.). Stamford, CN: Appleton & Lange.

Tseng, M., Everhart, J.E., & Sandler, R.S. (1999). Dietary intake and gallbladder disease: A review. *Public Health Nutrition, 2*(2), 161-172.

Uhl, W., et al. (1999). The role of Octreotide and Somatostatin in acute and chronic pancreatitis. *Digestion, 60* (Suppl. 2), 22-30.

Understanding gallstone formation. (1999). *Nursing, 29*(4), 14.

Interventions for Clients with Malnutrition and Obesity

DONNA D. IGNATAVICIUS

Learning Objectives

After studying this chapter, you should be able to:

1. Identify three anthropometric measurements that the nurse can use to evaluate a client's nutritional status.
2. Explain the potential consequences and complications associated with malnutrition.
3. Describe the risk factors for malnutrition, especially for older adults.
4. Discuss the role of laboratory testing in the diagnosis of malnutrition.
5. Analyze assessment data to determine common nursing diagnoses for the client with malnutrition.
6. Identify expected outcomes for clients who are malnourished.
7. Describe the nursing care of clients receiving total enteral nutrition (TEN).
8. Prioritize nursing care for clients receiving total parenteral nutrition (TPN).
9. Identify complications associated with TPN.
10. Explain the potential consequences and complications associated with obesity.
11. Discuss the role of culture and gender as factors in the prevalence of obesity.
12. Identify the role of drug therapy in the management of obesity.
13. Develop a postoperative teaching plan for clients having a gastroplasty or intestinal bypass.

Go to http://www.wbsaunders.com/SIMON/Iggy/ for self-assessment questions related to these Learning Objectives.

Nutrition plays a major role in promoting and maintaining health. Nutritional health not only contributes to positive care outcomes but also saves health care dollars. As part of a comprehensive health assessment, the nurse should include nutritional screening to identify clients who have nutritional deficits or are at risk for developing nutritional deficits. Nurses may also conduct a complete nutritional assessment (Grindel & Costello, 1996).

NUTRITION STANDARDS

Dietary Planning

Several national standards are available for planning and evaluating nutrition. The standard most widely accepted in the United States is the Recommended Dietary Allowance (RDA), established in 1943 by the Food and Nutrition Board (FNB) of the National Research Council/National Academy of Sciences. The most current revision in 1989 establishes recommendations for energy intake, protein, vitamins, and minerals for a healthy population. Healthy adults require approximately 1800 calories/day and 0.8 g of protein/kg of body weight to meet basal energy needs.

The RDA can be used to estimate the adequacy of nutrient intake over time. If a client does not meet 100% of the RDA, it is incorrect to assume that he or she is nutritionally deficient. The

risk of inadequate intake for any nutrient is not presumed to be increased until less than 70% of the RDA is consumed. It is also incorrect to assume that all clients in a specific population who meet 100% of the RDA are not at risk for malnutrition.

The FNB, with the involvement of Health Canada, has recommended Dietary Reference Intakes (DRI) replace the RDA. The first DRI released recommended the intake of nutrients related to bone health (Food and Nutrition Board, 1997). The established standard of Canada, the Recommended Nutrient Intake (RNI), is similar to that of the United States.

Disease Prevention and Health Promotion

The role of diet and nutrition in disease has been a subject of interest for many years. The current focus is on health promotion and the prevention of disease. In 1995, the Dietary Guidelines for Americans were revised by the U.S. Department of Agriculture (USDA) and the U.S. Department of Health and Human Services (DHHS). These seven guidelines emphasize the importance of selecting foods to maintain a healthful diet with balance, moderation, and variety (Figure 61-1). One of the most noticeable changes from previous editions occurs in the weight guideline. For the first time, diet and physical activity are emphasized in the second guideline with the goal of maintaining or improving body weight (Kennedy, Meyers, & Layden, 1996).

The Nutrition Recommendations for Canadians (Table 61-1) are similar to the Dietary Guidelines for Americans. In addition, they recommend limiting the caffeine content of the diet to no more than the equivalent of four cups of coffee per day, as well as adding fluoride to community water supplies to a level of 1 mg/L.

The USDA developed the Food Guide Pyramid in 1992 to translate food recommendations into a practical graphic format (Figure 61-2). A pyramid format was chosen to communicate three key dietary principles: variety, moderation, and proportionality. The pyramid design emphasizes building the diet on a base of grains, fruits, and vegetables. Moderate quantities of lean meats, protein sources, and dairy products are added, and the intake of fats and sweets is limited. This guide to daily food choices has replaced the basic four food groups as the standard for evaluating the nutritional adequacy of dietary intake. Table 61-2 suggests the daily servings of each food group and clarifies the size of a serving. Adhering to this pattern results in a nutritionally adequate intake if a variety of foods is chosen.

A variety of vegetarian diet patterns are being adopted by increasing numbers of people for health, environmental, and moral reasons. The **lacto-vegetarian** eats milk, cheese, and dairy foods but avoids meat, fish, poultry, and eggs. The **lacto-ovo-vegetarian** also includes eggs. The **vegan** eats only foods of plant origin. Vegans can develop megaloblastic anemia as a result of vitamin B_{12} deficiency. Vegans should include a daily source of vitamin B_{12} in their diets, such as a fortified breakfast cereal, fortified soy beverage, or meat analog (Messina & Burke, 1997). All vegetarians should ensure that they get adequate amounts of calcium, iron, zinc, and vitamins D and B_{12}. Well-planned vegetarian diets can provide adequate nutrition. The Vegetarian Food Pyramid, endorsed by the Vegetarian Resource Group, can assist vegetarians with daily food choices (Figure 61-3).

NUTRITIONAL ASSESSMENT

Malnutrition and obesity are common nutrition problems that occur as progressive changes within the client. When nutritional deficiencies or excesses develop, the body adapts through the use of homeostatic mechanisms. As the intake moves farther away from the accepted range, however, the body accommodates by reducing functional levels or changing the status or size of the affected body compartments. The nutritional status of a client can be determined by the presence or absence of these adaptations.

Nutritional status reflects the balance between nutrient requirements and nutrient intake. Factors affecting nutrient requirements include disease, infection, and psychologic stress. Nutrient intake is influenced by disease, eating behavior, economic factors, emotional stability, medication, and cultural factors.

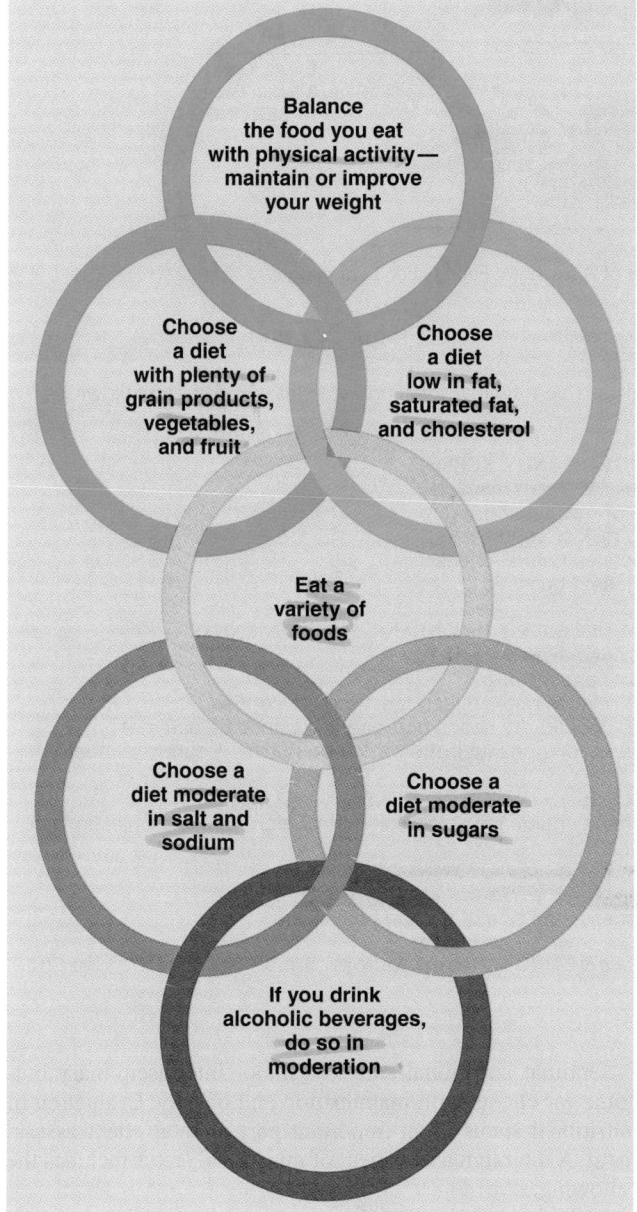

Figure 61-1 ● Dietary guidelines developed by the U.S. Department of Agriculture and the U.S. Department of Health and Human Services.

TABLE 61-1 • NUTRITION RECOMMENDATIONS FOR CANADIANS

- The sodium content of the Canadian diet should be reduced.
- The Canadian diet should include no more than 5% of total energy as alcohol, or two drinks daily, whichever is less.
- The Canadian diet should contain no more caffeine than the equivalent of four cups of regular coffee per day.
- Community water supplies containing less than 1 mg/L of fluoride should be fluoridated to that level.
- The Canadian diet should provide energy consistent with the maintenance of body weight within the recommended range.
- The Canadian diet should include essential nutrients in amounts specified in the Recommended Nutrient Intake.
- The Canadian diet should include no more than 30% of energy as fat (33 g/1000 kcal or 39 g/5000 kJ) and no more than 10% as saturated fat (11 g/1000 kcal or 13 g/5000 kJ).
- The Canadian diet should provide 55% of energy as carbohydrates (138 g/1000 kcal or 165 g/5000 kJ) from a variety of sources.

From Communications/Implementation Committee, Minister of National Health and Welfare. (1990). *Action towards healthy eating: Canada's guidelines for healthy eating and recommended strategies for implementation.* Cat. No. H39-166/1990E. Ottawa: Branch Publications Unit.

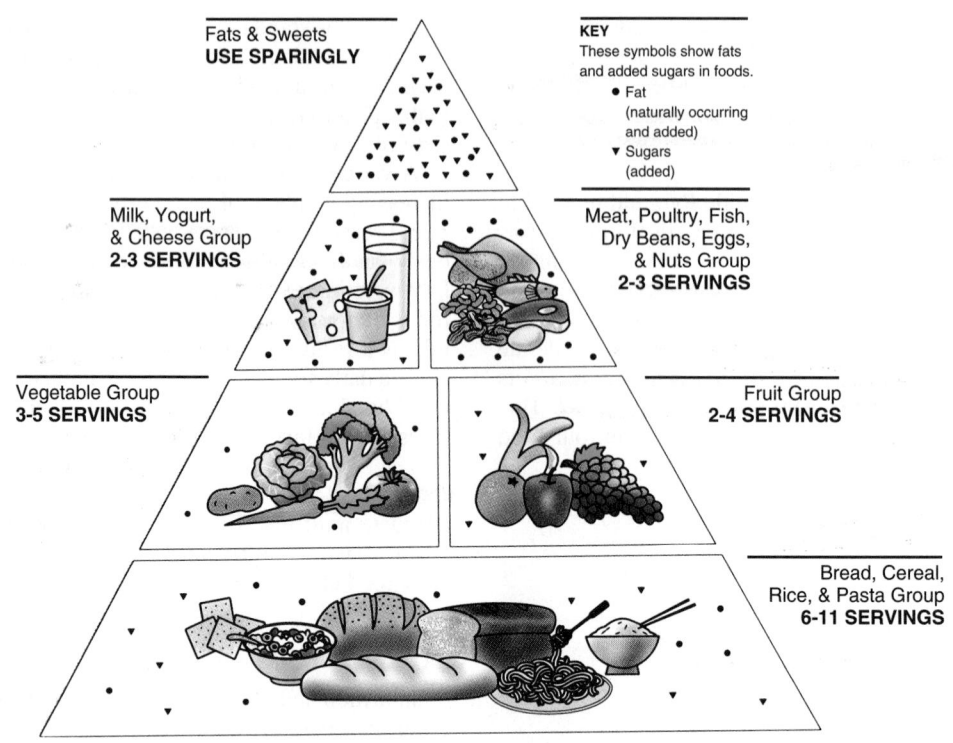

Figure 61-2 ● The U.S. Department of Agriculture Food Guide Pyramid.

TABLE 61-2 ● SERVING SIZES FOR EACH FOOD GROUP

With the Food Guide Pyramid, what counts as a "serving" may not always be a typical "helping" of what you eat. The following are some examples of servings.

BREAD, CEREAL, RICE, AND PASTA
6 to 11 servings recommended
Examples of one serving:
- 1 slice of bread
- 1 ounce ready-to-eat cereal
- ½ cup cooked cereal, rice, or pasta

VEGETABLES
3 to 5 servings recommended
Examples of one serving:
- 1 cup raw leafy vegetables
- ½ cup other vegetables, cooked or chopped raw
- ¾ cup vegetable juice

FRUITS
2 to 4 servings recommended
Examples of one serving:
- 1 medium apple, banana, or orange
- ½ cup chopped, cooked, or canned fruit
- ¾ cup fruit juice

MILK, YOGURT, AND CHEESE
2 to 3 servings recommended
Examples of one serving:
- 1 cup milk or yogurt
- 1½ ounces natural cheese
- 2 ounces processed cheese

MEAT, POULTRY, FISH, DRY BEANS, EGGS, AND NUTS
2 to 3 servings recommended
Examples of one serving:
- 2 to 3 ounces cooked lean meat, poultry, or fish
- ½ cup cooked dry beans or 1 egg = 1 ounce of lean meat
- 2 tablespoons peanut butter or ⅓ cup nuts = 1 ounce of meat

HOW MUCH IS AN OUNCE OF MEAT?
Here is a handy guide for determining the weight of meat, chicken, fish, or cheese:
- 1 ounce = the size of a matchbox
- 3 ounces = the size of a deck of cards
- 8 ounces = the size of a paperback book

Modified from Nutrition and your health: Dietary guidelines for Americans. (1995). *Home and Garden Bulletin No. 232* (4th ed.). Washington, D.C.: U.S. Department of Agriculture, U.S. Department of Health and Human Services.

CULTURAL CONSIDERATIONS

Lactose intolerance (inability to tolerate milk and milk products) is a relatively common condition that occurs in a number of ethnic groups. It is found in more than 66% of Mexican Americans and 79% of African Americans, as well as in some Native American tribes, Asian Americans, and Ashkenazic Jews (Giger & Davidhizar, 1999). A small percentage of Caucasians are also lactose intolerant. The cause of lactose intolerance is an insufficient amount of the lactase enzyme, which converts lactose into absorbable glucose.

Optimal nutritional care is a major interdisciplinary outcome for clients with malnutrition and obesity. Evaluation of nutritional status is an important part of total client assessment. A thorough assessment of nutritional status includes the following:

- Review of the diet history
- Food and fluid intake record
- Laboratory data
- Food-medication interactions
- Physical examination and health history

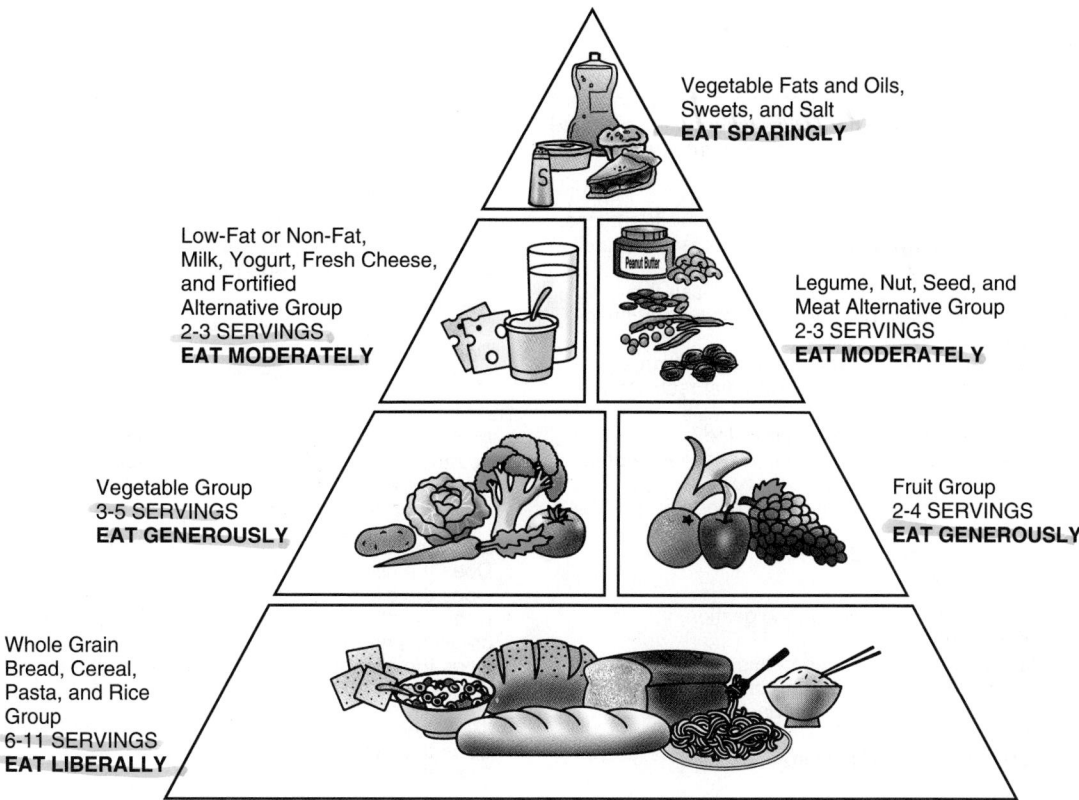

Figure 61-3 ● Food pyramid for a vegetarian diet. (Courtesy The Health Connection.)

- Anthropometric measurements
- Psychosocial assessment

Monitoring the nutritional care of a client is as important as the initial assessment. The health care provider, nurse, and dietitian collaborate to identify clients at risk for nutritional problems.

Initial Nutritional Screening

Not every client needs a complete nutritional assessment, but it is important to identify clients at risk for nutritional problems through screening. An initial nutritional screening provides the nurse with an inexpensive, quick way of determining which clients need more extensive nutritional assessment by the health care provider and dietitian.

The initial nutritional screening includes visual inspection, measured height and weight, weight history, usual eating habits, ability to chew and swallow, and any recent changes in appetite or food intake. Questions that may alert the nurse to clients at risk for nutritional problems can be incorporated into the history and physical assessment (Chart 61-1).

CONSIDERATIONS FOR OLDER ADULTS

Nutritional screening can take place in the home, ambulatory care setting, hospital, or nursing home. The Nutrition Screening Manual for Professionals Caring for Older Americans (1991) is a multidisciplinary project of the American Dietetic Association, the American Academy of Family Physicians, and the National Council on the Aging. The goal of this 5-year initiative was to use a collaboration of health care pro-

fessionals to promote routine nutrition screening to older Americans in all community health and medical care settings. Risk factors for malnutrition in older adults include inappropriate intake, poverty, social isolation, dependency or disability, acute or chronic diseases or conditions, and chronic medication use. The Nutrition Screening initiative developed a three-tiered approach to nutrition screening:

1. The *DETERMINE* Your Nutritional Health Checklist to alert older adults about the warning signs for poor nutritional health (Figure 61-4)
2. The Level I screen developed for use by professionals in health or social service settings, such as adult day-care centers, congregate meal programs, and assisted-living facilities
3. The Level II screen developed for use in medical settings such as acute care hospitals, physicians' offices, and long-term care facilities.

Another nutritional assessment tool, the Mini Nutritional Assessment (MNA), has recently been designed and tested worldwide to provide a single, rapid assessment of older adults in ambulatory care, hospitals, and nursing homes (Vellas et al., 1999). The MNA can be completed in about 10 minutes; a low score indicates malnutrition or a risk for malnutrition.

Anthropometric Measurements

Anthropometric measurements are noninvasive methods of evaluating nutritional status. These measurements include height and weight and assessment of body fat.

CHART 61-1

BEST PRACTICE *for*
Initial Nutrition Screening Assessment

The presence of one or more of the following conditions should alert the nurse that the client is at risk for malnutrition or has had a condition in the past requiring special nutritional care.

General
- Does the client have any conditions that cause nutrient loss, such as malabsorption syndromes, draining abscesses, wounds, fistulas, or protracted diarrhea?
- Does the client have any conditions that increase the need for nutrients, such as fever, burn, injury, sepsis, or antineoplastic therapies?
- Has the client been on NPO status for 3 days or more?
- Is the client receiving a modified diet or a diet restricted in one or more nutrients?
- Is the client being enterally or parenterally fed?
- Does the client describe food allergies, lactose intolerance, or limited food preferences?
- Has the client experienced a recent, unexplained weight loss?
- Is the client taking medications, either prescription, over-the-counter, or herbal/natural products?

Gastrointestinal
- Does the client complain of nausea, indigestion, vomiting, diarrhea, or constipation?
- Does the client exhibit glossitis, stomatitis, or esophagitis?
- Does the client have difficulty chewing or swallowing?
- Does the client have a partial or total gastrointestinal obstruction?
- What is the client's state of dentition?

Cardiovascular
- Does the client have ascites or edema?
- Is the client able to perform activities of daily living?
- Does the client have congestive heart failure?

Genitourinary
- Does fluid input approximately equal fluid output?
- Does the client have an ostomy?
- Is the client hemodialyzed or peritoneally dialyzed?

Respiratory
- Is the client receiving mechanical ventilatory support?
- Is the client receiving oxygen via nasal prongs?
- Does the client have chronic obstructive pulmonary disease (COPD) or asthma?

Integumentary
- Does the client have nail or hair changes?
- Does the client have rashes or dermatitis?
- Does the client have dry or pale mucous membranes or decreased skin turgor?
- Does the client have pressure areas on the sacrum, hips, or ankles?

Extremities
- Does the client have pedal edema?
- Does the client exhibit cachexia?

Modified with permission of Ross Products Division, Abbott Laboratories, Columbus, OH.
NPO, Nothing by mouth.

■ MEASUREMENT OF HEIGHT AND WEIGHT

Height and weight provide a baseline determination of nutritional status. The nurse or assistive nursing personnel obtains accurate measurements, because clients who report their own measurements tend to overestimate height and underestimate weight. Subsequent measurements may indicate an early change in nutritional status.

■ Height

Clients should be measured and weighed while wearing minimal clothing and no shoes. The nurse or assistive nursing personnel determines the client's height in inches or centimeters with the measuring stick of a weight scale. The client should stand erect and look straight ahead, with the heels together and the arms at the sides.

CONSIDERATIONS FOR OLDER ADULTS
Some older adults may have difficulty standing erect, and their actual height may be less than their height on recall. If height cannot be measured directly, it should be estimated by arm span or with use of a knee-height caliper, which provides a more precise height estimate.

■ Weight

The nurse or assistive nursing personnel weighs ambulatory clients with an upright balance beam scale. Nonambulatory clients can be weighed with a movable wheelchair balance beam scale or a bed scale. The manufacturer should calibrate weight scales twice yearly to ensure accurate readings. For daily or sequential weights, the nurse or assistive nursing personnel notes the time and obtains the weight at the same time each day, if possible. Conditions such as heart failure and renal disease affect fluid balance and, therefore, weight.

Normal weights for adult men and women are shown in the Metropolitan Life tables (Table 61-3). The latest U.S. Department of Agriculture (USDA) and U.S. Department of Health and Human Services (DHHS) Dietary Guidelines contain weight guidelines that emphasize both weight maintenance and weight loss. The same healthy weight guideline applies to all adults. Older adults are no longer permitted a higher weight standard. The weight range appears in the guidelines as a chart with three categories: healthy weight, moderate overweight, and severe overweight (Figure 61-5). Either the Metropolitan Life tables or the New Weight Guidelines from the USDA and the DHHS may be used for comparison with a client's height and weight. Some health care professionals prefer the Metropolitan Life tables because they consider body build differences by gender.

Changes in body weight can be expressed by three different formulas:

1. Weight as a percentage of ideal body weight (IBW):

$$\%IBW = \frac{Current\ weight \times 100}{Ideal\ weight}$$

2. Current weight as a percentage of usual body weight (UBW):

$$\%UBW = \frac{Current\ weight \times 100}{Usual\ weight}$$

3. Change in weight:

$$Weight\ change = \frac{Usual\ weight - Current\ weight}{Usual\ weight} \times 100$$

The Warning Signs of poor nutritional health are often overlooked. Use this checklist to find out if you or someone you know is at nutritional risk.

DETERMINE YOUR NUTRITIONAL HEALTH

Read the statements below. Circle the number in the yes column for those that apply to you or someone you know. For each yes answer, score the number in the box. Total your nutritional score.

	YES
I have an illness or condition that made me change the kind and/or amount of food I eat.	2
I eat fewer than 2 meals per day.	3
I eat few fruits or vegetables, or milk products.	2
I have 3 or more drinks of beer, liquor or wine almost every day.	2
I have tooth or mouth problems that make it hard for me to eat.	2
I don't always have enough money to buy the food I need.	4
I eat alone most of the time.	1
I take 3 or more different prescribed or over-the-counter drugs a day.	1
Without wanting to, I have lost or gained 10 pounds in the last 6 months.	2
I am not always physically able to shop, cook and/or feed myself.	2
TOTAL	

Total Your Nutritional Score. If it's —

0-2   **Good!** Recheck your nutritional score in 6 months.

3-5   **You are at moderate nutritional risk.** See what can be done to improve your eating habits and lifestyle. Your office on aging, senior nutrition program, senior citizens center or health department can help. Recheck your nutritional score in 3 months.

6 or more   **You are at high nutritional risk.** Bring this checklist the next time you see your doctor, dietitian or other qualified health or social service professional. Talk with them about any problems you may have. Ask for help to improve your nutritional health.

Remember that warning signs suggest risk, but do not represent diagnosis of any condition. Turn the page to learn more about the Warning Signs of poor nutritional health.

These materials developed and distributed by the Nutrition Screening Initiative, a project of:

AMERICAN ACADEMY OF FAMILY PHYSICIANS

 THE AMERICAN DIETETIC ASSOCIATION

 NATIONAL COUNCIL ON THE AGING, INC.

Figure 61-4 ● "DETERMINE Your Nutritional Health" checklist used to alert older adults to the warning signs of poor nutritional health. (Courtesy The Nutrition Screening Initiative, Washington, D.C.)

Continued

**The Nutrition Checklist is based on the Warning Signs described below.
Use the word <u>DETERMINE</u> to remind you of the Warning Signs.**

Disease

Any disease, illness or chronic condition which causes you to change the way you eat, or makes it hard for you to eat, puts your nutritional health at risk. Four out of five adults have chronic diseases that are affected by diet. Confusion or memory loss that keeps getting worse is estimated to affect one out of five or more of older adults. This can make it hard to remember what, when or if you've eaten. Feeling sad or depressed, which happens to about one in eight older adults, can cause big changes in appetite, digestion, energy level, weight and well-being.

Eating Poorly

Eating too little and eating too much both lead to poor health. Eating the same foods day after day or not eating fruit, vegetables, and milk products daily will also cause poor nutritional health. One in five adults skip meals daily. Only 13% of adults eat the minimum amount of fruit and vegetables needed. One in four older adults drink too much alcohol. Many health problems become worse if you drink more than one or two alcoholic beverages per day.

Tooth Loss/ Mouth Pain

A healthy mouth, teeth and gums are needed to eat. Missing, loose or rotten teeth or dentures which don't fit well or cause mouth sores make it hard to eat.

Economic Hardship

As many as 40% of older Americans have incomes of less than $6,000 per year. Having less—or choosing to spend less—than $25-30 per week for food makes it very hard to get the foods you need to stay healthy.

Reduced Social Contact

One third of all older people live alone. Being with people daily has a positive effect on morale, well-being and eating.

Multiple Medicines

Many older Americans must take medicines for health problems. Almost half of older Americans take multiple medicines daily. Growing old may change the way we respond to drugs. The more medicines you take, the greater the chance for side effects such as increased or decreased appetite, change in taste, constipation, weakness, drowsiness, diarrhea, nausea, and others. Vitamins or minerals when taken in large doses act like drugs and can cause harm. Alert your doctor to everything you take.

Involuntary Weight Loss/Gain

Losing or gaining a lot of weight when you are not trying to do so is an important warning sign that must not be ignored. Being overweight or underweight also increases your chance of poor health.

Needs Assistance in Self Care

Although most older people are able to eat, one of every five have trouble walking, shopping, buying and cooking food, especially as they get older.

Elder Years Above Age 80

Most older people lead full and productive lives. But as age increases, risk of frailty and health problems increase. Checking your nutritional health regularly makes good sense.

 The Nutrition Screening Initiative • 1010 Wisconsin Avenue, NW • Suite 800 • Washington, DC 20007

The Nutrition Screening Initiative is funded in part by a grant from Ross Laboratories, a division of Abbott Laboratories.

Figure 61-4, cont'd ● "DETERMINE Your Nutritional Health" checklist used to alert older adults to the warning signs of poor nutritional health. (Courtesy The Nutrition Screening Initiative, Washington, D.C.)

TABLE 61-3 • METROPOLITAN LIFE HEIGHT AND WEIGHT TABLES

Height*		Weight†			Height*		Weight†		
Feet	Inches	Small Frame	Medium Frame	Large Frame	Feet	Inches	Small Frame	Medium Frame	Large Frame
MEN					**WOMEN**				
5	2	128-134	131-134	138-150	4	10	102-111	109-121	118-131
5	3	130-136	133-143	140-153	4	11	103-113	111-123	120-134
5	4	132-138	135-145	142-156	5	0	104-115	113-126	122-137
5	5	134-140	137-148	144-160	5	1	106-118	115-129	125-140
5	6	136-142	139-151	146-164	5	2	108-121	118-132	128-143
5	7	138-145	142-154	149-168	5	3	111-124	121-135	131-147
5	8	140-148	145-157	152-172	5	4	114-127	124-138	134-151
5	9	142-151	148-160	155-176	5	5	117-130	127-141	137-155
5	10	144-154	151-163	158-180	5	6	120-133	130-144	140-159
5	11	146-157	154-166	161-184	5	7	123-136	133-147	143-163
6	0	149-160	157-170	164-188	5	8	126-139	136-150	146-167
6	1	152-164	160-174	168-192	5	9	129-142	139-153	149-170
6	2	155-168	164-178	172-197	5	10	132-145	142-156	152-173
6	3	158-172	167-182	176-202	5	11	135-148	145-159	155-176
6	4	162-176	171-187	181-207	6	0	138-151	148-162	158-179

Reprinted courtesy of Metropolitan Life Insurance Company, 1983.
*Shoes with 1-inch heels.
†Weight in pounds. Men: allow 5 pounds of clothing. Women: allow 3 pounds of clothing

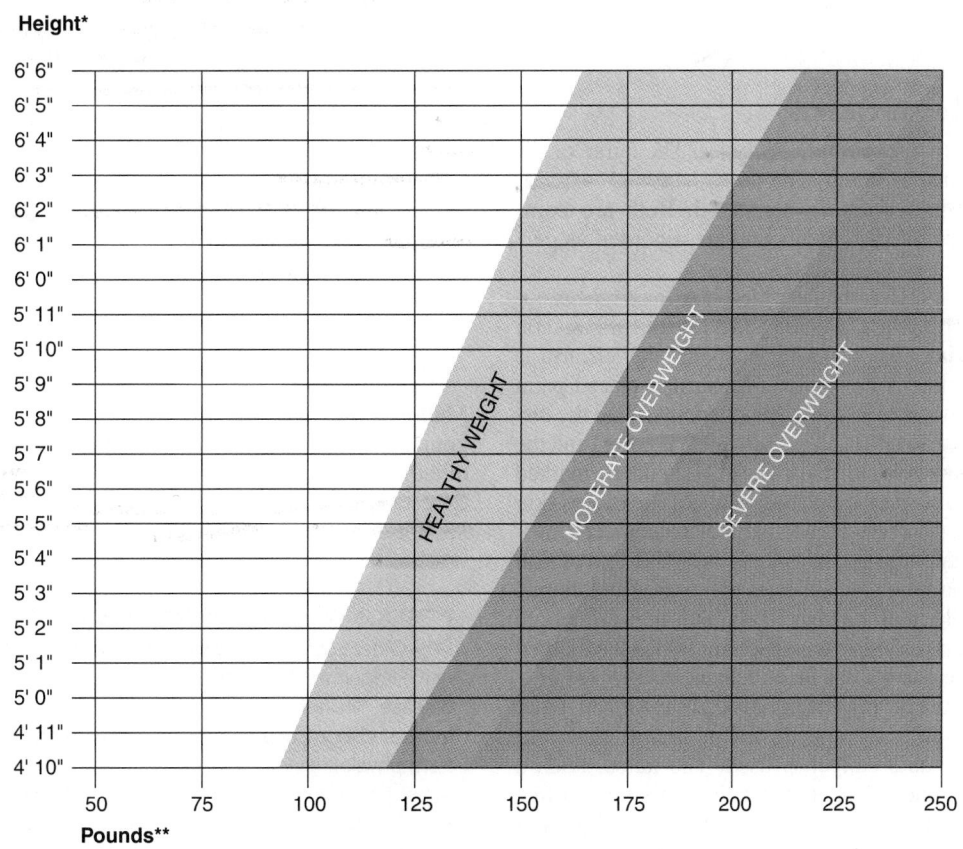

* Without shoes.
** Without clothes. The higher weights apply to people with more muscle and bone, such as many men.

Figure 61-5 ● The U.S Department of Agriculture and the U.S. Department of Health and Human Services guidelines for determining proper weight or degree of obesity. (Redrawn from http://www.nalusda.gov/fnic/Dietary/9dietgui.htm.)

An involuntary weight loss of 10% at any time significantly affects nutritional status. Weights may need to be taken daily, several times a week, or weekly for monitoring status and the effectiveness of nutritional support.

ASSESSMENT OF BODY FAT
Body Mass Index

The body mass index (BMI), or Quetelet index, is a measure of nutritional status that does not depend on frame size. The BMI indirectly estimates total fat stores within the body by the relationship of weight to height:

$$BMI = \frac{Weight\ (kg)}{Height^2\ (m^2)}$$

A simpler calculation for estimating BMI can be programmed into handheld computers:

$$BMI = \frac{Weight\ (lb)}{Height^2\ (inches^2)} \times 705$$

BMI can also be determined using a nomogram. The least risk of death from malnutrition is associated with scores between 20 and 25 (Mahan & Escot-Stump, 1996). BMIs above and below these values are associated with increased health risks. Older, healthy adults should have a BMI between 24 and 27.

Skin Fold Measurements

Skin fold measurements estimate body fat. The nurse or dietitian may measure the client. The triceps and subscapular skin folds are most commonly measured. Both are compared with standard measurements and are recorded as percentiles.

The nurse or dietitian can measure the triceps skin fold thickness by using a tape measure to locate and mark the midpoint on the client's upper arm. To obtain the midpoint, the left arm is bent 90 degrees at the elbow, and the forearm is placed palm down across the middle of the body. The midpoint is half the distance between the tip of the shoulder (acromion process) and the tip of the elbow (olecranon process). The skin should be marked at this point before any measurements are made. The triceps skin fold is measured on the back of the left arm over the triceps muscle at the marked midpoint. The nurse holds a double fold of skin and subcutaneous adipose tissue between the fingers and thumb. The skin fold is held until the jaws of the skin fold caliper are placed perpendicular to the length of the skin fold at the marked midpoint. The nurse records this measurement.

Subscapular skin fold thickness indirectly estimates body fat. The body position is the same as for triceps skin fold thickness, and the same caliper is used. The nurse holds a double fold of skin and subcutaneous adipose tissue in a line from the inferior angle of the left scapula to the left elbow, applies the calipers, and records the measurement.

Arm Circumference

The midarm circumference (MAC) can be obtained to measure muscle mass and subcutaneous fat. To measure MAC, the nurse or dietitian places a flexible tape around the arm at the same marked midpoint used to measure skin fold thickness, taking care to hold the tape firmly but gently to avoid compressing the tissue. This measurement is recorded in centimeters. The midarm muscle mass (MAMM) measures the amount of muscle in the body and is a more sensitive indicator of protein reserves. It can be computed from the MAC and the triceps skin fold measure.

MALNUTRITION
OVERVIEW

Carbohydrates, protein, and fat supply the body with energy. Under healthy conditions, the majority of this energy undergoes digestion and is absorbed from the gastrointestinal tract. Food energy is used to maintain body temperature, respiration, cardiac output, muscle function, protein synthesis, and the storage and metabolism of food sources.

Energy balance refers to the relationship between energy expended and energy stored. When energy expended exceeds energy intake, energy stores are used to supply the deficit; this results in weight loss. Body proteins are used for energy when calorie intake is insufficient. The body attempts to meet its calorie requirements even if it is at the expense of protein needs.

Many severely ill or traumatized hospitalized clients are at risk for **protein-calorie malnutrition (PCM),** also known as protein-energy malnutrition (PEM). PCM may present in three forms: marasmus, kwashiorkor, and marasmic-kwashiorkor. **Marasmus** is generally a calorie malnutrition in which body fat and protein are wasted. Serum proteins are often preserved. **Kwashiorkor** is a lack of protein quantity and quality in the presence of adequate calories. Body weight is more normal, and serum proteins are low. **Marasmic-kwashiorkor** is a combined protein and energy malnutrition. This problem often presents clinically when metabolic stress is imposed on a chronically starved client. The outcome of unrecognized or untreated PCM is often dysfunction or disability and increased morbidity and mortality.

Pathophysiology

Malnutrition is a multinutrient problem because foods that are good sources of calories and protein are also good sources of other nutrients. In the malnourished client, protein catabolism exceeds protein intake and synthesis, resulting in negative nitrogen balance, weight loss, decreased muscle mass, and weakness.

> ### CONSIDERATIONS FOR OLDER ADULTS
> Older adults are at a high risk for poor nutrition due to cognitive impairments, complicated physical conditions, or chronic disease. Malnutrition in older adults has been associated with increased complications from infections and slower recovery from physiologic stresses such as surgical wounds, bone fractures, pressure ulcers, and loss of functional capacity (Anderson, 2000). PCM has been shown to be a strong independent risk factor for 1-year posthospital discharge mortality.

The functional ability of the liver, heart, lungs, gastrointestinal tract, and immune system diminishes in the client with malnutrition. A decrease in serum proteins (**hypoproteinemia**) occurs as protein synthesis in the liver decreases. Vital capacity is also reduced as a result of respiratory muscle atrophy; cardiac output diminishes. Malabsorption occurs because of atrophy of gastrointestinal mucosa and the loss of intestinal villi.

Other complications of severe malnutrition in adults include the following:

- Leanness and cachexia (muscle wasting)
- Decreased effort tolerance
- Lethargy
- Intolerance to cold
- Edema
- Dry, flaking skin and various types of dermatitis
- Poor wound healing and a higher than usual number of infections, particularly postoperative infection

Etiology

Malnutrition results from inadequate nutrient ~~in~~creased nutrient losses, and increased nutrient re~~quirements~~. Inadequate nutrient intake can be linked to pov~~erty~~, education, substance abuse, decreased appetite, a ~~change~~ in functional ability to eat independently. Infecti~~ons~~ such as tuberculosis and human immunodefi~~ciency~~ (HIV) infection, are also precipitating factors i~~n dis~~eases that produce diarrhea and respiratory an ~~infec~~tions leading to anorexia result in negative calo~~rie~~ balance; anorexia then leads to poor food in~~take that~~ leads to decreased absorption with increased ~~losses.~~ Medical treatments such as chemotherapy can ~~impair~~ nutrition. In addition, catabolic processes incr~~ease re~~quirements and metabolic losses.

Inadequate nutrient intake can also result ~~in clients~~ admitted to the hospital or nursing home (D~~udek, 2000). De~~creased staffing may not allow time for clie~~nts to be~~ fed, especially older adults who may eat s~~lowly (Dudek,~~ 2000). Many diagnostic tests and surgery require a period of having nothing by mouth (NPO).

Unrecognized dysphagia is a common problem in nursing homes and can cause malnutrition, dehydration, and aspiration pneumonia. A study by Kayser-Jones and Pengilly (1999) found that 45 of 82 residents in one nursing home had some degree of dysphagia (difficulty swallowing) ranging from mild to profound. Only 10 of the 45 residents had been referred for dysphagia evaluation by a speech-language pathologist.

Eating disorders, such as anorexia nervosa and bulimia nervosa, also lead to malnutrition. **Anorexia nervosa** is a self-induced starvation resulting from a fear of fatness, even though the client is underweight. **Bulimia nervosa** is characterized by episodes of binge eating in which the client ingests a large amount of food in a short time. The binge eating is followed by some form of purging behavior, such as self-induced vomiting and/or an excessive use of laxatives and diuretics. If not treated, death can result from starvation, infection, or suicide. Information about eating disorders can be found in textbooks on mental health nursing.

Incidence/Prevalence

Malnutrition is present in many hospitalized clients (Dudek, 2000). In a review of eight studies with more than 1347 hospitalized adults, 40% to 55% were determined to be malnourished or at risk for malnutrition, and up to 12% were severely malnourished. Malnourished clients heal more slowly, suffer more complications, and have a higher mortality rate. Surgical clients with a likelihood of malnutrition were two to three times more likely to experience minor and major complications and excess mortality. Length of hospitalization in mal-

nourished medical-surgical clients can be extended by as much as 90%, which clearly increases health care costs (Gallagher-Allred et al., 1996).

The prevalence of PCM in long-term care facilities has been reported to range from 10% to 85% (Anderson, 2000). In one study, the prevalence of malnutrition in 100 clients admitted consecutively to a skilled nursing facility was 39%. The highest prevalence of malnutrition was found in clients admitted from acute care hospitals (Nelson et al., 1993).

Acute PCM may develop in clients who were adequately nourished before hospitalization if they experience starvation while in a catabolic state from infection, stress, or injury. ~~Chronic~~ PCM can occur in clients who have cancer, end-stage ~~renal disease, or chronic~~ neurologic disease.

CULTURAL CONSIDERATIONS

In Western countries, cultural factors do not seem to have a major influence on the development of malnutrition. However, newly arriving immigrants from developing countries may be at risk for malnutrition because of limited food supplies, poverty, and eating habits.

In the Native American population of the United States, poor nutrition has also been directly related to several leading causes of death, including heart disease and cirrhosis of the liver. The diets of many Native American tribes continue to be inadequate in protein, calcium, and vitamins A and C. These deficiencies may result from an unavailability of or a lack of money to purchase foods that are high in these nutrients (Giger & Davidhizar, 1999).

▶ COLLABORATIVE MANAGEMENT

SIMON
Activity Link

● Assessment

▦ HISTORY

The nurse reviews the medical history to determine the diagnosis, possibility of increased metabolic needs or nutritional losses, chronic disease, recent surgery of the gastrointestinal tract, drug and alcohol abuse, and recent, significant weight loss. Each of these conditions can contribute to malnutrition. For older adults, the nurse also explores mental status deterioration, poor eyesight or hearing, diseases affecting major organs, constipation or incontinence, slowed reactions, a review of prescription and over-the-counter medications (including herbal and natural supplements), and physical disabilities.

CHART 61-2

NURSING FOCUS on the OLDER ADULT
Risk Assessment for Malnutrition

- Recognize that clinical manifestations of malnutrition may not be apparent because they are similar to physiologic changes associated with aging (e.g., dry skin, decreased muscle tone, dry hair).
- Assess body weight and compare it with the usual body weight or ideal body weight.
- Be aware that multiple chronic diseases, especially gastrointestinal disorders such as malabsorption syndromes, predispose the client to malnutrition.
- Assess the client's financial ability to buy healthy food.
- Assess the client's physical and mental ability to prepare food.
- Inspect the client's oral cavity for the presence of teeth or dentures, gum disease, or oral lesions that could affect food intake.
- Review the client's medications, including prescription and over-the-counter (OTC) drugs. Many drugs interact with food or cause anorexia or nausea.
- Use the DETERMINE checklist and Level I or II screen, if appropriate.

For clients who live independently, the nurse or occupational therapist assesses the performance of instrumental activities of daily living (IADLs). Functional status can best be evaluated for institutionalized clients by assessing their performance of activities of daily living (ADLs). An inability to perform any of the eight IADLs or any of the six ADLs indicates a high level of dependence and the potential for disease and poor nutritional status (*Nutrition Screening Manual*, 1991). When functional status is evaluated with nutritional status, there appears to be a strong predictability of infections and complications among institutionalized adults. Chapter 10 describes functional assessment in detail.

The nurse interviews the client to obtain information about his or her usual daily food intake, eating behaviors, change in appetite, and recent weight changes. The client is asked to describe the usual foods eaten daily and the times of meals and snacks. This information is then compared with the Food Guide Pyramid for gross deficiencies. The dietitian can more thoroughly analyze the diet, if necessary.

The nurse explores with the client any changes in eating habits as a result of illness. Any change in appetite, taste, and weight loss is recorded. A weight loss of 5% or more in 30 days, a weight loss of 10% in 6 months, or a weight that is below ideal body weight is significant for malnutrition.

Difficulty or pain in chewing or swallowing is also assessed. The nurse asks the client whether any foods are avoided and why. The occurrence of nausea, vomiting, heartburn, or any other symptoms of discomfort with eating is also recorded. Finally, the client is asked about dental health problems, including the presence of dentures. Dentures or partial plates that do not fit well interfere with food intake.

■ PHYSICAL ASSESSMENT/CLINICAL MANIFESTATIONS

The nurse assesses for signs and symptoms of various nutrient deficiencies (Table 61-4). The nurse inspects the client's hair, eyes, oral cavity, nails, and musculoskeletal and neurologic systems. The condition of the skin, including any red-

TABLE 61-4 • SIGNS AND SYMPTOMS OF NUTRIENT DEFICIENCIES

Sign/Symptom	Potential Nutrient Deficiency
HAIR	
Alopecia	Zinc, essential fatty acids
Easy pluckability	Protein, essential fatty acids
Lackluster hair	Protein, zinc
"Corkscrew" hair	Vitamin C, vitamin A
Decreased pigmentation	Protein, copper
EYES	
Xerosis of conjunctiva	Vitamin A
Corneal vascularization	Riboflavin
Keratomalacia	Vitamin A
Bitot's spots	Vitamin A
GASTROINTESTINAL TRACT	
Nausea, vomiting	Pyridoxine
Diarrhea	Zinc, niacin
Stomatitis	Pyridoxine, riboflavin, iron
Cheilosis	Pyridoxine, iron
Glossitis	Pyridoxine, zinc, niacin, folic acid, vitamin B_{12}
Magenta tongue	Riboflavin
Swollen, bleeding gums	Vitamin C
Fissured tongue	Niacin
Hepatomegaly	Protein
SKIN	
Dry and scaling	Vitamin A, essential fatty acids, zinc
Petechiae/ecchymoses	Vitamin C, vitamin K
Follicular hyperkeratosis	Vitamin A, essential fatty acids
Nasolabial seborrhea	Niacin, pyridoxine, riboflavin
Bilateral dermatitis	Niacin, zinc
EXTREMITIES	
Subcutaneous fat loss	Calories
Muscle wastage	Calories, protein
Edema	Protein
Osteomalacia, bone pain, rickets	Vitamin D
Arthralgia	Vitamin C
HEMATOLOGIC	
Anemia	Vitamin B_{12}, iron, folic acid, copper, vitamin E
Leukopenia, neutropenia	Copper
Low prothrombin time, prolonged clotting time	Vitamin K, manganese
NEUROLOGIC	
Disorientation	Niacin, thiamine
Confabulation	Thiamine
Neuropathy	Thiamine, pyridoxine, chromium
Paresthesia	Thiamine, pyridoxine, vitamin B_{12}
CARDIOVASCULAR	
Congestive heart failure, cardiomegaly, tachycardia	Thiamine
Cardiomyopathy	Selenium

Used with permission of Ross Products Division, Abbott Laboratories, Columbus, OH.

dened or open areas, is observed. The anthropometric measurements previously described may also be obtained. The nurse or assistive nursing personnel monitors all food and fluid intake, observes the client at mealtime, and notes any mouth pain or difficulty in chewing or swallowing.

■ PSYCHOSOCIAL ASSESSMENT

The psychosocial history provides information about the client's economic status, occupation, educational level, living and cooking arrangements, and mental status. The nurse determines whether financial resources are adequate for providing the necessary food. If resources are inadequate, the social worker may refer the client to available community services.

■ LABORATORY ASSESSMENT

Routine laboratory tests provide additional information about nutritional status. These tests supply objective data that can support subjective data and identify preclinical deficiencies. Laboratory tests must be carefully interpreted with regard to the total client; an isolated value may yield an inaccurate conclusion.

HEMATOLOGY. Hemoglobin is measured to detect iron deficiency anemia. A low hemoglobin level may indicate anemia, recent hemorrhage, or hemodilution caused by fluid retention. Hemoglobin may be low secondary to conditions such as low serum albumin, infection, catabolism, or cancer. High hemoglobin levels may indicate hemoconcentration or dehydration, or they may be secondary to liver disease.

Hematocrit, a measure of cell volume, indicates iron status. Low hematocrit levels may reflect anemia, hemorrhage, excessive fluid, renal disease, or cirrhosis. High hematocrit levels may indicate dehydration or hemoconcentration.

PROTEIN STUDIES. Serum albumin, transferrin, and thyroxine-binding prealbumin can be measured in the laboratory. Serum albumin indicates the body's protein status but is not sensitive enough to detect early changes in nutritional status. The normal serum albumin level for men and women is greater than 3.5 g/dL. Table 61-5 indicates the level of protein depletion based on the serum albumin level.

Serum **transferrin,** an iron-transport protein, can be measured directly or calculated as an indirect measurement of total iron-binding capacity (TIBC) as follows:

$$\text{Calculated transferrin} = (0.68 \times \text{TIBC}) + 21$$

Serum transferrin has a shorter half-life of 8 to 10 days and therefore is a more sensitive indicator of protein status than is albumin. Table 61-6 indicates the level of protein depletion based on serum transferrin level.

Thyroxine-binding **prealbumin (PAB)** provides a more sensitive indicator of protein deficiency because of its short half-life of 2 days. Depending on the laboratory test used, the normal PAB range is 17 to 40 mg/dL. PAB can also assess improvement in nutritional status with refeeding; levels can increase by 1 mg/dL/day with adequate nutritional support. However, this test is expensive, and its cost may be prohibitive except at large facilities.

SERUM CHOLESTEROL. Cholesterol levels normally range between 160 and 200 mg/dL in adult men and women. Values are typically low with malabsorption, liver disease, pernicious anemia, terminal stages of cancer, sepsis, or stress. A cholesterol level below 160 mg/dL has been identified as a possible indicator of malnutrition.

TABLE 61-5 • METHOD OF ASSESSING VISCERAL PROTEIN MASS FROM SERUM ALBUMIN LEVELS	
When Serum Albumin (mg/dL) Is	**The Level of Visceral Protein Depletion Is**
>3.5	None
2.8-3.5	Mild
2.1-2.7	Moderate
<2.1	Severe

Modified with permission of Ross Products Division, Abbott Laboratories, Columbus, OH.
NOTE: Because the half-life of serum albumin is relatively long (about 20 days), albumin indicates initial visceral protein status but is not sensitive enough for detecting early changes in nutritional status.

TABLE 61-6 • METHOD OF ASSESSING VISCERAL PROTEIN MASS FROM SERUM TRANSFERRIN LEVELS	
Serum transferrin is measured or calculated from total iron-binding capacity (TIBC) by the following equation:	
Calculated transferrin = (0.68 TIBC) + 21	
When Serum Transferrin (mg/dL) Is	**The Level of Visceral Protein Depletion Is**
>200	None
151-200	Mild
100-150	Moderate
<100	Severe

Modified with permission of Ross Products Division, Abbott Laboratories, Columbus, OH.
NOTE: Serum transferrin has a half-life of approximately 8 days and therefore reflects acute changes in visceral protein status. The disadvantage of measuring serum transferrin is that the test is not routinely available in many clinical laboratories. Several formulas have been derived to calculate serum transferrin from TIBC, a measurement that is more readily available. However, measured transferrin is more accurate and is preferable when possible.

OTHER LABORATORY TESTS. Total lymphocyte count (TLC) can be used to assess immune function. Malnutrition suppresses the immune system and leaves the client more vulnerable to infection. When a client is malnourished, the TLC is usually decreased below 1500 mm³ (Bender et al., 2000).

● Analysis

■ COMMON NURSING DIAGNOSES AND COLLABORATIVE PROBLEMS

The most common diagnosis for the client with malnutrition is Imbalanced Nutrition: Less Than Body Requirements related to inadequate food intake or increased nutrient requirements.

■ ADDITIONAL NURSING DIAGNOSES AND COLLABORATIVE PROBLEMS

In addition to the common nursing diagnosis, clients with malnutrition may have one or more of the following:

- Risk for Impaired Skin Integrity related to depleted protein stores
- Risk for Infection related to suppressed immune system
- Risk for Disturbed Body Image related to physical changes from weight loss

Some clients with malnutrition are at risk for collaborative problems such as the following:

- Anemia
- Immunocompromised state

▶ Planning and Implementation

▓ IMBALANCED NUTRITION: LESS THAN BODY REQUIREMENTS

NOC **PLANNING: EXPECTED OUTCOMES.** The client with malnutrition is expected to (1) demonstrate an adequate nutrient intake, (2) maintain body mass and weight within normal limits (WNL), and (3) maintain laboratory values WNL (e.g., albumin).

INTERVENTIONS. The preferred route for feeding is through the gastrointestinal tract because it enhances the immune system and is safer, easier, less expensive, and more physiologically sound (Chart 61-3).

NIC **NUTRITION MANAGEMENT.** In collaboration with the health care provider and dietitian, the nurse provides high-calorie, high-protein foods (e.g., milkshakes, cheese and crackers). A feeding schedule of six small meals benefits many clients. If the client has difficulty chewing or is edentulous (toothless), a pureed or dental soft diet may facilitate food intake.

Malnourished ill clients often need to be encouraged to eat. The nurse provides a quiet environment, which is conducive to eating. Some clients, especially older adults, may take a long time to eat even small quantities of food.

Restorative feeding programs help nursing home residents who need special assistance. These residents eat in a separate dining area so that time and attention can be given to them. Chart 61-4 offers additional interventions to increase nutritional intake for older adults in any setting.

DRUG THERAPY. Medications may be given to some clients to stimulate appetite. For example, cyproheptadine (Periactin), an antihistamine, may be ordered for clients who are underweight, especially those with eating disorders. Megestrol acetate (Megace), an antineoplastic drug, may be used to increase appetite in clients who have cachexia, acquired immunodeficiency syndrome (AIDS), or unexplained weight loss. The mechanism for how these drugs work to increase appetite is unknown.

PARTIAL ENTERAL NUTRITION. The dietitian calculates the nutrients required daily and translates these requirements into meals for the client. If the client cannot ingest sufficient nutrients as food, **partial enteral nutrition** with fortified medical nutritional supplements (MNSs) (e.g., Ensure or Carnation Instant Breakfast) may be given, especially for older adults. Many commercial enteral products are available. For clients with medical diagnoses such as liver and renal disease, special products that meet their needs are also available. The client must enjoy the taste of the product for acceptability and optimal intake.

> ### ✤ CONSIDERATIONS FOR OLDER ADULTS
> Supplements used in acute care, long-term care, and home care are costly. In addition, older adults may refuse them, and the supplements are then wasted. Bender at al. (2000) found that a more successful alternative to having the MNS distributed by food service or nursing assistant staff in the nursing home was to have the supplements delivered by nurses during their usual medication passes. In this study, the nurses gave 60 mL or more of the MNS at least four times a day with the clients' medications. The subjects increased weight and had fewer pressure ulcers, thus making the program very cost-effective.

Nutritional supplements are supplied as liquid formulas, powders, bars, and puddings in a variety of flavors. They come in different degrees of sweetness and are also available as modular supplements that provide single nutrients. Examples of modular supplements are Polycose for carbohydrates and ProPac for protein. Carbohydrate modulars are useful only if additional calories are needed. Protein modulars are indicated when metabolic stress causes a need for higher protein intake.

The nurse bases adequate daily fluid intake on 30 mL of fluid per kilogram of body weight. This recommendation is

---

CHART 61-3

NIC **INTERVENTION ACTIVITIES for The Client with Malnutrition**

Nutrition Management: *Assisting with or providing a balanced dietary intake of foods and fluids*
- Ascertain client's food preferences.
- Determine, in collaboration with the dietitian, as appropriate, number of calories and type of nutrients needed to meet nutrition requirements.
- Encourage increased intake of protein, iron, and vitamin C, as appropriate.
- Offer snacks (e.g., frequent drinks, fresh fruits/fruit juice), as appropriate.
- Adjust diet to client's lifestyle, as appropriate.
- Weigh client at appropriate intervals.
- Encourage client to wear properly fitted dentures and/or acquire dental care.
- Assist client in receiving help from appropriate community nutritional programs, as needed.

NIC intervention activities selected from McCloskey, J.C., & Bulechek, G.M. (Eds.). (2000). *Nursing intervention classification (NIC)* (3rd ed.). St. Louis: Mosby. No part of this work is to be altered without prior written permission from the Publisher.

CHART 61-4

NURSING FOCUS *on the* **OLDER ADULT**
Promoting Nutritional Intake

- Observe the client during meals for food intake.
- Ask the client about food likes and dislikes.
- Encourage self-feeding, or feed the client slowly.
- Create an environment that is conducive to eating and socialization and relaxation, if possible.
- Serve snacks with activities, especially in long-term care settings.
- Document the percentage of food eaten at each meal and snack.
- Ensure that meals are visually appealing, appetizing, and properly prepared.
- Review the client's medication profile and discuss with the health care provider the use of drugs that may be suppressing appetite.
- If the client is depressed, be sure that the depression is treated by the health care provider.

not for clients with severe cardiac problems or fluid restrictions. The health care provider may also prescribe vitamin and mineral supplements.

The nurse or assistive nursing personnel maintains a daily calorie count and fluid intake to assess whether the client can meet the goals of nutritional therapy. The dietitian usually asks the nursing staff to keep the food intake record for at least 3 consecutive days. Accurate daily or weekly weights are also essential depending on the amount of depletion.

TOTAL ENTERAL NUTRITION. Clients often cannot meet the goals of nutritional therapy through their usual oral intake because of increased metabolic demands or a decreased ability to eat. In such cases, enteral tube feeding may be necessary to supplement oral intake or to provide total nutritional support.

CANDIDATES FOR TOTAL ENTERAL NUTRITION. Clients likely to receive **total enteral nutrition (TEN)** can be divided into three groups:

- Clients who can eat but cannot maintain adequate nutrition by oral intake of food alone
- Clients who have permanent neuromuscular impairment and cannot swallow
- Clients who do not have permanent neuromuscular impairment but are critically ill and cannot eat because of their condition

Clients in the first group are often older adults or clients receiving cancer treatment who cannot meet their calorie and protein needs (see the Legal/Ethical Issues in Health Care box below). Clients in the second group usually have permanent swallowing problems and require some type of feeding tube for delivery of the enteral product on a long-term basis. Examples of conditions that can cause permanent swallowing problems are strokes, severe head trauma, and advanced multiple sclerosis. Clients in the third group receive enteral nutrition for as long as their illness lasts. The feeding is discontinued when the client improves and can eat again. Total enteral nutrition is contraindicated for clients with diffuse peritonitis, severe pancreatitis, intestinal obstruction, intractable vomiting or diarrhea, and paralytic ileus (Bowers, 1996).

TYPES OF ENTERAL PRODUCTS. Many commercially prepared enteral products are available. An appropriate combination of carbohydrates, fat, vitamins, minerals, and trace elements is available in liquid form. Differences among products allow the dietitian to select the right formula for each client. An order from the health care provider is required for enteral nutrition, but the dietitian usually makes the recommendation and computes the amount and type of product needed for each client.

METHODS OF ADMINISTRATION OF TOTAL ENTERAL NUTRITION. TEN is administered as "tube feedings" through one of the available gastrointestinal tubes, either via a **nasoenteric tube (NET)** or an **enterostomal tube.**

Types of Tubes. A nasoenteric tube is any feeding tube inserted nasally and then advanced into the gastrointestinal tract. Commonly used NETs include the **nasogastric (NG) tube** and the **nasoduodenal tube (NDT).** A nasojejunal tube (NJT) is also available but is used less often than the other NETs. NDTs and NJTs are usually indicated for critically ill clients at risk for aspiration or delayed stomach emptying.

NETs are used for delivering short-term enteral feedings because they are easy to use and are safer for the client at risk for aspiration *if* the tip of the tube is placed below the pyloric sphincter of the stomach. Small-bore polyurethane or silicone tubes from 8 to 12 French external diameter are preferred over large-bore plastic or latex tubes. The smaller tubes are more comfortable and are less likely to cause complications such as nasal irritation, sinusitis, tissue erosion, and pulmonary compromise.

Enterostomal feeding tubes are used for clients who need long-term enteral feeding. The most common types are gastrostomies and jejunostomies. The physician directly accesses the gastrointestinal tract using various surgical, endoscopic, and laparoscopic techniques.

A **gastrostomy** is a stoma created from the abdominal wall into the stomach through which a short feeding tube is inserted by the physician. The gastrostomy may require a small abdominal incision or may be placed endoscopically; these tubes are called **percutaneous endoscopic gastrostomy (PEG)** or dual access gastrostomy-jejunostomy (PEG/J) tubes. The PEG does not require general anesthesia and is more secure and more durable than traditional gastrostomies. An alternative to either device is the **low-profile gastrostomy device (LPGD).** The LPGD is available with a firm or balloon-style internal bumper or retention disk. An antireflux valve keeps gastrointestinal contents from leaking onto the skin. This device is less irritating to the skin, longer lasting, and more cosmetically pleasing, and it allows greater client independence. However, skin-level devices do not allow easy access for checking residuals.

Jejunostomies are used less often than gastrostomies. A **jejunostomy** is used for long-term feedings when it is desirable to bypass the stomach, such as with gastric disease, upper gastrointestinal obstruction, and abnormal gastric or duodenal emptying.

ℒEGAL/ ℰTHICAL ℐSSUES IN HEALTH CARE

TOTAL ENTERAL NUTRITION FOR OLDER ADULTS

Total enteral nutrition provides a client's total daily nutrient and fluid requirements. In some cases, this artificial nutrition and hydration may not be desired by the older adult. For example, some clients have advance directives that state they do not want to be kept alive by artificial nutrition and hydration if certain conditions exist. However, questions arise when clients are not able to make their wishes known.

For many years it was believed that withholding food and fluids would cause discomfort. Recent cancer research indicates that clients who do not eat and drink do not suffer and in fact may be more comfortable if food and fluids are withheld. The decision to feed is complex, and there is no clear right or wrong answer. To compound this dilemma, medical complications (e.g., aspiration, pressure ulcers) are common in older adults who are tube fed.

When clinicians are making decisions about the desirability of tube feedings in these cases, the focus should be on achieving consensus by:

- Reviewing what is known about tube feedings, especially their risks and benefits
- Reviewing the medical facts about the client
- Investigating any available evidence that would help understand the client's wishes
- Obtaining the opinions of all stakeholders in the situation
- Delaying any action until consensus is achieved

Data from Daly, B.J. (2000). Special challenges of withholding artificial nutrition and hydration. *Journal of Gerontological Nursing. 26*(9), 25–31.

Types of Feedings. Tube feedings are administered by bolus feeding, continuous feeding, and cyclic feeding. **Bolus feeding** is an intermittent feeding of a specified amount of enteral product at specified times during a 24-hour period—typically every 4 hours. This method can be accomplished manually or by infusion through a mechanical pump or controller device. A more popular method of tube feeding is continuous enteral feeding. **Continuous feeding** is similar to IV therapy in that small amounts are continuously infused (by gravity drip or by a pump or controller device) over a specified time. **Cyclic feeding** is the same as continuous feeding except that the infusion is stopped for a specified time in each 24-hour period, usually 6 to 10 or more hours ("down time"). Down time typically occurs in the morning to allow bathing, bed making, and other treatments.

Infusion rates for continuous and cyclic feedings (and to some extent for intermittent bolus feeding) vary with the total amount of solution to be infused, the specific composition of the product, and the response of the client to the procedure.

The health care provider and dietitian usually decide the type, rate, and method of tube feeding, as well as the amount of additional water needed. If the client can swallow small amounts of food, he or she may also eat orally while the tube is in place.

The nurse is responsible for the care and maintenance of the feeding tube and the enteral feeding. Chart 61-5 lists the major nursing interventions for the client receiving an enteral feeding.

COMPLICATIONS OF TOTAL ENTERAL NUTRITION.

The nurse is responsible for the prevention, assessment, and management of complications associated with tube feeding. Some complications of therapy result from the type of tube used to administer the feeding, and other complications result from the enteral product itself. The most common problem associated with feeding tubes is the development of a clogged tube. Chart 61-6 lists nursing interventions for maintaining a patent tube.

A less common but more serious complication is dislodgement of the tube. Several techniques should be used to confirm proper placement. An x-ray study is the most accurate confirmation method and should always be done on initial tube insertion. After the initial placement is confirmed, the nurse checks the placement before each intermittent feeding or at least every 8 hours during continuous or cyclic feeding.

The traditional auscultatory method is not reliable, especially for clients with small-bore tubes (see the Evidence-Based Practice for Nursing box on p. 1371). In this method, the nurse instills 20 to 30 mL of air into the tube while listening over the stomach with a stethoscope. The whooshing sound that results does not guarantee correct tube placement. The nurse should instead aspirate a sample of the gastrointestinal content, observe its color, and test its pH. When aspirating fluid, the nurse waits at least 1 hour following medication administration, then flushes the tube with 20 mL of air to clear it. The aspirate is collected and tested with pH paper. The pH of gastric fluid ranges from 0 to 4.0. If the tube has migrated down into the intestines, the pH will be between 7.0 and 8.0. If the tube is in the lungs, the pH will be greater than 6.0 (Metheney at al., 1998). The pH may also be as high as 6 if the client takes certain medications, such as H_2 blockers (e.g., ranitidine [Zantac] and famotidine [Pepcid]).

CHART 61-5

BEST PRACTICE *for*
Tube Feeding Care and Maintenance

- If nasogastric or nasoduodenal feeding is ordered, use a soft, flexible, small-bore feeding tube (smaller than 12 French). The initial placement of the tube should be confirmed by x-ray study. Secure the tube with tape or a commercial attachment device after applying a skin protectant; change the tape regularly.
- Check tube placement by x-ray study when the correct position of the tube is in question; an x-ray study is the only reliable method. Checking the pH of the aspirant is a useful adjunct. Other traditional methods for determining tube placement have not proved to be reliable (see the Evidence-Based Practice for Nursing box on p. 1371).
- If a gastrostomy or jejunostomy tube is used, assess the insertion site for signs of infection or excoriation (e.g., excessive redness and drainage). Rotate the tube 360 degrees each day and check for in-and-out play of about $\frac{1}{4}$ in (0.5 cm). If the tube cannot be moved, notify the health care provider immediately, because the retention disk may be embedded in the tissue. Cover the site with a dry sterile dressing, and change the dressing at least once a day.
- Check and record the residual volume every 4 hours by aspirating stomach contents into a syringe. If residual feeding is obtained, check the physician's order for the appropriate intervention (usually to slow or stop the feeding for a time).
- Check the feeding pump or controller device (if used) to ensure proper mechanical operation.
- Ensure that the prescribed enteral product is infused at the ordered rate (mL/hr).
- Change the feeding bag and tubing every 24 hours; label the bag with the date and time of the change. Use an irrigation set for no more than 24 hours.
- For continuous or cyclic feeding, add only 4 hours of product to the bag each time to prevent bacterial growth; a closed system may be used for 24 hours.
- To prevent aspiration, keep the head of the bed elevated at least 30 degrees during the feeding and for 1 hour after the feeding.
- Monitor laboratory values, especially blood urea nitrogen (BUN), serum electrolytes, hematocrit, albumin, prealbumin, and glucose.
- Monitor for complications of tube feeding, especially diarrhea.
- Monitor and carefully record the client's weight and intake and output.

CHART 61-6

BEST PRACTICE *for*
Maintaining a Patent Feeding Tube

- Flush the tube with 30 to 60 mL of water (amount usually ordered by the health care provider or dietitian):
    At least every 4 hours during a continuous tube feeding
    Before and after each intermittent tube feeding
    Before and after medication administration (use warm water)
    After checking residual volume
- If the tube becomes clogged, use 30 mL of water for flushing, applying gentle pressure with a 50-mL piston syringe.
- Avoid the use of carbonated beverage, except for existing clogs *when water is not effective.* Do not use cranberry juice.
- Whenever possible, use liquid medications instead of crushed tablets.
- Do not mix medications with the feeding product. Crush tablets as finely as possible and dissolve in warm water.
- Consider use of automatic flush feeding pump such as Flexiflo, Quantum, or Kangaroo.

EVIDENCE-BASED PRACTICE
FOR NURSING

What is the best way to determine whether a nasogastric tube is in the right place?

Metheney, N., et al. (1998). pH, color, and feeding tubes. *RN, 61*(1), 25-27.

Next to x-ray studies, pH testing of aspirate is the most dependable method of confirming tube placement. In this study, the researchers aspirated gastrointestinal fluid from more than 1000 feeding tubes in acutely ill clients with new tubes. The pH of gastric contents ranged between 0 and 4. When the tube was in the small intestine, the pH increased to 7. The researchers also found that the color of gastric contents was different from aspirates from the pulmonary system or intestines. Gastric fluid was green, tan, off-white, bloody, or brown, whereas duodenal samples were a medium to golden yellow. Aspirates from the tracheobronchial tree in clients whose tubes were malpositioned were off-white in color and heavily tinged with mucus.

Critique. For more than 10 years the primary author of this study has been researching the most reliable methods for confirming proper placement of nasogastric tubes. This study replicated previous findings and added the assessment of color as another tool. A large sample of homogeneous clients was used to help generalize conclusions.

Implications for Nursing. The researchers clearly demonstrated that pH and color are more reliable indicators for ensuring proper placement of nasoenteric tubes than the auscultatory method, although the latter is common practice in clinical agencies. Nurses should use all of these methods to prevent enteral feeding into the lungs.

Fluid Imbalances. Clients receiving enteral nutrition therapy are at an increased risk for fluid imbalances. Clients who receive this therapy are often older or debilitated and may also have cardiac or renal problems. Fluid imbalances associated with enteral nutrition are usually related to the body's response to increased serum osmolarity.

Increased Osmolarity. Osmolarity is the amount or concentration of particles dissolved in solution. This concentration exerts a specific osmotic pressure within the solution. Normal osmolarity of extracellular fluid (ECF) ranges between 270 and 300 mOsm. Enteral feeding products range in osmolarity from isotonic (about 300 mOsm) to extremely hypertonic (600 mOsm). Electrolytes (including sodium) contribute to this hypertonicity, but more of the osmolarity is determined by the concentration of proteins and sugar molecules in the enteral product. Even when the product is isotonic, the ECF can become hyperosmolar unless some hypotonic fluids are also administered to the client. This situation is most likely to develop in clients who are unconscious, unable to respond to the thirst reflex, on fluid restrictions, or receiving hyperosmotic enteral preparations.

An increase in the osmolarity of the plasma increases the osmotic pressure of the plasma. Because this increased osmolarity is largely a result of extra glucose and proteins (which tend to remain in the plasma rather than move to interstitial spaces), the plasma osmotic pressure (water-pulling pressure) is increased. In this situation, intracellular and interstitial water move into and expand the plasma volume. This volume expansion results in an increased renal excretion of water (among clients with normal renal function) and leads to osmotic dehydration. If clients do not have normal renal and cardiac function, the expansion of the plasma volume can lead to circulatory overload and the formation of pulmonary edema, especially in older adults. The nurse assesses for signs and symptoms of circulatory overload and collaborates with the dietitian and physician in planning the correct amount of fluid to be provided to the client.

Dehydration. Excessive diarrhea may develop when hyperosmolar enteral preparations are delivered quickly. This situation can also lead to dehydration through excessive water loss. The nurse consults with the health care provider and dietitian for recommendations to prevent diarrhea.

First, the dietitian usually changes the feeding to a more iso-osmolar formula. Most of these formulas can be started full-strength but slowly at 15 to 20 mL/hr. The rate is gradually increased as the client tolerates and as the expected nutritional outcome is achieved. If diarrhea continues, the client should be evaluated for *Clostridium difficile* and its toxins.

In some cases, diarrhea may be the result of liquid medications, such as elixirs and suspensions that have a very high osmolality. Examples include acetaminophen, digoxin, furosemide, phenytoin, and potassium chloride. Clients receiving multiple liquid medications need to be evaluated to determine if their drug regimen can be changed to prevent diarrhea. Diluting these liquids may also be an option.

Another cause of diarrhea-related fluid imbalance among clients receiving enteral feeding preparations is lactose intolerance. Clients receiving milk-based enteral feeding preparations may become lactose intolerant. Most commercial enteral products, such as Ensure, are lactose free.

Vines et al. (1992) conducted a comprehensive review of research on diarrhea related to tube feeding. They concluded that diarrhea often results from bacterial contamination, and they implemented interventions for decreasing this risk.

Electrolyte Imbalances. Depending on the client's state of health, certain electrolyte imbalances can be avoided. This is achieved by the use of enteral preparations containing lower concentrations of the electrolytes that the client cannot handle well.

In addition to the client's specific electrolyte imbalances, the two most common electrolyte imbalances associated with enteral nutrition therapy are hyperkalemia and hypernatremia. Both of these conditions may be related to hyperglycemia-induced hyperosmolarity of the plasma and the resultant osmotic diuresis. Electrolyte imbalances are discussed in detail in Chapter 13.

CRITICAL THINKING CHALLENGE

An older adult in your nursing home has been eating less than 50% of her meals since admission the previous week. She has lost 3 pounds in 5 days. The nursing assistant reports to you today that the resident has a reddened area on her sacrum that does not blanch. When you speak to this client, she tells you that she is upset about being "put in a home."

- What other assessments should you perform at this time?
- What are her priority nursing diagnoses?
- What interventions are appropriate for her now?

For suggested answer guidelines, go to SIMON http://www.wbsaunders.com/SIMON/Iggy/.

PARENTERAL NUTRITION. When a client cannot effectively use the gastrointestinal tract for nutrition, parenteral nutrition therapy may maintain or improve his or her nutritional status. This form of IV therapy differs from standard IV therapy in that *all* nutrients (carbohydrates, proteins, fats, vitamins, minerals, and trace elements) are delivered to the client.

One liter of fluid containing 5% dextrose, which is often used as standard IV therapy, provides only 170 kcal. A hospitalized client typically receives 3 or 4 L a day for a total number of calories ranging between 500 and 700 a day. This calorie intake is not sufficient when the client requires IV therapy for a prolonged period and cannot eat an adequate diet or has increased calorie needs for tissue repair and building.

Parenteral nutrition (**hyperalimentation,** or "hyperal") is subdivided into two categories:

- Partial parenteral nutrition, or peripheral parenteral nutrition
- Total parenteral nutrition, or central parenteral nutrition

As suggested by the names, these categories differ by the site of administration and the content of the solutions.

PARTIAL PARENTERAL NUTRITION.

Partial parenteral nutrition (PPN) provides nutritional support to clients who are unable or unwilling to take a feeding via the gastrointestinal tract. PPN is typically used when a client has a prolonged post-operative ileus or when placement of a central IV line is not advised. It is used when nutritional support is needed less than 14 days. The client should be able to tolerate large fluid volumes and have readily accessible peripheral veins.

PPN is usually delivered through a cannula or catheter in a large distal vein of the arm. Two types of solutions are commonly used in various combinations for PPN: lipid (fat) emulsions and amino acid dextrose solutions.

Most lipid emulsions (20%) are isotonic, but the tonicity of commercially prepared amino acid dextrose solutions ranges from 300 mOsm to nearly 1200 mOsm. Amino acid dextrose solutions are considered more stable than the lipid emulsions, and therefore additives (e.g., vitamins, minerals, electrolytes, and trace elements) tend to be mixed with the amino acid dextrose solutions. The amino acid dextrose solution must be delivered through an in-line filter. Lipids and amino acid dextrose solutions are administered by a pump or controller device for accuracy and constancy in delivery rate.

A newer product for PPN is a *mixture* of lipids (10% or 20% fat emulsion) and an amino acid dextrose (usually 10%) solution. This mixture of three types of nutrients is referred to as a 3:1, total nutrient admixture (TNA), or triple-mix solution; it is available in 3-L bags.

TOTAL PARENTERAL NUTRITION.

When the client requires intensive nutritional support for an extended time, the health care provider prescribes centrally administered **total parenteral nutrition (TPN).** TPN is delivered through access to central veins, usually the subclavian or internal jugular veins. Central venous catheters and associated nursing care are described in detail in Chapter 14.

TPN solutions contain higher concentrations of dextrose and proteins, usually in the form of synthetic amino acids or protein hydrolysates (3% to 5%). These solutions are hyperosmotic (three to six times the osmolarity of normal blood). The base solutions are available as commercially prepared solutions. The hospital or community pharmacist adds components (specific electrolytes, minerals, trace elements, and insulin) according to the client's nutritional needs. This therapy provides needed calories and spares body proteins from catabolism for energy requirements.

TPN solutions are administered with a pump or an infusion controller device. The osmolarity of the fluid and the concentrations of the specific components make controlled delivery essential.

COMPLICATIONS OF PARENTERAL NUTRITION.

Clients receiving PPN or TPN are at risk for a wide variety of serious and potentially life-threatening complications. Complications may result from the PPN and TPN solutions or from the central venous catheter. The following discussion is limited to the complications of PPN and TPN that involve fluid or electrolyte balance. Complications of IV cannulas and central venous catheters are discussed in Chapter 14.

Fluid Imbalances. Clients receiving PPN or TPN are at increased risk for fluid imbalance. Not only is fluid delivered directly into the venous system, but the extreme hyperosmolarity of the solutions stimulates fluid shifts between body fluid compartments.

The hyperosmolarity of parenteral nutrition solutions is caused by their amino acid and dextrose concentrations. Increased dextrose causes hyperglycemia. As a result, some of the dextrose moves into the interstitial and intracellular spaces, where it is metabolized. However, dextrose remains in the plasma volume when the solutions are administered too rapidly, without enough insulin coverage, or in the presence of hyponatremia and hypokalemia. The result is a shift of water from the interstitial and intracellular spaces into the plasma. Expansion of the plasma volume together with hyperglycemia can cause osmotic diuresis and lead to serious dehydration and hypovolemic shock. If the client has an accompanying cardiac or renal dysfunction, the situation can lead to overhydration, congestive heart failure, and pulmonary edema.

The nurse monitors for these complications by taking daily weights and by recording accurate intake and output while the client is receiving parenteral nutrition. Serum glucose and electrolyte values are also monitored (Chart 61-7). Any major changes or abnormalities are reported to the health care provider.

CHART 61-7

BEST PRACTICE *for*
Care and Maintenance of Total Parenteral Nutrition

- Check each bag of total parenteral nutrition (TPN) solution for accuracy by comparing it with the physician's order.
- Monitor the IV pump for accuracy in delivering the prescribed hourly rate.
- If the TPN solution is temporarily unavailable, give 10% dextrose/water (D/W) or 20% D/W until the TPN solution can be obtained.
- If the TPN administration is not on time ("behind"), do not attempt to "catch up" by increasing the rate.
- Monitor the client's weight daily or according to agency protocol.
- Monitor serum electrolytes and glucose daily or per agency protocol. (Some agencies require finger stick blood sugars [FSBSs] every 4 hours, especially if the client is receiving insulin. Urine testing for ketones may also be ordered.)
- Monitor and carefully record the client's intake and output.
- Assess the client's IV site for signs of infection or infiltration (see Chapter 14).
- Change the IV tubing every 24 hours or per agency protocol.
- Change the dressing around the IV site every 48 to 72 hours or per agency protocol.

Electrolyte Imbalances. Clients receiving either PPN or TPN are at an increased risk for many different electrolyte imbalances, depending on the electrolyte composition of the solution and whether a fluid imbalance occurs. The health care provider usually orders daily determinations of serum electrolyte levels to detect these imbalances. The risk of metabolic and electrolyte complications is reduced when the rate of administration is carefully controlled and clients are closely monitored for response to treatment. Potassium and sodium imbalances are common among clients receiving PPN and TPN, especially when insulin is also administered as part of the therapy. Calcium imbalances, especially hypercalcemia, are associated with PPN and TPN, although immobility may play more of a role than the actual parenteral therapy in the development of this imbalance.

EFFECTS OF MEDICATION. There is no specific drug therapy for malnutrition, although multivitamins and an iron preparation may be prescribed to treat or prevent anemia. The nurse carefully reviews the client's medications because of food-medication interactions. Medications can affect nutritional status, and the foods ingested can affect the efficacy of medications.

Community-Based Care

Malnourished clients can be cared for in a variety of settings, including the acute care hospital, subacute unit, nursing home, or their own home. Malnutrition is often diagnosed when the client is admitted to the acute care hospital or as a consequence of events that occur after hospitalization, such as poor wound healing or sepsis. If the client is severely compromised, he or she may require admission to a subacute unit or traditional nursing home for either transitional or long-term care and be followed by a case manager. If adequate home support is available, the client may be discharged to home in the care of a family member, significant other, or other caregiver. Home care nurses may be needed to monitor and direct the care.

HEALTH TEACHING

The dietitian instructs the malnourished client and the family about high-calorie, high-protein diet and nutritional supplements. The pharmacist reviews any parenteral solutions with the client and family or significant others.

The nurse reinforces the importance of adhering to the diet and reviews any medications the client may be taking. If the client takes an iron preparation, the nurse teaches the importance of taking the medication immediately before or during meals. The nurse also cautions the client that iron tends to cause constipation. For the older adult already susceptible to constipation, the nurse stresses measures for prevention, including adequate fiber intake, adequate fluids, and exercise.

HOME CARE MANAGEMENT

The malnourished client needs a variety of resources at home to continue aggressive nutrition support. If the client can consume food by the oral route, the case manager or other discharge planner determines whether his or her financial resources are adequate for providing the necessary food and nutrition supplements. If the hospital provides ambulatory nutrition counseling services, the client is scheduled for follow-up after discharge for assessment of weight gain. The nurse assesses the ability of the client and family to understand and comply with instructions.

The malnourished client discharged to home on enteral or parenteral nutrition support needs the specialized services of a home nutrition therapy team. This team generally consists of the physician, nurse, dietitian, pharmacist, and social worker. Several commercial companies supply these services to clients in addition to the feeding supplies and formulas.

HEALTH CARE RESOURCES

The malnourished client may need help from community resources. Once nutrition therapy has progressed, the client may be discharged to the home setting or to a long-term care facility. The nurse collaborates with the case manager or discharge planner to find the best placement for each client. If the client is discharged to home, a home care nurse may visit until the client is stable.

Whether the client is discharged to home or to another facility, the dietitian provides written instructions about the diet and nutritional supplements. Communication with the new care provider is essential for continuity of care.

Evaluation: Outcomes

NOC The nurse evaluates the care of the malnourished client on the basis of the identified nursing diagnoses and collaborative problems. Expected outcomes include that the client:

- Has an adequate intake of all required nutrients on a daily basis
- Experiences no further weight loss or has a weight increase
- Has laboratory values within normal limits (WNL)

OBESITY

OVERVIEW

The terms **obesity** and **overweight** are often used interchangeably, but they refer to different conditions. Overweight is an increase in body weight for height compared with a reference standard, such as the Metropolitan Life height and weight tables (see Table 61-3) or 10% greater than ideal body weight. However, this weight may not reflect excess body fat. It is possible for well-developed athletes to appear overweight because of increased muscle mass; in such cases the proportion of muscle to fat is greater than average.

An obese person weighs at least 20% above the upper limit of the normal range for ideal body weight. **Morbid obesity** refers to a weight that has a negative effect on health—usually more than 100% above ideal body weight.

Pathophysiology

Obesity refers to an excess amount of body fat. It is possible to be obese at a weight that is within normal range according to a reference standard. The normal amount of body fat in *men* is between 15% and 20% of body weight. Obese young men have body fat greater than 22%, and older obese men have body fat greater than 25%. For *women*, the normal amount of body fat is 18% to 32%. Obese young women have body fat greater than 35% (Bray, 1994). Body fat can be measured in several ways. Height and weight are the easiest and most practical measurements for determining the degree of overweight.

OBESITY INDICES

To establish the percentage of ideal body weight (IBW), the height and weight of the client are compared with the midpoint of the desirable weight for a medium frame of the client's height and sex in the Metropolitan Life height and weight tables (see Table 61-3). The body mass index (BMI), as described previously on p. 1363, is a measure of heaviness and is only an indirect indicator of body fat. It reflects the combined effects of body build, proportions, lean body mass, and body fat. However, BMI has exhibited substantial correlations with fat mass for adult men and women and has been validated as a risk factor for cardiovascular disease. As a general rule, a BMI of 27 indicates obesity and an increased risk for health problems. Arm circumference and skin fold measurements more completely define body composition and adiposity.

The distribution of excess body fat rather than the degree of obesity has been used to predict increased health risks. The waist-to-hip ratio (WHR) or abdominal/gluteal ratio (AGR) differentiates a predominantly peripheral (gynecoid) lower body obesity from a central (android) upper body obesity. A WHR of 0.95 or greater in men (0.8 or greater in women) indicates android obesity with excess fat at the waist and abdomen; this pattern carries the greatest health risk. Two risk groups have been identified by location of abdominal fat: one with subcutaneous fat and one with intra-abdominal fat. The group with subcutaneous fat had fewer complications than did the group with excess intra-abdominal fat. Cross-sectional studies have shown that increased abdominal fat has been related to stroke, insulin resistance, hyperinsulinemia, and frank diabetes mellitus. Excessive abdominal fat may also enhance the risk for gallbladder disease (Pi-Sunyer, 1993).

COMPLICATIONS OF OBESITY

Obesity is a major public health problem and is associated with many complications, including death. As a result of this increasing problem, the Healthy People 2010 agenda addresses the need to reduce the proportion of children, adolescents, and adults who are obese. Nurses can help meet this goal through education and role modeling (see the Meeting Healthy People 2010 Objectives box above).

Complications of obesity that improve with weight loss include the following:
- Diabetes mellitus
- Hypertension
- Hyperlipidemia (increased serum lipids)
- Cardiac disease
- Sleep apnea
- Cholelithiasis
- Chronic back pain
- Early degenerative arthritis
- Certain types of cancer

TABLE 61-7 • CLASSIFICATION OF OBESITY BASED ON BODY MASS INDEX

Body Mass Index	Class	Risk for Disease Associated with Obesity
20-25	0	Low (not obese)
25-30	1	Low
30-35	2	Moderate
35-40	3	High
40+	4	Very high risk

Data from Bray, G.A. (1994). Etiology and prevalence of obesity. In C. Bouchard (Ed.). *The genetics of obesity* (pp. 17-33): Boca Raton, FL: CRC Press.

Obese people are also more susceptible to infectious diseases than are thinner people.

CLASSIFICATION

Bray (1994) has developed a classification of obesity based on BMI and the corresponding risk for disease (Table 61-7). This classification system eliminates describing obesity in unflattering and prejudicial terms such as *morbid* or *gross.*

Etiology

The cause of obesity involves complex interrelationships of many factors, including the following:
- Genetic
- Environmental
- Psychologic
- Social
- Cultural
- Pathologic
- Physiologic

Five major causes of both human and animal obesity have been identified (Bray, 1994). The first, neuroendocrine causes, include injury to the hypothalamus, Cushing's disease, polycystic ovary failure, hypogonadism, and growth hormone deficiency and insulinoma.

A second cause is dietary obesity associated with high-fat diets. Data suggest that obesity associated with a high-fat diet is more pronounced when the diet contains a significant amount of saturated fat.

Genetic factors are being studied as a third cause. They are found in clinically uncommon states, such as Prader-Willi syndrome. Genetic composition may predispose some people but not others to obesity. Researchers have recently identified the *ob* gene in mice, which helps to regulate energy balance. Leptin, the hormone encoded by the *ob* gene, appears to send a message to the brain that the body has stored enough fat; this serves as a signal to stop eating. For obese humans, a variant in this gene may mean that the body does not receive the signal to stop eating. More recent evidence suggests that energy balance and adiposity are regulated not only by the hormonal action of leptin and its receptors but also by the interaction of leptin and insulin with the hypothalamic neuropeptide Y system (Schwartz & Seeley, 1997).

The fourth cause of obesity is drug treatment. Drugs that promote obesity include the following:
- Corticosteroids
- Estrogens
- Nonsteroidal anti-inflammatory drugs
- Antihypertensives
- Antidepressants
- Antiepileptics
- Phenothiazines

Physical inactivity has been identified as the fifth cause. The major identified barriers to increasing physical activity include a lack of time and a lack of safe environments in which to be active. Regular exercise is associated with lower death rates for adults of any age. It also increases lean muscle, decreases body fat, aids in weight control, and enhances psychologic well-being. Regular exercise can also decrease the risk of falling in older adults.

Incidence/Prevalence

The number of overweight children, adolescents, and adults has continued to rise over the past four decades. In the United States, the total cost (medical cost and lost productivity) of obesity is more than $100 billion each year. Phase 1 of the third National Health and Nutrition Examination Survey (NHANES III) was conducted between 1988 and 1991 and concluded that 58 million adults in the United States were overweight. This figure represents 33.4% of Americans. "Overweight" in this study was a BMI equal to or greater than 27.8 for men (approximately 124% of IBW) and a BMI equal to or greater than 27.3 for women (approximately 120% of IBW) (Kuczmarski et al., 1994). In 2000, an estimated 107 million adults in the United States were overweight or obese.

Familial and genetic factors play an important role in obesity. When both parents are overweight, approximately 80% of their children will be overweight. If neither parent is overweight, fewer than 10% of the children will be overweight. In studies of identical twins, nonidentical twins, and parent-sibling relationships, about 50% of the difference in body fatness is transmitted to children, and approximately 50% of this amount is genetically controlled. A combination of improper diet and lack of physical activity produces obesity in genetically predisposed people.

Culture seems to be a factor in the prevalence of obesity. The prevalence of obesity among ethnic minorities, including African Americans, Hispanic Americans, Asian Americans and Pacific Islanders, Native Americans, Native Alaskans, and Native Hawaiians, is substantially higher than in Caucasians, especially among women (Kumanyika, 1993). A study by Harrell and Gore (1998) found that African-American women of low and middle socioeconomic status (SES) were much more likely to be obese and inactive than were African-American women of high SES. Among Caucasian women, those with low SES had the greatest prevalence of obesity and inactivity. After controlling for income and education, African-American women were twice as likely as Caucasian women to be obese and inactive.

Further research by Gore (1999) found that African Americans' frame of reference for "normal" body weight is much larger that the standard indicator for weight. Another factor contributing to larger body size in African-American women is that Caucasian women engage in weight loss methods for significantly longer periods of time than do African-American women (Tyler, Allan, & Alcozer, 1997).

A descriptive study of Hispanic women and their daughters demonstrated that daughters ate more fat than did their mothers (Garcia-Maas, 1999). The greater the fat intake, the more negatively women seemed to perceive their health status.

► COLLABORATIVE MANAGEMENT

► Assessment

HISTORY

The nurse or dietitian collects the following information about the client:
- Economic status
- Usual food intake
- Eating behavior
- Cultural background
- Attitude toward food
- Appetite
- Chronic diseases
- Medications
- Physical activity

A diet history usually incorporates a 24-hour recall of food intake and the frequency with which foods are consumed. The nurse or dietitian is objective but understands the personal nature of these questions. The adequacy of the diet can be rapidly evaluated by comparing the amount and types of foods consumed daily with the Dietary Guidelines for Americans (see Figure 61-1). Gross inadequacies for specific nutrients can be identified with this approach. The dietitian can provide a more detailed analysis of dietary intake.

Women have a unique risk for nutrition-related diseases and conditions and weight-related problems due to biologic, social, and political factors. The American Dietetic Association (ADA) and the Canadian Dietetic Association (CDA) issued a joint position paper on women's health and nutrition (ADA, 1995). Five of the leading causes of morbidity and mortality in North American women are cardiovascular disease, cancer, osteoporosis, diabetes, and overweight. Women are vulnerable to several weight-related health risks associated with being overweight. Recent estimates of North American women who are overweight range from 25% to 33%, with certain native and ethnic populations reporting even higher percentages.

Being overweight adds many risks for women, especially if the fat stores are located in the abdominal or truncal areas of the body. A waist/hip ratio of 0.85 puts women at higher risk for coronary heart disease, hypertension, dyslipidemia, diabetes, gallstone formation, and cancer of the reproductive organs. In addition to these medical risks, women are vulnerable to the social, economic, and emotional pressures associated with being overweight. Overweight women may find it difficult to feel good about themselves when challenged by society's discrimination against the overweight. The constant struggle for many women to lose weight often ends in failure and leads to patterns of weight cycling or disordered eating. Prevention and early intervention programs for overweight women and their families remain a critical need. The ADA and CDA will continue their efforts to include nutrition in clinical and preventive services for women because it is such a critical component of both risk reduction and treatment for weight-associated conditions.

■ PHYSICAL ASSESSMENT/CLINICAL MANIFESTATIONS

In collaboration with the dietitian, the nurse accurately obtains the client's height and weight and calculates the percentage of ideal body weight (% IBW) and the body mass index (BMI). The dietitian may:

- Calculate the waist/hip ratio
- Make the necessary skin fold measurements and record them in the chart

The nurse also examines the skin of the obese client for reddened or open areas; these may not be easily visible because of excess fat.

■ PSYCHOSOCIAL ASSESSMENT

The nurse obtains a psychosocial history to determine the client's circumstances and emotional factors that might prevent success of therapy or be worsened by it. The nurse or social worker interviews the client to determine his or her perception of current weight. The client may or may not view weight as a problem, which will affect treatment and outcome.

The nurse explores the client's past history to assess the following:

- Cause and duration of weight gain
- Family history of obesity
- Past attempts at weight reduction and outcomes

The nurse asks about the following:

- Current reasons for wanting to lose weight
- Stressors (e.g., home, employment, personal, financial, or community) that might prevent success
- Exercise patterns
- Current medications
- Perceptions of self-worth

The diet history provides a detailed analysis of the client's eating habits. As a member of the health care team, the nurse can evaluate the data to coordinate an interdisciplinary approach that incorporates diet, exercise, behavior modification, and psychologic support. The client may be referred to a community support group if one is available.

■ LABORATORY ASSESSMENT

There are no significant laboratory tests for obesity. However, the nurse should review all laboratory test results to assess the nutritional status of the client.

● Analysis

■ COMMON NURSING DIAGNOSES AND COLLABORATIVE PROBLEMS

The following are the most common nursing diagnoses for clients with obesity or overweight:

1. Imbalanced Nutrition: More Than Body Requirements related to a dysfunctional eating pattern or neuroendocrine disorder
2. Activity Intolerance related to a sedentary lifestyle

■ ADDITIONAL NURSING DIAGNOSES AND COLLABORATIVE PROBLEMS

In addition to the common nursing diagnoses, clients may have one or more secondary problems associated with obesity and overweight, which include the following:

- Situational Low Self-Esteem or Chronic Low Self-Esteem related to guilt associated with eating style
- Disturbed Body Image related to physical appearance
- Disturbed Thought Processes related to depression
- Ineffective Sexuality Patterns related to body image perception, rejection by partner, or difficulty assuming sexual positions
- Impaired Social Interaction related to poor self-esteem and rejection by others
- Impaired Physical Mobility related to decreased strength and endurance

Some clients with obesity are at risk for collaborative problems, which include the following:

- Diabetes mellitus
- Cardiovascular disease
- Hypertension

● Planning and Implementation

■ IMBALANCED NUTRITION: MORE THAN BODY REQUIREMENTS

NOC PLANNING: EXPECTED OUTCOMES. The client with obesity or overweight is expected to (1) participate in a structured weight loss program, (2) approach ideal body weight, and (3) establish a lasting, healthful dietary pattern that will result in permanent, sustained weight loss.

INTERVENTIONS. Weight is lost only when energy expended is greater than intake. Weight loss may be accomplished by dietary restriction with or without the aid of drugs. Clients who are candidates for surgical treatment:

- Repeatedly fail at nonsurgical techniques
- Have a body mass index (BMI) equal to or greater than 40 (class IV)
- Weigh more than 100% above ideal body weight (IBW)
- Have medically significant obesity

NONSURGICAL MANAGEMENT. The first clinical practice *Guidelines for Treatment of Adult Obesity* outlines treatment decisions based on risk assessment. Recommendations for appropriate weight reduction strategies or weight maintenance to prevent further weight gain are also included (Shape Up America and American Obesity Association, 1996). Various diet programs and medications have attempted to help obese clients achieve permanent weight loss.

DIET PROGRAMS. Modalities for helping people lose weight include fasting, very-low-calorie diets, balanced and unbalanced low-energy diets, and novelty diets.

Fasting. Short-term fasting programs have not been successful in treating morbidly obese clients, and prolonged fasting does not produce permanent benefits. Most clients regain the weight that was lost by this method. In addition, the risks associated with fasting (e.g., severe ketosis) require close medical supervision.

Very-Low-Calorie Diets. Very-low-calorie diets generally provide 200 to 800 calories/day. Two types of very-low-calorie diets are the *protein-sparing modified fast* and the *liquid formula diet.*

The protein-sparing modified fast provides protein of high biologic value (1.5 g/kg of desirable body weight/day) within a limited number of calories. The diet produces rapid weight loss while preserving lean body mass. The liquid formula diet provides between 33 and 70 g of protein daily.

Both diets require an initial cardiac evaluation, supervision by an interdisciplinary health team with monitoring by a physician, nutrition counseling by a registered dietitian, and supplementation with vitamins and minerals. These diets are only one part of a weight reduction program. Clients who are following these diets should receive nutrition education, psychologic counseling, exercise, and behavior therapy. Comparable weight losses have been achieved with both diets, but most clients do not sustain the weight loss and regain the weight.

Balanced and Unbalanced Low-Energy Diets. Nutritionally balanced diets generally provide 1200 calories/day with a conventional distribution of carbohydrate, protein, and fat. Vitamin and mineral supplements may be necessary if energy intakes fall below 1200 calories for women and 1800 calories for men. This diet provides conventional foods that are economical and easy to obtain; thus the goal of weight loss is facilitated, and that loss is maintained.

Unbalanced low-energy diets, such as the low-carbohydrate diet (e.g., Atkins diet), restrict one or more nutrients. No evidence supports the claim that the restricted nutrient increases or decreases weight loss beyond the calorie deficit it produces.

Novelty Diets. Novelty diets, such as the grapefruit diet, are often nutritionally *inadequate.* This type of diet implies that a certain food increases metabolic rate or accelerates the oxidation of body fat. Weight loss is achieved because energy is restricted by food choice, but clients do not sustain weight loss after terminating the diet.

DIET THERAPY. Diet recommendations for each client should be developed through close interaction between the client, physician, and dietitian. The diet should meet the client's needs and habits and should be realistic.

The dietitian develops a diet plan and instructs the client. At a minimum, the diet should:
- Have a scientific rationale
- Be nutritionally adequate for all nutrients except energy
- Have a low risk/benefit ratio
- Be practical and conducive to long-term success

Calorie estimates are easily calculated. Resting metabolic rate is determined using a gender-specific formula that incorporates the appropriate activity factor. This figure reflects the total calories needed daily for maintaining current weight. To encourage a weight loss of 1 pound (2.2 kg) a week, the dietitian subtracts 500 calories/day. To encourage a weight loss of 2 pounds (4.4 kg) a week, the dietitian subtracts 1000 calories/day. The amount of weight lost varies with the client's food intake, level of physical activity, and water losses. Carbohydrate, protein, and fat can be calculated as in Table 61-8. A reasonable goal of 5% to 10% loss of body weight has been shown to improve glycemic control and reduce cholesterol and blood pressure, and these benefits continue if the weight loss is sustained (Wing & Jeffery, 1995).

DRUG THERAPY. A BMI of 30, or a BMI of 27 with co-morbidities, is one indicator for the use of drug therapy (Shape Up America and American Obesity Association, 1996). Anorectic drugs suppress appetite, which reduces food intake and over time may result in weight loss. These drugs play a valuable role in a comprehensive weight reduction program but should be used only as part of such a program. Currently available drugs to treat obesity act on either the noradrenergic or serotonergic systems in the central nervous system. The most commonly used anorectic drug for the treatment of obesity is sibutramine (Meridia). Sibutramine is an anorectic drug that inhibits the reuptake of serotonin (which enhances satiety [feeling full when eating]) and norepinephrine (which raises metabolic rate). Adverse effects include dry mouth, constipation, and insomnia.

Orlistat (Xenical) is a different type of drug that inhibits lipase and leads to partial hydrolysis of triglycerides. Because fats are only partially digested and absorbed, calorie intake is decreased. Most clients taking orlistat experience gastrointestinal symptoms that include loose stools, abdominal cramps, and nausea.

TABLE 61-8 • NUTRIENT NEEDS DURING WEIGHT REDUCTION

Calorie Level	Protein	Carbohydrate	Fat	Multivitamin and Mineral Supplement
<600	1.5 g/kg/day*	50 g/day minimum	3-6 g/day linoleic acid minimum	Yes 100% of RDA or RNI
600-1200	1-1.5 g/kg/day	≥55% of calories	≤30% of calories	Yes 100% of RDA or RNI
1200	0.8-1.5 g/kg/day	≥55% of calories	≤30% of calories	Optional

Minimum at all calorie levels: Sodium, 500 mg/day; potassium, 2000 mg/day; calcium, 800 mg/day; iron, 15 mg/day; noncaloric fluids, 2 L/day.

Modified from Dwyer, J. T. (1991). Nutrient needs in weight management. *Contemporary Management of the Overweight Patient, 3,* 1-8.
*This requirement may necessitate more than 600 calories/day. Protein needs are based on ideal body weight.
RDA, Recommended Dietary Allowance; *RNI,* Recommended Nutrient Intake (Canada).

BEHAVIORAL TREATMENT. Behavioral treatment of obesity consists of various strategies to change daily eating habits to achieve weight loss. This ongoing process should produce a change in behavior. Self-monitoring techniques include keeping a record of foods eaten (food diary), exercise patterns, and emotional and situational factors. Stimulus control involves controlling the external cues that promote overeating. Reinforcement techniques are used to self-reward the behavior change. Cognitive restructuring involves modifying negative beliefs by learning positive coping self-statements.

Fairburn and Cooper (1996) have developed a cognitive behavioral approach to the acquisition of weight maintenance behavior skills. Clients are encouraged to accept modest weight loss goals and are further discouraged from losing more weight. The treatment focuses on the acquisition of weight maintenance skills and on cognitive factors and any tendency to evaluate self-worth in terms of body size. The client's focus is shifted from physical appearance to a concern for health.

> ### CRITICAL THINKING CHALLENGE
> You are caring for a 42-year-old female hospitalized client who is preparing to have bilateral knee replacements. She tells you that she has been obese her entire life and now has severe arthritis in both knees. She has tried every novelty diet available but regains the weight shortly after completing the diet. Her husband left her last year because he was embarrassed to be with her.
> - What are the priority nursing diagnoses related to her obesity?
> - What other options does she have for managing her nutritional problem?
> - What is the psychologic impact of being obese?
>
> For suggested answer guidelines, go to SIMON http://www.wbsaunders.com/SIMON/Iggy/.

SURGICAL MANAGEMENT. Clients who do not respond to traditional dietary intervention may be considered for a surgical procedure aimed at producing permanent weight loss. All clients with a body mass index (BMI) ≥40, or a BMI ≥35 with additional risk factors, should be considered for surgery (Shape Up America and American Obesity Association, 1996). Most surgical procedures fall into three categories:

1. Mechanical or physical (adipose tissue removal or intake restriction)
2. Malabsorptive (bypass of the gastrointestinal tract)
3. Regulatory (directly affecting hunger or thirst)

PREOPERATIVE CARE. The nurse reinforces health teaching before the client has surgery. Preoperative care is similar to that for any client undergoing abdominal surgery (see Chapter 17).

OPERATIVE PROCEDURES. Surgical procedures that physically restrict the intake of food include the following:
- Maxillomandibular fixation (jaw wiring)
- Esophageal banding
- Gastroplasty (banding or stapling the stomach)
- Intestinal bypass, in which the stomach and jejunum are connected

One of the most common procedures is gastroplasty, which decreases the size of the stomach. Stapling horizontally across the top of the stomach leaves only a small opening (0.8 to 1 cm) into the distal stomach. However, the fundic pouch created is often stretched too much, which inhibits weight loss. The vertical banded gastroplasty evolved from earlier forms of gastroplasty. It is designed with a less distensible vertical pouch that reduces the capacity for a meal by 100-fold. The small pouch outlet delays emptying and provides an internal cue for satiety.

Gastric restrictive operations sometimes produce maladaptive eating behaviors, such as the following:
- "Soft calorie syndrome" (consumption of excessive amounts of soft or liquid, calorically dense foods)
- Vomiting from inadequate chewing
- Inappropriate consumption of liquids after solids

An intestinal bypass reduces the size of the stomach with stainless steel staples but connects a small opening in the upper portion of the stomach to the small intestine by means of an intestinal loop (Figure 61-6). Complications of the intestinal bypass include bloating of the pouch. The incidence of nausea and vomiting is similar to that with gastroplasty. Intestinal bypass usually leads to greater weight loss that does gastroplasty, in part because of dumping syndrome as the use of the lower part of the stomach is omitted. Intestinal bypass operations have been modified to avoid blind loop bacterial overgrowth syndromes and are now performed as a biliointestinal bypass, jejunoileal bypass with ileogastrostomy, or duodenoileal bypass.

Surgical treatment of clinically severe obesity by either vertical banded gastroplasty or Roux-en-Y gastric bypass is a viable option for selected clients (NIH Consensus Development Conference Panel, 1991). Maximum weight loss from these procedures generally occurs 18 to 24 months after surgery. Two years after surgery, Roux-en-Y clients lost 60% to 70% of their weight, whereas gastroplasty clients lost 40% to 60%.

POSTOPERATIVE CARE. The client has a nasogastric (NG) tube put in place immediately after gastroplasty or intestinal bypass. In gastroplasty, the NG tube drains both the proximal pouch and the distal stomach. The nurse closely monitors the tube for patency. The tube is never repositioned because its movement can disrupt the suture line.

The NG tube is removed on the third day if the client has bowel sounds and is passing flatus. The nurse gives the client 1 ounce (30 mL) of water in a 1-ounce medicine cup and instructs the client to sip it slowly over 1 hour. Clear liquids are given if the client can tolerate water, and 1-ounce cups are used for each serving. Pureed foods, juice, and soups thinned with broth, water, or milk are added to the diet 24 to 48 hours after clear liquids are tolerated. Typically, the client can increase the volume to 1 ounce over 5 minutes or until satisfied, but the diet is limited to liquids or pureed foods for 6 weeks. The client then progresses to three meals a day, with an emphasis on nutrient-dense foods. Nausea, vomiting, or discomfort occurs if too much liquid is ingested.

Before discharge from the hospital, the nurse instructs the client to take liquid or chewable multivitamins daily and to consume adequate protein to promote wound healing. To avoid blockage of the pouch opening, clients are encouraged to eat slowly, chew foods well, and avoid swallowing chunks of food that cannot be liquefied completely.

ACTIVITY INTOLERANCE

PLANNING: EXPECTED OUTCOMES. The client with obesity or overweight is expected to (1) tolerate usual activity as evidenced by endurance, energy conservation, and self-care; and (2) incorporate daily exercise into his or her lifestyle.

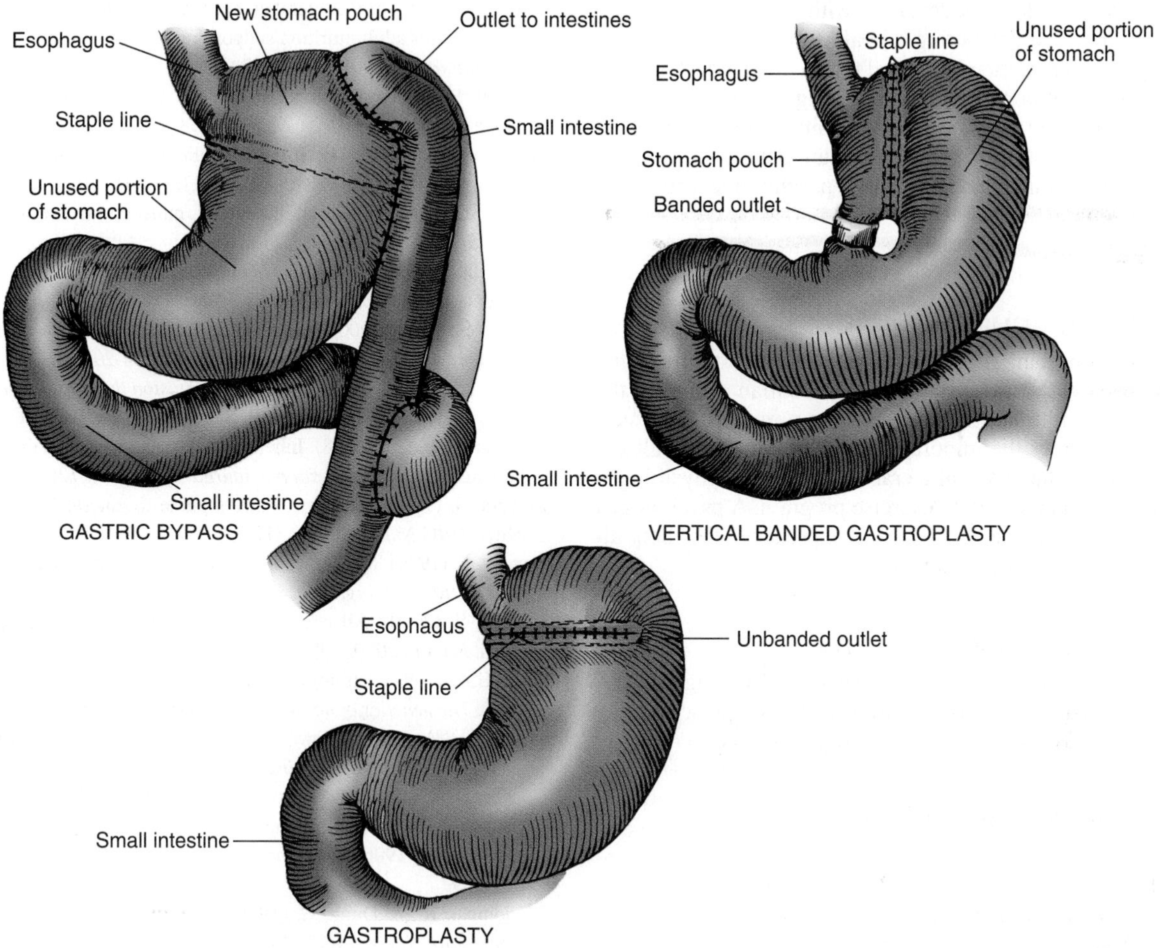

Figure 61-6 ● Surgical procedures for obesity. (Redrawn from Mahan, L.K., & Escott-Stump, S. [1996], *Krause's food, nutrition, & diet therapy* [9th ed.]. Philadelphia: W.B. Saunders.)

INTERVENTIONS. Management of the overweight or obese client is an interdisciplinary effort. The nurse collaborates with the physician, dietitian, and physical therapist or exercise physiologist to meet the goal of improving the client's physical activity tolerance. The major intervention is to increase the type and amount of daily exercise to create a calorie deficit along with modification of eating habits. Adding exercise to a diet intervention produces more weight loss than just dieting alone. More of the weight lost is fat, which preserves lean body mass. An increase in exercise produces a reduction in the waist/hip ratio.

Increasing and maintaining physical activity levels is important in maintaining weight loss. Many overweight or obese clients are so unfit that it may take several months of conditioning before they can exercise sufficiently to achieve weight loss.

The nurse or physical therapist or exercise physiologist first obtains a clinical exercise history. It is important to determine the client's current exercise pattern and exercise habits over a lifetime. The client should understand the importance of an exercise component in a weight loss program. The nurse also ascertains the client's desire to participate in an exercise program and his or her preferred types of exercise.

The health care provider evaluates the client by an exercise stress test. Not all clients need a stress test, but those with chronic disease may need a stress test and more specific exercise recommendations. The nurse counsels clients about unusual signs and symptoms during exercise (e.g., chest pain) and

what to do if they occur. The physical therapist or exercise physiologist first emphasizes the importance of exercising consistently and then stresses duration, intensity, and frequency.

A minimal-level workout should be developed for the client so that consistency can be achieved. The goal for the client is to maintain a lifetime of increased physical activity. The client is apt to be less fatigued and discouraged with a low-intensity, short-duration program. Sedentary clients are encouraged to increase their activity by walking 30 to 40 minutes daily (15 to 20 minutes/mile) or the equivalent. The activity may be performed all at once or divided over the course of the day. The nurse teaches the client to exercise only under the supervision of the physician. All members of the interdisciplinary team should provide encouragement and support for any increase in physical activity.

● Community-Based Care

Obese clients can be cared for in a variety of settings, including the acute care hospital and subacute unit (particularly following surgical treatment for obesity) or in their own home. Obesity is a chronic, lifelong problem. Diets, drug therapy, exercise, and behavior modification can produce short-term weight losses with reasonable safety. However, most clients who do lose weight often regain the weight. Treatment of obesity should focus on the long-term reduction of health risks and medical problems associated with obesity, improving quality of life, and promoting a health-oriented lifestyle. Interdisciplinary team members need to provide a nonjudgmental, supportive atmosphere that encourages the client to increase physical activity, decrease fat intake and reliance on medication use, establish a normal eating pattern in response to physiologic hunger, and address psychologic problems. Frequent, long-term ambulatory care follow-up coordinated by a case manager is essential for successful treatment.

HEALTH TEACHING

The most important features of client education focus on health-related behavior patterns. The dietitian counsels the client on a healthful eating pattern. The nurse provides support and reinforces the importance of maintaining a healthful eating pattern. The physical therapist or exercise physiologist recommends an appropriate exercise program. A psychologist recommends cognitive restructuring approaches that help alter dysfunctional eating patterns.

HOME CARE MANAGEMENT

The overweight or obese client needs proper weighing devices and measuring utensils to follow the diet prescribed by the physician. No other home care preparation is needed.

HEALTH CARE RESOURCES

The chances for success in a weight control program are enhanced if additional support is available. The nurse provides the client with a list of available community resources, such as Weight Watchers, Overeaters Anonymous, Take Off Pounds Sensibly (TOPS), comprehensive interdisciplinary treatment programs, and a list of professionals that includes a registered dietitian, psychologist, and exercise physiologist who may provide frequent follow-up in an ambulatory care setting.

● Evaluation: Outcomes

NOC The nurse evaluates the care of the client with obesity or overweight on the basis of the identified nursing diagnoses and collaborative problems. Expected outcomes include that the client:

- Establishes a lasting, healthful dietary pattern that results in permanent, sustained weight loss
- Slowly increases the amount of physical exercise to aid in promoting weight loss
- Incorporates daily exercise into lifestyle
- Participates in usual daily activities

ONLINE RESOURCES

For suggested readings and Internet resources, go to http://www.wbsaunders.com/SIMON/Iggy/.

SELECTED BIBLIOGRAPHY

Asterisk indicates a classic or definitive work on this subject.

*American Dietetic Association. (1995). Position of the American Dietetic Association and the Canadian Dietetic Association: Women's health and nutrition. *Journal of the American Dietetic Association, 95*(3), 362-366.

*American Society of Parenteral and Enteral Nutrition. (1993). Section II: Rationale for adult nutrition support guidelines. *Journal of Parenteral and Enteral Nutrition, 17*(4), 5SA-6SA.

Ammon, P.K. (1999). Individualizing the approach to treating obesity. *Nurse Practitioner, 24*(2), 27-31, 36-38, 41-43.

Anderson, E.B. (2000). Facilitating quality of life through nutrition. *Advance for Nurses (DC/Baltimore), 2*(11), 17-18, 30.

Andris, D.A. (1998). Total parenteral nutrition in surgical patients. *MEDSURG Nursing, 7*(2), 76-83.

*Bass, J.D., et al. (1996). The effect of dietary fiber on tube-fed elderly patients. *Journal of Gerontology Nursing, 22*(10), 37-44.

Bender, S., et al. (2000). Malnutrition: Role of the TwoCal® HN Med Pass Program. *MEDSURG Nursing, 9*(6), 284-296.

*Booker, M., & Ignatavicius, D. (1996). *Infusion therapy: Techniques and medications.* Philadelphia: W.B. Saunders.

*Bouchard, C., et al. (1988). Inheritance of the amount and distribution of human body fat. *International Journal of Obesity, 12*(3), 205-215.

*Bowers, S. (1996). Tubes: A nurse's guide to enteral feeding devices. *MEDSURG Nursing, 5*(5), 313-324.

Bowers, S. (1999). Nutrition support for malnourished, acutely ill adults. *MEDSURG Nursing, 8*(3), 145-166.

Bowers, S. (2000). All about tubes: Your guide to enteral feeding devices. *Nursing2000, 30*(12), 41-48.

*Bray, G.A. (1994). Etiology and prevalence of obesity. In C. Bouchard (Ed.), *The genetics of obesity* (pp. 17-33). Boca Raton, FL: CRC Press.

Cammon, S.A., & Hackshaw, H.S. (2000). Are we starving our patients? *American Journal of Nursing, 100*(5), 43-47.

*Conway, J.M. (1995). Ethnicity and energy stores. *American Journal of Clinical Nutrition, 62*(5 Suppl.), 1067S-1071S.

*Costello, M.C. (1996). Home health nutrition. *MEDSURG Nursing, 5*(4), 229-239.

*Davidhizar, R., & Dunn, C. (1996). Malnutrition in the elderly. *Home Healthcare Nurse, 14*(12), 948-956.

Dudek, S.G. (2000). Malnutrition in hospitals: Who's assessing what patients eat? *American Journal of Nursing, 100*(4), 36-43.

Edwards, S.J., & Metheney, N.A. (2000). Measurement of gastric residual volume: State of the science. *MEDSURG Nursing, 9*(3), 125-128.

Epley, D. (1999). Nutritional assessment in home care patients. *Home Care Provider, 4*(3), 102-105.

*Fairburn, C.G., & Cooper, Z. (1996). New perspectives on dieting and behavioural treatments for obesity. *International Journal of Obesity, 20*(Suppl. 1), S9-S13.

Fellows, L.S., et al. (2000). Evidence-based practice for enteral feedings: Aspiration prevention strategies, bedside detection, and practice change. *MEDSURG Nursing, 9*(1), 27-32.

Food and Nutrition Board, Institute of Medicine, National Academy of Sciences. (1997). *Dietary reference intakes: Calcium, phosphorus, magnesium, vitamin D, and fluoride.* Washington, D.C.: National Academy Press.

*Food and Nutrition Board, National Research Council/National Academy of Sciences. (1989). *Recommended dietary allowances* (10th ed.). Washington, D.C.: National Academy Press.

*Gallagher-Allred, C.R., et al. (1996). Malnutrition and clinical outcomes: The case for medical nutrition therapy. *Journal of the American Dietetic Association, 96*, 366-369.

Garcia-Maas, L.D. (1999). Intergenerational analysis of dietary practices and health perceptions of Hispanic women and their adult daughters. *Journal of Transcultural Nursing, 10*(3), 213-219.

Giger, J.N., & Davidhizar, R.E. (1999). *Transcultural nursing: Assessment and intervention* (3rd ed.). St. Louis: Mosby.

Goff, K.L. (1997). The nuts and bolts of enteral infusion pumps. *MEDSURG Nursing, 6*(1), 9-16.

*Goldstein, D.J., & Potvin, J.H. (1994). Long-term weight loss: The effect of pharmacologic agents. *American Journal of Clinical Nutrition, 60*(5), 647-657.

Gore, S.V. (1999). African-American women's perceptions of weight: Paradigm shift for advanced practice. *Holistic Nursing Practice, 13*(4), 71-79.

*Grindel, C.G., & Costello, M.C. (1996). Nutrition screening: An essential assessment parameter. *MEDSURG Nursing, 5*(3), 145-156.

Harrell, J.S., & Gore, S.V. (1998). Cardiovascular risk factors and socioeconomic status in African American and Caucasian women. *Research in Nursing and Health, 21*(4), 285-295.

Jones, S.A., & Guenter, P. (1997). Automatic flush feeding pumps. *Nursing97, 27*(2), 56-59.

Kayser-Jones, J., & Pengilly, K. (1999). Dysphagia among nursing home residents. *Geriatric Nursing, 20*(2), 77-84.

*Kennedy, E., Meyers, L., & Layden, W. (1996). The 1995 dietary guidelines for Americans: An overview. *Journal of the American Dietetic Association, 96*(3), 234-237.

Kohn-Keeth, C. (2000). How to keep feeding tubes flowing freely. *Nursing2000, 30*(3), 58-59.

*Kuczmarski, R. J., et al. (1994). Increasing prevalence of overweight among U.S. adults: The National Health and Nutrition Examination Surveys, 1960-1991. *Journal of the American Medical Association, 272*(3), 205-211.

*Kumanyika, S. (1993). Special issues regarding obesity in minority populations. *Annals of Internal Medicine, 119*(7 Pt. 2), 650-654.

*Lord, L.M., Lipp, J., & Stull, S. (1996). Adult tube feeding formulas. *MEDSURG Nursing, 5*(6), 407-420.

Lyman, B., & Marquardt, P. (1997). Nutrition screening tool development and utilization for home care patients. *Home Healthcare Nurse, 15*(12), 835-842.

Messina, V.K., & Burke, K.I. (1997). Position of the American Dietetic Association: Vegetarian diets. *Journal of the American Dietetic Association, 97*(11), 1317-1321.

*Metheney, N., et al. (1990). Effectiveness of the auscultatory method in predicting feeding tube location. *Nursing Research, 39,* 262-267.

Metheney, N., et al. (1998). pH, color, and feeding tubes. *RN, 61*(1), 25-27.

Metheney, N., et al. (1998). Testing feeding tube placement: Auscultation vs. pH method. *American Journal of Nursing, 98*(5), 37-43.

Miller, D. (2000). To crush or not to crush? *Nursing2000, 30*(2), 50-52.

*Nelson, K.J., et al. (1993). Prevalence of malnutrition in the elderly admitted to long-term care facilities. *Journal of the American Dietetic Association, 93*(4), 459-461.

*NIH Consensus Development Conference Panel. (1991). Gastrointestinal surgery for severe obesity. *Annals of Internal Medicine, 115*(12), 956-961.

*Nutrition and your health: Dietary guidelines for Americans. (1995). *Home and Garden Bulletin No. 232* (4th ed.). Washington, D.C.: U.S. Department of Agriculture and U.S. Department of Health and Human Services.

Nutrition Screening Manual for Professionals Caring for Older Americans: Nutrition Screening Initiative. (1991). Washington, D.C.: Greer, Margois, Mitchell, Grunwald & Associates. (Available from The Nutrition Screening Initiative, 2626 Pennsylvania Ave., N.W., Suite 301, Washington, D.C. 20037.)

*Pi-Sunyer, F.X. (1993). Medical hazards of obesity. *Annals of Internal Medicine, 119,*(7 Pt. 2), 655-660.

Pontieri-Lewis, V. (1997). The role of nutrition in wound healing. *MEDSURG Nursing, 6*(4), 187-192.

Rotkoff, N. (1999). Care of the morbidly obese patient in a long-term care facility. *Geriatric Nursing, 20*(6), 309-313.

Schwartz, M.W., & Seeley, R.J. (1997). The new biology of body weight regulation. *Journal of the American Dietetic Association, 97,* 54-58.

*Shape Up America and American Obesity Association. (1996). *Guidelines for treatment of adult obesity.* Bethesda, MD: Shape Up America.

Tyler, D.O., Allan, J.D., & Alcozer, F.R. (1997). Weight loss used by African American and Euro-American women. *Research in Nursing and Health, 20*(5), 413-423.

*Vegetarian food pyramid. (1994). *Vegetarian Journal, 13,* 21.

Vellas, B., et al. (1999). The Mini Nutritional Assessment (MNA) and its use in grading the nutritional state of elderly patients. *Nutrition, 15*(2), 159-161.

*Viall, C.D. (1996). Location, location, location. *Nursing96, 26*(9), 43-45.

*Vines, S.W., et al. (1992). Research utilization: An evaluation of the research related to causes of diarrhea in tube-fed patients. *Applied Nursing Research, 5,* 164-173.

*Webber-Jones, J., et al. (1992). How to declog a feeding tube. *Nursing, 22*(4), 62-64.

Wellman, N.S. (1997). A case manager's guide to nutrition screening and intervention. *The Journal of Care Management, 3*(2), 12-27.

*Wing, R.R. & Jeffery, R.W. (1995). Effect of modest weight loss on changes in cardiovascular risk factors: Are there differences between men and women or between weight loss and maintenance? *International Journal of Obesity, 19,* 67-73.

Yen, P.K. (1999). Cancer treatment compromises nutrition. *Geriatric Nursing, 20*(5), 278-279.

PROBLEMS OF REGULATION AND METABOLISM

Management of Clients with Problems of the Endocrine System

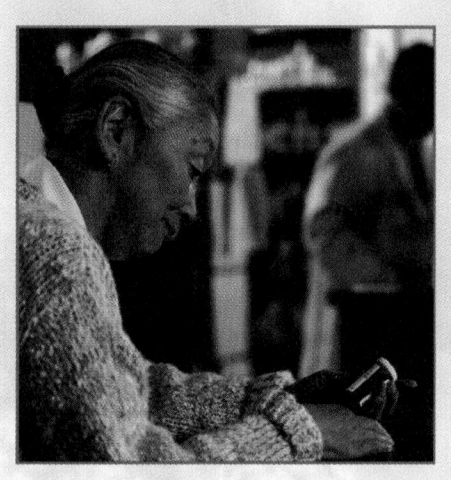

UNIT 13 PROBLEMS OF REGULATION AND METABOLISM: ENDOCRINE SYSTEM ■ Core Concepts Grid

Anatomy	Physiology	Pathophysiology	History	Physical Exam	Diagnostic Tests	Interventions	Pharmacology
• **Glands** Anterior pituitary Posterior pituitary Thyroid Parathyroid Pancreas Adrenal • **Hormones** Antidiuretic hormone (ADH) Thyroid-stimulating hormone (TSH) Adrenocorticotropic hormone (ACTH) Growth hormone (GH) Mineralocorticoids Glucocorticoids Androgens Epinephrine Norepinephrine Thyroxine Thyrocalcitonin Parathormone Insulin Glucagon	• **Neuroregulation** • **Hypothalamus** • **Regulation** Metabolism Fluids/electrolytes Glucose levels Stress response	• Inflammation • Hypersecretion • Hyposecretion • Infection • Diabetic ketoacidosis • Hyperglycemic hyperosmolar nonketotic syndrome (HHNKS) • Adrenal crisis	• **Client history** Energy level Elimination pattern Nutrition Reproductive function Libido • **Family history** Endocrine disease • **Social history** Drug/alcohol use Coping skills Age Gender • **Weight change**	• **Appearance** Skin Hair Body fat distribution Muscle mass Bruising Petechiae Edema Face Genitalia • **Size of thyroid** • **Vital signs** • **Weight**	• **Adrenocorticotropic hormone (ACTH) levels** • **Aldosterone assay** • **Antidiuretic hormone (ADH)** • **Blood glucose** • **Catecholamines** Vanillylmandelic acid (VMA) • **Cortisol** • **Glycosolated hemoglobin A$_{1c}$** • **17-hydroxycorticosteroids** • **Ketones** • **Parathyroid hormone level** • **T$_3$/T$_4$** • **Thyroid scan**	• **Hormone replacement** • **Nutrition** • **Fluid management** • **Stress management** • **Client education** Diet Exercise Hormone replacement regimen Overdose Underdose Foot care Signs of complications Need for carrying emergency medical information • **Postoperative care/monitoring for complications** Thyroidectomy Adrenalectomy Pancreas transplantation • **Monitoring for hypoglycemia and hyperglycemia**	• Glucagon • Insulin • Oral hypoglycemic agents • Thyroid replacement • Thyroid inhibitors • Pituitary hormone replacements • Pituitary hormone inhibitors • Parathyroid hormone replacement • Parathyroid hormone inhibitors • Calcium • Adrenal hormone replacements • Adrenal hormone inhibitors

62

Assessment of the Endocrine System

M. LINDA WORKMAN

Learning Objectives

After studying this chapter, you should be able to:

1. Describe the relationship between hormones and receptor sites.
2. Explain negative feedback as a control mechanism for hormone secretion.
3. Discuss the structure and function of the hypothalamus.
4. Discuss the structure and function of the anterior and posterior pituitary glands.
5. Discuss the structure and function of the adrenal glands.
6. Discuss the structure and function of the thyroid and parathyroid glands.
7. Discuss the structure and function of the pancreas.
8. Describe changes in the endocrine system associated with aging.
9. Identify laboratory tests that aid in determining endocrine function and dysfunction.

Go to http://www.wbsaunders.com/SIMON/Iggy/ for self-assessment questions related to these Learning Objectives.

The endocrine system is composed of glands in many tissues and organs in a variety of body areas (Figure 62-1). A key feature of all endocrine glands is the secretion of hormones. **Hormones** are biochemicals that exert their effects on specific tissues known as **target tissues.** Target tissues are usually located some distance from the endocrine gland, with no direct physical connection between the endocrine gland and its target tissue. For this reason endocrine glands are called "ductless" glands and must use the circulatory system to transport secreted hormones to the target tissues. Endocrine glands include the following:

- Pituitary gland
- Adrenal glands
- Thyroid gland
- Islet cells of the pancreas
- Parathyroid glands
- Gonads

The endocrine system works with the nervous system to regulate overall physiologic function. Such control is called **neuroendocrine regulation.** Many interactions must occur between the endocrine system and all other body systems to ensure that each system maintains a constant normal balance **(homeostasis)** in response to environmental changes. For example, neuroendocrine control of other body systems keeps the internal body temperature at or near 98.6° F (37° C), even when environmental temperatures are lower or higher. Other neuroendocrine actions help keep the serum sodium level between 136 and 145 mEq/L (mmol/L), regardless of whether a person eats 2 g or 12 g of sodium per day.

Table 62-1 lists the specific hormones secreted by various endocrine glands. Hormones usually travel through the bloodstream to all body areas but exert their actions only on target tissues. Hormones recognize their target tissues and exert their actions by binding to receptor sites on or within the target tissue cells. In general, each receptor site type is specific for only one hormone. Hormone-receptor interactions work in a "lock and key" manner in that only the correct hormone (key) can bind to and activate the receptor site (lock) (Figure 62-2). Binding a hormone to its receptor causes the target tissue to change its activity. In this way, hormones produce specific responses even though they circulate throughout the body. Table 62-2 lists the key features of hormones.

Disorders of the endocrine system are related to either an excess or a deficiency of a specific hormone or to a defect at its receptor site. The onset of these disorders can be either slow and insidious or abrupt and life threatening.

The nurse's observation and interviewing skills are especially important in assessing the endocrine system. Except for the thyroid gland and the testicles, the endocrine glands cannot be examined directly. A knowledge of the anatomy and physiology of the endocrine system together with data obtained from the history and laboratory diagnostic tests is essential in assessing the endocrine system.

ANATOMY AND PHYSIOLOGY REVIEW

The control of cellular function by any hormone depends on a series of reactions working through **negative feedback control mechanisms.** Hormone secretion is dependent on the need of the body for the final action of that hormone. When a body condition starts to move away from the normal range and a specific action or response is needed to correct this change,

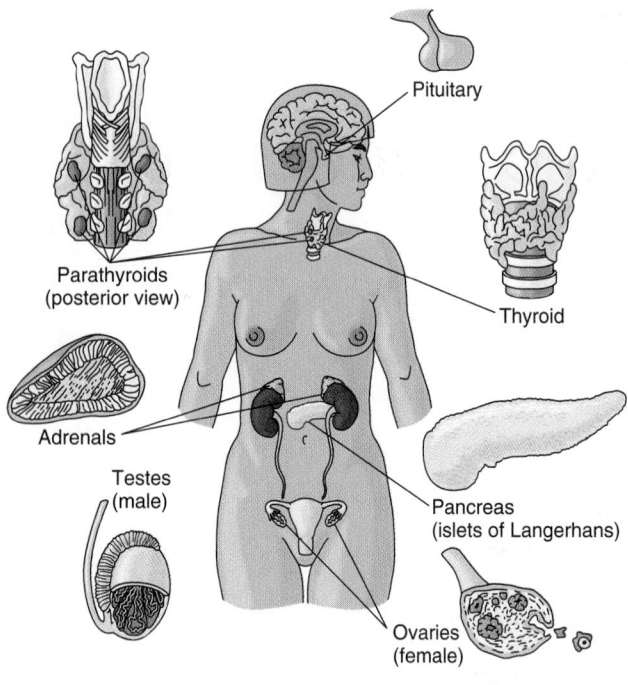

Figure 62-1 ● The endocrine system.

TABLE 62-1 • PRINCIPAL HORMONES OF THE ENDOCRINE GLANDS

Gland	Hormones
Anterior pituitary	Thyroid-stimulating hormone (TSH)
	Adrenocorticotropic hormone (ACTH, corticotropin)
	Luteinizing hormone (LH)
	Follicle-stimulating hormone (FSH)
	Prolactin (PRL)
	Growth hormone (GH)
	Melanocyte-stimulating hormone (MSH)
Posterior pituitary	Vasopressin (antidiuretic hormone [ADH])
	Oxytocin
Thyroid	Triiodothyronine (T_3)
	Thyroxine (T_4)
	Calcitonin
Parathyroids	Parathyroid hormone
Adrenal cortex	Glucocorticoids (cortisol)
	Mineralocorticoids (aldosterone)
Ovary	Estrogen
	Progesterone
Testes	Testosterone
Pancreas	Insulin _Beta_
	Glucagon _Alpha_
	Somatostatin _Delta_

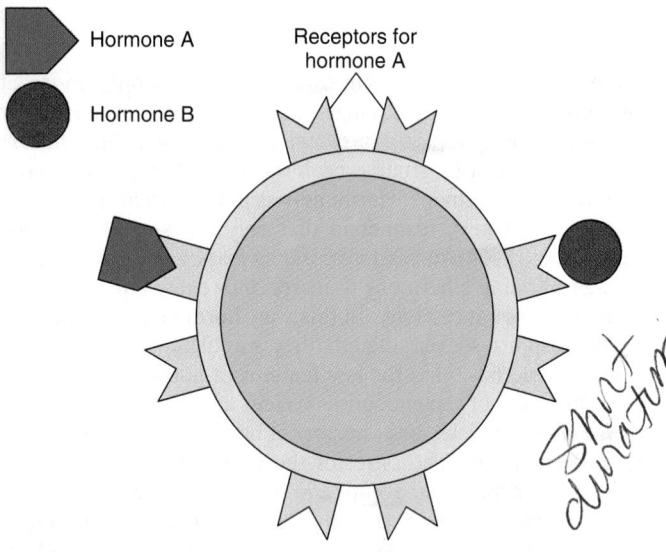

Figure 62-2 ● "Lock and key" hormone-receptor binding. Hormone A fits and binds to receptor sites, causing a change in cell action. Hormone B does not fit or bind to receptor sites, and therefore no change in cell action results.

TABLE 62-2 • COMMON KEY FEATURES OF HORMONES

- All hormones exert their effects at low blood concentrations.
- Receptors on or within target tissues are needed for *all* hormones to exert an effect.
- Most hormones (except for thyroid and adrenal medullary hormones) are not stored to any great extent and must be produced as needed.
- Hormones in the blood are bound to plasma proteins.
- Only free hormones (those not bound to plasma proteins) can bind to their receptor sites.
- Most hormones cause target tissues to increase or decrease their activity by changing gene activity either directly or indirectly. Exceptions are hormones that alter membrane permeability.
- The activity of most hormones is of short duration.
- Continued hormone activity requires continued production and secretion.
- The clearance of secreted hormones occurs through cellular uptake, enzymatic breakdown, gastrointestinal excretion, or urinary excretion.

secretion of the hormone capable of causing the correcting action or response is stimulated until the need (demand) is met. As the correction occurs, hormone secretion decreases (and may halt). This type of control for hormone synthesis is considered negative feedback because the hormone causes the opposite action of the initial condition change.

An example of a simple negative feedback hormone response is the control of insulin secretion. When blood glucose levels start to rise above normal, the hormone insulin is secreted. In-

sulin causes glucose to be taken up by the cells, causing a decrease in blood glucose levels. Thus the action of insulin (decreasing blood glucose levels) is opposite of the condition that stimulated insulin secretion (elevated blood glucose levels).

Some hormones that use negative feedback mechanisms have more complex interactions. These interactions involve a series of reactions in which more than one endocrine gland is stimulated as well as the final target tissues. In such a situation, the first hormone in the series may have another endocrine gland as its target tissue. For this type of mechanism to maintain homeostasis, the following series of interactions must occur:

- The central nervous system receives and reacts to various stimuli transmitted to the hypothalamus.

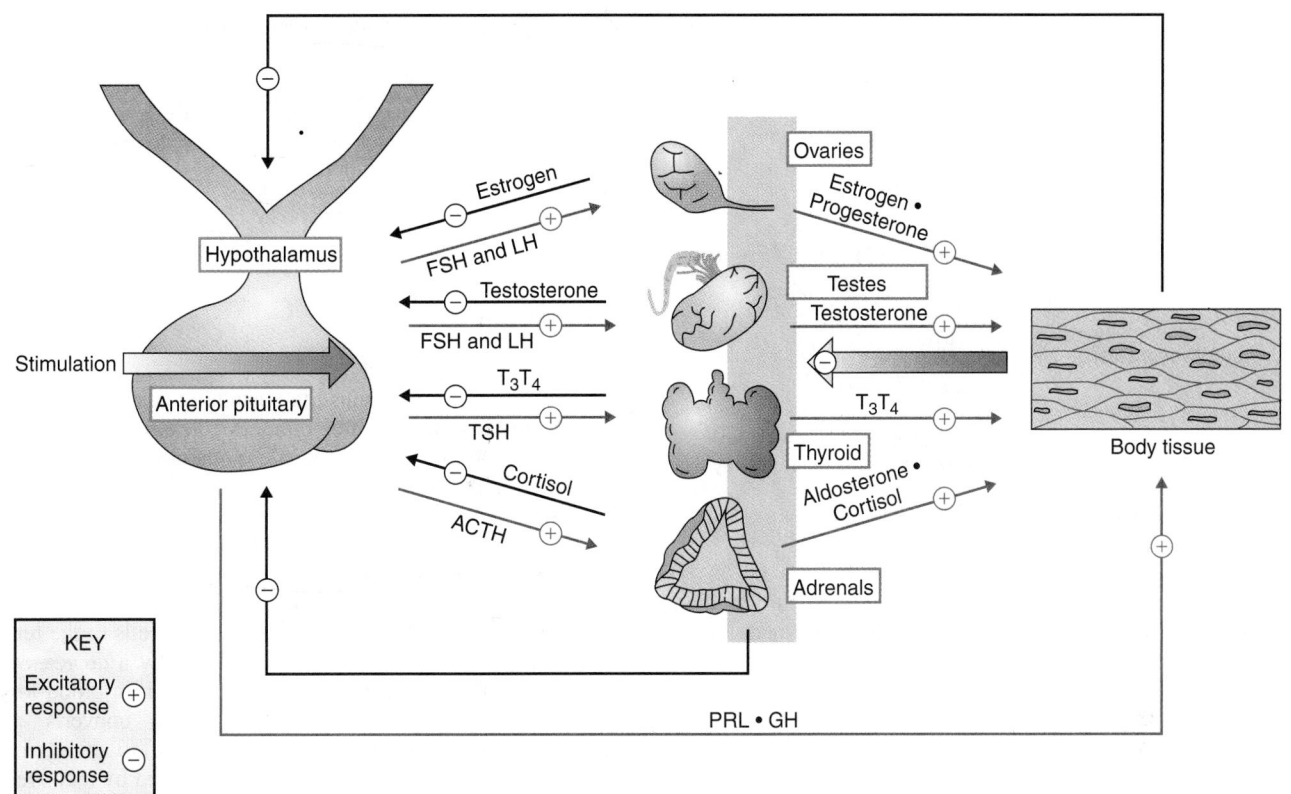

Figure 62-3 ● The feedback system of the hypothalamic-pituitary-target gland axis. (*ACTH,* Adrenocorticotropic hormone; *TSH,* thyroid-stimulating hormone; *T₃,* triiodothyronine; *T₄,* thyroxine; *FSH,* follicle-stimulating hormone; *LH,* luteinizing hormone; *PRL,* prolactin; *GH,* growth hormone.)

- The hypothalamus responds to the stimuli with the production and release of either releasing or inhibiting factors, which are transported to the pituitary.
- In the pituitary gland, the releasing or inhibiting factors either stimulate or inhibit the release of specific hormones.
- The anterior pituitary responds to these hormones by controlling the secretion of hormones from target organs or tissue.

This type of complex control is demonstrated by the interaction of the hypothalamus and the anterior pituitary with a target tissue (e.g., thyroid, adrenal cortex, or gonads) (Figure 62-3). The normal blood level range of each hormone is well defined. Excesses or deficiencies of hormone secretion can lead to pathologic conditions.

Hypothalamus and Pituitary Glands

Structure

The hypothalamus plays a major role in regulating endocrine function. The hypothalamus consists of nervous tissue located beneath the cerebral hemispheres and thalamus on each side of the third ventricle in the brain. Nerve fibers connect the hypothalamus to the rest of the central nervous system. The hypothalamus shares a miniature circulatory system with the anterior pituitary gland. This system is known as the **hypothalamic-hypophysial portal system** and allows hormones produced in the hypothalamus to travel directly to the anterior pituitary gland.

The pituitary gland is located at the base of the brain in an indentation of the sphenoid bone called the sella turcica (see Figure 62-1). The oval pituitary gland is about 1 cm in diameter and is divided into three lobes (Figure 62-4). The anterior lobe, or **adenohypophysis,** makes up about 70% of the gland. The posterior lobe, or **neurohypophysis,** stores hormones produced in the hypothalamus. Nerve fibers in the hypophysial stalk, a structure extending from the hypothalamus, connect the hypothalamus to the posterior pituitary. The area between the anterior and posterior lobes is the intermediate lobe **(pars intermedia).**

Function

The hypothalamus has both endocrine and nonendocrine functions. The endocrine function is to produce regulatory hormones (Table 62-3). Some of these hormones are released into the bloodstream and travel to the anterior pituitary, where they either stimulate or inhibit the release of anterior pituitary hormones.

In response to the releasing hormones of the hypothalamus, the anterior pituitary secretes **tropic hormones,** which stimulate various glands. Other anterior pituitary hormones, such as growth hormone (somatotropin) and prolactin, produce their primary effect directly on final target tissues (Table 62-4).

The hormones of the posterior pituitary, vasopressin (antidiuretic hormone [ADH]) and oxytocin, are produced in the hypothalamus and transported by the nerve tracts that connect the hypothalamus with the posterior pituitary. These hormones are stored in the nerve endings of the posterior pituitary and are released into the blood vessels when needed.

Other conditions or substances can affect the release of

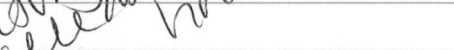

Stalk

Pars tuberalis

Capsule

Posterior lobe (neurohypophysis)

Intermediate lobe (pars intermedia)

Anterior lobe (adenohypophysis)

Figure 62-4 ● The pituitary gland.

TABLE 62-3 ● HYPOTHALAMIC HORMONES

- Thyrotropin-releasing hormone (TRH)
- Gonadotropin-releasing hormone (Gn-RH)
- Growth hormone–releasing hormone (GH-RH)
- Growth hormone–inhibiting hormone (somatostatin) (GH-IH)
- Corticotropin-releasing hormone (CRH)
- Prolactin-inhibiting hormone (PIH)
- Melanocyte-inhibiting hormone (MIH)

Function

MINERALOCORTICOIDS

The adrenal cortex maintains life-sustaining physiologic activities. **Aldosterone,** the chief mineralocorticoid produced by the adrenal cortex, plays a vital role in maintaining extracellular fluid volume. Aldosterone promotes sodium and water reabsorption and potassium excretion in the kidney tubules. Aldosterone secretion is regulated by the renin-angiotensin system, serum potassium ion concentration, and the presence of adrenocorticotropic hormone (ACTH or corticotropin).

Renin is produced by the juxtaglomerular cells of the renal afferent arterioles. Its release is stimulated by a decrease in extracellular fluid volume, which can occur from blood loss, sodium loss, or posture changes. Renin converts angiotensinogen (a plasma protein from the live) to angiotensin I. Angiotensin I undergoes a reaction catalyzed by a converting enzyme to form angiotensin II, the active form of angiotensin. In turn, angiotensin II stimulates the secretion of aldosterone. Chapters 11 (Figure 11-8), 12 (Figure 12-2), and 69 further describe the renin-angiotensin system. Aldosterone causes kidney reabsorption of sodium and water to bring the plasma volume and concentration back to normal.

Serum potassium ion concentration also has a regulatory effect on aldosterone secretion. The adrenal cortex secretes aldosterone when the serum potassium concentration increases above normal by as little as 0.1 mEq/L (Orth & Kovacs, 1998).

ACTH has a weak stimulatory effect on aldosterone secretion. When ACTH is administered, aldosterone secretion rapidly rises during the first hour then decreases rapidly to basal levels.

hormones from the pituitary gland (Table 62-5). Drugs, diet, lifestyle, and pathologic conditions can increase or decrease pituitary hormone secretion.

Gonads

The **gonads** are the male and female endocrine glands of reproduction. Male gonads are the testes, and female gonads are the ovaries. Although these glands are formed prenatally and are present at birth, their function does not begin until puberty.

During puberty in the male, the increased secretion of gonadotropins (luteinizing hormone [LH] and follicle-stimulating hormone [FSH]) from the anterior pituitary gland stimulates maturation of the testes, production of testosterone, and maturation of the external genitalia. During puberty in the female, increased secretion of the same gonadotropins stimulates ovarian maturation, estrogen production, ovulation, and maturation of the external genitalia. The structure and function of the testes and ovaries are detailed in Chapter 73.

Adrenal Glands

The adrenal glands are highly vascular, tent-shaped organs located at the top of each kidney (see Figure 62-1). Each gland is about 3.3 cm long and weighs $\frac{1}{16}$ to $\frac{1}{8}$ ounce (1.8 to 3.5 g).

The adrenal gland consists of an outer portion (**cortex**) and an inner portion (**medulla**); each has independent functions. The hormones of the adrenal glands have physiologic effects throughout the body.

ADRENAL CORTEX
Structure

The adrenal cortex makes up about 90% of the adrenal gland and consists of cells divided into three zones or layers (Figure 62-5). **Mineralocorticoids** are produced in the zona glomerulosa and help control the body's mineral content, especially sodium and potassium. Glucocorticoids, androgens, and estrogens are produced in the zona fasciculata and zona reticularis. The hormones produced and secreted by the cortex are often called **adrenal steroids** or **corticosteroids.**

GLUCOCORTICOIDS

The principal glucocorticoid secreted by the adrenal cortex is **cortisol.** Cortisol affects the following:

- Carbohydrate, protein, and fat metabolism
- The body's response to stress
- Emotional stability
- Immune function

Cortisol has a permissive effect on other physiologic processes. It must be present for other physiologic processes to occur, such as catecholamine action and the maintenance of normal excitability of the myocardium. Glucocorticoid functions are summarized in Table 62-6.

The release of glucocorticoids is regulated directly by the anterior pituitary hormone ACTH and indirectly by the hypothalamic corticotropin-releasing hormone (CRH). The release of CRH and ACTH is affected by the serum concentration of free cortisol, the diurnal sleep-wake cycle, and stress.

TABLE 62-4 • PITUITARY HORMONES: TARGET TISSUES AND SUBSEQUENT ACTIONS

Hormone	Target Tissue	Actions
ANTERIOR PITUITARY		
TSH (thyroid-stimulating hormone)	Thyroid	Stimulates synthesis and release of thyroid hormone
ACTH (adrenocorticotropic hormone, corticotropin)	Adrenal cortex	Stimulates synthesis and release of corticosteroids and adrenocortical growth
LH (luteinizing hormone)	Ovary	Stimulates ovulation and progesterone secretion
	Testes	Stimulates testosterone secretion
FSH (follicle-stimulating hormone)	Ovary	Stimulates estrogen secretion and follicle maturation
	Testes	Stimulates spermatogenesis
PRL (prolactin)	Mammary glands	Stimulates breast milk production
GH (growth hormone)	Bone and soft tissue	Promotes growth through lipolysis, protein anabolism, and insulin antagonism
MSH (melanocyte-stimulating hormone)	Melanocytes	Promotes pigmentation
POSTERIOR PITUITARY*		
Vasopressin (antidiuretic hormone [ADH])	Kidney	Promotes water reabsorption
Oxytocin	Uterus and mammary glands	Stimulates uterine contractions and ejection of breast milk

*These hormones are synthesized in the hypothalamus and are stored in the posterior pituitary gland. They are transported from the hypothalamus to the posterior pituitary while bound to neurophysins.

When levels of serum cortisol are low, the hypothalamus secretes CRH, which stimulates the pituitary to release ACTH. ACTH then stimulates the adrenal cortex to secrete cortisol. Conversely, adequate or elevated levels of circulating free cortisol *inhibit* the release of CRH and ACTH. This inhibitory effect is an example of a negative feedback system.

Glucocorticoid release peaks in the morning and reaches its lowest level 12 hours before and after each peak. Emotional, chemical, or physical stress results in an increased release of glucocorticoids.

■ SEX HORMONES

Small amounts of androgens and estrogens are secreted by the adrenal cortex in both genders. Adrenal secretion of these hormones is usually not significant because the **gonads** (ovaries and testes) secrete much larger amounts of estrogens and androgens. In women, however, the adrenal gland is the major source of androgens. Women who have adrenal insufficiency or who have undergone surgical removal of the adrenals may need a small amount of testosterone replacement.

■ ADRENAL MEDULLA

■ Structure

The adrenal medulla is actually a sympathetic nerve ganglion with glandular secretory cells. Stimulation of the sympathetic nervous system results in the release of adrenal medullary hormones, the **catecholamines.** Catecholamines travel to all areas of the body through the bloodstream and exert their effects on target cells. The adrenal medullary hormones are not essential for life but play a role in the physiologic stress response.

■ Function

The adrenal medulla secretes two catecholamines, **norepinephrine (NE)** and **epinephrine,** in proportions of 15% and

TABLE 62-5 • FACTORS AFFECTING SECRETION/RELEASE OF SELECTED PITUITARY HORMONES

VASOPRESSIN
Potential Causes of Increased Secretion
- Congestive heart failure
- Hemorrhage
- Diuretics
- Opioids
- Chlorpropamide
    Diabinese
    Novo-Propamide✦
- Cyclophosphamide
- Vincristine
- Nicotine
- Stress
- Hypoxia

Potential Causes of Decreased Secretion
- Alcohol consumption
- Phenytoin

GROWTH HORMONE
Potential Causes of Increased Secretion
- High-protein diet
- Deep sleep
- Hypoglycemia
- Fasting
- Estrogen
- Glucagon
- Dopamine

Potential Causes of Decreased Secretion
- REM sleep
- Hyperglycemia
- Obesity
- Hypothyroidism

PROLACTIN
Potential Causes of Increased Secretion
- Stress
- Nipple manipulation
- Estrogen
- Dopamine antagonists
- Chlorpromazine
    Thorazine
    Chlorpromanyl✦

Potential Causes of Decreased Secretion
- Dopamine
- Hyperthyroidism

OXYTOCIN
Potential Causes of Increased Secretion
- Nipple manipulation
- Orgasm
- Extracellular fluid hypertonicity

Potential Causes of Decreased Secretion
- Stress
- Opioids

Data from Wilson, J., et al. (Eds.). (1998). *William's textbook of endocrinology* (9th ed.). Philadelphia: W.B. Saunders.

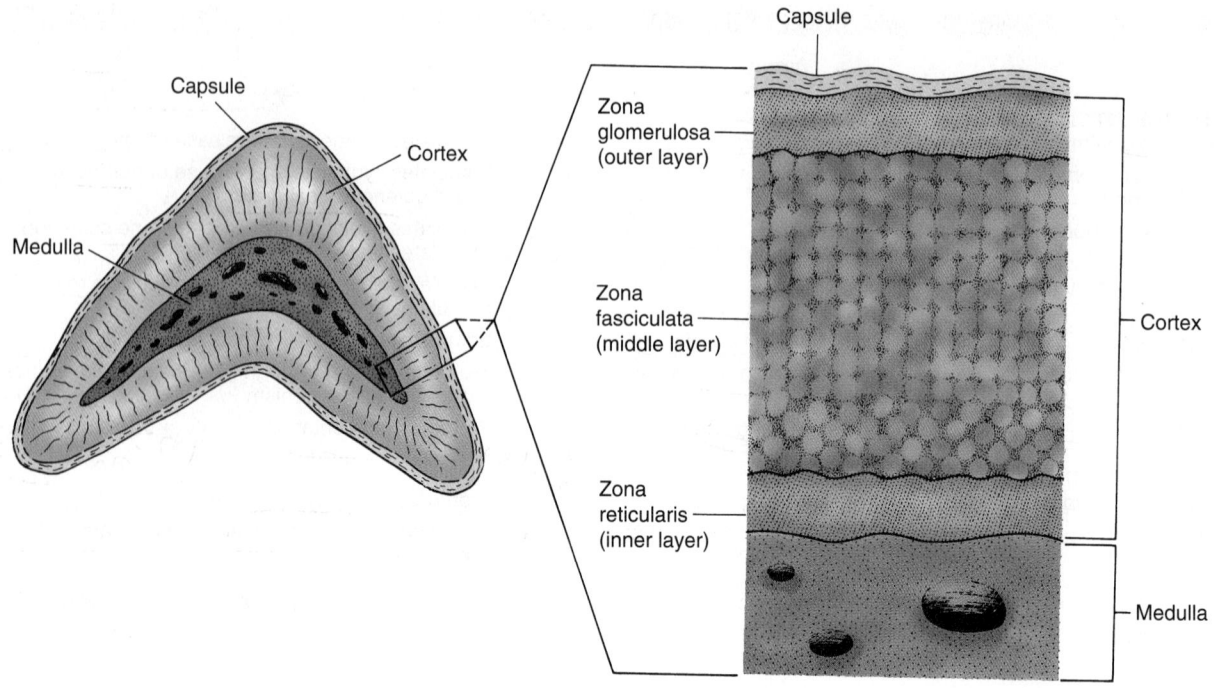

Figure 62-5 ● The structural detail of the adrenal gland.

TABLE 62-6 ● FUNCTIONS OF GLUCOCORTICOID HORMONES
• Maintain blood glucose level by increasing hepatic gluconeogenesis and inhibiting peripheral glucose use
• Increase lipolysis, releasing glycerol and free fatty acids
• Increase protein catabolism
• Degrade collagen and connective tissue
• Increase the number of polymorphonuclear leukocytes released from bone marrow
• Exert anti-inflammatory effects that decrease the migration of inflammatory cells to sites of injury
• Maintain behavior and cognitive functions

85%, respectively. The effects of catecholamines vary according to the specific receptor in the cell membranes of the target tissue.

These receptors are of two types: alpha adrenergic and beta adrenergic. Both types of receptors are further classified as alpha$_1$- and alpha$_2$-receptors and beta$_1$-, beta$_2$-, and beta$_3$-receptors. NE acts primarily on alpha-adrenergic receptors, whereas epinephrine most often stimulates beta-adrenergic receptors.

Catecholamines exert their actions on many target organs. Table 62-7 summarizes the effects of adrenal medullary hormone stimulation on body tissues and organs.

Activation of the sympathetic nervous system, with the subsequent release of adrenal medullary catecholamines, is an important component of the body's response to stress. Catecholamines are secreted in small amounts at all times to maintain homeostasis. Severe physical or psychologic stress triggers the increased secretion of catecholamines. This sympathetic activation results in the "fight-or-flight" response, a state of heightened physical and emotional awareness. (See Chapter 41 for more information on the sympathetic [adrenergic] nervous system.)

TABLE 62-7 ● CATECHOLAMINE RECEPTORS AND EFFECTS OF ADRENAL MEDULLARY HORMONE STIMULATION ON SELECTED ORGANS AND TISSUES		
Organ or Tissue	**Receptors**	**Effects**
Heart	Beta$_1$	Chronotropic action Inotropic action
Blood vessels	Alpha Beta$_2$	Vasoconstriction Vasodilation
Gastrointestinal tract	Alpha Beta	Increased sphincter tone Decreased motility
Kidney	Beta$_2$	Increased renin release
Bronchioles	Beta$_2$	Relaxation; dilation
Bladder	Alpha Beta$_2$	Sphincter contractions Relaxation of detrusor muscle
Skin	Alpha	Increased sweating
Fat cells	Beta	Increased lipolysis
Liver	Alpha	Increased gluconeogenesis and glycogenolysis
Pancreas	Alpha Beta	Decreased glucagon and insulin release Increased glucagon and insulin release
Eyes	Alpha	Dilation of pupils

Thyroid Gland

Structure

The thyroid gland is located anteriorly in the neck, directly below the cricoid cartilage (Figure 62-6). In the average adult, the thyroid weighs approximately ³⁄₅ of an ounce (18 g). It has

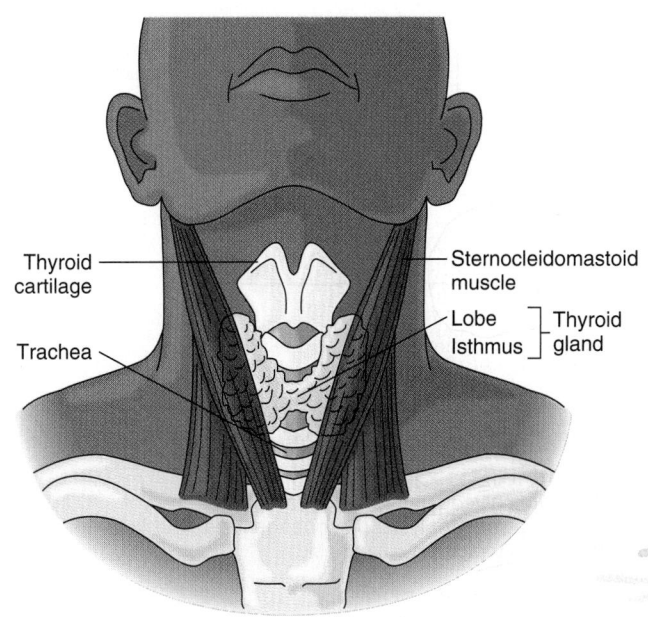

TABLE 62-8 • FUNCTIONS OF THYROID HORMONES

• Fetal development, particularly neural and skeletal systems
• Control metabolic rate of all cells
• Promote sufficient pituitary secretion of GH and
   gonadotropins
• Regulate protein, carbohydrate, and fat metabolism
• Exert chronotropic and inotropic cardiac effects
• Increase red blood cell production
• Affect respiratory rate and drive
• Increase bone formation and decrease bone resorption of
   calcium
• Act as insulin antagonists

GH, Growth hormone.

Figure 62-6 • Anatomic location of the thyroid gland.

two lobes joined by a thin **isthmus** that lies in front of the trachea.

The thyroid gland has a rich blood supply. The right lobe has a greater blood supply and is often larger than the left lobe. The thyroid is composed of follicular and parafollicular cells. Follicular cells produce and secrete the thyroid hormones **thyroxine (T_4)** and **triiodothyronine (T_3).** Parafollicular cells produce and secrete **thyrocalcitonin** (calcitonin), which plays a role in calcium regulation.

Function
REGULATION OF BASAL METABOLIC RATE

Both T_3 and T_4 increase the basal metabolic rate, which causes an increase in oxygen consumption and heat production. The two hormones differ not in function but rather in structure. Approximately 99.5% of circulating T_4 and T_3 is bound to plasma proteins, including prealbumin, albumin, and thyroid-binding globulin, but the proportion of bound hormone is in equilibrium with the free hormone. The free hormone is transported into the cell, where it binds to a specific receptor in the cell nucleus. Once in the cell, T_4 is converted to T_3—the most active form of the hormone. The cellular conversion of T_4 to T_3 is impaired by a number of factors that include stress, starvation, radiopaque dyes, beta blockers, and propylthiouracil (PTU); cold temperatures seem to increase conversion. Table 62-8 summarizes thyroid hormone function.

The secretion of T_3 and T_4 is regulated by a hypothalamic-pituitary-thyroid gland axis, or feedback mechanism. The anterior pituitary secretes thyroid-stimulating hormone (TSH), which stimulates the thyroid gland to release thyroid hormone. The circulating level of thyroid hormone is the major factor regulating the release of TSH: if thyroid hormone levels are high, TSH release is inhibited; if low, TSH release is increased. This is a classic example of a negative feedback system. Se-

cretion of TSH is also affected by the hypothalamic secretion of thyrotropin-releasing hormone (TRH). Cold and stress are two factors that cause the hypothalamus to secrete TRH, which then stimulates the anterior pituitary to secrete TSH.

The synthesis of thyroid hormones involves a series of steps. A sufficient dietary intake of protein and iodine in food and water is essential to produce thyroid hormones. Iodine is absorbed from the gastrointestinal tract as iodide. The thyroid gland withdraws iodide from the circulation and concentrates it. After its transport in the thyroid, iodide enters into a series of reactions that result in the formation of T_4 or T_3. The hormones are bound to thyroglobulin and are stored in the follicular cells of the thyroid gland. With stimulation, T_4 and T_3 break off from thyroglobulin and are released into the circulation.

CALCIUM AND PHOSPHATE REGULATION

Calcitonin is another thyroid hormone produced in the medullary portion of the thyroid. Calcitonin lowers serum calcium and serum phosphate levels by inhibiting bone resorption (breakdown). It works in opposition to parathyroid hormone (PTH).

The primary factor influencing calcitonin secretion is the serum calcium level. Low serum calcium levels suppress the release of calcitonin; elevated serum calcium levels increase its secretion. Additional factors that cause an increased release of calcitonin are pregnancy, a high-calcium diet, and an increased secretion of gastrin.

Parathyroid Glands
Structure

The parathyroid glands consist of four small glands located close to, embedded in, or attached to the posterior surface of the thyroid gland (see Figure 62-1). The parathyroid glands are composed of two types of cells: chief and oxyphil. Only the chief cells, which produce and secrete PTH, have endocrine function.

Function

PTH regulates calcium and phosphate metabolism as a result of its effect on three target organs: bone, kidney, and the gastrointestinal (GI) tract (Figure 62-7). Bone is the primary storage site of calcium in the body. PTH promotes increased bone resorption, thus increasing serum calcium. In the kidney

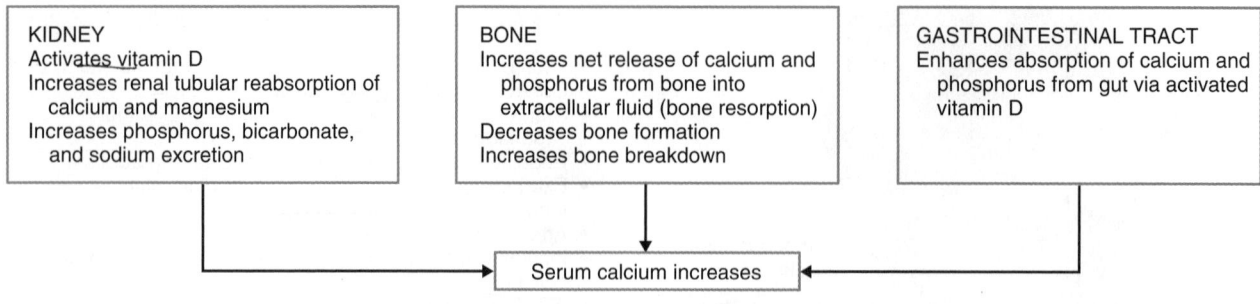

KIDNEY	BONE	GASTROINTESTINAL TRACT
Activates vitamin D Increases renal tubular reabsorption of calcium and magnesium Increases phosphorus, bicarbonate, and sodium excretion	Increases net release of calcium and phosphorus from bone into extracellular fluid (bone resorption) Decreases bone formation Increases bone breakdown	Enhances absorption of calcium and phosphorus from gut via activated vitamin D

Serum calcium increases

Figure 62-7 ● Effects of parathyroid hormone on target organs.

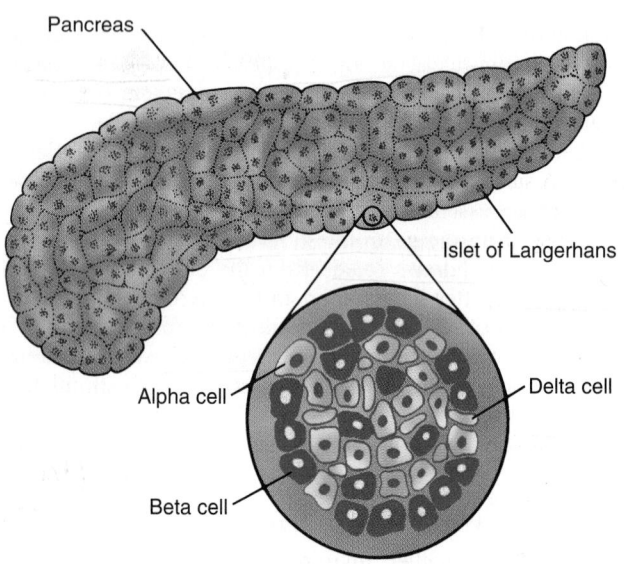

Figure 62-8 ● The islets of Langerhans of the pancreas.

tubules, PTH activates vitamin D, which increases the absorption of calcium and phosphate from the GI tract.

Calcium is the major controlling factor of PTH secretion. PTH secretion decreases when serum calcium levels are elevated, and it increases when serum calcium levels are low. Serum phosphate levels also affect PTH secretion, most likely because of its effect on serum calcium levels. PTH and calcitonin work together to maintain a normal level of ionic calcium in the extracellular fluid.

Pancreas
Structure

The pancreas lies behind the stomach and has endocrine and exocrine functions. The **islets of Langerhans** perform the endocrine functions of the pancreas (Figure 62-8). There are about 1 million islet cells throughout the pancreas.

The islets of Langerhans are composed of three distinct cell types: alpha cells, which secrete **glucagon;** beta cells, which secrete **insulin;** and delta cells, which secrete **somatostatin.** Glucagon and insulin affect carbohydrate, protein, and fat metabolism. Somatostatin, which is secreted not only in the pancreas but also in the gut and the brain, inhibits the release and action of glucagon and insulin from the pancreas. It also inhibits the release and action of gastrin, secretin, and other peptides in the gut.

TABLE 62-9 · ANABOLIC EFFECTS OF INSULIN

EFFECTS ON LIVER
- Promotes glycogen synthesis and storage
- Inhibits glycogenolysis, gluconeogenesis, and ketogenesis
- Increases triglyceride synthesis

EFFECTS ON MUSCLE
- Promotes protein synthesis
- Increases amino acid transport
- Promotes glycogenesis

EFFECTS ON FAT
- Increases fatty acid synthesis
- Promotes triglyceride storage
- Decreases lipolysis

Function

The exocrine function of the pancreas involves the secretion of digestive enzymes through ducts that empty into the duodenum (see Chapter 53). The primary endocrine function of the pancreas is to regulate blood glucose (sugar).

Glucagon increases blood glucose levels. Glucagon is stimulated by a decrease in blood glucose levels and an increase in blood amino acid levels. In conjunction with epinephrine, growth hormone (GH), and the glucocorticoids, glucagon maintains blood glucose levels. In the liver, the primary target organ of glucagon, glucagon causes **glycogenolysis** (the conversion of glycogen to glucose). In addition, glucagon enhances amino acid transport from muscle and promotes **gluconeogenesis** (the conversion of amino acids to glucose). In fat metabolism, glucagon enhances **lipolysis** (fat breakdown) and subsequent ketone formation.

Insulin, an **anabolic** hormone (one that stimulates growth), promotes the synthesis and storage of carbohydrate (CHO), protein, and fat (Table 62-9). Insulin lowers blood glucose levels by enhancing glucose diffusion across cell membranes in many tissues. Basal levels of insulin are secreted continuously in the fasting state to control metabolism. Insulin secretion rises in response to an increase in blood glucose levels. CHO is the major stimulus for insulin secretion; amino acids may produce an effect that is similar but not as potent. More information on insulin is presented in Chapter 65.

Endocrine Changes Associated with Aging

The effects of aging on the endocrine system vary considerably. It is difficult to distinguish normal from abnormal en-

CHART 62-1

NURSING FOCUS *on the* **OLDER ADULT**
Changes in the Endocrine System Related to Aging

Physiologic Change	Nursing Actions	Rationale
Decreased antidiuretic hormone (ADH)	Assess for diluted urine and polyuria.	Ongoing assessment helps to detect early signs of complications.
	Monitor fluid intake and output. Encourage fluid intake unless contraindicated.	A sufficient fluid intake may help prevent dehydration.
Decreased ovarian function	Teach the client the signs and symptoms of estrogen deficiency.	The client's ability to cope with changes may be enhanced with knowledge.
	Promote exercise and calcium intake.	Sufficient exercise and calcium intake delay bone loss and prevent osteoporosis.
Decreased glucose tolerance	Identify at risk clients by obtaining a family history of diabetes mellitus and obesity.	Identification of at-risk clients helps in early detection of complications and conditions such as diabetes.
	Assess for greater-than-ideal body weight or body mass index, little physical exercise, frequent yeast infections, polydipsia, polyuria.	
	Teach the client the signs and symptoms of hyperglycemia.	Knowledge helps improve the client's ability to recognize hyperglycemia.
Decreased peripheral metabolism	Assess for signs and symptoms of hypothyroidism, especially constipation, lethargy, dry skin, and mental deterioration.	Ongoing assessment helps differentiate hypothyroidism from the clinical features of aging.

docrine activity because of age-related variables such as the following:

- Acute and chronic illnesses
- Alterations in diet, activity, and lean body mass/fat ratio
- Disturbances in sleep patterns
- Decreased metabolic clearance rate of hormones
- Increased use of multiple drugs that may affect hormone function

The nurse considers these variables when assessing the client with endocrine dysfunction.

The nurse encourages the older adult client to participate in regular screening examinations, including fasting and postprandial blood glucose checks, calcium level determinations, and thyroid function testing. Chart 62-1 summarizes the endocrine changes that occur in the older adult and lists related nursing interventions.

ASSESSMENT TECHNIQUES

History

A systems approach is used for obtaining the history of clients with a suspected endocrine problem. This approach can be difficult because of the variety and combination of clinical symptoms. The information gathered from the history provides a basis for physical assessment and for planning care. The nurse identifies the client's response to actual or perceived changes and discusses the potential diagnostic and treatment plan. Chart 62-2 presents some assessment questions based on Gordon's Functional Health Patterns. Although endocrine problems can disturb any health pattern, the patterns most commonly affected are Nutritional-Metabolic, Activity, Elimination, Sleep-Rest, and Sexuality-Reproductive. These data are combined with

physical, psychosocial, and laboratory findings for a complete assessment of endocrine function.

■ DEMOGRAPHIC DATA

The age and gender of the client provide essential baseline assessment data. Certain disorders are more common in older than in younger clients, such as hyperosmolar states, loss of ovarian function, and decreased thyroid and parathyroid function. In particular, decreased glucose tolerance is common among older adults.

Manifestations of endocrine disorders can be gender related, such as the sexual effects of hyperpituitarism and hypopituitarism (see Chapter 63).

■ PERSONAL AND FAMILY HISTORY

The client is asked about any family history of obesity, growth or development difficulties, diabetes mellitus, infertility, or thyroid disorders. The nurse further assesses the client for a history of the following:

- Endocrine dysfunction
- Signs or symptoms that could indicate an endocrine disorder
- Hospitalizations

The client is asked about past and current medications, such as hydrocortisone, levothyroxine, oral contraceptives, and antihypertensive drugs.

■ DIET HISTORY

Nutritional changes or gastrointestinal (GI) tract disturbances may reflect a variety of endocrine problems. The nurse as-

CHART 62-2

ENDOCRINE ASSESSMENT
Using Gordon's Functional Health Patterns

Nutritional-Metabolic Pattern

What is your typical daily food intake? Describe a day's meals, snacks, and vitamins.

How much salt do you typically add to your food? Do you use salt substitutes?

How is your appetite?

Do you have any difficulty chewing or swallowing?

What is your typical daily fluid intake? What types of fluids (water, juices, soft drinks, coffee, tea)? How much?

Have you had any recent change in your weight? Weight gain? Weight loss? How much?

Have you noticed a change in the tightness of your rings or shoes? Tighter? Looser?

Elimination Pattern

What is your usual bowel elimination pattern? Frequency? Character? Discomfort? Laxatives?

What is your usual urinary elimination pattern? Frequency? Amount? Color? Odor? Control?

Have you noticed a change in the amount of urine?

Do you have any problem with excessive perspiration?

Do you have any other type of drainage?

Sleep-Rest Pattern

Do you have any difficulty falling asleep when you go to bed?

Is there a change in the number of hours you sleep per night?

Do you take any medication to help you sleep?

About how many times to you wake up during the night?

Do you have any difficulty getting back to sleep?

Are you bothered by nightmares or vivid dreams?

Do you have difficulty waking up in the morning?

Do you feel generally rested and ready for daily activities after sleep?

Do you take scheduled naps or rest periods during the day?

Do you find yourself falling asleep at work or at home while reading or watching television?

Sexuality-Reproductive Pattern

Are you sexually active?

Are you satisfied with your level of sexual activity?

Do you participate in sex as often as you would like?

Do you participate in sex as often as your partner would like?

Have you noticed a change in your interest in having sex over the past year?

Female:

At what age did menstruation start?

How regular are your periods?

Do you have any pain, cramping, or clotting during your periods?

Have you ever been pregnant? What was the outcome of the pregnancy(ies)?

Do you use contraceptives? What type? Have you had any problems with your chosen method of contraception?

Activity-Exercise Pattern

Do you feel you have sufficient energy to perform tasks or routines that are required of you?

Do you feel you have sufficient energy to do what you would like to do?

Do you exercise? How often? For how long each time? What type(s) of exercise do you perform?

What activities do you perform in your spare time?

What is your ability to perform the following tasks?

Feeding _____	Grooming _____
Bathing _____	General Mobility _____
Toileting _____	Cooking _____
Bed Mobility _____	Home Maintenance _____
Dressing _____	Shopping _____

Functional Levels Code

Level 0: Full self-care

Level I: Requires use of equipment or device

Level II: Requires assistance or supervision of another person

Level III: Requires assistance or supervision of another person and use of equipment or device

Level IV: Is dependent and does not participate

Based on Gordon, M. (2000). *Manual of nursing diagnosis* (9th ed.). St. Louis: Mosby.

sesses for a history of nausea, vomiting, and abdominal pain. An increase or decrease in food or fluid intake may also indicate specific disorders. For example, diabetes insipidus is characterized by excessive thirst, and primary adrenal hypofunction is characterized by salt craving. Hunger and thirst may also be increased in diabetes mellitus. Rapid changes in weight without accompanying changes in diet can signal the onset of a number of endocrine disorders, including diabetes mellitus and thyroid dysfunction.

SOCIOECONOMIC STATUS

Because the client's socioeconomic status can be a sensitive issue, the nurse explores with the client whether his or her resources are adequate to maintain a healthy diet, purchase needed medications, and seek consistent health care follow-up. This initial determination of socioeconomic status allows the nurse to involve social service and home care agencies at an early stage.

CURRENT HEALTH PROBLEMS

The nurse focuses on the client's reason for seeking health care, asking questions such as the following:

- Did the client's symptoms occur gradually, or was the onset sudden?
- Has the client been treated for this problem in the past?
- How have the current symptoms interfered with activities of daily living?

Such questioning provides clues to specific endocrine disorders. The nurse also explores changes in energy levels, elimination patterns, sexual and reproductive functions, and physical characteristics.

Energy Levels

Changes in energy levels are associated with a number of endocrine problems, particularly of the thyroid (see Chapter 64) and adrenal glands (see Chapter 63). The nurse asks the client about any change in ability to perform daily activities and assesses the client's current energy level. For instance, has the client been sleeping longer or experiencing fatigue or generalized weakness?

Elimination

Elimination patterns are also affected by the endocrine system. The nurse identifies the client's past pattern of elimination to determine deviations from the normal routine. The client is asked about urine amount and frequency. Does he or she urinate frequently in large amounts? Does the client wake during the night to urinate (**nocturia**), or does he or she experience pain on urination (**dysuria**)? Information about the frequency of bowel movements and their consistency and color may provide clues to problems in fluid balance or metabolic rate (i.e., thyroid function).

■ Sex and Reproduction

Sexual and reproductive functions are greatly affected by disturbances in the endocrine system. Women are asked about any changes in the menstrual cycle such as increased flow, duration, and frequency of menses; pain or excessive cramping; or a recent change in the regularity of menses. Men are asked whether they have experienced impotence. The nurse questions both men and women about a change in libido or any fertility problems.

■ Physical Appearance

The nurse discusses any changes in physical characteristics that the client perceives. Overt changes are identified during the physical assessment, but clients may be able to describe subtle changes that the nurse might miss. The client is asked about changes in the following:

- Hair texture or distribution
- Facial contours
- Voice quality
- Body proportions
- Secondary sexual characteristics

For example, the nurse might ask a man if he is shaving less often or a woman if she has noticed an increase in facial hair. These changes may be associated with pituitary, thyroid, parathyroid, or adrenal dysfunction.

⊙ CRITICAL THINKING CHALLENGE

The client is a 27-year-old woman who stopped having menstrual periods 6 months ago. She is not pregnant. At the beginning of the interview, the client shouts at you because she had to wait 15 minutes beyond her assigned appointment time. After the shouting, the client suddenly bursts into tears and apologizes to you.

- Given the client's age, gender, and initial presentation, are there any endocrine glands that do not need to be assessed? If so, which ones and why?
- What would be an appropriate response to this client's expressed anger and apology?
- What specific questions regarding her menstrual cycle should you ask?

For suggested answer guidelines, go to [SIMON] http://www.wbsaunders.com/SIMON/Iggy/.

Physical Assessment

■ INSPECTION

An endocrine problem can result in characteristic physical changes because of its effect on growth and development, regulation of sex hormone levels, fluid and electrolyte balance, and the body's use of nutrients. The nurse should be cautious, however, because many different clinical findings can be associated with multiple endocrine disorders or with nonendocrine pathologic processes.

Inspection of the client using a head-to-toe approach is often effective. The client's general appearance is observed, and height, weight, fat distribution, and muscle mass are assessed in relation to age. It is important to remember that heredity and age rather than a pathologic condition may be responsible for significant deviations (e.g., short stature).

When examining the head, the nurse focuses on abnormalities of facial structure, features, and expression, such as the following:

- Prominent forehead or jaw
- Round or puffy face
- Dull or flat expression
- Exophthalmos (protruding eyeballs and retracted upper lids)

The lower half of the neck is observed for a visible enlargement of the thyroid gland. In most instances the thyroid tissue cannot be observed. The isthmus may be noticeable when the client swallows. Jugular vein distention may be noted on inspection of the neck and can indicate fluid overload (see Chapter 12).

Skin abnormalities may reflect a dysfunction of specific endocrine glands. The nurse observes skin color and notes areas of hypopigmentation or hyperpigmentation. Fungal skin infections, slow wound healing, bruising, and petechiae are often seen in clients with adrenocortical hyperfunction. Skin infections, foot ulcers, and slow wound healing are common among clients with diabetes mellitus. In secondary hypofunction of the adrenal glands, the skin over the finger joints, elbows, and knees, as well as any scar tissue, may show increased pigmentation due to increased levels of ACTH and melanocyte-stimulating hormone.

Vitiligo (patchy areas of depigmentation with increased pigmentation at the edges) is seen with primary hypofunction of the adrenal glands and is due to autoimmune destruction of melanocytes in the skin. Areas of decreased pigmentation most often occur on the face, neck, and extremities. Mucous membranes can exhibit large areas of pigmentation. The nurse documents the location, distribution, color, and size of all skin discolorations and lesions.

The nurse inspects the client's fingernails for malformation, thickness, or brittleness, all of which may suggest thyroid gland difficulties. The extremities and the base of the spine are examined for edema, which suggests a disturbance in fluid and electrolyte balance.

Visual examination of the trunk can show signs of specific endocrine dysfunction. The nurse notes any abnormalities in chest size and symmetry. Truncal obesity, supraclavicular fat pads, and a "buffalo hump" may indicate adrenocortical excess. Hormonal imbalance may also change secondary sexual characteristics. The nurse inspects the breasts of both men and women for size, symmetry, pigmentation, and discharge. **Striae** (usually reddish purple "stretch marks") on the breasts or abdomen are often seen with adrenocortical excess.

The nurse assesses the client's hair distribution for indications of endocrine gland dysfunction, including **hirsutism** (abnormal growth of body hair, especially on the face, chest, and the linea alba of the abdomen of women), excessive hair loss, or changes in hair texture.

Examination of the genitalia may reveal a dysfunction in hormone secretion. The nurse notes the size of the scrotum and penis or of the labia and clitoris in relation to standards for the client's age. The distribution and quantity of pubic hair are often affected in hypogonadism.

PALPATION

The thyroid gland and the testes can be examined by palpation. Chapters 69 and 73 discuss examination of the testes. During the initial assessment, a specially trained nurse palpates the thyroid gland for size, symmetry, general shape, and the presence of nodules or other irregularities.

The nurse palpates the thyroid gland by standing either behind or in front of the client (Figure 62-9); the posterior approach may be easier. Offering the client sips of water to promote swallowing during the examination helps the clinician palpate the thyroid gland.

The client is asked to sit and to lower the chin. Using the posterior approach, the thumbs of both hands are placed on the back of the client's neck, with the fingers curved around to the front of the neck on either side of the trachea. The client is asked to swallow, and the nurse locates the isthmus of the thyroid and feels it rising. The anterior surface of the thyroid lobe is also identified. To examine the right lobe, the nurse:

* Turns the client's head to the right
* Displaces the thyroid cartilage to the right with the fingers of the left hand
* Palpates the right lobe with the right hand

This procedure is reversed for examination of the left lobe.

AUSCULTATION

The nurse auscultates the client's chest to establish baseline vital signs and to determine irregularities in cardiac rate and rhythm. A variety of endocrine disturbances can cause dehydration and volume depletion. Therefore the nurse documents any difference in the client's blood pressure and pulse in the lying, standing, or sitting positions (orthostatic vital signs).

If an enlarged thyroid gland is palpated, the area of enlargement is auscultated for bruits. Hypertrophy of the thyroid gland causes an increase in vascular flow, which may result in bruits.

Psychosocial Assessment

Information obtained from the history and physical examination aids the nurse in identifying potential or actual psychosocial problems. The nurse assesses the client's coping skills, support systems, and health-related beliefs.

A number of endocrine disorders seriously affect the client's perception of self. For example, body characteristics can change significantly in disorders of the pituitary, adrenal, and thyroid glands. Infertility, impotence, and other changes in sexual functioning may result from endocrine dysfunction. The nurse addresses any difficulty in coping with such changes. Additional support from social or counseling services may be appropriate when planning care.

Clients with endocrine problems may require lifelong medication and follow-up care. The nurse assesses the client's readiness to learn and his or her ability to carry out specific self-management skills. Clients may also face financial difficulties resulting from a prolonged medical regimen or interruption of employment. A referral to social service agencies may be necessary.

Diagnostic Assessment

LABORATORY TESTS

For the client with suspected endocrine dysfunction, laboratory tests are an essential part of the diagnostic process. The highly specialized testing for specific disorders is described in Chapters 63 to 65. Some generalizations can be made. Best practices for the collection of specimens for endocrine testing are listed in Chart 62-3.

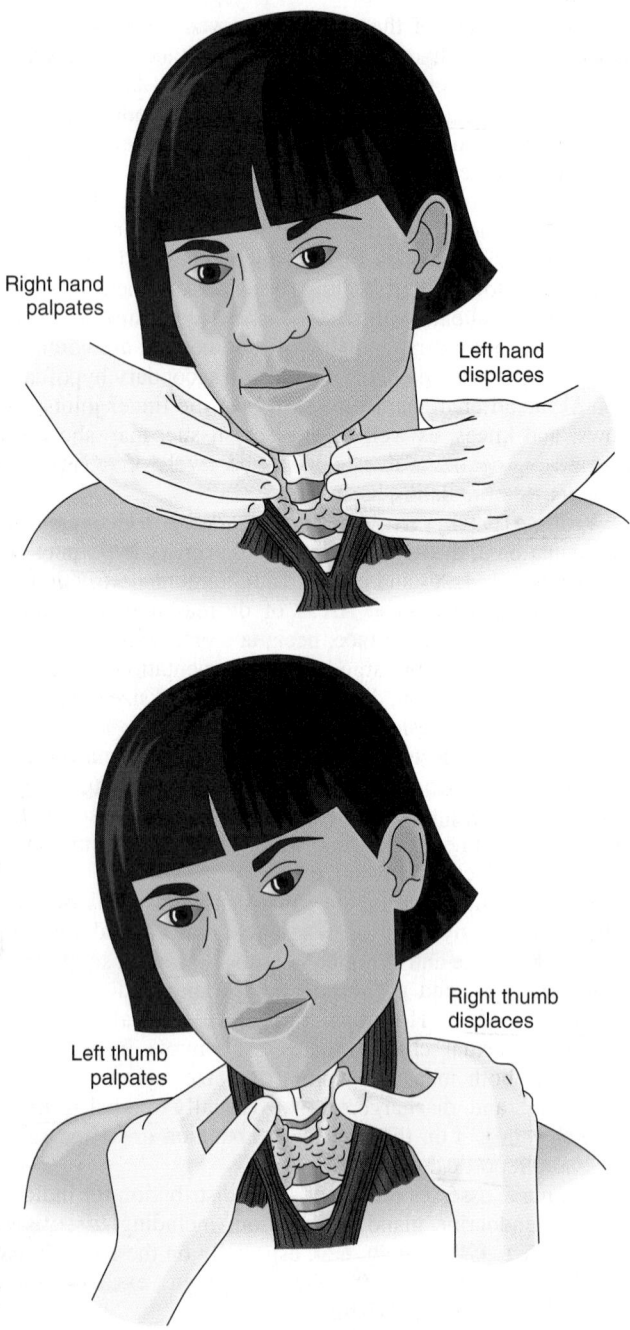

Right hand palpates

Left hand displaces

Left thumb palpates

Right thumb displaces

Figure 62-9 ● Palpation of the thyroid gland.

BEST PRACTICE *for*
Endocrine Testing

- Explain the procedure to the client.
- Emphasize the importance of taking a medication prescribed for the test on *time*. Tell the client to set an alarm if the medication is to be taken during the night.
- Instruct the client to begin the urine collection (whether for 2, 4, 8, 12, or 24 hours) by emptying his or her bladder. Tell the client *not* to save the urine specimen that begins the collection. The timing for the urine collection begins after this specimen. To end the collection, the client empties his or her bladder at the end of the timed period and adds that urine to the collection.
- Make sure that the preservative has been added to the collection container at the beginning of the collection, if necessary. Tell the client of its presence in the container.
- Check your laboratory's method of handling hormone test samples. Blood samples drawn for certain hormones (e.g., catecholamines) must be placed on ice and taken to the laboratory immediately.
- If you are drawing blood samples from a line, clear the IV line thoroughly. Do not use a double- or triple-lumen line to obtain samples; contamination or dilution from another port is possible.

Stimulation/Suppression Tests

Measurement of specific hormone levels does not always distinguish between the normal and the abnormal. The wide normal range for some hormones makes it necessary to elicit responses by stimulation or suppression tests.

In the client with suspected underactivity of an endocrine gland, a stimulus may be provided to determine whether the gland is capable of normal hormone production. This method is called *stimulation testing*. Measured amounts of selected hormones are given to stimulate the target gland to maximal production. Hormone levels are then measured and interpreted against a given norm. Failure of the hormone level to rise with stimulation denotes hypofunction.

Suppression tests are used when hormone levels are high or in the upper range of normal. Failure of hormone production to be suppressed during standardized testing indicates hyperfunction. (See the specific tests in Chapters 63 and 64.)

Radioimmunoassay

Radioimmunoassay is a competitive binding assay in which radioactively labeled amounts of hormone (antigen) compete with unlabeled hormones from the plasma or serum for antibody binding sites. Various techniques measure the amount of unbound and bound hormone. The unbound hormone is the active hormone.

Urine Tests

In addition to the measurement of hormones in the blood, hormone levels and the metabolites of specific hormones in the urine are often measured. Because many of the endocrine hormones are secreted in a pulsatile fashion, measurement of a specific hormone in a 24-hour urine collection better reflects the overall function of certain glands, such as the adrenal gland. The nurse teaches the client how to collect a 24-hour urine sample (see also Chart 62-3).

Certain hormones require additives in the container at the beginning of the collection. The nurse instructs the client not to discard the preservative from the container and to use caution when handling it, because some solutions are caustic. The client is also reminded that this collection is timed for *exactly* 24 hours. The nurse instructs the client to avoid taking any unnecessary medications during endocrine testing; drugs may interfere with the laboratory assays.

Tests for Glucose

Tests for functions of the islet cells of the pancreas are indirect; they measure the *result* of pancreatic islet cell function. Blood glucose values and the oral glucose tolerance test help the physician or nurse practitioner make a diagnosis of diabetes mellitus. The glycosylated hemoglobin (HbA_{1c}) value reveals the *average* blood glucose level over a period of 2 to 3 months. Its primary use is in assessing overall control of glucose level in diabetes mellitus. (See Chapter 65 for a full discussion of diabetes mellitus.)

RADIOGRAPHIC EXAMINATIONS

Anterior, posterior, and lateral skull x-ray studies may be used to visualize the sella turcica. Erosion of the sella turcica indicates invasion of the wall from an abnormal growth.

Computed tomography (CT) and magnetic resonance imaging (MRI) scans can show the extent of growth or locate a tumor buried within the pituitary. CT and MRI scans, sometimes using contrast media, also reveal the size and shape of other glands and nearby structures.

Angiography and venography may reveal structural abnormalities, such as aberrant blood vessels. Ultrasonography, especially of the thyroid gland, can indicate whether nodules or masses are solid or cystic.

OTHER DIAGNOSTIC TESTS

Needle biopsy is a relatively safe and quick outpatient procedure and can be used to indicate the composition of thyroid nodules. It is primarily used to determine whether surgical intervention is necessary.

CRITICAL THINKING CHALLENGE

The 27-year-old client with an absence of menses is scheduled to have blood drawn for follicle-stimulating hormone (FSH) levels, an ultrasound of the ovaries, a 24-hour urine collection for estradiol beta-17 levels, and a CT scan of the head. She is very anxious about the tests and the results.

- How should you prepare her physically for each test?
- What special instructions should you provide for the 24-hour urine test?
  The client is very concerned about pain and modesty.
- What reassurances can you provide for the level of pain expected?
- Is the client's modesty at risk with any of these procedures? If so, how? What precautions can be taken to reduce exposure?

For suggested answer guidelines, go to SIMON http://www.wbsaunders.com/SIMON/Iggy/.

ONLINE RESOURCES

For suggested readings and Internet resources, go to http://www.wbsaunders.com/SIMON/Iggy/.

SELECTED BIBLIOGRAPHY

Asterisk indicates a classic or definitive work on this subject.

Cook, L. (1999). The value of lab values. *American Journal of Nursing, 99*(5), 66-75.

Gordon, M. (2000). *Manual of nursing diagnosis* (9th ed.). St. Louis: Mosby.

Guyton, A., & Hall, J. (2001). *Textbook of medical physiology* (9th ed.). Philadelphia: W.B. Saunders.

Kelley, W. (Ed.). (1997). *Textbook of internal medicine* (3rd ed.). Philadelphia: Lippincott-Raven.

*Kokko, J., & Tannen, R. (1996). *Fluids and electrolytes* (3rd ed.). Philadelphia: W.B. Saunders.

Larsen, P.R., Davies, T., & Hay, I. (1998). In J. Wilson et al. (Eds.). *William's textbook of endocrinology* (9th ed., pp. 389-515). Philadelphia: W.B. Saunders.

*Mooradian, A. (1995). Normal age-related changes in thyroid hormone economy. *Clinics in Geriatric Medicine, 11*(2), 159-169.

Orth, D., & Kovacs, W. (1998). The adrenal cortex. In J. Wilson et al. (Eds.). *William's textbook of endocrinology* (9th ed., pp. 517-664). Philadelphia: W.B. Saunders.

Pagana, K., & Pagana, T. (1999). *Diagnostic testing and nursing implications: A case study approach.* St. Louis: Mosby.

Reeves, W.B., Bichet, D., & Andreoli, T. (1998). In J. Wilson et al. (Eds.). *William's textbook of endocrinology* (9th ed., pp. 341-387). Philadelphia: W.B. Saunders.

Sagre, G., & Brown, E. (1998). Measurement of hormones. In J. Wilson et al. (Eds.). *William's textbook of endocrinology* (9th ed., pp. 43-54). Philadelphia: W.B. Saunders.

Thorner, M., et al. (1998). The anterior pituitary. In J. Wilson et al. (Eds.). *William's textbook of endocrinology* (9th ed., pp. 249-340). Philadelphia: W.B. Saunders.

Wilson, J., et al. (Eds.). (1998). *William's textbook of endocrinology* (9th ed.). Philadelphia: W.B. Saunders.

*Winger, J., & Hornick, T. (1996). Age-associated changes in the endocrine system. *Nursing Clinics of North America, 31*(4), 827-844.

63

$\mathcal{I}$nterventions for Clients with Pituitary and Adrenal Gland Problems

M. LINDA WORKMAN

$\mathcal{L}$earning Objectives

After studying this chapter, you should be able to:

1. Compare and contrast the common clinical manifestations associated with pituitary hypofunction and pituitary hyperfunction.
2. Use clinical changes and laboratory data to determine the effectiveness of interventions for pituitary hypofunction.
3. Identify the teaching priorities for the client taking hormone replacement therapy for pituitary hypofunction.
4. Prioritize nursing care for the client immediately after a transsphenoidal hypophysectomy.
5. Use clinical changes and laboratory data to determine the effectiveness of interventions for pituitary hyperfunction.
6. Compare and contrast the problems associated with oversecretion and undersecretion of antidiuretic hormone.
7. Explain the effect of diabetes insipidus on blood and urine volumes and blood and urine osmolarity.
8. Explain the effects of the syndrome of inappropriate antidiuretic hormone (SIADH) on blood and urine volumes and blood and urine osmolarity.
9. Use clinical changes and laboratory data to determine the effectiveness of interventions for diabetes insipidus.
10. Identify teaching priorities for the client with diabetes insipidus.
11. Use clinical changes and laboratory data to determine the effectiveness of interventions for SIADH.
12. Identify teaching priorities for the client with SIADH.
13. Compare and contrast the clinical manifestations of Cushing's syndrome and Addison's disease.
14. Use clinical changes and laboratory data to determine the effectiveness of interventions for Cushing's syndrome.
15. Identify teaching priorities for the client with Cushing's syndrome.
16. Use clinical changes and laboratory data to determine the effectiveness of interventions for Addison's disease.
17. Identify teaching priorities for the client with Addison's disease.

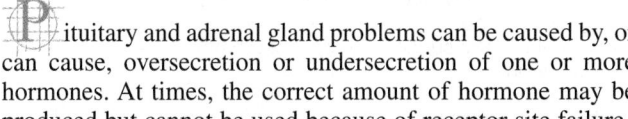

Go to http://www.wbsaunders.com/SIMON/Iggy/ for self-assessment questions related to these Learning Objectives.

$\mathcal{P}$ituitary and adrenal gland problems can be caused by, or can cause, oversecretion or undersecretion of one or more hormones. At times, the correct amount of hormone may be produced but cannot be used because of receptor site failure.

Hormones secreted from the anterior pituitary gland regulate growth, metabolism, and sexual development. These functions are affected when the pituitary gland secretes too much or too little of one or more hormones. The posterior pituitary gland secretes **vasopressin** (antidiuretic hormone [ADH]). Dysfunction of the posterior pituitary gland results in fluid and electrolyte imbalance. The adrenal gland produces and secretes hormones that influence homeostasis and are life sustaining.

The effects of endocrine problems occur throughout the body and may induce psychologic, as well as physical, changes. Nursing care for the client with pituitary or adrenal gland disorders includes the following:

- Performing a careful assessment
- Educating clients
- Evaluating responses to therapy
- Providing psychosocial support

A complete history and physical examination are performed during the assessment to detect specific clinical findings. The client also often undergoes a variety of diagnostic tests and relies on the nurse for specific instructions and explanations. Surgical intervention may be indicated. The client often needs hormone replacement therapy for the rest of his or her life. Physical and emotional support are critical.

DISORDERS OF THE PITUITARY GLAND

DISORDERS OF THE ANTERIOR PITUITARY GLAND

The anterior pituitary gland (adenohypophysis) controls growth, metabolic activity, and sexual development through the actions of the following hormones:

- Growth hormone (GH; somatotropin)
- Prolactin (PRL)
- Thyrotropin (thyroid-stimulating hormone [TSH])
- Corticotropin (adrenocorticotropic hormone [ACTH])
- Follicle-stimulating hormone (FSH)
- Luteinizing hormone (LH)
- Melanocyte-stimulating hormone (MSH)

Disorders of hormones secreted by the anterior pituitary gland can result from problems arising within the anterior pituitary gland itself (**primary pituitary dysfunction**) or from problems in the hypothalamus that change anterior pituitary function (**secondary pituitary dysfunction**). In either case, one or more hormones may be undersecreted (**pituitary hypofunction**) or oversecreted (**pituitary hyperfunction**).

Hypopituitarism

■ OVERVIEW
■ Pathophysiology

A person with hypopituitarism has a deficiency of one or more anterior pituitary hormones, resulting in metabolic abnormalities and sexual dysfunction. Decreased production of *all* of the anterior pituitary hormones is an extremely rare condition known as **panhypopituitarism.**

More commonly, there is a marked decrease in the secretion of one hormone and a lesser decrease in the other hormones. Deficiencies of adrenocorticotropic hormone (ACTH) and thyroid-stimulating hormone (TSH) are the *most* life threatening because they result in a corresponding decrease in the secretion of vital hormones from the adrenal and thyroid glands. Adrenal hypofunction is discussed on pp. 1412-1415; hypothyroidism is discussed in Chapter 64.

Deficiency of the **gonadotropins** (luteinizing hormone [LH] and follicle-stimulating hormone [FSH]—hormones that stimulate the ovaries and testes to produce sex hormones) changes sexual function in both men and women. In males, gonadotropin deficiency results in testicular failure, with decreased testosterone production from the Leydig cells and decreased or absent spermatogenesis from the seminiferous tubules. Decreased testosterone levels in males cause delayed onset of puberty and sterility. In females, gonadotropin deficiency results in ovarian failure, amenorrhea, and infertility.

Growth hormone (GH) deficiency changes tissue growth patterns indirectly. GH itself has little effect on tissues and cells. Rather, the presence of GH stimulates the liver to produce substances known as **somatomedins** (Guyton & Hall, 2000). These somatomedins, especially somatomedin C (insulin-like growth factor-1 [IGF-1]), then enhance growth activities in cells and tissues. Somatomedin C is responsible for bone and cartilage growth and maintenance.

GH deficiency may be a result of insufficient production of GH, failure of the liver to produce somatomedins, or a failure of the cells or tissues to respond to the presence of the somatomedins. GH deficiency in children leads to short stature and other manifestations of growth retardation. GH deficiency in adults produces no obvious anatomic changes but does increase the rate of bone destructive activity, leading to thinner, more fragile bones.

■ Etiology

The cause of hypopituitarism varies. Benign or malignant pituitary tumors can compress and destroy pituitary tissue. Pituitary function can be impaired by severe malnutrition or rapid loss of body fat, such as in people with **anorexia nervosa** (a disorder in which people see themselves as overweight and eat so little that excessive weight loss and starvation result). Poor circulation to the pituitary gland can cause hypoxia and infarction. Other causes of hypopituitarism are listed in Table 63-1. **Idiopathic hypopituitarism** may result in an isolated hormone deficiency, and often the cause is unknown.

Postpartum hemorrhage is the most common cause of pituitary infarction, which results in decreased hormone secretion. This clinical problem is known as **Sheehan's syndrome.** The pituitary gland normally enlarges during pregnancy, and when hypotension results from hemorrhage, ischemia and necrosis of the gland occur. Usually this condition develops immediately postpartum, although some cases have occurred several years after delivery.

➤ COLLABORATIVE MANAGEMENT
◖ Assessment

Some changes in physical appearance and target organ function are associated with deficiencies of specific pituitary hormones (Chart 63-1). Gonadotropin (LH and FSH) deficiency results in the loss of or change in secondary sex characteristics in men and women. While assessing the male client, the nurse notes the key signs and symptoms of facial and body hair loss. The nurse asks about episodes of impotence and decreased **libido** (sex drive). Female clients may report **amen-**

TABLE 63-1 • CAUSES OF HYPOPITUITARISM

CAUSES OF PRIMARY HYPOPITUITARISM
- Pituitary tumor (craniopharyngioma)
- Partial or total surgical hypophysectomy
- Radiation
- Infarction
- Metastatic disease
- Granulomatous process
- Trauma

CAUSES OF SECONDARY HYPOPITUITARISM
- Infection
- Trauma
- Brain tumor
- Congenital defects

orrhea (absence of menstrual periods), **dyspareunia** (painful intercourse), **infertility** (difficulty in achieving pregnancy), and decreased libido. While examining the female client, the nurse checks for dry skin, breast atrophy, and a decreased amount or absence of axillary and pubic hair.

Neurologic manifestations of hypopituitarism due to tumor growth often first occur as changes in visual perception. The nurse evaluates the client's visual acuity, particularly peripheral vision, for changes or loss. Bilateral temporal headaches are a common finding. Other manifestations may include **diplopia** (double vision) and ocular muscle paralysis, limiting eye movement.

Laboratory findings vary widely in people with hypopituitarism. Some pituitary hormone levels may be measured directly. Often, however, the *effects* of the hormones, rather than their actual levels, are assessed. Basal levels of triiodothyronine (T_3) and thyroxine (T_4) from the thyroid, as well as testosterone and estradiol from the gonads, are measured easily. If levels of one or all of these hormones are low or in the low-normal range, hypopituitarism is a possibility and further evaluation is necessary. Levels of pituitary gonadotropins (LH and FSH) and TSH are sufficient if function of the target organ is apparent. Function of LH and FSH is assessed by observing for the presence of secondary sexual characteristics; function of TSH is assessed by measuring circulating levels of thyroid hormones. ACTH levels may be normal or low, and prolactin (PRL) levels are low to high.

Some tests for pituitary function involve administering agents that are known to stimulate secretion of specific pituitary hormones and then measuring the response. Such tests are called **stimulation tests.** For example, the presence of insulin in people with normal pituitary function causes an increased release of GH and ACTH. The stimulation test for either GH or ACTH assessment involves injecting the client with regular insulin (0.05 to 1 units/kg of body weight) and checking the circulating levels of GH and ACTH. The stimulation test for TSH involves injecting thyrotropin-releasing hormone (TRH) and measuring the blood levels of thyroid hormones. The stimulation test for LH and FSH involves administering gonadotropin-releasing hormone (GnRH). In people with no pituitary problems, this injection results in a peak release of LH and FSH within 15 to 45 minutes after the injection. The stimulation test for PRL is the same as that for TSH.

Pituitary abnormalities may cause changes in the **sella turcica** (the bony nest where the pituitary gland rests) that can be seen with skull x-ray studies. Such changes may include enlargement, erosion, and calcifications in the area of the sella turcica as a result of pituitary tumors. Computed tomography (CT) and magnetic resonance imaging (MRI) can more distinctly define bone or soft-tissue lesions. An angiogram may be indicated to rule out the presence of an aneurysm or congenital vascular malformations, especially before any surgical intervention.

Interventions

Management of the adult with hypopituitarism focuses on replacement of deficient hormones. Older clients or those with a chronic disease often require a lower amount of hormone replacement. Men who have gonadotropin deficiency are treated with **androgens** (testosterone). The most widely used and most effective route of administration is intramuscular (IM), although use of transdermal testosterone patches is increasing. The nurse instructs the client in self-administration. Therapy is

CHART 63-1

KEY FEATURES of
Pituitary Hypofunction

Deficient Hormone	Clinical Manifestations
Anterior Pituitary Hormones	
Growth hormone (GH)	Decreased bone density Pathologic fractures Decreased muscle strength Increased serum cholesterol levels
Gonadotropins (luteinizing hormone [LH], follicle-stimulating hormone [FSH])	Women: • Amenorrhea • Anovulation • Low circulating estrogen levels • Breast atrophy • Loss of bone density • Decreased axillary and pubic hair • Decreased libido • Fine facial wrinkles Men: • Decreased facial hair • Decreased ejaculate volume • Reduced muscle mass • Loss of bone density • Decreased body hair • Decreased libido • Impotence • Fine facial wrinkles
Thyrotropin (Thyroid-stimulating hormone [TSH])	Decreased circulating TSH levels Decreased circulating thyroid hormone levels Weight gain Intolerance to cold Scalp alopecia Hirsuitism Menstrual abnormalities Decreased libido Slowed cognition Lethargy
Adrenocorticotropic hormone (ACTH)	Decreased serum cortisol levels Pale, sallow complexion Malaise and lethargy Anorexia Postural hypotension Headache Hypoglycemia Hyponatremia Decreased axillary and pubic hair (women)
Posterior Pituitary Hormones	

Vasopressin (antidiuretic hormone [ADH])	Diabetes insipidus
	• Greatly increased urine output
	• Low urine specific gravity (<1.005)
	• Hypovolemia
	  Hypotension
	  Dehydration
	• Increased plasma osmolarity
	• Increased thirst
	• Output does not decrease when fluid intake decreases

Data from Thorner, M., et al. (1998). The anterior pituitary. In J. D. Wilson et al. (Eds.), *Williams textbook of endocrinology* (9th ed., pp. 249-340). Philadelphia: W.B. Saunders; and Reeves, W.B., Bichet, D., & Andreoli, T. (1998). Posterior pituitary and water metabolism. In J.D. Wilson et al. (Eds.), *Williams textbook of endocrinology* (9th ed., pp. 341-387). Philadelphia: W.B. Saunders.

usually initiated with high-dose testosterone and is continued until **virilization** (presence of male secondary sex characteristics) is achieved. Maximal effects of treatment include increases in penis size, libido, muscle mass, bone size, and bone strength. Chest, facial, pubic, and axillary hair growth also increase, and the voice deepens. Clients usually report improved self-esteem and body image after therapy is initiated. The dose may then be decreased, but therapy continues throughout life.

Androgen therapy is avoided in men with prostate cancer. Side effects of testosterone therapy include **gynecomastia** (the development of breast tissue in men), baldness, and prostatic hypertrophy.

Achieving fertility in these clients is difficult and requires additional parenteral testosterone therapy. The nurse educates the client about the course of additional therapy and supports the client and family members emotionally because the outcome of fertility treatment is uncertain.

Women who have gonadotropin deficiency receive hormone replacement with a combination of estrogen and progesterone administered at their menstrual cycle, which causes withdrawal bleeding. The risk for hypertension or **thrombosis** (formation of blood clots in deep veins) is increased with estrogen therapy, especially among women who smoke. The nurse emphasizes measures to reduce risk and the need for regular health visits. For women who wish to become pregnant, clomiphene citrate (Clomid) may be given to induce ovulation. Menotropins in conjunction with human chorionic gonadotropin (hCG) are used to stimulate ovulation when therapy with clomiphene citrate has failed.

Adult clients who have GH deficiency may be treated with injections of GH, although this treatment is rare.

Hyperpituitarism

■ OVERVIEW

Hyperpituitarism is a condition of hormone oversecretion that occurs when a client has pituitary tumors or hyperplasias. Tumors usually arise from the somatotropic cells (growth hormone [GH]), the lactotropic cells (prolactin [PRL]), and the corticotropic cells (adrenocorticotropic hormone [ACTH[) of the anterior pituitary gland **(adenohypophysis).** An exception is the overproduction of PRL, which may occur in response to tumors that overproduce GH and ACTH. Hypersecretion of ACTH is sometimes associated with increased secretion of melanocyte-stimulating hormone (MSH).

■ Pathophysiology

A common reason for hyperpituitarism is the presence of a pituitary adenoma, a benign epithelial tumor. Adenomas are classified by size, the degree of invasiveness, and the hormone secreted. An invasive pituitary adenoma involves a portion or all of the sella turcica. When the sella turcica is not involved, the adenoma is "enclosed."

As an adenoma gets larger and compresses brain tissue, neurologic symptoms, as well as endocrine symptoms, may occur. Such symptoms may include visual changes, headache, and increased intracranial pressure.

PRL-secreting tumors are the most common of the pituitary adenomas. Excessive PRL secretion inhibits the secretion of gonadal steroids and gonadotropins in men and women, resulting in **galactorrhea** (production of breast milk), amenorrhea, and infertility.

Overproduction of GH results in **gigantism** (Figure 63-1) or **acromegaly** (Figure 63-2). The onset of the disease may be gradual with slow progression, and changes may remain unnoticed for years before diagnosis of the disorder. Early detection and treatment are essential to prevent irreversible changes in the soft tissues, such as those of the face, hands, feet, and skin. These changes are, to a certain extent, reversible after treatment, but skeletal changes are permanent.

In the client with gigantism, the onset of GH hypersecretion occurs *before* puberty, which causes rapid proportional growth in the length of all bones. In the client with acromegaly, excessive GH secretion occurs *after* puberty and produces increased skeletal thickness, hypertrophy of the skin,

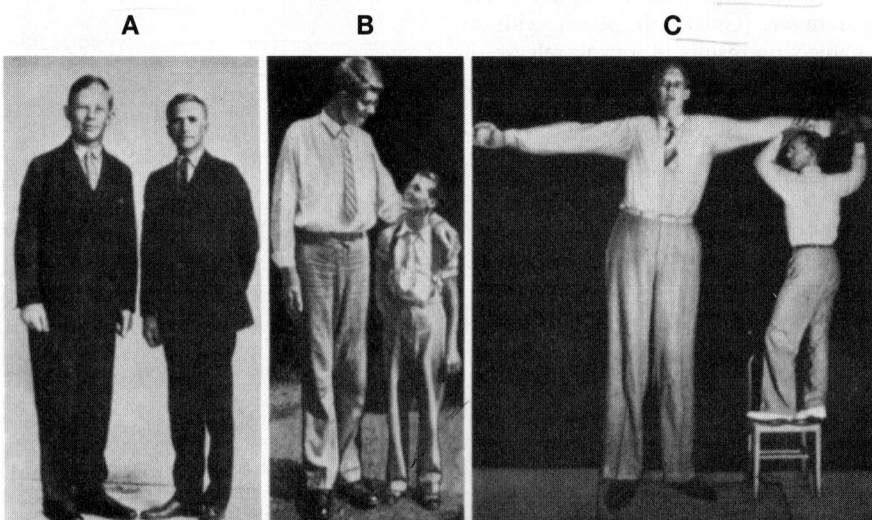

Figure 63-1 ● The clinical features of GH excess. Robert Wadlow, the "Alton giant," weighed 9 pounds at birth but grew to 30 pounds by the time he was 6 months old. By his first birthday, he had reached 62 pounds. At the time of his death at age 22 from cellulitis of the feet, he was 8 feet 11 inches tall and weighed 457 pounds. (**A** and **B** from Fadner, F. [1944]. *Biography of Robert Wadlow.* Courtesy Bruce Humphries, Publishers. **C** courtesy C.M. Charles and C.M. MacBryde.)

and enlargement of many visceral organs, such as the liver and heart.

Bony changes related to excessive GH occur slowly and include thickening, tufting of terminal phalanges (arrowhead fingertips), and bone cell overgrowth. Degeneration of joint cartilage and hypertrophy of ligaments, vocal cords, and eustachian tube mucosa are common. Nerve entrapment occurs because of tissue overgrowth with demyelinization of peripheral nerves. Because GH is an insulin **antagonist** (blocks the action of insulin), **hyperglycemia** (elevated blood glucose levels) is also common.

Hypersecretion of ACTH results in overstimulation of the adrenal cortex. This stimulation produces excessive amounts of glucocorticoids, mineralocorticoids, and androgens, which lead to the development of Cushing's disease (see Hypercortisolism [Cushing's Syndrome], p. 1416).

Etiology

Most cases of hyperpituitarism result from hormone-secreting adenomas arising from one pituitary cell type. Hyperpituitarism can also be caused by hypothalamic dysfunction in which excessive amounts of releasing hormones are produced and then overstimulate the normal pituitary gland.

Adenomas can develop in clients without a family history or as part of a syndrome known as **multiple endocrine neo-**

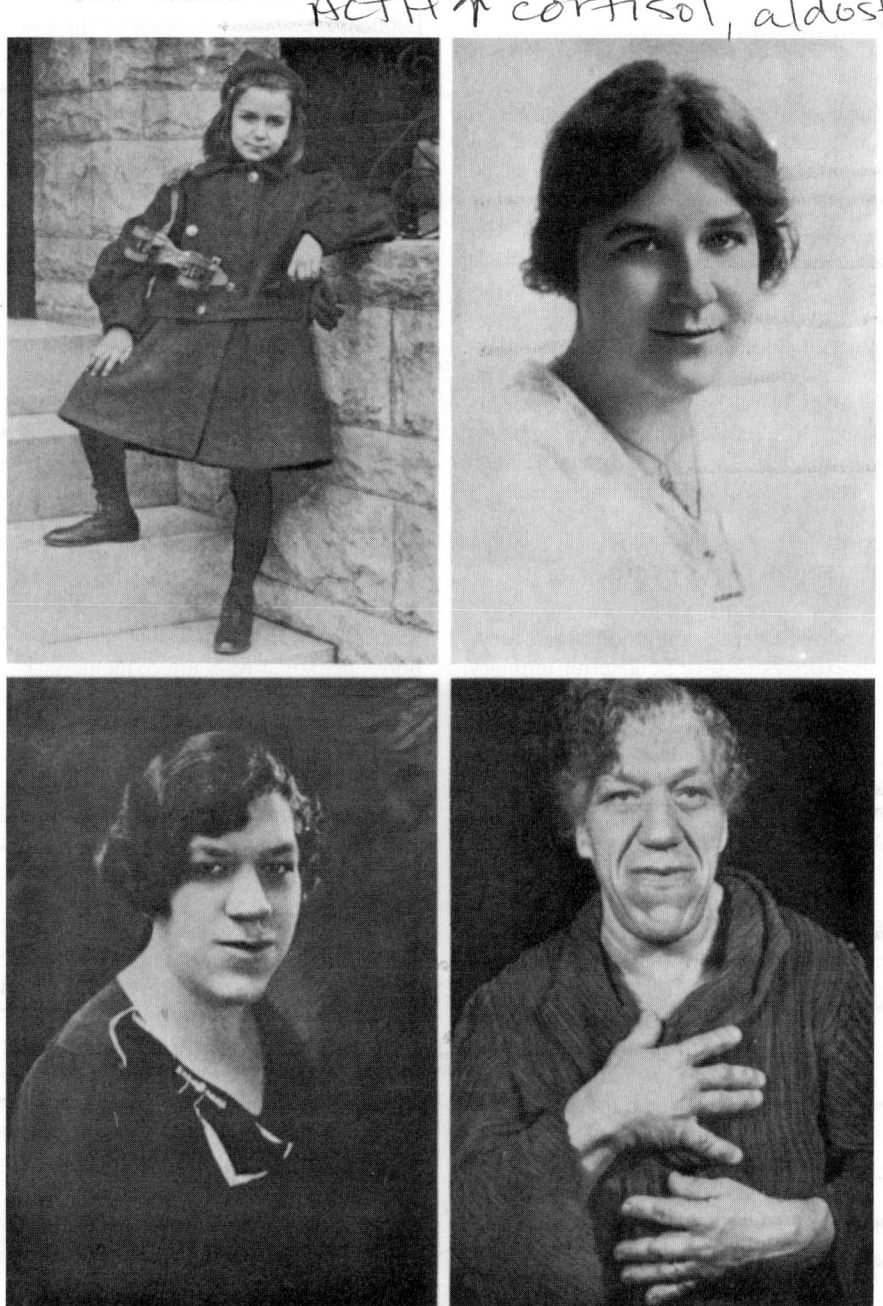

Figure 63-2 ● The progression of acromegaly. (From Mendelhoff, A., & Smith, D.E., [Eds.]. [1956]. Acromegaly, diabetes, hypermetabolism, proteinuria, and heart failure. Clinical Pathological Conference. *American Journal of Medicine, 20,* 133.)

plasia. This familial disorder, inherited as an autosomal dominant trait, may include parathyroid and pancreatic tumors.

Incidence/Prevalence

Hyperpituitarism is a rare disorder. The most common secretory tumors are prolactinomas, followed by GH-producing adenomas. Tumors secreting gonadotropin or thyroid-stimulating hormone (TSH) are the least common. Of all pituitary tumors for which surgery is performed, approximately 70% secrete one or more hormones.

► COLLABORATIVE MANAGEMENT

● Assessment

■ HISTORY

The symptoms of hyperpituitarism vary, depending on which hormone is produced in excess. The nurse obtains data about the client's age, gender, and family history. The client is asked about any change in hat, glove, ring, or shoe size. Fatigue and lethargy are common. The client with excessively high GH levels may have backache and **arthralgias** (joint pain) in response to bone changes. He or she is asked specifically about the presence of headaches and changes in vision.

The client with hypersecretion of PRL (hyperprolactinemia) often reports difficulties in sexual functioning. The nurse asks women about menstrual changes (e.g., amenorrhea, irregular menses, and difficulty in achieving pregnancy) and about decreased libido or **dyspareunia** (painful intercourse). Men may report decreased libido and impotence.

■ PHYSICAL ASSESSMENT/CLINICAL MANIFESTATIONS

Some changes in physical appearance and target organ function are associated with excesses of specific anterior pituitary hormones (Chart 63-2). Initial manifestations of GH hypersecretion are changes in the facial features, including increases in lip and nose sizes; increases in head, hand, and foot sizes; and a prominent supraorbital ridge. **Prognathism,** a projection of the jaw beyond the facial features, becomes marked. The client is assessed for difficulty in chewing and for dentures that no longer fit. Arthritic changes causing joint pain and decreased mobility may also be noted. Fingers and toes may have an "arrowhead" or tufted shape on x-ray films and a thickened appearance. At onset, acromegaly is characterized by increased metabolism and strength. As the disease progresses, these manifestations are replaced with lethargy and weakness.

The nurse assesses the client's vision for any changes related to compression of the optic nerves. The nurse also notes any increased perspiration and oil secretion on the skin. Other prominent features include the following:

- Organomegaly (cardiac or hepatic)
- Hypertension
- Dysphagia caused by an enlarged tongue
- Deepening of the voice caused by hypertrophy of the larynx

Hypersecretion of PRL is often observed, along with hypogonadism and galactorrhea (fluid leakage from the breast). Galactorrhea may be present in either gender but is predominant in females.

■ PSYCHOSOCIAL ASSESSMENT

The client with hyperpituitarism often seeks health care because of dramatic changes in physical appearance. The nurse assesses the impact of these physical changes on the client's interpersonal relationships.

In clients who are disturbed by an inability to conceive, the nurse identifies symptoms of emotional distress, such as crying, reports of depression, irritability, and hostility. They may express fear of the diagnosis, subsequent surgery, and prognosis, especially when a tumor is suspected.

■ LABORATORY ASSESSMENT

In a person with hyperpituitarism, usually only one hormone is produced in excess, because the cell types within the pituitary gland are so discretely organized. The most common hormones produced in excess are PRL, ACTH, and GH. Tumors producing TSH, luteinizing hormone (LH), or follicle-stimulating hormone (FSH) are extremely rare. Elevated levels of any of these hormones usually warrant further investigation. Elevations of LH and FSH, however, are normal in the postmenopausal woman.

■ RADIOGRAPHIC ASSESSMENT

Radiographic evaluation of the client with hyperpituitarism is identical to that for a client with hypopituitarism. Conventional skull x-ray films are made to identify abnormalities of the sella turcica. Computed tomography (CT) and magnetic resonance imaging (MRI) can define soft-tissue lesions, and angiography can rule out an aneurysm or congenital vascular malformations.

■ OTHER DIAGNOSTIC ASSESSMENT

Rather than just measuring the circulating level of a specific hormone, some tests are dynamic and measure how well the endocrine gland responds to stimulation changes. Suppression tests are a type of dynamic endocrine testing that can help in the diagnosis of hyperpituitarism. These tests involve administering agents that induce a suppressive response from the pituitary gland, and they can determine whether the normal negative feedback control mechanisms for hormonal regulation are intact. For example, high circulating levels of glucose have a suppressive effect on the release of GH. In a suppression test, 100 g of oral glucose or 0.5 g/kg of body weight is given intravenously. GH levels are measured serially for up to 120 minutes. GH levels that do not fall below 5 ng/mL indicate a positive (abnormal) result.

Another example of a suppression test is the administration of intravenous (IV) cortisol in the form of dexamethasone (Decadron). This agent should result in suppression of ACTH. When ACTH production continues in the presence of dexamethasone administration, the client may have pituitary Cushing's disease.

● Analysis

When hyperpituitarism is present, one or more of the anterior pituitary hormones are overproduced. The nursing diagnoses focus on the client's responses to excesses of prolactin (PRL) and growth hormone (GH).

CHART 63-2

KEY FEATURES *of*
Pituitary Hyperfunction

Excess Hormone	Clinical Manifestations
Anterior Pituitary Hormones	
Prolactin (PRL)	Hypogonadism (loss of secondary sexual characteristics) Decreased gonadotropin levels Galactorrhea Increased body fat Increased serum prolactin levels
Growth hormone (GH)	Acromegaly • Thickened, oily skin (facial) • Thickened lips • Folding of the scalp skin • Deepening of the voice • Enlarged hands and feet • Increasing head size • Protrusion of the lower jaw • Joint enlargement and pain (knees, hips, and shoulders) • Kyphosis and backache • "Barrel chest" • Excessive sweating (especially of the hands, feet, head, and face) • Coarse facial features • Tufting of the fingertips • Hyperglycemia • Airway narrowing, sleep apnea • Enlarged heart, lungs, and liver
Adrenocorticotropic hormone (ACTH)	Cushing's syndrome • Elevated plasma cortisol levels • Weight gain • Truncal obesity • "Moon face" • Extremity muscle wasting • Loss of bone density • Hypertension • Hyperglycemia • Purple striae • Acne • Thin, easily damaged skin • Hyperpigmentation
Thyrotropin (thyroid-stimulating hormone [TSH])	Elevated plasma TSH levels Elevated plasma thyroid hormone levels Weight loss Tachycardia Heat intolerance Increased gastrointestinal (GI) motility Fine tremors
Gonadotropins (luteinizing hormone [LH], follicle-stimulating hormone [FSH])	Men: • Elevated LH and FSH levels • Hypogonadism or hypergonadism Women: • Normal LH and FSH levels (The most common clinical manifestations in men and women are related to the physical presence of a tumor rather than to excessive hormone secretion.)
Posterior Pituitary Hormones	
Vasopressin (antidiuretic hormone [ADH])	Syndrome of inappropriate antidiuretic hormone (SIADH) • Decreased urine output • Increased urine osmolarity • Increased plasma volume • Decreased plasma osmolarity • Weight gain • Hyponatremia • Nonpitting edema • Central nervous system (CNS) changes (confusion, seizures)

Data from Thorner, M., et al. (1998). The anterior pituitary. In J.D. Wilson et al. (Eds.), *Williams textbook of endocrinology* (9th ed., pp. 249-340). Philadelphia: W.B. Saunders; and Reeves, W.B., Bichet, D., & Andreoli, T. (1998). Posterior pituitary and water metabolism. In J.D. Wilson et al. (Eds.), *Williams textbook of endocrinology* (9th ed., pp. 341-387). Philadelphia: W.B. Saunders.

■ COMMON NURSING DIAGNOSES AND COLLABORATIVE PROBLEMS

The following are common nursing diagnoses for clients with hyperpituitarism:

1. Disturbed Body Image related to altered physical appearance
2. Sexual Dysfunction related to actual limitation imposed by disease (e.g., loss of libido, infertility, impotence)

■ ADDITIONAL NURSING DIAGNOSES AND COLLABORATIVE PROBLEMS

In addition to the common nursing diagnoses, clients with hyperpituitarism may have one or more of the following:

- Acute Pain and Chronic Pain related to compression of tissues by tumor (e.g., discomfort, headache), backache, or arthralgia secondary to the effects of excessive GH levels; or to dyspareunia secondary to excessive PRL levels
- Fear related to a perceived threat of death from an intracranial tumor
- Anxiety related to a threat of or change in health status
- Ineffective Coping related to impaired self-concept and loss of control over the body
- Activity Intolerance related to the effects of excessive GH levels (e.g., pain or discomfort, lethargy, and weakness)
- Disturbed Sensory Perception (Visual) related to altered nerve transmission as a consequence of nerve compression from tumor or surrounding structures
- Deficient Knowledge (diagnosis and treatment regimen) related to unfamiliarity with information

▶ Planning and Implementation

■ DISTURBED BODY IMAGE

NOC **PLANNING: EXPECTED OUTCOMES.** The client with hyperpituitarism is expected to experience a sense of congruence between body reality, body ideal, and body presentation.

INTERVENTIONS. The goals of therapy for the client who has hyperpituitarism are to return hormone levels to normal or near normal, correct the problems of headache and visual disturbances, prevent complications, reverse as many of the body changes as possible, and preserve as much normal pituitary function as possible. The client who has excessive GH levels may have skeletal changes that cannot be reversed with treatment.

NONSURGICAL MANAGEMENT. The client is encouraged to verbalize concerns and fears about his or her altered physical appearance. The nurse helps the client identify personal strengths and positive characteristics, reinforcing each client's uniqueness and importance.

Galactorrhea, gynecomastia, and difficulties in sexual functioning can cause disturbances in body image and personal identity. The nurse reassures the client that treatment may alleviate some of these symptoms and encourages him or her to discuss his or her feelings.

DRUG THERAPY. Drug therapy may be used alone or in combination with surgery and/or radiation. The most common drugs used are dopamine agonists, especially bromocriptine

mesylate (Parlodel). This drug group stimulates dopamine receptors in the brain and inhibits the release of many pituitary hormones, most specifically GH and PRL. In most cases, small tumors (**microadenomas**) decrease until the pituitary gland is of normal size, and large pituitary tumors (**macroadenomas**) decrease to some extent. In clients with acromegaly, bromocriptine has reduced GH levels and decreased tumor size, especially when GH levels remain high after surgery or before the full effect of radiation therapy has occurred.

Side effects of bromocriptine include **orthostatic** (postural) hypotension, gastric irritation, nausea, headaches, abdominal cramps, and constipation. Bromocriptine is given with a meal or a snack to reduce some of these side effects. Treatment is usually initiated with a low dose and is gradually increased until the desired level (usually 7.5 mg/day) is reached. *If pregnancy occurs, the drug is stopped immediately.*

Other agents used for acromegaly are the somatostatin analogs, especially octreotide (Sandostatin). This drug group inhibits GH release through negative feedback. Although this therapy is effective in reducing GH levels, a disadvantage is the fact that it must be administered daily as a subcutaneous injection. A major side effect is gallbladder disease.

RADIATION THERAPY. Radiation therapy is not useful in the management of acute hyperpituitarism. Radiation therapy regimens take a long time to complete, and several years may pass before a therapeutic effect is evident. Side effects of radiation therapy include hypopituitarism, optic nerve damage, reduced coordinated eye movement, and visual field defects.

SURGICAL MANAGEMENT. Surgical removal of a microadenoma of the pituitary gland (**hypophysectomy**) is often indicated for clients with hyperpituitarism.

PREOPERATIVE CARE. The nurse explains that hypophysectomy decreases hormone levels, relieves headaches, and may reverse changes in sexual functioning. Body changes, visceral enlargement, and visual changes are not usually reversible. The nurse explains that because nasal packing is present for 2 to 3 days postoperatively, it will be necessary to breathe through the mouth, and a "mustache" dressing ("drip" pad) will be placed under the nose. The client is instructed not to brush teeth, cough, sneeze, blow the nose, or bend forward after surgery. These activities can open the muscle graft, increase intracranial pressure, and hinder healing of the incision. Nasal and oral mucous membrane swab specimens for bacterial culture and sensitivity are obtained preoperatively because surgery, especially the transsphenoidal approach, can cause infectious organisms from these areas to spread systemically.

OPERATIVE PROCEDURE. A transsphenoidal approach to the pituitary gland is most commonly used (Figure 63-3). Transsphenoidal hypophysectomy is microscopic surgery performed with the client under general anesthesia and in a semisitting position. The surgeon makes the initial incision just above the upper lip and reaches the pituitary gland through the sphenoid sinus. After the gland is removed, a muscle graft is taken, often from the anterior thigh, to support the area and prevent leakage of cerebrospinal fluid (CSF). The surgeon inserts nasal packing after the incision is closed and applies a mustache dressing. If the tumor cannot be reached by this approach, a craniotomy may be indicated (see Chapter 45).

POSTOPERATIVE CARE. The nurse monitors the client's neurologic response and documents any changes in vision, mental status, altered level of consciousness, or decreased strength of the extremities. The client is observed for postoperative complications (e.g., transient diabetes insipidus).

In a client with diabetes insipidus, urine specific gravity measurements are low and urine output is excessive. The nurse monitors the intake of IV fluid, encourages fluid intake in response to thirst, and administers vasopressin as indicated. A Foley catheter may be inserted for accurate measuring of urine output, and daily weights are taken.

The client is instructed to report any postnasal drip, which might indicate leakage of CSF. The head of the bed is elevated postoperatively. The nurse assesses nasal drainage for quantity, quality, and the presence of glucose (which indicates that the fluid is CSF). A light yellow color at the edge of the clear drainage on the dressing is called the "halo sign" and indicates CSF. If the client complains of persistent, severe headaches, CSF fluid may have leaked into the sinus area. Most CSF leaks resolve with bedrest. If the CSF leak persists, the physician may perform a spinal tap to reduce CSF pressure. Surgical intervention is rarely necessary.

Coughing is avoided postoperatively because it increases pressure in the incisional area and may lead to a CSF leak. The nurse reminds the client to perform deep breathing exercises frequently to prevent pulmonary complications. Clients may also have mouth dryness as a result of mouth breathing. The nurse or assistive nursing personnel performs frequent oral rinses and applies petroleum jelly to dry lips.

Infection can occur postoperatively as well. The nurse is particularly alert for symptoms of meningitis, such as headache, fever, and **nuchal** (neck) rigidity. The surgeon may prescribe antibiotics, analgesics, and antipyretics.

If the entire pituitary gland has been removed, thyroid hormones and glucocorticoids must be replaced. (Gonadotropin

deficiency is also noted in both male and female clients.) Best practices for postoperative care are reviewed in Chart 63-3.

SEXUAL DYSFUNCTION

PLANNING: EXPECTED OUTCOMES. The client with hyperpituitarism is expected to achieve a personal desired level of sexual functioning.

INTERVENTIONS. The nurse identifies the specific problems that the client is experiencing and encourages him or her to discuss any effect that sexual dysfunction has had on his or her sexual partner. Drug therapy with bromocriptine can decrease prolactin (PRL) levels in clients with PRL-secreting tumors. After PRL levels are decreased, gonadotropin function often returns to normal. Clients requiring hypophysectomy may experience sexual dysfunction as a result of postsurgical gonadotropin deficiency and require hormone replacement (discussed earlier under Interventions [Hypopituitarism], p. 1401).

> #### CRITICAL THINKING CHALLENGE
> The client is 24 hours postoperative from a transsphenoidal hypophysectomy. Her IV has been discontinued even though she still feels nauseated and does not want to eat or drink. She tells you that she would like to get up to use the bathroom because it seems like she has to use the bedpan every 15 minutes to urinate. She also asks you to change her moustache dressing because it is very wet and is irritating her skin.
> - What additional assessment data should you obtain?
> - Is it safe to let the client get up out of bed?
> - What information should you relay to the surgeon?
>
> For suggested answer guidelines, go to Ⓢ SIMON http://www.wbsaunders.com/SIMON/Iggy/.

● Community-Based Care

Clients who have advanced acromegaly may experience arthritic changes. The nurse assesses the degree of mobility impairment and identifies appropriate adaptations, such as the

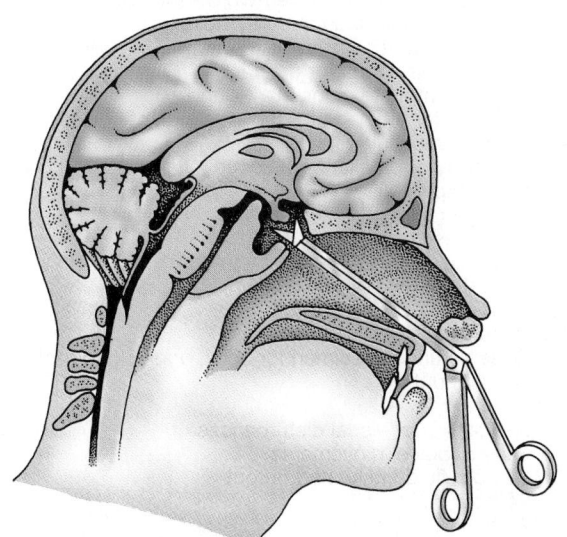

Figure 63-3 ● The transsphenoidal surgical approach to the pituitary gland. Selective adenomectomy leaves normal pituitary tissues undisturbed.

CHART 63-3
BEST PRACTICE *for*   **The Client After Hypophysectomy**

- Monitor the client's neurologic status.
- Monitor fluid balance, especially for output greater than intake, because transient diabetes insipidus can occur.
- Encourage the client to maintain pulmonary hygiene through deep breathing exercises.
- Instruct the client *not* to cough, blow the nose, or sneeze.
- Instruct the client to use dental floss and oral mouth rinses because brushing the teeth is not permitted until the incision heals sufficiently.
- Instruct the client to avoid bending at the waist for any reason, because this position increases intracranial pressure.
- Monitor the nasal drip pad for the type and amount of drainage. The presence of the halo sign may indicate a CSF leak.
- Monitor bowel movements to prevent constipation and subsequent "straining."
- Teach the client self-administration of the prescribed hormones.

CSF, Cerebrospinal fluid.

use of ambulatory aids (cane or walker) and the accessibility of bathroom facilities.

HEALTH TEACHING

After a transsphenoidal hypophysectomy, the nurse advises the client to avoid activities that might interfere with healing. Bending over from the waist to pick up objects or tie shoes must be avoided because doing so increases intracranial pressure. The client is instructed to bend the knees and then lower the body to retrieve fallen objects. Intracranial pressure also increases when the client strains to have a bowel movement. The nurse suggests techniques to prevent constipation, such as eating high-fiber foods, drinking additional fluids, and using stool softeners or laxatives. Both bending and straining with bowel movements should be avoided for up to 2 months after surgery.

The client must avoid toothbrushing for about 2 weeks after surgery until the incision has undergone significant healing. Frequent mouth care (every 4 to 6 hours) with mouthwash and daily flossing during this period provides adequate oral hygiene. Transient numbness in the area of the incision and a decreased sense of smell are expected after surgery and usually last 3 to 4 months. The nurse advises the client to use a mirror to check the gums for bleeding, because reduced sensation increases the risk for injury.

After a hypophysectomy, hormone replacement with vasopressin may be necessary to maintain fluid balance (see later discussion under Interventions [Diabetes Insipidus], p. 1410). If the anterior portion of the pituitary gland is removed, the client may require instruction in cortisol, thyroid, and gonadal hormone replacement. The nurse instructs the client to report the return of any symptoms of hyperpituitarism immediately to the primary health care provider.

HOME CARE MANAGEMENT

After treatment, the client who has hyperpituitarism may require daily self-management regimens and frequent checkups. The client may also need to develop strategies to minimize stress to prevent alterations of hormone production. The nurse performs a focused assessment during the first several home visits to a client who has undergone a hypophysectomy (Chart 63-4). Medication regimens, signs and symptoms of infection, and cerebral edema are reviewed with the family.

HEALTH CARE RESOURCES

The client with decreased mobility related to acromegaly or who has had recent surgery may require a home care aide or nurse to help maintain activities of daily living (ADLs). In addition, the client with hyperpituitarism must continue to have hormone levels monitored at regular intervals to detect any recurrence of tumor. Regularly scheduled follow-up with the health care team is essential.

● Evaluation: Outcomes

NOC The nurse evaluates the care of the client with hyperpituitarism on the basis of the identified nursing diagnoses and collaborative problems. The expected outcomes include that the client will:

- Experience an improvement in body image
- Achieve a personal desired level of sexual functioning
- Demonstrate adjustment to physical appearance
- Be willing to use strategies to enhance appearance and function

DISORDERS OF THE POSTERIOR PITUITARY GLAND

Disorders of the posterior pituitary (**neurohypophysis**) are directly related to a deficiency or excess of the hormone vasopressin (**antidiuretic hormone [ADH]**). Two disorders associated with ADH deficiency or excess are diabetes insipidus and the syndrome of inappropriate antidiuretic hormone (SIADH).

Diabetes Insipidus

OVERVIEW

Diabetes insipidus is a disorder of water metabolism caused by a deficiency of ADH—either a decrease in ADH synthesis or an inability of the kidneys to respond appropriately to ADH. ADH deficiency results in the excretion of large volumes of dilute urine. Without the presence of ADH, the distal tubules and collecting ducts of the kidney remain impermeable to water. Thus water is excreted as urine rather than being absorbed in these areas, which leads to **polyuria** (excessive urination with loss of free water).

Dehydration caused by this massive diuresis results in an increase in plasma osmolality, which stimulates the osmore-

---

CHART 63-4

FOCUSED ASSESSMENT *of*
Home Care Clients Who Have Undergone Transsphenoidal Hypophysectomy for Hyperpituitarism

Assess cardiovascular status.
- Vital signs, including apical pulse, pulse pressure, presence or absence of orthostatic hypotension, and the quality/rhythm of peripheral pulses.

Assess cognition and mental status.
- Level of consciousness
- Orientation to time, place, and person
- Accurately reading a seven-word sentence containing no words longer than three syllables

Assess condition of operative site.
- Observe nasal area for drainage
  If present, note color, clarity, and odor
    Test clear drainage for the presence of glucose

Assess neuromuscular status.
- Reactivity of patellar and biceps reflexes
- Oral temperature
- Handgrip strength
- Steadiness of gait
- Visual fields
- Distant and near visual acuity
- Pupillary responses to light

Assess renal system.
- Observe urine specimen for color, odor, cloudiness, and amount

Ask about:
- Headaches or visual disturbances
- Ease of bowel movements
- 24-hour fluid intake and output
- 24-hour diet recall
- 24-hour activity recall
- Over-the-counter and prescribed medications taken

Assess client's understanding of illness and compliance with treatment.
- Signs and symptoms to report to health care provider
- Medication plan (correct timing and dose)

ceptors to relay a sensation of thirst to the cerebral cortex. Normally, thirst promotes increased fluid intake and aids in maintaining water homeostasis. If the thirst mechanism is inadequate or absent, or if the person is unable to obtain water, dehydration becomes more severe.

ADH deficiency can be classified as nephrogenic, drug-related, primary, or secondary, depending on whether the problem is caused by insufficient production of ADH or an inability of the kidney to respond to the presence of ADH.

Nephrogenic diabetes insipidus is an inherited disorder. The renal tubules do not respond to the actions of ADH, which results in inadequate water reabsorption by the kidney. The actual amount of hormone produced is not deficient.

Primary diabetes insipidus is caused by a defect in the hypothalamus or pituitary gland, resulting in a lack of ADH production or release. Secondary diabetes insipidus results from tumors within or adjacent to the hypothalamus or pituitary gland, head trauma, infectious processes, surgical procedures (hypophysectomy), or metastatic tumors, usually from the lung or the breast. Less commonly, it is caused by brain hemorrhage, brain disease, or cerebral aneurysm. All of these problems can reduce the production of ADH.

Drug-related diabetes insipidus is caused by the administration of lithium carbonate (Eskalith, Lithobid, Carbolith♣) and demeclocycline (Declomycin). These drugs can interfere with the kidneys' response to ADH.

▶ COLLABORATIVE MANAGEMENT

● Assessment

Most of the clinical manifestations of diabetes insipidus are related to dehydration (Chart 63-5). The nurse notes the key symptoms of an increase in the frequency of urination and excessive thirst. The client is asked about a history of any known etiologic factors, such as recent surgery, head trauma, or medication use (e.g., lithium). Although increased fluid intake usually prevents serious dehydration and volume depletion, the client who is deprived of fluids or who cannot increase oral fluid intake may experience shock caused by fluid loss and plasma hyperosmolality. Signs of dehydration, such as poor skin turgor and dry or cracked mucous membranes or skin, may be present in varying degrees. (See Chapter 12 for further discussion of clients with dehydration.)

Loss of free water produces expected changes in blood and urine tests. The initial step in diagnosis is to measure a 24-hour fluid intake and output. The amount of the client's food and fluid is not restricted during this measurement. Urine output must be more than 4 L during this period for diabetes insipidus to be diagnosed. The amount of urine excreted in 24 hours may vary from 4 to 30 L/day. Urine is dilute and therefore has a low specific gravity (less than 1.005) and low osmolality (50 to 200 mOsm/kg). Fluid deprivation and hypertonic saline tests are also used for diagnosis of the disorder (Table 63-2).

CHART 63-5

KEY FEATURES of
Diabetes Insipidus

Cardiovascular Manifestations
- Hypotension
- Decreased pulse pressure
- Tachycardia
- Peripheral pulses weak, easily obliterated
- Hemoconcentration
    Increased hemoglobin
    Increased hematocrit

Renal/Urinary Manifestations
- Increased urine output
    Dilute, low specific gravity
    Hypo-osmolar

Integumentary Manifestations
- Poor turgor
- Dry mucous membranes

Neurologic Manifestations
- Increased sensation of thirst
    Irritability*
    Decreased cognition*
    Hyperthermia*
    Lethargy to coma*
    Ataxia*

*Occurs when access to water is limited and rapid dehydration results.

TABLE 63-2 • CARE OF THE CLIENT UNDERGOING SPECIAL TESTS FOR DIABETES INSIPIDUS	
Nursing Interventions	**Rationale**
FLUID DEPRIVATION TEST (TO IDENTIFY THE CAUSE OF POLYURIA)	
Obtain baseline vital signs; then check them hourly.	Assessment permits the nurse to detect changes, especially postural hypotension and tachycardia.
Deprive the client of fluid. Observe the client for compliance with fluid restriction.	Fluid restriction must be maintained for test results to be of diagnostic importance.
Measure urine output, specific gravity, and osmolality hourly.	Urine testing results determine whether testing can proceed.
Weigh the client hourly.	Testing can proceed if urine osmolality stabilizes for three samples and 3% weight loss is noted.
Give 5 units of aqueous vasopressin (subcutaneously), as ordered. Continue hourly urine measurements.	Vasopressin triggers—and ongoing assessment detects—changes in urine specific gravity and osmolality. Specific gravity and osmolality decrease with primary and secondary diabetes insipidus. No response is seen with nephrogenic diabetes insipidus.
HYPERTONIC SALINE TEST (TO STIMULATE RELEASE OF ADH)	
Administer a normal water load to the client, followed by infusion of hypertonic saline. Measure urine output hourly.	The procedure detects ADH release. A sudden decrease in urine output is a sign of ADH release.

ADH, Antidiuretic hormone.

● Interventions

Medical management is aimed at controlling the symptoms of the disease through drug therapy (Chart 63-6). If only a partial deficit of ADH is present, effective control can be achieved with oral chlorpropamide (Diabinese, Novo-Propamide ♣) or clofibrate (Atromid-S, Claripex ♣). These drugs increase the action of existing ADH and possibly have a direct stimulating effect on the production of ADH in the hypothalamus. They have some undesirable side effects, however, and are not used as often as synthetic vasopressin.

When ADH deficiency is severe, ADH is replaced in amounts sufficient to maintain water balance. Desmopressin acetate (DDAVP) is a synthetic form of vasopressin administered intranasally in a metered spray and is the drug of choice. The frequency of administration varies in different clients. Each metered spray delivers 10 g, and the client with mild diabetes insipidus may require only 1 to 2 doses in 24 hours. For the client with more severe diabetes insipidus, 1 to 2 metered doses two to three times per day may be needed. Lypressin (Diapid) is an older form of the drug and is given by nasal spray or subcutaneously when short-acting therapy is indicated. Subcutaneous injections last only 3 to 6 hours. During an acute exacerbation or severe dehydration, ADH may be given intravenously or intramuscularly. Ulceration of the mucous membranes, allergy, a sensation of chest tightness, and pulmonary inhalation of the spray may occur with use of the intranasal preparations. If side effects occur, or if the client has an upper respiratory tract infection, subcutaneous vasopressin is used.

Nursing management is aimed at the early detection of dehydration and the maintenance of adequate hydration. Interventions include accurately measuring fluid intake and output, checking urine specific gravity, and recording the client's weight daily.

The nurse encourages the client to consume amounts of oral fluids approximately equal to urine output. If fluids are administered intravenously, the nurse ensures the patency of the access catheter and pays meticulous attention to the amount infused each hour.

The client with permanent diabetes insipidus requires life-long vasopressin therapy. The nurse must assess the client's ability to follow instructions and willingness to participate in health care. The client using vasopressin preparations is instructed to recognize polyuria and polydipsia as signals for the need for another dose of medication. *All clients taking vasopressin need to record daily weight measurements to identify weight gain.* The nurse emphasizes the importance of using the same scale and weighing at the same time of day while wearing a similar amount of clothing. If weight gain occurs, the client is instructed to notify the health care provider. Clients with diabetes insipidus should also wear a medical alert bracelet identifying the disorder and current medication.

Syndrome of Inappropriate Antidiuretic Hormone

■ OVERVIEW

The **syndrome of inappropriate antidiuretic hormone (SIADH)** occurs when vasopressin (antidiuretic hormone [ADH]) is secreted even when plasma osmolality is low or normal. A decrease in plasma osmolality normally inhibits

CHART 63-6

DRUG THERAPY *for* **Diabetes Insipidus**

Drug	Usual Dosage	Nursing Interventions	Rationale
Lypressin (Diapid)	4-8 sprays (5-10 pressor units) (nasal spray) in divided doses	Monitor for upper respiratory tract infections or allergy.	The effectiveness of nasal sprays is affected by upper respiratory tract infections.
Desmopressin (DDAVP)	0.1-0.4 mL in single or divided dose (nasal spray)	Teach the client the proper method of administration.	Some clients may have difficulty with measuring and inhaling.
Aqueous vasopressin (Pitressin)	5-20 units in divided doses (SC, IM, or nasal spray)	Instruct the client to sit upright when spraying.	An upright position promotes effective absorption in the nasal mucosa.
		Instruct the client to hold his or her breath when using nasal spray.	Holding one's breath prevents nasal spray from entering the lungs and potentially causing pneumonia.
		Monitor the client's intake and output.	Intake and output measurement helps to guide dosage regulation.
		Have the client space fluid intake during waking hours.	Extra fluid intake at night can cause nocturia.
		Monitor the client frequently (every 3-4 hr) for a recurrence of symptoms.	Monitoring detects the need for additional doses of these short-acting medications.
		Monitor the client's weight.	Water retention can be detected by weight gain.
Clofibrate (Atromid-S, Claripex ♣)	6-8 g in 4 doses qod PO	Watch for signs of SIADH.	The drug can potentiate the action of vasopressin.
Chlorpropamide (Diabinese, Novo-Propamide ♣)	125-250 mg qod PO *Older adults:* 100-125 mg qod PO	Monitor the client for signs and symptoms of hypoglycemia.	Hypoglycemia is a potentially severe side effect.

SIADH, Syndrome of inappropriate antidiuretic hormone.

ADH production and secretion. SIADH is also known as the Schwartz-Bartter syndrome. SIADH is also discussed in Chapter 25 as a complication of cancer and cancer therapy.

In SIADH, the feedback mechanisms that regulate ADH do not function properly. ADH continues to be released even when plasma is hyposmolar. Water is *retained,* which results in dilutional **hyponatremia** (a decreased serum sodium level due to dilution) and expansion of the extracellular fluid volume. The increase in plasma volume causes an increase in the glomerular filtration rate and inhibits the release of renin and aldosterone. The combined effect is an increased sodium loss in urine, further contributing to hyponatremia.

SIADH is associated with a variety of pathologic conditions and specific drugs. Table 63-3 lists common causes of SIADH.

► COLLABORATIVE MANAGEMENT
● Assessment
■ HISTORY

The client is asked about his or her medical history, which may reveal conditions associated with the development of SIADH. The nurse pays particular attention to a history of the following:

- Recent trauma
- Cerebrovascular disease
- Tuberculosis or other pulmonary disease
- Cancer
- All past and current medication use

■ PHYSICAL ASSESSMENT/CLINICAL MANIFESTATIONS

Initially, the symptoms of SIADH are related to water retention. Gastrointestinal (GI) disturbances, such as loss of appetite, nausea, and vomiting, may occur first. The nurse weighs the client and documents any recent weight gain. In clients with SIADH,

free water (not salt) is retained and dependent edema is not usually present, even though water is retained.

Water retention, hyponatremia, and fluid shifts affect central nervous system function, especially when the serum sodium level drops below 115 mEq/L. The client may experience lethargy, headaches, hostility, and disorientation. A change in level of consciousness is an early sign of SIADH. Neurologic symptoms can progress from lethargy and headaches to decreased responsiveness, seizures, and coma. The nurse assesses deep tendon reflexes, which are often decreased or sluggish.

Vital sign changes include tachycardia (caused by the increased fluid volume) and hypothermia (caused by central nervous system disturbance). Chapter 13 presents other findings associated with hyponatremia.

■ DIAGNOSTIC ASSESSMENT

Water retention changes both plasma and urine osmolality. Urine volume decreases, and urine osmolarity increases. Plasma volume increases, and plasma osmolarity decreases. Elevated urine sodium levels and elevated specific gravity reflect increased urine concentration. Serum sodium levels are decreased, often as low as 110 mEq/L, because of volume expansion and sodium excretion.

Radioimmunoassay of ADH can diagnose SIADH when ADH levels are inappropriately elevated in relation to plasma osmolality. (When plasma osmolality is normal or decreased, ADH levels should be low.)

● Interventions

Interventions to treat SIADH focus on restricting fluid intake, promoting the excretion of water, replacing lost sodium, interfering with the action of ADH, and preventing injury if the client experiences increased cranial pressure or seizures.

FLUID RESTRICTION. Fluid restriction is essential in the management of the client with SIADH because fluid intake further dilutes the plasma sodium concentration. In some cases, fluid intake may be kept as low as 500 to 600 mL/24 hr. Tube feedings are diluted with a solution other than plain water, and saline is used to irrigate GI tubes. The nurse mixes any medications for GI tube administration with saline.

Measurement of intake, output, and daily weights determines the degree of fluid restriction necessary. A weight gain of 2 pounds (1 kg) or more per day or a gradual increase over several days is cause for concern. A 1-kg weight increase is equal to a 1000-mL fluid retention (1 kg = 1 L). The client is often uncomfortable during fluid restriction, and the nurse keeps mucous membranes moist by offering frequent oral rinsing (reminding the client not to swallow these rinses).

DRUG THERAPY. Diuretics are sometimes used to treat SIADH, particularly if congestive heart failure results from fluid overload. The nurse must be aware of the potential effect of electrolyte losses; sodium loss can be potentiated, further contributing to the problems caused by SIADH.

Hypertonic saline (i.e., 3% sodium chloride [3% NaCl]) is often used to treat SIADH. IV saline is given cautiously because it may add to existing fluid overload and promote congestive heart failure. If the client needs routine IV fluids, the physician orders a saline solution rather than a water solution.

TABLE 63-3	CONDITIONS CAUSING THE SYNDROME OF INAPPROPRIATE ANTIDIURETIC HORMONES

MALIGNANCIES	CNS DISORDERS
• Small cell carcinoma of the lung	• Trauma
• Pancreatic, duodenal, and GU carcinomas	• Infection
• Thymoma	• Tumors (primary or metastatic)
• Ewing's sarcoma	• Strokes
• Hodgkin's lymphoma	• Porphyria
• Non-Hodgkin's lymphoma	• Systemic lupus erythematosus
PULMONARY DISORDERS	**DRUGS**
• Viral and bacterial pneumonia	• Exogenous ADH
• Lung abscesses	• Chlorpropamide
• Active tuberculosis	• Vincristine
• Pneumothorax	• Cyclophosphamide
• Chronic lung diseases	• Carbamazepine
• Mycoses	• Opioids
• Positive-pressure ventilation	• Tricyclic antidepressants
	• General anesthetics

GU, Genitourinary; *CNS,* central nervous system; *ADH,* antidiuretic hormone.

The administration of drugs such as lithium carbonate (Eskalith, Lithobid, Carbolith♣) and demeclocycline (Declomycin) is associated with the development of diabetes insipidus. Their use has therefore been explored in the treatment of SIADH. Lithium is seldom used because of its toxicity; demeclocycline is more common.

PROVIDING A SAFE ENVIRONMENT. The nurse observes for and documents changes in the client's neurologic status. The nurse assesses for subtle changes, such as muscle twitching, before they progress to seizures or coma. Orientation to time, place, and person is checked every 2 hours because disorientation or confusion may be present. Environmental noise and lighting are reduced to prevent overstimulation.

Flow sheets with continuing information about the level of consciousness, motor and sensory neurologic assessments, and pertinent laboratory data are helpful in detecting neurologic trends. The frequency of neurologic checks depends on the status of the client: for the client with SIADH who is hyponatremic but alert, awake, and oriented, neurologic checks every 4 hours are sufficient. For the client who has had a change in level of consciousness, neurologic checks take place at least every hour. The nurse also inspects the environment at regular intervals, making sure that basic safety measures, such as siderails securely in place, are observed.

CRITICAL THINKING CHALLENGE

The client is a 63-year-old man with late-stage lung cancer who is being cared for at home by his wife. He has SIADH and is on a fluid restriction of 800 mL/day. During a home visit, the client seems to be more confused than when you last saw him. His wife tells you that his mouth is always dry and he does not want to eat. She also tells that you he would eat ice cream but that she has not given it to him because of the fluid restriction.

- What additional assessment data should you obtain?
- What comfort measures could you suggest?
- Should this client be permitted to have a serving of ice cream? Why or why not?

For suggested answer guidelines, go to 🖱️SIMON http://www.wbsaunders.com/SIMON/Iggy/.

DISORDERS OF THE ADRENAL GLAND

ADRENAL GLAND HYPOFUNCTION

OVERVIEW

Production of adrenocortical steroids may decrease as a result of inadequate secretion of adrenocorticotropic hormone (ACTH), dysfunction of the hypothalamic-pituitary control mechanism, and complete or partial destruction of the adrenal glands. Manifestations may develop gradually or occur quickly with stress. In acute adrenocortical insufficiency (**adrenal crisis**), life-threatening manifestations may appear without warning. Figure 63-4 outlines the normal pathway for adrenocortical hormone synthesis.

Loss of the adrenal medulla, which produces catecholamines (dopamine, norepinephrine, and epinephrine), does not upset the maintenance of homeostasis. This is because catecholamines are also synthesized and released from other areas in the sympathetic nervous system.

Pathophysiology

Insufficiency of adrenocortical steroids causes problems through the loss of mineralocorticoid (**aldosterone**) and glucocorticoid (**cortisol**) action. Impaired secretion of cortisol results in decreased **gluconeogenesis** (making glucose from proteins) along with depletion of liver and muscle glycogen, leading to **hypoglycemia** (low blood glucose levels). The glomerular filtration rate and gastric acid production decrease, leading to a reduction in urea nitrogen excretion, causing anorexia and weight loss.

Reduced aldosterone secretion causes potassium, sodium, and water imbalances. Potassium excretion is decreased, causing hyperkalemia; sodium and water excretion is increased, causing hyponatremia and hypovolemia. Potassium retention also promotes reabsorption of hydrogen ions, which can ultimately lead to acidosis.

Lower adrenal androgen levels result in the decrease or loss of body, axillary, and pubic hair, especially in women, because the adrenals produce most of the androgens in fe-

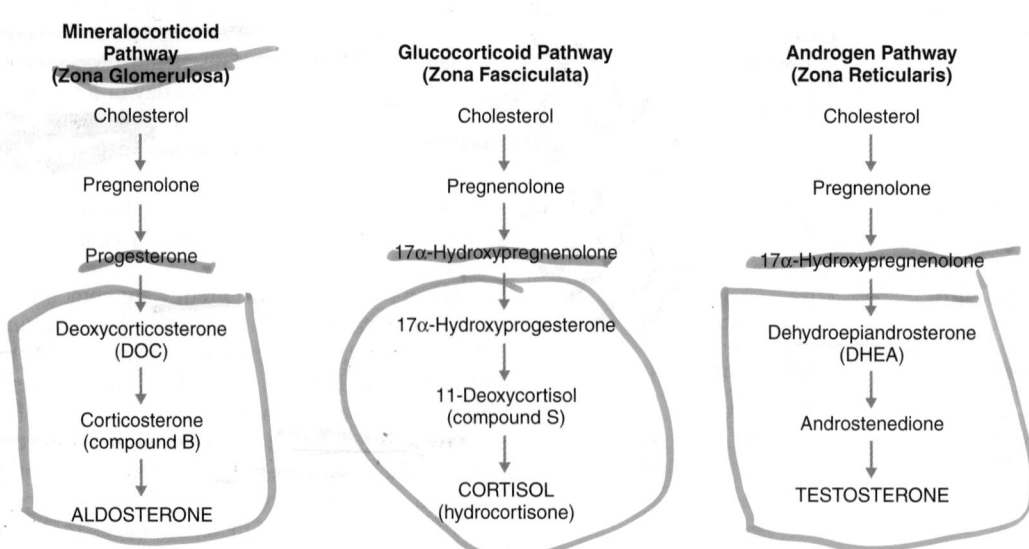

Mineralocorticoid Pathway (Zona Glomerulosa)	Glucocorticoid Pathway (Zona Fasciculata)	Androgen Pathway (Zona Reticularis)
Cholesterol	Cholesterol	Cholesterol
Pregnenolone	Pregnenolone	Pregnenolone
Progesterone	17α-Hydroxypregnenolone	17α-Hydroxypregnenolone
Deoxycorticosterone (DOC)	17α-Hydroxyprogesterone	Dehydroepiandrosterone (DHEA)
Corticosterone (compound B)	11-Deoxycortisol (compound S)	Androstenedione
ALDOSTERONE	CORTISOL (hydrocortisone)	TESTOSTERONE

Figure 63-4 ● A simplified explanation of the major pathways of adrenal steroidal synthesis from the adrenal cortex.

males. The severity of symptoms is related to the degree of deficiency in hormone secretion.

Acute adrenal insufficiency, or **Addisonian crisis,** is a life-threatening event in which the physiologic need for glucocorticoid and mineralocorticoid hormones is greater than the available supply. In most cases, acute adrenal insufficiency occurs in response to a stressful event (e.g., surgery, trauma, or severe infection), especially when the adrenal hormone output is already compromised. The pathophysiology of acute adrenal crisis is almost the same as that of chronic insufficiency; the one difference occurs in clients with acute adrenal crisis related to bilateral adrenal hemorrhage. These clients may have normal sodium and potassium levels because the time between the initial incident and the presentation may be too short for a change in electrolyte composition to occur. Unless intervention is initiated promptly, however, sodium levels fall and potassium levels rise rapidly. More severe hypotension results from the blood volume depletion that occurs with the loss of aldosterone. Best practices for emergency care of clients with acute adrenal insufficiency (Addisonian crisis) are outlined in Chart 63-7.

Etiology

Adrenal insufficiency may be classified as primary or secondary. Causes of primary and secondary adrenal insufficiency are listed in Table 63-4. One of the most frequent causes of secondary adrenal insufficiency is the sudden cessation of long-term, high-dose glucocorticoid therapy. This therapy suppresses production of glucocorticoids through negative feedback. Glucocorticoid drugs must be withdrawn gradually to allow for pituitary production of ACTH and adrenal production of cortisol.

▶ COLLABORATIVE MANAGEMENT
● Assessment
■ HISTORY

While taking a history from the client with suspected adrenal hypofunction, the nurse asks questions about symptoms and factors contributing to adrenal hypofunction. The client is also asked about any change in activity level, because lethargy, fatigue, and muscle weakness are often present. Questions about

salt intake are included because salt craving is often a symptom of adrenal hypofunction.

Gastrointestinal (GI) problems, such as anorexia, nausea, vomiting, diarrhea, and abdominal pain, often occur. The nurse asks about weight loss during the past weeks or months. Female clients report menstrual changes related to weight loss, and male clients may report impotence.

The medical history identifies potential causes of adrenal hypofunction. The nurse asks whether the client has had radiation to the abdomen or head. Significant medical problems (e.g., tuberculosis or previous intracranial surgery) and all past and current medications, especially steroids, anticoagulants, or cytotoxic drugs, are documented.

■ PHYSICAL ASSESSMENT/CLINICAL MANIFESTATIONS

The clinical manifestations of adrenal hypofunction vary, and the severity of symptoms is related to the degree of hormone deficiency (Chart 63-8). In clients with primary adrenal hypofunction, plasma ACTH and melanocyte-stimulating hormone (MSH) levels are elevated because of the loss of the adrenal-hypothalamic-pituitary feedback system. Elevated MSH levels result in areas of increased pigmentation (Figure 63-5). In primary autoimmune disease, areas of decreased pigmentation may occur because of destruction of pigment-producing cells in the skin (melanocytes). Body hair may also be decreased. In secondary disease, there is no increase in skin pigmentation.

TABLE 63-4 ● CAUSES OF PRIMARY AND SECONDARY ADRENAL INSUFFICIENCY	
PRIMARY CAUSES	**SECONDARY CAUSES**
• Idiopathic (autoimmune) disease*	• Pituitary tumors
• Tuberculosis	• Postpartum pituitary necrosis (Sheehan's syndrome)
• Metastatic cancer	• Hypophysectomy
• Fungal lesions	• High-dose pituitary radiation
• AIDS	• High-dose whole-brain radiation
• Hemorrhage	
• Gram-negative sepsis (Waterhouse-Friderichsen syndrome)	
• Adrenalectomy	
• Abdominal radiation therapy	
• Drugs (mitotane) and toxins	

*Most common cause.

CHART 63-7

BEST PRACTICE *for*
Nursing Care of the Client with Acute Adrenal Insufficiency

- Before initiating treatment, obtain a complete blood count and electrolyte, blood urea nitrogen, and plasma cortisol levels, as ordered by the physician.
- Give an initial dose of hydrocortisone sodium succinate (Solu-Cortef) 100 to 300 mg intravenously; then infuse 100 mg over an 8-hour period, as ordered by the physician.
- Give concomitant doses of hydrocortisone 50 mg intramuscularly every 12 hours, as ordered by the physician.
- After resolution of the crisis, adjust the dosage of medications, as ordered by the physician:
  Give oral glucocorticoids (e.g., hydrocortisone).
  Decrease the dosage of oral glucocorticoids during several days as maintenance levels are reached.
  Give supplemental mineralocorticoids, such as fludrocortisone (Florinef), as the glucocorticoid dosage is tapered.

CHART 63-8

KEY FEATURES *of*
Adrenal Insufficiency

Neuromuscular Manifestations
- Muscle weakness
- Fatigue
- Joint/muscle pain

Gastrointestinal Manifestations
- Anorexia
- Nausea, vomiting
- Abdominal pain
- Bowel changes (constipation/diarrhea)
- Weight loss
- Salt craving

Integumentary Manifestations
- Vitiligo
- Hyperpigmentation

Cardiovascular Manifestations
- Anemia
- Hypotension
- Hyponatremia
- Hyperkalemia
- Hypercalcemia

The nurse assesses the client for symptoms of hypoglycemia (e.g., sweating, headaches, tachycardia, and tremors) and volume depletion (postural hypotension and dehydration). **Hyperkalemia** (elevated blood levels of potassium) can cause dysrhythmias with an irregular heart rate and result in cardiac arrest.

PSYCHOSOCIAL ASSESSMENT

Depending on the degree of metabolic imbalance, clients may appear lethargic, apathetic, depressed, confused, and even

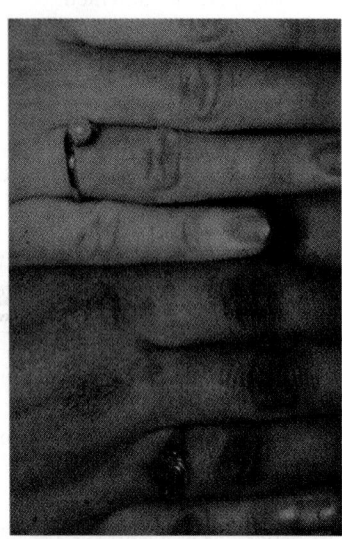

Figure 63-5 ● Hand of a client with hyperpigmentation related to adrenocortical insufficiency (bottom), shown alongside the hand of an unaffected person. Note the deep hyperpigmentation of the knuckles. (From Wilson, J.D, et al. (1998). *Williams textbook of endocrinology* (9th ed.). Philadelphia: W.B. Saunders. Courtesy Dr. H. Patrick Higgins.)

psychotic. The nurse observes the client and checks his or her orientation to person, place, and time. Families may report that the client has a decreased energy level, experiences wide mood swings, and is forgetful.

DIAGNOSTIC ASSESSMENT

Laboratory findings usually include low serum cortisol, decreased fasting blood glucose, low sodium, elevated potassium, and increased serum blood urea nitrogen (BUN) levels (Chart 63-9). In primary disease, the eosinophil count and ACTH level are elevated. Plasma cortisol levels fail to rise during stimulation tests.

Urinary 17-hydroxycorticosteroids are the glucocorticoid metabolites, and 17-ketosteroid levels reflect the adrenal androgen metabolites. Both levels are in the low or low-normal range in adrenal hypofunction. Table 63-5 lists drugs that can interfere with test results.

Skull x-ray films, computed tomography (CT), magnetic resonance imaging (MRI), and arteriography may aid in the search for a cause of pituitary problems leading to adrenal insufficiency.

Noninvasive procedures of the adrenal gland, such as CT scans without dye, may occasionally show atrophy of the gland. CT scans may help determine adrenal hypofunction.

An ACTH (cosyntropin [Cortrosyn], synthetic ACTH) stimulation test is the most definitive test for adrenal insufficiency. A rapid ACTH stimulation test may be administered on an outpatient basis. Cosyntropin 0.25 to 1 mg is given intramuscularly or intravenously, and plasma cortisol levels are obtained at 30-minute and 1-hour intervals after the baseline value is established. In primary insufficiency, the cortisol response is absent or markedly decreased; in secondary insufficiency, it is decreased.

A longer ACTH stimulation test uses a continuous infusion of 50 units of ACTH in saline for 24 hours or an 8-hour

CHART 63-9

LABORATORY PROFILE
Adrenal Gland Assessment

Test	Normal Range for Adults	Significance of Abnormal Findings	
		Hypofunction of the Adrenal Gland	**Hyperfunction of the Adrenal Gland**
Sodium	136-145 mEq/L	Decreased	Increased
Potassium	3.4-4.5 mEq/L	Increased	Decreased
Glucose	74-106 mg/dL *Older adults:* slightly increased	Normal to decreased	Normal to increased
Calcium	8.6-10.0 mg/dL (total) 4.6-5.08 mg/dL (ionized) *Older adults:* slightly decreased	Increased	Decreased
Leukocytes	20%-40%	Normal	Increased
Eosinophils	1%-4%	Increased	Decreased
Bicarbonate	22-29 mEq/L	Increased	Decreased
BUN	6-20 mg/dL *Older adults:* may be slightly higher	Increased	Normal
Cortisol	6 AM-8 AM 5-23 μg/dL or 138-635 SI units (nmol/L) 4 PM-6 PM 3-16 μg/dL or 83-441 SI units (nmol/L)	Decreased	Increased

BUN, Blood urea nitrogen; *SI,* System Internationale.

infusion daily for 4 to 5 days, with simultaneously collected 24-hour urine samples. Levels of urinary 17-hydroxycorticosteroids and urinary free cortisol are also measured. In clients with primary adrenal insufficiency, the response is low or absent; in those with secondary insufficiency, the value for 17-hydroxycorticosteroids fails to rise above 20 mg per total volume.

● Interventions

Nursing interventions are aimed at promoting fluid balance and monitoring for fluid deficit (Chart 63-10). The nurse or assistive nursing personnel weighs the client daily and records intake and output. Vital signs are assessed every 1 to 4 hours, depending on the client's condition and the occurrence of dysrhythmias or postural hypotension. Laboratory values are monitored to identify hemoconcentrations (e.g., increased hematocrit or BUN). Chapter 12 discusses fluid volume deficit in detail.

Glucocorticoid and mineralocorticoid deficiencies are completely corrected by replacement therapy. Hydrocortisone corrects glucocorticoid deficiency (Chart 63-11). Glucocorticoid replacement regimens vary. Generally, divided doses are given, with two thirds given in the morning and one third in the late afternoon to mimic the normal adrenal hormone secretion rhythm. Although most clients do well on this regimen, some may not tolerate the dosage or may need more.

An additional mineralocorticoid hormone, such as fludrocortisone (Florinef), may be needed to maintain correct electrolyte balance (especially sodium and potassium). Adjustments in dosage may be necessary in hot weather, when additional sodium is lost because of excessive perspiration. *Salt restriction or diuretic therapy should not be started without considering whether it might precipitate an adrenal crisis.*

ADRENAL GLAND HYPERFUNCTION

Unlike adrenal gland hypofunction, which results in a generalized deficiency of all adrenal hormones, the adrenal gland may oversecrete just one or all hormones. Hypersecretion by the adrenal cortex may result in excessive amounts of glucocorticoids, leading to **hypercortisolism** (e.g., **Cushing's syndrome**), **hyperaldosteronism** (excessive mineralocorticoid production), or excessive androgen production.

Hypersecretion of the adrenal medulla caused by a tumor (**pheochromocytoma**) results in excessive secretion of catecholamines, of which 80% is epinephrine and the remainder is norepinephrine.

TABLE 63-5 ● SOME DRUGS THAT INTERFERE WITH TESTS FOR URINARY 17-HYDROXYCORTICOSTEROIDS AND URINARY 17-KETOSTEROIDS

• Acetaminophen	• Hydralazine
• Acetazolamide	• Iodides
• Acetylsalicylic acid	• Medroxyprogesterone
• Amphetamines	• Meperidine
• Ascorbic acid	• Meprobamate
• Barbiturates	• Metyrapone
• Calcium gluconate	• Mitotane
• Carbon disulfide	• Morphine
• Chloral hydrate	• Nalidixic acid
• Chlordiazepoxide	• Oral contraceptives
• Chlormerodrin	• Paraldehyde
• Chlorothiazide	• Penicillin
• Chlorpromazine	• Pentazocine
• Chlorthalidone	• Perphenazine
• Colchicine	• Phenobarbital
• Corticotropin	• Phenothiazines
• Cortisone	• Phenylbutazone
• Dexamethasone	• Promazine
• Diazepam	• Propoxyphene
• Digitoxin	• Quinidine
• Digoxin	• Quinine
• Diphenhydramine	• Reserpine
• Diphenylhydantoin	• Secobarbital
• Erythromycin	• Spironolactone
• Estrogens	• Testosterone
• Fructose	• Vitamin K
• Glutethimide	

CHART 63-10

NIC INTERVENTION ACTIVITIES for Clients with Adrenal Insufficiency

Electrolyte Management: Hyperkalemia: *Promotion of potassium balance and prevention of complications resulting from serum potassium levels higher than desired*
- Administer electrolyte-binding and electrolyte-excreting resins (e.g., Kayexalate) as prescribed, if appropriate.
- Monitor lab values for changes in oxygenation or acid-base balance, as appropriate.
- Administer prescribed medications to shift potassium into the cell (e.g., 50% dextrose and insulin, sodium bicarbonate, calcium chloride, and calcium gluconate), as appropriate.
- Avoid potassium-sparing medications (e.g., spironolactone [Aldactone] and triamterene [Dyrenium]), as appropriate.
- Maintain potassium restrictions.
- Administer prescribed diuretics, as appropriate.
- Monitor fluid status, including intake and output, as appropriate.
- Monitor potassium levels after diuresis.
- Monitor cardiac manifestations of hyperkalemia (e.g., decreased cardiac output, heart blocks, peaked T waves, fibrillation, or asystole).
- Respond to cardiac arrest.

Hypoglycemia Management: *Preventing and treating low blood glucose levels*
- Determine recognition of hypoglycemia signs and symptoms.
- Monitor blood glucose levels, as indicated.
- Monitor for signs and symptoms of hypoglycemia (e.g., shakiness, tremor, sweating, nervousness, anxiety, irritability, impatience, tachycardia, palpitations, chills, clamminess, lightheadedness, pallor, hunger, nausea, headache, tiredness, drowsiness, weakness, warmth, dizziness, faintness, blurred vision, nightmares, crying out in sleep, paresthesias, difficulty concentrating, difficulty speaking, incoordination, behavior change, confusion, coma, seizure).
- Provide simple carbohydrate, as indicated.
- Administer glucagon, as indicated.
- Maintain IV access, as appropriate.
- Instruct client and significant others on signs and symptoms, risk factors, and treatment of hypoglycemia.
- Instruct client to have simple carbohydrate available at all times.
- Instruct client to obtain and carry/wear appropriate emergency identification.

NIC intervention activities selected from McCloskey, J.C., & Bulechek, G.M. (2000). *Nursing interventions classification (NIC)* (3rd ed.). St. Louis: Mosby. No part of this work is to be altered without prior written permission from the Publisher.

Hypercortisolism (Cushing's Syndrome)

■ OVERVIEW

■ Pathophysiology

Cushing's syndrome exaggerates the normal actions of glucocorticoids, causing widespread problems. Excessive stimulation of adrenocorticotropic hormone (ACTH) of either pituitary or ectopic origin causes adrenocortical hyperplasia, which results in loss of normal hormone secretion rhythms. The client's endocrine tissues have decreased responsiveness to releasing hormones, especially prolactin (PRL), thyrotropin, and gonadotropin. Many clients also experience abnormal sleep patterns. Most of these changes are due to excessive amounts of glucocorticoids.

The client with Cushing's syndrome has alterations of nitrogen, carbohydrate, and mineral metabolism. An increase in total body fat results from slow turnover of plasma fatty acids, and a redistribution of fat produces the typical body pattern of truncal obesity, "buffalo hump," and "moon face" (Figure 63-6). Increases in the breakdown of tissue protein and an increase in urine nitrogen excretion also occur, resulting in decreased muscle mass, **atrophic** (thin) skin, and bone density loss.

High levels of corticosteroids kill lymphocytes and shrink organs containing lymphocytes, such as the liver, the spleen, and the lymph nodes. Thus protection of the inflammatory and immune responses is reduced.

In most cases, increased androgen production causes acne, **hirsutism** (increased hair growth), and occasionally, clitoral hypertrophy. Increased androgen production can also interrupt the normal hormone feedback mechanism for the ovary, decreasing the ovary's production of estrogens and progesterone. **Oligomenorrhea** (scant or infrequent menses) occurs as a result.

■ Etiology

Cushing's syndrome is a group of clinical problems caused by an excess of cortisol, secreted by the adrenal cortex (**endogenous**) or administered for another clinical disorder (**exogenous** or **iatrogenic**). Table 63-6 lists causes of cortisol excess. Women are affected eight times more often than men.

➤ COLLABORATIVE MANAGEMENT

● Assessment

A thorough history and physical assessment aid in detecting clinical features of hypercortisolism, which result from glucocorticoid excess.

■ HISTORY

The client who has hypercortisolism has varied changes because of the widespread effect of excessive cortisol levels in the body. The nurse asks about changes in activity or sleep patterns, fatigue, and muscle weakness. Osteoporosis is common in hypercortisolism, and the client is asked about bone pain or a history of fractures. The nurse also questions the client about a history of frequent infections and easy bruising, which suggest hypercortisolism. Women may report a cessation of menses. Gastrointestinal (GI) complaints may indicate ulcer formation from increased hydrochloric acid secretion.

The nurse also refers to the client's medical history. Steroid or alcohol abuse can produce the clinical and biochemical features of Cushing's syndrome.

■ PHYSICAL ASSESSMENT/CLINICAL MANIFESTATIONS

The client with hypercortisolism has characteristic physical changes (see Figure 63-6). The general appearance of the client is observed. Changes in fat distribution may result in fat pads on the neck, back, and shoulders ("buffalo hump"); an enlarged trunk with thin arms and legs; and a round face ("moon face"). Other characteristics include generalized muscle wasting and weakness.

The nurse also inspects the client for skin changes resulting from increased blood vessel fragility, such as bruises, thin or translucent skin, and wounds that have not healed properly. Reddish purple **striae** ("stretch marks") are often present on

---

CHART 63-11

MAINTENANCE DRUG THERAPY *for* **Hypofunction of the Adrenal Gland**

Drug	Usual Dosage	Nursing Interventions	Rationale
Cortisone	25-50 mg PO either once daily in AM or daily in divided doses	Instruct the client to take the drug with meals or a snack.	Gastrointestinal irritation can occur
Hydrocortisone (Cortef, Hycort✦)	20-50 mg PO either once daily in AM or daily in divided doses	Instruct the client to report the following signs or symptoms of excessive drug therapy: • Rapid weight gain • Round face • Fluid retention	Cushing's syndrome, which indicates a need for dosage adjustment, can occur.
Prednisone (Winpred✦)	5-10 mg PO either once daily in AM or daily in divided doses	Instruct the client to report illness, such as:	Other conditions may indicate a need for dosage change. The usual daily dosage may not be adequate during periods of illness or severe stress
Fludrocortisone (Florinef)	0.05-0.2 mg PO daily	• Severe diarrhea • Vomiting • Fever	
		Monitor the client's blood pressure.	Hypertension is a potential side effect.
		Instruct the client to report weight gain or edema.	Sodium-related fluid retention is possible.

the abdomen, upper thighs, and upper arms because of the degradative effect of cortisol on collagen.

Excessive cortisol secretion may result in a fine coating of hair over the face and body and in acne. In the female client, the nurse looks for the presence of hirsutism, clitoral hypertrophy, and male pattern balding related to androgen excess.

Elevations in blood glucose levels are also a frequent finding. Hypertension from water and sodium retention is common.

PSYCHOSOCIAL ASSESSMENT

Hypercortisolism can result in emotional lability, and the nurse asks about mood swings, irritability, confusion, or depression. The client may become neurotic or psychotic as a result of changes in blood cortisol levels.

DIAGNOSTIC ASSESSMENT

Plasma cortisol levels are elevated in clients with hypercortisolism. Blood for cortisol assays is obtained at the same time of day because levels vary throughout the day. Further diagnostic testing is performed to confirm the diagnosis of hypercortisolism, because an increase in cortisol levels is also seen in acute illness and trauma. Plasma ACTH levels vary, depending on the cause of hypercortisolism. In ectopic (ACTH-producing) syndromes, ACTH levels are elevated. In Cushing's syndrome (primary disease of the adrenal gland), ACTH levels are low to immeasurable. Additional laboratory findings may include the following:

- Increased blood glucose level
- Elevated white blood cell count
- Elevated lymphocyte count
- Increased sodium level
- Decreased serum calcium level
- Decreased serum potassium level

Urine is tested to measure levels of free cortisol and the adrenal metabolites of cortisol and androgens (17-hydroxycorticosteroids and 17-ketosteroids). The client is instructed to save *all* urine for 24 hours. In Cushing's disease, basal levels of urinary free cortisol, 17-ketosteroids, and 17-hydroxycorticosteroids are all elevated, as are urine levels of calcium, potassium, and glucose.

Radiographic studies, computed tomography (CT) scans, magnetic resonance imaging (MRI), and arteriography may identify lesions of the adrenal or pituitary glands, lung, GI tract, or pancreas in a client with clinical manifestations of cortisol hypersecretion.

The *overnight dexamethasone suppression test* is an initial screening test for Cushing's syndrome. The client is instructed not to take medications, especially phenytoin (Dilantin) or phenobarbital, for at least 2 days before the test. Normally, plasma cortisol levels are lower than 5 µg/dL. Higher levels indicate that further, definitive testing is necessary.

For the *3-day, low-dose* dexamethasone suppression test, the client must take no medications for at least 2 days before the test (if possible) and have no stressful procedures (e.g., barium enema, myelogram, or an intense physical therapy session) performed during the test. Table 63-5 lists drugs that interfere with testing. A baseline 24-hour urine sample is collected on day 1. Dexamethasone 0.5 mg is administered every 6 hours on days 2 and 3, during which time 24-hour urine collections are taken. The 24-hour urine collections are tested for 17-ketosteroids, 17-hydroxycorticosteroids, creatinine, and urinary free cortisol. Normally, urinary 17-hydroxycorticosteroid excretion and free cortisol levels are suppressed by dexamethasone, and Cushing's syndrome is ruled out. If these levels are not suppressed, a higher-dose dexamethasone test is performed.

The *high-dose* (8-mg) dexamethasone suppression test distinguishes between bilateral adrenocortical hyperplasia (e.g., Cushing's syndrome) and an adrenocortical neoplasm as the cause of hypercortisolism. This test can be performed as an overnight test or a 2-day test and is similar to the tests previously discussed but uses higher doses of dexamethasone. In the overnight high-dose test, the client with Cushing's disease will have a reduced plasma cortisol level that is less than 50% of baseline. This test is more reliable than the 2-day high-dose test.

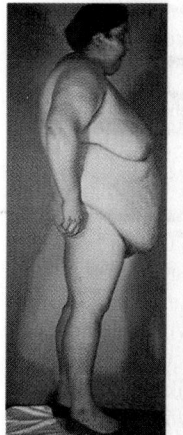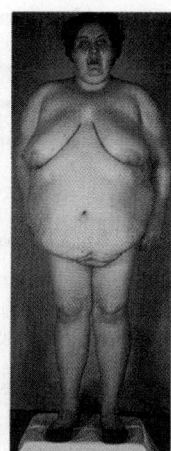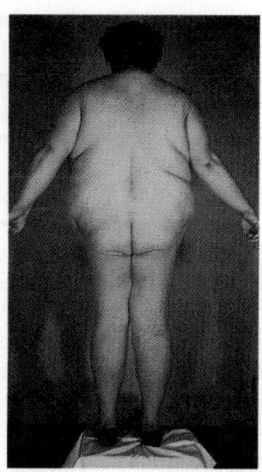

Figure 63-6 ● The typical appearance of a client with Cushing's disease or syndrome. Note truncal obesity, "moon face," "buffalo hump," thinner arms and legs, and abdominal striae. (From Wenig B.M., Heffess, C.S., & Adair, C.F. (1997). *Atlas of endocrine pathology*. Philadelphia: W.B. Saunders.

TABLE 63-6 ●	CONDITIONS CAUSING INCREASED CORTISOL SECRETION

ENDOGENOUS SECRETION
- Bilateral adrenal hyperplasia*
- Pituitary adenoma increasing the production of ACTH (pituitary Cushing's syndrome)
- Malignancies: carcinomas of the lung, gastrointestinal tract, pancreas
- Adrenal adenomas or carcinomas

EXOGENOUS ADMINISTRATION
- Therapeutic use of ACTH or glucocorticoids—most commonly for treatment of:
  Asthma
  Autoimmune disorders
  Organ transplantation
  Cancer chemotherapy
  Allergic responses
  Chronic fibrosis

ACTH, Adrenocorticotropic hormone.
*Most common cause.

● Interventions

Goals of treatment for hypercortisolism include reduction of plasma cortisol levels, removal of tumors, prevention of complications, and restoration of normal or acceptable body appearance. Specific nursing interventions and drug therapy address the problems of clients who have hypercortisolism. Preoperative and postoperative nursing care is an integral part of the management of the client with endogenous hypercortisolism because surgical intervention is usually necessary for the relief of symptoms.

NONSURGICAL MANAGEMENT. The nurse weighs the client daily and monitors intake and output to assess hydration status. Restriction of fluid intake is sometimes necessary to maintain fluid balance.

DRUG THERAPY. Most clients with endogenous hypercortisolism undergo surgery. Drugs that interfere with adrenocorticotropic hormone (ACTH) production or adrenal hormone synthesis, however, may be used for palliation. Mitotane (Lysodren) is an adrenal cytotoxic agent used for inoperable adrenal tumors. Aminoglutethimide (Elipten, Cytadren) is an adrenal enzyme inhibitor that decreases cortisol production. Trilostane (Modrastane), also an enzyme inhibitor, has not always been effective. Cyproheptadine (Periactin) is less commonly used to treat clients with adrenal hyperfunction resulting from pituitary-related Cushing's disease because it interferes with ACTH production. During all drug therapy, the nurse assesses the client for therapy effectiveness and side effects or symptoms of toxicity.

RADIATION THERAPY. Radiation, applied internally or externally, may be used to treat hypercortisolism caused by pituitary adenomas. However, radiation is not always effective and also may destroy normal tissue. The nurse observes for any changes in the client's neurologic status, such as headache, elevated blood pressure or pulse, disorientation, or changes in pupil size or reaction. The client may experience skin dryness, redness, flushing, or alopecia at the radiation site. The nurse reviews these possible side effects with the client. Chapter 45 specifically discusses radiation therapy to the head.

SURGICAL MANAGEMENT. The surgical treatment of adrenocortical hypersecretion depends on the cause of the disease. When adrenal hyperfunction is due to increased pituitary secretion of ACTH, transsphenoidal removal of an adenoma may be attempted. In many instances, small adenomas cannot be localized and **hypophysectomy** (surgical removal of the pituitary gland) is needed. Hypophysectomy is performed via the transsphenoidal or transfrontal craniotomy route. (See earlier discussion of hypophysectomy on pp. 1406 and 1407; see also Chapter 45 for nursing care of clients undergoing a craniotomy.)

If hypercortisolism is caused by adrenal adenomas or carcinomas, a partial or complete **adrenalectomy** (removal of the adrenal gland) may be needed.

PREOPERATIVE CARE. Electrolyte imbalances are corrected before surgery, and the nurse monitors potassium, sodium, and chloride values. Dysrhythmias from potassium imbalance may occur, and cardiac monitoring may be indicated. Hyperglycemia, if present, is controlled before surgery, and the nurse monitors blood glucose levels.

The client with hypercortisolism is susceptible to complications such as infections and fractures. The nurse and assistive nursing personnel attempt to prevent infection with handwashing and aseptic technique. The risk for falls is decreased by raising the siderails of the bed and encouraging the client to ask for assistance when getting out of bed. The physician orders a high-calorie, high-protein diet before surgery.

Glucocorticoid preparations are administered preoperatively as ordered. The client continues to receive glucocorticoids throughout the operative procedure to prevent adrenal crisis. The removal of the tumor results in a sudden drop in cortisol levels. The nurse discusses postoperative care and long-term medication therapy during preoperative teaching.

OPERATIVE PROCEDURES. A **unilateral adrenalectomy** is performed when one gland is involved. A **bilateral adrenalectomy** is necessary when ectopic ACTH-producing tumors cannot be treated by other means or when both adrenal glands are diseased.

Surgery can be abdominal or through the lateral flank. Abdominal surgery causes a higher degree of illness and risk. In the flank approach (the preferred approach), the abdominal cavity is not entered, and the morbidity and mortality rates are reduced. A new approach, laparoscopic adrenalectomy, may reduce the incidence of some postoperative complications.

POSTOPERATIVE CARE. After an adrenalectomy, the client is usually sent to a critical care unit. In the immediate postoperative period, the nurse assesses the client every 15 minutes to identify symptoms of cardiovascular collapse or shock (e.g., hypotension, a rapid, weak pulse, and a decreasing urine output) due to possible insufficient glucocorticoid replacement. The nurse monitors ongoing vital signs and other hemodynamic variables (central venous pressure, pulmonary wedge pressure), intake and output, daily weights, and serum electrolyte levels.

After a bilateral adrenalectomy, clients require lifelong glucocorticoid and mineralocorticoid replacement. The nurse administers glucocorticoid preparations as ordered. In unilateral adrenalectomy, glucocorticoid replacement continues until the remaining gland increases hormone production. This therapy may be required for up to 2 years after surgery.

PREVENTING COMPLICATIONS. The client who has hypercortisolism is prone to injury from skin breakdown, pathologic bone fractures, and gastrointestinal (GI) bleeding. Prevention of such injuries is a major nursing care focus.

Skin Breakdown. The nurse assesses the client's skin to detect reddened areas, excoriation, breakdown, and edema. If mobility is decreased, the client is turned frequently and bony prominences are padded to prevent skin breakdown.

The nurse instructs the client to avoid activities that can result in skin trauma. To minimize tissue injury, the client may use a soft toothbrush and electric razor. Proper hygiene is important, and clients are instructed to keep the skin clean and to dry it thoroughly after washing. Excessive dryness can be prevented by using a moisturizing lotion.

Adhesive tape frequently causes breakdown of the skin. This tape is used sparingly, and extreme caution is used when removing it. After venipuncture or arterial puncture, the client may experience an increase in bleeding because of blood vessel fragility. Pressure over the site is exerted for longer than normal to prevent excessive bleeding and **ecchymosis** (bruising).

Pathologic Fractures. Hypercortisolism results in demineralization of bone, which, if it persists, may lead to osteoporosis. The nurse instructs the client about safety issues and dietary needs. The client with osteoporosis is susceptible to fractures as a result of accidental falls or bumps. When helping the client to move in bed, the nurse uses a lift sheet instead of grasping him or her. The nurse instructs the client to call for assistance when ambulating. The nurse also reviews the use of ambulatory aids (walkers or canes), if needed. Rooms should be kept free of extraneous objects that might cause a fall. When assisting with daily activities, the nurse prevents the client from bumping into hard objects.

A dietitian is consulted to counsel the client about diet therapy. A high-calorie diet is ordered that includes items from all of the major food groups and increased amounts of calcium and vitamin D. Generous amounts of milk, cheese, yogurt, and green leafy and root vegetables add considerable amounts of calcium to the diet. The client is advised to avoid substances containing caffeine and alcohol.

Gastrointestinal Bleeding. Interventions are aimed at minimizing gastric irritation, usually through drug therapy. Drug therapy involves two different types of agents: those that protect the GI mucosa and those that decrease the secretion of hydrochloric acid.

Agents Protecting the Gastrointestinal Mucosa. Antacids are prescribed to buffer stomach acids and to protect the GI mucosa. The nurse teaches the client that these drugs should be taken on a regular schedule, rather than on a prn (asneeded) basis.

Agents Inhibiting the Secretion of Hydrochloric Acid. The most effective agents are those that block the H_2-receptor site in the gastric mucosa. When histamine binds to this receptor site, a series of membrane actions occur that result in the release of hydrochloric acid. Drugs that block the H_2-receptor site include cimetidine (Tagamet, Peptol✱, Novo-Cimetine✱), ranitidine (Zantac, Apo-Ranitidine✱), famotidine (Pepcid), and nizatidine (Axid). Omeprazole (Losec✱, Prilosec) inhibits the gastric proton pump and prevents the formation of hydrochloric acid.

Prevention of Irritation. The client is encouraged to reduce or eliminate habits that contribute to gastric irritation, such as consuming alcohol or caffeine, smoking, and fasting. The nurse discusses other prescribed and over-the-counter medications that the client may be taking. Nonsteroidal anti-inflammatory drugs (NSAIDs) and drugs that contain aspirin or other salicylates can cause gastritis and intensify any bleeding episode.

HEALTH TEACHING. Lifelong hormone replacement is required after bilateral adrenalectomy. The nurse educates the client and family members about compliance with the medication regimen and its side effects. Wearing a medical alert bracelet is essential. Education of clients after bilateral adrenalectomy and hypophysectomy is the same as that for those who have undergone cortisol replacement (Chart 63-12).

CHART 63-12

CLIENT EDUCATION GUIDE
Cortisol Replacement Therapy

- Take your medication in divided doses, the first dose in the morning and the second dose between 4 and 6 PM.
- Take your medication with meals or snacks.
- Weigh yourself daily.
- Increase your dosage as directed for increased physical stress or severe emotional stress, including surgery, dental work, influenza, fever, pregnancy, and family problems.
- Never skip a dose of medication. If you have persistent vomiting or severe diarrhea and cannot take your medication by mouth for 24 to 36 hours, call your physician. If you cannot reach your physician, go to the nearest emergency department. You may need an injection to take the place of your usual oral medication.
- Always wear your medical alert bracelet or necklace.
- Make regular visits for health care follow-up.
- Learn how to give yourself an intramuscular injection of hydrocortisone.

CRITICAL THINKING CHALLENGE

The client is a 76-year-old woman who has been taking 25 mg of prednisone daily for 2 years to treat a chronic inflammatory lung disease. She is now in an extended care facility recovering from a hip-pinning procedure following a fracture. The staff does not like working with her, because she claims she is hungry all the time and she has frequent spells of shouting at people that are intermixed with periods of weeping. She has many bruises, and her family is asking whether she is being physically abused.

- How should you approach the assistive nursing personnel about this "problem" client?
- What will you tell the family about the bruising?
- What interventions can you institute to reduce this client's risk for injury?
- How can her appetite be managed?

For suggested answer guidelines, go to ⓢⒾⓂⓄⓃ http://www.wbsaunders.com/SIMON/Iggy/.

Hyperaldosteronism

▮ OVERVIEW

In clients with hyperaldosteronism, increased secretion of aldosterone results in mineralocorticoid excess. **Primary hyperaldosteronism (Conn's syndrome)** is due to excessive secretion of aldosterone from one or both adrenal glands, which is most commonly caused by an adenoma. In a person with **secondary hyperaldosteronism,** the continuous excessive secretion of aldosterone is caused by high levels of angiotensin II that are due to high plasma renin activity. Causes of this renin activation include renal hypoxemia and the use of thiazide diuretics.

Increased aldosterone levels affect the renal tubules and cause sodium retention with potassium and hydrogen ion excretion. Hypernatremia, hypokalemia, and metabolic alkalosis result. Sodium retention increases blood and interstitial fluid volume, which elevates blood pressure and suppresses renin production. The elevated blood pressure may cause strokes and renal damage. Peripheral edema rarely occurs because of the "renal escape mechanism," in which the proximal tubule decreases sodium reabsorption. However, no compensatory mechanism exists to stop or reverse the loss of potassium. (See Chapter 13 for further discussion of electrolyte imbalances.)

Hyperaldosteronism occurs three times more frequently in women than in men and is most prevalent in clients between 30 and 60 years of age.

► COLLABORATIVE MANAGEMENT

● Assessment

Symptoms related to hypokalemia and elevated blood pressure are the most common problems of the client with hyperaldosteronism. The history may reveal nonspecific findings, such as headache, fatigue, muscle weakness, **nocturia** (excessive urination at night), and loss of stamina. **Polydipsia** (excessive fluid intake) and **polyuria** (excessive urine output) occur less frequently. **Paresthesias** (sensations of numbness and tingling) may occur if potassium depletion is severe. The client may have visual changes related to hypertension.

The diagnosis of primary hyperaldosteronism is made on the basis of laboratory studies and x-ray findings. Serum potassium levels are decreased, and sodium levels are elevated. Plasma renin levels are low; aldosterone levels are elevated. Increased hydrogen ion secretion results in metabolic alkalemia (elevated blood pH). Urine studies show low specific gravity and elevated aldosterone levels. Computed tomography (CT) scans reveal the presence and location of adrenal adenomas.

● Interventions

Surgery is the treatment of choice for hyperaldosteronism if the problem is identified in its early stages. Adrenalectomy may be unilateral or bilateral. Surgery is not performed, however, until the client's potassium levels are normal. The physician orders spironolactone (Aldactone, Novospiroton✦, Sincomen✦), a potassium-sparing diuretic and aldosterone antagonist, to promote fluid balance. Potassium supplements may be ordered to increase potassium levels before surgery. The client may also benefit from a low-sodium preoperative diet, but no dietary restrictions are needed after surgery because aldosterone levels should return to normal.

The client who has undergone a unilateral adrenalectomy may require temporary glucocorticoid replacement, and the client who has undergone a bilateral adrenalectomy needs lifelong replacement. Glucocorticoids are administered before surgery to prevent adrenal hypofunction. The client receiving long-term replacement therapy should wear a medical alert bracelet. (See the discussion of adrenalectomy under Hypercortisolism [Cushing's syndrome], pp. 1418 and 1419, for further postoperative care and client education.)

When surgery is inadvisable, spironolactone therapy is continued to control the symptoms of hypokalemia and hypertension. Because spironolactone is a potassium-sparing diuretic, hyperkalemia can occur in clients who have impaired renal function or excessive potassium intake. The nurse advises the client to avoid potassium supplements and foods rich in potassium (see Chart 13-6). Because hyponatremia can occur with spironolactone therapy, the client may require increased dietary sodium. He or she is instructed to report symptoms of hyponatremia, such as dryness of the mouth,

thirst, lethargy, or drowsiness. The nurse alerts clients to report any additional side effects of spironolactone therapy, including gynecomastia, diarrhea, drowsiness, headache, rash, **urticaria** (hives), confusion, inability to maintain an erection, hirsutism, and amenorrhea.

Pheochromocytoma

■ OVERVIEW

Pheochromocytoma is a catecholamine-producing tumor that arises in chromaffin cells. Pheochromocytomas usually occur as single, unilateral tumors on the right side; approximately 10% are bilateral tumors, and another 10% are found in the abdomen. Pheochromocytomas are most often benign, but about 10% are malignant. The tumors produce and store catecholamines.

Pheochromocytomas release the catecholamines epinephrine and norepinephrine (NE). Excessive epinephrine and NE stimulate alpha receptors and beta receptors and can have wide-ranging adverse effects mimicking stimulation of the sympathetic division of the autonomic nervous system.

Causes are unknown, but some are associated with inherited disorders such as neurofibromatosis and multiple endocrine neoplasia type II syndrome. Pheochromocytomas are rare and occur slightly more frequently in women. The tumors can occur at any age but appear most commonly in clients between 40 and 60 years of age.

► COLLABORATIVE MANAGEMENT

● Assessment

The history may include intermittent hypertensive episodes or attacks that vary in length from a few minutes to several hours. During these episodes, the client experiences severe headaches, palpitations, profuse diaphoresis, flushing, apprehension, or a feeling of impending doom. Pain in the chest or abdomen, with nausea and vomiting, can also occur. Certain stimuli, such as increased abdominal pressure, urination, and vigorous abdominal palpation, can provoke a hypertensive crisis. The client may also report heat intolerance, weight loss, and tremors.

Diagnostic tests include 24-hour urine collections for vanillylmandelic acid (VMA) (a product of catecholamine metabolism), metanephrine, and free catecholamines, all of which are elevated in the presence of a pheochromocytoma. Best practices for VMA testing are listed in Chart 63-13. Basal plasma catecholamine levels are elevated after the client has been at rest for at least 30 minutes. The clonidine suppression test is used in the diagnosis of a pheochromocytoma. When oral clonidine hydrochloride (Catapres, Dixarit✦) is given to a person who does not have a pheochromocytoma, the clonidine suppresses catecholamine release and reduces the serum catecholamine levels. The response is not seen in the client who has a pheochromocytoma.

When the client suspected of having a pheochromocytoma has severe hypertension, testing for the disorder may include alpha-adrenergic blockade with phentolamine. Phentolamine (Regitine, Rogitine✦) is administered intravenously at a dose of 5 mg, and blood pressure is measured every 30 seconds for 3 minutes, then every minute for 7 minutes. When a rapid drop of at least 35 mm Hg systolic pressure and 25 mm Hg diastolic pressure results, the test is considered positive.

CHART 63-13

BEST PRACTICE *for*
Vanillylmandelic Acid Testing

- Describe the test to the client and explain that his or her participation is needed for accurate test results.
- Instruct the client on the special vanillylmandelic acid (VMA)–restricted diet that starts 2 or 3 days before the 24-hour urine collection.
- Restricted foods include those containing caffeine (coffee, tea, cola, and chocolate or cocoa), certain fruits (citrus fruits and bananas), vanilla-containing foods, and licorice. Check your laboratory for a more inclusive food list.
- Confer with the physician about which medications should not be given during the 3- or 4-day test. Medications usually withheld include aspirin and antihypertensive agents.
- Be aware that strenuous physical activity, stress, and starvation can increase VMA levels; monitor, intervene, and teach the client as appropriate.
- Instruct the client about how to collect an accurate 24-hour urine sample: the collection is started with an empty bladder, and then all urine formed over the next 24 hours is collected in one container. At the end of the 24-hour period, the client voids and adds that urine to the collection.
- Obtain a urine collection container with preservative from the laboratory. Check with the laboratory about keeping the collection on ice.
- When the collection is complete, send the urine to the laboratory promptly.
- Help the client understand the test results; normal VMA excretion in 24 hours is 2 to 7 mg, or 10 to 35 μmol.

Catecholamine stimulation tests can be useful in the diagnosis of a pheochromocytoma; however, the danger of uncontrolled hypertension and effects on the heart limit the usefulness of this test. These tests involve the administration of histamine, glucagon, or tyramine to stimulate catecholamine release. Blood and urine catecholamine levels are measured. Catecholamine stimulation of **glycogenolysis** (breakdown of glycogen) and suppression of insulin may cause **hyperglycemia** (elevated blood glucose levels) and **glycosuria** (presence of glucose in the urine).

After diagnosis, computed tomography (CT) scans of the adrenal glands locate intra-adrenal tumors. Chest x-ray films and tomograms can locate tumors in the thoracic area; arteriograms can locate intra-abdominal tumors.

Interventions

Surgery is the treatment of choice for a pheochromocytoma. One or both adrenal glands are removed (depending on whether the tumor is bilateral). Preoperatively, the nurse focuses on adequate tissue perfusion, nutritional needs, and comfort measures.

Hypertension is the hallmark of the disease. The nurse monitors the blood pressure regularly and places the cuff consistently on the same arm, with the client in lying and standing positions. The nurse also identifies stressors that may precede a hypertensive crisis and attempts to minimize them. The client is instructed not to smoke, drink caffeine-containing beverages, or change position suddenly. The abdomen *should not be palpated.* A diet rich in calories, vitamins, and minerals is provided.

The client often benefits from preoperative hydration therapy because inadequate blood volume increases the risk for

intraoperative and postoperative hypotension. The nurse assesses the client's hydration status and notes symptoms of dehydration or fluid overload.

A calm, restful environment is provided because the client with a pheochromocytoma may experience incapacitating headaches. The client is instructed to limit activity. A private, darkened room helps to promote rest. If the client is sleeping, interruptions are avoided if possible.

The physician stabilizes the client with alpha-adrenergic blocking agents before surgery because of the increased risk for hypertension during surgery. Anesthetic agents and manipulation of the tumor during surgery can produce a release of catecholamines. The physician orders the short-acting alpha-adrenergic blocker phentolamine via IV bolus or drip for a hypertensive crisis. Oral phenoxybenzamine hydrochloride (Dibenzyline) produces long-acting alpha-adrenergic blockade and is used most frequently for preoperative management of hypertension and prevention of hypertensive crisis. It is also a drug of choice for long-term management of the client who is not a candidate for surgery.

The physician adjusts drug dosages for 2 to 3 weeks before surgery until blood pressure is controlled and no further hypertensive attacks occur. The blood volume expands, and blood pressure with the client in the supine position returns to normal.

The physician avoids using beta-adrenergic blocking agents in clients with a suspected or confirmed pheochromocytoma until after alpha-adrenergic blockade has been initiated, because these drugs may cause blood pressure to rise. After alpha-adrenergic blockade, low doses of propranolol hydrochloride (Inderal, Detensol✦) may be used to treat tachycardia and dysrhythmias.

Postoperative nursing care is similar to that for the client who has undergone an adrenalectomy (see Hypercortisolism [Cushing's Syndrome], pp. 1418 and 1419). The nurse closely monitors the client for hypotension related to the sudden decrease in catecholamine level and for hypovolemia, especially when the client was inadequately prepared for surgery. Hemorrhage and shock are possible, and the nurse administers plasma expanders and fluids as prescribed. Vital signs, as well as fluid intake and output, are monitored. If opioids are administered, the nurse observes their effect on blood pressure.

Tumors may be inoperable because of the client's other medical conditions. Treatment in these cases is medical, with alpha-adrenergic and beta-adrenergic blocking agents, because these tumors do not respond well to chemotherapy or radiation therapy. For clients who are medically managed, self-measurement of blood pressure with home monitoring equipment is essential.

ONLINE RESOURCES

For suggested readings and Internet resources, go to http://www.wbsaunders.com/SIMON/Iggy/.

SELECTED BIBLIOGRAPHY

Ahern-Gould, K., & Stark, J. (1998). Quick resource for electrolyte imbalance. *Critical Care Nursing Clinics of North America, 10*(4), 477-490.

Carson, P. (2000). Emergency: Adrenal crisis. *American Journal of Nursing, 100*(7), 49-50.

Castiglione, V. (2000). Emergency: Hyperkalemia. *American Journal of Nursing, 100*(1), 55-56.

Chmielewski, C. (1998). Hyperkalemic emergencies: Mechanisms, manifestations, and management. *Critical Care Clinics of North America, 10*(4), 449-457.

Clayton, L., & Dilley, K. (1998). Cushing's syndrome. *American Journal of Nursing, 98*(7), 40-41.

Cotran, RS., Kumar, V., & Collins, T. (1999). *Robbins' pathologic basis of disease* (6th ed.). Philadelphia: W.B. Saunders.

Eisenberg, A., & Redick, E. (1999). Caring for a patient after resection of pituitary adenoma. *Nursing99, 29*(12), 32cc1-32cc2, 32cc4-32cc6.

Ezzone, S. (1999). Clinical focus: SIADH. *Clinical Journal of Oncology Nursing, 3*(4), 187-188.

Fabius, D. (1998). How to recognize electrolyte imbalances on an ECG. *Nursing98, 28*(2), 32hn1-32hn6.

Goldberg, M. (2000). The diagnostic challenge—Hyperaldosteronism caused by bilateral adrenal hyperplasia. *Emergency Medicine, 32*(3), 55-56.

Guyton, A.C., & Hall, J.E. (2000). *Textbook of medical physiology* (10th ed.). Philadelphia: W.B. Saunders.

Heater, D. (1999a). If ADH goes out of balance: Diabetes insipidus. *RN, 62*(7), 44-46.

Heater, D. (1999b). If ADH goes out of balance: SIADH. *RN, 62*(7), 47-49.

Kearney, K. (2000). Emergency: Adrenal crisis. *American Journal of Nursing, 100*(7), 49-50.

Luken, K. (1999). Clinical manifestations and management of Addison's disease. *Journal of the American Academy of Nurse Practitioners, 11*(4), 151-154.

McCloskey, J.C, & Bulechek, G.M (2000). *Nursing interventions classification (NIC)* (3rd ed.). St. Louis: Mosby.

Nayback, A. (2000). Hyponatremia as a consequence of acute adrenal insufficiency and hypothyroidism. *Journal of Emergency Nursing, 26*(2), 130-133.

O'Donnell, M. (1997). Addisonian crisis. *American Journal of Nursing, 97*(3), 41.

Orth, D., & Kovacs, W. (1998). The adrenal cortex. In J.D. Wilson et al. (Eds.), *Williams textbook of endocrinology* (9th ed., pp. 517-664). Philadelphia: W.B. Saunders.

Reeves, W.B., Bichet, D., & Andreoli, T. (1998). Posterior pituitary and water metabolism. In J.D. Wilson et al. (Eds.), *Williams textbook of endocrinology* (9th ed., pp. 341-387). Philadelphia: W.B. Saunders.

Reincke, M. (2000). Subclinical Cushing's syndrome. *Endocrinology and Metabolism Clinics of North America, 29*(1), 43-56.

Thorner, M., et al. (1998). The anterior pituitary. In J.D. Wilson et al. (Eds.), *Williams textbook of endocrinology* (9th ed., pp. 249-340). Philadelphia: W.B. Saunders.

United States Pharmacopeia Dispensing Information (USP DI): Vol. I. Drug information for the health care professional. (20th ed.). (2000). Englewood, CO: Micromedix.

64

Interventions for Clients with Problems of the Thyroid and Parathyroid Glands

M. LINDA WORKMAN

Learning Objectives

After studying this chapter, you should be able to:

1. Compare and contrast the common clinical manifestations associated with hyperthyroidism and hypothyroidism.
2. Explain the pathophysiology of Graves' disease.
3. Use clinical changes and laboratory data to determine the effectiveness of interventions for hyperthyroidism.
4. Prioritize nursing care for the client during the first 24 hours following a total thyroidectomy.
5. Explain the pathophysiology of Hashimoto's thyroiditis.
6. Identify teaching priorities for the client taking thyroid hormone replacement therapy.
7. Use clinical changes and laboratory data to determine the effectiveness of interventions for hypothyroidism.
8. Compare and contrast the clinical manifestations associated with hyperparathyroidism and hypoparathyroidism.
9. Prioritize nursing care for the client during the first 24 hours following a parathyroidectomy.
10. Use clinical changes and laboratory data to determine the effectiveness of interventions for parathyroid problems.

Go to http://www.wbsaunders.com/SIMON/Iggy/ for self-assessment questions related to these Learning Objectives.

Hormones from the thyroid and parathyroid glands affect general metabolism, electrolyte balance, and excitable membrane activity. Therefore a disturbance in either thyroid or parathyroid function usually has widespread clinical manifestations. With mild disturbances, the problems are subtle. With more severe disturbances, the problems may be life threatening.

THYROID DISORDERS

Hyperthyroidism

OVERVIEW

Excessive thyroid hormone secretion results in **hyperthyroidism.** The clinical manifestations of hyperthyroidism are referred to as **thyrotoxicosis.** Thyroid hormones affect all metabolic processes in all body organs and therefore produce numerous and varied clinical manifestations. Hyperthyroidism can be temporary or permanent depending on the cause.

Pathophysiology

In hyperthyroidism, the normal feedback control over thyroid hormone secretion fails. Because thyroid hormones stimulate most body systems, excessive thyroid hormones produce a state of **hypermetabolism** with increased sympathetic nervous system activity. Many of the clinical manifestations of hyperthyroidism are caused by the body's response to the demands of hypermetabolism (Chart 64-1).

Thyroid hormones directly stimulate the heart. The increased heart rate and stroke volume in hyperthyroidism cause an increase in cardiac output and peripheral blood flow. This excessive or **hyperdynamic** circulatory state results from an increase in the number of adrenergic receptors on the heart muscle.

Elevated levels of thyroid hormones affect protein, carbohydrate, and lipid metabolism. Protein **synthesis** (buildup) and **degradation** (breakdown) are increased. Breakdown exceeds buildup, causing a net loss of protein known as a **negative nitrogen balance.** Glucose tolerance is decreased, and

---

CHART 64-1

KEY FEATURES *of*
Hyperthyroidism

Integumentary Manifestations
- Diaphoresis (excessive sweating)
- Fine, soft, silky hair (body)
- Smooth, warm, moist skin
- Thinning of scalp hair

Pulmonary Manifestations
- Shortness of breath with or without exertion

Cardiovascular Manifestations
- Palpitations
- Chest pain
- Increased systolic blood pressure
- Widened pulse pressure
- Tachycardia
- Dysrhythmias

Gastrointestinal Manifestations
- Weight loss
- Increased appetite
- Diarrhea

Musculoskeletal Manifestations
- Muscle weakness

Neurologic Manifestations
- Blurred or double vision
- Eye fatigue
- Corneal ulcers or infections
- Increased tears
- Injected (red) conjunctiva
- Photophobia
- Eyelid retraction, eyelid lag*
- Globe lag*
- Hyperactive deep tendon reflexes
- Tremors
- Insomnia

Metabolic Manifestations
- Increased basal metabolic rate
- Heat intolerance
- Low-grade fever

Psychologic/Emotional Manifestations
- Decreased attention span
- Restlessness
- Irritability
- Emotional lability
- Manic behavior

Reproductive Manifestations
- Amenorrhea
- Decreased menstrual flow
- Increased libido

Other Manifestations
- Goiter
- Wide-eyed (startled) appearance*
- Weakness, fatigue

*Present in Graves' disease only

TABLE 64-1 • CAUSES OF HYPERTHYROIDISM

Cause	Mechanism
Graves' disease (toxic diffuse goiter)	Autoimmune in nature. Antibodies (TSHAb) bind to TSH receptors and keep them activated, increasing the size of the gland and increasing the production of thyroid hormones.
Toxic multinodular goiter	Multiple thyroid nodules, resulting in thyroid hyperfunction.
Thyroid adenoma	Independent and inappropriate functioning of adenoma of follicular cells.
Pituitary hyperthyroidism	Pituitary adenoma resulting in excessive TSH secretion.
Thyroiditis (radiation-induced)	T_3 and T_4 secretion increased before destruction of gland. Hyperthyroid state usually transient.
T_3 thyrotoxicosis	Increase in thyroid secretion of T_3. Cause unknown.
Factitious hyperthyroidism	Ingestion of excessive amounts of thyroid hormone.
Jod-Basedow phenomenon (iodine induced)	Administration of iodine to an individual with endemic goiter, resulting in excessive production of thyroid hormone.
Struma ovarii	Dermoid tumor of the ovary that secretes thyroid hormone.
Thyroid carcinoma	Uncommon, usually occurs with large follicular carcinomas.
Trophoblastic tumors	Choriocarcinoma, hydatidiform mole, and embryonal carcinoma with high concentrations of chorionic gonadotropins that stimulate T_3 and T_4 secretion.

T_3, Triiodothyronine; T_4, thyroxine; *TSH,* thyroid-stimulating hormone.

---

the client has **hyperglycemia** (elevated blood glucose levels). Fat metabolism is increased, which results in decreased body fat stores. Although the client has an increased appetite, food intake does not meet energy demands, and the client loses weight. With prolonged hyperthyroidism, the client is in a state of chronic nutritional deficiency.

Thyroid hormones are produced in response to the stimulation hormones secreted by the hypothalamus and anterior pituitary glands. Thus oversecretion of thyroid hormones changes the secretion of hormones from the hypothalamus and anterior pituitary gland. In addition, thyroid hormones have some influence over sex hormone production in both men and women. If hyperthyroidism is present before puberty, sexual development is delayed. If hyperthyroidism develops after puberty, women experience menstrual irregularities and decreased fertility. Both

men and women with hyperthyroidism experience an increased **libido** (sexual urge or interest).

Etiology

The causes of hyperthyroidism are numerous (Table 64-1). The most common cause is **Graves' disease,** also called toxic diffuse goiter. The client with Graves' disease usually has hyperthyroidism, a **goiter** (enlargement of the thyroid gland), **exophthalmos** (abnormal protrusion of the eyes), and **pretibial myxedema** (dry, waxy swelling of the front surfaces of the lower legs). *Not all clients with a goiter have hyperthyroidism.*

Graves' disease is an autoimmune disorder in which antibodies (**immunoglobulins**) are made and attach to the thyroid stimulating hormone (TSH) receptor sites on the thyroid tissue. When these antibodies, known as thyroid-stimulating im-munoglobulins (TSIs), bind to the thyroid gland, the gland increases in size and overproduces thyroid hormones. In addition to the manifestations caused by hypermetabolism, the client with Graves' disease also has exophthalmos and pretibial edema.

Hyperthyroidism caused by multiple thyroid nodules is termed **toxic multinodular goiter.** Affected clients usually have had this goiter for years. The overproduction of thyroid hormone is usually milder than that seen in Graves' disease, and the client does not have exophthalmos or pretibial edema.

Hyperthyroidism also can be caused by overmedication with thyroid hormone (**exogenous hyperthyroidism**). Thyroid hormone has been abused by people trying to control weight or to increase their energy levels.

A condition called thyroid storm or thyroid crisis can occur when hyperthyroidism is untreated or poorly controlled or when the client is severely stressed. This condition is an extreme state of hyperthyroidism in which all clinical manifestations are more severe and life threatening.

Incidence/Prevalence

Hyperthyroidism is a common endocrine disorder. Graves' disease can occur at any age but is diagnosed most often in women between 20 and 40 years of age. Toxic multinodular goiter usually occurs after the age of 50 and affects women four times as often as men.

► COLLABORATIVE MANAGEMENT
● Assessment

▓ HISTORY

The client may have noticed many changes and problems, because hyperthyroidism can affect nearly all body systems. Age, gender, and usual weight are recorded. The client may report a recent weight loss and an increased appetite. Diarrhea is common.

A hallmark of hyperthyroidism is heat intolerance. The client may have **diaphoresis** (increased sweating) even when environmental temperatures are comfortable for others. The client often wears lighter clothing in cold weather. The client may also report palpitations or chest pain as a result of the cardiovascular effects. The nurse asks about changes in breathing patterns, because dyspnea (with or without exertion) is common.

Visual changes may be the earliest problem noted in the client with hyperthyroidism, especially ophthalmopathy with Graves' disease (Figure 64-1). The client is asked about changes in vision, such as blurring or double vision and tiring of the eyes.

The nurse inquires whether the client has noticed a change in energy level or his or her ability to perform activities of daily living (ADLs). Fatigue, weakness, and insomnia are common. Family and friends may report that the client has become more irritable or depressed.

Women are asked about changes in menses, because amenorrhea or a decreased menstrual flow is common. Initially, both men and women may experience an increase in libido.

The nurse explores the client's medical history. A history of thyroid surgery or radiation therapy to the neck is impor-

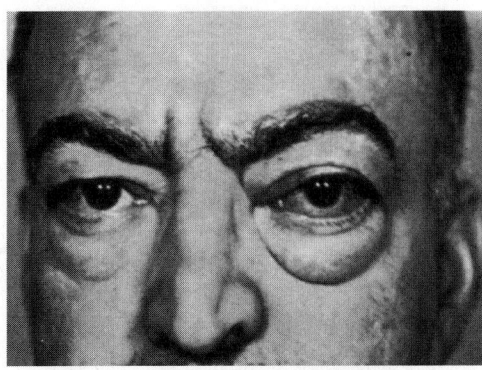

Figure 64-1 ● Ophthalmopathy. The client has proptosis.

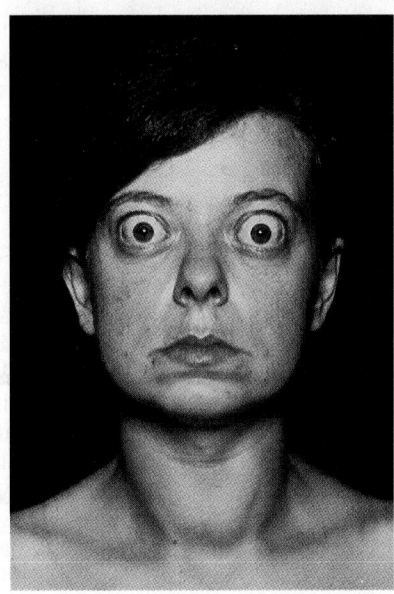

Figure 64-2 ● Exophthalmos. (From Seidel, H.M., et al. [1999]. *Mosby's guide to physical examination* [4th ed.]. St. Louis: Mosby.)

tant, because some people remain hyperthyroid after surgery or are resistant to radiation therapy. The client is asked about past and current medications, especially the use of thyroid hormone replacement or antithyroid drugs.

▓ PHYSICAL ASSESSMENT/CLINICAL MANIFESTATIONS

The nurse notes the client's general appearance. Two types of **ophthalmopathy** (abnormal eye appearance or function) are common with hyperthyroidism: eyelid retraction (eyelid lag) and globe (eyeball) lag. In eyelid lag, which occurs in all forms of thyrotoxicosis, the upper eyelid fails to descend when the client gazes slowly downward. In globe lag, the upper eyelid pulls back faster than the eyeball when the client gazes upward. During assessment, the client is asked to look down and then up, and the response is documented.

Infiltrative ophthalmopathy, which leads to exophthalmos, is common in clients with Graves' disease (Figure 64-2). The wide-eyed or "startled" look is due to edema in the extraocular muscles and increased fatty tissue behind the eye, which

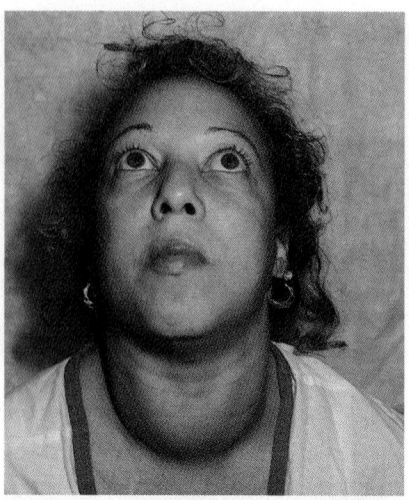

Figure 64-3 ● Goiter. (From Schwartz, M.H. [1998]. *Textbook of physical diagnosis: History and examination* [3rd ed.]. Philadelphia: W.B. Saunders.)

pushes the globe forward. Pressure on the optic nerve may impair vision. Swelling and shortening of the muscles may cause problems with focusing. If the eyelid fails to close completely and the eye is unprotected, the eye may become overdry and prone to corneal ulceration or infection. The nurse observes the client's eyes for excessive tearing and a bloodshot appearance and asks about sensitivity to light **(photophobia).**

The nurse palpates the thyroid gland to determine the presence of a mass or general enlargement, observing the size and symmetry of the gland. In goiter, a generalized thyroid enlargement in people with Graves' disease, the thyroid gland may increase to four times its normal size (Figure 64-3). **Bruits** (turbulence from increased blood flow) may be heard with a stethoscope. (See Chapter 62 for a full discussion of thyroid palpation and auscultation.)

The nurse inspects the client's hair and skin. Fine, soft, silky hair and smooth, moist skin are common with hyperthyroidism. The client may have extremity muscle weakness, hyperactive deep tendon reflexes, or tremors. Gross motor movements are observed for tremors, especially of the hands. Reflexes may be hyperactive. The client may appear extremely restless, irritable, and fatigued.

■ PSYCHOSOCIAL ASSESSMENT

The client with hyperthyroidism often experiences emotional **lability** (mood instability), irritability, decreased attention span, and manic behavior. Mild to severe hyperactivity often leads to a state of fatigue because of the inability to sleep well. The nurse asks the client whether he or she has been crying or laughing inappropriately or has had difficulty concentrating. The client's family members or significant other often report these changes in mental or emotional status.

■ LABORATORY ASSESSMENT

The diagnostic workup for hyperthyroidism includes measurement of the following serum values: triiodothyronine (T_3), thyroxine (T_4), T_3 resin uptake (T_3RU), and thyroid-stimulating hormone (TSH). Antibodies to TSH (TSHRAb) are measured to determine the presence of Graves' disease.

Laboratory findings in clients with hyperthyroidism are summarized in Chart 64-2.

■ OTHER DIAGNOSTIC ASSESSMENT

THYROID SCAN. The thyroid scan evaluates the position, size, and functioning of the thyroid gland. Radioactive iodine (RAI [^{123}I]) is given by mouth, and the uptake of iodine by the thyroid gland (RAIU) is measured. The half-life of ^{123}I is short, and radiation precautions are not necessary. Pregnancy, however, should be ruled out before the scan is performed.

Normally the thyroid has an uptake of 5% to 35% of the administered dose when measured at 24 hours. RAIU is increased in clients with hyperthyroidism. RAI not used by the thyroid is excreted by the kidney.

The nurse assesses whether the client has undergone procedures or has taken medications that might affect the results of the scan. Procedures that use iodine-containing dye (e.g., intravenous pyelogram [IVP]) should not be performed for at least 4 weeks before a thyroid scan. Any medication that contains iodine should be discontinued for 1 week before the scan.

ULTRASONOGRAPHY. Ultrasonography of the thyroid gland can be used to determine its size and the composition of any masses or nodules. This procedure takes approximately 30 minutes to perform, and the nurse reassures the client that it is painless.

ELECTROCARDIOGRAPHY. An electrocardiogram (ECG) usually shows tachycardia. Other ECG changes with hyperthyroidism include atrial fibrillation and alterations in P and T waveforms.

◎ CRITICAL THINKING CHALLENGE

The client is a 53-year-old woman who is brought to the emergency department after collapsing at her daughter's wedding rehearsal. She is 5' 8" tall and weighs 125 pounds. Her vital signs are as follows: blood pressure, 186/122; pulse, 104; respirations, 28. She has fine tremors of her hands.

The client is crying and yelling because the wedding rehearsal has been interrupted. Her daughter tells you that the client has not slept at all for the last three nights while finishing the dresses for the bridesmaids. The client insists that she is okay, only a little hungry after skipping lunch today. She says she has no health problems and is not being treated for any disorder. The health care team suspects hyperthyroidism and thyroid storm.

- What additional questions should you ask related to her weight?
- What diagnostic tests do you anticipate will be requested?
- What are your care priorities given the client's current clinical manifestations?
- The client insists that she must get back to the wedding rehearsal and threatens to leave immediately. How will you prevent her from leaving?

For suggested answer guidelines, go to SIMON, http://www.wbsaunders.com/SIMON/Iggy/.

● Interventions

Because Graves' disease is the most common form of hyperthyroidism, the interventions discussed in the following sections include those specific for the problems associated with Graves' disease as well as with other types of hyperthyroidism.

CHART 64-2

LABORATORY PROFILE
Thyroid Function

Test	Normal Range for Adults	Significance of Abnormal Findings	
		Hyperthyroidism	**Hypothyroidism**
Serum T_3	110-230 ng/dL, or 1.2-1.5 SI units	Increased	Decreased
Serum T_4	4.6-11 μg/dL, or 59-142 SI units	Increased	Decreased
Free T_4 index	0.8-2.8 ng/dL, or 10-30 SI units	Increased	Decreased
T_3 resin uptake	25%-35% (varies with different laboratories)	Increased	Decreased
TRH stimulation test	Doubling of baseline TSH 30 min after IV injection of 500 μg TRH (women have greater response)	Little or no TSH response	Delayed or poor TSH response in secondary hypothyroidism (pituitary failure) Elevated two or more times the normal in primary hypothyroidism (thyroid gland failure)
Thyroid suppression test	N/A	Fails to suppress RAIU or T_4 levels	No change in RAIU or T_4 levels
TSH stimulation test (thyroid stimulation test)	>10% in RAIU or >1.5 μg/dL	N/A (test differentiates primary from secondary hypothyroidism)	No response in primary hypothyroidism Normal response in secondary hypothyroidism
Thyroid antibodies (antithyroglobulin antibody)	Titer <1:100	High titer of antithyroglobulin antibodies	Increased titers
Thyrotropin receptor antibodies (TSH-RAb)	Titer <130% of basal activity	High titers indicate Graves' disease	No response

TSH, thyroid-stimulating hormone; *RAIU*, radioactive iodine uptake; *N/A*, not applicable; *T₃*, triiodothyronine; *T₄*, thyroxine; *TRH*, thyrotropin-releasing hormone, *SI*, System Internationale.

The cardiac problems of hyperthyroidism include increased systolic blood pressure, a widened pulse pressure, tachycardia, and other dysrhythmias. The goals of nonsurgical management are to decrease the effect of thyroid hormone on cardiac function and to reduce thyroid hormone secretion. Surgery may be necessary when nonsurgical interventions are unsuccessful.

NONSURGICAL MANAGEMENT. The nurse monitors the client's apical pulse, blood pressure, and temperature at least every 4 hours. The client is instructed to report any palpitations, dyspnea, vertigo, or chest pain immediately.

The nurse and other assistive nursing personnel minimize the client's discomfort from the clinical effects of hyperthyroidism. Fatigue is common, and the client is encouraged to rest. The environment is kept as quiet as possible. Frequent bed linen changes, sponge baths, and a cool environment decrease discomfort caused by diaphoresis and heat intolerance.

DRUG THERAPY. The most commonly ordered antithyroid drugs are the thioamides, including propylthiouracil (PTU) and methimazole (Tapazole), which block thyroid hormone production (Chart 64-3). The response to these drugs is delayed because the client may have large amounts of thyroid hormone stored that continues to be released. Other drugs are needed to control the manifestations (especially cardiac) of hyperthyroidism until hormone production and release are reduced.

Iodine preparations decrease blood flow through the thyroid gland. This action reduces the production and release of thyroid hormone. Improvement usually occurs within 2 weeks, but weeks may be needed before metabolism returns to normal. This treatment can result in hypothyroidism, and the client must be closely monitored for the need for medication changes.

Lithium carbonate also inhibits thyroid hormone release. However, its use is limited because of certain side effects such as depression, nephrogenic diabetes insipidus, tremors, nausea, and vomiting. Lithium may be prescribed when a client cannot tolerate other antithyroid drugs.

Beta-adrenergic blocking drugs, such as propranolol (Inderal, Detensol✣) and atenolol (Tenormin), relieve diaphoresis, anxiety, tachycardia, and palpitations.

RADIOACTIVE IODINE THERAPY. *Radioactive iodine (RAI) therapy is contraindicated in pregnant women because* ^{131}*I crosses the placenta and can adversely affect the fetal thyroid gland.* The client with hyperthyroidism may receive RAI in the form of oral ^{131}I. The dosage depends on the thyroid gland's size and sensitivity to radiation. The thyroid gland picks up the RAI, and some of the cells that produce thyroid hormone are destroyed by the local radiation. Because the thyroid gland stores thyroid hormone to some degree, the client may not experience complete symptom relief until 6 to 8 weeks after RAI therapy. The client usually needs drug therapy for hyperthyroidism during the first few weeks after RAI treatment.

RAI therapy usually involves one dose and can be performed on an outpatient basis. Occasionally a client needs a second or third dose. The radiation dose is usually low enough that radiation precautions are not required. The nurse reassures the client that the radioactivity is quickly eliminated. The de-

CHART 64-3

DRUG THERAPY *for* **Hyperthyroidism**

Drug	Usual Dosage	Nursing Interventions	Rationale
Propylthiouracil (PTU, Propyl-Thyracil♦)	100-150 mg tid PO	Give at 8-hr intervals around-the-clock	Spreading out dosage helps maintain suppression of hormone.
Methimazole (Tapazole)	5-15 mg tid PO	Monitor vital signs. Weigh the client weekly. Observe for sore throat, fever, headache, and skin eruptions.	Changes in vital signs or weight and appearance or other signs and symptoms may indicate adverse reactions, which may necessitate discontinuation of drug use.
Iodine products Strong iodine (Lugol's) solution Saturated solution of potassium iodide (SSKI) Potassium iodide tablets, solution, and syrup	Dosage varies, depending on the type of iodine prescribed, the manufacturer, and the form supplied (tablet, solution, or syrup)	Give in fruit juice or water. Observe for fever, rash, metallic taste, sore mouth, severe GI distress, and burning mouth and throat. Instruct the client to take tablets after meals.	Giving in fruit juice or water improves taste. Signs of iodism may necessitate discontinuation of drug use. Taking after meals enhances absorption.
Lithium carbonate (Lithobid, Carbolith♦, Lithizine♦)	Individualized 900-1200 mg/day PO in divided doses	Observe for signs of hypothyroidism. Instruct the client to drink 10-12 glassfuls of fluid a day Instruct the client to maintain normal sodium intake.	Signs of hypothyroidism may indicate drug-induced thyroid enlargement. Extra fluid intake helps to prevent dehydration. Reduced sodium intake can cause retention of the drug.
Propranolol (Inderal, Detensol♦) Atenolol (Tenormin)	20 mg/day qid in divided doses 25-50 mg PO qd	Weigh the client daily. Measure intake and output. Instruct the client to take the drug with food. Instruct the client to avoid smoking. Monitor the client's pulse.	Increased weight and decreased output may indicate congestive heart failure. Taking the drug with food enhances absorption. The drug's effect is reduced by smoking. Tachycardia is a sign of hyperthyroidism.

GI, Gastrointestinal.

gree of thyroid destruction is variable. Some clients become hypothyroid as a result of treatment. This complication may occur within a few weeks or may take several years to develop. The client then needs lifelong thyroid hormone replacement. All clients who have undergone RAI therapy should be monitored regularly for changes in thyroid function.

SURGICAL MANAGEMENT. Antithyroid drugs and RAI therapy are now the most common treatments for clients with hyperthyroidism. Surgery to remove all or part of the thyroid gland may be necessary for clients who have a large goiter causing tracheal or esophageal compression or who are unresponsive to antithyroid drugs. Removal of all (**total thyroidectomy**) or part (**subtotal thyroidectomy**) of the thyroid tissue decreases the production of thyroid hormones. Clients undergoing a total thyroidectomy must take lifelong thyroid hormone replacement. This surgery is also indicated in certain types of thyroid cancer.

PREOPERATIVE CARE. If possible, the client is treated with drug therapy first and experiences near-normal thyroid function (**euthyroid**) before thyroid surgery. The euthyroid state is achieved with antithyroid drugs that decrease the secretion of thyroid hormone. Iodine preparations are also used to decrease the size and vascularity of the gland, thereby re-

ducing the risk for hemorrhage and the potential for thyroid storm during surgery.

Cardiac problems of hypertension, dysrhythmias, and tachycardia must be controlled before surgery. The client with hyperthyroidism is often not at an optimal weight and may need to follow a high-protein, high-carbohydrate diet for days or weeks before surgery.

The nurse instructs the client to perform coughing and deep-breathing exercises. Teaching the client how to support the neck when coughing or moving is critical. Placing both hands behind the neck when moving reduces the strain on the suture line. The nurse explains that hoarseness may be present for a few days as a result of endotracheal tube placement during surgery.

Clients often fear thyroid surgery, perhaps because the incision is in the neck area. The nurse reassures the client by calmly explaining the surgery and postoperative care and by answering any questions the client and family may have.

OPERATIVE PROCEDURES. A thyroidectomy is performed with the client under general anesthesia. During surgery, the client's neck is extended and the surgeon makes a "collar" incision 1 to 2 cm above the clavicle. The surgeon identifies and avoids the parathyroid glands and recurrent laryngeal nerves to minimize complications and injury.

With a *subtotal thyroidectomy,* the remaining thyroid tissues are sutured to the trachea. With a *total thyroidectomy,* the surgeon leaves the parathyroid glands with an intact blood supply and removes the entire thyroid gland.

POSTOPERATIVE CARE. Vital signs are monitored every 15 minutes until the client is stable and are then monitored every 30 minutes. Monitoring of vital signs is increased or decreased depending on changes in the client's condition and on the physician's orders.

The nurse assesses the client's level of discomfort. Sandbags or pillows are used to support the head and neck. The client is placed in a semi-Fowler's position when awake. When positioning the client, the nurse decreases tension on the suture line by avoiding neck extension. Pain medications are administered as needed and as ordered.

Humidification of the air promotes easier respiration and thins respiratory secretions. The nurse assists the client in coughing and deep breathing every 30 minutes to 1 hour and also suctions oral and tracheal secretions when necessary.

Thyroid surgery can cause several complications, including hemorrhage, respiratory distress, parathyroid gland injury (resulting in **hypocalcemia** [low serum calcium levels] and **tetany** [hyperexcitability of nerves and muscles]), damage to the laryngeal nerves, and thyroid storm. The nurse is alert to the potential for complications and identifies manifestations early.

Hemorrhage. Hemorrhage is most likely to occur during the first 24 hours after surgery. After surgery, the nurse inspects the neck dressing and behind the client's neck for blood. A drain may be present with a moderate amount of serosanguineous drainage. Hemorrhage may also be seen as bleeding at the incision site or as respiratory distress caused by tracheal compression.

Respiratory Distress. Respiratory distress can also result from swelling or tetany. Laryngeal **stridor** (harsh, high-pitched respiratory sounds) is heard in acute respiratory obstruction. Emergency tracheostomy equipment is kept in the client's room. The nurse checks that oxygen and suctioning equipment are nearby and in working order. In some instances, nurses are instructed to remove clips or sutures when medical assistance is not immediately available.

Hypocalcemia and Tetany. The parathyroid glands can be damaged or their blood supply impaired during thyroid surgery. Hypocalcemia and tetany result when parathyroid hormone (PTH) levels decrease. The nurse assesses the client for symptoms of tingling around the mouth or of the toes and fingers and muscular twitching as signs of calcium deficiency. Calcium gluconate or calcium chloride for intravenous (IV) administration must be available in an emergency situation. (For information on the later signs of hypocalcemia, see Postoperative Care [Hyperparathyroidism], p. 1438, and Assessment [Hypoparathyroidism], p. 1438. The care of clients with hypocalcemia is discussed in Chapter 13.)

Laryngeal Nerve Damage. Hoarseness and a weak voice can result if the laryngeal nerve is injured during surgery. The nurse assesses the client's voice at 2-hour intervals and documents any changes. The client is reassured that hoarseness is usually temporary.

Thyroid Storm. Thyroid storm or **thyroid crisis** is a life-threatening event that occurs in clients with uncontrolled hyperthyroidism and is usually caused by Graves' disease. Signs and symptoms of crisis develop quickly. Thyroid storm is usu-

---

CHART 64-4

BEST PRACTICE *for*
Emergency Care of the Client During Thyroid Storm

- Maintain a patent airway and adequate ventilation.
- Give antithyroid drugs as ordered: propylthiouracil (PTU, Propyl-Thyracil✽), 300 to 900 mg/day; methimazole (Tapazole), up to 60 mg/day.
- Administer sodium iodide solution, 2 g/day IV as ordered.
- Give propranolol (Inderal, Detensol✽), 1 to 3 mg IV as ordered. Give slowly over 3 minutes; the client should be connected to a cardiac monitor, and a central venous pressure catheter should be in place.
- Give glucocorticoids as ordered: hydrocortisone, 100 to 500 mg/day IV; prednisone, 4 to 60 mg/day IV or IM.
- Monitor continually for cardiac dysrhythmias.
- Monitor vital signs every 30 minutes.
- Provide comfort measures, including a cooling blanket.
- Give nonsalicylate antipyretics as ordered.

---

ally triggered by a major stressor such as trauma or infection. Other conditions that can lead to thyroid storm include vigorous palpation of the goiter, exposure to iodine, and radioactive iodine (RAI) therapy. In the past, thyroid storm often occurred in the postoperative period when clients were not pretreated with antithyroid drugs and supportive drugs. Today postoperative thyroid storm is rare because clients receive antithyroid drugs, beta blockers, steroids, and iodides before thyroid surgery to prevent thyroid crisis.

The signs and symptoms of thyroid storm are caused by excessive thyroid hormone release that leads to a large increase in the metabolic rate. Symptoms include the following:

- Fever
- Tachycardia
- Systolic hypertension

The client may have gastrointestinal symptoms such as abdominal pain, nausea, vomiting, and diarrhea. Typically, the client with thyroid storm is agitated and anxious and has tremors. As the crisis progresses, he or she may become restless, confused, and psychotic and may have seizures, leading to coma. *Even with treatment, thyroid storm has a mortality rate of 25%.*

Emergency measures to prevent death vary with the intensity and type of specific symptoms. After the causative event has been identified, the following are primary concerns:

- Maintaining airway patency
- Providing adequate ventilation
- Stabilizing the hemodynamic status

Chart 64-4 outlines the best practices for the management of thyroid storm.

INFILTRATIVE OPHTHALMOPATHY. Treatment for hyperthyroidism does not affect the eye and vision problems of Graves' disease. Treatment of the client with infiltrative ophthalmopathy is symptomatic. The nurse instructs the client with mild symptoms to elevate the head of the bed at night and use an eye lubricant (artificial tears). If photophobia (sensitivity to light) is present, dark glasses or eye patches are often helpful. For the client who cannot close the eyelids completely, the nurse recommends gently taping the lids closed with nonallergic tape. These actions prevent irritation and injury. If pressure behind the eye continues and forces the eye forward, blood supply to the eye can be compromised, leading to ischemia and blindness. (See Chapter 46 for more discussion regarding eye protection.)

In severe cases the physician prescribes short-term steroid therapy to reduce swelling and halt the infiltrative process. Prednisone (Deltasone, Winpred✷) is often administered in high doses (often 120 mg/day) initially and then tapered down according to the client's response. The nurse explains the need to gradually reduce the prednisone and reviews its side effects with the client.

The physician may prescribe diuretics to decrease edema around the eye. Surgical intervention (orbital decompression) may be necessary if loss of sight or damage to the eyeball is possible.

HEALTH TEACHING. The signs and symptoms of hyperthyroidism are reviewed and the client is instructed to report an increase or recurrence of symptoms. The symptoms of hypothyroidism (discussed in the next section) and the need for thyroid hormone replacement are reviewed. The nurse reinforces the need for regular follow-up, because hypothyroidism can occur several years after radioactive iodine therapy.

If the client has had surgery, the surgeon usually removes the sutures on the third or fourth postoperative day. The client is instructed to inspect the incision area and to report redness, tenderness, drainage, or swelling to a member of the health care team.

The discharged client may continue to experience mood changes as a result of hyperthyroidism. The nurse explains the reason for emotional lability to the client and family and reassures them that it will decrease with continued treatment.

Hypothyroidism
■ OVERVIEW

The clinical manifestations of hypothyroidism (Chart 64-5) are the result of decreased metabolism from low levels of thyroid hormones. Hypothyroidism can occur at any time throughout the life span.

■ Pathophysiology

Thyroid cells may fail to produce sufficient levels of thyroid hormones for several reasons. Sometimes the cells themselves are damaged and no longer function normally. Other times the thyroid cells are functional but the person does not ingest enough of the substances needed to make thyroid hormones, especially iodide and tyrosine. When the production of thyroid hormones (THs) is too low or absent, the blood levels of TH are very low and the client has a decreased metabolic rate. This lowered metabolism causes the hypothalamus and anterior pituitary gland to make stimulatory hormones, especially thyroid-stimulating hormone (TSH), as compensation. The TSH binds to thyroid cells and causes the thyroid gland to enlarge, forming a **goiter.**

Most tissues and organs are affected by the low metabolic rate caused by hypothyroidism. Cellular energy production is decreased, and many metabolites build up. The metabolites are compounds of proteins and sugars called **glycosaminoglycans.** These compounds build up inside cells, which increases the mucous and water, forms cellular edema, and changes organ texture. The cellular edema is mucinous edema (called **myxedema**) rather than edema caused by water alone (Figure 64-4). This edema changes the appearance of the

---

CHART 64-5

KEY FEATURES *of*
Hypothyroidism

Integumentary Manifestations
- Cool, pale or yellowish, dry, coarse, scaly skin
- Thick, brittle nails
- Dry, coarse, brittle hair
- Decreased hair growth, with loss of eyebrow hair

Pulmonary Manifestations
- Hypoventilation
- Pleural effusion
- Dyspnea

Cardiovascular Manifestations
- Bradycardia
- Dysrhythmias
- Enlarged heart
- Decreased activity tolerance
- Hypotension

Metabolic Manifestations
- Decreased basal metabolic rate
- Decreased body temperature
- Cold intolerance

Musculoskeletal Manifestations
- Muscle aches and pains
- Delayed contraction and relaxation of muscles

Neurologic Manifestations
- Slowing of intellectual functions
  - Slowness or slurring of speech
  - Impaired memory
  - Inattentiveness
- Lethargy or somnolence
- Confusion
- Hearing loss
- Paresthesia (numbness and tingling) of the extremities
- Decreased tendon reflexes

Psychologic/Emotional Manifestations
- Apathy
- Agitation
- Depression
- Paranoia
- Withdrawal

Gastrointestinal Manifestations
- Anorexia
- Weight gain
- Constipation
- Abdominal distention

Reproductive Manifestations
Women
- Changes in menses (amenorrhea or prolonged menstrual periods)
- Infertility
- Anovulation
- Decreased libido

Men
- Decreased libido
- Impotence

Other Manifestations
- Periorbital edema
- Facial puffiness
- Facial coarseness
- Nonpitting edema of the hands and feet
- Hoarseness
- Goiter (enlarged thyroid gland)
- Thick tongue
- Increased sensitivity to opioids and tranquilizers
- Blank expression
- Weakness, fatigue
- Decreased urine output
- Anemia
- Easy bruising
- Iron deficiency
- Folate deficiency
- Vitamin B_{12} deficiency

client with full-blown hypothyroidism. Nonpitting edema forms everywhere and is especially evident around the eyes, in the hands and feet, and between the shoulder blades. These same compounds cause the tongue to thicken and edema to form in the larynx, making the voice more husky. It is likely that these metabolites build up in other tissues and organs, decreasing general physiologic function.

Myxedema coma is a rare but serious complication of untreated or inadequately treated hypothyroidism. The decrease in metabolism in cardiac tissue causes the heart muscle to become flabby and the chamber size to increase. The result is decreased cardiac output and decreased perfusion to the brain and other vital organs. The decreased perfusion makes the already slowed cellular metabolism worse, resulting in tissue and organ failure. *The mortality rate for myxedema coma is extremely high, and this condition is considered a life-threatening emergency.* Myxedema coma can be caused by a variety of events or conditions (Table 64-2).

Etiology

Most cases of hypothyroidism in the United States occur as a result of thyroid surgery and radioactive iodine (RAI) treatment of hyperthyroidism. Worldwide, hypothyroidism is common in areas where the soil and water have little natural iodide, causing **endemic goiter.** (This problem was common in the midwest region of the country before iodide was added to table salt and before fresh saltwater fish was widely available.) Hypothyroidism is also caused by a variety of other conditions and factors (Table 64-3).

Incidence/Prevalence

Hypothyroidism occurs most often in women between 30 and 60 years of age. Women are affected 7 to 10 times more often than men (Larsen, Davis, & Hay, 1998). A link between diabetes mellitus and the development of hypothyroidism has

been established. This link is supported by the finding of an increased incidence of hypothyroidism among minority populations at high risk for diabetes mellitus, such as Native Americans (see the Evidence-Based Practice for Nursing box on p. 1432).

► COLLABORATIVE MANAGEMENT

● Assessment

■ HISTORY

A decrease in thyroid hormone produces a variety of signs and symptoms related to decreased metabolic activity. The client often reports an increase in time spent sleeping, sometimes up to 14 to 16 hr/day. The client may also have generalized weakness, anorexia, muscle aches, and paresthesias. Constipation is common. The client often has cold intolerance, and the nurse asks if more blankets at night or sweaters and extra clothing in warm weather have been needed.

Both male and female clients may identify a decrease in libido. In addition, women with hypothyroidism may have had difficulty becoming pregnant or experienced changes in menses (heavy, prolonged bleeding or amenorrhea). Men can have problems with impotence and fertility.

TABLE 64-2 •	CONDITIONS OR EVENTS PRECIPITATING MYXEDEMA COMA

- Acute illness
- Anesthesia
- Surgery
- Hypothermia
- Chemotherapy
- Sedatives/opioids
- Rapid withdrawal of thyroid medications
- Untreated hypothyroidism
- Inadequately treated hypothyroidism

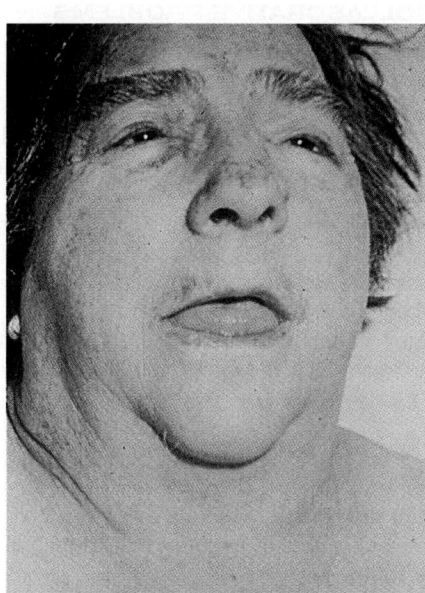

Figure 64-4 ● Myxedema. (From Seidel H.M., et al. [1999]. Mosby's guide to physical examination [4th ed.]. St. Louis: Mosby.)

TABLE 64-3 •	CAUSES OF HYPOTHYROIDISM

PRIMARY CAUSES
Decreased Thyroid Tissue
- Surgical removal of the thyroid
- Radiation-induced thyroid destruction
- Autoimmune thyroid destruction
- Congenital thyroid agenesis
- Congenital thyroid hypoplasia
- Congenital thyroid dysgenesis
- Cancer (thyroidal or metastatic)

Decreased Synthesis of Thyroid Hormone
- Endemic iodine deficiency
- Excessive exposure to iodine
- Medications
    Lithium
    Phenylbutazone
    Propylthiouracil
    Sodium or potassium perchlorate
    Aminoglutethimide

SECONDARY CAUSES
Inadequate Production of Thyroid-Stimulating Hormone
- Pituitary tumors, trauma, infections, or infarcts
- Congenital pituitary defects
- Hypothalamic tumors, trauma, infections, or infarcts

EVIDENCE-BASED PRACTICE
FOR NURSING

Native American diabetics more at risk for hypothyroidism

Michalek, A., Mahoney, M., & Calebaugh, D. (2000). Hypothyroidism and diabetes mellitus in an American Indian population, *Journal of Family Practice,* 49(7), 638-640.

A clinical relationship between the presence of diabetes mellitus and the development of hypothyroidism among the general population is beginning to be recognized, although the exact cause of this link is only speculated. Few minority populations have been examined for this phenomenon. During the past 30 years, the incidence and prevalence of both type I and type II diabetes mellitus among Native Americans has increased well beyond that of the general population. The incidence of hypothyroidism among this group is not known. The purpose of this study was to determine the incidence of hypothyroidism among members of a northeastern Native American nation who were also diabetic.

The researchers performed a chart review of 892 northeastern Native Americans living in an isolated area. All charts were from one clinic setting. Of the 892 charts reviewed, 156 clients were identified as having diabetes mellitus, and 25 of these clients also had hypothyroidism. Of particular interest was the fact that many more women than men had either or both of these disorders, especially women over the age of 60.

Critique. This descriptive survey included a large sample size, strengthening the validity of the findings. The retrospective nature of the design and the fact that data was obtained only from medical records clouds the issue of the true incidence and prevalence rates for either diabetes mellitus or hypothyroidism (many people with type II diabetes are unaware that they have the disease). It is likely that the actual incidence and prevalence for these disorders is even higher than the reported results. Nonetheless, the results of this study represent an important beginning for prevention and early detection strategies.

Implications for Nursing. When taking a history from any client, nurses need to obtain more specific racial/ethnic information to determine if a client has any degree of Native American heritage. Even more important, when a client is known to be Native American, the nurse needs to ask specific questions related to the clinical manifestations of both diabetes mellitus and hypothyroidism. The development of educational materials targeted to Native American populations regarding risk factors, early detection methods, and clinical manifestations can be a nursing priority.

The client is asked about his or her current or previous use of medications, such as lithium, aminoglutethimide, sodium or potassium perchlorate, thiocyanates, or cobalt. All of these drugs can impair the production of thyroid hormone. The client is asked whether he or she is taking any tranquilizers or opioids (hypothyroidism increases the sensitivity to these drugs as a result of decreased metabolism).

■ PHYSICAL ASSESSMENT/CLINICAL MANIFESTATIONS

The client's overall appearance is observed. Figure 64-4 shows the typical appearance of an adult with hypothyroidism. Common changes in appearance include coarse features, edema around the eyes and face, a blank expression, and a thick tongue. The client's overall muscle movement is slow.

■ PSYCHOSOCIAL ASSESSMENT

Hypothyroidism causes many problems in psychosocial functioning. Depression is the most common reason for seeking medical attention. Family members often bring the client for the initial evaluation. The client may be too lethargic, apathetic, or drowsy to recognize changes in his or her condition. Families may report that the client is withdrawn.

The nurse assesses the client's attention span and memory, both of which can be impaired by hypothyroidism. Paranoia and agitation may be additional findings.

■ LABORATORY ASSESSMENT

In general, laboratory findings for hypothyroidism are the opposite of those for hyperthyroidism. Triiodothyronine (T_3) and thyroxine (T_4) serum levels are decreased. TSH levels are elevated in primary hypothyroidism but can be decreased or near-normal in clients with secondary and tertiary hypothyroidism. More information is presented in Chart 64-2.

◎ CRITICAL THINKING CHALLENGE

The client is a 22-year-old college senior nursing student who has been brought to the student health service by her friends, who say she is not "acting right." This former straight-A student has been oversleeping and missing classes. Her grades have dropped to Bs and Cs. She has gained 40 pounds during the past semester and has not had a period for 5 months. Today she did not recognize her roommate's brother. She is not taking any prescribed or over-the-counter medications. She is wearing two sweaters and asking for a blanket even though the room is quite warm. The health care team suspects hypothyroidism.

- What assessment data should you obtain first?
- What comfort measures will you provide to this client?
- What questions will you ask the client, and what questions will you ask her friends?

For suggested answer guidelines, go to SIMON http://www.wbsaunders.com/SIMON/Iggy/.

● Analysis

■ COMMON NURSING DIAGNOSES AND COLLABORATIVE PROBLEMS

The following are common nursing diagnoses for clients with hypothyroidism:

1. **Decreased Cardiac Output** related to decreased stroke volume as a result of electrical or mechanical malfunction from bradycardia and arteriosclerotic coronary artery disease
2. **Ineffective Breathing Pattern** related to decreased energy, obesity, fatigue, and inactivity
3. **Disturbed Thought Processes** related to increased interstitial edema and water retention

The major collaborative problem is the Potential for Myxedema Coma.

■ ADDITIONAL NURSING DIAGNOSES AND COLLABORATIVE PROBLEMS

In addition to the common nursing diagnoses and collaborative problems, clients with hypothyroidism may have one or more of the following:

- **Imbalanced Nutrition: More than Body Requirements** related to decreased metabolic need
- **Hypothermia** related to decreased metabolic rate
- **Constipation** related to decreased gastrointestinal motility

- Impaired Physical Mobility related to fatigue, decreased strength and endurance, depression, obesity, and pain
- Disturbed Body Image related to changes in physical appearance
- Deficient Knowledge of condition, diagnosis, and treatment related to low energy level and fatigue

Additional collaborative problems for clients with hypothyroidism are Potential for Paralytic Ileus and Potential for Cardiomyopathy.

● Planning and Implementation

▦ DECREASED CARDIAC OUTPUT

NOC **PLANNING: EXPECTED OUTCOMES.** The client with hypothyroidism is expected to maintain normal cardiovascular function.

INTERVENTIONS. NIC interventions for the client with hypothyroidism are outlined in Chart 64-6. The client with hypothyroidism can have decreased blood pressure, bradycardia, and dysrhythmias. The nurse monitors blood pressure, heart rate, and rhythm and observes closely for signs of shock, such as hypotension, decreasing urine output, and mental status changes.

If hypothyroidism has been chronic, the client may have cardiovascular disease. The client is instructed to report episodes of chest pain or discomfort immediately.

The client with hypothyroidism requires lifelong thyroid hormone replacement. Synthetic hormone preparations are usually prescribed; the most common is levothyroxine sodium (Synthroid, T_4, Eltroxin✦). Therapy is started with low doses and gradually increased over a period of weeks. *The client with more severe symptoms of hypothyroidism is started on the lowest dose of thyroid hormone replacement.* This caution is especially important when the client has known cardiac problems. Starting at too high a dose or increasing the dose too rapidly can cause severe hypertension, heart failure, and myocardial infarction.

The nurse assesses the client for chest pain and dyspnea during initiation of therapy. The final dosage is determined by blood levels of TSH and the client's physical responses. The dosage and time required for symptom relief vary with each client. The nurse monitors for and teaches the client the signs and symptoms of hyperthyroidism, which can occur with replacement therapy.

▦ INEFFECTIVE BREATHING PATTERN

NOC **PLANNING: EXPECTED OUTCOMES.** The client with hypothyroidism is expected to have normal respiratory function as evidenced by respiratory rate and depth within normal limits (WNL) and pulse oximetry in expected range (IER).

INTERVENTIONS. The nurse observes and records the rate and depth of respirations. The lungs are auscultated for any abnormalities, such as a decrease in breath sounds. If hypothyroidism is severe, the client may have such severe respiratory distress that ventilatory support is required. Severe respiratory distress is usually associated with myxedema coma.

Sedating a client with hypothyroidism can make respiratory difficulties worse and is avoided, if possible. When a tranquilizer or sedative is needed, the dosage is reduced be-

CHART 64-6

NIC **INTERVENTION ACTIVITIES** *for*
The Client with Hypothyroidism

Respiratory Monitoring: *Collection and analysis of client data to ensure airway patency and adequate gas exchange*
- Monitor rate, rhythm, depth, and effort of respirations.
- Note chest movement, watching for symmetry.
- Monitor breathing patterns for bradypnea.
- Monitor for diaphragmatic muscle fatigue (paradoxical motion).
- Note changes in SaO_2 and SvO_2.
- Monitor client's ability to cough effectively.
- Monitor for dyspnea and events that improve and worsen it.

Shock Prevention: *Detecting and treating a client at risk for impending shock.*
- Monitor circulatory status: BP, skin color, skin temperature, heart sounds, heart rate and rhythm, presence and quality of peripheral pulses, and capillary refill.
- Monitor for signs of inadequate tissue oxygenation.
- Monitor for apprehension, increased anxiety, and changes in mental status.
- Monitor intake and output.
- Administer oxygen and/or mechanical ventilation, as appropriate.

Hypothermia Treatment: *Rewarming and surveillance of a client whose core body temperature is below 35° C.*
- Monitor client's temperature, using a low-recording thermometer if necessary.
- Place on a cardiac monitor, as appropriate.
- Cover with warmed blankets, as appropriate.
- Administer heated oxygen, as appropriate.
- Monitor vital signs, as appropriate.
- Monitor skin color and temperature.
- Monitor intake and output.
- Avoid giving IM or subcutaneous medications during the hypothermic state.
- Give client warm oral fluids, if alert and able to swallow.
- Teach client to consume a caloric intake sufficient to maintain a normal body temperature.
- Emphasize the importance of wearing warm, protective clothing when going into a cold environment.

NIC intervention activities selected from McCloskey, J.C., & Bulechek, G.M. (Eds.). (2000). *Nursing interventions classification (NIC)* (3rd ed.). St. Louis: Mosby. No part of this work is to be altered without prior written permission from the Publisher.
SaO_2, Arterial oxygen saturation; SvO_2, venous oxygen saturation.

cause hypothyroidism increases sensitivity to these drugs. The nurse assesses the client for signs of respiratory difficulty.

▦ ALTERED THOUGHT PROCESSES

PLANNING: EXPECTED OUTCOMES. The client with hypothyroidism is expected to have improved thought processes with correction of the hypothyroidism.

INTERVENTIONS. The nurse notes the presence and severity of symptoms, including lethargy, drowsiness, memory deficit, inattentiveness, and difficulty communicating. Symptoms should decrease with thyroid hormone treatment, and mental awareness usually returns to normal levels in adults within 2 weeks. The nurse orients the client to person, place, and time, explains all procedures slowly and carefully, and provides a safe environment.

Family members or significant others may have difficulty coping with the client's symptoms. The nurse encourages them to accept the mood changes and mental slowness as

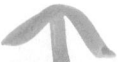

manifestations of the disease, which should improve with therapy.

MYXEDEMA COMA

Any client with hypothyroidism who has any other health problem or who is newly diagnosed is at risk for myxedema coma. Factors leading to myxedema coma are listed in Table 64-2. The following problems are associated with this condition:

- Coma
- Respiratory failure
- Hypotension
- Hyponatremia
- Hypothermia
- Hypoglycemia

Untreated myxedema coma leads to shock, organ damage, and death. The nurse assesses the client with hypothyroidism every shift for changes that indicate increasing severity of hypothyroid symptoms, especially changes in mental status.

The physician institutes treatment quickly according to the client's clinical presentation and history and without waiting for laboratory confirmation. Best practices for emergency care of the client with myxedema coma are outlined in Chart 64-7.

CONSIDERATIONS FOR OLDER ADULTS

Metabolic rate and thyroid hormone production decrease with advancing age, particularly among people older than 80 years (Chart 64-8). Until recently, however, data regarding normal levels of T_3 and T_4 were established only for adults between 20 and 30 years of age. By such criteria, older people with T_3 and T_4 levels 15% to 20% below the "normal levels" established for a younger population were considered to have hypothyroidism, and therapy with thyroid hormone was initiated. However, many of these clients were not truly hypothyroid, and therapy caused **pseudohyperthyroidism,** stressing many tissues and organs (Wallace & Hofmann, 1998). In addition, daily thyroid hormone therapy decreases the activity of the anterior pituitary gland and the thyroid gland, creating actual hypothyroidism. Health care providers need to assess more than just laboratory data to determine hypothyroidism in the older adult.

● Community-Based Care

Hypothyroidism is usually a chronic condition. Clients with hypothyroidism are managed on an outpatient basis and may reside in the home, in an assisted-living environment, or in a long-term care facility. Clients in acute care settings, subacute care settings, and rehabilitation centers may have long-standing hypothyroidism in addition to other acute or chronic health problems. The nurse needs to ensure that whoever is responsible for overseeing daily care is aware of the condition and understands its treatment.

HEALTH TEACHING

Most of the education needed by the client with hypothyroidism concerns hormone replacement therapy. The nurse emphasizes the need for lifelong medication and reviews the signs and symptoms of both hyperthyroidism and hypothyroidism. This information helps the client and family know when to seek medical interventions for dosage adjustment. All aspects of medication information are reviewed, including side effects. The client is instructed not to take any over-the-counter (OTC) medication because thyroid hormone preparations interact with many other drugs. The older adult client may need additional information about the effects of aging on the thyroid gland (see Chart 64-8).

The nurse advises the client to maintain a well-balanced diet with adequate fiber and fluid intake to prevent constipation. Excessive dietary fiber or fiber supplements may interfere with the absorption of thyroid hormone. The client is reminded of the importance of adequate rest periods before resuming a full schedule of daily activities. Family members are encouraged to voice their concerns to the health care provider.

The nurse discusses the necessity for follow-up care. All clients with hypothyroidism should wear a MedicAlert identification bracelet.

The time required for resolution of hypothyroidism symptoms varies; the nurse focuses on educating the family to be tolerant of any mental dullness or slowness in their loved one. Family members are instructed to orient the client frequently and to explain everything clearly and simply.

HOME CARE MANAGEMENT

The client with hypothyroidism does not usually require changes in the home unless cognition has decreased to the point that he or she poses a danger to self. Activity intolerance and fatigue may necessitate one-floor living for a short time. If symptoms have not cleared before discharge from the hospital, the nurse discusses the need for extra heat or clothing because of cold intolerance. The client who continues to have a decreased attention span may need assistance with the med-

---

CHART 64-7

BEST PRACTICE *for*
Emergency Care of the Client During Myxedema Coma

- Maintain a patent airway.
- Replace fluids as ordered.
- Give levothyroxine sodium IV as ordered.
- Administer glucose IV as ordered.
- Administer corticosteroids as ordered.
- Check the client's temperature frequently.
- Monitor blood pressure.
- Cover the client with warm blankets.
- Monitor for changes in mental status.

CHART 64-8

NURSING FOCUS *on the* **OLDER ADULT**
Thyroid Problems

Teach the client the following facts about changes in the thyroid gland related to aging:
- The thyroid gland decreases in size with increasing age.
- Thyroid hormone secretion decreases with age, but the hormone level remains stable because cellular clearance of the hormone also decreases with age.
- The basal metabolic rate decreases with age, usually as a result of decreased activity. This decrease changes the body composition from predominantly muscular to predominantly fatty.
- Older clients require lower doses of replacement thyroid hormone. Too large a dose may adversely affect the heart muscle.

ication regimen. The nurse discusses this issue with the family and client and develops a plan for medication administration. One person should be clearly designated as responsible for medication preparation and administration so that doses are neither missed nor duplicated.

■ HEALTH CARE RESOURCES

Immediately after returning home, the client may require a support person to stay and provide more attention than could be given by a visiting nurse or home care aide. Contact with the health care team is necessary for follow-up and identification of potential problems. The client taking thyroid medication may have symptoms of hypothyroidism if the dosage is inadequate or symptoms of hyperthyroidism if the dose is too high. The nurse performs a focused assessment at every home visit to the client under treatment for thyroid dysfunction (Chart 64-9).

CRITICAL THINKING CHALLENGE

The 22-year-old nursing student is started on oral levothyroxine (Synthroid). She tells you that she is scheduled to take the NCLEX exam in 10 days.

- What teaching priorities for her medication regimen will you establish?
- How will she be able to tell whether or not the medication is effective?
- Should she take the NCLEX as currently scheduled? Why or why not?

For suggested answer guidelines, go to SIMON http://www.wbsaunders.com/SIMON/Iggy/.

CHART 64-9

FOCUSED ASSESSMENT for
Home Care Clients with Thyroid Dysfunction

Assess cardiovascular status.
- Vital signs, including apical pulse, pulse pressure, presence or absence of orthostatic hypotension, and the quality and rhythm of peripheral pulses
- Presence or absence of peripheral edema
- Weight gain or loss

Assess cognition and mental status.
- Level of consciousness
- Orientation to time, place, and person
- Accurately reading a seven-word sentence containing no words greater than three syllables
- Can the client count backward from 100 by 3s?

Assess condition of skin and mucous membranes.
- Moistness of skin, most reliable on chest and back
- Skin temperature and color

Assess neuromuscular status.
- Reactivity of patellar and biceps reflexes
- Oral temperature
- Handgrip strength
- Steadiness of gait
- Presence or absence of fine tremors in the hand

Ask about the following:
- Sleep in the past 24 hours
- Client warm enough or too warm indoors
- 24-hour diet recall
- 24-hour activity recall
- Over-the-counter and prescribed medications taken
- Last bowel movement

Assess client's understanding of illness and compliance with treatment.
- Signs and symptoms to report to health care provider
- Medication plan (correct timing and dose)

● Evaluation: Outcomes

NOC The nurse evaluates the care of the client with hypothyroidism on the basis of the identified nursing diagnoses and collaborative problems. The expected outcome is that the client will:
- Maintain normal cardiovascular function
- Maintain adequate respiratory function as evidenced by respiratory rate and depth WNL and pulse oximetry IER
- Experience improvement in thought processes

Thyroiditis
■ OVERVIEW

Thyroiditis is an inflammation of the thyroid gland. There are three types: acute, subacute, and chronic. Chronic thyroiditis (Hashimoto's disease) is the most common type.

■ Acute Thyroiditis — *bacteria*

Acute thyroiditis, which is caused by bacterial invasion of the thyroid gland, is uncommon. Signs and symptoms include pain, neck tenderness, malaise, elevated temperature, and **dysphagia** (difficulty swallowing). This condition is treated symptomatically and usually responds to antibiotic therapy.

■ Subacute Thyroiditis *Viral*

Subacute or granulomatous thyroiditis results from a viral infection of the thyroid gland, occasionally after a cold or other upper respiratory tract infection. Manifestations include fever, chills, dysphagia, and muscle and joint pain. Pain can radiate to the ears and the jaw. The thyroid gland feels hard and moderately enlarged on palpation. Thyroid function can remain normal, although hyperthyroidism or hypothyroidism may develop.

The client with mild subacute thyroiditis is managed with rest, fluids, and acetylsalicylic acid (aspirin). In more severe cases, corticosteroids are given to reduce inflammation.

■ Chronic Thyroiditis *Auto Immune disorder*

Chronic thyroiditis (Hashimoto's disease) is a type of hypothyroidism that affects women more often than men, most commonly clients in their 30s to 50s. Hashimoto's disease is an autoimmune disorder. The thyroid becomes invaded with antithyroid antibodies and lymphocytes, causing thyroid tissue destruction. When large amounts of the gland are destroyed, serum thyroid hormone levels are low and secretion of thyroid-stimulating hormone is increased. *TH ↓ secretion TSH ↑*

▶ COLLABORATIVE MANAGEMENT

The clinical manifestations of Hashimoto's disease include dysphagia and painless enlargement of the gland. Diagnosis is based on the presence of circulating antithyroid antibodies and needle biopsy findings of the thyroid gland. Serum thyroid hormone levels, TSH levels, and radioactive iodine uptake (RAIU) vary depending on the stage of the disease.

The client is treated with thyroid hormone to prevent hypothyroidism and to suppress TSH secretion, thereby decreasing the size of the thyroid gland. Surgery (subtotal thyroidectomy) is necessary if the goiter does not respond to thyroid hormone, is disfiguring, or compresses other structures.

Nursing interventions focus on promoting client comfort and educating the client about hypothyroidism, medications, and surgery (see Surgical Management [Hyperthyroidism], p. 1428.)

Thyroid Cancer
OVERVIEW

There are four distinct types of thyroid cancer: papillary, follicular, medullary, and anaplastic. The initial clinical manifestation of thyroid cancer is a solitary, painless lump or nodule in the thyroid gland. Additional signs and symptoms depend on the presence and location of **metastasis** (spread of cancer cells).

Papillary Carcinoma

Papillary carcinoma, the most common type of thyroid cancer, is found more often in women and in clients younger than 40 years of age. It is a slow-growing tumor and can be present for years before spreading to nearby lymph nodes. When the tumor is confined to the thyroid gland, the chance for cure is good with a partial or total thyroidectomy.

Follicular Carcinoma

About 25% of all thyroid cancers are follicular carcinomas. This tumor primarily affects clients older than 50 years of age. The cancer invades blood vessels and spreads to bone and lung tissue. It rarely spreads to lymph nodes but can adhere to the trachea, neck muscles, great vessels, and skin, resulting in **dyspnea** (difficulty breathing) and **dysphagia** (difficulty swallowing). When the tumor involves the recurrent laryngeal nerves, the client may have a hoarse voice. The prognosis is fair when metastasis is minimal at the time of diagnosis.

Medullary Carcinoma

Medullary carcinoma accounts for 5% to 10% of all thyroid cancers and is more common in clients older than 50 years of age. Metastasis occurs through lymph nodes and invasion of surrounding structures. This tumor often occurs as part of multiple endocrine neoplasia (MEN) type II, a familial endocrine disorder. There is excessive secretion of calcitonin, adrenocorticotropic hormone (ACTH), prostaglandins, and serotonin.

Anaplastic Carcinoma

Anaplastic carcinoma is a rapid-growing, extremely aggressive tumor that directly invades nearby structures to cause symptoms of **stridor** (harsh, high-pitched respiratory sounds), hoarseness, and dysphagia. The prognosis is poor, and most clients die within a year after diagnosis. The client with anaplastic carcinoma may be treated with palliative surgery, radiation, or chemotherapy.

► COLLABORATIVE MANAGEMENT

Surgery is the treatment of choice for papillary, follicular, and medullary carcinomas. A total thyroidectomy is usually performed with a nodal neck dissection if regional lymph nodes are involved. The physician prescribes postoperative suppressive doses of thyroid hormone for 3 months. A radioactive iodine uptake (RAIU) study is performed after medication is withdrawn. If there is RAI uptake, the client is treated with **ablative** (enough

to destroy the tissue) amounts of RAI. If thyroid cancer does not respond to RAI, a course of chemotherapy is initiated.

PARATHYROID DISORDERS
Hyperparathyroidism
OVERVIEW

The parathyroid glands maintain calcium and phosphate balance (Figure 64-5). Serum calcium concentration is normally maintained within a narrow range; phosphate levels vary more widely. Increased levels of parathyroid hormone (PTH) act directly on the kidney, causing increased kidney reabsorption of calcium and increased phosphate excretion. These processes cause **hypercalcemia** (excessive calcium) and **hypophosphatemia** (inadequate phosphate) in the client with hyperparathyroidism.

In the bone, excessive PTH levels increase bone **resorption** (bone loss of calcium) by decreasing **osteoblastic** (bone production) activity and increasing **osteoclastic** (bone destruction) activity. This process releases calcium and phosphate into the circulation and demineralizes bone. When the normal solubility of calcium in the serum is exceeded, as in long-standing hypercalcemia, calcium is deposited in soft tissues.

Although the exact triggering mechanisms are unknown, *primary* hyperparathyroidism results when one or more parathyroid glands does not respond to the normal feedback of serum calcium. In 80% to 85% of the cases, the cause is a benign tumor in one parathyroid gland. Table 64-4 lists other causes of hyperparathyroidism.

► COLLABORATIVE MANAGEMENT
● Assessment

The nurse asks about the client's symptoms and any bone fractures, recent weight loss, arthritis, or psychologic distress. Any history of radiation treatment to the head or neck is also

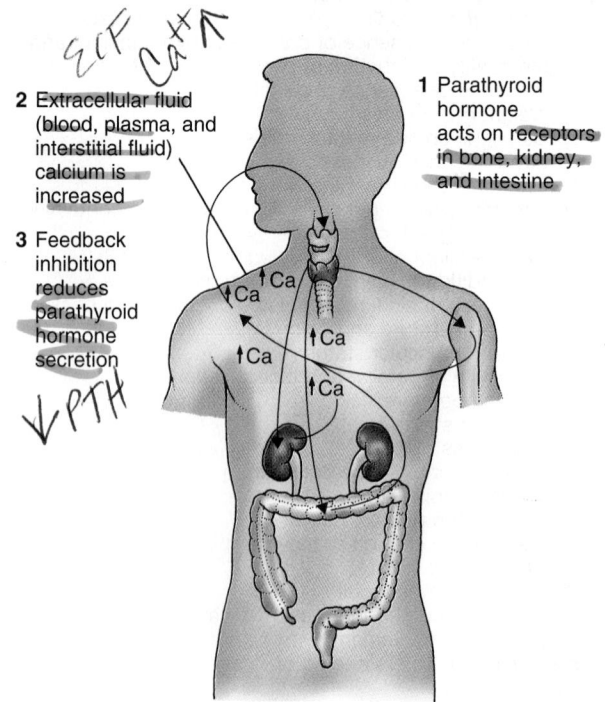

2 Extracellular fluid (blood, plasma, and interstitial fluid) calcium is increased

3 Feedback inhibition reduces parathyroid hormone secretion

1 Parathyroid hormone acts on receptors in bone, kidney, and intestine

Figure 64-5 ● The physiologic actions of parathyroid hormone.

obtained. The client with long-standing disease may have a waxy pallor of the skin and bone deformities in the extremities and back.

The clinical features of hyperparathyroidism may be related either to the effects of excessive PTH or to the effects of the accompanying hypercalcemia.

High levels of PTH cause **renal calculi** (kidney stones) and **nephrocalcinosis** (deposits of calcium in the soft tissue of the kidney). Bone lesions are due to an increased rate of bone destruction and result in pathologic fractures, bone cysts, and osteoporosis in advanced cases.

Gastrointestinal manifestations (e.g., anorexia, nausea, vomiting, epigastric pain, constipation, and weight loss) are common, particularly when serum calcium levels are high. **Hypergastrinemia** (elevated serum gastrin levels) is caused by hypercalcemia and leads to peptic ulcer disease. Fatigue and lethargy may be present and become more severe as the serum calcium levels increase. When serum calcium levels are greater than 12 mg/dL, the client may have psychosis with mental confusion, which leads to coma and death if left untreated. (See Chapter 13 for more information on the effects of hypercalcemia.)

Serum PTH, calcium, and phosphate levels and urine cyclic adenosine monophosphate (cAMP) are the most commonly used laboratory tests to detect hyperparathyroidism (Chart 64-10). X-rays may show kidney stones, calcium deposits, and bone lesions, such as cysts or fractures. Generalized bone demineralization and resorption in the long bones

occur in the client with chronic hyperparathyroidism. Other diagnostic tests include arteriography, computed tomography (CT), venous catheterization of the thyroid veins with sampling of the blood for PTH levels, and ultrasonography. The nurse explains the procedures and cares for the client undergoing diagnostic tests.

▶ Interventions

NONSURGICAL MANAGEMENT

DIURETIC AND FLUID THERAPY. The most common therapy for reducing serum calcium levels in clients who are not candidates for surgery is hydration and furosemide (Lasix, Uritol✚), a diuretic that increases kidney excretion of calcium. IV saline in large volumes also promotes renal calcium excretion.

The nurse monitors cardiac function and intake and output every 2 to 4 hours during hydration therapy. Continuous cardiac monitoring may be required. The nurse closely monitors serum calcium levels and immediately reports any precipitous drop to the physician. Sudden drops in calcium levels may cause tingling and numbness in the muscles.

DRUG THERAPY. When hydration and furosemide cannot reduce hypercalcemia, or if it becomes necessary to discontinue IV fluids, additional medications can help to reduce the clinical manifestations of hyperparathyroidism, especially those related to hypercalcemia.

Phosphates. Oral phosphates inhibit bone resorption and interfere with calcium absorption. IV phosphates are used only when serum calcium levels must be lowered rapidly.

Calcitonin. Calcitonin decreases skeletal calcium release and increases the kidney excretion of calcium. Calcitonin is not effective when used alone because of its short duration of action. Its therapeutic effects are greatly enhanced if given in conjunction with glucocorticoids.

Calcium Chelators. Some drugs lower calcium levels by binding (**chelating**) calcium, which reduces the levels of free calcium. Mithramycin, a cytotoxic agent, is the most effective and potent calcium chelator used to lower serum calcium levels. In most clients a single IV dose of 10 to 15 mg/kg of body weight by slow infusion can lower serum calcium levels within 48 hours. However, the toxic effects limit its use to two or three doses. **Thrombocytopenia** (decreased circulating platelets and an increased tendency to bleed) and kidney and

---

TABLE 64-4 • CAUSES OF PARATHYROID DYSFUNCTION

CAUSES OF HYPERPARATHYROIDISM
- Parathyroid adenoma
- Parathyroid carcinoma
- Congenital hyperplasia
- Neck trauma or radiation
- Vitamin D deficiency
- Chronic renal failure with hypocalcemia
- Parathyroid hormone-secreting carcinomas of the lung, kidney, or gastrointestinal tract

CAUSES OF HYPOPARATHYROIDISM
- Surgical or radiation-induced thyroid ablation
- Parathyroidectomy
- Congenital dysgenesis
- Idiopathic (autoimmune) hypoparathyroidism
- Hypomagnesemia

CHART 64-10

LABORATORY PROFILE
Parathyroid Function

Test	Normal Range for Adults	Significance of Abnormal Findings	
		Hyperthyroidism	Hypothyroidism
Serum calcium	Total: 8.6-10.0 mg/dL, or 2.20-2.55 SI units Ionized (active): 4.64-5.28 mg/dL, or 1.16-1.32 SI units	Increased in primary hyperparathyroidism	Decreased
Serum phosphate	2.7-4.5 mg/dL, or 0.87-1.45 SI units *Older adults:* May be slightly lower	Decreased	Increased
Serum parathyroid hormone	<2000 pg/mL	Increased	Decreased
Urinary cAMP	1-11.5 μmol/dL	Increased	Decreased

cAMP, Cyclic adenosine monophosphate; *SI,* System Internationale.

liver toxicity can result after only one dose. Liver function studies, blood urea nitrogen and creatinine, complete blood count (CBC), and serum calcium levels are closely monitored in the client receiving mithramycin. Another calcium chelator is penicillamine (Cuprimine, Pendramine).

SURGICAL MANAGEMENT. Surgical management of hyperparathyroidism involves a parathyroidectomy.

PREOPERATIVE CARE. Before parathyroidectomy, the client is stabilized and calcium levels are decreased to near-normal. If mithramycin has been used to lower serum calcium levels, the physician orders studies to determine bleeding and clotting times and orders a CBC to determine bone marrow function.

The nurse advises the client that coughing and deep-breathing exercises should be performed postoperatively and that talking may be painful for the first day or two after surgery. The nurse demonstrates neck support by having the client place both hands behind the neck to assist in elevating the head.

OPERATIVE PROCEDURES. Using general anesthesia and with the client's neck hyperextended, the surgeon makes a transverse incision in the lower neck. After the muscles are retracted, both sides of the neck are examined to evaluate all four parathyroid glands. Starting on one side, the surgeon examines the glands for enlargement. If only one gland on that side is enlarged, a frozen section is done on both glands. If a tumor is present on one side but the other side is normal, the surgeon removes the tumor and leaves the remaining gland intact.

POSTOPERATIVE CARE. The nurse observes the client for signs of respiratory distress, which may be due to compression of the trachea by hemorrhage or swelling of neck tissues. The nurse ensures that emergency equipment, including suction, oxygen, and tracheostomy equipment, is at the bedside. If severe swelling occurs, the surgeon may need to remove clips from the incision to preserve the airway. The nurse monitors vital signs, identifies any change in status, and checks the neck dressing for abnormal amounts of drainage or bleeding. A small amount (1 to 5 mL) of drainage is normal.

The remaining glands, which may be nonfunctional as a result of PTH overproduction, require several days to several weeks to return to normal function. A hypocalcemic crisis can occur during this critical period. Serum calcium levels are determined immediately after surgery and are monitored every 4 hours until calcium levels stabilize. The nurse monitors for signs and symptoms of hypocalcemia, such as tingling and twitching in the extremities and face. The nurse checks for Trousseau's and Chvostek's signs, either of which signal potential tetany (see Chapter 13).

Damage to the recurrent laryngeal nerve is rare, but the nurse assesses the client for persistent changes in voice patterns and hoarseness.

When hyperparathyroidism is due to **hyperplasia** (tissue overgrowth), three glands plus half of the fourth gland are usually removed; the remaining portion of the fourth gland is tagged to make it easy to find if future surgery is necessary. If all four glands are removed, a small portion of a gland may be implanted in the forearm, where it produces PTH and maintains calcium homeostasis. If all of these maneuvers fail, the client will need lifelong treatment with calcium and vitamin D because the resulting hypoparathyroidism is permanent.

Hypoparathyroidism

■ OVERVIEW

Hypoparathyroidism is an uncommon endocrine disorder in which parathyroid function is decreased. Problems are directly related to a lack of parathyroid hormone (PTH) secretion or to decreased effectiveness of PTH on target tissue. Whether the problem is a lack of PTH secretion or an ineffectiveness of PTH on tissues, the result is the same—hypocalcemia.

Iatrogenic hypoparathyroidism, the most common form, is caused by the removal of all parathyroid tissue during total thyroidectomy or by deliberate surgical removal of the parathyroid glands.

Idiopathic hypoparathyroidism is a rare condition that can occur spontaneously. The exact cause is unknown, but an autoimmune basis is suspected because antiparathyroid antibodies are present in many affected clients. In addition, hypoparathyroidism is often associated with the following autoimmune disorders: adrenal insufficiency, hypothyroidism, diabetes mellitus, pernicious anemia, gonadal failure, and vitiligo.

Hypomagnesemia (decreased serum magnesium levels) may also cause hypoparathyroidism. Hypomagnesemia is seen in alcoholics and in clients with malabsorption syndromes, chronic renal disease, and malnutrition. It causes impairment of PTH secretion and may interfere with PTH effects on the bones and kidneys.

► COLLABORATIVE MANAGEMENT
● Assessment

The nurse begins assessment of the client with suspected hypoparathyroidism by asking about any head or neck surgery or radiation therapy, because these treatments may cause hypoparathyroidism. The client is asked about the signs and symptoms of hypoparathyroidism, which may range from mild tingling and numbness to tetany. Tingling and numbness around the mouth or in the hands and feet reflect mild to moderate hypocalcemia. Severe muscle cramps, carpopedal spasms, and seizures (with no loss of consciousness or incontinence) reflect a more severe hypocalcemia. The client or caregiver may notice mental changes ranging from irritability to psychosis.

The physical assessment may show excessive or inappropriate muscle contractions that cause finger, hand, and elbow flexion; this can signal an impending attack of tetany. The nurse checks for Chvostek's sign and Trousseau's sign; positive responses indicate potential tetany. A parkinsonian-like syndrome may be evident. The presence of cataracts denotes chronic hypocalcemia. Bands or pits may encircle the crowns of the teeth, which indicates a loss of calcium from the teeth and causes enamel loss. The roots of the client's teeth may be defective.

Diagnostic tests for hypoparathyroidism include electroencephalography (EEG), blood tests, and computed tomography (CT). EEG changes are nonspecific and revert to normal with correction of hypocalcemia. Serum calcium, phosphate, magnesium, vitamin D, and urine cyclic adenosine monophosphate (cAMP) levels may be used in the diagnostic workup for hypoparathyroidism (see Chart 64-9). The CT scan can show brain calcifications, which indicate chronic hypocalcemia.

● Interventions

Management of hypoparathyroidism focuses on correcting hypocalcemia, vitamin D deficiency, and hypomagnesemia. For clients with acute and severe hypocalcemia, IV calcium is administered as a 10% solution of calcium chloride or calcium gluconate over 10 to 15 minutes. Acute vitamin D deficiency is treated with calcitriol (Rocaltrol), 0.5 to 2.0 mg/day. Acute hypomagnesemia is corrected with 50% magnesium sulfate in 2-mL doses (up to 4 g/day) either intramuscularly or intravenously. Long-term oral therapy for hypocalcemia involves the administration of calcium, 0.5 to 2.0 g/day in divided doses.

Long-term therapy for vitamin D deficiency is 50,000 to 400,000 units of ergocalciferol daily. The dosage is adjusted to keep the client's calcium level in the low-normal range (slightly hypocalcemic), enough to prevent symptoms of hypocalcemia. It must also be low enough to prevent increased urine calcium concentrations, which can lead to stone formation.

Nursing management includes teaching about the medication regimen and interventions to reduce anxiety. The client is instructed to eat foods high in calcium but low in phosphorus. Milk, yogurt, and processed cheeses are avoided because of their high phosphorus content. *The nurse stresses that therapy for hypocalcemia is lifelong.* The client is advised to use some form of identification, such as a MedicAlert bracelet or a wallet card. With adherence to the prescribed drug and diet regimen, the calcium level usually remains high enough to prevent a hypocalcemic crisis.

ONLINE RESOURCES

For suggested readings and Internet resources, go to http://www.wbsaunders.com/SIMON/Iggy/.

SELECTED BIBLIOGRAPHY

Asterisk indicates a classic or definitive work on this subject.

American Cancer Society. (2001). *Cancer facts and figures 2001.* Atlanta: Author; 01-300M-No. 5008.01.

Assessing thyroid disorder in women. (1998). *AWHONN Lifelines, 2*(5), 14.

Braverman, L., Dworkin, H., & Macindoe, J. (1997). Thyroid disease: When to screen, when to treat. *Patient Care, 31*(6), 18-20, 29, 34.

Clement, B. (1998). Parathyroid pathophysiology. *Seminars in Perioperative Nursing, 7*(3), 186-192.

Cotran, R., Kumar, V., & Collins, T. (1999). *Robbins' pathologic basis of disease* (6th ed.). Philadelphia: W.B. Saunders.

Elliott, B. (2000). Diagnosing and treating hypothyroidism. *The Nurse Practitioner, 25*(3), 92-105.

Goldsmith, C. (1999). Hypothyroidism. *American Journal of Nursing, 99*(6), 42-43.

Guyton, A., & Hall, J. (2000). *Textbook of medical physiology* (10th ed.). Philadelphia: W.B. Saunders.

*Kennedy, L.W., & Caro, J.F. (1996). The ABCs of managing hyperthyroidism in the older patient. *Geriatrics, 51*(5), 22-24, 27, 31, 32.

Klein, I., & Ojamaa, K. (2001). Thyroid hormone and the cardiovascular system. *New England Journal of Medicine, 344*(7), 501-509.

Larsen, P.R., Davies, T., & Hay, I. (1998). The thyroid gland. In J. Wilson et al. (Eds.). *William's textbook of endocrinology* (9th ed., pp. 389-515). Philadelphia: W.B. Saunders.

McCloskey, J.C., & Bulechek, G.M. (2000). *Nursing interventions classification (NIC)* (3rd ed.). St. Louis: Mosby.

Mead, M. (2000). Thyroid function tests. *Practice Nurse, 19*(6), 283.

Michalek, A., Mahoney, M., & Calebaugh, D. (2000). Hypothyroidism and diabetes mellitus in an American Indian population. *Journal of Family Practice, 49*(7), 638-640.

Mitchell, S. (1997). Thyroid eye disease: A patient's point of view. *Ophthalmic Nursing: International Journal of Ophthalmic Nursing, 1*(3), 14-16.

Payton, R., Gardner, R., & Reynolds, D. (1997). Pharmacologic considerations and management of common endocrine disorders in women. *Journal of Nurse-Midwifery, 42*(3), 186-206.

Sagre, G., & Brown, E. (1998). Measurement of hormones. In J. Wilson et al. (Eds.). *William's textbook of endocrinology* (9th ed.). (pp. 43-54). Philadelphia: W.B. Saunders.

Screening for thyroid disease: The latest guidelines. (1998). *Consultant, 38*(10), 2447-2448.

The thyroid "neck check": Thyroid blues. (1998). *ORL: Head and Neck Nursing, 16*(2), 31.

Trotto, N. (1999). Hypothyroidism, hyperthyroidism, hyperparathyroidism. *Patient Care, 33*(14), 186-188, 191, 195-200.

United States Pharmacopeia Dispensing Information (USP DI): Vol. I. Drug information for the health care professional (2000). (20th ed.). Englewood, CO: Micromedix.

Wallace, K., & Hofmann, M. (1998). Thyroid dysfunction: How to manage overt and subclinical disease in older patients. *Geriatrics, 53*(4), 32-41.

Walpert, N. (1998). The highs and lows of autoimmune thyroid disease. *Nursing98, 28*(12), 58-60.

Young, J. (1999). Myxedema coma. *Nursing99, 29*(1), 64.

Interventions for Clients with Diabetes Mellitus

M. ELAINE McLEOD

Learning Objectives

After studying this chapter, you should be able to:

1. Compare and contrast the age of onset, clinical manifestations, and pathologic mechanisms of type 1 and type 2 diabetes mellitus.
2. Identify clients at risk for developing type 2 diabetes mellitus.
3. Explain the effects of insulin on carbohydrate, protein, and fat metabolism.
4. Evaluate laboratory data to determine whether the client is using the prescribed dietary, medication, and exercise interventions for diabetes.
5. Explain the effect of aerobic exercise on blood glucose levels.
6. Describe the significance of the presence of ketone bodies in the urine of a diabetic client.
7. Use the exchange system to plan a menu for a client with diabetes who is prescribed to eat 1800 calories per day, divided into three meals and a snack, with 15% of calories from fat, 20% of calories from protein, and the remaining calories from carbohydrate sources.
8. Compare the mechanisms of action of the sulfonylureas, biguanides, alpha-glucosidase inhibitors, meglitinides, thiazolidinediones, and D-phenylalanine derivatives as antidiabetic agents.
9. Explain the effect of hypertension on the development of diabetic nephropathy and diabetic retinopathy.
10. Identify clients at risk for the development of hypoglycemia.
11. Prioritize nursing interventions for the client with mild to moderate hypoglycemia and moderate to severe hypoglycemia.
12. Identify clients at risk for developing diabetic ketoacidosis (DKA).
13. Prioritize nursing interventions for clients with DKA.
14. Identify clients at risk for developing hyperglycemic-hyperosmolar nonketotic syndrome (HHNS).
15. Prioritize nursing interventions for clients with HHNS.
16. Use laboratory data and clinical manifestations to determine the effectiveness of the interventions for DKA and HHNS.
17. Describe the steps required for subcutaneous insulin administration.
18. Describe the correct technique to use when mixing different types of insulin within the same syringe.
19. Compare and contrast the clinical manifestations of hyperglycemia and hypoglycemia.
20. Perform foot assessment and foot care for the client with diabetes.

Go to http://www.wbsaunders.com/SIMON/Iggy/ for self-assessment questions related to these Learning Objectives.

Diabetes mellitus is a common chronic disease requiring lifelong behavioral and lifestyle changes. Diabetes is best managed with an interdisciplinary team approach that helps empower the client to successfully manage his or her disease. As part of the team, the nurse plans, organizes, and coordinates care among the various health disciplines involved; provides care and education; and promotes the client's health and well-being. The Evidence-Based Practice for Nursing box on p. 1441 provides an example of the effects of team intervention on diabetes management.

■ OVERVIEW

Diabetes is a major public health problem worldwide. The complications of the disease cause many devastating health problems. The financial cost of diabetes is discussed in the Cost of Care box on p. 1441. In the United States, diabetes is the leading cause of new cases of blindness, end-stage renal disease requiring dialysis or transplantation, and lower limb amputations. A large percentage of the U.S. population with diabetes is undiagnosed, and many of those who are diagnosed have unacceptably high blood glucose levels. Studies

EVIDENCE-BASED PRACTICE
FOR NURSING

Teamwork for diabetes treatment pays off!

Koproski, J., Pretto, Z., & Poretsky, L. (1997). Effect of an intervention by a diabetes team in hospitalized patients with diabetes. *Diabetes Care, 20*(10): 1553-1555.

A randomized controlled trial was conducted to determine the effects of a diabetes team on length of hospital stay, glucose control, and readmission rates in hospitalized clients with diabetes. The study was conducted at a 492-bed community teaching hospital in New York City. Clients with concurrent or new-onset diabetes from November 1993 through November 1994 were selected for the study. There were 85 clients in the intervention group and 94 in the control group. A diabetes nurse educator and an endocrinologist visited clients in the intervention group daily. The client's plan of care was discussed with the primary care physician, and consultations were requested with a dietitian and social worker as needed. The control group received care in the "usual manner." Measures were obtained for length of stay, blood glucose control, insulin administration and blood glucose monitoring instructions, nutrition and social service consults, and readmission rates.

Clients in the intervention group received more education about diabetes. Documented instructions for blood glucose monitoring were present in 89% of cases in the intervention group as opposed to 57% in the control group. Documented instructions for insulin administration were present in 69% of the charts of the intervention group as opposed to 25% of the charts in the control group. Eighty-seven percent of clients had documentation of education of any kind in the intervention group as compared with 37% in the control group. Seventy-six percent of clients in the intervention group had nutrition consultation as compared with 40% in the control group. There was no difference in the amount of social worker contact.

Clients treated by the diabetes team had shorter lengths of stay, achieved better glycemic control early in the study, and demonstrated a significant reduction in readmission rates. Clients with a primary diagnosis of diabetes had a median length of stay of 5.5 days in the intervention group as compared with 7.5 days in the control group. The percentage of clients with "good" blood glucose control (75% of capillary blood glucose readings between 80 and 180 mg/dL) was 75% for the intervention group as compared with 46% in the control group during the first month of the program. In the intervention group 15% were readmitted within 3 months after discharge as compared with 32% in the control group.

Critique. Characteristics of the client population may have biased results of the study. There was a significant difference between the initial blood glucose levels between the two groups. The admission blood glucose levels were significantly higher in the intervention group, indicating that initial glycemic control was worse. Clients in the intervention group were younger. Younger diabetic clients tend to have acute illness that resolves quickly with treatment. They also tend not to have the number of chronic complications of diabetes. It is also difficult to prevent readmission of an older diabetic client with multiple chronic complications of diabetes.

Implications for Nursing. Clients in the intervention group clearly had more education documented and had more nutrition consultation than did the control group. Improved statistics for the implementation group are due in part to education provided by a multidisciplinary team. The nurse is an integral part of that team.

confirm that **glycemic** (blood glucose) control reduces complications of diabetes.

Today, interventions exist to reduce the incidence of blindness, drug therapy can reduce the incidence of kidney and coronary artery disease, and regular evaluation of the feet can reduce the incidence of amputation. The challenge for the

COST OF CARE
IMPLICATIONS FOR NURSING

DIABETES MELLITUS

Cost of Care

- The economic burden of diabetes mellitus in the United States is enormous. Direct medical expenses attributed to diabetes in 1997 totaled $44.1 billion. This figure includes $7.7 billion for diabetes and acute glycemic care, $11.8 billion for high prevalence of related chronic conditions, and $24.6 billion for high prevalence of general medical conditions (American Diabetes Association, 1999b).
- Medical care for diabetic clients accounts for 10% to 15% of all health care costs in the United States and 25% of all Medicare costs (Roman & Harris, 1997).
- The cost of diabetes is shared by all citizens, not just those with diabetes. In the United States, 60% of the medical costs for diabetic care are paid for with public money through agencies such as Medicare, Medicaid, and the Veterans Administration (Harris, 1998).
- Adults with diabetes are hospitalized more frequently and have longer hospital stays than nondiabetic individuals. Results of the National Medical Expenditure Survey indicated that the average per capita cost each year was over $11,000 for people with diabetes as compared with $2,600 for those without diabetes, with about 64% of the cost being due to inpatient hospitalization (Harris, 1998).

Implications for Nursing

If costs related to diabetes are to be reduced, attention must be directed to the prevention and treatment of chronic complications of diabetes. Therapies are available to reduce the incidence of blindness, medications are available to reduce the incidence of kidney and coronary artery disease, and regular sensory evaluation of the foot will reduce the incidence of amputation. The challenge for the nurse is to assist the diabetic client in achieving and maintaining meticulous glycemic control so that long-term chronic complications are prevented.

Data from American Diabetes Association. (1999). Reviews: Economic consequences of diabetes mellitus in the U.S. *Diabetes Care,* 22(2), 296-309; Harris, M. I. (1998). Diabetes in America: Epidemiology and scope of the problem. *Diabetes Care,* 21(suppl 3), 11-14; and Roman, S. H. & Harris, M. I. (1997). Management of diabetes mellitus from a public health perspective. *Endocrinology and Metabolism Clinics for North America,* 26(3), 443-474.

nurse is to assist the client with diabetes in achieving and maintaining tight glycemic control so that long-term chronic complications are prevented.

Pathophysiology

CLASSIFICATION OF DIABETES

For all types of diabetes mellitus, the main feature is chronic **hyperglycemia** (high blood glucose level) resulting from problems with insulin secretion, insulin action, or both. The disease is classified by age of onset, the underlying problem causing a lack of insulin, and the severity of the deficiency. Table 65-1 outlines the different types of diabetes.

THE ENDOCRINE PANCREAS

The endocrine portion of the pancreas consists of about 1 million small glands, the **islets of Langerhans,** scattered throughout the gland. The islet cells compose only a small portion of the gland, with most of the gland having exocrine functions for digestive processes. Four types of islet cells have been identified: alpha, beta, D, and F. Glucagon is produced by alpha cells, insulin is produced by beta cells, somatostatin is produced by D cells, and pancreatic polypeptide

TABLE 65-1 • CLASSIFICATION OF DIABETES MELLITUS

TYPE 1 DIABETES
- Primary beta-cell destruction leading to absolute insulin deficiency
  - Autoimmune process
  - Idiopathic

TYPE 2 DIABETES
- Ranges from insulin resistance with an insulin deficiency to secretory deficit with insulin resistance

OTHER SPECIFIC TYPES (CONDITIONS RESULTING IN HYPERGLYCEMIA)
- Genetic defects of beta-cell function
- Genetic defects in insulin action
- Diseases of the exocrine pancreas: pancreatitis, trauma, neoplasia, cystic fibrosis, hemochromatosis
- Endocrinopathies: acromegaly, Cushing's disease, glucagonoma, pheochromocytoma, hyperthyroidism, aldosteronoma
- Drug- or chemical-induced conditions (from use of pentamidine, nicotinic acid, glucocorticoids, thyroid hormone, diazoxide, beta-adrenergic agonists, thiazides, Dilantin, interferon-alpha, other drugs)
- Infections: congenital rubella, cytomegalovirus
- Uncommon forms of immune-related diabetes
- Other genetic syndromes associated with diabetes: Down syndrome, Klinefelter's syndrome, Turner's syndrome, Huntington's chorea, and others

GESTATIONAL DIABETES MELLITUS (GDM)
- Carbohydrate intolerance is first recognized during pregnancy.
- Children of mothers with GDM are at greater risk for neonatal mortality, congenital malformation, and macrosomia (large body size).
- Studies indicate that children of mothers with GDM have an increased risk of obesity and impaired glucose tolerance later in life.
- Clients with GDM are at high risk for developing diabetes after pregnancy.
- Diagnosis is based on the results of a 100-g oral glucose tolerance test during pregnancy.

Data from American Diabetes Association. (2000). Committee Report: Report of the Expert Committee on the Diagnosis and Classification of Diabetes Mellitus. *Diabetes Care,* 23(Suppl. 1), 4-19; and American Diabetes Association. (2000). Position statement: Gestational diabetes mellitus. *Diabetes Care, 23*(Suppl. 1), 77-79.

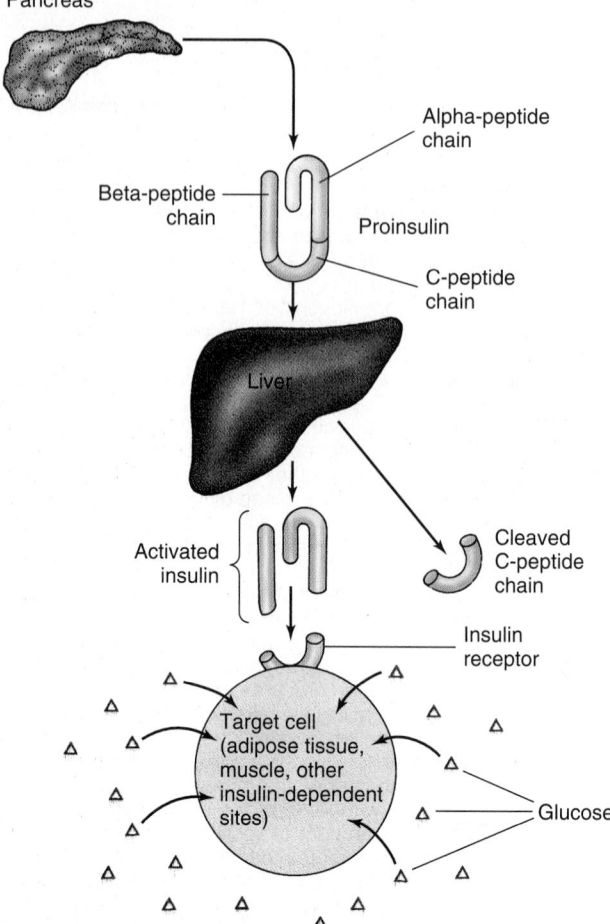

Figure 65-1 ● Proinsulin, secreted by and stored in the beta cells of the islets of Langerhans in the pancreas, is transformed by the liver into activated insulin. Insulin attaches to receptors on target cells, where it promotes glucose transport into the cells through the cell membranes.

is produced by F cells. This chapter focuses on the activity of glucagon and insulin. **Glucagon** is a major "counterregulatory" hormone that has actions opposite those of insulin and releases glucose from cell storage sites whenever blood glucose levels are low. **Insulin** plays a key role in allowing body cells to store and use carbohydrate, fat, and protein.

INSULIN PHYSIOLOGY

Insulin is a protein made up of 51 amino acids contained within two peptide chains: an alpha chain with 21 amino acids and a beta chain with 30 amino acids. **Preproinsulin** is produced initially. This protein is known as a **precursor molecule** because it is inactive and must be modified and made smaller to eventually become the active hormone insulin. Preproinsulin is cut by enzymes to proinsulin (a precursor that includes the alpha and beta chains of the insulin molecule) and an additional fragment called the C-peptide chain. In the islet cells, proinsulin is converted into equal amounts of insulin and C-peptide (Figure 65-1). C-peptide is not active and can

be used to measure the rate that pancreatic beta cells are secreting insulin.

The action of insulin allows glucose in the blood to move into cells to make energy. Thus insulin is like a key to unlock cell membrane entryways for glucose. Insulin action starts by binding to insulin receptors on the membranes of target cells. The liver is the first major organ to be reached by insulin in the blood. In the liver, insulin promotes tissue-building metabolism (**anabolism**) by causing both the production and storage of glycogen (**glycogenesis**) at the same time that it inhibits glycogen breakdown into glucose (**glycogenolysis**). Insulin increases protein and **lipid** (fat) synthesis and very-low-density lipoprotein (VLDL) formation. Insulin inhibits tissue-degrading metabolism (**catabolism**) by inhibiting liver glycogenolysis, **ketogenesis** (conversion of fats to acids), and **gluconeogenesis** (conversion of proteins to glucose). In muscle, insulin promotes protein and glycogen synthesis. In fat cells, insulin promotes the storage of triglycerides. Overall, insulin keeps blood glucose levels from becoming too high and also helps maintain blood lipid levels in the normal range.

The pancreas secretes about 40 to 50 units of insulin per day. Insulin is secreted directly into liver circulation in a **biphasic** (two-step) manner. Insulin is secreted at low levels during the fasting state (**basal insulin secretion**) and at increased levels after eating (**prandial**). There is an early burst of insulin secretion within 10 minutes of eating, followed by a progressively increasing phase of insulin release that lasts as long as hyperglycemia is present.

GLUCOSE HOMEOSTASIS

Glucose is the primary fuel for the central nervous system (CNS). Because the brain cannot produce or store much glucose, a continuous supply from the body's circulation is needed. Outside the CNS, fatty acids can be used as fuel for energy formation (Halperin & Goldstein, 1999). The circulating fuels of glucose and free fatty acids are stored inside cells as glycogen in the liver and muscles and as triglyceride in fat cells. Fat, in the form of triglyceride, is the most efficient means of storing energy. Fat has 9 calories of stored energy per gram, whereas protein and carbohydrate have only 4 calories per gram. Although protein can be degraded for fuel use during starvation, protein is not used for fuel under normal conditions.

The combined actions of insulin and counterregulatory hormones (discussed in the next section) keep blood glucose within the range of 65 to 105 mg/dL (3.6 to 5.8 mmol/L) to supply glucose for CNS functions. When glucose levels fall, insulin secretion stops and glucagon release is stimulated. Glucagon causes the release of glucose from the liver. Liver glucose is made available through **glycogenolysis** (breakdown of glycogen to glucose) and gluconeogenesis. When glucose is unavailable, **lipolysis** (breakdown of fat) and **proteolysis** (breakdown of amino acids) occur to provide fuel for energy.

Counterregulatory hormones increase blood levels of glucose by actions opposite those of insulin when more energy is needed. Glucagon is the main counterregulatory hormone. Other hormones that increase blood glucose levels are epinephrine, norepinephrine, growth hormone, and cortisol. In type 1 diabetes, glucagon secretion in response to hypoglycemia is lost, increasing the risk for severe hypoglycemic reactions.

ABSENCE OF INSULIN

The lack of insulin in diabetes, either from lack of insulin production or from a problem with the use of insulin at its cell receptor, prevents some cells from using glucose as an energy source. Insulin is needed to supply glucose to most of the body's tissues. Without insulin, the body enters a serious state of breaking down body fat and protein. Levels of counterregulatory hormones increase in an attempt to increase the availability of glucose from other sources. Table 65-2 outlines the body's response to insufficient insulin.

Without insulin, glucose builds up in the blood, causing **hyperglycemia** (high blood glucose levels). Hyperglycemia causes fluid and electrolyte imbalances, leading to the classic symptoms of diabetes: *polyuria, polydipsia,* and *polyphagia.*

Polyuria (frequent and excessive urination) results from an osmotic diuresis caused by excess glucose in the urine. As a result of diuresis, sodium, chloride, and potassium are excreted in the urine in large amounts, accompanied by severe water loss. The resulting dehydration stimulates the thirst mechanism, and **polydipsia** (excessive thirst) occurs. Because the cells are not receiving any food (glucose), the sense of cell starvation results in **polyphagia** (excessive eating). In spite of eating vast amounts of food, the person remains in a

TABLE 65-2 • PHYSIOLOGIC RESPONSE TO INSUFFICIENT INSULIN
• Decreased glycogenesis (conversion of glucose to glycogen) • Increased glycogenolysis (conversion of glycogen to glucose) • Increased gluconeogenesis (formation of glucose from non-carbohydrate sources, such as amino acids and lactate) • Increased lipolysis (breakdown of triglycerides to glycerol and free fatty acids) • Increased ketogenesis (formation of ketones from free fatty acids) • Proteolysis (breakdown of protein with amino acid release in muscles)

state of starvation until insulin is available to move glucose into the cells.

With insulin deficiency, fats break down (**lipolysis**), releasing free fatty acids. Conversion of free fatty acids to **ketone bodies** (small acids) provides a backup energy source. Because ketone bodies, or "ketones," are incomplete and abnormal degradation products of free fatty acids, they are not further metabolized and may accumulate in the blood when insulin is not available. This accumulation causes metabolic acidosis.

Because of the dehydration associated with diabetes mellitus, **hemoconcentration** (increased blood concentration) and **hypovolemia** (decreased blood volume) develop, leading to **hyperviscosity** (thick, concentrated blood) and **hypoperfusion** (decreased circulation) of tissues and poor tissue oxygenation (**hypoxia**). Hypoxic cells are unable to metabolize glucose efficiently, the Kreb's cycle is blocked, and lactic acid accumulates, causing more acidosis. Restoring tissue perfusion and oxygenation by treating the lack of insulin is the key to halting lactic acid production.

The excess acids present during a lack of insulin increase the hydrogen ion (H^+) and carbon dioxide (CO_2) concentrations of the blood and other extracellular fluids. These products stimulate the respiratory control areas of the brain to increase the rate and depth of respiration in an attempt to excrete more carbon dioxide and acid. This type of breathing is known as **Kussmaul respiration.** Acetone is exhaled, giving the breath a "fruity" odor. When the lungs can no longer offset acidosis, the pH drops. Arterial blood gas studies show a primary **metabolic acidosis** (decreased pH accompanied by decreased arterial bicarbonate [HCO_3] levels) and **compensatory respiratory alkalosis** (decreased partial pressure of arterial carbon dioxide [$PaCO_2$]) (see Chapter 16).

The absence of insulin causes total-body potassium depletion. Because of the increased fluid loss with hyperglycemia, excessive potassium is excreted in the urine, leading to *low* serum potassium levels. However, *high* serum potassium levels may occur in acidosis because of the shift of potassium from inside the cells to the blood and other extracellular fluids. Serum potassium levels in diabetes, then, may be low (**hypokalemia**), elevated (**hyperkalemia**), or even normal, depending on hydration, the severity of the acidosis, and the client's response to treatment. Chapters 15 and 16 discuss acid-base balance and acidosis in more detail.

ACUTE COMPLICATIONS OF DIABETES

Three emergencies related to abnormal blood glucose levels can occur in clients who have diabetes: **diabetic ketoacidosis**

(DKA) caused by lack of insulin and ketosis; **hyperglycemic-hyperosmolar nonketotic syndrome (HHNS)** associated with insulin deficiency, profound dehydration, and the absence of ketosis; and **hypoglycemia** occurring when too much insulin or too little glucose is present. *All three conditions require emergency treatment and can result in death if inappropriately treated or not treated at all.* The bases for these complications, along with the appropriate interventions, are described in the next section.

■ CHRONIC COMPLICATIONS OF DIABETES

Diabetes mellitus is a major risk factor for morbidity and mortality because of changes in the larger or generalized body blood vessels **(macrovascular),** as well as changes in small blood vessels **(microvascular)** within tissues and organs. These blood vessel changes lead to many complications as a result of poor tissue circulation and cell death. *Macrovascular* complications, including coronary heart disease, cerebrovascular disease, and peripheral vascular disease, are responsible for increased early death among diabetic clients as compared with the general population. *Microvascular* complications involve abnormalities of blood vessel wall structure and function, leading to nephropathy (kidney dysfunction), neuropathy (nerve dysfunction), and retinopathy (vision problems). Three theories have been used to explain the cause and progression of diabetic vascular complications:

* Chronic hyperglycemia causes irreversible structural changes resulting in basement membrane thickening and organ damage.
* Glucose toxicity directly or indirectly affects functional cell integrity.
* Chronic ischemia in microcirculatory branches results in connective tissue hypoxia and microischemia.

Strong evidence supports the association between chronic high blood glucose levels and the development of microvascular complications. The association between poor blood glucose control and the development of macrovascular complications is less clear. The development of macrovascular complications in people with type 2 diabetes seems to be more related to hypertension, a sedentary lifestyle, high blood lipid levels, and smoking than it does to hyperglycemia. The additional risk factor of obesity is important for people with type 2 diabetes. About 80% of clients with type 2 diabetes are obese, and cardiovascular events account for most of their deaths.

The National Diabetes Data Group of the National Institutes of Health estimates that the onset of type 2 diabetes may occur 9 to 12 years before the disorder is diagnosed. During the time that diabetes is not being treated, complications are developing. Up to 21% of clients are found to have retinopathy at the time of diagnosis (American Diabetes Association [ADA], 2000f). Many older diabetic clients do not develop classic signs of high blood glucose levels, and the diagnosis is made when the person seeks treatment for an acute illness or for complications caused by diabetes.

The Diabetes Control and Complications Trial (DCCT), an ongoing study involving 29 medical centers and more than 1400 people with type 1 diabetes, provides evidence that hyperglycemia is a critical factor in the development of long-term diabetic complications. Intensive therapy with good glucose control (maintaining blood glucose levels within identified ranges) delayed the onset and slowed the progression of retinopathy,

nephropathy, and neuropathy. Clients in the group receiving intensive treatment had a mean blood glucose level of less than 155 mg/dL (8.6 mmol/L) and a glycosylated hemoglobin (hemoglobin A_{1c} [HbA_{1c}]) concentration of 7.2% (ADA, 2000j).

The United Kingdom Prospective Diabetes Study (UKPDS) established that intensive therapy with lowered blood glucose levels reduced the onset of retinopathy, nephropathy, and possibly neuropathy in clients with type 2 diabetes. Analysis of UKPDS data showed a strong relationship between risks for microvascular complications and the blood glucose level. For every percentage point decrease in HbA_{1c}, there was a 35% reduction in the risk for kidney and eye complications. Lowering the blood glucose level was not shown to have an effect on cardiovascular complications (ADA, 2000k).

MACROVASCULAR COMPLICATIONS

CARDIOVASCULAR DISEASE. Cardiovascular disease is the major cause of death in clients with diabetes mellitus; it accounts for about 80% of all deaths in these clients. Three fourths of these deaths are from coronary artery disease (Herlitz & Malmberg, 1999). Death from coronary artery disease is about 3 to 10 times higher in clients with type 1 diabetes, and 2 to 4 times higher in clients with type 2 diabetes, than in people who do not have diabetes.

Diabetic clients have a greater incidence of acute myocardial infarction and a higher death rate from this complication than nondiabetic individuals (Herlitz & Malmberg, 1999). Several factors account for this difference. Diabetic clients tend to have extensive coronary artery disease, diabetic cardiomyopathy, and abnormal blood clotting. In addition, after myocardial infarction, complications of left ventricular dysfunction with cardiac failure and fatal cardiac dysrhythmias are more common in the diabetic population.

Complications from atherosclerosis in clients with diabetes are very common. Diabetic clients also have more extensive disease. Although clients with diabetes do not develop larger infarcts, they have a higher incidence of pump failure. Heart failure is increased 600% in men with diabetes and 900% in women with diabetes (Garber, 1998).

Risk factors for cardiovascular disease include hyperglycemia, hypertension, **hyperinsulinemia** (excessive blood insulin levels), **hyperlipidemia** (excessive blood levels of cholesterol and other fats), clotting abnormalities, and blood vessel problems (Sowers & Lester, 1999). In addition to being an early indication of nephropathy, **albuminuria** (presence of albumin in the urine) is associated with greater cardiovascular disease in both type 1 and type 2 diabetes. The finding of even microscopic amounts of albumin in the urine is used as an indication for further screening for vascular disease and aggressive intervention to reduce cardiovascular risk factors (ADA, 2000e).

Data from the DCCT strongly indicate that tight blood glucose control by strict insulin treatment is critical for prevention of cardiovascular disease in clients with diabetes. Studies indicate that cardiovascular disease complication rates with diabetes can be reduced through aggressive treatment of hypertension and hyperlipidemia. The American Diabetes Association (ADA) recommends that blood pressure be maintained at levels lower than 130/85 mm Hg and that low-density lipoprotein (LDL) cholesterol be lowered to less than 100 mg/dL (<2.60 mmol/L) (ADA, 2000t).

CEREBROVASCULAR DISEASE. Diabetes is a risk factor for cerebral infarction and stroke. The presence of other risk factors, such as hyperlipidemia, hypertension, coronary artery disease, nephropathy, peripheral vascular disease, and excessive alcohol and tobacco use, along with diabetes, greatly increases the risk for stroke (Davis et al., 1999).

Elevated blood glucose levels at the time of the stroke are associated with greater brain injury. In addition, some studies have shown that hyperglycemia worsens cerebral damage after a stroke.

MICROVASCULAR COMPLICATIONS

EYE AND VISION COMPLICATIONS. Legal blindness, defined as a corrected visual acuity of 20/200 or less, is 25 times more common in diabetic individuals than in nondiabetic individuals. In the United States, diabetic retinopathy is the most frequent cause of new cases of blindness among adults ages 20 to 74 years. Retinopathy is strongly related to the duration of diabetes. After 20 years of diabetes, nearly all clients with type 1 diabetes and 60% of those with type 2 diabetes have some degree of retinopathy.

The cause and progression of diabetic retinopathy are related to problems with retinal blood vessels that cause leakage and blockage of blood flow, leading to retinal hypoxia. **Nonproliferative diabetic retinopathy (NPDR)** (Figure 65-2) is characterized by structural abnormalities of retinal blood vessels, but growth of new blood vessels is not stimulated. With this problem, there are areas of poor retinal circulation, edema, hard fatty deposits in the eye, and retinal hemorrhages. **Microaneurysms** (small capillary wall dilations seen as red dots with an ophthalmoscope) form throughout the eye. They leak fluid and blood into the retina, causing retinal edema and hard exudates. Other abnormal retinal findings include intraretinal hemorrhages, nerve fiber atrophy from hypoxia, and venous beading. **Venous beading** is the abnormal appearance of retinal veins in which areas of swelling and constriction along a segment of vein resemble links of sausage. Venous beading occurs in areas of retinal ischemia and is a predictor of progression to proliferative diabetic retinopathy. NPDR develops slowly *over time* and rarely causes blindness. Clients with severe NPDR have a 50% chance of developing proliferative diabetic retinopathy (Neeley et al., 1998).

Proliferative diabetic retinopathy (PDR) is the growth of new retinal blood vessels (**neovascularization**). When circulation to the retina is poor and hypoxia develops, retinal cells secrete a "growth factor" that stimulates the formation of new blood vessels within the eye. These new vessels are thin, fragile, and prone to bleeding, resulting in eye hemorrhage and more vision loss (Figure 65-3). Reddish black particles floating across the field of vision indicate bleeding into vitreous fluid. Fibrous tissue bands, developing along with new blood vessels, cause retinal detachment and irreversible vision loss. Chapter 47 discusses treatment of retinal problems.

The incidence of retinopathy is associated with fasting blood glucose levels higher than 129 mg/dL. Hyperglycemia and hypertension have been found to predict progression of retinopathy in clients with type 1 diabetes (Cohen et al., 1999). A 1% increase in total glycosylated hemoglobin (HbA_{1c}) was associated with a 10% increase in risk for progression of retinopathy. The Diabetes Control and Complications Trial (DCCT) established that intensive diabetes management to obtain **near-euglycemic** (near-normal blood glucose levels) control could prevent or delay the progression of diabetic retinopathy (ADA, 2000f).

Vision loss can also occur from macular degeneration, corneal scarring, and changes in lens shape or clarity. Hyperglycemia may cause blurred vision, even through prescription eyeglasses. The diabetic client may report double vision during periods of hypoglycemia. Cataracts occur in diabetic clients at a younger age, progress at a faster rate, and occur with greater frequency than in nondiabetic individuals. Open-angle glaucoma is more common in clients with diabetes. The management and treatment of cataracts and glaucoma are the same as for nondiabetic clients (see Chapter 47).

CONSIDERATIONS FOR OLDER ADULTS

The older client with diabetic retinopathy has the additional effect of visual changes that occur with aging. As a result, the older diabetic client's ability to perform self-care activities may be more seriously affected than that of a younger person with diabetes (see Chapter 47). The ability to discriminate among blues, greens, and violets decreases with normal aging. This deterioration of color perception makes performing visual blood glucose monitoring more difficult.

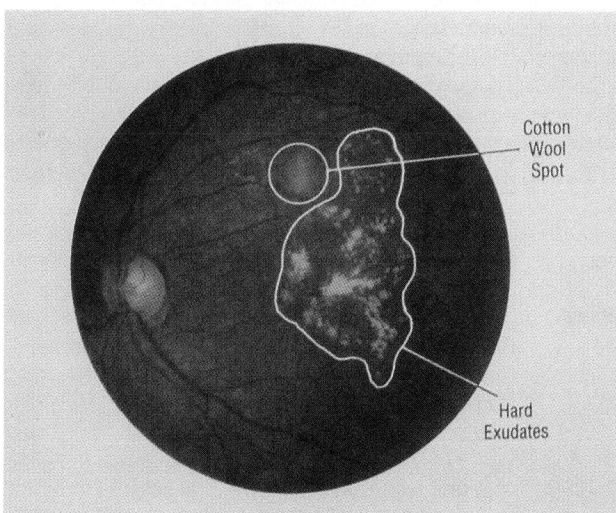

Figure 65-2 ● Select ophthalmic changes seen in nonproliferative diabetic retinopathy.

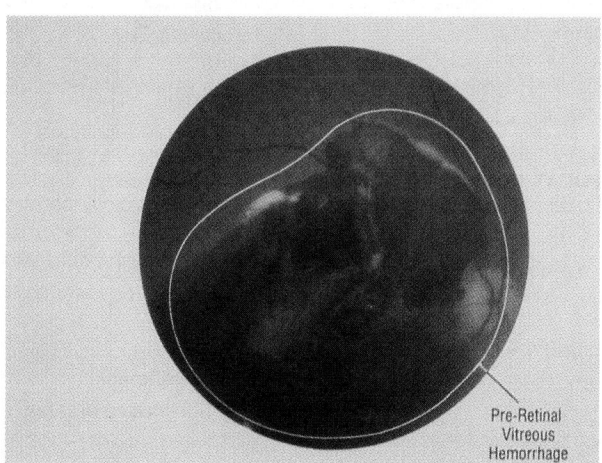

Figure 65-3 ● Ophthalmic hemorrhage that is possible with proliferative diabetic retinopathy.

DIABETIC NEUROPATHY. Neuropathy is a progressive deterioration of the nerves that results in loss of nerve function. Neuropathy is a common complication of diabetes and often involves all parts of the body. Damage to sensory nerve fibers results in either pain or loss of sensation. Damage to motor nerve fibers results in muscle weakness. Damage to nerve fibers in the autonomic nervous system results in widespread loss of many functions.

Diabetic neuropathy can be focal or diffuse, with each type having different causes, rates of progression, and treatments. The most common neuropathies among clients with diabetes are the diffuse neuropathies. **Diffuse neuropathies** involve generalized or widespread nerve function loss. These neuropathies have a slow onset, affect both sides of the body, involve motor and sensory nerves, progress slowly, and are usually irreversible. Diffuse neuropathies include autonomic nerve dysfunction. Late complications of diffuse neuropathies include foot ulcers and deformities.

Focal neuropathies are limited to a single nerve or nerve group. They are usually caused by a specific acute, ischemic event (ischemic neuropathy) or by the physical trapping of a nerve (entrapment neuropathy) within other tissues. Both types lead to nerve damage or nerve death. Ischemic neuropathies occur when the blood supply to a nerve or group of nerves is disrupted. The symptoms are sudden in onset, affect only one side of the body or body area, and are self-limiting in duration. Recovery time varies from nerve to nerve. Entrapment neuropathies occur because of compression of a nerve within a body compartment or between tissues. Symptoms are gradual in onset and can occur anywhere. They may be bilateral, having a waxing and waning course without spontaneous recovery. An example of focal entrapment neuropathy is carpal tunnel syndrome.

Insulin deficiency and hyperglycemia are thought to lead to neuropathy through blood vessel changes that cause inadequate oxygenation (hypoxia) to nerves. Both the axon and its myelin sheath are damaged by reduced blood flow, resulting in blocked nerve impulse transmission. Excessive glucose is converted to sorbitol, which accumulates in nerves. The increased sorbitol also slows motor nerve conduction. Commonly seen diabetic neuropathies are listed in Table 65-3. Neuropathy in the autonomic nervous system can lead to problems in cardiovascular, gastrointestinal (GI), and urinary function. Maintaining blood glucose levels within the normal range delays the onset and reduces the severity of diabetic neuropathies.

The cardiovascular problems of **orthostatic** (postural) hypotension and **syncope** (brief loss of consciousness), place the client with diabetes at risk for injury by falling. Common GI symptoms from diabetic neuropathy are **dysphagia** (difficulty swallowing), heartburn, nausea and vomiting, and bowel elimination problems. Diarrhea caused by diabetes is chronic, may be severe, often occurs at night, and may be associated with anal incontinence. Constipation, the most common GI symptom, is intermittent and may alternate with bouts of diarrhea. **Gastroparesis** (delay in gastric emptying) is a frequent cause of hypoglycemia. Loss of nerve input to the blad-

TABLE 65-3 • FEATURES OF DIABETIC NEUROPATHY		
	Complication	**Manifestation**
DIFFUSE NEUROPATHIES		
Distal symmetric polyneuropathy	Sensory alterations	Paresthesias: burning/tingling sensations, starting in toes and moving up legs Dysthesias: burning, stinging, or stabbing pain Anesthesia: loss of sensation
	Motor alterations in intrinsic muscles of foot	Foot deformities: high arch, claw toes, hammertoes; shift of weight bearing to metatarsal heads and tips of toes
Autonomic neuropathy	Anhidrosis	Drying, cracking of skin
	Gastroparesis	Delayed gastric emptying, constipation, nausea, anorexia
	Diabetic diarrhea	Diarrhea and bowel incontinence
	Neurogenic bladder	Atonic bladder, urinary retention
	Impotence	Erectile dysfunction
	Loss of cardiac reflexes	Orthostatic hypotension, resting tachycardia
	Defective counterregulation	Loss of warning signs of hypoglycemia
FOCAL NEUROPATHIES		
Focal ischemia	Thoracolumbar radiculopathy with sensory and reflex loss	Pain radiating across back, side, and front of chest or abdomen
	Cranial nerve palsies, third and sixth nerves	Sudden diplopia or ptosis; eye pain
	Amyotrophy	Pain; asymmetric weakness; wasting of iliopsoas, quadriceps, and adductor muscles
Entrapment neuropathies	Median nerve	Carpal tunnel syndrome
	Popliteal nerve/knee	Footdrop
	Posterior tibial nerve at tarsal tunnel	Tarsal tunnel syndrome: sensory impairment in sole of foot; weakness of intrinsic muscles of foot; burning pain and paresthesias at ankle and plantar surface

der results in incomplete emptying, which leads to urinary infection and kidney problems.

DIABETIC NEPHROPATHY. Nephropathy is the development of pathologic changes in the kidney that reduce kidney function and may lead to renal failure. Diabetes mellitus is the leading cause of end-stage renal disease (ESRD) and renal failure in the United States. Diabetic nephropathy develops in 40% of individuals with type 1 diabetes and in 50% of individuals with type 2 diabetes (Bell & Alele, 1999). Native Americans, Hispanics (especially Mexican Americans), and African Americans have much higher risks of developing ESRD than non-Hispanic whites. Renal failure is a common cause of death in clients with type 1 diabetes. Maintaining blood glucose levels within the normal range can delay the onset of diabetic nephropathy and, in some cases, may prevent it.

In addition to hyperglycemia, a genetic predisposition to kidney problems in a person with diabetes increases the risk for developing diabetic nephropathy. Examples of known or suspected genetic predisposition to kidney disease include a mutation of the gene for angiotensin-converting enzyme (ACE), polycystic kidney disease (see Chapter 71), and a family history of hypertension (Ravid, 1997). In addition, clients with diabetes who also produce excess collagen (such as people who form keloid scars) are at greater risk for developing diabetic nephropathy.

The earliest clinical sign of nephropathy is **microalbuminuria** (presence of very small amounts of albumin in the urine). The American Diabetes Association (ADA) recommends a test for microalbuminuria in clients who have had type 1 diabetes for at least 5 years and in all clients with type 2 diabetes.

Chronic high blood glucose levels cause hypertension in kidney blood vessels and excess kidney perfusion. The increased pressure damages the kidney in many ways. The blood vessels become more leaky, especially in the glomerulus. This leakiness allows filtration of larger particles (including albumin and other proteins), which then form deposits in the kidney tissue and blood vessels. Deposits narrow the vessels, decreasing kidney oxygenation and leading to kidney cell hypoxia and cell death. These processes worsen with the duration of diabetes. The blood vessels in the glomerulus become scarred and are unable to filter urine from the blood, leading to renal failure. After protein is found in the urine **(proteinuria),** progression to ESRD and renal failure is inevitable within the next 7 to 15 years.

Renal damage is also related to the mean arterial blood pressure increases seen as part of cardiovascular disease in diabetic clients. Both systolic and diastolic hypertension greatly accelerates the progression of diabetic nephropathy.

MALE ERECTILE DYSFUNCTION. Erectile dysfunction (ED) is defined as inability to achieve or maintain an erection sufficient for satisfactory sexual performance. ED occurs at a higher rate and at an earlier age among men with diabetes as compared with the general population. About half of diabetic men have ED. This occurs 10 to 15 years earlier than in the general population (Korenman, 1998). In diabetes, ED is related to poor blood glucose control, obesity, medically treated hypertension, heavy cigarette smoking, and the presence of other chronic microvascular and macrovascular complications of diabetes.

ED may be caused by neuropathy, vascular disease, psychologic factors, or accompanying endocrine disorders. Autonomic neuropathy and/or vascular changes are responsible for persistent ED in diabetes. Chapter 76 discusses erectile function problems in depth.

Etiology

TYPE 1 DIABETES

Type 1 diabetes is an autoimmune disorder in which beta-cell destruction in the pancreas occurs in a genetically susceptible individual (Table 65-4). In autoimmune disease, the immune

---

TABLE 65-4 • DIFFERENTIATION OF TYPE 1 AND TYPE 2 DIABETES

Features	Type 1	Type 2
Former names	Juvenile-onset diabetes Ketosis-prone diabetes Insulin-dependent diabetes mellitus (IDDM)	Maturity-onset diabetes Ketosis-resistant diabetes Non–insulin-dependent diabetes mellitus (NIDDM)
Age at onset	Usually under age 30 yr, occurs at any age	Peaks in 50s; may occur earlier
Symptoms	Abrupt onset, thirst, weight loss	Frequently none; thirst, fatigue, visual blurring, vascular or neural complications
Etiology	Viral infection	Not known
Pathology	Pancreatic beta-cell destruction	Insulin resistance Dysfunctional pancreatic beta cell
Antigen patterns	HLA-DR4, HLA-DR3	None
Antibodies	ICAs present at diagnosis	None
Endogenous insulin and C-peptide	None	Low, normal, or high
Inheritance	Recessive	Unknown
Nutritional status	Usually nonobese	60%-80% obese
Insulin	All dependent on insulin	Required for 20%-30%
Sulfonylurea therapy	None	Effective for most clients
Medical nutrition therapy	Mandatory	Mandatory

ICAs, Islet cell antibodies.

system fails to recognize normal body cells as "self" and takes destructive actions against them. In type 1 diabetes, immune system cells and cell products attack and destroy insulin-secreting cells within the islets. Although the exact cause or why a person's immune system would begin to attack normal body cells is not known, people with certain tissue types are more likely to develop autoimmune diseases, including type 1 diabetes. Specifically, people who have the tissue types HLA-DR3 and/or HLA-DR4 are at an increased risk for the development of type 1 diabetes. Certain viral infections, such as mumps, congenital rubella, and coxsackievirus infection, appear to be able to trigger autoimmune destruction of pancreatic beta cells.

Indicators, or **markers,** of immune damage to insulin-producing cells (a key feature of type 1 diabetes) are the presence of antibodies in the blood directed against the beta cells themselves or against substances made by the beta cells. Most clients with type 1 diabetes have islet cell antibodies (ICAs), autoantibodies to insulin (IAAs), autoantibodies to glutamic acid decarboxylase (GAD), and/or autoantibodies to tyrosine phosphates. Circulating ICA and IAA may be present before clinical manifestations of type 1 diabetes develop.

Risk for developing type 1 diabetes is determined by inheritance of the HLA-DR3 and HLA-DR4 genes. *It is important to remember, however, that although inheritance of these genes increases the risk, most people with these genes do not develop type 1 diabetes.* Development of the disease appears to be an interactive effect of genetic predisposition and exposure to the right environmental factors. In addition, it appears that the exposure must occur within a sensitive time period for it to enhance the predisposition. It is thought that the environmental exposure(s) insults or damages the beta cells of the pancreas, although time may be needed before the damage has the result of decreasing insulin production (Ilonen & Akerblom, 1999). The risk for developing type 1 diabetes in the general population ranges from 1 in 400 to 1 in 1000. The risk greatly increases for those people who have at least one parent with diabetes (from 1 in 20 to 1 in 50) (Funnell et al., 1998). It is unclear why some genetically susceptible people develop diabetes and others do not.

TYPE 2 DIABETES

Clients with type 2 diabetes have a reduction in the ability of most cells to respond to insulin **(insulin resistance),** poor control of liver glucose output, and decreased beta-cell function, eventually leading to beta-cell failure. Most people with type 2 diabetes are obese adults older than 40 years of age. The specific causes of type 2 diabetes are not known. Both insulin resistance and beta-cell failure have many genetic and nongenetic

Meeting
HEALTHY PEOPLE 2010
OBJECTIVES

DIABETES MELLITUS

Objective 18.4:   *Reduce the diabetes death rates (diabetes as the underlying cause) to no more than 12.0 per 100,000 persons.*

- Encourage all people to have a yearly screening physical examination that includes blood testing for diabetes.
- Inform all clients who have a sedentary lifestyle and who are overweight about the risk factors for and complications of diabetes.
- Assist diabetic clients who smoke to reduce or quit smoking.
- Instruct clients with diabetes mellitus to achieve and maintain body weight within 5 pounds of identified ideal weight for age and body size.
- Provide one-to-one education sessions, group education sessions, and printed and videotape information on diabetes treatment and care to clients diagnosed with diabetes.
- Educate clients about the specific medications prescribed to manage their disease.
- Demonstrate the use of the diet strategy individually planned for the client with diabetes.
- Encourage all clients with diabetes to participate in an individualized exercise program at least 3 days per week.
- Assist those clients with diabetes who also have hypertension to understand the importance of adhering to the prescribed drug therapies for both health problems.
- Instruct clients with diabetes to obtain annual vaccinations against influenza.
- Teach clients with type 2 diabetes to maintain adequate hydration, especially when any other illness is also present.
- Participate in mass screenings to identify people with undiagnosed type 2 diabetes among the general population.
- Develop culturally sensitive and literacy-appropriate education materials targeted to high-risk minority populations.

Objective 18.9:   *Reduce the frequency of foot ulcers in persons with diabetes.*

- Include foot assessment whenever caring for a client with diabetes.

- Include sensory testing of the feet for all clients with diabetes.
- Instruct the client with diabetes about proper foot care.
- Teach the client with diabetes the importance of always wearing protective footwear whenever the client is out of bed.
- Show the client the proper type of footwear to prevent foot injury.
- Find resources for those diabetic clients who are unable to afford properly fitting shoes.
- Teach the client how to monitor the circulatory status of his or her feet.
- Encourage the client to see a podiatrist twice a year.
- Refer the client with foot lesions to a wound management specialist.
- Encourage the client with diabetes who smokes to reduce or quit smoking.

Objective 18.23:   *Increase to 52% the proportion of persons with diabetes who have received formal diabetes education.*

- Evaluate the diabetes education materials and programs currently in place at your institution for currency, literacy, cultural sensitivity, and adequacy.
- Identify resources within your agency and community for diabetes education and support.
- Meet with the diabetes educator at your agency and establish means for collaboration and referral.
- If a diabetes educator is not available at your agency, work with existing personnel to enhance diabetes knowledge and awareness.
- Assist in policy-making decisions within your agency to develop a formalized teaching plan for all clients with diabetes, regardless of whether the clients are newly diagnosed or have had diabetes for a long time.
- Develop and offer diabetes education programs within your community in a variety of settings.

causes. Heredity plays a major role in the development of type 2 diabetes. Offspring of clients with type 2 diabetes have a 15% chance of developing the actual disease and a 30% risk of having impaired glucose tolerance. Specific gene defects have been identified in certain groups with high prevalence rates of type 2 diabetes. Pima Indians have a 50% prevalence of type 2 diabetes, with insulin resistance and hyperinsulinemia identified as a dominant trait (Funnell et al., 1998).

Incidence/Prevalence

Diabetes has become one of the most common chronic diseases in the United States. Diagnosed and undiagnosed diabetes affects 7% of all adults over the age of 20, with rates reaching 18.8% by age 60 (Harris et al., 1998).

The prevalence of diabetes has increased steadily over the past 40 years. In 1998 an estimated 10.5 million people had diabetes. About 90% of these individuals have type 2 diabetes. Diagnosed diabetes is most prevalent in middle-aged and older adult populations, affecting about 6% of people 45 to 64 years of age and 11% of those older than 65 years of age. Approximately 10% of clients diagnosed with diabetes are over 70 years of age. After the age of 40, new-onset diabetes is almost always non–insulin dependent. The prevalence of diabetes is similar for men and women.

Prevention

The fact that diabetes is a common disorder and causes many preventable but devastating complications makes the disease a major public health problem. The U.S. government has identified control of diabetes and its complications as a major focus for health promotion activities (see the Meeting Healthy People 2010 box on p. 1448).

Specific immune studies can accurately detect individuals who will develop immune-related type 1 diabetes. Measurement of ICA levels in relatives of clients with type 1 diabetes identifies those at risk for developing the disease. ICA measurement can predict 35% of relatives who will develop type 1 diabetes within 5 years and 60% to 70% of relatives likely to develop type 1 diabetes within 10 years (Dahlquist, 1999).

Treatment of increased blood glucose levels in clients who have glucose intolerance may help delay the onset of diabetes. Insulin therapy given to susceptible individuals appears to slow destruction of pancreatic beta cells. Sulfonylurea drugs decrease hyperglycemia and stimulate both insulin secretion and insulin action. Metformin (Glucophage), which inhibits intestinal absorption of glucose and improves insulin action, has been shown to be effective in preventing type 2 diabetes. Other interventions that prevent or delay diabetes include drug therapy to reduce the immune response and promote repair of deoxyribonucleic acid (DNA) damage. Immunosuppressive therapy can prolong the person's ability to secrete insulin. Nicotinamide (niacin) decreases the likelihood of diabetes caused by DNA damage.

Risk factors of obesity, physical inactivity, and a high-fat diet can be modified by behavioral changes. Weight reduction prevents type 2 diabetes. Reduced caloric intake improves insulin sensitivity, and weight reduction further improves insulin action. Low-fat diets, coupled with weight loss and increased exercise, have been shown to delay progression to type 2 diabetes in susceptible individuals. Studies are being conducted to determine if diabetes can be prevented or delayed through intervention with insulin during the "prediabetic" phase of the disease in high-risk relatives (ADA, 2000p).

CULTURAL CONSIDERATIONS

Certain ethnic groups have an increased risk of developing type 2 diabetes when compared with the U.S. population as a whole. African Americans have twice the risk of Caucasians for developing type 2 diabetes. The risk in Hispanics, especially those of Puerto Rican or Mexican origin, is approximately 2.5 times higher than the risk in Caucasians, whereas Native Americans show a fivefold increase in risk (Haffner, 1998a). Groups at high risk for type 2 diabetes are presented in Table 65-5.

The incidence and prevalence of type 2 diabetes have increased dramatically among Native Americans as a result of changes in physical activity and dietary habits. Obesity is a major risk factor for diabetes in Pima Indian tribes.

Harris et al. (1999) found racial and ethnic differences in glycemic control among U.S. adults with type 2 diabetes. Non-Hispanic black women and Mexican-American men were disproportionately represented among those with poor glycemic control. Minorities have a higher risk for complications even after adjusting for differences in blood glucose control.

CRITICAL THINKING CHALLENGE

You are caring for a 62-year-old woman who has had type 2 diabetes for more than 20 years. She is blind and has renal failure. Her 28-year-old daughter asks you what her own chances are for developing diabetes. The daughter reports that her 38-year-old sister has just been diagnosed with type 2 diabetes. You note that the daughter is 5 feet 8 inches tall and weighs about 140 pounds. She is a physical education teacher at a local high school and has a 1-year-old son.

- What personal questions should you ask the daughter to help determine her risk?
- Explain the genetics of type 2 diabetes.
- What tests (if any) might be helpful in determining this person's risk?
- How could the daughter reduce her risk or delay the development of the disease?

For suggested answer guidelines, go to SiMON http://www.wbsaunders.com/SIMON/Iggy/.

TABLE 65-5 • MAJOR RISK FACTORS FOR TYPE 2 DIABETES

- Family history of diabetes (parents or siblings)
- Obesity (more than 20% above a person's ideal body weight)
- Origin (African-American, Hispanic, Native American, or Asian-American)
- Age older than 45 years plus any of the preceding factors
- Previously identified impaired glucose tolerance or use of certain prescription drugs
- Hypertension (>140/90 mm Hg)
- High-density lipoprotein cholesterol levels <35 mg/dL (0.90 mmol/L) and triglyceride levels >250 mg/dL (2.82 mmol/L)
- History of gestational diabetes or delivery of infants weighing more than 9 pounds

Data from American Diabetes Association (2000). Position statement: Screening for type 2 diabetes. *Diabetes Care, 23*(Suppl. 1), 20-23.

► COLLABORATIVE MANAGEMENT
● Assessment

■ HISTORY

The nurse asks questions and collects data about risk factors, as well as symptoms related to diabetes. The client's age is important because type 2 diabetes is more common in older people, especially among African-American and Mexican-American clients. Women are asked how large their children were at birth because many women who develop type 2 diabetes had gestational diabetes or were glucose intolerant during pregnancy. These women often give birth to infants that weigh 9 pounds or more.

Assessing weight and weight change is important because excess weight and obesity are risk factors for type 2 diabetes. The client with type 1 diabetes often experiences weight loss with increased appetite during the weeks before diagnosis. For both types of diabetes, clients usually experience fatigue, polyuria, and polydipsia. They are asked about recent major or minor infections. In particular, women are asked about frequent vaginal yeast infections. All clients are asked if they have noticed whether small skin injuries become infected more easily or seem to take a longer time to heal.

The family history is explored for parents and siblings with diabetes. If the client has one or more relatives with diabetes, it is important to determine whether these relatives use insulin or control their disease with diet, exercise, and/or oral antidiabetic medications.

■ LABORATORY ASSESSMENT

BLOOD TESTS. The health care provider uses blood glucose values to diagnose diabetes. The nurse, the client, or a family member monitors the ongoing status of the disease by performing capillary blood glucose testing using a blood glucose meter. The physician and the nurse assess the overall result of treatment through review of glycosylated hemoglobin (hemoglobin A_{1c} [HbA_{1c}]) and fructosamine levels.

Instructions for blood glucose testing are presented in Chart 65-1. The American Diabetes Association (ADA) defines normal blood glucose values in Chart 65-2. ADA criteria for the diagnosis of adult diabetes mellitus are outlined in Table 65-6.

FASTING BLOOD GLUCOSE TEST. The results of the fasting blood glucose test are most accurate when the test is performed on blood obtained by venipuncture. The client should be fasting for at least 8 hours (water is permitted). The blood needs to be obtained before insulin or oral antidiabetic agents have been administered. A diagnosis of diabetes is made with two separate test results greater than 126 mg/dL (7 mmol/L) (ADA, 2000a).

ORAL GLUCOSE TOLERANCE TEST. The oral glucose tolerance test (OGTT) is the most sensitive test for the diagnosis of diabetes, although it is not routinely used, except in diagnosis of gestational diabetes. The test is inconvenient to clients, costly, and time consuming compared with the fasting plasma glucose measure. Before the test, the nurse reviews instructions from Chart 65-1 with the client. Carbohydrate intake restriction or bedrest before the test alters glucose tolerance. The client drinks a beverage containing a glucose load of 75 g, and blood samples are collected at 30-minute intervals for 2 hours. A di-

---

CHART 65-1

CLIENT EDUCATION GUIDE
Blood Glucose Testing

Fasting Plasma Blood Glucose
- Do not eat any food or drink any liquid for at least 8 hours.

Oral Glucose Tolerance Test
- Eat a balanced diet with carbohydrate intake of at least 150 g for a minimum of 3 days while maintaining normal physical activity.
- Carbohydrate restriction, bedrest, acute illness, and certain drugs interfere with the test. Phenytoin (Dilantin), anovulatory drugs, diuretics, nicotinic acid, and glucocorticoids adversely affect results.
- The test is performed in the morning after a 10- to 12-hour fast.
- A fasting blood sample is obtained.
- You will be asked to drink 300 mL (75 g) of a flavored beverage within 5 minutes of the fasting blood sample.
- Blood samples are drawn at 30-minute intervals for 2 hours.
- During the test, you will remain at rest and not be able to smoke or drink liquids.
- Report any signs suggesting hypoglycemia, such as weakness, dizziness, nervousness, and confusion.

CHART 65-2

LABORATORY PROFILE
Blood Glucose Values

Test	Normal Range for Adults	Significance of Abnormal Results
Fasting blood glucose test	<110 mg/dL (6.1 mmol/L) *Older Adults:* Levels rise 1 mg/dL per decade with age.	Levels >126 mg/dL (7.0 mmol/L) obtained on at least two occasions are diagnostic of diabetes, even in older adults.
Glucose tolerance test (2-hour post-load result)	<140 mg/dL (7.8 mmol/L)	Levels >140 mg/dL (7.8 mmol/L) and <200 mg/dL (11.1 mmol/L) indicate impaired glucose tolerance. Levels >200 mg/dL (11.1 mmol/L) indicate provisional diagnosis of diabetes.
Glycosylated hemoglobin (hemoglobin A_{1c} [HbA_{1c}]) test	4% to 6%	Levels over 8% indicate poor diabetic control with need for adherence to regimen or changes in therapy.

Data from American Diabetes Association. (2000). Committee report: Report of the Expert Committee on the Diagnosis and Classification of Diabetes Mellitus. *Diabetes Care, 23*(Suppl. 1), 4-19, and American Diabetes Association. (2000). Position statement: Tests for glycemia in diabetes. *Diabetes Care, 23*(Suppl. 1), 80-82.

---

agnosis of diabetes is made if the venous blood glucose is greater than 200 mg/dL (11.1 mmol/L) at 120 minutes.

GLYCOSYLATED HEMOGLOBIN ASSAYS. Glycosylated hemoglobin (HbA_{1c}) is the best indicator of the average blood glucose level. Because glucose attaches to the hemoglobin molecule, measurement of HbA_{1c} indicates the average blood glucose level during the previous 120 days—the life span of the average red blood cell. HbA_{1c} testing can be used

TABLE 65-6 • CRITERIA FOR THE DIAGNOSIS OF TYPE 2 DIABETES

Symptoms of diabetes plus casual blood glucose concentration greater than 200 mg/dL (11.1 mmol/L). Casual is defined as any time of day without regard to time since last meal. The classic symptoms of diabetes include polyuria, polydipsia, and unexplained weight loss.

Or

Fasting plasma glucose greater than 126 mg/dL (7.0 mmol/L). Fasting is defined as no caloric intake for at least 8 hours.

Or

2-hour plasma glucose greater than 200 mg/dL during an oral glucose tolerance test. The test should be performed using a glucose load containing the equivalent of 75 g glucose dissolved in water.

NOTE: Each test must be confirmed, on a subsequent day, under similar circumstances.

Data from American Diabetes Association. (2000). Committee report: Report of the Expert Committee on the Diagnosis and Classification of Diabetes Mellitus. *Diabetes Care,* 23(Suppl. 1), 4-19.

to assess long-term glycemic control, as well as to predict risk for the development of chronic complications. Unlike results of the fasting blood glucose test, HbA_{1c} test results are not influenced by changing one's eating habits the day before the test. It is recommended that HbA_{1c} testing be performed at the time of initial diagnosis and at intervals frequent enough to permit evaluation of the therapeutic plan. Hemolysis, blood loss, and pregnancy all increase red blood cell turnover and reduce HbA_{1c} levels. Triglycerides and bilirubin interfere with the assay, leading to overestimation of HbA_{1c} levels in clients with hypertriglyceridemia. The ADA recommends HbA_{1c} testing at least twice a year in clients who are meeting treatment goals and have stable blood glucose control, and quarterly assessments in clients whose therapy has changed and who are not meeting glycemic goals (ADA, 2000t).

GLYCOSYLATED SERUM PROTEINS AND ALBUMIN. Serum proteins and albumin become increasingly glycosylated with elevated blood glucose levels in the same way that HbA_{1c} does. However, because serum proteins and albumin turn over in 14 days, compared with the 120 days of red blood cells, glycosylated serum albumin (GSA) and glycosylated serum proteins (GSP) can be used to indicate blood glucose control over a shorter period. These measures are useful in conditions in which tight control of blood glucose levels is necessary (e.g., pregnancy) or in short-term follow up of treatment changes (ADA, 2000u).

URINE TESTS

URINE TESTING FOR KETONE BODIES. Ketones are a waste product of fat metabolism. The presence of urine ketones may indicate impending ketoacidosis. The ADA recommends testing urine for ketones during acute illness or stress, when blood glucose levels are consistently greater than 300 mg/dL (>16.7 mmol/L), during pregnancy, or when any symptoms of ketoacidosis are present (ADA, 2000u). Ketone testing is recommended for diabetic clients participating in a weight loss program.

TESTS FOR RENAL FUNCTION. The presence of urine protein when no symptoms of renal problems are present may

indicate microvascular changes in the kidney. Urine albumin excretion rates of 20 to 200 g/min (30 to 300 mg/hr) indicate microalbuminuria. Even minor elevations of albumin excretion are associated with increased mortality.

Once clinical proteinuria has been detected, kidney function (e.g., glomerular filtration rate) is assessed by creatinine clearance tests (see Chapter 69). In clients with known nephropathy, a rise in serum creatinine levels is related to both poor blood glucose control and hypertension.

URINE TESTING FOR GLUCOSE. Indirect measures of blood glucose may be obtained through urine testing for glucose, although this method is less precise than blood glucose testing. Fluid intake, urine concentration, time interval since last voiding, and certain drugs affect the results (ADA, 2000u).

OTHER DIAGNOSTIC ASSESSMENTS

The presence of certain autoantibodies can accurately indicate if a person will develop type 1 diabetes. Measurement of islet cell antibody (ICA) levels of relatives of clients with type 1 diabetes identifies those at high risk for diabetes development (Dahlquist, 1999). Insulin autoantibody (IAA) levels correlate with the rate of progression to diabetes and the age at which type 1 diabetes develops (the younger the age at which diabetes develops and/or the faster the progression to diabetes, the higher the level of IAA). Measurement of C-peptide levels indicates beta secretory function of the pancreas. C-peptide levels correlate well with insulin levels.

● Analysis

COMMON NURSING DIAGNOSES AND COLLABORATIVE PROBLEMS

The following are common nursing diagnoses for clients with diabetes:

1. Risk for Injury related to hyperglycemia
2. Risk for Injury related to stress of surgery
3. Risk for Injury related to sensory alterations (diabetic neuropathy)
4. Chronic Pain related to peripheral nerve dysfunction (diabetic neuropathy)
5. Risk for Injury related to visual sensory-perceptual alterations (diabetic retinopathy)
6. Ineffective Renal Tissue Perfusion related to the renal effects of vascular abnormalities (diabetic nephropathy)

The following are primary collaborative problems:

1. Potential for Hypoglycemia
2. Potential for Diabetic Ketoacidosis
3. Potential for Hyperglycemic-Hyperosmolar Nonketotic Syndrome

ADDITIONAL NURSING DIAGNOSES AND COLLABORATIVE PROBLEMS

In addition to the common nursing diagnoses and collaborative problems, clients with diabetes may have one or more of the following:

• Imbalanced Nutrition: More Than Body Requirements related to an imbalance of food intake and physical activity, lack of knowledge, and ineffective coping skills

- Risk for Deficient Fluid Volume related to fluid shifts, failure of regulatory mechanisms, hyperglycemic osmotic diuresis, polyuria, vomiting, diarrhea, decreased oral intake, and dehydration
- Acute Pain related to insulin injections or capillary blood glucose testing
- Impaired Oral Mucous Membrane related to microvascular circulatory changes and uncontrolled blood glucose levels
- Deficient Knowledge related to a lack of familiarity with information resources about the disease process, diet, exercise, medications, weight control, and mouth care
- Impaired Urinary Elimination and Urinary Retention (with Overflow Incontinence) related to diabetic neuropathy
- Constipation related to diabetic neuropathy
- Diarrhea related to diabetic neuropathy
- Risk for Impaired Skin Integrity related to decreased circulation, increased blood glucose levels, decreased mobility, and decreased sensation
- Risk for Infection related to increased blood glucose levels, decreased tissue perfusion, inadequate primary defenses (e.g., breaks in skin integrity), and the effects of chronic disease
- Risk for Infection related to wounds, urinary tract infection, intravenous (IV) access site, or oral mucous membranes
- Risk for Ineffective Sexuality Patterns (Male) related to autonomic neuropathy, decreased circulation, or psychologic problems
- Risk for Ineffective Sexuality Patterns (Female) related to the physical and psychologic stressors of diabetes
- Sexual Dysfunction related to impotence, impaired lubrication, painful intercourse with the changes in neurologic control of the genitalia, the effects of actual or perceived limitations imposed by the disease or therapy, and altered self-concept
- Situational Low Self-Esteem related to an inability to deal with the self-care demands of the diabetic regimen
- Anxiety related to the diagnosis of diabetes, potential complications of diabetes, and self-care regimens
- Fear related to the diagnosis of diabetes, potential complications of diabetes, and self-care regimens
- Ineffective Coping and Compromised Family Coping related to a chronic disease, a complex self-care regimen, and decreased social support
- Powerlessness related to the complications of diabetes (blindness, amputations, renal failure, and neuropathy)
- Social Isolation related to visual impairment or blindness
- Noncompliance with self-care related to the complexity and chronicity of the prescribed regimen
- Ineffective Health Maintenance related to insufficient knowledge of ADA exchange diet, weight control, weight maintenance, benefits and risks of exercise, self-monitoring of blood glucose, medications, sick-day care, foot care, hypoglycemia, and available resources

● Planning and Implementation

The management of diabetes mellitus is complicated and involves considerable client cooperation and education. The Concept Map on p. 1453 highlights care issues for the client with type 2 diabetes mellitus.

■ RISK FOR INJURY RELATED TO HYPERGLYCEMIA

NOC **PLANNING: EXPECTED OUTCOMES.** The client with diabetes is expected to maintain blood glucose levels in the expected range and avoid acute and chronic complications of diabetes.

INTERVENTIONS. The treatment of diabetes uses nonsurgical and surgical interventions.

NONSURGICAL MANAGEMENT. Nonsurgical management of diabetes mellitus involves dietary interventions, monitoring of blood glucose levels, a planned exercise program, and in some instances, medications to lower blood glucose levels. The nurse, in collaboration with the client, physician, dietitian, pharmacist, and in some cases, physical therapist, plans, organizes, and delivers care.

The American Diabetes Association (ADA) has proposed the following treatment goals in relation to glycosylated hemoglobin (HbA_{1c}) and blood glucose levels (ADA, 2000t):
- HbA_{1c} levels should be maintained at 7% or below.
- The majority of premeal blood glucose levels should be 80 to 120 mg/dL (4.4 to 6.7 mmol/L).
- Blood glucose values at bedtime should be between 100 and 140 mg/dL (5.6 to 7.8 mmol/L).

> ### 🌱 CONSIDERATIONS FOR OLDER ADULTS
> The primary aim of therapy in the older diabetic client is to maintain quality of life by maintaining blood glucose levels in the range that avoids both hypoglycemia and hyperglycemia. This precaution may require an aggressive therapy program with insulin in cases where the effects of uncontrolled hyperglycemia are greater than the risk of hypoglycemia occurring as a result of the therapy.

DRUG THERAPY. Medication administration is indicated when a client with type 2 diabetes does not have blood glucose control with dietary modification, regular exercise, and stress management. See Table 65-7 for the cost of diabetes medications.

Oral Therapy. Oral agents are prescribed only after dietary control has been shown to be insufficient.

Sulfonylurea Agents. Sulfonylurea agents are appropriate only for clients with some remaining pancreatic beta-cell function. These drugs stimulate insulin secretion (which reduces liver glucose output and increases cell uptake of glucose) and enhance the number or sensitivity of receptor sites on the cell for interaction with insulin. These drugs differ in strength, overall effects, metabolism, and risk for complications (Chart 65-3).

Hypoglycemia is the most serious complication of sulfonylurea therapy. Hypoglycemic episodes are more likely to occur with chlorpropamide (Diabinese, Novopropamide) because of its long duration of action. Underweight older clients with cardiovascular, liver, or kidney impairment are more susceptible to hypoglycemia.

Other, less common side effects include hematologic reactions (leukopenia, thrombocytopenia, hemolytic anemia), allergic skin reactions, and gastrointestinal (GI) effects (nausea, epigastric fullness, heartburn). In addition, many drugs can potentiate or interfere with the actions of sulfonylurea agents (Table 65-8).

Concept Map: Diabetes Mellitus Type 2

Key:

Interventions

Nursing diagnosis

Clinical manifestations

Pathophysiology

Ineffective tissue perfusion:
Cardiac
Renal
Peripheral
Cerebral

Risk for injury

Nutrition
Weight reduction
No concentrated sweets
Low fat
Low sodium

Control blood sugar with:
1. Second-generation sulfonylureas (Glipizide)
2. Biguanides (Metformin)
3. Alpha-glucosidase inhibitors (Acarbose)
Insulin if needed
Aspirin

Hyperglycemia
Hypoglycemia

Fasting blood sugar >128 mg/dL
Elevated postprandial blood sugar
Elevated triglycerides

Hemoglobin A$_{1C}$ 3-4 times/yr
Periodic lipid profiles
Routine blood glucose monitoring

Renal
Nephropathy
Male erectile dysfunction

Thirst
Fatigue
Weight loss

Visual blurring

Routine eye examinations

Diabetes Mellitus
Type 2

Excess production of glucose
Insulin deficiency
Insulin resistance
Age >45
>20% over ideal body weight
Family history of diabetes mellitus type 2
Hypertension
Race

Cardiovascular
Peripheral arterial disease
Cerebrovascular disease
Cardiovascular disease
Retinopathy

Control blood pressure
Stop smoking
Exercise 20-45 min/day,
3-4 times/week,
especially walking

Neurologic
Neuropathy
Neurogenic bladder
Vagal dysfunction

Pain

Foot care
Well-fitting shoes

Deficient knowledge

TABLE 65-7 • COST OF DIABETES MEDICATIONS

Medications	Specific Product	Size	Price
Humulin insulins	All products except Humulin R U-500:	100 units/mL, 10-mL vial	$20.81*
		1.5-mL cartridge, 5	$25.28*
	Humulin R U-500:	20-mL vial	$149.72*
Humalog insulin	Insulin lispro	100 units/mL, 10-mL vial	$28.55
		1.5-mL cartridge, 5	$35.32
Iletin insulins	Iletin I beef	100 units/mL, 10-mL vial	$19.44*
	Iletin II pork	100 units/mL 10-mL vial	$34.88*
Sulfonylurea agents	Chlorpropamide	100 mg, 100	$21.97 (generic brand)
		250 mg, 100	$35.37 (generic brand)
	Glipizide	5 mg, 100	$15.64 (generic brand)
	Glyburide	1.5 mg, 100	$24.96 (generic brand)
		3 mg, 100	$31.37 (generic brand)
	Glimepiride	1 mg, 100	$22.60
		4 mg, 100	$69.10
Nonsulfonylurea agents	Metformin	500 mg, 100	$54.82
	Repaglinide	0.5 mg, 100	$55.83
		2 mg, 100	$79.03
	Acarbose	100 mg, 100	$64.42
	Pioglitazone	15 mg, 90	$236.24
		30 mg, 90	$372.01
	Rosiglitazone	4 mg, 90	$191.75
		8 mg, 90	$348.08

Data from *1998 Drug Topics Red Book*. (1998). Montvale, NJ: Medical Economics Company; and http://www.planetrx. com.
*Average wholesale price.

CHART 65-3

DRUG THERAPY *for* **Diabetes Mellitus: Oral Blood Glucose Lowering Agents**

Drug	Dosage and Duration	Nursing Interventions	Rationale
FIRST-GENERATION SULFONYLUREA AGENTS			
Acetohexamide (Dymelor✦, Dimelor✦)	*Usual:* 0.25-1.5 g/day *Maximum:* 1.5 g/day *Duration:* 12-24 hr	Emphasize need for regular eating habits and patterns. Monitor renal function.	There is a high incidence of hypoglycemia in diabetic clients with renal impairment. Older clients can develop exaggerated hypoglycemia responses.
Chlorpropamide (Diabinese, Novo-propamide✦)	100-500 mg q24h *Maximum:* 500 mg/day *Duration:* 24-60 hr	Emphasize need for regular eating habits and patterns. Monitor weight and intake and output patterns.	The long half-life of the drug is associated with a high incidence of hypoglycemia. There is an increased potential for severe hyponatremia.
Tolazamide (Tolinase)	100-500 mg q12-24h *Maximum:* 2000 mg/day *Duration:* 12-24 hr	Administer with meals.	Taking with meals helps to avoid gastrointestinal upset.
Tolbutamide (Orinase, Mobenol✦)	750-1500 mg q12-24h *Maximum:* 3000 mg/day *Duration:* 6-10 hr	Administer 30 min before meals. Monitor weight and intake and output patterns.	Taking 30 min before meals gives the best reduction in postprandial hyperglycemia. Use with caution in patients with renal failure.
SECOND-GENERATION SULFONYLUREA AGENTS			
Glipizide (Glucotrol)	2.5-5 mg q12-24h *Maximum:* 40 mg/day *Duration:* 12-24 hr	Administer 30 min before meals.	The long half-life of the drug is associated with a high incidence of hypoglycemia.
Glyburide (DiaBeta✦)	1.25 to 20 mg/day *Maximum:* 20 mg/day *Duration:* 24 hr	Administer with first main meal. Emphasize need for regular eating habits and patterns.	Administration with food helps reduce gastrointestinal side effects. Hypoglycemia is more likely to occur with insufficient caloric intake.
Glimepiride (Amaryl)	1-4 mg once daily *Maximum:* 8 mg/day *Duration:* 24 hr	Administer with first main meal. Emphasize need for regular eating habits and patterns.	Individuals with impaired renal function are more sensitive to blood glucose–lowering effects of glimepiride.

CHART 65-3

DRUG THERAPY *for* Diabetes Mellitus: Oral Blood Glucose Lowering Agents—cont'd

Drug	Dosage and Duration	Nursing Interventions	Rationale
NONSULFONYLUREA AGENTS			
Metformin (Glucophage)	500 mg bid or 850 mg once a day *Maximum:* 2550 mg/day *Duration:* 12 hr	Administer with food. Monitor weight and intake and output patterns.	Primary side effects are nausea, diarrhea, and abdominal discomfort. Use with caution in patients with renal failure. Lactic acidosis occurs with greater frequency in patients with impaired renal function.
Repaglinide (Prandin)	0.5-2 mg *Maximum:* 16 mg/day *Duration:* 2-3 hr	Administer 30 min before meals.	Taking 30 min before meals gives the best reduction in postprandial hyperglycemia.
ALPHA-GLUCOSIDASE INHIBITORS			
Acarbose (Precose)	Individualized *Maximum:* 100 mg tid *Duration:* 2-4 hr	Instruct client to take with the first bite of each main meal.	Acarbose must be taken at the beginning of a meal to be fully effective.
Miglitol (Glyset)	Individualized Usual dose: 50 mg tid *Maximum:* 100 mg tid *Duration:* ≈1 hr	Instruct client to take with the first bite of each main meal. Monitor renal function.	Glyset must be taken at the beginning of a meal to be fully effective. Drug may accumulate in clients with renal dysfunction; not recommended for clients with serum creatinine greater than 2 mg/dL.
THIAZOLIDINEDIONES			
Pioglitazone (Actos)	15-30 mg once a day *Maximum:* 45 mg daily	Emphasize need for liver function tests as recommended. Emphasize need to report symptoms of unexplained nausea, vomiting, abdominal pain, fatigue, anorexia, or dark urine. Advise women of childbearing age to use adequate contraception.	Rare cases of liver failure have occurred with pioglitazone. Liver function tests are measured at start of therapy and at regular times thereafter. Administration of troglitazone with certain oral contraceptives may reduce the plasma concentration of the oral contraceptive.
Rosiglitazone (Advandia)	4 mg daily *Maximum:* 8 mg	Emphasize need for liver function tests as recommended. Instruct client to report signs and symptoms of nausea, vomiting, abdominal pain, fatigue, anorexia, or dark urine. Advise women of childbearing age to use adequate contraception.	Rare cases of liver failure have occurred with rosiglitazone. Liver function tests are measured at start of therapy and at regular times thereafter. Improved insulin sensitivity may allow ovulation to resume, increasing the chance of pregnancy.
D-PHENYLALANINE DERIVATIVES			
Nateglinide (Starlix)	*Usual:* 60-120 mg tid before meals *Maximum:* Optimal dose has not been defined *Duration:* 4 hr	Administer 1-30 min before meals. Instruct client to omit medication when skipping a meal.	Stimulates rapid secretion of insulin to reduce increases in blood glucose levels that occur soon after eating. Reduces the risk of hypoglycemia.

TABLE 65-8 • DRUG INTERACTIONS WITH SULFONYLUREA AGENTS

POTENTIATE HYPOGLYCEMIA	WORSEN HYPERGLYCEMIA
Allopurinol (Zyloprim)	Amphetamines
Ammonium chloride	Asparaginase (Elspar)
Androgens (testosterone [Testoderm])	Bumetanide (Bumex)
Angiotensin-converting agents (captopril [Capoten], enalapril [Vasotec])	Calcium channel blockers (diltiazem, nifedipine)
Anticoagulants, oral (dicumarol)	Cholestyramine (Questran)
Antifungal azoles, systemic (fluconazole [Diflucan], miconazole [Monistat])	Chlorthalidone (Hygroton)
Barbiturates	Clonidine (Catapres)
Beta-adrenergic blocking agents (atenolol, propranolol)	Corticosteroids (prednisone)
Bromocriptine	Corticotropin (ACTH)
Calcium channel blockers (verapamil)	Danazol (Danocrine)
Clofibrate (Atromid-S)	Diazoxide, parenteral (Hyperstat)
Disopyramide (Norpace)	Dextrothyroxine (Choloxin)
Ethanol	Diuretics, thiazide (hydrochlorothiazide)
Fenfluramine (Pondimin)	Estrogen (Estrace, Premarin)
Fluoroquinolone anti-infectives (ciprofloxacin)	Estrogen-progesterone–containing oral contraceptives (Brevicon, Depo-Provera, Estrostep)
Guanethidine (Ismelin)	Furosemide (Lasix)
Histamine H$_2$ antagonists (cimetidine [Tagamet], ranitidine [Zantac])	Gemfibrozil (Lopid)
MAO inhibitors (phenelzine [Nardil])	Glucagon
Methyldopa (Aldomet)	Isoniazid (INH)
NSAIDs (indomethacin [Indocin], ibuprofen [Advil])	Lithium (Lithobid)
Octreotide (Sandostatin)	Morphine (morphine sulfate)
Probenecid (Benemid, Probalan)	Nicotinic acid (Nicolar)
Pyridoxine (vitamin B$_6$)	Pentamadine (pentamadine isethionate)
Quinidine (quinidine gluconate)	Phenothiazines (prochlorperazine [Compazine], trifluoperazine [Stelazine])
Quinine (quinine sulfate)	Phenytoin (Dilantin)
Sulfinpyrazone (Anturane)	Rifampin (Rifadin)
Sulfonamides (trimethoprim/sulfamethoxazole [Bactrim], sulfisoxazole [Gantrisin])	Salicylates (large doses)
Tetracycline	Thyroid hormones (liothyronine [Cytomel], levothyroxine [Levothroid, Synthroid])

Meglitinides. Repaglinide (Prandin) is an agent that has actions and adverse effects similar to those of sulfonylureas, although it binds to a different receptor site. The drug is taken before meals, has a rapid onset, and has a limited duration of action. Adverse effects associated with Repaglinide (Prandin) include hypoglycemia, GI disturbances, upper respiratory tract infection, arthralgia or back pain, and headache.

Biguanides. Metformin (Glucophage) lowers glucose by decreasing liver glucose release and by decreasing cellular insulin resistance. This drug does not stimulate insulin release, and when given alone, it does not cause hypoglycemia. Its major route of excretion is through the kidney and should not be given to anyone with renal disease (creatinine ≥1.5 in males, ≥1.4 in females). The drug should be withheld for 48 hours after administration of contrast material (Mahler & Adler, 1999).

Metformin can cause lactic acidosis in diabetic clients with renal insufficiency and should not be used with conditions that decrease oxygenation or decrease drug clearance, such as renal insufficiency, liver disease, alcoholism, severe congestive heart failure, severe peripheral vascular disease, or severe chronic obstructive pulmonary disease (Samos & Roos, 1998). The symptoms of lactic acidosis are often subtle and nonspecific. The nurse teaches the client to report symptoms of fatigue, unusual muscle pain, difficulty breathing, unusual or unexpected stomach discomfort, dizziness, lightheadedness, or irregular heartbeats to the primary care provider. Clients are instructed to take metformin with meals to reduce GI effects. The nurse cautions against alcohol intake because alcohol potentiates the effects of metformin on lactate metabolism.

Alpha-Glucosidase Inhibitors. Alpha-glucosidase inhibitors reduce postprandial hyperglycemia by slowing digestion and absorption of carbohydrate within the intestine. These agents inhibit enzymes in the intestinal tract, delaying the digestion of carbohydrate. The prolonged digestion time reduces the rate of glucose absorption and lowers postprandial blood glucose levels. The most frequent side effects are flatulence, diarrhea, and abdominal discomfort. There are two drugs in this class. Acarbose (Precose) is well tolerated when dosing is started at a low range (25 mg once daily to three times daily with meals) and increased slowly. At higher doses, symptoms of carbohydrate malabsorption are common. Miglitol (Glyset) should be taken three times daily at the start (with the first bite) of each main meal. Clients using alpha-glucosidase inhibitors as combination therapy may experience hypoglycemia secondary to insulin or sulfonylureas. Because these drugs interfere with the conversion of complex sugars to glucose during digestion, only simple sugars or milk is used for oral correction of hypoglycemia.

Thiazolidinedione Antidiabetic Agents. Thiazolidinediones enhance insulin action, thus promoting glucose utilization in peripheral tissues. They are known as "insulin sensitizers" and include rosiglitazone (Avandia) and pioglitazone (Actos). These drugs improve sensitivity to insulin in muscle and fat tissue and inhibit gluconeogenesis. They can be used in combination with a sulfonylurea agent or insulin to improve blood glucose control because their mechanisms of action are different. Clients taking any drug of this class should have liver function studies performed at the start of therapy and regularly thereafter because of potential liver damage. Clients with liver enzyme values more than 2.5 times higher than normal should not start therapy, and those with values more than 3 times higher should have the drug discontinued (Rosiglitazone, 1999). All drugs in this class have effects on serum lipids.

Other side effects of this drug class include infection, headache, and pain. Administration of thiazolidinediones can reduce the effectiveness of oral contraceptives.

D-Phenylalanine Derivatives. Nateglinide (Starlix) lowers blood glucose by stimulating insulin secretion via interaction with the ATP-sensitive potassium channel on pancreatic beta cells. This action is dependent on functioning beta cells in the pancreatic islet cells. Nateglinide (Starlix) is rapidly absorbed and stimulates insulin secretion within 20 minutes of oral administration. It is taken just before meals to control mealtime hyperglycemia, resulting in improved overall glycemic control in clients with type 2 diabetes. Adverse effects include hypoglycemia, upper respiratory infection, and diarrhea. Clients who skip meals should also skip their scheduled dose of Starlix to reduce the risk of hypoglycemia.

Combination Agents. Newer oral agents combine drugs from two different classes. Glucovance, for example, combines the second-generation sulfonylurea glyburide with metformin. This combination of drugs is more efficient than either drug alone and decreases blood glucose levels at lower doses because these agents have different mechanisms of action.

Drug Administration. Drugs are started initially at the lowest effective dosage, and increases in dosage are made every 1 to 2 weeks until acceptable blood glucose control or maximal dosage is reached. If the maximal dosage does not control blood glucose levels, a different oral agent is used.

Antidiabetic drugs are not a substitute for dietary modification and exercise. The client is taught about the need for continuing dietary restrictions and regular exercise while taking antidiabetic medication. To avoid adverse drug interactions, the nurse teaches the client to consult with the primary care provider before using any over-the-counter drugs.

Drug Selection. The choice of oral antidiabetic drug is based on cost, the client's ability to manage multiple drug doses, and the client's age and response to the drugs. Sulfonylureas are less expensive than other oral antidiabetic agents, can be taken once daily, and are associated with few side effects. Metformin (Glucophage) is more expensive than sulfonylurea agents and is associated with GI side effects. Acarbose must be taken before each meal.

Beta-cell function often declines over time, reducing the effectiveness of oral antidiabetic drugs. The treatment regimen for the client with type 2 diabetes may eventually require insulin therapy either alone or in combination with oral agents.

Insulin Therapy. Insulin therapy is needed for type 1 diabetes and for moderate to severe type 2 diabetes. The safety of insulin therapy in older clients may be affected by decreasing vision, mobility and coordination problems, and decreased memory. There are many types of insulin and regimens, all aimed at achieving normal blood glucose levels.

Types of Insulin. Insulin is obtained from animal sources (beef or pork pancreas), combinations of animal sources and semisynthetic human insulin, and synthetic human insulin (made through recombinant DNA technology). There are differences in strength and onset of action between human insulin and animal-source insulin. Thus dose and timing adjustments are needed when a client changes from one type of insulin to the other. Human insulin tends to have a more rapid onset of action, a shorter peak action, and a shorter duration of action than animal-source insulin. Human insulin is preferred for pregnant women or women considering pregnancy, clients with allergies or resistance to animal-source insulins, clients beginning insulin therapy, and clients expected to use insulin only intermittently (ADA, 2000l).

Rapid-, short-, intermediate-, and long-acting forms of insulin can be injected separately or mixed in the same syringe. Insulin is available in concentrations of 100 units/mL (U-100) and 500 units/mL (U-500). U-500 is used only in rare cases of insulin resistance. U-500 and insulin lispro are the only insulins that require a prescription. Velosulin BR and Velosulin Human (both U-100 insulins) contain phosphate buffers for use with external insulin pumps. U-400 is being used in some implantable pumps on an experimental basis.

The nurse teaches the client that the insulin type and species, the injection technique, the site of injection, and the individual response can all affect the absorption, onset, degree, and duration of insulin activity. The nurse reinforces the information that changing insulins may affect blood glucose control and should be done only under careful supervision (ADA, 2000l). Table 65-9 reviews the types and sources of available insulin preparations, and Table 65-10 outlines the time activity of subcutaneous human insulin.

Insulin Regimens. Insulin regimens try to duplicate the normal release pattern of insulin from the pancreas. The pancreas produces a constant (basal) amount of insulin that balances liver glucose production with glucose use and maintains normal blood glucose levels between meals. The pancreas also produces additional (prandial) insulin, stimulated by food, that prevents postmeal blood glucose elevations. The insulin dose required for acceptable blood glucose control varies considerably among clients. A usual starting dose is between 0.5 and 1 units/kg of body weight per day. For multiple-dose regimens or continuous subcutaneous insulin infusion (CSII), basal insulin makes up about 40% to 50% of the total daily dosage, with the remainder divided into premeal doses of regular insulin. Dosage adjustments are based on the results of blood glucose monitoring. Because the rate of absorption is slowed by increasing the dosage, adjustments in dosage should be made no more often than every 3 to 4 days (Hirsh, 1998).

Most of the insulin regimens use NPH insulin for basal insulin coverage. Humulin U Ultralente insulin provides a lower basal rate and may be used instead of NPH insulin when frequent hypoglycemic episodes occur. Insulin glargine (Lantus), a long-acting insulin analog, is available for once-daily subcutaneous injection at bedtime to provide basal insulin coverage. The client determines the effect of long-acting insulin by monitoring fasting blood glucose values. Different insulin protocols (regimens or programs) are shown in Figure 65-4.

Single Daily Injection Protocol. Many clients inject insulin only once daily. This protocol may include only intermediate-acting insulin or a combination of short- and intermediate-

TABLE 65-9 • INSULIN PREPARATIONS

Type	Source
INSULIN ANALOG	
• Humalog (Lilly)	DNA technology
• Insulin aspart (Novo Nordisk)	DNA technology
SHORT-ACTING INSULINS	
Insulin injection (regular crystalline insulin):	
• Iletin II R (Lilly)	Pork (purified)
• Regular (Novo Nordisk)	Pork (purified)
Insulin human injection (regular human insulin):	
• Humulin R (Lilly)	DNA technology
• Novolin R (Novo Nordisk)	DNA technology
• Velosulin BR (Novo Nordisk)	Semisynthetic
• Velosulin BR (Novo Nordisk)	DNA technology
CONCENTRATED INSULIN	
Insulin injection (regular crystalline insulin):	
• Iletin II U-500 (Lilly)	Pork (purified)
INTERMEDIATE-ACTING INSULINS	
Isophane insulin suspension (NPH insulin):	
• Iletin II (Lilly)	Pork (purified)
• NPH pork (Novo Nordisk)	Pork (purified)
• Humulin N (Lilly)	DNA technology
• Novolin N (Novo Nordisk)	DNA technology
Insulin zinc suspension (Lente insulin):	
• Iletin II (Lilly)	Pork (purified)
• Lente L (Novo Nordisk)	Pork (purified)
• Humulin L (Lilly)	DNA technology
• Novolin L (Novo Nordisk)	DNA technology
FIXED-COMBINATION INSULINS	
• Humulin 50/50 (Lilly)	DNA technology
• Humulin 70/30 (Lilly)	DNA technology
• Novolin 70/30 (Novo Nordisk)	DNA technology
LONG-ACTING INSULINS	
• Humulin U (Lilly)	DNA technology
• Insulin Glargine (Aventis)	DNA technology
BUFFERED INSULINS FOR USE IN EXTERNAL PUMPS	
• Humulin BR (Lilly)	DNA technology
• Velosulin BR (Novo Nordisk)	Semisynthetic
• Velosulin BR (Novo Nordisk)	DNA technology

TABLE 65-10 • TIME ACTIVITY OF SUBCUTANEOUS HUMULIN INSULIN

Insulin	Onset	Peak	Duration
Rapid-acting (lispro insulin)	15-30 min	1-2 hr	3-4 hr
Short-acting (regular)	0.5-1 hr	2-4 hr	6-8 hr
Intermediate-acting (NPH, Lente)	1-4 hr	4-12 hr	18-24 hr
Long-acting (Ultralente)	4-8 hr	18 hr	24-36 hr

Three-Dose Protocol. A combination of short- and inter-mediate-acting insulin is given before breakfast, short-acting insulin is given before the evening meal, and intermediate-acting insulin is given at bedtime. Giving intermediate-acting insulin at bedtime results in lower fasting and after-breakfast blood glucose levels. This schedule avoids nighttime hypo-glycemia but may not provide enough coverage for the noon meal (Funnell et al., 1998).

Four-Dose Protocol. Giving short-acting insulin 30 min-utes before meals allows the greatest amount of insulin to be present during the greatest insulin need. Basal insulin is pro-vided by twice-daily injection of intermediate-acting insulin or a bedtime injection of long-acting insulin. Injection of pre-meal short-acting insulin based on anticipated carbohydrate intake allows some highly motivated clients with type 1 dia-betes to have more flexibility in meal timing and size. Insulin lispro should be given within 15 minutes of eating a meal; peak action usually occurs within 30 to 90 minutes. Because this insulin duration of action is short, the client taking insulin lispro also requires longer-acting insulin for basal insulin re-quirements.

Combination Therapy. A combination of oral agents and intermediate-acting insulin is given to clients with type 2 dia-betes who do not have reasonable control of blood glucose levels with oral agents alone. Obese diabetic clients with higher fasting C-peptide levels may be more likely to respond to combination therapy than to single therapy.

Intensified Therapy Regimens. Intensified regimens are composed of a basal dose of intermediate-acting insulin and a bolus dose of short-acting insulin designed to bring the next blood glucose value into the target range. The client's blood glucose patterns determine insulin dosage. The frequency of blood glucose monitoring is based on the timed action of short- and intermediate-acting insulins and may be required as often as eight times daily. Blood glucose testing 1 hour af-ter meals and within 10 minutes before the next meal helps determine the adequacy of the bolus dose. The client deter-mines the effects of basal insulin by monitoring pre-evening meal and fasting blood glucose values. Blood glucose values at 3 AM can detect nighttime hypoglycemia and indicate ade-quacy of both short- and intermediate-acting insulin doses.

Clients on intensified insulin regimens need extensive ed-ucation to achieve target blood glucose values. The client needs to understand clearly how to self-adjust insulin doses and must understand nutrition therapy so that dietary flexibil-ity can be maintained within target blood glucose values.

acting insulin. A single dose of intermediate-acting insulin may not match the blood insulin level with food intake. When fasting glucose levels become elevated, a multiple-injection protocol should be considered.

Two-Dose Protocol. Combinations of short- and interme-diate-acting insulin are injected twice daily. Two thirds of the daily dose is given before breakfast, and one third is given be-fore the evening meal. Initially, intermediate-acting and regu-lar insulin are usually given in a 2:1 ratio, and the evening (or bedtime) dose is given in a 1:1 ratio. Changes in these ratios are then based on results of blood glucose monitoring. Disad-vantages of this schedule are that nighttime hypoglycemia is common and the blood glucose value in the morning is higher than desired (Hirsh, 1998).

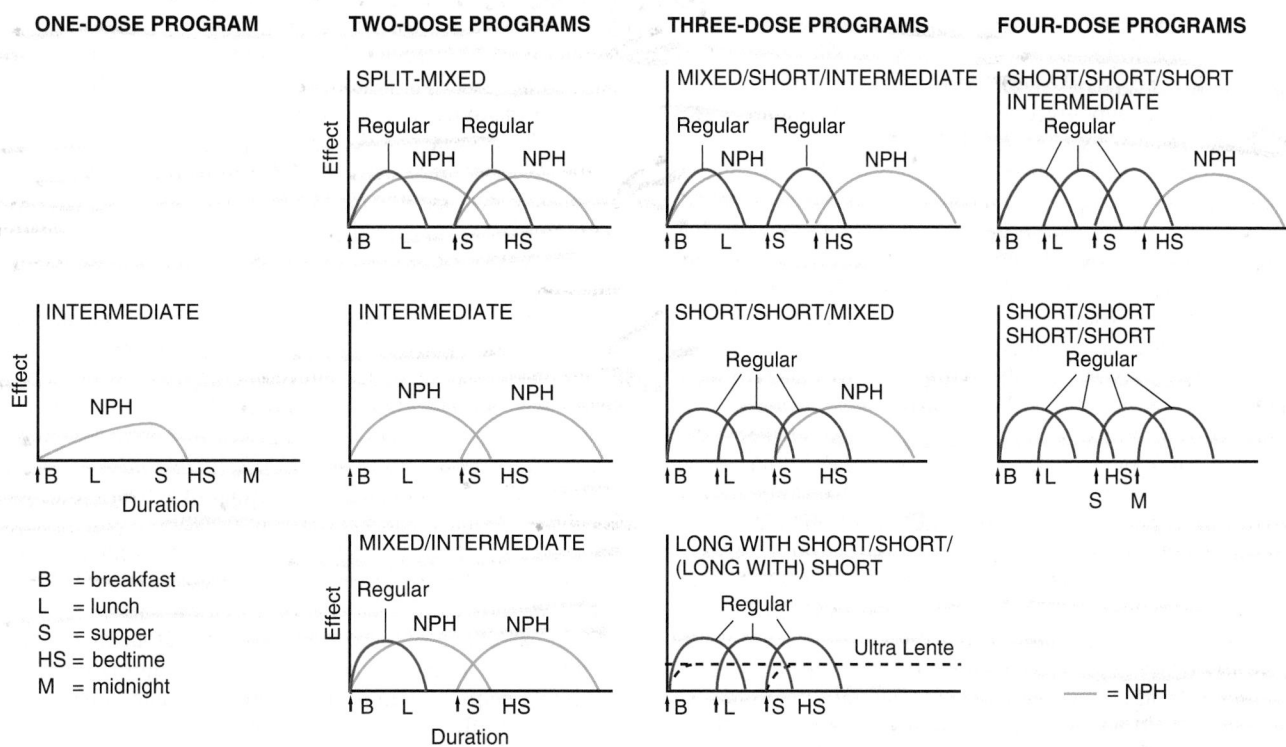

Figure 65-4 ● Insulin regimens. One injection a day of short-acting or intermediate-acting insulin may be enough to control blood glucose levels. However, split doses (two, three, or four injections of the daily dose) or split mixed doses (a mixture of short-acting and longer-acting insulins) may give better control.

Clients must also be able to perform blood glucose monitoring with precision so that therapy decisions can be based on accurate data.

Pharmacokinetics of Insulin. The action of insulin to move glucose into the cells after insulin injection depends on various factors, including physical factors and injection techniques.

Injection Site. Figure 65-5 shows common insulin injection sites. The site of injection affects the speed of insulin absorption. Absorption is fastest in the abdomen, followed by the deltoid, thigh, and buttocks. Rotating injection sites, either within one body area or between body areas, prevents **lipohypertrophy** (increased fat deposits in the skin) or **lipoatrophy** (loss of fatty tissue, leaving an uneven appearance). Rotation *within* one anatomic site is preferred to rotation from one site to another to prevent day-to-day changes in absorption. The abdomen (except for a 2-inch radius around the navel) is the preferred site of injection because it provides the most rapid insulin absorption.

Absorption Rate. Characteristics of insulin affect its absorption. The longer the duration of insulin action, the more unpredictable its absorption. Ultralente provides less consistent absorption than shorter-acting insulin preparations. The larger the dose of insulin, the more prolonged the absorption (Hirsh, 1998). Factors that increase blood flow from the injection site, such as local application of heat, massage of the area, and exercise of the injected area, increase insulin absorption. Scarred sites often become favorite injection sites because they are less sensitive to pain, but injection into scar tissue may delay absorption. Lipodystrophy does not affect the rate of insulin absorption (Burge & Schade, 1997).

Injection Depth. Injections are usually made into the subcutaneous tissue. Most individuals are able to lightly grasp a

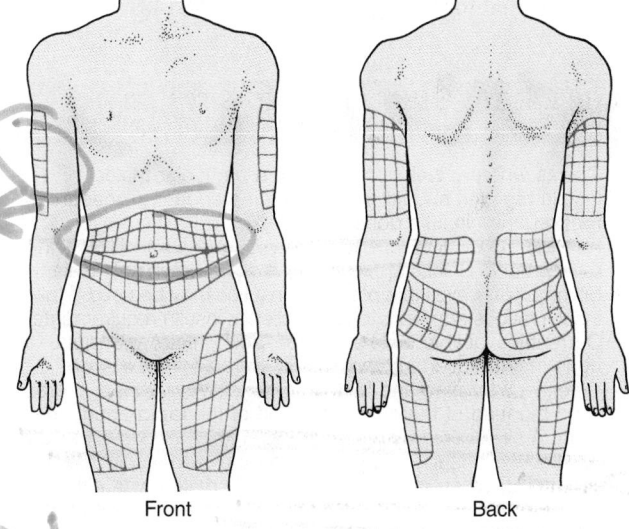

Figure 65-5 ● Common insulin injection sites.

fold of skin and inject at a 90-degree angle. Aspiration for blood is not necessary. Thin individuals may need to pinch the skin and inject at a 45-degree angle to avoid intramuscular (IM) injection. IM injection produces a slightly faster absorption than does subcutaneous injection but is not recommended for routine insulin administration because of the risk for hypoglycemia (ADA, 2000l). The nurse assesses the older client's ability to administer insulin and arranges for assistance when self-care is no longer possible.

Time of Injection. Injecting regular insulin 30 minutes before meals provides a greater amount of plasma free-insulin at

[handwritten annotation at top: Regular-short acting drawn 1st when mixed = long-acting insulin]

[handwritten annotation at left margin: I. lispro 15 min.]

mealtime. Eating within a few minutes after (or before) injecting short-acting insulin reduces insulin's ability to prevent rapid rises in postmeal blood glucose and may increase the risk of delayed hypoglycemia (Hirsh, 1998). Insulin lispro should be given 15 minutes before a meal.

Mixing Insulins. The nurse cautions clients that mixing different types of insulin can change the timing of peak insulin action. Mixtures of short- and intermediate-acting insulins produce a more normal blood glucose response in some clients than does a single dose of insulin. The client's response to mixed insulin may differ from the response to the same insulins given separately.

When rapid-acting (insulin lispro) or short-acting (regular) insulin is mixed with a longer-acting insulin, the shorter-acting insulin dose is drawn into the syringe first. This procedure prevents contamination of the shorter-acting insulin vial with the longer-acting insulin. Short-acting and NPH insulins may be used immediately when mixed, or they may be stored for future use. When rapid-acting insulin is mixed with either intermediate- or long-acting insulin, the mixture should be injected 15 minutes before a meal (ADA, 2001). *Insulin glargine (Lantus) must not be diluted or mixed with any other insulin or solution.* Mixing can result in a cloudy solution and an unpredictable alteration in both the onset of action and time to peak effect. The nurse follows American Diabetes Association (ADA) guidelines for mixing insulins (Table 65-11).

Complications of Insulin Therapy. Hypoglycemia, the result of excessive insulin levels, has a variety of causes. Manifestations and treatment of hypoglycemia are discussed later under Potential for Hypoglycemia, pp. 1478-1481.

TABLE 65-11 •	AMERICAN DIABETES ASSOCIATION GUIDELINES FOR THE MIXING OF INSULINS

- Clients who are well controlled on a particular mixed-insulin regimen should maintain their standard procedure for preparing insulin doses.
- No other medication or diluent should be mixed with any insulin product unless approved by the prescribing physician.
- Commercially available premixed insulins may be used if the insulin ratio is appropriate to the client's insulin requirements.
- Currently available NPH and short-acting insulin formulations may be used immediately or stored for future use.
- When rapid-acting and Ultralente insulins are mixed, there is no blunting of the onset of action of the rapid-acting insulin. A slight decrease in the absorption rate is seen when rapid-acting insulin and protamine-stabilized insulin (NPH) are mixed. When rapid-acting insulin is mixed with either an intermediate- or long-acting insulin, the mixture should be injected 15 minutes before a meal.
- Mixing of short-acting and Lente insulin is not recommended, except for a few clients already controlled on this mixture.
- On mixing, zinc present in Lente preparations binds with the regular insulin and delays its onset of action.
- Clients using Lente mixed with regular insulin should standardize the interval between mixing and injecting.
- Phosphate-buffered insulins (NPH) should not be mixed with Lente insulins. Zinc phosphate, present in NPH insulin, may precipitate and convert the longer-acting insulin to a short-acting insulin, with unpredictable results.
- There is no rationale for mixing animal insulins with human insulins.

Data from American Diabetes Association. (2000). Position statement: Insulin administration. *Diabetes Care, 23*(Suppl. 1), 86-89.

Hypertrophic lipodystrophy is a spongy swelling at or around the injection site. The condition occurs because of repeated injections in the same area. The overlying skin has decreased sensitivity, and the area can become large and unsightly. Treatment consists of rotating the injection site among different body areas. **Lipoatrophic lipodystrophy** is a loss of fat at or distant to the injection site and occurs as a reaction to beef or pork insulin. Treatment consists of injection of purified pork or human insulin at the edge of the lipoatrophic area.

Two conditions of fasting hyperglycemia can occur (Figure 65-6). **Dawn phenomenon** is thought to result from a nighttime release of growth hormone that causes blood glucose elevations at about 5 to 6 AM. Dawn phenomenon is treated by providing more insulin for the overnight period (e.g., administering the evening dose of intermediate-acting insulin at 10 PM). **Somogyi's phenomenon** is morning hyperglycemia secondary to an effective counterregulatory response to nighttime hypoglycemia. Somogyi's phenomenon is treated by ensuring adequate dietary intake at bedtime and evaluating the insulin dose and exercise programs to prevent conditions that precipitate hypoglycemia. Both phenomena are diagnosed by blood glucose monitoring during the night. The nurse helps to identify these problems and educates the client and family about management.

Alternative Methods of Insulin Administration. Many methods of insulin delivery are available in addition to traditional intermittent subcutaneous injections.

Continuous Subcutaneous Infusion of Insulin. Continuous subcutaneous infusion of a basal dose of insulin (CSII) with increases in insulin at mealtimes seems to be more effective in controlling blood glucose levels than a multiple-injection schedule. CSII allows for total flexibility in meal timing, because if a meal is skipped, the mealtime dose of insulin is not administered. CSII is administered by an externally worn pump containing a syringe and reservoir with rapid- or short-acting insulin and connected to the client by an infusion set. The nurse teaches the client to adjust the amount of insulin received on the basis of data from blood glucose monitoring.

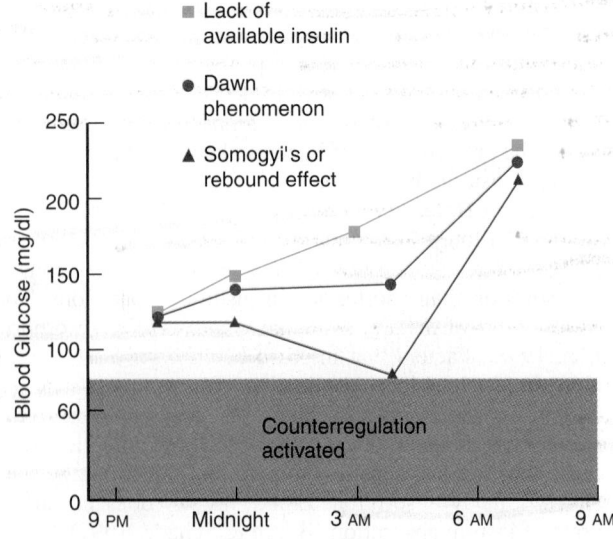

Figure 65-6 ● Three blood glucose phenomena in diabetic clients.

Lispro is an appropriate insulin for insulin infusion pumps. The stability of this insulin in both MiniMed and Disetronic pumps has been confirmed (Figure 65-7). Lispro is not approved for use in pregnancy (ADA, 2000c).

Skin infections may occur when the infusion site is not cleaned or the needle placement is not changed every 3 days. When the client is receiving rapid-acting insulin and has normal blood glucose levels, cessation of insulin administration quickly results in hyperglycemia. The use of CSII is associated with more frequent and more severe ketoacidosis than with other methods of insulin administration. Ketoacidosis is related to inexperience in using the pump, infection, accidental cessation of insulin infusion, infusion set obstruction, or mechanical problems related to the pump. Buffered insulin may be used to prevent the precipitation of insulin crystals within the catheter. The nurse stresses the importance of regular testing for the presence of ketones.

Intensive education for clients using CSII is necessary. Because of the potential for hypoglycemia, as well as hyperglycemia, the client must perform all necessary functions to ensure accurate insulin administration. The nurse teaches the client to operate the pump, make adjustments in settings, and respond appropriately to alarms. Removal of the pump for any length of time can result in hyperglycemia. The nurse provides supplemental insulin schedules for times when the pump is not operational. CSII is expensive, compared with traditional insulin injections, and not all costs are covered by insurance.

Implanted Insulin Pumps. Insulin pumps are implanted in the peritoneal cavity, where insulin can be absorbed by blood vessels in the peritoneum in a manner similar to that of natural insulin release (Figure 65-8). Absorption of insulin into the portal circulation is believed to reduce peripheral hyperinsulinemia. The pump is surgically implanted in a subcutaneous pocket in the lower abdomen. The pump reservoir is refilled with U-400 insulin every 1 or 2 months. The major complications of implanted insulin pumps (IIPs) have been catheter

blockage, inflammation in the subcutaneous pocket, and pump mechanical failure. Because mechanical problems associated with the pump, catheter, and insulin delivery have not been solved, the implantable pump is not widely available.

Injection Devices. In addition to traditional insulin syringes, injection devices include a needleless system and a pen-type injector. With a needleless device, the needle is replaced by an ultrathin liquid stream of insulin forced through the skin under high pressure. Insulin administered by jet injection is absorbed at a faster rate, with a resulting shorter duration of insulin action. How these changes affect overall metabolic control is yet to be determined. Cost is a primary drawback to this system.

Pen-type injectors hold small, lightweight, prefilled insulin cartridges. The injectors are easy to carry and make intensive insulin therapy with multiple injections easier to accomplish. These devices allow greater accuracy than traditional insulin syringes, especially when measuring doses lower than 5 units (Robertson, Glazer, & Campbell, 2000). The nurse discusses methods of maintaining the insulin cartridges at an appropriate temperature when using this device away from home. The nurse is cautious when recommending pen-type injectors for visually or neurologically impaired individuals. The packaging for all insulin pens includes a statement that they are not meant for independent use by visually impaired people (Williams, 1999b).

New Technology. Insulin absorption across the nasal mucosa is rapid, making nasal insulin delivery a possible alternative to parenteral injection. However only a small amount of insulin is actually absorbed through the mucosa, making blood glucose control inconsistent. A nasal spray, administered via nebulizer, is one new means of insulin administration. Studies are also underway to evaluate the effects of aerosolized insulin given by nebulized inhaler. Regular insulin (U-500) is delivered in an inhaler during inspiration (the lungs provide a large surface for absorption of insulin). Routine use of inhalers is imprecise and dependent on how the client times the dose with inhalation. Newer inhaler systems are being developed that trigger a precise dose of medication

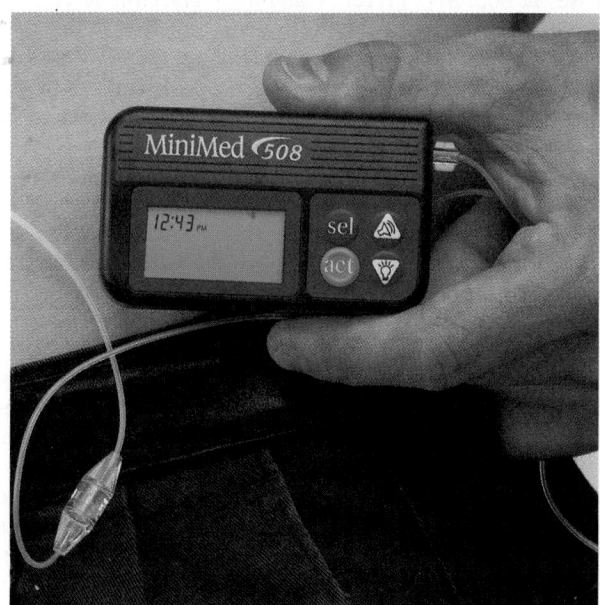

Figure 65-7 ● External insulin pump. (Courtesy MiniMed, Inc., Northridge, CA.)

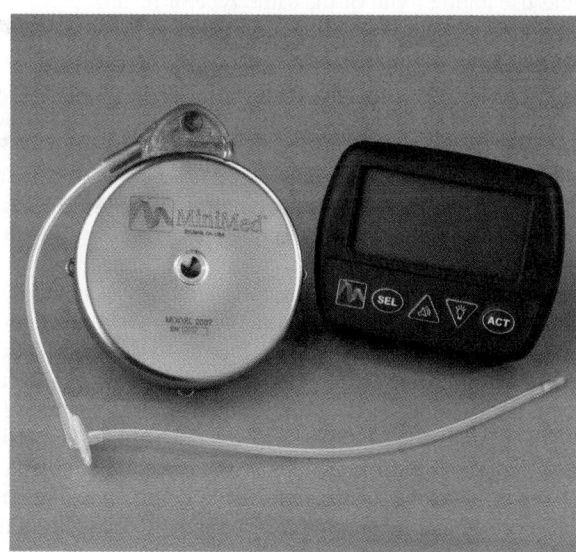

Figure 65-8 ● Internal insulin pump. (Courtesy MiniMed, Inc., Northridge, CA.)

at the time when airflow from inhalation reaches a certain rate (Saudek, 1997).

Transdermal (through the skin) delivery of insulin is being tested. This method of drug delivery appears to be predictable but slower than delivery with traditional injections (Robertson, Glazer, & Campbell, 2000).

NIC **Client Education: Prescribed Medication.** The nurse provides specific instructions to the client undergoing insulin therapy. Chart 65-4 lists NIC intervention activities for assisting with self-medication.

Storage. Insulin not in use should be refrigerated; refrigeration maintains potency, prevents exposure to sunlight, and inhibits bacterial growth. Insulin in use may be kept at room temperature to limit local irritation at the injection site, which may occur when cold insulin is used.

To prevent loss of drug potency, the client is taught to avoid subjecting insulin to temperatures less than 36° F (2.2° C) or greater than 86° F (30° C) or to excessive agitation. Ideally, insulin lispro is refrigerated but not frozen. The vial or cartridge of insulin lispro can be unrefrigerated for up to 28 days, as long as it is kept as cool as possible (not greater than 86° F [30° C]) and away from direct heat and light.

The client is instructed to always have a spare bottle of each type of insulin used. A slight loss in potency may occur after the bottle has been in use for more than 30 days even when the expiration date has not been passed. When refrigerated, prefilled syringes are stable up to 30 days. If possible, the syringes are stored in the vertical (upright) position, with the needle pointing upward, so that insulin particles do not clog the needle. The predrawn syringe should be rolled between the hands before administration. The primary care provider assesses the effect of premixing insulins on blood glucose control by examining blood glucose levels (ADA, 2000l).

Dose Preparation. The person administering the insulin inspects the bottle before each use for changes (e.g., clumping, frosting, precipitation, or change in clarity or color) that may signify loss in potency. Rapid- and short-acting insulins should be clear, and all other types of insulin should be uniformly cloudy after gently rolling the vial between the hands. If the potency of an insulin vial is questionable, the person should use another vial of the same type of insulin.

Syringes. Standard insulin administration involves subcutaneous injection with syringes marked in insulin units. Differences in the way units are indicated depend on the size of the syringe and the manufacturer. Some syringes are marked in 1-unit increments, and other syringes are marked in 2-unit increments. Syringes are manufactured in 0.25-, 0.3-, 0.5- and 1-mL capacity. The needle sizes range from 27 to 30 gauge. Needle lengths may be standard (12.7 mm), a very fine version (15.9 mm), or a short version (8 mm). Short needles are not used for obese clients because of variability of insulin absorption. To ensure accurate insulin measurement, the client is instructed to always buy the same type of syringes. Most insulin preparations have additives that inhibit growth of bacteria commonly found on the skin. Reuse of insulin syringes for the same client (*never between clients*) does not appear to increase the rate of skin infections at the injection site. Charts 65-5 and 65-6 review instructions for drawing up a single insulin injection and for mixing regular and NPH insulin in the same syringe (ADA, 2000l).

Client Education: Blood Glucose Monitoring. Self-monitoring of blood glucose levels (SMBG) provides information that allows the client to adjust therapy. The nurse teaches the client to use the physician's prescribed formulas to (1) self-adjust diet, exercise, or pharmacologic therapy; (2) identify and properly treat hyperglycemia and hypoglycemia; and (3) improve decision making and problem solving. See Table 65-12 for costs of blood glucose monitors and strips.

The American Diabetes Association (ADA) recommends SMBG for clients taking insulin or oral agent therapy. Ongoing knowledge of blood glucose levels is especially important for the following clients:

- Any diabetic client attempting to maintain glucose levels in the near-normal range
- Pregnant clients
- Clients with a tendency to develop severe ketosis or hypoglycemia
- Clients with hypoglycemic unawareness
- Clients undergoing intensive treatment programs, especially those using portable infusion devices, or taking multiple daily insulin injections

The operating principles of most self-monitoring systems are the same. The finger is pricked, and a drop of blood is made to flow over a reagent pad on a testing strip. Meters measure blood glucose by using color reflectance or sensor technology. With reflectance meters, the glucose in a drop of blood reacts with an enzyme in the strip, changing the color of the strip. The meter reads the color of the strip and gives a number for the blood glucose value. Meters that use sensor technology measure small electrical currents produced by the interaction between the glucose in the blood and the chemicals on the strip (Peragallo-Dittko, 1999). The client can also perform visual blood glucose monitoring by comparing the color on a test strip with the strip on the test strip vial.

There is some variation between glucose concentration in whole blood by SMBG systems and that measured by clinical laboratory procedures. The ADA has set the performance goal to be a total error of no more than 10% at glucose concentrations ranging between 30 and 400 mg/dL (1.6 and 22.2 mmol/L) (ADA, 1996). The accuracy of SMBG systems decreases at both hypoglycemic and hyperglycemic levels. The overall performance of SMBG systems depends on the accuracy of the specific blood glucose meter, operator proficiency, and test strip quality. Results may be influenced by the amount of blood on the strip; the meter's calibration to the strip currently in use; environmental conditions of altitude, temperature, and moisture; and client-specific conditions of hematocrit level, triglyceride concentration, and the presence of hypotension.

Most meters indicate blood glucose results as a number, but some have voice readouts, memories that can be displayed, or capabilities for graphic displays on a computer. A client's visual impairments, including color blindness, determine the method of SMBG selected. Some models have large, bold display screens and simple, user-friendly procedures. Other models use voice modules to announce the display messages.

The client and nurse follow Centers for Disease Control and Prevention (CDC) guidelines for infection control during SMBG. The chance of becoming infected from blood glucose monitoring processes can be reduced by handwashing before monitoring and not reusing lancets. Clients are instructed not to share their blood glucose monitoring equipment. Hepatitis B virus can survive in a dried state for at least 1 week. Infec-

CHART 65-4

NIC INTERVENTION ACTIVITIES *for*
The Diabetic Client with Hyperglycemia

Hyperglycemia Management: *Preventing and treating above-normal blood glucose levels*
- Monitor blood glucose levels, as indicated.
- Monitor for signs and symptoms of hyperglycemia: polyuria, polydipsia, polyphagia, weakness, lethargy, malaise, blurring of vision, or headache.
- Monitor urine ketones, as indicated.
- Monitor ABG, electrolyte, and β-hydroxybutyrate levels, as available.
- Monitor orthostatic blood pressure and pulse, as indicated.
- Administer insulin, as prescribed.
- Encourage oral fluid intake.
- Monitor fluid status (including I&O), as appropriate.
- Maintain IV access, as appropriate.
- Administer IV fluids, as needed.
- Administer potassium, as prescribed.
- Consult physician if signs and symptoms of hyperglycemia persist or worsen.
- Identify possible causes of hyperglycemia.
- Anticipate situations in which insulin requirements will increase (e.g., intercurrent illness).
- Restrict exercise when blood glucose levels are >250 mg/dL, especially if urine ketones are present.
- Instruct client and significant others on prevention, recognition, and management of hyperglycemia.
- Encourage self-monitoring of blood glucose levels.
- Instruct on urine ketone testing, as appropriate.
- Instruct client and significant others on diabetes management during illness, including use of insulin and/or oral agents, monitoring fluid intake, carbohydrate replacement, and when to seek health professional assistance, as appropriate.
- Provide assistance in adjusting regimen to prevent and treat hyperglycemia (e.g., increasing insulin or oral agent), as indicated.

Teaching: Prescribed Medication: *Preparing a client to safely take prescribed medications and monitor for their effects*
- Instruct the client to recognize distinctive characteristics of the medication(s), as appropriate.
- Inform the client of both the generic and brand names of each medication.
- Instruct the client on the purpose and action of each medication.
- Instruct the client on the dosage, route, and duration of each medication.
- Instruct the client on the proper administration/application of each medication.
- Evaluate the client's ability to self-administer medications.
- Instruct the client to perform needed procedures before taking a medication (e.g., check pulse, glucose), as appropriate.
- Inform the client what to do if a dose of medication is missed.
- Inform the client of consequences of not taking or abruptly discontinuing medication(s), as appropriate.
- Instruct the client on which criteria to use when deciding to alter the medication/dosage schedule, as appropriate.
- Instruct the client on possible adverse side effects of each medication.
- Instruct the client on how to relieve and/or prevent certain side effects, as appropriate.

- Instruct the client on appropriate actions to take if side effects occur.
- Instruct the client on the signs and symptoms of overdosage or underdosage.
- Inform the client of possible drug/food interactions, as appropriate.
- Instruct the client how to properly store the medication(s).
- Instruct the client on the proper care of devices used for administration.
- Instruct the client on proper disposal of needles and syringes at home, as appropriate, and where to dispose of the sharps container in their community.
- Provide the client with written information about the medication action, purpose, side effects, and so on.
- Assist the client to develop a written medication schedule.
- Instruct the client to carry documentation of his or her prescribed medication regimen.
- Instruct the client how to fill his or her prescription(s), as appropriate.
- Inform the client of possible changes in appearance and/or dosage when filling generic medication prescriptions.
- Warn the client of the risks associated with taking expired medications.
- Determine the client's ability to obtain required medications.
- Provide information on medication reimbursement, as appropriate.
- Provide information on cost savings programs/organizations to obtain medications and devices, as appropriate.
- Provide information on medication alert devices and how to obtain them.
- Reinforce information provided by other health care team members, as appropriate.
- Include the family/significant others, as appropriate.

Teaching: Prescribed Diet: *Preparing a client to correctly follow a prescribed diet*
- Appraise the client's current level of knowledge about prescribed diet.
- Determine the client's/significant other's feelings/attitude toward prescribed diet and expected degree of dietary compliance.
- Instruct the client on the proper name of the prescribed diet.
- Explain the purpose of the diet.
- Instruct the client about how to keep a food diary, as appropriate.
- Instruct the client on allowed and prohibited foods.
- Inform the client of possible drug/food interactions, as appropriate.
- Assist the client to accommodate food preferences into the prescribed diet.
- Assist the client in substituting ingredients to conform favorite recipes to the prescribed diet.
- Instruct the client about how to read labels and select appropriate foods.
- Observe the client's selection of foods appropriate to prescribed diet.
- Instruct the client about how to plan appropriate meals.
- Provide written meal plans, as appropriate.
- Reinforce information provided by other health care team members, as appropriate.
- Refer client to dietitian/nutritionist, as appropriate.
- Include the family/significant others, as appropriate.

NIC intervention activities selected from McCloskey J.C., & Bulechek, G.M. (2000). *Nursing interventions classification (NIC)* (3rd ed.). St. Louis: Mosby. No part of this work is to be altered without prior written permission from the Publisher.
ABG, Arterial blood gas; *I&O,* intake and output.

tion can be spread in the lancet holder even when the lancet itself has been changed. Small particles of blood can stick to the device and infect multiple users. Regular cleaning of the meter is important in infection control. Health care personnel who perform blood glucose testing and family members who assist with testing should wear gloves to provide protection from infection (American Association of Diabetes Educators, 1997).

Interpretation of Results. Accuracy of blood glucose measurements may be reduced by errors in technique, equip-

ment failure, or misrepresentation. The data obtained from SMBG are evaluated together with other measures of blood glucose levels (e.g., glycosylated hemoglobin, or hemoglobin A_{1c} [HbA_{1c}], values) or periodic laboratory blood glucose tests. Even when SMBG is performed correctly, the results are affected by hematocrit values (anemia falsely elevates hematocrit values; polycythemia falsely depresses them) and may be unreliable in the hypoglycemic or severe hyperglycemic ranges. Accuracy of the meter itself is also an issue. Even when highly trained personnel tested meters under optimal conditions, there was wide variation in accuracy and precision between capillary blood glucose monitoring devices approved for the clinical market. Laboratory glucose determinations are more accurate than SMBG.

Frequency of Testing. The frequency of monitoring varies with the complexity of the medication schedules and the goals of therapy. Diabetic clients with unstable blood glucose levels, as well as those undergoing intensive treatment regimens

---

CHART 65-5

CLIENT EDUCATION GUIDE
Subcutaneous Insulin Administration

- Wash your hands.
- Inspect the bottle for the type of insulin and the expiration date.
- Gently roll the bottle of intermediate-acting insulin in the palms of your hands to mix the insulin.
- Clean the rubber stopper with an alcohol swab.
- Remove the needle cover and pull back the plunger to draw air into the syringe. The amount of air should be equal to the insulin dose. Push the needle through the rubber stopper and inject the air into the insulin bottle.
- Turn the bottle upside down and draw the insulin dose into the syringe.
- Remove air bubbles in the syringe by tapping on the syringe or injecting air back into the bottle. Redraw the correct amount.
- Make certain the tip of the plunger is on the line for your dose of insulin. Magnifiers are available to assist in measuring accurate doses of insulin.
- Remove the needle from the bottle. Recap the needle if the insulin is not to be given immediately.
- Select a site within your injection area that has not been used in the past month.
- Clean your skin with an alcohol swab. Lightly grasp an area of skin and insert the needle at a 90-degree angle.
- Push the plunger all the way down. This will push the insulin into your body. Release the pinched skin.
- Pull the needle straight out quickly. Do not rub the place where you gave the shot.
- Dispose of the syringe and needle without recapping in a puncture-proof container.

Data from American Diabetes Association. (2000). Position statement: Insulin administration. *Diabetes Care, 23*(Suppl. 1), 86-89.

CHART 65-6

CLIENT EDUCATION GUIDE
How to Mix a Prescribed Dose of 10 Units of Regular Insulin and 20 Units of NPH Insulin

- Wash your hands.
- Inspect the bottles for the type of insulin and the expiration date.
- Gently roll the bottle of intermediate insulin in the palms of your hands to mix the insulin.
- Clean the rubber stopper with an alcohol swab.
- Inject 20 units of air into the NPH insulin bottle. The amount of air should be equal to the dose of insulin needed. Always inject air into the intermediate-acting insulin first. Withdraw the syringe.
- Inject 10 units of air into the regular insulin bottle. The amount of air is equal to the dose of insulin desired.
- Withdraw 10 units of regular insulin. Be sure that the syringe is free of air bubbles. Always withdraw the shorter-acting insulin first.
- Withdraw 20 units of NPH insulin with the same syringe, being careful not to inject any short-acting insulin into the bottle. (A total of 30 units should be in the syringe.)

Data from American Diabetes Association. (2001). Position statement: Insulin administration. *Diabetes Care, 23*(Suppl. 1), 86-89.

TABLE 65-12 • COST OF BLOOD GLUCOSE MONITORS AND STRIPS

Meter	Cost of Meter	Test Strips (50)	Test Strips (100)
Accu Chek Advantage:	Complete Care Kit: $97.99 (Rebate: $25.00, trade-in: $50.00)	Comfort Curve: $33.95	Comfort Curve: $59.44
One Touch Profile	One Touch Profile System: $97.99 (Rebate: $25.00, trade-in: $50.00)	$34.75	$61.29
Glucometer	Encore Diabetes Kit: $74.95 (Rebate: $30.00, trade-in: $10.00)	$31.99	
	Glucometer Elite XL Diabetes Care System: $49.95 (Rebate: $25.00, trade-in: $25.00)	$32.97	$59.99
Precision QID	QID: $54.99 (Rebate: $35.00, trade-in: $20.00)	$35.77	$56.95
Sure Step	Sure Step Blood Glucose System: $59.99 (Rebate: $40.00, trade-in: $20.00)	$33.95	$59.44
Exact Tech	R.S.G. Meter: $29.99 (Rebate: $20.00, Trade-in: $10.00)	$24.97	$43.99

Data from http://www.diabeteswebsite.com.

(continuous subcutaneous insulin infusions with pumps or more than three injections daily) require frequent blood glucose monitoring. Clients undergoing minimal treatment regimens designed to prevent symptomatic hyperglycemia or clients with type 2 diabetes receiving oral agents require less frequent monitoring.

Blood Glucose Therapy Goals. The nurse works with the client to reach set goals for blood glucose therapy. Target blood glucose levels are set individually for each client. On the basis of the Diabetes Control and Complications Trial (DCCT) results, a diabetes policy group recommends that clients with type 1 diabetes aim for premeal glucose levels of 80 to 120 mg/dL (4.4 to 6.7 mmol/L) and a bedtime level of 100 to 140 mg/dL (6.1 to 7.8 mmol/L) (Goldstein & Little, 1997).

Accuracy of Self-Monitoring of Blood Glucose Levels. All meters currently available are reasonably accurate when the manufacturer's directions are followed. Results are technique dependent regardless of whether test strips are read visually or with a meter. The nurse helps the client select a meter on the basis of the cost of the meter and strips, ease of use, availability of repair and maintenance service, and ability to discriminate color. The nurse provides training, including an explanation and demonstration of the procedures, assesses visual acuity, tests for color blindness as indicated, and checks the learner's ability to accurately perform the procedure through a return demonstration. Assessment of the diabetic client's ability to discriminate between colors is vital for those who do not use a blood glucose meter.

The most common error in SMBG is failure to follow instructions about properly applying blood on the test strip, timing, and removing blood samples from the monitor. Because performance accuracy deteriorates over time, continued retraining of clients performing SMBG is necessary to ensure that results are accurate.

CONSIDERATIONS FOR OLDER ADULTS

Visual interpretation of blood glucose values is affected by the normal changes of aging. The ability to discriminate shades of blue, violet, and green becomes less accurate. Older clients require three times as much light to see things as they did at age 20. It is more effective to place high-intensity light on the object or surface than to increase light for the entire room.

New Technology. Blood glucose measurements can be obtained "continuously" by means of a glucose sensor placed under the skin of the abdomen. The sensor measures glucose in interstitial fluid every 5 minutes. The information shows blood glucose fluctuations over the course of the day and allows adjustments in intensive insulin therapy to be made more accurately.

Several noninvasive monitoring systems that measure glucose in interstitial fluid are under development. The GlucoWatch received approval from the Advisory Panel of the Food and Drug Administration (FDA) in December 1999. The device sends a tiny electrical current through the skin and measures glucose from interstitial fluid just beneath the surface of the skin. Glucose measurements can be obtained every 20 minutes. The GlucoWatch is meant to supplement, not replace, finger stick tests. Because the reliability of this device has not yet been determined, the FDA recommends that insulin be given only after confirming the results of the GlucoWatch with a finger stick test (Trecroci, 1999) (Table 65-13).

Systems for obtaining blood without finger sticks are also being developed. The Professional Lancette uses a laser beam to vaporize a pinpoint of skin on the user's finger to get a drop of blood.

DIET THERAPY. Effective self-management of diabetes requires that the meal plan, education, and counseling program be individualized for each client (see Chart 65-4). Because of the complexity of nutrition issues, a registered dietitian should be a member of the treatment team. The nurse, dietitian, client, and family work together on all aspects of the meal plan. The meal plan must be realistic and as flexible as possible.

Goals of Diet Therapy. Diet therapy for clients with diabetes focuses on the following goals:

- Maintenance of as near-normal blood glucose levels as possible
- Achievement of optimal serum lipid levels: low-density lipoprotein (LDL) cholesterol less than 100 mg/dL (2.60 mmol/L) and triglyceride levels less than 200 mg/dL (<2.30 mmol/L) (ADA, 2000m, 2000t)
- Achievement of optimal blood pressure goals, usually less than 130/85 mm Hg (ADA, 2000t)
- Ensuring adequate calories for achieving reasonable weight for adults, meeting increased metabolic needs during pregnancy and lactation, or promoting recovery from illness
- Prevention and treatment of the acute complications of hypoglycemic medications, short-term illness, and exercise-related problems
- Prevention and treatment of complications of diabetes, such as renal disease, neuropathy, and cardiovascular disease
- Improvement of overall health through optimal nutrition (ADA, 2000n)

Principles of Nutrition in Diabetes. The dietitian formulates a meal plan based on the client's usual food intake. Day-to-day consistency in the timing and amount of food consumed helps control blood glucose. Clients receiving insulin therapy need to eat at consistent times that are coordinated with the timed action of insulin. Clients receiving in-

---

TABLE 65-13 • COST OF BLOOD GLUCOSE MONITORING PRODUCTS			
Product	**Cost**	**Cost of Supplies**	**Comments**
Lasette	$995	Disposable cartridge: $30 for a two-pack ($0.12 per test)	Cartridge is good for 120 uses. Battery is rechargeable, with 50 uses per charge.
GlucoWatch	$250-$350	Disposable pads: $4 to $5	Pads must be changed every 12 hours. Watch should last 2-3 yr.

Data from http://www.cellrobotics.com/perslasette.html; and http://www.glucowatch.com.

tense insulin therapy can be taught to adjust premeal insulin to allow for timing and quantity changes in their meal plan (ADA, 2000n).

Protein. The recommended protein intake for the client with diabetes is the same as that for the general population, with 10% to 20% of total caloric intake coming from protein. A dietary protein intake of 10% of calories (0.8 g/kg of body weight) is recommended for clients with nephropathy (ADA, 2000n).

Fat and Carbohydrate. The amount of calories from fat and carbohydrates is based on individualized nutritional goals. Of the remaining 80% to 90% of caloric intake, less than 10% should be from saturated fat and up to 10% should be from polyunsaturated fat. The remaining 60% to 70% of caloric intake is obtained from monounsaturated fat and carbohydrates (ADA, 2000n).

Further dietary fat restrictions for clients with diabetes are determined by a dietitian on the basis of specific lipid abnormalities. Adults with diabetes should be tested annually for lipid abnormalities. These tests include fasting serum cholesterol, triglyceride, high-density lipoprotein (HDL) cholesterol, and calculated LDL cholesterol levels (ADA, 2000m).

The percentage of calories obtained from carbohydrate sources is also individualized for each client. Various starches have different blood glucose responses. Emphasis is placed on the total amount of carbohydrate consumed each day rather than the source of the carbohydrate. Little scientific evidence supports the assumption that sugars are more rapidly absorbed than starches and cause blood glucose values to increase more rapidly.

Fiber. High-fiber diets seem to improve carbohydrate metabolism and lower cholesterol levels. The client is taught to select foods with moderate to high amounts of dietary fiber (e.g., legumes, lentils, roots, green leafy vegetables, all types of whole-grain cereals, and fruits). An intake of 20 to 35 g of dietary fiber per day is ideal.

The nurse teaches the client that incorporating high-fiber foods into the diet gradually can minimize abdominal cramping, discomfort, loose stools, and flatulence. An increase in fluid intake should accompany increased fiber intake. The nurse and the client pay careful attention to blood glucose levels because hypoglycemia can result when dietary fiber intake increases significantly.

Nonnutritive Sweeteners. The use of products to enhance the taste of food while not disturbing blood glucose control is desirable. The FDA has approved four nonnutritive sweeteners for use: saccharin, aspartame, acesulfame K, and sucralose.

Fat Replacers. Fat replacers are introduced into food processing to create good-tasting, lower-fat foods but may increase carbohydrate content. The dietitian and the nurse provide training to clients with diabetes on how to incorporate fat replacers into their meal plan. General guidelines regarding the use of fat replacers are as follows (ADA, 2000r):

- Fat replacer should be less than 20 calories or less than 5 g of carbohydrate per serving if it is a "free food."
- Limit fat replacer to three servings per day.
- From 6 to 10 g of carbohydrate per serving is one half of a carbohydrate choice.
- From 11 to 20 g of carbohydrate per serving is one carbohydrate choice.

Alcohol. Blood glucose levels will not be affected by *moderate* use of alcohol when diabetes is well controlled. The nurse teaches clients using insulin that two alcoholic beverages for men and one for women can be ingested with, and in addition to, the usual meal plan. (One alcoholic beverage = 12 ounces of beer, 5 ounces of wine, or 1.5 ounces of distilled spirits.) Because of the potential for alcohol-induced hypoglycemia, the client is instructed to ingest alcohol only with or shortly after meals. Because alcohol elevates plasma triglycerides, reducing or abstaining from alcohol may be recommended for diabetic clients with hyperlipidemia, a history of alcohol abuse, or during pregnancy. One alcoholic beverage is substituted for two fat exchanges when calculating caloric intake (ADA, 2000n).

Food Labeling. Nutrient and ingredient information help clients make appropriate food choices and select appropriate portions. For clients with diabetes, foods containing sucrose or other sugars are not restricted. These foods should be used sparingly and substituted for other carbohydrates in the individual meal plan. The client is instructed to use the food label to determine food carbohydrate content to aid in blood glucose control (ADA, 2000g).

Client Education: Prescribed Diet. The 1994 Nutrition Recommendations for Diabetes recognized that no one single meal plan is appropriate for all clients with diabetes. Each client's nutrition recommendations are based on blood glucose monitoring results, total blood lipid levels, and glycosylated hemoglobin. Results from self-monitoring of blood glucose levels (SMBG) help to determine whether current patterns of meals and exercise need adjustment or whether present habits need reinforcement. A specific dietary prescription is developed for each client.

The nurse supports and reinforces nutrition information provided by the dietitian. The diabetic client needs to understand how to make adjustments in nutritional intake during illness, planned exercise, and social occasions (such as restaurant meals) where the usual time of eating is delayed. The client may be unable to follow the prescribed diet because of an inability to see, read, or understand printed materials. Dietary information is shared with the person who prepares the meals. The dietitian sees each client at least yearly to note subtle changes in lifestyle and make appropriate diet therapy changes. The dietitian also sees those clients assessed by the case manager to be at *high risk* for nutritional problems. Some clients, such as those with weight control problems or low incomes, may require more frequent evaluation and counseling.

Meal Planning Strategies. A variety of meal planning approaches are available. Each approach emphasizes different aspects of nutrition.

Exchange System. The exchange system is based on three food groups: carbohydrates, meat and meat substitutes, and fat. The client's prescription identifies how many items from each food group are to be eaten at a meal or snack. Table 65-14 provides an example of the exchange system of diet therapy. The exchange list for meal planning assumes that foods with similar nutrient content affect blood glucose concentrations similarly. Diets based on the exchange system have been shown to produce predictable blood glucose responses.

Carbohydrate Counting. Carbohydrate (CHO) counting provides a simple approach to meal planning and is helped by the fact that the nutritional content of most packaged food items is listed on the label. Because fat and protein have little effect on postmeal blood glucose levels, CHO counting emphasizes the nutrient that has the greatest impact on these levels. CHO counting uses total grams of carbohydrate, regardless of the food source. The dietitian determines the number of grams of carbohydrate to be eaten at each meal and snack

TABLE 65-14 • EXCHANGE SYSTEM OF MEDICAL NUTRITION THERAPY

Food Content	Carbohydrate (g)	Protein (g)	Fat (g)	Calories	Examples
Carbohydrates	15	3	1 or less	80	1 slice bread, $\frac{1}{2}$ bagel, $\frac{1}{2}$ hamburger bun, $\frac{1}{2}$ cup corn, $\frac{1}{2}$ cup mashed potato
Fruit	15			60	1 apple, $\frac{1}{2}$ banana, $\frac{1}{2}$ grapefruit
Milk					
Skim	12	8	0-3	90	1 cup skim milk
Low-fat	12	8	5	120	1 cup 2% milk
Whole	12	8	5	150	1 cup whole milk
Other carbohydrates	Varies	Varies	Varies	Varies	1 glazed donut, 1 granola bar, 1 sweet roll
Vegetables	5	2		25	Carrots, green beans, spinach, $\frac{1}{2}$ cup cooked, 1 cup raw; 1 large tomato
Meat or meat substitutes					
Very lean		7	0.1	35	1 oz chicken (white meat, skinless), 1 oz fat-free cheese
Lean		7	3	55	1 oz lean beef, chicken (skinless), or fish; $\frac{1}{4}$ cup cottage cheese
Medium-fat		7	5	75	1 oz most beef, pork, lamb, or chicken with skin; $\frac{1}{4}$ cup tuna fish
High-fat		7	8	100	1 oz pork sausage, 1 tbsp peanut butter, 1 oz regular cheese
Fat			5	45	1 tsp butter or margarine, 1 strip bacon

Courtesy of Carole Colebanks.

and assists the client in making appropriate food choices. CHO counting is effective in achieving overall blood glucose control. Blood glucose control requires a consistent carbohydrate intake from day to day.

Clients who are receiving intensive insulin or pump therapies can use CHO counting to determine insulin coverage. After the amount of insulin needed to cover the usual meal is determined, insulin may be added or subtracted for changes in carbohydrate intake. The usual formula of 1 unit of short-acting insulin for each 15 g of carbohydrate provides flexibility to meal plans.

Special Considerations for Type 1 Diabetes. A meal plan based on the client's usual food intake is developed, and insulin therapy is integrated into the usual eating and exercises patterns. To prevent wide swings in blood glucose levels, day-to-day consistency in the timing and amount of food is important for a client using standard insulin therapy (one to two daily insulin injections). To match the effects of insulin, the daily caloric intake is distributed among three main meals, a bedtime snack, and one or more between-meal snacks. Clients receiving intensified insulin therapy with multiple daily injections of insulin or an insulin pump have more flexibility in the choice and timing of meals and snacks.

In addition to maintaining blood glucose levels within a target range, a second goal for the treatment of clients with type 1 diabetes is to avoid gaining weight. **Hyperinsulinemia** (chronic high blood insulin levels), which can occur with intensive treatment schedules, may result in weight gain. These clients may need to treat hyperglycemia by caloric restriction rather than by increases in insulin dosage. Weight gain can be minimized by adhering to the prescribed meal plan, consistently eating an evening snack, and avoiding overtreatment of hypoglycemia (Franz, 1997).

Special Considerations for Type 2 Diabetes. With type 2 diabetes, diet therapy is directed toward weight reduction and improvement in blood glucose and lipid levels in the obese

person. For clients in whom caloric reduction and exercise has not been successful in achieving long-term weight loss, emphasis is on reducing blood glucose and lipid levels. A moderate caloric restriction (250 to 500 calories less than the average daily intake) and an increase in physical activity improves diabetes control and weight control. Losing only as much as 10 to 20 pounds improves blood glucose control (Franz, 1997). Decreasing high dietary intake of cholesterol-raising fatty acids is important in reducing the risk for cardiovascular disease (ADA, 2000m).

CONSIDERATIONS FOR OLDER ADULTS

Older diabetic clients are at increased risk for malnutrition and hypoglycemia and are particularly prone to developing dehydration, a factor in the development of hyperglycemic-hyperosmolar nonketotic syndrome (HHNS). Many factors contribute to malnutrition. Older clients who prepare their own food or have tooth loss or poorly fitting dentures may not eat enough food. Neuropathy with gastric retention or diarrhea compounds poor food intake. Impaired cognition and depression may disrupt self-management. Older clients may have a marginal food supply because of inadequate income, may have poor understanding of meal planning goals, or may live alone and have reduced incentive to prepare or eat proper meals. They may eat in restaurants or live in situations where they have little control over meal preparation. Regular visits by home care nurses can assist the older client in following a diabetic meal plan.

A realistic approach to diet therapy is essential. Changing eating habits of 60 to 70 years' duration is very difficult. The nurse, the dietitian, and the client assess the usual eating patterns. The older client taking antidiabetic drugs is taught about the importance of eating meals and snacks at the same time every day, eating the same amount of food from day to day, and eating all food allowed on the diet.

EXERCISE THERAPY. Regular physical exercise is an essential part of a total diabetic treatment plan. Regular exercise has beneficial effects on carbohydrate metabolism and insulin sensitivity. In addition, exercise improves the client's sense of well-being and reduces the risk for atherosclerosis (ADA, 2000d).

In the person without diabetes, glucose use during exercise is matched by glucose production by the liver; thus exercise does not induce hyperglycemia or hypoglycemia. The client with type 1 diabetes is unable to make these hormonal adaptations. In the diabetic client without an adequate insulin supply, cells are unable to use glucose. Low insulin levels stimulate release of glucagon and epinephrine to increase hepatic glucose production, further raising blood glucose levels. In the absence of insulin, free fatty acids become the source of energy. Exercise in the client with uncontrolled diabetes results in further hyperglycemia and the formation of ketone bodies.

Exercise in the person with diabetes can cause hypoglycemia because of increased muscle glucose uptake and the inhibition of glucose release from the liver. Hypoglycemia can occur during exercise and for up to 24 hours after exercise. Replacement of muscle and liver glycogen stores, along with increased insulin sensitivity following exercise, causes insulin requirements to drop (Franz, 1997).

Diabetic clients may have prolonged elevated blood glucose levels after vigorous exercise periods. Liver glucose production increases to provide the energy needs for exercise. In nondiabetic clients, this increased glucose production is balanced by an increase in plasma insulin secretion so that fluctuations in blood glucose levels are avoided. The client with type 1 diabetes is unable to increase plasma insulin levels, and postexercise hyperglycemia develops.

Benefits of Exercise. Regular exercise of moderate intensity helps regulate blood glucose levels and results in lowered insulin requirements for clients with type 1 diabetes. Regular exercise improves diabetic control by increasing insulin sensitivity, improving cell uptake of glucose, and promoting weight loss.

Regular exercise decreases risk factors for cardiovascular disease. In response to training, clients with type 1 diabetes have decreases in most blood lipid levels and an increase in high-density lipoproteins (HDLs). Exercise decreases blood pressure and improves cardiovascular function. Regular vigorous physical activity appears to have an important role in the prevention of type 2 diabetes by reducing body weight, insulin resistance, and glucose intolerance.

Risks Related to Exercise. The client with diabetes is assessed for potential risk for injury related to exercise. Prolonged hypoglycemia or hyperglycemia can occur, particularly after sustained high-intensity exercise.

Several complications of diabetes can be made worse by exercise. The client with proliferative retinopathy is advised to avoid the **Valsalva maneuver** (breath holding while bearing down) and activities that increase blood pressure. Heavy lifting, rapid head motion, or jarring activities can cause vitreous hemorrhage or retinal detachment. Exercise may increase proteinuria in clients with diabetic nephropathy. The risk for foot and joint injury is increased for clients with peripheral neuropathy. Autonomic neuropathy can cause postexercise orthostatic hypotension (ADA, 2000d).

Screening Before Initiating an Exercise Program. The diabetic client is advised to have a complete history and physical examination before beginning a physical activity program. Regular physical activity increases the risk of both musculoskeletal injury and life-threatening cardiovascular events. The ability of the heart to respond to increasing levels of exercise on a treadmill, as well as the presence of other risk factors, forms the basis of the exercise prescription. For clients who are unable to perform vigorous exercise, the heart's ability to tolerate exercise is tested with cardiac stressor drugs (e.g., coronary vasodilators, dipyridamole thallium scans). The client needs to be carefully evaluated for the presence of macrovascular and microvascular complications that may be worsened by exercise (ADA, 2000d).

Guidelines for Exercise. The client determines blood glucose levels before exercise. When levels are greater than 250 mg/dL (13.8 mmol/L), the client tests the urine for ketones. The absence of urine ketones indicates that enough insulin is available to promote glucose transport and use, and that exercise should be effective in lowering blood glucose levels. The presence of ketones contraindicates exercise. Ketones indicate that current insulin levels are not adequate and that exercise would elevate blood glucose levels.

Low-intensity aerobic exercise for longer durations is most effective in achieving desired health effects for clients with diabetes. Such exercises are those that require slow, submaximal effort, continue for greater than 12 to 15 minutes, are rhythmic in nature, and result in a moderately elevated heart rate (above 50% of maximal heart rate). Examples of appropriate aerobic activities include walking briskly, running, jogging, stationary or regular bicycling, swimming, dancing, rowing, and cross-country skiing. These activities improve cardiac output.

For individuals with type 1 diabetes, the aerobic exercise should endure for 20 to 40 minutes and be performed 4 to 7 days per week. A 5- to 10-minute warm-up period with stretching and low-intensity exercise before aerobic exercise and a 5- to 10-minute cool-down period after aerobic exercise reduce the risk for dysrhythmias. Daily exercise increases total energy expenditure, facilitates weight loss, and improves blood glucose control.

NIC *Client Education: Exercise Promotion.* Chart 65-7 lists NIC intervention activities for exercise. The client is instructed to wear shoes with good traction and cushioning and to examine the feet daily and after exercise. Exercise in extreme heat or cold or during periods of poor control of diabetes is avoided. The client is advised to maintain hydration, especially during and after exercise in a warm environment.

Exercise is not performed within 1 hour of insulin injection or at the peak time of insulin action, because this activity can increase absorption of insulin from the injection site, causing an increase in blood insulin levels. The risk for hypoglycemia increases when insulin is injected into an area that is exercised.

The nurse makes certain that all diabetic clients engaging in exercise know the risks for hypoglycemia and teaches preventive measures. Clients taking oral medications or insulin should perform self-monitoring of blood glucose levels (SMBG) to determine the effects of their exercise program. The client is taught that supplemental snacks containing rapidly absorbable carbohydrate may be taken before and during exercise to maintain blood glucose levels within normal ranges. Additional carbohydrate may be taken for up to 24 hours after exercise to prevent postexercise hypoglycemia. The amount of additional carbohydrate intake is directed by

CHART 65-7

NIC INTERVENTION ACTIVITIES *for*
The Diabetic Client Needing to Increase Physical Activity

Exercise Promotion: *Facilitation of regular physical exercise to maintain or advance to a higher level of fitness and health*
- Appraise client's health beliefs about physical exercise.
- Encourage verbalization of feelings about exercise or need for exercise.
- Include client's family/caregivers in planning and maintaining the exercise program.
- Inform client about health beliefs and physiologic effects of exercise.
- Instruct client about appropriate type of exercise for level of health, in collaboration with physician and/or exercise physiologist.
- Instruct client about desired frequency, duration, and intensity of the exercise program.
- Instruct client about conditions warranting cessation of or alteration in the exercise program.
- Instruct client on proper warm-up and cool-down exercises.
- Instruct the client in techniques to avoid injury while exercising.
- Assist client to develop an appropriate exercise program to meet needs.
- Assist client to set short-term and long-term goals for the exercise program.
- Assist client to schedule regular periods for the exercise program into weekly routine.
- Monitor client's response to exercise program.
- Provide positive feedback for client's efforts.

Vital Signs Monitoring: *Collection and analysis of cardiovascular, respiratory, and body temperature data to determine and prevent complications*
- Monitor blood pressure, pulse, temperature, and respiratory response, as appropriate.
- Monitor for and report signs and symptoms of hypothermia and hyperthermia.
- Monitor presence and quality of pulses.
- Monitor cardiac rhythm and rate.
- Monitor heart tones.
- Monitor respiratory rate and rhythm (e.g., depth and symmetry).
- Monitor for abnormal respiratory patterns (e.g., Cheyne-Stokes, Kussmaul, Biot, apneustic, ataxic, and excessive sighing).
- Monitor skin color, temperature, and moisture.
- Identify possible causes of changes in vital signs.

NIC intervention activities selected from McCloskey J.C., & Bulechek, G.M. (2000). *Nursing interventions classification (NIC)* (3rd ed.). St. Louis: Mosby. No part of this work is to be altered without prior written permission from the Publisher.

the results of blood glucose monitoring. The nurse instructs the client to adjust insulin dosage before planned exercise as directed.

Clients with type 1 diabetes should perform vigorous exercise only if blood glucose levels are in the range of 80 to 250 mg/dL (4.4 to 13.8 mmol/L) and if there are no ketones present in the urine. In the nonobese client who is taking insulin, the nurse recommends a carbohydrate-containing snack before exercise if at least 1 hour has elapsed since the last food was eaten or if high-intensity exercise is planned. There is no need for additional carbohydrate intake when the blood glucose level is greater than 100 mg/dL (5.6 mmol/L) before exercise and the planned activity is of low intensity and short duration. When vigorous activity of long duration is planned,

the client should eat an additional 15 to 30 g of carbohydrate for every 30 to 60 minutes of exercise. Snacks such as fruit, fruit juice, bread products, and whole milk are effective in preventing hypoglycemia. The client is instructed to carry a simple sugar (hard candy) to eat if symptoms of hypoglycemia occur. The nurse also instructs the client to carry identifying information about having diabetes.

CONSIDERATIONS FOR OLDER ADULTS
With age, the ability of the heart and lungs to deliver oxygen to tissues and organs declines. These changes may be due more to a decline in muscle mass than to changes in cardiac output. Aerobic activities are thought to be important in maintaining muscle mass. Healthy older clients are able to maintain cardiac output by increasing stroke volume during exercise.

Specific exercise programs are beneficial for *frail older adults* who, because of weak muscles and poor balance, are at greater risk for falls and fractures. Clients who are limited to low-intensity programs can achieve benefits when exercise is performed at least three times per week. Some level of exercise is beneficial even to severely debilitated clients (Samos & Roos, 1998).

SURGICAL MANAGEMENT. Surgical interventions for diabetes mellitus include transplantation of all or part of the pancreas. Successful pancreas and islet cell transplantations are the only therapies that achieve blood glucose control by providing normal insulin secretion that responds to feedback regulation (Robertson et al., 2000). Clients' quality of life is improved when they no longer have to take insulin injections and are free of diabetic dietary restrictions.

WHOLE-PANCREAS TRANSPLANTATION. Improved surgical techniques and newer immunosuppressive therapies have improved outcomes in pancreatic transplantation. Simultaneous pancreas and kidney transplantation shows a 1-year client survival rate of greater than 90% and a 1-year **graft** (transplanted organ) survival rate of 82%. Pancreatic graft survival is defined as not needing insulin injections. The degree of tissue-type matching affects the results. Both graft and client survival are improved when a living related donor kidney is available (Manske, 1999). Pancreatic transplantation is performed in one of three situations: transplantation of the pancreas alone (PTA), transplantation of the pancreas after successful kidney transplantation (PAK), and simultaneous pancreas and kidney transplantation (SPK). The ideal procedure for diabetic clients with uremia is SPK. These clients are generally poor surgical candidates because of the presence of complications from the diabetes. The problems of diabetes must be severe enough to balance the expected toxicity of immunosuppressive drugs. Pancreatic transplantation is only partially successful in reversing the long-term complications of diabetes (ADA, 2000o).

Operative Procedure. The majority of pancreas transplants have been performed using the technique of **systemic venous delivery of insulin and bladder drainage of exocrine secretions (systemic-bladder).** This procedure involves attaching the donated pancreas to the client's urinary bladder. Because this procedure results in hyperinsulinemia and has urologic complications, techniques were developed to allow systemic venous delivery of insulin to the intestinal tract (systemic-enteric) and bladder drainage of pancreatic enzymes. Complications of this procedure include blood clot formation, duodenal leak, wound infections, and urologic problems.

Rejection Management. Transplant rejection accounts for 32% of graft failures in the first year after a pancreas transplant (Stratta, 1999). Most transplant centers use a combination of four drug and antibody types to reverse rejection. (See Chapter 20 for a listing of agents used to prevent or treat transplant rejection.) Clients undergoing immunosuppressive therapy initially receive drug therapy to prevent viral, bacterial, and fungal infection because of the risk of opportunistic infections.

Pancreatic transplantation is considered successful when the client is independent from insulin therapy, blood glucose levels are normal, and glycosylated hemoglobin values are normal. In nearly 90% of rejection episodes, kidney problems occur earlier than pancreatic problems. An increase in serum creatinine is an indication of rejection of both the transplanted kidney and the pancreas. In diabetic clients with urinary drained pancreas transplants, a decrease in the urine amylase level by 25% is used as an indication to treat rejection. High blood glucose levels are a later marker of rejection and usually indicate irreversible graft failure.

Long-Term Effects. Long-term immunosuppressive therapy is associated with increased risk for infections, cancer, and atherosclerosis. The transplanted pancreas does not duplicate all of the functions of a normal pancreas. Because the pancreas is transplanted into the peritoneal cavity, insulin drains into the systemic rather than the portal circulation, causing elevations in blood insulin levels **(hyperinsulinemia).** Hyperinsulinemia is a risk factor for both hypertension and macrovascular disease.

Complications. Complications are common in clients receiving organ transplants and requiring long-term immunosuppressive therapy. Major complications of a pancreas transplant include venous thrombosis, rejection, and infection. Careful monitoring of laboratory values, fluid and electrolyte status, physical signs and symptoms, and changes in vital signs can alert the nurse to possible complications and the need to notify the physician for therapy. Early removal of IV and intra-arterial lines, use of sterile technique with dressing changes and catheter irrigations, strict handwashing by health care personnel, and good pulmonary hygiene all help to prevent infection.

Thrombosis of blood vessels to the pancreas occurs in as many as 30% of clients who have had pancreas transplants. Changes in surgical technique have reduced the incidence of this complication. The nurse observes for, and reports to the physician, any sharp and sudden drop in urine amylase levels, rapid increases in blood glucose, gross hematuria **(bloody urine),** and tenderness or pain in the graft area (iliac fossa).

The nurse assesses the client for signs and symptoms of rejection. In acute rejection, decreased kidney function is indicated by increased serum creatinine of 0.3 mg/dL or greater (Stratta, 1999), decreased urine output, hypertension, increased weight, graft tenderness, and fever. Proteinuria is often the first indicator of chronic graft rejection. The nurse observes for signs and symptoms of rejection, including elevations of serum amylase, lipase, or glucose; decreased urine amylase; graft tenderness; hyperglycemia; and fever. It

is especially important to assess for signs and symptoms of infection and initiate appropriate treatment. Fever can be a sign of both infection and rejection.

The nurse monitors for side effects of the various immunosuppressive drugs. Cyclosporine (Neoral) is **nephrotoxic** (toxic to the kidney). Symptoms of nephrotoxicity include a rise in creatinine and a decrease in urine output. White blood cell counts are monitored daily, since azathioprine (Imuran) is associated with bone marrow suppression. Prednisone has multiple side effects, including elevated blood glucose levels. Common side effects of tacrolimus (Prograf) are nephrotoxicity, neurotoxicity, gastrointestinal (GI) toxicity, and glucose intolerance. Hypertension is a common adverse effect of tacrolimus.

The client's quality of life improves as a result of freedom from the need for insulin, a less restricted lifestyle, and a return to a normal diet. The nurse must stress, however, the potential for the need for insulin injections to treat hyperglycemia caused by immunosuppressive drugs.

ISLET CELL TRANSPLANTATION. Islet cell transplantation in rats and dogs successfully eliminates the requirement for insulin administration and provides protection from the complications of diabetes. Human transplantation of islet cells is limited by the technical inability to obtain a sufficient number of islet cells. Tissue type (HLA)–matched pancreas glands from cadavers are used, and isolated islet cells are injected into the portal vein or implanted beneath the kidney capsule or into the spleen. Successful transplantation has occurred in a small number of clients. Islet cell transplantation is currently considered an experimental procedure (ADA, 2000o).

■ RISK FOR INJURY RELATED TO STRESS OF SURGERY

PLANNING: EXPECTED OUTCOMES. The client with diabetes undergoing a surgical procedure is expected to have a satisfactory and complete postoperative recovery without complications.

INTERVENTIONS. Surgery is a physical and emotional stressor, and the diabetic client has a higher than average risk for complications. Acute stress increases the supply of glucose through the action of the counterregulatory hormones. These hormones suppress the action of insulin, increasing the risk for ketoacidosis and metabolic acidosis. Fasting contributes to the development of ketoacidosis. Diuresis from hyperglycemia can cause severe dehydration and loss of electrolytes.

Coronary artery disease, diabetic nephropathy, and autonomic neuropathy further increase the risk of surgical complications. Diabetic nephropathy makes fluid management more difficult. Cardiac dysrhythmias may result from the combined effect of anesthesia and autonomic neuropathy on the cardiovascular system. Autonomic neuropathy may cause paralytic ileus and urinary retention postoperatively.

Blood glucose must be controlled to prevent acute complications of hypoglycemia, diabetic ketoacidosis (DKA), and hyperglycemic-hyperosmolar nonketotic syndrome (HNNS). Blood glucose control is also necessary to reduce infection and promote wound healing. Keeping perioperative blood glucose levels between 120 and 200 mg/dL (6.7 and 11.1 mmol/L) has been found to prevent complications and promote wound healing (Hirsh & Paauw, 1997).

PREOPERATIVE CARE. Chlorpropamide (Diabinese) is discontinued for at least 36 hours before surgery. Metformin (Glucophage) is discontinued 48 hours before the surgical procedure and restarted only after renal function is normal. All other oral agents are discontinued the day of surgery. Adjustments in insulin therapy are based on preoperative blood glucose levels. When the client is admitted, the nurse starts IV fluids as ordered to maintain hydration, monitors blood glucose results, and administers insulin as ordered.

Operative procedures for clients with type 1 diabetes are performed early in the day to cause the least disruption in blood glucose control. Stable blood glucose levels can be achieved by administration of IV insulin when surgery is scheduled later in the day. Withholding normal insulin doses can cause hyperglycemia, ketosis, and electrolyte abnormalities. Moreover, giving a portion of the normal subcutaneous insulin dose involves guesswork and may cause a large, unpredictable release of insulin after surgery is underway (Hirsh & Paauw, 1997). The nurse performs frequent blood glucose monitoring throughout the perioperative period to determine the need for additional insulin.

Plans for postoperative pain control need to be made in the preoperative period. Pain, a stressor, stimulates the release of counterregulatory hormones, causing high blood glucose levels and increasing insulin needs. The older client who receives opioid analgesic drugs is more at risk for confusion, paralytic ileus, hypoventilation, and hypotension. The effects of opioid analgesics on slowing GI motility and the effects on blood glucose levels need to be considered. Many clients with long-standing diabetes have delayed gastric emptying. Compared with IM injections of opioids, patient-controlled analgesia (PCA) systems have fewer respiratory complications and a lower incidence of confusion. (See Chapter 7 for interventions related to pain and Chapter 17 for general preoperative care.)

INTRAOPERATIVE CARE. The frequency of blood glucose assessment depends in part on the type of anesthetic agent used. Epidural anesthesia minimally affects glucose metabolism. During general anesthesia, glucose levels increase early and remain elevated throughout the operative period. Surgery lasting 3 to 5 hours or longer leads to greater hyperglycemia, with these clients needing supplemental short-acting insulin.

IV administration of short-acting insulin in 5% to 10% glucose is recommended for all insulin-treated clients, as well as for clients with poorly controlled type 2 diabetes who are undergoing general anesthesia. Blood glucose levels less than 200 mg/dL during surgery reduce the incidence of wound infection during the postoperative period. Larger than normal doses of insulin may be needed during surgery because of stress-induced release of glucagon and epinephrine. The physician orders insulin/glucose infusion rates based on results of hourly capillary blood glucose tests.

NIC intervention activities for monitoring of vital signs are presented in Chart 65-7. The nurse monitors the client's temperature because body temperature is deliberately lowered in some operative procedures and inadvertently in others. Low operating room temperatures and large surgical incisions lower body temperature. Hypothermia decreases metabolic needs, depresses heart rate and contractility, causes vasoconstriction, and impairs insulin release, resulting in high blood glucose levels. The arterial blood gas values are monitored for acidosis.

POSTOPERATIVE CARE. The nurse continues glucose and insulin infusions, as ordered, until the client is stable and able to tolerate oral feedings. Supplemental short-acting insulin, with the dosage based on blood glucose monitoring, may be needed to control blood glucose levels until the client's usual medication regimen can be restarted. Short-term insulin therapy may be needed postoperatively for the client who usually uses oral agents alone. For the client receiving insulin therapy, changes in the usual insulin dosage may be needed until the stress of surgery subsides. To prevent the potential development of insulin allergy, only human insulin should be used for short-term therapy.

MONITORING. Clients with autonomic neuropathy or vascular disease require careful monitoring to avoid hypotension or respiratory arrest. Clients whose hypertension is well controlled with beta-blocking drugs must be monitored carefully for hypoglycemia (beta blocking agents mask hypoglycemia). Clients with **azotemia** (increased nitrogen waste products in the blood) may have problems with fluid management. The nurse monitors central venous pressure or pulmonary artery pressure as necessary.

Hyperkalemia (elevated blood potassium level) is often seen in clients with mild to moderate kidney failure and can lead to an acute cardiac dysrhythmia. In other clients, **hypokalemia** (low blood potassium levels) may be present and is made worse by insulin and glucose therapy given during surgical treatment. The nurse monitors the client's cardiac rhythm and serum potassium values as ordered.

Cardiovascular Monitoring. Serial electrocardiograms (ECGs) are recommended for older diabetic clients, those with long-standing type 1 diabetes, and those with known heart disease. Diabetic clients have a high incidence of postoperative myocardial infarctions that are associated with a high mortality rate. Alterations in ECGs or in potassium levels may indicate a silent myocardial infarction.

Renal Monitoring. Careful monitoring of fluid balance helps detect acute kidney failure. Diagnosis of renal impairment may require the use of x-ray studies using dyes, which may be nephrotoxic. Treatment of infections may require the use of nephrotoxic antibiotics. The physician and nurse ensure adequate hydration of the client when these drugs are used. The nurse monitors for impending renal failure through careful assessment of the client's fluid and electrolyte status.

NUTRITIONAL CARE. The use of **total parenteral nutrition (TPN)** in diabetic clients can result in severe metabolic changes. Frequent capillary blood glucose monitoring is used to determine the need for supplemental short-acting insulin. After a stable dose of insulin is reached, insulin can be added to the TPN solution and the frequency of capillary blood glucose monitoring decreased.

Returning to a normal meal plan as soon as possible after surgery promotes healing and re-establishes homeostasis. When oral foods are tolerated, the nurse ensures that the client takes at least 150 to 200 g of carbohydrate daily to prevent hypoglycemia.

150-200g of carbs

■ RISK FOR INJURY RELATED TO SENSORY ALTERATIONS

NOC **PLANNING: EXPECTED OUTCOMES.** The client with diabetes is expected to identify factors that increase the potential for injury, practice proper foot care to prevent injury (as evidenced by cleansing and inspecting the feet for cleanliness and healthy skin), and maintain intact skin on the feet.

INTERVENTIONS. Foot injury is the most common complication of diabetes leading to hospitalization. Diabetes is the leading cause of amputation worldwide. The overall risk of amputation is 15 times greater in diabetic clients than in nondiabetic clients. For clients who have had a previous amputation, the risk of amputation in the second leg is 10 to 20 times greater than the risk of amputation in the general population. The 5-year mortality rate after lower extremity amputation ranges from 39% to 68%.

Intensive education about foot care is needed for clients with diabetes. Low levels of high-density lipoprotein (HDL) cholesterol, high levels of plasma glucose and glycosylated hemoglobin (hemoglobin A_{1c} [HbA_{1c}]), and long duration of diabetes are associated with increased risk for amputation.

Sensory neuropathy, ischemia, and infection are the leading causes of foot disease associated with diabetes. Peripheral neuropathy is present in more than 80% of diabetic clients with foot ulcers (Abbott et al., 1998). Loss of pain, pressure and temperature sensation in the foot increases the chance of injury and development of ulcerations. Impaired blood flow to the foot limits healing of the wound.

Up to half of all people with diabetes have a hammertoe or claw toe deformity created by motor neuropathy (Mayfield et al., 1998). Toes become hyperextended, which increases pressure on the **metatarsal heads** ("ball" of the foot), resulting in ulceration. Thinning or shifting of the fat pad under the metatarsal heads decreases the cushioning and increases areas of pressure. These changes predispose the client to callus formation, ulceration, and infection. Figure 65-9 shows **hallux valgus** (turning of the great toe), and Figure 65-10 shows a hammertoe.

The **Charcot foot** is an example of a diabetic foot deformity. The Charcot foot is warm, swollen, and painful. Continued ambulation collapses the arch, shortens the foot, and gives the foot a "rocker bottom" shape.

Although sensory neuropathy may manifest as tingling or burning, it is more often evident as numbness and reduced sensation. Neuropathy causes loss of normal sweating and skin temperature regulation, resulting in dry and atrophic skin. Cracks and fissures in the skin increase the risk for infection.

The loss of sensation allows painless trauma to cause major foot problems. Because sensation is absent, the client does not notice physical, thermal, or chemical injuries to the foot. Thus the client does not take measures to treat these injuries. Foot injuries can be caused by walking barefoot, wearing ill-fitting shoes, sustaining thermal injuries from hot water (e.g., hot water bottles, heating pads, and baths), or receiving caustic burns caused by over-the-counter medications to treat corns. Because the blood supply to the diabetic foot is poor, these injuries sometimes lead to amputation.

Ulcers result from continued pressure. **Plantar** ulcers (ulcers on the bottom of the foot) are due to standing or walking, whereas ulcers on the top or sides of the foot are usually due to shoe pressure. The foot responds to increased pressure by callus formation. Most diabetic plantar ulcers are located under the metatarsal heads. Ulcerations usually occur over or around the great toe, under the metatarsal heads, and on the tops of claw toes.

The risk for infection increases whenever there is a break in the skin. Skin breaks tend to occur in areas of excessive or repetitive pressure. Infection is common in diabetic foot ulcers and, once present, is difficult to treat. Decreased immune function in diabetic clients increases the risk for infection. Infection also impairs glucose control, leading to higher blood glucose levels and reduced immune defense mechanisms.

PREVENTION OF HIGH-RISK CONDITIONS. Neuropathy of the lower extremities can be delayed by keeping blood glucose levels as near normal as possible. Poor blood glucose control increases the risk of neuropathy and amputation. Intensive therapy reduces the risk of development of peripheral

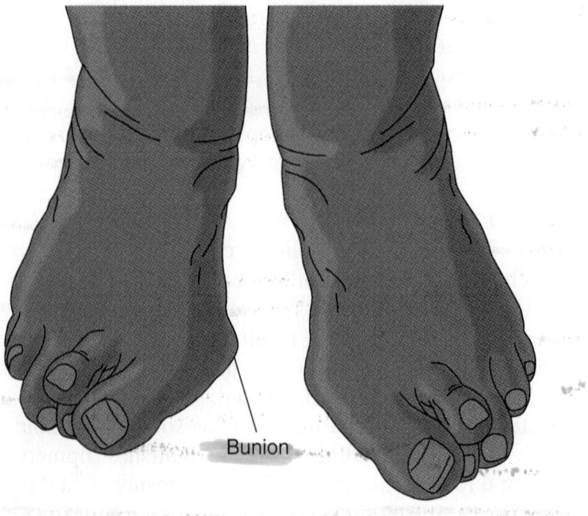

Figure 65-9 ● The appearance of hallux valgus with a bunion.

Bunion

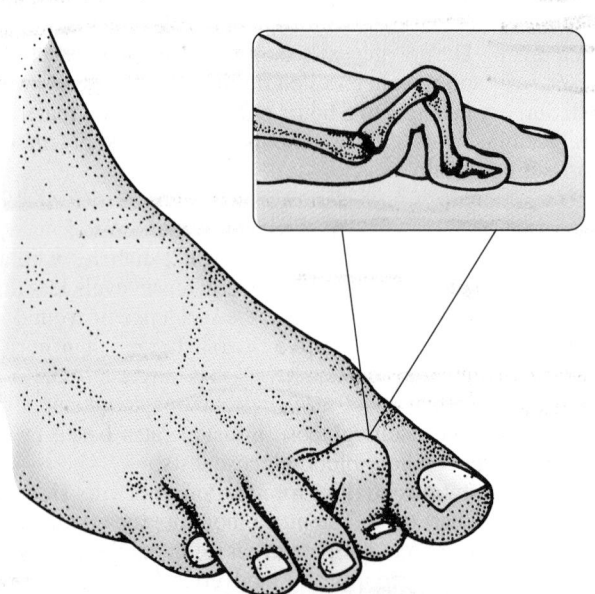

Figure 65-10 ● Hammertoe of the second metatarsophalangeal joint.

sensory neuropathy by 60%. Smoking cessation is encouraged to reduce the risk of vascular complications (ADA, 2000q).

The risk of ulcers or amputation is increased in clients who have had diabetes more than 10 years, are male, have poor glucose control, or have cardiovascular, retinal, or renal complications. Foot-related risks include poor gait and stepping mechanics, peripheral neuropathy, evidence of increased pressure (callus, erythema, hemorrhage under a callus, limited joint mobility, foot deformities, or severe nail pathology), peripheral vascular disease, and a history of ulcers or amputation (ADA, 2000q).

PERIPHERAL SENSATION MANAGEMENT. An in-depth circulatory, sensory, musculoskeletal, and skin evaluation of the feet should be done at least annually (ADA, 2000q). Chart 65-8 lists NIC intervention activities for peripheral sensation management and foot care, and Table 65-15 outlines foot risk categories. Sensory examination with Semmes-Weinstein monofilaments remains the single most practical measure of the risk for foot ulcers. The monofilaments are nylon wires of varying calibrated thickness. The threads are rigid but bend when pressure is applied. More pressure is needed to bend the thicker filaments. The client is asked to close his or her eyes. The nurse presses the tip of the thinnest filament to a defined area on the sole of the foot. The filament is pressed against the skin until either it bends or the client announces that he or she feels the pressure. If the filament bends before the client feels the sensation, the next-thicker filament is applied. Inability to feel the medium-size monofilament indicates high risk for injury. The nurse completes a full assessment of the diabetic foot as outlined in Chart 65-9.

FOOT CARE. All clients with diabetes need to wear shoes that protect the feet from injury. Shoes need to be fitted to the client by an experienced shoe fitter, such as a certified podiatrist. The shoe should be ½ to ⅝ inch longer than the longest toe. Heels should be less than 2 inches in height to avoid shifting the body weight onto the metatarsal heads, increasing the risk for foot ulcerations. Pressure from shoes that are too tight causes tissue damage when the shoes are worn for 4 hours or more with no relief. The nurse teaches the client to change his or her shoes by midday and again in the evening. Socks or stockings need to fit properly and be appropriate for the planned activity. Stockings should feel soft and not have thick seams, creases, or holes that can irritate the skin. Stockings should provide padding for the foot and be able to absorb excess moisture. Stockings that are tight or have constricting bands are to be avoided. Clients with toe deformities need to buy custom shoes with high, wide toeboxes and extra depth. Clients with severely deformed feet, such as Charcot feet, need specially molded shoes. All new shoes should have a slow break-in period, with periodic self-inspection of both feet for signs of irritation or blistering.

All clients with diabetes require education about preventive foot care and an examination of the feet and legs at each visit to a health care provider. The nurse or case manager identifies clients with *high-risk* foot conditions and provides education about foot care. Clients at risk are taught about the problems of the loss of protective sensation, the importance of monitoring their feet on a daily basis, the proper care of the feet (including nail and skin care), and how to select appropriate footwear. The client with neuropathy is advised to break in new shoes slowly to reduce blister formation (ADA, 2000q).

The nurse assesses the client's ability to inspect all areas of the foot and to perform appropriate care. Family members are taught principles of foot care for those clients with visual difficulties, physical limitations, or cognitive problems that prevent complete inspection of their feet (ADA, 2000q). Clients with diabetes are taught to inspect their feet daily. Chart 65-10 outlines foot care instructions.

CHART 65-8

NIC INTERVENTION ACTIVITIES *for*
The Diabetic Client with Reduced Sensation in the Lower Extremities

Peripheral Sensation Management: *Prevention or minimization of injury or discomfort in the client with altered sensation*
- Monitor for sharp/dull and/or hot/cold discrimination.
- Monitor for paresthesia: numbness, tingling, hyperesthesia, and hypoesthesia.
- Encourage client to use the unaffected body part to determine temperature of foods, liquids, bathwater, and so on.
- Instruct client or family to monitor position of body parts while bathing, sitting, lying, or changing position.
- Instruct client or family to examine skin daily for alteration in skin integrity.
- Monitor fit of bracing devices, prosthesis, shoes, and clothing.
- Instruct client or family to use thermometer to test water temperature.
- Encourage use of gloves or other protective clothing over affected body part when body part is in contact with objects that—because of their thermal, textural, or other characteristics—may be potentially hazardous.
- Avoid or carefully monitor use of heat or cold, such as heating pads, hot water bottles, and ice packs.
- Encourage client to wear well-fitting, low-heeled, soft shoes.
- Check shoes, pockets, and clothing for wrinkles or foreign objects.
- Instruct client to use timed intervals, rather than presence of discomfort, as a signal to alter position.
- Protect body parts from extreme temperature changes.
- Discuss or identify causes of abnormal sensation or sensation changes.
- Instruct client to visually monitor position of body parts, if proprioception is impaired.

Foot Care: *Cleansing and inspecting the feet for the purposes of relaxation, cleanliness, and healthy skin*
- Inspect skin for irritation, cracking, lesions, corns, calluses, deformities, or edema.
- Inspect client's shoes for proper fit.
- Dry carefully between toes.
- Apply lotion.
- Clean nails.
- Apply moisture-absorbing powder, as indicated.
- Discuss with client usual foot care routine.
- Instruct client/family on the importance of foot care.
- Offer positive feedback about self-care foot activities.
- Monitor client's gait and weight distribution on feet.
- Monitor cleanliness and general condition of shoes and stockings.
- Instruct client to inspect inside of shoes for rough areas.
- Monitor hydration level of feet.
- Monitor for arterial insufficiency in lower legs.
- Monitor legs and feet for edema.
- Instruct client to monitor temperature of feet using the back of the hand.
- Instruct client in the importance of inspection, especially when sensation is diminished.
- Cut normal-thickness toenails when soft, using a toenail clipper and using the curve of the toe as a guide.
- Refer to podiatrist for trimming of thickened nails, as appropriate.

NIC intervention activities selected from McCloskey J.C., & Bulechek, G.M. (2000). *Nursing interventions classification (NIC)* (3rd ed.). St. Louis: Mosby. No part of this work is to be altered without prior written permission from the Publisher.

TABLE 65-15 • FOOT RISK CATEGORIES

RISK CATEGORIES	MANAGEMENT CATEGORIES
Risk Category 0 • Has disease that leads to insensitivity • Has protective sensation • Has not had a plantar ulcer	*Management Category 0* • Examine feet at each visit, at least 4 times per year • Foot clinic once a year • Client education
Risk Category 1 • Does not have protective sensation • Has not had a plantar ulcer • Does not have a foot deformity	*Management Category 1* • Examine feet at each visit, at least 4 times per year • Foot clinic visit every 6 months • Soft insoles • Client education
Risk Category 2 • Does not have protective sensation • Has not had a plantar ulcer • Does have a foot deformity	*Management Category 2* • Examine feet at each visit, at least 4 times per year • Foot clinic visit every 3-4 months • Custom-molded insoles • Prescription footwear • Client education
Risk Category 3 • Does not have protective sensation • Has history of plantar ulcer	*Management Category 3* • Examine feet at each visit, at least 4 times per year • Foot clinic visit every 1-2 months • Custom-molded insoles • Prescription footwear • Client education

From Gillis W. Long Hansen's Disease Center Rehabilitation Branch (1992). *Foot screening: Care of the foot in diabetes: The Carville approach.* Carville, LA: Department of Health and Human Services.

CHART 65-9

FOCUSED ASSESSMENT *of*
The Diabetic Foot

Assess the client for risk of diabetic foot problems:
- History of previous ulcer
- History of previous amputation

Assess the foot for abnormal skin/nail conditions:
- Dry, cracked, fissured skin
- Ulcers
- Toenails: thickened, long nails; ingrown nails
- Tinea pedis; onychomycosis (mycotic nails)

Assess the foot for status of circulation:
- Symptoms of claudication
- Presence or absence of dorsalis pedis or posterior tibial pulse
- Prolonged capillary filling time (>25 seconds)
- Presence or absence of hair growth on the top of the foot

Assess the foot for evidence of deformity:
- Calluses, corns
- Prominent metatarsal heads (metatarsal head is easily felt under the skin)
- Toe contractures: clawed toes, hammertoes
- Hallux valgus or bunions
- Charcot foot ("rocker bottom")

Assess the foot for loss of strength:
- Limited ankle joint range of motion
- Limited motion of great toe

Assess the foot for loss of protective sensation:
- Numbness, burning, tingling
- Semmes-Weinstein monofilament testing at 10 points on each foot

CHART 65-10

CLIENT EDUCATION GUIDE
Foot Care Instructions

- Inspect your feet daily, especially the area between the toes.
- Wash your feet daily with lukewarm water and soap. Dry thoroughly.
- Apply moisturizing cream to your feet after bathing. Do not apply to the area between your toes.
- Change into clean cotton socks every day.
- Do not wear the same pair of shoes 2 days in a row, and wear only leather shoes.
- Check your shoes for foreign objects (nails, pebbles) before putting them on. Check inside the shoes for cracks or tears in the lining.
- Purchase shoes that have plenty of room for your toes. Buy shoes later in the day, when feet are normally larger. Break in new shoes gradually.
- Wear socks to keep your feet warm.
- Trim your nails straight across with a nail clipper. Smooth the nails with an emery board.
- See your physician or nurse immediately if you have blisters, sores, or infections. Protect area with a dry, sterile dressing. Do not use adhesive tape to secure dressing.
- Do not treat blisters, sores, or infections with home remedies.
- Do not smoke.
- Do not step into the bathtub without checking the temperature of the water with your wrist. Optimal temperature is 95° F (29.4° to 35° C).
- Do not use very hot or cold water. Never use hot water bottles, heating pads, or portable heaters to warm your feet.
- Do not treat corns, blisters, bunions, calluses, or ingrown toenails yourself.
- Do not go barefooted.
- Do not wear sandals with open toes or straps between the toes.
- Do not cross your legs or wear garters or tight stockings that constrict blood flow.
- Do not soak your feet.

WOUND CARE. The Wound Healing Society's standards of care for diabetic ulcers are a moist wound environment, debridement of necrotic tissue, and off-loading (Eaglstein & Falagna, 1997).

WOUND ENVIRONMENT. Dressings are used to reduce or prevent infection, allow painless debridement, reduce wound pain, and stimulate development of granulation tissue. Many commercial products achieve these purposes. Antiseptics such as povidone iodine, hydrogen peroxide, and chlorhexidine tend to be toxic to skin cells and interfere with wound healing. Research has not provided convincing evidence of their effectiveness (Lipsky, 1998). Dressings that keep the wound moist are essential.

DEBRIDEMENT. The value of debridement lies in removal of dead tissues that support bacterial growth. This is accomplished through surgical procedures, topically applied debriding agents, and dressing materials. Placing a wet dressing, letting it dry, and then tearing out the adherent tissue debrides the wound; however, this technique also delays wound repair (Hunt & Hopf, 1997).

ELIMINATION OF PRESSURE. The elimination of pressure on an infected area is essential to wound healing. Pressure is reduced through specialized orthotic devices; custom-molded shoe inserts, or shoe modifications that redistribute weight. Clients with foot ulcers are instructed not to wear a shoe on the affected foot while the ulcer is healing. Even the most ideally fitting prescription shoes will not take the pressure off a wound or ulcer nearly as well as a total-contact cast or removable cast walker (Armstrong & Lavery, 1998). Total-contact casts are used to aid in healing of ulcers. Casting material is molded to the foot and leg, allowing weight-bearing forces to be spread out along the entire surface of contact, thereby reducing vertical force. The almost complete elimination of motion of the total-contact cast reduces plantar shear forces. The cast is removed 24 to 48 hours after application and weekly thereafter until the ulcer is healed. The client must understand that unless measures are taken to redistribute weight on a permanent basis, foot ulcers will recur.

GROWTH FACTORS. Growth factors applied directly to wounds can increase the rate of healing by stimulating granulation tissue formation and enhancing cell growth (Steed, 1997). Diabetic foot ulcers that have been present for many months or even years are being healed with this treatment. Because treatment with growth factors is expensive and based on having other aspects of diabetes controlled, this treatment is generally performed in specialized treatment centers.

■ CHRONIC PAIN

NOC PLANNING: EXPECTED OUTCOMES. The client with diabetes who has neuropathic pain is expected to experience relief of pain, use preventive measures, and use available resources to increase comfort.

INTERVENTIONS. NIC intervention activities to manage pain are listed in Chart 65-11. Achieving and maintaining normal blood glucose levels may prevent neuropathy and relieve symptoms of acute nerve dysfunction. Anticonvulsant drugs are commonly used in the treatment of pain caused by diabetic neuropathy. Agents such as gabapentin (Neurontin) have been shown to reduce mean pain scores and improve the perceived quality of life in diabetic clients with neuropathic pain (Vinik, 1999). Tricyclic antidepressants, particularly amitriptyline hydrochloride (Elavil, Levate♣) and nortriptyline (Pamelor), also are beneficial in treating pain caused by neuropathy. These drugs have an analgesic effect, and smaller doses are required for analgesia than for antidepressant effects.

The burning typical of C-fiber neuropathy may respond to capsaicin cream 0.075% (Axsain♣, Zostrix-HP). This drug promotes depletion of neuropeptide substance P, which is involved in pain transmission (see Chapter 7). The nurse instructs the client in the application of capsaicin. Topical applications four times daily are needed for several weeks before relief is achieved. Neuropathic pain may often worsen for several days after therapy is initiated before improving.

■ RISK FOR INJURY RELATED TO VISUAL SENSORY-PERCEPTUAL ALTERATIONS

NOC PLANNING: EXPECTED OUTCOMES. The client with diabetes is expected to maintain optimal vision and be free of injury related to decreased visual acuity.

CHART 65-11

NIC INTERVENTION ACTIVITIES for
The Diabetic Client Experiencing Pain

Analgesic Administration: *Use of pharmacologic agents to reduce or eliminate pain*
- Determine pain location, characteristics, quality, and severity before medicating client.
- Check medical order for drug, dose, and frequency of analgesic prescribed.
- Attend to comfort needs and other activities that assist relaxation to facilitate response to analgesia.
- Set positive expectations regarding the effectiveness of analgesics to optimize client response.
- Document response to analgesic and any untoward effects.
- Teach about the use of analgesics, strategies to decrease side effects, and expectations for involvement in decisions about pain relief.

Teaching: Individual: *Planning, implementation, and evaluation of a teaching program designed to address a client's particular needs*
- Establish rapport.
- Determine the client's learning needs.
- Appraise the client's current level of knowledge and understanding of content.
- Appraise the client's educational level.
- Appraise the client's cognitive, psychomotor, and affective abilities/disabilities.
- Determine the client's ability to learn specific information (i.e., developmental level, physiologic status, orientation, pain, fatigue, unfulfilled basic needs, emotional state, and adaptation to illness).
- Set mutual, realistic learning goals with the client.
- Identify learning objectives necessary to reach goals.
- Determine the sequence for presenting the information.
- Appraise the client's learning style.
- Select appropriate teaching methods/strategies.
- Select appropriate educational materials.
- Tailor the content to the client's cognitive, psychomotor, and/or affective abilities/disabilities.
- Adjust instruction to facilitate learning, as appropriate.
- Provide an environment conducive to learning.
- Instruct the client, when appropriate.
- Evaluate the client's achievement of the stated objectives.
- Reinforce behavior, as appropriate.
- Correct information misinterpretations, as appropriate.
- Provide time for the client to ask questions and discuss concerns.
- Select new teaching methods/strategies, if previous ones were ineffective.
- Refer the client to other specialists/agencies to meet the learning objectives as appropriate.
- Document the content presented, the written materials provided, and the client's understanding of the information or client behaviors that indicate learning on the permanent medical record.
- Include the family/significant others, as appropriate.

NIC intervention activities selected from McCloskey J.C., & Bulechek, G.M. (2000). *Nursing interventions classification (NIC)* (3rd ed.). St. Louis: Mosby. No part of this work is to be altered without prior written permission from the Publisher.

INTERVENTIONS

BLOOD GLUCOSE CONTROL. Poor blood glucose control, proteinuria, diastolic hypertension, and long duration of diabetes are associated with the development of diabetic retinopathy. Retinopathy and vision loss can be markedly reduced with good control of blood glucose. Surgical intervention for retinal hemorrhage or new retinal blood vessel growth can also reduce vision loss.

Only about 10% of all clients with visual impairment are totally blind. The rest have reduced vision. In addition to regular eye examinations to evaluate retinopathy, the nurse encourages the client with diabetes and visual impairment to be examined by an optometrist or ophthalmologist for assessment of remaining vision and prescription of appropriate eyewear. A functional vision assessment, performed by a low-vision technician, rehabilitation teacher, or diabetes educator, is a task-specific evaluation that determines the client's use of lighting, contrast, nonoptical and low-vision devices, and large-print options. Included in the functional vision assessment is whether the client uses central or peripheral vision. Diabetic clients with macular edema have loss of central vision. This process causes difficulties with detail discrimination, reading printed materials, preparing insulin syringes for injection, and performing self-monitoring of blood glucose levels (SMBG).

ENVIRONMENTAL MANAGEMENT. Not all diabetic clients with visual impairment require the use of special devices. Adjustments in lighting, contrast, color, distance, type size of printed materials, and eye movement often improve visual abilities. The nurse recommends that the client supplement overhead fluorescent lighting with an incandescent lamp directed toward the workspace. Placing dark equipment against a white or yellow background (or vice versa) provides contrast to enhance vision. Coding objects such as vials of insulin with bright colors or with felt-tipped markers will aid in identification of the correct bottle to be used. Bringing the blood glucose lancet or insulin syringe close to the eye makes it easier to see. The nurse directs the client to sources of materials printed with a large type size or bold print to enhance ease of reading. The client is instructed to use peripheral fields of vision by learning how to move the eye to maximize vision.

Visually adapted devices make it possible for the client to self-administer insulin doses independently. Preset dose gauges (used to measure the space between the end of the syringe barrel and the plunger) allow a client to draw up the correct amount of insulin by feeling this distance. Variable dose gauges draw insulin in variable and mixed doses of 1-, 2-, and 10-unit increments. The client sets the desired dose by pressing a lever or turning a screw on the device. Critical points to stress when teaching the client to use an adaptive device include the following:

- Differentiating between bottles of fast-acting and slower-acting insulin (One commonly used method is to wrap a rubber band around the fast-acting insulin bottle.)
- Ensuring proper placement of the device on the syringe for correct measurements
- Holding the insulin bottle upright when measuring insulin
- Avoiding air bubbles in the syringe by pulling a small amount of insulin into the syringe, moving the plunger in and out three times, and measuring insulin on the fourth draw

A system to determine how many doses can be drawn from a bottle of insulin needs to be established so that the client does not inject air from an empty bottle rather than insulin (Williams, 1997, 1999b).

The nurse assists the diabetic client with visual impairment in maintaining blood glucose control to limit the amount of functional vision change that normally occurs with hypoglycemia and hyperglycemia.

CRITICAL THINKING CHALLENGE

The client has had diabetes mellitus for several years. He takes 30 units of NPH with 10 units of regular insulin in the morning before breakfast and 20 units of NPH insulin before the evening meal. He has recently undergone laser therapy for treatment of diabetic retinopathy. He wants to be independent in insulin administration, and your assessment indicates that he has the intellectual ability to learn the needed skills.

- List three methods for preventing both hypoglycemia and hyperglycemia that you would stress during your teaching sessions.
- Discuss four ways of altering the environment to aid in measurement of accurate insulin doses.
- List five critical points that would be included in a teaching session on adaptive devices for use with insulin syringes.

For suggested answer guidelines, go to SIMON http://www.wbsaunders.com/SIMON/Iggy/.

■ INEFFECTIVE RENAL TISSUE PERFUSION

PLANNING: EXPECTED OUTCOMES. The client with diabetes is expected to maintain a urine elimination pattern in the expected range and urine protein levels within normal limits.

INTERVENTIONS

PREVENTION. Tight control of blood glucose levels may reverse microalbuminuria and reduce the progression of renal disease in clients with type 1 diabetes. Control of hypertension also has been demonstrated to reduce the rate of progression of diabetic nephropathy and to reduce the complications of hypertensive nephropathy (ADA, 2000t).

The nurse stresses the need for yearly evaluation of kidney function according to American Diabetes Association (ADA) Standards of Care. Screening is performed by three methods: (1) measurement of the albumin-creatinine ratio in a random, spot urine collection; (2) 24-hour urine collection with creatinine, allowing for the simultaneous measurement of creatinine clearance; and (3) timed urine collection (e.g., 4 hours or overnight) (ADA, 2000t). The nurse explains the implications of the test and helps the client collect the specimen if necessary.

Aggressive control of blood glucose and hypertension in diabetic clients without microalbuminuria has been shown to avoid nephropathy. However, once microalbuminuria develops, end-stage renal disease is inevitable. Measures are then directed toward preventing progression of the disease. This is accomplished by treating hypertension, avoiding nephrotoxic agents, promptly treating urinary tract infections (UTIs), and preventing dehydration.

Control of blood pressure and blood glucose levels depends on the participation and cooperation of the client. Prescribed medications must be taken according to schedules, and dietary restriction must be maintained. All clients with diabetes must be aware of the roles of blood pressure and blood glucose levels in the development of renal disease. Nursing measures are directed toward assisting the client in maintaining normal blood glucose levels and blood pressure levels below 130/85 mm Hg (ADA, 2000e). In addition, the nurse stresses the need for yearly screening for microalbuminuria.

Any UTI has the potential to cause kidney infection and further irreversible decline in renal function. The nurse educates the client about the signs and symptoms of UTI. The client is instructed to take medications exactly as prescribed, making certain that the course of treatment is completed. The client needs to see the physician or nurse for follow-up urine cultures to reduce the risk of renal damage. Indwelling urinary catheters are avoided when possible.

Drugs can affect renal function either through toxic effects on the kidney or by an acute but reversible reduction in function. The most common nephrotoxic drugs are aminoglycoside antibiotics such as amikacin (Amikin), streptomycin, kanamycin (Kantrex), gentamicin (Garamycin), and tobramycin (Tobrex). Anticancer agents, such as cisplatin (Platinol); acetaminophen (Tylenol); other nonsteroidal anti-inflammatory drugs such as ibuprofen (Advil) or naproxen (Aleve); and antifungal agents (amphotericin B) should be avoided (Bell & Alele, 1999). Radiocontrast dyes and materials can also affect renal function. To prevent accidental ingestion of nephrotoxic drugs, the nurse cautions the client to check with his or her health care provider before taking any over-the-counter or prescription medication.

DIET THERAPY. Restriction of dietary protein to 0.8 g/kg of body weight per day is recommended for individuals with overt nephropathy. Once the glomerular filtration rate (GFR) begins to fall, further restriction to 0.6 g/kg may slow the decline in renal function (ADA, 2000e). Because of the difficulty in maintaining lifelong dietary restrictions, the nurse provides ongoing education to assist with dietary compliance.

NIC FLUID/ELECTROLYTE MANAGEMENT. The nurse institutes fluid and electrolyte management measures to prevent deterioration of renal status. NIC intervention activities for fluid and electrolyte management are listed in Chart 65-12. Avoiding dehydration is important in maintaining renal function. Any acute illness that causes dehydration is treated aggressively with IV fluids (Bell & Alele, 1999). The nurse assesses the status of fluid balance in the diabetic client and institutes measures to prevent dehydration. The most common cause of dehydration in clients with diabetic neuropathy is the overuse of diuretics. Clients are instructed to report edema or symptoms of orthostatic hypotension to their health care

---

CHART 65-12

NIC INTERVENTION ACTIVITIES for
The Diabetic Client Experiencing Fluid and Electrolyte and Acid-Base Imbalances

Fluid/Electrolyte Management: *Regulation and prevention of complications from altered fluid and/or electrolyte levels*
- Monitor for abnormal serum electrolyte levels, as available.
- Obtain laboratory specimens for monitoring of altered fluid or electrolyte levels (e.g., hematocrit, BUN, protein, sodium, and potassium levels), as appropriate.
- Weigh daily and monitor trends.
- Promote oral intake (e.g., provide oral fluids that are the client's preference, place in easy reach, provide a straw, and provide fresh water) as appropriate.
- Set an appropriate intravenous infusion (or blood transfusion) flow rate.
- Monitor laboratory results relevant to fluid balance (e.g., hematocrit, BUN, albumin, total protein, serum osmolality, and urine specific gravity levels).
- Monitor hemodynamic status, including CVP, MAP, PAP, and PCWP levels, if available.
- Keep an accurate record of intake and output.
- Monitor for signs and symptoms of fluid retention.
- Monitor vital signs, as appropriate.
- Maintain intravenous solution containing electrolyte(s) at a constant flow rate, as appropriate.
- Monitor client's response to prescribed electrolyte therapy.
- Monitor for manifestations of electrolyte imbalance.
- Assess client's buccal membranes, sclera, and skin for indications of altered fluid and electrolyte balance (e.g., dryness, cyanosis, and jaundice).
- Consult physician if signs and symptoms of fluid and/or electrolyte imbalance persist or worsen.
- Administer prescribed supplemental electrolytes, as appropriate.
- Monitor for fluid loss (e.g., bleeding, vomiting, diarrhea, perspiration, and tachypnea).

Acid-Base Management: Metabolic Acidosis: *Promotion of acid-base balance and prevention of complications resulting from serum HCO₃ levels lower than desired.*
- Obtain ordered specimens for laboratory analysis (e.g., ABG, urine, and serum levels), as appropriate.

- Monitor ABG levels for decreasing pH level, as appropriate.
- Maintain patent IV access.
- Monitor intake and output.
- Monitor determinants of tissue oxygen delivery (e.g., Pao₂, Sao₂, and hemoglobin levels and cardiac output), if available.
- Monitor for electrolyte imbalances associated with metabolic acidosis (e.g., hyponatremia, hyperkalemia or hypokalemia, hypocalcemia, hypophosphatemia, and hypomagnesemia), as appropriate.
- Monitor for decreasing bicarbonate from excessive nonvolatile acids (e.g., renal failure, diabetic ketoacidosis, tissue hypoxia, and starvation), as appropriate.
- Administer prescribed alkaline medications (e.g., sodium bicarbonate), as appropriate, based on ABG results.
- Prevent complications from excessive NaHCO₃ administration (e.g., metabolic alkalosis, hypernatremia, volume overload, decreased oxygen delivery, decreased cardiac contractility, and enhanced lactic acid production).
- Administer fluids as prescribed.
- Administer insulin and fluid hydration (isotonic and hypotonic) for diabetic ketoacidosis, causing metabolic acidosis, as appropriate.
- Institute seizure precautions.
- Monitor for CNS manifestations of metabolic acidosis (e.g., headache, drowsiness, decreased mentation, seizures, and coma), as appropriate.
- Monitor for cardiopulmonary manifestations of metabolic acidosis (e.g., hypotension, hypoxia, arrhythmias, and Kussmaul respiration), as appropriate.
- Monitor for GI manifestations of metabolic acidosis (e.g., anorexia, nausea, and vomiting), as appropriate.
- Provide comfort measures to deal with the GI effects of metabolic acidosis.
- Instruct the client and/or family on actions instituted to treat the metabolic acidosis.

NIC intervention activities selected from McCloskey J.C., & Bulechek, G.M. (2000). *Nursing interventions classification (NIC)* (3rd ed.). St. Louis: Mosby. No part of this work is to be altered without prior written permission from the Publisher.
BUN, Blood urea nitrogen; *CVP,* central venous pressure; *MAP,* mean arterial pressure; *PAP,* pulmonary artery pressure; *PCWP,* pulmonary capillary wedge pressure; *ABG,* arterial blood gas; *Pao₂,* partial pressure of arterial oxygen; *Sao₂,* arterial oxygen saturation; *NaHCO₃,* sodium bicarbonate; *CNS,* central nervous system; *GI,* gastrointestinal.

provider. The nurse also provides ongoing education to assist with dietary compliance.

Dialysis treatment for diabetic clients with renal failure is the same as for clients without diabetes (see Chapter 72). The dosage of insulin needs to be adjusted when dialysis is started.

■ POTENTIAL FOR HYPOGLYCEMIA

Proper central nervous system (CNS) function depends on a continuous supply of glucose in the blood. The brain cannot make glucose and stores only a few minutes' supply as glycogen. This needed continuous supply of glucose cannot be maintained when blood glucose concentration falls below critical levels.

The first defense against falling blood glucose levels in the nondiabetic client is decreased insulin secretion, decreased glucose use, and increased glucose production. Decreased insulin secretion normally occurs when blood glucose levels drop to about 83 mg/dL (4.5 mmol/L). Critical glucose counterregulatory hormones are activated at about 68 mg/dL (3.8 mmol/L), a blood glucose threshold well above the level for symptoms of hypoglycemia. The primary counterregulatory hormone is glucagon; epinephrine also becomes important in diabetic clients who have deficient glucagon levels. Both glucagon and epinephrine raise blood glucose levels by stimulating liver glycogenolysis and gluconeogenesis. In addition, epinephrine limits secretion of insulin.

Type 1 diabetes mellitus causes severe problems in the body's response to hypoglycemia. These changes are evident within 1 to 5 years of diagnosis. Regulation of circulating insulin levels is lost in clients with type 1 diabetes because the source of insulin is an injection rather than the pancreas. As blood glucose levels fall, insulin levels do not decrease. The ability of the pancreas to secrete glucagon in response to hypoglycemia is lost in clients with long-standing diabetes. After a few more years of type 1 diabetes, epinephrine response to falling blood glucose levels is also reduced. Epinephrine responses will occur but will require a lower blood glucose level to become active. These problems dramatically increase the risk for severe hypoglycemia.

A second problem found in clients with long-standing type 1 diabetes is **hypoglycemic unawareness.** These clients no longer have the warning symptoms of impending hypoglycemia that prompt them to take appropriate preventive action. Hypoglycemic unawareness is reported to occur in 50% of all clients with very-long-standing (>30 years) type 1 diabetes and in an estimated 25% of clients overall.

Symptoms of hypoglycemia are divided into two categories. **Neuroglycopenic** symptoms result directly from brain glucose deprivation and are associated with a more gradual decline in blood glucose. **Neurogenic** symptoms result from autonomic nervous system activation triggered by hypoglycemia and occur when there is a rapid decline in blood glucose (Table 65-16). Awareness of hypoglycemia is largely the result of perception of neurogenic symptoms (Cryer, 1999).

Blood glucose levels that cause symptoms of hypoglycemia vary among individuals. Many clients with diabetes have hypoglycemic symptoms when blood glucose levels are well above 50 mg/dL (2.8 mmol/L), especially if the level has dropped rapidly or if they are accustomed to sustained hyperglycemia. Thus clinical criteria are used to categorize hypo-

TABLE 65-16 · SYMPTOMS OF HYPOGLYCEMIA	
NEUROGLYCOPENIC SYMPTOMS	**NEUROGENIC SYMPTOMS**
• Headache	• Adrenergic:
• Confusion	Shaky/tremulous
• Slurred speech	Heart pounding
• Behavior changes	Nervous/anxious
• Coma	• Cholinergic:
• Warm	Sweaty
• Weak	Hungry
• Faint	Tingling
• Dizzy	
• Blurred vision	

Data from Towler, D.A., et al. (1993). Mechanism of awareness of hypoglycemia. Perception of neurogenic (predominantly cholinergic) rather than neuroglycopenic symptoms. *Diabetes, 42,* 1791.

glycemic severity. In mild hypoglycemia, the client remains totally alert and is able to treat symptoms. In severe hypoglycemia, neurologic function is so impaired that the assistance of another person is needed for treatment.

PLANNING: EXPECTED OUTCOMES. The client with diabetes is expected to have an optimal level of mental status functioning (e.g., alert and oriented to person, place, and time, with a Glasgow Coma Scale score greater than 7) and have decreased episodes of hypoglycemia.

INTERVENTIONS. Many diabetic clients have symptoms of hypoglycemia at levels above 50 mg/dL. A blood glucose level below 70 mg/dL alerts the nurse to assess for signs and symptoms of hypoglycemia (Funnell et al., 1998) (Table 65-17; see also Table 65-16).

HYPOGLYCEMIA MANAGEMENT. NIC intervention activities for hypoglycemia are listed in Chart 65-13. The nurse monitors blood glucose levels before administering antidiabetic agents, before meals, and before the hour of sleep, or when the client is symptomatic. All clients who take insulin or sulfonylurea agents to lower blood glucose levels are at risk for hypoglycemia, especially if they are older, have liver or kidney impairment, or are taking medications that potentiate the effects of oral antidiabetic drugs. Recognition of sulfonylurea-induced hypoglycemia is often delayed because the usual neurologic symptoms are often absent (Marks & Teale, 1999).

DIET THERAPY. When the client is hypoglycemic, the nurse starts treatment with carbohydrate replacement per physician orders or standing protocols. When the client can swallow, a liquid form of carbohydrate is administered, although virtually any low-fat source of carbohydrate can be used to treat hypoglycemia. Specific treatment recommendations are listed in Chart 65-14. The level of blood glucose being treated may determine the form of glucose to be used. Fluid is absorbed much more quickly from the gastrointestinal (GI) tract than solids. Highly concentrated sweetened fluids, such as juice with several spoonfuls of sugar added or a soft drink, may retard absorption. Commercially available products provide predictable amounts of glucose.

DRUG THERAPY. Glucagon administered subcutaneously or intramuscularly and 50% dextrose administered intravenously are given to diabetic clients who are unable to swal-

TABLE 65-17 • DIFFERENTIATION OF HYPOGLYCEMIA AND HYPERGLYCEMIA

Feature	Hypoglycemia	Hyperglycemia
Skin	Cool, clammy	Hot, dry*
Dehydration	Absent	Present
Perspiration	Profuse*	Absent
Respirations		Rapid, deep*; Kussmaul type; acetone odor to breath
Mental status	Anxious, nervous,* irritable, mental confusion,* seizures, coma	Varies from alert to stuporous, obtunded, or frank coma

Symptoms	Weakness,* double vision, blurred vision, hunger, tachycardia, palpitations	No specific symptoms for DKA
		  Acidosis: hypercapnea; abdominal cramps, nausea and vomiting
		  Dehydration: decreased neck vein filling, orthostatic hypotension, tachycardia, poor skin turgor

Glucose	50 mg/dL (2.8 mmol/L)	>250 mg/dL (13.8 mmol/L)
Ketones	Negative	Positive

DKA, Diabetic ketoacidosis.
*Classic symptoms.

CHART 65-13

NIC INTERVENTION ACTIVITIES *for*
**The Diabetic Client Experiencing or at Risk
for Hypoglycemia**

Hypoglycemia Management: *Preventing and treating low
blood glucose levels*
- Identify clients at risk for hypoglycemia.
- Monitor blood glucose levels, as indicated.
- Monitor for signs and symptoms of hypoglycemia (e.g., shakiness, tremor, sweating, nervousness, anxiety, irritability, impatience, tachycardia, palpitations, chills, clamminess, lightheadedness, pallor, hunger, nausea, headache, tiredness, drowsiness, weakness, warmth, dizziness, faintness, blurred vision, nightmares, crying out in sleep, paresthesias, difficulty concentrating, difficulty speaking, incoordination, behavior change, confusion, coma, seizure).
- Provide simple carbohydrate, as indicated.
- Provide complex carbohydrate and protein, as indicated.
- Administer glucagon, as indicated.
- Contact emergency medical services, as necessary.
- Administer intravenous glucose, as indicated.
- Maintain patent airway, as necessary.
- Maintain IV access, as appropriate.
- Protect from injury, as necessary.
- Review events prior to hypoglycemia to determine probable cause.
- Provide feedback regarding appropriateness of self-care management of hypoglycemia.
- Instruct client and significant others on signs and symptoms, risk factors, and treatment of hypoglycemia.
- Instruct client to have simple carbohydrates available at all times.
- Instruct client to obtain and carry/wear appropriate emergency identification.
- Instruct significant others on the use and administration of glucagon, as appropriate.
- Instruct on interaction of diet, insulin/oral agents, and exercise.
- Provide assistance in making self-care decisions to prevent hypoglycemia (e.g., reducing insulin/oral agents and/or increasing food intake for exercise).
- Encourage self-monitoring of blood glucose levels.
- Encourage ongoing telephone contact with diabetes care team for consultation regarding adjustments in treatment regimen.

NIC intervention activities selected from McCloskey J.C., & Bulechek, G.M. (2000). *Nursing interventions classification (NIC)* (3rd ed.). St. Louis: Mosby. No part of this work is to be altered without prior written permission from the Publisher.

CHART 65-14

CLIENT EDUCATION GUIDE
Treatment of Hypoglycemia at Home

For *mild* hypoglycemia (hungry, irritable, shaky, weak, headache, fully conscious; blood glucose usually less than 60 mg/dL [3.4 mmol/L]):
- Treat the symptoms of hypoglycemia with 10 to 15 g of carbohydrate. You may use one of the following:
   Glucose tablets or glucose gel (dosage is printed on the package)
   $1/2$ cup of fruit juice
   $1/2$ cup of regular (nondiet) soft drink
   8 ounces of skim milk
   6 to 10 hard candies
   4 cubes of sugar
   4 teaspoons of sugar
   6 saltines
   3 graham crackers
   1 tablespoon of honey or syrup
- Retest blood glucose in 15 minutes.
- Repeat this treatment if symptoms do not resolve.
- Eat a small snack of carbohydrate and protein if your next meal is more than an hour away.

For *moderate* hypoglycemia (cold and clammy skin; pale; rapid pulse; rapid, shallow respirations; marked change in mood; drowsiness; blood glucose usually less than 40 mg/dL [2.2 mmol/L]):
- Treat the symptoms of hypoglycemia with 15 to 30 g of rapidly absorbed carbohydrate.
- Take additional food, such as low-fat milk or cheese, after 10 to 15 minutes.

For *severe* hypoglycemia (unable to swallow; unconsciousness or convulsions; blood glucose usually less than 20 mg/dL [1.0 mmol/L]):
Treatment administered by family members:
- Administer 1 mg of glucagon as intramuscular or subcutaneous injection.
- Administer a second dose in 10 minutes if the person remains unconscious.
- Notify a primary care provider immediately, and follow instructions.
- If still unconscious, transport the person to the emergency department.
- Give a small meal when the person wakes up and is no longer nauseated.

low. Glucagon converts liver glycogen to glucose and is not effective in severely starved clients. The nurse takes care to prevent aspiration in clients receiving glucagon, since it often causes vomiting. The nurse gives 50% dextrose carefully to avoid extravasation. The effects of glucagon and dextrose are temporary, and after the client responds, the nurse administers a simple sugar followed by a small snack or meal. IV glucose may be ordered to maintain mild hyperglycemia. Diazoxide (Proglycem), a specific antidote to sulfonylurea-induced hypoglycemia, or octreotide (Sandostatin), which inhibits sulfonylurea-induced insulin release, may be required if there is difficulty keeping blood glucose levels up by infusion alone (Marks & Teale, 1999).

The nurse evaluates the results of treatment by monitoring blood glucose levels for several hours. Symptoms may persist for an hour or more after treatment of hypoglycemia. A target blood glucose level is 70 to 110 mg/dL (3.9 to 6.2 mmol/L).

PREVENTION STRATEGIES. The nurse teaches the diabetic client how to prevent future episodes of hypoglycemia. Four common causes of hypoglycemia are (1) excess insulin, (2) deficient intake or absorption of food, (3) exercise, and (4) alcohol.

INSULIN EXCESS. Even when insulin is injected in a consistent manner in a nonexercised body area, variations in absorption can cause hypoglycemia. Excess insulin can be caused by lowered insulin resistance, which occurs with termination of pregnancy or resolution of an infection. Increased insulin sensitivity can occur with weight loss or exercise programs and also leads to excess insulin. The nurse instructs the individual taking insulin not to change brands or change from animal-source to human insulin without medical supervision. Differences in formulation of insulin can result in hypoglycemia.

DEFICIENT FOOD INTAKE. Inadequate or incorrectly timed dietary intake can result in hypoglycemia. Irregularities in gastric absorption sometimes cause hypoglycemia in clients with delayed gastric emptying. This problem is more common in clients with diabetes of long duration, is more severe with solid than with liquid meals, and is made worse by illness or poor metabolic control. The nurse instructs the client about the importance of regularity in timing and quantity of food eaten.

EXERCISE. Blood glucose levels commonly decline during exercise in a client with type 1 diabetes. Severe and/or prolonged exercise can increase the rates of cellular glucose uptake and use for several hours after the exercise has been completed. The nurse instructs the client in blood glucose monitoring and carbohydrate supplementation during exercise.

ALCOHOL. The cause of alcohol-induced hypoglycemia is the inhibition of liver gluconeogenesis. Alcohol produces hypoglycemia only when fasting is prolonged and when glycogen stores are depleted before drinking begins (Marks & Teale, 1999). Alcohol cannot be converted to glucose and interferes with the counterregulatory response to hypoglycemia (Funnell et al., 1998). Alcohol may also impair glycogen breakdown and makes exercise-induced hypoglycemia more

severe. Alcohol also potentiates the effects of insulin and sulfonylurea-induced hypoglycemia. The nurse instructs the diabetic individual to ingest alcohol according to ADA guidelines—only with or shortly after eating a meal with enough carbohydrate to prevent hypoglycemia (ADA, 2000n). The client is cautioned about avoiding excess alcohol at bedtime to prevent nighttime hypoglycemia.

CLIENT EDUCATION. The cause of hypoglycemia may be subtle. At the onset of menses, a fall in progesterone level may decrease insulin requirements and contribute to hypoglycemia. When clients switch to a new bottle of insulin, hypoglycemia may be noted because the old bottle of insulin had lost its potency. Some clients report hypoglycemia when they change injection sites. Drugs such as propranolol (Inderal, Detensol✤) or other beta blockers mask the early warning signs and thus predispose clients to severe hypoglycemia. Some episodes of hypoglycemia occur without an obvious cause, and many are due to the erratic absorption of insulin, a problem that is not eliminated even in the most careful client.

The nurse can help each diabetic client to develop a personal treatment plan for hypoglycemia. Routine administration of 10 to 15 g of carbohydrate results in overtreatment of hypoglycemic episodes in some individuals and undertreatment in others. The exact glucose rise produced by a given amount of carbohydrate varies. Using the estimate that each 5 g of carbohydrate raises blood glucose about 20 mg/dL, a personal treatment plan can be developed that will provide direction for treatment of specific blood glucose levels. As an example, the client may be directed to take the following Farkas-Hirsh, 2000):

- 20 to 30 g of carbohydrate for a blood glucose level of 50 mg/dL (2.8 mmol/L) or less
- 10 to 15 g of carbohydrate for a blood glucose level of 51 to 70 mg/dL (2.9 to 3.9 mmol/L)

This treatment plan is revised or reinforced by blood glucose monitoring results.

The client is instructed to wear a medical alert bracelet to advise others of the diabetic status. This bracelet is helpful if clients become hypoglycemic and are unable to provide self-care. The nurse assists the client in obtaining the medical alert bracelet.

The nurse teaches the client and family about the signs and symptoms of hypoglycemia. Clients and family members must know that delaying a meal for more than 30 minutes increases the risk for hypoglycemia. The client should have a carbohydrate source with him or her at all times.

The cause of any episodes of hypoglycemia should be determined, and measures taken to prevent recurrence. Hypoglycemia is a major risk associated with exercise programs for clients receiving intensive insulin protocols. Nightmares or headaches on days after prolonged or severe exercise are associated with hypoglycemia, and this possibility should be understood by the client and his or her family.

ESTABLISHING TREATMENT PLANS. Blood glucose monitoring provides information on successful treatment of hypoglycemia. Treatment is continued until blood glucose target ranges have been achieved and maintained. Once treatment is successful and blood glucose control are regained, the specific cause of each hypoglycemic episode must be determined and measures taken to prevent further recurrences.

POTENTIAL FOR DIABETIC KETOACIDOSIS

Metabolic problems of diabetic ketoacidosis (DKA) are caused by a total or partial lack of insulin combined with the action of counterregulatory hormones (Figure 65-11). Laboratory diagnosis of DKA is shown in Table 65-18. DKA occurs in 2% to 5% of all clients with type 1 diabetes mellitus and is most often started by infection. *Death occurs in 1% to 10% of these clients even with appropriate treatment.* Mortality is highest for clients over 60 years of age. Most deaths in older clients occur when there are additional health problems, such as infection, stroke, myocardial infarction, vascular thrombosis, intestinal obstruction, or pneumonia, along with DKA.

Polyuria, polydipsia, and polyphagia start before the actual DKA. Central nervous system (CNS) depression results in changes in consciousness varying from lethargy to coma. The client is dehydrated and has signs and symptoms of severe fluid loss. Kussmaul respiration, abdominal pain, nausea, and vomiting are associated with the metabolic acidosis. Initial serum sodium levels may be low or normal. Initial potassium levels depend on how long DKA has existed before treatment. After therapy is initiated, serum potassium levels begin to drop quickly. Serum white blood cell counts of 20,000 cells/mm indicate dehydration; counts greater than 30,000 cells/mm^3 usually indicate infection.

PLANNING: EXPECTED OUTCOMES. The client with diabetes is expected to maintain a normal blood glucose level and have minimized episodes of hyperglycemia.

INTERVENTIONS

HYPERGLYCEMIA MANAGEMENT. The nurse monitors for signs and symptoms of DKA (see Table 65-18 and Figure 65-11). In the initial phases of treatment, the nurse checks the client's blood pressure, pulse, and respirations every 15 minutes until stable. The nurse records urine output, temperature, and mental status every hour. When a central venous catheter has been placed, the nurse assesses central venous pressure as ordered, usually every 30 minutes. Assessing the client's airway patency, level of consciousness, hydration status, status of fluid and electrolyte replacement, and levels of blood glucose are primary nursing measures. After treatment is underway and these variables are stable, monitoring vital signs and recording values every 4 hours is acceptable. Blood glucose values can be measured either by laboratory or bedside glucose monitoring. Results indicate the adequacy of insulin replacement and establish when to switch from saline to dextrose-containing solutions.

FLUID AND ELECTROLYTE MANAGEMENT. Close assessment of the *fluid status* of the diabetic client is essential. The kidneys are less able to respond to changes in pH or fluid and electrolyte balance, to concentrate urine, or to regulate blood osmolarity. The risk for kidney failure also rises with age. Impaired bicarbonate reabsorption and acid excretion in poorly functioning renal tubules can progress to acidosis. Car-

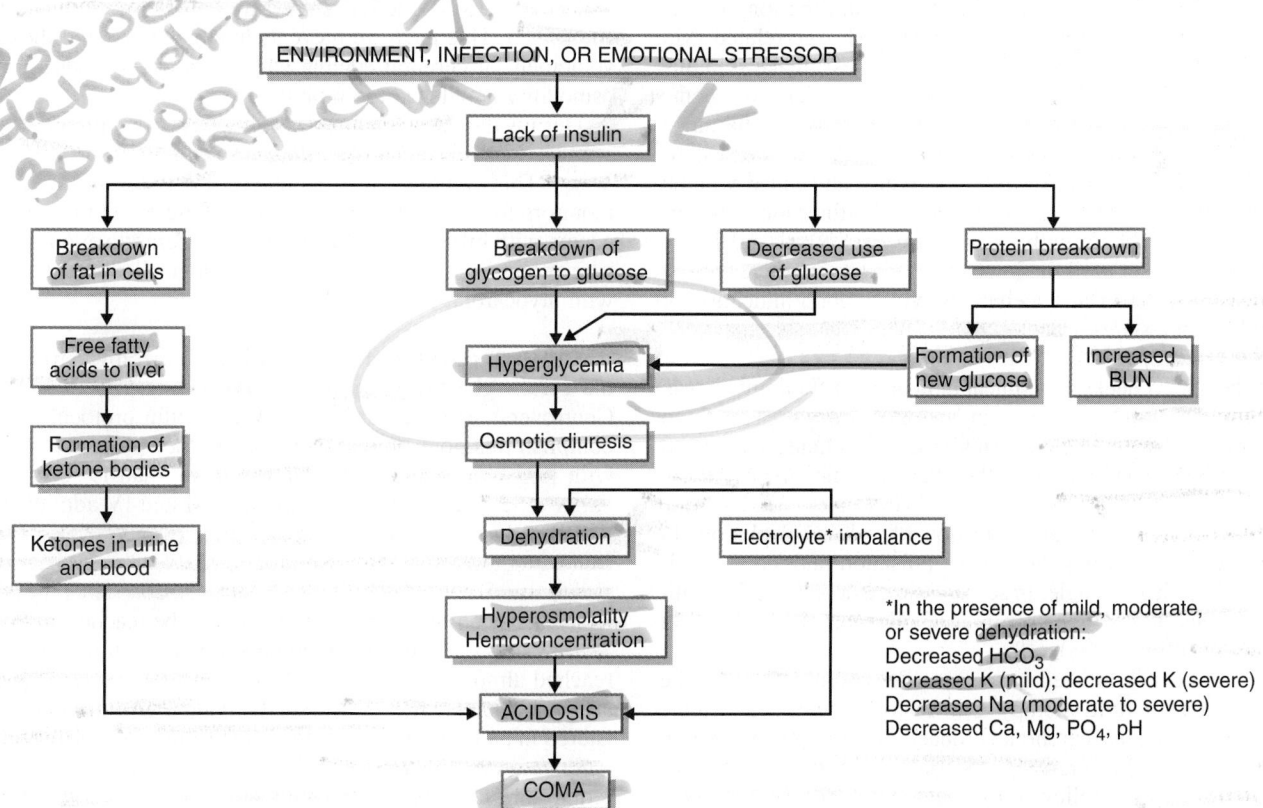

Figure 65-11 ● The pathophysiologic mechanism of diabetic ketoacidosis.

TABLE 65-18 • DIFFERENCES BETWEEN DIABETIC KETOACIDOSIS AND HYPERGLYCEMIC-HYPEROSMOLAR NONKETOTIC SYNDROME

	Diabetic Ketoacidosis (DKA)	Hyperglycemic-Hyperosmolar Nonketotic Syndrome (HHNS)
Onset	Sudden	Gradual
Precipitating factors	Infection Other stressors Inadequate insulin dose	Infection Other stressors Poor fluid intake
Manifestations	Ketosis: Kussmaul respiration, "fruity" breath, nausea, abdominal pain Dehydration or electrolyte loss: polyuria, polydipsia, weight loss, dry skin, sunken eyes, soft eyeballs, lethargy, coma	Altered central nervous system function with neurologic symptoms Dehydration or electrolyte loss: same as for DKA
LABORATORY FINDINGS		
Serum glucose	>300 mg/dL (16.7 mmol/L)	>800 mg/dL (44.5 mmol/L)
Osmolality	Variable	>350 mOsm/L
Serum ketones	Positive at 1:2 dilutions	Negative
Serum pH	<7.35	>7.4
Serum HCO$_3$	<15 mEq/L	>20 mEq/L
Serum Na	Low, normal, or high	Normal or low
Serum K	Normal; elevated with acidosis, low following dehydration	Normal or low
BUN	>20 mg/dL; elevated because of dehydration	Elevated
Creatinine	>1.5 mg/dL; elevated because of dehydration	Elevated
Urine ketones	Positive	Negative

HCO$_3$, Bicarbonate.

(handwritten margin note: generalized seizures, myoclonic jerking)

diovascular disease can cause fluid retention. The dehydrated client's lips and mouth may appear dry, and the tongue furrowed. Body temperature is often elevated. Age-related skin changes, such as loss of elasticity and dryness, make skin turgor a poor sign of dehydration in the older client. In clients with poor renal function and excess fluid volume, the nurse assesses for edema around the eyes and in the extremities, increasing abdominal girth, blood pressure and pulse volume increases, jugular venous distention, and orthostatic hypotension. Edema occurs with excess interstitial fluid and is not usually apparent until the interstitial volume has increased by at least 2 to 3 L. Daily weights provide a good indication of fluid volume status. One kilogram of body weight equals 1 L of fluid (Toto, 1998).

The nurse checks for clinical indicators of fluid imbalance. Volume overload can cause an increase in blood pressure to the point of hypertension. This is true in clients with renal failure who cannot excrete the extra volume. An increased jugular venous pressure occurs with volume overload. Orthostatic hypotension is an indication of volume depletion. In volume depletion, jugular venous pulsation may not be visible at a 45-degree angle. In severe volume depletion, the jugular venous pulsation may not be visible even with the client lying flat (Toto, 1998).

Treatment is initiated to correct a fluid volume deficit. The initial goal of fluid therapy is to restore circulating volume and protect against cerebral, coronary, or renal hypoperfusion. The nurse administers 1 L of isotonic saline over a period of 30 to 60 minutes, followed by a second liter in the next hour, or as ordered.

The second objective of fluid therapy, which is to replace total body and intracellular losses, is achieved more slowly, usually using 0.45% saline. When blood glucose levels reach 250 mg/dL (13.8 mmol/L), 5% dextrose in 0.45% saline is administered. This measure prevents hypoglycemia and the development of cerebral edema, which can occur when serum osmolality is reduced too rapidly.

During the first 24 hours of treatment, the client needs enough fluids to replace both the volume deficit and ongoing losses. This volume can be as much as 6 to 10 L. The nurse monitors for signs of congestive heart failure and pulmonary edema with infusions of this magnitude. Central venous pressure monitoring may be needed for older clients and those with myocardial disease.

DRUG THERAPY. The goal of insulin therapy is to lower the serum glucose by approximately 75 to 150 mg/dL/hr. Controversy exists regarding the best insulin protocol to accomplish this goal. "Low-dose" insulin therapy is associated with less hypokalemia and hypoglycemia than is seen with "high-dose" regimens. Although both IM and IV administration have been used, most protocols for treating DKA recommend continuous IV administration of regular insulin because absorption from intramuscular or subcutaneous sites may be erratic. A steady-state level of insulin can be reached in 25 to 30 minutes. Effective blood insulin concentrations are reached almost immediately when an IV bolus dose is given at the start of the infusion. Usually, regular insulin is administered in an initial IV bolus dose of 0.1 units/kg, followed by an IV drip of 0.1 units/kg/hr. Continuous infusion of insulin is required because of the 4-minute half-life of IV insulin. Subcutaneous insulin is started when the client can take oral nourishment and ketosis has stopped. The effects of insulin therapy are assessed by hourly blood glucose measurements.

ACIDOSIS MANAGEMENT. Regardless of the initial potassium value, there is a large total-body potassium deficit. With insulin therapy, the serum potassium level falls rapidly as potassium shifts into the cells. The nurse monitors the client for signs of hypokalemia, including fatigue, malaise, confusion, muscle weakness, shallow respirations, abdominal distention or paralytic ileus, hypotension, and weak pulse. An electrocardiogram (ECG) shows cardiac conduction changes related to potassium. Hypokalemia is a significant cause of death in the treatment of DKA. Before administering IV potassium, the nurse ensures that the client's urine output is at least 30 mL/hr.

Bicarbonate therapy is indicated only for *severe* acidosis. Inappropriate use of bicarbonate may reverse acidosis too rapidly and result in severe hypokalemia, which can cause fatal cardiac dysrhythmias. Rapid correction of acidosis can worsen the client's mental status. Metabolic acidosis is corrected with fluid replacement and insulin therapy. Sodium bicarbonate, administered by slow IV infusion over several hours, is indicated when the arterial pH is 7.0 or less or the serum bicarbonate level is less than 5 mEq/L (5 mmol/L).

After acid-base disturbances have been corrected, the health team's efforts are directed toward determining the cause of DKA. Infection is the most common precipitating cause (see Table 65-18).

CLIENT EDUCATION: PREVENTION. Investigation of the factors leading to DKA helps the nurse plan specific educational efforts. The nurse teaches the client to perform self-monitoring of blood glucose levels (SMBG) every 4 to 6 hours as long as symptoms such as anorexia, nausea, and vomiting are present and as long as SMBG results are greater than 250 mg/dL (13.8 mmol/L). The client checks urine ketone levels when blood glucose levels exceed 300 mg/dL (>16.7 mmol/L).

The client is taught to minimize the risk for dehydration by maintaining food and fluid intake. When nausea is present, the client is instructed to take liquids containing both glucose and electrolytes (e.g., soda pop, diluted fruit juice, and sports drinks [Gatorade]). Small amounts of fluid may be tolerated even when vomiting is present. The client should take 8 to 12 ounces (240 to 360 mL) of calorie-free and caffeine-free liquids every hour while awake.

Liquids containing carbohydrate can be taken when the diabetic client is unable to eat solid food. The risk of starvation ketosis is reduced by a minimum daily carbohydrate intake of 150 g. After consulting with the primary care provider, the nurse may instruct the client to take additional rapid-acting (lispro) or short-acting (regular) insulin on the basis of SMBG results.

The nurse instructs the client to consult the primary care provider when the following occur:
- SMBG results are greater than 250 mg/dL (13.8 mmol/L).
- Ketonuria is present for more than 24 hours.
- The client is unable to take food or fluids.
- Illness persists for more than 1 to 2 days.

The nurse also instructs the client or the primary caregiver to detect hyperglycemia by performing SMBG whenever the client is ill. Significant illness can result in dehydration with DKA, hyperglycemic-hyperosmolar nonketotic syndrome, or both. The sooner the client seeks treatment, the less severe is the degree of metabolic alteration. Chart 65-15 reviews guidelines for the ill client to follow.

CHART 65-15

CLIENT EDUCATION GUIDE
Sick-Day Rules

- Notify your health care provider that you are ill.
- Monitor your blood glucose at least every 4 hours.
- Test your urine for ketones when your blood glucose level is greater than 240 mg/dL (13.8 mmol/L).
- Continue to take insulin or oral antidiabetic agents.
- To prevent dehydration, drink 8 to 12 ounces of sugar-free liquids every hour that you are awake.
- Continue to eat meals at regular times.
- If unable to tolerate solid food because of nausea, consume more easily tolerated foods or liquids equal to the carbohydrate content of your usual meal.
- Call your primary care provider for any of the following danger signals:
  - Persistent nausea and vomiting
  - Moderate or large ketones
  - Blood glucose elevation after 2 supplemental doses of insulin
  - High (101.5° F [38.6° C]) or rising fever; fever for more than 24 hours.
- Treat your symptoms (e.g., diarrhea, nausea, vomiting, and fever) as directed by your primary care provider.
- Get plenty of rest.

POTENTIAL FOR HYPERGLYCEMIC-HYPEROSMOLAR NONKETOTIC SYNDROME AND COMA

Hyperglycemic-hyperosmolar nonketotic syndrome (HHNS) is a **hyperosmolar** (increased blood osmolarity) state caused by hyperglycemia of any origin. The pathophysiologic processes associated with HHNS are outlined in Figure 65-12. Although both HHNS and diabetic ketoacidosis (DKA) are associated with hyperglycemia, HHNS is different from DKA because of the absence of ketosis and the much higher than average blood glucose levels and osmolality. Often blood glucose levels are greater than 800 mg/dL (44.5 mmol/L) and blood osmolality is greater than 350 mOsL when HHNS is present. Other biochemical problems with HHNS tend to be more severe than those with DKA. Table 65-18 outlines the differences between DKA and HHNS.

CONSIDERATIONS FOR OLDER ADULTS

HHNS occurs most often in older clients and almost exclusively in people with type 2 diabetes mellitus, many of whom were previously undiagnosed. Mortality rates in older clients have been as high as 40% to 70%. The onset of HHNS is slow and may not be recognized. The older client typically seeks medical attention later and is sicker than the younger client. *HHNS does not occur in adequately hydrated individuals.* Older clients with diabetes are at greater risk for dehydration and HHNS because of age-related changes in thirst perception and poor urine-concentrating abilities.

Conditions such as myocardial infarction, sepsis, pancreatitis, and stroke, and drugs such as glucocorticoids, diuretics, phenytoin sodium (Dilantin), propranolol (Inderal), and calcium channel blockers also may precipitate HHNS. Central nervous system (CNS) changes range from confusion to complete coma. In contrast to clients with DKA, those with HHNS may have generalized seizures, myoclonic jerking, and reversible paralysis.

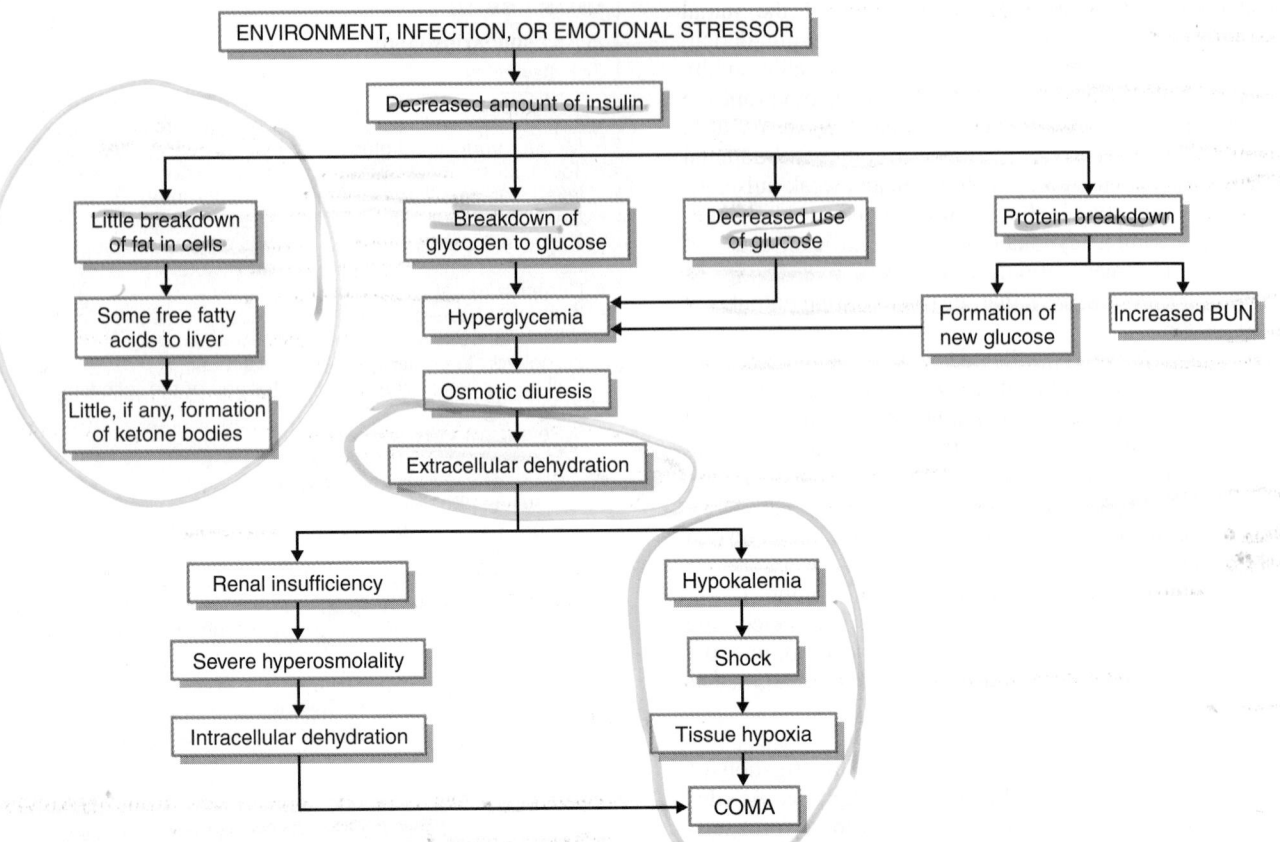

Figure 65-12 ● The pathophysiologic mechanism of hyperglycemic-hyperosmolar nonketotic syndrome.

The development of HHNS rather than DKA in any client is related to residual insulin secretion. In HHNS, the client secretes just enough insulin to prevent ketosis but not enough to prevent hyperglycemia. The hyperglycemia of HHNS is more severe than that of DKA, greatly increasing the blood osmolality and causing profound osmotic diuresis. Severe dehydration and electrolyte loss occur, and the client may lose 15% to 25% of body fluid. When dehydration is severe, glucose is not filtered into the urine, causing even greater hyperglycemia and hyperosmolality. Impairment of the thirst center in the brain occurs, making it impossible for the client to drink enough fluid to prevent dehydration.

PLANNING: EXPECTED OUTCOMES. The client with diabetes is expected to maintain a normal blood glucose level and have minimized episodes of hyperglycemia.

INTERVENTIONS

MONITORING. The nurse monitors for signs and symptoms of HHNS (see Tables 65-17 and 65-18 for symptoms of hyperglycemia). The nurse performs ongoing assessment of fluid status.

FLUID THERAPY. The goal of therapy is to complete rehydration and obtain normal blood glucose levels within 36 to 72 hours. The choice of fluid replacement and the rate of administration are critical in the management of HHNS. The severity of the CNS problems is related to the level of blood hyperosmolarity and cellular dehydration. Re-establishing fluid balance in brain cells is a difficult and slow process, and many clients do not recover baseline CNS function until several hours after blood glucose levels have returned to normal.

As with DKA, the *initial* objective for fluid replacement in HHNS is to increase circulating blood volume. If shock or severe hypotension is present, normal saline is given initially. Otherwise, half-normal saline is preferable because it more rapidly corrects the free-water deficit (Samos & Roos, 1998). The fluids are infused at a rate of 1 L/hr until central venous pressure or pulmonary capillary wedge pressure begins to rise or until the blood pressure and urine output are adequate. The rate is then reduced to 100 to 200 mL/hr. Half of the estimated water deficit is replaced in the first 12 hours, and the remainder is given during the next 36 hours. Body weight, urine output, kidney function, and the presence or absence of pulmonary congestion and jugular venous distention determine the rate of fluid administration. In clients with known congestive heart failure, renal insufficiency, or acute kidney failure, central venous pressure monitoring is indicated. The nurse assesses the client hourly for signs of cerebral edema. *Changes in the level of consciousness; changes in pupil size, shape or reaction; or seizures are reported immediately to the physician* (Konick-McMahan, 1999). Lack of any improvement in level of consciousness may indicate inadequate rates of fluid replacement or reduction in plasma osmolarity. Regression after initial improvement may indicate too rapid a reduction in plasma osmolarity. A slow but steady improvement in CNS function is the best evidence that fluid management is satisfactory.

CONTINUING THERAPY. IV insulin given at a rate of 10 units/hr is usually required to reduce blood glucose levels. Although fluid replacement reduces hyperglycemia, it cannot by itself return blood glucose levels to normal. A reduction of 10% per hour in the blood glucose level is a reasonable goal (Samos & Roos, 1998). Potassium loss occurs in HHNS, although not to the degree that it does in DKA. Because of the initial low urine output (**oliguria**) or absent urine output (**anuria**), potassium replacement may not be needed at the onset of therapy. Client education and interventions to minimize dehydration are similar to those for ketoacidosis.

● Community-Based Care

▓ HEALTH TEACHING

Education to attain blood glucose control must begin at the time of diagnosis of diabetes. Education is conducted in a hospital or outpatient setting, clinic, or primary care provider's office and involves the coordinated efforts of physicians, dietitians, nurses, pharmacists, social workers, and psychologists (see Chart 65-11).

ASSESSING LEARNING NEEDS. Although some education can be conducted in group settings, most will need to be done on a one-to-one basis. Continuing education will need to take place over time to master the knowledge, skills, and flexibility required to maintain long-term blood glucose control. The nurse or case manager assesses educational needs of the client and assures that education is provided by the appropriate disciplines.

The client's awareness of diabetes and the needs of the person and his or her family must be assessed before initiating teaching (Brink et al., 1995). This assessment includes the following:

* Age, occupation
* Likes, dislikes, fears
* Current lifestyle
* Evaluation of general health, attitudes about health, self-care behaviors
* Learning ability and style, willingness to learn
* Acceptance of diabetes, current knowledge of diabetes
* Skills needed, attitudes, goals
* Ethnic background, language
* Home situation

Before beginning actual diabetic education, the nurse assesses the client's baseline knowledge of diabetes and its treatment, determining what concerns the client the most about having diabetes. Adult learners are interested in information that applies directly to their situation. It is appropriate to ask what the client wants to learn. Starting with what he or she already knows and building on that base is a good way to increase knowledge and correct any errors in information that the client may have. To capture interest and motivate clients for further learning, the nurse presents material relevant to their first questions. Because they will be required to manage their own care after discharge, clients tend to focus on issues most important to them. Teaching about treatment measures that need to be started soon after diagnosis may be of more interest to the client than long-term control.

The client's physical condition dictates the timing of teaching efforts. When blood glucose levels are fluctuating, the client does not have the energy to learn complex information. Telling the client that good control of blood glucose levels improves the sense of well-being can help him or her accept the recommended therapy. An informal teaching program is started until the client feels able to attend a formal class. The nurse teaches and observes the client's technique for injections and blood glucose monitoring.

Individual clients learn in individual ways. A successful diabetic education program combines several different teaching methods. Some clients learn better when they read pamphlets; others learn better when they watch videotapes. Learning is enhanced when the equipment is handled, techniques are practiced, success is rewarded, and errors are corrected immediately.

ASSESSING PHYSICAL, COGNITIVE, AND EMOTIONAL LIMITATIONS. The nurse assesses the educational and reading levels of the client to determine what level of information to present. The client's visual ability to read printed information is assessed. In addition, the client taking insulin needs to be able to read the labels and markings on syringes and equipment. Many clients with type 2 diabetes have **presbyopia** (age-related far-sightedness) and baseline visual difficulties that are made worse by blurred vision caused by fluctuating blood glucose levels. The client must be able to understand the printed material that is presented. Even highly educated clients do not want to read complicated information when they are sick. Much of the printed material from drug companies is printed at the sixth- or seventh-grade level. The International Diabetes Center prepares printed diabetic education material at the second- and third-grade levels. The nurse develops creative teaching strategies for the client who cannot read.

The nurse also assesses the client's ability to conceptualize. The adjustment of insulin dosage on the basis of blood glucose monitoring is a difficult concept to understand and may not be appropriate for some clients who are unable to understand these concepts. Self-management of medication, exercise, and diet requires complex interpretation and behavior.

The nurse assesses manual dexterity and any physical limitations that may alter the teaching plan. A history of hand injury, the presence of hand tremors, or severe arthritis requires modification in insulin preparation instruction.

Information is best learned when the client is ready. Clients with newly diagnosed diabetes are facing a life crisis. Some may be more motivated to learn information that will be beneficial and are willing to change lifelong behaviors. Others may grieve the loss of their previous lifestyle and use denial as a means of coping with the diagnosis. In this instance, the client may not be able to learn needed information at this time.

EXPLAINING SURVIVAL SKILLS. The initial phase of diabetic education involves basic survival skills. The basic pathologic changes of diabetes and the relationship of diet, medication, and exercise to overall metabolic control are important.

A dietitian provides the initial diet instruction. The diabetic client needs to understand what food is to be eaten, how much food is to be eaten, and when the food is to be eaten. The nurse stresses the importance of eating meals on time, as well as the dangers of skipping meals. The client must be able to explain how to maintain food intake during illness. The nurse reinforces dietary instruction, answers questions, and refers questions to the dietitian or physician as indicated.

After the nurse provides medication instruction, the client should be able to identify the specific medication needed for control of blood glucose levels. When insulin administration is needed, the client must be able to prepare and administer the ordered dose accurately using sterile technique. The client must also be able to verbalize when insulin injections are to be taken, where insulin is to be injected, and how insulin is to be stored. The nurse stresses the dangers of skipping insulin doses. Possible drug interactions must be carefully reviewed with the client, particularly older individuals taking oral antidiabetic agents.

The diabetic client should be able to state a plan for regular physical activity. The client must be able to verbalize the relationship between exercise and blood glucose control and identify situations when activity is not appropriate. The nurse provides guidelines for additional carbohydrate intake to prevent hypoglycemia as a result of excessive exercise.

The diabetic client also must be able to verbalize the plan for monitoring blood glucose. The person performing self-monitoring of blood glucose levels (SMBG) must be able to do the procedure with accuracy and understanding of the results. The nurse provides guidelines for when SMBG is to be performed, acceptable ranges, and actions to be taken when results are out of these ranges. When the client is unable to perform SMBG, the nurse or case manager ensures that a resource (e.g., home care agency, health clinic, or primary care provider's office) will be available to do monitoring during times of illness).

The client must understand the significance, symptoms, causes, and treatment of hypoglycemia. It is essential for the diabetic client to verbalize the causes of hypoglycemia and the activities needed to prevent recurrence. He or she must be able to describe appropriate carbohydrate resources to have available and the intent to notify the physician regarding hypoglycemic episodes.

The client also must understand the significance of hyperglycemia and its relationship to illness. The client must describe actions to take during illness and when to communicate with the primary care provider.

Most of this survival information is retained when the client is ready to learn. Client education is a challenge to nurses because clients tend to be hospitalized for shorter periods. All of the diabetic education may be provided in an outpatient setting, where contact with the client is limited. It becomes necessary to squeeze important information into the time frames available. Many clients, regardless of the duration of their disease, do not progress in self-management beyond the survival level because of psychologic barriers.

COUNSELING. The major goal of in-depth counseling is to assist the client in becoming self-sufficient in diabetes management. Educational sessions with the client and family members are necessary in order to individualize the diabetes regimen to their particular needs, skills, and abilities. Education is often provided through the team efforts of a physician, a nurse educator, a dietitian, a social worker, a pharmacist, a psychologist, and other health care professionals as needed, and it occurs in a variety of outpatient settings.

In addition to knowledge gained at the survival level, the diabetic client should be able to discuss the action of insulin in the body and the effects of insulin deficiency on various body systems. The client should also be able to explain the effects of diet, medication, and activity on control of blood glucose levels. He or she should be able to relate the metabolic goals of maintaining normal blood glucose levels to the prevention of complications. This aspect involves being able to relate variations in SMBG results to the possible need for a change in insulin dosage.

The client must be able to describe the meal plan and explain what adjustments in dietary intake are needed to meet diabetic diet requirements. He or she should state how food intake needs to be altered when increased physical activity is planned and when he or she eats in restaurants or at family gatherings. It is essential that the client be able to list appropriate foods to be eaten to prevent and treat hypoglycemia, as well as adjustments to make when feeling ill.

The diabetic client must be able to demonstrate accuracy in insulin preparation and administration. He or she should be able to discuss the onset, peak, and duration of the specific insulin preparation. In reviewing insulin administration practices, the nurse stresses the importance of injection site selection and site rotation. The nurse carefully reviews guidelines for adjustment in insulin dosage on the basis of SMBG results (when permitted by the physician) and explains that follow-up SMBG results are needed to evaluate the effects of additional insulin. The client should explain the method of protecting insulin when traveling. For clients with the potential for severe hypoglycemia, the nurse observes a family member's ability to inject glucagon. When the client is taking oral diabetic medications, the nurse asks him or her to identify the medication and describe its schedule of administration. Because of the potential for drug interactions, the client must identify over-the-counter drugs with the potential to cause adverse drug interactions and the need to inform the primary care provider of the drug regimen.

Within the physical limitations imposed by the baseline health status, the client should be able to perform any desired physical activities. The diabetic client must state the SMBG levels that are safe for exercise, the frequency of performing SMBG during exercise, the food intake required before exercise, and what food to have available during exercise if symptoms of hypoglycemia occur. He or she should be aware of the potential for injury during exercise and explain the importance of protective footwear.

The goals of in-depth education are for the nurse to assist the diabetic client in solving problems of blood glucose fluctuation through the use of SMBG. The client should be able to identify practices, such as travel (Chart 65-16), that result in blood glucose fluctuations and to treat these problems with supplemental insulin administration, changes in physical activity levels, or changes in diet. The nurse asks the client to demonstrate urine ketone testing techniques and identify the conditions during which urine ketones should be measured.

The diabetic client must be able to describe a plan for periodic evaluation of the control of blood glucose levels by the primary care provider, as well as periodic dental and eye examinations. He or she must be able to demonstrate appropriate foot care, wear properly fitting shoes, and describe hazards related to foot care. The client must be able to relate plans to reduce specific risk factors, such as cigarette smoking and hypertension.

The client must verbalize that diabetes is a lifelong disease that necessitates lifestyle changes, describe the changes in progress, and indicate those that need to be made. He or she should be able to identify stress-producing situations and discuss methods for stress reduction.

■ PSYCHOSOCIAL PREPARATION

The diagnosis of diabetes may represent a loss of control. All but a few clients lose flexibility in routines. Life becomes ordered; time schedules and routines must be followed. Certain events surrounding diabetes are predictable. Taking an insulin injection and not eating for several hours causes hypoglycemia. Poorly controlled diabetes leads to complications and premature death. Tight control of blood glucose levels prevent these complications.

The stress of diabetes is in addition to the demands of normal daily life. The client must be able to integrate the demands of diabetes into daily and recreational schedules so as not to cause blood glucose alterations.

The nurse can assist in healthy psychologic adaptation to diabetes by providing successful educational experiences. The mastery of blood glucose monitoring assists the client in feeling that he or she has control over the disease. Knowledge of the effects of extra activities or extra food, as well as the result of taking additional insulin, is helpful in making future adjustments in regimens.

The client's feeling a sense of control over the condition does much to provide a positive psychologic attitude about diabetes. Success in self-injection of insulin provides concrete evidence that he or she is able to master the disease. The nurse breaks a task into small, achievable units to ensure mastery of techniques; for example, a client may begin learning how to administer an injection by first obtaining an accurate dose of insulin.

It is appropriate to devote as much time as possible to insulin injection and blood glucose monitoring techniques. Clients with newly diagnosed diabetes are often fearful of giving themselves injections. After insulin injection technique has been mastered, clients become less anxious and are able to attend to other tasks.

⊚ CRITICAL THINKING CHALLENGE

The client is a 60-year-old business man recently diagnosed with type 2 diabetes after developing hyperglycemic-hyperosmolar nonketotic syndrome (HHNS) following 2 days of vomiting and diarrhea. He has been started on a second-generation sulfonyl urea oral antidiabetic drug. Last week he attended a group class for clients with newly diagnosed diabetes. He tells you that he feels fortunate that his diabetes can be cured with oral medication instead of insulin injections. He also explains that eating in restaurants and having alcoholic cocktails with his customers are a major part of his occupation, and he wonders if the "pills will interfere with his drinking habits."

- How will you identify this client's most urgent educational needs?
- What, if any, referrals are most appropriate for this client?
- Do you have any suggestions for how this client could manage social contact with his customers without increasing his risk for diet- and alcohol-related changes in blood glucose levels?

CHART 65-16

CLIENT EDUCATION GUIDE
Travel Tips for Diabetic Clients

Before traveling visit your primary care provider and diabetes educator.
- See your physician to make certain you do not have any other health problems.
- Obtain a letter from your physician (typed on office letterhead) that indicates you have diabetes and lists the medications you are taking.
- Obtain any needed immunizations or inoculations.
- Obtain prescriptions from your physician for your medications, including glucagon if you take insulin, and prescriptions for motion sickness, nausea and vomiting, and traveler's diarrhea.
- Develop a plan for changing strengths of insulin if you are traveling to a country that does not carry the type of insulin you use. Learn how to use a U-100 syringe to draw up U-40 insulin.
- Develop a plan for meal and medication adjustment across time zones. Eastbound travel will shorten the day, requiring a reduction in the amount of medication needed. Westbound travel may add an extra meal to the day and require additional medication.
- Obtain a list of foods from your diabetes educator that you can substitute for food served in restaurants or airplanes.

If you are traveling by air, train, or boat, call ahead and request special meals for individuals with diabetes.
- Plan for delays in eating.
- Eat something every 4 hours.
- Drink a glass of water every 2 hours to prevent dehydration.
- Do not assume that special meals will be available; substitute items you cannot eat with foods you have in your travel kit.

Notify airline and hotel personnel that you have diabetes.
- Always wear medical alert identification and keep your medical alert card in your wallet.

While traveling:
- Check your blood glucose level frequently.
- Do not engage in activities when blood glucose levels are lower than 65 mg/dL.
- Stretch and walk around every 2 hours to help your circulation.
- Check your feet frequently for blisters and sores. You may be doing more walking than usual.
- Take extra shoes with you, and plan to change shoes often when walking more than normal.
- Protect your skin against exposure to the sun. Drug-induced photosensitivity can occur with some oral hypoglycemic agents.

Always have your travel kit with you; do not check your kit along with the rest of your luggage. Include these items in your travel kit:
- Twice as much medication and twice as many supplies as you think you will need (Pack medications separately from checked luggage.)
- Insulin stored in an insulated carrying case that will maintain temperatures according to the manufacturer's directions
- The letter from your physician (typed on office letterhead) that indicates you have diabetes and lists the medications you are taking
- A supply of fast-acting sugar (such as glucose tablets or gel, hard candy, and sugar cubes), as well as longer-acting foods (such as cheese and crackers and peanut butter and crackers)
- A self-monitoring diary

CHART 65-17

FOCUSED ASSESSMENT *of*
The Insulin-Dependent Diabetic Client During a Home or Clinic Visit

Assess overall mental status, wakefulness, ability to converse.
Take vital signs and weight:
- Fever could indicate infection.
- Are blood pressure and weight within target range? Why or why not?
Question client regarding any change in visual acuity; check current visual acuity.
Inspect oral mucous membranes, gums, and teeth.
Question client about injection areas used; inspect areas being used; assess whether client is utilizing areas and sites appropriately.
Inspect skin for intactness, wounds that have not healed, new sores, ulcers, bruises, or burns; assess any previously known wounds for infection, progression of healing.
Question client regarding foot care.
Assess lower extremities and feet for peripheral pulses, lack of or decreased sensation, abnormal sensations, breaks in skin integrity, condition of toes and nails.
Question client regarding color and consistency of stools and frequency of bowel movements; assess abdomen for bowel sounds.
Review client's home health diary:
- Is blood glucose within targeted range? Why or why not?
- Is glucose monitoring being recorded often enough?
- Is the client's food intake adequate and appropriate? Why or why not?
- Is exercise occurring regularly? Why or why not?
Assess client's ability to perform self-monitoring of blood glucose.
Assess client's procedures for obtaining and storing insulin and syringes, cleaning equipment, disposing of syringes and needles.
Assess client's insulin preparation and injection technique.

■ HOME CARE MANAGEMENT

Maintaining blood glucose control depends on the client's self-management skills. The primary role of the health care professional is to provide ongoing support and education and to empower the client to make informed decisions. Diabetes education aims to help the client acquire knowledge regarding the management of diabetes, behavior change skills, and communication skills to participate effectively as part of the health care team (Childs, 1998).

The nurse provides information about resources. The client must know whom to contact in case of an emergency. Older adults who live alone must have daily telephone contact with a friend or neighbor. The client may also need assistance with grocery shopping and meal preparation. He or she may have limited access to transportation out of the home and may not have sufficient supplies of food, particularly in bad weather. Because of the high frequency of visual problems in older clients, they may need assistance in preparing insulin syringes for injection or in performing blood glucose monitoring. The nurse or case manager initiates referrals to home care or public health agencies as appropriate. Such referral is especially important for older women with diabetes who are insulin dependent. Studies have reported that these women have greater cognitive decline with memory loss than do men with diabetes or women of the same age who do not have diabetes (Gregg et al., 2000). Chart 65-17 identifies areas for assessment during a home or clinic visit.

TABLE 65-19 • OUTCOME CRITERIA FOR DIABETIC TEACHING

Before being discharged to home, the diabetic client or the significant other should be able to:
- Tell why insulin or an oral hypoglycemic agent is being prescribed
- Name which insulin or oral hypoglycemic agent is being prescribed, and name the dosage and frequency of administration
- Discuss the relationship between mealtime and the action of insulin or the oral hypoglycemic agent
- Discuss plans to follow diabetic diet instructions
- Prepare and administer insulin accurately
- Test blood for glucose, or state plans for having blood glucose levels monitored
- Test urine for ketones, and state when this test should be done
- Verbalize how to store insulin
- List symptoms that indicate a hypoglycemic reaction
- Tell what carbohydrate sources are used to treat hypoglycemic reactions
- Tell what symptoms indicate hyperglycemia
- Tell what dietary changes are needed during illness
- Verbalize when to call the physician or the nurse (frequent episodes of hypoglycemia, symptoms of hyperglycemia)
- Verbalize the procedures for proper foot care

■ HEALTH CARE RESOURCES

A wide array of diabetic education material is available from drug companies. The American Diabetes Association (ADA) will refer a diabetic client to the appropriate agencies or resources (phone [800] 232-3472 in the United States; [703] 549-1500 in Canada). The American Association of Diabetes Educators can refer a diabetic client to a certified diabetes educator in his or her area for information about diabetes (phone [800] TEAM-UP-4). Additional resources are listed in the Selected Bibliography.

● Evaluation: Outcomes

NOC The nurse evaluates the care of the client with diabetes on the basis of the identified nursing diagnoses and collaborative problems. The ultimate evaluation of the success of survival-level and in-depth diabetic education is the ability of the client to maintain blood glucose levels within the normal range. Specific outcome criteria for client education are listed below and in Table 65-19. The expected outcomes include that the client will:

- Achieve blood glucose control as evidenced by maintaining blood glucose levels in the expected range
- Avoid acute and chronic complications of diabetes
- Have a satisfactory and complete postoperative recovery without complications
- Identify factors that increase the potential for injury
- Modify lifestyle to reduce the risk for injury
- Monitor health status changes
- Practice proper foot care to prevent injury, as evidenced by cleansing and inspecting the feet for cleanliness and healthy skin
- Maintain intact skin on the feet
- Experience relief of pain
- Recognize causal factors of pain
- Use preventive measures to avoid pain
- Use available resources to increase comfort
- Maintain optimal vision

- Be free of injury related to decreased visual acuity
- Maintain a urine elimination pattern in the expected range
- Maintain urine proteins within normal limits
- Have an optimal level of mental status functioning
- Have decreased episodes of hypoglycemia
- Have decreased episodes of hyperglycemia

ONLINE RESOURCES

For suggested readings and Internet resources, go to http://www.wbsaunders.com/SIMON/Iggy/.

SELECTED BIBLIOGRAPHY

Asterisk indicates a classic or definitive work on this subject.

Abbott, C.A., et al. (1998). Multicenter study of the incidence of and predictive risk factors for diabetic neuropathic foot ulceration. Diabetes Care, 21(12), 1071-1075.

Ahern-Gould, K. (1998). Quick resource for electrolyte imbalance. *Critical Care Nursing Clinics of North America, 10*(4), 477-490.

Aiello, L.P., Gardner, T.W., & King, G.L. (1998). Technical review: Diabetic retinopathy. *Diabetes Care, 21*(1), 143-156.

Alberts, M.J. (1999). Diagnosis and treatment of ischemic stroke. *American Journal of Medicine, 106*(2), 211-221.

Amanti, M., & Schumann, L. (1998). Coronary artery disease: A link between hypertension, diabetes, hyperlipidemia and obesity. *Journal of the American Academy of Nurse Practitioners, 10*(2), 77-81.

American Association of Diabetes Educators. (1997). Position statement: Blood glucose monitoring, http://www.aadenet.org.

*American Diabetes Association. (1996). Consensus statement: Self-monitoring of blood glucose. *Diabetes Care, 19*(Suppl. 1), 62-66.

American Diabetes Association. (1998). Consensus development conference on the diagnosis of coronary heart disease in people with diabetes. *Diabetes Care, 21*(9), 1551-1559.

American Diabetes Association. (1999a). Consensus development conference on diabetic foot wound care. *Diabetes Care, 22*(8), 1354-1399.

American Diabetes Association. (1999b). Reviews: Economic consequences of diabetes mellitus in the U.S. *Diabetes Care, 22*(2), 296-309.

American Diabetes Association. (2000a). Committee report: Report of the Expert Committee on the Diagnosis and Classification of Diabetes Mellitus. *Diabetes Care, 23*(Suppl. 1), 4-19

American Diabetes Association. (2000b). Position statement: Aspirin therapy in diabetes. *Diabetes Care, 23*(Suppl. 1), 61-62.

American Diabetes Association. (2000c). Position statement: Continuous subcutaneous insulin infusion. *Diabetes Care, 23*(Suppl. 1), 90.

American Diabetes Association. (2000d). Position statement: Diabetes mellitus and exercise. *Diabetes Care, 23*(Suppl. 1), 50-54.

American Diabetes Association. (2000e). Position statement: Diabetic nephropathy. *Diabetes Care, 23*(Suppl. 1), 69-72.

American Diabetes Association. (2000f). Position statement: Diabetic retinopathy. *Diabetes Care, 23*(Suppl. 1), 73-76.

American Diabetes Association. (2000g). Position statement: Food labeling, *Diabetes Care, 23*(Suppl. 1), 94-95.

American Diabetes Association. (2000h). Position statement: Gestational diabetes mellitus. *Diabetes Care, 23*(Suppl. 1), 77-79.

American Diabetes Association. (2000i). Position statement: Hospital admission guidelines for diabetes mellitus. *Diabetes Care, 23*(Suppl. 1), 83.

American Diabetes Association. (2000j). Position statement: Implications of the diabetes control and complications trial. *Diabetes Care, 23*(Suppl. 1), 24-26.

American Diabetes Association. (2000k). Position statement: Implications of the United Kingdom prospective diabetes study. *Diabetes Care, 23*(Suppl. 1), 27-31.

American Diabetes Association. (2000l). Position statement: Insulin administration. *Diabetes Care, 23*(Suppl. 1), 86-89.

American Diabetes Association. (2000m). Position statement: Management of dyslipidemia in adults with diabetes. *Diabetes Care, 23*(Suppl. 1), 57-60.

American Diabetes Association. (2000n). Position statement: Nutritional recommendations and principles for individuals with diabetes. *Diabetes Care, 23*(Suppl. 1), 43-46.

American Diabetes Association. (2000o). Position statement: Pancreas transplantation for patients with diabetes mellitus. *Diabetes Care, 23*(Suppl. 1), 85.

American Diabetes Association. (2000p). Position statement: Prevention of type 1 diabetes mellitus. *Diabetes Care, 23*(Suppl. 1), 108.

American Diabetes Association. (2000q). Position statement: Preventive foot care in people with diabetes. *Diabetes Care, 23*(Suppl. 1), 55-56.

American Diabetes Association. (2000r). Position statement: Role of fat replacers in diabetes medical nutrition therapy. *Diabetes Care, 23*(Suppl. 1), 96-97.

American Diabetes Association. (2000s). Position statement: Screening for type 2 diabetes. *Diabetes Care, 23*(Suppl. 1), 20-23.

American Diabetes Association. (2000t). Position statement: Standards of medical care for patients with diabetes mellitus. *Diabetes Care, 23*(Suppl. 1), 32-42.

American Diabetes Association. (2000u). Position statement: Tests for glycemia in diabetes. *Diabetes Care, 23*(Suppl. 1), 80-82.

Apfel, S.C. (1999). Neurotrophic factors in the therapy of diabetic neuropathy. *American Journal of Medicine, 107*(2B), 34-42.

Arezzo, J.C. (1999). New developments in the diagnosis of diabetic neuropathy. *American Journal of Medicine, 107*(2B), 9-16.

Armstrong, D., & Lavery, L.A. (1998). Shoes and the diabetic foot. *Practical Diabetology, 17*(1), 23-26.

Armstrong, D., Lavery, L.A., & Bushman, T.R. (1998). Peak foot pressures influence the healing time of diabetic foot ulcers treated with total contact casts. *Journal of Rehabilitation Research and Development, 35*(1), 1-5.

Armstrong, D., et al. (1998). Choosing a practical screening instrument to identify patients at risk for diabetic foot ulceration. *Archives of Internal Medicine, 158*(3), 289-292.

Bagley, M. (1998). Helping older adults to live better with hearing and vision loss. *Journal of Case Management, 7*(4), 147-152.

Bell, D.S., & Alele, J. (1999). Dealing with diabetic nephropathy. *Postgraduate Medicine, 105*(2), 83-94.

Bell, P.M., & Hadden, D.S. (1997). Metformin. *Endocrinology and Metabolism Clinics of North America, 26*(3), 523-537.

Bennett, G.A. (1998). Neuropathic pain: New insights, new interventions. *Hospital Practice, 33*(10), 95-114.

Bichler, L.M. (1999). Foot ulcers in diabetes. *ADVANCE for Nurse Practitioners, 7*(1), 49-52.

Bloomgarden, Z.T. (1999). New approaches to insulin treatment and glucose monitoring. *Diabetes Care, 22*(12), 2078-2082.

Bohannon, N.N.V. (1997). Benefits of lispro insulin. *Postgraduate Medicine, 101*(2), 73-80.

Bolli, G.B., & Fanelli, C.G. (1999). Physiology of glucose counterregulation to hypoglycemia. *Endocrinology and Metabolism Clinics of North America, 28*(3), 467-493.

Boulton, A.J.M., & Malik, R.A. (1998). Diabetic neuropathy. *Medical Clinics of North America, 82*(4), 909-929.

Brenner, Z.R. (1999). Preventing postoperative complications. *Nursing99, 29*(10), 34-39.

*Brink, S., et al. (1995). *Diabetes education goals.* Alexandria, VA: American Diabetes Association.

Brown, J.B., Pedula, K., & Bakst, A.W. (1999). The progressive cost of complications in type 2 diabetes mellitus. *Archives of Internal Medicine, 159*(16), 1873-1880.

Browne, A.C., & Sibbald, R.G. (1999). The diabetic neuropathic ulcer: An overview. *Ostomy/Wound Management, 45*(1A), 6-22.

Brunner, G., et al. (1998). Validation of home blood glucose meters with respect to clinical and analytical approaches. *Diabetes Care, 21*(4), 585-590.

Burge, M.R., & Schade, D.S. (1997). Insulins. *Endocrinology and Metabolism Clinics of North America, 26*(3), 575-598.

Burke, J., et al. (1999). Rapid rise in the incidence of type 2 diabetes from 1987 to 1996. *Archives of Internal Medicine, 159*(13), 1450-1456.

Capriotti, T., & McLeughlin. (1998). A revitalized battle against diabetes mellitus for the new millennium. *MEDSURG Nursing, 7*(6), 323-342.

Caspi, A. (1998). Sildenafil: A new drug treatment for male erectile dysfunction. *Pharmacy and Therapeutics, 23*(5), 233-240.

Childs, B.P. (1998). Diabetes care: Compliance versus empowerment. *Case Review, 4*(3), 14-20.

Clark, C.M. (1998). The burden of chronic hyperglycemia. *Diabetes Care, 21*(Suppl. 3), 32-34.

*Cleary, M.E. (Ed.). (1994). *Diabetes and visual impairment: An educator's resource guide.* Chicago: American Association of Diabetes Educators.

Cohen, R.A., et al. (1999). Determinants of retinopathy progression in type 1 diabetes. *American Journal of Medicine, 107*(1), 45-51.

Consensus development conference on diabetic foot wound care. (1999). *Ostomy/Wound Management, 45*(9), 32-47.

Culleton, J.L. (1999). Preventing diabetic foot complications. *Postgraduate Medicine, 106*(1), 74-83.

Cryer, P.E. (1997). *Hypoglycemia: Pathophysiology, diagnosis and treatment.* New York: Oxford University Press.

Cryer, P.E. (1999). Symptoms of hypoglycemia, thresholds for their occurrence and hypoglycemic unawareness. *Endocrinology and Metabolism Clinics of North America, 28*(3), 495-499.

Dagogo-Jack, S., & Santiago, J.V. (1997). Pathophysiology of type 2 diabetes and modes of action of therapeutic interventions. *Archives of Internal Medicine, 157*(16), 1802-1817.

Dahlquist, G. (1999). Primary and secondary prevention strategies of pre-type 1 diabetes. *Diabetes Care, 22*(Suppl. 2), 4-6.

Dahn, M.S. (1998). The role of growth factors in wound management of diabetic foot ulcers. *Federal Practitioner, 15*(Suppl. 7), 14-19.

Davidson, M.B. (1998). *Diabetes mellitus: Diagnosis and treatment.* Philadelphia: W.B. Saunders.

Davis, T.M.E., et al. (1999). Risk factors for stroke in type 2 diabetes mellitus. *Archives of Internal Medicine, 159*(10), 1097-1103.

Declair, V. (1999). The importance of growth factors in wound healing. *Ostomy/Wound Management, 45*(4), 64-80.

DePree, P.A. (1998). Lispro insulin. *Nursing98, 28*(11), 54-55.

Despres, J.P. (1999). Insulin resistance and hyperglycemic associated risk factors. *Diabetes Care, 22*(Suppl. 2), 38-40.

Dewey, C.M., & Riley, W.J. (1999). Have diabetes, will travel. *Postgraduate Medicine, 101*(2), 111-126.

Diabetes Prevention Program Research Group. (1999). The diabetes prevention program: Design and methods for a clinical trial in the prevention of type 2 diabetes. *Diabetes Care, 22*(4), 623-634.

Dinneen, S.F., & Gerstein, H.C. (1997). The association of albuminuria and mortality in non–insulin dependent diabetes mellitus. *Archives of Internal Medicine, 157*(13), 1413-1418.

Dinsmoor, R. (1999). Tools of the trade: New insulins, drugs and devices. *Diabetes Self-Management, 16*(6), 46-54.

Eaglstein, W.H., & Falanga, V. (1997). Chronic wounds. *Surgical Clinics of North America, 77*(3), 689-700.

Fagan, T., & Sowers, J. (1999). Type 2 diabetes mellitus: Greater cardiovascular risk factors and greater benefits of therapy. *Archives of Internal Medicine, 159*(10), 1033-1034.

Farkas-Hirsh, R. (Ed.). (2000). All about hypoglycemia. *Diabetes Self-Management, 17*(1), 21-27.

Feinglos, M.N., & Bethel, M.A. (1998). Treatment of type 2 diabetes. *Medical Clinics of North America, 82*(4), 757-790.

Fishman, L.M. (1999). The normal pathophysiology of aging. *Journal of Long-Term Home Health Care, 1*(2), 114-124.

Fleming, D.R. (1999). Challenging traditional insulin injection practices. *American Journal of Nursing, 99*(2), 72-73.

Franz, M.J. (1997). Lifestyle modifications for diabetes management. *Endocrinology and Metabolism Clinics of North America, 26*(3), 499-510.

Funnell, M., & Barlage, D. (2000). Saying a mouthful about oral diabetes drugs. *Nursing2000, 30*(11), 34-39.

Funnell, M.M., et al. (1998). *A core curriculum for diabetes education.* Chicago: American Association of Diabetes Educators.

Garber, A.J. (1998). Vascular disease and lipids in diabetes. *Medical Clinics of North America, 82*(4), 931-948.

Garg, S.K., et al. (1999). Correlation of fingerstick blood glucose measurements with GlucoWatch Biographer Glucose results in young subjects with type 1 diabetes. *Diabetes Care, 22*(10), 1708-1714.

Gaster, B., & Hirsh, I.B. (1998). The effects of improved glycemic control on complications of type 2 diabetes. *Archives of Internal Medicine, 158*(2), 134-140.

*Gillis W. Long Hansen's Disease Center Rehabilitation Branch. (1992). *Foot screening: Care of the foot in diabetes: The Carville approach.* (1992). Carville, LA: Department of Health and Human Services.

Goldberg, R.B. (1998). Prevention of type 2 diabetes. *Medical Clinics of North America, 82*(4), 805-821.

Goldstein, D.E., & Little, R.R. (1997). Monitoring glycemia in diabetes: Short term assessment. *Endocrinology and Metabolism Clinics of North America, 26*(3), 475-486.

Green, K., & Lydon, S. (1998). The continuum of patient care. *American Journal of Nursing, 98*(10), 16BBB-DDD.

Greene, D.A., Stevens, M.J., & Feldman, E.L. (1999). Diabetic neuropathy: The scope of the problem. *American Journal of Medicine, 107*(2B), 2-8.

Greenspan, F.S., & Strewler, G.J. (1997). *Basic and clinical endocrinology.* Stamford, CT: Appleton & Lange.

Gregg, E., et al. (2000). Is diabetes associated with cognitive impairment and cognitive decline among older women? *Archives of Internal Medicine, 160*(2), 174-180.

Grinslade, S., & Buck, E.A. (1999). Diabetic ketoacidosis: Implications for the medical-surgical nurse. *MEDSURG Nursing, 8*(1), 37-45.

Guerrero-Romero, F., & Rodriguez-Moran, M. (1999). Proteinuria is an independent risk factor for ischemic stroke in non–insulin dependent diabetes mellitus. *Stroke, 30*(9), 1787-1791.

Haffner, S.M. (1998a). Epidemiology of type 2 diabetes: Risk Factors. *Diabetes Care, 21*(Suppl. 3), 3-6.

Haffner, S.M. (1998b). Technical review: Management of dyslipidemia in adults with diabetes. *Diabetes Care, 21*(1), 160-178.

Halperin, M.L., & Goldstein, M.B. (1999). *Fluid, electrolyte and acid-base physiology.* Philadelphia, W.B. Saunders.

Halpin-Landry, J.E., & Goldsmith, S. (1999). Feet first: Diabetes care. *American Journal of Nursing, 99*(2), 26-33.

Harris, M.I. (1998). Diabetes in America: Epidemiology and scope of the problem. *Diabetes Care, 21*(Suppl. 3), 11-14.

Harris, M.I., Flegal, K.M., & Cowie, C.C. (1998). Prevalence of diabetes, impaired fasting glucose, and impaired glucose tolerance in U.S. adults. *Diabetes Care, 21*(4), 518-524.

Harris, M.I., et al. (1999). Racial and ethnic differences in glycemic control of adults with type 2 diabetes. *Diabetes Care, 22*(3), 403-408.

Hazlewood, F.J., Rodriguez, D.J. & Cypress, M. (1999). Exploring the roles of case managers in diabetes care. *Case Manager, 9*(2), 57-63.

Henry, R.R. (1997). Thiazolidinediones. *Endocrinology and Metabolism Clinics of North America, 26*(3), 553-573.

Herlitz, J., & Malmberg, K. (1999). How to improve the cardiac prognosis for diabetes. *Diabetes Care, 22*(Suppl. 3), 89-96.

Hernandez, D. (1998). Microvascular complications of diabetes: Nursing assessment and intervention. *American Journal of Nursing, 98*(6), 26-32.

Hirsh, I.B. (1998). Intensive treatment of type 1 diabetes. *Medical Clinics of North America, 82*(4), 689-719.

Hirsh, I.B., & Paauw, D.S. (1997). Diabetes management in special situations. *Endocrinology and Metabolism Clinics of North America, 26*(3), 631-645.

Hunt, T.K., & Hopf, H.W. (1997). Wound healing and wound infection. *Surgical Clinics of North America, 77*(3), 587-606.

Hunter, S.J., & Garvey, T. (1998). Insulin action and insulin resistance: Diseases involving defects in insulin receptors, signal transduction, and the glucose transport effector system. *American Journal of Medicine, 105*(4), 331-345.

Hussar, D.A. (2000). New drugs 2000. *Nursing2000, 30*(1), 55-56.

Ilonen, J., & Akerblom, H. (1999). New technologies and genetics of type 1 diabetes. *Diabetes Technology and Therapeutics, 1*(2), 205-207.

Inlow, S., Kalla, T. P., & Rahman, J. (1999). Downloading plantar foot pressures in the diabetic patient. *Ostomy/Wound Management, 45*(10), 28-38.

Jacober, S., & Sowers, J. (1999). An update on perioperative management of diabetes. *Archives of Internal Medicine, 159*(20), 2405-2411.

Janisse, D.J. (1998). Picking the shoe to fit the occasion. *Diabetes Self-Management, 15*, 30-33.

Jaremko, J., & Rorstad, O. (1998). Advances toward the implantable artificial pancreas for treatment of diabetes. *Diabetes Care, 21*(3), 444-450.

Joseph, S.E., Hopkins, D., & Korzon-Burokowska, A. (1998). The action profile of lispro is not blunted by mixing in the syringe with NPH insulin. *Diabetes Care, 21*(12), 2098-2102.

Kendall, D.M., & Robertson, R.P. (1997). Pancreas and islet transplantation. *Endocrinology and Metabolism Clinics of North America, 26*(3), 611-630.

Keown, P.A. (1999). Therapeutic strategies for optimal use of novel immunosuppressants. *Transplantation Proceedings, 31*(4), 1790-1793.

Kong, M.F., et al. (1999). Natural history of diabetic gastroparesis. *Diabetes Care, 22*(3), 503-507.

Konick-McMahan, J. (1999). Riding out a diabetic emergency. *Nursing99, 29*(9), 34-40.

Koproski, J., Pretto, Z., & Poretsky, L. (1997). Effect of an intervention by a diabetes team in hospitalized patients with diabetes. *Diabetes Care, 20*(10), 1553-1555.

Korenman, S.G. (1998). New insights into erectile dysfunction: A practical approach. *American Journal of Medicine, 105*(2), 135-144.

Kumar, A., et al. (1999). Combined kidney and pancreatic transplantation. *British Medical Journal, 318*(7188), 886-887.

Larsen, J. (1998). Dyslipidemia in diabetes. *ADVANCE for Nurse Practitioners, 6*(4), 36-43.

Lavery, L. (1998). Practical criteria for screening patients at high risk for diabetic foot ulceration. *Archives of Internal Medicine, 158*(2), 157-162.

Lebovitz, H.E. (1997). Alpha-glucosidase inhibitors. *Endocrinology and Metabolism Clinics of North America, 26*(3), 539-551.

LeRoith, D., Taylor, S., & Olefsky, J. (1997). *Diabetes mellitus.* Philadelphia: Lippincott-Raven.

*Letho, S., et al. (1996). Risk factors predicting lower extremity amputation in patients with NIDDM. *Diabetes Care, 19*(6), 607-612.

Lipsky, B.A. (1998). Overview of the diabetic foot: Epidemiology, pathophysiology and the role of infection. *Federal Practitioner, 15*(Suppl. 7), 2-7.

Lougheed, W.D., et al. (1997). Stability of insulin lispro in insulin infusion systems. *Diabetes Care, 20*(7), 1061-1065.

Mahler, R.J., & Adler, M.L. (1999). Type 2 diabetes mellitus: Update on diagnosis, pathophysiology and treatment. *Journal of Endocrinology and Metabolism, 84*(4), 1165-1171.

Malmberg, K. (1997). Intensive glucose control produced better long-term outcomes after myocardial infarction. *British Medical Journal, 314*(7093), 1512-1515.

Manske, C.L. (1999). Risks and benefits of kidney and pancreas transplantation for diabetic patients. *Diabetes Care, 22*(Suppl. 2), 114-120.

Marks, J.B., & Raskin, P. (1998). Nephropathy and hypertension in diabetes. *Medical Clinics of North America, 82*(4), 877-907.

Marks, V., & Teale, J.D. (1999). Drug-induced hypoglycemia. *Endocrinology and Metabolism Clinics of North America, 28*(3), 555-577.

Mayfield, J.A., et al. (1998). Technical review: Preventive foot care in people with diabetes. *Diabetes Care, 21*(12), 2161-2177.

Miettinen, H., et al. (1998). Impact of diabetes on mortality after first myocardial infarction. *Diabetes Care, 21*(1), 69-75.

Moss, S.E., Klein, R., & Klein, B. (1999). Risk factors for hospitalization in people with diabetes. *Archives of Internal Medicine, 159*(17), 2053-2057.

Muha, J. (1999). Local wound care in diabetic foot complications. *Postgraduate Medicine, 106*(1), 97-102.

*National Institute of Diabetes and Digestive and Kidney Diseases. (1995). *Diabetes in America.* NIH Pub. No. 95-1468, Bethesda, MD: National Institutes of Health.

Neeley, K.A., et al. (1998). Diabetic retinopathy. *Medical Clinics of North America, 82*(4), 847-876.

Nehra, A., Barrett, D.M., & Moreland, R.B. (1999). Pharmacologic advances in the treatment of erectile dysfunction. *Mayo Clinic Proceedings, 74*(7), 709-721.

O'Brien, T., Nguyen, T.T., & Zimmerman, B.R. (1998). Hyperlipidemia and diabetes mellitus. *Mayo Clinic Proceedings, 73*(10), 969-976.

O'Hanlon-Nichols. (1999). Neurologic assessment: The basis of a comprehensive examination. *American Journal of Nursing, 99*(6), 44-50.

O'Neill, K., & Ross-Kerr, J.C. (1999). Impact of an instructional program on nurse's accuracy in capillary blood glucose monitoring. *Clinical Nursing Research, 8*(2), 166-179.

Parry, G.J. (1999). Management of diabetic neuropathy. *American Journal of Medicine, 107*(2B), 27-33.

Peragallo-Dittko, V. (1999). Blood glucose meter roundup. *Diabetes Self-Management, 16*(2), 7-16.

Peters, S. (1998). Diabetic foot ulcers: Prevention is the key to successful management. *ADVANCE for Nurse Practitioners, 6*(6), 59-62.

Petronic, V., & Bhisitkul, R. (1999). Lasers and diabetic retinopathy: The art of gentle destruction. *Diabetes Technology and Therapeutics, 1*(2), 177-187.

Pieber, T., et al. (2000). Efficacy and safety of HOE 901 versus NPH insulin in patients with type 1 diabetes. *Diabetes Care, 23*(2), 157-162.

Pinzur, M.S. (1999). The American Orthopaedic and Foot and Ankle Society guidelines. *Practical Diabetology, 18*(1), 6-13.

Rabinovitch, A., & Skyler, J.S. (1998). Prevention of type 1 diabetes. *Medical Clinics of North America, 82*(4), 739-755.

Rassam, A., et al. (1999). Optimal administration of lispro insulin in hyperglycemic type 1 diabetes. *Diabetes Care, 22*(1), 133-136.

Ravid, M., et al. (1997). Main risk factors for nephropathy in type 2 diabetes mellitus are plasma cholesterol levels, mean blood pressure and hyperglycemia. *Archives of Internal Medicine, 158*(9), 998-1004.

Reddy, K.S., et al. (1999). Surgical complications after pancreas transplantation with portal-enteric drainage. *Transplantation Proceedings, 31*(1-2), 617-618.

Riddle, M.C. (1997). Tactics for type 2 diabetes. *Endocrinology and Metabolism Clinics of North America, 26*(3), 659-677.

Robbins, J. (1998). Foot ulcerations: Causes, therapy, prevention and care. *Federal Practitioner, 15*(Suppl. 7), 9-13.

Robertson, K., Glazer, N., & Campbell, R. (2000). The latest development in insulin injection devices. *Diabetes Educator, 26*(1), 135-152.

Robertson, R.P., et al. (2000). Technical review: Pancreas and islet transplantation for patients with diabetes. *Diabetes Care, 23*(1), 112-116.

Roman, S.H., Harris, M.I. (1997). Management of diabetes mellitus from a public health perspective. *Endocrinology and Metabolism Clinics of North America, 26*(3), 443-474.

Rosenbloom, A.L., et al. (1999). Emerging epidemic of type 2 diabetes in youth. *Diabetes Care, 22*(2), 345-354.

Rosiglitazone for type 2 diabetes mellitus. (1999) *Medical Letter, 41*(1059), 71-73.

Rosscamp, R.H., & Park, G. (1999). Long-acting insulin analogs. *Diabetes Care, 22*(Suppl. 2), 109-113.

*Ruderman, N., & Devlin, J.T. (Eds.). (1995). *The health professional's guide to diabetes and exercise.* Alexandria, VA: American Diabetes Association.

Ryan, A., et al. (2001). Insulin action after resistive training in insulin-resistant older men and women. *Journal of the American Geriatrics Society, 49*(3), 254-262.

Samos, L.F., & Roos, B.A. (1998). Diabetes mellitus in older persons. *Medical Clinics of North America, 82*(4), 791-803.

Saudek, C. (1997). Novel forms of insulin delivery. *Endocrinology and Metabolism Clinics of North America, 26*(3), 599-610.

Scheen, A.J., & Lefebvre, P.J. (1999). Troglitazone: Antihyperglycemic activity and potential role in the treatment of type 2 diabetes. *Diabetes Care, 22*(9), 1568-1577.

Schrier, R.W. (1997). *Renal and electrolyte disorders.* Philadelphia: Lippincott-Raven.

Service, F.J. (1999). Classification of hypoglycemic disorders. *Endocrinology and Metabolism Clinics of North America, 28*(3), 501-517.

Setter, S.M, Baker, D.E., & Campbell, R.K. (1999). Sildenafil (Viagra) for the treatment of erectile dysfunction in men with diabetes. *Diabetes Educator, 25*(1), 79-89.

Shorr, R.I., et al. (1997). Incidence and risk factors for serious hypoglycemia in older persons using insulin or sulfonylureas. *Archives of Internal Medicine, 157*(15), 1681-1686.

Simon, R.R., Aminoff, M.J., & Greenberg, D.A. (1999). *Clinical neurology.* Stamford, CT: Appleton & Lange.

Skyler, J.S. (1997a). Insulin therapy in type 11 diabetes. *Postgraduate Medicine, 101*(2), 85-96.

Skyler, J.S. (1997b). Tactics for type 1 diabetes. *Endocrinology and Metabolism Clinics of North America, 26*(3), 647-657.

Slovenkai, M.P. (1998). Foot problems in diabetes. *Medical Clinics of North America, 82*(3), 949-972.

Sollinger, H.W., et al. (1998). Experience with 500 simultaneous pancreas-kidney transplants. *Annals of Surgery, 228*(3), 284-293

Sowers, J.R., & Lester, M.A. (1999). Diabetes and cardiovascular disease. *Diabetes Care, 22*(Suppl. 3), 14-20.

Spollett, G.R. (1999). Assessment and management of erectile dysfunction in men with diabetes. *Diabetes Educator, 25*(1), 65-75.

Steed, D.L. (1997). The role of growth factors in wound healing. *Surgical Clinics of North America, 77*(3), 575-586.

Steiner, G. (1999). Risk factors for macrovascular disease in type 2 diabetes: Classic lipid abnormalities. *Diabetes Care, 22*(Suppl. 3), 6-9.

Stratta, R.J. (1999). Optimal immunosuppression in pancreas transplantation. *Transplantation Proceedings, 31*(1/2), 619-621.

Stratta, R.J., et al. (1999). Evolution in pancreas transplantation techniques: Simultaneous kidney-pancreas transplantation using portal-enteric drainage without antilymphocyte induction. *Annals of Surgery, 229*(5), 701-708.

Sutherland, D.E.R., Cecka, M., & Gruessner, A. (1999). Report from the International Transplant Registry—1998. *Transplantation Proceedings, 27*(1/2), 597-601.

Taub, L.F. (1998). The ADA's clinical practice recommendations in action. *American Journal of Nursing, 98*(10), 16B-16D.

Taylor, H.R. (1997). Diabetic retinopathy: A public health challenge. *American Journal of Ophthalmology, 123*(4), 543-545.

Tomky, D. (1997). Diabetes: Taking a new look at an old adversary. *American Journal of Nursing, 97*(11), 41-45.

Toto, K.H. (1998). Fluid balance assessment. *Critical Care Clinics of North America, 10*(4), 383-400.

Trecroci, D. (1999). FDA panel backs GlucoWatch monitor. *Diabetes Interview, 9*(1), 15.

Troglitazone for non-insulin dependent diabetes mellitus. (1997). *Medical Letter, 39*(1001), 49-51.

Vinik, A.I. (1999). Diabetic neuropathy: Pathogenesis and therapy. *American Journal of Medicine, 107*(2B), 17-26.

Ward, J.D. (1999). Improving prognosis in type 2 diabetes. *Diabetes Care, 22*(Suppl. 2), 84-87.

Wei, M., et al. (1998). Effects of diabetes and level of glycemia on all-cause and cardiovascular mortality. *Diabetes Care, 21*(7), 1167-1172.

White, J.R., Campbell, R.K., & Hirsh, I. (1997). Insulin analogues. *Postgraduate Medicine, 101*(2), 58-70.

Wierman, M.E. (1998). Erectile dysfunction: A multifaceted disorder. *Hospital Practice, 33*(10), 65-90.

Williams, A.S. (1997). Teaching nonvisual diabetes self-care: Choosing appropriate tools and techniques for visually impaired individuals. *Diabetes Spectrum, 10*(2), 128-134.

Williams, A.S. (1999a). Adjusting to vision loss. *Diabetes Self-Management, 16*(2), 45-51.

Williams, A.S. (1999b). Independent insulin management. *Diabetes Self-Management, 16*(5), 33-41.

Zimmerman, B.R. (1997). Sulfonylureas. *Endocrinology and Metabolism Clinics of North America, 26*(3), 511-522.

Zinman, B., et al. (1997). Insulin lispro in CSII. *Diabetes, 46*(3), 440-443.

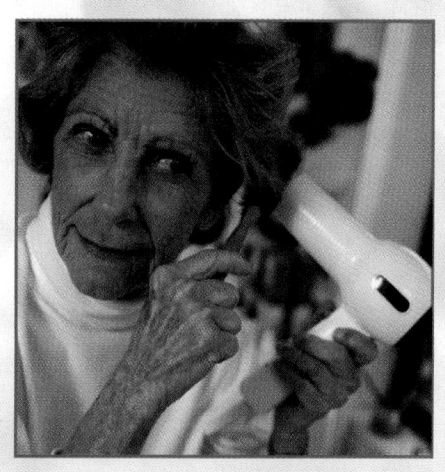

PROBLEMS OF PROTECTION

Management of Clients with Problems of the Skin, Hair, and Nails

UNIT

14

PROBLEMS OF PROTECTION: SKIN, HAIR, AND NAILS ■ Core Concepts Grid

Anatomy	Physiology	Pathophysiology	History	Physical Exam	Diagnostic Tests	Interventions	Pharmacology
Skin	**Protection**	**Inflammation**	**Client history**	**Skin**	**Cultures**	**Burn wound assessment**	**Topical antibiotics**
Subcutaneous fat	**Regulation**	**Infection**	Dermatologic problems	Color	**Skin tests**	Depth	**Topical antiin-flammatories**
Epidermis	Fluid balance	**Tumors**	Medications	Lesions	Patch	Area	**Keratolytic agents**
Dermis	Electrolyte balance	**Burns**	Liver, gallbladder, renal disease	Moisture	Scratch	Rule of Nines	**Antipsoriasis agents**
Hair	Temperature	Thermal	**Family history**	Vascular markings	**Biopsy**	**Burn fluid replacement formulas**	**Debriding agents**
Nails	**Vitamin synthesis**	Chemical	Chronic skin problems	Edema		**Graft care**	**Systemic antibiotics**
Glands		Electrical	**Social history**	Intactness		**Care of burn wounds**	
			Occupation	Tattoos		**Hypertrophy**	
			Nutritional status	Temperature		**Precautions for itching**	
			Sun exposure	Texture		**Emotional support**	
			Age	Turgor		**Debridement**	
			Race	Depth (stage) of wound		**Wound dressings**	
			Risk for pressure ulcers	Drainage		**Nutrition**	
				Hair/nails		**Prevention of pressure ulcers**	
				Shape		**Skin/wound ongoing assessment**	
				Distribution			
				Texture			

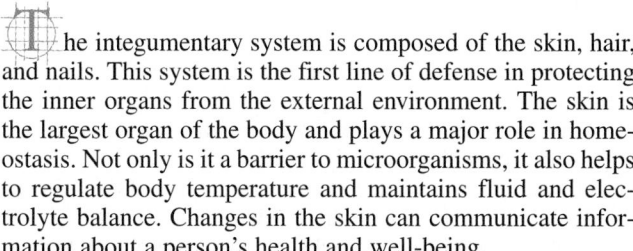

Assessment of the Skin, Hair, and Nails

JANICE CUZZELL

Learning Objectives

After studying this chapter, you should be able to:

1. Compare the structures and function of the dermis with those of the epidermis.
2. Describe the integumentary changes associated with aging.
3. Use proper terminology to describe different skin lesions.
4. Describe techniques to assess skin changes in clients with dark skin.
5. Distinguish between normal variations and abnormal skin manifestations with regard to skin color, texture, warmth, and moisture.
6. Explain the role of melanocytes in determining skin color.
7. Describe the ABCD method of assessing skin lesions for cancer.
8. Prioritize educational needs for the client undergoing an excisional biopsy for a skin lesion.

Go to http://www.wbsaunders.com/SIMON/Iggy/ for self-assessment questions related to these Learning Objectives.

The integumentary system is composed of the skin, hair, and nails. This system is the first line of defense in protecting the inner organs from the external environment. The skin is the largest organ of the body and plays a major role in homeostasis. Not only is it a barrier to microorganisms, it also helps to regulate body temperature and maintains fluid and electrolyte balance. Changes in the skin can communicate information about a person's health and well-being.

Emotional stress, systemic disease, and skin injury or disease can alter the function, appearance, and texture of the skin. Therefore the nurse examines the skin for important clues about the client's health. Because the skin has many sensory receptors, the client can report subjective skin sensations that may indicate specific health problems. The sensory function of the skin allows the nurse to use touch as a therapeutic intervention to provide comfort, relieve pain, and communicate caring.

ANATOMY AND PHYSIOLOGY REVIEW

Structure of the Skin

As shown in Figure 66-1, the skin has three distinct layers: fat, dermis, and epidermis. Each layer has unique properties that contribute to the skin's ability to maintain its complex functions.

SUBCUTANEOUS FAT (ADIPOSE TISSUE)

The innermost layer of the skin, which lies over muscle and bone, is the site for fat formation and storage. Fat cells act as heat insulators for the body. They absorb shock and protect against mechanical injury by padding internal structures. The distribution of fat varies with anatomic area, age, and gender. Many blood vessels perforate the fatty layer and extend into the dermal layer, forming capillary networks that supply nutrients and remove waste products.

DERMIS (CORIUM)

Above the subcutaneous fat lies the **dermis,** a layer of connective tissue that contains no cells. The dermis is composed of collagen and elastic fibers that are interwoven to give the skin both flexibility and mechanical strength.

Collagen, the main component of dermal tissue, is a protein formed by dermal cells called fibroblasts. The production of collagen increases in areas of tissue injury and helps form scar tissue. Fibroblasts also produce **ground substance,** a lubricating material composed of protein and sugar groups that surrounds the dermal cells and fibers and contributes to the skin's normal suppleness and turgor.

The elasticity of the skin depends on both the quantity and quality of the elastic fibers, which are scattered among the collagen fibers. The major component of the elastic fiber is **elastin.**

The dermis houses a network of capillaries and lymph vessels in which the exchange of oxygen and heat occurs. The dermis is also rich in sensory nerves that transmit the sensations of touch, pressure, temperature, pain, and itch.

EPIDERMIS

Anchored to the dermis by fingerlike projections of dermal tissue (**dermal papillae**) is the outermost layer of skin: the

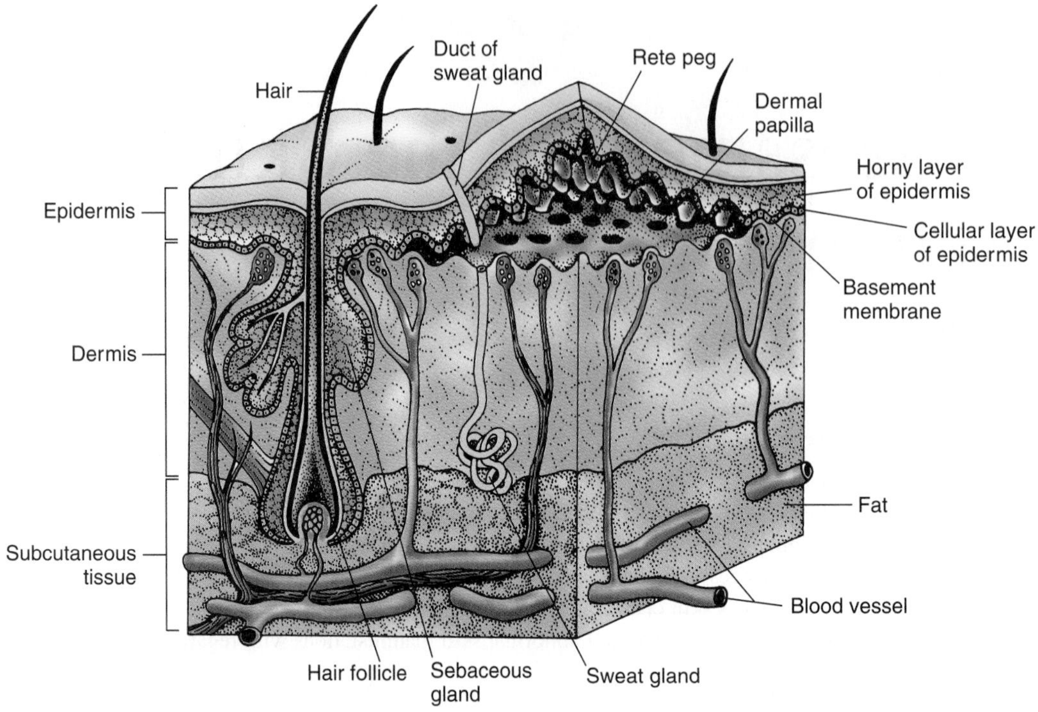

Figure 66-1 ● Anatomy of the skin.

epidermis. The fingers of epidermal tissue that project into the dermis are called **rete pegs.** The epidermis is less than 1 mm thick, but it is the protective barrier between the body and noxious stimuli in the environment.

The epidermis does not have a separate blood supply. It receives its nutrients by diffusion from the many blood vessels in the dermal layer through a porous basement membrane at the dermal-epidermal junction. Attached to the basement membrane are the keratinocytes. The basal cells (those keratinocytes capable of cell division and located closest to the basement membrane) continuously divide to form new cells. Older keratinocytes are pushed upward to form the stratified layers of the epithelium (**malpighian layers**). As keratinocytes move toward the surface, they flatten and eventually die. The outermost skin layer, the **stratum corneum** (horny layer), is composed of these dead cells. **Keratin,** the protein produced by keratinocytes, makes the horny layer relatively waterproof. A keratinocyte takes about 28 to 45 days to move from the basement membrane to the skin surface, where it is shed (**exfoliated).**

The final synthesis of vitamin D occurs primarily within the epidermis. Vitamin D is activated by ultraviolet (UV) light.

Melanocytes are found at the level of the basement membrane in a ratio of about 1 melanocyte for every 10 keratinocytes. These pigment-producing cells give color to the skin and account for the racial differences in skin tone. Darker skin tones are not caused by increased numbers of melanocytes; it is the size of the pigment granules (melanin) contained in each cell that determines the color. UV light stimulates the production of melanin, which protects against the harmful effects of sun exposure. Melanin production increases locally in response to endocrine changes or inflammation.

Structure of the Skin Appendages

HAIR

Hair, a remnant of the thick protective pelt worn by most mammals, is mainly a cosmetic feature for modern humans. Hair growth varies with race, gender, age, and genetic predisposition. Individual hairs can differ in both structure and rate of growth, depending on body location.

Hair follicles are located in the dermal layer of the skin but are actually extensions of the epidermal layer (see Figure 66-1). Within each hair follicle, a round column of keratin forms the mature hair shaft. The increased sulfur content of hair keratin (in contrast to that of keratin found in the cells of the stratum corneum) toughens the hair shaft as it forms. Hair color is genetically determined by a person's rate of melanin production.

Hair growth occurs in cycles; a growth phase (**anagen**) is followed by a resting phase (**telogen).** Local and systemic stressors can alter the growth cycle and result in temporary hair loss. Permanent baldness, such as common male pattern baldness, is genetic in origin and is seldom influenced by personal or environmental factors.

NAILS

Well-groomed fingernails and toenails have cosmetic value and serve as useful tools with which to scrape and grasp. Like hair follicles, the nails are extensions of the keratin-producing epidermal layers of the skin.

The white, crescent-shaped portion of the nail at the lower end of the nail plate (**lunula**) reflects the underlying nail matrix, where nail keratin is formed and nail growth begins (Figure 66-2). Unlike hair growth, which is cyclic, nail growth is a continuous but slow process. Total replacement of a fingernail

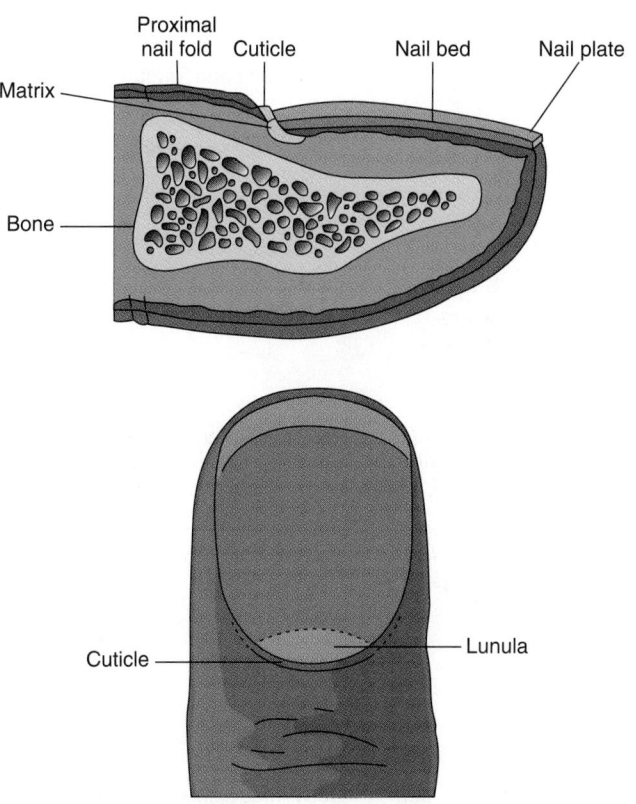

Figure 66-2 ● Anatomy of the nail.

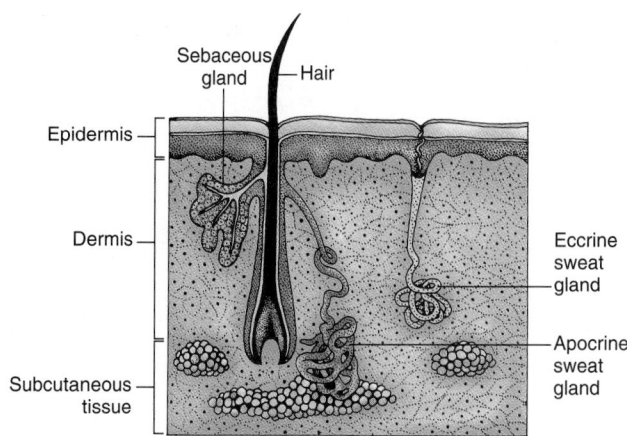

Figure 66-3 ● Anatomy of the hair follicle and sebaceous and sweat glands.

from the matrix to the end of the finger requires 3 to 4 months. Total replacement of a toenail may take up to 12 months.

The **cuticle,** a layer of keratin produced by the epithelial cells of the proximal nail fold, attaches the nail plate to the soft tissue of the nail fold. The nail body is largely translucent; the pinkish hue reflects a rich capillary blood supply beneath the nail surface. Nail growth and appearance are often altered during systemic disease or serious illness.

▓ GLANDS

SEBACEOUS GLANDS. The sebaceous glands are distributed over the entire skin surface, except for the palms of the hand and soles of the feet. Most sebaceous glands are directly connected to the hair follicles (Figure 66-3). The sebaceous glands of the eyelids, nipple areolae, and genitalia are freestanding.

Sebaceous glands continuously produce **sebum,** a mildly bacteriostatic, fat-containing substance. Sebum lubricates the skin and reduces water loss from the skin surface.

SWEAT GLANDS. The skin has two types of sweat glands: eccrine and apocrine. **Eccrine sweat glands** originate from the epithelial cells. They are found over the entire skin surface and are not associated with the hair follicle. The odorless, colorless, isotonic secretions of the eccrine glands are the single most important factor in the regulation of body temperature. Stimulation of the eccrine sweat glands and the resultant evaporative water loss enable the body to lose as much as 10 to 12 L of fluid in a single day.

Apocrine sweat glands are in direct contact with the hair follicle. They occur primarily in the areas of the axillae, perineum, nipple areolae, and periumbilicus. The interaction of skin bacteria with the secretions of the apocrine glands causes the characteristic body odor.

▓ Functions of the Skin

The skin is a complex organ responsible for the regulation of many body functions throughout the life span (Table 66-1). Although the skin has mainly protective and regulatory functions, the dynamic relationship between the skin and the outside world makes it an important way to communicate a client's state of health and body image.

▓ Skin Changes Associated with Aging

The process of aging begins at birth. As changes in physiology progress with aging, the skin undergoes age-related alterations in both structure and function (Chart 66-1). Figures 66-4 through 66-15 show some common age-related skin changes.

There are individual differences in how quickly and to what degree the skin ages. Although genetic background, hormonal changes, and systemic disease may change the appearance of the skin over time, chronic sun exposure is the single most important factor leading to degeneration of the skin components (Figure 66-16).

ASSESSMENT TECHNIQUES
History

Before examining the skin, the nurse obtains an accurate history from the client so that actual and potential skin problems can be readily identified. Chart 66-2 summarizes the best practices for obtaining a history from a client with a skin problem. The nurse begins by gathering information about integumentary changes and current skin care practices.

▓ DEMOGRAPHIC DATA

The nurse obtains demographic data from clients with actual or potential skin disorders. Age is important because many changes in the integumentary system are normal manifestations of the aging process.

TABLE 66-1 • FUNCTIONS OF THE SKIN

Epidermis	Dermis	Subcutaneous Tissue
PROTECTION Keratin provides protection from injury by corrosive materials Inhibits proliferation of microorganisms because of dry external surface Mechanical strength through intracellular bonds	Provides fibroblasts for wound healing Provides mechanical strength • Collagen fibers • Elastic fibers • Ground substance	Mechanical shock absorber
HOMEOSTASIS (WATER BALANCE) Low permeability to water and electrolytes prevents systemic dehydration and electrolyte loss	Lymphatic and vascular tissues respond to inflammation, injury, and infection	
TEMPERATURE REGULATION Eccrine sweat glands allow dissipation of heat through evaporation of sweat secreted onto the skin surface	Cutaneous vasculature, through dilation or constriction, promotes or inhibits heat conduction from the skin surface	Fat cells act as insulators and assist in retention of body heat
SENSORY ORGAN Transmits a variety of sensations through the neuroreceptor system	Encloses an extensive network of free and encapsulated nerve endings for relaying sensations to the brain	Contains large pressure receptors
VITAMIN SYNTHESIS 7-Dehydrocholesterol is present in large concentrations in malpighian cells; photoconversion to vitamin D takes place	No function	No function
PSYCHOSOCIAL Body image alterations with many epidermal diseases, such as generalized psoriasis	Body image alterations with many dermal diseases, such as scleroderma	Body image alterations may result from increases, decreases, and redistribution of body fat stores

Race and nationality can also be important. Some variations in skin appearance are normal among clients of specific races and nationalities but are abnormal for clients of other races or nationalities.

Information regarding the client's occupation and hobbies can provide clues to chronic skin exposure to chemicals, irritants, abrasive substances, and other environmental factors that may contribute to skin problems.

■ PERSONAL AND FAMILY HISTORY

The nurse obtains the client's medical history, including previous or current illnesses and surgical procedures. This information helps to determine whether skin changes are a manifestation of an underlying systemic disorder.

Because a predisposition to many skin diseases can be inherited, the nurse explores any family tendency toward chronic skin problems. An examination of the immediate family's current health status may identify a communicable disease that has been transferred between family members.

■ MEDICATION HISTORY

Because skin reactions to systemic medications are common, the client is asked about any recent use of prescription and over-the-counter (OTC) preparations (e.g., laxatives, antacids, and cold remedies). Information is obtained regarding when each medication was started, the dose and frequency of the

medication, and the time the last dose was taken. A medication history also helps identify skin changes that result from the treatment of other medical problems, such as the changes that occur with long-term steroid or anticoagulant therapy.

■ DIET HISTORY

The client's weight, height, body build, and food preferences are noted. Poor nutrition, especially protein deficiencies, vitamin deficiencies, and obesity, can predispose a client to skin lesions and delay wound healing. Fat-free diets and chronic alcoholism can lead to vitamin deficiencies and related skin changes. Some skin diseases, such as chronic urticaria and acne, may be worsened by certain foods or food additives.

■ SOCIOECONOMIC STATUS

The nurse asks the client about his or her social and economic background to identify environmental factors that might contribute to skin disease. Recent travel may be a source of skin infections or unusual lesions.

If the client is well tanned, the nurse asks about the amount of time spent in the sun and tanning booths and whether he or she has experienced any skin problems associated with sun exposure.

Skin problems related to poor hygiene are common. The client is asked about living conditions, bathing practices, and the availability of running water.

CHART 66-1

CHART 66-1

NURSING FOCUS *on the* **OLDER ADULT**
Changes in the Integumentary System Related to Aging

Physical Changes	Clinical Findings	Changes in Functional Ability
EPIDERMIS		
Decreased thickness in epidermal layer	Increased skin transparency and fragility	
Decreased epidermal mitotic activity	Delayed wound healing	Decreased cell replacement
Decreased epidermal mitotic homeostasis	Skin hyperplasia, such as hyperkeratoses and skin cancers (especially in sun-exposed areas)	
Increased epidermal permeability	Increased susceptibility to irritant reactions	Decreased barrier function
Decreased number of Langerhans cells	Decreased cutaneous inflammatory response	Decreased injury response
Decreased number of active melanocytes	Increased sensitivity to sun exposure	
Hyperplasia of melanocytes at the dermal-epidermal junction (especially in sun-exposed areas)	Mottled hyperpigmentation and hypopigmentation (e.g., liver spots and age spots)	
Decreased vitamin D production	Increased susceptibility to osteomalacia	Decreased vitamin D production
Flattening of the dermal-epidermal junction	Increased susceptibility to shearing forces, with resultant blisters, purpura, skin tears, and pressure-related skin problems	
DERMIS		
Decreased dermal blood flow	Increased susceptibility to dry skin (xerosis)	Decreased chemical clearance
Decreased vasomotor responsiveness	Increased thermoregulatory alterations (predisposition to heat stroke and hypothermia)	Decreased vascular responsiveness
Decreased dermal thickness	Paper-thin, transparent skin with an increased susceptibility to trauma	Decreased injury response
Degeneration of elastic fibers	Decreased tone and elasticity (wrinkles)	Body image alterations
Benign proliferation of capillaries	Cherry hemangiomas	
Abnormal nerve endings	Alterations in sensory perception	Decreased sensory perception
SUBCUTANEOUS LAYER		
Redistribution of adipose tissue	"Bags," cellulite, double chin, abdominal apron	Body image alterations
Thinning of subcutaneous fat layer	Increased susceptibility to hypothermia	Decreased thermoregulation
	Decreased resistance to mechanical injury (especially pressure necrosis)	Decreased injury response
HAIR		
Decreased number of hair follicles and rate of growth	Increased hair thinning	Decreased cell replacement
Decreased number of active melanocytes in follicle	Gradual loss of hair color (graying)	Body image alterations
NAILS		
Decreased rate of growth	Increased susceptibility to fungal infections	Decreased cell replacement
Decreased blood flow beneath the nail bed	Longitudinal nail ridges	
GLANDS		
Decreased sebum production despite sebaceous gland hyperplasia	Increased size of pores (especially on nose); large comedones in malar region	Decreased sebum production
Decreased eccrine and apocrine gland activity	Increased susceptibility to dry skin	Decreased sweat production
	Decreased perspiration, leading to decreased cooling effect	Decreased thermoregulation
	Decreased need for antiperspirants	

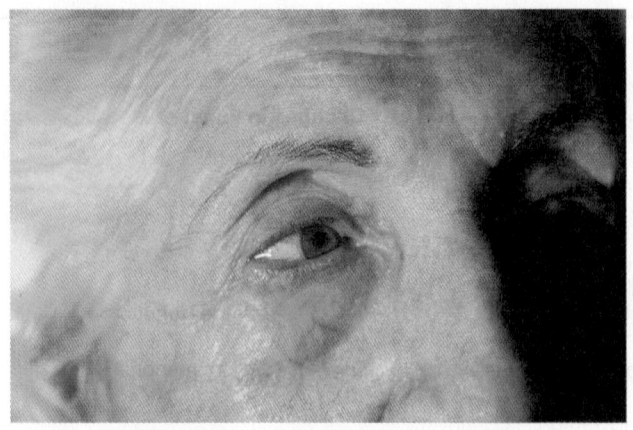

Figure 66-4 ● Eyelid eversion.

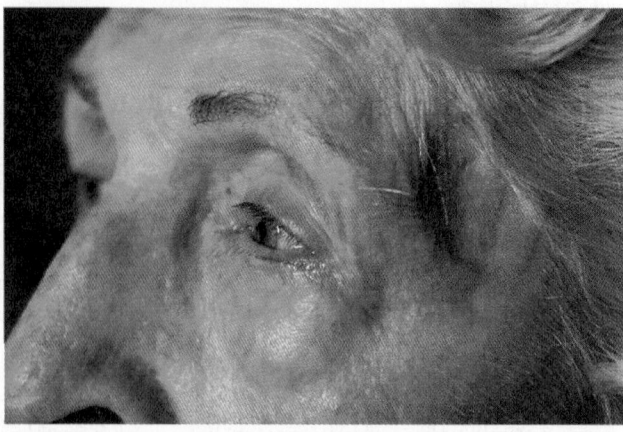

Figure 66-7 ● Changes in the body contour: "bags" under the eyes.

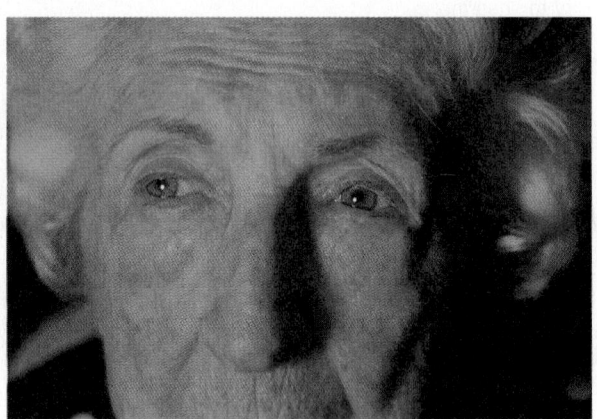

Figure 66-5 ● Deepening of the orbit.

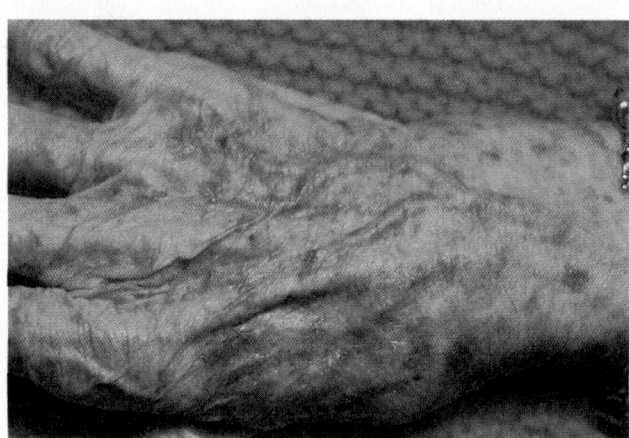

Figure 66-8 ● Paper-thin, transparent skin.

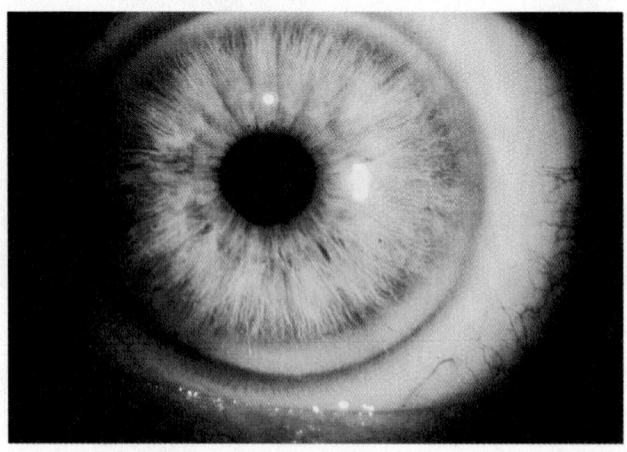

Figure 66-6 ● Arcus senilis of the iris.

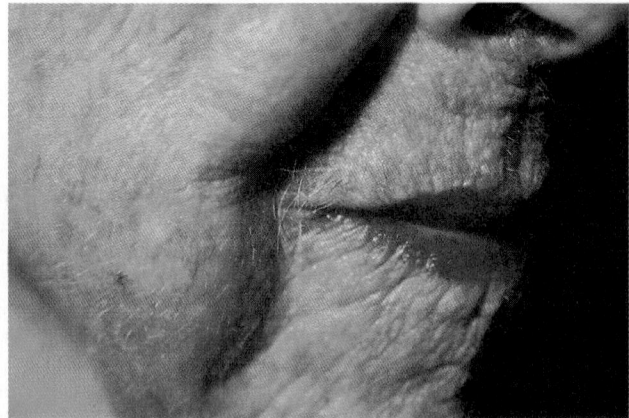

Figure 66-9 ● Wrinkles.

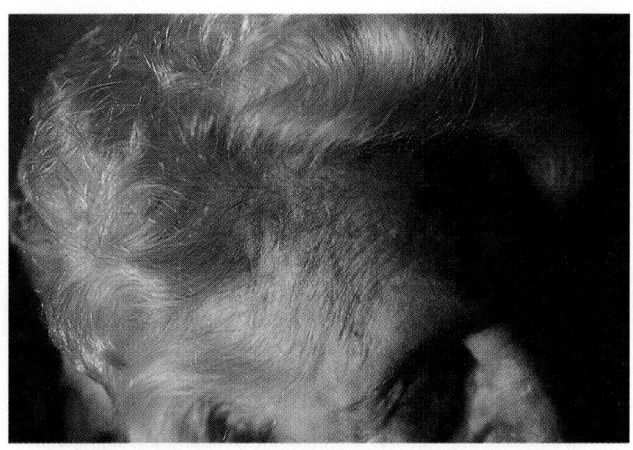

Figure 66-10 ● Graying and thinning of the hair.

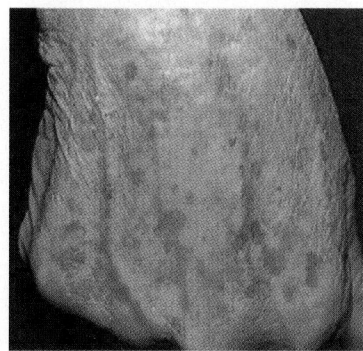

Figure 66-13 ● Actinic lentigo (liver spots).

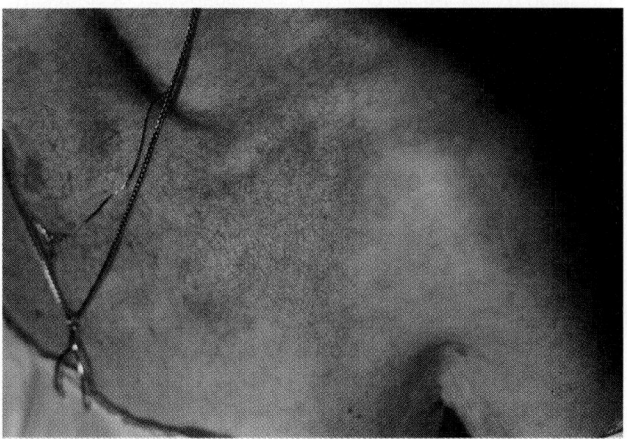

Figure 66-11 ● Xerosis (dry skin).

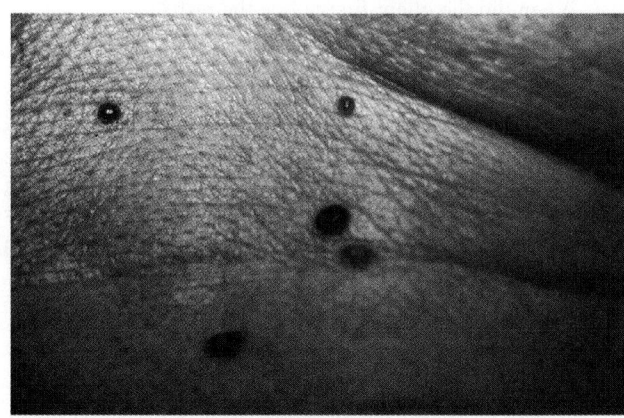

Figure 66-14 ● Senile (cherry) angiomas.

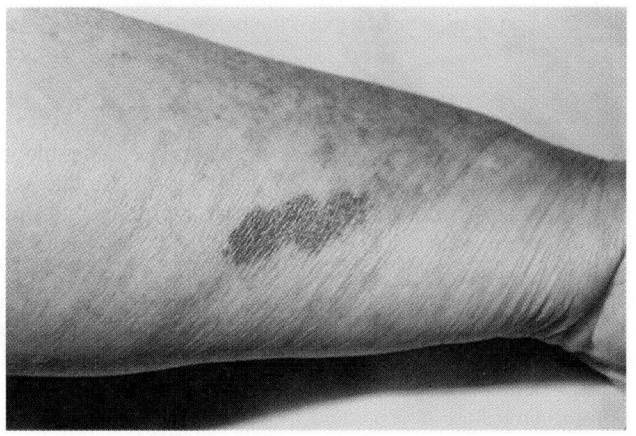

Figure 66-12 ● Actinic purpura.

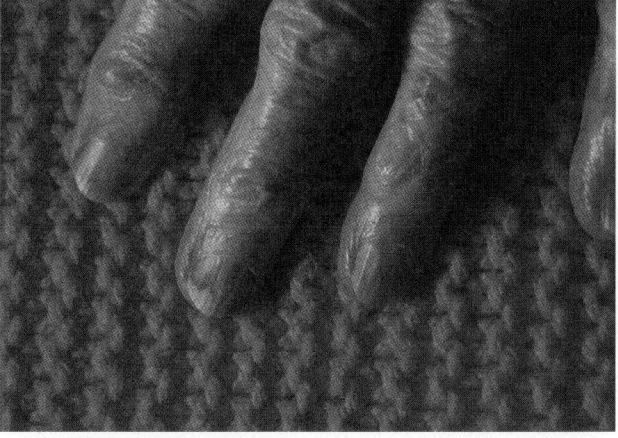

Figure 66-15 ● Nail changes, longitudinal ridges and thickening.

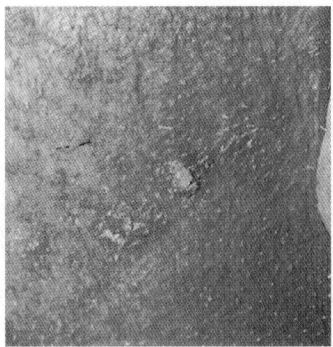

Figure 66-16 ● Actinic (solar) keratosis.

CURRENT HEALTH PROBLEM

If a skin problem is identified, the nurse obtains more information about the specific problem, such as the following:

- When did the client first notice the rash?
- Where on the body did the rash begin?
- Has the problem improved or become worse?

If a similar problem has occurred before, the client is asked to describe the course of the skin lesion and how it was treated. The nurse tries to link the problem with specific symptoms, such as itching, burning, numbness, pain, fever, sore throat, stiff neck, or nausea and vomiting. The client is asked to identify anything that seems to make the problem better or worse.

Physical Assessment

SKIN ASSESSMENT

Inspection

Skin changes may be related to specific skin diseases and may also reflect an underlying systemic disorder. By using skin assessment skills, the nurse is in a unique position to identify obvious and subtle clues about a client's state of wellness.

A thorough assessment of the skin is best accomplished with the client partially or completely disrobed. Skin examination for actual or potential impairments is incorporated as a routine part of daily care while bathing or assisting the client.

The nurse inspects the client's skin surfaces in a well-lighted room; natural or bright fluorescent lighting enhances the visibility of subtle skin changes. Although no special equipment is needed, a penlight is often helpful for close inspection of lesions and for illumination of the oral cavity.

Each skin surface is assessed systematically, including the scalp, hair, nails, and mucous membranes. Particular attention is given to the skin fold areas. The moist, warm environment of skin folds can harbor opportunistic microorganisms, such as yeast or bacteria. The following features are noted and documented:

- Obvious changes in color and vascularity
- The presence or absence of moisture
- Edema
- Skin lesions
- Skin integrity

In addition, the cleanliness of the various body areas may indicate a need for further evaluation of self-care activities.

CHART 66-2

BEST PRACTICE *for*
Obtaining an Accurate Nursing History of the Client with a Skin Problem

Medical-Surgical History
- Does the client have any current or previous medical problems?
- Has the client undergone any recent or previous surgical procedures?

Family History
- Is there any family tendency toward chronic skin problems?
- Do any members of the immediate family have recent skin complaints?

Medication History
- Is the client allergic to any systemic or topical medication? If so, have the client describe the reaction.
- What prescription drugs has the client taken recently? When was the drug started? What is the dose or frequency of administration? When was the last dose taken?
- What over-the-counter drugs has the client taken recently? When was the drug started? What is the dose or frequency of administration? When was the last dose taken?

Social History
- What is the client's occupation?
- What recreational activities does the client enjoy?
- Has the client traveled recently?
- What is the client's nutritional status?

Current Health Problem
- When did the client first notice the skin problem?
- Where on the body did the problem begin?
- Has the problem gotten better or worse?
- Has a similar skin condition ever occurred before? If so, have the client describe the typical course and how it was treated.
- Is the problem associated with any of the following: itching, burning, stinging, numbness, pain, fever, nausea and vomiting, diarrhea, sore throat, cold, stiff neck, new foods, new soaps or cosmetics, new clothing or bed linens, or stressful situations?
- Does anything seem to make the problem worse (e.g., sun exposure, medications, heat or cold, and menses)?
- Does anything seem to make the problem better?

COLOR

Skin color is affected by a number of factors, including blood flow, oxygenation, body temperature, and pigment production. In addition to these factors, the wide variability in natural skin tones often makes color assessment difficult, especially in clients with darker skin. (See Cultural Considerations, pp. 1510 and 1511, for suggestions for assessing clients with darker skin.)

Changes in skin color are described by their appearance (Table 66-2). The nurse documents alterations in color and notes whether the distribution is generalized or localized. Color changes are accentuated in the areas of least pigmentation, such as the buccal mucosa, sclera, nail beds, and the palms and soles. Therefore an inspection of these areas may help confirm more subtle color alterations of general body areas.

LESIONS

Skin disease is clinically described in terms of primary and secondary lesions (Figure 66-17). **Primary lesions** represent an initial reaction to an underlying problem that alters one of

TABLE 66-2 · COMMON ALTERATIONS IN SKIN COLOR

Alteration	Underlying Cause	Location	Significance
White (pallor)	Decreased hemoglobin level Decreased blood flow to the skin (vasoconstriction)	Conjunctivae Mucous membranes Nail beds Palms and soles Lips	Anemia Shock or blood loss Chronic vascular compromise Sudden emotional upset Edema
	Genetically determined defect of the melanocyte (decreased pigmentation)	Generalized	Albinism
	Acquired patchy loss of pigmentation	Localized	Vitiligo; tinea versicolor
Yellow-orange	Increased total serum bilirubin level (jaundice)	Generalized Mucous membranes Sclera	Increased hemolysis of red blood cells Liver disorders
	Increased serum carotene level (carotenemia)	Perioral Palms and soles Absent in sclera and mucous membranes	Increased ingestion of carotene-containing foods (carrots) Pregnancy Thyroid deficiency Diabetes
	Increased urochrome level	Generalized Absent in sclera and mucous membranes	Chronic renal failure (uremia)
Red (erythema)	Increased blood flow to the skin (vasodilation)	Generalized	Generalized inflammation (e.g., erythroderma)
		Localized (to area of involvement)	Localized inflammation (e.g., sunburn, cellulitis, trauma, and rashes)
		Face, cheeks, nose, and upper chest Area of exposure	Fever, increased alcohol intake Exposure to cold
Blue	Increase in deoxygenated blood (cyanosis)	Nail beds Mucous membranes Generalized	Cardiopulmonary disease Methemoglobinemia
	Bleeding from vessels into tissue: • Petechiae (1-3 mm) • Ecchymosis (>3 mm)	Localized	Thrombocytopenia Increased blood vessel fragility
Reddish blue	Increased overall amount of hemoglobin	Generalized	Polycythemia vera
	Decreased peripheral circulation	Distal extremities, nose	Inadequate tissue perfusion
Brown	Increased melanin production	Localized (to area of involvement) Pressure points, areolae, palmar creases, and genitalia Face, areolae, vulva, and linea nigra	Chronic inflammation Exposure to sunlight Addison's disease Pregnancy; oral contraceptives (melasma)
	Café au lait spots (tan-brown patches) • <6 spots • >6 spots Melanin and hemosiderin deposits (bronze or grayish tan color)	Localized Generalized Distal lower extremities Exposed areas or generalized	Nonpathogenic Neurofibromatosis Chronic venous stasis Hemochromatosis

the structural components of the skin. **Secondary lesions** are changes in the appearance of the primary lesion. These changes occur with normal progression of the underlying disease or in response to therapeutic intervention in the form of a topical or systemic treatment.

For example, acute dermatitis often occurs as primary vesicles with associated **pruritus** (itching). Secondary lesions in the form of crusts occur as the client scratches, the vesicles are opened, and the exudate dries. With chronic dermatitis, the skin often becomes **lichenified** (thickened) because of the client's continual rubbing of the epidermis to relieve itching.

Lesions are described in terms of their color, size, location, and configuration. The nurse notes whether the lesions occur as isolated changes or are grouped to form a distinct pattern. Table 66-3 defines terms commonly used to describe lesions.

The nurse assesses each lesion for the following ABCD characteristics associated with skin cancer:

A Asymmetry of shape
B Border irregularity
C Color variation within one lesion
D Diameter greater than 5 mm

A dermatologist or surgeon evaluates any lesion with one or more of the ABCD characteristics.

In describing the location of lesions, the nurse notes whether they are generalized or localized. If the lesions are localized, the specific body regions involved are identified. This information is important because some diseases are associated with a specific pattern of skin lesions. Involvement of only the sun-exposed areas of the body is important information when a possible cause is being considered. Rashes limited to the skin fold areas (e.g., on the axillae, beneath the

PRIMARY LESIONS

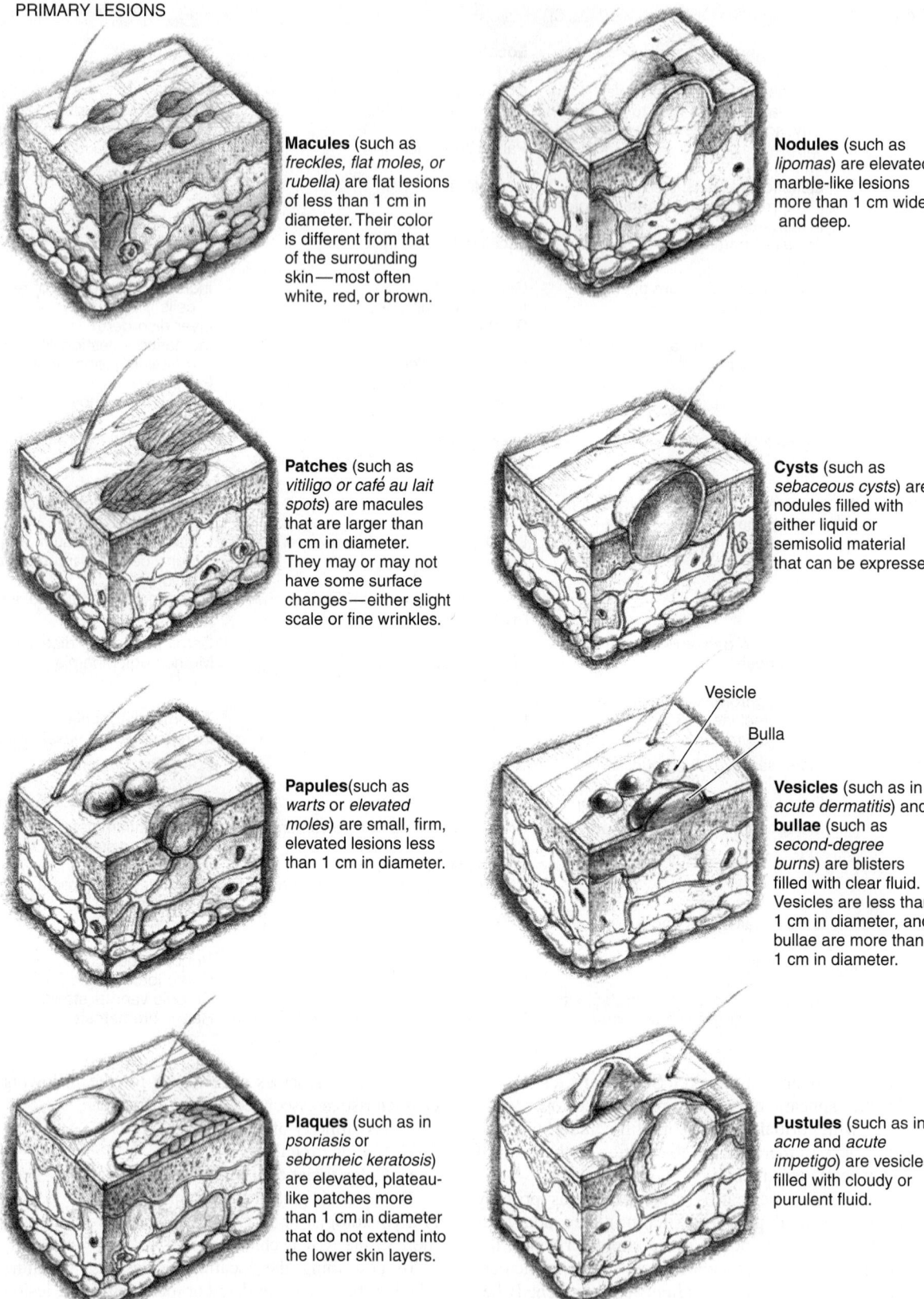

Macules (such as *freckles, flat moles, or rubella*) are flat lesions of less than 1 cm in diameter. Their color is different from that of the surrounding skin—most often white, red, or brown.

Nodules (such as *lipomas*) are elevated, marble-like lesions more than 1 cm wide and deep.

Patches (such as *vitiligo or café au lait spots*) are macules that are larger than 1 cm in diameter. They may or may not have some surface changes—either slight scale or fine wrinkles.

Cysts (such as *sebaceous cysts*) are nodules filled with either liquid or semisolid material that can be expressed.

Papules (such as *warts* or *elevated moles*) are small, firm, elevated lesions less than 1 cm in diameter.

Vesicle

Bulla

Vesicles (such as in *acute dermatitis*) and **bullae** (such as *second-degree burns*) are blisters filled with clear fluid. Vesicles are less than 1 cm in diameter, and bullae are more than 1 cm in diameter.

Plaques (such as in *psoriasis* or *seborrheic keratosis*) are elevated, plateau-like patches more than 1 cm in diameter that do not extend into the lower skin layers.

Pustules (such as in *acne* and *acute impetigo*) are vesicles filled with cloudy or purulent fluid.

Figure 66-17 ● Classification of skin lesions.

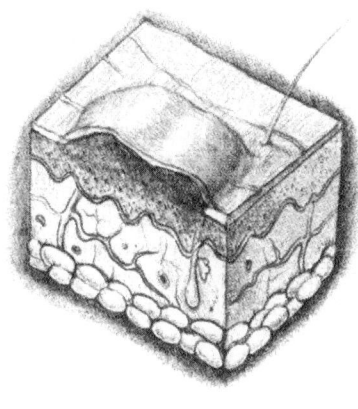

Wheals (such as *urticaria* and *insect bites*) are elevated, irregularly shaped, transient areas of dermal edema.

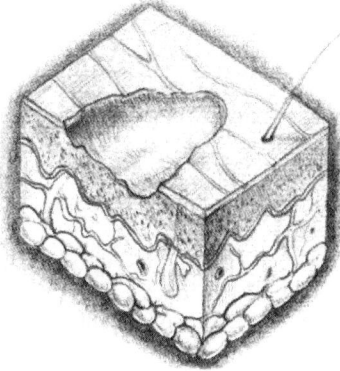

Erosions (such as in *varicella*) are wider than fissures but involve only the epidermis. They are often associated with vesicles, bullae, or pustules.

SECONDARY LESIONS

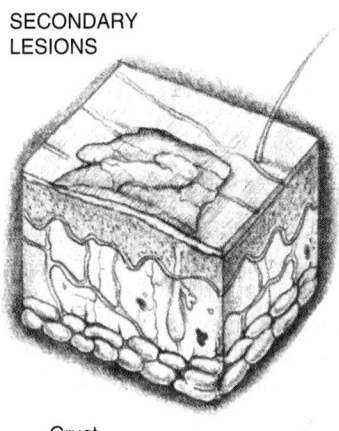

Scales (such as in *exfoliative dermatitis* and *psoriasis*) are visibly thickened stratum corneum. They appear dry and are usually whitish. They are seen most often with papules and plaques.

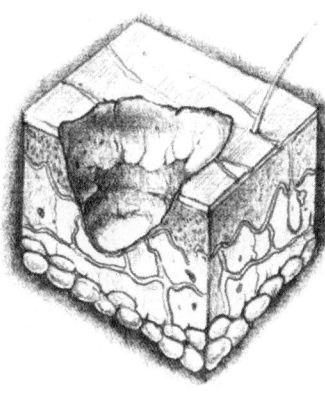

Ulcers (such as *stage 3 pressure sores*) are deep erosions that extend beneath the epidermis and involve the dermis and sometimes the subcutaneous fat.

Crust

Oozing

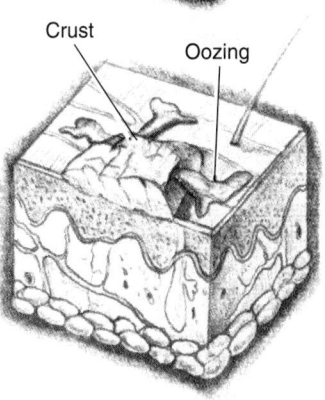

Crusts and oozing (such as in *eczema* and *late-stage impetigo*) are composed of dried serum or pus on the surface of the skin, beneath which liquid debris may accumulate. Crusts frequently result from broken vesicles, bullae, or pustules.

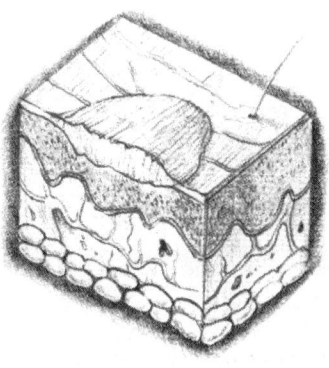

Lichenifications (such as in *chronic dermatitis*) are palpably thickened areas of epidermis with accentuated skin markings. They are caused by chronic rubbing and scratching.

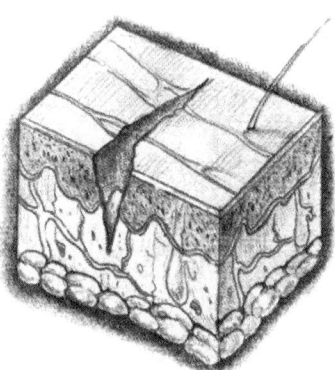

Fissures (such as in *athlete's foot*) are linear cracks in the epidermis, which often extend into the dermis.

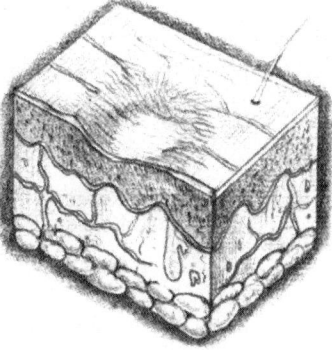

Atrophy (such as *striae* [stretch marks] and *aged skin*) is characterized by thinning of the skin surface with loss of skin markings. The skin is translucent and paper-like. Atrophy involving the dermal layer results in skin depression.

Figure 66-17, cont'd ● Classification of skin lesions.

breasts, in the groin) alert the nurse to problems associated with friction, heat, and excessive moisture.

EDEMA

The presence of edema causes the skin to appear shiny, taut, and paler than uninvolved skin. During skin inspection, the location, distribution, and color of any areas of edema are documented.

Skin elasticity is also affected by edema. Using moderate pressure, the nurse places the tip of the index finger against edematous tissue to determine the degree of indentation, or pitting (see Chapters 11 and 12).

MOISTURE

The skin is examined for moisture content. Normally, increased moisture in the form of perspiration can be expected with increased activity or elevated environmental temperatures. Dampness of the skin fold areas is common because of decreased air circulation where the skin surfaces touch. Excess moisture can cause eventual skin breakdown in bedridden and debilitated clients.

Overly dry skin can be caused by factors such as a dry environment, improper skin lubrication, inadequate fluid intake, and the normal processes of aging. Dry skin usually has scaling of the stratum corneum. Dry skin may be especially marked in areas of limited circulation, such as the feet and lower legs. Dry skin becomes a problem for most adults during the winter months, when the air contains less moisture, and in the hospital environment, where humidity is often poorly controlled.

VASCULAR MARKINGS

Vascular changes are classified as normal or abnormal depending on the cause. Normal vascular markings include birthmarks, cherry angiomas (see Figure 66-14), spider angiomas, and venous stars (Table 66-4). Bleeding into the tissue results in purpuric lesions: petechiae and ecchymosis.

Petechiae are small vascular lesions (<0.5 mm in diameter) that do not fade or blanch when pressure is applied (Figure 66-18). They often indicate increased capillary fragility. Petechiae of the lower extremities are commonly associated with stasis dermatitis, a condition commonly seen in clients with a history of chronic venous insufficiency.

Ecchymoses (bruises) are larger areas of hemorrhage that range in size from several millimeters to many centimeters. In older adults, bruising is common after minor trauma to the skin, especially on sun-exposed areas of the body.

INTEGRITY

The nurse thoroughly examines areas with actual breaks in skin integrity. For example, skin tears are a common finding in older people as a result of a flattening of the dermal-

---

TABLE 66-3 • TERMS COMMONLY USED TO DESCRIBE SKIN LESION CONFIGURATIONS

annular Ringlike with raised borders around flat, clear centers of normal skin
circinate Circular
circumscribed Well defined with sharp borders
clustered Several lesions grouped together
coalesced Lesions that merge with one another and appear confluent
diffuse Widespread, involving most of the body with intervening areas of normal skin; generalized
linear Occurring in a straight line
serpiginous With wavy borders, resembling a snake
universal All areas of the body involved, with no areas of normal-appearing skin

---

TABLE 66-4 • COMMON VASCULAR SKIN LESIONS

Lesion	Clinical Findings	Location	Significance
Cherry angioma (senile angioma)	Bright to dusky red, dome-shaped papule 2-5 mm in diameter Adjacent lesions may vary in size and color Partial blanching on palpation	Chest and back	Normal skin change with aging
Spider angioma	Bright red, starlike lesion varying in size from small to 2 cm Center of "star" is sometimes raised and may pulsate when palpated	Face, neck, and upper trunk	Associated with liver disease, pregnancy (change in estrogen level), and vitamin B deficiency May be normal finding
Telangiectasia	Reddish blue linear or star-like lesion caused by enlargement of the superficial blood vessels	Face and trunk	Associated with sun exposure and prolonged alcohol intake May be seen in systemic scleroderma and after continued use of potent topical steroids
Venous star	Spider-like, blue marking varying in size from small to several inches May have a "cascading" appearance Does not blanch with pressure	Legs (near veins) and anterior chest Face, scalp, and groin	Associated with increased pressure in superficial veins (varicose veins)
Port-wine stain	Large, dark red to purple area of discoloration Does not blanch with pressure		Congenital abnormality If on the face, may be associated with neurologic disorders and ocular abnormalities

epidermal junction with aging. The thin, fragile skin is easily disrupted by friction or shearing forces, especially if areas of ecchymosis are already present. The nurse looks for skin tears in the following areas:

- In areas where constricting clothing rubs against the skin surface
- On the upper extremities, where the skin is grasped when assisting a client to ambulate
- In areas where adhesive tapes or dressings have been applied and removed

The nurse remains alert to the presence of multiple abrasions or early pressure-related skin changes. These may signal previously unrecognized impairments in physical mobility or alterations in sensory perception.

Breaks in skin integrity are described by their location, size, color, and distribution, as well as by the presence of drainage or any signs of infection. The evaluation of partial-thickness and full-thickness wounds, including objective criteria that describe progress toward healing, is discussed in Chapter 68.

CLEANLINESS

The nurse evaluates the cleanliness of the skin to gain information about self-care needs. The hair, nails, and skin are inspected closely for excessive soiling and offensive odor. Depending on a client's degree of self-care deficit, hard-to-reach areas (e.g., perirectal and inguinal skin folds, axillae, feet) may be less clean than other skin surface areas.

Palpation

Because skin inspection alone can be misleading, palpation is performed to gather additional information about skin lesions, moisture, temperature, texture, and turgor (Table 66-5).

Palpation confirms the size of the lesions and determines whether they are flat or slightly raised. The consistency of larger lesions can vary from soft and pliable to firm and solid. With eyes closed, the nurse can detect more subtle changes, such as the difference between a fine **macular** (flat) rash and a **papular** (raised) rash. The client is asked whether he or she experiences pain or tenderness during palpation of the skin.

The nurse touches areas of excess moisture to determine the thickness and consistency of secretions. In areas of excess

dryness, a finger is rubbed against the skin surface to determine the degree of flaking or scaling.

Both generalized and localized changes in skin temperature can be detected by placing the back of a hand on the skin surface. Before assessing for changes in skin temperature, the nurse makes certain to have warm hands. Cold hands interfere with accurate assessment and are uncomfortable for the client.

The skin surfaces are palpated to assess texture, which differs according to body region and exposure to environmental irritants. For example, areas of long-term sun exposure have a rougher texture than that of protected skin surfaces. The client whose occupation requires repeated exposure to harsh soaps or chemicals may show skin changes related to this exposure. Increased skin thickness from scarring, lichenification, or edema usually decreases elasticity.

Turgor indicates the amount of skin elasticity. The turgor of the skin can be altered by a number of factors, including water content and age. The skin is gently pinched between the thumb and forefinger and released. If skin turgor is normal, the skin immediately returns to its original state when released. Poor skin turgor is evidenced by "tenting" of the skin, with a gradual return to the original state (see Chapter 11). A normal loss of elasticity with aging makes the assessment of skin turgor difficult in an older client. If the client is in a supine position, the forehead or chest tissue gives the best indication of skin hydration.

HAIR ASSESSMENT

During the skin assessment, the hair is inspected and palpated for cleanliness, distribution, quantity, and quality. Hair is normally found in an even distribution over most of the body surfaces, with the hair on the scalp, in the pubic region, and in the axillary folds thicker and coarser than hair on the trunk and extremities. Although color and growth patterns vary widely, sudden or marked changes in hair characteristics may reflect an underlying disease process. As with skin changes, the nurse investigates any abnormal findings by obtaining an in-depth history of the circumstances surrounding any change.

How well the hair is groomed, including the cleanliness of areas of thicker hair growth, can confirm information already gathered about a client's social history and health care needs. If the client has intense itching or scratches continually, the scalp and pubis are examined for lice and **nits** (lice eggs). The scalp is inspected for excessive scaling, redness, lesions, excoriation, crusting, and tenderness.

Dandruff, an accumulation of patchy or diffuse white or gray scales that appear on the surface of the scalp, is common. Dandruff is mainly a cosmetic problem, but an excessively oily scalp can result in inflammatory changes with erythema and pruritus. Severe inflammatory dandruff can extend to involve the eyebrows and the skin of the face and neck. *If severe dandruff is not treated, hair loss can occur.*

Although gradual hair loss is associated with aging, sudden asymmetric or patchy hair loss at any age is of concern. The nurse assesses the scalp for distribution and thickness of the hair and notes variations.

Hirsutism is excessive body hair growth or hair growth in abnormal body areas. Increased hair growth across the face and anterior chest in women is a sign of hirsutism. Hirsutism is one manifestation of hormonal imbalance. If hirsutism is apparent, the nurse looks for changes in fat distribution and

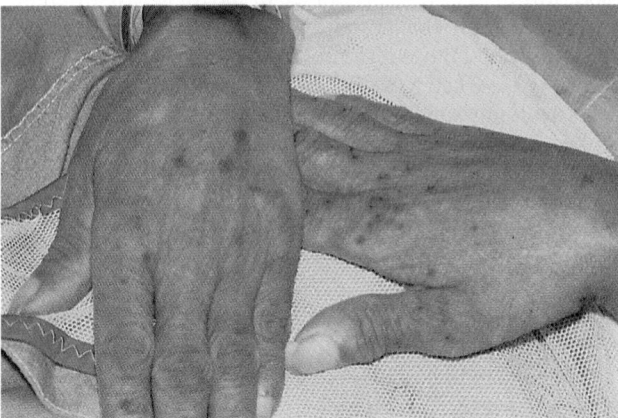

Figure 66-18 ● Petechiae.

TABLE 66-5 · COMMON CLINICAL FINDINGS IN SKIN PALPATION

Clinical Findings	Cause	Location	Examples of Predisposing Conditions
EDEMA			
Localized	Inflammatory response	Area of injury or involvement	Trauma
Dependent or pitting	Fluid and electrolyte imbalance	Ambulatory: dorsum of foot and medial ankle	Congestive heart failure
	Venous and cardiac insufficiency		Renal disease
		Bedridden: buttocks, sacrum, and lower back	Hepatic cirrhosis
			Venous thrombosis or stasis
Nonpitting	Endocrine imbalance	Generalized, but more easily seen over the tibia	Hypothyroidism (myxedema)
MOISTURE			
Increased	Autonomic nervous system stimulation	Face, axillae, skin folds, palms, and soles	Fever, anxiety, activity
			Hyperthyroidism
Decreased	Dehydration	Buccal mucous membranes with progressive involvement of other skin surfaces	Fluid loss
	Endocrine imbalance		Postmenopausal status
			Hypothyroidism
			Normal aging
TEMPERATURE			
Increased	Increased blood flow to the skin	Generalized	Fever, hypermetabolic states
		Localized	Inflammation
Decreased	Decreased blood flow to the skin	Generalized	Impending shock, sepsis, anxiety
			Hypothyroidism
		Localized	Interference with vascular flow
TURGOR			
Decreased	Decreased elasticity of the dermis (tenting when pinched)	Abdomen, forehead, or radial aspect of the wrist	Severe dehydration
			Sudden, severe weight loss
			Normal aging
TEXTURE			
Roughness or thickness	Irritation, friction	Pressure points (e.g., soles, palms, and elbows)	Calluses
			Chronic eczema
			Atopic skin diseases
	Sun damage	Areas of sun exposure	Normal aging
	Excessive collagen production	Localized or generalized	Scleroderma
			Keloids
Softness or smoothness	Endocrine disturbances	Generalized	Hyperthyroidism

capillary fragility, which can occur in Cushing's disease; and for clitoral enlargement and deepening of the voice, which may indicate ovarian dysfunction.

■ NAIL ASSESSMENT

Dystrophic (abnormal) nails often reflect a serious systemic illness or local skin disease involving the epidermal keratinocytes. The fingernails and toenails are evaluated for color, shape, thickness, texture, and the presence of lesions.

Many variations in color, texture, and grooming of the nails are influenced by factors unrelated to disease, such as occupation. When assessing the older adult, the nurse notes minor variations associated with the aging process (see Figure 66-15), such as a gradual thickening of the nail plate, the presence of longitudinal ridges, or a yellowish-gray discoloration.

■ COLOR

The color of the nail plate depends on many factors, including thickness and transparency of the nail, blood composition, adequacy of arterial blood flow, and pigment deposits (Table 66-6). Figure 66-19 shows normal variations in nail color. Changes in color can be attributed to external factors, such as the chemical damage encountered in some occupations and in the long-term use of nail polish.

During examination, the client's fingers and toes should be free of any surface pressure that might interfere with local blood flow or alter the appearance of the digits. To differentiate between color changes attributable to the underlying vascular supply and those resulting from pigment deposition, the nail bed is blanched to see whether a significant color change occurs with pressure. This technique involves gently squeezing the end of the finger or toe, exerting downward pressure on the nail bed, and then releasing the pressure. Color caused by vascular alterations changes as pressure is applied and returns to the original state when pressure is released. Color caused by pigment deposition remains unchanged.

■ SHAPE

Nail shape may indicate early or late changes consistent with systemic disease. For example, fingernail clubbing is diagnostic for impaired gas exchange.

TABLE 66-6 • COMMON ALTERATIONS IN NAIL COLOR

Alteration	Clinical Findings	Significance
White	Horizontal white banding or areas of opacity	Chronic hepatic or renal disease (hypoalbuminemia)
	Generalized pallor of nail beds	Shock
		Anemia
		Early arteriosclerotic changes (toenails)
		Myocardial infarction
Yellow-brown	Diffuse yellow to brown discoloration	Jaundice
		Peripheral lymphedema
		Bacterial or fungal infections of the nail
		Psoriasis
		Diabetes
		Cardiac failure
		Staining from tobacco, nail polish, or dyes
		Long-term tetracycline therapy
		Normal aging (yellow-gray color)
	Vertical brown banding extending from the proximal nail fold distally	Normal finding in African-American clients
		Nevus or melanoma of nail matrix in Caucasian clients
Red	Thin, dark red vertical lines 1-3 mm in length (splinter hemorrhages)	Bacterial endocarditis
		Trichinosis
		Trauma to the nail bed
		Normal finding in some clients
	Red discoloration of the lunula	Cardiac insufficiency
	Dark red nail beds	Polycythemia vera
Blue	Diffuse blue discoloration that blanches with pressure	Respiratory failure
		Methemoglobinuria
		Venous stasis disease (toenails)

The nail shape is evaluated by examining the curve of the nail plate and surrounding soft tissue from all angles. The fingertips are palpated to define areas of sponginess, tenderness, or marked edema. Table 66-7 describes common variations in nail shape.

■ THICKNESS

The nail plate can thicken as a result of trauma, chronic dermatologic disease, or decreased arterial blood flow. In older clients, the nurse looks for a "heaped-up" appearance of the toenails, which is commonly associated with fungal infection **(onychomycosis).**

■ CONSISTENCY

Nail consistency is described as hard, soft, or brittle. Nail plates may become hard, with increased thickening. A warm-water soak or lubrication with petroleum jelly is required to soften the nail plates before they can be trimmed.

Soft nail plates, which are thin and bend easily with pressure, have been associated with malnutrition, chronic arthritis, myxedema, and peripheral neuritis.

Brittle nails can split, as in the client with onychomycosis or advanced psoriasis. Splitting of the nail plate is also caused by repeated exposure to water and detergents, which damage the plate over time.

■ LESIONS

Separation of the nail plate from the nail bed **(onycholysis)** creates an air pocket beneath the nail plate. The pocket first appears as a grayish white opacity. The color may change as

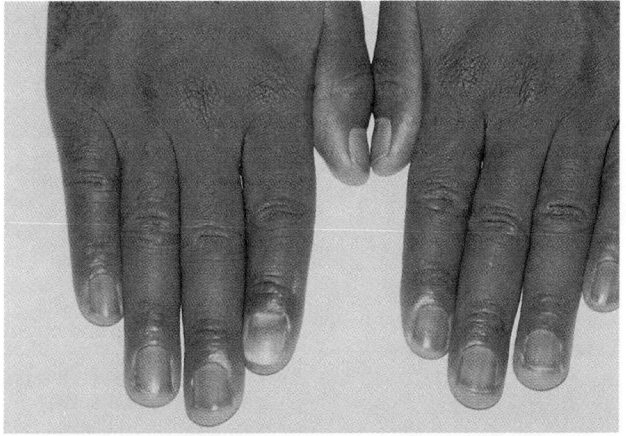

A

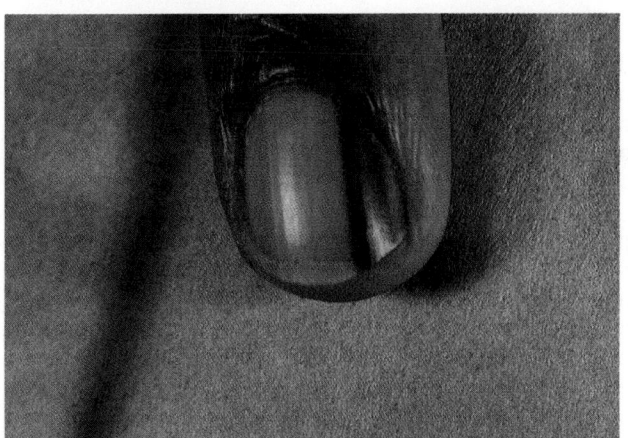

B

Figure 66-19 ● **A,** Diffuse nail pigmentation. **B,** Linear nail pigmentation.

TABLE 66-7 • COMMON VARIATIONS IN NAIL SHAPE

Nail Shape	Clinical Findings		Significance
Normal	Angle of 160 degrees between the nail plate and the proximal nail fold • Nail surface slightly convex • Nail base firm when palpated		Normal finding
Clubbing Early clubbing	Straightening of angle between the nail plate and the proximal nail fold to 180 degrees • Nail base spongy when palpated		Hypoxia Lung cancer
Late clubbing	Angle between the nail plate and the proximal nail fold exceeds 180 degrees • Nail base visibly edematous and spongy when palpated • Enlargement of the soft tissue of the fingertips gives a "drumstick" appearance when viewed from above		Prolonged hypoxia Advanced lung cancer
Spoon nails (koilonychia) Early koilonychia	Flattening of the nail plate with an increased smoothness of the nail surface		Iron deficiency (with or without anemia) Poorly controlled diabetes >15 yr in duration
Late koilonychia	Concave curvature of the nail plate		Local injury Psoriasis Chemical irritants Developmental abnormality
Beau's grooves	1-mm wide horizontal depressions in the nail plates caused by growth arrest (involves all nails)		Acute, severe illness Prolonged febrile state Isolated periods of severe malnutrition
Pitting	Small, multiple pits in the nail plate • May be associated with plate thickening and onycholysis • Most often involves the fingernails (several or all)		Psoriasis Alopecia areata

dirt and keratin collect in the pocket, and the area begins to have a bad odor. Onycholysis is common with fungal infections and after trauma. Separation of the nail plate may also occur with psoriasis or as a result of prolonged contact with chemicals.

The nurse inspects the soft-tissue folds around the nail plate for localized redness, heat, swelling, and tenderness. Inflammation of the skin around the nail (**acute paronychia**) is usually associated with a torn cuticle or an ingrown toenail. If acute paronychia occurs in an immunocompromised client, an opportunistic infection caused by the *Staphylococcus* organism is probable.

Chronic paronychia is more common and is characterized by inflammation that persists for months. People at risk for chronic paronychia are men and women with frequent exposure to water, such as homemakers, bartenders, and laundry workers.

■ CULTURAL CONSIDERATIONS

Pallor, erythema, cyanosis, and other color changes reflective of the physical state are more difficult to recognize in clients with naturally dark skin tones. Although physiologic processes are the same for both light-skinned and dark-skinned clients, the amount of skin pigmentation greatly alters how the skin appears in response to physiologic alterations. Consequently, the nurse develops assessment skills to detect the more subtle color changes. He or she becomes familiar with the normal appearance of a dark-skinned client's mucous membranes, nail beds, and skin tone so that variations from normal can be identified.

■ Assessment of Pallor in Dark-Skinned Clients

To detect generalized pallor, the nurse inspects the mucous membranes for an ash gray color. If the lips and the nail beds are not heavily pigmented, they appear paler than normal for that client. The skin is examined under appropriate lighting for the absence of the underlying red tones that normally give heavily pigmented skin a healthy glow. With generalized decreased blood flow to the skin, brown skin appears yellow-brown, and very dark brown skin is ash gray.

Assessment of Cyanosis in Dark-Skinned Clients

Cyanosis is even more difficult to detect in a client with dark skin. If impaired gas exchange is suspected, the nurse examines the lips, tongue, nail beds, conjunctivae, and palms and soles at regular intervals for subtle color changes. In a client with cyanosis, the lips and tongue are gray, and the palms, soles, conjunctivae, and nail beds have a bluish tinge. To support these observations, the nurse assesses for the more obvious manifestations of hypoxia, including tachycardia, hypotension, changes in respiratory rate or rhythm, decreased breath sounds, changes in level of consciousness, and any increase in the amount or viscosity of secretions.

Assessment of Inflammation in Dark-Skinned Clients

If areas of acute inflammation are suspected, the back of the examiner's hand is used to palpate for the increased warmth that occurs when blood flow to the skin increases. With the fingertips, the nurse palpates for hardened areas deep in the tissue, which may give the skin a "woody" feeling. Inflamed skin is tender and edematous. If edema is extensive, the skin is taut and shiny.

Areas of the body where inflammation (e.g., inflammatory rash or cellulitis) has recently resolved appear darker than the normal skin tone. This is due to stimulation of the melanocytes during the inflammatory process and to the increased pigment production that continues after inflammation subsides. More extensive injury to the skin with destruction of melanocytes (e.g., deep ulcer, full-thickness burn) may heal with color changes that are lighter than the normal skin tone. Unlike acute changes, chronic inflammatory changes seldom produce tenderness on palpation. If scar tissue is present, the skin may feel less supple, especially over the joints. If chronic inflammatory changes are suspected, the nurse asks the client about a history of skin problems in that area of the body.

Assessment of Jaundice in Dark-Skinned Clients

Jaundice in a client with dark skin is best assessed by inspecting the oral mucosa, especially the hard palate, for yellow discoloration. Inspection of the conjunctivae and adjacent sclera may be misleading, because normal deposits of subconjunctival fat produce a yellowish hue that is visible in contrast to the dark periorbital skin. Therefore the nurse examines the sclera closest to the cornea for a more accurate determination of jaundice. The palms and soles of dark-skinned clients may appear yellow if they are callused; a callus should not be mistaken for jaundice.

Assessment of Skin Bleeding in Dark-Skinned Clients

Purpuric lesions may be difficult to detect depending on the degree of skin pigmentation. Areas of ecchymosis appear darker than normal skin; they may be tender and easily palpable, depending on whether hematoma is present. In most cases, the client relates a history of trauma to the area that confirms the assessment. Petechiae are rarely visible in dark skin and may be seen only in the oral mucosa and conjunctiva.

Psychosocial Assessment

Actual impairments in skin integrity are commonly associated with altered perceptions in body image, especially when more visible skin surfaces (e.g., face, hair, hands) are involved. The nurse assesses the client's body language for clues indicating a disturbance in self-concept. For example, the avoidance of eye contact or the use of garments to cover the affected areas communicates concern about physical appearance. Clients with chronic skin diseases often relate a history of social isolation that is attributable to a fear of rejection by others or a belief that the skin problem is contagious.

Skin changes linked to poor hygiene are common in clients from low socioeconomic backgrounds. The nurse assesses the client's overall appearance for excessive soiling, matted hair, body odor, or other self-care deficits. The nurse confirms unsanitary living conditions by obtaining a social history. Clients may relate similar skin problems among family members, friends, and sexual contacts.

If skin problems related to poor hygiene are identified in older clients, the nurse also evaluates any physical limitations that may be contributing to poor health maintenance. For example, visual problems or limited mobility can make it difficult for clients to see or reach skin surfaces to clean them.

> **CRITICAL THINKING CHALLENGE**
> The client is a 75-year-old Caucasian woman who shows you an area on the left side of her chest—over her ribs and under the arm—that has numerous small red lesions. The lesions are macular and do not blanche with pressure.
> - What additional physical assessment techniques should you use?
> - What specific questions should you ask this client?

For suggested answer guidelines, go to SIMON http://www.wbsaunders.com/SIMON/Iggy/.

Diagnostic Assessment

LABORATORY TESTS

When a fungal, bacterial, or viral pathogen is suspected as the cause of certain skin changes, confirmation by microscopic examination is necessary.

Cultures for Fungal Infections

When superficial fungal (**dermatophyte**) infections are suspected, scales are gently scraped from the skin lesions into a Petri dish or a similar clean container and taken to the laboratory for culture. Fingernail clippings and hair are collected in a similar manner. Unfortunately, waiting for culture results can delay treatment of a superficial fungal infection. For this reason, the specimen is also treated with a potassium hydroxide (KOH) preparation and examined microscopically. Fungal infections show branched hyphae when viewed under a microscope after treatment with KOH. A positive KOH test often eliminates the need for a culture.

For deeper fungal infections, a piece of tissue is obtained for culture. The physician obtains the specimen by punch biopsy (see Skin Biopsy, below). The biopsy specimen may be sent for cell analysis and special fungal stains; the tissue specimen is bisected, or two separate biopsy specimens are obtained.

Cultures for Bacterial Infections

Specimens for bacterial culture are obtained from intact primary lesions (bullae, vesicles, or pustules), if possible. Material is expressed from the lesion, collected with a cotton-tipped applicator, and placed in a bacterial culture medium. For intact lesions, **unroofing** (lifting or puncturing of the outer surface) may be required with a sterile small-gauge needle before the material can be easily expressed. If secondary lesions in the form of crusts are present, the nurse removes the crusts and swabs the underlying exudate.

A biopsy of deep bacterial infections may be required to obtain a specimen for culture. If bacterial cellulitis is suspected, nonbacteriostatic saline can be injected deep into the tissue and aspirated; the aspirant is sent for culture.

Cultures for Viral Infections

Viral cultures are indicated if a herpes virus infection is suspected. The physician uses a cotton-tipped applicator to obtain vesicle fluid from intact lesions. Unlike bacterial and fungal specimens, which can remain at room temperature until being transported to the laboratory, viral culture tubes are placed on ice immediately after the specimen is obtained and are transported to the laboratory as soon as possible.

OTHER DIAGNOSTIC TESTS

Skin Biopsy

To establish an accurate diagnosis or assess the effectiveness of an intervention, the physician must often obtain a small piece of skin tissue for histopathologic study. Before preparing the client, the nurse checks with the physician to determine the number, location, and type of skin biopsies to be performed.

TYPES OF BIOPSIES. Depending on the size, depth, and location of the skin changes, the physician may perform a punch biopsy, shave biopsy, or scalpel excision (excisional biopsy).

PUNCH BIOPSY. The punch biopsy is the most basic technique. A small circular cutting instrument, or punch, ranges in diameter from 2 to 6 mm. After the site is injected with a local anesthetic, a small plug of tissue is cut to the depth of the subcutaneous fat and removed with forceps and scissors. The biopsy site may be closed with one or two sutures if it is on the face or lower extremity. Some physicians allow the biopsy site to heal without suturing.

SHAVE BIOPSY. A shave biopsy removes only that portion of the skin elevated above the surrounding tissue by injection of the local anesthetic. A scalpel or razor blade is moved parallel to the skin surface to remove the tissue specimen. Shave biopsies are usually indicated for superficial or raised lesions. Suturing is not necessary.

EXCISIONAL BIOPSY. In rare instances, larger or deeper specimens are obtained by excision with a scalpel. Deep incisions are made and then sutured after the specimen is removed. In contrast to punch and shave biopsies, excisional biopsies usually involve more discomfort for the client while the site is healing.

CLIENT PREPARATION. As with any invasive procedure, the nurse prepares the client for a biopsy by briefly explaining what to expect. The nurse emphasizes that a biopsy is a minor procedure with few, if any, complications. If a punch or shave biopsy is planned, the client is reassured that scarring is minimal because of the small size of the tissue removed. If an excisional biopsy is planned, the nurse tells the client to expect a cosmetic result similar to that of a healed surgical incision.

PROCEDURE. The nurse establishes a sterile field and assembles all necessary supplies and instruments. A syringe with the physician's choice of local anesthetic is available. A small-gauge needle (No. 25) is attached to the syringe to minimize discomfort during injection. Although preparation of the biopsy site differs according to the physician's preference, the skin is simply wiped with alcohol in most cases.

The most uncomfortable time for the client is during the injection of a local anesthetic agent, which produces a burning or stinging sensation. The nurse reassures the client that the discomfort will subside as the anesthetic takes effect. Talking the client through the procedure with a quiet voice, in combination with a gentle touch, has a calming effect.

After removal, tissue specimens for routine pathologic study are placed directly in 10% formalin for fixation. Specimens for culture are placed in sterile saline solution. Bleeding of the biopsy site is sometimes controlled with Monsel's solution, a topical hemostatic agent. If topical treatment does not stop the bleeding, suturing is considered.

FOLLOW-UP CARE. After bleeding is under control and any sutures have been placed, the site is covered with an adhesive bandage or a dry gauze dressing. The nurse instructs the client to keep the dressing dry and in place for a minimum of 8 hours. After the dressing is removed, the site is cleaned once a day with tap water or saline to remove any dried blood or crusts. The physician may also prescribe an antibiotic ointment to minimize local bacterial colonization. The biopsy site may be left open unless a covering is preferred for cosmetic reasons or because the site is an area often soiled. The nurse instructs the client to report any erythema or excessive drainage at the site. Sutures are usually removed 7 to 10 days after biopsy.

Wood's Light Examination

A handheld, long-wave length ultraviolet (black) light or Wood's light is sometimes used during physical examination. Areas of blue-green or red fluorescence are associated with certain skin infections. Hypopigmented skin becomes more prominent when it is viewed under black light, which greatly facilitates the evaluation of pigment changes in fair-skinned clients.

Examination of the skin under a Wood's light is always carried out in a darkened room. The nurse reassures the client that no discomfort is associated with a Wood's light examination.

Diascopy

Diascopy is a noninvasive and painless technique that eliminates erythema caused by increased blood flow to the skin, thereby facilitating the inspection of skin lesions. A glass slide or lens is pressed down over the area to be examined, blanching the skin and revealing the shape of the underlying lesions.

Skin Testing

If a client's rash is thought to be an allergic contact dermatitis, patch testing may identify the responsible allergen. The technique for allergy testing of the skin is described in Chapter 23.

CRITICAL THINKING CHALLENGE

The client is a 45-year-old Asian woman who speaks no English. She has a large, black, papular lesion with irregular borders on her left cheek. Her daughter is serving as the interpreter. You are concerned that this lesion may be a melanoma. The daughter tells you that this mark has been on her mother's face for at least 20 years and that her mother considers it a "mark of beauty."

- Should this lesion be examined by a surgeon or dermatologist? Why or why not?
- What additional information should you obtain from the mother (with the daughter's assistance)?
- What additional physical assessment data should you obtain regarding this lesion?

For suggested answer guidelines, go to ⟨SiMON⟩ http://www.wbsaunders.com/SIMON/Iggy/.

ONLINE RESOURCES

For suggested readings and Internet resources, go to http://www.wbsaunders.com/SIMON/Iggy/.

SELECTED BIBLIOGRAPHY

Asterisk indicates a classic or definitive work on this subject.

Ebersole, P., & Hess, P. (1998). *Toward healthy aging* (5th ed.). St. Louis: Mosby.

*Gaskin, F.C. (1986). Detection of cyanosis in the person with dark skin. *Journal of the National Black Nurses Association, 1*(1), 52-60.

Guyton, A., & Hall, J. (2000). *Textbook of medical physiology* (10th ed.). Philadelphia: W.B. Saunders.

Jarvis, C. (2000). *Physical examination and health assessment* (3rd ed.). Philadelphia: W.B. Saunders.

Lookingbill, D.P., & Marks, J.G., Jr. (2000). *Principles of dermatology* (3rd ed.). Philadelphia: W.B. Saunders.

Matteson, M. (1997). Age-related changes in the integument. In M.A. Matteson, E.S. McConnell, & A.D. Linton (Eds.), *Gerontological nursing: Concepts and practice* (2nd ed., pp. 174-195). Philadelphia: W.B. Saunders.

Interventions for Clients with Skin Problems

JANICE CUZZELL

Learning Objectives

After studying this chapter, you should be able to:

1. Prioritize nursing care for a client with dry skin.
2. Compare and contrast wound healing by first, second, and third intention.
3. Identify clients at risk for pressure ulcer development.
4. Plan an individualized strategy for pressure ulcer prevention for a specific client at increased risk.
5. Differentiate the clinical manifestations for stage I through stage IV pressure ulcers.
6. Prioritize the nursing interventions for a client with a stage III pressure ulcer.
7. Evaluate the effectiveness of interventions for pressure ulcer management.
8. Compare the clinical manifestations and modes of transmission for bacterial, viral, and fungal skin infections.
9. Prioritize nursing care and educational needs for clients who have parasitic skin infections.
10. Explain the rationale for drug therapy for psoriasis.
11. Explain the rationale for ultraviolet therapy for psoriasis.
12. Identify interventions for prevention of skin cancer.
13. Describe the clinical manifestations of melanoma.

SIMON

Go to http://www.wbsaunders.com/SIMON/Iggy/ for self-assessment questions related to these Learning Objectives.

Skin problems are common, and the causes of many skin disorders are often not clear. The skin, in addition to having unique functions, can also reflect other body conditions. Thus skin problems may truly arise in the skin or may have their origin in a systemic disease or injury. Drugs and other interventions for any health problem can trigger a skin response or reaction. Skin problems can interfere with the medical or surgical treatment of other conditions. Age-related skin changes, as well as problems arising from immobility, chronic disease, debility, and change in immune function, place the older client at increased risk for skin damage.

MINOR IRRITATIONS

Dryness

▌ OVERVIEW

Dry skin is a common problem, especially in older clients. Dry skin is a fine flaking of the **stratum corneum** (outermost skin layer), which is more pronounced over the distal lower extremities. Dehydration of the stratum corneum (**xerosis**) is often accompanied by a generalized **pruritus** (itching). In clients with chronic skin conditions, unrelieved pruritus may result in secondary skin lesions, excoriations, **lichenification** (thickening), and infection as they scratch and rub the skin in an attempt to relieve the intense itching.

Xerosis is worse in dry climates. Central heating and air-conditioning reduce the humidity in the air and increase skin dryness. Wind, cold, and sunlight also contribute to the problem. Frequent bathing with harsh soap and hot water and poor application of moisturizers further dries the skin; however, frequent bathing with moisturizing soaps, oils, and lotions may reduce dryness.

► COLLABORATIVE MANAGEMENT

Immediate nursing intervention is aimed at rehydration of the skin and relief of itching. A 20-minute soak in a mildly warm bath, followed by application of an emollient cream or lotion, can rehydrate the skin and promote comfort. If the client is bedridden or if tub baths are contraindicated, the trunk and extremities can be wrapped in warm, moist towels covered by plastic sheeting and additional blankets to prevent chilling. Skin creams or lotions are always applied to slightly damp skin after these procedures or within 2 to 3 minutes after routine bathing.

Contrary to popular belief, the cream or lotion is *not* what makes the skin soft and supple. Water is the agent that softens the outer skin layers. Lubricating creams and lotions seal in the moisture provided by water, promoting suppleness and preventing flaking. Some skin lotions are **hydrophilic** (water seeking) and actually draw moisture from the skin, making the dryness worse if they are not applied directly to damp skin.

The nurse educates clients and family members or significant others in measures to maintain healthy skin. Chart 67-1 lists practical ways to avoid drying the skin.

Pruritus
OVERVIEW

Pruritus, or itching, is a distressing symptom that may or may not be associated with skin disease. Pruritus is caused by stimulation of itch-specific nerve fibers at the dermal-epidermal junction. Physical or chemical agents either act directly on these nerve fibers or activate chemical mediators, such as histamine, which then act on the itch receptors.

As a subjective sensation similar to pain, pruritus varies among clients in location and severity. Regardless of the underlying cause, clients usually report that pruritus is worse at night. Pruritus can be made worse by poor skin hydration, increased skin temperature, perspiration, and emotional stress.

► COLLABORATIVE MANAGEMENT

Clients usually seek relief from pruritus by scratching or rubbing the skin, a response that further stimulates the itch receptors and causes a pattern referred to as the **"itch-scratch-itch" cycle.** When the pruritus is associated with skin lesions, relief can usually be obtained by treatment of the underlying dermatologic disorder with appropriate topical and systemic medications. Systemic diseases, such as liver and venous disorders, can also cause pruritus without skin lesions.

The nurse plans care to promote comfort and prevent alterations in skin integrity that can result from vigorous scratching. Because dry skin is often a contributing factor, proper bathing and skin lubrication techniques are emphasized (see Chart 67-1). Clients are encouraged to keep the fingernails trimmed short, with rough edges filed, to minimize skin excoriation. They may wear mittens or splints at night to prevent inadvertent scratching during sleep.

A cool sleeping environment combined with a larger dose of sedating antihistamines at bedtime (when the side effect of drowsiness is welcome) may provide an uninterrupted night's sleep. Therapeutic baths **(balneotherapy)** containing colloidal oatmeal preparations or tar extracts may provide temporary relief (Table 67-1).

If antihistamines are ordered, the nurse closely monitors the client's response to therapy so that the dosage can be adjusted as needed. The anti-inflammatory properties of many topical steroid preparations can be maximized if the ointment or cream is applied to slightly damp skin.

Sunburn
OVERVIEW

Sunburn is a first-degree or superficial burn and one of the most common skin injuries. Excessive exposure to ultraviolet (UV) light injures the superficial dermis, with subsequent di-

---

CHART 67-1
CLIENT EDUCATION GUIDE
Prevention of Dry Skin

- Use a room humidifier during the winter months or whenever the furnace is in use.
- Take a complete bath or shower only every other day (wash face, axillae, perineum, and any soiled areas daily).
- Use tepid water.
- Use a superfatted, nonalkaline soap instead of deodorant soap.
- Rinse the soap thoroughly from your skin.
- If you like bath oil, add the oil to the water at the end of the bath.
- Pat rather than rub skin surfaces dry.
- Avoid clothing that continuously rubs the skin, such as tight belts, nylon stockings, or pantyhose.
- Maintain a daily fluid intake of 3000 mL unless contraindicated for another medical condition.
- Do not apply rubbing alcohol, astringents, or other drying agents to the skin.
- Avoid caffeine and alcohol ingestion.

TABLE 67-1 • USES OF THERAPEUTIC BATHS

Agents	Disease	Purpose
ANTIBACTERIAL BATHS Potassium permangenate (1:32,000; 1:64,000)	Infected eczema Pemphigus Multiple infected ulcerations	To lower skin bacterial load
COLLOIDAL BATHS Starch and baking soda (1 cup each per tub) Aveeno colloidal oatmeal (1 cup per tub) Aveeno oilated colloidal oatmeal	Atopic eczema Psoriasis Chickenpox	To relieve itching To soothe To lubricate
EMOLLIENT BATHS* Bath oils; Alpha Keri Lubath Mineral oil	Any dry skin condition	To clean and hydrate the skin
TAR BATHS* Bath oils with tar: Balnetar, Zetar, Polytar Coal tar concentrate (liquor carbonis, detergents)	Scaly dermatosis Psoriasis Eczema	To loosen scale To relieve itching To potentiate ultraviolet A or ultraviolet B light therapy

Modified from Rosen, T., Lanning, M.B., & Hill, M.J. (1983). *The nurse's atlas of dermatology.* Boston: Little, Brown & Co. ©1983 by Theodore Rosen and Marilyn B. Lanning.
*For emollient and tar baths, add 3 to 6 capfuls of therapeutic agent per standard bathtub.

lation of the capillaries, erythema, tenderness, edema, and occasional blister formation. Involvement of large areas of the body may also produce systemic symptoms, such as headache, nausea, and fever.

► COLLABORATIVE MANAGEMENT

Redness (erythema) and pain begin within a few hours after sunburn has occurred and gradually increase in intensity for 1 to 2 days before subsiding. Treatment is directed toward symptomatic relief and includes cool baths and soothing lotions, such as bland lubricants or refrigerated moisturizing lotions. Antibiotic ointments are used only if blistering of the skin causes secondary infection. If pain is severe, topical corticosteroids may decrease the inflammation temporarily.

Urticaria

■ OVERVIEW

Urticaria (hives) is the presence of white or red edematous papules or plaques of varying sizes. Urticaria is usually caused by exposure to a specific noxious stimulus, which releases histamine in the dermal tissue, causing vasodilation and leakage of plasma protein to form lesions or wheals. Unfortunately, the exact cause of urticaria is identified in only a small number of cases. The following factors are thought to cause urticaria: drugs, foods, infections, autoimmune diseases, malignancies, physical stimuli, and psychogenic responses.

► COLLABORATIVE MANAGEMENT

Treatment is aimed at removal of the potential stimulus and relief of symptoms. Because the skin reaction is caused by histamine release, antihistamines are the drugs of choice. The nurse instructs the client to avoid overexertion, alcohol consumption, and warm environments, which contribute to vasodilation and make the symptoms worse.

TRAUMA

■ OVERVIEW

Skin trauma can vary from a neat, aseptic surgical incision performed in a controlled environment to a grossly infected, draining pressure ulcer with tissue destruction. Injury to the skin stimulates a series of events for repair and re-establishment of the body's protective barrier.

■ Phases of Wound Healing

Wound healing occurs in three phases: the inflammatory, or "lag," phase; the fibroblastic, or connective tissue repair phase; and the maturation, or remodeling, phase. Table 67-2 summarizes the key events of normal wound healing. The length of each phase depends on the type of injury and whether the wound is allowed to heal by first, second, or third intention (Figure 67-1).

A wound without tissue loss, such as a clean laceration or a surgical incision, can be closed with sutures or staples. The wound edges are brought together, with the skin layers approximated and held in place until healing is complete. Because the wound can be easily corrected and dead space elim-

---

TABLE 67-2 · NORMAL WOUND HEALING

INFLAMMATORY PHASE
- Begins at the time of injury or cell death and lasts 3-5 days.
- Immediate responses are vasoconstriction and clot formation.
- After 10 minutes, vasodilation with increased capillary permeability and leakage of plasma (and plasma proteins) into the surrounding tissue.
- Migration of white blood cells (especially macrophages) into the wound.
- Clinical manifestations of local edema, pain, erythema, and warmth.

FIBROBLASTIC PHASE
- Begins about the fourth day after injury and lasts 2-4 weeks.
- Fibrin strands form a scaffold or framework.
- Mitotic fibroblast cells migrate into the wound, attach to the framework, divide, and stimulate the secretion of collagen.
- Collagen, together with ground substance, builds tough and inflexible scar tissue.
- Capillaries in areas surrounding the wound form "buds" that grow into new blood vessels.
- Capillary buds and collagen deposits form the "granulation" tissue in the wound, and the wound contracts.
- Epithelial cells grow over the granulation tissue bed.

MATURATION PHASE
- Begins as early as 3 weeks after injury and may continue for a year.
- Collagen is reorganized to provide greater tensile strength.
- Scar tissue gradually becomes thinner and paler in color.
- The mature scar is firm and inelastic when palpated.

---

inated, healing by **first intention** shortens the phases of tissue repair. Inflammation resolves quickly, and connective tissue repair is minimal, resulting in a thin scar.

Deeper tissue injuries or wounds with tissue loss, such as a chronic pressure ulcer or venous stasis ulcer, result in a cavity-like defect that requires gradual filling in of the dead space with connective tissue. Consequently, healing by **second intention** prolongs the repair process.

Wounds with a high potential for infection, such as surgical incisions that enter a nonsterile body cavity or traumatic wounds that occur under unclean conditions, may be intentionally left open for several days. After debris and exudate have been removed and inflammation has subsided, the wound is closed by first intention. Healing by delayed primary closure, or **third intention,** results in a scar similar to that found in wounds that heal by first intention. As shown in Table 67-3, healing can be impaired by a number of factors.

■ Mechanisms of Wound Healing

The body restores skin integrity through the processes of epithelialization and contraction. The degree to which these processes can close the wound depends on the depth of injury and the extent of tissue loss. The mechanisms of epithelialization and contraction can be easily understood if two categories of injury are considered: partial-thickness wounds and full-thickness wounds.

■ PARTIAL-THICKNESS WOUNDS

Partial-thickness, or superficial, wounds heal by **epithelialization,** the production of new skin cells by epithelial cells re-

The Process of Wound Healing

▶ Healing by First Intention

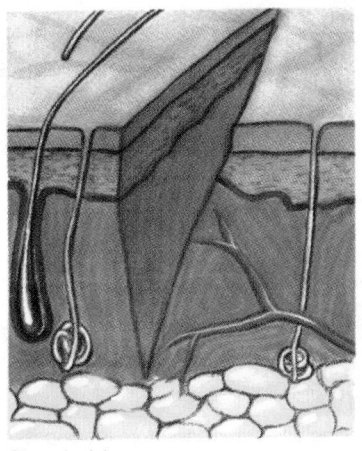 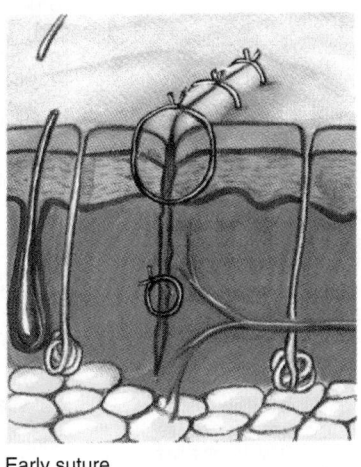 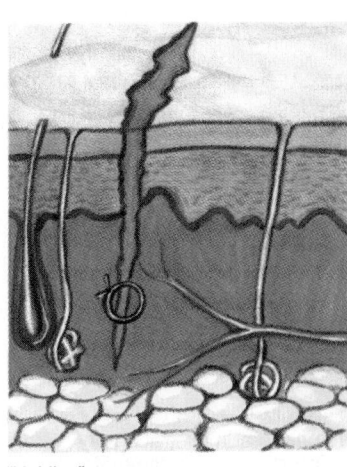

Clean incision   Early suture   "Hairline" scar

An aseptically made wound with minimal tissue destruction and minimal tissue reaction begins to heal as the edges are approximated by close sutures or staples. No open areas or dead spaces are left to serve as potential sites of infection.

▶ Healing by Second Intention (Granulation) and Contraction

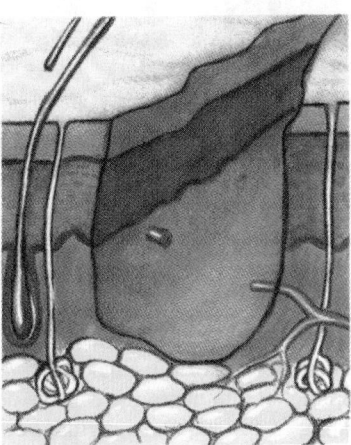 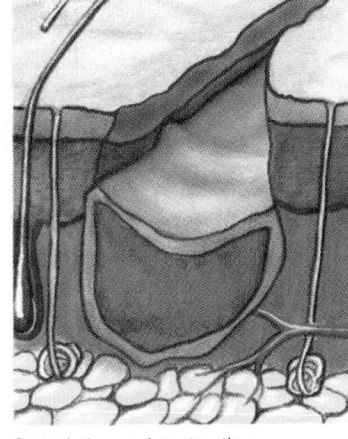 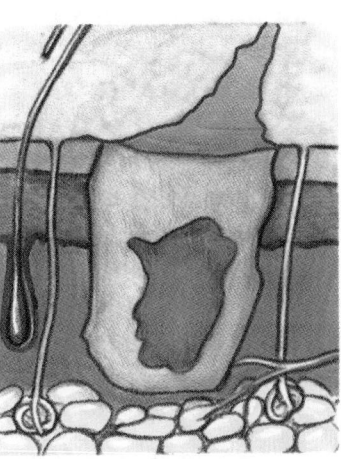

Gaping, irregular wound   Granulation and contraction   Growth of epithelium over scar

An infected or chronic wound or one with tissue damage so extensive that the edges cannot be smoothly approximated is usually left open and allowed to heal from the inside out. The nurse periodically cleans and assesses the wound for healthy tissue production. Scar tissue is extensive, and healing is prolonged.

▶ Healing by Third Intention (Delayed Closure)

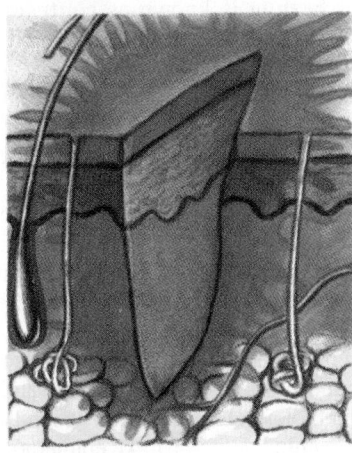 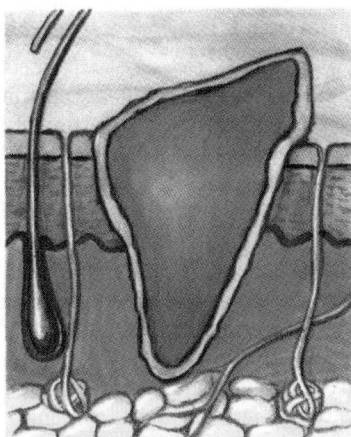 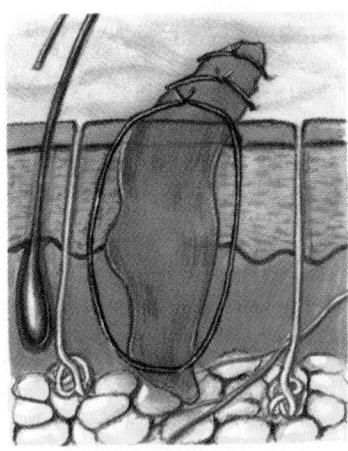

Infected wound   Granulation   Closure with wide scar

A potentially infected surgical wound may be left open for several days. If no clinical signs of infection occur, the wound is then closed surgically.

Figure 67-1 ● The process of wound healing.

TABLE 67-3 • CAUSES OF IMPAIRED WOUND HEALING

Cause	Mechanism
ALTERED INFLAMMATORY RESPONSE	
Local	
Arteriosclerosis	Altered local tissue circu-
Diabetes	lation, resulting in is-
Vasculitis	chemia, impaired leuko-
Thrombosis	cytic response to
Venous insufficiency	wounding, and in-
Lymphedema	creased probability of
Pharmacologic vasoconstriction	wound infection
Irradiated tissue	
Crush injuries	
Primary closure under tension	
Systemic	
Leukemia	Systemic inhibition of
Prolonged administration of	leukocytic response, re-
high-dose anti-inflammatory	sulting in impaired host
drugs	resistance to infection
• Corticosteroids	
• Aspirin	
IMPAIRED CELLULAR PROLIFERATION	
Local	
Wound infection	Prolonged inflammatory
Foreign body	response, which can re-
Necrotic tissue	sult in low tissue oxy-
Repeated injury or irritation	gen tension and further
Movement of wound	tissue destruction
(e.g., across a joint)	
Wound desiccation	
or maceration	
Systemic	
Aging	Impaired cellular prolifera-
Chronic stress	tion and collagen
Nutritional deficiencies	synthesis
• Calories	Decreased wound
• Protein	contraction
• Vitamins	
• Minerals	
• Water	
Impaired oxygenation	
• Pulmonary insufficiency	
• Heat failure	
• Hypovolemia	
Cirrhosis	
Uremia	
Prolonged hypothermia	
Coagulation disorders	
Cytotoxic drugs	

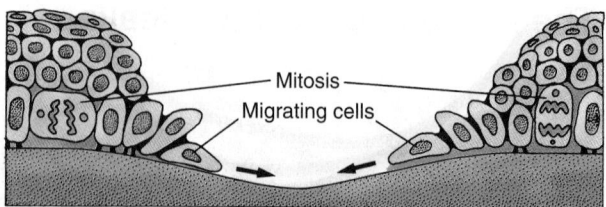

Skin cells at the edge of the wound begin multiplying and migrate toward the center of the wound.

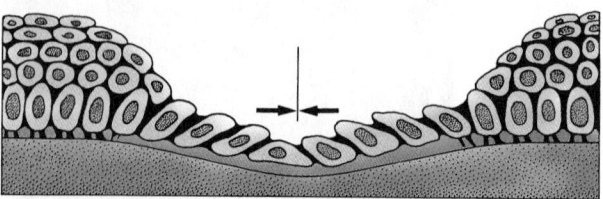

Once advancing epidermal cells from the opposite sides of the wound meet, migration halts.

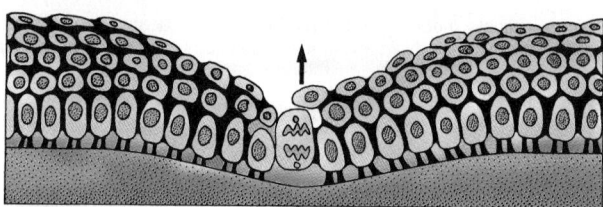

Epithelial cells continue to divide until the thickness of the new skin layer approaches normal.

Figure 67-2 • Epithelialization. (Modified from Swaim, S.F. (1980). *Surgery of traumatized skin.* Philadelphia: W.B. Saunders.)

■ FULL-THICKNESS WOUNDS

In a client with a deeper, or full-thickness, wound, most if not all of the epithelial remnants have been destroyed, except those remaining at the wound margins. For a full-thickness wound to heal, the **nonviable** (dead) tissue must be removed so that gradual filling in of the defect with granulation tissue can progress.

Drawing together of the wound edges occurs at the same time as collagen synthesis and wound revascularization. This type of healing is known as **contraction** (see Figure 67-1). Unlike epithelialization, in which new tissue is formed, wound contraction decreases the surface area of a full-thickness wound by stretching and thinning the existing tissue surrounding the wound. Fibroblastic cells in the wound bed exert a mechanical force on the wound edges, causing the wound to decrease in size at a uniform rate of about 0.6 to 0.75 mm/day. Complete closure of a wound by contraction depends on the mobility of the surrounding skin as tension is applied to it. Necrotic tissue provides a physical obstacle to wound contraction and must be removed for healing to occur.

If tension in the surrounding skin exceeds the force of contraction, wound closure does not occur, and the wound remains open until epithelial cells at the wound edges eventually bridge the remaining defect. Unlike epithelialization in partial-thickness wounds, in which the skin integrity soon returns to normal, the movement of epithelial cells from wound edges over fibrous connective tissue results in an unstable epithelial surface that is poorly attached to the underlying tissue and thus

maining in the dermal layer of the skin and at the base of the epidermal appendages (Figure 67-2). On injury, a fibrin clot forms. Undamaged epithelial cells at the basement membrane and at the base of the hair follicles and glands undergo a burst of cell division (mitosis). The new skin cells move into "cell-free" spaces on the wound surface, where the fibrin clot acts as a frame. Regrowth across the open area (**resurfacing**), initially only one cell layer thick, proceeds with thickening or layering of the new epidermis and, eventually, rete peg formation and keratin production.

In a healthy client, healing of a partial-thickness wound by epithelialization takes 5 to 7 days. Epithelialization occurs best in tissue that is well hydrated, is well oxygenated, and has few microorganisms.

is susceptible to reinjury. A venous stasis leg ulcer is one example of a skin defect in an area where effective movement of the surrounding skin is usually not sufficient to allow wound healing by contraction. As a result, the thin epithelial covering cannot withstand environmental hazards and abrades easily.

Epithelialization and contraction do not continue indefinitely. Natural healing processes can slow down or even be halted by the presence of infection, pressure, or mechanical obstacles, such as a poorly applied dressing. In the case of chronic wounds, healing can cease spontaneously and without a clearly defined cause.

➤ COLLABORATIVE MANAGEMENT

Specific treatment of skin trauma varies with the depth and circumstances of the injury. The focus of all treatment for any type of skin trauma is to enhance wound healing, prevent infection, and restore function to the area. Management for pressure ulcers presents common interventions, as does treatment for burns (see Chapter 68).

PRESSURE ULCERS

■ OVERVIEW

A **pressure ulcer** is any lesion caused by unrelieved pressure resulting in damage of underlying tissue or a lesion that is a clearly localized area of cellular necrosis due to vascular insufficiency in an area of tissue under pressure. This type of injury most commonly occurs over bony prominences. These skin lesions are a specific type of skin trauma that occurs almost exclusively in people with limited mobility. Once formed, pressure ulcers are slow to heal, requiring weeks to years, and result in increased morbidity and health care costs. The term *pressure ulcer* matches the guidelines provided by the Agency for Healthcare Research and Quality (formerly the Agency for Health Care Policy and Research) of the U.S. Department of Health and Human Services.

■ Pathophysiology

Mechanical forces exerted to or on the skin lead to the formation of pressure ulcers. These forces—pressure, friction, and shear—lead to direct and ischemic tissue damage. Although injury occurs more often to skin over bony prominences, pressure ulcers may occur anywhere. Excessive skin moisture increases the susceptibility of the skin to damage when mechanical forces are exerted.

■ PRESSURE

Pressure occurs as a result of gravity. Dependent tissues in contact with a fixed surface experience varying degrees of pressure. Pressure is determined by the amount of weight exerted at the point of contact, the distribution of weight at the point of contact, and the density of the contacting surface. Excessive or prolonged pressure can compress blood vessels at the point of contact, leading to ischemia, inflammation, and tissue necrosis. Pressure occurs when the client is positioned on a hard, unyielding surface that does not diffuse the weight or when he or she remains in the same position too long.

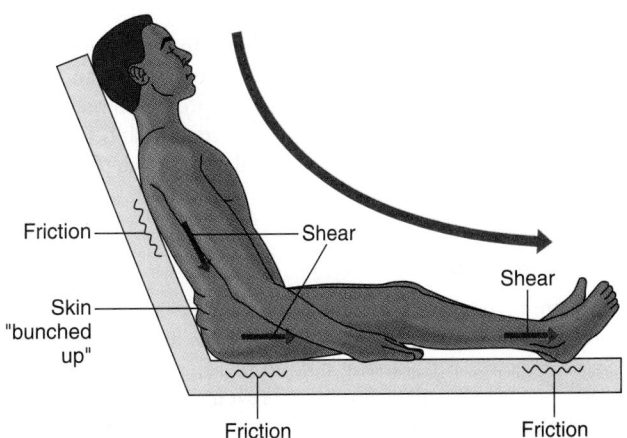

Figure 67-3 ● Shearing forces pulling skin layers away from deeper tissue. The skin is "bunched up" against the back of the mattress while the rest of the bone and muscle in the area press downward on the lower part of the mattress. Blood vessels become kinked, obstructing circulation and leading to tissue death.

■ FRICTION

Friction occurs when surfaces rub the skin and irritate or directly pull off epithelial tissue. Such forces are generated when the client is dragged or pulled across bed linen.

■ SHEAR

Shear or shearing forces are generated when the skin itself remains stationary and the tissues below the skin (such as fat and muscle) shift or move (Figure 67-3). The movement of the deeper tissue layers reduces the blood supply to the skin, leading to skin hypoxia, anoxia, ischemia, inflammation, and necrosis.

Gravity plays a role in the development of shearing forces. A shear injury commonly occurs when a client is in bed in a semisitting position and gradually slides downward. Often, the skin over the sacrum does not slide down at the same pace as the deeper tissues; thus the skin is mechanically "sheared," causing blood vessels to stretch and leading to soft-tissue ischemia, although no break in external skin integrity is observed.

■ Etiology

Pressure ulcers occur as a result of mechanical trauma and tissue anoxia.

> ### ❀ CONSIDERATIONS FOR OLDER ADULTS
> Older adults are at particular risk for pressure ulcers because of the presence of age-related skin changes. Progressive flattening of the dermal-epidermal junction predisposes older people to skin tears from mechanical shearing forces, such as the removal of adhesive tape and friction from tightly applied restraints. In addition, skin moisture and irritation from incontinence and friction over bony prominences can lead to partial-thickness skin destruction and early pressure ulcer formation. *If pressure is unrelieved, tissue destruction progresses to full-thickness injury.*

Incidence/Prevalence

Pressure ulcer development is a problem found among clients in the acute care setting, long-term care facility, and home care setting. Although client care has improved in many ways and new products are available for prevention and treatment, 3% to 14% of hospitalized clients still experience pressure ulcer formation.

Prevention

Pressure ulcers can be prevented if the risk is recognized and intervention begins early (see Chart 67-2 and the Evidence-Based Practice for Nursing box on p. 1521). Key health care team members for pressure ulcer prevention and management are the enterostomal therapist (ET), the certified wound specialist, and the registered dietitian (RD).

A pressure ulcer prevention program consists of two steps: (1) identification of high-risk clients and (2) implementation of aggressive intervention for prevention with the use of pressure relief/reduction devices. Many facilities do not recognize the value of preventing pressure ulcers with appropriate consultation, use of pressure relief/reduction products, and ensuring adequate nutrition. The costs of implementing such prevention strategies is more than justified by the savings seen in comparison with the costs of intervention for care when actual ulceration is present (see the Cost of Care box on p. 1521).

Risk identification and prevention measures must include education of the client and the caregiver. Documentation of risk assessment, prevention measures implemented, and education of all individuals involved in the care of the client at risk for pressure ulcer formation is key to the plan's success. Periodic reassessment of risk and continuing evaluation of the implemented plan are necessary as client conditions change.

■ IDENTIFICATION OF HIGH-RISK CLIENTS

All clients admitted to a health care facility or home care agency should be assessed for pressure ulcer risk, as recommended by the Agency for Healthcare Research and Quality (AHRQ). The use of a risk assessment tool increases the chances of identifying those clients at greater risk for skin breakdown. The two risk assessment tools recommended by the AHRQ guidelines are the Norton Scale and the Braden Scale (Figure 67-4).

Other factors to consider when determining the risk category for pressure ulcer formation are mental status, activity/mobility, nutritional status, and incontinence.

MENTAL STATUS. The client's mental status determines whether he or she is a partner in the prevention of pres-

---

CHART 67-2

NIC INTERVENTION ACTIVITIES *for*
The Client at Risk for or with Pressure Ulcers

Pressure Ulcer Prevention: *Prevention of pressure ulcers for a client at high risk for developing them*
- Use an established risk assessment tool to monitor client's risk factors (e.g., Braden scale).
- Document skin status on admission and daily.
- Monitor any reddened areas closely.
- Remove excessive moisture on the skin resulting from perspiration, wound drainage, and fecal or urinary incontinence.
- Apply protective barriers, such as creams or moisture-absorbing pads, to remove excess moisture, as appropriate.
- Turn every 1 to 2 hours, as appropriate.
- Turn with care to prevent injury to fragile skin.
- Post a turning schedule at the bedside, as appropriate.
- Inspect skin over bony prominences and other pressure points when repositioning at least daily.
- Avoid massaging over bony prominences.
- Position with pillows to elevate pressure points off the bed.
- Keep bed linens clean, dry, and wrinkle free.
- Utilize specialty beds and mattresses, as appropriate.
- Use devices on the bed (e.g., sheepskin) that protect the client.
- Moisturize dry, unbroken skin.
- Avoid hot water and use mild soap when bathing.
- Apply elbow and heel protectors, as appropriate.
- Facilitate small shifts of body weight frequently.
- Ensure adequate dietary intake, especially protein, vitamins B and C, iron, and calories, using supplements, as appropriate.
- Instruct family member/caregiver about signs of skin breakdown, as appropriate.

Pressure Ulcer Care: *Facilitation of healing in pressure ulcers*
- Describe characteristics of pressure ulcers at regular intervals, including size (L × W × D), stage (I to IV), location, exudate, granulation or necrotic tissue, and epithelialization.
- Monitor color, temperature, edema, moisture, and appearance of surrounding skin.
- Keep ulcer moist to aid in healing.
- Cleanse the skin around the ulcer with mild soap and water.
- Debride ulcer, as needed.
- Cleanse the ulcer with the appropriate nontoxic solution, working in a circular motion from the center.
- Note characteristics of any drainage.
- Apply dressings, as appropriate.
- Monitor for signs and symptoms of infection in the wound.
- Position every 1 to 2 hours to avoid prolonged pressure.
- Use specialty beds and mattresses, as appropriate.
- Ensure adequate dietary intake.
- Monitor nutritional status.
- Teach client/family member(s) wound care procedures.
- Initiate consultation services of the enterostomal therapy nurse, as needed.

Pressure Management: *Minimizing pressure to body parts*
- Place on appropriate therapeutic mattress/bed.
- Place on a polyurethane foam pad, as appropriate.
- Refrain from applying pressure to the affected body part.
- Elevate injured extremity.
- Turn the immobilized client at least every 2 hours, according to a specific schedule.
- Facilitate small shifts of body weight.
- Monitor skin for areas of redness and breakdown.
- Use an established risk assessment tool to monitor client's risk factors (e.g., Braden scale).
- Monitor the client's nutritional status.
- Monitor for sources of pressure and friction.

NIC intervention activities selected from McCloskey J.C., & Bulechek, G.M. (2000). *Nursing interventions classification (NIC)* (3rd ed.). St. Louis: Mosby. No part of this work is to be altered without prior written permission from the Publisher.

sure. When the client understands that turning and shifting of weight prevents tissue damage, the risk for pressure ulcer formation decreases. When he or she has a mental status problem because of stroke, head injury, organic brain disease, Alzheimer's disease, or other problem with cognition, the risk for pressure ulcer formation increases.

ACTIVITY/MOBILITY. The level of the client's independent mobility is a direct factor in the risk for pressure ulcer formation. Those clients who have unimpaired mobility and can respond to physical sensation changes are at low risk for pressure ulcer formation. Any client, regardless of age, who requires assistance with turning and positioning or who is less aware of physical sensation changes is at high risk for pressure ulcer formation. A client who must be confined to bed or a chair is at higher risk than a client who requires assistance with ambulation.

NUTRITIONAL STATUS. Nutritional status is a critical risk factor for the development of pressure ulcers. Maintenance of skin integrity and wound healing are dependent on a positive nitrogen balance and adequate serum protein levels. The client in a negative nitrogen balance not only heals more slowly but also is at greater risk for tissue destruction. In addition, draining wounds are a route of protein loss.

Attaining and maintaining adequate nutrition is as important as pressure reduction in the prevention of pressure ulcer formation. A dietitian or other nutrition specialist should be a part of the pressure reduction team or program.

Nutritional status assessment includes laboratory studies, evaluation of weight and weight change, ability of the client to consume an adequate diet, and the need for vitamin, mineral, or protein supplementation. Nutrition is considered inadequate when the client's serum albumin level is lower than 3.5 mg/dL or the lymphocyte count is less than 1800/mm^3. Other indicators of inadequate nutrition include a weight loss of 15% of total body weight or greater.

A positive nitrogen balance requires an intake of 30 to 35 calories/kg of body weight per day with a protein intake of 1.25 to 1.5 g/kg/day. Up to 2 g/kg/day of protein may be required when nutritional deficits are severe or protein loss is ongoing. Vitamin supplementation is individualized according to the client's nutritional status.

INCONTINENCE. Incontinence results in prolonged contact of the skin with such substances as urea, bacteria, yeast, and enzymes carried in urine and feces. These substances are irritants and lead to skin breakdown. The excessive moisture associated with incontinence macerates intact skin, increasing the risk for breakdown. Daily inspection of the skin for any areas of redness or skin breakdown is a major part of pressure ulcer prevention. Maintenance of clean, intact skin also assists in the prevention process. The skin should be washed with a pH-balanced soap to maintain the normal acid level. Creams or lotions are used to lubricate and moisturize the skin. Barrier ointment protection is needed

EVIDENCE-BASED PRACTICE FOR NURSING

Assess and reassess for accurate predictability

Bergstrom, N., et al. (1998). Predicting pressure ulcer risk. *Nursing Research, 47*(5), 261-269.

This prospective, investigator-controlled/coordinated study of 843 randomly selected subjects conducted at multiple sites sought to test the Braden Scale for predictive validity and established cutoff points in assessing pressure ulcer risk. Sites of the study included two tertiary care hospitals, two Veterans Administration Medical Centers, and two skilled nursing facilities. Subjects ranged in age from 19 to 102 years, with a mean age of 63 years. Research staff were trained in scoring the Braden Scale, staging ulcers, and recording data on the skin assessment tool. Videotapes were used in initial and refresher training. The inter-rater reliability was established at .95 and maintained throughout the study. The Braden Scale has six subscale items for rating with a possible score ranging from 6 to 23 points. The critical cutoff point in previous studies was established at 16. Subjects were assessed on admission and every 48 to 72 hours until discharge for a maximum of 4 weeks.

None of the subjects had observable pressure ulcers on admission. One hundred eight subjects (12.8%) developed one or more pressure ulcers during their stay at the facility. The critical cutoff score in this study was higher than that of previous studies: 18 rather than 16. The Braden Scale was determined to be predictive on admission but even more predictive for the assessments completed at 48 to 72 hours after admission. The subjects who developed pressure ulcers had a mean age 10 years greater than those who did not develop pressure ulcers. Women were more likely to develop pressure ulcers than men.

Critique. This clinical study was well designed and well controlled. The methods of study were appropriate for the questions asked.

Implications for Nursing. The Braden Scale has demonstrated reliability, validity, sensitivity, and specificity in predicting pressure ulcer risk. The study underscores the importance of risk reassessment beyond admission, when client conditions can change and risk increases. This scale should be used for ongoing evaluation of pressure ulcer risk throughout the client's stay in the facility.

COST OF CARE IMPLICATIONS FOR NURSING

PRESSURE ULCER PREVENTION

Cost of Care
- Medicare reimbursement for medically complex residents of long-term care decreased from an average of $408 to $231 per day, beginning in 1997.
- Most residents with complex wounds and stage III or IV pressure ulcers fall into the category of medically complex.
- Pressure relief/reduction devices and appropriate dressing materials cost more than the available reimbursement.
- Many long-term care facilities made product choices based on cost alone.
- Use of pressure relief/reduction devices for prevention of pressure ulcers was limited.
- The number and severity of pressure ulcers among residents of long-term care facilities increased during this budget reduction period.

Implications for Nursing
An ounce of prevention may be worth tons rather than pounds of cure. Although on the surface, pressure relief/reduction devices, high-protein diets, and appropriate dressing materials appear expensive, the actual cost in nursing hours, equipment, devices, and consumable supplies when caring for a client with even one pressure ulcer is far greater. New legislation, signed in late 1999, will allow prevention costs, as well as care costs, to be justly reimbursed. Nurses need to consider pressure ulcer prevention in the care setting as a number one priority of care.

Data from Motta, G. (2000). Reimbursement relief. *Continuing Care, 19*(4), 14-16.

Client's name _____ Evaluator's name _____ Date of assessment

Category		1	2	3	4
Sensory perception Ability to respond meaningfully to pressure-related discomfort		**1. Completely limited** Unresponsive to painful stimuli (does not moan, flinch, or grasp) because of diminished level of consciousness or sedation OR limited ability to feel pain over most of body surface	**2. Very limited** Responds only to painful stimuli; cannot communicate discomfort except by moaning or restlessness OR has a sensory impairment that limits the ability to feel pain or discomfort over half of the body	**3. Slightly limited** Responds to verbal commands but cannot always communicate discomfort or need to be turned OR has some sensory impairment that limits ability to feel pain or discomfort in one or two extremities	**4. No impairment** Responds to verbal commands; has no sensory deficit that would limit ability to feel or voice pain or discomfort
Moisture Degree to which skin is exposed to moisture		**1. Constantly moist** Skin is kept moist almost constantly by perspiration, urine; dampness is detected every time the client is moved or turned	**2. Very Moist** Skin is often but not always moist; linen must be changed at least once a shift	**3. Occasionally moist** Skin is occasionally moist, requiring an extra linen change approximately once a day	**4. Rarely moist** Skin is usually dry; linen requires changing only at routine intervals
Activity Degree of physical activity		**1. Bedfast** Confined to bed	**2. Chairfast** Ability to walk severely limited or nonexistent; cannot bear own weight and must be assisted into chair or wheelchair	**3. Walks occasionally** Walks occasionally during the day but for very short distances, with or without assistance; spends the majority of each shift in bed or chair	**4. Walks frequently** Walks outside the room at least twice a day and inside the room at least once every 2 hours during waking hours
Mobility Ability to change or control body position		**1. Completely immobile** Does not make even slight changes in body or extremity position without assistance	**2. Very limited** Makes occasional slight changes in body or extremity position but unable to make frequent or significant changes independently	**3. Slightly limited** Makes frequent though slight changes in body or extremity position independently	**4. No limitations** Makes major and frequent changes in position without assistance
Nutrition Usual food intake pattern		**1. Very poor** Never eats a complete meal; rarely eats more than a third of any food offered; eats two servings or less of protein (meat or dairy products) per day; takes fluids poorly; does not take a liquid dietary supplement OR is NPO or maintained on clear liquids or IV for more than 5 days	**2. Probably inadequate** Rarely eats a complete meal and generally eats only about half of any food offered; protein intake includes only three servings of meat or dairy products per day; occasionally will take a dietary supplement OR receives less than optimal amount of liquid diet or tube feeding	**3. Adequate** Eats over half of most meals; eats a total of four servings of protein (meat, dairy products) each day; occasionally will refuse a meal, but will usually take a supplement if offered OR is receiving tube feeding or total parenteral nutrition, which probably meets most nutritional needs	**4. Excellent** Eats most of every meal; never refuses a meal; usually eats a total of four or more servings of meat and dairy products; occasionally eats between meals; does not require supplementation
Friction and shear		**1. Problem** Requires moderate to maximum assistance in moving; complete lifting without sliding against sheets is impossible; frequently slides down in bed or chair, requiring frequent repositioning with maximum assistance; spasticity, contractures, or agitation leads to almost constant friction	**2. Potential problem** Moves feebly or requires minimum assistance during a move; skin probably slides to some extent against sheets, chair, restraints, or other devices; maintains relatively good position in chair or bed most of the time but occasionally slides down	**3. No apparent problem** Moves in bed and in chair independently and has sufficient muscle strength to lift up completely during move; maintains good position in bed or chair at all times	
					Total score

Scoring system: 15-16 = mild risk, 12-14 = moderate risk, <11 = severe risk

Figure 67-4 ● The Braden Scale for predicting pressure ulcer risk. (From Barbara Braden and Nancy Bergstrom. Copyright 1988. Reprinted with permission.)

whenever incontinence is present. Absorbent pads or garments must be changed quickly with each incontinence episode to avoid prolonged skin contact with urine and/or feces. Reddened areas are *never* massaged, since this action can damage capillary beds and increase tissue necrosis.

PRESSURE RELIEVING TECHNIQUES

The cornerstone in the prevention (and treatment) of pressure ulcers is the provision of adequate pressure relief. A consideration in pressure relief is the **capillary closing pressure,** the amount of pressure needed to occlude skin capillary blood flow, in the area at risk. The normal capillary closing pressure ranges from 12 to 32 mm Hg. Any device used must provide pressure relief below the capillary closing pressure in order to prevent tissue ischemia. *Most devices have a standardized guaranteed pressure relief reading; however, these readings do not ensure that capillary blood flow for any given client is adequate. Therefore the nurse must use observation of skin color, integrity, and temperature to determine capillary flow adequacy.*

Devices are categorized according to whether they relieve pressure or merely reduce pressure. In addition, devices are further categorized as dynamic or static. Dynamic systems alternate air inflation and deflation of the device through the use of electricity. Static devices, made of gel, water, foam, or air, are in a constant state of inflation that distributes the client pressure load over a larger area, thus reducing the pressure any one area experiences.

Pressure relief/reduction products come in many forms, such as specialty beds, mattress replacements, overlays, and assistive devices. Choosing the correct product is important in the success of the prevention or management plan. The product selected is re-evaluated daily for effectiveness in reducing pressure, comfort, and elimination of "bottoming out," wherein the client's bony prominences sink into the mattress or cushion, causing him or her to have pressure even with the product in place.

PRESSURE RELIEF DEVICES. Pressure relief devices consistently reduce pressure below capillary closing pressure. These devices are recommended for clients who:

* Need prevention of skin breakdown because they cannot turn
* Need prevention of extension of skin breakdown that has already occurred
* Need promotion of healing of breakdown present on several turning surfaces

PRESSURE REDUCTION DEVICES. Pressure reduction devices lower pressure below that provided by a standard hospital mattress or chair surface but do not consistently reduce pressure below the capillary closing pressure. Such devices must be used in conjunction with an individualized turning schedule.

POSITIONING. A good plan for positioning is the 30-degree rule. This rule involves ensuring that the client is positioned and propped so that whatever part of the body is elevated is tilted back at least 30 degrees to the mattress, rather than resting directly on a dependent bony prominence. This rule applies to side-lying, as well as head-of-bed elevation,

positions. The client who must be elevated to a full 90 degrees because of respiratory difficulties should be tilted forward even more than 90 degrees, with pillows behind the back to keep pressure off of the sacral/coccyx area.

The client at risk for pressure ulcer formation in bed is also at risk while sitting. Careful assessment for proper wheelchair or regular chair cushioning is essential for pressure ulcer prevention. Physical therapists and rehabilitation specialists may be consulted for selection of these products.

Even with an appropriate mattress or cushion, the client must change or be assisted in changing positions periodically. Many facilities require turning and positioning every 2 hours. *However, pressure can occur in less time, and the actual turning/repositioning schedule for each client should be individualized.*

Pillows and other positioning/padding devices are used to keep heels pressure free at all times for high-risk clients. Frequent assessment of heel positioning is needed to ensure that pressure is not redistributed to another high-risk area, such as the sides of the feet. Assessment is needed even more frequently when devices that hide the feet, such as boots, are used, especially if the client has a peripheral vascular problem.

► COLLABORATIVE MANAGEMENT
● Assessment
HISTORY

When taking a history from the client with a pressure ulcer, the nurse identifies the underlying cause of skin loss, as well as factors that may impair healing. The specific circumstances of the skin loss are investigated. In general, clients with chronic pressure ulcerations usually have a history of delayed healing or recurrence of the ulcer after healing has occurred. Because pressure-related skin loss is common among the severely debilitated, the nurse remains alert to the following contributing factors:

* Prolonged bedrest
* Immobility
* Incontinence
* Inadequate nutrition or hydration
* Altered mental status (decreased sensory perception)

PHYSICAL ASSESSMENT/CLINICAL MANIFESTATIONS

The nurse inspects the entire body, including the back of the head, for areas of skin injury or pressure. Special attention is given to bony prominences (such as the heels, sacrum, elbows, trochanter, and posterior and anterior iliac spines) and areas that are vulnerable to excessive moisture. In addition, the nurse assesses the client's general appearance for issues related to skin health. Such issues include body weight and the proportion of weight to height, because obese persons, as well as thin persons, are at increased risk for pressure ulcer formation. Overall cleanliness of the skin, hair, and nails is noted, as is any alteration in mobility or range of joint motion.

WOUND ASSESSMENT

The appearance of pressure ulcers changes with the depth of the injury. Chart 67-3 lists the characteristics of the four stages of pressure ulceration, and Figures 67-5 to 67-8 show examples.

Wounds are assessed for location, size, color, extent of tissue involvement, cell types in the wound base and margins, exudate, condition of surrounding tissue, and presence of foreign bodies. This initial assessment is documented to serve as a starting point for determining the nature of the intervention plan and its effectiveness. How often a wound is assessed is determined by the written policies and procedures at the facility or agency. Weekly documented assessment is the standard in many facilities. *However, the wound should be assessed at each dressing change, with the existing parameters compared with previous documentation to determine the current state of healing or deterioration.*

The location and size of the wound are the first two clinical parameters recorded. Wounds are sized by length, width, and depth, using millimeters or centimeters. In standardizing the wound size for documentation and communication purposes, the wound is assessed as a clock face with 12 o'clock in the direction of the client's head and 6 o'clock in the direction of the client's feet. The length is always measured from 12 o'clock to 6 o'clock, and the width is measured at 9 o'clock and 3 o'clock. The depth is the distance from the deepest portion of the wound base to skin level. When all caregivers use this format, measurement is accurate and wound progress can be determined.

The nurse inspects the wound margins for **cellulitis** (inflammation of the skin cells) extending beyond the area of injury. Progressive tissue destruction, as reflected by an increase in the size or depth of the ulcer and accompanied by increased wound drainage, usually indicates an impairment in the client's ability to resist infection if proper measures have been taken to relieve pressure.

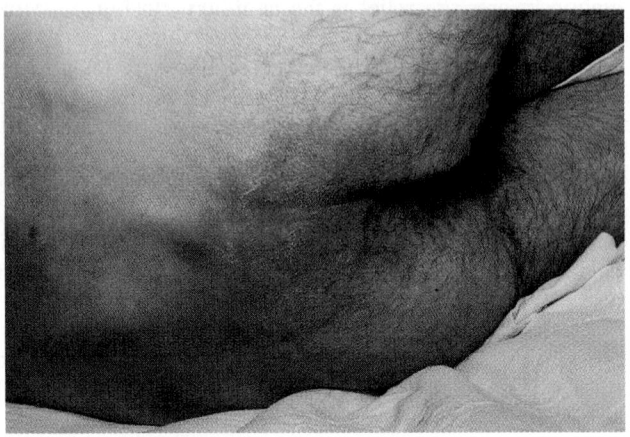

Figure 67-5 ● A stage I pressure ulcer.

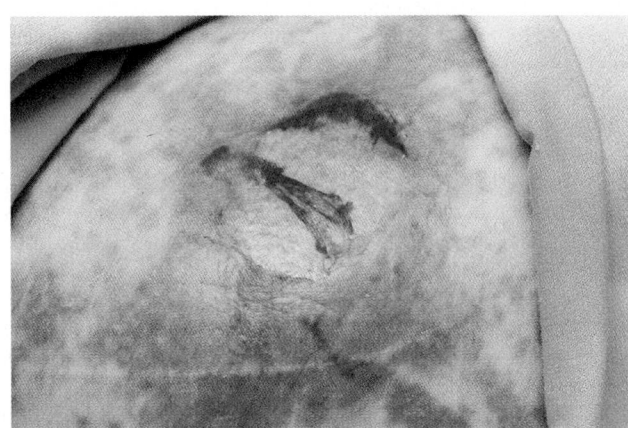

Figure 67-6 ● A stage II pressure ulcer.

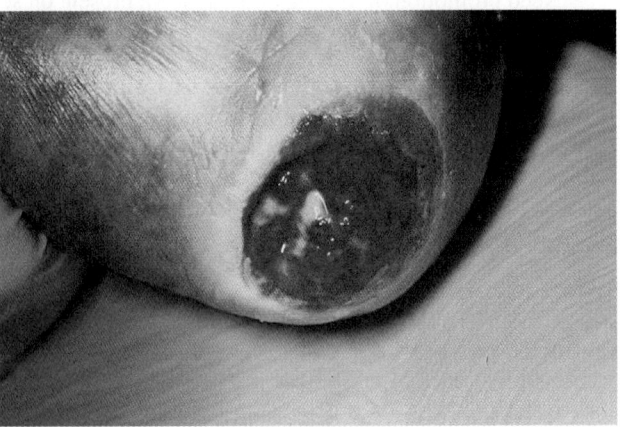

Figure 67-7 ● A stage III pressure ulcer.

CHART 67-3

KEY FEATURES *of*
Pressure Ulcers

Stage I
- Skin is intact.
- Area is red and does not blanch with external pressure.
- For clients with darker skin that does not blanch†:

Observable pressure-related alteration of intact skin—changes are compared with an adjacent or opposite area and include one or more of the following:
  - Skin temperature (warmth or coolness)
  - Tissue consistency (firm or boggy)
  - Sensation (pain, itching)

The ulcer appears as a defined area of persistent redness in lightly pigmented skin, whereas in darker skin tones, the ulcer may appear with persistent red, blue, or purple hues.

Stage II
- Skin is not intact.
- There is partial-thickness skin loss of the epidermis or dermis.
- Ulcer is superficial and may be characterized as an abrasion, a blister, or a shallow crater.

Stage III
- Skin loss is full thickness.
- Subcutaneous tissues may be damaged or necrotic.
- Damage extends down to but not through the underlying fascia.
- There is a deep crater-like appearance or eschar present.
- Undermining may or may not be present.

Stage IV
- Skin loss is full thickness with extensive destruction, tissue necrosis, or damage to muscle, bone, or supporting structures.
- Undermining is present.
- Sinus tracts may develop.

Data from U.S. Department of Health and Human Services. (1992). *Pressure ulcers in adults: Prediction and prevention, Clinical Practice Guideline, No. 3.* Rockville, MD: Agency for Health Care Policy and Research, Public Health Service, U.S. Department of Health and Human Services.
†Data from Henderson, C., et al. (1997). Draft definition of stage I pressure ulcers: Inclusion of persons with darkly pigmented skin. *Advances in Wound Care, 10*(5), 16-19.

The nurse inspects the wound for the presence or absence of necrotic tissue. Because of the depth of tissue destruction, a full-thickness pressure ulcer is initially covered by a layer of black, gray, or brown, nonviable, denatured collagen called wound **eschar.**

In the early stages of wound healing, the eschar is dry, leathery, and firmly attached to the wound surface. As the inflammatory phase of wound healing begins and removal of wound debris progresses, the eschar starts to lift up and separate from the tissue beneath. When disrupted, this nonviable eschar is an excellent breeding ground for bacteria normally found on the skin surface, as well as those inadvertently introduced by other means. As bacteria increase in number, they release enzymes, which increase the liquefaction of necrotic tissue. This tissue becomes softer and more yellow. In the presence of bacterial colonization, wound exudate increases substantially; the color and odor of wound exudate indicate the predominant microorganism present. The characteristics of wound exudate are presented in Table 67-4.

Beneath the separating dead tissue, granulation tissue appears. Early granulation is pale pink, progressing to a beefy red color as it grows and fills the wound. A wound with poor local arterial blood supply appears dry, with pale immature granulation tissue present. Venous obstruction causes an excessively moist ulcer surface with a deep red color (reflective of the deoxygenated blood beneath the ulcer surface).

The nurse palpates the ulcerated area or wound to determine the texture of the granulations. Healthy granulations have a slightly spongy texture. Pressure ulcers may involve more extensive tissue destruction than is first evident on inspection. Separation of the skin layers at the wound margins from the underlying granulation tissue is known as **undermining.** The nurse inspects undermined areas for gradual filling with healthy granulations and for wound healing progress. The nurse palpates the bony prominences for deep hardening of the surrounding soft tissue, which often suggests tissue ischemia well beneath the surface of the skin.

After ischemia has occurred, continued pressure over the area of injury results in the progression of tissue destruction from the deep tissue layers toward the surface. This "hidden" wound may first appear as a small opening in the skin through which purulent drainage exudes. If such an opening is observed, the nurse uses a cotton-tipped applicator to probe gently for a much larger pocket of necrotic tissue beneath the opening.

▪ PSYCHOSOCIAL ASSESSMENT

The client with one or more pressure ulcers may have an altered body image. Ineffective coping patterns emerge as the client and family or significant others strive to comply with changes in lifestyle that are necessary to facilitate healing. In addition, chronic, slow-healing ulcers are often painful and costly to treat.

The nurse assesses the client's and family's or significant others' knowledge of the treatment goals at each stage of the healing process, as well as compliance with the prescribed treatment regimen. The client's skills in cleaning the wound and applying a dressing are assessed as well. Noncompliance with pressure ulcer care procedures may reflect an inability to accept the diagnosis or to cope with the pain, cost, or potential scarring associated with prolonged healing. Depending on his or her activity level and the location of the ulcer, the client may need the assistance of a family member or home care nurse to care adequately for the pressure ulcer at home.

The nurse explores with the client specific changes in activities of daily living (ADLs) that are needed to relieve pressure and promote healing. Increased activity is promoted whenever possible to enhance circulation to the affected tissue. Frequent bedrest with elevation of the legs may be necessary for healing when ulcers occur on the lower legs, particularly in the client with venous insufficiency and lower leg edema. When the client is bedridden, frequent repositioning to relieve pressure (every 2 hours in bed; every 1 hour in a chair) can be labor intensive. In the home environment, repositioning, incontinence management, and dressing changes are often required around the clock, disrupting family routines and contributing to stress.

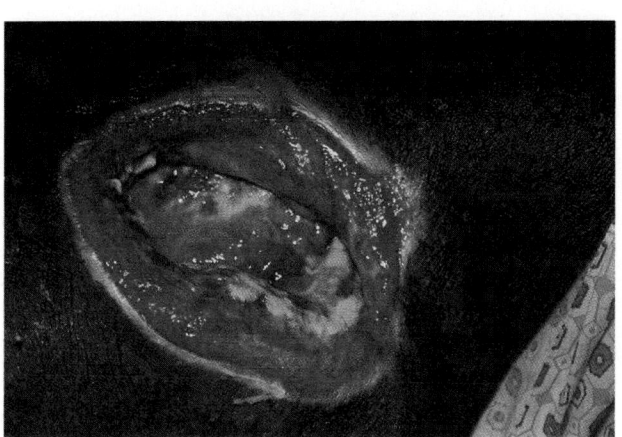

Figure 67-8 ● A stage IV pressure ulcer.

TABLE 67-4 • TYPES OF WOUND EXUDATE	
Characteristics	**Significance**
SEROSANGUINEOUS EXUDATE	
Blood-tinged amber fluid consisting of serum and red blood cells	Normal for first 48 hr after injury
	Sudden increase in amount precedes wound dehiscence in wounds closed by first intention
PURULENT EXUDATE	
Creamy yellow pus	Colonization with *Staphylococcus*
Greenish-blue pus, causing staining of dressings and accompanied by a "fruity" odor	Colonization with *Pseudomonas*
Beige pus with a "fishy" odor	Colonization with *Proteus*
Brownish pus with a "fecal" odor	Colonization with aerobic coliform and *Bacteroides* (usually occurs after intestinal surgery)

▓ LABORATORY ASSESSMENT

A wound that is exposed is always *contaminated* but not always *infected.* **Contamination** is the presence of microorganisms without any clinical manifestation of infection. The normal body immune defenses keep the number of bacteria to a minimum and prevent infection. **Wound infection** is contamination with pathogenic microorganisms to the degree that growth and spread cannot be controlled by the body's immune defenses. Wounds that exhibit inflammation, induration, odor, erythema, and moderate to heavy exudate should be evaluated by culture and sensitivity studies for infection to identify the causative microorganism. The presence of pus as exudate alone does not indicate an infection, since pus formation occurs when necrotic tissue debrides and liquifies through autolysis.

If wounds are extensive, if the client is severely immunocompromised, or if local blood supply to the wound is impaired, bacterial growth may exceed the body's ability to defend against invasion into deeper tissue layers. The result is deep wound infection and, eventually, bacteremia and sepsis (systemic infection).

Swab cultures are helpful only in identifying the types of bacteria present on the ulcer surface and may be misleading when trying to identify or quantify bacteria in the underlying tissues. Tests such as quantitative wound biopsies allow the numbers of bacteria to be analyzed. Unfortunately, these tests are time consuming, costly, and unavailable in many medical laboratories. Therefore the clinical indicators of infection—cellulitis, progressive increase in ulcer size or depth, changes in the quantity and quality of exudate, and systemic signs of bacteremia—are important criteria in the diagnosis and subsequent treatment of an infection.

▓ OTHER DIAGNOSTIC ASSESSMENT

Any additional laboratory studies are performed on the basis of the suspected cause of the wound. For pressure ulcers to show progress toward healing, the underlying factors contributing to delayed healing must be diagnosed and treated. For example, noninvasive and invasive arterial blood flow studies are indicated if arterial occlusion is suspected in delayed healing of a pressure ulcer on the heel or ankle. Similarly, blood tests to establish specific nutritional deficiencies are helpful in treating the debilitated, malnourished client with a pressure ulcer.

> ◎ **CRITICAL THINKING CHALLENGE**
> The client is a 78-year-old woman admitted preoperatively for a total right hip replacement. She has been donating her own blood for several weeks before the surgery to reduce the need for an unknown donor blood transfusion. This woman is 5 feet tall and weighs 98 pounds. She has some degenerative joint disease in her left hip as well.
> - What risk factors does this client have for pressure ulcer development?
> - What additional assessment data should you obtain?
> - What (if any) preoperative interventions could be made to reduce her risk for pressure ulcer formation?

For suggested answer guidelines, go to [SIMON] http://www.wbsaunders.com/SIMON/Iggy/.

● Analysis

▓ COMMON NURSING DIAGNOSES AND COLLABORATIVE PROBLEMS

The most common nursing diagnosis for clients with pressure ulcers is Impaired Skin Integrity related to vascular insufficiency and traumatic circumstances. The most common collaborative problem is Risk for Infection and Wound Extension related to disruption of the skin's protective barrier and impaired local blood supply.

▓ ADDITIONAL NURSING DIAGNOSES AND COLLABORATIVE PROBLEMS

In addition to the common nursing diagnoses and collaborative problems, clients with pressure ulcers may have one or more of the following:
- Acute Pain or Chronic Pain related to skin trauma, wound infection, and wound treatment
- Disturbed Body Image related to loss of skin and altered appearance
- Ineffective Coping related to the chronicity of the ulcer, alteration in body image, and changes in lifestyle required to promote healing
- Imbalanced Nutrition: Less Than Body Requirements related to inadequate intake of calories, protein, vitamins, and minerals
- Ineffective (Peripheral) Tissue Perfusion related to vascular disease and prolonged alterations in fluid volume
- Deficient Knowledge related to lack of information about or unclear explanation of the treatment regimen

● Planning and Implementation

▓ IMPAIRED SKIN INTEGRITY

[NOC] **PLANNING: EXPECTED OUTCOMES.** The client with a pressure ulcer is expected to (1) protect the viable cells on the wound surface until healing is completed; (2) experience complete ulcer healing by second intention as evidenced by granulation, epithelialization, and resolution of wound size; (3) have skin thickness in the expected range in the pressure ulcer area; and (4) not experience the formation of other pressure ulcers.

INTERVENTIONS. Wound care techniques for pressure ulcers vary according to each client's needs and the physician's preference. Although aggressive removal of necrotic tissue by surgical excision may be indicated in a severely immunosuppressed client who is susceptible to a life-threatening wound infection, a nonsurgical approach to ulcer debridement is preferred for an older client who has adequate host defenses but is too ill or debilitated to undergo surgery.

NONSURGICAL MANAGEMENT. NIC interventions for pressure ulcer prevention and management are listed in Chart 67-2. Nonsurgical intervention of pressure ulcers is often left to the discretion of the nurse, who collaborates with the physician to select a method of wound dressing on the basis of the identified goal of wound management.

DRESSINGS. A properly designed dressing can expedite healing by removing unwanted debris from the ulcer surface, protecting exposed viable tissues, and re-establishing a temporary barrier between the body and the environment until ulcer closure is complete. For a client with a draining, necrotic ulcer, the dressing must be designed to remove excessive exudate and loose debris without damaging migrating epithelial cells or newly formed granulation tissue. If necrosis is extensive and the eschar is thick, nonviable (dead) tissue must be surgically or chemically removed before further debridement with dressings will be effective. Depending on the dressing material used, dressings help to remove debris either through mechanical entrapment and detachment of dead tissue or by creating an environment that promotes self-digestion of necrotic material by the bacterial enzymes (Table 67-5).

After all of the nonviable tissue has been removed, protection of any exposed vital structures, such as tendon, bone, and newly formed collagen, becomes a primary objective of pressure ulcer care. The ideal environment for healing by epithelialization and contraction is a clean, *slightly* moist ulcer surface with minimal bacterial colonization. Heavy moisture from an excessively secreting ulcer or a dressing that is too wet can interfere with healing by promoting the growth of microorganisms and causing maceration of healthy tissue. Likewise, if a clean ulcer surface is exposed to air or if highly absorbent dressing materials are used for prolonged periods, the subsequent drying effect can lead to dehydration of viable surface cells, scab formation, or conversion to a deeper injury.

The nurse assesses the ulcer for the presence or absence of nonviable tissue and the quantity of exudate. A dressing material with properties that promote an optimal environment for healing is selected (Table 67-6). For example, a material that does not stick to the wound surface and does not remove fragile epithelial cells when it is changed is the dressing of choice for protecting new tissue. Depending on the amount of drainage, the nurse selects either a hydrophobic or a hydrophilic material:

- A **hydrophobic** (nonabsorbent, waterproof) material is beneficial when the wound is relatively free of drainage and the objective is to protect the ulcer from external contamination, such as urine or feces.
- A **hydrophilic** (absorbent) material draws excessive drainage away from the ulcer surface, preventing maceration.

A variety of synthetic materials with hydrophilic and hydrophobic properties are available. Unlike cotton gauze dressings, these may be left intact for extended periods. Some biologic skin substitutes can also prevent tissue dehydration and promote healing (see Chapter 68). These substances include **homograft** (human cadaver skin), **heterograft** (pigskin), collagen material, amniotic membrane, and cultured human skin cells (epithelium).

The frequency of dressing changes depends on the amount of necrotic material or exudate. Dry gauze dressings are changed when "strike through" occurs or when the outer layer of the dressing first becomes saturated with exudate. Gauze dressings used for debridement, such as those placed on a wound wet, allowed to dry, and then removed, are changed frequently enough to take off any loose debris or exudate, usually every 4 to 6 hours. Synthetic dressings are changed when accumulation of exudate causes the adhesive seal to break and leakage to occur.

Before reapplying any dressing, the nurse gently cleans the ulcer surface with saline or a nontoxic wound cleanser as prescribed. If an antibacterial cleanser is ordered, the nurse dilutes the agent to minimize tissue toxicity and then rinses and dries the surface thoroughly before applying the dressing.

PHYSICAL THERAPY. As an adjunct to the use of dressings for ulcer debridement, the use of daily whirlpool treatments can facilitate mechanical removal of dead tissue. The ulcerated area is immersed in warm tap water to which an antibacterial cleansing agent has been added. Continuous agitation of the water mechanically loosens the debris and washes away exudate and particulate matter. During treatment, the ulcer surface is cleaned with a gauze pad. After treatment, the therapist or certified wound specialists often uses instruments to trim away any obvious bits of dead tissue that are still loosely attached to the ulcer surface.

DRUG THERAPY. Clean, healthy granulation tissue is vascular and capable of providing white blood cells and antibodies to the ulcer surface to combat infection. However, if extensive necrosis is present or local tissue defenses are impaired, topical antibacterial agents are often needed to control bacterial growth. (Chapter 68 details the advantages and uses of topical antimicrobial agents.) In the absence of established ulcer infection, prophylactic antibiotics are usually avoided because of the danger of the development of resistant strains of bacteria.

DIET THERAPY. Successful healing of pressure ulcers depends on adequate nutritional stores of calories, protein, vitamins, minerals, and water. Nutritional deficiencies are common among older adults and chronically ill clients. Such deficiencies contribute to an increased risk of skin breakdown

---

TABLE 67-5 • COMMON DRESSING TECHNIQUES FOR WOUND DEBRIDEMENT

Technique	Mechanism of Action
Wet-to-dry saline-moistened gauze	Dry, necrotic debris is softened by the saline, allowing it to become more effectively entrapped in the interstices as the gauze dries and shrinks. Dressing may also entrap healing tissue.
Wet-to-damp saline-moistened gauze	As with the wet-to-dry technique, necrotic debris is mechanically removed, but with less trauma to healing tissue.
Continuous wet gauze	The wound surface is continually bathed with a wetting agent of choice, promoting dilution of viscous exudate and softening of dry eschar.
Topical enzyme preparations	Proteolytic action on thick, adherent eschar causes breakdown of denatured protein and more rapid separation of necrotic tissue.
Moisture-retentive dressing	Spontaneous separation of necrotic tissue is promoted by autolysis.

TABLE 67-6 • COMMONLY USED DRESSING MATERIALS

	Alginates	Biologic Dressings	Cotton Gauze Dressing	Foams	Hydrocolloidal Wafers	Hydrogel Dressing	Transparent Films
Indications	Absorption Protection	Debridement after eschar removal* Protection Test before skin grafts (pigskin and cadaver skin) Burns Dormant, nonhealing wounds that do not respond to other topical therapies	*Continuous Dry* Absorption Protection (nonadherent contact layer) *Continuous Wet* Delivery of topical agent Debridement (autolysis) Protection *Wet to Damp* Atraumatic mechanical debridement *Wet to Dry* Aggressive mechanical debridement	Absorption Protection	Debridement* Absorption Protection	Debridement* Absorption Protection	Debridement* Protection (partial-thickness lesions) Secondary (cover) dressing
Advantages	Highly absorbent Biodegradable Easy application Nonadhesive Can be used as packing for deep wounds Can be used for infected wounds	Most "natural" wound covering Reduces pain Conforms to uneven wound surfaces Acts as a catalyst for healing Alternative to autograft	Readily available Good mechanical debridement *if used properly* Effective delivery of topical agents	Absorbent Insulates wound Easy application Nonadhesive (most products) Conforms to uneven wound surfaces	Absorbent Excludes bacteria Waterproof Reduces pain Easy application Easy to store	Absorbent Nonadhesive Reduces pain Conducive to use with topical agents Conforms to uneven wound surfaces Amorphous form can be used as a filler Easy to store	Wound visualization Good adhesion Waterproof Reduces pain Cost-effective Easy to store
Disadvantages	Requires secondary dressing to secure Can cause desiccation of tissue if drainage is minimal	Requires secondary dressing to secure Very expensive Skin substitutes require skill to apply	Delayed healing if used improperly Pain on removal Requires frequent dressing changes	Poor barrier function Requires secondary dressing to secure	Nontransparent Softening and loss of shape with pressure, heat, and friction Odor with dressing removal Expensive Requires use of "fillers" for deep, draining lesions	Poor barrier function Only partial wound visualization Requires secondary dressing to secure Can promote growth of *Pseudomonas* and other microorganisms	Difficult to apply properly Nonabsorbent Adhesive to normal and healing tissue Limited to superficial lesions
Dressing changes	When dressing is saturated (q3-5 days) or more frequently	Topical growth factors: Daily skin substitutes: Varies (similar to grafts)	Necrotic base: q4-6h Clean base: q12-24h	When dressing is saturated or more frequently	Necrotic base: q24h Clean base: on leakage of exudate	Necrotic base: q6-8h Clean base: q24h	Necrotic base: q24h Clean base: on leakage of exudate

*Use with caution in patients with leukopenia or vascular disease.

and delayed healing of wounds already present (see Nutritional Status, p. 1521). Severe protein deficiency inhibits all stages of the healing process and impairs local host defenses against bacterial invasion.

To promote healing, the nurse encourages the client to eat a well-balanced diet, emphasizing foods containing nutrients vital to epidermal proliferation and collagen synthesis (Table 67-7). If the client cannot eat sufficient amounts of food, na-sogastric feedings and hyperalimentation via a central venous catheter may be needed to increase protein and caloric intake. Vitamin and mineral supplements also are indicated.

SURGICAL MANAGEMENT. Surgical management of a pressure ulcer includes sharp debridement of nonviable tissue and skin grafting to re-establish skin integrity in wounds that cannot heal by epithelialization and contraction.

TABLE 67-7 • FOODS THAT PROMOTE WOUND HEALING

Food	Function	Food	Function
PROTEIN SOURCES Meat Fish Poultry Milk Cheese Eggs Soybeans Legumes Nuts Nutritional supplements	Maintenance and healing of body tissues Antibody production Energy	**IRON SOURCES*—cont'd** Eggs Dark green leafy vegetables Blackstrap molasses Whole-grain breads and cereals **SOURCES OF VITAMIN B$_{12}$** Liver Organ meats Muscle meats Fish Eggs Shellfish Milk Yogurt Cheese	Protein synthesis
CARBOHYDRATE SOURCES Whole grains (preferable to enriched because of higher nutritional and fiber content) Enriched grain and cereal products Fruit Juices Vegetables (especially starchy ones: corn, peas, potatoes) Milk Desserts and sweets	Energy Sparing of protein (if diet does not contain sufficient nonprotein calories, protein from body tissues will be broken down to supply energy) Wound healing	**SOURCES OF VITAMIN B$_6$** Meats Liver Some vegetables (including potatoes) Wheat germ Wheat bran Whole-grain cereals and breads Fish Brewer's yeast Dried beans	Amino acid metabolism
SOURCES OF VITAMIN C Berries Broccoli Brussels sprouts Cabbage Citrus fruits and juices Green peppers Kale Melons Spinach and dark green vegetables Tomatoes Vitamin C–enriched juices	Collagen synthesis Immunity	**FOLATE SOURCES** Liver Yeast Leafy vegetables Dried beans Green vegetables Nuts Fresh oranges Whole-wheat cereals and breads	Protein synthesis
ZINC SOURCES Same as protein sources Beef Organ meat Shellfish Salmon Poultry Cheese Whole grains Dried beans	Tissue repair (zinc-deficient diet causes poor wound healing, decreased ability to taste, and poor appetite) Protein synthesis	**WATER SOURCES** Water Milk Juices Gelatin Tomatoes Citrus fruit Melons Vegetables Berries Broths Soups Tea Coffee Carbonated beverages	Maintain condition of the skin (dehydration can lead to tissue breakdown, poor appetite, and constipation)
IRON SOURCES* Liver Meat Baked beans Dried fruits Legumes	Cellular respiration Hemoglobin synthesis		

From Ross, R., & Noe, J. (1983). *Chronic problem wounds*. Boston: Little, Brown & Co.
*Iron cooking utensils add iron to the diet.

PREOPERATIVE CARE. Preoperative care is focused on preparing the ulcer to accept a skin graft. The nurse monitors potential donor sites, taking care to maintain the integrity of the donor skin and to avoid minor injuries that may result in infection and graft loss.

OPERATIVE PROCEDURES. The operative procedures commonly used for surgical management of pressure ulcers include debridement and grafting. One or both of these procedures may be done.

Debridement, or sharp excision of thick, adherent wound eschar using a scalpel or scissors, is sometimes undertaken to hasten the removal of the dead tissue, a potential source of infection. Surgical debridement is indicated for severely immunosuppressed clients or those with large, full-thickness ulcers, because the extensive time required for spontaneous separation of eschar places the client at risk for systemic sepsis or prolonged hospitalization. Depending on the size and depth of the ulcer and the projected blood loss, the surgeon can perform the excision at the bedside, in the treatment room, or in an operating room.

Grafting or autografting is used for wound closure when full-thickness ulcers cannot close by second intention because of the extent of the injury or forces inhibiting contraction and when natural healing results in loss of joint function, an unacceptable cosmetic appearance, or a high potential for wound recurrence. Successful grafting of skin requires a clean and granulating or freshly excised ulcer bed. Partial-thickness (split-thickness) or full-thickness strips of skin are removed from the donor area (Figure 67-9), transferred to the ulcer, and sutured or stapled in place. Full-thickness free grafts and myocutaneous flaps are used to cover deep, massive ulcers or ulcers in which vital structures, such as bone or tendon, are exposed.

Unlike free grafts, a pedicle flap is a full-thickness flap of skin that is raised and rotated to cover the defect, with one edge of the flap still attached to the site of origin to provide a blood supply (Figure 67-10). Because all skin layers are removed, full-thickness donor sites are closed primarily or covered with additional split-thickness skin grafts. Partial-thickness donor sites heal by epithelialization if infection is avoided.

POSTOPERATIVE CARE. Postoperative graft sites are immobilized with bulky cotton pressure dressings for 3 to 5 days to allow vascularization, or "take," of the newly grafted skin. The nurse does not disturb the dressing and encourages elevation and complete rest of the grafted area. Any activity that might cause movement of the dressing against the body and separation of the graft from the wound is prohibited.

After dressings are removed, the nurse monitors the graft for indications of failure to vascularize—nonadherence to the wound or graft necrosis. If a pedicle flap has been used to cover the wound, the nurse inspects the edges of the flap frequently for changes in color. A pale flap with delayed capillary filling when blanched may have inadequate arterial perfusion. A dusky color or sharp line of color demarcation suggests inadequate venous or lymphatic drainage. Other techniques to monitor trends of blood flow in the graft, depending on the graft's location, include pulse oximetry, Doppler ultrasonography, and transcutaneous oxygen determination.

Postoperative care of donor sites aims to protect the area from injury and infection until healing can occur and to promote comfort. The client usually returns from surgery with a pressure dressing in place over the donor area to promote hemostasis. After 24 to 48 hours, this outer dressing is removed, revealing a single wound contact layer of fine-mesh gauze or synthetic mesh material.

If the donor site is treated with dry exposure, the nurse promotes air circulation to the wound by positioning the client to avoid pressure on the site and using an overbed cradle to tent the sheets. In the rare instance when heat lamps are ordered, the nurse places the 60- to 100-watt bulb at least 2 feet from the wound to prevent thermal injury to the skin. After the dressing has dried and formed a "scab," the wound is kept dry and left undisturbed until healing is evident (at 10 to 14 days). As the donor site heals, the gauze and dried blood lift away from the new epithelium beneath. Trimming the separating gauze close to the skin surface minimizes the chance of the client's catching the loose end of the dressing on an object and removing the still adherent gauze before healing is complete. Today, most surgeons prefer to dress donor sites with moisture-retentive dressings, such as synthetic transparent films, instead of the traditional dry exposure method of treatment (see Table 67-6).

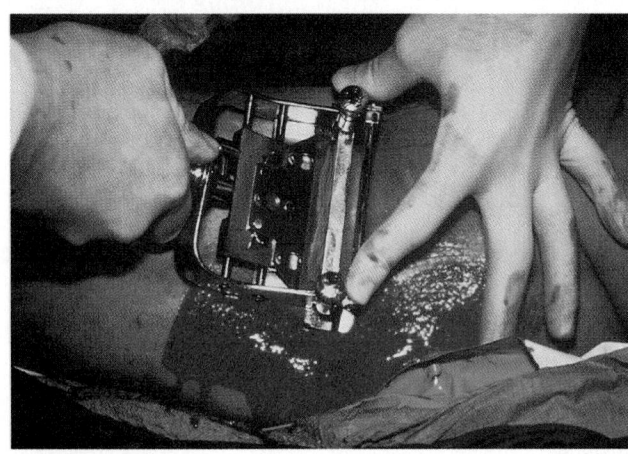

Figure 67-9   ● Removal of a partial-thickness (split-thickness) skin graft.

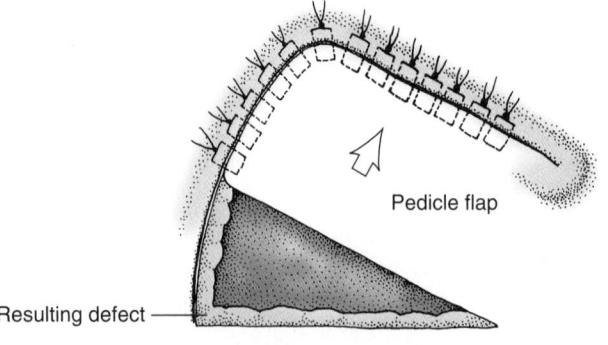

Pedicle flap

Resulting defect

Figure 67-10   ● A full-thickness pedicle flap of skin is separated and rotated to cover the wound. Blood vessels are left intact. The resultant defect is either primarily closed or covered with skin grafts. The flap is held in place with staples or sutures.

Because exposed donor sites are initially more painful than graft sites, pain medication is administered as ordered and other comfort measures are provided as needed. The client is repositioned during the immediate postoperative period to promote comfort only if movement of the graft site can be avoided. The nurse may offer back rubs to help relieve muscle spasms that occur with bedrest and immobility. Attention must also be paid to relieving pressure over unaffected bony prominences that may lead to additional ulcers.

Graft and donor sites involving the posterior body surfaces present a particular problem. For the graft or flap to become fully vascularized or for the donor sites to dry, the client must be immobilized in a side-lying or prone position for 7 to 10 days.

An alternative to difficult positioning is the use of special low-pressure or air-fluidized beds, which not only minimize ischemia of the graft or flap while the client is supine but also help prevent breakdown of intact skin. A major limitation to the use of these beds is cost, which is usually outweighed by the potential for decreased morbidity and length of hospital stay.

RISK FOR INFECTION AND WOUND EXTENSION

PLANNING: EXPECTED OUTCOMES. The client with a pressure ulcer is expected to remain free of wound infection or systemic sepsis and to experience healing of the pressure ulcer.

INTERVENTIONS. Because of the many intrinsic factors that can affect a client's resistance to infection, the nurse closely monitors the ulcer's progress so that timely treatment with topical and systemic antibiotics can be initiated if ulcer deterioration occurs. Steps are taken to minimize introduction of pathogenic organisms to the ulcer through direct contact.

MONITORING ULCER PROGRESS. Frequent monitoring of the ulcer's appearance using objective criteria allows the nurse to evaluate response to treatment and recognize early signs of impending infection. If an ulcer shows no progress toward healing within 3 weeks, the treatment plan should be re-evaluated. Table 67-8 outlines objectives of local infection for wounds with and without tissue loss. Clients who are at highest risk for infection may have a reduced inflammatory response to infection. These clients include those who are older, have white blood cell disorders, are receiving steroid therapy, or have wounds with a compromised blood supply.

PREVENTION OF INFECTION AND WOUND EXTENSION. Complications of infection and wound extension are avoided by diligent monitoring of the ulcer's progress and by prevention of new ulcer formation. The nurse reports the following signs to the physician:

- Sudden deterioration of the ulcer, as evidenced by an increase in the size or depth of the lesion
- Changes in the color or texture of the granulation tissue
- Changes in the quantity, color, or odor of exudate

The nurse also remains alert for the classic signs of wound infection: increased erythema, edema, purulent and malodorous drainage, and tenderness of the wound margins, which

may or may not be accompanied by clinical signs of bacteremia, such as fever, an elevated white blood cell count, and positive blood cultures. The nurse uses appropriate interventions to prevent the formation of new pressure ulcers and to prevent early-stage ulcers from progressing to deeper wounds (Chart 67-4; see also Chart 67-2).

MAINTAINING A SAFE ENVIRONMENT. Because of the variety of microorganisms in the hospital environment, keeping an ulcer totally free of bacteria is impossible. Optimal ulcer management is based on maintaining acceptably low levels of microorganisms through meticulous local wound care and minimizing contamination with pathogenic organisms. The nurse and assistive nursing personnel use standard precautions to prevent direct contact with ulcer secretions and cross-contamination among clients. All health care providers and assistive nursing personnel practice thorough handwashing before and after dressing changes and properly dispose of soiled dressings and linens.

● Community-Based Care

Clients with pressure ulcers may be in acute care, subacute care, long-term care, or home care settings. If pressure ulcer therapy requires hospitalization, most clients with pressure ulcers are discharged before complete wound closure is obtained. Discharge may be to the home setting or to a long-term care facility, depending on the degree of debilitation and other client factors.

HEALTH TEACHING

Before the client is discharged, the client or family member or significant other who will be performing the wound care should demonstrate facility in removing the dressing, cleaning the wound, and applying the dressing. When choosing a dressing to be used at home, the nurse considers the client's or caregiver's ability to apply the dressing properly. If the client's finances are limited, the nurse also addresses the cost of the dressing material. Some dressings may be easier to apply and less expensive than other materials. At times, the more expensive dressing materials that require less frequent changing may be preferred. The nurse explains the signs and symptoms of wound infection.

The nurse encourages the client to eat a balanced diet with frequent high-protein snacks. The nurse discusses diet preferences with the client and suggests foods that promote wound healing (see Table 67-7). The physician may order vitamin and mineral supplements if there are dietary deficiencies.

If the client is incontinent, the nurse emphasizes the need to keep the skin clean and dry. If bowel and bladder training is not possible, the use of absorbent underpads, briefs, and topical moisture barrier creams and ointments is discussed as a method to reduce skin exposure to urine and feces.

HOME CARE MANAGEMENT

Care of the ulcer in the client's home is similar to care in the hospital. Most dressing supplies and pressure relief devices can be easily obtained at the local pharmacy or medical supply store. If mechanical debridement of the ulcer is still needed, a handheld shower device or forceful irrigation of the

TABLE 67-8 • MONITORING THE WOUND

Variable	Frequency of Assessment	Rationale
WOUNDS WITHOUT TISSUE LOSS		
Examples		
Surgical incisions and clean lacerations closed primarily by sutures or staples		
Observations (Using First Postoperative Dressing Change as Baseline)		
Check for the presence or absence of increased: • Localized tenderness • Swelling of the incision line • Erythema of the incision line >1 cm on each side of wound • Localized heat	At least every 24 hr until sutures or staples are removed	To detect cellulitis (bacterial infections)*
Check for the presence or absence of: • Purulent drainage from any portion of the incision site • Localized fluctuance (from fluid accumulation) and tenderness beneath a *portion* of the wound when palpated	At least every 24 hr until sutures or staples are removed	To detect abscess formation related to presence of foreign body (suture material) or deeper wound infection*
Check for the presence or absence of approximation (sealing) of wound edges with or without serosanguineous drainage.	At least every 24 hr until sutures or staples are removed	To detect potential for wound dehiscence
WOUNDS WITH TISSUE LOSS		
Examples		
Partial- or full-thickness skin loss caused by pressure necrosis, vascular disease, trauma, etc., and allowed to heal by secondary intention		
Observations		
Wound Size		
Measure wound size at greatest length and width using a metric ruler or, for asymmetric ulcers, by tracing the wound onto a piece of plastic film or sheeting (plastic template). Compare all subsequent measurements against the initial measurement.	At least every week	To detect increase in wound size and depth secondary to infectious process
Ulcer Base		
Check for the presence or absence of: • Necrotic tissue (loose or adherent) • Presence or absence of foul odor from wound when dressing is changed Note the frequency of dressing changes or dressing reinforcements owing to drainage.	At least every 24 hr	To detect the need for debridement or the response to treatment (necrotic tissue) and to detect local wound infection (frequent dressing changes and foul odor)
Wound Margins		
Check for the presence or absence of: • Erythema and swelling extending outward >1 cm from wound margins • Increased tenderness at wound margins	At least every 24 hr or at each dressing change	To detect wound infection*
Systemic Response		
Check for the presence or absence of elevated body temperature, WBCs, or positive blood culture	As needed	To detect bacteremia

WBCs, White blood cells.
*The wounds of clients who are severely immunosuppressed or those wounds with compromised blood supply may not exhibit a typical inflammatory response to local wound infection.

wound with a 35-mL syringe and 19-gauge angiocatheter can be substituted for whirlpool therapy.

Clients with chronic pressure ulcers are often depressed about their debilitated state, which may affect their compliance with wound care measures. Many clients cannot change their own dressings because of distress over an altered body image or the pain experienced with dressing removal. Others are totally dependent on family members or significant others

or support personnel because of limited physical mobility or inability to reach the wound.

For some clients, drastic changes in daily activities are necessary to promote healing. Clients with pressure ulcers on the lower extremities may need frequent rest periods with leg elevation to minimize edema. Immobile clients with pressure ulcers require around-the-clock repositioning as often as every 2 to 4 hours to prevent further breakdown, which takes

CHART 67-4

BEST PRACTICE *for*
Preventing Pressure Ulcers

Positioning
- Pad contact surfaces with foam, silicon gel, or air pads.
- Do not keep the head of the bed elevated above 30 degrees.
- Use a lift sheet to move client in the bed. Avoid dragging or sliding the client.
- When positioning a client on his or her side, do not position directly on the trochanter.
- Reposition an immobile client every 2 hours while in bed and every 1 hour while sitting in a chair.
- Do not place a rubber ring or doughnut under the client's sacral area.
- When moving an immobile client from a bed to another surface, use a designated slide board well lubricated with talc.
- Place pillows or foam wedges between two bony surfaces.
- Keep the client's skin directly off plastic surfaces.
- Keep the client's heels off the bed surface.

Nutrition
- Ensure a fluid intake between 2000 and 3000 mL/day.
- Help the client maintain an adequate intake of protein and calories.

Skin Care
- Use moisturizers daily on dry skin, and apply when skin is damp.
- Keep moisture from prolonged contact with skin.
  - Dry areas where two skin surfaces touch, such as the axilla and under the breasts.
  - Place absorbent pads under areas where perspiration collects.
  - Use moisture barriers on skin areas where wound drainage or incontinence occurs.
- Do not massage bony prominences.
- Humidify the room.

Skin Cleaning
- Clean the skin as soon as possible after soiling occurs and at routine intervals.
- Use a mild, heavily fatted soap.
- Use tepid rather than hot water.
- While cleaning, use the minimal scrubbing force necessary to remove soil.
- Gently pat rather than rub the skin dry.

CHART 67-5

FOCUSED ASSESSMENT *of*
Home Care Clients at Risk for Pressure Ulcer

Assess cardiovascular status:
- Presence or absence of peripheral edema
- Hand vein filling in the dependent position
- Neck vein filling in the recumbent and sitting positions
- Weight gain or loss

Assess cognition and mental status:
- Level of consciousness
- Orientation to time, place, and person
- Can the client accurately read a seven-word sentence containing no words greater than three syllables?

Assess condition of skin:
- Assess general skin cleanliness.
- Observe all skin areas, paying particular attention to bony prominences and those areas in greatest contact with the bed and other firm surfaces.
- Measure and record any areas of redness or loss of integrity.
- If possible, photograph areas of concern.
- Note presence or absence of skin tenting over the sternum or the forehead.
- Note moistness of skin and mucous membranes.
- If wounds are present, remove dressings (noting condition of dressings), cleanse the wound, and compare with previous notations of wound condition.
  - Presence, amount, and nature of exudate
  - Use a ruler to measure wound diameter and depth
  - Amount (%) and type of necrotic tissue
  - Presence of granulation/epithelium
  - Presence or absence of cellulitis
  - Presence or absence of odor

Take client's temperature.

Assess client's understanding of illness and compliance with treatment:
- Signs and symptoms to report to health care provider
- Mediation plan (correct timing and dose)
- Ambulation or positioning schedule
- Dressing changes/skin care
- Diet modifications (24-hour diet recall)

Assess client's nutritional status:
- Change in muscle mass
- Lackluster nails, sparse hair
- Recent weight loss >10% of usual weight
- Impaired oral intake
- Difficulty swallowing
- Generalized edema

its toll on family members or caregivers. The nurse explains the rationale for activity changes to the client and family or significant others and explores alternative ways of coping with these changes.

■ **HEALTH CARE RESOURCES**

A home care nurse may be needed to follow wound progress after the client is discharged. The hospital nurse provides details of ulcer size and appearance and any special wound care needs to the nurse in the home, who can then accurately judge changes in ulcer appearance. Chart 67-5 provides a guideline for focused assessment of the client with pressure ulcers.

To minimize waste and to help decrease the overall cost of treatment, the nurse emphasizes proper use of dressing materials. Clean tap water and nonsterile supplies are acceptable for treatment of chronic wounds in the home and are less costly than sterile products. Nonsterile dressing materials can often be purchased in bulk from a local medical supply store at reduced cost.

The client with activity restrictions may require daily assistance from a home care aide. Consultation with a physical therapist may be appropriate to help the client and family or significant others continue rehabilitation efforts in the home.

CRITICAL THINKING CHALLENGE
In spite of preventive care, the client who had a hip replacement is being discharged to an extended care facility with a stage I pressure ulcer on her coccyx.
- What should you teach this client regarding ways to prevent extension of this ulcer?
- What information should be communicated to the new facility?
- Is there anything else you can think of to do to help this client when she leaves your unit?

▶ Evaluation: Outcomes

NOC The nurse evaluates the care of the client with a pressure ulcer on the basis of the identified nursing diagnoses and collaborative problems. The expected outcomes include that the client will:

- Demonstrate skills necessary to care for the wound in the home environment
- Incorporate modifications of lifestyle related to promotion of healing in activities of daily living (ADLs)
- List the signs and symptoms of wound infection
- Make the necessary changes in dietary intake to correct any nutritional deficiencies
- Demonstrate an understanding of measures needed to prevent future episodes of skin breakdown and pressure ulcer formation
- Experience wound healing by secondary intention as evidenced by granulation, epithelialization, and resolution of wound size
- Develop skin thickness in expected range at ulcer area
- Remain tissue lesion free

COMMON INFECTIONS

▌ OVERVIEW
▌ Bacterial Infections

Bacterial skin lesions usually start at the hair follicle, where bacteria easily accumulate and grow in the warm, moist environment. **Folliculitis** is a superficial infection involving only the upper portion of the follicle and is usually caused by *Staphylococcus* (Figure 67-11). **Furuncles** (boils) are also caused by *Staphylococcus,* but the infection is much deeper in the follicle (Figure 67-12). **Cellulitis** is a generalized nonfollicular infection with either *Staphylococcus* or *Streptococcus* and involves the deeper connective tissue.

Minor skin trauma usually precedes the appearance of folliculitis and furuncles and may or may not be associated with the development of cellulitis. Clients may spread the infection to other parts of their bodies by scratching or rubbing the skin with fingernails that have microorganisms under them. Furuncles are more likely to occur in the presence of heat and moisture, such as in the hair-bearing skin fold areas. Cellulitis can occur as a result of secondary bacterial infection of an open wound, or it may be unrelated to skin trauma.

▌ Viral Infections
▌ HERPES SIMPLEX VIRUS

Herpes simplex virus (HSV) infection is the most common viral infection of adult skin. HSV infections are of two types. Type 1 (HSV 1) infections cause the classic recurring cold sore. The severity of the disease increases with age and immunosuppression. Genital herpes, caused by type 2 infection (HSV 2), is also recurrent (see Chapter 77).

After a primary infection, the virus remains in the body in a dormant state in the nerve ganglia, and the client is asymptomatic. Reactivation of the infection stimulates the virus to travel the pathway of sensory nerves to the skin, where lesions reappear. In healthy people, recurrence of HSV infection is triggered by physical or psychologic stressors, such as sunburn, trauma, fever, menses, and fatigue. The virus can also be spread by direct contact between an actively infected person and a susceptible host. *Autoinoculation,* or transfer of either viral type from one part of the body to another, is also possible.

The time span between episodes and the severity of individual attacks varies. Outbreaks of oral herpes simplex usually last 3 to 10 days, and active shedding of the virus and contagion are possible for the first 3 to 5 days. The client may experience tingling or burning of the lip before any lesion is evident.

The most common clinical presentation of HSV 1 infection is isolated or grouped vesicles on an erythematous base (Figure 67-13). The infection can occur anywhere on the skin and may be spread by respiratory droplets or by direct contact with an active lesion or virus-containing fluid (such as saliva).

Herpetic whitlow is a form of herpes simplex infection occurring on the fingertips of medical personnel who have come in contact with viral secretions. This form of herpes is a potential source of client inoculation. Immunosuppressed clients are at a particular risk for severe and persistent eruptions that can lead to life-threatening complications.

▌ HERPES ZOSTER

Herpes zoster (shingles) is caused by reactivation of the latent varicella-zoster virus in clients who have previously had chickenpox. The dormant virus resides in the dorsal root ganglia of the sensory cranial and spinal nerves. The individual lesions of herpes zoster infections are similar to those of herpes simplex, but they have a different distribution pattern (Figure

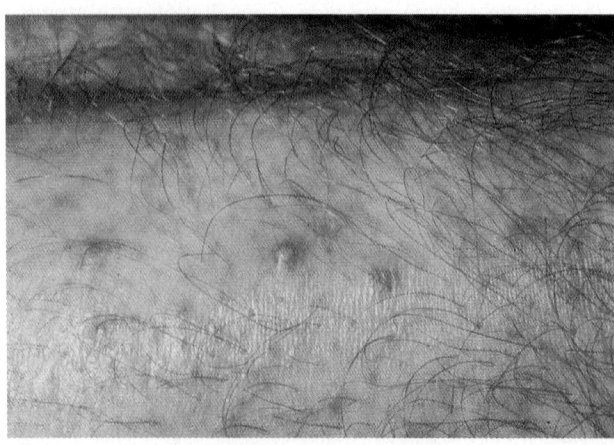

Figure 67-11 ● Folliculitis.

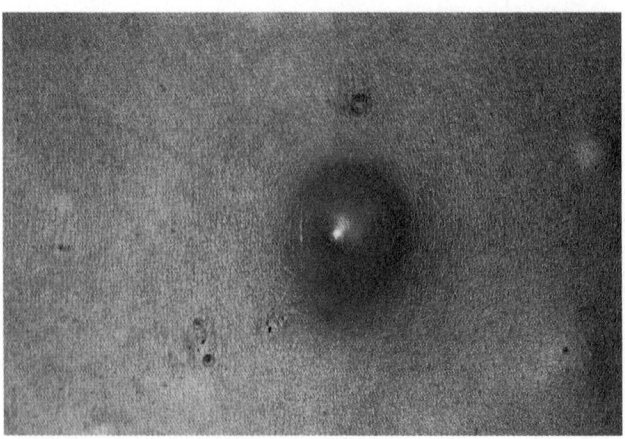

Figure 67-12 ● A furuncle.

67-14). Multiple lesions occur in a segmental distribution on the skin area innervated by the infected nerve. Herpes zoster eruptions are preceded by several days of discomfort, which may vary from minor irritation and itching to severe, deep pain. The course of eruption usually lasts several weeks. **Postherpetic neuralgia,** pain persisting after the lesions have resolved, is a common complication in older clients.

Herpes zoster is essentially a disease of immunosuppression, occurring with increased frequency and severity in older people or in anyone who is immunosuppressed for any reason. Dissemination of the virus can be accompanied by fever and malaise, often progressing to visceral involvement. Herpes zoster is contagious to people who have not been previously exposed to chickenpox.

Complications can include full-thickness skin necrosis, Bell's palsy, or ophthalmic infection and scarring if the virus is introduced into the eye.

Fungal Infections

Superficial fungal (dermatophyte) infections can differ in lesion appearance, anatomic location, and species of the in-

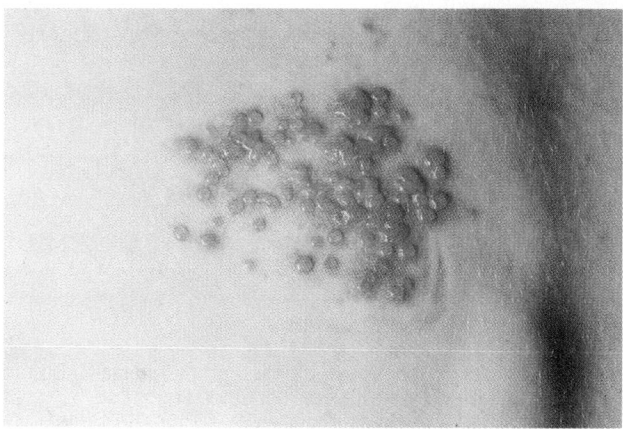

Figure 67-13 ● Herpes simplex.

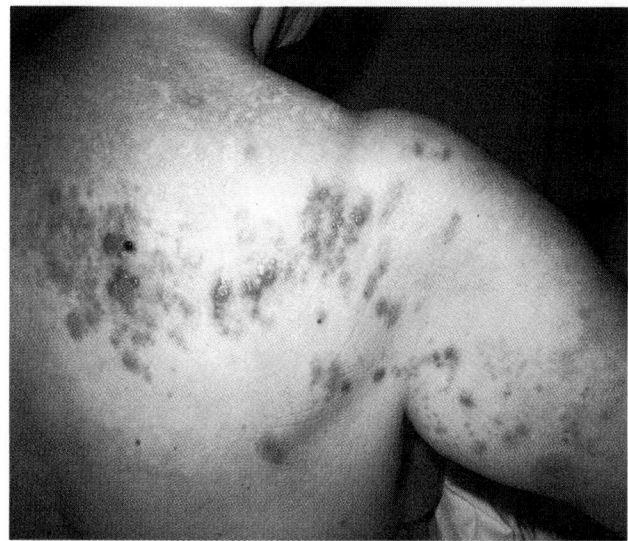

Figure 67-14 ● Herpes zoster.

fecting organism. The term *tinea* is used to describe dermatophytoses. Table 67-9 lists the corresponding anatomic locations of the various categories of infection.

Depending on the species, dermatophytes reside mainly in the soil, on animals, and on humans. Superficial infection can start only if suitable conditions exist for inoculation and maintenance of the organism in the outer layers of the skin.

Dermatophyte infections occur when the infecting organism comes in contact with an impaired skin surface in a susceptible host. Most infections are spread by direct contact with infected humans or animals. Certain types of dermatophytoses, such as tinea capitis and tinea corporis, can be transmitted by means of inanimate objects. For example, tinea capitis is associated with poor personal hygiene and the subsequent sharing of contaminated combs, brushes, hats, pillowcases, and similar objects.

➤ COLLABORATIVE MANAGEMENT

● Assessment
■ HISTORY

The clinical manifestations of the skin infection provide direction for collection of data to confirm a suspected diagnosis. To differentiate among the possible causes of the lesions, the nurse concentrates on risk factors associated with each type of infection. If the location and appearance of lesions suggest a bacterial infection, the nurse explores any recent history of skin trauma, as well as past or current staphylococcal or streptococcal infections. Associated symptoms of fever and malaise are also noted.

Lesions appearing on the lips, in the oral cavity, or in the genital region alert the nurse to a possible viral infection. The nurse seeks information about the following:
- A history of similar lesions in the same location
- Signs of burning, tingling, or pain
- Recent stress factors that may have precipitated the outbreak
- Recent contact with an infected person

Acknowledgment by the client of the recurrent nature of the lesions is often important in helping to differentiate viral from bacterial lesions. If herpes zoster is suspected, the nurse confirms *previous exposure to chickenpox* and asks whether the client has a history of shingles.

The type of information asked of a client with probable dermatophyte infection depends on the anatomic location of the lesions. The presence of tinea corporis and tinea capitis requires further assessment of social and environmental factors that may have contributed to inoculation, such as direct contact with an infected person, poor personal hygiene practices, or frequent contact with animals. If tinea cruris and tinea

TABLE 67-9 ● TINEA INFECTIONS	
Infection	**Location**
Tinea pedis	Feet (athlete's foot)
Tinea manus	Hands
Tinea cruris	Groin (jock itch)
Tinea corporis	Smooth skin surfaces (ringworm)
Tinea capitis	Scalp
Tinea barbae	Beard

pedis are suspected, the nurse asks the client about the type and frequency of athletic activities.

■ PHYSICAL ASSESSMENT/CLINICAL MANIFESTATIONS

Because most skin infections are contagious, the nurse takes necessary precautions to prevent the spread of infection when performing a physical assessment. Chart 67-6 lists the clinical manifestations of common skin infections.

■ LABORATORY ASSESSMENT

When pustules are present in bacterial infections, the infecting organism is confirmed by swab culture of the purulent material. Blood cultures may be helpful, especially if the client is showing clinical signs of bacteremia.

Viral infections are confirmed by *Tzanck's smear* and viral culture. **Tzanck's smear** is a cytologic examination in which cells from the base of a lesion are examined under a microscope. The presence of multinucleated giant cells confirms a viral infection.

CHART 67-6

KEY FEATURES *of* Common Skin Infections

Clinical Manifestations	Distribution
Bacterial Infections	
Folliculitis	
Isolated erythematous pustules occur singly or in groups; hairs grow from centers of many of the lesions. Occasional papules are present. There is little or no associated discomfort. There is no residual scarring.	Areas of hair-bearing skin, especially buttocks, thighs, beard area, and scalp
Furuncle	
Small, tender erythematous nodules become pus filled and more tender over time. Lesions may be single or multiple and also recurrent. Regional lymphadenopathy is sometimes present; fever is rare. Occasional scarring results.	Areas of hair-bearing skin, especially buttocks, thighs, abdomen, posterior neck regions, and axillae
Cellulitis	
Localized area of inflammation may enlarge rapidly if not treated. Redness, warmth, edema, tenderness, and pain are present. On rare occasions, blisters are present. Cellulitis is often accompanied by lymphadenopathy and fever.	Lower legs, areas of persistent lymphedema, and areas of skin trauma (leg ulcer, puncture wound, and so forth)
Viral Infections	
Herpes Simplex	
Grouped vesicles are present on an erythematous base. Vesicles evolve to pustules, which rupture, weep, and crust. Older lesions may appear as punched-out, shallow erosions with well-defined borders. Lesions are associated with itching, stinging, or pain. Secondary bacterial infection with necrosis is possible in immunocompromised clients.	Type 1 classically on the face and type 2 on the genitalia, but either may develop in any area where inoculation has occurred; recurrent infections occur repeatedly in the same skin area
Herpes Zoster	
Lesions are similar in appearance to herpes simplex and also progress with weeping and crusting. Grouped lesions present unilaterally along a segment of skin following the pathway of a spinal or cranial nerve (dermatomal distribution). Eruption is preceded by deep pain and itching. Postherpetic neuralgia is common in older adults. Secondary infection with necrosis is possible in immunocompromised clients.	Anterior or posterior trunk following involved dermatome; face, sometimes involving trigeminal nerve and eye
Fungal Infections	
Dermatophytosis	
Annular or serpiginous patches are present with elevated borders, scaling, and central clearing. Pruritus is common. Lesions may be single or multiple.	Anywhere on the body
Candidiasis	
Erythematous macular eruption occurs with isolated pustules or papules at the border (satellite lesions). Candidiasis is associated with burning and itching. Oral lesions (thrush) appear as creamy white plaques on an inflamed mucous membrane. Cracks or fissures at the corners of the mouth may be present.	Skin fold areas: perineal and perianal region, axillae, beneath breasts, and between the fingers; under wet or occlusive dressings
	Lesions possibly present on the oral or vaginal mucous membranes

Fungal infections are confirmed by a potassium hydroxide (KOH) test. Scrapings of scales from the lesions are obtained and, after preparation with KOH, examined under a microscope. The presence of fungal hyphae confirms the diagnosis. In addition to a KOH test, a fungal culture is sometimes indicated. Occasionally, a skin biopsy is performed to obtain microorganisms for identification.

Interventions

Most skin infections heal well with nonsurgical management. Surgical intervention may be required when an infectious agent is present in deep tissue layers.

NONSURGICAL MANAGEMENT. The nurse is concerned with meticulous skin care to the involved areas to facilitate resolution of lesions and adherence to general isolation precautions. In some instances, drug therapy is needed.

SKIN CARE. Clients with bacterial infections should bathe daily with an antibacterial soap. The nurse instructs the client to remove any pustules or crusts gently so that topical medications are more easily absorbed. The application of warm compresses twice a day to furuncles or areas of cellulitis often increases comfort.

The application of astringent compresses, such as Burow's solution, to viral lesions for 20 minutes three times a day promotes crust formation and healing. Compresses also relieve the irritation and pain associated with herpetic infection. The client is instructed to avoid constricting garments that might rub the lesions and increase irritation.

Most superficial skin infections resolve more quickly if the involved skin is allowed to dry between treatments. Excessive moisture, especially under occlusion, promotes growth of microorganisms. If the client is bedridden, the nurse or other assistive nursing personnel positions the client for optimal air circulation to the area and avoids occlusive dressings or garments.

ISOLATION PRECAUTIONS. The nurse takes precautions to minimize the spread of pathogenic organisms to other people. For most superficial bacterial infections, attention to proper handwashing is sufficient to prevent cross-contamination. However, when hospitalized clients are colonized with *Staphylococcus* that is resistant to antibiotic therapy, strict adherence to isolation procedures is necessary.

Of the dermatophyte infections, tinea capitis, tinea corporis, and tinea pedis show the highest rates of cross-transmission. The nurse instructs clients to avoid sharing potentially contaminated personal items, such as hairbrushes, articles of clothing, or footwear. Repeated infections transmitted by dogs or cats may mean that clients might have to get rid of a family pet to control infections.

DRUG THERAPY. Commonly used topical medications for the treatment of bacterial, viral, and fungal skin infections are listed in Chart 67-7.

Mild bacterial infections of the skin usually resolve with topical antibacterial treatment. Clients with extensive infections, including those with associated fever or lymphadenopathy, require systemic antibiotic therapy.

Acyclovir (Zovirax) is the drug of choice for the treatment of viral infections. Topical acyclovir ointment decreases the numbers of active virus on the skin surface and reduces pain in primary herpetic infections and localized lesions in immunocompromised clients. Topical treatment is of little benefit in recurrent infection. Intravenous (IV) administration is limited to severe primary infections and immunosuppressed clients with symptoms of systemic involvement.

Topical antifungal agents are indicated for clients with dermatophyte and yeast infections. An imidazole cream is applied to the infected skin at least twice a day until the lesions have cleared. To prevent recurrence, the therapy is usually continued for 1 to 2 weeks after clearing. In some instances, antifungal powders may also help to suppress fungal growth. For widespread or resistant fungal infections, systemic antifungal agents, such as ketoconazole (Nizoral), are administered.

SURGICAL MANAGEMENT. Surgery is not usually performed for a superficial skin infection, except for incision and drainage of furuncles. In severely immunocompromised clients, superficial lesions can progress to full-thickness wounds requiring surgical excision.

PARASITIC DISORDERS

Parasitic skin disorders are most often associated with poor hygiene and substandard living conditions. The nurse examines clients who show obvious signs of a self-care deficit for these contagious parasitic infections.

Pediculosis

OVERVIEW

Pediculosis refers to infestation by human lice—*pediculosis capitis* (head lice), *pediculosis corporis* (body lice), and *pediculosis pubis* (pubic, or crab, lice). Human lice are oval and measure approximately 2 to 4 mm. The female louse lays hundreds of eggs, called *nits,* which are deposited at the base of the hair shaft in hair-bearing areas.

► COLLABORATIVE MANAGEMENT

The most prominent symptom of pediculosis is pruritus, which may or may not be accompanied by excoriation. In addition to causing discomfort, these parasites can also be vectors of systemic disease (e.g., typhus and recurrent fever).

Assessment

Pediculosis capitis occurs more commonly in women than in men, especially on the sides and back of the scalp. Pruritus, the result of biting of the scalp by the parasites, is intense. With severe infestation, it is possible for a secondary infection to develop from scratching.

Because the louse is difficult to see on inspection, the nurse examines the scalp for visible white flecks, the nits of the female louse. Matting and crusting of the scalp accompanied by a foul odor alert the nurse to the probability of secondary infection.

Pediculosis corporis is caused by lice that live and lay eggs in the seams of clothing. The parasites also cause itching. The only visible sign of infestation may be excoriations on the trunk, abdomen, or extremities.

Pediculosis pubis causes intense pruritus of the vulvar or perirectal region. Pubic lice, which are more compact and crablike in appearance than body lice, can be contracted from

CHART 67-7

DRUG THERAPY *for* **Skin Disorders**

Drug	Usual Dosage	Nursing Interventions	Rationale
ANTIBACTERIAL DRUGS			
Ointments			
Neomycin sulfate Combination antibiotics (Neosporin, Bacitracin, Polysporin, Mycitracin) Gentamicin (Garamycin) Chloramphenicol (Chloromycetin) Povidone-iodine (Betadine) Bactroban	Apply a thin layer to the affected area tid. Dressing is optional.	Gently clean affected areas with saline, half-strength peroxide, or tap water before applying ointments.	Atraumatic cleaning promotes healing by preventing further injury to skin cells. Cleaning helps to remove exudate, crusts, and residual medication and increases the effectiveness of therapy.
		Avoid rubbing ointment into skin. Apply with downward strokes in direction of hair growth.	Ointments can irritate hair follicles and lead to folliculitis.
		Assess for worsening of problem in spite of topical therapy. Discontinue use if rash appears.	Client may become allergic to active ingredients, the ointment base, or added preservatives.
Creams			
Silver sulfadiazine Silvadene, SSD, Flamazine✤)	Apply in layer approximately $1/16$-inch thick to affected areas tid and prn. Dressing is optional.	Assess for allergy to sulfa drugs.	Use should be avoided in clients with a suspected or known sulfa allergy.
		Gently clean affected areas with saline, half-strength hydrogen peroxide, or tap water before reapplying.	Cleaning removes crusts, exudate, and caked-on medication while promoting percutaneous absorption of drug.
		If affected areas are left open without dressings, reapply cream prn between cleanings to maintain a layer of cream at all times.	Cream base melts with increase in body or room temperature and is easily rubbed off with movement if left uncovered.
		Monitor white blood cell count for drop to <5000/mm³.	Use of silver sulfadiazine over large skin surface areas has been associated with a transient leukopenia (cause unknown).
ANTIFUNGAL DRUGS			
Ointments and Creams			
Clotrimazole (Lotrimin, Mycelex, Canesten✤) Nystatin (Mycolog II, Mycostatin, Nilstat) Ciclopirox olamine (Loprox) Miconazole nitrate (Monistat-Derm 2%) Econazole (Spectazole, Ecostatin✤) Tolnaftate (Tinactin, Pitrex✤) Haloprogin (Halotex✤) Undecylenic acid (Desenex) Ketoconazole (Nizoral)	Apply a thin layer to the affected area tid.	Teach the importance of thoroughly drying the skin before applying medication. Position bedridden clients for maximal air circulation to involved areas. Emphasize wearing of nonconstricting cotton garments to absorb perspiration.	Moist environment promotes the growth of fungal organisms. Increasing air circulation to the affected areas promotes drying. Cream base is easily removed with perspiration, decreasing the effectiveness of therapy.
Powders			
Nystatin (Mycostatin) Tolnaftate (Zeasorb-AF 1%)	Apply a thin dusting of powder to the affected area tid.	Teach the client to thoroughly dry skin before applying powder.	In addition to discouraging the growth of fungal organisms, a dry skin surface minimizes caking of powder in skin fold areas.

CHART 67-7

DRUG THERAPY *for* Skin Disorders—cont'd

Drug	Usual Dosage	Nursing Interventions	Rationale
ANTIFUNGAL DRUGS—cont'd			
Oral Preparations			
Nystatin (Mycostatin oral suspension, Nilstat oral suspension)	Rinse the mouth qid with 4-6 mL (400,000-600,000 units) and swallow.	Teach the client to coat the entire oral cavity with medication and hold the suspension in the mouth for several minutes before swallowing.	Effectiveness of medication is dependent on good contact of medication with mucous membrane surfaces.
Clotrimazole (Mycelex troche)	Take 1 troche 5 times/day.	Teach the client to let troche dissolve slowly in the mouth.	
ANTI-INFLAMMATORY DRUGS			
Potent Fluorinated Steroid Preparations			
Clobetasol propionate (Temovate 0.05%) Triamcinolone acetonide (Aristocort 0.5%, Kenalog 0.5%, Triaderm✤ 0.5%) Amcinonide (Cyclocort 0.1%) Betamethasone dipropionate (Diprosone 0.05%, Betaderm✤ 0.5%) Diflorasone diacetate (Maxiflor 0.05%, Florone 0.05%) Halcinonide (Halog 0.025%) Fluocinonide (Lidex 0.05%, Topsyn gel✤ 0.05%, Lidemol✤ 0.05%, Topsyn✤ 0.05%) Fluocinolone acetonide (Synalar-HP 0.2%, Fluoderm✤ 0.2%) Desoximetasone (Topicort 0.25%) Betamethasone benzoate (Uticort 0.025%, Novobetamet✤ 0.025%)	Apply a small amount to affected areas no more than 4 times in 24 hr.	Teach the client to use the least amount of medication possible to cover the treatment site and to use the medication *only* under the direction of a physician. Never apply highly potent steroid preparations to the face, genital area, or skin fold areas.	Overuse of topical steroid preparations can cause serious side effects, including skin thinning (atrophy), superficial dilated blood vessels (telangiectasia), acnelike eruptions, and adrenal suppression. The incidence of side effects increases proportionately with the potency of the steroid and is most common with prolonged widespread use of the high-potency preparations. Absorption of topical steroids is much higher in these areas, and the associated side effects are more severe.
Medium-Potency Fluorinated Steroid Preparations			
Triamcinolone acetonide (Kenalog 0.025%, 0.1%; Aristocort 0.025%, 0.1%) Flurandrenolide (Cordran 0.5%, 0.025%) Fluocinolone acetonide (Fluonid 0.025%, Synalar 0.025%) Desoximetasone (Topicort LP 0.05%) Betamethasone valerate (Valisone 0.1%)			
Low-Potency Nonfluorinated Steroid Preparations			
Hydrocortisone 0.5%, 1.0%, 2.5% Desonide (Tridesilon) Hydrocortisone valerate (Westcort)		Teach the client to hydrate the skin before applying a topical steroid.	Skin hydration increases percutaneous absorption and maximizes the effectiveness of topical treatment.
Antiviral Drugs			
Ointments			
Acyclovir (Zovirax)	Apply to affected areas 6 times/day.	Teach the client to use topical acyclovir only under the direction of a physician for primary infections. Emphasize precautionary measures to prevent transmission of infection while the lesion is present.	Topical acyclovir has no proven clinical benefit in the prevention or treatment of recurrent infections. There is no evidence that topical treatment prevents transmission of infection.

infested bed linen or during sexual intercourse. Although the louse is usually confined to the genital region, it can also infest the axillae, the eyelashes, and the chest.

Interventions

The treatment of pediculosis is chemical killing of the parasites with agents such as lindane (Bio-Well, Kwell, Kwellada) or topical malathion (Ovide, Prioderm). In the case of pediculosis capitis, areas where the client's head has rested (such as on pillows or chair backs) should also be treated. Clothing and bed linens should be washed in hot water or dry cleaned. The use of a fine-toothed comb can help remove nits from an infested scalp. In all cases of louse infestation, social contacts are treated when possible.

Scabies

OVERVIEW

Scabies is a contagious skin disease caused by mite infestations. Scabies infections are transmitted by close and prolonged contact with an infested companion or infested bedding. Infestation is common among clients of lower socioeconomic status. The scabies mite is also carried by pets and is found among schoolchildren and institutionalized older clients.

► COLLABORATIVE MANAGEMENT

Scabies is characterized by epidermal curved or linear ridges and follicular papules. The pruritus experienced by clients with scabies infestation is more intense than in those with pediculosis, and clients often report that the itching becomes unbearable at night.

The visible white epidermal ridges are formed by burrowing of the mite into the outer skin layers. The nurse closely examines the skin between the fingers and on the palms and volar aspects of the wrists, where these ridges are most common. A hypersensitivity reaction to the mite results in excoriated erythematous papules, pustules, and crusted lesions found primarily on the elbows, nipples, lower abdomen, buttocks, and thighs and in the axillary folds. Male clients can also have excoriated papules on the penis.

Suspected infestation is confirmed by taking a scraping of a lesion and examining it under the microscope for mites and eggs. Close contacts are also monitored for the possibility of infestation.

Treatment consists of chemical disinfection with scabicides, such as lindane (Kwell, Kwellada) or topical sulfur preparations, with one or two daily applications. Clothes and personal items are laundered but do not need to be disinfected.

COMMON INFLAMMATIONS

OVERVIEW

The inflammatory skin conditions are characterized by a variety of nonspecific epidermal manifestations, including marked pruritus, lesions with indistinct borders, and different distribution patterns. The cause of the eruption may or may not be identifiable. Inflammatory rashes can evolve from acute to chronic conditions.

Most inflammatory rashes are related to allergic immune responses. The responses may be triggered by external skin exposure to allergens or by exposure of the internal environment to allergens and irritants. The result is tissue destruction or epidermal alteration induced by antibodies or cellular mediators of the immune system. (A more detailed description of these immune mechanisms is presented in Chapter 20.)

The specific cause of inflammatory rashes is not always known. When this is the case, the catchall diagnosis of nonspecific eczematous dermatitis, or *eczema,* is often used.

Contact dermatitis is an acute or chronic eczematous rash caused by either direct contact with an irritant substance, resulting in toxic injury to the skin, or by contact with an allergen, resulting in a cell-mediated immune reaction.

Atopic dermatitis is a chronic rash associated with a genetic predisposition to respiratory allergies and atopic skin disease. Although the exact mechanism is unknown, atopic dermatitis is exacerbated by a number of factors, including dry or irritated skin, food allergies, chemicals, or stress. (Atopic inflammatory reactions are described in Chapter 23.)

► COLLABORATIVE MANAGEMENT

● Assessment

Because all of the inflammatory skin eruptions have similar clinical presentations, data collected from the client are often the determining factor in identifying the cause. Although the clinical appearance of eczematous dermatitis lesions is similar, the chronicity of the disease, the distribution of lesions, and associated symptoms may vary. Chart 67-8 lists the clinical manifestations of the various types of inflammatory skin conditions. Diagnosis is based on historical and clinical data.

● Interventions

If the cause of the rash is identified, avoidance therapy is used in an attempt to reverse the reaction and clear the rash. Even when the cause is unclear, certain irritants in the environment may cause the rash to worsen and increase discomfort. Additional interventions are aimed at promoting comfort through suppression of the inflammatory response.

STEROIDS. Topical, intralesional, or systemic steroids are prescribed to suppress inflammation. The vehicle used to deliver a topical steroid generally depends on the body area involved. Because a side effect of oral corticosteroid administration is adrenal suppression, clients receiving long-term therapy must taper their drug dosages rather than come to an abrupt halt.

Corticosteroids never cure. During active disease, these agents keep the disease from manifesting itself and relieve associated discomfort. The nurse can moisten dressings with warm tap water to place over topical steroid preparations for short periods to facilitate absorption.

OIL-BASED PRODUCTS. Oil-based ointments and pastes are not applied in the sweaty skin fold areas because increased maceration and blocking of pores may result in folliculitis. Instead, water-soluble creams are the vehicle of choice for these areas. Lotions and gels prevent matting of the hair and are more appropriate for hairy areas, such as the scalp. Stiff pastes are used to apply therapy to localized areas

CHART 67-8

KEY FEATURES *of*
Common Inflammatory Skin Conditions

Clinical Manifestations	Distribution
Nonspecific Eczematous Dermatitis Evolution of lesions from vesicles to weeping papules and plaques. Lichenification occurs in chronic disease. Oozing, crusting, fissuring, excoriation, or scaling may be present. Pruritus is common.	Anywhere on the body; localized eczema commonly involves the hands or feet
Contact Dermatitis Localized eczematous eruption with well-defined, geometric margins that are consistent with contact by an irritant or allergen. Usually seen in the acute form, but may become chronic if exposure is repeated. Allergy to plants (e.g., poison ivy or oak) classically occurs as linear streaks of vesicles or papules.	Cosmetic/perfume allergy: head and neck Hair product allergy: scalp Shoe/rubber allergy: dorsum of feet Nickel allergy: earlobes Mouthwash/toothpaste allergy: perioral region Airborne contact allergy (e.g., paint and ragweed): generalized
Atopic Dermatitis Hallmark in adults is lichenification with scaling and excoriation. Extremely pruritic. Face involvement is seen as dry skin with mild to moderate erythema, perioral pallor, and skin folds beneath the eyes (Dennie-Morgan lines). Associated with linear markings on the palms.	Face, neck, upper chest, and antecubital and popliteal fossae
Drug Eruption Bright red erythematous macules and papules are found. Skin blisters in extreme cases. Lesions tend to be confluent in large areas. Moderately pruritic. Fever is rare. Dehydration and hypothermia can occur with extensive involvement. Condition clears only after offending medication has been discontinued.	Generalized Involvement begins on trunk, proceeds distally (legs are the last to be involved)

because this vehicle clings to the skin where it is applied and resists spreading to uninvolved skin.

Cream preparations are indicated in clients with acute dermatitis with oozing and weeping. Chronic dermatitis responds more favorably to oil-based ointments that seal in moisture and help combat dryness and scaling.

ANTIHISTAMINES. Antihistamines provide some relief of pruritus but may fail to keep the client totally symptom free. The sedative effects of antihistamines can be minimized if the client takes most of the daily dose near bedtime.

COMPRESSES AND BATHS. Cool, moist compresses and tepid baths with bath additives have a soothing effect, decrease inflammation, and help debride crusts and scales. Colloidal oatmeal preparations, tar extracts, cornstarch, or oils are often added to baths to relieve pruritus (see Table 67-1).

PSORIASIS

■ OVERVIEW

Psoriasis is a lifelong disorder characterized by exacerbations and remissions. Even though psoriasis cannot be cured, clients can usually achieve control of symptoms with proper treatment.

■ Pathophysiology

Psoriasis is a scaling disorder with underlying dermal inflammation. The problem involves an abnormality in the proliferation of epidermal cells in the outer skin layers. Normally, cells at the basement membrane of the epidermis take about 27 days to reach the outermost stratum corneum, where they are shed. In a person with psoriasis, the rate of cell division is speeded up so that cells are shed every 4 to 5 days.

■ Etiology

The cause of psoriasis is not known. A genetic predisposition has been recognized in some cases; however, often there is no family history of the disease. Many environmental factors precipitate outbreaks and influence the severity of clinical symptoms, but these vary significantly from person to person. Triggering factors may be local or systemic. A psoriatic lesion may appear after skin trauma (Koebner's phenomenon), such as surgery, sunburn, or excoriation.

Clients with psoriasis seem to improve in warmer climates, where there is more exposure to sunlight. Systemic factors that can aggravate the disease include infections (severe streptococcal throat infection, *Candida* infection, upper respiratory tract infection), hormonal changes (during puberty and menopause), psychologic stress, drugs (lithium, beta-blocking agents, indomethacin, antimalarials), obesity, and the presence of other diseases.

➤ COLLABORATIVE MANAGEMENT

● Assessment

■ HISTORY

In addition to collecting routine epidemiologic data, the nurse asks the client about any family history of psoriasis, including the age at onset, a description of the disease progression, and the pattern of recurrences. The nurse asks the client to describe the current flare-up of psoriasis, including whether the onset was gradual or sudden, where the lesions first appeared, whether the client observed any changes in severity over time, and whether associated symptoms (e.g., fever and pruritus) are present. Possible precipitating factors are explored, including recent skin trauma, upper respiratory tract infection, recent surgeries, menopause status, past and current use of medication, and recent stress-provoking occurrences. Previous treatment modalities and the effectiveness of each in initiating and maintaining remission of the disease are investigated.

■ PHYSICAL ASSESSMENT/CLINICAL MANIFESTATIONS

The appearance of psoriasis and its course vary among clients. Typically, during flare-ups of the disease, lesions thicken and extend to involve new areas of the body. As psoriasis responds to treatment, individual lesions become thinner with less scaling.

PSORIASIS VULGARIS. Psoriasis vulgaris, the most common type of psoriasis, is characterized by thick erythematous papules or plaques surmounted by silvery white scales (Figure 67-15). Borders between the lesions and normal skin are sharply defined. As a result of maceration from perspiration, patches appear less red and more moist in skin fold areas. Lesions are usually distributed symmetrically; the more common sites are the scalp, elbows, trunk, knees, sacrum, and extensor surfaces of the limbs. The facial skin is rarely affected. The client may have only a few isolated lesions, or the entire skin surface may be affected.

EXFOLIATIVE PSORIASIS. Exfoliative psoriasis (erythrodermic psoriasis) is an explosively eruptive form of the disease characterized by generalized erythema and scaling without obvious lesions. The nurse examines for signs of dehydration and hypothermia or hyperthermia related to this severe inflammatory reaction. The vasodilation and increased blood flow to the skin that occur with inflammation can alter fluid volume as a result of increased evaporative water loss from the skin surface.

● Interventions

The several approaches to therapy are based on the extent of disease, the client's distress, the physician's preference, and the resistance of the psoriasis to treatment. Clients must understand that no cure for psoriasis yet exists. Therapy is aimed at decreasing epidermal proliferation and underlying inflammation.

TOPICAL THERAPY. The pharmacologic and physical topical agents used to treat psoriasis are topical steroids, topical tar and anthralin preparations, and ultraviolet (UV) light.

TOPICAL STEROIDS. Corticosteroids have anti-inflammatory properties. When they are applied to psoriatic lesions, they suppress mitotic activity. The effectiveness of a topical steroid depends on its potency and ability to be absorbed into the skin. The more potent preparations are generally used to treat clients with psoriasis.

A simple procedure for enhancing the skin penetration of these agents is for the steroid to be applied directly to the skin. This step is followed by warm, moist dressings and an occlusive outer wrap of plastic film, plastic gloves, booties, or similar garments. When large surface areas are involved, occlusive therapy is limited to 12 hours per day because of the increased risk of local and systemic side effects.

TAR PREPARATIONS. When a tar preparation is applied to the skin, it suppresses mitotic activity and produces an anti-inflammatory effect. Preparations containing crude coal tar and derivations of crude coal tar are available as solutions, ointments, lotions, gels, and shampoos. The use of crude coal tar ointments is usually limited to inpatient care and special-

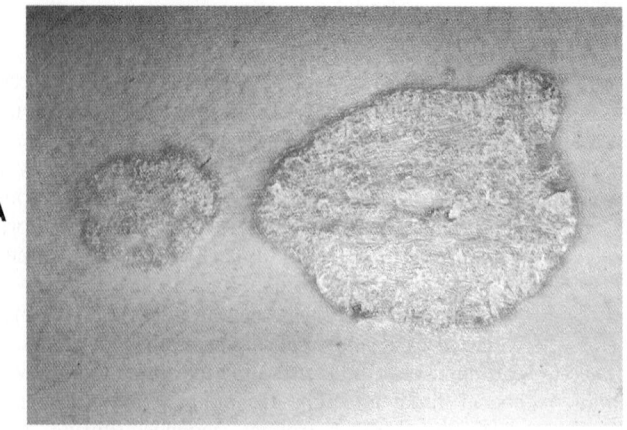
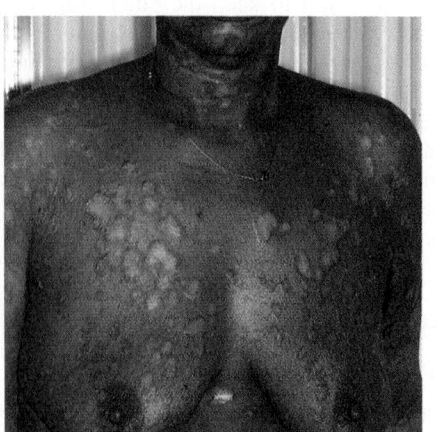

A **B**

Figure 67-15 ● **A,** Psoriasis vulgaris in a Caucasian client. **B,** Psoriasis vulgaris in an African-American client.

ized outpatient treatment clinics because these ointments are messy, cause staining, and have an unpleasant odor.

Topical therapy with anthralin (Anthraforte✤, Drithocreme, Lasan), a hydrocarbon with action similar to that of tar, also relieves chronic psoriasis. Topical therapy is used in a variety of potencies alone and in combination with coal tar baths and UV light.

The nurse applies high-potency anthralin, suspended in a stiff paste, to individual lesions for short periods (not exceeding 2 hours). Because anthralin is a strong irritant and can cause chemical burns, the nurse observes for local tissue reaction and prevents inadvertent contact with uninvolved skin. Anthralin is not indicated for the treatment of acute, spreading psoriasis, because it tends to induce Koebner's phenomenon (see Skin Cancer, pp. 1546 and 1548).

Newer topical therapy with calcipotriene (Dovonex) as a cream, ointment, or lotion has proved to be effective for many clients with mild to moderate psoriasis. This drug is a synthetic form of vitamin D and is thought to regulate skin cell reproduction. Tazarotene (Tazorac), a vitamin A derivative primarily used for acne, has been helpful for treatment of psoriasis in those clients who have lesions on less than 20% of the body surface. This drug is teratogenic (can cause birth defects) even when administered topically. In addition, methotrexate delivered as a topical agent directly to lesions is undergoing study for its effectiveness in controlling psoriasis. Other immunosuppressive agents are being tested for effectiveness in a topical form.

ULTRAVIOLET LIGHT THERAPY. UV radiation is a physical agent commonly used as a topical treatment in many skin conditions, including psoriasis. Ultraviolet B (UVB) light, which produces more energy, is responsible for the obvious biologic effects of the sun, such as burning. Ultraviolet A (UVA) light emits a lower level of energy, requiring longer exposure time before cellular destruction occurs. Although the sun is the least expensive source of UV radiation, control of availability and intensity in skin treatment is best obtained with artificial light sources. These sources include high-intensity mercury vapor lamps or specially constructed cabinets containing UV tubes. *The use of commercial tanning beds is not recommended for the client with psoriasis.*

In general, UV therapy is limited by the potency and distance of the source from the skin, as well as the exposure time. Potency and distance remain constant, and the time of exposure is gradually increased to achieve a mild sunburn effect without burning or tenderness. The client's skin type, ranging from fair to darkly pigmented, affects his or her susceptibility to burning and determines the initial and subsequent exposure times. Because of the extremely high intensity of most artificial UVB light sources, daily treatments are measured in seconds of exposure; clients must wear eye protection during treatment.

The nurse teaches clients to inspect the skin carefully each day for signs of overexposure. If clients complain of tenderness on palpation and have clinical signs of severe erythema or vesicle and bullae formation, the physician must be notified promptly before therapy is resumed.

Psoralen and UVA (PUVA) treatments are more common on an outpatient basis (Figure 67-16). Clients ingest psoralen, a photosensitizing agent, 2 hours before exposure to UVA light. Because UVA light produces less energy than UVB light, the onset of erythema and skin darkening may be delayed as long as 96 hours after exposure. Treatments are limited to two to three times a week and are not given on consecutive days. Exposure is gradually increased until tanning occurs. As with UVB exposure, dosage corrections are adjusted according to the erythema reaction of normal skin, as well as the response of psoriatic lesions.

The nurse observes for generalized erythema with edema and tenderness. Treatment must be interrupted until symptoms subside. Because of the strong photosensitizing properties of psoralen, clients must wear dark glasses during treatment and for the remainder of the day.

Long-term side effects of both UVB and PUVA therapies include premature aging of the skin, actinic keratosis, and an increased incidence of skin cancer.

SYSTEMIC THERAPY. Some clients have severe psoriasis that is resistant to topical therapy. In these instances, systemic treatment with a cytotoxic agent, such as methotrexate (Folex, Mexate), is warranted. Because of the hepatotoxic side effects of methotrexate, a liver biopsy is recommended before therapy is initiated and yearly thereafter. Relatively small doses are required to obtain clearing of lesions. This treatment of last resort is contraindicated if clients have liver damage, bone marrow suppression, or impaired renal function.

Because psoriasis has an autoimmune basis, some systemic agents that induce immunosuppression are used occasionally when lesions do not respond to other therapies. Such agents include cyclosporin (Sandimmune) and azathioprine (Imuran). The many health risks associated with these therapies must be considered along with the potential benefits.

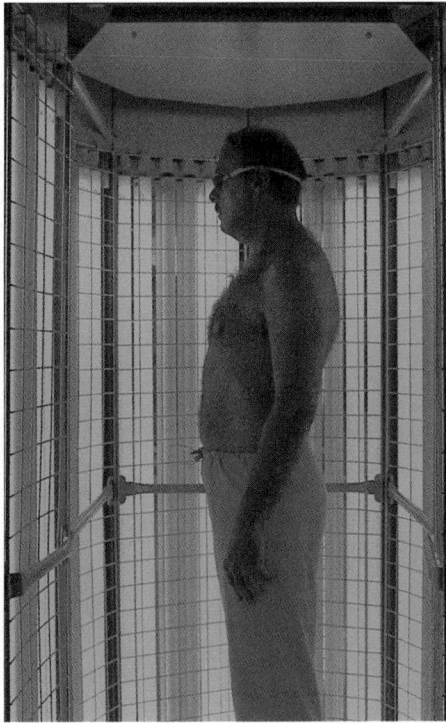

Figure 67-16 ● A client receiving psoralen and ultraviolet A treatment. (Courtesy the Department of Dermatology, Baylor College of Medicine, Houston, TX.)

EMOTIONAL SUPPORT. Often clients' self-esteem suffers not only because of the presence of skin lesions but also because of the unpleasantness associated with some of the treatment modalities. Tar not only looks dirty but also has a very unpleasant odor. Bed linen and pajamas become stained, further discouraging social interaction.

The nurse encourages contact with other clients who have similar problems. Group discussions involving family members or significant others can increase the socialization process.

The use of touch takes on an added significance for clients with psoriasis. For example, the nurse shakes the client's hand during an introduction or places a hand on the client's shoulder when explaining a procedure. The nurse does not wear gloves during these social interactions. Touch, more than any other gesture, communicates acceptance of the person and the skin problem.

BENIGN TUMORS
Cysts
OVERVIEW

Cysts are firm, flesh-colored nodules that contain liquid or semisolid material. Unlike malignant growths, which are hard and firmly attached to underlying structures, a cyst is characterized by fluctuance and mobility on palpation. Often there is a central pore through which the material can be expressed if the lesion is squeezed.

The most common cyst is an epidermal inclusion cyst. These benign growths often occur spontaneously and are asymptomatic. They can be located anywhere on the body but occur most often on the head and trunk (Figure 67-17). The most common cyst on the scalp is the sebaceous, or pilar, cyst.

► COLLABORATIVE MANAGEMENT

Therapy to remove cysts is rarely indicated. If the client prefers that the cyst be removed, surgical excision with primary closure is performed with a local anesthetic agent. The surgeon removes the entire cyst wall during excision to prevent recurrence.

A pilonidal cyst is a lesion of the sacral area that is often associated with a sinus track extending into deeper tissue structures. Because the lesion's proximity to the perineum may result in secondary infection, surgical incision and drainage are necessary.

Seborrheic Keratoses
OVERVIEW

Seborrheic keratoses are a common problem of older people. These benign epidermal neoplasms are gradually acquired after middle age and are often mistaken for actinic keratoses or pigmented skin cancers. These growths may occur anywhere on the body but are more commonly found on the face, neck, upper trunk, and arms.

► COLLABORATIVE MANAGEMENT

On inspection, seborrheic keratoses appear as multiple "pasted-on" papules or plaques ranging in color from flesh tones to brown or black. The surface of the lesion has a rough, greasy, wartlike texture on palpation.

Seborrheic keratoses should be removed only for cosmetic reasons or if a lesion becomes irritated from friction or excoriation. Cryosurgery or curettage with or without a local anesthetic is performed.

Keloids
OVERVIEW

A keloid is overgrowth of a scar resulting from an excessive accumulation of collagen and ground substance after skin trauma. Keloids are more common in darker-skinned people and often arise at sites of surgical incisions, burns, and ear piercing (Figure 67-18).

► COLLABORATIVE MANAGEMENT

On physical examination, a keloid appears as an elevated, protruding lesion that extends well beyond the boundaries of the original injury. Treatment of these cosmetically disfiguring lesions is difficult and not always successful. Because surgical excision alone can result in a larger, more protuberant

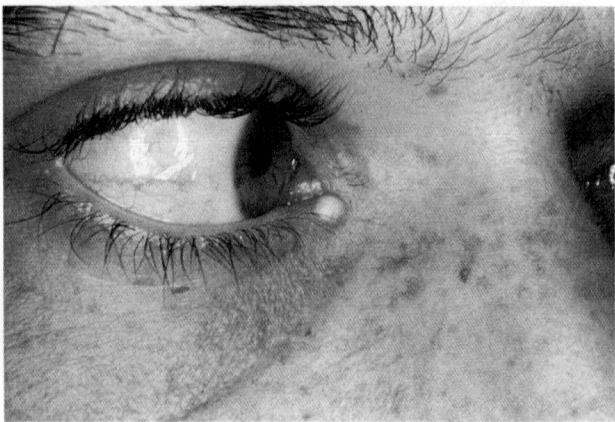

Figure 67-17 ● An epidermal inclusion cyst.

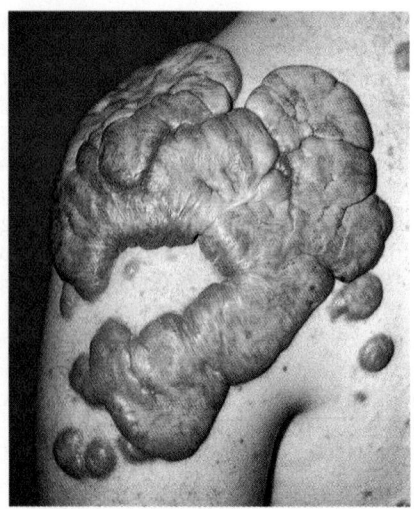

Figure 67-18 ● A keloid.

scar, surgery is usually combined with another form of therapy, such as intralesional steroid injections or low-dose radiotherapy. Pressure dressings or elastic garments worn over the skin for 1 year after excision or steroid injection may also help to keep the lesion flat.

Nevi
▓ OVERVIEW

A **nevus,** or mole, is a benign neoplasm of the pigment-forming cells. These lesions are classified according to their location within the layers of the skin.

➤ COLLABORATIVE MANAGEMENT

Normal nevi have regular, well-defined borders and are uniform in color, ranging from light colors to dark brown. The lesion's surface may be rough or smooth. Because about 50% of malignant melanomas arise from moles, nevi with irregular or spreading borders and those with multiple colors should be considered highly suspicious. Other abnormal findings include sudden changes in the size of the lesion and complaints of itching or bleeding.

Unsightly nevi or those subject to repeated irritation or trauma can be removed. Biopsy of any suspicious lesions is performed to rule out malignancy.

Warts
▓ OVERVIEW

Warts, or **verrucae,** are small tumors caused by papillomavirus infection of the skin cells. They may occur singly or in groups and are classified according to their anatomic location.

Common warts are raised, flesh-colored papules with a rough surface (Figure 67-19). Although they may grow anywhere on the skin surface, they often occur on the hands and fingers.

Flat warts range in size from 2 to 4 mm. They appear as slightly elevated reddish brown or flesh-colored papules with flat tops and minimal scale. These warts often multiply and affect the hands and the face.

An often painful wart occurring on the bottom of the foot is the plantar wart. Plantar warts are covered with a thick cal-

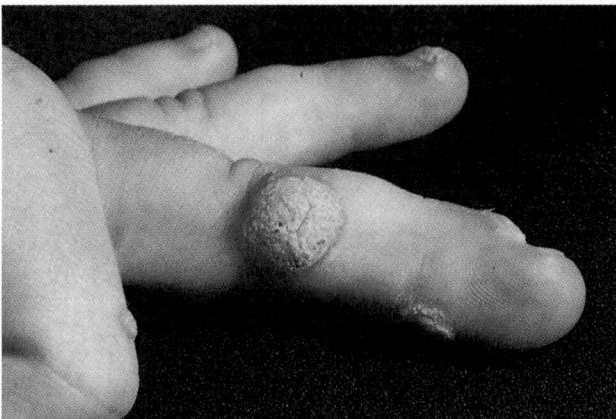

Figure 67-19 ● A common wart.

lus that when removed reveals tiny black dots (thrombosed capillaries).

➤ COLLABORATIVE MANAGEMENT

The treatment of warts is aimed at destroying the skin cells containing the virus, a process that can be destructive and painful. Treatment modalities include surgical excision, electrodesiccation and curettage, and cryosurgery. Cryosurgery is usually preferred because a local anesthetic is not required and scarring is less likely. Topical caustic agents, including salicylic acid and lactic acid, are also used. These agents are painted onto the surface of the lesion and result in destruction of the cells and peeling of the infected skin area.

Hemangiomas

Hemangiomas (angiomas) are blood vessel tumors and are one of the most common types of benign tumors. The clinical appearance varies from lesions that appear shortly after birth and gradually regress to those that are present at birth and gradually expand in size with growth.

Nevus flammeus is a congenital hemangioma involving the mature capillaries. These lesions are usually found on the face and the upper body. They appear as well-demarcated macular patches ranging in color from pink to bluish purple. Although nevus flammeus may gradually fade during the first years of life, a form of this neoplasm, the port-wine stain, grows with the child and remains unchanged in adult life. Port-wine stains usually occur as solitary lesions that vary in size.

The problem of nevus flammeus is cosmetic. Depending on the size of the lesion, surgical excision with or without skin grafting may be indicated. Treatment with laser therapy also is an alternative to surgery. Noninvasive treatment consists of masking the lesion by covering it with an opaque makeup.

Cherry hemangiomas are often seen in older adults. These lesions are small, dome-shaped papules ranging in color from red to purple (see Figure 66-14). Treatment is not indicated except when the client is unhappy with his or her appearance.

SKIN CANCER
▓ OVERVIEW

Overexposure to sunlight is the major cause of skin cancer, although other factors are associated. Because sun damage is an age-related skin finding, screening for suspicious lesions is an integral part of routine physical assessment of the older adult. The most common skin cancers are actinic or solar keratosis, squamous cell carcinoma, basal cell carcinoma, and melanoma.

▓ Pathophysiology

Actinic keratoses are premalignant lesions involving the cells of the epidermis. These lesions are common in people with chronically sun-damaged skin (see Figure 66-16). Progression to squamous cell carcinoma may occur if lesions are untreated.

Squamous cell carcinomas are cancers of the epidermis. They can invade locally and are potentially metastatic. Lesions on the ear, lip, and external genitalia are more likely to invade and metastasize than those found elsewhere on the body (Figure 67-20). Chronic skin damage from repeated injury or irritation also predisposes to this malignancy.

Basal cell carcinomas arise from the basal cell layer of the epidermis (Figure 67-21). Early malignant lesions often go unnoticed, and although metastasis is rare, underlying tissue destruction can progress to include vital structures. Genetic predisposition and chronic irritation are risk factors; however, ultraviolet (UV) radiation remains the primary carcinogen.

Melanomas are pigmented cancers originating in the melanin-producing cells of the epidermis (Figure 67-22). Risk factors include genetic predisposition, excessive exposure to UV light, and the presence of one or more precursor lesions that resemble unusual moles. *This skin cancer is highly metastatic, and a person's survival depends on early diagnosis and treatment.*

Incidence/Prevalence

The incidence of skin cancer is highest among light-skinned races and people older than 60 years of age (American Cancer Society, 2001). The incidence is higher among people who work outdoors and live at higher altitudes or lower latitudes. Occupational exposure to arsenic or other chemical carcinogens also increases risk. The incidence of malignant melanoma has rapidly increased during the past 30 years, accounting for 2% of all cancers and 1% of all cancer deaths (American Cancer Society, 2001).

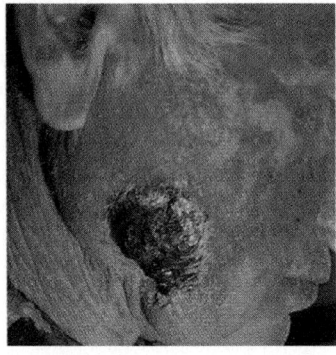

Figure 67-20 ● Squamous cell carcinoma.

The single most effective prevention strategy for skin cancer is avoiding or reducing skin exposure to sunlight. However, even when people understand the cause of skin cancer and the seriousness of the disease, preventive behaviors are not always practiced (see the Evidence-Based Practice for Nursing box on p. 1547).

► COLLABORATIVE MANAGEMENT

● Assessment

In addition to age and race, the nurse asks the client about any family history of skin cancer and any past surgery for removal of skin growths. Recent changes in the size, color, or sensation of any mole, birthmark, wart, or scar are also significant. The client is asked about which geographic regions he or she has lived in and where he or she currently resides. The nurse obtains information about occupational and recreational activities in relation to sun exposure, as well as any occupational history of exposure to chemical carcinogens (e.g., arsenic, coal tar, pitch, radioactive waste, and radium). The client is asked about any skin growths that are repeatedly irritated by the rubbing of clothes against them.

The skin cancers vary in their appearance and distribution. Although most skin cancers appear in sun-exposed areas of the body, the entire skin surface is inspected. The nurse systematically examines the skin for any unusual lesions, particularly moles, warts, birthmarks, and scars. Hair-bearing areas of the body, such as the scalp and genitalia, are also examined. Lesions are palpated to determine their surface texture. The location, size, color, and surface characteristics of all lesions are documented, as are any subjective reports of associated tenderness or itching.

Table 67-10 summarizes important facts about common skin cancers. Chart 67-9 lists methods of prevention that clients can use to reduce their risk for skin cancer.

Punch, shave, or excisional biopsy of suspicious lesions is necessary to confirm the diagnosis of a malignancy.

● Interventions

Nonsurgical and surgical interventions are combined for the most effective management of skin cancer. Specific treatment is determined by the size and severity of the malignancy, the

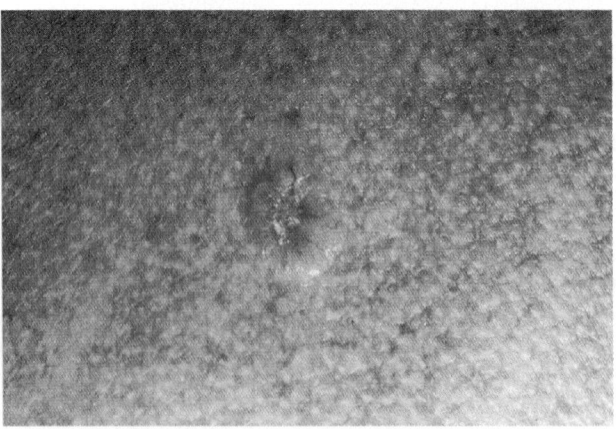

Figure 67-21 ● Basal cell carcinoma.

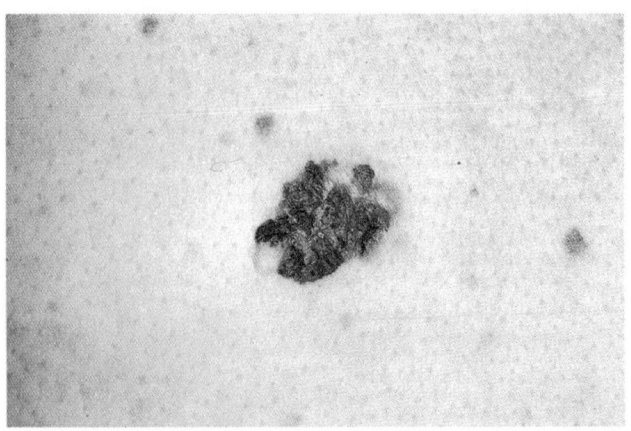

Figure 67-22 ● Melanoma.

location of the lesion, and the age and general health of the client.

NONSURGICAL MANAGEMENT

DRUG THERAPY. Topical chemotherapy with 5-fluorouracil cream is reserved for treatment of clients with multiple actinic keratoses or, in rare instances, widespread superficial basal cell carcinoma that would require several surgical procedures to eradicate. Therapy is continued for several weeks; during this time, the treated areas become increasingly tender and inflamed as the lesions crust, ooze, and erode. The nurse prepares the client for an unsightly appearance during therapy and reassures the client that the cosmetic result will be positive.

After treatment is discontinued, cool compresses and topical corticosteroid preparations help to decrease inflammation and promote comfort.

Systemic chemotherapeutic agents are rarely indicated in the treatment of cutaneous malignancy. These agents may be used, however, when the prognosis is poor, as in advanced metastatic melanoma.

Drug therapy with interferon, a biological response modifier, is now an accepted treatment after surgery for melanomas that are stage III or more advanced cancer. The client is initially started on high-dose (20,000,000 units/m²) interferon intravenously daily for 5 days per week for 4 weeks after the surgical wound is well healed. Maintenance doses of 10,000,000 units/m² are continued three times per week for 1 year. The maintenance doses are administered subcutaneously, and the client must learn to self-inject the drug.

RADIATION THERAPY. Radiation therapy for malignant skin lesions is limited to older clients with large, deeply invasive basal cell tumors and to those who are poor risks for surgery. Primary malignant melanoma is resistant to radiation therapy; however, radiation therapy has proved to be of some value for clients with metastatic disease when used in combination with systemic corticosteroids.

IMMUNOTHERAPY. An experimental treatment available at some centers for clients with melanoma that has metastasized to distant sites is a melanoma vaccine. This treatment takes advantage of distinctive cell surface proteins found on some melanomas that can act like antigens. Although this form of cancer therapy is new and as yet unapproved, it shows promise for this type of cancer.

SURGICAL MANAGEMENT. Surgical intervention ranges from local treatment of individual lesions, with minimal discomfort and positive cosmetic results, to massive excision of large areas of the skin.

CRYOSURGERY. Cryosurgery involves the local application of liquid nitrogen ($-200°$ C) to isolated lesions, causing cell death and tissue destruction. Local anesthesia is seldom needed because clients experience only minor discomfort during the procedure. The nurse prepares clients for swelling and increased tenderness of the treated area when the skin thaws. Tissue freezing is followed in 1 or 2 days by hemorrhagic blister formation. The nurse instructs clients to clean the treatment sites with hydrogen peroxide to prevent infection. A topical antibiotic may also be ordered.

CURETTAGE AND ELECTRODESICCATION. For clients who have small lesions with well-defined borders, curettage and electrodesiccation are used to destroy the cancerous cells while minimizing damage to the surrounding uninvolved tissue. After a local anesthetic is administered, the surgeon uses a semisharp dermal curette to scrape away the cancerous tissue. After curettage is complete, the surgeon places an electric probe on the wound surface, and malignant remnants of the tumor are destroyed by thermal and mechanical energy.

Wounds treated by curettage and electrodesiccation are allowed to heal by second intention. Scarring is usually minimal. The nurse instructs clients in caring for the wound, including cleaning the wound, using prescribed antibacterial medications, and applying prescribed dressings.

EXCISION. For clients with large or poorly defined skin cancers, recurrent tumors, and deeply invasive cancers, wide excision is required to remove the malignancy. If the size and location of the lesion permit, surgical excision with primary closure is the procedure of choice. If the tumor has already been removed several times or if radiation therapy has damaged the surrounding skin, healing by second intention is indicated. This procedure allows the wound to be carefully monitored for cancer recurrence. Skin grafts and flaps are used to repair large defects with deep-tissue destruction.

EVIDENCE-BASED PRACTICE
FOR NURSING

Good role modeling requires knowing your risk!

Grubbs, L., & Tabano, M. (2000). Use of sunscreen in health care professionals. *Cancer Nursing, 23*(1), 164-167.

The purpose of this descriptive study was to examine the relationship between perceived risk for skin cancer and use of sunscreen among a convenience sample of 98 health care professionals living in a high sun exposure area of the United States. The health care professionals group was made up of registered nurses, pharmacists, psychologists, nurse practitioners, and physicians. The level of education in this group was high, with 63% having postgraduate or professional degrees. Most of the participants were Caucasian women.

The study involved completion of a questionnaire that included demographic and skin cancer risk assessment questions. A total of 90 questionnaires were returned (92% response rate). The perceived risk for skin cancer among this group was 50% low perceived risk, 44% high perceived risk, and 6% neutral. The actual risk for skin cancer, based on family history, burn history, and skin type, was 7% low risk, 48% average risk, and 45% high risk. Statistical analysis confirmed that subjects at high risk and those at low risk had an accurate perception of actual risk. The subjects at average risk overwhelmingly reported their perceived risk as low. There was no relationship between perceived risk and consistent use of sunscreen.

Critique. The study was appropriately designed as a descriptive pilot study. Subject homogeneity limits the generalizability of the study results beyond this group.

Implications for Nursing. Nurses and other health care professionals are perceived by the general public as role models of healthy behaviors. With a preventable cancer, such as skin cancer, nurses can have the greatest impact by encouraging preventive practices. An inaccurate perception of personal risk and inconsistent use of protective or preventive practices reduce this positive impact.

TABLE 67-10 • COMMON SKIN CANCERS

Clinical Manifestations	Distribution	Course
ACTINIC KERATOSIS (PREMALIGNANT) Small (1-10 mm) macule or papule with dry, rough, adherent yellow or brown scale Base may be erythematous Associated with yellow, wrinkled, weatherbeaten skin Thick, indurated keratoses more likely to be malignant	Cheeks, temples, forehead, ears, neck, backs of hands, and forearms	May disappear spontaneously or reappear after treatment. Slow progression to squamous cell carcinoma is possible.
SQUAMOUS CELL CARCINOMA Firm, nodular lesion topped with a crust or with a central area of ulceration Indurated margins Fixation to underlying tissue with deep invasion	Sun-exposed areas, especially head, neck, and lower lip Sites of chronic irritation or injury (e.g., scars, irradiated skin, burns, and leg ulcers)	Rapid invasion with metastasis via the lymphatics occurs in 10% of cases. Larger tumors are more prone to metastasis.
BASAL CELL CARCINOMA Pearly papule with a central crater and rolled, waxy borders Telangiectasias and pigment flecks visible on close inspection	Sun-exposed areas, especially head, neck, and central portion of face	Metastasis is rare. May cause local tissue destruction. 50% recurrence rate related to inadequate treatment.
MELANOMA Irregularly shaped, pigmented papule or plaque Variegated colors, with red, white, and blue tones	Can occur anywhere on the body, especially where nevi (moles) or birthmarks are evident Commonly found on upper back and lower legs Soles of feet and palms in Asians and African-Americans	Horizontal growth phase followed by vertical growth phase. Rapid invasion and metastasis with high morbidity and mortality.

CHART 67-9

CLIENT EDUCATION GUIDE
Prevention of Skin Cancer

- Avoid sun exposure between 11:00 AM and 3:00 PM.
- Use sunscreens with the appropriate skin protection factor for your skin type.
- Wear a hat, opaque clothing, and sunglasses when you are out in the sun.
- Examine your body monthly for possibly cancerous or precancerous lesions.
- Seek medical advice if you note any of the following:
  - A change in the color of a lesion, especially if it darkens or shows evidence of spreading
  - A change in the size of a lesion, especially rapid growth
  - A change in the shape of a lesion, such as a sharp border becoming irregular or a flat lesion becoming raised
  - Redness or swelling of the skin around a lesion.
  - A change in sensation, especially itching or increased tenderness of a lesion
  - A change in the character of a lesion, such as oozing, crusting, bleeding, or scaling

A specialized form of excision, Mohs' surgery, is used to treat basal and squamous cell carcinomas. The cancerous tissue is sectioned horizontally in layers, and each layer is examined histologically to determine the exact location of residual tumor cells. Although the procedure is long and tedious, cure rates are higher and there is less sacrifice of healthy tissue compared with other surgical methods.

PLASTIC OR RECONSTRUCTIVE SURGERY

■ OVERVIEW

The aim of plastic or reconstructive surgery is to correct functional defects and alter physical appearance—processes that directly influence a person's concept of self. Unlike a medical illness that is unexpected, plastic surgery is usually an elective procedure. Surgical intervention is sought by clients who cannot perform activities of daily living (ADLs) as a result of an anatomic malformation or by those who are unsatisfied with their body image. In the United States the decision to undergo plastic surgery is often a response to established social and cultural norms. Clients become self-conscious about unsightly scars, obvious facial lesions, disproportionate anatomic features, or changes in physical features associated with aging. In some instances, severe trauma or extensive surgical excision of soft tissue leads to acquired functional defects that warrant surgical correction. For example, breast reconstruction is commonly performed after a radical mastectomy. This type of surgery not only serves an aesthetic purpose for some clients but also replaces lost anatomy and negates the need for a prosthesis.

Clients may request plastic surgery as a remedy for the normal changes in skin appearance that occur with aging. Loss of skin elasticity and redistribution of adipose tissue is progressive and especially noticeable around the eyes, near the cheeks, and on the neck. Fine facial wrinkles around the eyes and mouth are one of the first signs of aging and are followed by gradual stretching and downward displacement of the soft tissue of the lower two thirds of the face. Similar changes in skin texture contribute to wrinkling and flaccidity of the skin on the upper extremities and the chest, abdomen, buttocks, and thighs—a problem also seen after dramatic weight loss. Gradual appearance of skin lesions associated with chronic sun exposure may trouble the aging client.

► COLLABORATIVE MANAGEMENT

● Assessment

■ HISTORY

When taking a history from a client who elects to have plastic surgery, the nurse uses a nonjudgmental approach and is careful not to assume the reason for surgery on the basis of physical appearance. Often what might appear to be unsightly to the nurse is of little concern to the client, who wishes to change something else. The nurse also observes for any nonverbal communication that might establish the emotional state of the person or reveal feelings of embarrassment or guilt. The nurse encourages the client to describe the problem, including why it is bothersome and what he or she expects as a result of the change. The client is asked about both his or her health history and recent medical problems, including obesity and trauma, to predict the amount of surgery needed to correct the defect and potential complications.

■ PHYSICAL ASSESSMENT/CLINICAL MANIFESTATIONS

The client seeking plastic surgery may have alterations in appearance ranging from minor to significant deformity. Depending on the location of the deformity, the client may need to disrobe before the examination. The client may be embarrassed by the problem, and the nurse ensures privacy.

The nurse begins the physical assessment by closely examining the area of involvement to determine the extent of the deformity or problem. Having the client assume different normal sitting and standing postures may provide better visibility of nonfacial defects. The nurse notes any asymmetry of anatomic features, wrinkling or skin redundancy, scars or disfiguring skin marks, and obvious skin lesions.

■ PSYCHOSOCIAL ASSESSMENT

The nurse addresses the client's expectations of plastic surgery. Often people who seek plastic surgery have unrealistic expectations or are uncertain about what they actually want. For example, the client with minor deformities who is seeking perfection is sure to be disappointed. The client who wants an operation mainly to please the spouse or partner is also a poor candidate. His or her psychologic outlook before surgery should be positive if results are to be therapeutic.

> **CRITICAL THINKING CHALLENGE**
> The client is a 28-year-old woman admitted for breast augmentation surgery. After she has had her preoperative medication, she tells you that she is having this surgery because her fiance insists that she have it before their marriage. She also tells you that she is afraid to be put to sleep.

- Whom should you notify about this revelation?
- How should you document the client's concerns?
- What is your role in this situation?

For suggested answer guidelines, go to SIMON, http://www.wbsaunders.com/SIMON/Iggy/.

● Interventions

SURGICAL MANAGEMENT. Depending on the planned intervention, surgery is performed either in the outpatient setting with the client under local anesthesia or in the hospital. Most clients scheduled for plastic surgery will have had several office consultations with their physician to discuss the planned intervention, possible complications, and postoperative expectations. The indications and complications of common cosmetic procedures are summarized in Table 67-11.

Many plastic surgeons use photography both as a visual aid when discussing clients' problems and as a means of documentation before and after surgical intervention. Pictures taken of clients are confidential. Showing clients pictures of other clients is done only after proper consent is obtained.

PREOPERATIVE CARE. Because of the large amount of blood loss associated with skin (particularly facial) surgery, the nurse instructs the client to avoid ingestion of salicylates for several weeks before and after the procedure. Immediate preoperative care is focused on collection of any routine laboratory test data required before general anesthesia and preparation of the operative site. In most cases, the procedure for shaving and washing the skin is dictated by the physician's preference.

Clients undergoing facial surgery, specifically **rhytidectomy** (face-lift), are often asked to wash their hair several times with antibacterial soap to decrease bacterial flora near the incision site. The nurse instructs clients to remove any makeup and avoid using face creams before surgery. If a **rhinoplasty** (reconstruction of the nose) is scheduled, the nurse prepares clients for the early postoperative period by explaining the need for nasal packing to control bleeding and by reviewing mouth-breathing techniques.

OPERATIVE PROCEDURES. Reconstructive procedures vary extensively depending on the location, purpose, and extent of reconstruction. Ironically, in performing plastic surgery, the surgeon must inflict a potentially disfiguring wound to correct existing skin deformities.

POSTOPERATIVE CARE. Postoperative care focuses on monitoring for complications associated with surgical intervention (see Chapter 19). Pressure dressings may be applied at the time of surgery and left in place for several days to control hemorrhage and edema formation. The nurse checks dressings and any nasal packing for bright red bleeding and monitors changes in vital signs and level of consciousness indicating active hemorrhage.

Repeated swallowing followed by belching after rhinoplasty is a sign of postnasal bleeding, and this sign is reported immediately to the surgeon. The client who has had breast surgery may have drains in place postoperatively, and the nurse monitors the amount and color of drainage. When the client has had any facial reconstruction, he or she is placed in a semi-Fowler's position to minimize edema and promote comfort.

Additional comfort measures, such as the application of ice packs or cold compresses, are instituted as ordered. Spe-

TABLE 67-11 • COMMON PLASTIC SURGICAL PROCEDURES

Description	Indications	Complications
BLEPHAROPLASTY Excision of bulging fat and redundant skin of the periorbital area with primary closure	Bags under the eyes	Hematoma Ectropion Corneal injury Visual loss (rare) Wound infection (rare)
BREAST AUGMENTATION (AUGMENTATION MAMMOPLASTY) Insertion of synthetic breast-shaped implants through a skin incision	Inadequate breast volume or contour	Hematoma or hemorrhage Wound infection (with gram-positive organisms) Phlebitis
BREAST REDUCTION (REDUCTION MAMMOPLASTY) Excision of excessive breast tissue and skin with primary closure	Hypertrophy of breast tissue caused by elevated hormone levels, endocrine abnormalities, or obesity	Hematoma or hemorrhage Nipple, areola, and skin flap necrosis Wound infection Fat necrosis Wound dehiscence
DERMABRASION Abrasive removal of the facial epidermis and a portion of the dermis followed by healing by second intention	Moderate to severe acne scars Deep wrinkling Multiple actinic keratoses Hyperpigmentation (postinflammatory or after the use of estrogens)	Hypertrophic scarring Altered skin pigmentation Acne flare Wound infection (rare)
RHINOPLASTY Removal of excessive cartilage and tissue from the nose with correction of septal defects if indicated	Disproportionate anatomy Post-traumatic nasal deformity	Hematoma or hemorrhage Ecchymosis and edema (temporary) Wound infection (with gram-positive organisms) Septal perforation Minor skin irritation
RHYTIDECTOMY (FACE-LIFT) Removal of excess skin and tissue from the face at the level of the hairline followed by primary closure	Excessive wrinkling or sagging of facial skin	Hematoma or hemorrhage Facial nerve damage (temporary or permanent) Wound infection Ecchymosis and edema (temporary) Skin necrosis Hair loss
LIPOSUCTION (SUCTION LIPECTOMY) Removal of subcutaneous fat from localized areas of accumulation such as the hips, abdomen, neck, and arms	Disproportionate distribution of adipose tissue	Hematoma Severe pain Infection Emboli Sagging of skin (if skin is not elastic enough to contract after fat removal)

cial support garments are often indicated after breast augmentation surgery to minimize edema and tension on the suture line from the weight of the breast tissue.

The nurse monitors for signs and symptoms of wound infection and progress toward healing. Of particular concern are any areas of skin necrosis or eschar formation near the operative site, a complication related to excessive tension on the suture line from edema and subsequent obstruction of microcirculation. (For a description of criteria used to monitor wound infection, see Table 67-8.)

Regardless of the planned procedure, the nurse prepares the client preoperatively for edema and discoloration of the operative site. Swelling and ecchymosis alter the facial fea-tures and may not resolve for several weeks after surgery. The client is reminded that the true results of surgery will not be visible until healing is complete, usually 6 months to a year or longer postoperatively.

OTHER SKIN DISORDERS

Acne

■ OVERVIEW

Acne is a red pustular eruption affecting the sebaceous glands of the skin. It is a common condition that, despite popular belief, is not confined to adolescents. Lesions result from in-

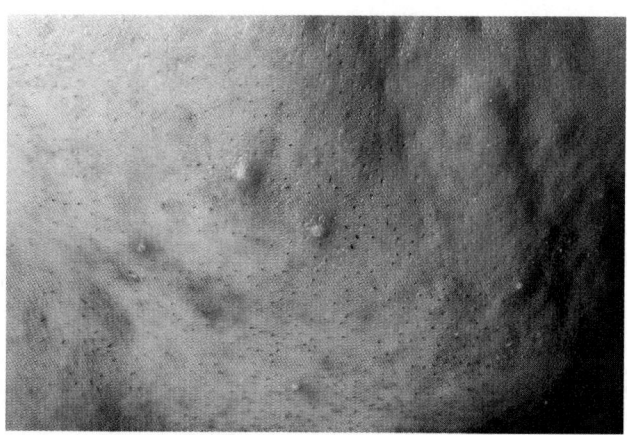

Figure 67-23 ● Acne.

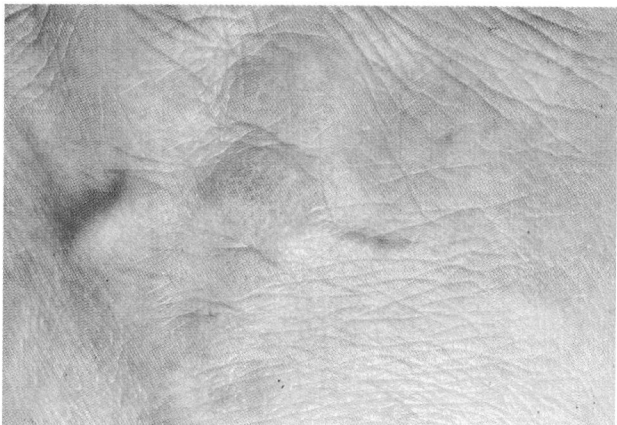

Figure 67-24 ● Lichen planus.

creased sebum production, which is stimulated by elevated androgenic hormones and obstruction of the sebaceous canal outlet. Accumulation of debris promotes bacterial growth and eventual rupture of the sebaceous gland into the surrounding dermis with inflammation.

➤ COLLABORATIVE MANAGEMENT

Acne is a progressive disorder that results in the clinical appearance of several types of lesions, including noninflammatory **comedones** (blackheads and whiteheads), inflammatory papules, pustules, and cysts. Distribution of lesions is usually limited to the face and upper trunk (Figure 67-23).

Control of the disorder is possible, with spontaneous remission occurring over time. However, severe eruptions or chronic inflammation can lead to extensive scarring.

For clients with superficial lesions and comedones, topical agents (retinoic acid, benzoyl peroxide, antibiotic solutions) are used. Systemic antibiotics, with tetracycline being the drug of choice, are indicated for those with inflammatory disease. Clients with severe acne have undergone dramatic improvement after receiving isotretinoin (Accutane, Accutane Roche✚). Side effects include elevated liver function test results; dry, chapped skin; and depression in some clients. The most important concern, however, is the teratogenic effect of systemic retinoic acid. A pregnancy test is required before therapy, and strict birth control measures must be used during therapy.

Lichen Planus
▮ OVERVIEW

Lichen planus is a fairly common skin disorder characterized by purple, flat-topped papules that are itchy. Although viral infections and emotional stress may be possible causes, lichen planus remains an idiopathic disorder. The course of the disease can be chronic, or it can resolve spontaneously.

➤ COLLABORATIVE MANAGEMENT

Lesions of lichen planus are usually distributed over the wrists and the inner surfaces of the forearms, but they may also be present on the lower legs, genitalia, and other body areas. Oral lesions may occur alone or in combination with

skin changes. Unlike the skin lesions, mucosal lesions have a characteristic white lacelike appearance; they usually occur on the buccal mucosa and are often confused with thrush (Figure 67-24).

Treatment is symptomatic. Topical steroids help to reduce inflammation, and antihistamines help to relieve itching. Occasionally, systemic steroids are prescribed when involvement is widespread, but long-term use is avoided because of the associated toxicity.

Pemphigus Vulgaris
▮ OVERVIEW

Pemphigus vulgaris is a rare, chronic blistering disease with high morbidity and mortality. It is caused by an autoimmune disorder that occurs predominantly during middle and old age.

➤ COLLABORATIVE MANAGEMENT

The acute lesions of pemphigus vulgaris occur on nonerythematous, normal-appearing skin or mucous membrane surfaces as fragile, flaccid bullae (Figure 67-25). Disruption of the bullae leaves partial-thickness wounds that bleed, weep, and eventually form crusts.

Distribution is generalized; the initial lesions usually occur on the oral mucosa; later lesions form on the trunk. Spread of the disease is characterized by the appearance of new lesions, particularly on the face and in skin fold areas, whereas older lesions are in the process of healing. Oral lesions are common and can interfere with chewing and swallowing.

Treatment of pemphigus vulgaris is aimed at suppressing the immune response that causes the blister formation. Systemic steroids and cytotoxic agents are used to bring about remission. Topical antibiotic creams or ointments are used to minimize bacterial infection of the unhealed lesions.

Toxic Epidermal Necrolysis
▮ OVERVIEW

Toxic epidermal necrolysis (TEN) is a rare, acute drug reaction of the skin characterized by diffuse erythema and bullae formation. Mucous membranes are often involved, and marked systemic toxicity is evident. The drugs most often im-

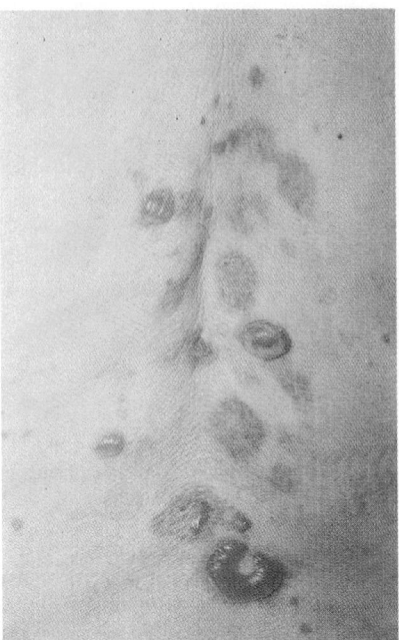

Figure 67-25 ● Pemphigus vulgaris.

plicated in triggering this disease are sulfonamides, pyrazolones, barbiturates, and antibiotics. Removal of the offending agent is usually followed by gradual healing in 2 to 3 weeks, with widespread peeling of the epidermis.

➤ COLLABORATIVE MANAGEMENT

The drug thought to be causing a toxic reaction is discontinued, and therapy is aimed at systemic support and prevention of secondary infection. Clients with TEN are often admitted to burn units, where fluid and electrolyte balance, caloric intake, and potential problems with hypothermia can be closely monitored. Topical antibacterial agents are used to suppress bacterial growth until healing occurs. Systemic steroids are not beneficial in the treatment of clients with TEN and, because of the increased risk for infection, are avoided.

Frostbite
■ OVERVIEW

Cold injury of the skin depends on the intensity of the external temperature, the duration of exposure to cold temperatures, and the relative hypoxia of the tissues at the time of exposure. Cell death occurs as a result of inadequate tissue oxygenation owing to cold-induced blood vessel constriction. With continued exposure to the cold, vascular necrosis and gangrene are imminent. Factors that increase the risk for cold injury are age, immobility, alcohol use, vascular disease, and psychiatric disorders.

➤ COLLABORATIVE MANAGEMENT

Acute frostbite is treated in the hospital setting, with rapid and continuous rewarming of the tissue in a water bath (90° to 107° F [32° to 42° C]) for 15 to 20 minutes or until flushing

of the skin occurs. Slow thawing or interrupted periods of warmth are avoided because they can contribute to increased cellular damage. Thawing can cause considerable pain, and analgesics are administered as ordered.

After thawing, the extremity is left exposed so that local tissue changes can be monitored. Blisters are left intact. With time, the degree of actual tissue destruction becomes evident as an eschar forms. After an eschar is evident, local care of the wound is similar to that for skin trauma. Complications of cold injury include amputation, scarring, depigmentation, and thickened nail plates.

Leprosy
■ OVERVIEW

Leprosy (Hansen's disease) is a chronic, contagious, systemic mycobacterial infection of the peripheral nervous system with secondary skin involvement. The clinical course of the disease is either progressive or self-limiting, depending on the immunologic status of the host. Although often thought to be extinct, Hansen's disease is found in the United States; most cases are reported in Florida, Louisiana, Texas, New York, California, and Hawaii.

The exact mechanism of transmission to a susceptible host remains unknown. Clinical studies suggest transmission via the airborne route, by insects, or through direct contact with skin lesions.

➤ COLLABORATIVE MANAGEMENT

Clinical manifestations of leprosy, including any skin changes, are directly related to the degree of individual resistance to the mycobacteria:

- Localized (high-immunity) leprosy is characterized by one or two isolated, erythematous, anesthetic plaques that are hairless and sometimes scaly in texture.
- Generalized (low-immunity) leprosy involves widespread, faintly erythematous macules, papules, nodules, and plaques.
- Varying degrees of diminished skin sensation of the lesions are caused by the concomitant peripheral nerve damage.

Modern treatment is available on an outpatient basis. The aim is to control bacterial proliferation and minimize associated physical deformities. The drug of choice is dapsone (DDS; Avlosulfon), a sulfone with relatively few side effects that clients must take for life. In clients with sulfone-resistant disease, clofazimine (Lamprene) is indicated. This drug has a slow bactericidal effect on the microorganism that causes leprosy. The major side effects include severe abdominal symptoms and skin discoloration (pink to brownish black).

NAIL DISORDERS
Ingrown Toenail
■ OVERVIEW

Although seemingly a minor problem, an ingrown toenail **(unguis incarnatus)** can be troublesome. Pain and local infection result when the edge of the nail plate grows into the soft pulp of the toe.

► COLLABORATIVE MANAGEMENT

Conservative management is aimed at controlling local infection while encouraging the nail edges to grow beyond the level of the pulp, where the nail plate can be trimmed transversely. The client soaks the foot in warm water (to which an antiseptic has been added) for 20 to 30 minutes. The softened nail plate is gently lifted, and a small piece of gauze is inserted between the nail and the flesh on each side. This procedure is repeated twice daily until the nail has grown beyond the flesh so that it can be cut.

An ingrown toenail can be treated more aggressively with surgical removal of the nail plate. However, the pain of surgical removal can be severe, and recurrence is possible if the nail bed is not completely destroyed.

ONLINE RESOURCES

For suggested readings and Internet resources, go to http://www.wbsaunders.com/SIMON/Iggy/.

SELECTED BIBLIOGRAPHY

Asterisk indicates a classic or definitive work on this subject.

Alfonso, L., & Hogan, D. (1999). Contact dermatitis for primary care providers. *Nurse Practitioner Forum, 10*(2), 67-73.

American Cancer Society. (2001). *Cancer facts and figures—2001.* Report No. 01-300M-No. 5008.01. Atlanta: Author.

Anderson, S. (1998). Laser resurfacing: A survey of pre- and postoperative care. *Plastic Surgery Nursing, 18*(4), 229-232.

Baranoski, S. (2000). Skin tears: The enemy of frail skin. *Advances in Skin and Wound Care, 13*(3), 123-126.

Beitz, J., Fey, J., & O'Brien, D. (1998). Perceived need for education vs. actual knowledge of pressure ulcer care in a hospital nursing staff. *MEDSURG Nursing, 7*(5), 293-301.

Bergstrom, N., et al. (1998). Predicting pressure ulcer risk. *Nursing Research, 47*(5), 261-269.

Bielan, B. (2000). What's your assessment? *Dermatology Nursing, 12*(5), 350-351.

Bjorgen, S. (1998). Clinical snapshot: Herpes zoster. *American Journal of Nursing, 98*(2), 46-47.

Black, J. (1999). Malignant melanoma: An update on treatments, *Plastic Surgical Nursing, 19*(3), 143-147.

Cloote, H. (2000). Psoriasis. *Nursing Standard, 14*(45), 47-42.

Cooper, D. (1999). Wound healing: New understandings. *Nurse Practitioner Forum, 10*(2), 74-86.

Crossland, M., Shawler, L., & Boykin, J. (1998). The chronic wound. *ADVANCE for Nurse Practitioners, 6*(8), 61-65.

D'Epiro, (1999). Psoriasis: New clues to causation, new ways to treat. *Patient Care for the Nurse Practitioner, 2*(5), 42-44, 46-50.

DeBoer, S., & Zeglin, D. (2001). Necrotizing fasciitis. *American Journal of Nursing, 101*(4), 37-38.

*Fewkes, J., & Mohs, F.E. (1987). Dermatologic surgery: Microscopically controlled surgical excision (the Mohs technique). In T.B. Fitzpatrick et al. (Eds.), *Dermatology in general medicine* (3rd ed., pp. 2557-2563). New York: McGraw-Hill.

Fishman, T. (2000). Wound assessment and evaluation. *Dermatology Nursing, 12*(3), 194-195.

Goolsby, M.J. (1998). The elusive itch: Assessment, diagnosis, and management of pruritus. *ADVANCE for Nurse Practitioners, 6*(11), 61-64.

Grubbs, L., & Tabano, M. (2000). Use of sunscreen in health care professionals. *Cancer Nursing, 23*(1), 164-167.

Guyton, A., & Hall, J. (2000). *Textbook of medical physiology* (10th ed.). Philadelphia: W.B. Saunders.

Hallett, C., Caress, A., & Luker, K. (2000). Wound care in the community setting: Clinical decision-making in context. *Journal of Advanced Nursing, 31*(4), 783-793.

Harris, J. (2000). A plan to promote the prevention and early detection of melanoma. *Dermatology Nursing, 12*(5), 329-333.

Henderson, C., et al. (1997). Draft definition of stage I pressure ulcers: Inclusion of persons with darkly pigmented skin. *Advances in Wound Care, 10*(5), 16-19.

Hess, C. (2000). Skin care basics. *Advances in Skin and Wound Care, 13*(3), 127-128.

Hilton, D., Williams, L., & Nesbitt, L. (2000). Systemic glucocorticosteroid therapy in dermatology. *Dermatology Nursing, 12*(4), 258-263.

Johnson, M., Maas, M., Moorhead, S. (Eds.). (2000). *Nursing outcomes classification (NOC)* (2nd ed.). St. Louis: Mosby.

Klassen, A. (1999). Problems reported by people who request cosmetic surgery. *Plastic Surgical Nursing, 19*(4), 193-197.

Lang, P. (2000). Dermatoses in African-Americans. *Dermatology Nursing, 12*(2), 87-98.

Lapka, D. (2000). Oncology today: Skin cancer. *RN, 63*(7), 32-39.

Leber, K., Perron, V., Sinni-McKeehen, B. (1999). Common skin cancers in the United States: A practical guide for diagnosis and treatment. *Nurse Practitioner Forum, 10*(2), 106-112.

Levine, N. (2000). Exfoliative erythroderma: Skin biopsy is required to determine the cause of this pruritic eruption. *Geriatrics, 55*(8), 25.

Lookingbill, D.B., & Marks, J.G., Jr. (2000). *Principles of dermatology* (3rd ed.). Philadelphia: W.B. Saunders.

Matteson, M.A. (1997). Age-related changes in the integument. In M.A. Matteson, E.S. McConnell, & A.D. Linton (Eds.), *Gerontological nursing: Concepts and practice* (2nd ed., pp. 174-195). Philadelphia: W.B. Saunders.

McCloskey, J.C., & Bulechek, G.M. (2000). *Nursing interventions classification (NIC)* (3rd ed.). St. Louis: Mosby.

McKay, S. (2000). Why we need to worry about warts. *RN, 63*(9), 68-72.

Moss, R., Moss, C., & Broadway, D. (2000). Body contouring with ultrasound-assisted lipoplasty. *AORN Journal, 71*(2), 370-385.

Motta, G. (1997). Setting the stage for healing. *Continuing Care, 16*(3), 14-18.

Motta, G. (2000). Reimbursement relief. *Continuing Care, 19*(4), 14-16.

Nicol, N., & Boguniewicz, M. (1999). Understanding and treating atopic dermatitis. *Nurse Practitioner Forum, 10*(2), 48-55.

Palmisano, C., & Norman, R. (2000). Geriatric dermatology in chronic care and rehabilitation. *Dermatology Nursing, 12*(2), 116-123.

Peters, J. (2000). Toxic epidermal necrolysis. *Nursing Times, 96*(36), 43-44.

Pieper, B. (1998). Pressure ulcer management. *ADVANCE for Nurse Practitioners, 6*(10), 55-59.

Pirrung, M. (2001). Management of toxic epidermal necrolysis. *Journal of Intravenous Nursing, 24*(2), 107-113.

Rapaport, M. (2000). Eyelid dermatitis. *Dermatology Nursing, 12*(5), 352-354.

Rayner, V. (2000). Cosmetic rehabilitation. *Dermatology Nursing, 12*(4), 267-271.

Rivera, E., Walsh, A., & Bradley, M. (2000). Using behavior modification to promote wound healing. *Home Healthcare Nurse, 18*(9), 579-586.

Scholl, D., & Langkamp-Henken, B. (2001). Nutrient recommendations for wound healing. *Journal of Intravenous Nursing, 24*(2), 124-132.

Sheppard, C., & Brenner, P. (2000). The effects of bathing and skin care practices on skin quality and satisfaction with an innovative product. *Journal of Gerontological Nursing, 25*(10), 36-45.

Sibbald, G., et al. (2000). Preparing the wound bed: Debridement, bacterial balance, and moisture balance. *Ostomy Wound Management, 46*(11), 14-35.

*U.S. Department of Health and Human Services. (1992a). *Pressure ulcers in adults: Prediction and prevention. Clinical Practice Guideline No. 3.* Rockville, MD: Agency for Health Care Policy and Research, Public Health Service, U.S. Department of Health and Human Services.

*U.S. Department of Health and Human Services. (1992b). *Preventing pressure ulcers: A patient's guide. Clinical Practice Guideline No. 3.* Rockville, MD: Agency for Health Care Policy and Research, Public Health Service, U.S. Department of Health and Human Services.

United States Pharmacopeia Dispensing Information (USP DI): Vol. I. Drug information for the health care professional (20th ed.). (2000). Englewood, CO: Micromedix.

Whitney, J., & Heitkemper, M. (1999). Modifying perfusion, nutrition, and stress to promote wound healing in patients with acute wounds. *Heart and Lung, 28*(2), 123-133.

Interventions for Clients with Burns

ERIC MARSH

Learning Objectives

After studying this chapter, you should be able to:

1. Identify burn clients at risk for inhalation injury.
2. Compare and contrast the clinical manifestations of superficial, partial-thickness, and full-thickness burn injuries.
3. Explain the expected clinical manifestations of neural and hormonal compensation during the emergent phase of burn injury.
4. Calculate the total body surface area involved in a burn injury.
5. Prioritize nursing care for the client during the emergent phase of burn injury.
6. Use laboratory data and clinical manifestations to determine the effectiveness of fluid resuscitation during the emergent phase of burn injury.
7. Use the Parkland formula to establish the correct rate and timing of fluid replacement.
8. Prioritize nursing care for the client during the acute phase of burn injury.
9. Explain the alteration of nutritional needs for the burn client during the acute phase of burn injury.
10. Evaluate wound healing in the client during the acute phase of burn injury.
11. Compare and contrast pain management strategies for clients in the emergent and acute phases of burn injury.
12. Describe the characteristics of infected burn wounds.
13. Explain the positioning and range-of-motion interventions for the prevention of mobility problems in the client with burns.
14. Prioritize nursing care for the client during the rehabilitation phase of burn injury.
15. Discuss the potential psychosocial problems associated with burn injury.

SIMON

Go to http://www.wbsaunders.com/SIMON/Iggy/ for self-assessment questions related to these Learning Objectives.

Burn injuries of the skin and other tissues cause clients to experience many physiologic, metabolic, and psychologic changes. Burn injuries can range from a minor loss of small segments of the outermost layers of the skin to complex injuries involving all layers of the skin. When the skin is injured, significant fluid loss and large inflammatory responses result in altered function in most, if not all, body systems. The burn client requires complex, comprehensive care for weeks to months in order to survive the injury, reduce complications, and return to his or her best possible functional status. Collaboration with a multidisciplinary team of health care providers is essential to ensure optimal care and improve client outcomes.

INTRODUCTION TO THE BURN PROBLEM
Pathophysiology of Burn Injury

The tissue destruction caused by a burn injury can cause many local and systemic problems, including fluid and protein losses, sepsis, and disturbances of the metabolic, endocrine,

respiratory, cardiac, hematologic, and immune systems. The extent of local and systemic disruption is related to many factors, including age, general health status, extent of injury, depth of injury, and area of body injured. Even after healing, the burn injury can cause late complications such as contracture formation and extensive scarring. Therefore the prevention of infection and closure of the burn wound are vitally important. A lack of or delay in healing is a key factor for all systemic disturbances and is responsible for much morbidity and mortality among clients who are burned.

▇ INTEGUMENTARY CHANGES RESULTING FROM BURN INJURY
▇ Anatomic Changes

The skin is the largest organ of the body (see Chapter 66). Each of its two major layers, the epidermis and dermis, has several sublayers. The epidermis, the outer layer of skin, is a superficial layer of stratified epithelial tissues approximately

0.15 mm thick (somewhat thinner in older adults and younger children). This layer can regenerate after a significant injury because the epidermal cells surrounding sweat and oil glands and hair follicles extend into dermal tissue and are responsible for the healing of partial-thickness wounds. Collectively, the sweat and oil glands and the hair follicles are referred to as **dermal appendages.** The depth of the dermal appendages varies considerably across body areas. The sweat and oil glands in the palm of the hand and the sole of the foot, for example, extend deep into the dermis. This allows for healing of fairly deep burns in these areas. The epidermis has no blood vessels and receives nutrients by diffusion from the second layer of skin, the dermis.

The basement membrane, a thin noncellular protein surface, separates the dermis from the epidermis. The dermis is sometimes called the "true skin" because it is not constantly shed and replaced; it is thicker than the epidermis and ranges in thickness from 0.60 to 1.2 mm. The dermis makes up the bulk of the skin and is composed of collagen meshes, fibrous connective tissue, and elastic fibers. Within the dermis are the functional elements of the skin: blood vessels, sensory nerves, hair follicles, lymph vessels, sebaceous glands, and sweat glands.

When burn injury occurs, the skin can regenerate as long as parts of the dermis are present. When the entire layer of dermis is burned, all epithelial cells or dermal appendages are destroyed, and the skin can no longer regenerate spontaneously. The subcutaneous tissue, or superficial fascia, varies in thickness and lies below the dermis. With deep burns, the subcutaneous tissues may be damaged, leaving bones, tendons, and muscles exposed.

Functional Changes

The skin serves multiple functions (see Table 66-1). The skin is primarily a protective barrier against injury and microbial invasion from the environment. A burn injury breaks this barrier, greatly increasing the risk for infection.

The skin also helps maintain the delicate fluid and electrolyte balance essential for life. After a burn injury, massive fluid loss occurs through evaporation. Water vapor can evaporate through burn-injured skin four times as rapidly as from intact skin. The rate of evaporation is proportional to the total body surface area burned and the depth of injury.

Skin is important in thermoregulation. Normally the body can adjust to most fluctuations in environmental temperatures because subcutaneous fat provides insulation and because blood flow to the skin changes with these fluctuations in environmental temperature. When the skin is damaged, the body cannot adjust to the loss of heat as readily, and body temperature tends to decrease.

The skin functions as an excretory organ through perspiration. Full-thickness burns destroy the sweat glands, which results in a loss of excretory ability.

The skin is the largest sensory organ of the body. Pain, pressure, temperature, and touch are sensed on the skin in normal daily activities, which allows a person to react to changes in the environment. All burn injuries are painful. With partial-thickness burns, nerve endings are exposed to the surface, which causes an increased sensitivity and a subsequent increase in pain. With full-thickness burns, nerve endings are completely destroyed. Initially these wounds are completely **anesthetic** (do not transmit sensation) when a sharp stimulus is applied. Despite this destruction, clients often complain of a dull or pressure-type of pain in these areas.

Skin exposed to sunlight produces vitamin D. The conversion of cholesterol derivatives into the active form of vitamin D is completed in the skin. Partial-thickness burns reduce the activation of vitamin D; this conversion is lost completely in full-thickness burns.

The skin is an important determinant of physical identity. The skin's cosmetic quality contributes to each person's unique appearance. With a change in appearance through a major burn, severe psychologic problems may develop.

■ TEMPERATURE

The temperature of the body's internal environment falls within a narrow range (approximately 84.2° to 109.4° F [29° to 43° C]) compared with the wide temperature fluctuations in the external environment. The body has several mechanisms to compensate for wide variations in external temperature. Circulating blood both provides and dissipates heat. Heat dissipation is efficient under normal conditions. When heat is applied to the skin, the temperature of the immediate subdermal layer rises rapidly. As soon as the heat source is removed, the body's compensatory mechanisms quickly return the area to a normal temperature. If the heat source is not removed, or if it is applied at a rate or level that exceeds the skin's capacity to dissipate it, cellular destruction occurs.

The skin can tolerate temperatures up to 104° F (40° C) without sustaining injury. At temperatures of 158° F (70° C) and above, cell destruction is so rapid that brief periods of exposure damage the skin down to and including the subcutaneous level. Figure 68-1 shows the relationship between temperature and exposure time for an experimental model of burn injury.

■ DEPTH OF BURN INJURY

The magnitude of a burn injury is based on the depth and extent of the total body surface burn. The degree of tissue destruction is determined by what agent specifically caused the burn and by the temperature and duration of exposure to the heat source.

Variations in skin thickness over different parts of the body also influence burn depth. In areas where the epidermis and dermis are thin (e.g., eyelids, ears, nose, genitalia, tops of the hands and feet, fingers, and toes), a short exposure to extreme temperatures can result in a deep burn injury. The skin is thinner in older adults, which predisposes them to increased burn severity, even at lower temperatures of shorter duration.

Burn wounds are classified as superficial-thickness wounds, partial-thickness wounds, full-thickness wounds, and deep full-thickness wounds. The partial-thickness wounds are further separated into superficial and deep subgroups. Table 68-1 characterizes the clinical differences of these burns.

The American Burn Association (ABA) describes burns as minor, moderate, or major depending on the depth, extent, and location of injury (Table 68-2). Figure 68-2 shows specific tissue layers involved with different depths of injury and describes the criteria for referral to a burn center.

SUPERFICIAL-THICKNESS WOUNDS. Of all burn types, superficial-thickness wounds have the least destruction because the epidermis is the only portion of the skin that is injured. The basal epithelial cells and basement membrane—structures necessary for the total regeneration of epithelial cells—remain present.

Superficial-thickness wounds often result from prolonged exposure to low-intensity heat (e.g., sunburn) or short (flash) exposure to high-intensity heat. Erythema with mild edema,

pain, and increased sensitivity to heat occurs as a result. Peeling of dead skin (**desquamation**) occurs for 2 to 3 days after the burn, and the area rapidly heals in 3 to 5 days without a scar. No significant clinical consequences occur at this level of injury.

PARTIAL-THICKNESS WOUNDS. A partial-thickness wound involves the entire epidermis and varying depths of the dermis. Depending on the amount of dermal tissue damaged, partial-thickness wounds are further subdivided into superficial partial-thickness and deep partial-thickness injuries.

SUPERFICIAL PARTIAL-THICKNESS WOUNDS. Superficial partial-thickness wounds result from either increased duration or increased intensity of exposure. These wounds are typically erythematous and moist (Figure 68-3). The classic **vesicle** (blister) forms as the stratum corneum and stratum granulosum are destroyed. When intact, the blister forms a sterile environment, which protects the wound from potential infection and excess water loss. However, large or numerous blisters are opened to promote healing and prevent immunosuppression.

Superficial partial-thickness wounds result in increased pain sensation. Nerve endings are exposed to the surface, and any stimulation (touch or temperature change) causes intense pain. With standard treatment these burns heal in 10 to 14 days with no scar, but some minor pigment changes may occur.

DEEP PARTIAL-THICKNESS WOUNDS. Deep partial-thickness wounds extend deeper into the dermal layer of the skin, and fewer healthy epidermal cells remain. The wounds usually appear red and waxy white without blisters (Figure 68-4). Edema is moderate; pain is present to a lesser degree than with superficial burns because more of the nerve endings have been destroyed. Blisters are absent because the dead tissues adhere to the underlying dermal collagen fibers.

The remaining blood supply to these areas is greatly reduced due to intense vasoconstriction. Progression to deeper injury can occur through hypoxia and ischemia. Ad-

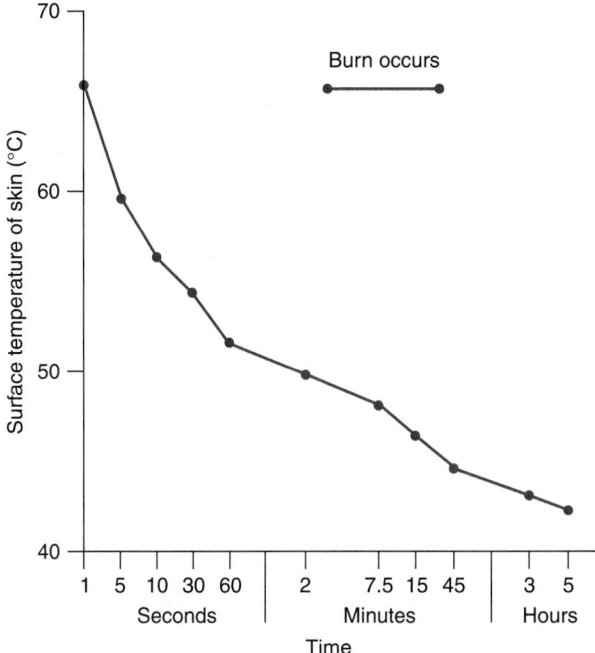

Figure 68-1 ● Relationship between intensity of heat and duration of exposure. Exposure for prolonged periods causes burns, even with milder temperatures. At more extreme temperatures, tissue damage results after only seconds. (Modified from Moritz, A.R. [1947]. Studies of thermal injuries: II. The relative importance of time and surface temperature in causation of cutaneous burns. *American Journal of Pathology, 23,* 695.)

TABLE 68-1 ● CLASSIFICATION OF BURN DEPTH

Characteristic	Superficial	Partial-Thickness Superficial	Deep Partial-Thickness	Full-Thickness	Deep Full-Thickness
Color	Pink to red	Pink to red	Red to white	Black, brown, yellow, white, red	Black
Edema	Mild	Mild to moderate	Moderate	Severe	Absent
Pain	Yes	Yes	Yes	Yes and no	Absent
Blisters	No	Yes	Rare	No	No
Eschar	No	No	Yes, soft and dry	Yes, hard and inelastic	Yes, hard and inelastic
Healing time	3-5 days	~2 wk	2-6 wk	Weeks to months	Weeks to months
Grafts required	No	No	Can be used if healing is prolonged	Yes	Yes
Example	Sunburn, flash burns	Scalds, flames, brief contact with hot objects	Scalds; flames; prolonged contact with hot objects, tar, grease, chemicals	Scalds; flames; prolonged contact with hot objects, tar, grease, chemicals, electricity	Flames, electricity, grease, tar, chemicals

TABLE 68-2 • CLASSIFICATION OF BURN INJURY AND BURN CENTER REFERRAL CRITERIA

Characteristics	Comments
MINOR BURNS Deep partial-thickness burns <15% TBSA Full-thickness burns <2% TBSA No burns of eyes, ears, face, hands, feet, or perineum No electrical burns No inhalation injury No complicated concomitant injury Patient is under 60 yr and has no chronic cardiac, pulmonary, or endocrine disorder	Clients in this category should receive emergency care at the scene and be taken to a hospital emergency department. A special expertise hospital or designated burn center is not necessary.
MODERATE BURNS Deep partial-thickness burns 15%-25% TBSA Full-thickness burns 2%-10% TBSA No burns of eyes, ears, face, hands, feet, or perineum No electrical burns No inhalation injury No complicated concomitant injury Patient is under 60 yr and has no chronic cardiac, pulmonary, or endocrine disorder	Clients in this category should receive emergency care at the scene and be transferred either to a special expertise hospital or to a designated burn center.
MAJOR BURNS Partial-thickness burns >25% TBSA Full-thickness burns >10% Any burn involving the eyes, ears, face, hands, feet, perineum Electrical injury Inhalation injury Client over 60 yr of age Burn is complicated with other injuries (e.g., fractures) Client has cardiac, pulmonary, or other chronic metabolic disorders	Clients who meet *any one* of the criteria for a major burn should receive emergency care at the nearest emergency department and then be transferred to a designated burn center as soon as possible.

TBSA, Total body surface area.

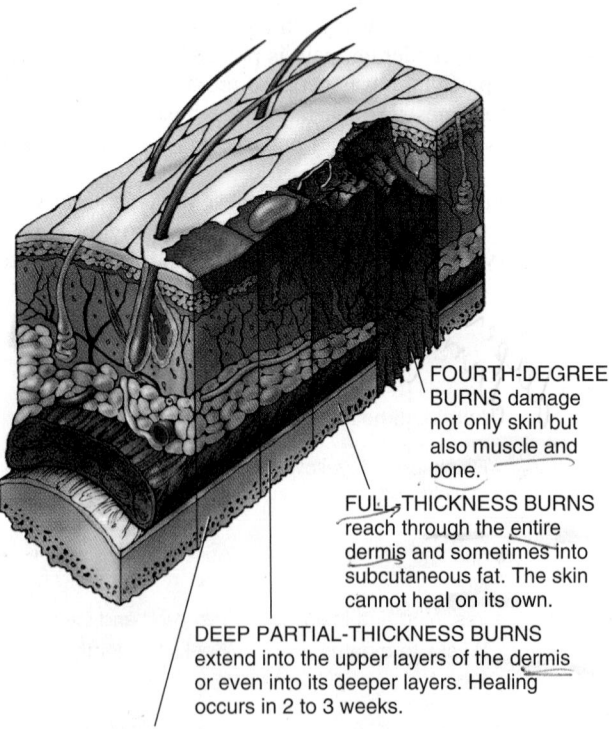

FOURTH-DEGREE BURNS damage not only skin but also muscle and bone.

FULL-THICKNESS BURNS reach through the entire dermis and sometimes into subcutaneous fat. The skin cannot heal on its own.

DEEP PARTIAL-THICKNESS BURNS extend into the upper layers of the dermis or even into its deeper layers. Healing occurs in 2 to 3 weeks.

SUPERFICIAL PARTIAL-THICKNESS BURNS are those in which the epidermis is the only layer of skin destroyed. Uncomplicated healing occurs in 3 to 5 days.

Figure 68-2 ● The tissue involved in burns of various depths.

equate hydration, nutrients, and oxygen are necessary for spontaneous re-epithelialization of the wound and the prevention of conversion to deeper burns. Partial-thickness wounds can convert to full-thickness wounds when tissue damage increases with infection, hypoxia, or ischemia. Deep partial-thickness wounds generally heal in 3 to 6 weeks, but a large amount of scar formation results. Surgical intervention with skin grafting is required if healing will be prolonged.

FULL-THICKNESS WOUNDS. A full-thickness wound involves the entire epidermal and dermal layers of the skin (Figure 68-5). No living **(viable)** epidermal cells remain for re-epithelialization, and skin grafts are required in areas larger than approximately 12 to 16 cm^2. In smaller areas, secondary wound closure occurs by the growth of collagen-based scar tissue from the unburned edges inward (see Chapter 67).

The area of full-thickness injury has a hard, dry, leathery **eschar** (burn crust) that forms from coagulated particles of destroyed dermis. *The eschar is dead tissue; it must slough off or be removed from the burn wound before healing can occur.* The thick, coagulated particles often adhere to the subcutaneous layer by collagen fibers, which makes the removal of eschar difficult. Edema is a significant problem in burns and is pronounced under the eschar in a full-thickness wound. When the injury completely surrounds an extremity or the thorax **(circumferential),** circulation and ventilation may be compromised by tight eschar. **Escharotomies** (incisions through the eschar) or **fasciotomies** (incisions through eschar

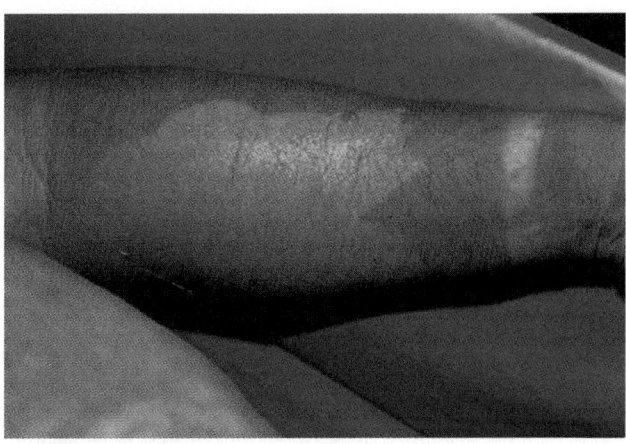

Figure 68-3 ● The typical appearance of a superficial partial-thickness burn injury.

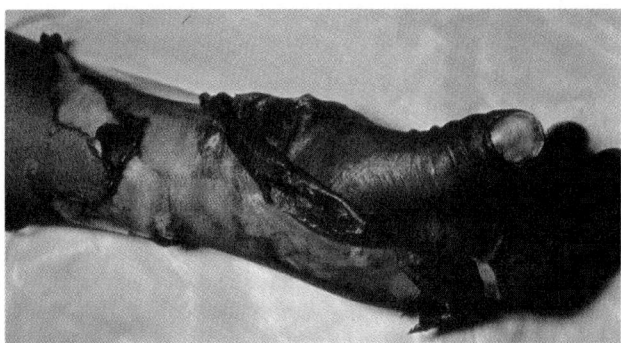

Figure 68-5 ● The typical appearance of a full-thickness burn injury.

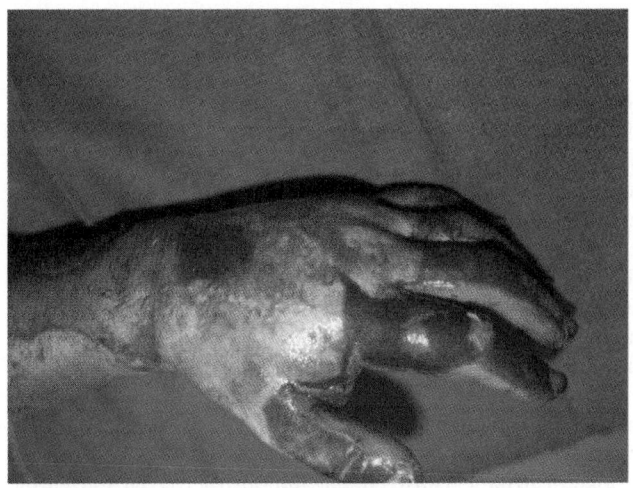

Figure 68-4 ● The typical appearance of a deep partial-thickness burn injury.

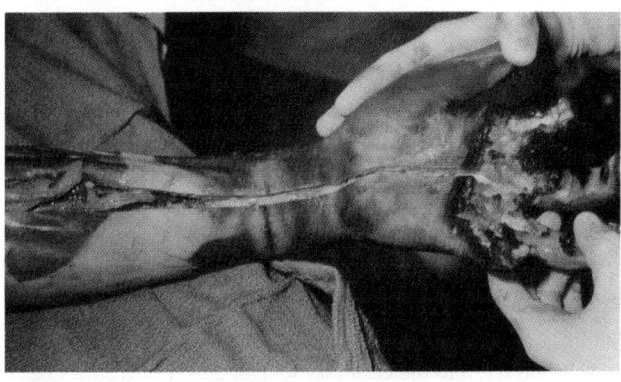

Figure 68-6 ● The typical appearance of a deep full-thickness burn injury.

and fascia) may be required to relieve pressure and allow normal perfusion and breathing (see Surgical Management [Ineffective Tissue Perfusion], p. 1572).

The color of a full-thickness burn wound may be waxy white, deep red, yellow, brown, or black. Thrombosed vessels may be present and visible beneath the surface of the burn because the dermal blood vessels are heat coagulated, causing the burned tissue to be without a blood supply **(avascular).** Sensation is minimal or absent in these areas of injury due to the destruction of nerve endings. Healing time depends on the re-establishment of an adequate blood supply within the injured areas and can range from weeks to months.

DEEP FULL-THICKNESS WOUNDS. Deep full-thickness wounds extend beyond the skin into underlying fascia and tissues. These deep injuries damage muscle, bone, and tendons and leave them exposed to the surface. These burns occur with flame, electrical, or chemical injuries. The wound is blackened and depressed, and sensation is completely absent (Figure 68-6). All full-thickness burns benefit from early excision and grafting. Grafting decreases

pain and length of stay and accelerates recovery (Ramzy et al., 1999). Amputation may be required when an extremity is involved.

◼ VASCULAR CHANGES RESULTING FROM BURN INJURIES

Major circulatory disruption occurs at the burn site immediately after a burn injury. The vessels supplying the burned skin are occluded, and blood flow through the arterial and venous channels decreases or ceases completely. Damaged macrophages within the tissues release chemicals (mediators) that initially produce vasoconstriction. Peripheral vessel thrombosis may occur; this decrease in tissue perfusion can cause necrosis, which can lead to deeper injuries in the already damaged areas.

◼ Fluid Shift

After the initial vasoconstriction, vessels adjacent to the burn injury dilate. This leads to increased capillary hydrostatic pressure and is accompanied by increased capillary permeability (Figure 68-7). This fluid shift, also known as *third spacing* or *capillary leak syndrome,* involves a continuous leak of plasma from the intravascular space into the interstitial space. The loss of plasma fluids and proteins results in a decreased colloidal osmotic pressure in the vascular space. Leakage of fluid and electrolytes from the vascular space continues, causing significant edema formation. Fluid shift usually occurs in the first 12 hours after the burn but can continue for 24 to 36 hours.

The amount of plasma to interstitial fluid shift depends on the extent and severity of injury. Capillary leak occurs in both burned and unburned tissues when tissue damage is extensive (i.e., greater than 20% to 30% total body surface area [**TBSA**]). Peripheral edema develops as the protein-rich fluids, plasma, and electrolytes escape into the interstitial space. Tissue colloidal osmotic pressure increases as a result of the movement of proteins, increasing the third-spacing fluid shift.

Profound imbalances of fluid, electrolytes, and acid-base occur as a result of the fluid shift and other physiologic disruptions caused by injury. These imbalances usually include hypovolemia, metabolic acidosis, **hyperkalemia** (elevated blood potassium levels), and **hyponatremia** (decreased blood sodium levels). Hyperkalemia occurs as a result of direct tissue damage that releases large amounts of intracellular potassium into the vascular space; it is generally self-limiting. **Hemoconcentration** (elevated blood osmolarity, hematocrit, and hemoglobin) develops from the circulatory dehydration. Hemoconcentration increases blood viscosity, which reduces flow through small vessels and contributes to generalized tissue hypoxia.

Fluid Remobilization

The inflammatory responses gradually subside 24 to 36 hours after the injury, and the capillary leak abates. Fluid shifts back into the circulation. This fluid remobilization phase restores fluid and electrolyte levels and renal blood flow, resulting in increased urine formation and diuresis. Body weight returns to normal over several days as peripheral edema subsides.

During this phase, hyponatremia is likely to develop because of increased renal sodium excretion and the loss of sodium from wounds. Hypokalemia can occur now as potassium returns to the intracellular compartment. Anemia often develops as a result of hemodilution, but it is generally not severe enough to require blood transfusions. Transfusions are

indicated if the client's hematocrit is less than 20% to 25% and is accompanied by clinical signs and symptoms of hypoxia. The exact laboratory value is not as critical as the clinical signs and symptoms. The timing of transfusions is controversial, and the trend is to limit transfusion unless absolutely necessary.

CARDIAC FUNCTION CHANGES RESULTING FROM BURN INJURY

Because of the initial fluid shifts and hypovolemia that occur after a burn injury, cardiac output decreases in spite of an increased heart rate. Cardiac output may remain depressed until 18 to 36 hours after the burn injury occurs. Cardiac output increases with adequate fluid resuscitation and reaches normal levels before plasma volume is restored completely. Appropriate fluid resuscitation and support with adequate oxygenation prevent further complications.

PULMONARY CHANGES RESULTING FROM BURN INJURY

Respiratory insufficiency (inhalation injury) rarely occurs from direct contact with flames but is caused by superheated air, steam, toxic fumes, or smoke. It is a major cause of morbidity and mortality in thermally injured clients. Pulmonary complications cause or contribute to death in 77% of clients with a combined inhalation and cutaneous burn injury (Flynn, 1999). Respiratory failure associated with burn injuries can also result from airway edema during fluid resuscitation, increased alveolar capillary permeability, circumferential chest burns that compromise breathing, and carbon monoxide toxicity.

Damage to the respiratory system from an inhalation injury can occur in the upper and major airways and the lung parenchyma. The upper airway is affected when inhaled smoke or irritants cause edema and obstructive closure of the trachea. Irritants coming in contact with the upper airway cause a reflex closure of the vocal cords. This protective mechanism results in a decrease in the amount of smoke and toxic gases entering the lungs. Although air is a poor conductor of heat, some heat does reach the upper airway, causing an inflammatory response that leads to oropharyngeal edema and potentially dangerous airway obstruction.

Major airway injury results from chemicals and toxic gases, rather than heat, that are produced from incomplete combustion. The ciliated, mucus-secreting epithelial cells lin-

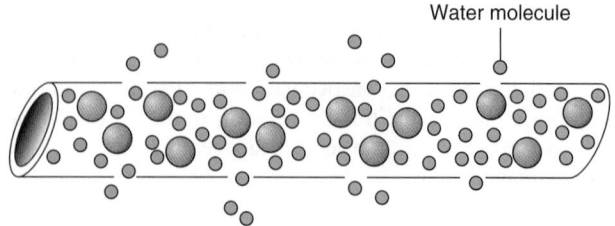

NORMAL BLOOD CAPILLARY

Water molecule

Water is the smallest molecule that can pass through the capillary pores.

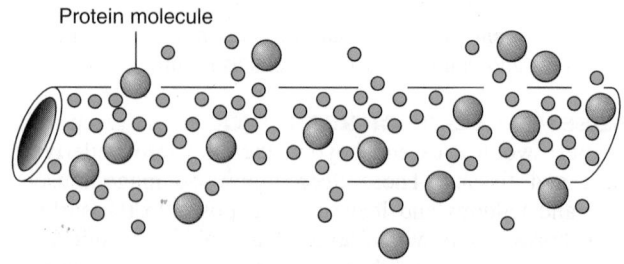

POSTBURN BLOOD CAPILLARY

Protein molecule

Permeability is drastically increased, which allows large molecules such as proteins to pass through the capillary pores easily.

Figure 68-7 ● The vascular capillary response to burn injury (early phase).

ing the trachea normally trap bacteria and foreign materials. Smoke and products of combustion slow this activity, which allows foreign particles to enter the bronchi. The lining of the trachea and bronchi may slough 48 to 72 hours after injury, enter the airway, narrow the tracheal lumen, and obstruct the lower airways.

Parenchymal injuries result from damage to the alveolar epithelium and capillary endothelium by toxic irritants. Increased alveolar-capillary membrane permeability results in intra-alveolar edema. This edema can occur immediately or as late as 1 week after the injury. The fluid that diffuses across the membrane settles in the interstitial spaces; fibrinous membranes eventually form, which leads to respiratory distress. Progressive pulmonary failure develops with acute pulmonary insufficiency and infection.

■ GASTROINTESTINAL CHANGES RESULTING FROM BURN INJURY

Because of the fluid shifts and decreased cardiac output that occur after injury, blood flow is shifted to the brain, heart, and liver. Consequently other organs, including the gastrointestinal (GI) tract, have decreased perfusion. Gastric mucosal integrity and motility are impaired. The sympathetic nervous system stress response causes increased secretion of catecholamines (especially epinephrine and norepinephrine), which inhibit GI motility and reduce the flow of blood to the area. Peristalsis decreases, and a paralytic ileus may develop. Mucosal secretions and gases collect in the intestines and stomach, causing abdominal distention.

Curling's ulcer, or acute ulcerative gastroduodenal disease, may develop within 24 hours after a severe burn injury because of reduced GI perfusion and mucosal damage. The mucosal membrane normally acts as a barrier to the absorption of hydrogen ions secreted into the gastric lumen. With an alteration in gastric mucosal function, this barrier is compromised and hydrogen ion production is increased. Ulcerations may develop as a result. However, this complication has become extremely uncommon in recent years because of the use of H_2 histamine blockers such as cimetidine (Tagamet) and ranitidine (Zantac), mucoprotectants such as sucralfate (Carafate), and early enteral nutrition.

■ METABOLIC CHANGES RESULTING FROM BURN INJURY

A significant burn injury places the client in a hypermetabolic state. Increased secretion of catecholamines, antidiuretic hormone, aldosterone, and cortisol increase metabolism. With hypermetabolism, oxygen and calorie requirements are high.

The secreted catecholamines activate the stress response. The increased production (and loss) of heat results in protein and fat breakdown **(catabolism),** the rapid use of glucose and calories, and increased urinary nitrogen losses. The evaporated heat and water from the burn also increase metabolic and catabolic rates, which increase calorie expenditure. Depending on the extent of injury, the client's calorie requirements may be double or triple normal energy needs. These increased rates peak 4 to 12 days after the burn and can remain elevated for months until all wounds are closed.

The hypermetabolic condition also results in an increase in core body temperature. The client loses heat through the burned skin surfaces because the protective barrier is lost. Core body temperature increases as a response to the adjustment in the hypothalamus. Central thermoregulation is altered to compensate for the hypermetabolic state. There is an impaired shift in temperature; a low-grade fever can develop, which is common among clients with burn injuries. Essentially what occurs is a resetting of the body's normal temperature-regulating mechanism.

■ IMMUNOLOGIC CHANGES RESULTING FROM BURN INJURY

Thermal injury results in a loss of the protective barrier of the skin, which increases the risk for infection. The burn injury activates the inflammatory response but can also suppress immune function (see Chapter 20). Antibody-mediated immunity and cell-mediated immunity are both suppressed. All immune responses are therefore reduced. Topical antimicrobial agents, systemic antibiotics, general anesthesia, blood component transfusion, and the stress of surgical procedures further compromise immune function.

■ COMPENSATORY RESPONSES TO BURN INJURY

Any tissue injury is a threat to homeostasis and is a physiologic stressor. Two compensatory responses have immediate benefit: the inflammatory response and the sympathetic nervous system stress response. Together these responses cause the physiologic changes that result in many of the clinical manifestations seen in the first 2 to 3 days after a burn injury.

■ Inflammatory Compensation

The inflammatory compensatory response can be helpful by initiating healing in the injured tissues. It also is responsible for some of the serious problems that occur with the fluid shift. Inflammatory compensation causes blood vessels to leak fluid into the interstitial space and white blood cells to release chemicals that generate local tissue reactions. The inflammatory compensatory mechanisms cause the massive fluid shift, edema formation, and hypovolemia that characterize the emergent phase (first 48 hours) after a burn injury. The extent and intensity of the inflammatory response depend on the severity of the burn injury. Chapter 20 explains the inflammatory compensatory mechanisms in detail.

The inflammatory compensatory response is immediately helpful to the body when injury occurs. These actions are intended to function on a relatively local and short-term basis. When these actions are widespread and/or persistent, the tissue-damaging consequences can be severe.

■ Sympathetic Nervous System Compensation

The sympathetic nervous system stress response is generated by the sympathetic division of the autonomic nervous system and some components of the endocrine system when any physical or psychologic stressors are present. Changes resulting from sympathetic compensation are most evident in the cardiovascular, respiratory, and gastrointestinal systems. Fig-

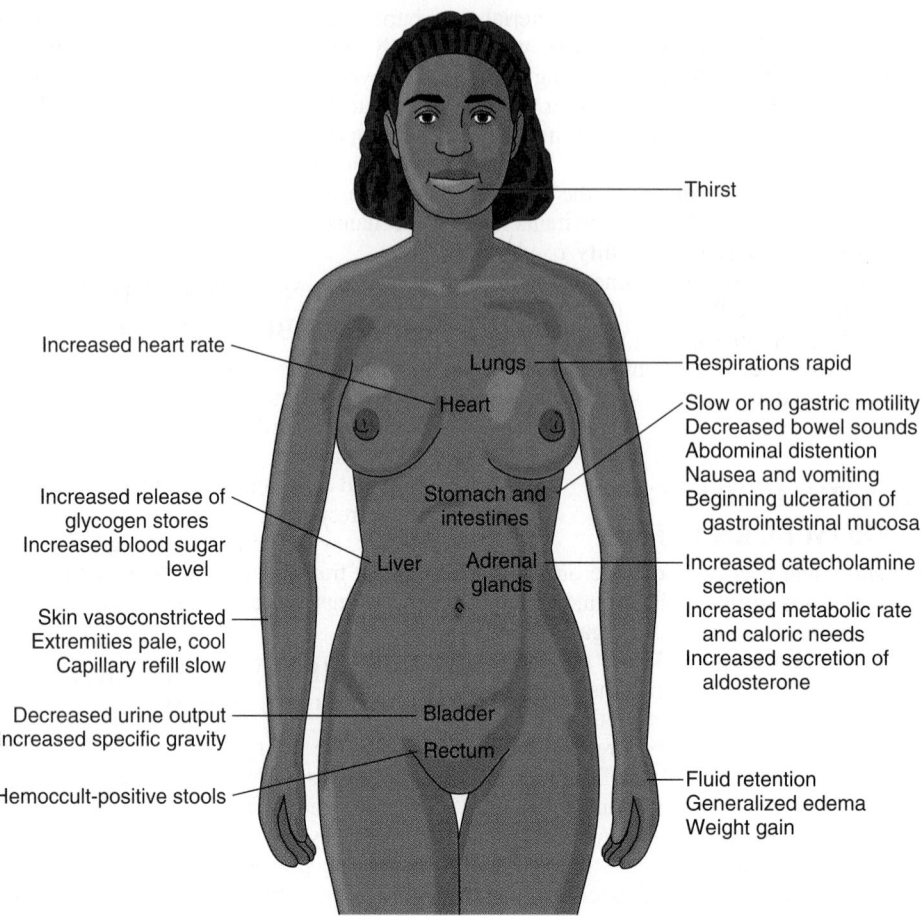

Figure 68-8 ● The physiologic actions of the sympathetic nervous system compensatory responses to burn injury (early phase).

ure 68-8 summarizes the physical consequence of sympathetic nervous system stimulation.

Etiology of Burn Injury

Burn injuries are caused by a variety of sources, including dry heat (flame), moist heat (scald), contact with hot surfaces, chemicals, electricity, and ionizing radiation. The causative agent of the injury affects both the prognosis and the treatment.

DRY HEAT

Dry heat injuries are caused by open flame. The most common causes of flame injuries are house fires and explosions. Ignited clothing from an open flame accounts for most of the injuries. Explosions usually result in flash burns because they produce a brief exposure to very high temperatures.

MOIST HEAT

Moist heat (scald) injuries are caused by contact with hot liquids. Scald injuries are most common among adults older than 65 years (Stone, Ahmed, & Evans, 2000). Hot liquid spills usually burn the upper, frontal surfaces of the body,

whereas immersion scald injuries usually involve the lower portions of the body.

CONTACT BURNS

Hot metal, tar, and grease can cause full-thickness burns when they contact the skin. Hot metal injuries occur when a client places a part of the body against a hot surface, such as a space heater or iron. They also can occur in industrial settings from molten metals. Tar and asphalt temperatures usually are greater than 400° F, and significant deep injuries occur within seconds when the skin is immersed in or splashed with the agent. Hot grease injuries result from cooking agents and are usually deep because of the temperature of the grease.

CHEMICAL INJURY

A burn injury occurs when chemicals come in direct contact with the skin and epithelial tissues or are ingested. The severity of the injury depends on the duration of contact, the concentration of the chemical, the amount of tissue exposed, and the mechanisms of action of the chemical.

Chemical burns to the skin usually occur in adults in industrial settings, but they may also occur in the home from contact with products such as drain cleaner and toilet bowl cleaner.

Strong acids (e.g., hydrochloric acid, sulfuric acid) and strong alkalis (e.g., sodium hydroxide) destroy tissue by precipitation of chemical compounds in the cell, cellular dehydration, protoplasmic poisoning, and dissolution of tissue proteins. Acids cause coagulation necrosis and pain. Alkalis cause liquefaction necrosis, with deeper penetration and less pain.

ELECTRICAL INJURY

An electrical injury is considered a nonthermally induced burn; it is caused when an electrical current enters the body (Figure 68-9). Electrical injuries are serious because they damage deep structures and organs and can even result in the loss of one or more limbs. The amount of damage depends on amperage, voltage, resistance to flow, type of current, duration of contact, and the current's path through the body.

Resistance (impedance to flow) varies in different parts of the body. Nerve, muscle, and blood vessels have very low resistance and are susceptible to deep injuries. Tendons, fat, and bone have the most resistance. Skin has intermediate resistance. Wet skin has less resistance to current flow than dry, calloused areas. The higher the resistance, the greater the heat generated by the current flow and the greater the potential for soft-tissue injury.

The longer the electricity is in contact with the body, the greater the damage. The duration of contact may be increased by tetanic contractions of the strong flexor muscles in the forearm, which can prevent the person from releasing the electrical source. Severe tetanic muscle contractions have been associated with fractures of the spine and long bones, necessitating immobilization of the client with a cervical collar and backboard.

It is difficult to know the exact path a current takes in the body. The course of flow is generally defined by the locations of the "entrance" and "exit" wounds. Initially, the wounds may not be obvious. When visible, the entrance site is usually well defined and rounded. The exit site is usually explosive and surrounded by charred tissue.

Burn injuries from electricity can occur in one of three ways: *thermal burns, flash burns,* or *true electrical injury.* Thermal burns may occur when clothes ignite from heat or flames produced by electrical sparks. External burn injuries can occur when the electrical current jumps, or "arcs," between two charged surfaces. Injuries usually are severe and deep and are associated with high-tension current. True electrical injury can occur when the body makes direct contact with an electrical source. Internal damage results, and the injuries can be devastating. Damage starts on the inside and goes out; deep-tissue destruction may not be apparent initially after injury. Organs in the path of the current may become ischemic and necrotic.

RADIATION INJURY

Clients incur radiation injuries when they are exposed to large doses of radioactive material. The most common type of radiation exposure leading to tissue injury occurs in conjunction with therapeutic radiation. This injury is usually minor and rarely causes extensive skin damage.

Radiation exposure is more serious in industrial settings where radioactive energy is produced or radioactive isotopes are used. The injury depends on the amount and type of energy deposited over time. Chapter 25 discusses the penetrating ability and potential for tissue damage of alpha, beta, and gamma radiation. The severity of injury is determined by the

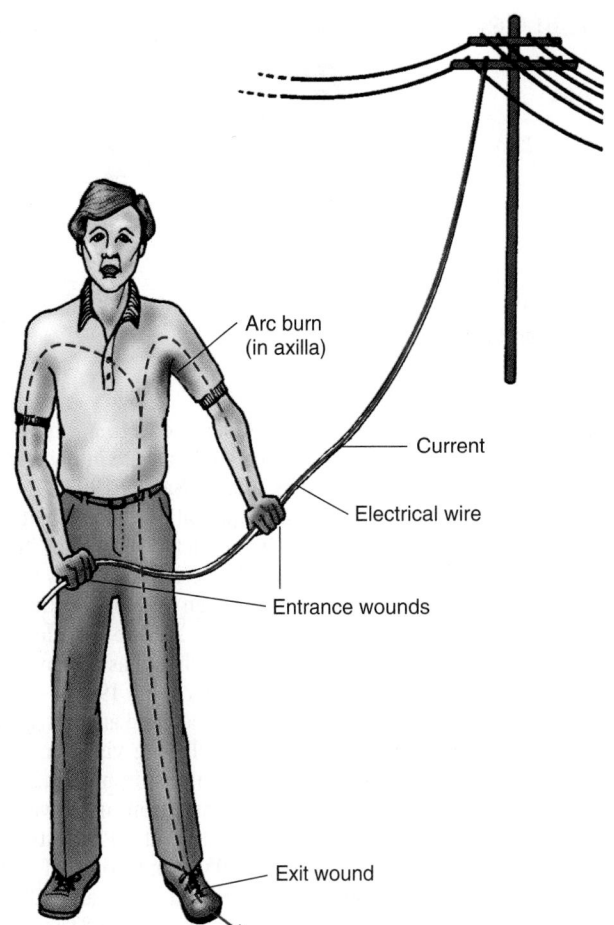

Figure 68-9 ● The mechanism of electrical injury. Currents passing through the body follow the path of least resistance to the ground.

type of radiation, distance from the source, duration of exposure, absorbed dose, and depth of penetration into the body.

Incidence/Prevalence of Burn Injury

Approximately 1.25 million burn injuries occur each year in the United States, leading to 600,000 emergency department visits. Of the clients who seek medical attention, approximately 45,000 require inpatient care; most are now being treated in a burn unit or center. The rest of the injuries are minor, and treatment with basic first aid at home is adequate. Approximately 3761 deaths were attributed to fires, burns, and fire-related injuries in 1996 (American Burn Association [ABA], 1999). The vast majority of these burns are attributable to house fires, and the remainder result from multiple other causes (Burn Foundation, 1999). According to the National Center for Health Statistics, there was a 40% decrease in burn deaths from 1971 to 1995.

Burns remain the sixth leading cause of accidental death in the United States. Causes vary among different age-groups (Table 68-3). The highest risk is among those 75 years and older. Males are at slightly higher risk for both fatal and nonfatal injuries resulting from fires and burns.

The probability of survival after a burn injury has improved steadily over the past 50 years. In 1945 only 50% of clients survived burns involving 40% of the total body surface. In

TABLE 68-3 • PERCENTAGE OF BURN INJURIES BY AGE IN THE UNITED STATES

Age	Dry Heat (Flame)	Moist Heat (Scalds)	Contact	Chemical	Electrical	Ionizing Radiation
Birth-23 mo	10	72	15	1	2	<1
2-4 yr	34	54	8	1	3	<1
5-12 yr	70	23	4	1	2	<1
13-18 yr	69	20	5	2	4	<1
19-35 yr	56	26	10	4	4	<1
36-54 yr	44	33	13	4	6	<1
55 yr and older	73	21	4	1	1	<1

1998 more than 50% of all clients survived burns involving 80% of their total body surface. The survival rate may be even higher for adolescents and young adults (Saffle, 1998).

With appropriate intervention, the probability of death after a burn injury is low. Mortality can be predicted soon after injury on the basis of simple, objective clinical criteria. Factors with a significant impact on mortality include an age greater than 60 years, a burn greater than 40% total body surface area, and the presence of an inhalation injury. When a client has all three risk factors, the risk of mortality is 90% (Ryan et al., 1998).

The success of modern day burn care can be attributed to a wide array of therapeutic advances, including vigorous fluid resuscitation, early excision of burn wounds, improvement in critical care monitoring, early enteral nutrition, improved efficacy of topical and systemic antibiotics, and the evolution of specialized burn centers (Saffle, 1998). The costs of these treatments are significant, with $2 billion spent annually in the United States on burn care (Ryan et al., 1998) (see the Cost of Care box at right).

WOMEN'S HEALTH CONSIDERATIONS

Burn injury during pregnancy has adverse effects on both maternal and fetal survival. The problems affecting the fetus include spontaneous labor and an increase in intrauterine fetal death due to compromised circulation. The signs of shock may not be evident until 30% to 35% of the circulating blood volume is lost. Placental-fetal perfusion depends on maternal blood pressure. Therefore if the mother has sustained a significant burn injury and develops significant hypovolemia, fetal circulation is likely to be compromised. Fetal monitoring is then necessary to determine fetal stability and/or viability.

In addition, respiratory injuries to the mother can result in trauma to the fetus due to respiratory exchange disturbances across the placental barrier, leading to hypoxia. Cesarean delivery may be indicated depending on the condition of the mother and the fetus. Each case is different, and the decision must be based on the gestational age of the fetus and the available data obtained through complete assessments of both the mother and fetus.

EMERGENT PHASE OF BURN INJURY

OVERVIEW

Burns are often described as the most severe devastating and dehumanizing injury that a human can endure. Events within the first hour after injury can make the difference between life and death in a thermally injured client. Immediate care fo-

COST OF CARE

IMPLICATIONS FOR NURSING

BURN DRESSINGS AND WOUND MANAGEMENT

Cost of Care
• Burn wound dressing materials, especially biologic materials, are expensive (range in price from $150 to more than $500 per square foot)
• Biologic materials and artificial skin are easily damaged by rough handling, nonadherence to recommended storage and use procedures, inappropriate client positioning, and contamination.
• Most burn wound dressing procedures are labor intensive and require one or more experienced burn nurses.

Implications for Nursing
Nurses need to consider the cost of materials when planning a burn wound dressing change. Only the necessary amount of materials should be prepared (thawed, etc.) for the specific individual procedure to avoid material wastage. Careful documentation at each change can assist in the communication for materials needed at the next burn wound dressing change.

Data from Burn Foundation (1999). Burn incidence and treatment in the United States, http://www.burnfoundation.org/adultfact.html; Rakel, B.A., et al. (1999). Split-thickness skin graft donor site care: A quantitative synthesis of the research. *Applied Nursing Research, 11*(4), 174-182; Ryan, C.M., et al. (1998). Estimates of the probability of death from burn injuries. *New England Journal of Medicine, 338*(6), 362-66; Winfrey, M. Cochran, M., & Hegarty, M. (1999). A new technology in burn therapy: Integra artificial skin. *Dimensions of Critical Care Nursing, 18*(1), 14-20.

cuses on maintaining an open airway, ensuring adequate breathing and circulation, limiting the extent of injury, and maintaining the function of vital organs. Chart 68-1 outlines the emergency management of a burn injury.

The emergent phase is the first phase of a burn injury. It begins at the onset of injury and continues to approximately 48 hours. During this phase the injury is evaluated and immediate problems resulting from the burn, including fluid loss, edema formation, and the potential for peripheral circulatory impairment, are assessed. Interventions are initiated to resolve and/or prevent potential complications.

► **COLLABORATIVE MANAGEMENT**

● **Assessment**

■ **HISTORY**

During the emergent phase, the nurse obtains a history of the mechanism of injury and other pertinent information from the client if possible. If information cannot be obtained from the client, questions should be directed to significant others and those present at the scene of the injury. Important infor-

CHART 68-1

BEST PRACTICE *for*
Emergency Management of Burns

General Management for All Types of Burns
- Assess for airway patency.
- Administer oxygen as needed.
- Cover the client with a blanket.
- Keep the client on NPO status.
- Elevate the extremities if no fractures are obvious.
- Obtain vital signs.
- Initiate an IV line and begin fluid replacement.
- Administer tetanus toxoid for prophylaxis.
- Perform a head-to-toe assessment.

Specific Management
Flame Burns
- Smother the flames.
- Remove smoldering clothing and all metal objects.

Chemical Burns
- Brush off any dry chemicals present on the skin or clothing.
- Remove the client's clothing.
- Ascertain the type of chemical causing the burn.
- Do not attempt to neutralize the chemical unless it has been positively identified and the appropriate neutralizing agent is available.

Electrical Burns
- At the scene, separate the client from the electrical current.
- Smother any flames that are present.
- Initiate cardiopulmonary resuscitation.
- Obtain an electrocardiogram (ECG).

Radiation Burns
- Remove the client from the radiation source.
- If the client has been exposed to radiation from an unsealed source, remove the client's clothing (using tongs or lead protective gloves).
- If the client has radioactive particles on his or her skin, send the client to the nearest designated radiation decontamination center.
- Help the client to bathe or shower.

CHART 68-2

NURSING FOCUS *on the* **OLDER ADULT**
Age-Related Changes That Increase Mortality and Morbidity from Burns

- The skin of an older person is thinner and more easily damaged than that of a younger person. Therefore burn injuries tend to be more extensive in older clients, even when exposure to causative agents is short.
- Healing time is slower in the older adult, which increases the risk for infection and other complications.
- Cardiac impairment in the older client with burns limits the amount and type of fluids used in resuscitation. As a result, older clients are more likely to develop complications from hypovolemic shock and inadequate renal perfusion.
- The immune responses of the older client may be reduced, which increases the risk for infection and sepsis. In addition, the older adult may not have a fever when an infection is present.
- Older adults are more likely to have a pre-existing medical condition (e.g., diabetes mellitus, cardiovascular disorders, pulmonary or renal impairment, or immunosuppression) that may further compromise vital organ function or interfere with resuscitation and treatment.

mation about the circumstances of the injury includes the time of injury, the source and cause of injury, a detailed description of how the burn occurred, and the events occurring from the time of injury until help arrived. Additional demographic data, health history (including pre-existing illness), medication use, the presence of concomitant injuries, and pain information are obtained. Potential complications associated with burn injuries must constantly be considered.

Demographic data include age, weight, and height. The rate of serious complications and death from burn injuries is greatly increased among adults over 50 years of age. Chart 68-2 summarizes the age-related differences in the older adult in response to a burn injury. The client's preburn weight is used to calculate fluid rates, energy requirements, and drug doses. The preburn weight often is referred to as "dry weight." Calculations based on a weight obtained after the initiation of fluid replacement are not accurate because of water-induced weight gain. Height is important in determining body surface area (BSA), which is used to calculate nutritional needs.

A health history, including any pre-existing illnesses, must be known for appropriate treatment to be given. The client is asked specifically about his or her history of cardiac or renal impairment and diabetes mellitus; any of these problems influence fluid resuscitation. A medication history that includes allergies,

current medications, and immunization status is obtained from the client or significant other. The dose and time of the last medication taken are determined. An assessment is obtained regarding whether or not the client smokes or drinks alcohol daily; these factors can influence treatment and physical responses.

Other injuries are unusual but may occur at the time of the burn. The most common causes of associated injuries are falls and motor vehicle accidents. Such injuries often increase the morbidity and mortality of the client. A determination is made as to whether additional injuries such as fractures, chest injuries, and abdominal trauma are causing pain or discomfort.

■ PHYSICAL ASSESSMENT/CLINICAL MANIFESTATIONS

Physical assessment findings in the emergent phase may vary greatly from findings later in the course of the injury. A systems approach is used to ensure that no problem is missed. The systems assessed first are those that can have immediate, life-threatening alterations in function.

RESPIRATORY ASSESSMENT. Clients with major burn injuries and those with inhalation injury are at risk for respiratory complications. Respiratory manifestations commonly associated with a burn injury are presented in Chart 68-3.

DIRECT AIRWAY INJURY. The degree of inhalation damage depends on the fire source, temperature, environment, and types of toxic gases generated. Information is obtained about the source of the fire, duration of exposure, and history of being in an enclosed space. The respiratory system is assessed by visual inspection of the mouth, nose, and pharynx. Burns of the lips, face, ears, neck, eyelids, eyebrows, and eyelashes are strong indicators of exposure to flames; these burns increase the possibility of an inhalation injury. Intraoral burns and singed nasal hairs indicate potentially serious injuries. Black carbon particles in the nose and mouth along with congestion and edema of the nasal septum are indicative of smoke inhalation.

CHART 68-3

KEY FEATURES *of*
Upper Airway Obstruction and Inhalation Injury

Upper Airway Obstruction
- Edema, erythema, and ulceration of airway mucosa, especially the posterior pharynx
- Increased hoarseness
- Stridor
- Any face or neck burn with edema formation
- Heat-induced intraoral injury

Inhalation Injury
- Airway injury
- Carbonaceous sputum
- Singed nasal hairs
- Bronchorrhea
- Wheezing
- Pulmonary vasoconstriction
- Reduced cardiac output
- Bronchospasm

TABLE 68-4 • PHYSIOLOGIC EFFECTS OF CARBON MONOXIDE POISONING	
Carbon Monoxide Level	**Physiologic Effects**
1%-10% (normal)	Increased threshold to visual stimuli Increased blood flow to vital organs
11%-20% (mild poisoning)	Headache Decreased cerebral function Decreased visual acuity Slight breathlessness
21%-40% (moderate poisoning)	Headache Tinnitus Nausea Drowsiness Vertigo Altered mental state Confusion Stupor Irritability Decreased blood pressure and increased heart rate Depressed ST segment on electrocardiogram and dysrhythmias on palpation Pale to reddish purple skin
41%-60% (severe poisoning)	Coma Convulsions Cardiopulmonary instability
61%-80% (fatal poisoning)	Death

An alteration in respiratory pattern may be indicative of pulmonary injury. The client may:
- Become progressively hoarse
- Exhibit a brassy cough
- Drool or have difficulty swallowing
- Produce expiratory sounds that include grossly audible wheezes, crowing, and stridor

Upper airway edema and inhalation injury are most notable in the trachea and mainstem bronchi. Auscultation of these areas may reveal wheezes, which are a sign of obstruction. Clients with severe inhalation injuries may sustain such progressive obstruction that within a short time they cannot force air through the narrowed airways. As a result, the wheezing sounds disappear. *This finding indicates impending airway obstruction and demands immediate intubation.* Many clients are intubated prophylactically based on suspicion of inhalation injury rather than waiting until there is significant obstruction that may make endotracheal or nasotracheal intubation difficult or impossible.

CARBON MONOXIDE POISONING. Carbon monoxide is a colorless, odorless, tasteless gas produced as a by-product of combustion. Inhalation injury presents a simultaneous risk for carbon monoxide poisoning.

When carbon monoxide is inhaled, it binds to the hemoglobin molecule 200 to 250 times more tightly than does oxygen, and carboxyhemoglobin (CoHb) is formed. This situation impairs tissue oxygen availability. CoHb reduces the oxygen-carrying capacity of hemoglobin, which results in impaired oxygen transport, decreased oxygen delivery, and an inability of the cells to use oxygen. Even though the oxygen-carrying capacity of the hemoglobin is reduced, the partial pressure of arterial oxygen (PaO_2) is normal. The vasodilating action of carbon monoxide causes the "cherry red" color in these clients. Clinical manifestations vary with the concentration of CoHb. Table 68-4 summarizes the physiologic effects of carbon monoxide poisoning.

THERMAL (HEAT) INJURY. Thermal injury to the respiratory tract results from the inhalation of superheated air or steam. The client inhales the hot air, which is rapidly cooled by the upper airway, where the most severe damage from superheated air is confined.

Inhaled steam can injure the lower respiratory tract because water holds heat better than does dry air. The entire respiratory tract, up to the major bronchioles, can be damaged by steam. Ulcerations, erythema, and edema of the mouth and epiglottis are usually the first manifestations, with rapid edema formation progressing to upper airway obstruction. Stridor, hoarseness, and shortness of breath result.

SMOKE POISONING. Smoke poisoning, or chemical injury from the inhalation of combustion by-products, is the most common mechanism of inhalation injury. Toxic by-products, especially hydrogen cyanide, are produced when various structural materials (e.g., plastics) or home furnishings are burned. The most significant effects of smoke poisoning are atelectasis, pulmonary edema, and tissue anoxia.

PULMONARY FLUID OVERLOAD. Pulmonary edema can result even when the lung tissues have not sustained any direct damage. Other damaged tissues release such large quantities of vasoactive amines, leading to increased capillary permeability, that even pulmonary capillaries leak fluid into the pulmonary interstitial spaces.

Circulatory overload from fluid resuscitation may cause left-sided congestive heart failure. The circulatory overload creates such high hydrostatic pressure within pulmonary vessels that even more fluid is lost from the pulmonary vascular space into the interstitial spaces. Excess interstitial fluid makes gas exchange difficult. The client is extremely short of breath and experiences increased dyspnea in the supine position. Crackles are heard on auscultation.

EXTERNAL FACTORS. In addition to pulmonary problems, clients with burn injuries may experience respiratory difficulties as a result of external factors. The most common external factor affecting respiration is tight eschar from deep circumferential chest burns. The eschar either restricts chest movement or compresses anatomic structures in the neck and throat to such an extent that ventilation is impaired. The chest is visually inspected for ease of respiration, amount of chest movement, rate of breathing, and effort required to breathe.

CARDIOVASCULAR ASSESSMENT. Changes in the cardiovascular system begin immediately after the burn injury and include shock from various causes. Shock is a common cause of death in the immediate postburn period in clients with significant injuries. Chapter 37 discusses the pathophysiologic and compensatory mechanisms for all types of shock.

The initial cardiovascular clinical manifestations reflect hypovolemia and decreased cardiac output. The nurse notes the presence of edema and assesses cardiovascular status by measuring central and peripheral pulses, blood pressure, capillary refill, and pulse oximetry. Noninvasive blood pressure readings are inaccurate in clients with large burns involving the upper extremities (Ahrns & Harkins, 1999). This situation necessitates invasive monitoring for blood pressure measurement. Initially, tachycardia, decreased blood pressure, and diminished peripheral pulses are present. Peripheral capillary refill is slow or absent as tissue perfusion decreases. With fluid resuscitation in the initial postburn period, peripheral edema increases, as does the client's body weight.

Electrocardiographic (ECG) changes indicate electrical damage to the heart. These changes are commonly associated with electrical burn injuries or with stress that induces a myocardial infarction. Baseline ECG tracings are obtained at the time of admission to the hospital or burn center.

RENAL/URINARY ASSESSMENT. Changes in renal function with burn injury are related to decreased renal perfusion and to the presence of cellular debris. During the fluid shift of the emergent period, perfusion may not be adequate for glomerular filtration. As a result, urine output is greatly diminished compared with intravenous (IV) fluid intake. The urine is highly concentrated and has a high specific gravity.

As a result of specific tissue damage, other substances may be present in the blood that perfuses the kidney. Destroyed red blood cells release hemoglobin and potassium. When muscle damage occurs from a major burn or electrical injury, a large oxygen-carrying protein called **myoglobin** is released from damaged muscle and circulates to the kidney. Most damaged cells release protein products that form uric acid. All of these large molecules in the blood may precipitate in the kidney tubular system. This precipitation blocks filtrate flow and may contribute to severe renal dysfunction.

Renal function is assessed by accurately measuring urine output and comparing this value with fluid intake. Urine output is decreased during the first 24 hours of the emergent phase. The rate of resuscitation fluid administration should maintain adult urine output at 30 to 50 mL or 0.5 ml/kg/hr. Adequate response to fluid resuscitation is further assessed by

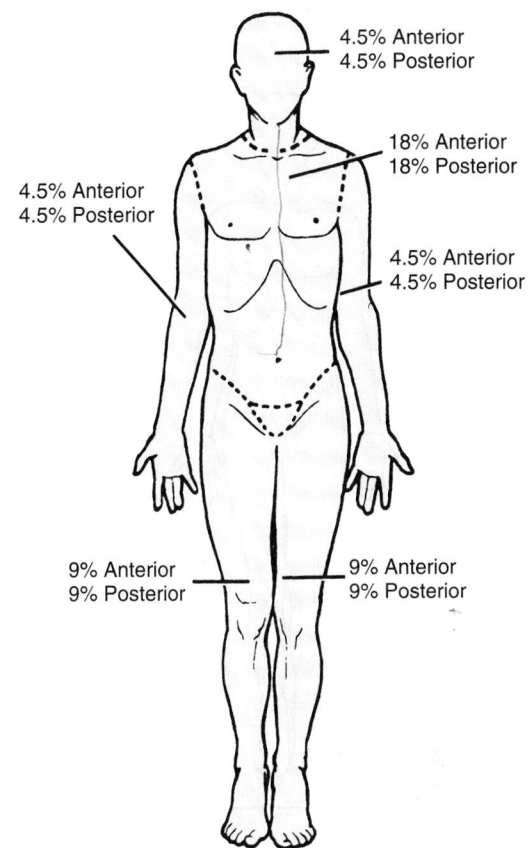

Figure 68-10 ● The rule of nines for estimating burn percentage.

measuring urine specific gravity and blood urea nitrogen (BUN), serum creatinine, and serum sodium levels. The urine is examined for color, odor, and the presence of particulate matter or foam.

INTEGUMENTARY ASSESSMENT. The skin is assessed to determine the size and depth of burn injury. The size of the injury is first estimated in comparison to the total body surface area (TBSA). For example, a burn that involves 40% of the TBSA is a 40% burn. The size of the injury is important not only for diagnosis and prognosis but also for calculating specific interventions such as drug dose, fluid replacement volumes, and caloric requirements.

The skin is inspected to identify injured areas and changes in color and appearance. Except with electrical burns, this initial size assessment usually can be made accurately with specific assessment tools and charts.

The most rapid method for calculating the size of a burn injury in adult clients whose weights are in normal proportion to their heights is the *rule of nines* (Figure 68-10). With this method, the body is divided into areas that are multiples of 9%. Although the rule of nines is useful at the site of injury and in emergency departments, overestimation of the percentage of TBSA involved can easily occur.

The Lund-Browder and Berkow methods are more accurate for evaluating the size of the injury (Figure 68-11). These methods take into account changes in body surface area from birth through adulthood.

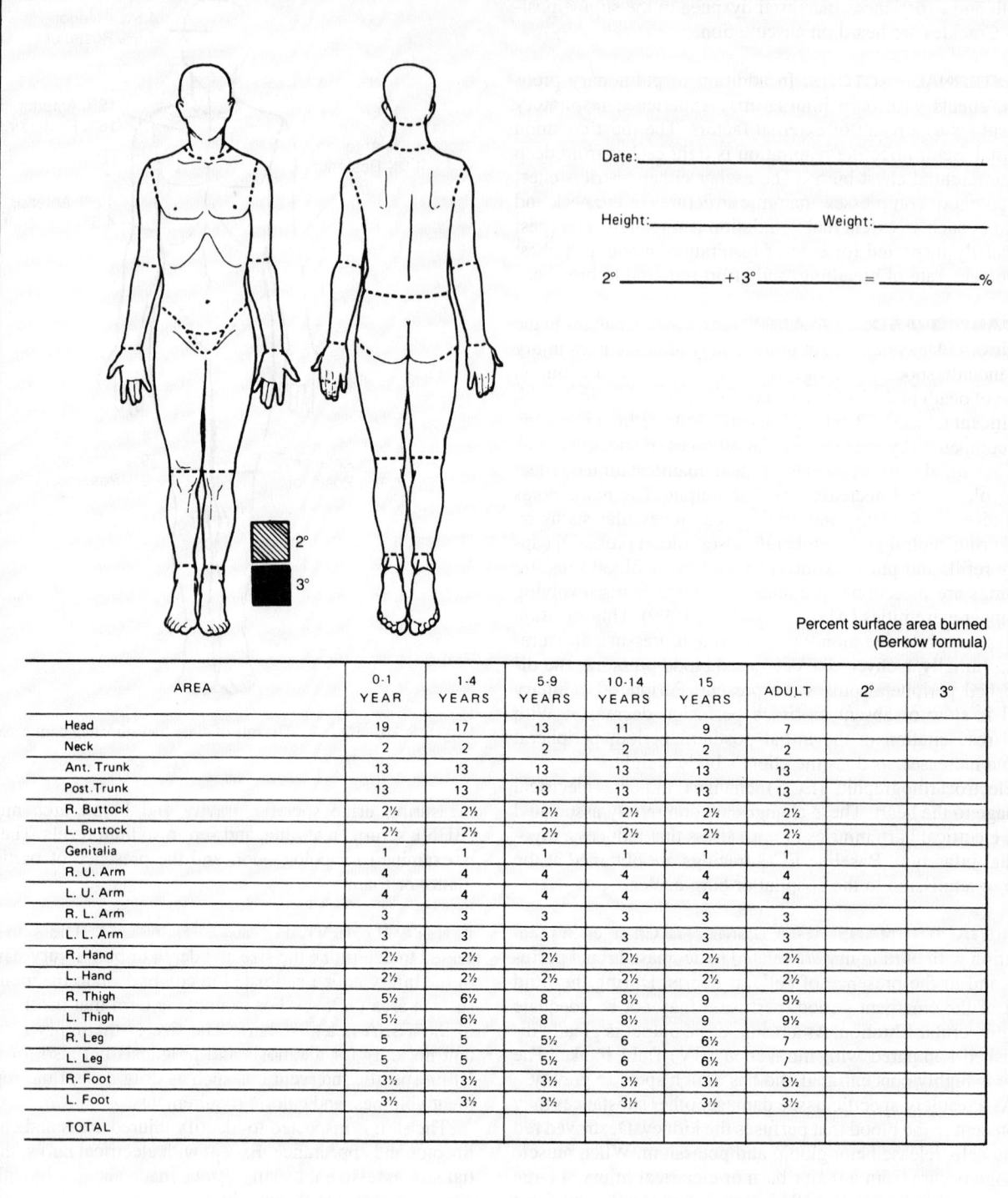

Date:_____

Height:_____ Weight:_____

$2° \underline{\hspace{3cm}} + 3° \underline{\hspace{3cm}} = \underline{\hspace{3cm}}\%$

Percent surface area burned
(Berkow formula)

AREA	0-1 YEAR	1-4 YEARS	5-9 YEARS	10-14 YEARS	15 YEARS	ADULT	2°	3°
Head	19	17	13	11	9	7		
Neck	2	2	2	2	2	2		
Ant. Trunk	13	13	13	13	13	13		
Post.Trunk	13	13	13	13	13	13		
R. Buttock	2½	2½	2½	2½	2½	2½		
L. Buttock	2½	2½	2½	2½	2½	2½		
Genitalia	1	1	1	1	1	1		
R. U. Arm	4	4	4	4	4	4		
L. U. Arm	4	4	4	4	4	4		
R. L. Arm	3	3	3	3	3	3		
L. L. Arm	3	3	3	3	3	3		
R. Hand	2½	2½	2½	2½	2½	2½		
L. Hand	2½	2½	2½	2½	2½	2½		
R. Thigh	5½	6½	8	8½	9	9½		
L. Thigh	5½	6½	8	8½	9	9½		
R. Leg	5	5	5½	6	6½	7		
L. Leg	5	5	5½	6	6½	7		
R. Foot	3½	3½	3½	3½	3½	3½		
L. Foot	3½	3½	3½	3½	3½	3½		
TOTAL								

Figure 68-11 ● Estimation of the extent of burn injury by the Lund-Browder (Berkow) method. (*Ant.*, Anterior; *Post.*, posterior; *R.*, Right; *L.*, left; *R.U.*, right upper; *L.U.*, left upper; *R.L.*, right lower; *L.L.*, left lower.)

CHART 68-4

LABORATORY PROFILE
Burn Assessment During the Emergent Period

Test	Normal Range for Adults	Significance of Abnormal Findings
SERUM STUDIES		
Hemoglobin	11.7-15.5 g/dL (women) 13.2-17.3 g/dL (men)	Elevated as a result of fluid volume loss
Hematocrit	34%-45% (women) 39%-59% (men)	Elevated as a result of fluid volume loss
Urea nitrogen	10-20 mg/dL	Elevated as a result of fluid volume loss
Glucose	70-105 mg/dL	Elevated as a result of the stress response and increased uptake across injured tissues
ELECTROLYTES		
Sodium	136-145 mEq/L (mmol/L)	Decreased; sodium is trapped in edema fluid and lost through plasma leakage
Potassium	3.5-5.0 mEq/L (mmol/L)	Elevated as a result of disruption of the sodium-potassium pump, tissue destruction, and red blood cell hemolysis
Chloride	90-110 mEq/L (mmol/L)	Elevated as a result of fluid volume loss and reabsorption of chloride in urine
ARTERIAL BLOOD GAS STUDIES		
Pao_2	83-108 mm Hg	Slightly decreased
$Paco_2$	32-48 mm Hg	Slightly increased from respiratory injury
pH	7.35-7.45	Low as a result of metabolic acidosis
Carboxyhemoglobin	0%-10%	Elevated as a result of inhalation of smoke and carbon monoxide
OTHER		
Total protein	6-8.3 g/dL	Low; protein exudate is lost through the wound
Albumin	3.5-5.5 g/dL	Low; protein is lost through the wound and through vascular membranes because of increased permeability

Pao_2, Partial pressure of arterial oxygen; $Paco_2$, partial pressure of arterial carbon dioxide.

Because specific treatments are related to the depth of the burn injury, initial assessment of the integumentary system includes estimations of burn depth. Criteria for establishing the depth of injury are based on appearance and associated characteristics (see Depth of Burn Injury, pp. 1556-1559).

GASTROINTESTINAL ASSESSMENT. Although the gastrointestinal (GI) tract usually is not directly injured in most burn clients (except in those with chemical burns), alterations in GI function are expected. The decreased blood flow during the emergent phase may result in a loss of GI motility and paralytic ileus. The abdomen is auscultated for the presence of bowel sounds to assess GI motility. Bowel sounds are commonly diminished or absent in a client with severe burns. Associated clinical manifestations include nausea, vomiting, and abdominal distention. To prevent aspiration and remove gastric secretions, a nasogastric (NG) tube is usually placed and assessed for proper placement and patency.

Because of the potential for ulcer formation in the GI tract, the nurse examines the stool and vomitus for the presence of gross blood or other material indicative of partially digested blood. Tests for the presence of occult blood are performed.

■ LABORATORY ASSESSMENT

Alterations in laboratory test values are found in different phases of postburn recovery and usually indicate direct tissue damage and expected compensatory mechanisms. However, other alterations in specific laboratory findings suggest complications.

During the emergent phase and before the initiation of fluid resuscitation, venous blood analysis reflects the fluid shift and direct tissue damage. Baseline laboratory test values and early postburn variations are presented in Chart 68-4.

Changes in the total white blood cell (WBC) count and differential count reflect immune function responses to the trauma of burn injury. The burn client's total WBC count, especially the neutrophil percentage, initially rises and then drops rapidly, with a "left shift" (see Chapter 20) as the immune system becomes unable to sustain its defenses. If sepsis occurs, the total WBC count may be as low as 2000 cells/mm³.

Additional laboratory tests that provide useful information about the burn client's status may include urine electrolyte assays, urine cultures, liver enzyme studies, and clotting studies. Drug and alcohol screens are obtained if drug or alcohol intoxication is suspected.

CULTURAL CONSIDERATIONS
For African-American clients, a sickle cell preparation may be appropriate if sickle status is unknown. Trauma often triggers a sickle cell crisis in clients who have the disease and in those who carry the trait.

■ RADIOGRAPHIC ASSESSMENT

Standard x-ray studies and scans do not provide direct assessment data about the burn wound. Such an assessment is not performed unless additional trauma is suspected.

OTHER DIAGNOSTIC ASSESSMENT

In addition to routine laboratory tests and examinations, specific studies of involved organs are performed. For example, when burn injuries involve the eye, an ophthalmic evaluation detects corneal damage (see Chapters 46 and 47 for specific ophthalmic evaluation procedures).

Specific diagnostic examinations can be performed when visceral organ trauma is suspected. Such examinations include intravenous pyelography (IVP), computed tomography (CT), ultrasonography, bronchoscopy, and magnetic resonance imaging (MRI) studies.

CRITICAL THINKING CHALLENGE

The client is a 22-year-old man admitted directly to the burn center after sustaining a high voltage electrical injury while attempting to remove copper at an electrical substation. He is awake and alert. He states he has a great deal of pain in his back and right arm. He has what appears to be a deep, puncture-type wound on his right thumb, and his right hand is extremely edematous. When you check his peripheral pulses, you discover an absence of the right radial and ulnar pulses. Further assessment shows a large charred exit wound in his right lower flank. The client has a 20-gauge IV line in the left hand.

- Is this client at risk for an inhalation injury? Why or why not?
- What initial consideration must be given in moving the client from the stretcher to the bed?
- Once the client is found to have an adequate airway and level of consciousness, what is your next priority?
- The client asks, "Will I lose my arm?" What is your response?

For suggested answer guidelines, go to SIMON, http://www.wbsaunders.com/SIMON/Iggy/.

▶ Analysis

A burned client experiences dramatic changes not only in the directly damaged tissues but also in many other body systems. During the course of the illness, most burn clients experience all of the common and many of the additional nursing diagnoses listed in the following sections.

COMMON NURSING DIAGNOSES AND COLLABORATIVE PROBLEMS

The following are common nursing diagnoses for clients with burn injuries in the emergent phase who have sustained a burn injury greater than 25% of the total body surface area (TBSA):

1. Decreased Cardiac Output related to an increase in capillary permeability
2. Deficient Fluid Volume related to electrolyte imbalance, a loss of plasma volume, and inadequate fluid resuscitation
3. Ineffective Tissue Perfusion (Cerebral, Cardiopulmonary, Renal, Gastrointestinal, and Peripheral) related to decreased cardiac output, extravascular fluid shifts, hypovolemia, constriction of eschar, and edema
4. Ineffective Breathing Pattern related to respiratory distress from upper airway edema, pulmonary edema, airway obstruction, or pneumonia
5. Acute Pain and Chronic Pain related to damaged or exposed nerve endings, debridement, dressing changes, invasive procedures, and donor sites

The following are primary collaborative problems:

1. Potential for Pulmonary Edema
2. Potential for Acute Respiratory Distress Syndrome (ARDS)

ADDITIONAL NURSING DIAGNOSES AND COLLABORATIVE PROBLEMS

In addition to the common nursing diagnoses and collaborative problems, clients with burn injuries in the emergent phase may have one or more of the following:

- Excess Fluid Volume related to massive IV fluid administration
- Risk for Ineffective Thermoregulation related to hypermetabolism and a loss of the protective barrier
- Disturbed Sensory Perception related to periorbital edema or ulcerations, hospital environment, noise, infections, and dressings
- Anxiety related to initial burn trauma, threat of death, situational crisis, painful procedures, unfamiliar environment, separation from significant others, and loss of control
- Fear related to pain, knowledge deficit, therapeutic procedures, hospitalization, separation, and social re-entry

▶ Planning and Implementation

DECREASED CARDIAC OUTPUT; DEFICIENT FLUID VOLUME; INEFFECTIVE TISSUE PERFUSION

NOC PLANNING: EXPECTED OUTCOMES. Following appropriate intervention, the client with a burn injury in the emergent phase is expected to (1) have cardiac output restored to normal as evidenced by blood pressure and heart rate in expected ranges and strong peripheral pulses; and (2) maintain adequate oxygenation and circulation to all vital organs as evidenced by oxygen saturation, partial pressure of arterial oxygen (Pao_2), partial pressure of arterial carbon dioxide ($Paco_2$), and arterial pH within normal limits.

INTERVENTIONS. Interventions are aimed at increasing intravascular fluid volume, supporting compensatory mechanisms, and preventing complications. Chart 68-5 lists some NIC intervention activities for the burn client with decreased cardiac output, deficient fluid volume, and ineffective tissue perfusion. Nonsurgical management is often sufficient for achieving these aims. Surgical management is required most often for full-thickness burns.

NONSURGICAL MANAGEMENT. Restoration of fluid volume and tissue perfusion can be accomplished through IV fluid therapy, plasma exchange therapy, and drug therapy.

INTRAVENOUS FLUID THERAPY. Appropriate infusion of IV fluids maintains a circulating volume sufficient for normal cardiac output, mean arterial pressure, and tissue oxygenation. Clients with burns involving 15% to 20% of the TBSA generally require IV fluid resuscitation (Shirani et al., 1996). Many formulas for calculating fluid requirements exist. Table 68-5 summarizes the formulas most commonly used for the therapy of adult clients. Although the types and amounts of electrolytes, crystalloids, and colloids vary, the ultimate purpose of all of these formulas is to prevent shock by maintaining an adequate intravascular fluid volume. The optimal formula and administration schedules remain controversial.

Resuscitation from a severe burn requires large fluid loads in a short time to maintain vital organ perfusion. The Parkland formula recommends that half of the calculated fluid volume be given in the first 8 hours after injury. The other half is administered over the next 16 hours for a total of 24 hours. In general, fluid boluses are avoided because they increase capillary hydrostatic pressure and worsen edema. In the second 24-hour period after a burn injury, the volume and content of the IV fluids are based on the client's

specific volume and electrolyte imbalances and his or her response to treatment.

Most fluid replacement formulas are calculated from the time of injury and not from the time of arrival at the hospital. For example, if a burn injury occurred at 8 AM but the client was not admitted to the hospital until 10 AM, the first 8-hour period would be completed at 4 PM, or 8 hours after the injury. Thus, if resuscitation were delayed until admission to the hospital, calculated fluids would need to be administered over a 6-hour period rather than an 8-hour period. All burn resuscitation formulas are used as *guides,* with the understanding that the client's response to therapy determines ultimate fluid requirements. No single formula has been found to provide superior results over another.

The management of extensive burns may necessitate the placement of a large-bore central venous catheter so that massive fluid loads can be administered. Peripheral lines sometimes become dislodged or fluid flow is cut off because massive peripheral edema compresses the IV catheter.

PLASMA EXCHANGE THERAPY. Shock may persist in the postburn period despite adequate fluid resuscitation. The cause of this persistent shock is unknown, but toxic serum factors have been theorized. Plasma exchange therapy is occasionally used in some burn centers for clients with massive burns who fail to respond to conventional resuscitation from burn shock.

The plasma exchange process either removes the client's plasma and replaces it with fresh frozen plasma (**plasmapheresis**) or removes the client's blood and replaces it with whole banked blood (**exchange transfusion**). Plasma exchange can decrease the amount of required fluid and increase urine output, thus helping those clients who do not respond to conventional fluid therapy.

MONITORING. Clinical criteria are monitored to determine the adequacy of fluid resuscitation. These parameters are indications of hydration and adequate tissue perfusion to the brain, heart, and kidneys. In animal studies, a 50% decrease in renal blood flow was observed while perfusion to the vital organs was preserved. These findings suggest that urine output diminishes before the compromise or loss of vital organ perfusion. During resuscitation, deviation from any of the desirable parameters suggests an inadequate or excessive amount of fluid.

Urine output is the most common and most sensitive noninvasive assessment parameter for cardiac output and tissue per-

---

CHART 68-5

NIC **INTERVENTION ACTIVITIES** *for*
The Burn Client with Decreased Cardiac Output, Deficient Fluid Volume, and Ineffective Tissue Perfusion

Fluid Monitoring: *Collection and analysis of client data to regulate fluid balance*
- Monitor serum and urine electrolyte values, as appropriate.
- Monitor BP, heart rate, and respiratory status.
- Monitor orthostatic blood pressure and change in cardiac rhythm, as appropriate.
- Monitor weight.
- Keep an accurate record of intake and output.
- Note presence or absence of vertigo on rising.
- Monitor color, quantity, and specific gravity of urine.

Fluid Resuscitation: *Administering prescribed intravenous fluids rapidly*
- Obtain and maintain a large-bore IV.
- Administer IV fluids, as prescribed.
- Monitor hemodynamic response.
- Monitor oxygen status.
- Monitor for fluid overload.
- Monitor output of various body fluids (e.g., urine, nasogastric drainage, and chest tube).
- Monitor BUN, creatinine, total protein, and albumin levels.
- Monitor for pulmonary edema and third spacing.

Fluid Management: *Promotion of fluid balance and prevention of complications resulting from abnormal or undesired fluid levels*
- Administer IV therapy, as prescribed.
- Give fluids, as appropriate.
- Distribute the fluid intake over 24 hours, as appropriate.

NIC intervention activities selected from McCloskey, J.C., & Bulechek, G.M. (Eds.). (2000). *Nursing interventions classification (NIC)* (3rd ed.). St. Louis: Mosby. No part of this work is to be altered without prior written permission from the Publisher.
BP, Blood pressure; *BUN,* blood urea nitrogen.

TABLE 68-5 • COMMON FLUID RESUSCITATION FORMULAS FOR THE FIRST 24 HOURS AFTER A BURN INJURY

	Formula	Solution	Rate of Administration
Modified Brooke	0.5 mL/kg/% TBSA burn	Protenate or 5% albumin in isotonic saline	$1/2$ given in first 8 hr $1/2$ given in next 16 hr
	1.5 mL/kg/% TBSA burn	Lactated Ringer's without dextrose	
Parkland (Baxter)	4 mL/kg/% TBSA burn for 24-hr period	Crystalloid only (lactated Ringer's)	$1/2$ given in first 8 hr $1/2$ given in next 16 hr
Monafo		Crystalloid (hypertonic saline: sodium = 250 mEq/L)	Adjust to maintain urine output of 30 mL/hr
Modified Parkland	4 mL/kg/% TBSA burn + 15 mL/m² of TBSA	Crystalloid only (lactated Ringer's)	$1/2$ given in first 8 hr $1/2$ given in next 16 hr
Winski	2 mL/kg/% burn + maintenance fluid	Crystalloid only (lactated Ringer's)	$1/2$ given in first 8 hr $1/2$ given in next 16 hr

fusion (see Chapters 12 and 37). Regardless of the total amount of fluid calculated as appropriate to meet the fluid needs of the client, the amount of fluid administered depends on how much IV fluid per hour is required to maintain the hourly urine output at 0.5 mL/kg (30 mL/hr). Adjustment of the IV fluid rate on the basis of urine output plus serum electrolyte values is known as the **titration** of fluid to meet the perfusion needs of the client. *In clients with burns larger than 35% TBSA, the use of urine output and vital signs to guide resuscitation may be insufficient. Additional invasive monitoring of cardiopulmonary function is necessary to ensure optimal fluid resuscitation.*

Burn clients often develop severe hypovolemic shock and require invasive cardiac monitoring. With the use of modern electronic equipment (see Chapter 37), vital parameters such as central venous pressure, pulmonary artery pressures, and cardiac output can be obtained on a frequent to continuous basis. Because an adequately functioning cardiovascular system is imperative, the nurse monitors the electrocardiographic activity of clients who have sustained large burns. Rhythms that affect the mechanics of the heart (e.g., atrial fibrillation) are often present in older clients.

DRUG THERAPY. A common mistake in treatment is administering diuretics to increase urine output rather than changing the amount and rate of fluid administration. *Diuretics do not increase cardiac output; they actually decrease circulating volume and cardiac output by pulling fluid from the circulating blood volume to enhance diuresis.* This effect can cause a dangerous reduction in perfusion to other vital organs (especially the heart, lungs, and brain) and greatly increases the probability of developing a state of severe hypovolemic shock. Therefore diuretics are not generally used to improve urine output for burn clients. An exception is the client with a burn injury caused by electrical energy. Muscle and deep tissue damage can cause the release of large protein molecules (myoglobin), which precipitate in and obstruct the renal tubules. Although the diuretic mannitol (Osmitrol) is often used in this situation, it should always be given after adequate urine output has been established and is accompanied by the alkalinization of urine with sodium bicarbonate supplementation.

In some clients, particularly older adults or those with a history of cardiac disease, a complicating factor in reduced cardiac output may be congestive heart failure or myocardial infarction. Drugs that increase cardiac output, such as dopamine (Intropin), or that strengthen the force of myocardial contraction, such as digoxin (Lanoxin), may be used along with fluid therapy.

SURGICAL MANAGEMENT. The primary surgical procedure for the treatment of inadequate tissue perfusion is *escharotomy.* An incision through the burn eschar with an electrocautery device or scalpel relieves pressure caused by the restricting force of circumferential burns on the extremity or chest and improves circulation. If the pressure is not relieved, arterial compression can occur with a resultant compromise of extremity perfusion, ischemia, and possibly necrosis. Incisions are made along the medial and lateral sides of the extremity and extend into the subcutaneous tissue (Figures 68-6 and 68-12). This procedure relieves the tourniquet effect of the eschar. If tissue pressure measurements remain elevated after escharotomies, a *fasciotomy* (an incision extending through the subcutaneous tissue and fascia) may be required.

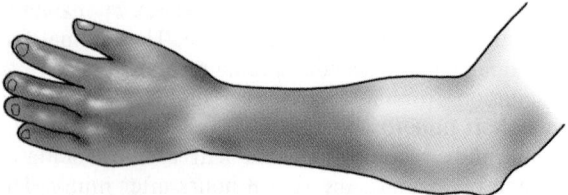

Tight, circumferential eschar restricting outward swelling as edema forms in the tissues beneath the eschar. Edema compresses blood vessels, which inhibits blood flow to the distal extremity.

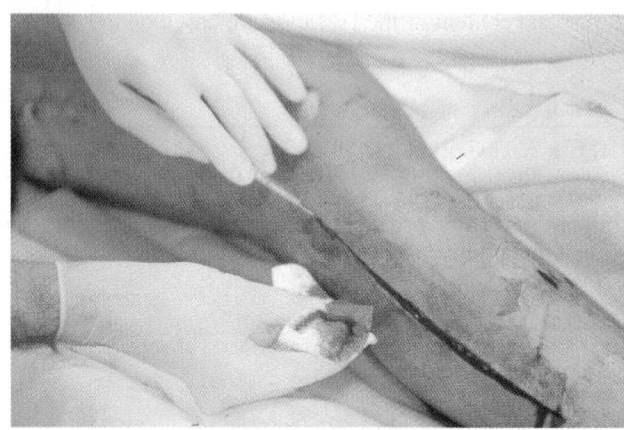

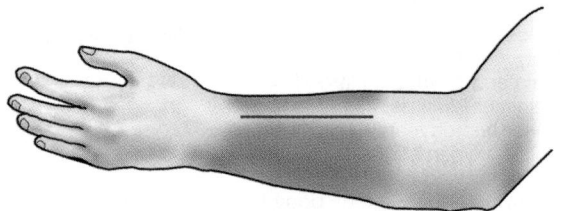

An escharotomy incision allows outward swelling of edematous tissues. Restricted blood flow through the vessels to the distal extremity is relieved.

Figure 68-12 ● Escharotomy to release circumferential burn eschar and improve circulation to a distal extremity.

Escharotomies and fasciotomies are often performed at the bedside. No anesthesia is required for escharotomy because nerve endings have been destroyed by the burn injury, but sedation and analgesia are commonly given to reduce anxiety. The nurse prepares the client by providing verbal assurance that the client will be made as comfortable as possible during the procedure. Preparation for escharotomy requires removing the dressings and thoroughly cleansing the areas to be incised. Following the procedure, topical antimicrobial agents and dressings are reapplied to the area. Escharotomy sites are carefully monitored for excessive bleeding. Fasciotomies generally require large doses of narcotics or anesthesia for pain management.

■ INEFFECTIVE BREATHING PATTERN

NOC PLANNING: EXPECTED OUTCOMES. With appropriate intervention, the client with a burn injury in the emergent phase is expected to maintain a patent airway, and have an effective breathing pattern as evidenced by maintaining oxygen saturation, PaO_2, $PaCO_2$, and arterial pH within normal limits.

INTERVENTIONS. Interventions are aimed at supporting normal pulmonary mechanisms and preventing pulmonary problems. Specific plans for pulmonary management depend on the cause of the insult and the status of the respiratory tract.

NONSURGICAL MANAGEMENT. Appropriate interventions include airway maintenance, promotion of ventilation, monitoring gas exchange, oxygen therapy, drug therapy, and positioning and deep breathing.

AIRWAY MAINTENANCE. Maintenance of the airway begins at the incident scene in an unconscious victim and may involve only a chin lift or a head tilt maneuver. Upper airway edema becomes pronounced 8 to 12 hours after the initiation of fluid resuscitation. These clients often require immediate nasal or oral intubation once signs of crowing, stridor, and dyspnea are present.

The physician performs a bronchoscopy to examine the vocal cords and airways of clients at risk for obstruction. Clients with severe smoke inhalation or poisoning may require a bronchoscopy when admitted to the hospital and routinely thereafter for examination of the respiratory tract, accurate diagnoses, deep suctioning of the lungs, and removal of sloughing necrotic tissue. The endotracheal tube is assessed frequently to ensure patency in intubated clients.

Other causes of airway obstruction are excessive secretions and sloughed tissue from damaged lungs. Suctioning is performed as indicated based on clinical assessment or clinician order. Vigorous endotracheal or nasotracheal tube suctioning is commonly performed after chest physiotherapy and aerosol treatments. Clients have reported that deep endotracheal suctioning is extremely painful. Therefore suctioning the endotracheal tube often requires increased analgesia and/or sedation.

PROMOTION OF VENTILATION. Respiration depends on skeletal muscle contractions and movement of the thoracic cavity for ventilation. Movement of the thoracic cavity can be restricted by tight dressings that cover the neck, thorax, and abdomen. The nurse observes the client for effectiveness and ease of respiratory movements and loosens tight dressings as needed to assist with ventilation.

MONITORING GAS EXCHANGE. The effectiveness of gas exchange is monitored by using laboratory tests (e.g., arterial blood gas, carboxyhemoglobin levels) and by noting physical signs such as cyanosis, disorientation, and increased pulse rate. Other data to monitor in critically ill clients include chest x-ray studies, pulmonary artery catheters, and central venous pressure measurement.

The possibility of cyanide poisoning must be considered in clients involved in house fires. An elevated plasma lactate level is a useful indicator of cyanide toxicity in clients who do not have severe burns.

OXYGEN THERAPY. Management of impaired breathing patterns includes administering humidified oxygen by face mask, cannula, or hood. Arterial oxygenation less than 60

(PaO_2 <60 mm Hg) is an indication for intubation, and mechanical ventilation is instituted. Emergency airway equipment should be located at or near the client's bedside and include oxygen, masks, cannulas, ambu bags, laryngoscope, endotracheal tubes, and equipment for tracheostomy. Chapter 32 addresses specific nursing actions for clients during mechanical ventilation.

DRUG THERAPY. When pneumonia or other pulmonary infections further impair breathing, the physician prescribes antibiotics. Antibiotic selection is based on known culture and sensitivity reports or is empirically based on a knowledge of the specific microflora of the burn unit. Impaired breathing patterns resulting from cardiac failure and increased pulmonary pressures may be treated with drugs that improve cardiac output and enhance renal excretion.

When a client's activity severely compromises respiratory mechanics, it may be necessary to use a paralytic drug, such as Atracurium (Tracrium) or Vecuronium (Norcuron). This situation is often referred to as "bucking" the ventilator. Paralytic agents remove all ventilatory control from the client and allow uninterrupted administration of artificial ventilation. *These drugs do not prevent the client from seeing and hearing or from experiencing fear, pain, and loss of control. Any client receiving neuromuscular blockade drugs must also receive agents for sedation, analgesia, and antianxiety unless clinically contraindicated. Extreme care must be taken to ensure that all alarms are operative and that clients are checked frequently, because they cannot call for help should they become extubated.*

POSITIONING AND DEEP BREATHING. To improve breathing patterns and oxygenation, the client is turned frequently and assisted out of bed to a chair as much as possible. Pulmonary hygiene techniques such as coughing and deep breathing exercises and incentive spirometry must be taught to the client and encouraged frequently. Chest physiotherapy may be helpful to facilitate the mobilization of pulmonary secretions based on the client's clinical condition and the clinician's order.

SURGICAL MANAGEMENT. A tracheostomy may be necessary in clients for whom long-term intubation is expected. A tracheostomy carries a greater risk for infection in burn clients than in nonburned clients. Emergency tracheostomies are performed when an airway becomes occluded and oral or nasal intubation cannot be achieved.

Other common surgical procedures for improving the burn client's breathing pattern include inserting chest tubes and performing an escharotomy. Chest tubes are used to re-expand the lung when a pneumothorax or hemothorax has occurred (see Chapter 30).

Tight eschar on the neck, chest, or abdomen can restrict respiratory movement. Escharotomies (described on p. 1572) can relieve this restriction and permit greater respiratory movement.

■ ACUTE PAIN; CHRONIC PAIN

The pain associated with burn injuries is both chronic and acute. Many factors contribute to burn pain and may be manipulated to alter the response to pain. Pain from the actual injury is compounded when painful procedures are performed. Nurses working with burn clients must often inflict pain on clients during the course of treatment. They must cope with this problem by developing strategies that allow them to rationalize the necessity for inflicting pain during procedures. One common coping mechanism is to distance oneself from the client's pain (Nagy, 1999). Accurate assessment of the client's pain before and during procedures is an essential part of pain management. In addition to more standard visual analog scales, pain assessment scales that use color or faces have been used successfully to assess pain in the client with burns (see the Evidence-Based Practice for Nursing box at right).

NOC **PLANNING: EXPECTED OUTCOMES.** The pain level of a client with a burn injury in the emergent phase is expected to be alleviated or reduced as evidenced by a decreased report of pain and a decreased length of pain episodes.

INTERVENTIONS. The plan for pain management is tailored to the client's tolerance for pain, coping mechanisms, and physical status.

NONSURGICAL MANAGEMENT. Interventions for the client experiencing pain include drug therapy, complementary therapy measures, and environmental manipulation.

DRUG THERAPY. Opioid and nonopioid analgesics, such as morphine sulfate, meperidine (Demerol), and nalbuphine (Nubain), are given with relative frequency throughout hospitalization. However, these drugs rarely offer more than moderate relief during acutely painful procedures, and they produce side effects of respiratory depression and diminished gastrointestinal motility.

During the emergent postburn phase, the IV route is the preferred route for administration of narcotics because of potential problems with absorption from the muscle and stomach. When these agents are administered by the intramuscular route, they remain in the spaces and do not relieve pain. In addition, when edema is present, cumulative subcutaneous or intramuscular doses are rapidly reabsorbed when the fluid shift is resolving. This delayed reabsorption can result in lethal blood levels of analgesics.

Anesthetic agents, such as ketamine (Ketalar), pentobarbital sodium (Nembutal, Novopentobarb✤), and nitrous oxide, also reduce pain. Strict protocols must be used when administering these agents to prevent serious complications.

COMPLEMENTARY AND ALTERNATIVE THERAPY. Complementary and alternative therapy measures include relaxation techniques, meditative breathing, guided imagery, music therapy, massage, and healing or therapeutic touch. Hypnosis and autohypnosis of lucid, cooperative clients can be attempted by trained therapists. Therapeutic touch, acupuncture, and acupressure are used to a limited extent for burn clients; the results are variable. Nontraditional and complementary therapy types of pain intervention are detailed in Chapter 7.

ENVIRONMENTAL MANIPULATION. The nurse can increase the client's comfort by providing a quiet environment, using nonpainful tactile stimulation, and increasing the client's control. Sleep deprivation is a significant issue for victims of burn injury. Increasing sleep or rest time in a quiet

EVIDENCE-BASED PRACTICE FOR NURSING

What pain assessment tool is preferred by clients with burns?

Gordon, M., et al. (1998). Use of pain assessment tools: Is there a preference? *Journal of Burn Care and Rehabilitation, 19*(5), 451-454.

Pain is a major issue for clients with burns. The most commonly used method of assessing pain among burn clients is the Visual Analog Scale (VAS). This prospective, descriptive study of 40 clients with burn injuries sought to determine what pain assessment tool is perceived as most useful by clients having pain related to burn injury and burn care procedures.

Four pain assessment tools were tested: Faces Pain Rating Scale (FPRS), Adjective Pain Rating Scale (APRS), Visual Analog Scale (VAS), and Analog Chromatic Continuous Scale (ACCS). The ACCS incorporates properties of two types of scales: (1) a calibrated measure similar to the VAS ranging from "no pain" to "severe pain," and (2) a color scale ranging from light pink (no pain) through a shade of red and black (severe pain). Forty adult clients who were inpatients with burn injuries were asked to use two of the pain assessment tools for 3 consecutive days twice daily. Pain was assessed at a "quiet time" and at a time immediately following a painful activity. The 3-day assessment cycle was repeated with the remaining two pain assessment scales. Clients were asked to select the preferred type of pain assessment tool after each 3-day cycle and at the end of the test period. Most clients (35) were male; the average age was 36 years, and the average total body surface area (TBSA) injured was 20%. Overall, clients preferred the FPRS and the ACCS to the VAS and the ARPS. However, when results were compared by gender, the five women always preferred the VAS over the ACCS.

Critique. The authors initiated study in an important area of care for the client with burns. Although this study concluded that adult clients with burn injuries preferred the FPRS and ACCS to the more commonly used VAS, the results are not generalizable to all adult clients with burn injuries. The sample size was small, with a preponderance of men (35) compared to women (5). No attempt was made to correlate severity of pain with pain assessment tool preference. The study could have been strengthened by including client education or literacy level as well as by ensuring that the painful activities were similar for all clients.

Implications for Nursing. Pain management and client comfort remain important issues when caring for clients with burns. Pain assessment may not be accurate if the client experiencing the pain either does not understand the assessment tool used or finds it inadequate. Because pain is a subjective experience and pain assessment is critical to pain management, nurses could seek to individualize pain assessment by determining which pain assessment tool each client prefers and then consistently use the client-identified tool.

environment helps reduce the adverse effects of sleep deprivation, replenishes catecholamine stores, helps prevent critical care unit psychosis, and restores the diurnal effects of endorphins. Health care providers need to perform as many procedures as possible during the client's waking hours.

Tactile stimulation can reduce pain. The client's position is changed routinely to reduce pressure on any specific area; repositioning improves circulation to painful areas and eases pain. Massaging nonburn areas may reduce pain transmission on thick pain-sensory nerve fibers by stimulating an increased release of endorphins. Applying heat and maintaining warm room temperatures prevent shivering and stimulate the production of serotonin, which triggers the relaxation response.

To reduce anxiety and increase feelings of confidence and independence, the client is encouraged to participate in pain control measures. For example, the nurse and client make a contract that specifies how long a painful procedure will last. This helps clients deal with the pain for that particular period. Patient-controlled analgesia (PCA) also reduces pain in burned clients. Important issues and techniques for the best use of PCA include the following: giving an initial bolus of 5 to 10 mg of morphine (or equivalent drug), increasing the PCA dose as needed to achieve pain relief, and planning for a change in dosing regimens at night (e.g., giving a bolus dose at bedtime).

SURGICAL MANAGEMENT. A technique of early surgical excision of the burn wound is used in many burn centers (see Surgical Excision, pp. 1578 and 1579). Early excision under anesthesia can reduce the pain associated with daily debridement at the bedside or during hydrotherapy.

■ POTENTIAL FOR PULMONARY EDEMA

PLANNING: EXPECTED OUTCOMES. With intervention, the client with a burn injury in the emergent phase is expected to be free of pulmonary edema.

INTERVENTIONS. Pulmonary edema can arise from pulmonary injury; however, pulmonary edema in the emergent phase is associated with fluid resuscitation and myocardial overload. Even a young healthy person may have some degree of ventricular insufficiency. These clients usually receive digoxin or another inotropic agent to improve left ventricular function and prevent or treat pulmonary edema. Diuretics, a mainstay of therapy for pulmonary edema from other causes, may or may not be used in the emergent phase depending on the client's vascular hydration status and renal function.

■ POTENTIAL FOR ACUTE RESPIRATORY DISTRESS SYNDROME

PLANNING: EXPECTED OUTCOMES. The client with a burn injury in the emergent phase is expected to have arterial blood gases (ABGs) within normal limits, maintain normal lung compliance, and be free of respiratory distress.

INTERVENTIONS. Clients who have developed acute respiratory distress syndrome (ARDS) as a result of burn injury require thorough assessments and interventions. The interventions are aimed at increasing lung compliance and improving PaO_2 (partial pressure of arterial oxygen) levels.

In collaboration with the physician and respiratory therapist, the client receives positive end-expiratory pressure (PEEP) to augment the decreased lung volume by providing a continuous positive pressure in the airways and alveoli. This procedure optimizes the diffusion of oxygen across the alveolar-capillary membrane. PEEP can be combined with intermittent mandatory volume (IMV) to enhance its effectiveness.

The client's response is assessed and documented so that appropriate ventilator changes can be made. Any signs of respiratory distress and changes in respiratory patterns are documented and reported to the physician. Pulse oximetry and arterial blood gas (ABG) levels also are monitored for changes in respiratory status.

Neuromuscular blocking agents (atracurium) can be used in clients requiring mechanical ventilation to reduce or elimi-

nate spontaneous breathing efforts and to reduce oxygen consumption (see the discussion of specific nursing care under Drug Therapy [Ineffective Breathing Pattern], p. 1573).

> **⊚ CRITICAL THINKING CHALLENGE**
> The client who sustained the electrical injury described earlier is started on fluid resuscitation. You notice that his urine is becoming darker and has a high specific gravity.
> - Do you expect that this client needs as much fluid for resuscitation as a person who has a flame burn? Why or why not?
> - What should be your first action upon viewing the change in the character of this client's urine?
> - What additional medications or adjustment(s) in resuscitation should you expect to be ordered?

For suggested answer guidelines, go to ⌢SiMON⌣ http://www.wbsaunders.com/SIMON/Iggy/.

ACUTE PHASE OF BURN INJURY

■ OVERVIEW

The acute phase of burn injury begins approximately 48 hours after injury and lasts until wound closure is complete. During this phase, an intense collaborative approach to care is directed toward continued assessment and maintenance of the cardiovascular and respiratory systems, as well as toward gastrointestinal and nutritional status, burn wound care, pain control, and psychosocial interventions.

➤ COLLABORATIVE MANAGEMENT
● Assessment

■ PHYSICAL ASSESSMENT/CLINICAL MANIFESTATIONS

CARDIOPULMONARY ASSESSMENT. In the acute phase of burn injury, the physical assessment findings related to the cardiovascular and respiratory systems are directed at maintaining these systems and treating potential complications as they occur. Although airway injuries should be resolved, the client may experience pneumonia that can compromise the airway and result in respiratory failure requiring mechanical ventilation. Any cardiovascular system problems also should be resolved. However, the client is at risk for infection, which can lead to septic shock and affect cardiovascular function. The assessment and clinical interventions undertaken in the emergent phase should also be used in these isolated clinical situations.

NEUROENDOCRINE ASSESSMENT. The increased metabolic demands placed on the body after a severe burn injury can severely compromise nutritional status. The client's weight is obtained as ordered and is compared with his or her preburn weight. Body weight measurements are obtained without dressings or splints, if possible. A loss of 2% in body weight indicates a mild deficit; a weight loss of 10% or more is significant and requires the evaluation of caloric and fluid intake and appropriate modifications.

Indirect calorimetry often is used to obtain accurate calorie requirements for burn clients. This technique determines kilocalories of energy expenditure by measuring oxygen consumption (V_{O_2}) and carbon dioxide production (V_{CO_2}). Measurements are performed while the client is at rest and preferably at least 30 minutes after the most recent dressing changes or other stressful procedures. Indirect calorimetry generally is performed shortly after admission and at least once each week until the wounds are closed.

IMMUNOLOGIC ASSESSMENT. The client with a burn injury is susceptible to infection as a result of the inflammatory response and the compromise in immune function. Burn wound sepsis is a serious complication of burn injury, and infection remains the leading cause of morbidity and mortality during the acute phase of recovery. The nurse must continually assess the client for signs of local and systemic infections (Table 68-6), including changes in wound appearance, changes in neurologic and gastrointestinal function, and subtle changes in vital signs. Gram-positive, gram-negative, and fungal infections produce a variety of clinical signs and symptoms, and the nurse monitors for these differences (Table 68-7). A strict policy of meticulous handwashing for all health care providers is enforced. Aseptic technique in caring for wounds and during invasive monitoring or therapy is important in preventing hospital-acquired infections.

MUSCULOSKELETAL ASSESSMENT. Clients with a burn injury are at risk for musculoskeletal problems as a result of other injuries, immobility, healing processes, and treatment. The client's musculoskeletal status is initially evaluated within the first few hours of admission to the hospital or burn center and throughout the acute phase of injury. An assessment of active and passive range of motion for all joints, including the neck, is performed. Special attention is given to joints within the burn area. Ranges and limitations are noted for future reference.

● Analysis

During the acute phase of the burn injury, the client with a burn injury experiences a resolution of some earlier problems, may have initial problems that extend into the acute phase, and experiences new problems in many body systems.

■ COMMON NURSING DIAGNOSES AND COLLABORATIVE PROBLEMS

The following are common nursing diagnoses for clients with burn injuries in the acute phase who have sustained a burn injury greater than 25% of the total body surface area (TBSA):

1. Impaired Skin Integrity related to burn wound, graft site, or donor site
2. Risk for Infection related to impaired skin integrity, the presence of multiple invasive catheters, compromise in immune function, and nutritional compromise
3. Imbalanced Nutrition: Less than Body Requirements related to increased metabolic rate; reduced calorie intake; altered glucose, fat, and protein metabolism; and increased urinary nitrogen losses
4. Impaired Physical Mobility related to open burn wounds, pain, and scars and contractures
5. Disturbed Body Image related to changes in physical appearance and lifestyle, as well as alterations in sensory and motor function

The primary collaborative problem is Wound Care Management.

TABLE 68-6 ● LOCAL AND SYSTEMIC SIGNS OF INFECTION

LOCAL SIGNS
- Conversion of a partial-thickness injury to a full-thickness injury
- Ulceration of healthy skin at the burn site
- Erythematous, nodular lesions in uninvolved skin and vesicular lesions in healed skin
- Edema of healthy skin surrounding the burn wound
- Excessive burn wound drainage
- Pale, boggy, dry, or crusted granulation tissue
- Sloughing of grafts
- Wound breakdown after closure
- Odor

SYSTEMIC SIGNS
- Altered level of consciousness
- Changes in vital signs (tachycardia, tachypnea, temperature instability, hypotension)
- Increased fluid requirements for maintenance of a normal urine output
- Hemodynamic instability
- Oliguria
- Gastrointestinal dysfunction (diarrhea, vomiting, abdominal distention, paralytic ileus)
- Hyperglycemia
- Thrombocytopenia
- Change in total white blood cell count (above normal or below normal)
- Metabolic acidosis
- Hypoxemia

TABLE 68-7 ● SIGNS AND SYMPTOMS OF SEPSIS CAUSED BY DIFFERENT ORGANISMS

Sign/Symptom	Gram-Positive	Gram-Negative	Fungal
Onset	Insidious, 2-6 days	Rapid, 12-36 hr	Delayed
Sensorium	Severe disorientation and lethargy	Mild disorientation	Mild disorientation
Ileus	Severe	Severe	Mild
Diarrhea	Rare	Severe	Occasional
Temperature	Hyperpyrexia	Hypothermia	Hyperpyrexia
Hypotension	Late	Early	Late
White blood cell count	Neutrophilia	Neutropenia	Neutrophilia
Platelets	Normal	Low	Low

ADDITIONAL NURSING DIAGNOSES AND COLLABORATIVE PROBLEMS

In addition to the common nursing diagnoses and collaborative problems, clients with burn injuries in the acute phase may have one or more of the following:

- Anticipatory Grieving related to loss of significant others, loss of possessions, physical disfigurement, and changes in body image
- Disabled Family Coping related to loss of home, family, or significant others; crises resulting from burn injury; disturbances in normal functions; role changes; and prolonged hospitalization and rehabilitation
- Ineffective Coping related to situational crises, disfigurement, separation, and sensory overload
- Self-Care Deficits (Feeding, Bathing/Hygiene, Dressing/Grooming, Toileting) related to pain; contractures; and loss of function in the hands, extremities, and other body parts
- Sexual Dysfunction related to perineal, genital, and breast burns; immobility, fatigue, and depression; and disturbance in body image
- Disturbed Sleep Pattern related to pain, treatment regimen, and environmental noise
- Social Isolation related to the protective isolation treatment regimen and alterations in physical appearance
- Deficient Knowledge related to the treatment regimen and healing process
- Potential for Pneumonia
- Potential for Septicemia

● Planning and Implementation

IMPAIRED SKIN INTEGRITY; WOUND CARE MANAGEMENT

NOC PLANNING: EXPECTED OUTCOMES. With appropriate intervention, the client with a burn injury in the acute phase is expected to experience no further loss of skin integrity, have skin integrity restored without complications, and have skin thickness in the expected range in the burn wound area.

INTERVENTIONS. Interventions aim to preserve the integrity of nonburned skin, enhance wound healing of burned skin, and prevent complications.

NONSURGICAL MANAGEMENT. Nonsurgical burn wound management, or conservative treatment, involves removing exudates and necrotic tissue, cleaning the area, stimulating granulation and revascularization, and applying dressings. Restoration of skin, whether by natural healing or grafting, starts with the removal of eschar and other cellular debris from the burn wound. This removal is called **debridement.** Conservative treatment allows noninvasive debriding of the wound through mechanical and enzymatic actions that stimulate the separation of eschar over time. The goal is to have the wound slowly prepare itself for grafting and wound closure by a natural process.

MECHANICAL DEBRIDEMENT. Burn wounds are debrided and cleaned a minimum of once, and usually two to three times, each day during hydrotherapy (the application of water for treatment). Nurses, assistive nursing personnel, and physical therapists perform hydrotherapy daily to debride necrotic tissue and to examine the wounds. Hydrotherapy can be accomplished by immersing the client in a tub, showering the client on a specially designed table, or successively washing only small areas of the wound at the bedside if the client is too unstable to be moved. Showering enhances visualization of the wounds and allows water temperature to be kept constant.

Nurses and skilled technicians use forceps and scissors to remove loose, nonviable tissue during hydrotherapy. The care of intact blisters is controversial. At most institutions, small blisters are left alone because they serve as a protective barrier that assists with wound healing and re-epithelialization. Because the protein-filled fluid within blisters can cause some degree of immunosuppression, many institutions open larger blisters. Washcloths or gauze sponges also can facilitate the debridement of "cheesy" eschar or pseudoeschar. During hydrotherapy, the burn areas are washed thoroughly and gently with mild soap or detergent and water. The areas are then rinsed with water at room temperature.

ENZYMATIC DEBRIDEMENT. Enzymatic debridement can occur naturally by autolysis or artificially by the application of exogenous agents. **Autolysis** is the spontaneous disintegration of tissue by the action of the client's own cellular enzymes. This process is seldom used in North America for larger burns because it is slow and results in a prolonged hospital stay.

Exogenous agents, such as collagenase (Santyl), are topical enzymes used for rapid wound debridement. When these agents are applied directly to the burn wound in a once-a-day dressing change, the enzymes digest native and denatured collagen in necrotic tissues. Because collagen accounts for 75% of the dry weight of skin tissue, the ability of collagenase (Santyl) to digest collagen in the physiologic pH range makes it an important debriding agent for burn wounds. Polysporin powder is often used with this topical agent to prevent infection.

DRESSING THE BURN WOUND. After burn wounds are cleaned and debrided, topical antibiotics are reapplied to prevent infection (see Risk for Infection, p. 1579). Some type of dressing is then applied to the burn wound. Burn dressings include standard wound dressings, biologic dressings, and synthetic dressings and artificial skin. (Table 67-6 describes the characteristics of many types of dressings.)

Standard Wound Dressings. Standard wound dressings consist of multiple layers of gauze applied over the topical agent or antibiotic on the burn wound. The number of gauze layers depends on the following:

- Depth of the injury
- Amount of drainage expected
- Area injured
- Client's mobility
- Frequency of dressing changes

The gauze layers are held in place with roller-type gauze bandages applied in a distal to proximal direction or with circular net fabrics. On the client's extremities, the nurse covers gauze dressings with elastic wraps, especially if the client is ambulatory. Based on assessed needs or clinician orders, nursing personnel generally change and reapply the dressings every 8 to 24 hours after thoroughly cleaning the areas.

Biologic Dressings. Biologic dressings are materials obtained from human tissue donors (homograft or allograft) or animals (heterograft or xenograft). When applied over open wounds, a biologic dressing rapidly adheres and promotes healing or prepares the wound for permanent skin graft coverage.

Biologic materials are used in healing partial-thickness and granulating full-thickness wounds that are clean and free of eschar. Table 68-8 outlines the advantages and disadvantages of biologic dressings. The type of biologic dressing selected depends on the type of wound to be covered and the availability of the material.

Homograft. Skin for a **homograft** (**allograft**) is usually obtained from a cadaver and provided through a skin bank. It is fresh or frozen; frozen skin is thawed in a warm bath of sterile normal saline before application. Disadvantages to the use of homografts are the excessive costs ($750 to $1000 per square foot) and the risk of transmitting a bloodborne infection.

Heterograft. Skin for a **heterograft** (**xenograft**) is obtained from another species. Pigskin is the most common heterograft because of its relative compatibility with human skin. The pigskin is replaced on a continual basis until the wound heals naturally or is closed with autograft. Because pigskin does not control bacterial proliferation, it is changed frequently, usually daily.

Amniotic Membrane. Amniotic membrane is another form of biologic dressing used on burn wounds. Its large size, low cost, and availability have helped with its success. In full-thickness injuries, the amniotic membrane immediately adheres to the wound. With partial-thickness areas, the amniotic membrane is effective as a dressing until re-epithelialization occurs. The membrane may require frequent changes because it does not vascularize and has the tendency to disintegrate in 48 hours.

Cultured Skin. Cultured skin can be grown from a small biopsy specimen of epidermal cells from an unburned portion of the client's body. The cells are grown in a laboratory to produce larger epithelial sheets that can be grafted on the client to generate a permanent epidermal surface. The length of time for culturing and growing the skin is prolonged, and the epithelial sheets are not durable. Extreme care must be taken when these sheets are applied to ensure adherence and prevent sloughing. This process is also extremely costly.

Artificial Skin. Artificial skin, first developed in 1980, is an alternative approach to closure of the burn wound. This substance has two layers composed of a Silastic epidermis and a porous dermis made from bovine hide collagen and shark cartilage (Winfrey, Cochran, & Hegarty, 1999).

After the artificial skin is applied to a clean, excised wound surface, fibroblasts move into the collagen part of the artificial skin and create a fibrinous structure similar to normal dermis. The artificial dermis slowly dissolves and is replaced with normal blood vessels and connective tissue (*neodermis*). The neodermis will support a standard split-thickness autograft that is placed over it when the Silastic layer is removed.

Synthetic Dressings. Synthetic dressings consisting of solid silicone and plastic membranes (e.g., polyvinyl chloride and polyurethane) may be substituted for antimicrobial, standard, or biologic dressings. Synthetic dressings are applied directly to the surface of a clean or surgically prepared wound and remain in place until they fall off or are removed due to nonadhesion. Because many of these dressings are transparent or translucent, the nurse can inspect the wound without removing the dressing. The client experiences pain reduction at the site because these agents also prevent contact of the wound with air. These dressings may also be used to cover donor sites where skin was obtained for autografting.

A recent review of the literature found transparent film to be the best dressing for the care of donor site wounds (see the Evidence-Based Practice for Nursing box on p. 1579). Transparent film was associated with one of the fastest healing rates, a low infection rate, the least amount of associated pain, and minimal cost (Rakel et al., 1998). An additional strategy that merits consideration has been used to manage donor site pain. Topical lidocaine applied to donor harvest sites produced an analgesic effect that reduced narcotic requirements, significantly lowered pain scores, and did not produce toxic blood concentrations in clients undergoing grafting for burns involving less than 15% of the total body surface area (TBSA) (Jellish et al., 1999).

SURGICAL MANAGEMENT. Surgical management of burn wounds focuses on surgical excision and wound covering. Surgical excision usually occurs early in the postburn period. Grafting procedures for skin covering may be performed throughout the acute phase as burn wounds are made ready and donor sites are available. Grafting may improve function or appearance in the rehabilitative phase.

Wound covering is achieved through autografting. With autografting, viable skin from an area of the client's intact, healthy skin is transplanted to the area where a full-thickness burn wound was excised.

SURGICAL EXCISION. Surgical excision is a widely used method for managing full-thickness injuries; it is the treatment of choice for most deep partial-thickness wounds. The client is taken to the operating room as early as possible within the first 5 days after injury and as needed until complete permanent coverage has been achieved.

TABLE 68-8 • BIOLOGIC DRESSINGS

USES
- Debridement of untidy wounds after separation of eschar
- Promotion of re-epithelialization of deep partial-thickness wounds
- Temporary coverage after excision of the burn wound
- Protection of granulation tissue between autografts
- Test graft before autografting

ADVANTAGES
- Early adherence to the wound
- Reduction of evaporative heat loss
- Reduction of evaporate water loss
- Prevention of desiccation of granulation tissue
- Reduction of exudate protein losses
- Reduction of pain
- Assistance in wound debridement
- Enhancement of healing with partial-thickness injuries
- Protection of exposed neovascular tissue
- Inhibition of bacterial proliferation

DISADVANTAGES
- Early lysis resulting in bacterial proliferation
- Expensive
- Rejection responses
- Possible burn wound sepsis if applied over eschar
- Not readily available
- Storage (some may require refrigeration)
- Possible transmission of diseases, such as hepatitis

The burn wound is excised by either a tangential or a fascial excision technique. In the tangential technique, the surgeon excises very thin layers of the necrotic burn surface until bleeding tissue is encountered. Bleeding indicates that a viable bed of dermis or subcutaneous fat has been reached for application of the graft.

In the fascial technique, the surgeon excises the burn wound to the level of superficial fascia. Fascial excision usually is reserved for very deep and extensive burns. Blood loss is minimal, and grafting is usually successful.

WOUND COVERING. Permanent skin coverage for extensive full-thickness injuries is achieved by applying an autograft. Skin for an autograft is taken from the client's own body. The surgeon usually removes a piece of skin from a remote unburned area of the body and transplants it to cover the burn wound. Skin grafts are generally of split thickness (0.015 inch); a partial-thickness injury is formed at the site of surgical removal (the donor site). Grafts are placed either on a clean granulated bed or over a surgically excised area of burn (see also Chapter 67).

The availability of donor sites for larger burns is small. Clients with burns of a large surface area may have a mere 5% to 20% of the skin surface available to cover the 80% to 95% burned area. Coverage is accomplished in the following ways:

- Successive reharvesting of the available donor site, with time allowed between harvests for re-epithelialization and healing

- Meshing the split-thickness skin grafts (Figure 68-13) to allow a small graft to cover a larger area; although small open spaces (interstices) are present uniformly throughout the graft, healing time is slower for a meshed graft because the skin must fill in the interstices as well as attach to the granulation bed

■ RISK FOR INFECTION

Burn wound infection occurs through *autocontamination,* in which the client's own normal flora overgrows and penetrates the internal environment; and *cross-contamination,* in which microorganisms from another person or the environment are transferred to the client.

PLANNING: EXPECTED OUTCOMES. The client with a burn injury in the acute phase is expected to remain free from infection by cross-contamination and not experience septicemia.

INTERVENTIONS. Interventions aim to prevent infection and remove infected tissue.

NONSURGICAL MANAGEMENT. Nonsurgical management of clients at high risk for infection consists of minimizing exposure of the burn client to exogenous microorganisms, reducing the risk of autocontamination, and recognizing the signs and symptoms of infection early. Drug therapy, isolation therapy, and environmental manipulation are appropriate strategies for preventing and managing infection.

DRUG THERAPY FOR INFECTION PREVENTION. Burn wound conditions favor the growth of *Clostridium tetani.* All burn clients are at risk for this potentially fatal infectious complication. Tetanus toxoid, 0.5 mL administered intramuscularly, enhances previously acquired immunity to *C. tetani;* this is a routine prophylactic procedure when the client is admitted to the hospital. The additional administration of tetanus immune globulin (human) (Hyper-Tet) is recommended when the history of tetanus immunization is questionable.

The use of topical antimicrobial agents is one of the most important interventions for infection prevention in burn

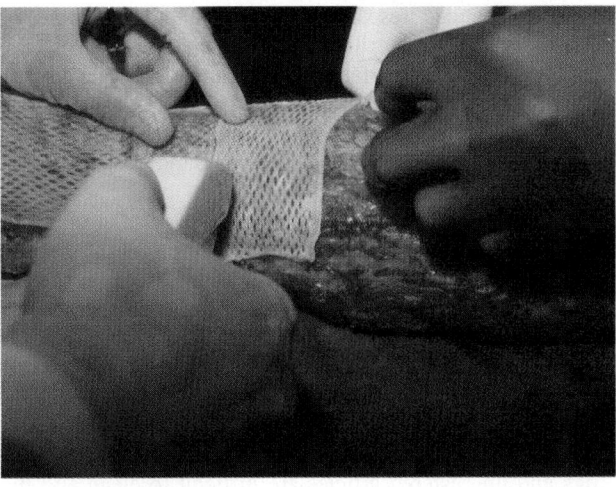

Figure 68-13 ● The typical appearance of meshed autografts.

wounds. The primary goal of topical antimicrobial therapy is to minimize bacterial proliferation into the wound and prevent systemic sepsis.

Topical antibiotics are applied by either the *open* or the *closed* technique. With the open technique, the nurse uses either aseptic or clean methods to apply the agent directly to the burn wound without further dressing the wound. The nurse cleans the wound every 8 to 24 hours and applies fresh antimicrobial agents. With the more common closed technique, the burn wound is dressed after applying the topical agents.

Topical antimicrobial drugs are not applied to freshly grafted areas because many of these agents inhibit cell growth. Chart 68-6 summarizes the characteristics of various topical antimicrobial agents; two of the more commonly used agents are silver sulfadiazine (Silvadene, Flamazine✚) and mafenide acetate (Sulfamylon).

DRUG THERAPY FOR THE TREATMENT OF INFECTION.
Systemic antibiotics are ordered when burn clients experience symptoms of an actual infection, including septicemia. Broad-spectrum antibiotics are administered until the results of blood cultures and sensitivity status are available. At that time, more specific antibiotics, including the aminoglycosides such as amikacin (Amikin) or gentamicin (Garamycin, Alcomicin✚) and cephalosporins such as cephalothin (Keflin) or ceftriaxone (Rocephin), are used. Because of increased metabolism, burn clients generally require a larger than normal dose of these drugs to maintain therapeutic serum levels. If aminoglycosides are used, serial peak and trough serum levels are obtained to monitor the efficacy of treatment and evaluate potential renal toxicity.

ISOLATION THERAPY.
Some clinicians believe that isolation therapy significantly reduces the incidence of cross-contamination; however, methods of isolation are varied and controversial. Some burn centers practice virtually no isolation, whereas others use near-total sterile conditions. All isolation methods for the client with burns emphasize proper and consistent handwashing as the single most effective technique for preventing the transmission of infection.

ENVIRONMENTAL MANIPULATION.
All health care providers wear gloves during all contact with open wounds. The use of sterile versus clean gloves for noninvasive, routine wound care procedures varies by agency and is a matter of debate. Regardless of sterility, the nurse changes gloves when handling wounds on different areas of the body and between handling old and new dressings.

The equipment on burn units is not shared among clients. Disposable items (e.g., pillows, syringes, and dishes) are used as much as possible. The nurse assigns to each client any equipment used in daily routine care (e.g., thermometers, blood pressure cuffs, and stethoscopes). Daily cleaning of the equipment and general housekeeping are essential for environmental infection control. All equipment must be cleaned after use on one client and before use on another. Because *Pseudomonas* has been shown to sequester in plants, the presence of plants and flowers is prohibited. Some burn units do not permit clients to eat raw foods (such as salads, fruit, and pepper) to minimize exposure to exogenous microorganisms. Rugs and upholstered articles are difficult to clean and may harbor organisms; their use is also restricted.

Visitors are restricted when the client is immunosuppressed. Ill people, small children, and other clients should not come into direct contact with the burn client. Some burn units recommend that all visitors wear protective clothing (gowns, gloves, masks, and shoe and hair covers) in the room of the immunosuppressed client, but no conclusive data are available to support this approach.

SECONDARY PREVENTION/EARLY DETECTION.
The burn wounds are carefully monitored on admission and at each dressing change. The wounds are examined for the following signs of infection:
- Pervasive odor
- Color changes
- Change in texture
- Purulent drainage
- Exudate
- Sloughing grafts
- Redness at the wound edges extending to nonburned skin

Laboratory cultures and biopsies are recommended. Quantitative biopsies of the eschar and granulation tissue are performed routinely and as needed to monitor the proliferation of organisms and are considered the gold standard for wound monitoring.

SURGICAL MANAGEMENT.
Infected burn wounds with colony counts of or approaching 10^5 colonies per gram of tissue are life threatening, even with antibiotic therapy. Aggressive surgical excision of the burn wound may be necessary.

◼ IMBALANCED NUTRITION: LESS THAN BODY REQUIREMENTS

NOC **PLANNING: EXPECTED OUTCOMES.** The client with a burn injury in the acute phase is expected to maintain adequate nutrient intake for meeting the body's calorie requirements as evidenced by the maintenance of normal body weight, serum albumin within expected range, and tissue healing.

INTERVENTIONS. Interventions aim to calculate the client's calorie needs and provide an adequate daily source of calories and nutrients that the client can ingest and metabolize.

Diet therapy begins with calculating the client's current daily metabolic needs and calorie requirements. Several formulas and charts are used for this calculation. Nutritional requirements for a client with a relatively large burn area can exceed 5000 kcal/day. In addition to a high-calorie intake, the burn client requires a diet high in protein for wound healing. The nurse collaborates with the dietitian and the client to plan alternatives to conventional nutritional patterns.

Oral diet therapy may be delayed for several days after the injury until the client has sufficient gastrointestinal motility. As a result, nasoduodenal tube feedings are often initiated soon after admission. The provision of early enteral feeding helps to decrease weight loss, gut atrophy, bacterial translocation, and subsequent sepsis. These feedings often are initiated within 4 hours of commencing fluid resuscitation. This type of nutritional supplement prevents nutritional deficits in critically burned clients.

CHART 68-6

TOPICAL DRUG THERAPY *for* Burns

Agent	Description	Action	Advantages	Disadvantages	Interventions
Silver sulfadiazine (Silvadene, Flamazine✦)	Nontoxic salt of silver sulfadiazine in water-based cream	Binds to bacterial cell membranes and interferes with DNA synthesis	Does not cause hypochloremia, hyponatremia, electrolyte imbalance, or kidney disease Painless Wide-spectrum antimicrobial action against gram-positive and gram-negative organisms Long shelf life Delays eschar separation to a lesser degree than do many other topical agents	Absorbed into eschar less than other agents May cause rash, pruritus, burning, and leukopenia Not consistently effective for burns covering more than 60% of the body Not effective against *Pseudomonas*	Watch for signs of infection, such as soupiness of wound area. Watch for allergic reaction causing drop in white blood cell count. Do not use if reaction to sulfonamide has occurred.
Collagenase (Santyl) with polysporin powder	Topical enzymatic debriding agent with 250 collagenase units/g of white petroleum	Digests collagen in necrotic tissue	Painless Daily dressing changes No side effects Quick debridement action Easy to apply	Expensive Use only on partial-thickness injuries	Apply only once a day.
Mafenide acetate (Sulfamylon)	Soft, white, non-staining water-based cream	Bacteriostatic action against many gram-positive and gram-negative organisms	Effective against *Pseudomonas* Long shelf life Excellent for treating electrical burns Penetrates thick eschar	May lead to infection May cause metabolic acidosis, hyperpnea, and rash When applied, may cause pain that lasts 30-40 min	Premedicate for pain before application. Monitor blood gas and serum electrolyte levels. Do not use if sulfa drug allergy or respiratory or kidney disease is present.
Nitrofurazone (Furacin)	Cream, solution, or water-soluble powder	Wide-spectrum anti-bacterial	Effective against *Staphylococcus aureus* and some antibiotic-resistant organisms Causes neither pain nor maceration	May cause contact dermatitis (rare) Messy to apply in cream form May cause renal problems if used for extensive burns	Observe carefully for signs of allergic reaction and evidence of super-infections.
Povidone-iodine (Betadine)	Iodine complex available as solution, ointment, or foam	Microbicidal against gram-positive and gram-negative organisms	Effective against many infections not well controlled by silver sulfadiazine	May cause metabolic acidosis and elevated serum iodine levels May form crusts if burns are not cleaned properly Causes rash and burning in some clients Stains clothes and linen Deactivated by wound proteins	Check serum electrolyte and serum iodine levels frequently.
Gentamicin sulfate (Garamycin, Gentamar)	Available as cream or solution for topical use	Antibiotic action against organisms resistant to other agents	Effective against *Pseudomonas* Does not cause pain	May have ototoxic and nephrotoxic effects May result in resistance by certain organisms	Use with caution in clients with decreased renal function. Monitor serum and urine creatinine clearance before and during treatment.
Polymyxin B–bacitracin	Topical cream	Wide-spectrum anti-bacterial	Painless Effective against many gram-positive and gram-negative organisms Can be used on the face Can be placed on healed grafts to lubricate	May cause urticaria, burning, and inflammation Does not penetrate eschar	Apply q2-8h to keep areas moist.

The nurse encourages clients who can eat solid foods to ingest as many calories as possible. The client's preferences are taken into consideration for diet planning and food selection. Clients are encouraged to request food whenever they feel they can eat—not just according to the hospital's standard meal schedule. The nurse also offers frequent high-calorie, high-protein supplemental feedings. Care is taken to keep an accurate calorie count for foods and beverages that are actually ingested by the client.

Clients who cannot swallow but who have adequate gastric motility may meet calorie and nutrition needs through enteral tube feedings (see Chapter 61). Parenteral nutrition may be administered by the intravenous route when the gastrointestinal tract is not functional or when the client's nutritional requirements cannot be met by oral and enteral feeding. This method is used as a last resort because it is invasive and can lead to infectious and metabolic complications.

■ IMPAIRED PHYSICAL MOBILITY

NOC **PLANNING: EXPECTED OUTCOMES.** The client with a burn injury in the acute phase is expected to regain and maintain an optimal ability to move purposefully.

INTERVENTIONS. Interventions aim to maintain the client's preburn range of joint motion and prevent contracture formation.

NONSURGICAL MANAGEMENT. Nonsurgical management includes positioning, range-of-motion exercises, ambulation, and pressure dressings.

POSITIONING. Positioning is critical for clients with burn injuries because the position of comfort for the client is often one of joint flexion, which predisposes him or her to the development of contractures. Care is taken to maintain the client in a neutral body position with minimal flexion. Best practice for the prevention of contractures is presented in Chart 68-7.

Splints and other conforming devices may assist in maintaining position. These devices are used most frequently on the joints of the hands, elbows, knees, neck, and axillae.

RANGE-OF-MOTION EXERCISES. Range-of-motion exercises are performed actively at least three times a day. If the client cannot move a joint actively, the nurse performs passive range-of-motion exercises. Burned hands are given special attention. The client is encouraged to perform active range-of-motion exercises for the hand, thumb, and fingers every hour while awake.

AMBULATION. Ambulation is started as soon as possible after the fluid shifts have resolved. Clients with a variety of attached equipment (IV catheters, nasogastric tubes, electrocardiographic leads, extensive dressings) can ambulate with preparation and assistance. Ambulation is performed two or three times a day and progresses in length each time. Ambulation inhibits the loss of bone density, strengthens muscles, stimulates immune function, promotes ventilation, and prevents a wide variety of complications.

PRESSURE DRESSINGS. After the graft heals, pressure dressings are implemented to assist in the prevention of contractures and tight hypertrophic scars, which can inhibit mobility. These dressings also inhibit venous engorgement and edema formation in areas with decreased lymphatic outflow. Pressure dressings may be elastic wraps or specially designed, custom-fitted, elasticized clothing that provide continuous and uniform pressure over burned surfaces. Figure 68-14 illustrates such garments. For maximal effectiveness, pressure garments should be worn at least 23 hours a day, every day, until the scar tissue is mature (12 to 24 months). Pressure garments generally cause an increase in warmth and itchiness and often are seen as very uncomfortable by the client. The nurse must reinforce to the client that wearing pressure garments is extremely beneficial in maintaining mobility and reducing hypertrophic scarring.

CHART 68-7		
BEST PRACTICE *for* **Positioning to Prevent Contractures**		
AFFECTED BODY PART	**POSITION OF FUNCTION**	**INTERVENTIONS**
Head and neck	Hyperextension	Place a towel roll under the client's neck or shoulder, or use a double mattress.
Posterior neck	Flexion	Have the client turn the head from side to side.
Upper chest and chest	Shoulder retraction	Place the client supine. Do not allow pillows. Place a folded towel under the spine, between the scapulae.
Lateral trunk	Flexion to uninvolved side	Place the client supine with the arm on the affected side up over the head.
Anterior shoulder	Abduction and external rotation	Maintain the upper arm at 90 degrees of abduction from the lateral aspect of the trunk.
Posterior shoulder	Slight flexion and interior rotation	Keep the arm slightly behind the midline.
Elbow	Extension and supination	Keep the joint in the extended position.
Wrist	30-45 degrees of extension	Use a splint.
Fingers		
MP joints	70-90 degrees of flexion	Use a splint.
PIP and DIP joints	Extended	Use a splint.
Ankle	90 degrees of dorsiflexion	Use a footboard or splint.
Legs	15-20 degrees of abduction	Place a small pillow between the legs.

MP, Metacarpal-phalangeal; *PIP,* proximal interphalangeal, *DIP,* distal interphalengeal.

SURGICAL MANAGEMENT. Surgical management is restorative rather than preventive. Surgical techniques for contracture release are most commonly performed in the neck, axilla, elbow flexion areas, and hand. Specific surgical procedures to improve movement vary for each client.

Postoperative nursing responsibilities include nonsurgical interventions to prevent contractures from reforming as well as the care of new grafts and suture lines. The nurse constantly reinforces the need for the client to comply with exercise and splinting regimens to prevent the recurrence of joint immobility.

DISTURBED BODY IMAGE

NOC PLANNING: EXPECTED OUTCOMES. Following intervention, the client with a burn injury in the acute phase is expected to have a positive perception of his or her own appearance and body functions as evidenced by a willingness to touch the affected body part, adjustment to changes in body function, a willingness to use strategies to enhance appearance and function, a successful progression through the grieving process, and the use of support systems.

INTERVENTIONS. Nonsurgical and surgical interventions can assist clients who experience body image disturbances as a result of burn injury.

NONSURGICAL MANAGEMENT. Understanding the stages of grief is helpful for the client, family, and nurse. The nurse assesses which stage of grief the client is currently experiencing and helps interpret his or her behaviors. The client often is unaware of or is confused by his or her feelings. The nurse reassures him or her that feelings of grief, loss, anxiety, anger, fear, and guilt are normal. The client may be grieving the loss of body parts, appearance, role identity, and social identity. The nurse seeks the help of other health care team members (e.g., psychologist, psychiatrist, social worker, or clergy or religious leader) in addressing these problems.

The nurse accepts the physical and psychologic characteristics of the client. Clients and families are presented with realistic expected outcomes for the client's functional capacity and physical appearance. Information sessions and counseling for the family or significant others can identify previous and current patterns of support that are effective for the client and family. The nurse facilitates their use of these systems and the development of new support systems and makes referrals to specific support groups. To identify the effectiveness of such assistance and possible gaps in support, the nurse continually evaluates support resources throughout the course of illness.

Engaging in decision making and independent activities fosters feelings of self-worth, which are closely linked to body image. To this end, the nurse plans and encourages the client's participation in self-care activities. Family members are assisted in understanding that it is more beneficial for the client to perform these activities than to have them performed by someone else. Families are encouraged to include the client in family decision making to the same degree that he or she participated in this process before the injury.

SURGICAL MANAGEMENT. Reconstructive and cosmetic surgery can be performed for many years after the burn injury. Restoration of function and improvement of physical appearance through surgical techniques often increase the client's feelings of self-worth and promote a positive body image. Many clients have unrealistic expectations of reconstructive surgery and envision an appearance identical or equal in quality to the preburn state. The nurse educates the client and family about expected cosmetic outcomes.

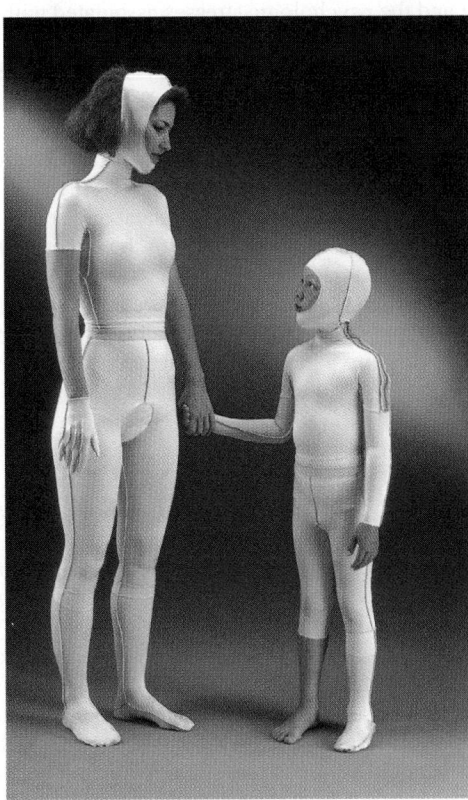

Figure 68-14 ● Models wearing pressure garments. (Courtesy Beiersdorf-Jobst, Inc., Charlotte, NC.)

CRITICAL THINKING CHALLENGE

The 22-year-old client who experienced an electrical injury has had his thumb and part of his right hand amputated and has had his right kidney removed. His right arm, above and below the elbow, was grafted with a split-thickness meshed graft taken from his left thigh. When you change the dressing, you note that the graft has a dusky appearance and that the edges of the graft are beginning to curl. The margins of the wound are firm and red with some purulent drainage. You also note a greenish blue color in the burned area next to the graft.

- What is your first action?
- Should range-of-motion exercises be performed for the right elbow at this time? Why or why not?
- What additional assessment data should you obtain about the graft and the surrounding burn wound?

For suggested answer guidelines, go to **SIMON** http://www.wbsaunders.com/SIMON/Iggy/.

REHABILITATIVE PHASE OF BURN INJURY

OVERVIEW

Although rehabilitation efforts are started from the time of admission, the technical rehabilitative phase begins with wound closure and ends when the client returns to the highest possible level of functioning. The emphasis during this phase is the psychosocial adjustment of the client, the prevention of scars and contractures, and the resumption of preburn activity, including work, family, and social roles. This phase may take years or even last a lifetime as clients adjust to permanent limitations that may not be apparent until long after the initial injury.

► COLLABORATIVE MANAGEMENT

Although attention initially is placed on the physical interventions for and clinical manifestations of the burn injury, psychologic care is equally important. The nurse provides psychosocial support to the client and family throughout hospitalization but more extensively throughout the rehabilitative phase.

Information from the client and family aids in the assessment and diagnosis of psychologic problems and allows treatment to be instituted. The nurse explores the client's feelings about the burn injury. It is extremely difficult for clients to concentrate on the many tasks before them when obstacles such as guilt and grief are in the forefront.

The client or family member is asked whether there is a history of psychologic or organic impairment. The type of coping mechanisms the client has used successfully during times of stress is assessed and documented to assist with a future plan of care. The nurse also assesses the client's family unit and the family members' history of interaction. The nurse determines cultural and ethnic factors and takes these into consideration when planning psychosocial interventions.

Throughout the hospitalization the client progresses through a variety of stages and exhibits a myriad of feelings, including denial, regression, and anger. The nurse accurately assesses the client's feelings during each stage so appropriate plans of care can be developed and carried out.

◗ Community-Based Care

Discharge planning for the client with a burn injury begins at the time of admission to the hospital or burn center. In most burn centers, the multidisciplinary team meets regularly to plan for discharge. In helping the client to reach mutually established discharge goals, the team evaluates the progress of each discipline. Table 68-9 summarizes the usual discharge needs of the client with burns.

■ PSYCHOSOCIAL PREPARATION

During the recovery period and for some time after discharge from the hospital, clients with severe burn injuries are likely to experience psychologic problems that require psychosocial assistance. Such problems include posttraumatic stress disorder, sexual dysfunction, and severe depression. Assistance is coordinated with the client, family, and health care team. Psychosocial assistance is best provided by a professional counselor with previous experience in helping burn clients.

One specific area to be addressed with the client is the reaction of others to the sight of healing wounds and disfiguring scars. Clients with facial burns are especially subjected to stares and other forms of disquieting behavior from the general public. Visits from friends and short public appearances before discharge may help the client begin adjusting to this problem. Community reintegration programs can assist the psychosocial and physical recovery of the client with serious burns.

TABLE 68-9 • NEEDS TO BE ADDRESSED BEFORE DISCHARGE OF THE CLIENT WITH BURNS

- Early client assessment
- Financial assessment
- Evaluation of family resources
- Weekly discharge planning meeting
- Psychologic referral
- Client and family teaching (home care)
- Designation of principal learners (specific family members or significant others who will help with care)
- Development of teaching plan
- Training for wound care
- Rehabilitation referral
- Home assessment (on-site visit)
- Medical equipment
- Public health nursing referral
- Evaluation of community resources
- Visit to referral agency
- Re-entry programs for school or work environment
- Nursing home placement
- Environmental interventions
- Auditory testing
- Speech therapy
- Prosthetic rehabilitation

■ HOME CARE MANAGEMENT

The client with severe burns is often discharged from the acute care setting when life-threatening complications are resolved and minimal wound areas remain open. During the initial weeks at home after discharge, the client usually continues to require at least daily wound care, rehabilitative therapy, nutritional support, symptom management, and drug therapy.

Although the client usually views the prospect of going home in a positive light, the difficulties associated with physical care and the psychologic stresses associated with changes in appearance, role, function, and lifestyle are numerous and may overwhelm the client and family. Successful discharge depends on extensive planning and preparation of the client, family, and home environment through education and the involvement of appropriate support agencies and services.

Preparation for discharge includes assessment of the family and home care situation from physical and social perspectives. The nurse considers the needs of the client when evaluating the environment for cleanliness; access to bathing facilities, electricity, and running water; stairways; number of occupants; temperature control; and safety. If the burn injuries are a result of a fire at home, a new residence may need to be established.

■ HEALTH TEACHING

Education about burn care and living with the consequences of burn injuries begins when the client is admitted to the hospital or burn center. A weekly plan for client education is outlined; the primary goal is progression toward independence for the client and family. Critical for this goal is teaching clients, family members, or significant others to perform specific care tasks, such as dressing changes. Clients and family members first observe the nurse changing the dressings, then assist in performing the changes, and finally change the dressings independently under the supervision of the burn care nurse.

Before discharge, all people who will be involved in the client's home care participate in discharge planning and teaching sessions. In addition to details about dressing changes, the nurse explains the following:

- Signs and symptoms of infection
- Medication regimens
- Proper use of prosthetic and positioning devices
- Correct application and care of pressure garments
- Comfort measures to reduce pruritus
- Dates for follow-up appointments

■ HEALTH CARE RESOURCES

The nurse and health care team evaluate the family in terms of capacity and willingness to assist in providing care to the client after discharge. A visiting nurse or case manager referral can assist the family with care problems arising at home. In addition, the visiting nurse can help the family determine what special equipment, supplies, or services will be needed. The frequency of home visits depends on the client's condition and the ability of family members to function as care providers. It is imperative that the visiting nurse have extensive experience in providing burn care. The home care nurse may benefit from a brief visit to the client while in the hospital and from observing burn wound care.

The home care of a client after an extensive burn often involves daily physical therapy and rehabilitation sessions at special centers. Transportation problems are addressed and resolved before the client is discharged. In some instances, the burn center has arrangements for transportation. Some community volunteer agencies provide transportation by private car.

When rehabilitation is expected to be prolonged, the client may be discharged to a special rehabilitation facility. Before this point, the burn care nurse consults with the rehabilitation nurse or team and provides copies of the care and teaching plans used with the client.

◎ CRITICAL THINKING CHALLENGE

The 22-year-old client who sustained an electrical injury and had his right thumb and part of his right hand amputated is being prepared for discharge. He tells you he is afraid that he will not be accepted by his friends or ever get married because of his appearance and the disability resulting from the amputation.

- Are this client's fears justified? Why or why not?
- What is your immediate response to his statements?
- What resources or referrals would be most appropriate for this client at this time?

For suggested answer guidelines, go to ⌂⌐SiMON⌐ http://www.wbsaunders.com/SIMON/Iggy/.

▶ Evaluation: Outcomes

NOC The nurse evaluates the care of the client with a burn injury on the basis of the identified nursing diagnoses and collaborative problems. The expected outcomes may include that the client will:

- Have cardiac output restored to normal as evidenced by blood pressure and heart rate in expected ranges and by strong peripheral pulses
- Maintain adequate oxygenation and circulation to all vital organs as evidenced by oxygen saturation, partial pressure of arterial oxygen (PaO_2), partial pressure of arterial carbon dioxide ($PaCO_2$), and arterial blood pH within normal limits
- Have arterial blood gases (ABGs) within normal limits
- Have normal lung compliance
- Be free of respiratory distress
- Be free of pulmonary edema
- Be free of visceral organ damage
- Maintain stable cardiac rhythms
- Maintain a patent airway
- Have an effective breathing pattern as evidenced by maintaining oxygen saturation, PaO_2, $PaCO_2$, and an arterial blood pH within normal limits
- Have pain alleviated or reduced as evidenced by a decreased report of pain and a decreased length of pain episodes
- Experience no further loss of skin integrity
- Have skin integrity restored without complications
- Have skin thickness in the expected range in the burn wound area
- Remain free from infection by cross-contamination
- Not experience septicemia
- Maintain an adequate nutrient intake for meeting the body's calorie requirements as evidenced by maintenance (achievement) of normal weight, serum albumin within expected range, and tissue healing
- Regain and maintain an optimal ability to move purposefully
- Have a positive perception of his or her own appearance and body functions
- Willingly touch affected body parts
- Accept altered appearance as a result of the burn injury
- Successfully progress through the grieving process
- Use support systems

ONLINE RESOURCES

For suggested readings and Internet resources, go to http://www.wbsaunders.com/SIMON/Iggy/.

SELECTED BIBLIOGRAPHY

Asterisk indicates a classic or definitive work on this subject.

Ahrns, K.A., & Harkins, D.R. (1999). Initial resuscitation after burn injury: Therapies, strategies and controversies. *AACN Clinical Issues: Advanced Practice in Acute and Critical Care, 10*(1), 46-60.

American Burn Association. (1999). U.S. trauma and burn statistics; http://www.ameriburn.org.

Atkins, S. (1999). Burns assessment and initial management. *Nursing Times, 95*(35), 46-48.

*Baud, F.J., et al. (1991). Elevated blood cyanide concentrations in victims of smoke inhalation. *New England Journal of Medicine, 325*(25), 1761-1766.

Burn Foundation. (1999). Burn incidence and treatment in the United States; http://www.burnfoundation.org/adultfact.html.

*Cadier, M., & Shakespear, P. (1995). Burns in octogenarians. *Burns, 21*(3), 200-204.

*Covington, D., Wainwright, D., & Parks, D. (1996). Prognostic indicators in the elderly patient with burns. *Journal of Burn Care and Rehabilitation, 17*(3), 222-230.

*Dries, D.J., & Waxman, K. (1991). Adequate resuscitation of burn patients may not be measured by urine output and vital signs. *Critical Care Medicine, 19*(3), 327-329.

Flynn, M. (1999). Identifying and treating inhalation injuries in fire victims. *DCCN: Dimensions of Critical Care Nursing, 18*(4), 18-23.

Fowler, A. (1998). Nursing management of minor burn injuries. *Nursing Standard, 12*(49), 47-52, 55-56.

Gordon, M., et al. (1998). Use of pain assessment tools: Is there a preference? *Journal of Burn Care & Rehabilitation, 19*(5), 451-454.

Greenfield, E., & McManus, A. (1997). Infectious complications: Prevention and strategies for their control. *Nursing Clinics of North America, 32*(2), 297-309.

*Hansbrough, J., et al. (1995). Wound healing in partial-thickness burn wounds treated with collagenase ointment versus silver sulfadiazine cream. *Journal of Burn Care and Rehabilitation, 16*(3), 241-247.

Hunt, J., et al. (2000). Occupation-related burn injuries. *Journal of Burn Care: Rehabilitator 21*(4), 327-332.

Iraniha, S., et al. (2000). Determination of burn depth with noncontact ultrasonography. *Journal of Burn Care and Rehabilitation, 21*(4), 333-338.

Jellish, W.S., et al. (1999). Effect of topical local anesthetic application to skin harvest sites for pain management in burn patients undergoing skin-grafting procedures, *Annals of Surgery, 229*(1), 115-120.

Jordan, B., & Harrington, D. (1997). Management of the burn wound. *Nursing Clinics of North America, 32*(2), 251-273.

Kagan, R., & Smith, S. (2000). Evaluation and treatment of thermal injuries. *Dermatology Nursing, 12*(5), 334-335, 338-344, 347-350.

*Kealey, G. (1995). Pharmacologic management of background pain in burn victims. *Journal of Burn Care and Rehabilitation, 16*(3), 358-362.

Kraft, P. (2000). The osmotic shift. *Journal of Intravenous Nursing, 23*(4), 220-224.

*Kravitz, M., et al. (1989). A randomized trial of plasma exchange in the treatment of burn shock. *Journal of Burn Care and Rehabilitation, 10*(1), 17-26.

*Latarjet, J., & Choinere, M. (1995). Pain in burn patients. *Burns, 21*(5), 344-348.

Lawrence, J.W., et al. (1998). Sleep disturbance after burn injury: A frequent yet understudied complication. *Journal of Burn Care & Rehabilitation, 19*(6), 480-486.

*Marvin, J.A., et al. (1996). Pain response and control. In D.L. Herndon (Ed.), *Total Burn Care,* Philadelphia: W.B. Saunders.

Mayes, T., Gottschlich, M., & Warden, G. (1997). Clinical nutrition protocols for continuous quality improvements in the outcomes of patients with burns. *Journal of Burn Care and Rehabilitation, 18*(4), 365-368.

McCain, D., & Sutherland, S. (1998). Skin grafts for patients with burns. *American Journal of Nursing, 98*(7), 34-38.

Mertens, D., Jenkins, M., & Warden, G. (1997). Outpatient burn management. *Nursing Clinics of North America, 32*(2), 343-364.

*Moritz, A.R. (1947). Studies of thermal injuries: II. The relative importance of time and surface temperature in the causation of cutaneous burns. *American Journal of Pathology, 23,* 695.

Nagy, S. (1999). Strategies used by burn nurses to cope with the infliction of pain on patients. *Journal of Advanced Nursing, 29*(6), 1427-1433.

*Nguyen, T.T., et al. (1996). Current treatment of severely burned patients. *Annals of Surgery, 223*(1), 14-25.

The physiology of burns. (1999). *Nursing Times, 95*(34), 30.

Rakel, B.A., et al. (1998). Split-thickness skin graft donor site care: A quantitative synthesis of the research, *Applied Nursing Research, 11*(4), 174-182.

Ramzy, P.I., Barret, J.P., & Herndon, D.N. (1999). Thermal injury. *Critical Care Clinics, 15*(2), 333-352.

*Rodriguez, D. (1996). Nutrition in patients with severe burns: State of the art. *Journal of Burn Care and Rehabilitation, 17*(1), 62-70.

Ryan, C.M., et al. (1998). Estimates of the probability of death from burn injuries. *New England Journal of Medicine, 338*(6), 362-66.

Saffle, J.R. (1998). Predicting outcome of burns. *New England Journal of Medicine, 338*(6), 387-388.

Scholl, D., & Langkamp-Henken, B. (2001). Nutrient recommendations for wound healing. *Journal of Intravenous Nursing, 24*(2), 124-132.

Sheridan, R. (2000). Evaluating and managing burn wounds. *Dermatology Nursing, 12*(1), 17-28.

*Shirani, K.Z., et al. (1996). Update on current therapeutic approaches in burns. *Shock, 5*(1), 4-16.

Sibbald, G., et al. (2000). Preparing the woundbed: Debridement, bacterial balance, and moisture balance. *Ostomy Wound Management, 46*(4), 14-35.

Stone, M., Ahmed, J., & Evans, J. (2000). The continuing risk of domestic hot water scalds to the elderly. *Burns, 26*(4), 347-350.

Wiebelhaus, P., & Hansen, S. (2001). What you should know about managing burn emergencies. *Nursing2001, 31*(1), 36-41.

Winfree, J., & Barillo, D. (1997). Nonthermal injuries. *Nursing Clinics of North America, 32*(2), 275-296.

Winfrey, M. Cochran, M., & Hegarty, M. (1999). A new technology in burn therapy: Integra artificial skin. *Dimensions of Critical Care Nursing, 18*(1), 14-20.

PROBLEMS OF EXCRETION

Management of Clients with Problems of the Renal/Urinary System

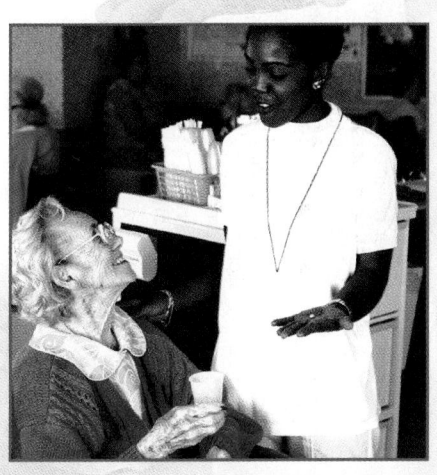

PROBLEMS OF EXCRETION: RENAL/URINARY ■ Core Concepts Grid

Anatomy	Physiology	Pathophysiology	History	Physical Exam	Diagnostic Tests	Interventions	Pharmacology
Macro-structures Kidneys Ureters Bladder Urethra **Micro-structures** Cortex Medulla Pelvis Glomerulus Nephron	**Regulation** Water balance Waste products Acid-base balance **Synthesis of hor-mones** Erythropoietin Renin Activated vitamin D **Glomerular filtration**	**Obstruction** **Inflammation** **Infection** **Trauma** **Tumors** **Metabolic acidosis**	**Client history** Past renal problems Difficulty with urination Change in urinary elimination pattern Pain Hypertension **Family history** Diabetes mellitus Hypertension **Social history** Alcohol/drug use Occupation Age	**Skin** Color/turgor Moisture **Eyes** Conjunctiva **Mouth** Moisture/color Ulceration **Chest** Shape Pulsation **Periphery** Color Hair distribution Striae/edema Pulses/rashes **Abdomen** Striae/tenderness over kidney Bruits over renal artery	• Urinalysis • Specific gravity • Sediment • Serum creatinine • Blood urea nitrogen (BUN) • Uric acid • Scans • Renal arteriogram • Kidney, ureter, and bladder (KUB) • Sonograms • Intravenous pyelography (IVP) • Biopsy • Creatinine clearance • Serum pH • Cystoscopy	• Fluid regulation • Dialysis Hemodialysis Peritoneal dialysis Continuous ambu-latory peritoneal dialysis (CAPD) • Renal transplantation • Extracorporeal shock wave lithotripsy (ESWL) • AV fistula • AV shunt • Therapeutic diet • Fluids, as appropriate • Lithotripsy • Health teaching • Bladder training • Skin care • Urinary catheter care	• Diuretics • Anti-inflammatories • Antibiotics • Immunosup-pressive agents • Calcium replacement agents • Hormone re-placement agents • Chelating agents • Phosphorus-binding agents • Anticholinergics • Skin barrier topical agents

69

Assessment of the Renal/Urinary System

CHRIS WINKELMAN

Learning Objectives

After studying this chapter, you should be able to:

1. Compare and contrast kidney function with functions of the ureters, bladder, and urethra.
2. Describe the roles of the afferent and efferent arterioles in glomerular filtration.
3. Explain the influence of antidiuretic hormone and aldosterone on urine formation and composition.
4. Describe age-related changes in the renal/urinary system.
5. Use laboratory data to distinguish between dehydration and renal impairment.
6. Describe how to obtain a sterile urine specimen from a client with a Foley catheter.
7. Identify teaching priorities for a client who needs to obtain a 24-hour urine specimen.
8. Identify teaching priorities for a client who needs to obtain a "clean catch" urine specimen.
9. Describe the correct techniques to use in physically assessing the renal system.
10. Prioritize nursing care for the client during the first 24 hours following a renal arteriogram.

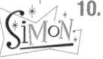

Go to http://www.wbsaunders.com/SIMON/Iggy/ for self-assessment questions related to these Learning Objectives.

Kidneys contribute to health in several ways. Their primary role is to maintain body fluid volume and composition and to filter waste products for elimination. The kidneys also help regulate blood pressure, participate in acid-base balance, produce erythropoietin for red blood cell synthesis, and metabolize vitamin D to an active form.

The renal system includes the kidneys and the entire urinary tract. The ureters, bladder, and urethra provide a drainage route for the excretion of urine. Structural or functional problems in the kidney or urinary tract usually alter fluid, electrolyte, and acid-base balance.

Assessment of the client at risk for or with actual problems of the renal system begins with a history and physical assessment. A clear understanding of the anatomy, physiology, and diagnostic tests of the renal system will help the nurse in problem solving about renal function in the clinical setting. It will also assist the nurse in teaching the client about the purpose of tests or procedures and in physically and emotionally preparing the client for assessment.

ANATOMY AND PHYSIOLOGY REVIEW

Kidneys

Structure

GROSS ANATOMY

Normally, two kidneys are located in the **retroperitoneal space** (behind the peritoneum, not really in the abdominal cavity), one on either side of the vertebral column (Figure 69-1).

The adult kidney is 4 to 5 inches (11 to 13 cm) long, 2 to 3 inches (5 to 7 cm) wide, and about 1 inch (2.5 to 3 cm) thick. It weighs about 8 ounces (250 g). The left kidney is slightly longer and narrower than the right kidney. Kidney size is usually determined via ultrasound. Larger-than-usual kidneys may indicate renal obstruction or polycystic disease, whereas smaller-than-usual kidneys may indicate chronic renal disease.

Several layers of protective, supportive tissue surround the kidney. On the outer surface of the kidney is a layer of fibrous tissue called the **renal capsule** (Figure 69-2). This capsule covers most of the kidney except the **hilum,** the area in which the renal artery enters and the renal vein and ureter exit. The renal capsule is surrounded by layers of fat and connective tissue (Gerota's fascia).

Lying beneath the renal capsule is functional renal tissue composed of two distinct sections: the cortex and the medulla. The **renal cortex,** or outer tissue layer, is in direct contact with the renal capsule. The **medulla,** or medullary tissue, lies below the cortex in the shape of many fans. Each "fan" is called a **pyramid,** and there are 12 to 18 pyramids per kidney. The **renal columns** (columns of Bertin) are cortical tissue that dip down into the interior of the kidney and separate the pyramids.

The tip, or end, of each pyramid is called the **papilla.** The papillae drain urine into the collecting system. A cuplike structure called a **calyx** collects the urine at the end of each papilla. The calices merge together to form the **renal pelvis,** which narrows to become the ureter.

The kidneys receive 20% to 25% of the total cardiac output. Renal blood flow per minute varies from about 600 to 1300 mL/min. The blood supply to each kidney is usually delivered by a single **renal artery,** which branches from the abdominal aorta (Table 69-1). The renal artery separates into progressively smaller arteries, supplying all areas of the renal tissue **(parenchyma)** and the nephrons. The smallest arteries, the afferent arterioles, feed the nephrons directly to form urine.

Venous blood from the kidneys starts with the capillaries surrounding each nephron. These capillaries drain into progressively larger veins, with blood eventually returned to the inferior vena cava through the renal vein.

MICROSCOPIC ANATOMY

The **nephron** is the functional unit of the kidney, and it is here that urine is actually formed from blood. There are about 1 million nephrons per kidney, and each nephron separately makes urine from blood.

There are two types of nephrons: cortical nephrons and juxtamedullary nephrons. The cortical nephrons are short, with all parts located in the renal cortex. The juxtamedullary nephrons (about 20% of all nephrons) are longer, and their tubes and associated blood vessels dip deeply into the

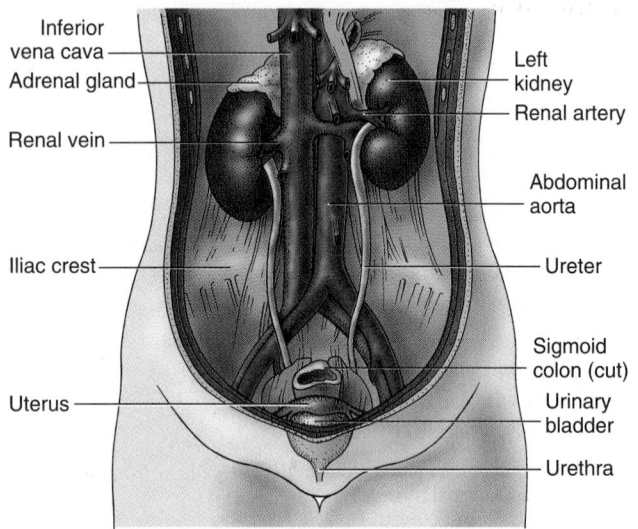

Figure 69-1 ● Anatomic location of organs of the renal/urinary system.

TABLE 69-1 ● THE SEQUENCE OF RENAL BLOOD FLOW FROM THE RENAL ARTERY TO THE RENAL VEIN
1. Renal artery
2. Interlobar artery
3. Arcuate artery
4. Interlobular artery
5. Afferent arteriole — *blood supply to nephron*
6. Glomerulus
7. Efferent arteriole *blood exits glomerulus*
8. Peritubular capillaries or vasa recta
9. Stellate vein
10. Interlobular vein
11. Arcuate vein
12. Interlobar vein
13. Renal vein

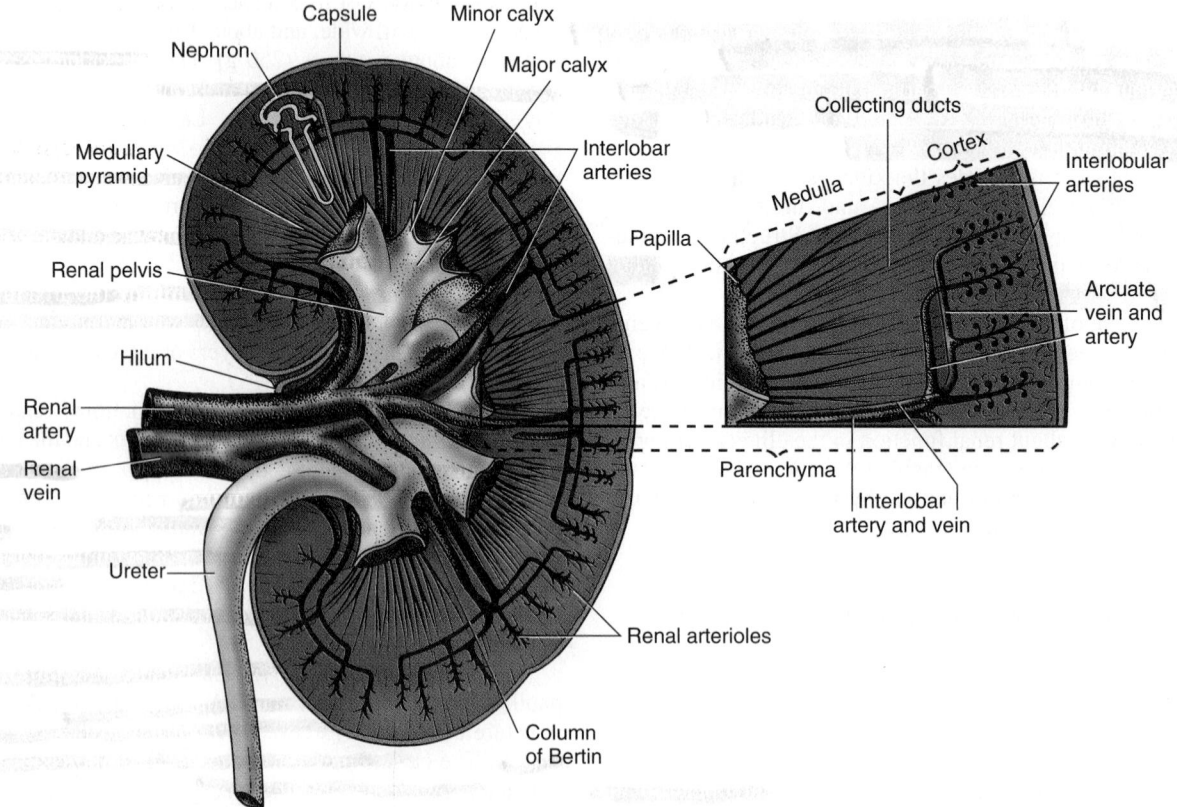

Figure 69-2 ● Bisection of the kidney showing the major structures of the kidney.

medulla. The purpose of the juxtamedullary nephrons is to concentrate urine during times of low fluid intake. The ability to concentrate urine allows for the maximum excretion of waste products with less fluid loss.

Blood supply to the nephron is delivered via the **afferent arteriole,** the smallest, most distal portion of the renal arterial system. From the afferent arteriole, blood flows into the **glomerulus,** a series of specialized capillary loops. It is through these capillaries that water and small particles are filtered from the blood to make urine. The remaining blood exits the glomerulus via the **efferent arteriole.** From the efferent arteriole, blood exits into one of two additional capillary systems:

- The **peritubular capillaries** around the tubular component of cortical nephrons
- The **vasa recta** around the tubular component of juxtamedullary nephrons

Each nephron is a tubular structure with distinct parts (Figure 69-3). The tubular component of the nephron begins with **Bowman's capsule,** a saclike structure that surrounds the glomerulus. The tubular tissue of Bowman's capsule narrows into the **proximal convoluted tubule (PCT).** The PCT twists and turns, finally straightening into the descending limb of the **loop of Henle.** The descending loop of Henle dips in the direction of the medulla but forms a hairpin loop and comes back up into the cortex.

As the loop of Henle changes direction, two segments are identified in the ascending limb of the loop of Henle: the thin and thick segments. The **distal convoluted tubule (DCT)** is formed from the thick segment of the ascending limb of the loop of Henle. The DCT ends in one of many **collecting ducts** located in the kidney tissue. The urine in the collecting ducts passes through the papillae and empties into the renal pelvis.

A series of specialized cells located in the afferent arteriole, efferent arteriole, and DCT are collectively known as the **juxtaglomerular complex** (Figure 69-4). The specialized cells in this area are the **renin-producing cells,** which produce and store renin. **Renin** is a hormone that helps to regulate blood flow, glomerular filtration rate (GFR), and systemic blood pressure. Renin is secreted when special cells in the DCT called the **macula densa** sense changes in blood volume and pressure. The macula densa lies next to the renin-producing granular cells of both afferent and efferent arterioles. Renin is secreted when the macula densa cells sense that blood volume, blood pressure, or blood sodium levels are low. Renin then converts angiotensinogen into angiotensin I. This leads to a series of reactions that cause secretion of the hormone **aldosterone** (Figure 69-5). Aldosterone increases kidney reabsorption of sodium and water, restoring blood pressure, blood volume, and blood sodium levels. (See Chapter 11 for a more complete description of the renin-angiotensin-aldosterone pathway).

Microscopically, the glomerular capillary wall has three layers (Figure 69-6): the endothelium, the basement membrane, and the epithelium. The endothelial and epithelial cells lining the glomerular capillary are separated by pores that filter water and small particles from the blood into Bowman's capsule. This fluid is called the **filtrate,** or early urine.

Function

The kidneys have both regulatory and hormonal functions. The regulatory functions control fluid, electrolyte, and acid-base balance. The hormonal functions control red blood cell formation, blood pressure, and vitamin D activation.

REGULATORY FUNCTIONS

The physiologic processes responsible for maintaining fluid, electrolyte, and acid-base balance are glomerular filtration,

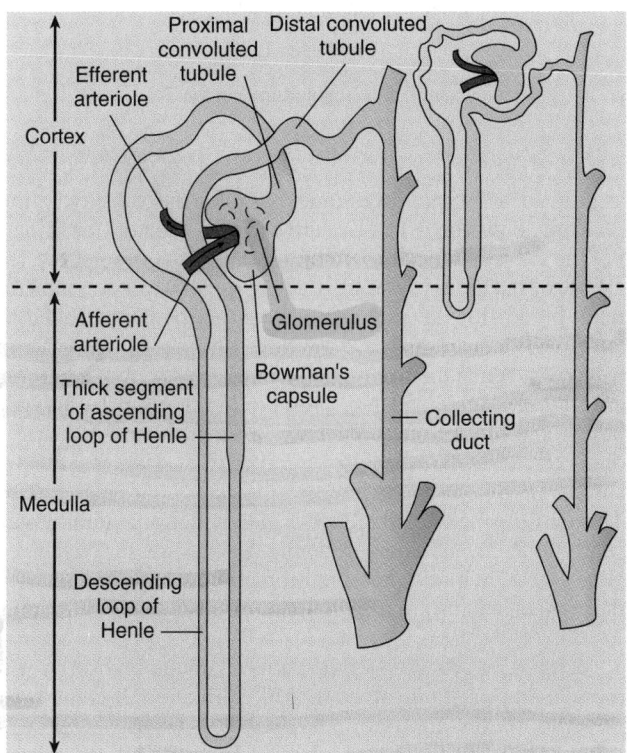

Figure 69-3 ● Anatomy of the nephron, the functional unit of the kidney. Note that the particular nephron labeled here is a juxtamedullary nephron.

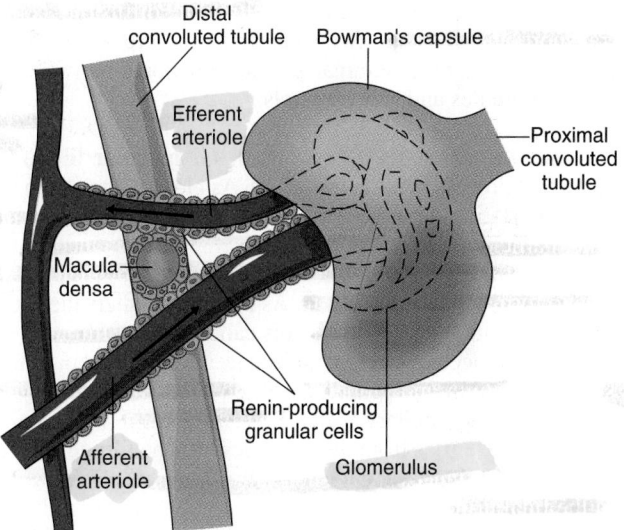

Figure 69-4 ● The juxtaglomerular complex showing juxtaglomerular cells and the macula densa.

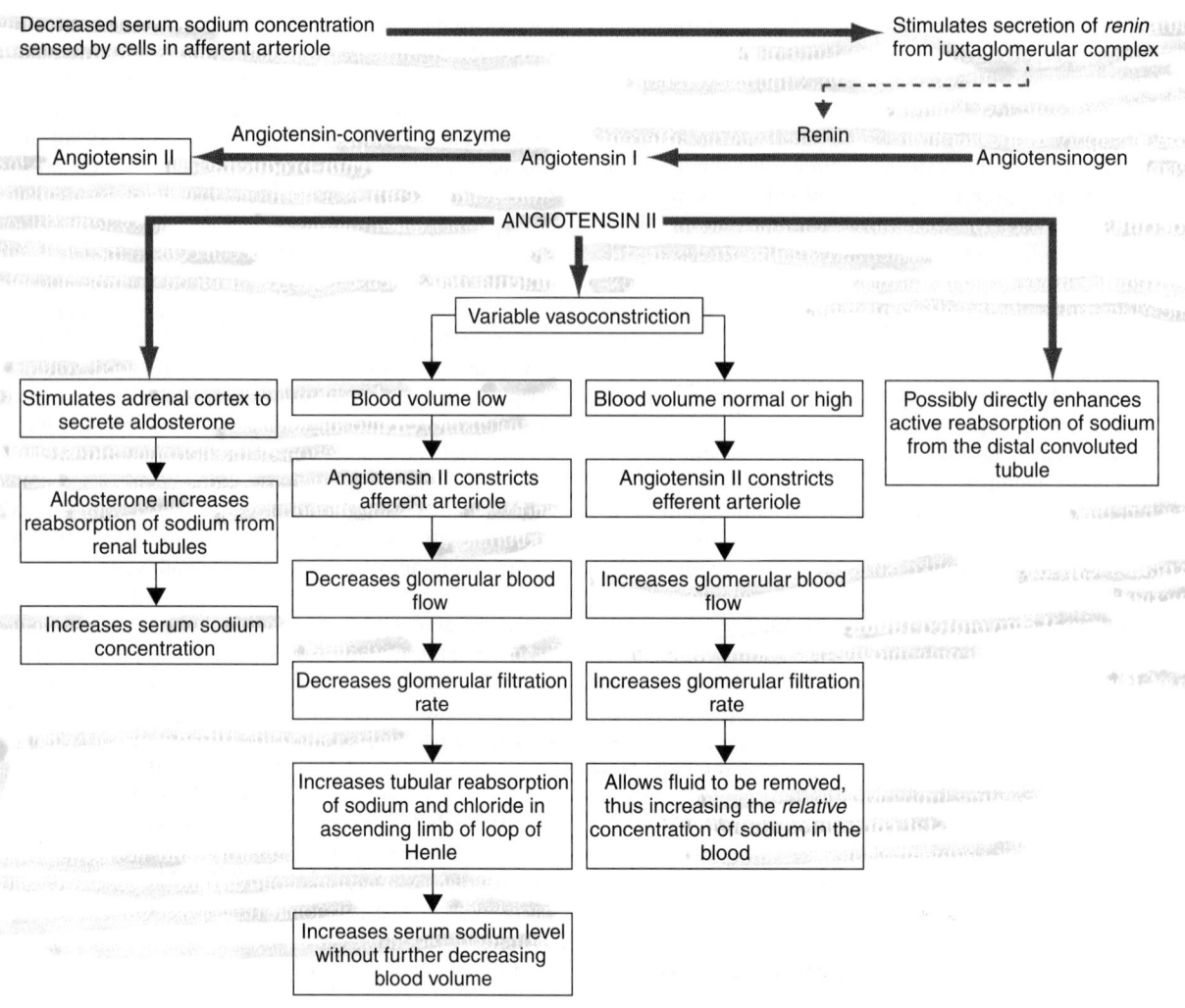

Figure 69-5 ● The role of aldosterone, angiotensinogen, angiotensin I, and angiotensin II in the renal regulation of water and sodium.

tubular reabsorption, and tubular secretion (Figure 69-7). These processes occur through filtration, diffusion, active transport, and osmosis. (See Chapter 11 for a review of these actions.) Table 69-2 summarizes the functional activities of nephron tubules and blood vessels.

GLOMERULAR FILTRATION. Glomerular filtration is the first process in urine formation. As blood passes from the afferent arteriole into the glomerulus, water, electrolytes, and other particles (e.g., creatinine, urea nitrogen, and glucose) are filtered across the glomerular membrane into Bowman's capsule to form *glomerular* filtrate. As the filtrate enters the proximal convoluted tubule (PCT), it is called *tubular* filtrate.

Large–molecular weight substances (>69,000 daltons), such as albumin and globulin, are too large to filter through the glomerular capillary walls. Red blood cells (RBCs) also are too large to pass from the arterioles into the filtrate. Therefore these substances are not normally present in the filtrate or in the final urine.

Approximately 180 L of glomerular filtrate is formed from the blood each day. The rate of filtration is often expressed in milliliters per minute. A normal glomerular filtration rate (GFR) averages 125 mL/min. If all filtrate were to be excreted

as urine, death would occur quickly from massive dehydration. Actually, only about 1 to 3 L are excreted each day as urine.

The GFR is related to blood pressure and blood flow. The ability of the kidneys to self-regulate renal blood pressure and renal blood flow keeps GFR constant. GFR is controlled by selectively constricting and dilating the afferent and efferent arterioles. When the afferent arteriole is constricted and/or the efferent arteriole is dilated, pressure in the glomerular capillaries falls and filtration decreases. When the afferent arteriole is dilated and/or the efferent arteriole is constricted, pressure in the glomerular capillaries rises and filtration increases. Through this self-regulation the kidney can maintain a constant GFR, even when systemic blood pressure changes. When systolic blood pressure drops below about 70 mm Hg, these mechanisms are unable to compensate, and GFR stops.

TUBULAR REABSORPTION. Tubular reabsorption is the second process involved in urine formation. It is the tubular reabsorption of most of the filtrate that keeps normal urine output at 1 to 3 L/day and prevents dehydration. As the filtrate passes through the tubular component of the nephron, the kidney reabsorbs variable amounts of water and electrolytes. Reabsorption returns particles (**solutes**) and water to the blood.

BOWMAN'S CAPSULE

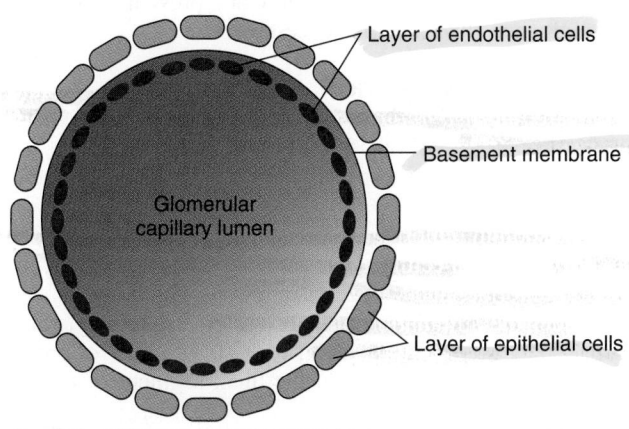

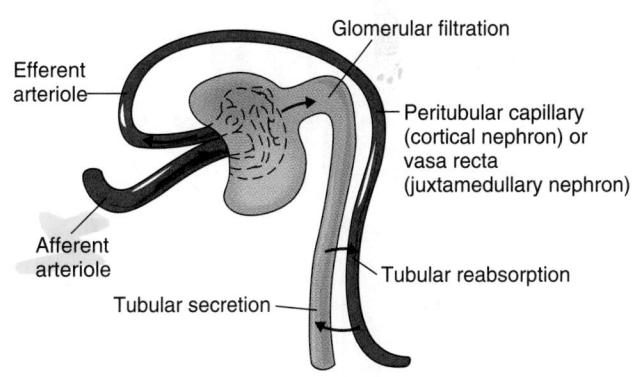

Figure 69-6 ● Glomerular capillary wall.

Figure 69-7 ● Glomerular filtration, tubular reabsorption, and tubular secretion.

TABLE 69-2 • VASCULAR AND TUBULAR COMPONENTS OF THE NEPHRON

Structure	Anatomic Features	Physiologic Aspects
VASCULAR COMPONENTS		
Afferent arteriole	Delivers arterial blood from the branches of the renal artery into the glomerulus	Autoregulation of renal blood flow via vaso-constriction or vasodilation Renin-producing granular cells
Glomerulus	Capillary loops with thin semipermeable membrane	Site of glomerular filtration Glomerular filtration occurs when hydrostatic pressure (blood pressure) is greater than opposing forces (tubular filtrate and on-cotic pressure)
Efferent arteriole	Delivers arterial blood from the glomerulus into the peritubular capillaries or the vasa recta	Autoregulation of renal blood flow via vaso-constriction or vasodilation Renin-producing granular cells
Peritubular capillaries (PTCs) and vasa recta (VR)	PTCs: surround tubular components of cortical nephrons VR: surround tubular components of jux-tamedullary nephrons	Tubular reabsorption and tubular secretion allow movement of water and solutes to or from the tubules, interstitium, and blood
TUBULAR COMPONENTS		
Bowman's capsule (BC)	Thin membranous sac surrounding $^{7}/_{8}$ of the glomerulus	Collects glomerular filtrate (GF) and funnels GF into the tubule
Proximal convoluted tubule (PCT)	Evolves from and is continuous with Bow-man's capsule Specialized cellular lining facilitates tubular re-absorption	Site for reabsorption of sodium, chloride, water, glucose, amino acids, potassium, calcium, bicarbonate, phosphate, and urea
Loop of Henle Descending limb (DL)	Continues from PCT Juxtamedullary nephrons dip deep into the medulla Permeable to water, urea, and sodium chloride	Regulation of water balance
Ascending limb (AL)	Emerges from DL as it turns and is redirected up toward the renal cortex	Potassium and magnesium reabsorption in the thick segment Thin segment is impermeable to water
Distal convoluted tubule (DCT)	Evolves from AL and twists so the macula densa cells lie adjacent to the juxtaglomeru-lar cells of afferent arteriole	Site of additional water and electrolyte reab-sorption, including bicarbonate Potassium and hydrogen secretion
Collecting ducts	Collects formed urine from several tubules and delivers it into the renal pelvis	Receptor sites for antidiuretic hormone regu-lation of water balance

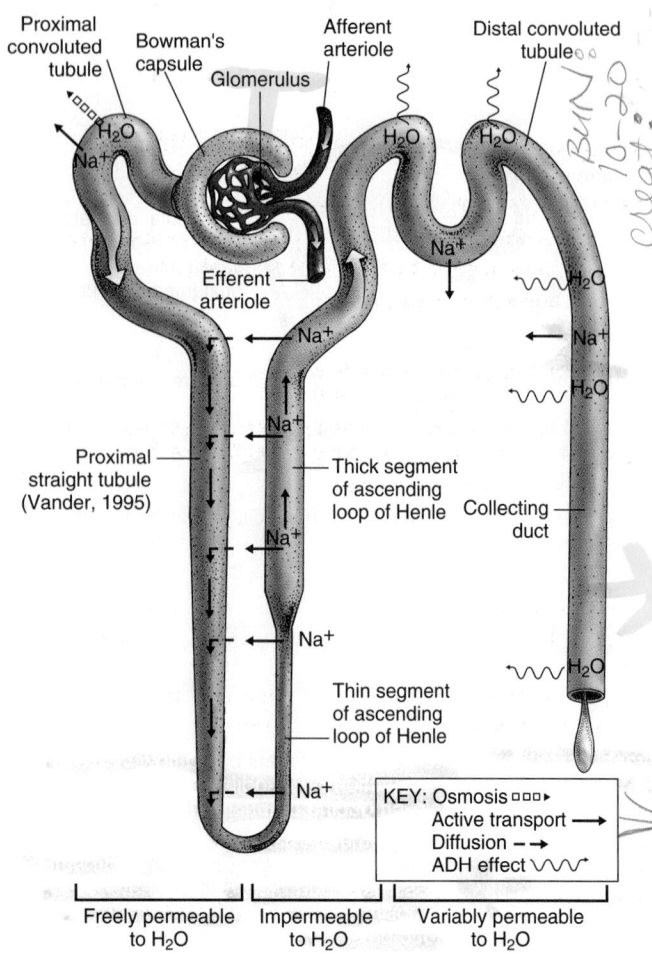

Figure 69-8 ● Sodium and water reabsorption by the tubules of a cortical nephron.

Reabsorption occurs *from the filtrate* across the tubular lumen of the nephron and into the blood of the peritubular capillaries. The PCT reabsorbs approximately 65% of the total glomerular filtrate.

WATER REABSORPTION. The tubules reabsorb more than 99% of all filtered water back into the body (Figure 69-8). Most water reabsorption from the filtrate into the plasma occurs as the filtrate passes through the PCT. Water reabsorption continues as the filtrate flows down the descending loop of Henle. The thin segment of the ascending loop of Henle is *not* permeable to water.

The distal convoluted tubule (DCT) is potentially permeable to water, and therefore water reabsorption can occur as the filtrate continues to flow through the tubule. The membrane of the DCT may be made more permeable to water through the influence of the hormones **antidiuretic hormone (ADH)** and aldosterone. ADH increases the permeability of the membrane to water and enhances water reabsorption. Aldosterone promotes the reabsorption of sodium in the DCT; water reabsorption occurs as a result of the movement of sodium (where sodium goes, water follows).

The ability of the kidneys to vary the volume or concentration of urine helps regulate total water balance regardless of water intake. In this way, the healthy kidney can prevent dehydration when fluid intake is low and prevent circulatory overload when fluid intake is excessive.

SOLUTE REABSORPTION. Some particles in the tubular filtrate are *returned to the blood.* This process is called **tubular reabsorption.** About 50% of all urea present in the glomerular filtrate is reabsorbed, but virtually no creatinine is reabsorbed.

Most sodium, chloride, and water reabsorption occurs in the PCT. The collecting ducts are the other major site of sodium, chloride, and water reabsorption, which usually occurs under the stimulation of aldosterone. Potassium is also primarily reabsorbed in the PCT, with 20% to 40% of potassium reabsorption occurring in the thick segment of the ascending loop of Henle.

Bicarbonate, calcium, and phosphate are reabsorbed in the PCT, with a little additional reabsorption occurring in the ascending loop of Henle and the DCT. The reabsorption of bicarbonate helps neutralize acids and maintain a normal blood pH. Calcium reabsorption and excretion is controlled by circulating calcitonin and parathyroid hormone (PTH) levels (see Chapter 13).

The kidney reabsorbs some of the glucose filtered from the blood. However, there is a limit to how much glucose the kidney can reabsorb. This limit is called the **renal threshold** for glucose reabsorption or the **transport maximum** for glucose reabsorption. The usual renal threshold for glucose is about 220 mg/dL. This means that at a blood glucose level of 220 mg/dL, all glucose is reabsorbed from the filtrate and returned to the blood. When blood glucose levels are greater than 220 mg/dL, some glucose stays in the filtrate and is present in the urine. Normally, almost all glucose and any filtered amino acids or proteins are reabsorbed.

TUBULAR SECRETION. Tubular secretion is a third process involved in urine formation. Like glomerular filtration, it is a process by which substances may move *from the blood* into the tubular filtrate. During tubular secretion, molecules pass from the peritubular capillaries, across capillary membranes, and into the cells that line the tubules. From the cells these substances are moved into the urine to be excreted from the body. Potassium (K^+) and hydrogen ions (H^+) are some of the substances moved in this way to maintain homeostasis of electrolytes and pH.

■ HORMONAL FUNCTIONS

The kidneys produce renin, prostaglandins, bradykinin, erythropoietin, and activated vitamin D (Table 69-3). Other secretions, such as the kinins, influence renal blood flow and capillary permeability. The kidneys also have a role in the breakdown and excretion of insulin.

RENIN PRODUCTION. As discussed earlier under Microscopic Anatomy (pp. 1590 and 1591), renin assists in the regulation of blood pressure. Renin is formed and released when there is a decrease in blood flow, volume, or pressure through the renal arterioles or when a decrease in the sodium ion concentration of the tubular filtrate is detected through the receptors of the juxtaglomerular complex.

TABLE 69-3 • RENAL HORMONE PRODUCTION AND HORMONES INFLUENCING RENAL FUNCTION

	Site	Action
RENAL HORMONE PRODUCTION		
Renin	Renin-producing granular cells	Raise blood pressure as result of angiotensin (local vasoconstriction) and aldosterone (volume expansion) secretion
Prostaglandins	Renal tissues	Regulate intrarenal blood flow by vasodilation or vasoconstriction
Bradykinins	Juxtaglomerular cells of the arterioles	Increases blood flow (vasodilation) and vascular permeability
Erythropoietin	Renal parenchyma	Stimulates bone marrow to make red blood cells
Activated vitamin D	Renal parenchyma	Promotes absorption of calcium in the gastrointestinal tract
HORMONES INFLUENCING RENAL FUNCTION		
Antidiuretic hormone (ADH, vasopressin)	Released from posterior pituitary	Makes DCT and CD permeable to water to maximize reabsorption and produce a concentrated urine
Aldosterone	Released from adrenal cortex	Promotes sodium reabsorption and potassium secretion in DCT and CD; water and chloride follow sodium movement
Natriuretic hormones	Cardiac atria, brain	Cause tubular secretion of sodium

DCT, Distal convoluted tubule; *CD,* collecting ducts.

The release of renin stimulates the production of *angiotensin II* through a series of metabolic steps (see Figure 69-5). Angiotensin II increases systemic blood pressure through powerful vasoconstrictive effects and stimulates the release of aldosterone from the adrenal cortex. Aldosterone increases the reabsorption of sodium in the distal tubule of the nephron. Therefore more water is reabsorbed and blood pressure is increased because of increases in blood volume expansion. When renal blood flow is diminished, this renin-angiotensin-aldosterone system of blood pressure regulation influences the autoregulatory blood pressure processes within the nephron as well as systemic blood pressure (see also Chapter 11).

PROSTAGLANDIN PRODUCTION. Prostaglandins are produced in a variety of tissues, including the kidney. Specific prostaglandins produced in the kidney are prostaglandin E_2 (PGE_2) and prostacyclin (PGI_2). These prostaglandins help regulate glomerular filtration, kidney vascular resistance, and renin production. PGE_2 acts on the distal tubule and collecting duct to inhibit ADH secretion, decrease membrane permeability, and promote sodium and water excretion.

BRADYKININ PRODUCTION. The presence of angiotensin II, prostaglandins, and ADH stimulates the release of bradykinin in the renal system. **Bradykinin** dilates the afferent arteriole and increases capillary membrane permeability to some solutes. These actions maintain kidney blood flow and tubular function even when other conditions cause systemic vasoconstriction.

ERYTHROPOIETIN PRODUCTION. Erythropoietin is produced and released in response to decreased oxygen tension in the renal blood supply. Erythropoietin stimulates red blood cell (RBC) production in the bone marrow. When kidney tissue is destroyed or nonfunctional, erythropoietin production decreases and the person becomes anemic.

VITAMIN D ACTIVATION. A series of metabolic changes are necessary for vitamin D, a hormone, to become active. Metabolic conversions take place in the skin through exposure to ultraviolet light and then in the liver. From there, vitamin D is converted to its active form (1,25-dihydroxycholecalciferol) in the kidney. Activated vitamin D is necessary to absorb calcium in the gastrointestinal tract and is critical in the regulation of calcium balance.

Ureters

Structure

Each kidney has a single ureter, a hollow tubelike structure that connects the renal pelvis with the urinary bladder. The ureter is about ½ inch (1.25 cm) in diameter and about 12 to 18 inches (30 to 45 cm) in length.

The diameter of the ureter narrows in three areas:
- In the upper third of the ureter, at the point at which the renal pelvis becomes the ureter, is a narrowing known as the **ureteropelvic junction (UPJ).**
- The ureter also narrows as it arches toward the abdominal wall (aortoiliac bend).
- Each ureter then narrows upon entering the posterior wall of the urinary bladder at an oblique angle; this point is referred to as the **ureterovesical junction (UVJ).**

The ureter tunnels through bladder tissue for a few centimeters before opening into the bladder in an area referred to as the **trigone** (Figure 69-9).

The ureter is composed of three layers: an inner lining of mucous membrane (**urothelium**), a middle layer of smooth muscle fibers, and an outer layer of fibrous tissue. The outer layer of the ureter contains the blood supply. The middle layer of ureteral tissue contains longitudinal and circular muscle fibers. These muscle fibers are under the control of a variety of nerve pathways from the lower spinal cord.

Function

Rapid peristaltic contractions of the smooth muscle in the ureter move urine from the renal pelvis of the kidney to the bladder. Stretch receptors in the renal pelvis regulate ureteral peristalsis. For example, a large volume of urine in the renal pelvis stimulates the stretch receptors, which respond by causing an increase in ureteral peristalsis.

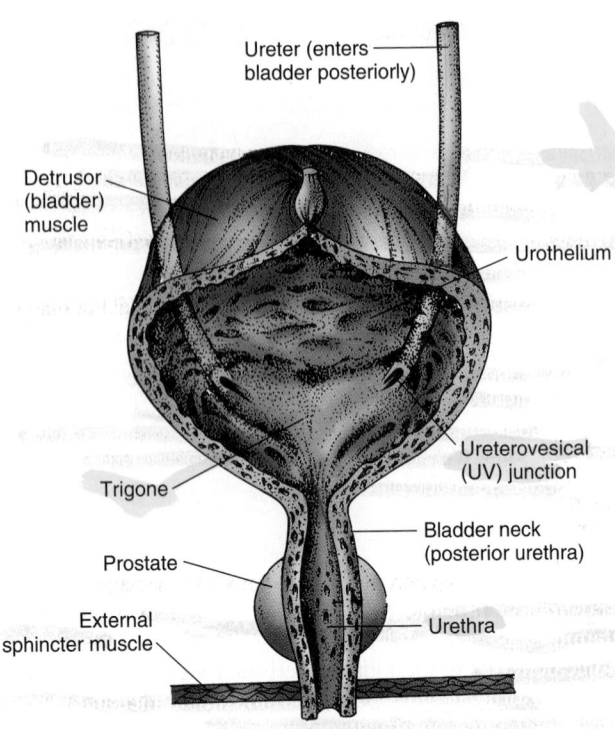

Figure 69-9 ● Gross anatomy of the urinary bladder.

Urinary Bladder

Structure

The urinary bladder is a muscular sac. The upper surface lies next to the peritoneal cavity. In men, the bladder is in front of the rectum. In women, the bladder is in front of the vagina. The bladder lies directly behind the pubic symphysis, the connecting point for pelvic bone structures.

The bladder is composed of the **body** (the rounded sac portion) and the **bladder neck** (posterior urethra), which connects to the bladder body. The bladder has three linings, an inner lining of epithelial cells (**urothelium**), middle layers of smooth muscle (**detrusor muscle**), and an outer lining. The **trigone** is an area on the inner aspect of the posterior bladder wall between the points of ureteral entry (ureterovesical junctions [UVJs]) and the urethra.

The **internal urethral sphincter** is composed of the smooth detrusor muscle of the bladder neck and elastic tissue. The **external urethral sphincter** is composed of skeletal muscle that surrounds the urethra. In men, the external sphincter surrounds the urethra at the base of the prostate gland. In women, the external sphincter is at the base of the bladder. The pudendal nerve from the spinal cord controls the external sphincter.

Function

The urinary bladder is a site for the temporary storage of urine. The bladder also provides continence and enables micturition (voiding). The secretions of the bladder lining resist bacteria.

Bladder continence is achieved during filling through the combination of detrusor muscle relaxation, internal sphincter muscle tone, and external sphincter contraction. As the bladder fills with urine, stretch sensations are transmitted to segments of spinal sacral nerves S2 and S3.

■ MAINTAINING CONTINENCE

Continence is maintained by the interaction of the nerves that control the muscles of the bladder, bladder neck, urethra, the pelvic floor, as well as by factors that close the urethra. During bladder filling, the sympathetic nervous system fibers prevent detrusor muscle contraction. These control centers are located in the cerebral cortex, the brainstem, and the sacral part of the spinal cord. For urethral closure to be adequate for continence, the mucosal surfaces must be in contact and must be adhesive. Contact depends on the structural and functional integrity of the involved nerves and muscles. Adhesion depends on the adequate secretion of mucus-like substances.

■ MICTURITION

Micturition (voiding) is a reflex of parasympathetic control that stimulates contraction of the detrusor muscle at the same time as relaxation of the external sphincter and the muscles of the pelvic floor. With detrusor muscle contraction, the UVJ of the ureter closes, and the normally round bladder assumes the shape of a funnel. Voiding is a voluntary act as the result of a learned response and is controlled by the cerebral cortex and the brainstem. Contraction of the external sphincter inhibits the micturition reflex and prevents voiding.

Urethra

■ Structure

The urethra is a narrow, tubelike structure lined with mucous membranes and epithelial cells. The **urethral meatus,** or opening, is the terminal point of the urethra. In men, the urethra is about 6 to 8 inches (15 to 20 cm) long, with the urethral meatus is located at the tip of the penis. Three sections make up the male urethra:

- The prostatic urethra, which traverses the prostate gland from the urinary bladder
- The membranous urethra, which traverses the wall of the pelvic floor
- The cavernous urethra, which is external and extends through the length of the penis

In women, the urethra is about 1 to 1.5 inches (2.5 to 3.75 cm) long and exits the urinary bladder through the pelvic floor. The urethral meatus lies slightly below the clitoris and directly in front of the vagina and rectum.

■ Function

The urethra is a tube for eliminating urine from the body. The passing of urine normally removes bacteria from the urethra.

Renal/Urinary System Changes Associated with Aging

■ Renal Changes

Structural and functional changes occur in the kidney as a result of the aging process. These changes often have clinical significance. The kidney loses cortical mass and gets smaller by 80 years of age. This cortical loss is caused by reduced re-

CHART 69-1

NURSING FOCUS *on the* **OLDER ADULT**
Changes in the Renal/Urinary System Related to Aging

Physiologic Change	Nursing Implications	Rationale
Decreased glomerular filtration rate (GFR)	Monitor hydration status. Ensure adequate fluid intake. Administer potentially nephrotoxic agents or medications carefully.	With aging, the ability of the kidneys to regulate water balance is decreased. The kidneys are less able to conserve water when necessary. Dehydration results in decreased renal blood flow and increases the nephrotoxic potential of many agents. Acute or chronic renal failure may result.
Nocturia	Ensure adequate nighttime lighting and a hazard-free environment. Ensure the availability of a toilet, bedpan, or urinal. Discourage excessive fluid intake for 2-4 hr before the client retires for the evening.	Nocturia may occur from decreased renal concentrating ability associated with aging. The desire to maintain continence prompts individuals to seek the bathroom. Falls and injuries are common among older clients seeking bathroom facilities. Excessive fluid intake at nighttime may increase nocturia.
Decreased bladder capacity	Encourage the client to use the toilet, bedpan, or urinal at least q2h. Respond as soon as possible to the client's indication of the need to void.	By emptying the bladder on a regular basis, urinary incontinence from overflow may be avoided.
Weakened urinary sphincter muscles and shortened urethra in women	Respond as soon as possible to the client's indication of the need to void. Provide thorough perineal care after each voiding.	A quick response may alleviate episodes of urinary stress incontinence. The shortened urethra increases the potential for bladder infections. Good perineal hygiene may prevent skin irritations and urinary tract infection (UTI).
Tendency to retain urine	Observe the client for urinary retention (e.g., bladder distention) or urinary tract infection (e.g., dysuria, foul odor, confusion). Provide privacy, assistance, and voiding stimulants such as warm water over the perineum as needed.	Urinary stasis may result in a UTI. UTIs may become bloodstream infections, resulting in septicemia or septic shock. Nursing interventions can help to initiate voiding.

nal blood flow. The medulla appears not to be affected by aging, and the juxtamedullary nephrons are generally preserved. However, the glomerular and tubular basement membranes thicken, reducing filtrating ability. Both the number of glomeruli and their surface area decrease with aging. The length of the tubules also decreases.

Kidney function also changes with aging (Chart 69-1). Blood flow to the kidney decreases by about 10% per decade as blood vessels thicken and become more rigid. Glomerular filtration rate (GFR) decreases with advancing age and more rapidly after 45 years of age. By age 65 years, the GFR decreases to approximately 65 mL/min (roughly half the rate in a young adult). This decline is more rapid in clients with diabetes or hypertension.

Tubular changes with aging are shown by a decreased ability to concentrate urine, resulting in **nocturia** (increased need to urinate at night). The excretion and regulation of sodium, acids, and bicarbonate remain effective but are less efficient because homeostasis is slower. Along with an age-related impairment in the thirst mechanism, these changes may be associated with an increased incidence of dehydration and hypernatremia (increased blood sodium levels) in the older adult (Brenner, 2000). Hormonal changes include a

decrease in renin secretion, aldosterone levels, and activation of vitamin D.

CULTURAL CONSIDERATIONS

African Americans experience more rapid age-related decreases in GFR than do Caucasians (Brenner, 2000). The renal excretion of sodium is less effective in hypertensive African Americans who have high sodium intake, and the kidneys have approximately 20% less blood flow as a result of anatomic changes in small renal vessels (Shulman & Hall, 1991).

■ Urinary Changes

Changes in the elasticity of the detrusor muscle may cause decreased bladder capacity and a decreased ability to retain urine. The sensation of the urge to void may cause immediate bladder emptying because the urinary sphincters lose muscle tone and often become weaker with age. In women, weakening muscles shorten the urethra, which contributes to incontinence. In men, an enlarged prostate gland causes difficulty in starting the urine stream and may cause urinary retention.

ASSESSMENT TECHNIQUES

History

One way to assess renal and urologic function is to use Gordon's Functional Health Patterns (Gordon, 2000). The patterns most pertinent to the renal system are Nutritional/Metabolic and Elimination (Chart 69-2).

▮ DEMOGRAPHIC DATA

Age, gender, race, and ethnicity are important in the overall history of the client with suspected renal or urinary dysfunction. A sudden onset of hypertension in clients older than 50 years of age suggests possible kidney disease. Clinical evidence of adult polycystic kidney disease typically occurs in clients in their 40s or 50s. In men older than 50 years, altered urine patterns suggest prostatic disease.

Anatomic gender differences make some disorders worse or more common. For example, men rarely have urinary tract infections unless there are abnormalities, such as ureteral reflux or prostatic enlargement. Women have a shorter urethra and therefore more commonly experience **cystitis** (bladder infection) because bacteria pass more readily into the bladder.

> ≋ CULTURAL CONSIDERATIONS
> End-stage renal disease (ESRD) is three to four times more common in African Americans, Native Americans, and Mexican Americans than in Caucasians. A history of hypertension or diabetes mellitus (both associated with renal disease) is also common in these groups.

▮ PERSONAL AND FAMILY HISTORY

The family history of the client with a suspected kidney or urologic problem is significant because some disorders have a familial inheritance pattern. The client is asked whether his or her siblings, parents, parents' siblings, or grandparents have had renal problems. Past terms used for kidney disease include Bright's disease, nephritis, and nephrosis. Clients may use these terms to describe kidney disease as it was known by their parents or grandparents in the earlier part of the twentieth century. Adult polycystic kidney disease can occur in clients of either gender.

The client is asked about any previous renal or urologic disorders, including tumors, infections, stones, or urologic surgery. A history of any chronic health problems, such as diabetes mellitus or hypertension, may contribute to the development of renal disease.

The nurse identifies all of the client's prescription medications. The client is asked about their duration of use and whether any recent changes in medications have been prescribed. Drugs prescribed for diabetes mellitus, hypertension, cardiac disorders, hormonal disorders, cancer, arthritis, and psychiatric disorders are potential causes of renal dysfunction. Antibiotics taken for infections, such as gentamicin (Garamycin, Cidomycin✤), may also produce sudden renal dysfunction.

The use of over-the-counter (OTC) drugs or agents, including vitamin and mineral supplements and replacements, laxatives, analgesics, and nonsteroidal anti-inflammatory drugs (NSAIDs) is explored. Many of these drugs affect renal

---

> **CHART 69-2**
>
> **RENAL/URINARY ASSESSMENT**
> **Using Gordon's Functional Health Patterns**
>
> **Nutritional/Metabolic Pattern**
> What is your typical daily food intake? Describe a day's meals, snacks, and vitamins.
> How much salt do you typically add to your food? Do you use salt substitutes?
> How is your appetite?
> Have you experienced any nausea or vomiting?
> What is your typical daily fluid intake?
> What types of fluids do you drink (water, juices, soft drinks, coffee, tea)?
> How much fluid do you drink each day?
> Have you had any recent change in your weight? Weight gain? Weight loss? How much?
> Have you noticed a change in the tightness of your rings or shoes? Tighter? Looser?
> Have you noticed any skin changes lately? More dry? Less Dry? Itchy?
>
> **Elimination Pattern**
> What is your usual bowel elimination pattern? Frequency? Character? Discomfort? Laxatives?
> What is your usual urinary elimination pattern? Frequency? Amount? Color? Odor? Control?
> Have you noticed a change in the amount of urine?
> Do you have any problem with excessive perspiration?
> Do you have any other type of drainage?

Based on Gordon, M. (2000). *Manual of nursing diagnosis* (9th ed.). St. Louis: Mosby.

function. The long-term use of NSAIDs, especially combination agents, can seriously reduce renal function.

The client is specifically asked whether he or she has ever been told about the presence of protein or albumin in the urine. The question "Have you ever been told that your blood pressure is high?" may prompt a vastly different response than "Do you have high blood pressure?" The nurse also asks female clients about health problems associated with pregnancy (e.g., proteinuria, high blood pressure, gestational diabetes, and urinary tract infections). Additional information is obtained about the following:

- Chemical or environmental toxin exposure in occupational or other settings
- Recent travel to geographic regions that pose infectious disease risks
- Recent physical injuries
- Trauma
- Sexual contacts
- A history of altered patterns of urinary elimination

▮ DIET HISTORY

The client with known or suspected renal or urologic disorders is asked about his or her usual diet and any recent changes in the diet. The excessive intake or omission of certain categories of foods is noted. Information about food and fluid intake is obtained. If the client has followed a diet for weight reduction, the details of the diet plan are pertinent. A high-protein intake can result in temporary renal problems. Clients susceptible to **calculi** (stone) formation who ingest large amounts of calcium-containing products or have an insufficient fluid intake may form new stones.

Changes in appetite, alterations in taste acuity, and an inability to discriminate tastes are important. These symptoms are associated with the accumulation of nitrogenous waste products from renal failure. Changes in thirst or fluid intake may also produce changes in urine output or other evidence of urologic disorders. Endocrine disorders may also produce changes in thirst, fluid intake, and urine output (see Chapter 63).

SOCIOECONOMIC STATUS

The socioeconomic status of the client may influence health care practices. People with limited income or no health insurance often ignore physical ailments or delay seeking health care because they lack the funds to pay for diagnostic tests or treatment. They may also have difficulty following medical advice, having prescriptions filled, and keeping follow-up appointments.

The information that a client has about the disease and its symptoms may relate to educational level. Educational level may also affect health-seeking practices. Recurring urinary tract infections often result from inadequate or incomplete treatment, including lack of follow-up to ensure eradication. The lack of money to pay for antibiotics or nutritious foods or the lack of knowledge or motivation to select healthful foods may inhibit full recovery.

The client's health beliefs affect the approach to health and illness. Cultural background or religious affiliation may influence the belief system.

The language used by clients may be different from that used by the health care professional. Anatomic or medical terms may have no meaning for the client (Table 69-4). When obtaining a history, the nurse listens to and explores the terms used by the client. By using the client's own terms, the nurse may help him or her to provide a more complete and thorough description of the problem. This technique may increase the amount of information communicated and decrease the client's discomfort when discussing bodily functions.

CURRENT HEALTH PROBLEMS

The effects of renal failure result in changes in all body systems. Therefore all of the client's current health problems are documented. The client is encouraged to describe all health concerns, because some renal and urologic disorders are associated with symptoms that are related to other body systems or that occur as generalized problems. Recent upper respiratory problems, generalized musculoskeletal discomfort, or gastrointestinal (GI) problems may be related to problems of kidney function.

The kidney and urologic system are assessed specifically. The client is asked about any changes in the appearance (color, odor, clarity) of the urine, pattern of urination, ability to initiate or control voiding, and other unusual symptoms. Urine that is reddish, dark brown or black, greenish, or otherwise different from the usual yellowish, straw color usually prompts the client to seek health care assistance. Urine typically has a mild but distinct odor of ammonia. An increase in the intensity of color, a change in odor quality, or a decrease in urine clarity may suggest infection.

The client is asked about changes in urination patterns, such as nocturia, frequency, or an increase or decrease in the amount of urine. The normal urine output for adults is 1 mL/kg/hr, or approximately 1500 to 2000 mL/day. The client usually does not know the exact amount of urine produced; a bladder diary may provide useful data (see the Evidence-

TABLE 69-4 · COMMONLY USED RENAL AND URINARY TERMS
anuria   Total urine output of less than 100 mL in 24 hours
azotemia   Increased blood urea nitrogen and serum creatinine levels suggestive of renal impairment but without outward symptoms of renal failure
dysuria   Discomfort or pain associated with micturition
frequency   Feeling the need to void often, usually voiding small amounts of urine each time; may void every hour or even more frequently than hourly
hesitancy   Difficulty in initiating the flow of urine, even when the bladder has sufficient urine to initiate a void and the sensation of the need to void is present
micturition   The act of voiding
nocturia   Awakening prematurely from sleep because of the need to empty the bladder
oliguria   Decreased urine output; total urine output between 100 and 400 mL in 24 hours
polyuria   Increased urine output; total urine output usually greater than 2000 mL in 24 hours
uremia   Full-blown signs and symptoms of renal failure; sometimes referred to as the uremic syndrome, especially if the cause of the renal failure is unknown
urgency   A sudden onset of the feeling of the need to void immediately; may result in incontinence if the client is unable to locate or get to toileting facilities quickly

EVIDENCE-BASED PRACTICE
FOR NURSING

How does one assess a urinary elimination problem?

Pfister, S.M. (1999). Bladder diaries and voiding patterns in older adults. *Journal of Gerontological Nursing, 25*(3), 36-41.

The purpose of this article is to describe how a bladder diary was used in research with residents of retirement settings. Bladder diaries are similar to intake and output records but are self-recorded by clients. It reviews different methods of collecting information about fluid consumed and urine eliminated. The narrative details the written record used by 51 subjects in a self-care community of retired individuals and the instructions given to participants so as to yield specific and accurate information.

The author concludes that bladder diaries were used successfully and allow both the client and health care provider to visualize daily voiding patterns. Based on bladder diary data, nurses can diagnose, plan, and intervene to manage voiding problems such as incontinence.

Critique. The clients in this study were physically mobile, able to write, and cognitively intact. Although self-reported bladder diaries may not apply to all clients with elimination problems, the forms and techniques described in this report specify a useful assessment tool that can be used in a variety of community settings.

Implications for Nursing. Bladder diaries can assist the nurse and client in determining the patterns of intake and voiding. Diaries can also be used to evaluate responses to interventions.

Based Practice for Nursing box above). The nurse also asks the following:

- If the client has difficulty initiating urine flow
- If a burning sensation or other discomfort is present on urination
- If the force of the urine stream is decreased (in men)

The nurse asks about any loss of urinary continence. Situations that increase intra-abdominal pressure (e.g., coughing and sneezing) may result in the involuntary passage of urine. Clients may also report a persistent dribbling of urine.

The onset of pain in the flank, in the lower abdomen or pelvic region, or in the perineal area is often of great concern and usually prompts the client to seek assistance. The nurse inquires about the onset, intensity, and duration of the pain, its location, and its association with any activity or event.

Pain associated with renal or ureteral irritation is often severe and spasmodic. Pain that radiates into the perineal area, groin, scrotum, or labia is described as **renal colic.** Renal colic pain is usually associated with distention or spasm of the ureter, such as in an obstruction or the passing of a stone. Renal colic pain may be intermittent or continuous and may even be systemic with pallor, diaphoresis, and hypotension. These general symptoms occur because of the location of the nerve tracts associated with the kidneys and ureters.

Because the kidneys are close to the GI organs and the nerve pathways are similar, GI symptoms may be part of the client's presenting history. These **renointestinal reflexes** often complicate the detailed description of the renal problem.

Uremia results from the accumulation of nitrogenous waste products in the blood, a result of renal failure. Symptoms include anorexia, nausea and vomiting, muscle cramps, **pruritus** (itching), fatigue, and lethargy.

Physical Assessment

The physical assessment of the client with a known or suspected renal or urologic disorder includes an assessment of general appearance, a general review of body systems, and specific structure and functions of the renal/urinary systems.

The nurse assesses the general appearance of the client and checks for a yellowish skin color and the presence of any rashes, bruising, or other discoloration. The skin and tissues may show edema, which with renal disorders may be detected in the **pedal** (foot), **pretibial** (shin), sacral tissues, and around the eyes. The lungs are auscultated to determine whether fluid is present. Weight and blood pressure measurements are obtained for comparison purposes.

The nurse assesses the client's general level of consciousness and level of alertness, noting deficits in concentration, thought processes, or memory. Family members may report subtle changes. Such cognitive changes may be the result of an insufficient clearance of waste products when renal disease is present.

ASSESSMENT OF THE KIDNEYS, URETERS, AND BLADDER

Assessment of the kidneys, ureters, and bladder is performed in conjunction with an abdominal assessment. Auscultation is performed before percussion and palpation because these activities can enhance bowel sounds and obscure abdominal vascular sounds.

Inspection

The nurse inspects the abdomen and the flank regions with the client in both the supine and the sitting position. The client is observed for asymmetry (e.g., swelling) or discoloration (e.g., bruising or redness) in the flank region, especially in the area of the **costovertebral angle (CVA).** The CVA is located between the lower portion of the twelfth rib and the vertebral column.

Auscultation

The nurse listens for a bruit over each renal artery on the midclavicular line. A **bruit** is an audible swishing sound produced when the volume of blood or the diameter of the blood vessel changes. A bruit is usually associated with blood flow through a narrowed vessel, as in renal artery stenosis.

Palpation

Renal palpation identifies masses and areas of tenderness in or around the kidney. The abdomen is lightly palpated in all quadrants. The nurse asks about areas of tenderness or discomfort and examines nontender areas first. The outline of the bladder may be seen as high as the umbilicus in clients with severe bladder distention. Special training and practice under the guidance of a qualified practitioner are necessary; therefore appropriate education is essential before attempting the procedure. If tumor or aneurysm is suspected, palpation may harm the client.

Because the kidneys are deep, posterior structures, palpation is easier in thin clients who have little abdominal musculature. For palpation of the right kidney, the client assumes a supine position while the nurse places one hand under the right flank and the other hand over the abdomen below the lower right part of the rib cage. The lower hand raises the flank, and the upper hand depresses the anterior abdomen as the client takes a deep breath (Figure 69-10). The left kidney is deeper and rarely palpable. A transplanted kidney is readily palpable in either the lower right or left abdominal quadrant. The kidney should feel smooth, firm, and nontender.

Percussion

A distended bladder sounds dull when percussed. After gently palpating to determine the general outline of the distended bladder, the nurse begins percussion on the skin of the lower abdomen and continues in the direction of the umbilicus until dull sounds are no longer produced.

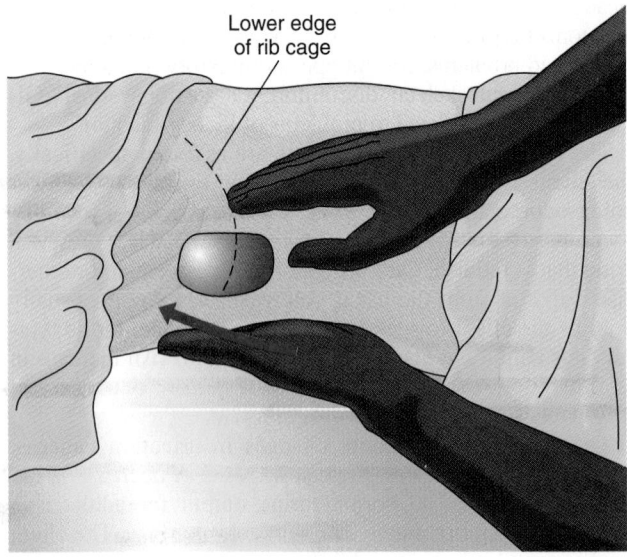

Lower edge of rib cage

Figure 69-10   Advanced technique for palpation of the kidney.

If the client identifies flank pain or tenderness, the nontender flank is percussed first. The client assumes a sitting, side-lying, or supine position, and the nurse forms one hand into a clenched fist. The heel of the other hand and the little finger form a flat area with which a firm thump to the CVA area can be quickly administered. Costovertebral tenderness is highly suggestive of kidney infection or inflammation. Clients with inflammation or infection in the kidney or adjacent structures may describe their pain as severe or as a constant, dull ache.

ASSESSMENT OF THE URETHRA

Using a good light source and wearing gloves, the nurse inspects the urethra by examining the meatus and surrounding tissues. Any unusual discharge such as blood, mucus, and purulent drainage is noted. The skin and mucous membranes of surrounding tissues are inspected, and the presence of lesions, rashes, or other abnormalities of the penis or scrotum or of the labia or vaginal orifice is documented. Urethral irritation is suspected when the client reports discomfort with urination.

Psychosocial Assessment

Concerns about the urologic system may evoke fear, anger, embarrassment, anxiety, guilt, or sadness in the client. Childhood learning often includes privacy with regard to urination habits. Urologic disorders may stimulate previously forgotten memories of difficult toilet training and bedwetting or of childhood experiences of exploring one's body. The client may ignore symptoms or delay seeking health care because of emotional responses or cultural taboos about the urogenital area.

> ### CRITICAL THINKING CHALLENGE
> The client is a 62-year-old woman who has had a backache in the lower left flank area for a month. She has been seen by an orthopedic specialist, who has determined the pain is not from a strained muscle or spinal problem. This women is about 5 feet tall and weighs 95 pounds.

- What personal or demographic data should you obtain?
- What additional questions should you ask this client regarding her pain?
- How would you proceed in gathering physical assessment data?

For suggested answer guidelines, go to SIMON http://www.wbsaunders.com/SIMON/Iggy/.

Diagnostic Assessment

LABORATORY TESTS

Blood Tests

SERUM CREATININE

Serum creatinine is a measurement of the end product of muscle and protein metabolism. Creatinine is filtered by the kidneys and excreted in the urine. Because muscle mass and metabolism are usually constant, the serum creatinine level is an excellent indicator of kidney function. Normal serum creatinine levels vary with age, gender, and body muscle mass. The normal serum creatinine value is slightly higher in adult men than in adult women (Chart 69-3). In general, men have a larger muscle mass than do women, but there are exceptions. Muscle mass and the amount of creatinine produced diminish with age. Because of decreased rates of creatinine clearance, however, the serum creatinine level remains relatively constant in older adults unless renal disease is present.

No common pathologic condition other than renal disease results in an increase in serum creatinine level. The serum creatinine level does not increase until at least 50% of the renal function is lost, and therefore *any* elevation of serum creatinine values is important.

BLOOD UREA NITROGEN

Blood urea nitrogen (BUN) measures the renal excretion of urea nitrogen, a by-product of protein metabolism in the liver. Urea nitrogen is produced primarily from food sources of pro-

---

CHART 69-3

LABORATORY PROFILE
Renal Function Blood Studies

Test	Normal Range for Adults	Significance of Abnormal Findings
Serum creatinine	*Males:* 0.6-1.2 mg/dL (80-115 mmol/L) *Females:* 0.5-1.1 mg/dL (44-97 mmol/L) *Older Adults:* may be decreased	An *increased level* indicates renal impairment. A *decreased level* may be caused by a decreased muscle mass.
Blood urea nitrogen (BUN)	10-20 mg/dL (2.1-7.1 mmol/L) *Older Adult:* 60-90 yr: 8-23 mg/dL (2.9-8.2 mmol/L); over 90 yr: 10-31 mg/dL (3.6-11.1 mmol/L)	An *increased level* may indicate hepatic or renal disease, dehydration or decreased renal perfusion, a high-protein diet, infection, stress, steroid use, GI bleeding, or other situations in which there is blood in body tissues. A *decreased level* may indicate malnutrition, fluid volume excess, or severe hepatic damage.
BUN/creatinine ratio	Mass ratio: 12:1 to 20:1; mole ratio: 48.5:1 to 80.8:1	An *increased ratio* may indicate fluid volume deficit, obstructive uropathy, catabolic state, or a high-protein diet. A *decreased ratio* may indicate fluid volume excess or acute renal tubular acidosis. *No change* in the ratio with increases in both the BUN and creatinine levels indicates renal impairment.

Data from Pagana, K.D., & Pagana, T.J. (1999). *Diagnostic testing and nursing implications: A case study approach* (5th ed.). St. Louis: Mosby.
GI, Gastrointestinal.

tein, which undergo metabolism by the liver. The kidneys filter urea nitrogen from the blood and excrete the nitrogenous waste in urine. BUN levels indicate the extent of renal clearance of this nitrogenous waste product.

Other factors may influence the BUN level, and therefore an elevation does not always represent renal disease (see Chart 69-3). For example, rapid cell destruction from infection or steroid therapy may elevate BUN level. In addition, blood is a protein. If blood is present in body tissues, the reabsorption of the blood protein is processed by the liver, resulting in an increased BUN level.

The liver must function properly to produce urea nitrogen. When liver and kidney dysfunction are both present, urea nitrogen levels are actually decreased; this decrease reflects the liver failure but not the kidney failure. The BUN level is not always elevated with kidney disease and is not the most reliable indicator of kidney function. However, an elevated BUN level is highly *suggestive* of kidney dysfunction.

RATIO OF BLOOD UREA NITROGEN TO SERUM CREATININE

The BUN/creatinine ratio determines whether factors such as dehydration or lack of renal perfusion are causing the elevated BUN level. When a blood volume deficit (dehydration) or hypoperfusion exists, the BUN level rises more rapidly than the serum creatinine level. As a result, the ratio of BUN to creatinine is *increased.*

When both the BUN and serum creatinine levels increase at the same rate, the BUN/creatinine ratio remains normal. However, the elevated serum creatinine and BUN levels suggest renal dysfunction that is not related to acute volume depletion or hypoperfusion.

Urine Tests

URINALYSIS

Urinalysis is a usual part of any complete physical examination but is particularly useful for clients with suspected kidney or urologic disorders (Chart 69-4). Ideally, the urine specimen is collected at the first morning's voiding; specimens obtained at other times may not be adequately concentrated. The specimen may be collected by several techniques (Table 69-5).

COLOR, ODOR, AND TURBIDITY. The color of urine is derived from urochrome pigment. Variations in color may result from increased levels of urochrome or other pigments, changes in the concentration or dilution of the urine, and the presence of drug metabolites in the urine. Urine smells faintly like ammonia and is normally clear without **turbidity** (cloudiness) or haziness.

SPECIFIC GRAVITY. The specific gravity of urine measures the concentration or density of urine compared to water. The specific gravity of urine ranges from 1.000 (the specific gravity of water) to greater than 1.035. In kidney disease, increases and decreases in specific gravity may not reflect systemic fluid volume. For example, dilute urine with a decreased specific gravity may occur in a dehydrated client who has a lack of nephron receptors for antidiuretic hormone.

An *increase* in specific gravity occurs with dehydration, decreased kidney perfusion, or the presence of antidiuretic hormone (ADH). (ADH production is normally increased with stress, surgery, anesthetic agents, and certain drugs such as morphine and oral antidiabetic agents.) In each of these situations the expected kidney response is to reabsorb water and decrease urine output. As a result, the urine produced is more concentrated.

A *decrease* in specific gravity occurs with increased fluid intake, diuretic administration, and diabetes insipidus. In each of these situations, the normal kidney response is to excrete more water; thus urine output is increased. In kidney disease, the specific gravity decreases because there is less solute, and it does not vary with changes in plasma osmolality (e.g., it becomes fixed).

pH. A pH value less than 7 is considered acidic, and a value greater than 7 is considered alkaline. Various factors influence the acidity or alkalinity of urine. A diet high in certain fruits and vegetables results in a more alkaline urine, whereas a high-protein diet produces a more acidic urine. The presence of *Escherichia coli* in the urine also results in an acidic urine.

Urine specimens become more alkaline when left standing unrefrigerated for more than 1 hour, if urea-splitting bacteria are present, or if a specimen is left uncovered. Alkaline urine increases cell breakdown; thus the presence of red blood cells may be missed on analysis. The nurse ensures that urine specimens are covered and delivered to the laboratory promptly or refrigerated. During metabolic or respiratory acidosis or alkalosis, the kidneys, along with blood buffers and the lungs, should respond appropriately to maintain a normal serum pH. Chapters 15 and 16 discuss acid-base balance and imbalance.

GLUCOSE. Glucose is filtered at the glomerulus and is reabsorbed in the proximal tubule of the nephron. When the blood glucose level rises above 220 mg/dL, the renal threshold for reabsorption is usually exceeded, and glucose is excreted in the urine. Variations in the renal threshold for glucose occur in many clients, such as those who experience any infection or those who have had diabetes mellitus for a number of years. It is possible that their serum glucose level may be high (e.g., greater than 400 mg/dL), and glucose may still not be present in the urine.

KETONE BODIES. Three types of ketone bodies are acetone, acetoacetic acid, and beta-hydroxybutyric acid. **Ketone bodies** are by-products of the incomplete metabolism of fatty acids. Normally there are no ketones in urine. Ketone bodies are produced when fat sources are used instead of glucose to provide cellular energy. When ketones are present in the blood, they are partially excreted in the urine.

PROTEIN. Protein, such as albumin, is not normally present in the urine. Levels greater than 300 mg/24 hr, or 200 µg/min, are abnormal. The glomerular membrane is semipermeable to small molecules; protein molecules are too large to pass through this semipermeable membrane. When permeability of the glomerular membrane is increased, protein molecules pass through and are excreted in the urine. Increased glomerular membrane permeability may be caused by infection, inflammation, or immunologic problems. Certain systemic processes result in the production of abnormal proteins, such as globulin. These proteins are not detected with routine

CHART 69-4

LABORATORY PROFILE
Urinalysis

Test	Normal Range for Adults	Significance of Abnormal Findings
Color	Pale yellow	*Dark amber* indicates concentrated urine. *Very pale yellow* indicates dilute urine. *Dark red or brown* indicates blood in the urine; brown also may indicate increased urinary bilirubin level; red may also indicate the presence of myoglobin. *Other color changes* may result from diet or medications.
Odor	Specific aromatic odor, similar to ammonia	*Foul smell* indicates possible infection, dehydration, or ingestion of certain foods or drugs.
Turbidity	Clear	*Cloudy urine* indicates infection or sediment or high levels of urinary protein.
Specific gravity	Usually 1.010-1.025; possible range 1.000-1.030; after 12-hr fluid restriction >1.025 *Older adult:* Decreased because of decreased concentrating ability	*Increased* in decreased renal perfusion, inappropriate antidiuretic hormone secretion, or congestive heart failure. *Decreased* in chronic renal insufficiency, diabetes insipidus, malignant hypertension, diuretic administration, and lithium toxicity.
pH	Average: 6; possible range: 4.6-8	*Changes* are caused by diet, the administration of medications, infection, freshness of the specimen, acid-base imbalance, and altered renal function.
Glucose	<0.5 g/day (<2.78 mmol/L)	*Presence* reflects hyperglycemia or a decrease in the renal threshold for glucose.
Ketones	None	*Presence* reflects incomplete metabolism of fatty acids, as in diabetic ketoacidosis, prolonged fasting, anorexia nervosa.
Protein	8-18 mg/dL (10-140 mg/L)	*Increased amounts* may indicate stress, infection, recent strenuous exercise, or glomerular disorders.
Bilirubin (urobilinogen)	None	*Presence* suggests hepatic or biliary disease or obstruction.
Red blood cells (RBCs)	0-2 per high-power field	*Increased* amounts are normal with indwelling or intermittent catheterization or menses but may reflect tumor, stones, trauma, glomerular disorders, cystitis, or bleeding disorders.
White blood cells (WBCs)	Males: 0-3 per high-power field Females: 0-5 per high-power field	*Increased* amounts may indicate an infectious or inflammatory process anywhere in the renal/urinary tract, renal transplant rejection, fever, or exercise.
Casts	A few or none, composed of RBC or WBC, protein, or tubular cell casts	*Increased amounts* indicate the presence of bacteria or protein, which is seen in severe renal disease and could also indicate urinary calculi.
Crystals	None	*Presence* of normal or abnormal crystals may indicate that the specimen has been allowed to stand.
Bacteria	<1000 colonies/mL	*Increased amounts* indicate the need for urine culture to determine the presence of urinary tract infection.
Parasites	None	*Presence* of *Trichomonas vaginalis* indicates infection, usually of the urethra, prostate, or vagina.
Nitrates	None	*Presence* suggests bacteria, usually *Escherichia coli.*

urinalysis procedures; urine protein electrophoresis or other tests are necessary to detect these unusual proteins.

A random finding of proteinuria followed by a series of negative (normal) findings does not imply renal disease. If infection is suspected to be the cause of the proteinuria, urinalyses after elimination of the infection should be negative for protein. Persistent proteinuria needs further investigation.

Microalbuminuria is the presence of albumin in the urine that is not measurable by a urine dipstick or conventional urinalysis procedures. Specialized immunoassay tests can quickly analyze a freshly voided urine specimen for microscopic levels of albumin. The normal microalbumin levels in a freshly voided random specimen should range between 2.0 to 20 mg/mmol for men and 2.8 to 28 mg/mmol for women. Higher levels indicate microalbuminuria and could mean the presence of very early kidney disease, especially in clients

with diabetes mellitus. For 24-hour urine specimens, levels of 30 to 300 mg/24 hr, or 20 to 200 µg/min, indicate microalbuminuria.

SEDIMENT. Urine sediment refers to particles in the urine. These particles include cells, casts, crystals, and bacteria.

CELLS. Types of cells abnormally present in the urine may include tubular cells (from the tubule of the nephron), epithelial cells (from the lining of the urinary tract), red blood cells (RBCs), and white blood cells (WBCs).

CASTS. Casts are structures formed around other particles. There may be casts of cells, bacteria, or protein. When casts are formed, there is a clumping or agglutination of the element, and gelatinous substances form the surrounding

TABLE 69-5 • COLLECTION OF URINE SPECIMENS

Nursing Interventions	Rationale
VOIDED URINE Collect the first specimen voided in the morning. Send the specimen to the laboratory as soon as possible. Refrigerate the specimen if a delay is unavoidable.	Urine is more concentrated in the early morning. After urine is collected, cellular breakdown results in more alkaline urine. Refrigeration delays the alkalinization of urine. Bacteria are more likely to multiply in an alkaline environment.
CLEAN-CATCH SPECIMEN Explain the purpose of the procedure to the client. Instruct the client to self-clean before voiding. Instruct the female client to separate the labia and use the sponges and solution provided to wipe with three strokes over the urethra. The first two wiping strokes are over each side of the urethra; the third wiping stroke is centered over the urethra (from front to back). Instruct the male client to retract the foreskin of the penis and to similarly clean the urethra, using three wiping strokes with the sponge and solution provided (from the head of the penis downward). Instruct the client to initiate voiding after cleaning. The client then stops and resumes voiding into the container. Only 1 ounce (30 mL) is needed; the remainder of the urine may be discarded into the commode. Ensure that the client understands the procedure. Assist the client as needed.	Correct technique is needed to obtain a valid specimen. Surface cleaning is necessary to remove secretions or bacteria from the urethral meatus. A midstream collection further removes secretions and bacteria because urine flushes the distal portion of the internal urethra. An improperly collected specimen may result in inappropriate or incomplete treatment. The client's understanding and the nurse's assistance ensure proper collection.

CATHETERIZED SPECIMEN
For nonindwelling (straight) catheters:
 	
   Avoid routine use.
   Follow the facility's procedures for catheterization technique.
For indwelling catheters:
 	
Apply a clamp to the drainage tubing, distal to the injection port.
 	
Clean the injection port cap of the catheter drainage tubing with an appropriate antiseptic. Povidone-iodine solution or alcohol is acceptable.
Insert a sterile 5-mL syringe into the port and aspirate the quantity of urine required.
Inject the urine sample into a sterile specimen container.
Remove the clamp to resume drainage.
Properly dispose of the syringe.
	The one-time passage of a urinary catheter may be necessary to obtain an uncontaminated specimen for analysis or to measure the volume of residual urine.
	These procedures minimize bacterial entry.
	
	Collection of urine from an indwelling catheter or tubing is performed when clients have catheters for continence or long-term urinary drainage.
	Clamping allows urine to collect in the tubing at the location where the specimen is obtained.
	Surface contamination is prevented by following the cleaning procedures.
	
	A minimum of 5 mL is needed for culture and sensitivity (C&S) testing.
	A sterile container is used for C&S specimens.

24-HOUR URINE COLLECTION Instruct the client thoroughly. Provide written materials to assist in instruction. Place signs appropriately. Inform all personnel or family caregivers of test in progress. Check laboratory or procedure manual on proper technique for maintaining the collection (e.g., on ice, in a refrigerator, or with a preservative). On initiation of the collection, ask the client to void, discard the urine, and note the time. If a Foley catheter is in use, empty the tubing and drainage bag at the start time and discard the urine. Collect all urine for the next 24 hr. 24 hr after initiation, ask the client to empty the bladder and add that urine to the container. Do not remove urine from the collection container for other specimens.	A 24-hr collection of urine is necessary to quantify or calculate the rate of clearance of a particular substance. Instructional materials for clients, signs, and so on remind clients and staff to ensure that the total collection is completed. Proper technique prevents breakdown of elements to be measured. Proper techniques ensure that *all* urine formed within the 24-hr period is collected. Urine in the container is not considered a "fresh" specimen and may be mixed with preservative.

CHART 69-5

LABORATORY PROFILE
24-Hour Urine Collections

Component	Normal Range for Adults	Significance of Abnormal Findings
Creatinine	0.8-2 g/24 hr *Males:* 1-2 g/24 hr or 14-26 mg/kg/24 hr (124-230 μmol/kg/24 hr or 7.1-17.7 mmol/24 hr) *Females:* 0.6-1.8 g/24 hr or 11-20 mg/kg/24 hr (97-177 μmol/kg/24 hr or 5.3-15.9 mmol/24 hr) *Older adults:* 10 mg/kg/24 hr (88.4 μmol/kg/24 hr) at 90 yr	*Decreased amounts* indicate a deterioration in renal function caused by renal disease, shock, hypovolemia, or any condition affecting muscle. *Increased amounts* occur with infections, exercise, diabetes mellitus, and meat meals.
Urea nitrogen	12-20 g/24 hr (0.43-0.71 mmol/24 hr)	*Decreased amounts* occur when renal damage or liver disease is present. *Increased amounts* commonly result from a high-protein diet, dehydration, trauma, or sepsis.
Sodium	40-220 mEq/24 hr (40-220 mmol/24 hr)	*Decreased amounts* are seen in hemorrhage, shock, hyperaldosteronism, and prerenal acute renal failure. *Increased amounts* are common with diuretic therapy, excessive salt intake, hypokalemia, and acute tubular necrosis.
Chloride	110-250 mEq/24 hr (110-250 mmol/24 hr) *Older adults:* 95-195 mEq/24 hr (95-195 mmol/24 hr)	*Decreased amounts* are seen in certain renal diseases, malabsorption syndrome, pyloric obstruction, prolonged nasogastric tube drainage, diarrhea, diaphoresis, congestive heart failure, and emphysema. *Increased amounts* are seen with hypokalemia, adrenal insufficiency, and massive diuresis.
Calcium	100-400 mg/24 hr (2.50-7.50 mmol/kg/24 hr)	*Decreased amounts* are often associated with hypocalcemia, hypoparathyrodism, nephrosis, and nephritis. *Increased amounts* are commonly seen with calcium renal stones, hyperparathyroidism, sarcoidosis, certain cancers, immobilization, and hypercalcemia.
Total catecholamines*	<100 μg/24 hr (<591 mmol/24 hr)	*Increased amounts* occur with pheochromocytoma, neuroblastomas, stress, or strenuous exercise.
Protein	1-14 mg/dL (10-140 mg/L) or 50-80 mg/24 hr at rest	*Increased amounts* indicate glomerular disease, nephrotic syndrome, diabetic nephropathy, urinary tract malignancies, and irritations.

*Epinephrine and norepinephrine only; dopamine is not measured.

structure, a cast. Casts are described by the type of element in the structure (e.g., RBC cast, WBC cast, tubular epithelial cast) or the stage of degeneration. The degeneration of casts refers to the stage of breakdown of the internal element. Casts are described as "granular" (coarse or fine) and "waxy."

CRYSTALS. Crystals in the urine come from various salts. These particles may be a result of diet, drugs, or disease. The salts may be composed of calcium, oxalate, urea, phosphate, magnesium, or other substances. Certain drugs, such as the sulfates, can also produce crystals.

BACTERIA. Bacteria in a urine sample multiply quickly, so the specimen must be analyzed promptly. Normally urine is sterile, but it can be contaminated easily by perineal bacteria or airborne pathogens during collection.

■ URINE FOR CULTURE AND SENSITIVITY

The nurse may collect a sample of urine for laboratory determination of the number and types of pathogens present. The presence of clinical symptoms and unexplained bacteria in a urinalysis specimen are indications for urine culture and sensitivity

testing. When bacterial colonies are present, they are placed in a medium containing different antibiotic drugs to determine which drugs are effective in killing or stopping the growth of the bacteria (sensitivity). Those drugs to which the microorganisms are sensitive or resistant are reported to guide decisions about needed therapy. A clean-catch or catheter-derived specimen is always preferred for culture and sensitivity testing.

■ COMPOSITE URINE COLLECTIONS

When ordered, urine collections are made for a number of hours (e.g., 24 hours) for laboratory quantitative and qualitative analysis of one or more substances. Collections are often ordered to measure levels of urinary creatinine or urea nitrogen, sodium, chloride, calcium, catecholamines, or other components (Chart 69-5). For a composite urine specimen, *all* urine within the designated time frame must be collected (see Table 69-5). If other voided or catheterized specimens must be obtained while the collection is in progress, the nurse measures and appropriately documents the amount collected but not added to the timed collection.

The urine collection may need to be refrigerated or stored on ice to prevent changes in the urine during the collection time. The nurse follows the procedure from the laboratory for urine storage. The urine collection must be free from fecal contamination. Menstrual blood and toilet tissue also contaminate the specimen and can invalidate the results.

The collection of urine for a 24-hour period is often more difficult than it seems. With hospitalized clients, the cooperation of staff personnel, the client, family members, and visitors is essential. Placing signs in the bathroom, instructing the client and family, and emphasizing the need to save the urine are helpful.

■ CREATININE CLEARANCE TEST

Creatinine clearance is a calculation of glomerular filtration rate. It is the best indication of overall kidney function. The amount of creatinine cleared from the blood (e.g., filtered into the urine) is measured in the total volume of urine excreted in a defined period. A urine specimen for a creatinine clearance test is usually collected for 24 hours, but it can be collected for shorter periods (e.g., 8 or 12 hours). The calculation requires a comparison with the blood creatinine level, and therefore a blood specimen for creatinine must also be collected.

The laboratory or the physician calculates the creatinine clearance. Because the client's age, gender, height, weight, diet, and activity level influence the expected amount of creatinine to be excreted, these variables are considered in the interpretation of creatinine clearance test results.

The following formula is used to calculate creatinine clearance:

$$\text{Creatinine clearance} = U \times V/P \times T$$

where U is creatinine in urine (mg/dL), V is volume of urine (mL/24 hr), P is creatinine in plasma or blood (mg/dL), and T is time (minutes).

The rate of creatinine clearance is expressed as milliliters per minute per 1.73 m² of body surface area. The range for normal creatinine clearance is 90 to 139 mL/min for adult males and 80 to 125 mL/min for females.

Creatinine clearance measurements are necessary to determine the client's current kidney function. Decreases in the creatinine clearance rate may require modification of drug dosing and often signifies the need for further investigation of the cause of kidney deterioration.

■ URINE ELECTROLYTES

Urine samples may be collected for the analysis of urine electrolyte levels (e.g., sodium and chloride). Normally the amount of sodium excreted in the urine is nearly equal to that consumed. Urine sodium levels of less than 10 mEq/L indicate that the tubules are functioning to conserve (reabsorb) sodium.

■ OSMOLALITY

Osmolality is a measure of the concentration of particles in solution, in this case the concentration of solutes in urine. These solutes include electrolytes and solutes such as glucose, urea, and creatinine.

BLOOD/PLASMA OSMOLALITY. The kidneys excrete or reabsorb water to maintain a blood osmolality in the range of 285 to 295 mOsm/kg. Osmolality is slightly higher in older adult clients (285 to 301 mOsm/kg). When blood osmolality is decreased, the release of antidiuretic hormone (ADH) is inhibited. Without ADH, the distal tubule and collecting ducts are *not* permeable to water. As a result, water is *excreted*, not reabsorbed, and blood osmolality increases. When blood osmolality increases, ADH is produced. With ADH production, the distal tubule is made permeable to water. Consequently, water is reabsorbed, and blood osmolality decreases.

URINE OSMOLALITY. Urine osmolality can vary from 50 to 1400 mOsm/kg water, depending on the clinical and hydration status of the client and the functional status of the kidneys. With average fluid intake, the range for urine osmolality is 300 to 900 mOsm/kg water. The fixed acids and other wastes that are continually produced constitute a solute load that must be excreted in the urine on a regular basis. This is referred to as *obligatory solute excretion*. If the client has lost excessive fluids, the renal response is to conserve water, preserve blood osmolality, and excrete small amounts of highly concentrated urine. Many factors such as diet, medications, and activity can influence urine osmolality. Thus increased urine osmolality reflects a concentrated urine with less water than solutes. A decreased urine osmolality reflects a dilute urine with more water than solutes.

■ RADIOGRAPHIC EXAMINATIONS

Radiographic and other special procedures are used to diagnose abnormalities within the genitourinary system (Table 69-6). The nurse explains the procedures thoroughly to the client, prepares the client, and provides postprocedural care.

■ Kidney, Ureter, and Bladder X-Ray Examination

Radiographic examination of the kidneys, ureters, and bladder (KUB) is a plain film of the abdomen taken without any specific client preparation. The KUB study shows gross anatomic features and may show obvious stones, strictures, calcifications, or obstructions in the urinary tract. This test identifies the organs' shape, size, and relationship to other parts of the urinary tract. Other tests are necessary for diagnosis of functional or structural abnormalities.

There is no discomfort or risk from this procedure. The nurse tells the client that the films will be taken while the client is in a supine position. No specific postprocedure care is necessary.

■ Intravenous Urography

Other names for intravenous urography include excretory urography and (the older term) intravenous pyelography (IVP).

CLIENT PREPARATION. Before urography, the nurse assesses the client (Chart 69-6), institutes bowel preparation, and teaches the client. Allergy information is reported to the physician. Contrast reactions can be minor (nausea and vomiting, urticaria, itching, sneezing), moderate (nephrotoxic effects, congestive heart failure, pulmonary edema), or severe

TABLE 69-6 • COMMON RADIOLOGIC AND SPECIAL DIAGNOSTIC TESTS FOR CLIENTS WITH DISORDERS OF THE RENAL/URINARY SYSTEM

Test	Purpose	Comments
Radiography of kidneys, ureters, and bladder (KUB) (plain film of abdomen)	To screen for the presence of two kidneys To measure the kidneys' size To detect gross obstruction	
Excretory urography	To measure the kidneys' size To detect obstruction To assess parenchymal mass	Radiopaque contrast media may cause an allergic (hypersensitivity) reaction in iodine-sensitive clients. Contrast agent is also hypertonic and increases the risk of acute renal failure in adults with serum creatinine levels greater than 1.5 mg/dL, diabetes mellitus, multiple myeloma, or dehydration. Nephrotoxic complications can be prevented by parenteral fluid administration, the use of mannitol, and daily monitoring of serum creatinine levels.
Nephrotomography	To assess various planes of kidney tissue for cysts, tumors, or calculi	Same as for excretory urogram.
Computed tomography (CT)	To measure the size of the kidneys To evaluate contour to assess for masses or obstruction	Contrast medium may provoke acute renal failure. See comments with excretory urography for high-risk clients and preventive measures related to contrast. May be performed without contrast medium and still obtain adequate visualization.
Cystography and cystoscopy	To identify abnormalities of the bladder wall and urethral and ureteral occlusions To treat small obstructions or lesions via fulguration, lithotripsy, or removal with a stone basket	Instrumentation of the urinary tract increases the risk of infection. Monitor for infection for 48-72 hr after the procedure.
Voiding cystourethrography (VCUG)	To outline the bladder's contour and to detect urinary reflux from vesicourethral junctions	The risk of infection is similar to that in cystography because urinary catheterization is necessary. Monitor for postprocedure infection.
Renal arteriography	To identify vascular abnormalities within each kidney and adjacent aorta	Contrast medium may provoke acute renal failure. See comments with excretory urography for high-risk clients and preventive measures related to contrast. Essential for diagnosis and treatment of some vascular abnormalities, such as renal artery stenosis. Monitor for bleeding after the procedure.
Ultrasonography (US)	To identify the size of the kidneys or obstruction in the kidneys or the lower urinary tract May detect tumors or cysts	Ultrasonography entails minimal risk to the client. Ultrasonography is a good alternative to excretory urography.
Renography (Renal scan)	To assess renal blood flow	Radioactive material is used for this test. Captopril or another angiotensin-converting enzyme (ACE) inhibitor may be used, placing the client at risk for severe hypotensive reactions during and following this procedure.

(bronchospasm, anaphylaxis). If the diagnostic test is to be performed in the presence of minor allergy, the physician orders preprocedural medications such as a steroid (methylprednisolone or prednisone), and an antihistamine (diphenhydramine hydrochloride [Benadryl, Allerdryl♣]) to suppress the allergic response (Cohan & Ellis, 1997). The nurse explains the rationale for the procedure to the client.

Procedures to ensure that films provide adequate visualization vary according to the radiologist's preferences. Some radiologists recommend a light evening meal or clear liquids, then fasting (NPO status) from midnight on the night before

the procedure. Others recommend increased fluid intake to prevent dehydration up until the time of the procedure. Because of the possibility of a vomiting reaction to the intravenous (IV) contrast, however, the physician may prefer the client to remain on NPO status at least a few hours before the procedure. The physician orders hydration with IV fluids as indicated.

The physician orders a bowel preparation to remove fecal contents, fluid, and air from the gut, which permits an adequate outline of the lower poles of the kidneys, ureters, and bladder. Bowel preparation procedures vary but usually include the use

---

CHART 69-6

BEST PRACTICE *for*
Assessing the Client About to Undergo a Diagnostic Test or Interventional Procedure Using Contrast Media

Before the procedure:
- Ask the client if he or she has ever had a reaction to contrast media. (Such a client has the highest risk for having another reaction.)
- Ask the client about a history of asthma. (Clients with asthma have been shown to be at greater risk for contrast reactions than the general public; when reactions do occur, they are more likely to be severe.)
- Ask the client about known hay fever or food or medication allergies, especially to seafood, eggs, milk, or chocolate. (Contrast reactions have been reported to be as high as 15% in these clients.)
- Ask the client to describe any specific allergic reactions (e.g., hives, facial edema, difficulty breathing, bronchospasm).
- Assess for a history of renal insufficiency and for conditions that have been implicated in increasing the chance of developing renal failure after contrast media (e.g., diabetic nephropathy, class IV heart failure, dehydration, concomitant use of potentially nephrotoxic medications such as the aminoglycosides or NSAIDs, and cirrhosis).
- Ask the client if he or she is taking metformin (Glucophage). (Metformin must be discontinued at least 48 hours before any study using contrast media because the life-threatening complication of lactic acidosis, although rare, could occur.)
- Assess hydration status by checking blood pressure, heart and respiratory rates, mucous membranes, skin turgor, and urine concentration.
- Ask the client when he or she last ate or drank anything.

From Cohan, R.H., & Ellis, J.H. (1997). Iodinated contrast material in uroradiology. Choice of agent and management of complications. *Urologic Clinics of North America, 24*(3), 471-491. *NSAIDS,* Nonsteroidal anti-inflammatory drugs.

of laxatives the day before the procedure. Enemas also may be prescribed but are controversial because air and fluid can be introduced with inadequate expulsion of fecal contents.

🐚 CONSIDERATIONS FOR OLDER ADULTS

Bowel preparation procedures increase the risk for dehydration, especially in older clients. To help prevent dehydration, the nurse contacts the testing department and requests that urograms be scheduled early in the day for older clients.

The contrast medium (dye) is potentially nephrotoxic. The risk for *contrast-induced renal failure* is greatest in clients who are older or dehydrated, who have some renal insufficiency (e.g., serum creatinine levels greater than 1.5 mg/dL), or who are also taking other nephrotoxic drugs. These clients usually require additional IV fluids before the procedure to maintain hydration and to decrease the nephrotoxic risk. Diuretics may be administered immediately after the dye is injected to enhance its excretion.

The nurse instructs the client in the preparation procedures for the urogram and explains the procedure so he or she knows what to expect in the examination room (Chart 69-7). The nurse intervenes on behalf of the client to ensure that questions are answered *before* the procedure.

CHART 69-7

CLIENT EDUCATION GUIDE
Excretory Urogram

- The urogram outlines your urinary tract and helps determine any problems there.
- Notify your nurse or physician if you have had any reactions (allergic or otherwise) to any food or drugs, especially shellfish (shrimp, scallops, crab, lobster, and so on) or iodine, or to x-ray "dyes" such as contrast media; if you have a history of asthma; or if you are taking metformin (Glucophage) or Glucovance.
- The day before the test, follow the instructions about changes in your diet and fluid intake to be sure that as much information as possible is gained from the test.
- After you start the bowel preparation, you may need to be close to toileting facilities. The preparation medications usually work quickly.
- You will be lying on an x-ray table with the x-ray machine above you for most of the procedure.
- A pressure band, similar to a large blood pressure cuff, may be placed around your stomach or abdomen to help obtain better x-ray pictures.
- If you do not already have an IV access site, one will be started to give you the contrast agent.
- After the contrast is injected, you may feel a sense of warmth or heat as it travels throughout your body. You also may have a taste in your mouth that is sometimes described as metallic. These sensations last only a few seconds or minutes.
- When the pressure band is inflated, you may feel some tightness around your abdomen. The sensation is similar to the feeling on your arm when you have your blood pressure taken.
- A series of x-ray pictures will be taken. You may be asked to empty your bladder and return to the table for more films. You also may be asked to have a standing film taken.
- After the test is completed, you are usually able to resume your normal activities and diet.
- The contrast will be excreted normally in your urine. You will not notice any change in the color or characteristics of your urine.
- Please do not hesitate to ask your nurse, physician, or x-ray technologist any question, no matter how slight the question may seem to you. It is important that you have as much understanding as possible.

PROCEDURE. A radiopaque contrast medium (dye) is injected intravenously with the client in a supine position. As blood (with the dye) rapidly circulates into the kidney blood vessels and is filtered by the glomeruli, the dye is excreted in the urine. A series of x-ray films are taken at various times after injection. When ordered, nephrotomograms are taken at the same time as the urogram. Tomograms provide images of different planes of tissue and show any abnormalities present at varying depths. The technologist then asks the client to empty the bladder and return for a few more films. An outline of the kidneys, ureters, and bladder results as urine containing the dye is excreted.

The urogram provides information about the following:
- The number, size, shape, and location of the kidneys
- The adequacy of uptake (filling) and the rate of excretion of contrast medium
- The number, size, location, appearance, and patency of the calices, pelves, and ureters
- The size, location, and nature of the urinary bladder

FOLLOW-UP CARE. After the urogram, the nurse monitors the client for altered renal function and other effects from the dye. Adequate hydration is ensured by encouraging the client to take fluid orally or by administering IV fluids. Hydration decreases the risk for renal deterioration. Blood creatinine levels are monitored to determine ongoing renal function.

Computed Tomography

CLIENT PREPARATION. The nurse informs the client that a computed tomography (CT) scan is performed to provide three-dimensional information about the kidneys, ureters, bladder, and surrounding tissues. A CT scan is usually performed after other diagnostic procedures and can provide information about tumors, cysts, abscesses, other masses, obstruction, and certain blood vessel abnormalities.

A bowel preparation with laxatives or an enema and a light meal the evening before the procedure is needed. The client is given nothing by mouth (NPO status) after midnight on the night before the examination. For clients having the CT scan with dye, the physician orders preprocedural IV hydration. The nurse assesses for any allergy to dye and intervenes as with IV urography.

PROCEDURE. The CT scan is performed in a special room, usually in the radiology department. An IV injection of radiopaque dye may be administered before starting the imaging procedures. The use of dye may be eliminated in clients at risk for contrast media–induced acute renal failure, but the images produced are less distinct. Tomograms are obtained at various levels.

FOLLOW-UP CARE. No special follow-up care is necessary unless a dye was used. In that case, the follow-up care is the same as for IV urography.

Cystography and Cystourethrography

CLIENT PREPARATION. The nurse explains the procedure to the client undergoing a cystography or cystourethrography. A urinary catheter is temporarily needed to instill a contrast medium (dye). The dye is necessary for visualization of the lower urinary tract.

PROCEDURE. In both cystography and cystourethrography, dye is instilled into the bladder via a urethral catheter. After bladder filling, a variety of films are obtained from the front, back, and side positions. For the voiding cystourethrogram (VCUG), the client is requested to void, and films are taken during the voiding. A VCUG is obtained to determine whether a vesicoureteral reflux is present. The cystogram is often indicated in cases of trauma when urethral or bladder injury is suspected.

FOLLOW-UP CARE. The nurse monitors for the development of infection as a result of catheterization. In this test, the dye is not nephrotoxic because it is not injected into the bloodstream. Fluid intake is encouraged to dilute the urine and reduce the burning sensation from catheter irritation after removal. Because pelvic or urethral trauma may be present, the nurse also monitors for changes in urine output.

OTHER RENAL DIAGNOSTIC TESTS
Renal Arteriography (Angiography)

CLIENT PREPARATION. The nurse informs the client that an arteriography is used to assess the arterial blood supply of the kidneys. A bowel preparation is given to remove fecal contents, gas, and fluid. A light evening meal is given, and the client is on NPO status until after the procedure. An IV may be placed before the procedure. IV fluids are often given to ensure adequate hydration because a contrast medium (dye) is used as part of the procedure.

The nurse reviews the procedure with the client, answers questions, and reviews the medication regimen and blood study results as indicated. For example, the nurse reviews the prothrombin time if the client has been taking warfarin sodium (Coumadin, Warfilone✦). The client also signs an informed consent statement. Renal arteriography is performed to explore suspected causes of decreased renal function such as renovascular hypertension, other vessel abnormalities, and bleeding from trauma.

PROCEDURE. The injection of a radiopaque dye into the renal arteries requires entry into an artery, usually the femoral artery in the groin. After the client is sedated and the skin is prepared and draped, the radiologist injects a local anesthetic. An arterial puncture is then performed through which the angiographic catheter is inserted.

Using fluoroscopy, the radiologist guides the catheter into the abdominal aorta and the renal artery. When the tip of the catheter is positioned at each renal artery, the radiologist injects dye and films are taken. The speed of distribution of the dye and any areas of blood vessel narrowing are noted. Arterial blockage is noted when the dye fails to circulate within the kidney. **Extravasation** (infiltration) of dye into surrounding tissue indicates vessel rupture, which could be present after trauma.

Visualization of the renal vessels can be improved by using a digital subtraction technique. In the digital subtraction arteriogram (DSA), a computer is used to "subtract out" loops of bowel, ribs, and other structures normally seen on the x-ray film. As a result, even the small-vessel images are improved. In addition, the use of a smaller amount of dye means less risk for nephrotoxicity. DSA procedures may not provide sufficient detail for surgical intervention when used without full arteriography.

FOLLOW-UP CARE. Bleeding from the catheter insertion site and dye-induced reactions are the two most common complications of renal arteriography. The nurse monitors the catheter insertion site for signs of bleeding or swelling. A pressure dressing may have been placed as a preventive measure before the client returned to the nursing area. The nurse ensures that a 5-pound sandbag and ice are available in case of emergency.

The vital signs are monitored as per the physician's order or according to the agency's policy, usually every 15 minutes for 1 hour, then every 30 minutes for 2 hours, then every hour for 4 hours, and then every 4 hours. The nurse checks the temperature and color of the extremities and distal pulses. A sudden absence of pulses in the catheterized vessel may reflect hematoma formation or embolization. Hemoglobin and hematocrit levels are monitored closely for 24 hours after the procedure, usually every 6 hours.

The period of absolute bedrest (to prevent bleeding) after arteriography varies. In general, bedrest is maintained for 4 to 6 hours. The nurse instructs the client about the importance of keeping the leg in a straight position for those 4 to 6 hours. A restraint may be used on the leg with the client's consent. Ankle flexing and weight shifting are encouraged to prevent deep vein thrombosis. If there is no evidence of bleeding after 4 to 6 hours, the client may be permitted to stand to void or may use a bedside commode.

Serum creatinine tests are ordered for several days after the arteriogram to determine whether the procedure has affected kidney function. For some clients with renal insufficiency, the administration of dye may cause an episode of acute renal failure sufficient to require short-term dialysis. Because the test is used to provide information for interventions to restore blood flow and thus preserve kidney function, many clients are willing to accept the risk of short-term dialysis to prevent the need for permanent dialysis. The client is urged to drink fluids after the procedure to ensure adequate excretion of the dye.

Renal Biopsy

CLIENT PREPARATION. The nurse explains that a biopsy of the kidney is performed to determine a pathologic reason for unexplained renal dysfunction and to direct or change a course of therapy. The client signs an informed consent or operative permit.

In a closed biopsy, the physician obtains kidney tissue samples **percutaneously** (through the skin and other tissues). In an open biopsy, the tissues are obtained surgically. Factors to consider include the number of kidneys, the ability of the client to cooperate, and the need for abdominal surgical exploration. If a percutaneous biopsy is selected, the client must have two kidneys, be able to breathe comfortably in a prone position for 30 to 45 minutes, and be able to hold his or her breath on request for several seconds. The client is on NPO status for 4 to 6 hours before the procedure in case a major complication requires immediate surgery.

An open renal biopsy is performed when cancer is suspected or when the client has only one kidney, cannot hold his or her breath, or is unable to tolerate a prone position. If abdominal surgery is necessary for other reasons and a renal biopsy is also needed, the nephrologist may request the surgeon to perform the biopsy, thereby eliminating the need for a second procedure. If an open biopsy is performed, client preparation is the same as for general surgery and anesthesia (see Chapter 17).

Because of the risk for postprocedure bleeding, coagulation studies such as platelet count, activated partial thromboplastin time (aPTT), prothrombin time (PT), and bleeding time are performed before surgery. A blood transfusion may be needed to correct a low hemoglobin level before biopsy. Hypertension and uremia increase the risk for bleeding and the physician may order antihypertensive medications or dialysis before a biopsy.

PROCEDURE. Immediately before a percutaneous biopsy, the nurse asks the client to void to decrease the possibility of puncturing the bladder. The left kidney is biopsied because it is closer to the skin and is not near the liver. The exact position of the kidney is determined via fluoroscopic or ultrasonographic examination or by radionuclide scan. In some clients the nephrologist may locate the kidney by using landmarks from previous images. In other clients the closed biopsy is performed directly during fluoroscopy or ultrasonographic examination.

For a closed biopsy, the client is placed in a prone position. A roll of padding is placed under the client's abdomen to angle the kidney closer to the skin. The skin is prepared and draped, and a local anesthetic is injected. The depth of the kidney is identified by inserting a thin-gauge spinal needle. Movement of the spinal needle with breathing helps to determine that the capsule of the kidney has been located. A specially designed trocar is inserted in the path established by the spinal needle. While the client holds his or her breath, tissue is obtained by inserting the biopsy needle through the trocar and capsule into the kidney cortex. Automated spring-loaded and smaller biopsy needles have improved the tissue samples obtained. Ideally, three tissue specimens are obtained.

FOLLOW-UP CARE. After a closed percutaneous biopsy, the major risk is bleeding from the biopsy site. For 24 hours after the biopsy, the nurse monitors the dressing site, vital signs, urinary output, hemoglobin level, and hematocrit (as for postarteriography protocols). Even if the dressing is dry and there is no hematoma, the client could be bleeding from the site. An internal bleed is not readily visible but is suspected with flank pain, decreasing blood pressure, decreasing urine output, or other signs of hypovolemia or shock.

The client follows a plan of strict bedrest, lying in a supine position with a back roll for additional support for at least 6 hours after the biopsy. The head of the bed may be elevated, and the client may resume oral intake of food and fluids. After 6 hours, the client may have limited bathroom privileges if there is no evidence of bleeding.

The nurse monitors for hematuria, the most common complication of a percutaneous renal biopsy. Hematuria occurs microscopically in almost all clients, whereas 5% to 9% have gross hematuria. This problem usually resolves spontaneously 48 to 72 hours after the biopsy but can persist for 2 to 3 weeks. In rare cases, transfusions and surgery are required. There should be no obvious blood clots in the urine.

The client may have some local discomfort after the percutaneous renal biopsy. If aching originates at the biopsy site and begins to radiate to the flank and around the front of the abdomen, the nurse suspects an onset of bleeding or the development of a perinephric hematoma. This pattern of discomfort with bleeding occurs because blood in the perirenal tissues and musculature increases pressure on local nerve tracts.

If bleeding occurs, IV fluid, packed red blood cells, or both may need to be administered to restore blood pressure. In general, a small amount of bleeding creates enough pressure to compress bleeding sites; this is called a **tamponade effect.** If tamponade does not occur and bleeding becomes extensive, surgical intervention for hemostasis or even nephrectomy may be necessary. A perinephric hematoma may become infected, requiring treatment with antibiotics and surgical drainage.

If no bleeding occurs, the client can resume general activities after 24 hours. The nurse instructs him or her to avoid lifting heavy objects, exercising, or performing other strenuous activities for 1 to 2 weeks after the biopsy procedure. Driving may also be restricted.

Refer to Chapter 19 for general postoperative care for the client undergoing an open renal biopsy.

Renography (Kidney Scan)

CLIENT PREPARATION. The nurse explains to the client that a kidney scan is performed to provide general information about renal blood flow. A small amount of radioactive material, a radionuclide, is used. The nurse reassures the client that there is generally no danger from the small amount of radioactive material present in the agent.

PROCEDURE. For a kidney scan, the radionuclide is injected intravenously. After injection, the radionuclide is absorbed into kidney tissue and gives off low-level radioactive emissions **(scintillations).** The amount of emission is measured by a scintillator or a scintillation counter. A specially designed camera records the emissions and produces an image. At the same time, the rate and location of the emissions are recorded by computer, and information about renal blood flow, or glomerular filtration, is provided.

In some cases captopril (Capoten), an antihypertensive agent, is administered at the start of the procedure to change blood flow in the kidney. This procedure is known as a Captopril Renal Scan. The drug can cause severe hypotension during and after the procedure.

FOLLOW-UP CARE. If the client is able, urination into a commode is acceptable without risk from the small amount of radioactive material to be excreted. If the client is incontinent, the nurse changes the bed linens promptly and wears gloves to maintain standard precautions. If captopril was used during the procedure, the client's blood pressure is assessed frequently. The client is cautioned about rapid position changes and the risk for falling associated with orthostatic (positional) hypotension.

Ultrasonography

CLIENT PREPARATION. The nurse informs the client that ultrasonography does not cause discomfort and is without risk. This test involves applying sound waves to structures of different densities to produce images of the kidneys, ureters, and bladder and surrounding tissues. Ultrasonography allows assessment of kidney size, cortical thickness, and status of the calices. The test can be used to identify obstruction in the urinary tract, tumors, cysts, and other masses without the use of nephrotoxic contrast material (dye).

PROCEDURE. The client undergoing renal ultrasound is usually placed on a table in a prone position. A sonographic gel is applied to the skin over the back and flank areas to promote the conduction of sound waves. A transducer in contact with and moving across the skin delivers sound waves and measures the echoes. Images of the internal structures are produced.

FOLLOW-UP CARE. Skin care to remove the gel is all that is necessary after ultrasonography.

OTHER URINARY TRACT DIAGNOSTIC TESTS

Cystoscopy and Cystourethroscopy

CLIENT PREPARATION. Cystoscopy and cystourethroscopy are considered operative procedures and thus require completion of a preoperative checklist and an informed consent statement. The nurse provides a complete description of and reasons for the procedure. Cystoscopy may be performed for diagnosis or treatment. Diagnostic indications include examination for bladder trauma (cystoscopy) or urethral trauma (cystourethroscopy) and identification of the causes of urinary tract obstruction from stones or tumors. Cystoscopy may be indicated to remove bladder tumors or an enlarged prostate gland.

Cystoscopy may be performed under general or local anesthesia with sedation. The client's age, general health, and expected duration of the procedure are some of the considerations in the decision about anesthesia. A light evening meal may be eaten. Usually the client is on NPO status after midnight on the night before the cystoscopy. A bowel preparation with laxatives or enemas is performed the evening before the procedure.

PROCEDURE. The cystoscopic examination is performed in a specially designed cystoscopic examination room. If the procedure is performed in a surgical suite under general anesthesia, traditional surgical support personnel are present. This procedure is more often performed in outpatient settings, such as a clinic, an ambulatory surgery or short-procedure unit, or a urologist's office.

The client is assisted onto a table and, after sedation, is placed in the lithotomy position. After the administration of anesthesia, skin cleaning, and draping, a cystoscope is inserted via the urethra into the urinary bladder. If visualization of the urethra is also indicated, a urethroscope is used. Examinations commonly include the use of both the cystoscope and the urethroscope.

FOLLOW-UP CARE. After cystoscopic examination with general anesthesia, the client is returned to a postanesthesia care unit (PACU) or area. If local anesthesia and sedation were used, the client may be returned directly to the hospital room. Clients undergoing cystoscopic examinations as outpatients are transferred to an area for monitoring before discharge to home. The nurse monitors the client for airway patency and breathing, alterations in vital signs (including temperature), and changes in urine output. The nurse also observes for the complications of bleeding and infection.

A catheter may or may not be present after cystoscopy. The client without a catheter has urinary frequency due to irritation from the catheter. The urine may be pink tinged, but gross bleeding is not expected. Bleeding or the presence of clots may obstruct the catheter and decrease urine output. The nurse monitors urine output and notifies the physician of obvious blood clots or a decreased or ceased urine output. The Foley catheter is irrigated with sterile saline, as ordered. The physician is notified if the client has a fever (with or without chills) or an elevated white blood cell (WBC) count, which suggests infection. The client is encouraged to take oral fluids to promote adequate urine output (which helps prevent clotting) and to reduce the burning sensation on urination.

Retrograde Procedures

CLIENT PREPARATION. The client is prepared for retrograde procedures (retrograde pyelography, retrograde cystography, and retrograde urethrography) in a manner similar to that for the cystoscopic examination. **Retrograde** means going against the normal flow of urine. The nurse explains that a retrograde examination of the ureters and pelves (**pyelogram**), the bladder (**cystogram**), and the urethra (**urethrogram**) involves the direct injection of radiopaque contrast medium (dye) into the lower urinary tract. Because the dye is instilled directly to obtain an outline of the structures desired, the dye does not enter the bloodstream. Therefore the client is not at risk for dye-induced acute renal failure or a systemic allergic response.

PROCEDURE. Retrograde films are obtained during the cystoscopic examination. After placement of the cystoscope by the urologist, catheters are placed into each ureter, and contrast medium is instilled into each ureter and renal pelvis. The catheters are removed by the urologist, and films are taken by the radiology technician to outline these structures as the dye is excreted. The procedure identifies any obstruction or structural abnormality.

For clients undergoing retrograde cystoscopy or urethrography, contrast medium is instilled similarly into the bladder or urethra. Cystography and urethrography also identify structural abnormalities, such as fistulas, diverticula, and tumors.

FOLLOW-UP CARE. After retrograde procedures, the nurse monitors the client for the development of infection as a result of instrumentation of the urinary tract. Because these procedures are performed during cystoscopic examination, follow-up care is the same as that for cystoscopy.

Urodynamic Studies

Urodynamic studies describe the processes of voiding and include the following:
- Tests of bladder capacity, pressure, and tone
- Studies of urethral pressure and urine flow
- Examination of the function of perineal voluntary muscles

These tests are often used along with excretory urographic or cystoscopic procedures to evaluate problems with urine flow.

■ CYSTOMETROGRAPHY

CLIENT PREPARATION. The nurse explains that the purpose of a cystometrogram (CMG) is to determine the effectiveness and sensitivity of the bladder wall (detrusor) muscle. Determinations about bladder capacity, bladder pressure, and voiding reflexes may be made with these measurements of detrusor muscle quality. A urinary catheter may be needed temporarily during the procedure.

PROCEDURE. The nurse asks the client to void normally. The nurse records measurements of the amount, rate of flow, and time of voiding. A urinary catheter is inserted to

measure the residual bladder urine volume. The cystometer is attached to the catheter, and fluid is instilled via the catheter into the bladder. The point at which the client first notes a feeling of the urge to void and the point at which the client notes a strong urge to void are recorded. Bladder capacity and bladder pressure readings are recorded graphically. The client is asked to void when the bladder instillation is complete (about 500 mL). The urinary residual after voiding is noted, and the catheter is removed. Electromyography of the perineal muscles may also be performed during the cystometric examination.

FOLLOW-UP CARE. As with any instrumentation of the urinary tract, the nurse monitors for infection. The client's temperature, the characteristics of the urine, and the amount of urine output are recorded.

■ URETHRAL PRESSURE PROFILE

CLIENT PREPARATION. The nurse explains that a urethral pressure profile (also called a urethral pressure profilometry [UPP]) can provide information about the nature of urinary incontinence or urinary retention. A urinary catheter may be temporarily placed during the procedure.

PROCEDURE. A special catheter with pressure-sensing capabilities is inserted into the bladder. Variations in the pressure of the smooth muscle of the urethra are recorded as the catheter is slowly withdrawn.

FOLLOW-UP CARE. As with other studies involving instrumentation of the urinary tract, the client is monitored for the development of infection.

■ ELECTROMYOGRAPHY

CLIENT PREPARATION. The nurse explains that electromyography (EMG) of the perineal muscles may be useful in evaluating the strength of the muscles used in voiding. This information may assist in identifying methods of improving continence. The nurse informs the client that some temporary discomfort may accompany placement of the electrodes.

PROCEDURE. In EMG of the perineal muscles, electrodes are placed in either the rectum or the urethra to measure muscle contraction and relaxation.

FOLLOW-UP CARE. After the completion of EMG, the nurse administers analgesics to promote the client's comfort. Any discomfort is usually mild and of short duration.

■ URINE STREAM TEST

CLIENT PREPARATION. The nurse explains that a urine stream test evaluates pelvic muscle strength and the effectiveness of pelvic muscles in interrupting the flow of urine. It is useful in evaluating urinary incontinence.

PROCEDURE. Three to five seconds after urination begins, the examiner gives the client a signal to stop urine flow. The length of time required to interrupt the flow of urine is recorded.

FOLLOW-UP CARE. Cleansing of the perineal area, as after any voiding, is all that is necessary after the urine stream test.

CRITICAL THINKING CHALLENGE

The client, a 62-year-old woman with type 2 diabetes, is scheduled to have a percutaneous biopsy of the left kidney. She asks you whether she should take her oral antidiabetic medicine in the morning before the procedure. She also asks if the procedure will be painful and if she can attend her card party the evening after the procedure.

- Should this client take her usual antidiabetic medication before the procedure? Why or why not?
- What will you tell this client about activity restrictions?
- How will you reassure this client about pain management during and after the procedure?

For suggested answer guidelines, go to http://www.wbsaunders.com/SIMON/Iggy/.

ONLINE RESOURCES

For suggested readings and Internet resources, go to http://www.wbsaunders.com/SIMON/Iggy/.

SELECTED BIBLIOGRAPHY

Asterisk indicates a classic or definitive work on this subject.

Beck, L.H. (1998). Changes in renal function with aging. *Clinics in Geriatric Medicine, 14*(2), 199-209.

Brenner, B.M. (Eds.). (2000). *Brenner & Rector's The kidney* (6th ed.). Philadelphia: W.B. Saunders.

Cohan, R.H., & Ellis, J.H. (1997). Iodinated contrast material in uroradiology: Choice of agent and management of complications. *Urologic Clinics of North America, 24*(3), 471-491.

*Driver, D.S. (1996). Renal assessment: Back to basics. *American Nephrology Nurses' Association Journal, 23*(4), 361-368.

Duthrie, E.H., & Katz, P.R. (1998). *Practice of geriatrics* (3rd ed.). Philadelphia: W.B. Saunders.

Gordon, M. (2000). *Manual of nursing diagnosis* (9th ed.). St. Louis: Mosby.

Guyton, A.C., & Hall, J.E. (2000). *Textbook of medical physiology* (10th ed.). Philadelphia: W.B. Saunders.

*Holechek, M.J. (1992). Glomerular filtration and renal hemodynamics. *American Nephrology Nurses' Association Journal, 19*(3), 237-245.

Jarvis, C. (2000). *Physical examination and health assessment* (3rd ed.) Philadelphia: W.B. Saunders.

Krop, J.S., et al. (1999). A community-based study of the explanatory factors for the excess risk for early renal function decline in blacks vs whites with diabetes: The atherosclerosis risk in communities study. *Archives of Internal Medicine, 159*(15), 1777-1783.

*Lancaster, L.E. (Ed.). (1995). *Core curriculum for nephrology nursing* (3rd ed.). Pitman, NJ: A.J. Janetti.

Little, C. (2000). Renovascular hypertension. *American Journal of Nursing, 100*(2), 46-51.

Pagana, K., & Pagana, T. (1999). *Diagnostic testing and nursing implications: A case study approach.* St. Louis: Mosby.

Pfister, S.M. (1999). Bladder diaries and voiding patterns in older adults. *Journal of Gerontological Nursing, 25*(3), 36-41.

*Preisig, P. (1994). Renal acidification. *American Nephrology Nurses' Association Journal, 21*(4), 251-257.

*Radke, K.J. (1994). The aging kidney: Structure, function, and nursing practice implications. *American Nephrology Nurses' Association Journal, 21*(4), 181-193.

Shinopulos, N. (2000). Bedside urodynamic studies: Simple testing for urinary incontinence. *The Nurse Practitioner, 25*(6), 19-20, 22, 25-26, 28, 33-34, 37.

*Shulman, N.B., & Hall, W.D. (1991). Renal vascular disease in African-Americans and other racial minorities. *Circulation, 83*(4), 1477-1479.

Stanton, B.A., & Koeppen, B.M. (1998). The kidney. In R.M. Berne et al. (Eds.), *Physiology* (4th ed.). St. Louis: Mosby.

Stark, J. (1998). Interpretation of BUN and creatinine. *Critical Care Nursing Clinics of North America, 10*(4), 491-496.

U.S. Renal Data Systems. (1999). *USRDS 1999 annual data report.* Bethesda, MD: The National Institutes of Health, National Institute of Diabetes and Digestive and Kidney Diseases.

*Valtin, H., & Schafer, J.A. (1995). *Renal function* (3rd ed.). Boston: Little, Brown.

Walsh, P.C., et al. (1998). *Campbell's urology* (7th ed.). Philadelphia: W.B. Saunders.

*Yucha, C., & Keen, M. (1996). Renal regulation of extracellular fluid volume and osmolality. *American Nephrology Nurses' Association Journal, 23*(5), 487-497.

Interventions for Clients with Urinary Problems

CHRIS WINKELMAN

Learning Objectives

After studying this chapter, you should be able to:

1. Describe the clinical manifestations of cystitis.
2. Prioritize educational needs for a person at risk for cystitis.
3. Compare and contrast the pathophysiology and manifestations of stress incontinence, urge incontinence, overflow incontinence, mixed incontinence, and functional incontinence.
4. Prioritize educational needs for the client taking sulfonamide antibiotics for a urinary tract infection.
5. Describe the techniques used to assess pelvic floor strength in the client who is experiencing some incontinence.
6. Explain the proper application of exercises to strengthen pelvic floor muscles.
7. Explain the drug therapy for different types of incontinence.
8. Prioritize nursing care for the client with renal colic.
9. Describe the common clinical manifestations of bladder cancer.
10. Develop a teaching plan for a client who has had a urinary diversion for bladder cancer.

Go to http://www.wbsaunders.com/SIMON/Iggy/ for self-assessment questions related to these Learning Objectives.

Urinary disorders affect the storage or elimination of urine. Both acute and chronic urinary problems are common and costly. More than 20 million people in the United States annually experience urinary tract infections, cystitis, kidney and ureter stones, or urinary incontinence (U.S. Renal Data Systems, 1999). Although life-threatening complications are rare with urinary disorders, clients experience significant functional, physical, and psychosocial changes that adversely affect quality of life. Nursing interventions are directed toward prevention, detection, and management of urologic disorders.

INFECTIOUS DISORDERS

Infections of the urinary tract and kidneys occur often. Symptoms of urinary tract infection (UTI) account for more than 6.5 million health care visits annually in the United States, and 1.5 million hospital discharges involve a diagnosis of UTI (Centers for Disease Control and Prevention [CDC], 2001). In the hospital, UTIs are the most prevalent nosocomial infection (Warren, 1997). Total direct and indirect costs for urologic disorders are estimated at nearly $200 million dollars each year.

The primary site of the infectious process describes infections in the urinary tract. Acute infections in the lower urinary tract include urethritis (urethra), cystitis (bladder), and **prostatitis** (prostate gland). **Acute pyelonephritis** is an upper urinary tract (kidney) infection. It is important to determine the site of infection, since both the site of infection and the specific type of bacteria present determine treatment. A number of structural or functional abnormalities of the urinary tract and characteristics of the urine are thought to predispose clients to UTIs (Table 70-1).

Cystitis

■ OVERVIEW

Cystitis is an inflammation of the urinary bladder. It can be caused by infection from bacteria, viruses, fungi, or parasites. Infectious cystitis is the most common of the UTIs. Noninfectious cystitis is caused by chemicals or radiation. Interstitial cystitis is an inflammatory process of unknown etiology.

■ Pathophysiology

Infectious agents, most commonly bacteria, typically move up the urinary tract from the external urethra to the bladder. Less typically, spread of infection through the blood and lymph fluid can occur. Once bacteria enter the urinary tract, several factors influence the outcome (Table 70-2).

Asymptomatic bacteriuria is more common in older adults and is generally considered a benign condition. No studies have demonstrated a relationship between asymptomatic bacteriuria and progression to acute infection or renal insuffi-

TABLE 70-1 • FACTORS CONTRIBUTING TO URINARY TRACT INFECTIONS

Factor	Mechanism	Interventions
Obstruction	Incomplete bladder emptying creates a continuous pool of urine where bacteria can grow, prevents flushing out of bacteria, and allows bacteria to ascend more easily to higher structures.	Relieve or bypass the obstruction to promote complete bladder emptying.
	Bacteria have a greater chance of multiplying the longer they remain in residual urine.	Increase liquids to dilute urine and encourage more frequent voiding.
	Overdistention of the bladder damages the mucosa and allows bacteria to invade the bladder wall.	Use intermittent catheterization to keep the bladder from becoming distended.
Calculi	Large calculi can cause obstruction to urine flow.	Remove calculi and/or treat the underlying condition that causes the calculi to form.
	The rough surface of a calculus irritates mucosal surfaces and creates a spot where bacteria can establish and grow.	
	Bacteria can live within calculi and cause reinfection.	
Vesicoureteral reflux	Bacteria-laden urine is forced backward from the bladder up into the ureters and kidneys, where pyelonephritis can develop.	The affected ureters may be able to be surgically reimplanted in the bladder to eliminate the reflux.
	Reflux of sterile urine can cause renal scarring, which may promote renal dysfunction.	
Diabetes mellitus	Excess glucose in urine provides a rich medium for bacterial growth.	Maintain good glucose control in clients with diabetes.
	Peripheral neuropathy affects bladder innervation and leads to a flaccid bladder and incomplete bladder emptying.	
Characteristics of urine	Alkalotic urine promotes bacterial growth.	Acidify urine by taking vitamin C tablets, not citrus fruits. Such fruits make the urine alkaline.
	Concentrated urine promotes bacterial growth.	Increase urine dilution by increasing fluid intake.
Gender	Female clients are susceptible to periurethral colonization with coliform bacteria.	Explain the importance of perineal hygiene (wiping front to back) to prevent large amounts of coliform bacteria from remaining in the perineal area.
	Bladder displacement during pregnancy predisposes women to cystitis and the development of pyelonephritis.	Routine monitoring of pregnant women for UTIs prevents complications.
	A diaphragm or pessary that is too large can cause an obstruction to urine flow or trauma to the urethra.	Be sure diaphragms and pessaries are properly fitted.
Age	Obstruction may be caused by incomplete bladder emptying as a result of an enlarged prostate in men and cystocele and prolapse in women.	Do not rush older clients during toileting; provide regular and private toileting times to promote complete bladder emptying.
	Neuromuscular conditions that cause incomplete bladder emptying, such as Parkinson's disease and strokes, affect older adults more frequently.	Straight catheter for residual and Credé maneuver to promote more complete emptying.
	The use of anticholinergic medications in older adults contributes to delayed bladder emptying.	Monitor and report this medication side effect.
	Fecal incontinence contributes to poor perineal hygiene.	Promptly clean clients after episodes of incontinence.
	Hypoestrogenism in older women adversely affects the cells of the vagina and urethra, making them more susceptible to infections.	Give vaginal estrogen cream as directed to improve the health of the client's vaginal and urethral cells.
Sexual activity	Irritation of the perineum and urethra during intercourse can promote migration of bacteria from the perineal area to the urinary tract in some women.	Empty the bladder before and after intercourse. Drink 8 oz of fluid (especially water) after intercourse.
	Spermicides can alter vaginal pH, increasing potential numbers of pathogens.	Consider alternate method of birth control if experiencing repeated UTIs.
	Inadequate vaginal lubrication may exacerbate potential urethral irritation.	Use an artificial vaginal lubricant.
	Bacteria may be introduced into the man's urethra during anal intercourse or during vaginal intercourse with a woman who has a bacterial vaginitis.	Use a condom.

TABLE 70-2 • IMPORTANT FACTORS INFLUENCING THE OUTCOME OF URINARY TRACT INFECTIONS

Facilitating Aspects	Protective Aspects
ANATOMY	
Females: Short length of the urethra and its proximity to the vagina and rectum facilitate colonization of coliform bacteria.	*Males:* Long length of the urethra and its distance from the rectum provide protection from colonization with coliform bacteria.
Males: With age, the prostate enlarges and may obstruct the normal flow of urine, producing stasis.	
PHYSIOLOGY	
Females: Pregnancy predisposes a woman to ureteral reflux and subsequent pyelonephritis; with age the decline in estrogen facilitates colonization of *E. coli*.	*Females:* Well-estrogenized mucosa in the urethra and trigone may inhibit bacterial colonization.
Males: With age, prostatic secretions lose their antibacterial characteristics and predispose to bacterial proliferation in the urine.	*Males:* Normal prostatic secretions inhibit bacterial growth.
	Both males and females: Mucin is produced by urothelial cells lining the bladder—this helps to maintain mucosal integrity and prevent cellular damage; mucin may also prevent bacteria from adhering to urothelial cells.
TRAUMA	
Females: Vaginal penetration with sexual intercourse may traumatize the urethra and bladder base, leading to postcoital (or honeymoon) cystitis; a vaginal diaphragm that is too large can place pressure on the urethra, causing trauma; vaginal childbirth can cause permanent damage to the urethra.	*Females:* Adequate lubrication, either natural or artificial, with intercourse may prevent any trauma.
Males: Sexually transmitted diseases may cause urethral strictures that obstruct the flow of urine and predispose to urinary stasis.	
Both males and females: Urethral instrumentation (such as catheterization) may disturb the urothelial surface and predispose to adherence of bacteria that would ordinarily not be pathogenic.	
INFECTIOUS AGENT	
Some organisms are better able to adhere to host cells and secrete substances that induce inflammation.	A small inoculum (number of microorganisms introduced into the body) is more easily flushed away by the flow of urine.

ciency in clients without obstructive conditions, reflux, stones, or diabetes mellitus.

Etiology

The most common pathogens in infectious cystitis are organisms from the gastrointestinal (GI) tract. It is estimated that 90% of UTIs are caused by *Escherichia coli*. Other, less common infective organisms include *Staphylococcus saprophyticus, Klebsiella pneumoniae,* and organisms from the *Proteus* and *Enterobacter* species.

In most cases, GI organisms first grow in the perineal area; then move into the urethra as a result of irritation, trauma, or instrumentation of the urinary tract (i.e., catheterization); and ascend to the bladder. Catheters are the most common predisposing factor for UTIs in the hospital setting. Within 48 hours of catheter insertion, bacterial colonization begins. About 50% of clients with indwelling catheters become infected within 1 week of catheterization. The etiology of catheter-related infections varies between genders. Bacteria from a female client's perineal area are more likely to adhere to the outer surface of the catheter and then ascend to the bladder. In male clients, bacteria tend to gain access to the bladder from inside the lumen of the catheter (Warren, 1997). Any break in the closed urinary drainage system provides an opportunity for bacteria to adhere to and migrate through the urinary tract. Best practices to minimize the risk of catheter contamination are listed in Chart 70-1.

Organisms other than bacteria can cause cystitis. Fungal infections, such as those caused by *Candida*, may develop during long-term antibiotic therapy, since antibiotics alter normal flora. Clients who are severely immunocompromised and have decreased resistance to infection, are receiving glucocorticosteroids or other immunosuppressive agents, or have diabetes mellitus or acquired immunodeficiency syndrome (AIDS) are also at risk for fungal UTIs.

Viral and parasitic infections are rare and usually accompany an infection in another site. For example, *Trichomonas,* a parasite found in the vagina, can also be found in the urine. Treatment of the vaginal infection (see Chapter 75) is usually sufficient to treat the UTI.

Noninfectious cystitis may result from chemical exposure, such as to drugs (e.g., cyclophosphamide [Cytoxan, Procytox❖]), from radiation therapy, and from immunologic responses, as with systemic lupus erythematosus (SLE).

Interstitial cystitis is a relatively rare, chronic inflammation of the bladder. The condition affects women more often than men (in a 12:1 ratio), and the diagnosis is difficult to make. The symptoms are identical to those of simple cystitis, but the urgency and bladder pain are more intense (Thompson & Christmas, 1996).

Although cystitis is not life threatening, infectious cystitis can lead to life-threatening complications, including pyelonephritis and sepsis. There is considerable debate about the risk for kidney tissue damage and subsequent kidney failure as a result of bacteria ascending from the bladder to the kidney. Most experts believe that severe deterioration of renal function is a rare complication without one or more predisposing factors, such as anatomic abnormalities, pregnancy, obstruction, reflux, calculi, or diabetes mellitus.

The spread of the infecting agent from the urinary tract to systemic circulation is termed **urosepsis. Sepsis** from any

CHART 70-1

BEST PRACTICE *for*
Minimizing Catheter-Related Infection

- Avoid long-term use (>3 days) during active illness or perioperatively.
- Use aseptic routine when handling catheter devices; manipulation can promote an environment favorable to pathogens.
- Use strict sterile technique to insert the catheter (in the hospital setting); a break in technique can introduce pathogens into the urinary tract.
- Ensure that catheter tubing connections are sealed securely; disconnections can introduce pathogens into the urinary tract.
- Keep urine collection bags below the level of the bladder at all times; elevating the collection bag above the bladder causes reflux of pathogens from the bag into the urinary tract.
- Secure the catheter to the client's thigh (female) or lower abdomen (male); catheter movement can cause urethral friction and irritation.
- Perform daily catheter care by washing the perineum and proximal portion of the catheter with soap and water, drying gently (removes pathogens and reduces pathogenic population).
- *Application of antiseptic solutions or antibiotic ointments to the perineal area of catheterized clients has not been demonstrated to have any beneficial effect.*

CHART 70-2

KEY FEATURES *of*
Urinary Tract Infection

Common Clinical Manifestations
- Frequency
- Urgency
- Dysuria
- Hesitancy or difficulty in initiating urine stream
- Low back pain
- Nocturia
- Incontinence
- Retention
- Suprapubic tenderness or fullness
- Feeling of incomplete bladder emptying

Rare Clinical Manifestations
- Fever
- Chills
- Nausea
- Vomiting
- Malaise
- Flank pain

Atypical Clinical Manifestations That May Occur in the Older Adult
- The only symptom may be something as vague as increasing mental confusion or frequent, unexplained falls.
- A sudden onset of incontinence or a worsening of incontinence may be the only symptom of an early UTI.
- Fever, tachycardia, tachypnea, and hypotension, even without any urinary symptoms, may be signs of urosepsis.
- Loss of appetite, nocturia, and dysuria are common symptoms.

UTI, Urinary tract infection.

source is a systemic infection that can lead to overwhelming organ failure, shock, and death. The most common cause of sepsis in the hospitalized client is a UTI (Warren, 1997). Sepsis is associated with high mortality and prolonged hospitalization (see Chapter 37).

Incidence/Prevalence

The incidence of UTI is second only to that of upper respiratory infections in primary care. Clients who have the symptoms of **frequency** (an urge to urinate frequently in small amounts), **dysuria** (pain and/or burning with urination), and **urgency** (the feeling that urination will occur immediately) account for more than 5 million health care visits annually. Approximately 50% of these clients will have a confirmed UTI. Recurrent infections account for an unknown number of these visits (CDC, 2001).

WOMEN'S HEALTH CONSIDERATIONS
The prevalence of UTIs varies with age and gender. Generally, women are more commonly affected with UTIs than men. In men 65 to 70 years old, the incidence of UTI is 3%; after age 70, however, the incidence is 20%. In women over the age of 80, the prevalence rises from 20% to 50% (Duffield, 1997). It is believed that skin and mucous membrane changes from a lack of estrogen account for much of the increased risk.

► COLLABORATIVE MANAGEMENT
● Assessment
■ PHYSICAL ASSESSMENT/CLINICAL MANIFESTATIONS

Frequency, urgency, and dysuria are the primary clinical manifestations of a urinary tract infection (UTI), but other signs and symptoms may be present (Chart 70-2). Urine may be cloudy, foul smelling, or blood tinged. Identifying risk factors contributing to UTI are included in the assessment (see Table 70-1).

Before performing the physical assessment, the nurse asks the client to void so that the urine can be examined and the bladder emptied before palpation. The nurse assesses vital signs to help rule out sepsis, inspects the lower abdomen, and palpates the urinary bladder. Distention after voiding indicates incomplete bladder emptying.

Using standard precautions (see Chapter 26), the nurse notes inflammation and any skin lesions around the urethral meatus and vaginal introitus (opening). Female clients often report "burning with urination" when normal, acidic urine touches labial tissues that are inflamed and ulcerated by vaginal infections or sexually transmitted diseases (STDs). Privacy is maintained with drapes during the examination.

The prostate is palpated by rectal examination for size, alteration in contour, and any evidence of tenderness. The physician or advanced-practice nurse performs the rectal prostate assessment.

■ LABORATORY ASSESSMENT

Laboratory evaluation for a UTI is usually a urinalysis with a microscopic count of bacteria, white blood cells (WBCs), and red blood cells (RBCs). The presence of 100,000 colonies/mL and/or the presence of WBCs (**pyuria**) indicate an infection. A urinalysis is performed on a clean-catch midstream specimen. If the client cannot produce a clean-catch specimen, the nurse may need to obtain the specimen with a small-caliber (6 Fr) urethral catheter. For a routine urinalysis, 10 mL of urine is required; smaller quantities are sufficient for culture.

A urine culture confirms the type of microorganism and the number of colonies. Urine culture is expensive and takes 48 hours to obtain results. It is indicated when the UTI is complicated or not responsive to usual therapy or if the diagnosis is uncertain. The presence of a UTI is confirmed when there are more than 10^5 colony-forming units in the urine from any client, although in a symptomatic client as few as 10^3 colony-forming units may be diagnostic. Multiple organisms in low colony counts generally indicate a contaminated specimen.

Sensitivity testing follows culture results, especially when complicating factors are present, such as stones or recurrent infection, or when the client is older.

Occasionally the serum WBC count may be elevated, with the differential WBC count showing "left shift." This shift indicates that the number of immature WBCs is increasing in response to the infectious organisms. Consequently, the number of bands, or immature WBCs, is elevated. Left shift most commonly occurs with urosepsis and rarely occurs with uncomplicated cystitis.

■ OTHER DIAGNOSTIC ASSESSMENT

The clinician usually bases the diagnosis of cystitis on the history, physical examination, and laboratory data. If urinary retention and obstruction to urinary outflow are suspected, urography, abdominal sonography, or computed tomography (CT) may be needed to determine the site of obstruction or the presence of calculi. Voiding cystourethrography (see Chapter 69) is used for the diagnosis of suspected cases of vesicoureteral reflux.

Cystoscopy (see Chapter 69) is often performed when there is a history of recurrent UTIs (more than three or four a year). The urine is sterilized with antibiotic therapy before the procedure so that the risk of sepsis is not increased. Cystoscopy can identify abnormalities that may have contributed to the development of cystitis. These abnormalities include bladder calculi, bladder diverticula, urethral strictures, foreign bodies (such as sutures from previous surgery), and **trabeculation** (an abnormal thickening of the bladder wall caused by urinary retention and obstruction). Retrograde pyelography, along with the cystoscopic examination, produces outlines and images of the drainage tract. Areas of obstruction or malformation and the presence of reflux are then identified early.

Cystoscopy is the only means of accurately diagnosing interstitial cystitis. A urinalysis may show WBCs and RBCs but no bacteria. Classic findings in interstitial cystitis include a small-capacity bladder, the presence of **Hunner's ulcers** (a type of bladder lesion), and small hemorrhages after bladder distention.

● Interventions

NONSURGICAL MANAGEMENT

DRUG THERAPY. Medications prescribed to treat bacteriuria and promote comfort in the client with cystitis include urinary antiseptics or antibiotics, analgesics, and antispasmodics. The clinician prescribes antibiotics to treat any infection (Chart 70-3). Antifungal agents are administered when the infecting organism is a fungus. Amphotericin B is most often given in daily bladder instillations, and ketoconazole (Nizoral) is given in oral or parenteral form. The antispasmodic agents decrease bladder spasm and promote complete bladder emptying.

Antibiotic therapy is the usual prescription for a UTI (see Chart 70-3). Guidelines for UTIs in women indicate that a 3-day course of trimethoprim/sulfamethoxazole or fosfomycin is effective in eradicating an uncomplicated, community-acquired UTI (Houston, 1999). These shorter courses increase compliance and reduce cost. A longer treatment course of 7 to 21 days with oral or parenteral antibiotics is required for hospitalized clients; those with complicating factors, such as indwelling catheters or calculi; and those with a history of diabetes or immunosuppression.

> **WOMEN'S HEALTH CONSIDERATIONS**
> Pregnant women require vigorous intervention when bacteriuria is identified because of the tendency of simple cystitis to lead to acute pyelonephritis. Pyelonephritis in pregnancy can cause preterm labor and deleterious effects on the fetus.

Long-term antibiotic therapy is recommended for the treatment of chronic, recurring infections caused by structural abnormalities or calculi. Trimethoprim 100 mg daily may be prescribed for long-term management of the older client with frequent UTIs (Duffield, 1997). For women who experience recurrent UTIs after sexual intercourse, 1 low-dose tablet of nitrofurantoin (Macrodantin, Nephronex✿, Novofuran✿) after intercourse is often recommended.

URINARY ELIMINATION. The goal is to maintain an optimal urinary elimination pattern. Interventions for the management of cystitis are highlighted in Chart 70-4.

DIET THERAPY. The diet should include all food groups and include a number of calories for the increased metabolic processes associated with infection. Unless medically contraindicated, fluid intake needs to be at least 2 to 3 L/day for adequate flushing of urine through the system. Evidence suggests that 300 mL of cranberry juice consumed daily decreases bacterial adherence to the urinary tract, decreasing the incidence of UTIs in some clients. Cranberry juice must be consumed for 3 to 4 weeks to be effective (Walsh et al., 1998).

OTHER PAIN RELIEF MEASURES. A warm sitz bath taken two or three times a day for 20 minutes may provide comfort and some relief of local symptoms. If burning with urination is severe or urinary retention occurs, the nurse instructs the client to sit in the sitz bath and urinate into the warm water.

SURGICAL MANAGEMENT. Surgical interventions for clients with cystitis treat the conditions that predispose to recurrent UTIs (e.g., removal of obstructions, treatment of calculi, and repair of vesicoureteral reflux). Procedures may include cystoscopy (see Chapter 69) to identify and remove calculi or obstructions.

● Community-Based Care

The nurse assesses the client's level of understanding from his or her description of the problem. The client's knowledge about factors contributing to the development of cystitis is the basis on which further teaching interventions are planned.

CHART 70-3

DRUG THERAPY *for* Urinary Tract Infection

Drug	Usual Dosage	Nursing Interventions	Rationale
ANTIMICROBIALS			
Quinolones		Avoid use in pregnancy and those <18 yr.	Can interfere with cartilage formation in weight-bearing joints.
Ciprofloxacin (Cipro)	250 mg bid PO for 3 days with uncomplicated cystitis, for 7 days with complicated cystitis, and for 10-14 days with uncomplicated pyelonephritis	Avoid taking with aluminum- or magnesium-containing antacids. Give 1 hr before or 2 hr after food or drink.	Food, calcium, and antacids interfere with drug adsorption.
		Avoid caffeinated beverages, and use with caution in clients receiving theophylline.	Quinolones prolong the half-life of caffeine and theophylline.
Lomefloxacin (Maxaquin)	400 mg qd PO for 3 days for uncomplicated cystitis, for 7 days for complicated cystitis, and for 10-14 days for uncomplicated pyelonephritis	As above. Avoid the sun.	As above. Drug causes photosensitivity.
Levofloxacin (Levaquin)	250 mg qd PO for 3 days for uncomplicated cystitis, for 7 days for complicated cystitis, and for 10-14 days for uncomplicated pyelonephritis	As above. Avoid the sun.	As above. Drug causes photosensitivity.
Norfloxacin (Noroxin)	400 mg bid PO for 3 days for uncomplicated cystitis, for 7 days for complicated cystitis, and for 10-14 days for uncomplicated pyelonephritis	As above.	As above.
Ofloxacin (Floxin)	200 mg bid PO for 3 days for uncomplicated cystitis, for 7 days for complicated cystitis, and for 10-14 days for uncomplicated pyelonephritis	As above.	As above.
Sparfloxacin (Zagam)	400 mg PO for 1 day, then 200 mg/day for 2 days for uncomplicated cystitis, for 7 days for complicated cystitis, and for 10-14 days for uncomplicated pyelonephritis	As above.	As above.
Penicillins		Inquire about penicillin allergy.	
Amoxicillin (Amoxil)	500 mg bid PO for 3 days	Give with food.	Food reduces GI upset.
Amoxicillin/clavulanate (Augmentin, Clavulin✦)	500 mg bid PO for 3 days	Give with food.	Food reduces GI upset.
Cephalosporins		Inquire about allergy to cephalosporin or penicillin.	There is a 1% to 20% cross-reactivity between penicillin and cephalosporins.
Cefadroxil (Duricef)	1000 mg qd PO for 3 days for uncomplicated cystitis, or 1000 mg bid for 10 days for complicated cystitis		
Cefixime (Suprax)	400 mg PO qd for 3 days for uncomplicated cystitis, for 7 days for complicated cystitis, and for 10-14 days for uncomplicated pyelonephritis		
Fosfomycin (Monurol)	3 g PO (1 packet) as a single dose	Avoid use of GI drugs during dosing.	Less effective if given with drugs that increase GI motility.

GI, Gastrointestinal; *G6PD,* glucose-6-phosphate dehydrogenase deficiency.

Continued

CHART 70-3

DRUG THERAPY *for* Urinary Tract Infection—cont'd

Drug	Usual Dosage	Nursing Interventions	Rationale
SULFONAMIDE Trimethoprim/ sulfamethoxazole (Bactrim, Septra, Sulfatrim Roubac♣)	1 double-strength tablet (DS or 160/800 mg), for 3 or 10 days for uncomplicated cystitis, or single-strength PO (80/400 mg) after coitus for prophylaxis	Provide adequate fluid intake. Avoid ascorbic acid and ammonium chloride that acidify the urine. Use with caution in clients with asthma, G6PD deficiency, or multiple allergies.	Sulfa can crystallize in acidic or concentrated urine. Sulfa allergies are relatively common; monitor client for potential reaction.
URINARY ANTISEPTIC Nitrofurantoin (Macrobid Macrodantin, Nephronex♣, Novofuran♣)	*Macrobid:* 100 mg bid PO for 7 days *Macrodantin:* 100 mg qid PO for 7 days	Give with food or milk. Monitor for flu-like symptoms in older clients and in those with pulmonary disease.	Food or milk decreases GI upset. Rare case of interstitial pneumonitis can occur in susceptible clients.
ANALGESIC Phenazopyridine (Pyridium, Phenazo♣)	100-200 mg PO tid for 2-3 days	Give with food. Advise client that urine will become red or orange. Help the client to understand the difference between a urinary analgesic and antibiotic.	Food helps reduce GI upset. Urine discoloration is normal. A complete dosing schedule is not necessary.
ANTISPASMODIC Hyoscyamine (Anaspaz, Cystospaz-M, others)	0.125-0.5 PO tid and hs	Assess for safety, constipation, and urinary retention.	Anticholinergics cause drowsiness, blurred vision, dry mouth, constipation, and urinary retention.

GI, Gastrointestinal; *G6PD,* glucose-6-phosphate dehydrogenase deficiency.

CHART 70-4

NIC **INTERVENTION ACTIVITIES** *for*
The Client with a Urinary Tract Infection

Urinary Elimination Management: *Maintenance of an optimum urinary elimination pattern*
- Monitor urinary elimination, including frequency, consistency, odor, volume, and color, as appropriate.
- Teach client signs and symptoms of urinary tract infection.
- Obtain midstream voided specimen for analysis, as appropriate.
- Refer to physician if signs and symptoms of urinary tract infection occur.
- Instruct to respond immediately to urge to void, as appropriate.
- Teach client to drink 8 ounces of liquid with meals, between meals, and in early evening.
- Assist client with development of toileting routine, as appropriate.

NIC intervention activities selected from McCloskey, J.C., & Bulechek, G.M. (Eds.). (2000). *Nursing interventions classification (NIC)* (3rd ed.). St. Louis: Mosby. No part of this work is to be altered without prior written permission from the Publisher.

The client is instructed in self-administration of medications. Appropriate spacing of doses throughout the day and the need to complete all of the prescribed medication are stressed. If the drug will change the color of the urine, as it does with phenazopyridine (Pyridium, Pyronium), the nurse informs the client to expect this occurrence. The nurse offers techniques for remembering the medication schedule, such as the use of a daily calendar or the association of medications with usual activities (e.g., mealtimes).

Clients may associate symptoms of discomfort with sexual activities and experience feelings of guilt and embarrassment. Frank and sensitive discussions with a woman who experiences frequent recurrences of UTI after sexual intercourse can help her find appropriate techniques to handle the problem (see Table 70-1). The nurse explores with the woman the factors that contribute to her postcoital infections, such as diaphragm use and her general resistance to infection. The client is reminded that vigorous cleaning of the perineum with harsh soaps and vaginal douching may irritate the perineal tissues and actually increase the risk of UTI. At the client's request, the nurse discusses the problem with the client and her partner to help them find ways of maintaining their intimate relationship. Chart 70-5 gives other specific instructions for preventing UTIs.

Urethritis

■ OVERVIEW

Urethritis is an inflammation of the urethra that causes symptoms similar to urinary tract infection (UTI). In male clients, signs and symptoms of urethritis are burning or difficulty with urination and usually a discharge from the urethral meatus. The most common cause of urethritis in men is sexually transmitted diseases (STDs): gonorrhea or nonspecific urethritis caused by *Ureaplasma* (a gram-negative bacterium),

CHART 70-5

CLIENT EDUCATION GUIDE
Preventing a Urinary Tract Infection

- Drink 2 to 3 L of fluid every day.
- Drink 300 mL of cranberry juice daily.
- Be sure to get enough sleep, rest, and nutrition daily.
- [For women] Clean your perineum (the area between your legs) from front to back.
- [For women] Avoid irritating substances, such as bubble bath, nylon underwear, and scented toilet tissue. Wear loose-fitting cotton underwear.
- [For women] Empty your bladder before and after intercourse.
- If you experience burning when you urinate, if you have to urinate frequently, or if you find it difficult to begin urinating, notify your physician or other health care provider right away, especially if you have a chronic medical condition (such as diabetes).
- Empty your bladder as soon as you feel the urge to urinate.
- Empty your bladder regularly (e.g., every 4 hours), even if you do not feel the urge to urinate.
- You may try the following home therapies:
    Apple cider vinegar, 2 tablespoons three times per day in juice.
    Echinacea (herb), one dropperful three times per day in juice or herbal tea (Duffield, 1997).
    Vitamin C 500 mg/day to acidify the urine.
- To prevent recurrent infection:
    Take your medication as directed even after the symptoms go away.
    Schedule a follow-up appointment for 10 to 14 days after you finish taking your medication. At your follow-up visit, another urine sample may be taken for analysis or culture.

Chlamydia (a prevalent sexually transmitted gram-negative bacterium), or *Trichomonas vaginalis* (a protozoan found in both the male and female genital tract).

In female clients, urethritis causes symptoms similar to those of bacterial cystitis. Urethritis is known by several synonyms: *pyuria-dysuria syndrome, frequency-dysuria syndrome, trigonitis syndrome,* and *urethral syndrome.* Urethritis is most common in postmenopausal women and is probably caused by tissue changes related to low estrogen levels.

➤ COLLABORATIVE MANAGEMENT
● Assessment

The nurse asks the client about a history of STD, painful or difficult urination, discharge from the penis or vagina, and internal discomfort in the lower abdomen. Urinalysis may show **pyuria** (white blood cells [WBCs]) without a significant number of bacteria; however, results of urethral culture may indicate an STD. In female clients, the diagnosis may be made by exclusion when urinalysis and urethral culture are negative for bacteria and symptoms persist. In such cases, pelvic examination may show symptoms of **hypoestrogenism** (tissue changes from low estrogen levels) in the vagina; cystourethroscopy may show hypoestrogenism with inflammation of urethral tissues.

● Interventions

STDs and infectious processes are treated with appropriate antibiotic therapy. Further information on STDs can be found in Chapter 74.

Postmenopausal women with urethral syndrome often have improvement in their urethral symptoms with the use of estrogen vaginal cream. Estrogen cream applied locally to the vagina increases the amount of estrogen in the urethra as well, and irritating symptoms are reduced.

NONINFECTIOUS DISORDERS
Urethral Strictures
■ OVERVIEW

Urethral strictures are narrowed areas of the urethra. These problems may be caused by complications of an STD (usually gonorrhea) and from trauma during catheterization, urologic instrumentation, or childbirth. Strictures occur more often in men than in women and may be an important factor in other urologic conditions, such as recurrent UTIs, urinary incontinence, and urinary retention.

➤ COLLABORATIVE MANAGEMENT

The most common symptom of urethral stricture is obstruction to the flow of urine; strictures rarely cause pain. Because stasis of urine can result when flow is obstructed, the client with a stricture is more likely to develop a UTI and have overflow incontinence. **Overflow incontinence** is the involuntary loss of urine when the bladder is overdistended. The nurse assesses the client for these two problems.

A urethral stricture is usually treated surgically. Dilation of the urethra (using a local anesthetic) is a temporary measure, not a curative one. The best chance of long-term cure is with **urethroplasty,** a surgical procedure in which the affected area is removed or grafted to create a larger opening for the passage of urine. The recurrence rate with surgical interventions is still high, and most clients need repeated procedures.

Urinary Incontinence
■ OVERVIEW

Continence (control over the time and place of urination) is a unique accomplishment of humans and certain domestic animals. Continence is a learned behavior whereby a person can suppress the urge to urinate until a socially appropriate (culturally prescribed) location is available (e.g., a toilet). Efficient bladder emptying (i.e., coordination between bladder contraction and urethral relaxation) is required for continence. Continence is learned in early childhood through toilet training and is generally accomplished by age 5 years.

Incontinence is an involuntary loss of urine severe enough to cause social or hygienic problems. Incontinence is *not* a normal consequence of aging or childbirth. Because of the stigma associated with incontinence and the belief that it is normal in the older adult, incontinence is one of the most underreported health problems. Many people suffer in silence, socially isolated and unaware that treatment is available.

The Agency for Healthcare Research and Quality (AHRQ) (formerly the Agency for Health Care Policy and Research [AHCPR]) chose urinary incontinence as one of its first topics for Clinical Practice Guidelines. The agency's goal is to educate the public and health care professionals about assessment and management of this condition (AHCPR, 1992, 1996).

TABLE 70-3 • TYPES OF URINARY INCONTINENCE

Type	Definition/Description	Cause	Clinical Manifestations
Stress incontinence	The involuntary loss of urine during activities that increase abdominal and detrusor pressure. Clients cannot tighten the urethra sufficiently to overcome the increased detrusor pressure; leakage of urine results	Weakening of bladder neck supports; associated with childbirth. Intrinsic sphincter deficiency caused by such congenital conditions as epispadias (abnormal location of the urethra on the dorsum of the penis) or myelomenigocele. Acquired anatomic damage to the urethral sphincter (from repeated incontinence surgeries, prostatectomy, radiation therapy, and trauma)	Urine loss with physical exertion, cough, sneeze, or exercise. Usually only small amounts of urine are lost with each exertion. Normal voiding habits ($\leq$8 times per day, 2 or fewer times per night). Postvoid residual usually $\leq$50 mL. Pelvic examination shows hypermobility of the urethra or bladder neck with Valsalva maneuvers
Urge incontinence	The involuntary loss of urine associated with a strong desire to urinate. Clients cannot suppress the signal from the bladder muscle to the brain that it is time to urinate	Unknown	An abrupt and strong urge to void. May have loss of large amounts of urine with each occurrence
Detrusor hyperreflexia (reflex incontinence)	The abnormal detrusor contractions result from neurologic abnormalities	Central nervous system (CNS) lesions from stroke, multiple sclerosis, and parasacral spinal cord lesions. Local irritating factors such as caffeine, medications, or bladder tumor	Postvoid residual >50 mL
Detrusor	No associated neurologic abnormality	Unknown	Postvoid residual $\leq$50 mL
Overflow incontinence	The involuntary loss of urine associated with overdistention of the bladder when the bladder's capacity has reached its maximum. The urethra is obstructed, so it fails to relax sufficiently to allow urine to flow, resulting in incomplete bladder emptying or complete urinary retention, causing overflow incontinence	Diabetic neuropathy; side effects of medication; after radical pelvic surgery or spinal cord damage; outlet obstruction. Causes external to the mechanism of the urethra include an enlarged prostate (male clients) and large genital prolapse (female clients). When the cause is intrinsic to the urethra, abnormal contraction of the skeletal muscle occurs, causing obstruction; this condition, called *detrusor dyssynergia,* is seen in clients with spinal cord injuries and multiple sclerosis	Bladder distention, often up to the level of the umbilicus. Constant dribbling of urine

Pathophysiology

Continence occurs when pressure in the urethra is greater than pressure in the bladder. For normal voiding to occur, the urethra must relax and the bladder must contract with sufficient pressure and duration to empty completely. Voiding should occur in a smooth and coordinated manner under a person's conscious control. The symptom of urinary incontinence has several possible causes and can be either temporary or chronic (Table 70-3). Temporary causes of incontinence are usually external to the urinary tract and involve no disorder of the urinary tract itself. The most common forms of urinary incontinence in adults are stress incontinence, urge incontinence, overflow incontinence, functional incontinence, and a mixed form.

STRESS INCONTINENCE

The urethra can be relaxed and tightened under conscious control because skeletal muscles of the pelvic floor surround it. When a person feels the urge to urinate, the conscious contraction of the urethra can override a bladder contraction if the urethral contraction is strong enough.

Clients who suffer from *stress incontinence* cannot tighten the urethra sufficiently to overcome the increased detrusor pressure. Stress incontinence is common after childbirth, when the pelvic muscles are stretched and weakened from pregnancy and delivery. The weakened pelvic floor contributes to mobility and displacement of the urethra during exertion. If the pelvic muscles are not properly strengthened, this condition continues. Decreasing amounts of estrogen after menopause also contribute to stress incontinence. Vaginal, urethral, and pelvic floor muscles become thin and weak without estrogen. Stress incontinence is the most common form of incontinence in women.

URGE INCONTINENCE

Bladder contractions are perceived as an urge to urinate. When the bladder is full, contraction of the smooth muscle fibers of the

TABLE 70-3 • TYPES OF URINARY INCONTINENCE—cont'd

Type	Definition/Description	Cause	Clinical Manifestations
Mixed incontinence	A combination of stress, urge, and overflow incontinence	As with each separate disorder	As with each separate disorder
Functional incontinence	Leakage of urine caused by factors other than disease of the lower urinary tract		Quantity and timing of urine leakage vary; patterns are difficult to discern
Transient causes	Transient causes will improve with treatment of the underlying condition	Loss of cognitive functioning Loss of awareness that urination is to occur in a socially acceptable place	Altered mental state, as in delirium, confusion, depression, dementia, sepsis, mental illness, or severe psychologic stress
		Abnormal openings in the urinary tract, such as a fistula or diverticulum	Urinary drainage noted from areas other than the urinary meatus
		Medications, such as sedatives, hypnotics, diuretics, anticholinergics, decongestants, antihypertensives, and calcium channel blockers	Some medications cause altered mental state; others cause increased urine production
		Diabetes insipidus or psychogenic polydipsia	Increased urine output
		Inability to get to toileting facilities	Restraints, restricted mobility
		Direct bladder pressure or urethral obstruction	Constipation or fecal impaction
Permanent causes	Permanent causes are organic but may be improved with treatment	Cognitive impairment Traumatic or surgical effects Those factors contributing to stress incontinence, urge incontinence, and overflow incontinence Structural or functional defects of the bladder or the sphincters Injuries or diseases of the spinal cord, brainstem, or cerebral cortex (neurogenic bladder) Congenital defects, including exstrophy of the bladder (bladder turned "inside out") and spina bifida	Clinical manifestations depend on the cause

bladder detrusor muscle normally signals the brain that it is time to urinate. Continent persons override that signal and relax the detrusor muscle for the time it takes to locate a toilet. Those who suffer from urge incontinence cannot suppress the signal. Abnormal detrusor contractions may be a result of neurologic abnormalities or may occur with no known abnormality.

■ OVERFLOW INCONTINENCE

When the detrusor muscle fails to respond by contracting, the bladder becomes overdistended. Overflow incontinence (also known as reflex incontinence) occurs when the bladder has reached its absolute maximal capacity and some urine must leak out to prevent bladder rupture. Causes for the underactive (**acontractile**) bladder may or may not be determined.

The urethra can also be obstructed so that it fails to relax enough to allow urine flow. Incomplete bladder emptying or complete urinary retention due to urethral obstruction results in overflow incontinence.

■ MIXED INCONTINENCE

Many clients with urinary incontinence fall into the mixed category. Their signs and symptoms have aspects of more than one of the major subtypes. This category is more common in older women.

■ FUNCTIONAL INCONTINENCE

Factors other than the abnormal function of the bladder and urethra also result in functional incontinence. The most common factor is a loss of cognitive function in clients affected by dementia. To maintain continence, a person must be aware that urination needs to occur in a socially acceptable place; clients with dementia may not have that awareness.

■ Etiology

Incontinence may have temporary or permanent causes. Evaluation of the incontinent client means considering all possible causes, beginning with those that are temporary and correctable. Surgical and traumatic causes of urinary incontinence are usually related to procedures or surgery in the lower pelvic structures, areas that are richly supplied by complex nerve pathways. Radical urologic, prostatic, and gynecologic procedures associated with pelvic cancers may result in postsurgical urinary incontinence. Trauma that injures segments S2 to S4 of the spinal cord may cause incontinence from interruption of normal nerve pathways.

Inappropriate bladder contraction may result from disorders of the brain and nervous system or from bladder irritation due to chronic infection, stones, chemotherapy, or radiation therapy. Failure of bladder contraction accompanies the autonomic neuropathy associated with diabetes mellitus and syphilis.

Costs associated with incontinence are enormous. The Cost of Care box below gives information about the individual and institutional considerations in providing continence care.

> **CONSIDERATIONS FOR OLDER ADULTS**
>
> Numerous factors contribute to the increased incidence of urinary incontinence in older adults (Chart 70-6). An older person may have decreased mobility from disease, neurologic dysfunction, or musculoskeletal degeneration. In the hospital or extended care setting, mobility is further limited when the older client is restrained or placed on bedrest. Vision and hearing impairments may also prevent the client from locating a call bell to notify the nurse or assistive nursing personnel of the need to void. The nurse assesses for these factors and, if possible, minimizes them to prevent urinary incontinence.

Incidence/Prevalence

Urinary incontinence is a significant health problem that affects more than 13 million people of all ages in the United States (AHCPR, 1996); about 85% are women. The disorder is particularly common in older adults, including 15% to 30% of community-dwelling older people and at least one half of all nursing home residents (AHCPR, 1996).

In adult clients under 65 years of age, urinary incontinence occurs twice as often in women as in men. Incontinence in

women of this age may occur after one or more pregnancies. Men in this age-group rarely experience urinary incontinence unless they have prostate disease or a spinal cord injury.

► COLLABORATIVE MANAGEMENT

● Assessment

■ HISTORY

The nurse asks, "Do you ever leak urine?" If the answer is yes, the nurse proceeds with a focused assessment (Chart 70-7). Incontinence may be underreported because health care professionals do not question clients about urine loss. It is not safe to assume that clients will volunteer the information without specifically being asked.

■ PHYSICAL ASSESSMENT/CLINICAL MANIFESTATIONS

The nurse assesses the abdomen to estimate suprapubic fullness, to rule out palpable hard stool, and to evaluate bowel sounds. With a physician's order, the nurse determines the amount of postvoid residual urine by catheterizing the client immediately after voiding. In some facilities, the nurse estimates the postvoid residual amount with a pelvic ultrasonographic scanner (AHCPR, 1996). Urinary incontinence is confirmed by evaluating the force and character of the urine stream during voiding by the client. Asking the client to cough while wearing a perineal pad may be useful in evaluating stress incontinence; a wet pad with forceful coughing may indicate stress incontinence (see the Evidence-Based Practice for Nursing box on p. 1625). A cystometrogram (see Chapter 69) is used as the basic diagnostic study in most cases (Walsh et al., 1998).

COST OF CARE
IMPLICATIONS FOR NURSING

INCONTINENCE

Cost of Care
- $16.4 billion is spent every year in the United States on incontinence-related care
  - $11.2 billion is spent for community-based programs and at-home care.
  - $5.2 billion is spent in long-term care facilities.
- $1.1 billion is spent every year on disposable continence care products for adults.
- The urologic diagnostic evaluation for incontinence ranges between $400 and $2000.
- Implementation of the Agency for Healthcare Research and Quality (AHRQ) Clinical Practice Guidelines for Urinary Incontinence has yielded significant cost savings.
  - Over a 14-month period, use of the guidelines helped one nursing home reduce the number of incontinent residents by 65%.
  - Diagnostic tests recommended by the guidelines average $100.
  - One nurse practitioner reported a cure of or improvement in incontinence problems in 98% of her clients through use of the behavioral methods recommended in the guidelines.

Implications for Nursing
Because of the high cost and prevalence of incontinence in the United States, nurses need to become familiar with the evidence-based Clinical Practice Guidelines for Urinary Incontinence. Competence in implementing the guidelines can reduce the financial, functional, and psychosocial burden of this common disorder.

Data from Jirovec, M.M., Wyman, J.F., & Wells, T.J. (1998). Addressing urinary incontinence with educational continence-care competencies. *Image: The Journal of Nursing Scholarship, 30*(4), 375-378; and Agency for Health Care Policy and Research. (1996). *Urinary incontinence in adults: Acute and chronic Management. Clinical practice guideline.* AHCPR Pub. No. 96-0682. Rockville, MD: Agency for Health Care Policy and Research, Public Health Service, U.S. Department of Health and Human Services; http://www.ahcpr.gov/clinic/uhistory.html (Clinical Practice Guidelines Online Urinary Incontinence Guideline: Real World Examples of Use).

CHART 70-6

NURSING FOCUS *on the* OLDER ADULT
Factors Contributing to Urinary Incontinence*

MEDICATIONS
- Central nervous system depressants, such as opioid analgesics, decrease the client's level of consciousness and the urge to void, and they contribute to constipation.
- Diuretics cause frequent voiding, often of large amounts of urine.
- Multiple medications can contribute to changes in mental status or mobility, and they can irritate the bladder.

DISEASE
- Cerebrovascular accidents and other neurologic disorders decrease mobility, sensation, or cognition.
- Arthritis decreases mobility and causes pain.
- Parkinson's disease causes muscle rigidity and an inability to initiate movement.

DEPRESSION
- Depression decreases the energy necessary to maintain continence.
- Decreased self-esteem and feelings of self-worth decrease the importance to the client of maintaining continence.

INADEQUATE RESOURCES
- Clients who have glasses or use a cane, walker, or slippers may be afraid to ambulate.
- Products that help clients manage incontinence are often costly.
- No one may be available to assist the client to the bathroom or help with incontinence products.

*These factors are in addition to the physiologic changes of aging given in Chapter 5.

For women, the nurse inspects the external genitalia to determine whether there is apparent urethral or uterine prolapse, **cystocele** (herniation of the bladder into the vagina), or **rectocele.** These conditions occur because of pelvic floor muscle weakness. An advanced-practice nurse puts on an examination glove and inserts two fingers into the vagina to assess the strength of these muscles. Strength is described as weak, adequate, or strong on the basis of the amount of pressure felt by the nurse as the client tightens her vaginal muscles. The color, consistency, and odor of any secretions from the genitourinary orifices are described and documented. The urine stream interruption test (see Chapter 69) is another method of determining pelvic muscle strength. For men, the nurse inspects the urethral meatus for any discharge.

A digital rectal examination is performed on both male and female clients. The digital rectal examination may provide information about the integrity of the nerve supply to the bladder. The examiner determines whether there is tactile sensation in the anorectal area by noting whether the rectal sphincter is relaxed or contracted on digital insertion. Because nerve supply to the bladder is similar to nerve supply to the rectum, the presence of tactile sensation and a rectal sphincter that contracts suggest that the nerve supply to the bladder is intact. During rectal examination, the nurse also notes any fecal impaction. Enlargement of the prostate is assessed in men by the physician or advanced-practice nurse.

LABORATORY ASSESSMENT

A urinalysis is inexpensive and useful to rule out infection. This test is the first step in the assessment of incontinent clients of any age. The presence of red blood cells (RBCs), white blood cells (WBCs), leukocyte esterase, or nitrites is an indication for culturing the urine. Any infection is treated before further assessment of incontinence.

RADIOGRAPHIC ASSESSMENT

Radiographic assessment is rarely indicated unless surgery is being considered. Excretory urography is the most useful for locating the kidneys and ureters. A voiding cystourethrogram (VCUG) may be performed to assess the size, shape, support, and function of the bladder; look for obstruction (especially prostate obstruction in men); and assess for postvoid residual (PVR) with a postvoid film. An assessment of PVR also can be made with a portable ultrasonographic bladder scanner.

OTHER DIAGNOSTIC ASSESSMENT

Clients who have unusual symptoms, medical complications, or a history of failed incontinence surgery often undergo urodynamic studies to determine the cause of their incontinence. A urodynamic evaluation is not a standardized procedure and may consist of any combination of the following tests:

- Cystourethroscopy to examine the inside of the bladder and urethra directly
- Cystometrogram (CMG) to measure the pressure inside the bladder as it fills
- Urethral pressure profilometry (UPP) to measure the pressure in the urethra in relation to the bladder pressure during various activities

---

CHART 70-7

FOCUSED ASSESSMENT *of*
The Client with Urinary Incontinence

Note the presence of risk factors for urinary incontinence:
- Age
- If female, menopausal status
- Neurologic disease
    Parkinson's disease
    Dementia
    Multiple sclerosis
    Stroke
    Spinal injury
- Diabetes mellitus
- Childbirth
- Urologic procedures
- Medications
- Bowel patterns
- Stress/anxiety level

Detail the symptoms of urinary incontinence:
- Leakage
- Frequency
- Urgency
- Nocturia
- Sensation of full bladder before leakage

Obtain a 24-hour intake and output record:
- Time and amount of oral intake and continent voidings
- Time and estimated amount of incontinent leakages
- Activity around the time of leakage

Assess client's:
- Mobility
- Self-care ability
- Cognitive ability
- Communication patterns

Assess the environment for barriers to toileting:
- Privacy
- Restrictive clothing
- Access to toilet

Data from Jirovec, M.M., Wyman, J.F., & Wells, T.J. (1998). Addressing urinary incontinence with educational continence-care competencies. *IMage: The Journal of Nursing Scholarship, 30*(4), 375-378; and Agency for Health Care Policy and Research. (1996). *Urinary incontinence in adults: Acute and chronic management. Clinical practice guideline.* AHCPR Pub. No. 96-0682. Rockville, MD: Agency for Health Care Policy and Research, Public Health Service, U.S. Department of Health and Human Services; http://www.ahcpr.gov/clinic/uhistory.html (Clinical Practice Guidelines Online: Urinary Incontinence Guideline: Real World Examples of Use).

EVIDENCE-BASED PRACTICE
FOR NURSING

"Low-tech" tests can be reliable

Swift, S.E., & Yoon, E.A. (1999). Test-retest reliability of the cough stress test in the evaluation of urinary incontinence. *Obstetrics and Gynecology, 94*(1), 99-102.

The goal of this descriptive study was to determine whether a forceful cough initiated in a standing woman with a full bladder would reliably demonstrate results of urine leakage at two different times. Of the 50 women studied, 35 had a positive cough stress test initially and 33 (91%) had a positive cough stress test 1 to 4 weeks later (no treatment occurred between tests). The reliability was highest in those subjects with pure stress incontinence, but the test was also fairly reliable (80%) in those subjects with mixed incontinence.

Critique. The sample size was adequate for the design of the study. No attempt was made to ensure that the bladder volumes were the same at the time of the two testing periods for each subject.

Implications for Nursing. A cough stress test is inexpensive and does not rely on technology or site. It can aid the clinician in differentiating between stress and urge incontinence. Knowing that the test is reliable in assessing the presence of stress and mixed incontinence, it may also be useful in determining client response to treatment. That is, after intervention, if a cough test is negative, one may be more likely to consider the intervention successful and continue that plan of care.

- Uroflowmetry to measure speed and completeness of bladder emptying

Testing may take several hours and more than one visit (see Chapter 69).

Electromyography (EMG) of the pelvic muscles may be a part of the urodynamic studies. A perineometer is a tampon-shaped instrument inserted into the vagina to measure the strength of pelvic muscle contractions. The graph can be used to demonstrate the amplitude of muscle contraction to the client as a method of biofeedback.

> ### CRITICAL THINKING CHALLENGE
> You are assigned to care for an older client in the community who is recovering from right total hip replacement surgery. She has a history of diabetes mellitus. She is able to care for herself but is using a walker for ambulation as she recovers. When you ask how things are going, she confides that she has a terrible rash on her "bottom" because "I leak urine so terribly since the surgery."
> - What is your next step?
> - How might this client's other medical diagnosis and her current health status affect the physical assessment?

For suggested answer guidelines, go to SIMON http://www.wbsaunders.com/SIMON/Iggy/.

Analysis

COMMON NURSING DIAGNOSES AND COLLABORATIVE PROBLEMS

The following are priority nursing diagnoses for clients with urinary incontinence (AHCPR, 1996):

1. Stress Urinary Incontinence related to weak pelvic muscles and structural supports
2. Urge Urinary Incontinence related to decreased bladder capacity, bladder spasms, and neurologic impairment
3. Reflex Urinary Incontinence related to incomplete bladder emptying
4. Mixed or Total Urinary Incontinence related to multiple causes
5. Functional Urinary Incontinence related to cognitive, motor, or sensory deficits

ADDITIONAL NURSING DIAGNOSES AND COLLABORATIVE PROBLEMS

In addition to the common nursing diagnoses, clients with urinary incontinence may have one or more of the following:

- Social Isolation related to altered state of wellness or fear of embarrassment
- Risk for Impaired Skin Integrity related to external risk factors, such as urinary excretions
- Disturbed Body Image related to odor, need to alter clothing selections, or need to wear protective briefs or supplies
- Risk for Infection related to retained or refluxing urine

Planning and Implementation

Several interventions are useful for each type of incontinence and for mixed incontinence. Collaborative management uses these interventions, as well as medication, surgical repair, and diet therapy.

STRESS URINARY INCONTINENCE

PLANNING: EXPECTED OUTCOMES. The client with urinary incontinence is expected to have fewer episodes of stress incontinence or a decreased amount of urine lost with each episode.

INTERVENTIONS. Initial interventions for clients with stress incontinence include diary keeping, behavioral interventions, and medications. Surgery is reserved as an option. The nurse explains the purpose of a detailed diary in which the client records times of urine leakage, activities, and foods eaten. The diary is then used by the health care practitioner to plan and evaluate interventions. Collection devices, absorbent pads, and undergarments may be used during the sometimes lengthy process of assessment and treatment and by those clients who elect not to pursue further interventions.

NONSURGICAL MANAGEMENT. Drug therapy and behavioral interventions (primarily diet and exercise) for stress incontinence require active participation on the part of the client for success. The ongoing availability of a nurse to provide encouragement, clarification, and support is extremely valuable for maximizing the effects of all interventions.

EXERCISE THERAPY. Pelvic floor (**Kegel**) exercises for female clients with stress incontinence are designed to strengthen the muscles of the pelvic floor (circumvaginal muscles). These muscles become strengthened, as any other skeletal muscle does, by frequent, systematic, and repeated contractions.

The most important step in teaching pelvic muscle exercises is to help the client become aware of which muscle to exercise. During the pelvic examination in women and the rectal examination in men or women, the nurse instructs the client to tighten the pelvic muscles around the examiner's fingers. The nurse then provides feedback about the strength of the contraction. Biofeedback devices, such as electromyography (EMG) or perineometers (see earlier discussion), measure the strength of contraction. Retention of a vaginal weight is also evidence that the client has identified the proper muscle. The ability to start and stop the urine stream or stop the passage of flatus is further evidence that the client has correctly identified the pelvic muscles.

Instructions for pelvic muscle exercises are given in Chart 70-8. Although improvement may take several months, most clients notice a significant change after 6 weeks. Clients may need to continue the exercises to maintain the improvement (AHCPR, 1996).

DIET THERAPY. A diet plan to encourage weight reduction is helpful for obese clients because stress incontinence is made worse by increased abdominal pressure from obesity. The nurse instructs the client to avoid alcohol and caffeine (bladder irritants) and refers him or her to the dietitian as needed.

DRUG THERAPY. Because bladder pressure is greater than urethral resistance in clients with stress incontinence, medications may be prescribed to increase the resistance of the urethra (Chart 70-9). Beta-adrenergic blocking agents, such as propranolol (Inderal, Detensol✦), have not been ade-

CHART 70-8

CLIENT EDUCATION GUIDE
Pelvic Muscle Exercises

- The pelvic muscles are composed of a sling of muscles that support your bladder, urethra, and vagina. Like any other muscles in your body, you can make your pelvic muscles stronger by alternately contracting (tightening) and relaxing them in regular exercise periods. By strengthening these muscles, you will be able to stop your urine flow more effectively.
- *To identify your pelvic muscles,* sit on the toilet with your feet flat on the floor about 12 inches apart. Begin to urinate, then try to stop the urine flow. Do not strain down, lift your bottom off the seat, or squeeze your legs together. When you start and stop your urine stream, you are using your pelvic muscles.
- *To perform pelvic muscle exercises,* tighten your pelvic muscles for a slow count of 10, then relax for a slow count of 10. Do this exercise 15 times while you are lying down, sitting up, and standing (a total of 45 exercises). Repeat, this time rapidly contracting and relaxing the pelvic muscles 10 times. This should take no more than 10 to 12 minutes for all three positions, or 3.5 to 4 minutes for each set of 15 exercises.
- Begin with 45 exercises a day in three sets of 15 exercises each. You will notice faster improvement if you can do this twice a day, or a total of 20 minutes each day. Remember to exercise in all three positions so your muscles learn to squeeze effectively despite your position. At first, it is helpful to have a designated time and place to do these exercises because you will have to concentrate to do them correctly. After you have been doing them for several weeks, you will notice improvement in your control of urine; however, many people report that improvement may take as long as 3 months.

quately tested in controlled trials and thus are not recommended for the treatment of incontinence (AHCPR, 1996).

Estrogen is used to treat postmenopausal women with stress incontinence, although its exact mechanism of action is unknown. Estrogen may increase the blood flow and tone of the circumvaginal and periurethral muscles, thus improving the client's ability to contract those muscles during times of increased intra-abdominal stress.

VAGINAL CONE THERAPY. Vaginal cones are a set of five small, cone-shaped weights. They are of equal size but of varying weights and are used with pelvic muscle exercise. The woman inserts the lightest cone, labeled 1, into her vagina (Figure 70-1), with the string to the outside, for a 1-minute test period. If she can hold the first cone in place without its slipping out while she walks around, she proceeds to the second cone, labeled 2, and repeats the procedure. The client begins her treatment with the heaviest cone she can comfortably hold in her vagina for the 1-minute test period. Treatment periods are 15 minutes twice a day. When she can comfortably hold the cone in her vagina for the 15-minute period, the client progresses to the next heaviest weight. Treatment is completed with the cone labeled 5.

Several studies have shown weighted vaginal cones to be helpful in strengthening the pelvic muscles and decreasing stress incontinence (AHCPR, 1996). Further research is needed, however, before recommending the weights to clients with pelvic prolapse. Vaginal cones are available without prescription, and the cost may be reimbursable by some health insurance companies.

OTHER THERAPY. Other types of interventions for stress incontinence include behavior modification, psychotherapy,

CHART 70-9

DRUG THERAPY *for* Urinary Incontinence

Drug	Usual Dosage	Nursing Interventions	Rationale
Estrogen (Premarin, C.E.S.✣)	0.3-1.25 mg daily PO 1-2 g qod per vagina	Report any unusual vaginal bleeding or calf pain.	Estrogen use can increase the risk of endometrial cancer and thrombophlebitis.
Anticholinergics/ antispasmodics		Check the client's intraocular pressure before starting the regimen.	Anticholinergics can increase intraocular pressure and are contraindicated in the presence of narrow-angle glaucoma.
Propantheline (Pro-Banthine, Propanthel✣)	7.5-30 mg tid/qid PO		
Oxybutynin (Ditropan)	2.5-5 mg tid/qid PO	Offer fluids and hard candy to moisten the mouth.	Anticholinergics cause extreme dryness of the mouth.
Dicyclomine hydrochloride (Bentyl, Di-Spaz, Bentylol✣, Formulex✣, Lomine✣)	10-20 mg tid PO	Give the drug between meals.	Food interferes with absorption of the drug.
		Increase fluids and fiber in the client's diet.	Anticholinergics decrease GI motility and can cause constipation.
Tricyclic antidepressants		Administer the full dose at bedtime if possible and warn clients that dizziness may occur on arising in the morning.	Tricyclics have a high potential to cause postural hypotension.
Imipramine (Tofranil, Novo-Pramine✣)	25-100 mg daily PO		
Desipramine (Norpramin)	10-25 mg tid PO	Warn clients about other anticholinergic and alpha-adrenergic side effects.	Tricyclics have a combination of anticholinergic and alpha-adrenergic effects.
Nortriptyline (Pamelor)	10-25 mg tid PO		

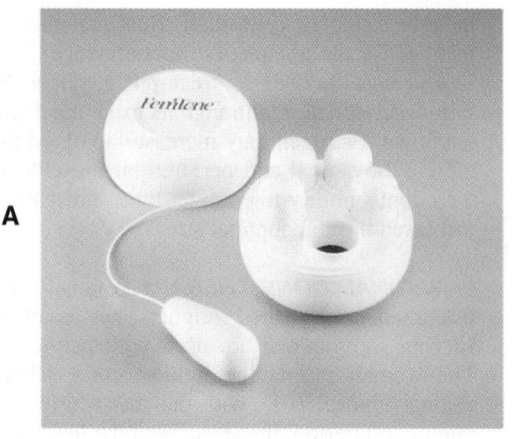
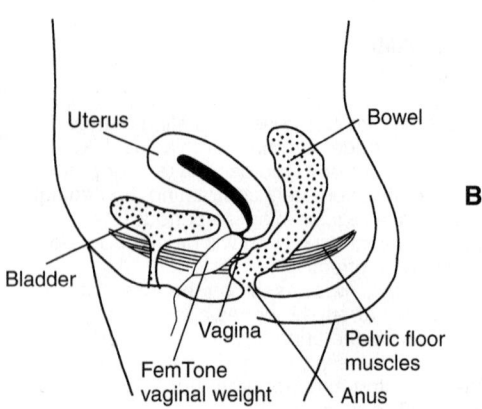

Figure 70-1 ● **A,** FemTone vaginal weights, or cones. The number on the top of each cone represents increasing weight up to the heaviest cone, a *5.* **B,** Diagram showing the correct positioning of a vaginal weight, or cone, in place. (**A** courtesy Convatec, a Bristol-Myers Squibb Company, a division of E.R. Squibb & Sons, Inc., Princeton, NJ; **B** from Convatec [1996]. *FemTone vaginal weights: A training aid for pelvic floor exercises* [brochure]. Princeton, NJ: Author.)

and electrical stimulation devices to strengthen urethral contractions. A variety of intravaginal and intrarectal electrical stimulation devices have been used to treat neurologically and nonneurologically impaired clients with varying degrees of success. More research is needed to determine the ideal level of stimulation and methods of reducing the associated discomfort before electrical stimulation becomes a standard treatment for incontinence.

The Reliance insert is like a tiny tampon that the client inserts into the urethra. After insertion, the client inflates a tiny balloon, which rests at the bladder neck and prevents the flow of urine. To void, the client pulls a string to deflate the balloon and removes the device. The applicator is reusable, although the tampon part is disposed of after each void (Gallo, 1997).

SURGICAL MANAGEMENT. Stress incontinence may be surgically corrected by vaginal, abdominal, or retropubic procedures. Success rates vary between 50% and 90% for most procedures, but these rates are difficult to evaluate because of the varying definitions of "cure" in the studies. Furthermore, cure may vary between short-term and long-term (over 5 years) results. In addition, published complication rates are significant, ranging from less than 2% for collagen or siloxane injection to 50% for bladder neck suspension.

PREOPERATIVE CARE. The nurse instructs the client about the surgical procedure and clarifies events surrounding the surgery. Extensive urodynamic testing (see Chapter 69) is often performed before surgery, and the need for such thorough assessment should be explained to the client.

OPERATIVE PROCEDURES. The surgical procedures used for women are designed to reposition the urethra and bladder, change the structure of the involved tissues, or insert artificial devices to improve function (Table 70-4).

POSTOPERATIVE CARE. After surgery, the nurse assesses for and intervenes to prevent or detect complications. For prevention of unnecessary movement or traction on the bladder neck, the urethral catheter is secured with tape or a

tube holder. If a suprapubic catheter is present instead of a urethral catheter, the dressing is monitored for leakage of urine, as well as serosanguineous drainage. Catheters are usually in place until the client can urinate easily and has postvoid residual urine of less than 50 mL. (See Chapters 17 and 19 for a thorough discussion of general preoperative and postoperative care.)

▧ URGE URINARY INCONTINENCE

PLANNING: EXPECTED OUTCOMES. The client with urinary incontinence is expected to use techniques to prevent or manage urge incontinence.

INTERVENTIONS. Interventions for clients with urge incontinence, sometimes called "overactive bladder" by the lay public, include behavioral interventions and medications. Surgery is not recommended for treatment of this condition. Collection devices and absorbent pads and undergarments may be used.

DRUG THERAPY. Because the hypertonic bladder contracts involuntarily in clients with urge incontinence, medications that relax the smooth muscle and increase the bladder's capacity are prescribed (see Chart 70-9).

The most effective medications are anticholinergics, such as propantheline (Pro-Banthine, Propanthel✤), and anticholinergics with smooth muscle relaxant properties, such as oxybutynin (Ditropan) and dicyclomine hydrochloride (Bentyl, Formulex✤, Spasmoban✤, Viscerol✤). Anticholinergics have serious side effects and are therefore used in conjunction with behavioral interventions. These agents inhibit the cholinergic fibers that stimulate bladder contraction. Tricyclic antidepressants with anticholinergic and alpha-adrenergic agonist activity, such as imipramine (Tofranil, Novopramine✤), have been used successfully. Other drugs, such as flavoxate (Urispas) and the antihistamines, nonsteroidal anti-inflammatory agents, beta-adrenergic agonists, and calcium channel blockers, have not been studied well enough for their use to be recommended (AHCPR, 1996).

TABLE 70-4 • SURGICAL PROCEDURES FOR STRESS INCONTINENCE

Procedure	Purpose	Nursing Considerations
Anterior vaginal repair (colporrhaphy)	Elevates the urethral position and repairs any cystocele	Because the operation is performed by vaginal incision, it is often done in conjunction with a vaginal hysterectomy. Recovery is usually rapid, and a urethral catheter is in place for 24-48 hr.
Retropubic suspension (Marshall-Marchetti-Krantz or Burch colposuspension)	Elevates the urethral position and provides longer-lasting results	The operation requires a low abdominal incision and a urethral or suprapubic catheter for several days postoperatively. Recovery takes longer, and urinary retention and detrusor instability are the most frequent complications.
Needle bladder neck suspension (Pereyra or Stamey procedure)	Elevates the urethral position and provides longer-lasting results without a long operative time	The combined vaginal approach with a needle and a small suprapubic skin incision does not allow direct vision of the operative site; however, the high complication rates may be due to the selection of clients who, because of their medical condition, are not good candidates for longer retropubic procedures.
Pubovaginal sling procedures	A sling made of synthetic or fascial material is placed under the urethrovesical junction to elevate the bladder neck	The operation uses an abdominal, vaginal, or combined approach to treat intrinsic sphincter deficiencies. Temporary or permanent urinary retention is common postoperatively.
Artificial sphincters	A mechanical device to open and close the urethra is placed around the anatomic urethra	The operation is done more frequently in men. The most common complications include mechanical failure of the device, erosion of tissue, and infection.
Periurethral injection of collagen or siloxane	Implantation of small amounts of an inert substance through several small injections provides support around the bladder neck	The procedure can be done in an ambulatory care setting and can be repeated as often as necessary. Certain compounds may migrate after injection; an allergy test to bovine collagen must be performed before implantation.

Data from Schultz, J.A., & Drutz, H.P. (1999). The surgical management of recurrent urinary stress incontinence. *Current Opinions in Obstetrics and Gynecology, 11*(5), 489-494; and Lightner, D.J., & Itano, N.M. (1999). Treatment options for women with stress urinary incontinence. *Mayo Clinic Proceedings, 74*(11), 1149-1156.

DIET THERAPY. The nurse instructs the client to avoid foods that have a direct bladder-stimulating or diuretic effect, such as caffeine and alcohol. Spacing fluids at regular intervals throughout the day (e.g., 120 mL every hour or 240 mL every 2 hours) and limiting fluids after the dinner hour (e.g., only 120 mL at bedtime) help avoid placing a fluid overload on the bladder and allow urine to accumulate at a steady pace.

BEHAVIORAL INTERVENTIONS. Behavioral interventions for urge incontinence include bladder training, habit training, exercise therapy, and electrical stimulation.

NIC interventions for urinary bladder training and urinary habit training are presented in Chart 70-10. It can be difficult for clients to understand these interventions because they involve a significant amount of participation on their part. The ongoing availability of a nurse to provide encouragement, clarification, and support is extremely valuable for maximizing the effects of all interventions. Behavioral interventions are often combined with drug therapy for maximal effect.

NIC **BLADDER TRAINING.** Bladder training is primarily an education program for the client that begins with a thorough explanation of the problem of urge incontinence. Instead of the bladder being in control of the client, the client learns to control the bladder. For the program to succeed, he or she must be alert, aware, and able to resist the urge to urinate.

A regular schedule for voiding is established, beginning with the longest interval that is comfortable for the client, even if the interval is only 30 minutes. The nurse instructs the client to void every 30 minutes and ignore any urge to urinate between the mandated intervals. Once the client is comfort-able with the initial schedule, the interval is increased by 15 to 30 minutes; the new schedule is followed until the client again achieves success. As he or she progressively increases the voiding interval, the bladder gradually tolerates more volume. The client is taught relaxation and distraction techniques to maximize success in the retraining. The nurse provides positive reinforcement for maintaining the prescribed schedule.

NIC **HABIT TRAINING.** Habit training (scheduled toileting) is a variation of bladder training that has been successful in reducing incontinence in cognitively impaired clients. To use habit training, caregivers assist the client in voiding at specific times (e.g., every 2 hours on the even hours) in an effort to get him or her to the toilet before incontinence can occur. There is no effort to increase bladder capacity by gradually lengthening the voiding intervals.

Prompted voiding, a supplement to habit training, attempts to increase the client's awareness of the need to void and to prompt him or her to ask for toileting assistance. Habit training otherwise relies completely on a time schedule.

EXERCISE THERAPY. Pelvic muscle exercises for urge incontinence have been helpful and are taught in the same way as for stress incontinence (see Chart 70-8). Improved urethral resistance enhances the client's ability to overcome abnormal detrusor contractions long enough to get to the toilet.

ELECTRICAL STIMULATION. A variety of intravaginal and intrarectal electrical stimulation devices have been used to treat both urge and stress incontinence.

CHART 70-10

(NIC) INTERVENTION ACTIVITIES *for*
The Client with Urinary Incontinence

Urinary Bladder Training: *Improving bladder function for those with urge incontinence by increasing the bladder's ability to hold urine and the client's ability to suppress urination*
- Determine ability to recognize urge to void.
- Keep a continence specification record for 3 days to establish voiding pattern.
- Establish interval of initial toileting schedule, based on voiding pattern.
- Establish beginning and ending time for toileting schedule if not for 24 hours.
- Establish interval for toileting of not less than 1 hour and preferably not less than 2 hours.
- Toilet client or remind client to void at prescribed intervals.
- Provide privacy for toileting.
- Use power of suggestion (e.g., running water or flushing toilet) to assist client to void.
- Avoid leaving client on toilet for more than 5 minutes.
- Reduce toileting interval by $1/2$ hour if client is unable to void at two or more scheduled toileting times.
- Increase toileting interval by 1 hour if client has no incontinence episodes for 3 days until optimal 4-hour interval is achieved.
- Teach the client to consciously hold urine until the scheduled toileting time.
- Discuss daily record of continence with client to provide reinforcement.

Urinary Habit Training: *Establishing a predictable pattern of bladder emptying to prevent incontinence for persons with limited cognitive ability who have urge, stress, or functional incontinence*
- Keep a continence specification record for 3 days to establish voiding pattern.
- Establish interval of initial toileting schedule based on voiding pattern and usual routine (e.g., eating, rising, and retiring).
- Establish beginning and ending time for toileting schedule if not for 24 hours.
- Establish interval for toileting of preferably not less than 2 hours.
- Assist client to toilet and prompt to void at prescribed intervals.
- Provide privacy for toileting.
- Use power of suggestion (e.g., running water or flushing toilet) to assist client to void.

- Avoid leaving the client on the toilet for more than 5 minutes.
- Reduce toileting interval by $1/2$ hour if there are more than two incontinence episodes in 24 hours.
- Maintain toileting interval if there are two or fewer incontinence episodes in 24 hours.
- Increase toileting interval by $1/2$ hour if client has no incontinence episodes for 48 hours until optimal 4-hour interval is achieved.
- Discuss daily record of continence with staff to provide reinforcement and encourage compliance with toileting schedule.
- Maintain scheduled toileting to assist in establishing and maintaining voiding habit.
- Give positive feedback or positive reinforcement (e.g., 5 minutes of social conversation) to client when voids at scheduled toileting times, and make no comment when client is incontinent.

Urinary Catheterization: Intermittent: *Regular periodic use of a catheter to empty the bladder*
- Teach client/family the purpose, supplies, method, and rationale of intermittent catheterization.
- Teach client/family clean intermittent catheterization technique.
- Provide quiet private room for the procedure.
- Demonstrate procedure and have a return demonstration, as appropriate.
- Determine catheterization schedule based on comprehensive urinary assessment.
- Adjust frequency of catheterization to maintain output of 300 mL or less.
- Maintain client on prophylactic antibacterial therapy for 2 to 3 weeks at initiation of intermittent catheterization, as appropriate.
- Complete a urinalysis about every 2 weeks to 1 month.
- Establish a catheterization schedule based on individual needs.
- Maintain a detailed record of catheterization schedule, fluid intake, and output.
- Teach client/family signs and symptoms of urinary tract infection.
- Monitor color, odor, and clarity of urine.

NIC intervention activities selected from McCloskey, J.C., & Bulechek, G.M. (Eds.). (2000). *Nursing interventions classification (NIC)* (3rd ed.). St. Louis: Mosby. No part of this work is to be altered without prior written permission from the Publisher.

■ REFLEX URINARY INCONTINENCE

PLANNING: EXPECTED OUTCOMES. The client with urinary incontinence is expected to achieve continence by keeping urine volume in the bladder within normal limits, preventing bladder overdistention.

INTERVENTIONS. Interventions for the client with reflex (overflow) incontinence caused by obstruction of the bladder outlet may include surgery to relieve the obstruction. The most common surgical procedures are removal of the prostate (see Chapter 76) and repair of genital prolapse (see Chapter 75). For overflow incontinence related to detrusor muscle inadequacy, the most effective method of treatment is intermittent catheterization. Behavioral interventions such as bladder compression and intermittent self-catheterization are the primary management techniques for urinary retention leading to overflow incontinence.

DRUG THERAPY. Medications are prescribed for short-term management of urinary retention, often postoperatively. They are not indicated in long-term management of the hypotonic bladder resulting in overflow incontinence. The most commonly used medication is bethanechol chloride (Urecholine), a cholinergic agent that increases bladder pressure.

BEHAVIORAL INTERVENTIONS. The mainstays of behavioral interventions include methods for bladder compression and intermittent self-catheterization.

BLADDER COMPRESSION. Techniques that promote bladder emptying include the Credé method, the Valsalva maneuver, double-voiding, and splinting.

In the Credé method, the nurse instructs the client in external compression of the urinary bladder or parasympathetic stimulation via tugging at pubic hair or massaging the genital area. These techniques manually assist the bladder in emptying. In the Valsalva maneuver, breathing techniques increase intrathoracic and intra-abdominal pressure. This increased pressure is then directed toward the bladder during exhalation. With the technique of double-voiding, the client empties the bladder and then, within a few minutes, consciously attempts a second bladder emptying.

For women who have a severe cystocele (prolapse of the bladder into the vagina), a technique called *splinting* both compresses the bladder and moves the obstruction out of the way. The woman inserts her own fingers into her vagina, gently pushes the cystocele back into the vagina, and begins to urinate.

⬤ INTERMITTENT SELF-CATHETERIZATION. NIC interventions for intermittent urinary catheterization are presented in Chart 70-10. The nurse teaches intermittent self-catheterization to clients with long-term problems of incomplete bladder emptying. Techniques of self-catheterization are well established and can be learned fairly easily. The nurse remembers the following important points in teaching this technique:

- Proper handwashing and cleaning of the catheter reduce the frequency of infection.
- A small lumen and adequate lubrication of the catheter prevent urethral trauma.
- A regular schedule for bladder emptying prevents overdistention of the bladder with subsequent mucosal trauma.

Clients must be able to understand instructions and have the manual dexterity to manipulate the catheter. Caregivers or family members in the home can also be taught to perform straight catheterization using a clean (rather than sterile) technique with good outcomes.

▧ FUNCTIONAL URINARY INCONTINENCE

PLANNING: EXPECTED OUTCOMES. The client with urinary incontinence is expected to use methods of urine containment or collection that ensure dryness until the underlying cause of the incontinence is treated.

INTERVENTIONS. Causes of functional (or chronic intractable) incontinence vary greatly; some are reversible, and others are not. The primary focus of intervention is treatment of reversible causes. When incontinence is not reversible, urinary habit training (see Habit Training, p. 1629) is done to establish a predictable pattern of bladder emptying to prevent incontinence regardless of the cause(s). A final strategy focuses on containment of the urine and protection of the client's skin. Nonsurgical interventions include applied devices, containment, and urinary catheterization.

APPLIED DEVICES. Applied devices include intravaginal pessaries for women and penile clamps for men. The intravaginal pessary supports the uterus and vagina and helps maintain the correct position of the bladder. (See Chapter 75 for further discussion of pessaries.) The penile clamp is applied externally to compress the urethra and prevent leakage of urine.

The dangers of pessaries and penile clamps include damage to the tissues and infection from constant pressure in sensitive areas. Both devices require that the client have manual dexterity or a caregiver who applies and removes the device. The clinician prescribes the device, and the nurse instructs the client or caregivers in its use. Male clients may use an external collecting device, such as a condom catheter. Design of a suitable external collecting device for women has not been as successful.

CONTAINMENT. Absorbent pads and briefs are designed to collect urine and keep the client's skin and clothing dry. A variety of types and sizes of pads are available:

- Shields or liners inserted inside a panty
- Undergarments consisting of full-sized pads with waist straps
- Plastic-lined protective underpants with or without elastic legs
- Combination pad and pant systems
- Absorbent bed pads

A major concern with the use of protective pads is the risk that skin breakdown will occur. Materials and costs vary; some are reusable, and others are disposable. The disposal of these products raises ecologic concerns. Newer, more absorbent products are coming on the market as manufacturers take advantage of the growth of the "adult diaper" market. The nurse avoids use of the word "diaper," however, because of the usual association of diapers with a baby.

URINARY CATHETERIZATION. Catheterization for the control of incontinence may be intermittent or involve placement of an indwelling catheter. Intermittent self-catheterization is preferred to placement of an indwelling catheter because of the decreased likelihood of infection. Indwelling urinary catheters should be used temporarily and only when all other alternatives have been tried and have been unsuccessful. A long-term indwelling urinary catheter is appropriate for clients with skin breakdown who need a dry environment for healing, clients who are terminally ill and need comfort, and clients who are acutely or critically ill and require careful measurement of urine output.

> **⟳ CRITICAL THINKING CHALLENGE**
> Your client is diagnosed with mixed stress and urge incontinence. Her environment has no barriers to toileting, and she is able to ambulate in her home with the walker. Your client reports drinking about four cups of coffee daily.
> - What effect does coffee have on continence?
> - What exercises can you teach and reinforce in relation to continence care?
> - How can you help evaluate your client's response to exercise and/or prescribed medication to improve continence?
>
> For suggested answer guidelines, go to ⟨SIMON⟩ http://www.wbsaunders.com/SIMON/Iggy/.

⬤ Community-Based Care

Community-based care for the client with urinary incontinence considers his or her personal, physical, emotional, and social resources. Important personal resources for self-care include mobility, vision, and manual dexterity. The nurse considers who will be the primary caregiver and what environmental circumstances or factors will influence the effectiveness of the plan.

HEALTH TEACHING

The nurse teaches the client and family or significant others about the cause of the identified type of urinary incontinence and discusses treatment options available for its management. The teaching plan addresses the prescribed medications (purpose, dosage, method and route of administration, and expected and potential side effects). The client and family are also instructed about the importance of weight reduction and dietary modification to assist with control of urinary incontinence.

When external devices or protective pads are needed, the nurse describes the possible options, discusses the advantages and disadvantages of each, and helps the client make a selection that considers lifestyle and resources. For clients who will use intermittent catheterization or those with artificial urinary sphincters, the nurse demonstrates the appropriate technique to the client or caregiver. Return demonstrations are evaluated for correct technique. Chart 70-11 also addresses teaching.

The embarrassment experienced by incontinent clients can be devastating to their self-esteem, body image, and interpersonal relationships. The unpredictability of incontinence creates anxiety. Clients are often embarrassed to seek help, and even when resources are identified, they may need assistance to feel comfortable in using the resources. Even buying supplies in the local drugstore or grocery store can be perceived as a threat to their privacy.

The nurse assists in psychosocial preparation by accepting and acknowledging the personal concerns of the client and caregiver. These concerns must never be minimized or made to seem trivial. The nurse helps the client learn methods of controlling or managing the fear or anxiety. As the client learns the specifics of the plan that will allow control of urinary incontinence, the confidence to resume psychosocial interactions should return.

HOME CARE MANAGEMENT

The home environment is assessed for barriers that impede access to the toileting facilities. Environmental hazards that might slow walking or contribute to injury are eliminated. These hazards might include small area rugs (throw rugs), tables or chairs with legs that extend into the walking area, slippery waxed or polished floors, and inadequate lighting.

If the client must climb stairs to reach a bathroom, handrails should be installed and stairs should be kept free of obstacles. Toilet seat extenders may help provide the appropriate level of seating so that maximal abdominal pressure may be applied to encourage voiding. Portable commodes may be obtained for homes in which ambulatory access to toilets is impractical or impossible. Physical and occupational therapists are valuable resources for assisting with home care management.

HEALTH CARE RESOURCES

Referral to home care agencies for assistance with personal care and to continence clinics that specialize in evaluation and treatment may be helpful. In many continence clinics, nurses collaborate with physicians and other health care professionals to evaluate and manage clients. The treatment plan is specific for each client; supplies and products are custom selected.

Clients benefit emotionally from education and from the support of others who experience similar concerns. The National Association for Continence (NAFC) and the Simon Foundation for Continence publish newsletters with informative articles and educational materials written with simple, easy-to-understand explanations. The Agency for Healthcare Research and Quality (AHRQ) has also published a caregiver guide (AHCPR Pub. No. 96-0683) for the public that is available on the Internet or by calling (800) 358-9295. Local hospitals, in collaboration with the NAFC, may conduct local support groups.

Evaluation: Outcomes

The nurse evaluates the care of the client with urinary incontinence on the basis of the identified nursing diagnoses and collaborative problems. The expected outcomes are that the client will:

- Describe the type of urinary incontinence experienced
- Demonstrate knowledge of proper use of medications and correct procedures for self-catheterization, use of the artificial sphincter, or care of an indwelling urinary catheter
- Demonstrate effective use of the selected exercise or bladder training program
- Select and use incontinence devices and products
- Have a reduction in the number of incontinence episodes

Urolithiasis

OVERVIEW

Urolithiasis is the presence of **calculi** (stones) in the urinary tract. Stones are generally asymptomatic until they pass into the lower urinary tract, where they can cause excruciating

---

CHART 70-11

CLIENT EDUCATION GUIDE
Urinary Incontinence

- Maintain a normal body weight to reduce the pressure on your bladder.
- Do not try to control your incontinence by limiting your fluid intake. Adequate fluid intake is necessary for kidney function and health maintenance.
- If you have a catheter in your bladder, follow the instructions given to you about maintaining the sterile drainage system.
- If you are discharged with a suprapubic catheter in your bladder, inspect the entry site for the tube daily, clean the skin around the opening gently with warm soap and water, and place a sterile gauze dressing on the skin around the tube. Report any redness, swelling, drainage, or fever to your physician.
- Do not put anything into your vagina, such as tampons, medications, hygiene products, or exercise weights, until you check with your physician at your 6-week checkup after surgery.
- Do not have sexual intercourse until after your 6-week postoperative checkup.
- Do not lift or carry anything heavier than 5 pounds or participate in any strenuous exercise until your physician gives you postoperative clearance. In some cases, this could be as long as 3 months.
- Avoid exercises, such as running, jogging, step or dance aerobic classes, rowing, cross-country ski or stairclimber machines, and mountain biking. Brisk walking without any additional hand, leg, or body weights is allowed. Swimming is allowed after all drains and catheters have been removed and your incision is completely healed.
- If Kegel exercises are recommended, ask your nurse for specific instructions.

pain. The term **nephrolithiasis** describes a condition in which stones form in the kidney. Formation of stones in the ureter is **ureterolithiasis.**

Pathophysiology

Urologic stones result from a variety of metabolic disorders. However, the exact mechanism of stone formation, commonly referred to as stone disease, is not entirely understood. Everyone excretes crystals in the urine at some time, but fewer than 10% of people form calculi. About 75% of calculi contain calcium as one component of the stone complex, which may be calcium oxalate or calcium phosphate (Hruska, 1996). Struvite (15%), uric acid (8%), and cystine (3%) make up the less common stones (Balaji & Menon, 1997).

Formation of stones seems to involve three conditions:

- Slow urine flow, resulting in supersaturation of the urine with the particular element (such as calcium) that first becomes crystallized and later becomes the stone
- Damage to the lining of the urinary tract (i.e., from crystals)
- Decreased inhibitor substances in the urine that would otherwise prevent supersaturation and crystal aggregation

High urine acidity (as with uric acid and cystine stones) or alkalinity (as with calcium phosphate and struvite stones) also contributes to stone formation.

One example of a metabolic problem causing stone formation begins when excessive amounts of calcium are absorbed through the intestinal tract (the most common cause of hypercalciuria). As blood circulates through the kidneys, the excess calcium is filtered into the urine, causing supersaturation of calcium in the urine. If fluid intake is inadequate, such as when a client is dehydrated, supersaturation is more likely to occur, and there is an increased risk of calcium combining with another compound to form a larger molecule. The calcium complex often serves as a center for additional deposition, and eventually a stone forms.

Stones that form in the kidney and then pass into the ureter often lodge in the ureteropelvic angle, the aortoiliac bend, or the ureterovesical angle. When the calculus occludes the ureter and blocks the flow of urine, the ureter dilates. An enlargement of the ureter is called **hydroureter.**

The pain associated with ureteral spasm is excruciating and may cause the client to go into shock from stimulation of nearby sympathetic nerves. In addition, **hematuria** (bloody urine) may result from damage to the urothelial lining. If the obstruction is not removed, urinary stasis may result in infection and impair kidney function on the side of the blockage. As the blockage persists, **hydronephrosis** (enlargement of the kidney caused by blockage of urine lower in the tract and filling of the kidney with urine) and irreversible kidney damage, although rare, may develop.

Etiology

The cause of urolithiasis is unknown, although several hypotheses have been suggested. At least 90% of clients with calculi have a contributing metabolic risk factor. Table 70-5 summarizes the known metabolic defects that commonly cause stone formation.

A diet high in calcium is not believed to cause stones unless a metabolic defect or renal tubular defect already exists. Even in clients with a history of nephrolithiasis, taking calcium citrate supplements does not cause new stone formation (Parivar, Low, & Stoller, 1996). Urinary stasis, urinary retention, immobilization, and dehydration all contribute to a calculus-forming environment. Except for the use of the thiazides for calcium oxalate stones, diuretics can cause volume depletion and thus may promote the formation of calculi.

Incidence/Prevalence

The incidence of stone disease in the adult population is relatively high and varies with geographic location, race, and family history. About 12% of adults will have at least one episode of renal stone disease. Overall, the incidence is higher in men; however, struvite calculi are twice as common in women. Recurrence rates vary, depending on the type of treatment. The recurrence rate of untreated calcium oxalate stones is 35% to 50% in 5 to 10 years. A higher recurrence of stones is found in those clients with a family history of stone disease and those who had their first occurrence by age 25 years.

> ### CULTURAL CONSIDERATIONS
> There is an increased incidence of stone disease in the southeastern United States and a rising incidence in Japan and Western Europe. Calcium stone disease is more common in men than in women and tends to occur in young adults or during early middle adulthood. Stone disease in African Americans is uncommon (Hruska, 1996). Cystinuria is more common among Jews of Libyan extraction (Rutchik & Resnick, 1997).

TABLE 70-5 • METABOLIC DEFECTS THAT COMMONLY CAUSE CALCULI	
Metabolic Deficit	**Etiology**
Hypercalcemia	
Primary	Absorptive: increased intestinal calcium absorption
	Renal: impaired renal tubular resorption of calcium
Secondary	Resorptive: hyperparathyroidism, vitamin D intoxication, renal tubular acidosis, prolonged immobilization
Hyperoxaluria	
Primary	Genetic: autosomal recessive trait resulting in high oxalate production
Secondary	Dietary: excess oxalate from foods such as spinach, rhubarb, Swiss chard, cocoa, beets, wheat germ, pecans, peanuts, okra, chocolate, and lime peel
Hyperuricemia	
Primary	Gout is an inherited disorder of purine metabolism (20% of clients with gout have uric acid calculi)
Secondary	Increased production or decreased clearance of purine from myeloproliferative disorders, thiazide diuretics, carcinoma
Struvite	Made of magnesium ammonium phosphate and carbonate apatite; formed by urea splitting by bacteria, most commonly, *Proteus mirabilis;* needs an alkaline urine to form
Cystinuria	Autosomal recessive defect of amino acid metabolism that precipitates insoluble cystine crystals in the urine

► COLLABORATIVE MANAGEMENT
● Assessment
▣ HISTORY

The client is asked about a personal or family history of urologic stones. A diet history, including fluid intake patterns, is also obtained. If the client has a history of calculus formation, the nurse asks about past treatment, whether chemical analysis of the stone was performed, and what preventive measures the client follows.

▣ PHYSICAL ASSESSMENT/CLINICAL MANIFESTATIONS

The major clinical manifestation of calculi is severe pain, commonly called **renal colic.** Flank pain suggests that the stone is in the kidney or upper ureter. Flank pain that radiates abdominally or into the scrotum and testes or the vulva suggests that stones are in the ureters or bladder. Pain is most intense when the stone is moving or when the ureter is obstructed (Walsh et al., 1998).

Renal colic begins suddenly and is usually described as "unbearable." Nausea, vomiting, pallor, and diaphoresis often accompany the pain. A large stationary stone in the kidney (staghorn calculus), however, rarely causes much pain. Frequency and dysuria occur when a stone reaches the bladder.

Hematuria is a common finding; blood may make the urine appear smoky or rusty. Increased turbidity and odor are associated with infectious processes that may accompany urolithiasis. **Oliguria** (scant urine output) or **anuria** (absence of urine output) suggests obstruction, possibly at the bladder neck or urethra. Obstruction of the urinary tract is an emergency and must be treated immediately to preserve kidney function.

The nurse examines the client to detect bladder distention. The physical examination may reveal pale, ashen, diaphoretic skin; the client may suffer from excruciating pain. Vital signs may be moderately elevated with pain; body temperature and pulse are elevated with infection. Blood pressure may decrease markedly if the severe pain causes shock.

▣ LABORATORY ASSESSMENT

Urinalysis may show red blood cells (RBCs), white blood cells (WBCs), and bacteria. RBCs are most likely the result of direct trauma, caused by the stone, on the endothelial lining of the ureter, bladder, or urethra. WBCs and bacteria may be present as a result of urinary stasis. Urine culture reveals infection (associated with struvite stones); sensitivity studies of the culture identify antibiotic effectiveness. Microscopic examination of the urine may identify crystals from which stones could form. Urinary pH is measured to determine acidity or alkalinity.

The serum WBC count is elevated with infection. Increases in the serum calcium, serum phosphate, or serum uric acid levels suggest that excess minerals are present and may contribute to stone formation.

▣ RADIOGRAPHIC ASSESSMENT

Stones are easily seen on x-ray films of the kidneys, ureters, and bladder (KUB); IV urograms; or computed tomography (CT) scans. The primary purpose of these radiographic procedures is to confirm the presence and location of the calculi.

The urogram is useful for identifying whether urinary tract obstruction is present; however, because of the risk of acute renal failure induced by contrast media, other diagnostic tests may be chosen for high-risk clients (older adults and clients who have diabetes mellitus, multiple myeloma, or elevated serum creatinine levels). CT is generally needed to identify cystine or uric acid stones, neither of which are visible on x-ray examination.

▣ OTHER DIAGNOSTIC ASSESSMENT

Renal ultrasonography produces images from sound waves. Structures of varying density are reproduced. Solid structures, such as stones, are extremely dense; therefore the images of stones are clear. The identification of small stones and their exact location, however, may not be as precise as desired.

● Interventions

Nursing interventions are focused on pain management and prevention of infection and urinary obstruction. The majority of clients will be able to expel the stone without invasive procedures. The most important factors regarding whether a stone will pass on its own are its composition, size, and location. The larger the stone and the higher up in the urinary tract it is, the less likely it is to be passed. Other interventions may be necessary when the client does not pass the stone spontaneously (Figure 70-2).

PAIN RELIEF MEASURES. Nonsurgical and surgical approaches are used to assist the client with a kidney stone in achieving an acceptable degree of pain relief.

NONSURGICAL MANAGEMENT

DRUG THERAPY. Pain is usually most severe in the first 24 to 36 hours. Opioid analgesics are often required to control the moderately severe to severe pain caused by stones in the urinary tract. Opioid agents, such as morphine sulfate (Statex✦), are often administered intravenously so that prompt and adequate absorption is ensured. Nonsteroidal anti-inflammatory drugs such as ketorolac (Toradol) in the acute phase may be quite effective.

Control of pain is more effective when medications are given at regularly scheduled intervals or via a constant delivery system (e.g., skin patch) instead of as needed (prn). Spasmolytic agents, such as oxybutynin chloride (Ditropan) and propantheline bromide (Pro-Banthine, Propanthel✦), are extremely important for the relief and control of pain (see Chart 70-9). The nurse administers the medication and assesses the response by asking the client to rate the discomfort on a rating scale.

COMPLEMENTARY AND ALTERNATIVE THERAPY. Relaxation techniques, such as hypnosis and imagery, therapeutic or healing touch, and acupuncture, can relieve pain. Clients often have great difficulty finding a comfortable position in which to relax; assisting the client with positioning can often aid in relaxation. Breathing techniques, such as those used in childbirth, can also help clients to relax.

OTHER MANAGEMENT TECHNIQUES. Avoiding overhydration in the acute phase helps to make the spontaneous passage of a stone less painful (Singal & Denstedt, 1997). The nurse strains the urine to monitor for excretion of the calcu-

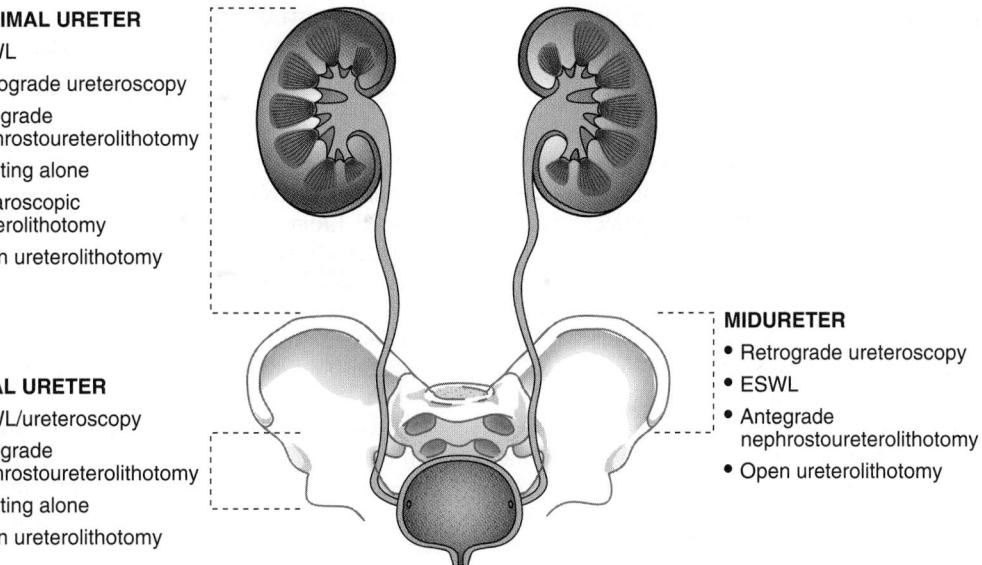

PROXIMAL URETER
- ESWL
- Retrograde ureteroscopy
- Antegrade nephrostoureterolithotomy
- Stenting alone
- Laparoscopic ureterolithotomy
- Open ureterolithotomy

DISTAL URETER
- ESWL/ureteroscopy
- Antegrade nephrostoureterolithotomy
- Stenting alone
- Open ureterolithotomy

MIDURETER
- Retrograde ureteroscopy
- ESWL
- Antegrade nephrostoureterolithotomy
- Open ureterolithotomy

Figure 70-2 ● Treatment options for ureteral stones. (ESWL, Extracorporeal shock wave lithotripsy.) (From Singal, R.K., & Denstedt, J.D. [1997]. Contemporary management of ureteral stones. *Urologic Clinics of North America, 24*[1], 59-70.)

lus. Any stones obtained are sent to the laboratory for analysis; preventive therapy is based on stone composition.

EXTRACORPOREAL SHOCK WAVE LITHOTRIPSY. **Lithotripsy,** also known as extracorporeal shock wave lithotripsy (ESWL), is the application of sound, laser, or dry shock wave energies (electrohydraulic, electromagnetic, or piezoelectric) to break the stone into small fragments. The client receives conscious sedation and lies on a flat x-ray–type table with the lithotriptor aimed at the stone, which is visualized by fluoroscopy. A local anesthetic cream is applied to the skin focal site 45 minutes before the procedure.

During the procedure, cardiac rhythm is monitored by electrocardiography (ECG), and the shock waves are administered in synchrony with the R wave; 500 to 1500 shock waves are administered in 30 to 45 minutes. Continuous ECG monitoring for dysrhythmia and fluoroscopic observation for destruction of the stone are maintained.

After lithotripsy, the nurse may strain the urine to monitor the elimination of stone fragments. Some bruising may occur on the flank of the affected side after extracorporeal shock wave lithotripsy (ESWL).

Occasionally a stent is placed in the ureter before ESWL to facilitate passage of the stone fragments. Cystine stones are generally resistant to ESWL.

SURGICAL MANAGEMENT. Various minimally invasive surgical and open surgical procedures are indicated if urinary obstruction occurs or if the stone is too large to be passed spontaneously.

MINIMALLY INVASIVE SURGICAL PROCEDURES. Minimally invasive surgical (MIS) procedures include stenting, retrograde ureteroscopy, percutaneous antegrade nephrostoureterolithotomy, and laparoscopic ureterolithotomy.

Stenting. A stent is a small tube that is placed in the ureter through the endoscopic procedure of ureteroscopy. The stent dilates the ureter and creates a passageway for the stone or stone fragments. This procedure prevents the passing stone from coming in contact with the ureteral mucosa, thereby reducing pain. A Foley catheter also may be placed to facilitate passage of the stone through the urethra.

Retrograde Ureteroscopy. Retrograde ureteroscopy is an endoscopic procedure. The ureteroscope is passed through the urethra and bladder into the ureter. Once the stone is seen, it can be removed using grasping baskets, forceps, or loops. Through the ureteroscope, lithotripsy also can be performed. A Foley catheter also may be placed to facilitate passage of the stone fragments through the urethra.

Percutaneous Antegrade Nephrostoureterolithotomy. In percutaneous antegrade nephrostoureterolithotomy, the client lies prone or laterally and receives general anesthesia. The physician identifies the ideal kidney entry point with fluoroscopy and then passes a needle into the collecting system of the kidney. Once a tract has been made in the kidney, other equipment, such as an **intracorporeal** (inside the body) ultrasonic or laser lithotriptor, can be used to break up and remove the stone. An endoscope with a special attachment to grasp and extract the stone also could be used. Often a nephrostomy tube is left in place initially to prevent the stone fragments from passing through the normal urinary tract.

The nurse provides routine nephrostomy tube care and monitors the client for complications after the procedure. Possible complications include bleeding at the site or through the tube, pneumothorax, and infection.

Laparoscopic Ureterolithotomy. Laparoscopic ureterolithotomy uses a laparoscope to access the ureters. The surgeon enters the ureter and removes, fragments, and vaporizes the stone with the laser. Preoperative and postoperative care is the same as for any laparoscopic procedure.

OPEN SURGICAL PROCEDURES. After failed attempts to remove the stone through other methods, or when risk of a lasting injury to the ureter or kidney is possible, an **open ureterolithotomy** (into the ureter), **pyelolithotomy** (into the kidney pelvis), or **nephrolithotomy** (into the kidney) procedure may be indicated. These procedures are used for a large or impacted stone.

Preoperative Care. The nurse prepares the client for the selected procedure by explaining how, when, and where the procedure will be performed. The nurse describes what the client can expect before and after the procedure. The client receives nothing by mouth and also receives preoperative bowel preparation. (See Chapter 17 for routine preoperative care.)

Operative Procedures. The retroperitoneal area is entered through a large flank incision, as for nephrectomy (see Chapter 71), for pyelolithotomy or nephrolithotomy and through a lower abdominal incision for ureterolithotomy. The urinary tract is entered surgically and the stone removed. Before closure, various tubes and drains may be placed (e.g., nephrostomy tube, ureteral stent, Penrose or other wound drainage device, and Foley catheter).

Postoperative Care. The nurse follows routine procedures for assessment of the client who has received anesthesia. (See Chapter 19 for routine postoperative care.) The concerns after urologic surgery are monitoring the amount of bleeding from incisions and in the urine, maintaining adequate urine output, straining the urine to monitor the elimination of stone fragments, and assisting the client in preventing future stones through dietary modification.

INFECTION PREVENTION. Control of infections before invasive and noninvasive procedures is critical for the prevention of urosepsis. Interventions include the administration of appropriate antibiotics, either to eliminate an existing infection or to prevent new infections, and the maintenance of adequate nutrition and fluid intake. Because infection is always a component of struvite stone formation, the health care team plans for long-term prevention.

DRUG THERAPY. The clinician initially prescribes broad-spectrum antibiotics, such as the aminoglycosides (e.g., gentamicin [Garamycin]) and cephalosporins (e.g., cephalexin [Keflex, Novo-Lexin❖]), for treatment of infections occurring with urologic stone disease. The broad coverage is effective against gram-negative bacilli. After the results of the culture and sensitivity (C&S) studies are obtained, the clinician can select more specific antibiotics. C&S studies may be done 48 hours after the initiation of antibiotic therapy and again 48 hours after the conclusion of the prescribed course of therapy.

Blood levels of certain antibiotics, such as the aminoglycosides, are measured to ensure that appropriate levels of the antibiotic have been reached. If the desired blood level of these antibiotics is exceeded, toxic effects and kidney damage may result. If the blood level of the antibiotic is inadequate, microorganisms may not be completely eliminated. New clinical evidence of an infection (such as chills, fever, or altered mental status) warrants the collection of a urine sample for repeated C&S tests.

For the client with struvite stones, the primary care provider prescribes periodic and long-term monitoring of the urine for infection. Commonly, urine cultures are ordered monthly for 3 months, then quarterly for 1 year. Drugs that prevent bacteria from splitting urea, such as acetohydroxamic acid (Lithostat) and hydroxyurea (Hydrea), are often prescribed on a long-term basis for clients with struvite stones. The primary care provider monitors the serum creatinine with acetohydroxamic acid; its administration is contraindicated for levels above 2 mg/dL. The nurse reviews interventions aimed at preventing urinary tract infection (UTI) (see Interventions [Cystitis], p. 1618).

DIET THERAPY. The client's diet ideally includes adequate calorie intake representing a balance of all food groups. Unless medically contraindicated, the nurse encourages fluid intake of 2 to 3 L/day.

PREVENTION OF OBSTRUCTION. Measures to prevent urinary obstruction by stones include a high intake of fluids (3 L/day or more) and careful measures of intake and output. A liberal but not excessive fluid intake assists in preventing dehydration, promotes the flow of urine, and decreases the chance of crystals forming a stone. Interventions also depend on the type of stone. Medications, diet modification, and fluid intake are the major strategies available.

DRUG THERAPY. The selection of drugs for the prevention of obstruction depends on what is promoting the formation of stones and the type of stone formed. The nurse teaches the client the reason for the medication and assesses for side effects or adverse drug reactions.

CALCIUM-CONTAINING STONES. Drugs to treat **hypercalciuria** (high levels of calcium in the urine) may include thiazide diuretics (e.g., chlorothiazide [Diuril] or hydrochloro-thiazide [HydroDiuril, Natrimax❖, Urozide❖]), orthophosphate, and sodium cellulose phosphate. The thiazide diuretics promote calcium resorption from the renal tubules back into the body, thereby preventing excess calcium loads in the urine. Orthophosphate affects normal calcium-phosphorus metabolism, resulting in decreased urinary saturation of calcium oxalate. Sodium cellulose phosphate reduces intestinal absorption of calcium.

OXALATE-CONTAINING STONES. For clients with **hyperoxaluria** (high levels of oxalic acid in the urine), allopurinol (Zyloprim) and vitamin B_6 (pyridoxine) are used.

URIC ACID–CONTAINING STONES. For clients with chronic gout, allopurinol helps prevent the formation of **urate** (uric acid) stones. To alkalinize the urine, medications such as potassium citrate, 50% sodium citrate, and sodium bicarbonate may be used. The desired urinary pH is 6 to 6.5. Because the normal urinary pH averages 5 to 6, these desired values are termed "alkaline."

CYSTINE-CONTAINING STONES. For clients with **cystinuria** (high levels of cystine in the urine), alpha-mercaptopropionylglycine (AMPG) and captopril (Capoten) have both been found to lower urinary cystine levels. Their use is reserved for when hydration and alkalinization of the urine have not been successful.

DIET THERAPY. Diet modification depends on the type of stone formed (Table 70-6). The nurse consults the dietitian to plan the appropriate diet for the client.

OTHER MEASURES. The nurse encourages the client to ambulate frequently. Ambulation promotes passage of stones and reduces the possibility of calcium resorption from the bones. The nurse checks the pH of the urine daily and strains the urine with filter paper to collect passed fragments of stones.

HEALTH TEACHING. Key points of health teaching are described in Chart 70-12. The client often experiences tremendous anxiety and fear that a stone and its related pain may re-

TABLE 70-6 • DIETARY TREATMENT FOR RENAL STONES

Stone Type	Dietary Interventions	Rationale
Calcium oxalate	Avoid oxalate sources, such as spinach (see also Table 70-5).	Reduction of urinary oxalate content may help prevent these stones from forming. Urinary pH is not a factor.
Calcium phosphate	Decrease intake of foods high in protein.	Reduction of protein intake reduces acidic urine and prevents calcium precipitation.
	Some clients may benefit from a reduced calcium intake (milk, other dairy products).	Reduction of urine calcium concentration may prevent calcium precipitation and crystallization.
Struvite (magnesium ammonium phosphate)	Limit high-phosphate foods, such as dairy products, red and organ meats, and whole grains.	Reduction of urinary phosphate content may help prevent these stones from forming.
Uric acid (urate)	Decrease intake of purine sources, such as organ meats, poultry, fish, gravies, red wines, and sardines.	Reduction of urinary purine content may help prevent these stones from forming.
Cystine	Encourage PO fluids, up to 3 L/day.	Increased fluid helps dilute the urine and prevent the cystine crystals from forming.

CHART 70-12

CLIENT EDUCATION GUIDE
Urinary Calculi

- Finish your entire prescription of antibiotics to ensure that you will not get a urinary tract infection.
- You may resume your usual daily activities.
- Remember to balance regular exercise with sleep and rest.
- You may return to work 2 days to 6 weeks after surgery, depending on the type of intervention, your personal tolerance, and your physician's directives.
- Depending on the type of stone you had, your diet may be restricted to prevent further stone formation.
- Remember to drink at least 3 L of fluid a day to dilute potential stone-forming crystals, prevent dehydration, and promote urine flow.
- Monitor urine pH as directed (may be up to three times per day).
- You can expect bruising after lithotripsy. The bruising may be quite extensive and may take several weeks to resolve.
- Your urine may be bloody for several days after surgery.
- Pain in the region of the kidneys or bladder may signal the beginning of an infection or the formation of another stone. Report any pain, fever, chills, or difficulty with urination immediately to your physician or nurse.
- Keep follow-up appointments to check on infection, have repeat cultures done, and so forth.

TABLE 70-7 • STAGING OF BLADDER CANCER

PRIMARY TUMOR (T)

T_X	Primary tumor cannot be assessed
T_0	No evidence of primary tumor
T_{is}	Carcinoma in situ: "flat tumor"
T_1	Tumor invades submucosa (subepithelial connective tissue)
T_2	Tumor invades superficial muscle (inner half)
T_3	Tumor invades deep muscle or perivesical fat
T_{3a}	Tumor invades deep muscle (outer half)
T_{3b}	Tumor invades perivesical fat
T_4	Tumor invades any of the following: prostate, uterus, vagina, pelvic wall, abdominal wall
T_{4a}	Tumor invades prostate, uterus, vagina
T_{4b}	Tumor invades pelvic or abdominal wall

LYMPH NODE (N)

N_X	Regional lymph nodes cannot be assessed
N_0	No regional lymph node metastasis
N_1	Metastasis in a single lymph node, 2 cm or less in greatest dimension
N_2	Metastasis in a single lymph node, more than 2 cm but not more than 5 cm in greatest dimension, or multiple lymph nodes, none more than 5 cm in greatest dimension; pelvic only

DISTANT METASTASIS (M)

M_X	Presence of distant metastasis cannot be assessed
M_0	No distant metastasis
M_1	Distant metastasis or nodes positive above aortic bifurcation

Modified from American Joint Committee on Cancer. (1992). In O.H. Beahrs (Ed.), *Manual for staging of cancer* (4th ed.). Philadelphia: Lippincott-Raven; and Bennett, J.C., & Plum, F. (Eds.). (1996). *Cecil textbook of medicine* (20th ed.). Philadelphia: W.B. Saunders.

---

cur. In addition to anxiety about the pain, the possibility of repeated surgical interventions or permanent and serious kidney damage is of tremendous concern. Psychosocial preparation is generally enhanced when clients know what to expect and what actions to take should the unexpected develop. The nurse reassures the client that preventive and health promotion activities are designed to prevent recurrence.

Urothelial Cancer

OVERVIEW

Urothelial cancers are malignant tumors of the urothelium, which is the lining of transitional cells in the kidney, renal pelvis, ureters, urinary bladder, and urethra. Most urothelial tumors occur in the urinary bladder. Consequently, the general term *bladder cancer* is sometimes used to describe this pathologic condition.

In the United States, approximately 72% of urinary tract cancers occur as transitional cell carcinomas in the bladder (American Cancer Society [ACS], 2001). The second most common site of urinary tract cancer is the kidney and renal pelvis (27%). Squamous cell carcinoma accounts for approximately 5% of all bladder cancers.

Urothelial tumors are generally low grade, have multiple points of origin (**multifocal**), and are recurrent. Once the tumors spread beyond the transitional cell layer, they tend to be highly invasive and metastatic. Because of the multifocal, recurrent nature of the disease, clients with superficial tumors may experience recurrence up to 10 years after being tumor free.

Table 70-7 shows the staging of bladder cancer. Tumors confined to the mucosa are treated by simple excision, whereas carcinoma in situ (CIS), or stage T_{IS}, is generally treated with excision plus **intravesical** (inside the bladder) chemotherapy. Disease that has spread beyond CIS is treated with more extensive resection, often a **radical cystectomy** (removal of the bladder and surrounding tissue) with urinary diversion. Chemotherapy and radiotherapy are used in addition to surgery. When the tumor remains unchecked, it can invade surrounding structures, metastasize to distant sites (liver, lung, and bone), and ultimately lead to death.

Exposure to environmental toxins, particularly the chemicals used in the rubber, paint, electric cable, and textile industries, is highly associated with bladder cancer. The greatest risk factor for bladder cancer is tobacco use. Other risks include *Schistosoma haematobium* (a parasite) infection, excessive use of phenacetin compounds, and long-term administration of cyclophosphamide (Cytoxan, Procytox✤).

There are approximately 54,300 new cases of bladder cancer diagnosed each year in the United States and approximately 12,400 deaths per year from the disease (ACS, 2001). The condition is rare in adults younger than age 40, and there is a substantial increase in incidence after age 60.

➤ COLLABORATIVE MANAGEMENT
▐▶ Assessment

▐ PHYSICAL ASSESSMENT/CLINICAL MANIFESTATIONS

The nurse inquires about the client's perception of general health. The gender and age of the client are documented. The nurse inquires about active and passive exposure to cigarette smoke. To detect potentially harmful environmental agents, the nurse asks the client to describe his or her occupation in detail. He or she is also asked to describe any change in the color, frequency, or amount of urine and any abdominal discomfort.

The overall appearance of the client is observed, especially skin color and general nutritional status. The nurse inspects, percusses, and palpates the abdomen for asymmetry, tenderness, and bladder distention.

The urine is examined for color and clarity. Hematuria is the predominant sign associated with bladder cancer; it may be gross or microscopic and is usually painless and intermittent. Dysuria, frequency, and urgency are usual symptoms when infection or obstruction is also present.

▐ PSYCHOSOCIAL ASSESSMENT

The nurse assesses the client's emotions, including his or her response to known or suspected bladder cancer, and notes anxiety, fear, sadness, anger, or guilt. Early symptoms are painless, and many clients ignore hematuria because it is intermittent. Clients also may be reluctant to seek treatment because they suspect a sexually transmitted disease (STD). Consequently, they may experience guilt or anger about their own delays in seeking medical attention.

The nurse assesses the client's personal methods of coping and the degree of evident support from family or significant others. Social interaction and active role relationships with others may provide support and motivation for coping with convalescence.

▐ DIAGNOSTIC ASSESSMENT

The only significant finding on a routine urinalysis is generally gross or microscopic hematuria. Cytologic testing on voided urine specimens is not usually helpful. Bladder-wash specimens and bladder biopsies are the most sensitive and specific tests for cancer.

Cystoscopy with retrograde pyelography is the primary method for evaluation of painless hematuria. A closed biopsy of a visible bladder tumor can be performed during cystoscopy. This is essential for staging and is usually performed in a day-surgery unit before admission to the hospital for treatment. Excretory urography is useful in identifying obstructions, especially at the ureterovesical junction. The computed tomography (CT) scan shows tumor invasion of surrounding tissues.

Ultrasonography shows masses but is less valuable for tumor staging. Magnetic resonance imaging (MRI) may help in the assessment of deep, invasive tumors.

▐▶ Interventions

Therapy for the client with bladder cancer usually begins with surgical removal of the tumors for diagnosis and staging of disease. For tumors extending beyond the mucosa, surgery is followed by intravesical chemotherapy or immunotherapy. High-grade or recurrent tumors are treated with more radical surgery plus intravesical chemotherapy and/or radiotherapy. Systemic chemotherapy is reserved for clients with distant metastases. (See Chapter 25 for general care of the client receiving chemotherapy or radiation therapy.)

NONSURGICAL MANAGEMENT. Prophylactic immunotherapy with intravesical instillation of bacille Calmette-Guérin (BCG), a compound used to vaccinate against tuberculosis in some countries, is used to prevent tumor recurrence of superficial cancers (stage T_1 or lower). This procedure has been more effective than single-agent chemotherapy; side effects, however, are comparable.

Multiagent systemic chemotherapy is successful in prolonging life after distant metastasis has occurred but is rarely curative. Radiation therapy has also been successful in prolonging life.

SURGICAL MANAGEMENT. The type of surgery for bladder cancer depends on the type and stage of the cancer and the client's general health status. Complete cystectomy with extensive surgical removal of surrounding muscle and tissue offers the best chance of a cure for large, invasive bladder cancers.

PREOPERATIVE CARE. Specific client education depends on the type and extent of the planned surgical procedure. The nurse coordinates preoperative education with the physician and enterostomal (ET) therapist. The nurse discusses the type of urinary diversion and the selection of a site for the stoma. The goal is for the client to have a positive attitude about body image and a positive self-image. The nurse intervenes with educational counseling to ensure accurate understanding about self-care practices, methods of pouching, control of urine drainage, and minimization of odor.

The site selected for the stoma should be visible and avoid folds of skin, bones, and scar tissue. When possible, the client's waistline or belt area is avoided. The nurse prepares the client for the number and type of drains that will be present postoperatively. General preoperative care is discussed in Chapter 17.

OPERATIVE PROCEDURES. Transurethral resection of the bladder tumor (TURBT) or partial cystectomy is performed for small, early, superficial tumors. In a partial (segmental) cystectomy, a portion of the urinary bladder is removed. This procedure is generally used when there is only a single isolated bladder tumor.

When the entire bladder must be removed (complete cystectomy), the ureters are diverted into a collecting reservoir. Techniques for urinary diversion are illustrated in Figure 70-3. With an ileal conduit, the ureters are surgically implanted in a portion of the ileum, and urine is collected in a pouch on the skin around the stoma. Increasingly, continent reservoirs are being used. With cutaneous ureterostomy or ureteroureterostomy, the ureter opening is brought out onto the skin. The cutaneous ureterostomies may be located on either side of the abdomen or side by side.

POSTOPERATIVE CARE. After cutaneous ureterostomy, as with the ileal conduit, an external pouch covers the ostomy to collect urine. The nurse collaborates with the enterostomal therapist and focuses care on the wound, the skin, and urinary drainage. (See Chapters 56 and 57 for ostomy care.)

The client with a Kock's pouch, a continent reservoir, may have a Penrose drain and a plastic Medena catheter in the stoma. The drain removes lymphatic fluid or other secretions; the catheter ensures urine drainage so that suture lines may heal. The physician orders irrigation of the catheter to ensure patency. General postoperative care is discussed in Chapter 19.

● Community-Based Care

■ HEALTH TEACHING

The nurse educates the client and family or significant others about medications, diet and fluid therapy, the use of external pouching systems, and the technique for catheterization of a continent reservoir.

With some procedures, the client may require electrolyte replacements to prevent long-term deficits. The nurse instructs the client to avoid foods that are known to produce gas if the urinary diversion uses the gastrointestinal (GI) tract. When the intestinal production of gas is minimized, flatus will not result in incontinence.

The nurse also instructs the client and family or significant others about any changes in self-care activities related to the urinary diversion. In conjunction and collaboration with the enterostomal therapist, the nurse demonstrates external pouch application, local skin care, pouch care, methods of adhesion, and drainage mechanisms. If a Kock's pouch has been created, the client is instructed about the technique of catheterization. For all instruction, the nurse observes at least one return demonstration by the client or the family caregiver. The client ideally assumes responsibility for self-care before discharge.

The nurse assists the client in preparing psychologically for the impact of urinary diversion on self-image, body image, sexual functioning, and self-esteem. Counseling provides information and support so that the feelings of powerlessness may be minimized.

Through discussions with the client about usual social situations, the nurse helps the client gain control over new toileting practices. Men with a urinary diversion into the sigmoid colon need to learn a new habit of sitting to urinate. For clients of either gender, the nurse promotes confidence in social situations by encouraging frequent emptying of urinary collection devices before traveling or attending social functions or events. Resumption of sexual activity is a major concern for many adult clients, regardless of age; this topic needs to be addressed openly and with sensitivity. Cystectomy causes physiologic impotence in men, but treatment is available (see Chapter 76).

■ HEALTH CARE RESOURCES

The United Ostomy Association and the American Cancer Society units and chapters have educational materials that may be useful to clients. In some areas, local support groups have meetings to assist others and to send visitors to provide peer counseling and support. Home care personnel may assist with follow-up, easing the transition from hospital to home. The Wound, Ostomy, and Continence Nurses Society provides educational programs and a journal devoted to the care of clients with ostomies.

Bladder Trauma
■ OVERVIEW

Bladder trauma can be caused by penetrating or blunt injury to the lower abdomen. Penetrating lower abdominal injury may occur by stabbing, gunshot wound, or other trauma in which objects pierce the abdominal wall. A fractured pelvis with puncture of the bladder by bone fragments is the most common cause of bladder trauma. Bladder trauma may also be a result of sexual assault.

Blunt trauma compresses the abdominal wall and the bladder. A seat belt may compress the bladder hard enough to cause injury, especially if the bladder is full or distended.

▶ COLLABORATIVE MANAGEMENT
● Assessment

Clients with a penetrating bladder wound often have anuria or hematuria. In the emergency department, initial assessment includes inspection of the urinary meatus for blood.

Diagnostic tests include cystography and voiding cystourethrography (VCUG). If renal or ureteral trauma is suspected, IV urography is scheduled before cystography so that any leakage of bladder contrast medium does not mask the outlines of the kidneys or ureters. The cystogram shows whether there is a defect in bladder filling; the voiding cystourethrogram defines bladder emptying.

● Interventions

Bladder trauma, other than a simple contusion, requires surgical intervention. Stabilization of any fractures usually precedes bladder repair. Surgical interventions include procedures to repair the anterior or posterior bladder wall and peritoneal membrane. In general, repairs of the bladder are accomplished by closure procedures.

The client with an anterior bladder wall injury commonly has a Penrose drain and a Foley catheter in place postoperatively; the client with a posterior bladder wall injury has a

Ureterostomies divert urine directly to the skin surface through a ureteral skin opening (stoma). After ureterostomy, the client must wear a pouch.

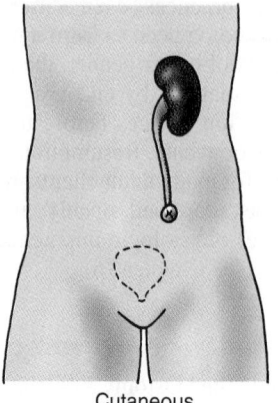

Cutaneous ureterostomy

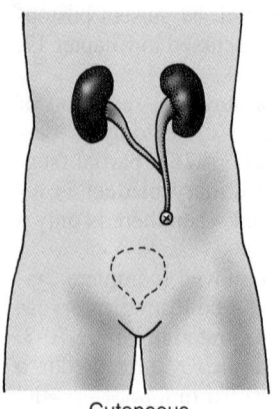

Cutaneous ureteroureterostomy

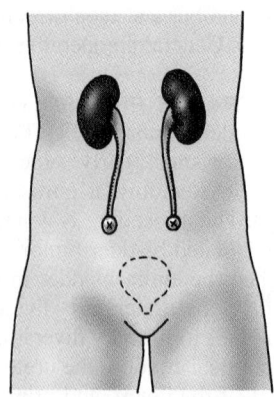

Bilateral cutaneous ureterostomy

Conduits collect urine in a portion of the intestine, which is then opened onto the skin surface as a stoma. After the creation of a conduit, the client must wear a pouch.

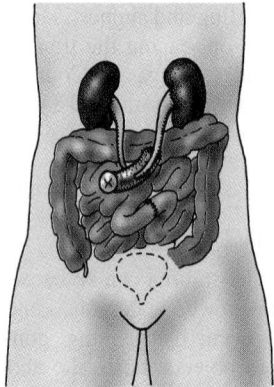

Ileal (Bricker's) conduit

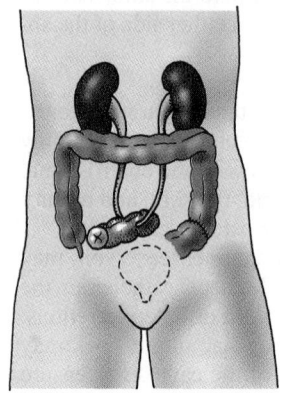

Colon conduit

Ileal reservoirs divert urine into a surgically created pouch, or pocket, that functions as a bladder. The stoma is continent, and the client removes urine by regular self-catheterization.

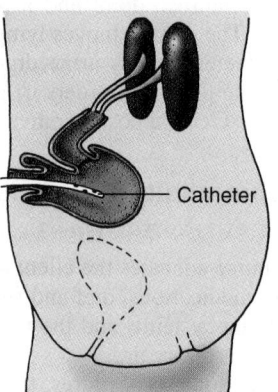

Continent internal ileal reservoir (Kock's pouch)

Sigmoidostomies divert urine to the large intestine, so no stoma is required. The client excretes urine with bowel movements, and bowel incontinence may result.

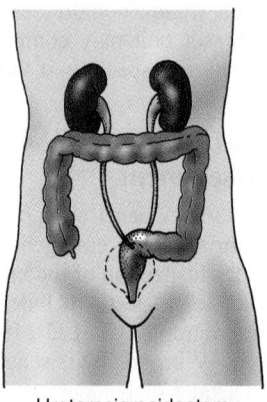

Ureterosigmoidostomy

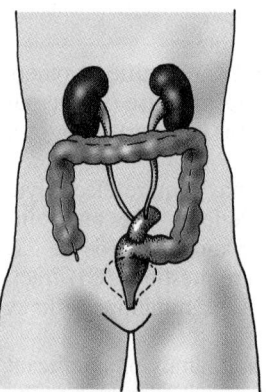

Ureteroiliosigmoidostomy

Figure 70-3 ● Urinary diversion procedures used in the treatment of bladder cancer.

Penrose drain and Foley or suprapubic catheter. In some instances, vaginal or rectal fistulas may also require repair.

Psychosocial support is critical for clients who have sustained traumatic injuries. The nurse refers the client to appropriate resources to assist in dealing with potential psychosocial issues.

ONLINE RESOURCES

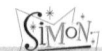

For suggested readings and Internet resources, go to http://www.wbsaunders.com/SIMON/Iggy/.

SELECTED BIBLIOGRAPHY

Asterisk indicates a classic or definitive work on this subject.

*Adams, D.H., & Abernathy, B.B. (1996). Laser ureterolithotripsy for cystine calculi. *AORN Journal, 64*(6), 924, 926-927, 929-930.

*Agency for Health Care Policy and Research. (1992). *Urinary incontinence in adults. Clinical practice guideline.* AHCPR Pub. No. 92-0038. Rockville, MD: Agency for Health Care Policy and Research, Public Health Service, U.S. Department of Health and Human Services.

*Agency for Health Care Policy and Research. (1996). *Urinary incontinence in adults: Acute and chronic management. Clinical practice guideline.* AHCPR Pub. No. 96-0682. Rockville, MD: Agency for

Health Care Policy and Research, Public Health Service, U.S. Department of Health and Human Services.

American Cancer Society. (2001). *Cancer facts and figures—2001.* Report No. 01-300M-No. 5008.01. Atlanta: Author.

Balaji, K.C., & Menon, M. (1997). Mechanism of stone formation. *Urologic Clinics of North America, 24*(1), 1-11.

Centers for Disease Control and Prevention. (May 2001); www.cdc.gov/nchs.

Cohen, M., & Rothmann, M. (2001). Gemcitabine and cisplatin for advanced metastatic bladder cancer. *Journal of Clinical Oncology, 19*(4), 1229-1231.

Diering, C., & Palmer, M. (2001). Professional information about urinary incontinence on the World Wide Web: Is it timely? Is it accurate? *Journal of Wound, Ostomy, and Continence Nursing, 28*(1), 55-62.

Duffield, P. (1997). Urinary tract infections in the elderly. *ADVANCE for Nurse Practitioners, 5*(4), 30-32.

Gallo, M. (1997). Quality of life improvement and the reliance urinary control insert. *Urologic Nursing, 17,* 146-153.

Houston, M. (1999). Uncomplicated urinary tract infection in women: Diagnostic and therapeutic recommendations by the Institute for Clinical Systems Integration. *Postgraduate Medicine, 105*(5), 181-183, 187-188.

*Hruska, K. (1996). Renal calculi. In J.C. Bennett & F. Plum (Eds.), *Cecil textbook of medicine* (20th ed.). Philadelphia: W.B. Saunders.

Jay, J., & Staskin, D. (1998). Urinary incontinence: Strategies for effective diagnosis and management. *ADVANCE for Nurse Practitioners, 6*(10), 32-37.

Jirovec, M.M., Wyman, J.F., & Wells, T.J. (1998). Addressing urinary incontinence with educational continence-care competencies. *Image: The Journal of Nursing Scholarship, 30*(4), 375-378.

Johnson, S. (2000). From incontinence to confidence. *American Journal of Nursing, 100*(2), 69-76.

Johnson, V. (2001). Effects of a submaximal exercise protocol to recondition the pelvic floor musculature. *Nursing Research, 50*(1), 33-41.

Kee, J.L. (1998). *Handbook of laboratory and diagnostic tests with nursing implications* (3rd ed.). Stamford, CN: Appleton & Lange.

Kincade, J., Peckous, B., & Busby-Whitehead, J. (2001). A pilot study to determine predictors of behavioral treatment completion for urinary incontinence. *Urologic Nursing, 21*(1), 39-44.

Kirton, C.A. (1997). Assessing for bladder distension. *Nursing97, 27*(4), 64.

Krautschick, A.W. (1999). Metabolic evaluation and medical therapy for stone formation. *Current Opinions in Urology, 9*(4), 335-338.

Lightner, D.J., & Itano, N.M. (1999). Treatment options for women with stress urinary incontinence. *Mayo Clinic Proceedings, 75*(11), 1149-1156.

Lingappa, V. (2000). Renal disease. In S. McPhee, V. Lingappa, & W. Ganong (Eds.), *Pathophysiology of disease* (3rd ed.). New York: Lange Medical Books/McGraw-Hill.

*Lowe, A., & Gabriel, L.S. (1993). Laser lithotripsy: Patient care, staff education. *AORN Journal, 58*(5), 961-964, 966, 968-969.

Lyons, S., & Specht, J. (2000). Prompted voiding protocol for individuals with urinary incontinence. *Journal of Gerontological Nursing, 20*(6), 5-13.

Marchiondo, K. (1998). A new look at urinary tract infection. *American Journal of Nursing, 98*(3), 34-39.

McCloskey, J.C., & Bulechek, G.M. (2000). *Nursing interventions classification (NIC)* (3rd ed.). St. Louis: Mosby.

*Parivar, F., Low, R.K., & Stoller, M.L. (1996). The influence of diet on urinary stone disease. *Journal of Urology, 155,* 432-440.

Parker, S.L., et al. (1997). Cancer statistics, 1997. *CA: A Cancer Journal for Clinicians, 47*(1), 5-27.

Renner, C., & Rassweiler, J. (1999). Treatment of renal stones by extracorporeal shock wave lithotripsy. *Nephron, 81*(Suppl. 1), 71-81.

Resnick, M.I. (Ed.). (1997). Urolithiasis. *Urologic Clinics of North America, 24*(1), entire issue.

Ruml, L.A., Pearle, M.S., & Pak, C.Y.C. (1997). Medical therapy: Calcium oxalate urolithiasis. *Urologic Clinics of North America, 24*(1), 117-133.

Rutchik, S.D., & Resnick, M.I. (1997). Cystine calculi. *Urologic Clinics of North America, 24*(1), 163-171.

Scheinman, S.J. (1999). Nephrolithiasis. *Seminars in Nephrology, 19*(4), 381-388.

Schulz, J.A., & Drutz, H.P. (1999). The surgical management of recurrent stress urinary incontinence. *Current Opinions in Obstetrics and Gynecology, 11*(5), 489-494.

Schwartz, B.F., & Stoller, M.L. (1999). Nonsurgical management of infection-related renal calculi. *Urologic Clinics of North America, 26*(4), 765-778.

Singal, R.K., & Denstedt, J.D. (1997). Contemporary management of ureteral stones. *Urologic Clinics of North America, 24*(1), 59-70.

Sirls, L.T., & Rashid, T. (1999). Geriatric urinary incontinence. *Geriatric Nephrology and Urology, 9*(2), 87-99.

Smith, D. (1998). A continence care approach for long-term care facilities. *Geriatric Nursing, 19*(2), 81-86.

Stockert, P.A. (1999). Getting UTI patients back on track. *RN, 62*(3), 49-54.

Strangio, L. (1997). Interventional uroradiologic procedures. *AORN Journal, 66*(2), 286-290, 292-294.

Suchinski, G.A., et al. (1999). Treating urinary tract infections in the elderly. *Dimensions in Critical Care Nursing, 18*(91), 21-27.

Swift, S.E., & Yoon, E.A. (1999). Test-retest reliability of the cough stress test in the evaluation of urinary incontinence. *Obstetrics and Gynecology, 94*(1), 99-102.

*Thompson, A.C., & Christmas, T.J. (1996). Interstitial cystitis: An update. *British Journal of Urology, 78*(6), 813-820.

United States Pharmacopeia Dispensing Information (USP DI): Vol. I. Drug information for the health care professional (20th ed.). (2000). Englewood, CO: Micromedix.

U.S. Renal Data Systems. (1999). *USRDS 1999 annual data report.* Bethesda, MD: The National Institutes of Health, National Institute of Diabetes and Digestive and Kidney Diseases.

Vaughn, D., & Malkowicz, S. (2001). Recent advances in bladder cancer chemotherapy. *Cancer Investigation, 19*(1), 77-85.

Walsh, P.C., et al. (1998). *Campbell's urology* (7th ed.). Philadelphia: W.B. Saunders.

Warren, J.W. (1997). Catheter-associated urinary tract infections. *Infectious Disease Clinics of North America, 11*(93), 609-622.

Warren, J.W., et al. (1999). Guidelines for antimicrobial treatment of uncomplicated acute bacterial cystitis and acute pyelonephritis in women. *Clinics in Infectious Disease, 29*(4), 745-758.

Young-McCaughan, S. (1999a). Invasive bladder cancer. In C. Miaskowski & P. Buchsel (Eds.), *Oncology nursing: Assessment and clinical care* (pp. 1055-1087), St. Louis: Mosby.

Young-McCaughan, S. (1999b). Superficial bladder cancer. In C. Miaskowski & P. Buchsel (Eds.), *Oncology nursing: Assessment and clinical care* (pp. 1031-1055), St. Louis: Mosby.

Zagoria, R.J. (Ed.). (1997). Uroradiology. *Urologic Clinics of North America, 24*(3), entire issue.

Interventions for Clients with Renal Disorders

CHRIS WINKELMAN

Learning Objectives

After studying this chapter, you should be able to:

1. Prioritize nursing care for the client with polycystic kidney disease.
2. Describe the clinical manifestations of hydronephrosis.
3. Identify clients at risk for pyelonephritis.
4. Use laboratory data and clinical manifestations to determine the effectiveness of therapy for pyelonephritis.
5. Compare and contrast the pathophysiology and clinical manifestations of acute glomerular nephritis and nephrotic syndrome.
6. Prioritize nursing care for the client during the first 24 hours after a nephrectomy.
7. Explain how diabetic nephropathy can affect glucose metabolism and control in the client with diabetes mellitus.
8. Develop a teaching plan for the client who has had a nephrectomy for renal cell carcinoma.

Go to http://www.wbsaunders.com/SIMON/Iggy/ for self-assessment questions related to these Learning Objectives.

Renal disorders interfere with the ability of the kidney to filter wastes and to balance fluid and solutes. The kidneys work in an integrated way with so many other organ systems; therefore a renal disorder can significantly affect systemic health and lead to life-threatening outcomes. Renal disorders can be categorized as congenital, obstructive, infectious, glomerular, and degenerative. Renal tumors and renal trauma are also described in this chapter.

CONGENITAL DISORDERS

Polycystic Kidney Disease

OVERVIEW

Polycystic kidney disease (PKD) is one of the most common inherited disorders and affects 250,000 to 500,000 people in the United States. It can be inherited as either an autosomal dominant trait or, less commonly, as an autosomal recessive trait. People who inherit the recessive form of PKD usually die in early childhood. The 5% to 10% incidence of PKD in clients with no family history occurs as a result of a spontaneous genetic mutation. PKD is more common in Caucasians than in people of other races.

Pathophysiology

Fluid-filled cysts in the epithelial cells of the nephron characterize PKD. In the dominant form only 5% to 10% of nephrons

may be involved until the fourth decade of life, whereas in the autosomal recessive form nearly 100% of nephrons are involved at birth. Cysts develop as a result of kidney cell proliferation, altered secretion, and abnormal cell matrix biology (Avner, et al., 1999; Calvet & Grantham, 2001).

Cysts can develop anywhere in the nephron. Over time, small cysts become progressively larger (up to a few centimeters in diameter) and more widely distributed; the glomerular and tubular membranes are damaged. As the cysts become filled with fluid, the nephron functions of filtration, reabsorption, and secretion become less effective.

The kidney tissue is eventually replaced by nonfunctioning cysts, which look like a cluster of grapes (Figure 71-1). The kidneys are grossly enlarged; each cystic kidney may enlarge to two or three times its normal size, becoming as large as a football. Other abdominal organs are displaced, and the client has considerable discomfort. The fluid-filled cysts are also prone to infection, rupture, and bleeding.

More than 60% of clients with PKD have high blood pressure. The cause of hypertension in this disorder is thought to be related to renal ischemia from the enlarging cysts. As the vessels are compressed and renal blood flow decreases, the renin-angiotensin system is activated, raising blood pressure. Control of hypertension is a top priority because proper treatment can interrupt the vasoconstriction that leads to renal ischemia.

Cysts may also occur in other tissues, such as the liver, blood vessels of the brain, and cardiac blood vessels. Cysts may alter liver function or result in spontaneous rupture of

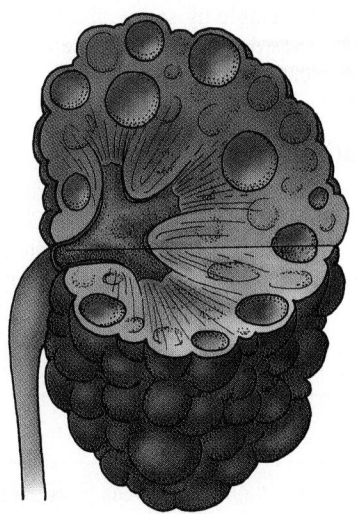

Figure 71-1 ● Polycystic kidney.

vascular cysts (*berry aneurysms*) in the brain, causing sudden death. For reasons as yet unknown, kidney stones occur in 8% to 36% of the clients with PKD. Heart valve abnormalities (e.g., mitral valve prolapse), left ventricular hypertrophy, and colonic diverticuli also are more prevalent in clients with PKD.

■ Etiology

PKD has at least two inherited forms. Men and women have an equal chance of inheriting the disease because the gene responsible for PKD is not located on the sex chromosomes. The offspring of parents who have PKD have a 50% probability of inheriting the gene that causes the autosomal dominant form of the disease.

Manifestations of autosomal dominant polycystic kidney disease (ADPKD) usually do not appear until the fourth decade of life. Half of the affected people develop renal failure by age 50 years. ADPKD-1 is the most severe form both in disease progression and in mortality. ADPKD-2 involves a slower rate of cystic formation and growth, resulting in a delayed progression to renal failure and other complications.

At present, there is no way to prevent PKD, although early detection and management of hypertension may slow the progression of renal impairment. Genetic counseling and evaluation may be useful for adults who have one parent or both parents with PKD. For those whose clinical symptoms do not appear until after the childbearing years, offspring can be included in genetic counseling sessions.

➤ COLLABORATIVE MANAGEMENT
● Assessment
■ HISTORY

The nurse explores the family history of a client with suspected or actual PKD and asks whether either parent was known to have PKD or whether there is any family history of kidney disease. The age at which signs and symptoms developed in the parent and any related complications may have prognostic significance. The client is asked about constipation, abdominal discomfort, a change in urine color or fre-

quency, high blood pressure, headaches, and a family history of sudden death from a stroke.

■ PHYSICAL ASSESSMENT/CLINICAL MANIFESTATIONS

Chart 71-1 lists key features of PKD. Pain is the presenting symptom in 20% to 30% of clients and is noted in at least 60%. The nurse inspects the abdomen. A protruding and distended abdomen is common as the cystic kidneys swell and push the abdominal contents forward. Polycystic kidneys are easily palpated because of their increased size. The nurse proceeds with *gentle* abdominal palpation because the cystic kidneys and nearby tissues may be tender, and palpation is uncomfortable.

The client also may have flank pain as a dull ache or as sharp and intermittent discomfort. Dull and aching pain is caused by increased kidney size with distention or from infection within the cyst. Sharp, intermittent pain occurs in response to a ruptured cyst or the presence of a stone. When a cyst ruptures, the client may notice bright red or cola-colored urine. The nurse suspects infection if the urine is cloudy or foul smelling or if there is **dysuria** (pain on urination).

Nocturia (the need to urinate excessively at night) may be an early disease sign and occurs because of decreased renal concentrating ability. As renal function further declines, the client experiences increasing hypertension, edema, and uremic symptoms such as anorexia, nausea, vomiting, pruritus, and fatigue (see Chapter 72). Because berry aneurysms often occur in clients with PKD, a severe headache with or without neurologic or vision alterations deserves particular attention.

■ PSYCHOSOCIAL ASSESSMENT

As an inherited disorder, PKD may cause complex psychosocial responses. The client often has had direct experience with the effects and consequences of the disease in other close family members. He or she may have had a parent who died or other close relatives who required dialysis or transplantation. While obtaining the family history, the nurse listens carefully for spoken and unspoken feelings of anger, resentment, hostility, futility, sadness, or anxiety; such feelings may need further exploration. The focus may be one or both parents or the process of diagnosis and treatment. Feelings of guilt and concern for the client's own children may further complicate the adjustment.

■ DIAGNOSTIC ASSESSMENT

Urinalysis usually reveals **proteinuria** (protein in the urine) once the glomeruli are involved. Hematuria may be gross or microscopic. Bacteria in the urine suggest an infection, usually in the cysts. A urine sample for culture and sensitivity testing is obtained when there is clinical or laboratory evidence of infection. As kidney function deteriorates, serum creatinine and blood urea nitrogen (BUN) levels rise. With worsening kidney function, the 24-hour creatinine clearance decreases. Renal handling of sodium may cause either sodium losses or sodium retention.

Diagnostic studies include renal sonography, computed tomography (CT), and magnetic resonance imaging (MRI).

Small cysts are detectable by sonography, CT, or MRI. Renal sonography provides diagnostic evidence of PKD, with minimal risk in most cases.

● Interventions

Common nursing diagnoses for the client with polycystic kidney disease (PKD) include Acute Pain, Chronic Pain, and Constipation. Common collaborative problems include Potential for Infection, Hypertension, Stone Formation, or Renal

---

CHART 71-2

NIC INTERVENTION ACTIVITIES *for*
The Client with Renal Problems

Pain Management: *Alleviation of pain or a reduction in pain to a level of comfort that is acceptable to the client.*
- Observe for nonverbal cues of discomfort, especially in those unable to communicate effectively.
- Assure client attentive analgesic care.
- Consider cultural influences on pain response.
- Utilize a developmentally appropriate assessment method that allows for monitoring of change in pain (e.g., flow sheet, daily diary).
- Control environmental factors that may influence the client's response to discomfort.
- Consider type and source of pain when selecting pain relief strategy.
- Provide the person optimal pain relief with prescribed analgesics.
- Implement the use of patient-controlled analgesia (PCA), if appropriate.
- Use pain control measures before pain becomes severe.
- Evaluate the effectiveness of the pain control measures used through ongoing assessment of the pain experience.
- Institute and modify pain control measures on the basis of the client's response.

Bowel Management: *Establishment and maintenance of a regular pattern of bowel elimination.*
- Note pre-existent bowel problems, bowel routine, and use of laxatives.
- Teach client about specific foods that are assistive in promoting bowel regularity.
- Initiate a bowel training program, as appropriate.
- Instruct client in foods high in fiber, as appropriate.
- Evaluate medication profile for gastrointestinal side effects.

Medication Management: *Facilitation of safe and effective use of prescription and over-the-counter drugs.*
- Monitor client for the therapeutic effect of the medication.
- Monitor for signs and symptoms of drug toxicity.
- Monitor for adverse effects of the drug.
- Develop strategies with the client to enhance compliance with prescribed medication regimen.
- Teach the client and/or family members the expected action and side effects of the medication.
- Instruct client when to seek medical attention.

Energy Management: *Regulating energy use to treat or prevent fatigue and optimize function.*
- Determine client's physical limitations.
- Determine client's/significant other's perceptions of causes of fatigue.
- Encourage verbalization of feelings about limitations.
- Determine what and how much activity is required to build endurance.
- Monitor nutritional intake to ensure adequate energy resources.

- Monitor client for evidence of excess physical and emotional fatigue.
- Monitor cardiorespiratory response to activity (e.g., tachycardia, other dysrhythmias, dyspnea, diaphoresis, pallor, hemodynamic pressures, and respiratory rate).
- Monitor location and nature of discomfort or pain during movement/activity.
- Promote bedrest/activity limitation (e.g., increase number of rest periods).
- Encourage alternate rest and activity periods.
- Provide calming diversional activities to promote relaxation.
- Plan activities for periods when the client has the most energy.
- Assist with regular physical activities (e.g., ambulation, transfers, turning, and personal care), as needed.
- Encourage physical activity (e.g., ambulation or performance of activities of daily living, consistent with client's energy resources).

Fluid Monitoring: *Collection and analysis of client data to regulate fluid balance.*
- Monitor weight.
- Monitor intake and output.
- Monitor serum and urine electrolyte values, as appropriate.
- Monitor serum albumin and total protein levels.
- Monitor serum and urine osmolality levels.
- Keep an accurate record of intake and output.
- Monitor for distended neck veins, crackles in the lungs, peripheral edema, and weight gain.
- Restrict and allocate fluid intake, as appropriate.
- Administer pharmacologic agents to increase urine output, as appropriate.
- Administer dialysis, as appropriate, noting client response.

Urinary Retention Care: *Assistance in relieving bladder distension.*
- Provide privacy for elimination.
- Provide Credé maneuver, as necessary.
- Use double voiding technique.
- Insert urinary catheter, as appropriate.
- Monitor degree of bladder distension by palpation and percussion.
- Catheterize for residual, as appropriate.
- Implement intermittent catheterization, as appropriate.

Infection Protection: *Prevention and early detection of infection in a client at risk.*
- Monitor for systemic and localized signs and symptoms of infection.
- Maintain asepsis for client at risk.
- Inspect condition of any surgical incision/wound.
- Instruct client to take antibiotics as prescribed.
- Obtain cultures, as needed.

Failure. Chart 71-2 lists some NIC interventions for clients with renal disorders. (See Chapter 70 for information on renal infections and stone formation. See Chapter 72 for care of the client with renal failure.)

PAIN

PAIN MANAGEMENT; ANALGESIC ADMINISTRATION. Comfort strategies include pharmacologic, physical, and integrative approaches. A combination may be most effective. Non-steroidal anti-inflammatory agents (NSAIDs) are used cautiously because of their tendency to adversely affect renal function. Aspirin-containing compounds are avoided to prevent an increased potential for bleeding.

If cyst infection is the cause of discomfort, the physician orders a lipid-soluble antibiotic such as trimethoprim/sulfamethoxazole (Bactrim, Septra, Trimpex) or ciprofloxacin (Cipro), which penetrate the cyst wall. Monitoring serum creatinine levels is necessary because antibiotic therapy can be nephrotoxic. Applying dry heat to the abdomen or flank may promote comfort when renal cysts are infected. When pain is severe or debilitating, cysts can be decompressed with percutaneous needle aspiration and drainage.

The nurse teaches the client methods of enhancing relaxation and promoting comfort via deep breathing, guided imagery, or other relaxation strategies. The overall goal is client self-management. (See Chapter 7 for pain management.)

CONSTIPATION

BOWEL MANAGEMENT. The nurse also teaches the client how to prevent constipation. The teaching plan covers adequate fluid intake, the role of increased dietary fiber when fluid intake is more than 2500 mL/24 hr, and the need for regular exercise to achieve regular bowel elimination. The nurse explains that pressure on the large intestine may further impede peristalsis as the polycystic kidneys increase in size. Consequently, the client should know that these recommendations for bowel management might change, particularly if renal failure also develops. The nurse also advises about the appropriate use of stool softeners and bulk agents, including the careful use of laxatives, to prevent complications related to chronic constipation.

HYPERTENSION AND RENAL FAILURE

TEACHING: DISEASE PROCESS; TEACHING: PRESCRIBED MEDICATION. Blood pressure control is necessary to minimize cardiovascular complications and slow the progression of renal dysfunction. Nursing interventions include education to promote self-management and understanding (see Chapter 36 for more information on hypertension). When renal impairment is evident through a decreased concentrating ability (e.g., nocturia, low urine specific gravity), the nurse encourages the client to drink at least 2 L of fluid per day to prevent fluid volume deficit, which could further affect renal function. Restricting excess dietary sodium intake may control blood pressure. Because fluid volume intake is not restricted, intravascular volume depletion and decreased renal perfusion does not occur.

Medications for blood pressure control include antihypertensive agents and diuretics. Antihypertensive agents include angiotensin-converting enzyme (ACE) inhibitors, calcium channel blockers, beta blockers, and vasodilators (see Chart 36-2). ACE inhibitors show promise in controlling the

epithelial-proliferative aspects of PKD and in reducing microalbuminuria (Torra, 1999). If PKD progresses to chronic renal failure or end-stage renal disease, treatment approaches are similar to those in Chapter 72.

The nurse teaches the client, family, or significant other how to measure and record blood pressure. The nurse also helps the client establish a schedule for self-administering medications, monitoring daily weights, and keeping blood pressure records (Chart 71-3). The potential side effects of the medications are explained. The nurse makes written materials, such as medication teaching cards and booklets, available.

A low-sodium diet is often prescribed to control the hypertension that usually accompanies PKD. However, some clients may experience salt wasting and do not require a sodium-restricted diet. As the disease progresses, the physician may limit the client's protein intake to slow the development of renal failure. The nurse assists the client, family, or significant other in understanding the recommended diet plan and clarifies its rationale. The nurse works closely with the dietitian to foster the client's understanding. The nurse may also initiate a referral for nutritional counseling.

■ Health Care Resources

The Polycystic Kidney Research Foundation conducts research and provides education about PKD. Many publications are available on request; there is a fee for some materials. Chapters of the National Kidney Foundation (NKF) and the American Association of Kidney Patients (AAKP) may also provide resources for client information and support.

OBSTRUCTIVE DISORDERS
Hydronephrosis, Hydroureter, and Urethral Stricture
■ OVERVIEW

Hydronephrosis and hydroureter are disorders usually associated with the obstruction of urine outflow. Urethral strictures also obstruct outflow. Prompt recognition and treatment are crucial to prevent permanent renal damage.

In **hydronephrosis,** the kidney becomes enlarged as urine accumulates in the pelvis and kidney tissue. Because the ca-

---

CHART 71-3

CLIENT EDUCATION GUIDE
Polycystic Kidney Disease

- Measure and record your blood pressure daily.
- Take your temperature if you suspect you have a fever.
- Weigh yourself every day at the same time of day and with the same amount of clothing, notify your physician or nurse if you have a sudden weight gain.
- Limit your intake of salt to help control your blood pressure.
- Notify your physician or nurse if your urine is foul smelling or if there is blood in your urine.
- Notify your physician or nurse if you have a headache that does not go away or if you have visual disturbances.
- Monitor bowel movements to prevent constipation.

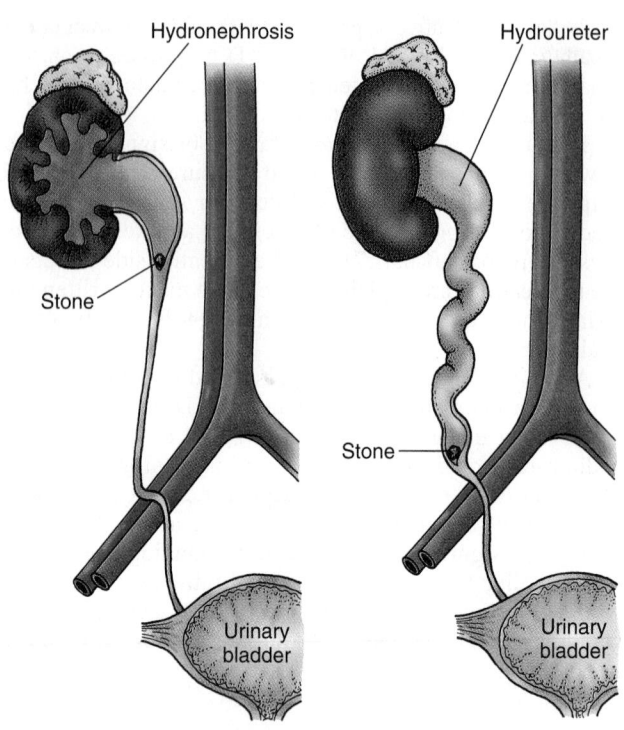

Figure 71-2 ● Hydronephrosis is caused by obstruction in the upper part of the ureter; hydroureter is caused by obstruction in the lower part of the ureter.

pacity of the renal pelvis is normally 5 to 8 mL, obstructions within it or at the ureteropelvic junction (UPJ) quickly result in renal pelvic distention. Kidney medullary pressure increases as the volume of urine increases. Over time, sometimes in only a matter of hours, the blood vessels and renal tubules can be damaged extensively (Figure 71-2).

In clients with **hydroureter,** the pathophysiologic effects are similar but the obstruction is lower in the urinary tract. The ureter is most likely to become obstructed where the iliac vessels cross or at the ureterovesical entry. Dilation of the ureter above the point of obstruction results in enlargement as urine continues to accumulate (see Figure 71-2).

In a client with a **urethral stricture,** the obstruction is very low in the urinary tract; this causes bladder distention to occur before hydroureter and hydronephrosis. The problems and kidney damage are similar without prompt treatment.

A urinary obstruction can cause structural damage when pressure builds up directly on tissue. Tubular filtrate pressure also increases within the nephron as drainage through the collecting system is impaired. With this added pressure, glomerular filtration decreases or ceases, and renal failure results. Nitrogenous waste products (urea, creatinine, and uric acid) and electrolytes (sodium, potassium, chloride, and phosphorus) are retained in the serum, and renal regulation of acid-base balance is impaired.

Disorders that can cause hydronephrosis or hydroureter include tumors, stones, trauma, congenital structural defects, and retroperitoneal fibrosis. Early treatment of the causes can prevent hydronephrosis and hydroureter and thus prevent permanent renal damage. The specific time needed to prevent permanent damage varies and depends on the client's underlying renal status. Permanent damage may occur in less than 48 hours in some clients and after several weeks in other clients.

► COLLABORATIVE MANAGEMENT

● Assessment

The nurse obtains a history from the client, focusing on known renal or urologic disorders. A history of childhood urinary tract problems may signal the presence of previously unidentified structural defects. The nurse inquires about the client's pattern of urination, especially its amount, frequency, color, clarity, and odor. The client is asked about recent flank or abdominal pain. Chills, fever, and malaise may be present with a urinary tract infection (UTI).

The nurse inspects each flank to identify asymmetry, which may occur with a renal mass, and *gently* palpates the client's abdomen to identify any areas of tenderness. The urinary bladder is also palpated and percussed to detect distention. Gentle pressure on the abdomen may cause urine leakage, which reflects a full urinary bladder and possible obstruction of the bladder/urethral junction.

Urinalysis may show bacteria or white blood cells if infection is present. When urinary tract obstruction is prolonged, microscopic examination may reveal tubular epithelial cells. The chemical analysis of serum is normal unless decreased glomerular filtration has occurred; serum creatinine and blood urea nitrogen (BUN) levels increase with a decreased glomerular filtration rate (GFR). Serum electrolyte levels may also be altered and indicate hyperkalemia, hyperphosphatemia, hypocalcemia, and metabolic acidosis (bicarbonate deficit).

Intravenous urography reveals ureteral or renal pelvis dilation. Urinary outflow obstruction may be revealed by sonography (renal echography) or computed tomography (CT).

● Interventions

NIC FLUID MONITORING; URINARY RETENTION CARE; INFECTION PROTECTION. Urinary retention and potential for infection are the primary problems. Failure to treat the cause of urinary obstruction may lead to infection and renal failure. Surgery is usually required to remove or reduce the cause of the obstruction.

INFECTIOUS DISORDERS

The urinary system is normally one in which a sterile body fluid (urine) is excreted. The unobstructed and complete passage of urine from the renal and urinary systems is critical to the sterility of the urinary tract. When a structural abnormality (either congenital or acquired) is present, the potential for degenerative changes from infection is dramatically increased. **Urinary tract infection (UTI)** usually refers to infections in this sterile system. **Pyelonephritis** is a bacterial infection within the kidney and renal pelvis—the *upper* urinary tract. Infections within the *lower* urinary tract are described in Chapter 70.

Pyelonephritis

■ OVERVIEW

With improved diagnostic techniques and a better understanding of the inflammatory response, pyelonephritis has come to refer to active microorganisms or the effects of kidney infections. **Acute pyelonephritis** is the condition resulting from an active bacterial infection, whereas **chronic pyelonephritis** results from repeated or continued upper urinary tract infections or infectious sequelae. Chronic pyelonephritis is usually associated with an anatomic urinary tract anomaly, urinary obstruction or, most commonly, vesicoureteral reflux. The vesicoureteral junction is the point at which the ureter joins the bladder. Reflux refers to the reverse (e.g., backward, upward, ascending) flow of urine toward the renal pelvis and kidney.

Pathophysiology

In pyelonephritis, microorganisms usually ascend from the lower urinary tract into the renal pelvis. Infection from organisms carried in the blood (**hematogenous**) may occur, but they occur with much less frequency. Bacteria activate the inflammatory response, and local edema results.

Acute pyelonephritis involves acute interstitial inflammation, tubular cell necrosis, and a tendency for abscess formation. Abscesses, pockets of localized infection, can appear in the capsule, cortex, or medulla. The pattern of infection within the kidney is not uniform; normal tissue and tubules can lie next to infected areas. Fibrosis or scar tissue develops as the inflammatory process subsides. The calices become blunted, and scars develop in the interstitial tissue.

Vesicoureteral and intrarenal reflux of infected urine are the major mechanisms responsible for chronic pyelonephritis. Some papillae in the kidney do not close with increased intracaliceal pressure, causing intrarenal reflux. Refluxing papillae are most often located in the upper and lower poles of the kidney and therefore are more susceptible to chronic pyelonephritis. Inflammation, fibrosis, and deformity of the renal pelvis and calices are evident. Repeated or continuous infectious produce additional scar tissue. Vascular, glomerular, and tubular changes within the scars can occur. Filtration, reabsorption, and secretion are eventually impaired, and renal function is diminished (Figure 71-3).

Etiology

Single episodes of *acute* pyelonephritis may result from the entry of bacteria associated with pregnancy, obstruction, or reflux. *Chronic* pyelonephritis is usually associated with structural abnormalities and/or obstruction with reflux. Vesicoureteral reflux or obstruction leading to chronic pyelonephritis is often due to stones, obstruction, or neurogenic impairment involving the voiding mechanism. Reflux is more common in children, who as adults often have scarring associated with chronic pyelonephritis. Clients who develop chronic pyelonephritis without having reflux as a child are usually adults with a history of spinal cord injury, bladder tumor, prostatic hypertrophy, or urinary tract stones.

Acute or chronic pyelonephritis is more likely to occur in clients who have undergone manipulation of the urinary tract (e.g., placement of a urinary catheter), those who have diabetes mellitus or chronic renal calculi, or those who overuse analgesics. In clients with diabetes mellitus, the development and progression of bladder atony increase the tendency to develop pyelonephritis. In clients with chronic stone disease, calculi provide a site for ongoing infection and resultant renal scarring. Nonsteroidal anti-inflammatory drug (NSAID) use has been associated with papillary necrosis, which then permits reflux.

The most common pyelonephritis-causing organism is *Escherichia coli*. *Enterococcus faeclus* is typical in hospitalized clients. Both are organisms of the gastrointestinal tract. Non–*E. coli* organisms such as *Proteus mirabilis, Klebsiella,*

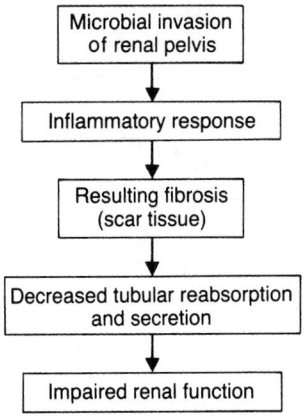

Figure 71-3 ● Pathophysiology of pyelonephritis.

and *Pseudomonas aeruginosa* and the more antibiotic-resistant organisms are also causes of pyelonephritis in hospitalized clients. When the infection is bloodborne, common infecting organisms include *Staphylococcus aureus* and the *Candida* and *Salmonella* species.

Theories of noninfectious or idiopathic causes of intrarenal scarring and the eventual outcome of pyelonephritis include an antibody reaction, cell-mediated immunity against the bacterial antigens, or an autoimmune reaction.

Incidence/Prevalence

The exact incidence and prevalence of pyelonephritis are not known; this diagnosis is not separately reported from all urinary tract infections. Acute urinary conditions of the kidneys or urinary tract, nephritic syndrome, urethral stricture, and cystitis account for more than 7 million new cases annually in noninstutionalized Americans (NIDDK National Kidney and Urologic Diseases Information Clearinghouse, 1999). Women overall have more cases of pyelonephritis. After age 65, rates for men increase greatly because of the increased incidence of prostatitis.

► COLLABORATIVE MANAGEMENT
● Assessment

HISTORY

The nurse asks about a history of urinary tract infections (UTIs), diabetes mellitus, stone disease, and other structural or functional abnormalities of the genitourinary tract. The nurse attempts to determine whether the UTIs were associated with pregnancy and asks the client about any previous experiences with pyelonephritis or similar symptoms. Recurrences are common and may lead to a deterioration of renal function.

PHYSICAL ASSESSMENT/CLINICAL MANIFESTATIONS

The nurse asks the client about specific symptoms associated with acute pyelonephritis (Chart 71-4). Chronic pyelonephritis has a less dramatic clinical presentation; signs and symptoms are usually related to the infection or renal function. The nurse asks the client to describe any vague or nonspecific urinary symptoms or abdominal discomfort and inquires about any history of repeated, low-grade fevers. The client with chronic pyelonephritis often has asymptomatic bacteremia. Chart 71-5 outlines the renal effects of chronic pyelonephritis.

The nurse inspects the flanks and gently palpates in the **costovertebral angle (CVA).** Each CVA is inspected to determine any enlargement or asymmetry, edema, or erythema, all of which are possible manifestations of inflammation. If there is no local tenderness to light palpation in either CVA, a specially trained nurse firmly percusses each area. Tenderness or discomfort reflects evidence of infection or inflammation.

■ PSYCHOSOCIAL ASSESSMENT

As with any disorder associated with the genitourinary tract, the client may have feelings of anxiety, embarrassment, or guilt. The nurse listens carefully to the client's description for evidence of generalized anxiety or specific fears and prevents embarrassment during assessment. Feelings of guilt, often associated with sexual habits or practices, may be masked through denial (e.g., delay in seeking treatment) or through vague, nonspecific responses to specific or direct questions. The nurse encourages clients to tell their own story in familiar, comfortable language.

■ LABORATORY ASSESSMENT

A urinalysis shows white blood cells and bacteria. The urine is analyzed to determine whether gram-positive or gram-negative organisms are responsible for the infection. The urine sample for culture and sensitivity testing, obtained by the clean-catch method, reveals the bacterial species and susceptibility or resistance of the specific organism to various antibiotics. In clients with recurrent episodes of pyelonephritis or upper UTIs, more specific testing of bacterial antigens and antibodies may help determine whether the same organism is responsible for the recurrent infections.

Blood cultures are examined for specific pathogenic microorganisms. Nonspecific serologic tests include the C-reactive protein and erythrocyte sedimentation.

■ RADIOGRAPHIC ASSESSMENT

An x-ray examination of the kidneys, ureters, and bladder (KUB) and intravenous (IV) urography are performed initially to determine the presence of stones or obstructions. A cystourethrogram is also indicated for some clients. These radiographic procedures define urinary tract structures and identify any structural defects. Specific defects to be identified include foreign bodies, such as stones; obstruction to the outflow of urine, such as tumors, structural defects, or prostate enlargement; and urine reflux associated with incompetent ureterovesical valve closure. (See Chapter 69 for more information on radiographic diagnostic assessment.)

■ OTHER DIAGNOSTIC ASSESSMENT

Several other diagnostic tests are currently being researched, including examining antibody-coated bacteria in urine, certain enzymes (e.g., lactate dehydrogenase isoenzyme 5), and radionuclide scintillation (e.g., gallium scan). Examining urine for antibody-coated bacteria is useful in identifying clients who may need long-term antibiotic therapy. High-molecular-weight enzymes in urine, such as lactate dehydrogenase isoenzyme 5, are present with any process associated with renal tissue deterioration and give trend data. The gallium scan can identify active pyelonephritis or abscesses in the perinephric region.

> ### CRITICAL THINKING CHALLENGE
>
> You are assigned to admit a 28-year-old woman who is 26 weeks pregnant. She complains of flank and CVA pain, dysuria, urgency, nocturia, and frequency: "I have to pee all the time, all night long, too, and it hurts!" She complains of nausea: "I thought morning sickness would be gone by now." She also reports fatigue: "Usually I can work a 10-hour day without even a bathroom break. I stayed in bed the past two days. My husband insisted I go to the emergency department this morning." She states, "I hope you can help me; I've never had anything like this before." Her vital signs are: heart rate, 110; blood pressure, 110/50; respirations, 20; and temperature 38° C. Her urinalysis is cloudy, amber, and foul smelling, with white blood cells and gram-negative bacteria.
>
> • What signs and symptoms support a diagnosis of a lower UTI (e.g., cystitis)? Pyelonephritis? Both?
> • What risk factors for pyelonephritis are present for this client?

For suggested answer guidelines, go to SIMON http://www.wbsaunders.com/SIMON/Iggy/.

▶ Analysis

■ COMMON NURSING DIAGNOSES AND COLLABORATIVE PROBLEMS

The primary common nursing diagnosis for the client with pyelonephritis is Acute Pain (Flank and Abdominal) related to inflammation and infection. A common collaborative problem is Potential for Renal Failure.

CHART 71-4
KEY FEATURES *of* **Acute Pyelonephritis**

- Fever
- Chills
- Tachycardia and tachypnea
- Flank, back, or loin pain
- Tender costal vertebral angle (CVA)
- Abdominal, often colicky, discomfort
- Nausea and vomiting
- General malaise or fatigue
- Burning, urgency, or frequency of urination
- Nocturia

CHART 71-5
KEY FEATURES *of* **Chronic Pyelonephritis**

- Hypertension
- Inability to conserve sodium
- Decreased concentrating ability (nocturia)
- Tendency to develop hyperkalemia and acidosis

ADDITIONAL NURSING DIAGNOSES AND COLLABORATIVE PROBLEMS

In addition to the common nursing diagnoses and collaborative problems, clients with pyelonephritis may have one or more of the following:

- Infection or Risk for Infection related to inadequate primary defenses (urinary stasis) or instrumentation
- Deficient Knowledge regarding the medical diagnosis and therapy related to lack of information resources
- Activity Intolerance related to fatigue, debilitation, and generalized weakness associated with the infection
- Fear of development of chronic renal failure related to an inability to control recurrent infections
- Hyperthermia related to increased metabolic rate from infection

An additional collaborative problem is Potential for Sepsis and Septic Shock.

● Planning and Implementation

ACUTE PAIN

NOC **PLANNING: EXPECTED OUTCOMES.** The client with pyelonephritis is expected to report that he or she has achieved a state of comfort that allows for adequate rest, nutrition, and activity.

INTERVENTIONS

NIC **PAIN MANAGEMENT.** Interventions may be nonsurgical or surgical. The availability and success of several noninvasive techniques that result in stone crushing, such as extracorporeal shock wave lithotripsy and percutaneous ultrasonic pyelolithotomy (see Chapter 70), have decreased the need for surgery.

NONSURGICAL MANAGEMENT. Nonsurgical interventions include the use of medications, diet and fluid therapy, and educational counseling to ensure the client's understanding about the treatment.

DRUG THERAPY

NIC *Medication Management.* Antibiotics are ordered to treat the infection. Initially, the antibiotics are broad spectrum. With urine and blood culture and sensitivity results, the physician may order a more specific antibiotic. Urinary antiseptic medications (e.g., nitrofurantoin [Macrodantin]) may also be prescribed to provide comfort.

DIET THERAPY

Fluid Monitoring; Teaching: Prescribed Diet. For healing to occur, the client's nutritional intake must include adequate numbers of calories and all food groups. Fluid intake is recommended at 2 to 3 L/day unless medically contraindicated.

SURGICAL MANAGEMENT. Surgical interventions may be needed to correct structural abnormalities causing urine reflux or obstruction of urine outflow or to eradicate the source of intractable infection.

PREOPERATIVE CARE. Antibiotics are given, usually intravenously, to achieve adequate blood levels or sterile blood culture results. The nurse also teaches the client the nature and purpose of the proposed surgery, the expected outcome, and expectations of how the client can participate.

OPERATIVE PROCEDURES. The surgical procedures may be one of the following: **pyelolithotomy** (stone removal from the renal pelvis), **nephrectomy** (removal of the kidney), ureteral diversion, or reimplantation of ureter to restore proper bladder drainage.

A pyelolithotomy is indicated for removal of a large stone in the renal pelvis that blocks urine flow and causes infection. Nephrectomy is considered a last resort when all other measures to eradicate infection have failed. For clients with incompetent ureterovesical valve closure or dilated ureters, **ureteroplasty** (repair or revision) or ureteral reimplantation (through another site in the posterior bladder wall) preserves renal function and eliminates infections.

POSTOPERATIVE CARE. See Chapter 70 for postoperative nursing care for the client undergoing urologic surgery.

POTENTIAL FOR RENAL FAILURE

PLANNING: EXPECTED OUTCOMES. It is expected that the client under treatment for pyelonephritis will conserve existing renal function for as long as possible and then experience a slow progression of renal failure once the process of renal failure begins.

INTERVENTIONS. The physician or nurse practitioner orders specific antibiotics to treat the infection. The nurse stresses the importance of taking all the medication as directed. The nurse also discusses with the client and family the importance of regular follow-up examinations and completing diagnostic tests as recommended.

Control of blood pressure is necessary to minimize the progression of renal dysfunction. When renal impairment is evident through a decreased concentrating ability (e.g., nocturia, low urine specific gravity), the nurse encourages the client to drink at least 2 L of fluid per day to prevent fluid volume deficit, which could further affect renal function. When dietary protein is restricted to delay the onset of renal failure, the nurse refers the client to the dietitian as needed. Other interventions related to the progression of chronic renal failure are covered in Chapter 72.

● Community-Based Care

Acute or chronic pyelonephritis causes fear and anxiety in the client and family. The severity of the acute process and its potential to develop into a chronic process are quite frightening. Both the client and the family require reassurance that treatment and preventive measures can be accomplished.

HEALTH TEACHING

After assessing the client's and family's understanding of pyelonephritis and the suggested treatment, the nurse explains the following:

- Medication administration (purpose, timing, frequency, duration, and possible side effects)
- The role of nutrition and adequate fluid intake
- The need for a balance between rest and activity, including any limitations after surgery
- The signs and symptoms of disease recurrence
- The use of previously successful coping mechanisms

The nurse advises the client to complete all prescribed antibiotic regimens and instructs the client to report any side effects or unusual symptoms to the prescribing health team member rather than suspend the regimen. The client and family are referred for nutritional counseling as needed, because many clients have special nutritional requirements, such as those caused by diabetes mellitus or pregnancy.

▓ HOME CARE MANAGEMENT

If no surgery is performed, the client may need assistance with self-care, nutrition, and medication administration at home. If surgical intervention is necessary, the client may require help with incision care, self-care, and transportation for follow-up medical appointments.

▓ HEALTH CARE RESOURCES

The client may also briefly need a community health nurse to help administer medications or nutrition at home. Housekeeping services may also be helpful while the client is regaining strength.

● Evaluation: Outcomes

NOC The nurse evaluates the care of the client with pyelonephritis on the basis of the identified nursing diagnoses and collaborative problems. Expected outcomes may include that the client will:

- Demonstrate methods of enhancing comfort
- Report that pain is controlled
- Express satisfaction with pain control
- Describe the role of antibiotics and self-administration of medications
- Explain and offer techniques to ensure adequate nutrition and hydration
- Describe the plan for posttreatment follow-up, including knowledge of recurrent symptoms
- Modify the prescribed regimen as directed by a health care professional

---

CRITICAL THINKING CHALLENGE

Your client is prescribed IV ciprofloxacin (Cipro) for pyelonephritis. She is also prescribed 25 mg meperidine every 3 hours prn for her pain. Radiographic studies are deferred at this time because of her pregnancy. A urine culture indicates that the infecting organism is *E. coli*, and the sensitivity of the bacteria to ciprofloxacin is confirmed. After 3 days her pain is absent, her fever is resolved, and her urinary symptoms are clearing. She is to be discharged today and is to continue taking her antibiotic orally at home. A follow-up medical visit is scheduled in 7 days.

- What discharge planning and health care teaching are indicated at this time?

For suggested answer guidelines, go to SIMON http://www.wbsaunders.com/SIMON/Iggy/.

Renal Abscess

▓ OVERVIEW

An **abscess** is a collection of fluid and cells caused by an inflammatory response to bacteria. An abscess may occur within the renal parenchyma (renal abscess), in the renal and Gerota's fascia (perinephric abscess), or in the flank. An abscess is suspected when fever and symptoms are not relieved promptly by antibiotic therapy.

▶ COLLABORATIVE MANAGEMENT

A renal or perirenal abscess is readily diagnosed via sonography or a computed tomography (CT) scan. Arteriography and radionuclide scintillation methods (e.g., gallium scan) also may be useful for diagnosis. Symptoms of renal abscess include fever, flank pain, and general malaise. Local flank edema and erythema may be observed.

Drainage by surgical incision or needle aspiration is often necessary. Appropriate broad-spectrum antibiotics are also prescribed.

Renal Tuberculosis

▓ OVERVIEW

The genitourinary tract is the most common extrapulmonary site of tuberculosis. Approximately 10% of new cases of tuberculosis are extrapulmonary (Tolkoff-Rubin, Cotran, & Rubin, 2000). Tuberculosis of the kidney is sometimes called *granulomatous nephritis*. After *Mycobacterium tuberculosis* invades the kidneys, usually by a bloodborne route, an inflammatory response is activated and forms scar tissue (**granuloma**) that replaces normal kidney tissue.

▶ COLLABORATIVE MANAGEMENT

Clients may experience urinary frequency, dysuria, hematuria and/or proteinuria, flank pain or renal colic secondary to the passage of clots or stones, pyuria, and hypertension. Skin test (e.g., purified protein derivative [PPD]) or chest x-ray film evidence of tuberculosis may or may not be present.

Clients with current or previous pulmonary tuberculosis who show signs of unexplained fever, hematuria, and sterile pyuria are at high risk for renal tuberculosis. The diagnosis is made through a urine culture of three clean-catch, first-morning specimens. Other genitourinary sites for tuberculosis include the prostate, epididymis, ureters, testes, bladder, and seminal vesicles.

Antitubercular therapy is the primary treatment. Recommendations include a 2-month course of rifampin, isoniazid, and pyrazinamide followed by 4 months of rifampin and isoniazid. Three to six more months of rifampin and isoniazid may be recommended for men who may be harboring the organism in the prostate (Tolkoff-Rubin, Cotran, & Rubin, 2000).

Complications include the loss of renal function, nephrolithiasis, obstructive uropathy, and bacterial superinfection of the urinary tract. Surgical excision of diseased tissue may be indicated to preserve renal function.

IMMUNOLOGIC RENAL DISORDERS

Glomerulonephritis is the third leading cause of end-stage renal disease (ESRD). Approximately 1% of all ESRD cases are attributed to one of the primary or secondary causes of glomerulonephritis (NIDDK, 1999).

Both primary and secondary diseases or syndromes result in glomerular injury. Glomeruli are usually involved in primary disease (Table 71-1); the extrarenal effects of primary disease stem from the glomerular injury. Most primary diseases and syndromes have an immunologic component, and many have an underlying genetic basis. Secondary glomerular disease refers to the situation in which glomerular involvement is part of another disease. For example, certain systemic diseases and infections can have renal effects and cause glomerular injury (Table 71-2). Some of the conditions causing secondary glomerular disease include systemic lupus erythematosus and diabetic nephropathy.

Each primary or secondary disease or syndrome has a specific pathophysiology and associated clinical manifestations. Their *glomerular* effects are caused by injury to the glomeruli and result in proteinuria, hematuria, decreased glomerular filtration rate (GFR), edema, and hypertension due to sodium retention. The extent and duration of renal injury, prognosis, and specific known cause vary considerably among these syndromes.

Immunologic changes may result in injury to the glomeruli, interstitium, and/or tubules, and the effects may be acute or chronic. Both antibody and cellular immune responses are involved. The resultant renal disorder may be a systemic disease or localized in the kidneys.

Most forms of glomerulonephritis are associated with an accumulation of immune complexes in the glomeruli (Figure 71-4). An immune complex is made up of antigen and antibody. The antigen can be normal kidney tissue such as the glomerular basement membrane, tubular basement membrane, or mesangium, or it can be dissolved in a body fluid (e.g., blood). Bacteria and viruses are also examples of antigens. Increasingly, exposure to bacteria, viruses, drugs, or other toxins is believed to be the trigger for glomerular injury.

Antibody reaction with antigen can lead to immune complex formation either directly in or deposited in glomerular tissue. The immune complexes activate many mediators—including complement, leukocytes, and coagulation proteins—that are re-

sponsible for the resultant renal tissue injury. Some of the major responses causing tissue injury include damage to cell membranes, local edema, movement of white blood cells to the site of inflammation, and activation of platelets.

Acute Glomerulonephritis
▊ OVERVIEW

An infection often occurs before the renal manifestations of acute glomerulonephritis (GN). The onset of symptoms averages 10 days from the time of infection; there is a broad range of illness severity but recovery is usually complete and quick. The term *acute nephritic syndrome* also describes this disorder.

Most causes of acute GN are postinfectious (Table 71-3) or are related to other systemic diseases (see Table 71-2). The incidence of acute GN is unknown, but poststreptococcal GN is more common in males.

➤ COLLABORATIVE MANAGEMENT
▶ Assessment
▊ HISTORY

The nurse asks about recent infections, particularly of the skin or upper respiratory tract, and about recent travel or other activities with possible exposure to viruses, bacteria, fungi, or parasites. Recent illnesses, surgery, or other invasive procedures may suggest infections. The nurse also asks about any known systemic diseases, such as systemic lupus erythematosus (SLE), which could cause acute GN.

▊ PHYSICAL ASSESSMENT/CLINICAL MANIFESTATIONS

The nurse inspects the client's skin for lesions or recent incisions and the face, eyelids, hands, and other areas for edema (present in approximately 75% of the clients with acute GN).

TABLE 71-1 •	PRIMARY GLOMERULAR DISEASES AND SYNDROMES

- Acute glomerulonephritis
- Rapidly progressive glomerulonephritis (RPGN)
- Chronic glomerulonephritis
- Nephrotic syndrome
- Persisting urinary abnormalities with few or no symptoms

TABLE 71-2 •	SECONDARY GLOMERULAR DISEASES AND SYNDROMES

- Systemic lupus erythematosus (SLE)
- Schönlein-Henoch purpura
- Goodpasture's syndrome
- Systemic necrotizing vasculitis
- Wegener granulomatosis
- Periarteritis nodosa (also called polyarteritis nodosa)
- Amyloidosis
- Diabetic glomerulopathy
- HIV-associated nephropathy
- Alport syndrome
- Multiple myeloma
- Viral hepatitis B
- Viral hepatitis C
- Cirrhosis
- Sickle-cell disease
- Nonstreptococcal postinfectious acute glomerulonephritis (GN)
- Infective endocarditis
- Hemolytic-uremic syndrome
- Thrombotic thrombocytopenic purpura (TTP)

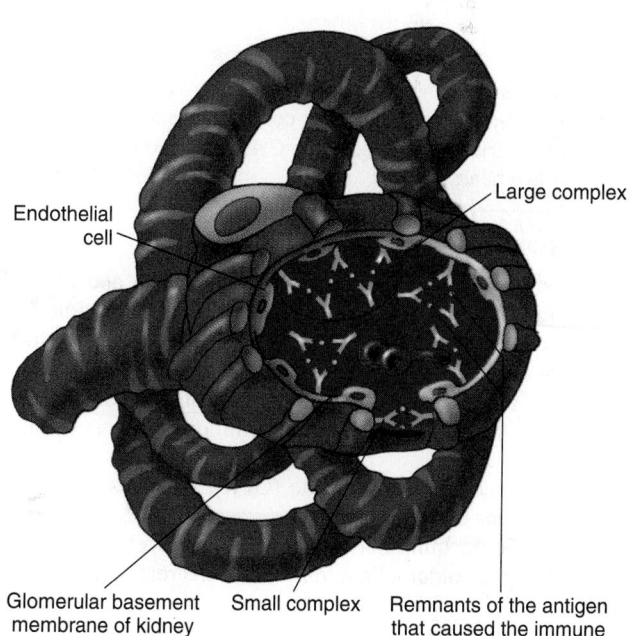

Figure 71-4 ● An immune complex precipitating in the glomerulus of a client with glomerulonephritis.

Endothelial cell

Large complex

Glomerular basement membrane of kidney   Small complex   Remnants of the antigen that caused the immune complexes to form

TABLE 71-3 • INFECTIOUS CAUSES OF ACUTE GLOMERULONEPHRITIS

- Group A beta-hemolytic *Streptococcus*
- Staphylococcal or gram-negative bacteremia or sepsis
- Pneumococcal, *Mycoplasma,* or *Klebsiella* pneumonia
- Syphilis
- Visceral abscesses
- Infective endocarditis
- Hepatitis B
- Infectious mononucleosis
- Measles
- Mumps
- Rocky Mountain spotted fever
- Cytomegaloviral (CMV) infection
- Histoplasmosis
- Toxoplasmosis
- Varicella
- *Chlamydia psittaci* infection
- Coxsackievirus infection
- Any bacterial, parasitic, fungal, or viral infection (potentially)

In assessing for circulatory congestion and fluid overload (which often accompanies the sodium and fluid retention associated with acute GN), the client is asked about any difficulty in breathing, nocturnal or exertional dyspnea, or orthopnea. The nurse also assesses for crackles in the lung fields, an S₃ heart sound (gallop rhythm), and neck vein distention.

The nurse asks about changes in urination pattern and any change in urine color. Microscopic hematuria occurs up to 66% of the time, and clients often describe their urine as smoky, reddish-brown, rusty, or cola colored. The client is asked about dysuria or oliguria. He or she is weighed because changes in urine output may result in fluid retention.

The blood pressure is measured and compared with the client's baseline blood pressure. Mild to moderate hypertension often accompanies acute GN due to sodium and fluid retention. The client may have symptoms of fatigue, a lack of energy, anorexia, nausea, and/or vomiting if uremia from renal failure is present.

CONSIDERATIONS FOR OLDER ADULTS
The less common signs of acute GN are especially common in older adults. Circulatory congestion often dominates the client's clinical picture. Acute GN is easily confused with congestive heart failure.

LABORATORY ASSESSMENT

Urinalysis reveals red blood cells (**hematuria**) and protein (**proteinuria**). Examination of an early morning specimen of urine is preferred because the urine is most acidic and formed elements are more intact at that time. Further microscopic examination often reveals red blood cell casts as well as casts from other substances. The urine sediment assay is usually positive.

The glomerular filtration rate (GFR), which is measured by the 24-hour urine test for creatinine clearance, may be decreased to 50 mL/min. Serum urea nitrogen levels are usually increased. The older client may have a greater decline in GFR.

A 24-hour urine collection for total protein assay is also obtained. The protein excretion value for clients with acute GN may be increased to values of 500 mg to 3 g/24 hr in more

than 75% of clients. Serum albumin levels may be decreased because of the large amount of protein lost in the urine and because of fluid retention (dilutional value).

Specimens from the blood, skin, or throat are obtained for culture, if indicated. Other serologic tests include antistreptolysin-O titers, C3 complement levels, cryoglobulins (immunoglobulin G [IgG]), antinuclear antibodies (ANAs), and circulating immune complexes.

Antistreptolysin-O titers are increased after group A beta-hemolytic *Streptococcus* infections. Complement levels are decreased when the complement system is activated. Type III cryoglobulins may be found during acute illness. ANAs suggest an autoimmune response, and SLE is only one possibility. Circulating immune complexes containing IgG and C3 are often detected.

OTHER DIAGNOSTIC ASSESSMENT

A percutaneous renal biopsy may provide a precise diagnosis of the pathologic condition, assist in determining the prognosis, and help outline treatment (see Chapter 69). The specific tissue morphology is determined by light microscopy, immunofluorescent stains, and electron microscopy to identify the type of cellular proliferation (light microscopy), the presence of immunoglobulins (immunofluorescence), or the specific type of tissue deposits (electron microscopy).

▶ Interventions

Interventions focus on treating the underlying infectious process, preventing complications, and providing appropriate client education.

MANAGEMENT OF INFECTION

MEDICATION MANAGEMENT. Treatment for cases of acute GN with an infectious cause would be the appropriate anti-infective. Penicillin, erythromycin, or azithromycin are usually prescribed for poststreptococcal GN. The nurse checks the client's known allergies before administering any medication. To prevent infection spread, the physician may order anti-infective drugs for persons in immediate close contact with the client. The nurse stresses personal hygiene and basic infection control principles (e.g., handwashing) to prevent spread of the organism.

PREVENTION OF COMPLICATIONS. For clients with circulatory congestion, hypertension, and edema, the physician orders diuretics and a sodium and water restriction. Antihypertensive medications may be needed to control hypertension (see Chart 36-3). The usual fluid allowance is equal to the 24-hour urine output plus 500 to 600 mL for insensible fluid losses. Clients with oliguria also usually have increased serum levels of potassium and blood urea nitrogen (BUN). Potassium and protein intake may be restricted to prevent hyperkalemia and additional uremic manifestations of the elevated BUN.

Nausea, vomiting, or anorexia indicates that uremia is interfering with nutrition. Dialysis is necessary if uremic symptoms or fluid volume excess cannot be controlled (see Chapter 72). **Plasmapheresis** (removal and filtering of the plasma to eliminate antibodies) also may be attempted (see Chapter 40); steroids are not usually helpful.

NIC *ENERGY MANAGEMENT.* To conserve and maintain the client's energy, the nurse assists him or her in maintaining a restful environment, balancing activity and rest, and coordinating necessary assessments and treatments. The client also needs to minimize emotional stress, and the nurse encourages him or her to practice relaxation techniques and to participate in diversional activities.

CLIENT EDUCATION. The nurse instructs the client, family, or significant other about the purpose and desired effects of prescribed medications, the dosage and route of administration, and potential adverse side effects. The nurse ensures that the client and family understand dietary or fluid modifications, including methods of detecting fluid retention. The client is advised to measure his or her weight and blood pressure daily at the same time each day and to notify the primary care provider of sudden increases in weight or of any increase in blood pressure.

If short-term dialysis is required to control fluid volume excess or uremic symptoms, the nurse explains peritoneal or vascular access care and dialysis schedules and routines (also see Chapter 72).

Rapidly Progressive Glomerulonephritis

Rapidly progressive glomerulonephritis (RPGN), a variant of acute nephritis, is also called *crescentic glomerulonephritis* because of the usual accumulation of crescent-shaped cells in Bowman's capsule. RPGN develops over several weeks or months and is associated with a significant loss of renal function. Clients can become quite ill quickly and have signs and symptoms of renal failure: fluid volume excess with hypertension and oliguria, electrolyte imbalances, and uremic symptoms.

A previous infection or multisystem disease, such as systemic lupus erythematosus (SLE), is sometimes identified in the client's recent history. The renal deterioration often progresses to nonreversible end-stage renal disease (ESRD).

Chronic Glomerulonephritis

OVERVIEW

Chronic glomerulonephritis, or *chronic nephritic syndrome,* refers to renal deterioration or failure that develops over 20 to 30 years or even longer. The exact onset of the disorder is rarely identified. In many instances the cause of the disease is not known because the kidneys are atrophied and tissue is not available for biopsy or diagnosis. Mild proteinuria and hematuria, hypertension, and occasional edema are often the only manifestations.

Although the exact pathogenesis is not known, changes in the renal parenchyma may result from hypertension, intermittent or recurrent parenchymal infections and inflammation, and altered metabolism and hemodynamics. Kidney tissue atrophies, and the functional mass of nephrons decreases significantly. The cortex of the parenchyma is thinned, but the calices and pelves are normal. Tissue obtained by renal biopsy in the late stages of atrophy may reveal hyalinization of the glomeruli, loss of tubules, and fibrosis of the kidney tissue. Immunofluorescent examination and electron microscopy may reveal residual effects of immune complex deposition.

The loss of nephrons results in decreased glomerular filtration. Hypertension with sclerosis of the renal arterioles is often present. The glomerular injury also causes proteinuria because of increased permeability of the glomerular capillaries. Chronic glomerulonephritis eventually results in chronic renal failure (see Chapter 72).

► COLLABORATIVE MANAGEMENT
● Assessment
HISTORY

The nurse asks the client about previously identified health problems, including systemic diseases, renal or urologic disorders, childhood infectious diseases (e.g., streptococcal infections), and recent exposures to infections. The client is asked about his or her overall health status and whether increasing fatigue and lethargy have been experienced.

The client's pattern of voiding is noted; the nurse asks whether the frequency of voiding has increased or the quantity of urine has decreased. The client is asked about changes in urine color, odor, or clarity and is asked about dysuria and continence.

Because edema can result from oliguria and fluid volume excess, the nurse also asks about the client's general comfort and any dyspnea at rest or with exertion.

The nurse asks about and observes changes in mental functioning, such as irritability or an inability to read or to perform job-related functions or other processes requiring mental concentration. Changes in memory and the ability to concentrate occur with the waste product accumulation that accompanies renal failure.

PHYSICAL ASSESSMENT/CLINICAL MANIFESTATIONS

The nurse assesses for signs of systemic circulatory overload by auscultating lung fields to detect crackles, observing the quality of respirations, measuring blood pressure and weight, and auscultating the heart to describe rate, rhythm, and the presence of an S_3 heart sound. The nurse inspects the neck veins to identify venous engorgement and checks for edema in the pedal, pretibial, and presacral tissues.

The nurse notes changes due to uremia, such as slurred speech, ataxia, tremors, or **asterixis** (flapping tremor of the fingers or the inability to maintain a fixed posture with the arms extended and wrists hyperextended). The nurse inspects the client's skin for a yellowish color, texture, ecchymoses, rashes, or eruptions. Areas of dryness and breaks that may have resulted from scratching are noted.

DIAGNOSTIC ASSESSMENT

Urine output may decrease, but gross visual changes in urine are unusual unless there is an associated urinary tract infection (UTI). Urinalysis commonly shows proteinuria, usually less than 2 g in a 24-hour collection; the specific gravity is usually fixed at a constant level of dilution (around 1.010). There may be red blood cells and casts in the urine, which suggests chronic renal disease processes.

The glomerular filtration rate (GFR) is measured by creatinine clearance and is reduced from the normal range of 105 to 120 mL/min. The serum creatinine level is elevated and varies depending on the client's muscle mass. Serum creatinine levels are usually greater than 6 mg/dL but may be as high as 30 mg/dL or more. Blood urea nitrogen (BUN) is increased and varies in relation to the dietary protein intake; BUN levels are often between 100 and 200 mg/dL.

Serum electrolyte levels may be abnormal as a result of decreased renal function. Sodium retention is common, but dilution of the plasma from excess fluid results in an apparently normal serum sodium level (135 to 145 mEq/L) or a dilutional hyponatremia (<135 mEq/L). When oliguria develops, potassium retention occurs; hyperkalemia is present when levels exceed 5.4 mEq/L. Hyperphosphatemia develops with serum levels greater than 4.7 mg/dL. Serum calcium levels are usually at the lower end of the normal range or are slightly below normal.

A base deficit with a decrease in serum carbon dioxide (CO_2) occurs with respiratory compensation by hyperventilation in response to metabolic acidosis. If respiratory compensation is present, the pH of arterial blood is between 7.35 and 7.45. A pH of less than 7.35 signifies inadequate respiratory compensation for metabolic acidosis (see Chapter 16).

In clients with chronic glomerulonephritis, the kidneys appear to be small when observed by x-ray or IV urography and when measured by sonography or computed tomography (CT).

A renal biopsy is important in the early stages of glomerulonephritis, when proteinuria or hematuria is initially present. Changes include an increase in the number and types of cells infiltrating the glomerular tissue, deposition of immune complexes, and vessel sclerosis. A renal biopsy (percutaneous or open) is rarely performed for clients once glomerulonephritis progresses to ESRD because the kidneys are too small to obtain tissue.

● Interventions

Interventions focus on slowing the progression of the disease and preventing complications. Treatment consists of dietary modification, fluid intake sufficient to prevent reduced blood flow volume to the kidneys, and medication therapy to temporarily control the symptoms of uremia. Eventually, the client requires dialysis or transplantation to prevent death from the numerous potential systemic effects of uremia. (Nursing care for the client with ESRD requiring dialysis or transplantation is discussed in Chapter 72.)

Nephrotic Syndrome
■ OVERVIEW

Nephrotic syndrome (NS) is a condition of increased glomerular permeability that causes massive proteinuria, edema, and hypoalbuminemia. Many agents, diseases, and physiologic processes are implicated as possible causes of NS.

Glomerular membrane changes from immune processes permit protein loss into urine. With this loss, plasma albumin levels decrease and edema develops. Altered liver activity results in elevated lipid production.

► COLLABORATIVE MANAGEMENT

The primary feature of nephrotic syndrome is severe proteinuria (>3.5 g of protein in 24 hours). Clients diagnosed with NS also often have hypoalbuminemia (serum albumin <3 g/dL), hyperlipidemia, lipiduria, edema, and hypertension (Chart 71-6). Renal vein thrombosis often occurs at the same time as

---

CHART 71-6

KEY FEATURES *of*
Nephrotic Syndrome

- Massive proteinuria
- Hypoalbuminemia
- Edema
- Hyperlipidemia
- Increased coagulation
- Infection

NS—either as a cause or as an effect. Clot development is not clearly understood. NS may progress to ESRD, but progression is not inevitable.

Treatment varies depending on the specifics of the glomerulopathy identified by renal biopsy. Some immunologic processes may respond to steroids or cytotoxic agents. Dietary modification is often prescribed. If the glomerular filtration rate (GFR) is normal, proteins should contain all essential amino acids; if the GFR is decreased, dietary protein intake is decreased. Mild diuretics (Chart 71-7) and dietary sodium restriction may be needed to control edema and hypertension. The nurse assesses the client to ensure that plasma volume depletion does not occur; hemodynamic changes and acute renal failure may be avoided if renal perfusion can be maintained.

IMMUNOLOGIC INTERSTITIAL AND TUBULOINTERSTITIAL DISORDERS

Interstitial and tubulointerstitial disorders in the kidney may be immunologically mediated; renal changes may be acute or chronic. The acute effects are often associated with medications such as penicillin-like antibiotics, sulfonamides, or nonsteroidal anti-inflammatory drugs (NSAIDs). Chronic interstitial nephritis has many causes, including analgesic nephropathy, complement activation, the medication cyclosporin, polycystic kidney disease, systemic lupus erythematosus, sarcoidosis, multiple myeloma, sickle cell disease, obstructive disorders, and radiation nephritis. Drug-induced problems are often associated with rash or eosinophilia. Fever is common in idiopathic forms of interstitial nephritis. Progression to ESRD is likely unless the offending agent can be identified and removed.

DEGENERATIVE DISORDERS

Degenerative disorders that cause changes in renal function are usually associated with the damage or effects caused by a multisystem disorder. Many of these degenerative disorders result from changes in kidney blood vessels.

Nephrosclerosis
■ OVERVIEW

Nephrosclerosis is a problem of changes in the nephron blood vessels. Vessel walls thicken, and the vessel lumen narrows. As a result, renal blood flow is decreased and kidney tissue is chronically hypoxic. Ischemia and fibrosis develop over time.

Nephrosclerosis is associated with all types of hypertension, atherosclerosis, and a history of diabetes mellitus. The more severe the hypertension, the greater the risk for extensive kidney damage. Nephrosclerosis is rarely seen when blood pressure is consistently below 160/110 mm Hg. The changes associated with hypertension may be reversible or

CHART 71-7

DRUG THERAPY *for* **Diuretics Used to Increase Urine Output**

Drug	Usual Dosage	Indication	Nursing Interventions	Rationale
OSMOTIC DIURETICS (act on glomerulus and renal tubular system)				
Mannitol (Osmitrol✦), urea	50-100 g IV as a 5%-25% solution	Causes rapid diuresis (e.g., after contrast media infusion)	Measure fluid intake and output.	Severe dehydration is possible. Mannitol may crystallize while on the shelf.
			Check vial for crystals. If crystals are present, warm vial between the hands.	Crystals will dissolve with body warmth.
			Administer through a filter.	This will prevent remaining crystals from entering the body.
THIAZIDE AND THIAZIDE-LIKE DIURETICS (act on cortical diluting site of ascending limb of loop of Henle)				
Chlorothiazide (Diuril)	250 mg PO, IV once to four times/day	Hypertension	Observe for signs and symptoms of electrolyte imbalance	Common complications include hypokalemia and hypercalcemia.
Hydrochlorothiazide (HydroDIURIL, Apo-Hydro✦, Urozide✦)	25-100 mg PO once or twice daily	Congestive heart failure (CHF) with edema	Monitor heart sounds for S_3, lung sounds for crackles and other signs of CHF.	Ongoing monitoring detects complications and helps ensure prompt treatment.
Chlorthalidone (Hygroton, Uridon✦)	25-100 mg PO daily	Edema, hypertension	Do not give with NSAIDs.	An increased diuretic effect is seen with concomitant use of NSAIDs.
Metolazone (Zaroxolyn)	5-20 mg PO daily	Edema, hypertension	Do not give with NSAIDs.	
LOOP DIURETICS (act on ascending limb of loop of Henle)				
Furosemide (Lasix, Furoside✦)	20-80 mg PO, IV once or twice daily; maximum dose 600 mg/day	Hypertension	Observe for orthostatic hypotension.	An early sign of rapid fluid volume depletion may be orthostatic hypotension.
Bumetanide (Bumex)	0.5-2 mg PO daily	CHF	Monitor for possible hyponatremia and hypokalemia.	These agents increase excretion of both sodium and potassium.
Ethacrynic acid (Edecrin)	50-200 mg PO daily	Edema (when creatinine clearance is <25-50 mL/min)	Monitor older clients closely for excessive diuresis.	Older adults are susceptible to the effects of rapid fluid changes.
POTASSIUM-SPARING DIURETICS (act on distal convoluted tubule)				
Spironolactone (Aldactone, Novospiroton✦)	25-200 mg PO once or twice daily	Primary aldosteronism	Observe for signs and symptoms of electrolyte imbalance.	Hyperkalemia with cardiac manifestations is a common complication.
Triamterene (Dyrenium)	25-100 mg once or twice daily; maximum dose 300 mg/day	Hypertension (with other drugs to decrease potassium loss)	Teach client to avoid unprotected sun exposure.	Photosensitivity reactions are possible.
Amiloride (Midamor✦)	5-10 mg daily	Edema, hypertension	Give with food or milk.	Stomach upset is possible.

NSAID, Nonsteroidal anti-inflammatory drug.

may progress to end-stage renal disease (ESRD) within months or years.

Hypertension is the second leading cause of ESRD. Approximately 30% of clients requiring lifesaving renal replacement therapy (e.g., dialysis or transplantation) have hypertension as the cause of their renal failure (NIDDK, 1999).

at risk for ESRD from hypertension is nearly 20:1 (Richardson & Piepho, 2000). These findings do not suggest that ESRD from nephrosclerosis does not occur in Caucasians but rather that affected Caucasians are likely to be older.

► COLLABORATIVE MANAGEMENT

Treatment aims to control high blood pressure and preserve renal function. Although many antihypertensive drugs may lower blood pressure, the client's response is important in ensuring long-term adherence to the prescribed therapy. Factors promoting adherence include regimen simplicity (e.g., once-a-day dosing), low cost, and minimal side effects.

Lack of basic knowledge or misinformation about hypertension poses additional challenges to nurses and all health care providers working with hypertensive clients. When evidence of renal disease occurs, adherence to therapy is even more important for preserving health.

Many medications can control high blood pressure (see Chart 36-2); more than one agent may be necessary. Angiotensin-converting enzyme (ACE) inhibitors are particularly useful in reducing hypertension and preserving renal function. Diuretics can maintain fluid and electrolyte balance in the presence of renal insufficiency. Caution is required to prevent hyperkalemia when potassium-sparing diuretics (e.g., triamterene or spironolactone) or combination agents containing a potassium-sparing diuretic are used for clients with known renal disease.

Renovascular Disease

▌ OVERVIEW

Pathologic processes affecting the renal arteries may result in severe lumen narrowing and drastically reduced blood flow to the renal parenchyma. Uncorrected renovascular disease, such as renal artery stenosis or thrombosis, causes ischemia and atrophy of renal tissue.

Renovascular disease is suspected with a sudden onset of hypertension, particularly in clients older than 50 years. Clients with high blood pressure but with a negative family history for hypertension may also be considered potential candidates for renal artery stenosis (RAS).

RAS from atherosclerosis or fibromuscular hyperplasia (increased amount of tissue) is the primary cause of renovascular disease. Other causes include thrombosis and renal aneurysms.

Atherosclerotic changes in the renal artery are often associated with sclerosis in the aorta and other major vessels. Changes in the renal artery are close to where the renal artery and aorta meet. Fibrotic changes of the vessel wall occur throughout the length of the renal artery.

► COLLABORATIVE MANAGEMENT

▐● Assessment

Key features of renovascular disease are listed in Chart 71-8. The onset of hypertension is usually after age 40 to 50 years, and the family history is often negative for hypertension. Diagnosis is made by renal arteriography; measurement of renal vein renin levels provides additional evidence but may not be confirmatory. A renal arteriogram visualizes the renal vasculature and offers critical information for invasive treatment. The comparison of renal vein renin levels *may* reveal which kidney is producing more renin.

▐● Interventions

Visualization of the type of defect, extent of narrowing, and surrounding vasculature is critical to decide treatment intervention. The client's overall condition and the size of the atrophied kidney further influence decisions about intervention.

RAS may be treated by drugs to control high blood pressure and by percutaneous transluminal balloon angioplasty or by surgical bypass procedures to restore the renal blood supply. Drugs may control high blood pressure but may not lead to long-term preservation of kidney function. In young and

---

CHART 71-8

KEY FEATURES *of*
Renovascular Disease

- Significant, difficult to control blood pressure
- Elevated serum creatinine
- Decreased creatinine clearance

---

middle-aged adults, a lifetime of treatment with multiple agents for high blood pressure may make treatment difficult and the outcomes uncertain.

Balloon angioplasty is considered less risky and requires much less time for recovery than does renal artery bypass surgery (see Chapter 36). Renal artery bypass surgery is a major procedure and involves at least 2 months for convalescence. A bypass may be performed for either one or both renal arteries. The surgeon inserts a synthetic graft that redirects blood flow from the abdominal aorta into the renal artery, beyond the area of stenosis. Increasingly, splenorenal bypass procedures can also restore renal blood flow. Technically, the process is similar to other arterial bypass procedures (see Chapter 36).

For clients with RAS, the diagnostic and treatment alternatives present tremendous decisional conflict. Clients often experience a deterioration of renal function, as noted by elevated serum creatinine levels and decreased creatinine clearance. These clients are at increased risk for acute renal failure from the administration of nephrotoxic agents such as radiopaque contrast media and from possible intraoperative hypotensive episodes. However, no treatment probably means that dialysis is inevitable.

Diabetic Nephropathy

▌ OVERVIEW

Diabetes mellitus is the leading cause of end-stage renal disease (ESRD) among Caucasians in the United States. Approximately 36% of clients requiring dialysis or renal transplantation have diabetes mellitus as the primary contributing factor (NIDDK, 1999). The cost of preventing or reducing renal problems among clients with diabetes is offset by the high cost of treating severe renal disease (see the Cost of Care box on p. 1657). Diabetic nephropathy may result from type 1 or type 2 diabetes mellitus. Diabetic renal disease is influenced by the extent, duration, and effects of atherosclerosis, hypertension, and autonomic neuropathy, which promotes bladder atony, urinary stasis, and urinary tract infection.

Immunologic response mechanisms have also been implicated in glomerular basement membrane thickening and other changes in clients with diabetic renal disease. Investigations continue to explore if defects are the result of genetic or metabolic disturbances.

► COLLABORATIVE MANAGEMENT

Diabetic nephropathy is a *microvascular* complication of diabetes defined by persistent albuminuria (as shown by dipstick or a urinary albumin excretion rate above 0.3 g/dL), without evidence of other renal disease. A diagnosis of renal disease in clients with diabetes mellitus is made on the basis of the history and clinical examination. Diabetic renal disease is progressive (Table 71-4).

COST OF CARE
IMPLICATIONS FOR NURSING

DIABETES AND RENAL DISEASE

Cost of Care

- A common complication of both type I and type 2 diabetes mellitus (DM) is nephropathy leading to end-stage renal disease.
- Diabetic clients are five times more likely to develop end-stage renal disease than others in their cohort.
- Abnormal renal function increases diabetes treatment costs by $1337 and advanced renal disease by $3979 per individual treated.
- Intensive therapy was shown by the Diabetes Control and Complications Trial to avert complications in type 1 DM; a similar trial is examining the effects of tight control on type 2 DM clients.

Implications for Nursing

Although the cost of maintaining tight control is two to three times the costs of conventional therapy, economic modeling predicts that tight control could reduce end-stage renal disease from 24% to 7%. Thus the costs of maintaining tight control are offset by the savings related to a reduced need for the diagnosis and treatment of DM-related renal disease.

Renal disease is an expensive diagnosis, not only in dollar costs but also in social, psychologic, and functional costs as patients undergo extensive diagnostic workups and work-limiting treatments. Preventing the renal complications of DM saves money; it also saves individuals from a heavy biopsychosocial burden.

Data from Brown, J.B., Pedula, K.L., & Baskt, A.W. (1999). The progressive cost of complications in type 2 diabetes mellitus. *Archives of Internal Medicine, 159*(16), 1873-1880; Herman, W.H. & Eastman, R.C. (1998). The effects of treatment on the direct costs of diabetes. *Diabetes Care, 21*(Suppl. 3), C19-C24; Nathan, D.M. (1993). Diabetes Control and Complications Trial Research Group. The effect of long-term intensified insulin treatment on development of microvascular complications of diabetes. *New England Journal of Medicine, 329*,(14) 977-986; and Ramsy, S.D., et al. (1999). Patient-level estimates of the cost of complications in diabetes in a managed-care population. *Pharmacoeconomics, 16*(3), 285-295.

TABLE 71-4 •	THE STAGES OF PROGRESSION OF TYPE 1 DIABETIC RENAL DISEASE

- **Stage I, at the time diabetes is diagnosed.** Kidney size and glomerular filtration rate are increased. Blood sugar control can reverse the changes.
- **Stage II, 2 to 3 years after diagnosis.** Glomerular and tubular capillary basement membrane changes result in microscopic changes, with loss of filtration surface area and scar formation. Glomerular changes are referred to as glomerulosclerosis.
- **Stage III, 7 to 15 years after diagnosis.** Microalbuminuria is present. The glomerular filtration rate (GFR) may still be normal or may be increased.
- **Stage IV.** Albuminuria is detectable by dipstick. GFR is decreased. Blood pressure is increased, and retinopathy is present.
- **Stage V.** GFR decreases at an average rate of 10 mL/min/yr.

Structural and functional changes occur in the kidneys of diabetic clients. Initially, kidney size is slightly increased and glomerular filtration rates (GFR) are higher than normal. A radioimmunoassay of urine detects the microlevels of albumin associated with albuminuria. Progressive renal damage occurs before dipstick procedures can detect protein in the urine. For most clients, proteinuria (albuminuria) indicates the need for a renal biopsy for further diagnosis. For the client with diabetes, observed microvascular changes in the retina

EVIDENCE-BASED PRACTICE
FOR NURSING

Does a multidisciplinary case management approach affect patient outcomes?

Harris, L.E., et al. (1998). Effects of multidisciplinary case management in patients with chronic renal insufficiency. *American Journal of Medicine, 195*(6), 464-471.

Case management has been recommended to improve clients' outcomes. In one setting, 437 clients with chronic renal insufficiency were enrolled in an intensive, multidisciplinary case management program for 2 years. A similar number received usual care in an urban, academic, general medicine practice. There were no differences in renal function, health services use, and mortality in the first, second, third, or fifth year of enrollment. The authors conclude that the intensive, multidisciplinary case-management intervention had no effect on the outcomes of care among primary care clients with established chronic renal insufficiency.

Critique. Both clients and practitioners knew which clients were receiving intensive case management; those in the control group may have modified their interventions (either client initiated or practitioner initiated) to demonstrate "equal" competence in care and practice. Most clients in the United States do not receive care in an urban, academic setting; these findings may not be reproducible in a community or rural setting.

Implications for Nursing. The potential benefits of assembling a multidisciplinary team to evaluate and manage the care of clients with chronic renal insufficiency were not supported. Individual practices may be a key factor in influencing the early diagnosis and accurate treatment of renal insufficiency. Further examination is essential to identify provider differences that positively influence client outcomes.

---

correlate well with the renal microvascular changes. Examination of the retina showing capillary leakage, fibrosis, and the typical changes of diabetic retinopathy eliminates the need for a risky renal biopsy.

As with nephrotic syndrome, proteinuria may be mild, moderate, or severe. Clients with diabetes mellitus are always considered to be at risk for renal failure. If possible, nephrotoxic agents (e.g., radiopaque contrast media or aminoglycosides) and fluid volume deficit are avoided. Clients with worsening renal function may begin to have frequent hypoglycemic episodes and a decreased need for insulin or oral antihyperglycemic agents. The nurse explains to the client that the kidneys metabolize and excrete insulin. When renal function deteriorates, the insulin is available for a longer time and thus less of it is needed. Unfortunately, many clients believe this means their diabetes mellitus is improving. The result is accelerated progression to ESRD. (See Chapter 65 for more information on diabetic nephropathy.)

Care of the client with chronic renal insufficiency is thought to be more effective when a multidisciplinary case management approach is used. Research has not demonstrated a clear advantage to such an approach (see the Evidence-Based Practice for Nursing box above).

TUMORS

Cysts and Benign Tumors

■ OVERVIEW

Benign urinary tract growths include cysts and tumors of the renal parenchyma or urinary bladder. Because malignant growths may occur within cystic structures, a thorough evaluation is essential.

A simple renal cyst grows out of renal parenchymal tissue, usually the *cortical* tissue. The cyst is filled with fluid and can cause local tissue destruction as it enlarges. Many cysts cause no symptoms and are discovered accidentally during fluoroscopic examination or autopsy.

Although the exact cause is unknown, cysts are usually considered a structural defect that occurs prenatally. The etiology and incidence of benign tumors is also unknown. Thus far there are no recognized methods of prevention.

► COLLABORATIVE MANAGEMENT

Diagnosis of a simple renal cyst involves IV urography, sonography, and computed tomography (CT). If the cyst appears to be filled with fluid at urographic examination, a sonography is generally recommended; if the cyst appears denser, a CT scan is needed.

Treatment may consist of percutaneous aspiration of a fluid-filled cyst or surgical exploration with the potential for total or subtotal nephrectomy.

Renal Cell Carcinoma

■ OVERVIEW

Renal cell carcinoma is also referred to as *adenocarcinoma of the kidney*. As with other malignancies, the healthy tissue of the kidney is replaced and displaced by cancer cells. Although the exact mechanism is not known, the tumor cells are thought to originate in the proximal convoluted tubules of the nephron.

Systemic effects occurring with the cancer are called **paraneoplastic syndromes** and include anemia, erythrocytosis, hypercalcemia, liver dysfunction with elevated liver enzymes, hormonal effects, increased sedimentation rate, and hypertension.

Anemia and erythrocytosis may appear contradictory: There is some blood loss from hematuria, but the amount lost is not sufficient to cause anemia. Erythrocytosis may be caused by erythropoietin production in the tumor cells. Hypertension may result from increased renin.

Parathyroid hormone produced by tumor cells may be the cause of hypercalcemia; other hormone alterations include increased renin levels (causing hypertension) and increased human chorionic gonadotropin (hCG) levels, which are accompanied by decreased libido and changes in secondary sex characteristics. The cause of the increased sedimentation rate and changes in liver function studies is not known.

Renal tumors are categorized into four stages (Table 71-5). Complications include metastasis and urinary tract obstruction. Metastasis usually occurs via the blood or lymph to the adrenal gland, liver, lungs, long bones, or the other kidney. When the tumor surrounds a ureter, hydroureter and urinary tract obstruction may result.

The exact cause of renal cell carcinoma is unknown, but links to tobacco use and exposure to chemicals such as lead, phosphate, and cadmium have been observed. Other studies suggest the possibility of hereditary influences.

Renal malignancies account for approximately 2% of reported cancers, with about 28,800 new cases and 11,300 deaths annually in the United States. The 5-year survival rate is 60% in the United States (Bonsib, 1999). Renal cell carcinoma usually affects clients between 55 and 60 years of age.

TABLE 71-5 • STAGING RENAL TUMORS

- **Stage I.** Tumors of up to 2.5 cm within the capsule of the kidney; the renal vein, perinephric fat, and adjacent lymph nodes have no tumor.
- **Stage II.** Tumors are larger than 2.5 cm and extend beyond the capsule but are within Gerota's fascia; the renal vein and lymph nodes are not involved.
- **Stage III.** Tumors extend into the renal vein and/or lymph nodes.
- **Stage IV.** Tumors include invasion of adjacent organs beyond Gerota's fascia or metastasis to distant tissues.

► COLLABORATIVE MANAGEMENT

● Assessment

■ HISTORY

The nurse asks the client for specific information, including age, known risk factors (e.g., smoking or environmental exposures), history of weight loss, changes in urine color, abdominal or flank discomfort, and fever. The cause of fever is unknown, but pyrogens produced by the tumor cells have been implicated.

■ PHYSICAL ASSESSMENT/CLINICAL MANIFESTATIONS

Presentations of renal carcinoma are seen only in 5% to 10% of clients and include flank pain, gross hematuria, and a palpable renal mass. The nurse asks about the nature of the flank or abdominal discomfort; clients typically describe the pain as dull and aching. The pain may be more intense if bleeding into the tumor occurs. The nurse inspects the flank, noting asymmetry or obvious protrusions. An abdominal mass may be detected through *gentle* palpation. A renal bruit may be heard on auscultation.

Hematuria is a *late* common sign. Blood in the urine may be grossly observable as bright red flecks or clots, or the urine may appear smoky or cola colored. Without gross hematuria, microscopic examination may or may not reveal red cells.

The skin is inspected for pallor, darkening of the nipples and breast enlargement (in men). Other findings may include muscle wasting, weakness, generally poor nutritional status, and weight loss. All tend to occur late in the disease.

■ DIAGNOSTIC ASSESSMENT

Urinalysis may reveal red blood cells. Hematologic studies reveal decreased hemoglobin and hematocrit values, hypercalcemia, increased erythrocyte sedimentation rate, and increased levels of adrenocorticotropic hormone, human chorionic gonadotropin (hCG), cortisol, renin, and parathyroid hormone.

Renal masses may be detected by surgical exploration, IV urogram with nephrograms, or sonography. The mass and surrounding structures may be further delineated by CT with contrast or magnetic resonance imaging (MRI). Staging or determining the extent of tumor spread is best accomplished with renal arteriography and renal venography.

● Interventions

Interventions focus on controlling the cancer and preventing metastasis.

NONSURGICAL MANAGEMENT. Chemotherapy with a variety of agents has had limited effectiveness. The Food and Drug Administration (FDA) has approved expanded clinical trials for the study of interleukin-2 (IL-2), a biologic response modifier (see Chapters 20 and 25). Interferon (INF) and tumor necrosis factor (TNF) are also being used investigationally. Studies with lymphokine-activated killer (LAK) cells and tumor-infiltrating lymphocytes (TIL) are in the clinical trial stage.

SURGICAL MANAGEMENT. Renal cell carcinoma is usually treated surgically by **nephrectomy** (kidney removal) when pain, bleeding, or tumor spread cannot be controlled otherwise.

PREOPERATIVE CARE. The client is instructed about surgical routines (see Chapters 17, 18, and 19). The nurse explains the probable site of incision and the postoperative dressings, drains, or other equipment needed and reassures the client about pain relief. Preoperative care includes administering blood and fluids to achieve hemodynamic stabilization.

OPERATIVE PROCEDURE. The client is placed in the lateral position with the operative kidney uppermost; after positioning the arms and legs, the client's trunk area is flexed to increase exposure of the kidney area. Removal of the eleventh or twelfth rib is needed to provide better access to the kidney. The surgeon removes the entire kidney, renal artery and vein, and surrounding Gerota's fascia after ligation of the ureter. The adrenal gland is left intact. A drain may be placed in the wound before closure.

When a *radical* nephrectomy is performed, the periaortic lymph nodes are also removed. the surgical approach may be transthoracic (as discussed in the previous paragraph), lumbar, or transabdominal depending on the size and location of the lesion. Radiation therapy may follow a radical nephrectomy. Studies are ongoing to identify the effectiveness of adjuvant therapy (e.g., chemotherapy).

POSTOPERATIVE CARE. Refer to Chapter 19 for postoperative care. Assessment of urologic and renal function is essential to determine function in the remaining kidney.

Monitoring. The nurse observes the client's abdomen for distention from bleeding and symptoms of adrenal insufficiency. The nurse observes the bed linens under the supine client, because bleeding may be present. Hemorrhage or adrenal insufficiency may be accompanied by hypotension, a decrease in urine output, and an altered level of consciousness.

A decrease in blood pressure is one of the earliest signs of both hemorrhage and adrenal insufficiency; in clients with hypotension, urine output also decreases immediately. Large water and sodium losses in the urine occur in clients with adrenal insufficiency; consequently, a large urine output is followed by hypotension and subsequent oliguria (<400 mL/24 hr or less than 25 mL/hr). The physician may prescribe IV replacement of fluids and the administration of packed red blood cells.

The second kidney is expected to provide adequate renal function. The nurse assesses urine output hourly for the first 24 hours postoperatively; a urine flow of 30 to 50 mL/hr is acceptable. Flow rates of less than 25 to 30 mL/hr suggest a decrease in renal perfusion. Initially, the postoperative hemo-

globin level, hematocrit values, and white blood cell count may be measured every 6 to 12 hours.

The nurse monitors the client's temperature, pulse rate, and respiratory rate at least every 4 hours; careful measurement and recording of fluid intake and output are critical. The client is weighed daily.

The client may be in a special care unit for 24 to 48 hours postoperatively for monitoring of bleeding and/or adrenal insufficiency. A drain placed near the site of incision removes residual fluid. Because of the discomfort associated with lung expansion, the client is susceptible to atelectasis. Fever, chills, thick sputum, or decreased breath sounds suggest pneumonia.

Pain Management. After surgery, opioid analgesics (e.g., meperidine [Demerol], hydromorphone [Dilaudid], and morphine sulfate [Statex♣]) are given parenterally. The incision site, in which the major muscle groups associated with breathing and movement are involved, necessitates the liberal use of analgesic agents. These medications may be required for 3 to 5 days for pain management. Oral analgesic agents may be considered when the client is permitted to eat and drink.

Prevention of Complications. One or more antibiotics may be prescribed for intraoperative and postoperative prophylaxis. These agents are usually given as single-dose prescriptions. The need for additional antibiotics is based on clinical and laboratory evidence of infection. Steroid replacements may be necessary in adrenal insufficiency.

RENAL TRAUMA

OVERVIEW

Trauma to one or both kidneys is always a concern in penetrating wounds or blunt injuries to the back, flank, or abdomen. Injury to the kidney can be minor, major, or pedicle (Figure 71-5). Strategies to prevent trauma are reviewed in Chart 71-9.

Minor injuries include contusions, small lacerations, and disruption of the integrity of the parenchyma and the calyx (forniceal disruption). In a person with a contusion, one or both kidneys sustained a bruise because of the major impact. Small blood vessels may be damaged, causing some hematuria. One or more small lacerations may result in small, localized hematomas. There may also be a small hematoma at the site of forniceal disruption. Common causes include falls, contact sports, and blows to the back and torso.

Major injuries involve lacerations to the cortex, medulla, or one of the segmental branches of the renal artery or vein. Deep parenchymal injuries may extend throughout the kidney and result in hematomas contained within or disrupting the capsule. Other parenchymal injuries involve the cortex and cause shattering of tissue, resulting in either an intact or a disrupted capsule.

A major injury is most likely to follow a penetrating abdominal, flank, or back wound (such as seen with gunshot wounds, knife wounds, or motor vehicle accidents). Bleeding is extensive, and surgical exploration is often required. Because of the hemorrhage, hypoperfusion of renal parenchyma can produce short-term or long-term renin-induced hypertension.

Pedicle injuries involve a laceration or disruption of the renal artery and/or renal vein. Hemorrhage is extensive and rapid, and death may ensue quickly unless diagnosis and intervention are prompt.

MINOR TRAUMA

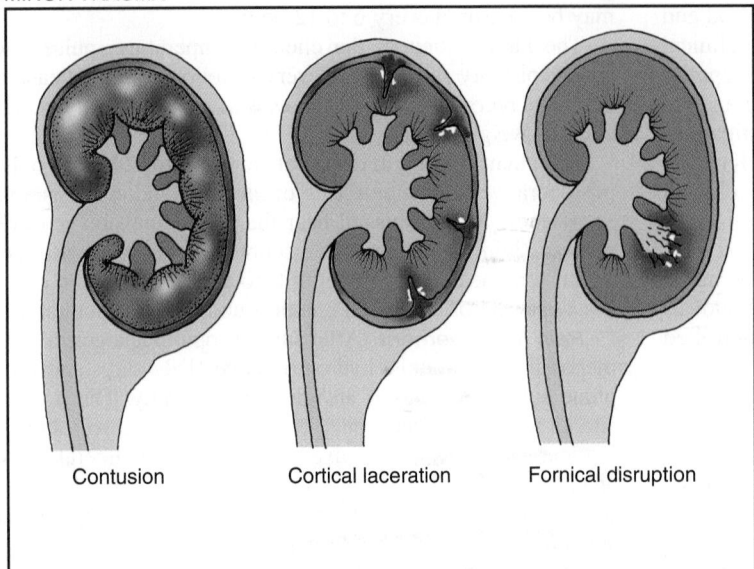

Contusion   Cortical laceration   Fornical disruption

PEDICLE INJURY

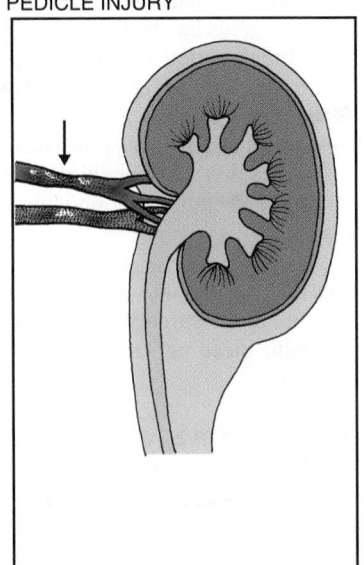

MAJOR TRAUMA

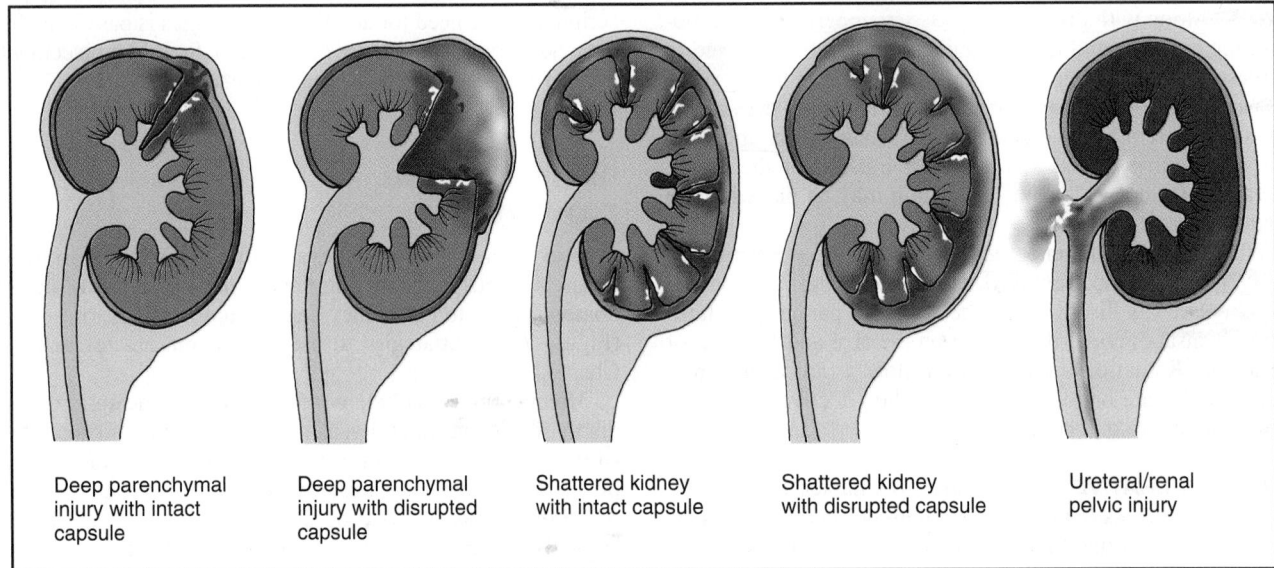

Deep parenchymal   Deep parenchymal   Shattered kidney   Shattered kidney   Ureteral/renal
injury with intact   injury with disrupted   with intact capsule   with disrupted capsule pelvic injury
capsule   capsule

Figure 71-5 ● Common types and locations of renal trauma.

► COLLABORATIVE MANAGEMENT
▶ Assessment

The nurse obtains a history of the client's usual health status and the events surrounding the trauma from the client, a witness, or emergency personnel. Critical assessment information includes a history of renal or urologic disease, surgical intervention, or systemic health problems (e.g., diabetes mellitus or hypertension).

Ureteral and/or renal pelvic injury may cause diffuse abdominal pain, local collections of urine, and infection. The nurse asks the client about pain, specifically flank or abdominal pain, and solicits a description: Is the pain dull? Sharp? Constant? Intermittent? Aggravated by coughing?

The nurse measures the client's blood pressure and apical and peripheral pulse rates, respiratory rate, and temperature. The right and left flanks are inspected to determine asymmetry or penetrating injuries of the lower thorax or back. Similarly, the nurse inspects the abdomen for ecchymoses, percusses the abdomen for distention, and observes for penetrating wounds. The urethra is inspected for gross bleeding.

Urinalysis commonly reveals hemoglobin or red blood cells from the rupture of small or large renal blood vessels.

Microscopic examination of the urine may also show red blood cell casts, which suggest tubular damage. Hemoglobin and hematocrit values decrease with blood loss; the white blood cell count is elevated with inflammation or infection.

Fluoroscopic procedures include IV urography, renal arteriography, and computed tomography (CT). A urogram reveals the number of kidneys and the integrity and patency of the collecting system. Renal sonography is an alternative diagnostic procedure to a urogram that avoids radiopaque contrast media exposure to clients with elevated serum creatinine levels.

Renal arteriography reveals the number of kidneys and, more specifically, the blood supply to each. In clients with pedicle injuries, the contrast media used in arteriography extravasates from the ruptured vessels, and the renal parenchyma is not visualized. The CT scan shows the location of the injury and vascular and tissue integrity. Intracapsular and extracapsular hematomas are readily observable on the CT scan.

◗ Interventions

Nursing diagnoses for the client with renal trauma include Ineffective (Renal) Tissue Perfusion, Anxiety, Pain, Impaired Urinary Elimination, Post-Trauma Syndrome, and Risk for Infection. Interventions include medications for vascular support, fluids to restore fluid volume, and surgery when indicated.

NONSURGICAL MANAGEMENT

DRUG THERAPY. Prescribed IV dopamine (Revimine♣, others) supports renal perfusion. Coagulation factors such as vitamin K and platelets are assessed and administered as needed.

FLUID THERAPY. Fluid administration to restore circulating blood volume is critical for renal tissue perfusion. *Crystalloid* solutions replace water and some electrolytes and include 0.9% sodium chloride (NSS), 5% dextrose in 0.45% sodium chloride, and Ringer's solution. When significant bleeding has occurred, whole blood or packed red cell replacement restores the oxygen-carrying capacity of hemoglobin. *Plasma volume expanders,* such as dextran or albumin, help re-establish plasma oncotic pressure and minimize fluid shift from the intravascular to the interstitial fluid space.

During fluid resuscitation or restoration, the nurse administers fluid at the prescribed rate and monitors the client for hemodynamic instability. The nurse also monitors vital signs as often as every 5 to 15 minutes and measures and records urine output hourly. Urine output should be greater than 25 to 30 mL/hr.

SURGICAL MANAGEMENT. Surgical interventions may include nephrectomy and partial nephrectomy. For clients with major vascular tearing, the kidney may be surgically removed, repaired through revascularization techniques, and then reimplanted. The repair of kidney tissue outside the client is called *bench surgery.* Autotransplantation is transplantation of one's own kidney.

◗ Community-Based Care

The nurse instructs the client, family, or significant other about the effects of the injury and how to assess for infection or other complications, such as the onset of bleeding or urinary retention. The client is instructed to observe the pattern and frequency of urination and to note whether the color, clarity, and amount appear normal. The nurse also instructs the client to seek medical attention if these characteristics change significantly and if a feeling of bladder distention or inadequate bladder emptying occurs, which suggests an obstruction. Chills, fever, lethargy, and/or cloudy, foul-smelling urine may suggest a urinary tract infection. The nurse warns the client not to ignore these symptoms and to seek medical care promptly if they occur.

ONLINE RESOURCES

For suggested readings and Internet resources, go to http://www.wbsaunders.com/SIMON/Iggy/.

SELECTED BIBLIOGRAPHY

Asterisk indicates a classic or definitive work on this subject.

*Adler, S.G., Cohen, A.H., & Glassock, R.J. (1996). Secondary glomerular diseases. In B.M. Brenner & F.C. Rector (Eds.), *Brenner & Rector's the kidney* (5th ed., pp. 1498-1596). Philadelphia: W.B. Saunders.

Agodoa, L. (1998). African-American study of kidney disease and hypertension (AASK): Clinical trial update. *Ethnic Disease, 8*(2), 249-253.

American Cancer Society. (2001). *Cancer facts and figures 2001.* 01-300M-NO.5008.01. Atlanta: Author.

Avner, E.D., et al. (1999). Cellular pathophysiology of cystic kidney disease: Insight into future therapies. *International Journal of Developmental Biology, 43*(5 Spec. No.), 457-461.

Bakris, G. et al. (2000). Preserving renal function in adults with hypertension and diabetes: A consensus approach. National Kidney Foundation Hypertension and Diabetes Executive Committees Working Group. *American Journal of Kidney Disease, 36*(3), 646-661.

Bernini, G., et al. (1998). Treatment of renovascular disease and of renovascular hypertension. *Journal of Nephrology, 11*(6), 311-317.

Bleyer, A.J., & Appel, R.G. (1999). Risk factors associated with hypertensive nephrosclerosis. *Nephron, 82*(30), 193-198.

Bonsib, S.M. (1999). Risk and prognosis in renal neoplasms. A pathologists prospective. *Urologic Clinics of North America, 26*(3), 643-660, viii.

Brater, D.C. (1999). The use of diuretics in cirrhosis and nephrotic syndrome. *Seminars in Nephrology, 19*(6), 575-580.

Brown, J.B., Pedula, K.L., Baskt, A.W. (1999). The progressive cost of complications in type 2 diabetes mellitus. *Archives of Internal Medicine, 159*(16), 1873-1880.

Calvet, J., & Grantham, J. (2001). The genetics and physiology of polycystic kidney disease. *Seminars in Nephrology, 21*(2), 107-123.

Connolly, A., & Thorp, J.M. (1999). Urinary tract infections in pregnancy. *Urology Clinics of North America, 26*(4), 779-787.

Coresh, J., & Jaar, B. (1997). Further trends in the etiology of end-stage renal disease in African-Americans. *Current Opinions in Nephrology & Hypertension, 6*(3), 243-249.

Crook, E.D. (1999). The role of hypertension, obesity, and diabetes in causing renal vascular disease. *American Journal of Medical Science, 17*(3), 183-188.

*Duley, I., & Gabow, P. (1990). *PKD patient's manual: Understanding and living with autosomal dominant polycystic kidney disease.* Kansas City, MO: PKD Foundation.

Falk, J., Jennett, J., & Nachman, S. (2000). Primary glomerular disease. In B.M. Brenner & S.A. Levine (Eds.), *Brenner & Rector's the kidney* (6th ed., pp. 1263-1349). Philadelphia: W.B. Saunders.

Fliser, D., & Ritz, E. (1998). Does essential hypertension cause progressive renal disease? *Journal of Hypertension Supplement, 16*(4), S13-S15.

Fogo, A.B. (1999). Current concepts in glomerulosclerosis. *American Journal of Kidney Disease, 34*(5), liv-lvi.

Germino, G.G. (1997). Autosomal dominant polycystic kidney disease: A two-hit model. *Hospital Practice, 32*(3), 81-82, 85-88, 91-92, 95-97, 102.

Golan, L., Birkmeyer, J.D., Welch, H.G. (1999). The cost-effectiveness of treating all patients with type 2 diabetes with angiotensin-converting enzyme inhibitors. *Annals of Internal Medicine, 131*(9), 660-667, editorial 707-708.

Gonzalez, R.P., et al. (1999). Surgical management of renal trauma: Is vascular control necessary? *Journal of Trauma, 47*(6), 1039-1042, discussion 1042-1044.

Grist, T.M. (1999). Magnetic resonance angiography of renal artery stenosis. *Coronary Artery Disease, 10*(3), 151-156.

Harris, L.E., et al. (1998). Effects of multidisciplinary case management in patients with chronic renal insufficiency. *American Journal of Medicine, 195*(6), 464-471.

Hartman, D.S., & Stagg, P.L. (1998). Diagnosis please. Case 3: Renal tuberculosis. *Radiology, 209*(1), 69-72.

Hartmann, J.S. & Bokemeyer, C. (1999). Chemotherapy for renal cancer. *Anticancer Research, 19*(2C), 1541-1543.

Herman, W.H. & Eastman, R.C. (1998). The effects of treatment on the direct costs of diabetes. *Diabetes Care, 21*(Suppl. 3), C19-C24.

Ichigi, Y., et al. (1999). Significance of hematoma size for evaluating the grade of blunt renal trauma. *International Journal of Urology, 6*(10), 502-508.

Kelly, C.J., & Neilson, E.G. (2000). Tubulointerstitial diseases. In B.M. Brenner & S.A. Levine (Eds.), *Brenner & Rector's the kidney* (6th ed., pp. 1506-1536). Philadelphia: W.B. Saunders.

Knudson, M.M., & Maull, K.I. (1999). Nonoperative management of solid organ injuries: Past, present, and future. *Surgery Clinics of North America, 79*(6), 1357-1371.

Krautschick, A.W. (1999). Metabolic evaluation and medical therapy for stone formation. *Current Opinion in Urology, 9*(4), 335-338.

*Lancaster, L.E. (Ed.). (1995). *Core curriculum for nephrology nursing* (3rd ed.). Pitman, NJ: A.J. Jannetti.

Laragh, J.H., & Blumenfeld, J.D. (2000). Essential hypertension. In B.M. Brenner & S.A Levine (Eds.), *Brenner & Rector's the kidney* (6th ed., pp. 1967-2006). Philadelphia: W.B. Saunders.

*Letizia, M., & Conway, A.M. (1996). Interleukin-2 therapy for renal cell cancer. *Critical Care Nurse, 16*(5), 20-26, 30-32, 34-35.

Levy, A.S., et al. (1999). Dietary protein restriction and the progression of chronic renal disease: What have all the results of the MDRD study shown? Modification of Diet in Renal Disease Study Group. *Journal of the American Society of Nephrology, 10*(11), 2426-2439.

Lewis, J.B., et al. (1999). Effect of intensive blood pressure control on the course of type 1 diabetic nephropathy: Collaborative Study Group. *American Journal of Kidney Disease, 34*(5), 809-817.

Little, C. (2000). Renovascular hypertension. *American Journal of Nursing, 100*(2), 46-51.

Losito, A., et al. (1999). Survival of patients with renovascular disease and ACE inhibition. *Clinics in Nephrology, 52*(6), 339-343.

McCarthy, S., & McMullen, M. (1997). Autosomal dominant polycystic kidney disease: Pathophysiology and treatment. *American Nephrology Nurses' Association Journal, 24*(1), 45-53.

McCloskey, J., & Bulechek, G. (2000). *Nursing interventions classification (NIC)* (3rd ed.). St. Louis: Mosby.

*McKinney, B. (1996). When this rare cancer strikes: Renal cell carcinoma. *RN, 59*(12), 36-41, 51.

Mihara, S., et al. (1999). Early detection of renal cell carcinoma by ultrasonographic screening based on the results of 13 years of screening in Japan. *Ultrasound in Medicine and Biology, 25*(7), 1033-1039.

Morganti, A., et al. (1999). Renovascular hypertension: Clinical and diagnostic clues. *Annals of Urologie, 33*(3), 137-143.

Nangaku, M., Pippin, J., & Couser, W.G. (1999). Complement membrane attack complex (C5b-9) mediates interstitial disease in experimental nephrotic syndrome. *Journal of the American Society of Nephrology, 10*(11), 2323-2331.

*Nathan, D.M. (1993). Diabetes Control and Complications Trial Research Group: The effect of long-term intensified insulin treatment on development of microvascular complications of diabetes. *New England Journal of Medicine, 329*(14), 977-986.

Nickeleit, V., et al. (1999). Nephrotic syndrome in an adult: The ongoing saga of fibrils versus microtubules. *American Journal of Kidney Disease, 34*(6), 1146-1151.

Nicolau, C., et al. (1999). Autosomal dominant polycystic kidney disease types 1 and 2: Assessment of US sensitivity for diagnosis. *Radiology, 213*(1), 273-276.

NIDDK National Kidney and Urologic Diseases Information Clearinghouse. (1999). *Kidney and Urologic Diseases Statistics for the United States.* Bethesda, MD: U.S. Government NIH Pub. No. 99-3895.

Parker, S.L., et al. (1997). Cancer statistics, 1997. *CA: A Cancer Journal for Clinicians, 47*(1), 5-27.

*Pasternack, M.S., & Rubin, R.H. (1993). Urinary tract tuberculosis. In R.W. Schrier & C.W. Gottschalk (Eds.), *Diseases of the kidney* (5th ed., pp. 909-928). Boston: Little, Brown.

Ramsy, S.D., et al. (1999). Patient-level estimates of the cost of complications in diabetes in a managed-care population. *Pharmacoeconomics, 16*(3), 285-295.

Rees, C.R. (1999). Stents for atherosclerotic renovascular disease. *Journal of Vascular Interventional Radiology, 10*(6), 689-705.

Richardson, A., & Piepho, R. (2000). Effect of race on hypertension and antihypertensive therapy. *International Journal of Clinical Pharmacology, 38*(2), 75-79.

Ritz, E., et al. (1999). End-stage renal failure in type 2 diabetes: A medical catastrophe of worldwide dimensions. *American Journal of Kidney Disease, 34*(5), 795-808.

Roberts, J.A. (1999). Management of pyelonephritis and upper urinary tract infections. (1999). *Urology Clinics of North America, 26*(4), 753-763.

Rodriguez-Itrube, B. (2000). Post-infectious glomerulonephritis. *American Journal of Kidney Disease, 35*(1), xlvi-xlviii.

Rosenberg, M. (1999). Pharmacoeconomics of treating uncomplicated urinary tract infections. *International Journal of Antimicrobial Agents, 11*(3-4), 247-251, discussion 261-264.

*See, W.A., & Williams, R.D. (1992). Tumors of the kidney, ureter, and bladder. *Western Journal of Medicine, 156*(5), 523-534.

Seedat, Y.K. (1999). Improvement in treatment of hypertension has not reduced the incidence of end-stage renal disease. *Journal of Human Hypertension, 13*(11), 747-751.

Sessa, A., et al. (1999). Renal-retinal diabetic syndrome. *Nephron, 83*(3), 285-286.

*Smith, M.F. (1990). Renal trauma: Adult and pediatric considerations. *Critical Care Nursing Clinics of North America, 2*(10), 67-77.

*Sommers, M. S. (1990). Blunt renal trauma. *Critical Care Nurse, 10*(3), 38-49.

Sorcini, A., & Libertino, J.A. (1999). Vascular reconstruction in urology. *Urologic Clinics of North America, 26*(1), 219-234, x-xi.

Stuart, R. & Nigam, S. (2000). Developmental biology of the kidney. In B.M. Brenner and S.A. Levine (Eds.), *Brenner & Rector's the kidney* (6th ed., pp. 68-92). Philadelphia: W.B. Saunders.

Tolkoff-Rubin, N., Cotran, R., & Rubin, R. (2000). Urinary tract infection, pyelonephritis, and reflux nephropathy. In B.M. Brenner & S.A. Levine (Eds.), *Brenner & Rector's the kidney* (6th ed., pp. 1449-1508). Philadelphia: W.B. Saunders.

Torra, R. (1999). Autosomal dominant polycystic kidney disease, type 2 (PKD2 disease). *Advances in Nephrology Necker Hospital, 29*(11), 277-287.

*Torres, V.E. (1996). Polycystic kidney disease: Guidelines for family physicians. *American Family Physician, 53*(3), 847-850.

Torres, V.E. (1999). Extrarenal manifestations of autosomal dominant polycystic kidney disease. *American Journal of Kidney Disease, 34*(6), xlv-xlvii.

U.S. Renal Data Systems. (1999). *USRDS 1999 annual data report.* Bethesda, MD: The National Institutes of Health, National Institute of Diabetes and Digestive and Kidney Diseases.

*Watson, M., & Torres, V. (Eds.). (1996). *Polycystic kidney disease.* New York: Oxford University Press.

Weir, M.R., & Dzau, V.J. (1999). The renin-angiotensin-aldosterone system: A specific target for hypertension management. *American Journal of Hypertension, 12*(12 Pt. 3), 105S-213S.

*Wong, J.M., et al. (1991). Surgery after failed percutaneous renal artery angioplasty. *Journal of Vascular Surgery, 30*(3), 468-482.

Zuccala, A., & Zucchelli, P. (1998). Ischemic nephropathy: Diagnosis and treatment. *Journal of Nephrology, 11*(6), 318-324.

Interventions for Clients with Acute and Chronic Renal Failure

CONSTANCE VISOVSKY

Learning Objectives

After studying this chapter, you should be able to:

1. Compare and contrast the pathophysiology and causes of chronic renal failure (CRF) and acute renal failure (ARF).
2. Identify clients at risk for development of ARF.
3. Identify clients at risk for development of CRF.
4. Use laboratory data and clinical assessment to determine the effectiveness of therapy for renal failure.
5. Discuss interventions to prevent ARF.
6. Prioritize nursing care for the client with ARF.
7. Compare the clinical manifestations of stage I, stage II, and stage III CRF.
8. Discuss the mechanisms of peritoneal dialysis (PD) and hemodialysis (HD) as renal replacement therapies.
9. Prioritize nursing care for the client with end-stage renal disease.
10. Prioritize teaching needs for the client using continuous ambulatory PD.
11. Prioritize teaching needs for the client with a permanent vascular access for long-term HD.
12. Compare and contrast the dietary modifications needed for the client undergoing HD with those for the client undergoing PD.
13. Plan prevention strategies for the complications of PD.
14. Discuss the criteria for kidney donation.
15. Prioritize nursing care for the client during the first 24 hours after kidney transplantation.

Go to http://www.wbsaunders.com/SIMON/Iggy/ for self-assessment questions related to these Learning Objectives.

Acute and chronic renal failure have become increasingly more common in the United States, resulting in considerable morbidity and mortality. Acute renal failure is responsible for 7% of all hospital admissions, and the prevalence of end-stage renal disease has virtually doubled in the last decade (Stark, 1998; U.S. Renal Data Systems, 1999). There are many causes of renal failure, but complications related to poorly controlled diabetes remain the most common cause.

The functions of the kidney are excretion of waste, water and salt regulation, maintenance of acid balance, and hormone secretion. When renal function deteriorates gradually, as occurs with most causes of chronic renal failure, 90% to 95% of the nephrons must be destroyed before significant renal failure is evident. The client may have many years of decreased renal reserve and chronic renal insufficiency before the uremia of end-stage renal failure develops. During this

time of decreased renal reserve and chronic renal insufficiency, the client is at increased risk for acute renal failure because of the diminished availability of functioning nephrons.

When renal deterioration is sudden, the capacity of the functioning nephrons is exceeded more quickly, and renal failure may develop with the loss of only 50% of functioning nephrons. Acute renal failure and chronic renal failure are compared in Table 72-1. Acute renal failure affects *many* body systems; chronic renal failure affects *every* body system. The abnormalities are primarily related to the effects of the following:

- Fluid volume excess
- Electrolyte and acid-base abnormalities
- Accumulated nitrogenous wastes
- Hormonal inadequacies

When renal function decreases to the point where the kidneys can no longer meet the body's homeostatic demands, re-

TABLE 72-1 • CHARACTERISTICS OF ACUTE AND CHRONIC RENAL FAILURE

Characteristic	Acute Renal Failure	Chronic Renal Failure
Onset	Sudden (hours to days)	Gradual (months to years)
Percentage of nephron involvement	~50%	90%-95%
Duration	2-4 wk; less than 3 mo	Permanent
Prognosis	Good for return of renal function with supportive care; high mortality in some situations	Fatal without a renal replacement therapy, such as dialysis or transplantation

nal replacement therapy is required to prevent death from potentially life-threatening consequences.

ACUTE RENAL FAILURE

■ OVERVIEW

Acute renal failure (ARF) is a rapid decrease in renal function, leading to the accumulation of metabolic waste in the body. ARF can result from conditions that cause inadequate kidney perfusion (**prerenal failure**); damage to the glomeruli, interstitium, or tubules (**intrarenal failure**); or obstruction (**postrenal failure**) (Kelly, 1997). ARF in clients with chronic renal insufficiency (CRI) may result in **end-stage renal disease (ESRD)** or may resolve to nearly the pre-ARF level of renal function. Many factors contribute to renal insults resulting in ARF, but the acute syndrome may be reversible.

■ Pathophysiology

The pathophysiologic process of ARF is related to the cause of the sudden decrease in kidney function and the involved site or sites of the kidney. Hypoperfusion, toxins, tubular ischemia, infections, and obstruction have different effects on the renal system. Any of these processes can result in a decreased glomerular filtration rate (GFR), alterations in renal tubular cell membrane integrity, and tubular lumen obstruction.

With acute hypoperfusion, autoregulatory responses (i.e., renal vasoconstriction, activation of renin-angiotensin-aldosterone, and release of antidiuretic hormone [ADH]) increase blood volume and improve renal perfusion. However, these compensatory mechanisms cause urine volume to fall, resulting in **oliguria** (urine output less than 400 mL/day). Tubular cell injury is more likely to occur from the increasing ischemia related to hypoperfusion. Toxins can cause vasoconstrictive responses in the kidney, leading to reduced renal blood flow and renal ischemia.

Interstitial inflammatory changes resulting from infection, drugs, or infiltrating tumors result in immune-mediated changes in renal tissue. With extensive tubular damage, sloughing of tubular cells and other formed elements (e.g., red blood cell [RBC] casts) may obstruct the tubular lumen and prevent the formation or outflow of urine. Obstruction anywhere within the genitourinary tract eventually results in full or partial obstruction to the formation and outflow of urine.

When intratubular pressure exceeds glomerular hydrostatic pressure, glomerular filtration ceases. This process causes a progressive elevation of the serum blood urea nitrogen (BUN) and creatinine levels. When the BUN rises faster than the serum creatinine level, the cause is usually related to protein catabolism or volume depletion. When both the BUN and creatinine levels rise and the ratio between the two remains constant, renal failure is present.

■ TYPES OF ACUTE RENAL FAILURE

Several syndromes describe the types of ARF. These include prerenal azotemia, intrarenal (intrinsic) ARF, and postrenal azotemia. Table 72-2 summarizes the pathologic changes and causes of ARF.

Prerenal azotemia can be reversed by establishing normal intravascular volume, increasing blood pressure and cardiac output. Prolonged, untreated hypoperfusion can lead to severe ischemic injury and intrarenal failure.

The term *intrarenal ARF* is often shortened to just *ARF* in the clinical setting. Other terms include **acute tubular necrosis (ATN)** and **lower nephron nephrosis.** Infections (bacteria, viral, fungal, or endotoxin), drugs (especially aminoglycoside antibiotics and nonsteroidal anti-inflammatory drugs [NSAIDs]), and infiltrating tumors (e.g., lymphomas or leukemias) can cause acute interstitial nephritis. Inflammation of the glomeruli (glomerulonephritis) or of the small vessels of the kidneys (vasculitis) or a major obstruction to blood flow can also cause intrarenal ARF.

Postrenal azotemia develops from obstruction to the outflow of formed urine anywhere within the genitourinary tract.

■ PHASES OF ACUTE RENAL FAILURE

When a client's renal function has been compromised, the phases of ARF begin (Table 72-3). Increasing numbers of clients have a *nonoliguric* form of ARF. The description of the phases of this form of ARF are similar to those described in Table 72-3 except for the references to urine output. In addition, the treatment of these clients is less complicated because renal replacement therapy is rarely needed. Interventions to restore circulating volume, improve cardiac output, or reestablish blood pressure may prevent progression of the phases when renal hypoperfusion is present.

■ Etiology

Many types of renal insults can lead to reduced renal function. Severe hypotension from excessive blood loss or dehydration results in hypoperfusion of blood to the kidneys and can lead to prerenal ARF. Cardiac disease or heart failure also results in decreased renal perfusion. The client may be oliguric, or even anuric (less than 100 mL/24 hr), if the dehydration or renal blood flow obstruction is severe. The following are other conditions that precipitate ARF:

- Nephrotoxic agents (antibiotics, NSAIDs) (Table 72-4)
- Disseminated intravascular coagulation (DIC)

TABLE 72-2 • CAUSES OF THE THREE TYPES OF ACUTE RENAL FAILURE

Pathologic Change	Causes

PRERENAL
Decreased blood flow to the kidneys leading to ischemia in the nephrons; prolonged hypoperfusion can lead to tubular necrosis and ARF
	Conditions that cause decreased cardiac output
	   Shock
	   CHF
	   Pulmonary embolism
	   Anaphylaxis
	   Pericardial tamponade
	   Sepsis

INTRARENAL (INTRINSIC) Actual tissue damage to the kidney caused by inflammatory or immunologic processes or from prolonged hypoperfusion	Acute interstitial nephritis Exposure to nephrotoxins Acute glomerulonephritis Vasculitis Hepatorenal syndrome ATN Renal artery or vein stenosis/thrombosis
POSTRENAL Obstruction of the urine collecting system anywhere from the calyces to the urethral meatus Obstruction of the bladder must be bilateral to cause postrenal failure unless only one kidney is functional	Urethral or bladder cancer Renal calculi Atony of bladder Prostatic hyperplasia or cancer Cervical cancer Urethral stricture

ARF, Acute renal failure; *CHF,* congestive heart failure; *ATN,* acute tubular necrosis.

TABLE 72-3 • THE PHASES OF OLIGURIC ACUTE RENAL FAILURE

Phase	Description	Characteristics	Duration
Onset phase	Begins with the precipitating event and continues until oliguria develops.	The gradual accumulation of nitrogenous wastes, such as serum creatinine and BUN, may be noted.	Can last hours to several days.
Oliguric phase	Characterized by a urine output of 100-400 mL/24 hr that does not respond to fluid challenges or diuretics.	Laboratory data include increasing serum creatinine and BUN levels, hyperkalemia, bicarbonate deficit (metabolic acidosis), hyperphosphatemia, hypocalcemia, and hypermagnesemia. Sodium retention occurs, but this is masked by the dilutional effects of water retention. Urinary indices are typically low and fixed; regulation of water balance by the kidneys is impaired, so urine specific gravity and urine osmolality will not vary as plasma osmolality changes.	Typically lasts 8-15 days but can last for several weeks, especially in older clients or those having pre-existing renal insufficiency.
Diuretic phase (high-output phase)	Often has a prompt onset, with urine flow increasing rapidly over a period of several days. The diuresis can result in an output of up to 10 L/day of dilute urine.	Electrolyte losses typically precede clearance of nitrogenous wastes. Later in the diuretic phase, the BUN level starts to fall and continues to fall until the level reaches normal limits or reaches a plateau. Normal renal tubular function is reestablished during this phase.	Usually occurs 2-6 wk after the onset of oliguric acute renal failure and continues until the BUN level ceases to rise.
Recovery phase (convalescent phase)	In this phase, the client begins to return to normal levels of activity.	The client functions at a lower energy level and has less stamina than before the illness. Residual renal insufficiency may be noted through regular monitoring of renal function. Renal function may never return to preillness levels, but renal function sufficient for a long and healthy life is likely.	Renal function may continue to improve for up to 12 mo after oliguric acute renal failure began. The client is particularly vulnerable to additional renal injury during this time.

BUN, Blood urea nitrogen.

- Obstruction by thrombosis or stenosis
- Uric acid crystals or other obstructing precipitates
- Acute hemolytic transfusion reactions
- Complications of infection (e.g., endotoxins or sepsis)
- Acute glomerulonephritis
- Vasculitis
- Severe hypertension
- Hepatorenal syndrome of cirrhosis

Incidence/Prevalence

ARF affects 20% of all critically ill clients and carries a 50% to 80% mortality rate (Stark, 1998). Eighty percent of ARF episodes are due to ATN and exacerbations of CRI. Volume depletion leading to prerenal azotemia is the most common cause of acute renal deterioration and is reversible in most cases with prompt intervention.

For clients surviving the precipitating event, the opportunity for return of renal function is good. Complications during the course of ARF can vastly increase mortality. Bloodstream infections associated with central and peripheral lines and the pulmonary system are most often involved in complications. However, the highest mortality occurs with trauma (70%) and surgery. ARF caused by nephrotoxic substances is associated with the lowest rates (10% to 26%) of recovery. The prognosis for ARF caused by obstruction or glomerulonephritis is much better.

▶ COLLABORATIVE MANAGEMENT
Prevention

Nurses have an essential role in the prevention of acute renal failure (ARF). The nurse notes the signs of impending renal dysfunction through careful physical assessment and close monitoring of laboratory values. Prompt recognition and correction of extrarenal problems usually restore renal function

TABLE 72-4 • SOME POTENTIALLY NEPHROTOXIC SUBSTANCES

DRUGS	
Antibiotics/Anti-infectives	• Fluorinate anesthetics
• Amphotericin B	• Indomethacin
• Colistimethate	• D-Penicillamine
• Methicillin	• Phenazopyridine
• Polymyxin B	hydrochloride
• Rifampin	• Quinine
• Sulfonamides	
• Tetracycline hydrochloride	**OTHER SUBSTANCES**
• Vancomycin	*Organic Solvents*
	• Carbon tetrachloride
Aminoglycoside Antibiotics	• Ethylene glycol
• Gentamicin	
• Kanamycin	*Nondrug Chemical Agents*
• Neomycin	• Radiographic contrast dye
• Netilmicin sulfate	• Pesticides
• Tobramycin	• Fungicides
	• Myoglobin (from break-
Antineoplastics	down of skeletal muscle)
• Cisplatin	
• Cyclophosphamide	*Heavy Metals and Ions*
• Methotrexate	• Arsenic
	• Bismuth
Other Drugs	• Copper sulfate
• Acetaminophen	• Gold salts
• Captopril	• Lead
• Cyclosporine	• Mercuric chloride

before tissue damage can occur. Careful physical assessment is required to evaluate the client's fluid status. Intake and output records and body weights can assist in identifying trends in fluid balance. If vascular volume is depleted, decreased urine output, postural hypotension, and tachycardia will be present. Prompt fluid resuscitation for clients in the prerenal stage can prevent intrarenal problems that can lead to renal tissue damage and renal failure.

The nurse also monitors laboratory values for any changes that reflect compromised renal function. Decreased urine specific gravity indicates a loss of urine-concentrating ability and is the earliest sign of renal tubular damage. Other laboratory values that are helpful in monitoring renal function include serum creatinine, urine and serum electrolytes, and blood urea nitrogen (BUN).

The nurse is aware of nephrotoxic substances that the client may ingest or be exposed to (see Table 72-4). The nurse questions orders for potentially nephrotoxic drugs, and the ordered dose is validated before the client receives the drug. Antibiotics are the most likely drug group to have nephrotoxic side effects. NSAIDs may cause or potentiate the risk for ARF. Combinations of drugs can cause synergistic reactions, further increasing the risk for ARF. If a client must receive a potentially nephrotoxic drug, the nurse monitors laboratory values, including BUN, creatinine, and drug peak and trough levels, closely for indications of actual or potential renal dysfunction.

● Assessment
HISTORY

The accurate diagnosis of ARF, including its type and its cause, largely depends on a detailed history. The history must include questions relating to the potential causes of ARF. The client is asked about exposure to nephrotoxins, recent surgery or trauma, transfusion, or other factors that might lead to renal ischemia. A medication history is also important, since treatment with certain anti-infectives, aminoglycoside antibiotics, angiotensin-converting enzyme (ACE) inhibitors, and NSAIDs can cause prerenal failure. Exposure to radiographic contrast medium can precipitate ARF, especially in older clients with reduced renal reserve. In some situations, ARF must be differentiated from chronic renal insufficiency (CRI). In these cases, the nurse asks about known renal diseases; systemic diseases, such as diabetes mellitus and systemic lupus erythematosus and other connective tissue diseases; and chronic hypertension.

To identify possible acute glomerulonephritis, questions about acute illnesses such as influenza, colds, gastroenteritis, and sore throats or pharyngitis, as well as the presence of cocoa-colored urine (hematuria), are included.

Reversible prerenal azotemia may be suspected after hypotension, hemorrhage or shock, burns, congestive heart failure (CHF), or any situation in which the client experiences intravascular volume depletion. Phosphorus-containing bowel preparations and being allowed nothing by mouth (NPO) preoperatively, in conjunction with the fluid losses of most surgical procedures, are sufficient to cause prerenal azotemia in many clients (Orias, Mahnensmith, & Perazella, 1999).

Postrenal azotemia can be identified by focusing on any history of obstructive disease processes that would be manifested as difficulty in starting the urine stream, changes in the amount or appearance of the urine, narrowing of the urine stream, nocturia, urgency, or symptoms of renal calculi. The nurse also notes any history of malignant carcinoma that may cause bilateral obstruction.

Because of the widely varied causes and the potentially reversible nature of the illness, the nurse obtains or validates a detailed history when ARF is suspected.

■ PHYSICAL ASSESSMENT/CLINICAL MANIFESTATIONS

The clinical manifestations of ARF are related to azotemia, as well to as the underlying cause (Chart 72-1). Signs and symptoms of *prerenal* azotemia are hypotension, tachycardia, decreased urine output, decreased cardiac output, decreased central venous pressure (CVP), and lethargy. The general clinical appearance of a client with prerenal azotemia is similar to that of a client with heart failure or dehydration, depending on the cause of the renal compromise.

Intrarenal (intrinsic) ARF usually involves damage to the glomeruli, interstitium, or tubules. Classic manifestations include oliguria or **anuria** (absence of urine), edema, hypertension, tachycardia, shortness of breath, jugular venous distention, elevated CVP, weight gain, rales or crackles, anorexia, nausea, vomiting, and lethargy or varying levels of consciousness. Clinical manifestations of electrolyte abnormalities, such as electrocardiographic (ECG) changes, may also be present.

CHART 72-1

KEY FEATURES *of*
Acute Renal Failure

Prerenal Azotemia
- Hypotension
- Tachycardia
- Decreased cardiac output
- Decreased central venous pressure
- Decreased urine output
- Lethargy

Intrarenal (Intrinsic) ARF and Postrenal Azotemia
- Renal manifestations
    Oliguria or anuria
    Increased urine specific gravity
- Cardiac manifestations
    Hypertension
    Tachycardia
    Jugular venous distention
    Increased central venous pressure
    ECG changes: tall T waves
- Respiratory manifestations
    Shortness of breath
    Orthopnea
    Rales or crackles
    Pulmonary edema
    Friction rub
- Gastrointestinal manifestations
    Anorexia
    Nausea
    Vomiting
    Flank pain
- Neurologic manifestations
    Lethargy
    Headache
    Tremors
    Confusion
- General manifestations
    Generalized edema
    Weight gain

ARF, Acute renal failure; *ECG,* electrocardiogram.

In clients with *postrenal* azotemia, the nurse monitors for oliguria or intermittent anuria, symptoms of uremia, and lethargy. The nurse reports changes in the character of the urine stream or difficulty starting urination.

■ LABORATORY ASSESSMENT

The numerous alterations in laboratory values in the client with ARF are similar to those occurring in chronic renal failure (CRF) (Chart 72-2; see also Laboratory Assessment [Chronic Renal Failure], p. 1681). The nurse can expect to find rising BUN and creatinine levels, and abnormalities in serum electrolytes. Table 72-5 shows the effects of renal failure on electrolyte values. Clients with ARF, however, typically do *not* experience the anemia associated with CRF unless there is hemorrhagic blood loss. However, uremic hemolysis secondary to severe azotemia can develop and may be the cause of anemia in the early phase of ARF.

In the early phases of ARF, urinalysis and microscopic examination of urine may provide diagnostic information. Urine sodium levels are often less than 10 to 20 mEq/L in clients with prerenal azotemia. In prerenal azotemia, the urine is often concentrated, with a specific gravity greater than 1.020. The presence of urine sediment (red blood cells [RBCs], RBC casts, tubular cells), myoglobin, or hemoglobin; a urinary sodium level lower than 40 mEq/L; and a specific gravity of 1.010 are indicative of intrarenal failure. In postrenal failure, urinary sodium levels may be normal to 40 mEq/L, with a specific gravity of 1.000 to 1.010.

■ RADIOGRAPHIC ASSESSMENT

X-ray studies help to determine the cause of ARF. A flat-plate x-ray film of the abdomen is obtained to determine the size of the kidneys. In the absence of underlying renal disease, normal-size kidneys are expected. Enlarged kidneys, possibly due to obstruction, may result from hydronephrosis. This x-ray finding may also illustrate obstructing calculi in the renal pelvis, ureters, or bladder.

Renal ultrasonography is a noninvasive procedure using high-energy sound waves. It is useful in the diagnosis of urinary tract obstruction. Dilation of the renal calyces and collecting ducts, as well as calculi, can be detected.

Computed tomography (CT) scans without contrast dye can be obtained to identify obstruction or tumors. Contrast media are usually avoided to prevent further renal damage. A sonogram is generally preferred to the intravenous pyelogram (IVP) to determine kidney size and the patency of the ureters.

Aortorenal angiography may be used to examine renal blood vessels and blood flow. The procedure involves the necessary risk of using contrast media but can reveal any occlusion of major renal vessels by thrombus, embolus, or stenosis. Cystoscopy or retrograde pyelography may be indicated to identify possible obstructive lesions in the urinary tract.

■ OTHER DIAGNOSTIC ASSESSMENT

Renal biopsy may be performed if the primary cause is uncertain, an immunologic disease is suspected, or the reversibility of the renal failure needs to be determined after ARF has persisted for an extended period. The nurse assists with many of the diagnostic studies, prepares the client before

CHART 72-2

LABORATORY PROFILE
Renal Failure

Test	Normal Range for Adults	Values in Renal Failure	Comments
TESTS TO EVALUATE REMOVAL OF NITROGENOUS WASTES			
Serum creatinine	0.6-1.1 mg/dL (women) 0.9-1.3 mg/dL (men) *Older adults:* Decreased	*In Chronic Renal Failure* May increase by 0.5-1.0 mg/dL every 1-2 yr May be as high as 15-30 mg/dL *before* symptoms of CRF are present *In Acute Renal Failure* Gradual increase of 1-2 mg/dL every 24-48 hr May increase 1-6 mg/dL in 1 wk or less	Consistently elevated levels indicate decreased renal function. Serum creatinine levels are used to evaluate the effectiveness of dialysis treatments.
Blood urea nitrogen	6-20 mg/dL *Older adults:* May be slightly increased	*In Chronic Renal Failure* May reach 180-200 mg/dL *before* symptoms develop *In Acute Renal Failure* Often increases by 10-20 mg/dL at same pace as serum creatinine level May reach 80-100 mg/dL within 1 wk	Increases depend on protein intake and other factors (see text). Rate of increase is controlled by limiting protein intake. This intervention is believed to decrease the rate of onset of systemic symptoms, such as anorexia, nausea, and vomiting. Elevations have multiple causes, including diminished renal function, excessive protein intake, sepsis, GI bleeding, dehydration, and tissue catabolism.
ELECTROLYTE STUDIES			
Serum sodium	136-145 mEq/L; 136-145 mmol/L (SI units)	Normal or decreased	Clients with renal failure retain sodium. With associated water retention, serum sodium levels seem normal. With excessive water retention, serum sodium levels seem decreased owing to hemodilution. Assess the client for evidence of fluid volume excess: edema, weight increase, or elevation of diastolic blood pressure. Limit fluid intake as directed. Avoid excessive sodium intake. Monitor for signs of hypernatremia: dry skin, excessive thirst, dry mucous membranes, elevated body temperature, and flushed skin. Client may need diuretics or dialysis.
Serum potassium	*Male:* 3.5-5.0 mmol/L (SI units) *Female:* 3.4-4.4 mmol/L (SI units)	Increased	Advise the client to avoid salt substitutes and to limit potassium-containing foods. Monitor for rapidly increasing serum potassium levels in ARF. ECG changes occur with serum potassium levels ≥6.5. Monitor for signs of hyperkalemia: dizziness, weakness, cardiac irregularities, muscle cramps, diarrhea, and nausea. May require administration of sodium polystyrene sulfonate (Kayexalate) or other treatment.

GI, Gastrointestinal; *ARF,* acute renal failure; *ECG,* electrocardiogram; *CRF,* chronic renal failure; *RBCs,* red blood cells; *WBCs,* white blood cells; *GFR,* glomerular filtration rate.

Continued

CHART 72-2

LABORATORY PROFILE
Renal Failure—cont'd

Test	Normal Range for Adults	Values in Renal Failure	Comments
Serum phosphorus (phosphate)	3.0-4.5 mg/dL; 0.97-1.45 mmol/L (SI units) *Older adults:* May be slightly decreased	Increased	Short-term increases have potential to cause rapid decrease in serum calcium level and cardiac rhythm disturbances. Long-term increases demineralize bones of calcium and enhance fracture potential. Phosphate-binding medications help control hyperphosphatemia and prevent calcium depletion from the bones.
Serum calcium	Total calcium: 9.0-10.5 mg/dL; 2.25-2.75 mmol/L (SI units) Ionized calcium: 4.60-5.08 mg/dL; 1.15-1.27 mmol/L (SI units) *Older adults:* Slightly decreased	Decreased	Decreases in ARF may necessitate replacement. Decreases in CRF may only be slight and may or may not necessitate replacement. As the serum phosphate level increases, the serum calcium level decreases. Chronic calcium deficiency leads to renal osteodystrophy. Control of phosphate excess is usually essential before calcium replacement is initiated. Monitor for signs and symptoms of hypocalcemia: abdominal cramps, hyperactive reflexes, tingling in fingertips, and spasms in feet and wrists (see also Chapter 13).
Serum magnesium	1.2-2.0 mEq/L; 0.66-1.07 mmol/L (SI units)	Increased	Advise the client to avoid compounds containing magnesium (e.g., laxatives).
Serum carbon dioxide combining power (bicarbonate)	23-29 mEq/L (venous); 23-29 mmol/L (SI units)	Decreased	Replace bicarbonate. Monitor respiratory rate and depth. Monitor for decreased orientation.
Arterial blood pH	7.31-7.42	Decreased (in metabolic acidosis) or normal	The respiratory system attempts to compensate by hyperventilation (increased rate and depth of respiration). Values are within the normal range if blood buffers and lungs can compensate. Monitor breathing rate and depth. Monitor level of consciousness.
Arterial blood bicarbonate (HCO_3^-)	21-28 mEq/L	Decreased	Provide replacement PO, IV, or by hemodialysis or peritoneal dialysis.
Arterial blood $Paco_2$	*Male:* 35-48 mm Hg *Female:* 32-45 mm Hg	Decreased	Monitor for respiratory fatigue (the client breathes more rapidly and deeply to "blow off" carbon dioxide).
OTHER BLOOD STUDIES Hemoglobin	11.7-15.5 g/dL (women); 7.4-9.9 mmol/L (SI units) 13.2-17.3 g/dL (men); 8.7-11.2 mmol/L (SI units) *Older adults:* Slightly decreased	Decreased	Decreased levels indicate anemia. Monitor for pallor, weakness, lethargy, dizziness, possible shortness of breath, and activity intolerance.
Hematocrit	*Female:* 35%-45% *Male:* 39%-49% *Older adults:* May be slightly decreased	Decreased to 20%	Same as for hemoglobin. With erythropoietin therapy, may be able to obtain levels as high as 36%.

GI, Gastrointestinal; *ARF,* acute renal failure; *ECG,* electrocardiogram; *CRF,* chronic renal failure; *RBCs,* red blood cells; *WBCs,* white blood cells; *GFR,* glomerular filtration rate.

CHART 72-2

LABORATORY PROFILE
Renal Failure—cont'd

Test	Normal Range for Adults	Values in Renal Failure	Comments
URINALYSIS*			
Specific gravity	Usually 1.016-1.022; possible range: 1.001-1.035	Usually decreased and fixed	Reflects inability of the tubules to produce a concentrated or diluted urine in response to changes in plasma osmolality. Monitor for fluid volume deficit or excess.
pH	Average: 5.5-6; possible range: 4.5-8	May be fixed; pH does not change with dietary changes	Collect a freshly voided specimen for testing
Glucose	None or <15 mg/dL Usually detectable in urine of nondiabetic clients when blood level is 160-180 mg/dL	Increased	The renal threshold is often increased; therefore the blood glucose level may be >160-180 mg/dL before glucose is detectable in the urine. Monitor *blood* glucose levels.
Protein	2-8 mg/dL	Increased when there is glomerular damage or disease	Increases may be an incidental and benign finding. Transient increases occur with extreme exercise, fever, stress, or infection. Persistent proteinuria requires 24-hr collection for determination of total quantity excreted. Persistent proteinuria may indicate a serious renal problem. Instruct the client about the need for follow-up. Instruct the client in the correct procedure for collection of 24-hr specimen (see Chapter 69).
Occult blood	No RBCs or occasionally 2 or 3 RBCs per high-power field No hemoglobin	More than 2 or 3 RBCs per high-power field Detectable hemoglobin	Hemoglobin is detectable when hemolysis of RBCs has occurred. Intact RBCs are only detectable with microscopic examination. Collect a freshly voided specimen for testing.
WBCs	0-5 per high-power field	Increased in urinary tract infection	Often indicates need for urine culture.
Bacteria	Less than 1000 colonies/mL	Increased in the presence of infection, with or without an increase in WBCs	Obtain urine culture.
Casts	None or a few; composed of RBCs, WBCs, protein, or tubular cell casts such as hyaline	Casts present	Casts may be a benign occurrence or may signify that some renal injury or disease is present. Collect a freshly voided specimen for direct microscopic examination.
Creatinine clearance	97-137 mL/min (men) 88-128 mL/min (women) *Older adults:* Progressively decreased with advancing age	Decreased	Change reflects decreases in GFR. Creatinine clearance is determined from a 24-hr urine collection and a serum creatinine value.

GI, Gastrointestinal; *ARF,* acute renal failure; *ECG,* electrocardiogram; *CRF,* chronic renal failure; *RBCs,* red blood cells; *WBCs,* white blood cells; *GFR,* glomerular filtration rate.
*Urine may become cloudy with heavy sediment. Urine output and appearance vary, depending on remaining renal function.

TABLE 72-5 • EFFECTS OF RENAL FAILURE ON ELECTROLYTE BALANCE

Electrolyte	Effects of Renal Failure	Problems	Treatments

Potassium	Retained with oliguria	Hyperkalemia
		  Cardiac dysrhythmias
		  Asystole
			Kayexalate, PO or rectal
			Regular IV insulin with 5% to 50% dextrose
			IV calcium gluconate
			Dialysis

Sodium	Retained	Dilutional hyponatremia Fluid volume excess Hypertension Congestive heart failure Pulmonary edema	Diuretics until no longer responsive Dialysis Fluid restriction Sodium restriction
Phosphate	Retained	Hyperphosphatemia Metastatic calcium phosphate deposits Renal bone disease	Phosphate-binding agents Limit phosphorus intake Vitamin D analogs
Calcium	Decreased gastrointestinal absorption Binds to phosphate	Bone demineralization Pathologic fractures	Replace vitamin D Calcium supplements
Hydrogen	Retained	Binds with bicarbonate for excretion through respiratory compensation	Dialysis Bicarbonate supplements
Bicarbonate	Depleted	Used for blood buffering to prevent metabolic acidemia	Dialysis Bicarbonate supplements
Magnesium	Retained	Potential for hypermagnesemia	Avoid magnesium-containing antacids and laxatives

the test, and provides follow-up care. The nurse must be aware of all test results and understand how they may affect the treatment regimen. (See Chapter 69 for a detailed discussion of renal diagnostic tests.)

• Interventions

The primary nursing diagnosis and collaborative problems for the client with acute renal failure (ARF) are Excess Fluid Volume, Potential for Pulmonary Edema, and Potential for Electrolyte Imbalances. The client with ARF may pass from the oliguric phase (in which fluid and electrolytes are retained) to the diuretic phase. If the client moves to the diuretic phase, hypovolemia and electrolyte *loss* are the primary problems. As a result, the client in the diuretic phase of ARF needs a plan of care that focuses on fluid and electrolyte *replacement* and monitoring.

These examples of output variation reflect the continually changing nature of ARF and the need for the plan of care to be constantly updated to reflect the client's movement through the stages of the disease process. Drug therapy, diet therapy, and renal replacement therapy (peritoneal dialysis [PD], hemodialysis [HD], or hemofiltration) are commonly employed in the management of ARF.

DRUG THERAPY. Clients with ARF receive numerous medications. As kidney function changes, the physician often modifies drug doses. The nurse is knowledgeable about the site of drug metabolism and is especially careful when administering medications. The nurse constantly monitors for possible side effects and interactions of the drugs the client with ARF is receiving (Chart 72-3; see also Drug Therapy under Chronic Renal Failure, p. 1685). Diuretics may be used to increase urine output.

In clients with prerenal azotemia, fluid challenges and diuretics are often used to promote renal perfusion. In clients

without signs and symptoms of fluid volume excess, 500 to 1000 mL of normal saline may be infused over a 1-hour period. In prerenal azotemia, the client should respond to the fluid challenge by producing urine soon after the initial bolus. Diuretics such as furosemide (Lasix) may also be ordered in conjunction with a fluid bolus. If oliguric renal failure is diagnosed, the fluid challenges and diuretics are discontinued. The physician may prescribe low-dose (1 to 3 µg/kg) dopamine in a continuous infusion to enhance renal perfusion and/or increase blood pressure (Zellner, 1999) (Chart 72-4). These clients often require central venous pressure (CVP) monitoring or measurement of pulmonary arterial pressure by means of a Swan-Ganz catheter for a more exact evaluation of their hemodynamic status. They also require constant nursing supervision for assessment of the response to fluid and drug administration. The nurse carefully monitors for signs of possible fluid overload.

Calcium channel blockers may be used to treat ARF resulting from nephrotoxic acute tubular necrosis (ATN) by preventing the influx of calcium into the kidney cells, thereby maintaining cell integrity and improving the glomerular filtration rate (GFR).

DIET THERAPY. Clients who have ARF often have a high rate of catabolism. The exact mechanism for this state is not well understood. Increases in catabolism may be related to the stress of a critical illness, causing an increase in levels of circulating catecholamines, cortisol, and glucagon, all of which stimulate catabolism. The rate of catabolism is correlated with the severity of uremia and azotemia. This hypercatabolic state causes the breakdown of muscle for protein, which leads to an increase in azotemia and an even more elevated serum blood urea nitrogen (BUN) level.

If the client with ARF has an adequate dietary intake (see Imbalanced Nutrition: Less Than Body Requirements [Chronic Renal Failure] , p. 1682), nutritional support may

CHART 72-3

DRUG THERAPY *for* Renal Failure

Drug	Usual Dosage	Indications	Nursing Interventions	Rationale
CARDIOTONICS				
Digoxin (Lanoxin, Novodigoxin✤)	0.125-0.25 mg PO or IV daily or every other day *Older adults:* 0.0625-0.125 PO or IV daily or every other day	Decreased stroke volume Decreased strength of cardiac contractions	Monitor for signs of digoxin toxicity and hypokalemia. Monitor for bradycardia (pulse <50-60 beats/min). Monitor serum drug levels.	Digoxin remains in the body longer when renal function is impaired. Bradycardia is a sign of digoxin toxicity. A toxic digoxin level is >2.5 ng/mL.
VITAMINS AND MINERALS				
Folic acid (vitamin B_9, Folvite, Novofolacid✤)	0.1 mg PO, SC, or IM daily	Dietary supplement	Usually given after dialysis.	Water-soluble vitamins are removed during dialysis.
Ferrous sulfate (Feosol, Novoferrosulfa✤)	325 mg tid or qid PO	Anemia	Monitor for constipation. Note any change in the stools, which normally become blackish green.	Constipation is a frequent and uncomfortable side effect associated with oral iron supplements. The color is caused by the presence of unabsorbed iron and is harmless.
BIOLOGIC RESPONSE MODIFIERS				
Erythropoietin alpha (Epogen, Procrit)	50-100 units/kg IV or SC 3 times/wk	Anemia associated with CRF	Monitor hematocrit twice weekly until maintenance dose is achieved. Monitor blood pressure.	The dose is based on response as measured by hematocrit changes. Rapid rise in hematocrit can cause hypertension.
PHOSPHATE BINDERS				
Aluminum hydroxide gel (Amphojel, AlternaGEL, Alu-Cap, Nephrox) Aluminum carbonate gel (Basaljel)	500 mg-2 g bid-qid PO as tablets, capsules, or oral suspension	Phosphate binder Prevention of renal osteodystrophy	Monitor for constipation, which occurs frequently. Monitor for signs of hypophosphatemia. Monitor serum aluminum levels.	Constipation is a frequent side effect of many drugs that bind phosphorus. These drugs can prevent intestinal absorption of phosphorus to the extent that the client develops hypophosphatemia. Aluminum toxicity may cause bone disease and dementia.
Sevelamer hydrochloride (Renagel)	Serum phosphorus 6.0-7.5 mg/dL; 2 capsules tid Serum phosphorus 7.6-8.9 mg/dL; 3 capsules tid Serum phosphorus >9.0 mg/dL; 4 capsules tid	Hyperphosphatemia	Give with meals Tell client to swallow capsule whole; do not chew. Monitor serum phosphorus levels.	Drug binds with phosphorus in food, preventing absorption. Drug expands when capsule is broken. Drug can cause hypophosphatemia.
Calcium carbonate (Tums, OsCal, CalciChew)	1-3 PO daily in divided doses tid or qid	Dietary supplement Phosphate binder	Give only when serum phosphate levels are normal. Monitor for hypercalcemia, constipation, and soft-tissue calcifications Give after meals.	Calcium supplements may cause a *decrease* in serum phosphate levels because these two minerals exist in blood in a balanced, *reciprocal* relationship. Giving binders after meals enhances binding capacity.
STOOL SOFTENERS AND LAXATIVES				
Docusate sodium (Colace) Bisacodyl (Dulcolax, Bisco-Lax, Laxit✤)	100-300 mg daily 5-10 mg PO or PR daily or every other day	Prevention of constipation caused by limited fluid intake, iron supplements, and phosphate binders	Observe for abdominal cramps and diarrhea. Monitor bowel movements.	These gastrointestinal effects indicate drug overdose. Monitoring bowel movements is a way of determining medication effectiveness.

CHART 72-4

BEST PRACTICE *for*
Administering Renal-Dose Dopamine

- Take an accurate weight because the dose is ordered according to the client's weight.
- Know the hospital's policy regarding who is responsible for calculating the rate of infusion (i.e., physician, pharmacist, or nurse). Renal-dose dopamine is 1 to 5 μg/kg body wt/min but is converted to mL/min for an IV infusion.
- Before hanging the dopamine infusion, double-check the amount of dopamine added to the solution, the total volume of solution (usually 250 mL), and the calculation milliliters per minute.
- Do not hang the dopamine infusion until all questions about the calculation are clarified.
- If dopamine is to be infused into a peripheral vein, be sure that the line is intact and secured.
- Once the infusion is started, check the client's blood pressure and pulse per hospital policy or the physician's orders, usually at least every 2 hours.
- Notify the physician of changes in vital signs per policy or the physician's orders.
- Monitor the IV site frequently for clinical manifestations of infiltration.
- If infiltration occurs, stop the infusion but do not discontinue the IV catheter. Prepare for phentolamine (Regitine, Rogitine♣) administration through the IV catheter and subcutaneously into the infiltrated tissue.

not be necessary. The health care provider may order a consultation with a dietitian, who will calculate the client's caloric requirements. In conjunction with the dietitian, the health care provider will order a diet with specific levels of protein and sodium and the amount of fluids required. If the client does not require dialysis, 0.6 g/kg of body weight or 40 g/day of protein is ordered. For clients needing dialysis, the protein level needed will range from 1 to 1.5 g/kg. The amount of dietary sodium ranges from 60 to 90 mEq. In the presence of hyperkalemia, dietary potassium is restricted to 60 to 70 mEq. The amount of fluid permitted is generally calculated to equal the urine volume plus 500 mL. The nurse continually assesses oral intake to make certain that sufficient calories are consumed.

Many clients with ARF are too ill or too anorexic to eat sufficient food. For these clients, some form of nutritional support (e.g., total parenteral nutrition [TPN] or hyperalimentation) must be initiated to avoid catabolism. The goals of nutritional support in ARF are to provide sufficient nutrients to maintain or improve nutritional status, to preserve lean body mass, to restore or maintain fluid balance, and to preserve renal function.

If TPN is administered, the solutions may be formulated to meet the client's specific needs. Because kidney function is unstable in ARF, the nurse constantly monitors the serum electrolyte concentrations and facilitates revisions in the hyperalimentation solution as needed. In addition to TPN, intravenous (IV) fat emulsion (Intralipid) infusions provide a nonprotein source of calories. In uremic clients, fat emulsions can be used in place of glucose to avoid the problems associated with excessive sugars.

DIALYSIS THERAPIES. Hemodialysis (HD) and peritoneal dialysis (PD) may be implemented for clients with ARF if necessary. Until recently, intermittent hemodialysis

(IHD) has been the most common treatment of ARF. The following are indications for dialysis in ARF:

- Uremia nitrogenous waste in blood
- Persistent hyperkalemia
- Uncompensated metabolic acidosis
- Fluid volume excess unresponsive to diuretics
- Uremic pericarditis
- Uremic encephalopathy

Immediate vascular access for HD in clients with ARF is established by placement of a dual- or triple-lumen catheter specifically designed for HD. For HD that is expected to be necessary for several weeks, the catheter is usually placed into the subclavian or internal jugular vein. If only one or two treatments are expected to be necessary, as for removal of drugs or toxins by hemoperfusion, a femoral site may be selected. Longer use of the femoral site is generally discouraged because of positioning limitations (i.e., required immobility) and other potential complications, such as hematomas and infection. Repeated cannulation of the femoral site also increases the risk for hematoma formation and makes repeated use of the vein impossible.

The subclavian vein is often preferred over femoral vein cannulation because the catheter can be left in place between dialysis treatments. This placement is also a disadvantage, however, because the longer the catheter is left in place, the greater is the chance for infection. The subclavian dialysis catheter (Figure 72-1) is inserted at the bedside. A physician performs the sterile procedure, and then the catheter is covered with a sterile dressing. Catheter placement is checked by chest x-ray examination before its use.

HD catheters have two lumens separating the outflow and inflow extensions of the catheter. Consequently, the continuous outflow of blood to be dialyzed is separated from the dialyzed blood returned through the inflow port and lumen. A triple-lumen catheter for HD is now available. The third lumen provides a port for drawing venous blood or administering medication and fluid without interruption of the dialysis lumens.

PD may also be used in the treatment of ARF, but its use may be limited in the critically ill, since mechanically ventilated clients may not be able to tolerate the accompanying abdominal distention, and since its use requires an intact, uninfected abdominal cavity (Giuliano & Pysznik, 1998). PD uses the peritoneum as a semipermeable membrane for which dialysate is infused through a catheter implanted in the peritoneum. A more complete discussion of PD is provided later in this chapter under Chronic Renal Failure, pp. 1694-1697).

CONTINUOUS RENAL REPLACEMENT THERAPIES. Currently, continuous renal replacement therapies (CRRTs) have become the standard treatment for ARF. Renal replacement therapies in the form of hemofiltration may be better tolerated than HD for clients who are critically ill, since rapid shifts of fluids and electrolytes associated with HD are avoided (Giuliano & Pysznik, 1998).

Continuous arteriovenous hemofiltration (CAVH) and continuous arteriovenous hemodialysis and filtration (CAVHD) provide additional renal replacement therapies for clients with ARF. These procedures share some similarities with HD, but their use and indications are specific and limited.

CAVH is indicated for clients who are fluid volume overloaded, resistant to diuretics, and hemodynamically unstable. The implementation of CAVH requires the placement of both arterial and venous catheters to provide adequate filtration

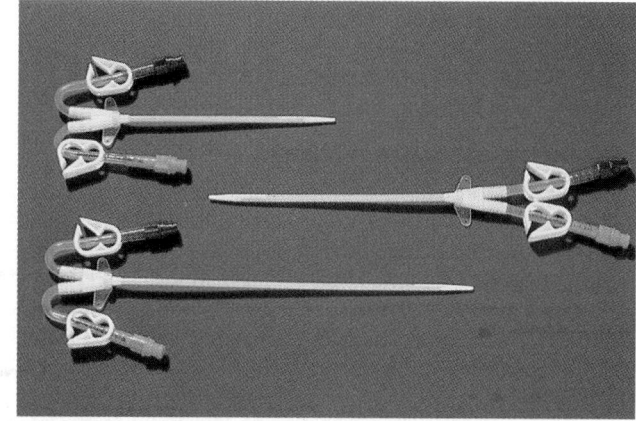

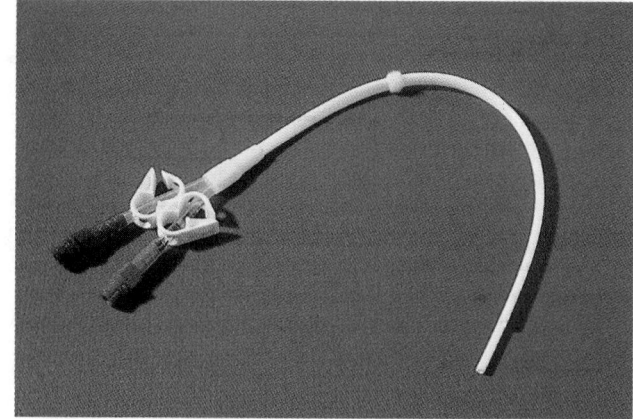

Figure 72-1 ● Subclavian dialysis catheters. These catheters are radiopaque tubes that can be used for hemodialysis access. The Y-shaped tubing allows arterial outflow and venous return through a single catheter. **A,** Mahurkar catheters, made of polyurethane and used for short-term access. **B,** A PermCath catheter, made of silicone and used for long-term access. (Courtesy Kendall Company, Bothell, WA.)

and a mean arterial pressure of at least 60 mm Hg. CAVH removes large amounts of plasma water and solutes on a continuous basis. When large volumes of plasma water are removed, electrolytes are also removed. Electrolytes are replaced through prescribed amounts of IV electrolyte solution. The most significant disadvantage of arteriovenous (AV) filtration is the risk of bleeding associated with anticoagulants used to prevent membrane clotting (Craig, 1998).

A double-lumen dialysis catheter inserted into a large vein (subclavian, jugular) provides access for CAVHD. CAVHD uses a **dialysate** (a solution composed of water, glucose, sodium chloride, potassium, magnesium, calcium, and bicarbonate) delivery system to remove nitrogenous or other waste products in addition to fluid in clients with limited cardiac output, those with significant hypotension, or those who have been unresponsive to diuretic therapy. The conventional form of HD would not be tolerated, and PD would probably be inadequate for the fluid removal required.

Continuous venovenous hemofiltration (CVVH) is often considered to be the treatment of choice for critically ill clients. CVVH requires only a double-lumen venous catheter for access and is powered by a pump, making the rate of filtration more reliable than that of the mean arterial pressure (Giuliano & Pysznik, 1998). There is a risk of air embolus as-

sociated with the pump, but most pumps are equipped with alarms that detect air. These systems also require the use of anticoagulants, but at lower doses than needed for AV systems. These procedures are performed in a critical care unit, and clients require continuous nursing care.

POSTHOSPITAL CARE. The posthospital care for a client with ARF varies widely, depending on the status of the disease when the client is discharged. The course of ARF varies, with recovery lasting up to several months. If the renal failure is resolving, follow-up care is often provided by a nephrologist or by the family physician in consultation with the nephrologist. On occasion, however, ARF results in permanent renal damage and the need for chronic dialysis or even transplantation. In these cases, the posthospital care may be as extensive and multifaceted as it is for any other client with chronic renal failure (CRF) (see Community-Based Care [Chronic Renal Failure] , p. 1700).

If the ARF is in the process of resolving, the follow-up care may involve a variety of services. Frequent medical visits are necessary, as are routine laboratory blood and urine tests to monitor renal function. Consultation with a dietitian may be needed to modify the client's diet according to the degree of renal function and ongoing nutritional requirements. Clients continuing dialysis after discharge must be taught to limit foods high in potassium and sodium and to observe protein restrictions. In addition, education concerning the need for limited fluid intake may be necessary.

Some clients may need some form of temporary dialysis until their kidneys can metabolize fluid and waste products independently. The dialysis begun while the client was hospitalized may be continued at an outpatient dialysis center for as long as necessary. Teaching concerning the type of dialysis, care of vascular access sites, dietary restrictions, fluid restrictions, and prevention of complications is ongoing throughout the recovery phase. Depending on their level of independence and family support, some clients may also need home care nursing or social work assistance.

CHRONIC RENAL FAILURE

■ OVERVIEW

In contrast to the ability of the kidneys to regain function following acute renal failure (ARF), chronic renal failure (CRF) represents a clinical syndrome of progressive, irreversible kidney injury. When kidney function is inadequate for sustaining life, CRF is referred to as end-stage renal disease (ESRD). Terms associated with renal failure include **azotemia** (accumulation of nitrogenous waste products in the bloodstream), **uremia** (azotemia with clinical symptoms [Chart 72-5]), **uremic syndrome** (the diverse systemic clinical and laboratory manifestations associated with ESRD), and *renal replacement therapy* (hemodialysis [HD], peritoneal dialysis [PD], renal transplantation; necessary to sustain life in clients with renal failure). ARF and CRF are compared in Table 72-1.

■ Pathophysiology

■ STAGES OF RENAL FAILURE

The kidneys tend to fail in an organized fashion. The client's progression toward ESRD usually begins with a gradual decrease in renal function of 30% to 50% (Table 72-6). Initially,

---

CHART 72-5

KEY FEATURES *of*
Uremia

- Metallic taste in the mouth
- Anorexia
- Nausea
- Vomiting
- Muscle cramps
- Itching

- Fatigue and lethargy
- Hiccups
- Edema
- Dyspnea
- Muscle cramps
- Paresthesias

TABLE 72-6 • PROGRESSION TOWARD CHRONIC RENAL FAILURE

STAGE I: DIMINISHED RENAL RESERVE
- Renal function is reduced, but no accumulation of metabolic wastes occurs.
- The healthier kidney compensates for the diseased kidney.
- Ability to concentrate urine is decreased, resulting in nocturia and polyuria.
- A 24-hour urine collection for creatinine clearance is necessary to detect that renal reserve is less than normal.

STAGE II: RENAL INSUFFICIENCY
- Metabolic wastes begin to accumulate in the blood because the unaffected nephrons can no longer compensate.
- Responsiveness to diuretics is decreased, resulting in oliguria and edema.
- The degree of insufficiency is determined by decreasing the GFR and is classified as mild, moderate, or severe.
- Treatment is medical.

STAGE III: END-STAGE RENAL DISEASE
- Excessive amounts of metabolic wastes such as urea and creatinine accumulate in the blood.
- The kidneys are unable to maintain homeostasis.
- Treatment is by dialysis or other renal replacement therapy.

GFR, Glomerular filtration rate.

---

there is a *diminished renal reserve*. A 24-hour urine specimen for monitoring creatinine clearance is necessary to detect that renal reserve is less than normal. In this stage, reduced renal function occurs without any measurable accumulation of metabolic wastes in the serum because of the ability of the unaffected nephrons to compensate for the decreased functioning of the diseased nephrons. Renal damage is accompanied by an elevation in the systemic blood pressure, resulting in an increase in the pressure within the glomerular apparatus and the remaining unaffected nephrons. Eventually, the unaffected nephrons may be damaged by long-term exposure to this increased pressure, leading to the progressive renal damage characteristic of CRF. However, under stressful conditions, such as infection, fluid overload, or dehydration, renal function at this stage can appear compromised.

In the next stage, *renal insufficiency,* metabolic wastes begin to accumulate in the blood because the healthier kidney tissue can no longer compensate for the loss of nonfunctioning nephrons. Levels of blood urea nitrogen (BUN), serum creatinine, uric acid, and phosphorus are increasingly elevated in relation to the degree of renal function loss. Careful nursing and medical management of fluid volume, blood pressure, electrolytes, dietary intake, and medication administration may slow the progression of renal failure.

Many clients ultimately progress to *end-stage renal disease (ESRD)*. Excessive amounts of nitrogenous wastes, such as urea and creatinine, accumulate in the blood, and the kidneys cannot maintain homeostasis. Initially, severe fluid overload and electrolyte and acid-base imbalances occur. Without renal replacement therapy, fatal complications are likely.

■ PATHOLOGIC ALTERATIONS

Renal dysfunction causes multiple pathologic situations, including disruptions in the glomerular filtration rate (GFR), abnormalities of urine production and water excretion, electrolyte imbalances, and metabolic abnormalities. The kidneys can maintain an effective GFR until 70% to 80% of renal function is lost. Homeostasis is maintained until late in the course of renal failure. When less than 20% of the nephrons are functional, the GFR is altered despite hypertrophy of the remaining nephrons. This alteration occurs because the hypertrophied nephrons can maintain the excretion of solutes or waste products only by decreasing water reabsorption. As a result, **hyposthenuria** (the loss of urine concentrating ability) and *polyuria* (increased urine output) occur. Both hyposthenuria and polyuria are early signs of CRF and, if the problem is untreated at this stage, can cause severe dehydration.

As the disease progresses, the ability to dilute the urine is increasingly diminished, resulting in urine with a fixed osmolality **(isosthenuria).** As renal function continues to diminish, the concentration of urea is increased in the blood, and urine output decreases. When renal function deteriorates to this level, the client is at risk for fluid overload because of loss of adequate urine output.

■ METABOLIC ALTERATIONS

UREA AND CREATININE. Renal failure also causes disturbances in urea and creatinine excretion. Creatinine is derived from creatine and phosphocreatine, which are present in skeletal muscle. The normal rate of creatinine excretion depends on muscle mass, physical activity, and diet. Without major alterations in the diet or physical activity, the serum creatinine level remains relatively constant. Creatinine is partially excreted by the renal tubules, and a decrease in renal function leads to a buildup of serum creatinine. Urea is the primary product of protein metabolism and is excreted by the kidneys. The BUN level normally varies directly with protein intake.

An important method for accurately estimating the GFR is to monitor the creatinine clearance of the kidneys. As renal function and glomerular filtration diminish, creatinine clearance decreases and the serum creatinine level rises (see Chapter 69).

SODIUM. In addition to decreased BUN and creatinine excretion, alterations in sodium excretion are common. Early in chronic renal failure (CRF), the client is particularly susceptible to hyponatremia (sodium depletion) because, although a diminishing number of nephrons are reabsorbing sodium at their maximal ability, there is an obligatory loss of sodium in urine production. Thus the polyuria often seen in early renal failure also causes sodium depletion.

In the later stages of renal failure, the capacity of the kidneys to excrete sodium diminishes as urine production decreases. As a result, sodium retention can occur with only modest increases in dietary sodium intake and can lead to severe fluid and electrolyte imbalances (see Chapters 12 and 13). Sodium retention manifests as hypertension and edema.

Despite the sodium retention, the concurrent retention of water results in an *apparently* normal serum sodium level; dilutional hyponatremia is likely, since fluid volume excess develops (see Table 72-5).

POTASSIUM. The kidney is the primary organ responsible for potassium excretion. Any increase in potassium load during the later stages of renal disease can lead to hyperkalemia (excessive potassium retention). Normal serum potassium levels of 3.5 to 5 mEq/L are maintained until the 24-hour urine output falls below 500 mL with a decreased GFR. When hyperkalemia develops, serum levels are quickly elevated and may be 7 to 8 mEq/L or higher. Severe electrocardiographic (ECG) changes result from this elevation, increasing the risk of fatal dysrhythmias. Other factors contributing to hyperkalemia in renal failure include ingestion of potassium in medications, failure to restrict potassium in the diet, excessive tissue breakdown secondary to the hypercatabolic state, blood transfusions, and excessive bleeding or hemorrhage. (See Chapter 13 for further discussion of hyperkalemia.)

ACID-BASE BALANCE. In the early stages of renal disease, loss of functioning nephrons causes little change in blood pH because the remaining nephrons increase their rate of acid excretion. As the loss of nephrons continues, the kidneys cannot compensate and acid excretion is restricted; a *bicarbonate deficit* or *metabolic acidosis* results (see Chapter 16).

Many factors contribute to metabolic acidosis in renal failure. First, the kidney becomes unable to excrete excessive hydrogen ions. Normally, renal tubular cells secrete hydrogen ions into the tubular lumen for excretion, but ammonia and bicarbonate are required in order for excretion to take place. In clients with renal failure, the kidney's ability to produce ammonia is decreased, and the normal reabsorption of filtered bicarbonate does not occur. This process leads to a buildup of hydrogen ions for which the supply of bicarbonate and other buffering bases is inadequate. As a result, there is a base (bicarbonate) deficit in an environment with excess acid. In the presence of hyperkalemia, renal ammonium production and excretion are inhibited further.

As renal failure advances and acid retention increases, respiratory compensation is essential for maintenance of a blood pH compatible with life. The respiratory system compensates for the decreased pH by increasing the rate and depth of breathing to excrete carbon dioxide through the lungs. This pattern of breathing, called **Kussmaul respiration,** is increasingly apparent when worsening renal failure results in respiratory alkalosis. Serum bicarbonate measures the extent of metabolic acidosis (bicarbonate deficit). Individuals with CRF usually require treatment with alkali replacement to counteract acidosis.

CALCIUM AND PHOSPHATE. A complex, balanced reciprocal relationship between calcium and phosphate is influenced by vitamin D (see Chapter 13). Vitamin D facilitates calcium absorption in the intestines, and the kidney produces 1,25-dihydroxycholecalciferol, a hormone needed to create active vitamin D.

In renal failure, phosphate retention and a deficiency of active vitamin D contribute to the disruption in calcium and phosphate balance and metabolism. Normally, excessive dietary phosphate is excreted by the kidneys in the urine.

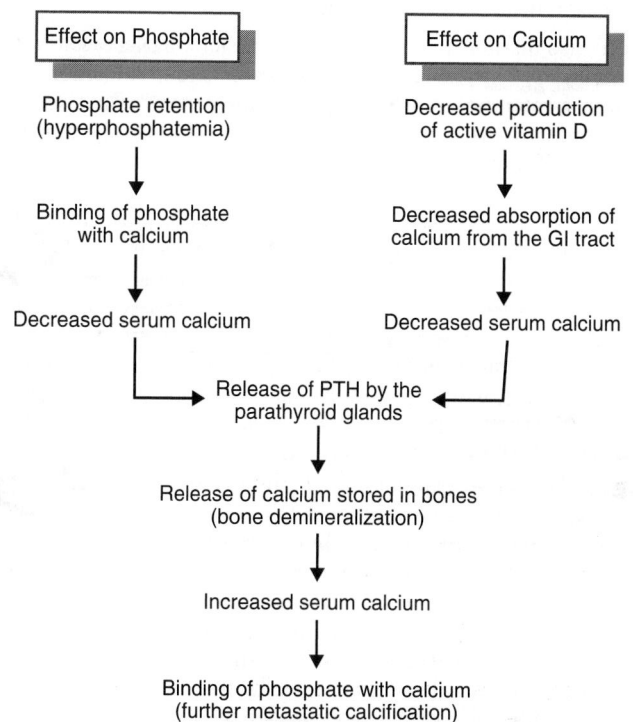

Figure 72-2 ● The effects of renal failure on phosphate and calcium balance. (*GI,* Gastrointestinal; *PTH,* parathyroid hormone.)

Parathyroid hormone (PTH) regulates the amount of phosphate in the blood by causing tubular excretion of phosphate when there is a serum phosphate excess. One of the initial effects of decreased renal function is decreased phosphate excretion due to a diminished GFR (Figure 72-2). As plasma phosphate levels increase (causing hyperphosphatemia), calcium levels decrease (causing hypocalcemia). Chronic hypocalcemia results in chronic stimulation, hyperplasia, and hypertrophy of the parathyroid glands. Under the influence of additional PTH, calcium is released from storage areas in bones (**bone resorption**), which results in demineralization. The additional calcium is needed to compensate, or balance, excess plasma phosphate concentration. The problem of hypocalcemia is compounded because decreased renal function also causes decreased production of active vitamin D. Thus less calcium is absorbed through the intestinal mucosa in the absence of sufficient vitamin D.

The pathologic process in bone metabolism and structure caused by hypocalcemia and hyperphosphatemia is called **renal osteodystrophy.** Skeletal demineralization resulting from hyperparathyroidism may be manifested as bone pain, sclerosis of the spine, pseudofractures, demineralization of parts of the skull, osteomalacia, resorption of bone, or loss of the lamina dura in the teeth.

Metastatic calcifications, crystals formed from excessive calcium phosphate, may precipitate in various parts of the body. When the plasma concentration of the calcium-phosphate product (serum calcium concentration times serum phosphate concentration) exceeds 70 mg/dL, the crystals may lodge in the kidneys, heart, lungs, major blood vessels, joints, eyes (causing conjunctivitis), and brain. Uremic pruritus is also believed to be the result of calcium-phosphate imbalances and excess PTH production.

■ CARDIAC ALTERATIONS

CRF also disrupts the cardiovascular system. Excess fluid retention associated with uremia leaves the client vulnerable to congestive heart failure (CHF) and pulmonary edema. Excess metabolic toxins are thought to be responsible for the development of uremic pericarditis.

HYPERTENSION. Approximately 80% to 90% of clients with CRF have hypertension. Hypertension may be either the cause or the result of CRF. The elevation in blood pressure results from fluid and sodium overload and the malfunction of the renin-angiotensin-aldosterone system. The retention of sodium and water in renal disease causes circulatory overload, which leads to an elevated blood pressure. The kidneys respond to a decrease in renal blood flow or low serum sodium levels by trying to improve the renal blood flow. The release of renin further stimulates the production of angiotensin and aldosterone. Angiotensin causes vasoconstriction and an elevation in blood pressure. Aldosterone, a mineralocorticoid released by the adrenal glands, stimulates the distal convoluted tubule to reabsorb sodium and water. Consequently, plasma volume is expanded, and the blood pressure is elevated. As a result of this malfunction of the renin-angiotensin-aldosterone system, the blood pressure is elevated either by vasoconstriction or by volume expansion. The kidneys do not recognize the increase in blood pressure and continue to produce renin. The result is severe hypertension that is difficult to treat and that ultimately worsens renal function. Many clients with CRF also have cardiomyopathy and left ventricular hypertrophy as a consequence of prolonged hypertension.

HYPERLIPIDEMIA. CRF is associated with alterations in the metabolism of lipoproteins. Increased triglyceride, total cholesterol, and low-density lipoprotein levels are seen with a corresponding reduction in high-density lipoprotein levels. CRF renders individuals at increased risk for coronary artery disease and acute cardiac events.

CONGESTIVE HEART FAILURE. Many clients with renal failure have some form of myocardial dysfunction. CRF causes an increased workload on the heart because of anemia, hypertension, and fluid overload. Left ventricular hypertrophy and CHF are common manifestations of late end-stage renal disease (ESRD). Uremia itself may cause uremic cardiomyopathy, the uremic toxin effect on the myocardium. CHF is also common in these clients because of the presence of hypertension and coronary artery disease. Cardiac disease is the leading cause of death in clients with ESRD (U.S. Renal Data Systems, 1999).

UREMIC PERICARDITIS. Pericarditis also occurs in clients with CRF. If it is not treated effectively, this inflammation of the pericardium can lead to pericardial effusion, cardiac tamponade, and death. The pericardial sac becomes inflamed and irritated by uremic toxins or infection. Signs and symptoms include localized, severe chest pain, an increased pulse rate, a low-grade fever, and an intermittent and transient pericardial friction rub that can be heard on auscultation.

As the pericarditis continues and the pericardial effusion worsens, dysrhythmias may develop; heart tones become softer and less audible, the blood pressure decreases, and the client may experience shortness of breath. Progressive pericardial effusion results in cardiac tamponade, a medical and surgical emergency in which pulse pressure diminishes and bradycardia or asystole results. Treatment of pericardial tamponade involves removal of pericardial fluid by placement of a needle, catheter, or drainage tube into the pericardium or pericardiectomy with pericardial drainage. The incidence of uremic pericarditis has diminished with the initiation of early, aggressive dialysis.

■ HEMATOLOGIC ALTERATIONS

Anemia is the primary hematologic abnormality in clients with CRF. Normochromic, normocytic anemia is a common manifestation of CRF and contributes to the client's symptoms. The causes include a decreased erythropoietin level with resulting decreased red blood cell (RBC) production, decreased RBC survival time resulting from uremia, iron and folic acid deficiencies, and impaired platelet function as a result of uremic toxins.

■ GASTROINTESTINAL ALTERATIONS

Uremia can affect all levels of the gastrointestinal (GI) system. The normal flora of the oral cavity is altered in uremia. The mouth normally contains the enzyme urease, which hydrolyzes urea. The ammonia generated from this reaction contributes to uremic halitosis and may also cause uremic **stomatitis** (mouth inflammation).

Anorexia, nausea, vomiting, and hiccups are relatively common in clients with uremia. The specific cause of these symptoms is uncertain but may be related to increased nitrogenous waste levels (i.e., blood urea nitrogen [BUN] and creatinine levels) and metabolic acidosis.

Peptic ulcer disease is also common in clients with uremia; however, the exact cause is unclear. Uremic colitis with profound watery diarrhea or constipation may also be present in clients with uremia. Ulcerations may occur in the stomach or small or large intestine, causing erosion of blood vessels. The blood loss caused by these erosions may result in melena or, in more serious cases, may progress to hemorrhagic shock from severe GI bleeding.

■ Etiology

The etiology of CRF is complex (Table 72-7). There are more than 100 different disease processes that can result in progressive loss of renal function (see also Chapter 71). However, diabetes and hypertension are the most common causes of CRF.

■ Incidence/Prevalence

The number of clients with CRF is continually increasing. The 1999 U.S. Renal Data Systems annual report suggests that more than 307,000 people in the United States are receiving treatment for ESRD. In 1999 the reported incidence of renal disease (i.e., new clients requiring renal replacement therapy) was 79,102. There were more than 57,000 deaths in 1999 related to ESRD. Three primary causes of ESRD include diabetes mellitus (40%), hypertension (27%), and

TABLE 72-7 • SELECTED CAUSES OF CHRONIC RENAL FAILURE

MORPHOLOGIC

Glomerular Disease
- Glomerulonephritis
- Basement membrane disease
- Goodpasture's syndrome
- Intercapillary glomerulosclerosis

Tubular Disease
- Chronic hypercalcemia
- Chronic potassium depletion
- Franconi's syndrome
- Heavy metal (lead) poisoning

Vascular Disease of the Kidney
- Ischemic disease of the kidney
- Bilateral renal artery stenosis
- Nephrosclerosis
- Hyperparathyroidism

Urinary Tract Disease
- Obstructive uropathy

Congenital Anomalies
- Hypoplastic kidneys
- Medullary cystic disease
- Polycystic kidney disease

ETIOLOGIC

Infection
- Pyelonephritis
- Tuberculosis

Systemic Vascular Disease
- Intrarenal renovascular hypertension
- Extrarenal renovascular hypertension

Metabolic Renal Disease
- Amyloidosis
- Gout (hyperuricemic nephropathy)
- Diabetic nephropathy
- Milk-alkali syndrome
- Sarcoidosis

Connective Tissue Disease
- Progressive systemic sclerosis
- Systemic lupus erythematosus
- Polyarteritis

NOTE: List is not all-inclusive.

CHART 72-6

CLIENT EDUCATION GUIDE
Prevention of Renal and Urinary Problems

- Be alert to the general appearance of your urine. Note any changes in its color, clarity, or odor.
- Changes in the frequency or volume of urine passage occur with changes in fluid intake. More frequent, or infrequent, voiding not associated with changes in fluid intake may signal potential problems.
- Any discomfort or distress with the passage of urine is not normal. Pain, burning, urgency, aching, or difficulty with initiating urine flow or complete bladder emptying is of some concern.
- The kidneys need $1\frac{1}{2}$ to 2 quarts of fluid a day to flush out your body wastes. Water is the ideal flushing agent.
- Changes in kidney function are often silent for many years. Periodically ask your health care provider to measure your kidney function with a blood test (serum creatinine) and a urinalysis.
- If you have a history of renal disease, diabetes mellitus, or hypertension (high blood pressure), or a family history of kidney disease, you should know your serum creatinine level and your 24-hour creatinine clearance. At least one checkup per year that includes laboratory blood and urine testing of kidney function is recommended.
- If you are identified as having decreased kidney function, ask about whether any prescribed medication, diet, diagnostic test, or therapeutic procedure will present a risk to your current kidney function. Check out all nonprescription medications with your physician or pharmacist before using them.

glomerulonephritis (11%). There is a higher incidence of ESRD in men than in women (U.S. Renal Data Systems, 1999). The greatest increase in ESRD is in those 65 years of age and older. More than 221,000 people were estimated to be receiving renal replacement therapy in the United States in 1999 (U.S. Renal Data Systems, 1999). Chart 72-6 addresses prevention of renal and urinary problems.

CULTURAL CONSIDERATIONS

Significant racial differences can be observed in the incidence of ESRD. The highest incidence of ESRD is in African Americans, followed by Native Americans and Asians. Caucasians have the lowest incidence of the disease (U.S. Renal Data Systems, 1999).

► COLLABORATIVE MANAGEMENT
● Assessment

■ HISTORY

When taking a history from a client with suspected chronic renal failure (CRF), the nurse focuses on the signs and symptoms of CRF. The client's age and gender are noted. The nurse obtains accurate weight and height measurements and inquires about usual weight and recent weight gain or loss. Weight gain may indicate cardiovascular overload and fluid retention caused by poorly functioning kidneys. Weight loss may be the result of anorexia associated with the uremic syndrome.

The nurse also obtains a complete history of known renal or urologic disorders, long-term health problems, medication use, and current health conditions. The client is asked about knowledge of any existing renal disease or family history of renal disease, which might indicate a hereditary disorder. A history of kidney infection or renal calculi could imply past kidney damage. It is important to explore long-term health problems because illnesses such as hypertension, diabetes, systemic lupus erythematosus, arthritis, cancer, and tuberculosis can contribute to decreased renal function.

The nurse documents use of both prescription and over-the-counter medications because many medications are potentially nephrotoxic and can cause renal damage.

The nurse examines the client's dietary or nutritional habits and discusses any present GI problems. A change in the taste of foods often accompanies renal failure. Clients may note that sweet foods are not as appealing or that certain foods, especially meats, leave a metallic taste in the mouth. The client is asked specifically about a history of GI problems, such as nausea, vomiting, anorexia, hiccups, diarrhea, or constipation. Any of these manifestations can be the result of the buildup of nitrogenous or other metabolic wastes that the body cannot excrete because of renal malfunction.

The nurse questions the client about his or her current energy level and any recent injuries or bleeding. Changes in the client's daily routine are explored as a possible *result* of physical fatigue. Weakness, drowsiness, and shortness of breath are typical and suggest impending pulmonary edema or neurologic degeneration. The nurse asks specifically about abnormal bruising or bleeding, which may be the result of hematologic changes associated with uremia.

The nurse discusses the client's urinary elimination in detail, including frequency of urination, appearance of the urine, and any difficulty starting or controlling urination. This information can help identify existing urologic disorders that may influence the preservation of existing renal function.

PHYSICAL ASSESSMENT/CLINICAL MANIFESTATIONS

Chronic renal failure (CRF) results in many multisystem manifestations (Chart 72-7). Clinical manifestations of CRF or uremia are associated with changes in fluid volume and chemical composition. The specific causes of many of these manifestations are not known.

NEUROLOGIC MANIFESTATIONS. Neurologic manifestations of the uremic syndrome of CRF are numerous (see Chart 72-7) and vary widely, depending on nitrogenous waste products, acid-base imbalances, and electrolyte imbalances. The nurse observes for neurologic signs, ranging from lethargy to seizures or coma, indicating uremic encephalopathy. In addition, the nurse assesses for sensory changes that generally appear in a glove and stocking distribution over the lower extremities and examines for weakness in the upper or lower extremities (i.e., uremic neuropathy).

If untreated, uremic encephalopathy progresses to seizures and coma. Dialysis is the treatment of choice for neurologic disturbances associated with CRF. The manifestations of uremic encephalopathy resolve with the initiation of dialysis. However, improvement in uremic neuropathy is limited if the neuropathy is severe and motor function is already impaired.

CARDIOVASCULAR MANIFESTATIONS. The clinical manifestations of CRF and uremia lead to specific cardiovascular abnormalities of fluid volume excess, hypertension, congestive heart failure (CHF), uremic pericarditis, and cardiac

dysrhythmias associated with hyperkalemia. The nurse assesses for signs of a diminished ability to excrete salt and water. The resulting circulatory fluid overload, if untreated, can lead to CHF, pulmonary edema, peripheral edema, and hypertension.

The nurse assesses heart rate and rhythm, listening for extra beats (particularly an S_3), irregular patterns, or a pericardial friction rub. Unless a hemodialysis (HD) vascular access has been previously created, blood pressure is measured in each arm. The nurse assesses the jugular veins for distention and assesses for the presence of pedal, pretibial, presacral, and periorbital edema. Shortness of breath with exertion and paroxysmal nocturnal dyspnea (PND) suggest fluid volume excess.

RESPIRATORY MANIFESTATIONS. Respiratory manifestations of CRF vary widely among clients (e.g., breath that smells like urine [*uremic fetor* or uremic halitosis], deep sighing, yawning, shortness of breath). The nurse notes the rhythm, rate, and depth of breathing. Tachypnea (increased rate of breathing) and hyperpnea (increased depth of breathing) are respiratory compensation mechanisms for worsening metabolic acidosis.

With severe metabolic acidosis, the nurse may observe extreme hyperventilation or Kussmaul respiration. A few clients have hilar pneumonitis, or *uremic lung*. In these clients, the nurse assesses for thick sputum, minimal coughing, an increased respiratory rate, and an elevated temperature. A pleural friction rub may be heard with a stethoscope. Clients often have pleuritic pain with breathing. The nurse auscultates the lungs for crackles, which indicate fluid volume overload.

HEMATOLOGIC MANIFESTATIONS. Hematologic abnormalities include anemia and abnormal bleeding. The nurse notes indicators of anemia, including fatigue, pallor, lethargy, weakness, shortness of breath, and dizziness. The

---

CHART 72-7

KEY FEATURES *of*
Chronic Renal Failure

Neurologic Manifestations
- Lethargy and daytime drowsiness
- Inability to concentrate or decreased attention span
- Seizures
- Coma
- Slurred speech
- Asterixis
- Tremors, twitching, or jerky movements
- Myoclonus
- Ataxia (alteration in gait)
- Paresthesias

Cardiovascular Manifestations
- Cardiomyopathy
- Hypertension
- Peripheral edema
- Congestive heart failure
- Uremic pericarditis
- Pericardial effusion
- Pericardial friction rub
- Cardiac tamponade

Respiratory Manifestations
- Uremic halitosis
- Tachypnea
- Deep sighing, yawning
- Kussmaul respirations
- Uremic pneumonitis
- Shortness of breath
- Pulmonary edema
- Pleural effusion
- Depressed cough reflex
- Crackles

Hematologic Manifestations
- Anemia
- Abnormal bleeding and bruising

Gastrointestinal Manifestations
- Anorexia
- Nausea
- Vomiting
- Metallic taste in the mouth
- Changes in taste acuity and sensation
- Uremic colitis (diarrhea)
- Constipation
- Uremic gastritis (possible GI bleeding)
- Uremic fetor
- Stomatitis
- Diarrhea

Urinary Manifestations
- Polyuria, nocturia (early)
- Oliguria, anuria (later)
- Proteinuria
- Hematuria
- Diluted, strawlike appearance

Integumentary Manifestations
- Decreased skin turgor
- Yellow-gray pallor
- Dry skin
- Pruritus
- Ecchymosis
- Purpura
- Soft-tissue calcifications
- Uremic frost (late, premorbid)

Musculoskeletal Manifestations
- Muscle weakness and cramping
- Bone pain
- Pathologic fractures
- Renal osteodystrophy

Reproductive Manifestations
- Decreased fertility
- Infrequent or absent menses
- Decreased libido
- Impotence

GI, Gastrointestinal.

presence of abnormal bleeding is assessed by observing for bruising, petechiae, purpura, ecchymoses (confluent bruises), mucous membrane bleeding in the nose or gums, abnormal vaginal bleeding, or gastrointestinal (GI) bleeding (often demonstrated by black tarry stools [melena]).

GASTROINTESTINAL MANIFESTATIONS. The nurse assesses for a foul odor to the breath, mouth ulceration, or mouth inflammation and notes any vomiting. Abdominal pain or cramping may be associated with uremic colitis. Stools may test positive for blood.

URINARY MANIFESTATIONS. The urinary findings in renal failure reflect the kidneys' decreasing functioning. At first, changes occur in the amount, frequency, and appearance of the urine. Many etiologic features of chronic renal disease result in proteinuria; some cause hematuria.

The quantity and composition of the urine change as renal function deteriorates. With the onset of end-stage renal disease (ESRD), the urine may become more dilute and clearer, reflecting a diminished glomerular filtration rate (GFR). The nurse must be aware that the actual urine output in a client with CRF varies with the amount of remaining renal function. The client with ESRD usually has oliguria, but some clients will remain relatively nonoliguric, producing 1 L or more per 24 hours. Urine volume produced per day will probably change again after dialysis is initiated.

INTEGUMENTARY MANIFESTATIONS. There are several dermatologic manifestations of CRF. In clients with uremia, deposition of urochrome pigment in the skin results in a yellowish coloration. Some African Americans report a darkening of the skin. The anemia of CRF causes a sallowness to the quality of the color, which some people describe as a faded suntan. This is most noticeable in lighter-skinned clients.

Skin oils and turgor are decreased in clients with uremia. One of the most uncomfortable problems of uremia is severe **pruritus** (itching). The nurse also assesses for bruises (**ecchymoses**), purple patches (**purpura**), and occasionally, drug-induced rashes.

Uremic frost, a layer of urea crystals from evaporated perspiration, may appear on the face, eyebrows, axilla, and groin in clients with advanced uremic syndrome.

■ PSYCHOSOCIAL ASSESSMENT

CRF and its treatment disrupt more aspects of a client's life than almost any other illness. Nurses are in a unique position to evaluate the client with newly diagnosed renal failure and to assist with these adjustments.

Psychosocial assessment and support are part of the nurse's role from the time that CRF is first diagnosed. Initially, the nurse asks about the client's understanding of the diagnosis and its implications for treatment regimens (e.g., diet, medication, and dialysis). The nurse assesses for any signs of anxiety and for the coping mechanisms used by the client or family members. Some of the psychosocial aspects altered by CRF include family relations, social activity, work patterns, body image, and sexual activity. The chronicity of ESRD, the variety of treatment options, and the uncertainties surrounding the course of the disease and its treatment necessitate an ongoing psychosocial assessment.

■ LABORATORY ASSESSMENT

CRF results in serious abnormalities in many laboratory values (see Chart 72-2). The following blood values are routinely monitored in clients with CRF: creatinine, blood urea nitrogen (BUN), sodium, potassium, calcium, phosphate, bicarbonate, hemoglobin, and hematocrit.

Initially, a urinalysis is performed, and a 24-hour urine specimen for creatinine and urea clearance is obtained. In the early stages of renal insufficiency, urinalysis can reveal key indicators of kidney function. Urinalysis may show excessive protein, glucose, red blood cells (RBCs), white blood cells (WBCs), and decreased or fixed specific gravity. Urine osmolality is usually decreased. A 24-hour creatinine clearance is calculated after serum and urinary creatinine levels are collected and quantified. These data, along with information on body weight and height, are used to calculate renal creatinine clearance. As renal failure progresses, the urine output may decrease dramatically.

Trends in renal function and progressive deterioration are typically monitored by measurements of the serum creatinine and BUN levels. Serum creatinine levels may increase gradually over a period of years, reaching levels of 15 to 30 mg/dL or more, depending on the client's muscle mass. Urea nitrogen levels are directly related to dietary protein intake. Without dietary protein restriction, BUN levels are typically 10 to 20 times the value of the serum creatinine level. As dietary protein is increasingly restricted in an attempt to slow the rate of progression of renal failure, BUN levels remain elevated but less than the 10:1 to 20:1 ratio of nonprotein-restricted clients. Other factors affect the level of BUN, and the nurse must consider these for a complete assessment. Chapter 69 describes the factors influencing BUN levels, as well as the interpretation of serum creatinine and creatinine clearance.

■ RADIOGRAPHIC ASSESSMENT

X-ray findings in clients with CRF are few. Bone radiographs of the metacarpals and phalanges of the hand can reveal the presence of renal osteodystrophy. With established ESRD, the kidneys are atrophic and may be 8 to 9 cm or less. This diminished size is usually the result of renal tubular atrophy and fibrosis. If obstructive uropathy is a possible factor contributing to deterioration of renal function that is more rapid than expected, a renal ultrasound or computed tomography (CT) scan without contrast media may be obtained. (See Chapter 69 for a complete description of renal diagnostic tests.)

CRITICAL THINKING CHALLENGE

You are gathering the initial history for a 67-year-old African-American client admitted to your unit with suspected CRF. The client tells you that he has a history of diabetes, gout, and peptic ulcer disease. He also states that he has noted a 7-pound weight gain over the last 4 weeks.

- What other questions should you ask this client regarding his symptoms?
- What risk factors for the development of CRF are noted in his past medical history?
- What cardiac and respiratory manifestations may you find on physical examination of this client?

For suggested answer guidelines, go to ![SIMON] http://www.wbsaunders.com/SIMON/Iggy/.

▶ Analysis

The client with chronic renal failure (CRF) has usually experienced a progressive degeneration of renal function and is often hospitalized for evaluation and modification of the treatment plan. The focus of care is to control or manage symptoms and prevent complications.

▧ COMMON NURSING DIAGNOSES AND COLLABORATIVE PROBLEMS

The following are priority nursing diagnoses for clients with CRF:

1. Imbalanced Nutrition: Less Than Body Requirements related to nausea and vomiting, decreased appetite, effects of a catabolic state, decreased level of consciousness, altered taste sensations, or dietary restrictions
2. Excess Fluid Volume related to compromised regulatory mechanisms (inability of the kidneys to maintain body fluid balance)
3. Decreased Cardiac Output related to reduction in stroke volume as a result of electrical malfunction (dysrhythmias) and mechanical malfunction (increased preload [volume excess] and increased afterload [increased peripheral vascular resistance])
4. Risk for Infection related to inadequate primary defenses (broken skin), chronic disease, or malnutrition
5. Risk for Injury related to internal biochemical risk factors associated with renal failure (increased susceptibility to bleeding, falls, and pathologic fractures) and external risk factors, such as drugs
6. Fatigue related to altered metabolic energy production, imbalance between oxygen supply and demand, and anemia
7. Anxiety related to threat to or change in health status, socioeconomic status, relationships, role functioning, support systems, or self-concept; situational crisis; threat of death; lack of knowledge (procedures, diagnostic tests, disease process, renal replacement therapy); loss of control; feelings of failure; or disrupted family life

The primary collaborative problem is Potential for Pulmonary Edema.

▧ ADDITIONAL NURSING DIAGNOSES AND COLLABORATIVE PROBLEMS

In addition to the common nursing diagnoses and collaborative problems, clients with CRF may have one or more of the following:

* Diarrhea related to chemical or electrolyte imbalances, fear, anxiety, or side effects of medications
* Impaired Oral Mucous Membrane related to parotid gland changes, limited fluid intake, malnutrition, and elevated levels of uremic toxins
* Impaired Skin Integrity related to altered chemical balance and uremic toxins
* Social Isolation related to illness or alterations in physical appearance
* Interrupted Family Processes related to situational crisis, reduced income, unemployment, or effects of chronic illness
* Sexual Dysfunction related to altered body function (decreased libido and/or impotence) from disease and/or effects of medications, depression, or disturbance in self-esteem or body image
* Disturbed Thought Processes related to irritation, central nervous system (CNS) depression, side effects of medications, sleep deprivation, or clinical depression
* Deficient Knowledge (disease process, care regimen, and follow-up care) related to lack of informational resources and magnitude of the care issues
* Potential for Sepsis
* Potential for Malnutrition
* Potential for Electrolyte Imbalances
* Potential for Metabolic Acidosis
* Potential for Gastrointestinal (GI) Bleeding

▶ Planning and Implementation

The Concept Map on p. 1683 addresses assessment and nursing care issues related to clients who have renal failure that has progressed to end-stage renal disease (ESRD).

▧ IMBALANCED NUTRITION: LESS THAN BODY REQUIREMENTS

PLANNING: EXPECTED OUTCOMES. The client with CRF is expected to attain and maintain the following:

* Adequate nutritional status
* Ideal body weight for age, height, and body build
* Laboratory values within safe levels

INTERVENTIONS. The nutritional requirements and dietary restrictions for the client with renal failure vary according to the degree of decrease in renal function and the type of dialysis performed, if any (Table 72-8).

NIC **NUTRITION THERAPY.** The purpose of nutrition therapy is the administration of food and fluids to support the metabolic processes of a client who is malnourished or at high risk of becoming malnourished. Clients begun on hemodialysis (HD) have an increase in catabolism and subsequent decrease in intake that often results in a loss of lean body mass. NIC interventions for nutrition therapy are summarized in Chart 72-8.

The client is referred to a registered dietitian for dietary teaching and planning. The nurse in collaboration with the dietitian instructs the client about alterations in the diet that are necessary as a result of CRF. Dietary alterations include control of protein intake; limitation of fluid intake; restriction of potassium, sodium, and phosphorus intake; administration of appropriate vitamin and mineral supplements; and provision of adequate calories to meet metabolic demand.

If adequate calories are not supplied, the body will use tissue protein for energy, which leads to a negative nitrogen balance and malnutrition. The dietitian assists in determining the number of calories and types of nutrients needed to meet nutritional requirements.

PROTEIN RESTRICTION. There is some evidence to suggest that early implementation of a protein-restricted diet prevents some of the symptoms associated with CRF and may preserve kidney function. Dietary protein is restricted on the basis of the degree of renal insufficiency and the severity of the symptoms in accordance with the belief that the accumulation of waste products from protein metabolism is the pri-

Concept Map: End-Stage Renal Disease

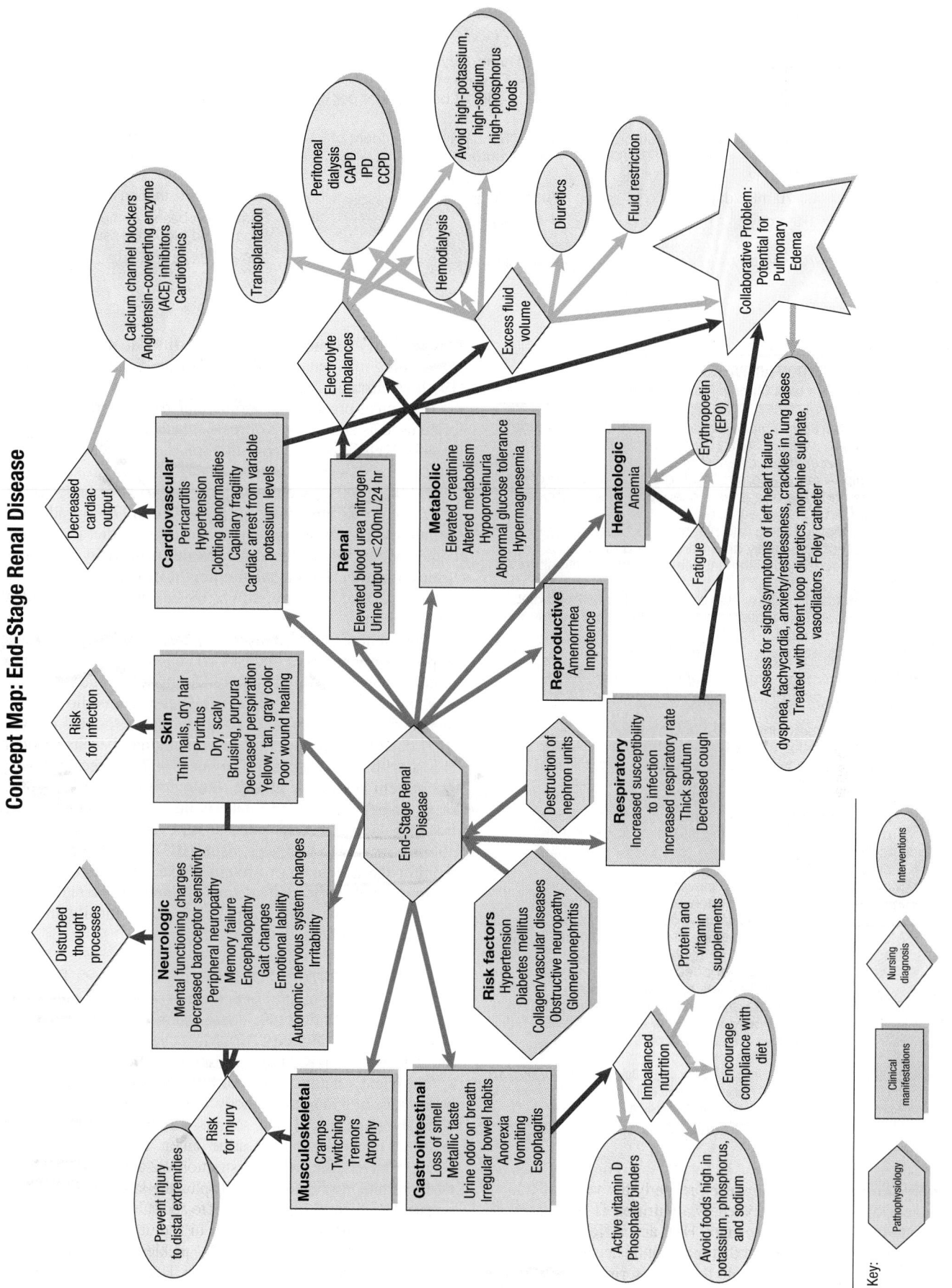

TABLE 72-8 • DIETARY RESTRICTIONS FOR THE CLIENT WITH RENAL FAILURE

Dietary Component	With Chronic Uremia	With Hemodialysis	With Peritoneal Dialysis
Protein	0.55-0.60 g/kg of body weight per day	1.0-1.5 g/kg of body weight per day	1.2-1.5 g/kg of body weight per day
Fluid	Depends on urine output, but may be as high as 1500-3000 mL/day	500-700 mL/day plus amount of urine output	Restriction based on fluid weight gain and blood
Potassium	60-70 mEq/day	70 mEq/day	Usually no restriction
Sodium	1-3 g/day	2-4 g/day	Restriction based on fluid weight gain and blood pressure
Phosphorus	700 mg/day	700 mg/day	800 mg/day

CHART 72-8

NIC INTERVENTION ACTIVITIES for The Client with Chronic Renal Failure

Nutrition Therapy: *Administration of food and fluids to support metabolic processes of a client who is malnourished or at high risk of becoming malnourished*
- Determine—in collaboration with dietitian—number of calories and type of nutrients needed to meet nutritional requirements.
- Refer to diet teaching and planning, as needed.
- Teach client and family about prescribed diet.
- Provide needed nourishment within limits of prescribed diet.
- Give client and family written examples of prescribed diet.
- Monitor food/fluid ingested and calculate daily caloric intake, as appropriate.
- Offer herbs and spices as an alternative to salt.

Fluid Management: *Promotion of fluid balance and prevention of complications resulting from abnormal or undesired fluid levels.*
- Maintain accurate intake and output record.
- Monitor hydration status (e.g., moist mucous membranes, adequacy of pulses, and orthostatic blood pressure), as appropriate.
- Monitor for indications of fluid overload/retention (e.g., crackles, elevated CVP or pulmonary capillary wedge pressure, edema, neck vein distention, and ascites), as appropriate.
- Weigh daily and monitor trends.
- Monitor laboratory results relevant to fluid retention (e.g., increased specific gravity, increased BUN, decreased hematocrit, and increased urine osmolality levels).
- Monitor client's weight change before and after dialysis, if appropriate.
- Assess location and extent of edema, if present.
- Administer prescribed diuretics, as appropriate.
- Distribute the fluid intake over 24 hours, as appropriate.
- Consult health care provider if signs and symptoms of fluid volume excess persist or worsen.

NIC intervention activities selected from McCloskey J.C., & Bulechek, G.M. (2000). *Nursing interventions classification (NIC)* (3rd ed.). St. Louis: Mosby. No part of this work is to be altered without prior written permission from the Publisher.
CVP, Central venous pressure; *BUN,* blood urea nitrogen.

---

mary cause of uremia. However, recently the value of a low-protein diet has been debated. Malnutrition is often seen in clients undergoing maintenance HD, and at least one study suggests that a low-protein diet may not be necessary in renal failure. Some studies indicate that a prescription of 1.5 g of protein/kg of body weight per day may be necessary for weight gain and improvement in nutritional status in clients undergoing maintenance HD (Kuhlmann, Schmidt, & Kohler, 1999; Mehrotra & Nolph, 1999).

In clinical practice the glomerular filtration rate (GFR) is often used as an indicator of renal function and can be a guide to safe levels of protein consumption. A client with a severely reduced GFR who is *not* undergoing dialysis is usually permitted 0.55 to 0.60 g of protein per kilogram of body weight (e.g., 40 g of protein daily for a 150-pound [70-kg] adult). If proteinuria is present, protein is added to the diet in amounts equal to that lost in the urine, as determined by a 24-hour urine collection. The calculation for the protein requirement is based on actual body weight (corrected for edema), not ideal body weight.

The client receiving dialysis requires more protein because of protein loss through dialysis. HD clients have their protein requirements individually tailored according to their postdialysis, or "dry," weight. Typically, HD clients are allowed protein in the amount of 1 to 1.5 g/kg/day; peritoneal dialysis (PD) clients are allowed 1.2 to 1.5 g/kg/day because protein is lost with each exchange (Levine, 1997). Three fourths of the protein should be of high biologic value, such as milk, meat, or eggs. If protein intake is inadequate, a negative nitrogen balance develops and causes muscle wasting. Serum albumin and blood urea nitrogen (BUN) levels are used to monitor the adequacy of protein intake. Decreases in serum albumin levels indicate inadequate protein intake and malnutrition. Excessive protein intake can dramatically increase BUN levels in clients with renal failure.

SODIUM RESTRICTION. The nurse monitors fluid and sodium intake. In clients with little or no urine output, fluid and sodium retention can cause edema, hypertension, and congestive heart failure (CHF). Most clients with renal failure retain sodium; a few cannot conserve sodium.

The client's status in terms of fluid and sodium retention can be estimated by monitoring body weight and blood pressure. In nondialyzed uremic clients, sodium is limited to 1 to 3 g daily, and fluid intake depends on urine output. In oliguric clients receiving dialysis, the sodium restriction is 2 to 4 g daily; fluid intake is limited to 500 to 700 mL plus the amount of any urine output. The client is instructed not to add salt at the table or during food preparation. Foods high in sodium (processed foods, fast foods, potato chips, pretzels, pickles, ham, bacon, and sausage) are permitted in moderation. Herbs and spices can be used as an alternative to salt for enhanced flavoring of food.

POTASSIUM RESTRICTION. The nurse monitors potassium intake because hyperkalemia can cause dangerous cardiac dysrhythmias. Cardiac rhythm is monitored for the tall, peaked T waves characteristic of hyperkalemia; the serum potassium level is also documented. The client with advanced CRF is instructed to limit potassium intake to 60 to 70 mEq/day. The labels of seasoning agents are carefully inspected for sodium and potassium content. Clients are instructed to avoid salt substitute agents, many of which are composed of potassium chloride, if oliguria is present. Clients receiving PD or who are producing urine may not need dietary potassium restrictions.

PHOSPHORUS RESTRICTION. Control of phosphate levels is begun early in renal failure to avoid osteodystrophy. The nurse monitors serum phosphate levels, and the physician may order dietary phosphorus restrictions and medications to assist with phosphate control. Phosphate binders must be taken at mealtime. Most clients with kidney disease already restrict their protein intake, and because high-protein foods are high in phosphorus, their phosphorus consumption is also reduced. Chapter 11 lists foods high in potassium, sodium, and phosphorus.

VITAMIN SUPPLEMENTATION. Most clients with renal failure require daily vitamin and mineral supplementation. Low-protein diets are usually deficient in vitamins, and water-soluble vitamins are removed from the blood during dialysis. In addition, anemia is a chronic problem in clients with renal failure because of the limited iron content of low-protein diets and decreased erythropoietin production by the kidneys. Thus supplemental iron is needed. Calcium and vitamin D supplements may also be required, depending on the client's serum levels and bone status.

INDIVIDUALIZATION OF THE DIET. Clients undergoing PD require a slightly different diet from those undergoing HD. Because protein is lost with the dialysate in PD, a major nutritional problem for these clients is replacing lost protein. In many cases, 1.2 to 1.5 g of protein per kilogram of body weight per day is recommended. The anorexia that often accompanies advanced renal disease requires clients to consume a diet with sufficient protein that includes high-calorie enteral supplements. The amount of sodium restriction varies with fluid weight gain and blood pressure. There is usually no need to restrict dietary potassium because the dialysate is potassium free. The potassium restriction, if any, is determined by the serum potassium level.

The nurse plays a vital role in managing the client's diet. In collaboration with the dietitian, the nurse provides teaching and performs ongoing assessments of the client's comprehension of and compliance with dietary regimens. Written examples of the prescribed diet can be given to the client and family. The nurse and dietitian can help clients adapt the diet to their budget, ethnic background, and food preferences to maximize caloric intake within the diet's restrictions.

■ EXCESS FLUID VOLUME

PLANNING: EXPECTED OUTCOMES. The client with chronic renal failure (CRF) is expected to:
- Achieve and maintain an acceptable fluid balance
- Minimize the risk of complications from fluid imbalances

INTERVENTIONS. Management of the client with CRF includes drug therapy, diet therapy, fluid restriction, and dialysis. Diet therapy is discussed under Imbalanced Nutrition: Less Than Body Requirements, p. 1682, and dialysis is discussed under Renal Replacement Therapies, p. 1688).

NIC **FLUID MANAGEMENT.** The purpose of fluid management is the promotion of fluid balance and the prevention of complications resulting from abnormal or undesired fluid levels (see Chart 72-8). The nurse monitors the client's intake and output and hydration status. In addition, the nurse assesses for signs and symptoms indicative of fluid volume excess, such as crackles in the bases of the lungs, edema, and distended neck veins.

DRUG THERAPY. Diuretics are prescribed for clients with renal insufficiency when needed for treatment of fluid retention or to help control blood pressure. The diuresis produced from these drugs is useful in treating fluid overload in clients who still have some urine output. Diuretics are seldom used in clients with end-stage renal disease (ESRD) after dialysis has been initiated because, as kidney function diminishes, these drugs can have harmful side effects, including nephrotoxic and ototoxic effects.

The nurse uses daily weight measurements and intake and output records as important sources of assessment data. Daily weight gain generally indicates fluid retention rather than true body weight gain. The nurse estimates the amount of fluid retained: 1 kg of weight equals approximately 1 L of fluid retained. Daily weights are taken at the same time each day, on the same scale, with the client wearing the same amount of clothing, and after the bladder has been emptied if the client is not anuric. The weight is monitored for changes before and after dialysis.

FLUID RESTRICTION. The amount of fluid restriction ordered is discussed under Sodium Restriction, p. 1684. The nurse considers all forms of intake, including oral, intravenous, and fluid or medication administration through gastrointestinal (GI) tubes, when calculating fluid intake. The nurse assists the client in distributing fluid intake by mouth over a 24-hour period. The client's response to fluid restriction is monitored, and the health care provider is notified if signs and symptoms of fluid volume excess persist or worsen.

■ DECREASED CARDIAC OUTPUT

NOC **PLANNING: EXPECTED OUTCOMES.** The client with CRF is expected to attain and maintain normal sinus rhythm, adequate cardiac output, and blood pressure in expected ranges.

INTERVENTIONS. Many clients with long-standing hypertension have renal insufficiency, and some progress to CRF and ESRD. Therefore the control of hypertension is an essential factor in preserving renal function. To control hypertension, the physician may order calcium channel blockers, angiotensin-converting enzyme (ACE) inhibitors, alpha-adrenergic and beta-adrenergic blockers, and vasodilators. Recent studies have documented the effectiveness of ACE inhibitors, as compared with other antihypertensives, in slowing the progression of renal failure (Levine, 1997). More information on the specific medications can be found in Chapter 36. Indications vary, depending on the client, and these drugs are used carefully to avoid hyperkalemia and hypotension. Various combinations and doses may be tried until blood pressure control is adequate and side effects are minimized. Calcium channel blockers seem to improve the GFR and renal blood flow.

The client and family or significant others are instructed to measure blood pressure. The nurse evaluates the client's ability to measure and record blood pressure accurately using the client's own equipment. The nurse periodically rechecks measurement accuracy. In addition to accurate measurement of blood pressure, the client and family must understand the relationship of blood pressure control and regulation to diet and medication therapy. The nurse further instructs the client to measure weight daily and to bring records of blood pressure measurements and weights for discussion with the physician, nurse, or dietitian.

The nurse assesses and monitors, on an ongoing basis, for signs and symptoms of decreased cardiac output, heart failure, congestive heart failure (CHF), and dysrhythmias. These topics are discussed in Chapters 33 through 35.

■ RISK FOR INFECTION

PLANNING: EXPECTED OUTCOMES. The client with CRF is expected to remain free of infection.

INTERVENTIONS. The nurse or assistive nursing personnel provides meticulous care to any areas where skin integrity has been broken (incisions, site of drains, puncture sites, cracked or excoriated skin, pressure sores) and provides good basic preventive skin care. For clients undergoing dialysis, the nurse also inspects the vascular access site or PD catheter insertion site. These areas are assessed on an ongoing basis for redness, swelling, pain, and drainage. Vital signs are monitored for any signs or symptoms of infection.

■ RISK FOR INJURY

PLANNING: EXPECTED OUTCOMES. The client with chronic renal failure (CRF) is expected to remain free of injury (will not fall or experience injury from a fall and will not experience pathologic fractures, bleeding, or toxic effects of medications administered in the presence of CRF).

INTERVENTIONS. Managing drug therapy in clients with CRF is a complex and ongoing clinical problem. Many over-the-counter drugs contain ingredients that may affect renal function. Therefore it is important to obtain a detailed drug history. The nurse must be aware of the use of each drug, its side effects, and the site of metabolism. The nurse, in conjunction with the physician and pharmacist, monitors the client closely for drug-related complications and adjusts dosages accordingly.

Certain medications must be avoided, and the dosages of others must be adjusted according to the degree of remaining renal function. As the client's renal function decreases, repeated dosage adjustments are necessary. The nurse assesses for side effects and signs of drug toxicity and notifies the physician as appropriate.

A number of medications are routinely administered to clients with renal failure (see Chart 72-3). The nurse giving these medications understands the rationale for administration and the nursing interventions for each drug. Many clients have some degree of cardiac disease and may require cardiotonic drugs, such as digoxin. Clients with decreased renal function are particularly susceptible to digoxin toxicity because the drug is excreted by the kidneys. The nurse caring for clients with CRF who are receiving any digitalis derivative, including digoxin, monitors for signs of toxicity, such as nausea, vomiting, anorexia, visual disturbances, restlessness, headache, fatigue, confusion, cardiac irregularities (particularly bradycardia [pulse rate, 50 to 60 beats/min] and tachycardia [pulse rate, 100 beats/min]), and serum drug levels above therapeutic range. In addition, serum levels of potassium are monitored closely in any client receiving cardiotonic medications.

Drugs to control an excessively high phosphate level include phosphate-binding compounds. Calcium acetate, calcium carbonate, and aluminum hydroxide are used as phosphate-binding agents in clients with renal failure. These drugs treat the metabolic complications that if untreated may lead to renal osteodystrophy and related injuries. To prevent further complications, the nurse stresses the importance of these and all medications.

Hypercalcemia (excessively high serum calcium levels) is a possible complication for clients taking calcium-containing compounds to control phosphate excess. **Hypophosphatemia** (low serum phosphorus levels) is also a possible outcome of phosphate binding but is typically also associated with phosphate depletion in clients who are not eating adequately but are continuing to take phosphate-binding medications. In clients taking aluminum-based phosphate binders for prolonged periods, retention and deposition of aluminum may cause bone disease or neurologic manifestations that may not be reversible. The nurse monitors the client for evidence of muscle weakness, anorexia, malaise, tremors, or bone pain.

Clients with renal disease should avoid antacid compounds containing magnesium. Clients with renal failure cannot excrete magnesium and thus should avoid additional intake.

In addition to the drugs used to treat renal failure, the use of other medications requires special consideration. These medications include antibiotics, opioids, antihypertensives, diuretics, insulin, and heparin.

Many antibiotics are safe for clients with renal failure, but those excreted primarily by the kidneys require dose modification. To prevent complications of bloodstream infections from oral cavity bacteria, prophylactic antibiotic treatment is routinely given to clients with CRF before any dental procedures. The antibiotic and protocol used vary with the client's needs and the physician's preference.

The nurse administers opioid analgesics cautiously in clients with renal failure because the effects often last much longer than in people with healthy kidneys. Clients with uremia are particularly sensitive to the respiratory depressant effects of these drugs. Because opioids are metabolized by the liver and not the kidneys, the dose recommendations are often the same regardless of the level of renal function. The nurse monitors these clients closely after opioid administration and evaluates the need for additional administration on the basis of the client's reaction to the drug.

As renal disease progresses, the client with diabetes mellitus often requires modification of an insulin or oral antidiabetic drug dose because of decreased insulin metabolism by failing kidneys. Frequent blood glucose determinations are obtained to evaluate the client's insulin or oral agent needs. Urine glucose measurements are less accurate when renal disease is present.

Because of poor platelet function and capillary fragility in renal failure, heparin and other anticoagulants are used cautiously.

■ FATIGUE

NOC **PLANNING: EXPECTED OUTCOMES.** The client with chronic renal failure (CRF) is expected to conserve energy by balancing activity and rest in order to be able to perform self-care and activities of daily living.

INTERVENTIONS. All clients with renal dysfunction are given some type of vitamin and mineral supplement. Because of diet restrictions and vitamin losses associated with both peritoneal dialysis (PD) and hemodialysis (HD), water-soluble vitamins must be replaced. The nurse avoids giving the client these vitamin supplements before HD treatment because they will be dialyzed out of the body and the client will receive no benefit.

The anemic client with CRF is treated with recombinant erythropoietin (erythropoietin alfa [Epogen, Procrit]). The goal of erythropoietin therapy is to achieve a hematocrit of 30% to 35%. For erythropoietin to stimulate bone marrow to produce red blood cells (RBCs), clients must have adequate iron stores. In addition, chronic administration of erythropoietin can deplete iron stores, necessitating iron supplementation. Many who receive epoetin alfa report improved appetite and sexual function along with decreased fatigue; in some clients, hypertension associated with a rise in hematocrit has been reported. The improved appetite may challenge clients in their attempts to maintain dietary protein, potassium, and fluid restrictions and necessitates additional education.

■ ANXIETY

NOC **PLANNING: EXPECTED OUTCOMES.** The client with CRF is expected to eliminate or reduce feelings of apprehension and tension from an unidentified source as evidenced by:

- Seeking information to reduce anxiety
- Using effective coping strategies
- Reporting an absence of physical manifestations of anxiety

INTERVENTIONS. The nurse has the most frequent contact with the client with CRF when the client is hospitalized or undergoing in-center dialysis treatments. Thus nurses perform an ongoing assessment of the client's anxiety level to determine the level of nursing intervention required. The nurse observes the client's behavior for physical cues indicating anxiety (e.g., an anxious facial expression or gestures and an increased pulse rate). In addition, the nurse evaluates the support systems, as evidenced by the involvement of family and friends with the client's care.

Unfamiliar settings and situations, and lack of knowledge about treatments and tests can increase the client's anxiety level. The nurse explains all procedures, tests, and treatments. The client's knowledge deficits concerning normal renal func-

tion and renal failure are identified. Evaluating the client's current knowledge avoids needless repetition during teaching sessions. The nurse provides instruction appropriate to the client's needs and ability to understand. By explaining the disease process, the nurse enhances the client's acceptance and decreases anxiety.

The nurse provides continuity of care, whenever possible, to establish a consistent nurse-client relationship to decrease anxiety and promote discussions of client and family concerns. As the nurse-client relationship develops, the client is encouraged to discuss current problems or concerns. A multidisciplinary team of professionals participates to provide support and counseling for the client and family, often over many years of treatment.

The nurse encourages the client to ask questions and discuss fears about the diagnosis of renal failure. An open atmosphere that allows for discussion can decrease anxiety level. Nurses also facilitate discussions with family members or significant others concerning the prognosis and the potential impact on the client's lifestyle.

■ POTENTIAL FOR PULMONARY EDEMA

PLANNING: EXPECTED OUTCOMES. The client with CRF is expected to remain free of pulmonary edema. A secondary outcome is to maintain optimal fluid volume balance through dialysis and pharmacologic measures, thus preventing the onset of pulmonary edema.

INTERVENTIONS. In the client with CRF, pulmonary edema can result from either of two distinct mechanisms: left-sided heart failure or microvascular injury. In left-sided heart failure, the heart is unable to adequately eject blood from the left ventricle, leading to an increase in hydrostatic pressure. The increased pressure allows fluid to cross the capillaries into the pulmonary interstitium. Pulmonary edema can also occur from injury to the vascular endothelium or alveolar epithelial cells secondary to uremia. Fluids then leak into the interstitial space and ultimately into the alveoli.

The nurse assesses the client for early signs of pulmonary edema, such as restlessness, heightened anxiety, tachycardia, dyspnea, and crackles that begin at the base of the lungs. As pulmonary congestion worsens, the level of fluid in the lungs rises. Auscultation will reveal increased rales, decreased air exchange, and dullness to percussion at the upper limits of fluid collection. The client may expectorate frothy, blood-tinged sputum. With further cardiac and respiratory compromise, the client can become diaphoretic and cyanotic.

The client who develops pulmonary edema is often admitted to the intensive care unit for aggressive treatment, which includes continuous cardiac monitoring. The client is placed in a high Fowler's position and given oxygen to maximize lung expansion and improve gas exchange. Drug therapy with renal failure and pulmonary edema is difficult at best because of the potential adverse effects of drugs on the kidneys. Treatment of pulmonary edema involves the administration of potent loop diuretics, such as furosemide (Lasix). Furosemide dosing usually begins at 40 mg, administered intravenously over a 1- to 2-minute period. This dose may be repeated in 30 minutes if no response is elicited. For clients already receiving maintenance doses of furosemide, an IV dose equivalent to the oral maintenance dose is given; it is doubled in 30 minutes if no response is seen (Johnson & Lalonde, 1997). Renal impairment multiplies the risk of ototoxicity with the use of furosemide; thus IV doses are given cautiously.

Morphine sulfate 1 to 2 mg administered intravenously is usually prescribed to reduce myocardial oxygen demand by reducing ventricular preload and to provide vasodilation and sedation. The dose is adjusted to achieve the desired response, but the potential for respiratory depression exists. Therefore the nurse monitors the client's respiratory rate and blood pressure closely. To further decrease hydrostatic pressure, a continuous infusion pump may administer a vasodilator, such as nitroglycerin. Vital signs are monitored vigilantly, since these drugs in combination may result in severe hypotension.

Nursing interventions include Foley catheter placement and frequent assessment of urine output to gauge the effectiveness of diuretic therapy. Diuresis usually begins within 5 minutes of administration of IV furosemide. Urine output is measured every 15 to 30 minutes during the acute episode and every hour thereafter until the client is stabilized. In addition, the nurse assesses breath and heart sounds for improvement in crackles and for the presence of an S_3, indicating fluid overload.

The nurse monitors serum chemistry results for electrolyte imbalances and reports abnormalities to the appropriate health care provider so that correction of imbalances can be initiated. Continuous cardiac monitoring is initiated to identify potential dysrhythmias. Oxygen saturation levels are monitored by pulse oximetry and arterial blood gas values. The oxygen delivery system is adjusted to maintain adequate oxygen saturation levels. The nurse monitors the client for deterioration, manifested as increasing pulmonary congestion and hypoxemia. It may be necessary to intubate the client and mechanically ventilate the lungs at this point to prevent death.

Clients with CRF are at increased risk for developing pulmonary edema, since they may present with precipitating fluid volume overload and existing cardiac compromise secondary to hypertension and volume overload. Such clients are less likely to respond quickly to treatment and are more likely to develop adverse effects from pharmacologic agents as a result of renal impairment. Occasionally, ultrafiltration may be used to further reduce fluid volume.

■ Renal Replacement Therapies

Renal replacement therapy is required only when the clinical and laboratory manifestations of renal failure present complications that are potentially life threatening or that pose continuing discomfort to the client. When the client can no longer be managed with conservative therapies, such as diet, medication, and fluid restriction, dialysis is indicated. Transplantation may be discussed at any time.

▓ HEMODIALYSIS

Hemodialysis (HD) is one of several renal replacement therapies used for the treatment of renal failure (Table 72-9). Dialysis removes excess fluids and waste products and restores chemical and electrolyte balance. HD involves the extracorporeal (outside of the body) passage of the client's blood through a semipermeable membrane that serves as an artificial kidney.

CLIENT SELECTION. Any client may be considered for HD therapy. Initiation of renal replacement therapy de-

TABLE 72-9 • A COMPARISON OF HEMODIALYSIS AND PERITONEAL DIALYSIS AS RENAL REPLACEMENT TREATMENT OPTIONS	
Hemodialysis	**Peritoneal Dialysis**
ADVANTAGES	
More efficient clearance	Easy access
Short time needed for treatment	Few hemodynamic complications
COMPLICATIONS	
Disequilibrium syndrome	Protein loss
Muscle cramps	Peritonitis
Hemorrhage	Hyperglycemia
Air embolus	Respiratory distress
Hemodynamic changes (hypotension, cardiac dysrhythmias, and anemia)	Bowel perforation
CONTRAINDICATIONS	
Hemodynamic instability	Extensive peritoneal adhesions
	Peritoneal fibrosis
	Recent abdominal surgery
ACCESS	
Vascular access route	Intra-abdominal catheter
PROCEDURE	
Complex	Simple
Specially trained registered nurses required	Training less complex than for hemodialysis
NURSING IMPLICATIONS	
Vascular access care	Abdominal catheter care
Restrict diet	More flexible diet

pends on the symptoms of the client, not on the creatinine clearance. Dialysis is initiated immediately for clients who exhibit the following: fluid overload refractory to diuretics, presence of pericarditis, uncontrolled hypertension, neurologic manifestations, and development of bleeding diathesis. More commonly, dialysis is started when clients have signs of symptom progression, such as nausea and vomiting, decreased attention span, decreased cognition, worsening anemia, and pruritus (Levine, 1997).

The duration of survival after HD depends on the client's age, the cause of renal failure, and the presence of other diseases, such as coronary artery disease, hypertension, or diabetes. The following are general guideline requirements for appropriate client selection:

- Presence of fatal, irreversible renal failure when other therapies are unacceptable or ineffective
- Absence of illnesses that would prevent or seriously complicate HD
- Expectation of rehabilitation
- The client's acceptance of the regimen

DIALYSIS SETTINGS. Clients may receive HD treatments in any of several settings, depending on specific needs. They may be dialyzed in an acute care (hospital-based) center if they have recently begun treatment or have complicating conditions that require close nursing or medical supervision. Stable clients with chronic renal failure (CRF) may be hemodialyzed in a freestanding HD center in the community when they no longer require intensive supervision. Stable clients may participate in complete or partial self-care in an outpatient center or with in-home HD.

In-home HD offers the least disruptive form of therapy and allows for the most adaptation of the regimen to the client's lifestyle. Unfortunately, many clients cannot participate in in-home dialysis because they lack a reliable and consistent partner to administer the therapy and manage the dialysis machine. For some clients and partners, the responsibilities of in-home dialysis are extremely stressful, so that this option is less desirable. In addition, a water treatment system must be installed in the home to provide a safe, clean water supply for the dialysis process.

Regardless of the setting for therapy, the client needs ongoing nursing support and intervention to maintain this complex and lifesaving treatment.

PROCEDURE. The principles of HD are based on the passive transfer of toxins, which is accomplished by diffusion. **Diffusion** is the movement of molecules from an area of higher concentration to an area of lower concentration. The rate of diffusion is affected by numerous factors. Diffusion during dialysis occurs more rapidly when the membrane pores are large, there is a large surface area of membrane, the temperature of the solutions is higher, and there is a greater difference in the solute concentrations. Molecules that are too large, such as RBCs and plasma proteins, cannot pass through the membrane.

When HD is initiated, blood and dialysate flow in opposite directions from their respective sides of an enclosed semipermeable membrane. The dialysate is a balanced mix of electrolytes and water that closely resembles human plasma. On the other side of the membrane is the client's blood, which contains metabolic waste products, excess water, and excess electrolytes. During HD, the waste products move from the blood into the dialysate because of the difference in their concentrations (diffusion). Excess water is also removed from the blood into the dialysate (**osmosis**). Electrolytes can move in either direction, as needed, and take some fluid with them. Potassium and sodium typically move out of the plasma into the dialysate, whereas bicarbonate and calcium move from the dialysate into the plasma. This process continues as the blood and the dialysate are circulated past the membrane for a preset length of time. Water volume may be removed from the plasma by applying positive or negative pressure to the system.

The components of an HD system include a dialyzer, dialysate, vascular access routes, and an HD machine. The artificial kidney, or **dialyzer** (Figure 72-3), has four components: a blood compartment, a dialysate compartment, a semipermeable membrane, and an enclosed structure to support the membrane.

Dialysate is made from clear water and chemicals and is free of any metabolic waste products or drugs. Because bacteria and other microorganisms are too large to pass through the membrane, dialysate does not need to be sterile. The water used in dialysate must meet specific standards, and water treatment systems are used to ensure a safe water supply. The dialysate composition may be altered according to the client's needs for treatment of electrolyte imbalances. During HD, the dialysate is warmed to approximately 100° F (37. 8° C) to increase the efficiency of diffusion and to prevent a decrease in blood temperature.

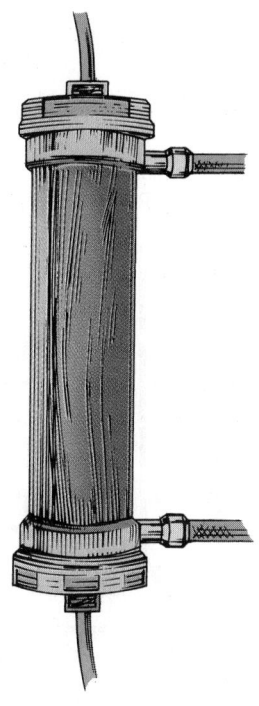

Hollow fiber
dialyzer

Figure 72-3   ●   Artificial kidney (dialyzer) used in hemodialysis.

An essential function of an HD machine is the monitoring for potential problems, including the following:
- Changes in dialysate temperature
- Presence of air in the blood tubing
- A blood leak in the dialysate compartment
- Changes in the pressure or composition within the blood and the dialysate compartments

If any of these problems are detected, an alarm alerts the nurse. The monitoring systems protect the client from life-threatening complications that can result if these technical problems are not corrected.

All models of HD machines function, in principle, as illustrated in Figure 72-4. Figure 72-5 shows one type of machine. The duration and frequency of HD treatments depend on the amount of metabolic waste to be cleared, the clearance capacity of the dialyzer, and the amount of fluid to be removed. Most dialyzers provide sufficient clearance to limit the total number of hours of dialysis to about 12 hours a week. This time is usually divided into three 4-hour treatments a week. For clients with less muscle or more ongoing urine production, two 5- to 6-hour treatments a week may be adequate. If the client gains large amounts of fluid weight, a longer treatment time may be needed to remove the fluid without hypotension or severe side effects.

ANTICOAGULATION. To prevent blood clots from forming within the dialyzer membrane and the blood tubing, anticoagulation with heparin is necessary during HD treatments. Heparin, a short-acting anticoagulant, inhibits the tendency of blood to clot when it comes in contact with foreign surfaces. There is considerable variability among clients in

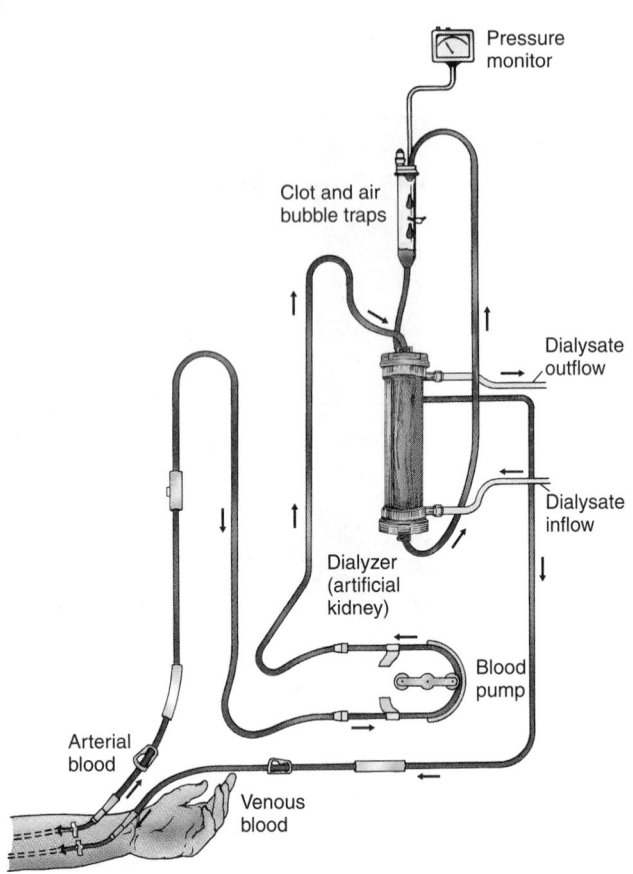

Figure 72-4 ● A hemodialysis circuit.

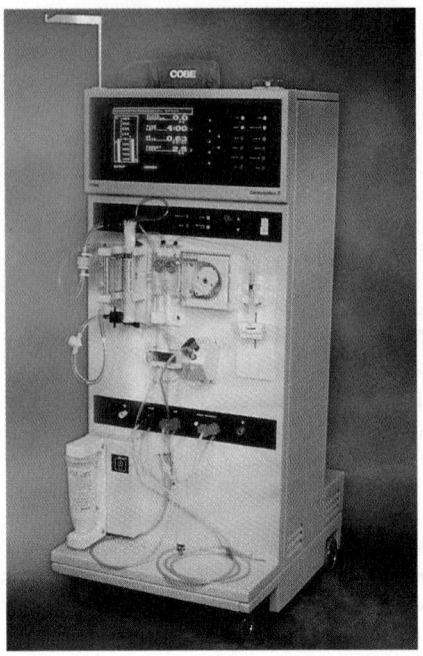

Figure 72-5 ● A hemodialysis machine. (Courtesy Gambro Healthcare.)

their anticoagulation response and elimination of heparin. The heparin dose must be adjusted on the basis of each client's need. Clients receiving erythropoietin may need more heparin.

Heparin remains active in the body for 4 to 6 hours after administration, making the client at risk for hemorrhage during and immediately after HD treatments. The client must avoid any invasive procedures during that time. Thus the nurse monitors closely for any signs of bleeding or hemorrhage. Clotting tendencies can be monitored during HD with a bedside machine (such as the Hemochron), by whole-blood clotting times (Lee-White clotting test), or by activated partial thromboplastin times (aPTT) during and after HD. Protamine sulfate is given as an antidote to neutralize heparin's anticoagulant activity when necessary.

VASCULAR ACCESS. For hemodialysis (HD) to be performed, a vascular access route is required (Table 72-10). Dialysis treatments necessitate the easy availability of a large amount of blood flow—at least 250 to 300 mL/min, usually for a period of 3 to 4 hours. Normally, the body cannot provide this type of circulatory access without surgical revision of blood vessels.

LONG-TERM VASCULAR ACCESS. An internal access is preferred for most clients undergoing long-term HD (see Table 72-10). There are two common choices: an internal arteriovenous (AV) fistula or an AV graft (Figure 72-6). *AV fistulas* are formed by connecting (**anastomosis**) an artery to a vein. The most commonly used vessels are the radial or brachial ar-

tery and the cephalic vein of the nondominant arm. This process increases the blood flow through the vein to 250 to 400 mL/min, the amount required for dialysis to be effective.

Some time is necessary for an AV fistula to develop, and the amount of time required for the fistula to "mature" varies. Primary AV fistulas may not be suitable for use for as long as 4 months. Therefore vascular access must be planned accordingly. As the fistula matures, the increased pressure of the arterial blood flow into the vein causes the vessel walls to thicken. This thickening increases their strength and suitability for repeated cannulation.

To obtain access to a fistula, the nurse cannulates it or inserts two needles, one toward the venous blood flow and one toward the arterial blood flow. This procedure allows the HD machine to draw the blood out through the arterial needle and return it through the venous needle. The client may require a temporary vascular access (AV shunt or HD catheter) for HD treatments until the fistula is ready for use.

AV grafts are used when the AV fistula does not develop or when complications of the AV fistula limit continued use. The polytetrafluoroethylene (PTFE) graft is a synthetic material (Gore-Tex). This type of graft is commonly used in older clients undergoing HD.

PRECAUTIONS. Several precautions must be observed to ensure the functioning of an internal AV fistula or AV graft. First, the nurse assesses for adequate circulation in the fistula or graft, as well as in the distal portion of the extremity. The nurse then checks for a bruit or a thrill by auscultation or palpation over the access site. Repeated compression can result in the loss of the vascular access; therefore the nurse avoids taking the blood pressure in the arm with the vascular access unless absolutely necessary. The AV fistula or graft is *not* used for administration of IV fluids; venipuncture is avoided anywhere in the arm used for HD access. Chart 72-9 lists best practices for care of the client with an HD access.

TABLE 72-10 • TYPES OF VASCULAR ACCESS FOR HEMODIALYSIS

Access Type	Description	Location	Initial Use
PERMANENT			
AV fistula	An internal anastomosis of an artery to a vein	Forearm	2-4 mo or longer
AV graft	Synthetic vessel tubing tunneled beneath the skin, connecting an artery and a vein	Forearm Upper arm Inner thigh	1-2 wk
Dual-lumen hemodialysis catheter	An extended-use catheter, surgically tunneled under the skin with a barrier cuff	Subclavian vein	Immediately postoperatively and after x-ray confirmation of placement
TEMPORARY			
Hemodialysis catheter (dual- or triple-lumen)	A specially designed catheter with two or three lumens Two lumens are for blood outflow and inflow for hemodialysis; a third lumen allows venous access without accessing dialysis lumens	Subclavian, internal jugular, or femoral vein	Immediately after insertion and x-ray confirmation of placement
AV shunt (relatively uncommon)	An external loop of Silastic tubing connecting an artery and a vein Each section of tubing is sutured into a vessel and brought through a skin stab wound	Forearm	Immediately after insertion

AV, Arteriovenous.

COMPLICATIONS. Complications can occur regardless of the type of access. The most common problems include thrombosis or stenosis, infection, aneurysm formation, ischemia, and high-output heart failure.

Thrombosis, or clotting, is the most frequent complication. Some clients are more susceptible to clotting than are others and may be given anticoagulants. Surgical declotting or revision of stenotic areas is typically performed in the surgical suite with the use of local anesthesia.

Most infections that occur in clients undergoing long-term HD involve the vascular access. The most common organism causing infection is *Staphylococcus aureus,* which can be introduced by punctures for dialysis access. The nurse limits the incidence of infections by using careful sterile technique before needle cannulation (Table 72-11).

Aneurysms can form in any internal fistula and are caused by repeated needle punctures at the same site. Aneurysms that appear to be increasing in size may cause loss of the fistula's function and require surgical repair.

Ischemia occurs in a few clients with vascular access when the formation of the fistula causes a decrease in arterial blood flow to areas distal to the fistula. Ischemic symptoms *(steal syndrome)* vary from cold or numb fingers to gangrene. If the collateral circulation is inadequate, the existing fistula may need to be ligated and a new fistula created in another area for circulation to be preserved in the extremity.

The shunting of blood directly from the arterial system to the venous system, through the fistula, can cause high-output heart failure in clients with a limited cardiac reserve (see Chapter 35). This complication occurs rarely, but if it does, the fistula may need to be revised to decrease the blood flow from the arterial supply.

TEMPORARY VASCULAR ACCESS. The first type of vascular access developed was the external *arteriovenous (AV) shunt* (Figure 72-7; see also Table 72-10), but it is rarely

used today. To create a shunt, the surgeon places a piece of silicone rubber (Silastic) tubing into an artery and a second piece into an adjacent vein. The tubings are connected externally to provide a readily available vascular access. The arterial limb is used to obtain the blood for passage through the artificial kidney (dialyzer membrane), and the venous limb is used to return the blood to the client's body after each pass through the dialyzer.

Temporary vascular access with special catheters has replaced the use of the AV shunt for most clients requiring immediate HD. A catheter designed for HD may be inserted into the subclavian, internal jugular, or femoral vein if no permanent vascular access is available for use (see Dialysis Therapies, pp. 1674 and 1675). The lumens of these devices are considerably smaller than the permanent accesses, and the duration of each dialysis session is increased (usually requires 4 to 8 hours).

POSTDIALYSIS NURSING CARE. The nurse closely monitors the client immediately after dialysis and for several hours afterward for any side effects from the treatment. The more common clinical manifestations of complications include hypotension, headache, nausea, malaise, vomiting, dizziness, and muscle cramps.

The nurse obtains vital signs and weight for comparison with predialysis measurements. Blood pressure and weight are expected to be reduced as a result of fluid removal. Excessive hypotension may require rehydration with IV fluids, such as normal saline. The client's temperature may also be elevated, because the dialysis machine warms the blood slightly. If the temperature is elevated excessively, sepsis is suspected and a blood sample is obtained, as ordered, for culture and sensitivity determinations.

The heparinization required for hemodialysis (HD) increases the clotting time and thus the risk for excessive bleeding. *All invasive procedures must therefore be avoided for 4 to 6 hours after dialysis, and the nurse continually monitors the*

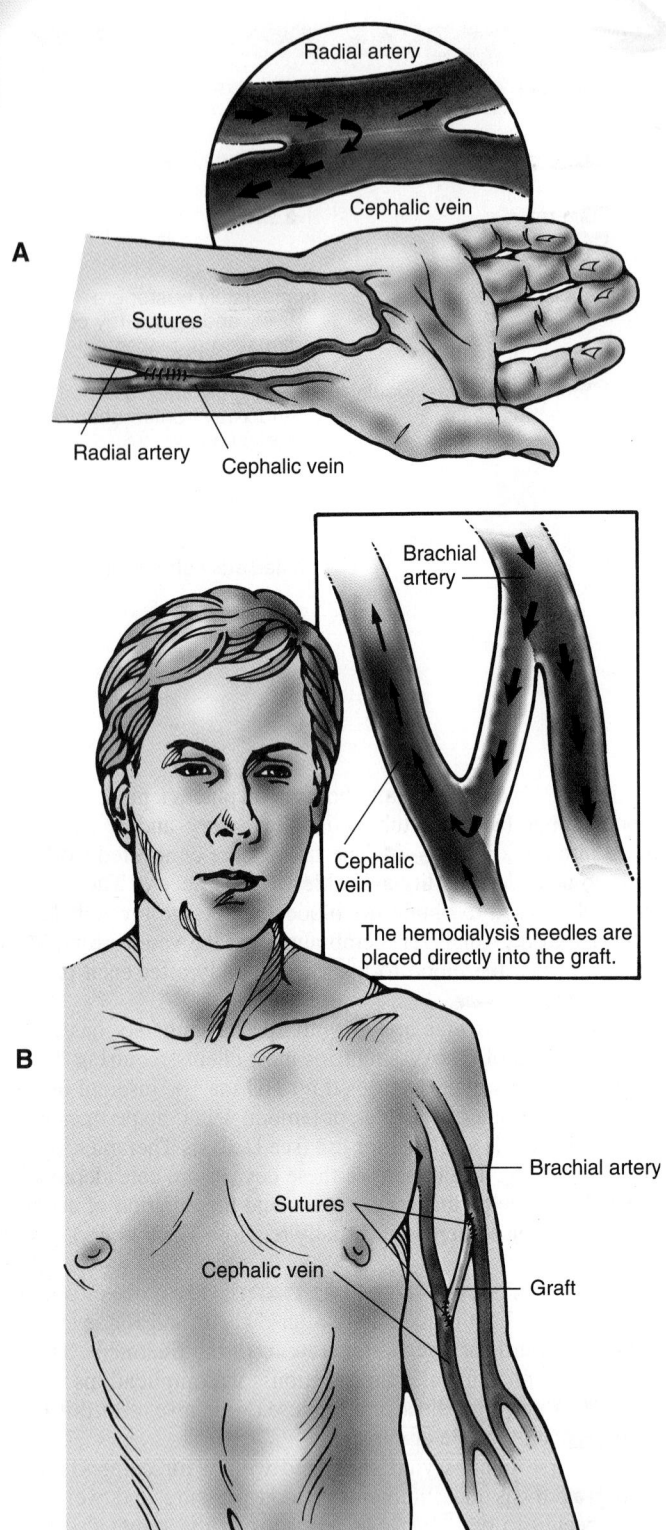

Figure 72-6 ● Options for long-term vascular access for hemodialysis. **A,** A surgically created venous fistula. The increased pressure from the artery forces blood into the vein. This process causes the vein to dilate enough for fistula needles to be placed for hemodialysis. When the vein dilates in this matter, the fistula is said to be "developed." **B,** A surgically placed straight vascular graft in the upper arm. The graft creates a shunt between arterial and venous blood.

client for signs of hemorrhage during dialysis and for 1 hour after dialysis (Chart 72-10).

COMPLICATIONS. A variety of fluid-related and infectious complications can occur from HD. The most common complications include disequilibrium syndrome and acquisition of viral infections.

Dialysis disequilibrium syndrome may develop during HD or after HD has been completed. The cause is unknown but may be due to the rapid decrease in blood urea nitrogen (BUN) levels during HD. These changes in urea levels can cause cerebral edema, which leads to increased intracranial pressure. Neurologic complications can result (headache, nausea, vomiting, restlessness, decreased level of consciousness, seizures, coma, or death).

Early recognition by the nurse of the signs of the syndrome and appropriate treatment with anticonvulsant medications and barbiturates may prevent a life-threatening situation. Dialysis disequilibrium syndrome may be avoided, or minimized, by introducing HD for short periods initially with low blood flows so that rapid changes in plasma composition are avoided.

Infectious diseases transmitted by blood transfusion are another serious complication associated with long-term HD. Two of the most serious blood-transmitted infections are hepatitis and human immunodeficiency virus (HIV).

Hepatitis infection in clients with chronic renal failure (CRF) has decreased in recent years, paralleling the decrease in blood transfusion requirement for these clients because of the availability of erythropoietin therapy. Yet, because of the blood access and the risk of microscopic exposure, hepatitis continues to be a problem for clients undergoing HD. The hepatitis B virus can be transmitted through the use of contaminated needles or instruments, by entry of contaminated blood through open wounds in the skin or mucous membranes, or through transfusion of blood contaminated with the virus.

CHART 72-9

BEST PRACTICE for
Caring for the Client with an Arteriovenous Fistula,
Arteriovenous Graft, or Arteriovenous Shunt

- Do not take blood pressure readings using the extremity in which the vascular access is placed.
- Do not perform venipunctures or start an IV line in the extremity in which the vascular access is placed.
- Palpate for thrills and auscultate for bruits every 4 hours while the client is awake.
- Assess the client's distal pulses and circulation.
- Elevate the affected extremity postoperatively.
- Encourage routine range-of-motion exercises.
- Check for bleeding at needle insertion sites or shunt tubing insertion sites. (Keep small clamps handy on the dressing of the AV shunt.)
- Assess for signs and symptoms of infection at needle sites and shunt tubing insertion sites.
- Instruct the client not to carry heavy objects or anything that compresses the extremity in which the vascular access if placed.
- Instruct the client against sleeping with his or her body weight on top of the extremity in which the vascular access is placed.

AV, Arteriovenous.

The incubation period for acute hepatitis is 6 weeks to 6 months. Thus the nurse continually monitors the client undergoing HD who is receiving frequent transfusions for signs of hepatitis virus infection (see Chapter 59).

HIV is a bloodborne and body fluid–borne virus with some potential threat to clients undergoing HD. Fortunately, the risks of HIV transmission are minimized by the consistent practice of standard precautions (blood and body fluids), routine screening of donated blood for HIV, and decreased numbers of blood transfusions for clients with end-stage renal disease (ESRD). Despite this progress, however, an unknown number of clients may have already been infected with the HIV virus. Clients who have been undergoing HD and who received frequent transfusions during the early to mid-1980s are at risk for acquired immunodeficiency syndrome (AIDS) (see also Chapter 22).

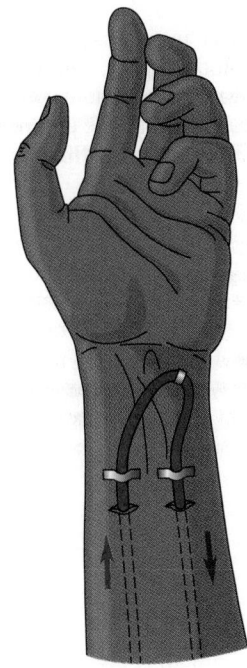

Figure 72-7 ● An arteriovenous shunt in the forearm. One part of the shunt cannula is placed in an artery; the other part in a vein. The ends of the shunt cannula are joined when dialysis is not in progress.

CRITICAL THINKING CHALLENGE

Your client has been diagnosed as having ESRD. The health care provider has ordered dietary teaching. In addition, your client will begin outpatient HD three times per week.

- What instructions should you provide regarding the dietary and fluid needs for this client?
- What complications should you monitor the client for during and immediately following dialysis?

For suggested answer guidelines, go to SIMON http://www.wbsaunders.com/SIMON/Iggy/.

CONSIDERATIONS FOR OLDER ADULTS

There is a greater occurrence of ESRD in individuals 65 to 69 years of age. In the past decade there has been an 8% increase in the incidence of ESRD in individuals ages 45 to 65, and a 14% increase in those 75 years of age and older (USRSD, 1999). In addition, clients over age 65 who are receiving dialysis treatments are more at risk for dialysis-induced hypotension.

CHART 72-10

BEST PRACTICE *for*
Caring for the Client Undergoing Hemodialysis

- Weigh the client before and after dialysis.
- Know the client's dry weight.
- Discuss with the physician whether any of the client's medications should be withheld until after dialysis.
- Be aware of events that occurred during the dialysis treatment.
- Measure blood pressure, pulse rate, respirations, and temperature.
- Assess for symptoms of orthostatic hypotension.
- Assess the vascular access site.
- Observe for bleeding.
- Assess the client's level of consciousness and assess for headache, nausea, and vomiting.

TABLE 72-11 • NURSING MEASURES FOR PREVENTION OF COMPLICATIONS IN HEMODIALYSIS VASCULAR ACCESS			
Access Type	**Bleeding**	**Infection**	**Clotting**
AV fistula or AV graft	Apply pressure to the needle puncture sites.	Ensure adequate site cleaning before cannulation.	Avoid constrictive devices. Rotate needle insertion sites with each hemodialysis treatment. Assess for thrill and bruit.
AV shunt	Keep clamps available.	Perform exit site care 3 times/wk.	Avoid constrictive devices. Assess for thrill and bruit.
Hemodialysis catheters (temporary and permanent)	Monitor the access site.	Use aseptic technique. Change the dressing 3 times/wk.	Place a heparin or heparin/saline dwell solution after hemodialysis treatment. Not used between treatments.

AV, Arteriovenous.

◾ PERITONEAL DIALYSIS

Peritoneal dialysis (PD) takes place within the peritoneal cavity. PD is slower than hemodialysis (HD), however, and more time is needed for the same effect to be obtained.

CLIENT SELECTION. Most clients with chronic renal failure (CRF) can select either HD or PD. For clients who are hemodynamically unstable and for those who cannot tolerate systemic anticoagulation, PD is less hazardous than HD. The lack of vascular access due to inadequate vessels may eliminate HD as an option. In addition, some clients with a new arteriovenous (AV) fistula receive PD while waiting for the access to mature for HD. PD is also often the treatment of choice in the older adult and pediatric populations because it offers more flexibility if the client's status changes frequently.

In some relatively rare situations, PD cannot be performed, usually because of peritoneal adhesions or intra-abdominal surgery in the peritoneal cavity. In these cases, the peritoneal membrane's surface area has been reduced too much to allow for adequate dialysis exchange. In other cases, peritoneal membrane fibrosis may occur after repeated infections, which decreases membrane permeability despite adequate surface area.

PROCEDURE. The surgical insertion of a siliconized rubber (Silastic) catheter into the abdominal cavity is required to allow the infusion of dialyzing fluid (dialysate) (Figure 72-8). According to the physician's order, 1 to 2 L of dialysate is infused by gravity (*fill*) into the peritoneal space over a 10- to 20-minute period, according to the client's tolerance. The fluid *dwells* in the cavity for a specified time ordered by the physician. The fluid then flows out of the body (*drain*) by gravity into a drainage bag. The peritoneal outflow contains the dialysate in addition to the excess water, electrolytes, and nitrogenous waste products that have accumulated in the body. The dialyzing fluid is called peritoneal *effluent* on outflow. The three phases of the process (infusion, or "fill"; dwell; and outflow, or drain) are considered one PD exchange. The number and frequency of PD exchanges are prescribed by the physician, depending on the clinical manifestations and laboratory data.

PROCESS. PD occurs through diffusion and osmosis across the semipermeable peritoneal membrane and adjacent capillaries. The peritoneal membrane is large and porous. It allows solutes, which carry fluid with them, to move by an osmotic gradient from an area of higher concentration in the body (blood) to an area of lower concentration in the dialyzing fluid.

The peritoneal cavity is rich in capillaries and provides a ready access to the blood supply. The fluid and waste products dialyzed from the client move through the blood vessel walls, the interstitial tissues, and the peritoneal membrane and are removed when the dialyzing fluid is drained from the body.

The efficiency of PD can be affected by numerous situations, such as changes in the peritoneal membrane's permeability caused by infection or irritation, and changes in the capillary blood flow resulting from vasoconstriction, vascular disease, or decreased perfusion of the peritoneum. Excess water removal (ultrafiltration) in HD is accomplished by use of hydrostatic positive pressure or transmembrane negative pressure on the dialysis machine. In PD, the amount of water removed from the client depends on the

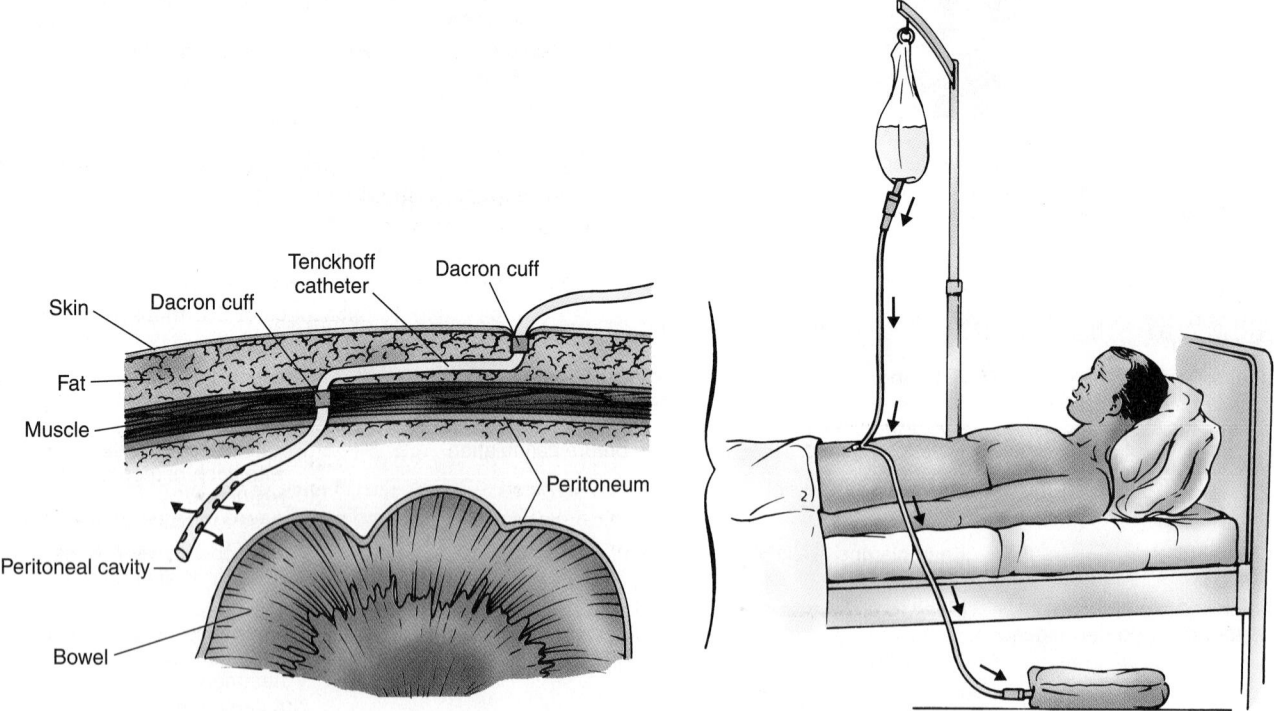

Figure 72-8 ● Manual peritoneal dialysis via an implanted abdominal catheter (Tenckhoff catheter).

concentration of the dialysate. Increasing the glucose concentration of the dialysate makes the solution increasingly more hypertonic. The more hypertonic the solution, the greater the osmotic pressure for ultrafiltration and thus the greater the amount of fluid removed from the client during an exchange. The physician orders the dialysate concentration on the basis of the client's fluid status.

MEDICATION ADDITIVES. Heparin may be added to the dialysate to prevent fibrin clot formation in the catheter or tubing; this intraperitoneal (IP) heparin administration is necessary only after new catheter placement or with the occurrence of peritonitis. There is no systemic absorption of heparin with IP administration, so clotting studies are not needed.

Other agents that may be administered by the IP route include potassium chloride and antibiotics. Commercially prepared dialysate does not contain potassium chloride. Some clients will need potassium chloride added to the dialysate so that the dialysate does not excessively deplete potassium from the plasma. Oral potassium supplements may be prescribed in selected clients. The physician may order IP administration of antibiotics (e.g., gentamicin, vancomycin, cephalosporins) when peritonitis is present or suspected. The combination of potassium chloride and antibiotics in the same bag of dialysate is not recommended, because chemical interactions may limit effectiveness.

TYPES OF PERITONEAL DIALYSIS. Many types of PD are available, including continuous ambulatory PD, multiple-bag continuous ambulatory PD, automated PD, intermittent PD, and continuous-cycle PD. The selection of the type depends on the client's ability and lifestyle.

CONTINUOUS AMBULATORY PERITONEAL DIALYSIS. In continuous ambulatory peritoneal dialysis (CAPD), the client performs self-dialysis by infusing four 2-L exchanges of dialysate into the peritoneal cavity, where the dialysate remains for 4 to 8 hours, 7 days a week. During the dwell period, the client can choose a continuous connect system or a disconnect system.

With the continuous *connect* system (straight transfer set), the dialysate bag is usually attached to the catheter by 48-inch (122-cm) tubing; the empty bag and tubing are folded and worn beneath the clothing until they are used for outflow. After draining, the client removes the bag and connects a new bag to repeat the process.

With the *disconnect system* (Y-transfer set), the client removes the connecting tubing and empty dialysate bag after inflow and attaches a protective cap to the PD catheter junction. The disconnect system eliminates the need to wear the tubing and bag but requires opening the system two extra times with each exchange. This opening of the system increases the potential for contamination and infection.

With CAPD treatment, no machine is necessary, and client independence is encouraged. Theoretically, no partner is required. However, many home training programs suggest that a partner be trained in CAPD as a support for the client should illness or temporary disability occur. Devices to assist in the safe, uncontaminated connection of the tubing spike with the dialysate bag are increasingly in use. These devices

can be considered for clients with impaired vision, limited manual dexterity, or decreased upper extremity strength. CAPD offers the advantage of constant removal of fluid and wastes and more nearly resembles renal function than does HD. Some clients continue to perform their own exchanges while hospitalized.

MULTIPLE-BAG CONTINUOUS AMBULATORY PERITONEAL DIALYSIS. For those who are unable to perform self-CAPD in the acute care setting, a multiple-bag CAPD (MB-CAPD) system allows continuation of CAPD. With MB-CAPD, a manifold of tubing connected to the dialysate and hanging on a portable pole is attached to the PD catheter by connecting tubing (see Figure 72-8). The nurse inflows the dialysate at the prescribed time, allows the dwell, and initiates the outflow for each exchange. The MB-CAPD system permits mobility for the ambulatory client and provides for continuous PD.

AUTOMATED PERITONEAL DIALYSIS. An automated cycling machine that provides for dialysate inflow, dwell, and outflow according to preset times and volumes may be used. A warming chamber for dialysate is part of the machine. Automated peritoneal dialysis (APD) may be used in the acute care setting, the outpatient dialysis center, or the client's home. The functions are performed in response to machine programming that can be individualized for the client's specific needs. A typical prescription calls for 30-minute exchanges (10/10/10 for inflow, dwell, and outflow) for a period of 8 to 10 hours. The machines have numerous safety monitors and alarms and are relatively simple to learn to use.

APD has several distinct advantages. It permits the performance of in-home dialysis while the client sleeps, allowing him or her to be dialysis free during waking hours. Also, because the number of connections and disconnections are fewer with APD, the incidence of peritonitis has been reduced. Finally, APD provides a means by which increased volumes of dialysis solution can be administered to clients who require higher clearances (Levine, 1997).

INTERMITTENT PERITONEAL DIALYSIS. Intermittent peritoneal dialysis (IPD) combines the principles of an osmotic pressure gradient and true dialysis. The client usually requires exchanges of 2 L of dialysate at 30- to 60-minute intervals, allowing 15 to 20 minutes of drain time. For most anuric clients, 30 to 40 exchanges of 2 L three times weekly are sufficient. IPD treatments can be automated or manual.

CONTINUOUS-CYCLE PERITONEAL DIALYSIS. Continuous-cycle peritoneal dialysis (CCPD) also uses an automated cycling machine. Exchanges occur at night while the client sleeps. The final exchange of the night is left to dwell through the day and is drained the next evening as the process is repeated. CCPD offers the advantage of 24-hour dialysis, as in CAPD, but the sterile catheter system is less often violated.

COMPLICATIONS. Complications are possible with PD, but many can be treated or prevented with careful nursing care.

PERITONITIS. The major complication of PD is peritonitis. The most common cause of peritonitis is contamination of the connection site during an exchange. This infection of the peritoneum is manifested by cloudy dialysate outflow (effluent), fever, rebound abdominal tenderness, abdominal pain, general malaise, nausea, and vomiting.

When peritonitis is suspected, the nurse sends a specimen of the dialysate outflow for culture and sensitivity study, Gram stain, and cell count to identify the infecting organism so that an appropriate antibiotic can be ordered. Procedures for routine or periodic culturing of PD effluent vary with institutional practice. In today's era of cost containment, routine practices are less likely to be the norm. Cloudy or opaque effluent is the earliest sign of peritonitis. Thus nursing observations are key to the detection and identification of peritonitis. The best treatment of peritonitis is prevention. The nurse must maintain meticulous sterile technique when caring for the PD catheter and when hooking up or clamping off dialysate bags (Chart 72-11).

PAIN. Pain during the inflow of dialysate is common during the first few exchanges because of peritoneal irritation; however, it disappears after a week or two. Cold dialysate aggravates discomfort. Thus the dialysate bags should be warmed before instillation by use of a heating pad to wrap the bag or by use of the warming chamber of the automated cycling machine. *Microwave ovens are not recommended for the warming of dialysate because of their unpredictable warming patterns and temperatures.*

EXIT SITE AND TUNNEL INFECTIONS. The normal exit site from a PD catheter should be clean, dry, and without pain or evidence of inflammation. Exit site infections (ESIs) are associated with all types of PD catheters. Such infections can be difficult to treat and can become chronic. Exit site and tunnel infections cause increased morbidity, since they can lead to peritonitis, catheter failure, and hospitalization. Dialysate leakage and pulling or twisting of the catheter can predispose the client to ESIs. A Gram stain and culture should be performed when exit sites have purulent drainage.

Tunnel infections occur in the path of the catheter from the skin to the cuff. Signs of infection include redness, tenderness, and pain. ESIs are treated with antimicrobials; however, deep cuff infections usually require catheter removal.

INSUFFICIENT FLOW OF THE DIALYSATE. Constipation is the primary cause of inflow or outflow problems. To prevent constipation, the physician orders a bowel preparation before placing the PD catheter. Colon evacuation before the initiation of PD may also prevent constipation. A high-fiber diet and stool softeners are often needed for ongoing prevention. Other causes of inflow or outflow difficulty include kinking or clamped connection tubing, the client's positioning, fibrin clot formation, and PD catheter migration.

Because outflow drainage is by gravity, the nurse ensures that the drainage bag is lower than the client's abdomen. The nurse inspects the connection tubing and PD system for kinking or twisting and rechecks to make sure that clamps are open. If inflow or outflow drainage is still inadequate, the nurse attempts to stimulate inflow or outflow by repositioning the client. Turning the client to the other side or making sure that he or she is in good body alignment may help. Having the client in a supine low-Fowler's position seems to minimize the buildup of intra-abdominal pressure. Increased intra-abdominal pressure that occurs in the sitting or standing position, or with coughing, contributes to leakage at the PD catheter site.

Fibrin clot formation may occur after PD catheter placement or with the onset of peritonitis. Careful milking of the tubing may dislodge the fibrin clot and facilitate inflow and outflow. Radiographic examination is needed to identify PD catheter migration out of the pelvic area. If migration has occurred, the physician repositions the PD catheter.

DIALYSATE LEAKAGE. When dialysis is initiated, small volumes of dialysate are used. It may take clients 1 to 2 weeks to tolerate a full 2-L exchange without leakage around the catheter site. Leakage tends to occur most often in obese or diabetic clients, older adults, and those on long-term steroid therapy (Levine, 1997). Dialysate leakage presents as clear fluid emitting from the catheter exit site. During this time, clients may require hemodialysis (HD) support.

OTHER COMPLICATIONS. The PD effluent (outflow drainage) is expected to be relatively clear and light yellow. The nurse notes any change in the color of the outflow. With the initial exchanges, the outflow may be bloody. The physician may order several in-and-out exchanges of unwarmed dialysis solution in an effort to clear the dialysate of blood. In these cases, the client's hematocrit, pulse, and blood pressure are closely monitored. If the drainage return is brown, a bowel perforation must be suspected. Similarly, if the outflow is the same color as urine and has the same glucose concentration, a possible bladder perforation should be investigated. If the drainage is cloudy or opaque, an infection is suspected.

NURSING CARE DURING PERITONEAL DIALYSIS. In the hospital setting, peritoneal dialysis (PD) is routinely initiated and monitored by the nursing staff. Before the treatment, the nurse evaluates baseline vital signs, including blood pressure, apical and radial pulse rates, temperature, quality of respirations, and breath sounds. The client is weighed, always on the same scale, before beginning the procedure and at least every 24 hours while receiving treatment. Baseline laboratory value determinations, such as electrolyte

---

CHART 72-11

BEST PRACTICE *for*
Caring for the Client with a Peritoneal Dialysis Catheter

- Mask yourself and your client. Wash your hands.
- Put on sterile gloves. Remove the old dressing. Remove the contaminated gloves.
- Assess the area for signs of infection, such as swelling, redness, or discharge around the catheter site.
- Use aseptic technique:
    Open the sterile field on a flat surface and place two precut 4 × 4 inch gauze pads on the field.
    Place three cotton swabs soaked in povidone-iodine on the field. Put on sterile gloves.
- Use cotton swabs to clean around the catheter site. Use a circular motion starting from the insertion site and moving away toward the abdomen. Repeat with all three swabs.
- Apply precut gauze pads over the catheter site. Tape only the edges of the gauze pads.

and glucose levels, are also essential and are repeated at least daily during the PD treatment.

During PD, the nurse continually monitors the client. Vital signs are taken regularly and recorded on a flow sheet. For the first few exchanges, the nurse records the vital signs every 15 minutes. The nurse also performs an ongoing assessment of the client for signs of respiratory distress, pain, or discomfort. The abdominal dressing around the catheter exit site is checked frequently for wetness. The nurse monitors dwell time and initiates outflow. The physician orders dwell time according to the client's needs for fluid removal and electrolyte balance.

For hourly exchanges, dwell time usually ranges from 20 to 40 minutes. Glucose absorption may occur in some clients, and blood glucose assessment is necessary. The outflow should be a continuous stream after the clamp is completely open. The total amount of outflow is recorded accurately after each exchange. Accurate inflow and outflow records are maintained when hourly PD exchanges are done. When outflow is less than inflow, the difference is equal to the amount absorbed or retained by the client during dialysis and should be counted as intake. For clients performing self-CAPD, or when the MB-CAPD system is used, a daily weight is used to monitor fluid status. A visual inspection of the outflow bag and daily weights may be sufficient to note the adequacy of the return.

■ RENAL TRANSPLANTATION

Dialysis and transplantation are life-sustaining treatments for end-stage renal disease (ESRD); transplantation is not considered a "cure." It is up to each client, in consultation with nephrology personnel, to determine which type of therapy is best suited to that client's physical condition and lifestyle. In 2001, 13,290 kidney transplants were performed. Currently, more than 48,000 people are awaiting renal transplantation in the United States alone (United Network for Organ Sharing [UNOS], 2001).

CANDIDATES. Candidates for transplantation must be free of medical problems that might increase the risks associated with the procedure. The usual age range for clients undergoing transplantation is 2 to 70 years of age. In clients older than 70 years of age, the risk of complications increases, but clients older than 70 years of age are considered on an individual basis. A thorough body systems assessment of the client is performed before the client is considered for transplantation (see the Legal/Ethical Issues in Health Care box at right). The process of transplantation can place a life-threatening stress on the cardiac system in clients with advanced, uncorrectable cardiac disease. Thus these clients are usually excluded from consideration for transplantation. Contraindications for transplantation include metastatic malignant neoplasms, chronic infection, severe cardiovascular disease unresponsive to treatment, and severe psychosocial problems such as chemical dependency (Bartucci, 1999). In addition, long-standing disease of the pulmonary system increases the risk of morbidity and mortality owing to respiratory tract infections after transplantation. Clients with diseases of the gastrointestinal (GI) system may require treatment before consideration for transplantation. Such problems as peptic ulcer and diverticulosis can be severely aggravated by the large doses of steroids used after transplantation.

The urinary system must be completely evaluated to ensure its ability to manage normal urine flow. Many clients with ESRD have not used their lower urinary tract for extended periods, and ureteral or bladder abnormalities may require surgical correction before renal transplantation.

Metabolic diseases, such as diabetes mellitus, gout, and hyperparathyroidism, cause even greater risks. These clients can still accept a renal transplant, but careful observation and management are necessary to limit complications. Other conditions that may complicate transplantation include malignant neoplasm and inflammatory disease. Clients with a recent history of a malignant tumor are usually treated with dialysis because of the shortage of donor organs, the possibility that the cancer could attack the transplanted kidney, and the limited life expectancy of these clients. In addition, the immunosuppressive agents used after transplantation increase the risk for cancer recurrence. If more than 2 to 5 years have passed since eradication of the cancer, the client can be considered for a transplant.

Other complicating conditions are considered on an individual basis, depending on the client's current health status. Renal transplantation can be considered for most of those with ESRD and may prove to be the optimal therapy for many people (see the Evidence-Based Practice for Nursing box on p. 1698).

DONORS. The sources of donor kidneys are living donors, non–heart-beating donors (NHBDs), and cadaveric donors. The available kidneys are matched on the basis of immunologic similarity between the donor and the recipient. Living donors are most often blood relatives, but in recent years, unrelated donors have been used. NHBDs are persons declared dead by cardiopulmonary criteria. Kidneys from NHBDs are harvested immediately after death in cases where clients have previously given consent for organ donation and

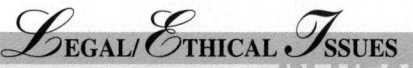

LEGAL/ETHICAL ISSUES IN HEALTH CARE

UNEQUAL ACCESS TO KIDNEY TRANSPLANTATION

There is evidence to suggest that individuals who are insured by Medicaid alone may not be placed on the kidney transplant waiting list. Medicare covers most, but not all, Americans with end-stage renal disease (ESRD). In a retrospective study of all California ESRD clients under 65 years of age who were eligible for Medicare or Medicaid, an analysis was done to determine the importance of health insurance status in relation to kidney transplantation.

The findings of this study suggest that placement on the kidney transplant waiting list is associated with insurance status. In California, clients undergoing dialysis who are ineligible for Medicare coverage are more likely to be poor, female, and members of a minority group. These individuals are also much less likely to be placed on a kidney transplant waiting list. However, once placed on the waiting list, insurance status does not affect access to cadaveric transplantation. It is possible that potential loss of insurance following transplantation, cultural barriers, and educational factors are explanatory factors.

Data from Thamer, M. et al. (1999). Unequal access to cadaveric kidney transplantation in California based on insurance status. *Health Services Research, 34*(4), 879-898.

EVIDENCE-BASED PRACTICE
FOR NURSING

Does race or gender affect quality of life in nondiabetic kidney transplant recipients?

Johnson, C., et al. (1998). Racial and gender differences in quality of life following kidney transplantation. *Image: The Journal of Nursing Scholarship, 30*(2), 125-130.

The purpose of this descriptive, prospective clinical study was to determine if race or gender affected changes in quality of life (QOL) reported by nondiabetic kidney transplant recipients before transplantation and 6 and 12 months after transplantation. The convenience sample obtained for this study consisted of 90 subjects (63 men, 27 women), of whom 36 were African Americans and 55 were Caucasians ages 19 to 67 years. None of the subjects had a history of diabetes.

The Sickness Impact Profile (SIP), Ferrans and Powers Quality of Life Index (QLI), and Adult Self-Image Scales (ASIS) were administered to clients before transplantation and 6 months and 12 months after transplantation. The SIP was used to capture dimensions of QOL related to functional disability, the QLI was used to assess health-focused QOL, and the ASIS was used to determine the psychoemotional aspects of QOL.

QOL scores improved overall for both racial and gender groups after kidney transplantation. African Americans appeared to improve less than Caucasians in such areas as self-image and emotional behavior; however, they had higher baseline scores in these areas as compared with Caucasians. African Americans appeared to suffer more functional impairment before transplantation and demonstrated less improvement following transplantation as compared with Caucasians. Overall, women's scores on QOL measures tended to be lower than those of men.

Possible explanations for the racial differences observed in baseline functional status may relate to poorer socioeconomic status and less access to health care. The higher affective scores of African Americans may be related to spiritual factors. Whereas men seemed to regain independence and improved self-image after transplantation, women may have had more difficulty in adjusting to physical changes and the immunosuppressant regimen. The authors suggest that nurses should consider sociocultural influences and functional concerns of African Americans and women.

Critique. Quality of life has become an important consideration for many individuals in making health care decisions. It is also an important outcome in the evaluation of new therapies. The convenience sample makes it difficult to generalize the results to other kidney transplant recipients, particularly since the majority of transplants are performed on people with diabetes. In addition, the relatively higher baseline scores of the African Americans on the ASIS and QLI may have made comparing QOL scores between races unreliable. Additional studies are needed to lend support to these findings.

Implications for Nursing. Sociocultural and economic factors and gender need to be considered in preparing clients for transplant surgery. Nurses may need to design education interventions that prepare clients for what to expect and how to manage their differing recovery trajectories.

no longer seek active treatment or by in situ preservation in which a cool preservation solution is infused via a catheter inserted into the abdominal aorta after death is declared. Cadaveric donors are usually individuals who suffered irreversible brain injury, typically as a result of trauma. This type of donor must be maintained on a ventilator and have sufficient cardiovascular functioning in order for the kidneys to remain transplantable (Bartucci, 1999).

The size of the kidney is seldom a problem in adults. Pediatric cadaveric kidneys hypertrophy to accommodate adult needs within a few months.

Organs from living *related* donors (LRDs) provide the highest rates of renal graft survival (90%). Donors are usually at least 18 years old because of legal requirements and are seldom older than 65 years of age. General physical criteria for donors include the following:

- Absence of systemic disease and infection
- No history of cancer
- Absence of hypertension and renal disease
- Adequate renal function as evidenced by diagnostic studies

In addition, LRDs must express a clear understanding of the associated surgery and a willingness to give up a kidney. Some transplant centers also require a psychiatric evaluation to determine the motivation of the donor.

Because of advances in immunosuppressant therapy and medical management, the United Network of Organ Sharing (UNOS) reported 1-year renal transplant graft survival to be 90% for all centers in the United States (UNOS, 2001).

PREOPERATIVE CARE. Many issues must be decided before transplantation. Some issues are related to client health and others to the actual transplant procedure. The Clinical Pathway on pp. 1848-1851 highlights care needs for the client undergoing renal transplantation.

IMMUNOLOGIC STUDIES. The major barrier to successful renal transplantation after a suitable donor kidney is available is the body's ability to identify and reject tissue that is not its own. This immunologic process attacks the transplanted kidney and renders it nonfunctional. For immunologic contraindications to be overcome, in-depth tissue typing is done on all candidates for transplantation. These studies include simple ABO blood group typing for compatible blood transfusions and human leukocyte antigen (HLA) studies, as well as other tests. The HLAs have become the principal histocompatibility system used to match transplant recipients with compatible donors. The more similar the antigens of the donor are to those of the recipient, the more likely it is that the transplant will be successful and immunologic rejection will be avoided. Research is ongoing in immunology, and new information in this area could increase the success rate of organ transplantations in the future (see Chapter 20).

SURGICAL TEAM. The surgical team is a group of specialists trained in transplantation procedures. The team includes operating room nurses (circulating and scrub nurses), clinical nurse specialists, and preoperative nurses, as well as transplant surgeons, anesthesiologists, and nephrologists. The role of the preoperative nurse includes the following:

- Teaching about the procedure and postoperative care
- In-depth client assessment
- Coordination of diagnostic tests
- Development and implementation of treatment plans

The transplant recipient usually requires dialysis within 24 hours of the surgery. In addition, the recipient often receives a blood transfusion before surgery. Current research favors donor-specific transfusions, in which blood from the kidney donor is transfused into the recipient. This procedure has resulted in increased graft survival, especially of organs from LRDs.

OPERATIVE PROCEDURES. The donor nephrectomy procedure varies depending on whether the donor is an

NHBD, cadaveric donor, or living donor. The NHBD or cadaveric donor nephrectomy is conducted as a sterile autopsy in the operating room. All arterial and venous vessels and as long a piece of ureter as possible are carefully preserved. After removal, the kidneys are preserved until time for implantation into the recipient. The technique for kidney removal from living donors requires greater surgical care and is a delicate procedure lasting 3 to 4 hours. A flank incision is used, and care is taken to avoid scarring. Donors usually experience more pain than do recipients. They also need special nursing care and support for the psychologic adjustment to loss of a body part.

The transplantation surgery usually takes 4 to 5 hours. The transplanted kidney is usually placed in the right anterior iliac fossa (Figure 72-9) instead of the usual anatomic position. This placement allows easier anastomosis of the ureter and the renal artery and vein, and it also allows for assessment by palpation. The recipient's own nonfunctioning kidneys are not usually removed unless chronic infection in one or both kidneys would compromise overall recovery. The client is then taken to the postanesthesia unit and then, when stable, to a designated surgical unit in the transplant center or to a critical care unit.

POSTOPERATIVE CARE. Postoperative care of the kidney transplant recipient requires that nurses be knowledgeable about the expected clinical findings and potential complications unique to this population. Nursing care includes ongoing physical assessment with an emphasis on evaluation of renal function. The transplant recipient requires particularly close attention because the immunosuppressive drug therapy to prevent tissue rejection causes impaired healing and an increased susceptibility to infection. Careful urologic management is essential to graft success. These clients always have a large indwelling (Foley) catheter for accurate measurements of urine output and decompression of the bladder and to prevent stretch on suture and anastomosis sites on the bladder. An abrupt decrease in urine output is significant, since it can herald the onset of complications such as rejection, acute tubular necrosis (ATN), thrombosis, or obstruction. The urine color is carefully monitored (usually hourly). The urine is initially pink and bloody, but it gradually returns

to normal over a period of several days to several weeks, depending on renal function. A continuous bladder irrigation is occasionally prescribed to decrease the formation of blood clots, which could increase pressure in the bladder and jeopardize the graft. Routine catheter care is performed to minimize contamination of the catheter; the nurse adheres to the agency's policy. The catheter is removed as soon as possible to avoid infection, usually 3 to 7 days postoperatively. The nurse is also responsible for obtaining daily urine tests, including urinalysis, glucose determinations, tests for the presence of acetone, culture, and specific gravity measurement.

During the postoperative period, the function of the transplanted kidney (renal graft) can result in either oliguria or diuresis. Oliguria may occur as a result of ischemia and ATN, rejection, or other complications. To increase urine output, the physician may order diuretics and osmotic agents, such as mannitol. The nurse and the physician carefully monitor the client's fluid status because fluid overload can cause hypertension, congestive heart failure (CHF), and pulmonary edema. Daily weight measurement, frequent blood pressure readings, and careful intake and output measurements are required to evaluate fluid status.

Instead of oliguria, the client may have diuresis, especially with a transplanted kidney from a living related donor (LRD). The nurse carefully monitors fluid intake and output and observes for electrolyte imbalances, such as hypokalemia and hyponatremia. Hypovolemia from excessive diuresis may cause hypotensive episodes. The nurse strives to prevent this situation because decreased blood pressure also decreases the oxygen and blood supply to the new kidney, which can threaten graft survival.

COMPLICATIONS. Unfortunately, numerous potential complications are associated with transplantation surgery.

REJECTION. The most common and the most threatening complication of renal transplantation is rejection. Rejection is the leading cause of graft loss. A reaction occurs between the antigens in the transplanted kidney and the antibodies and cytotoxic T-cells in the recipient's blood. These immunologic substances treat the new kidney as a foreign invader and cause tissue destruction, thrombosis, and eventual necrosis of the kidney. The three types of rejection are hyperacute, acute, and chronic. Acute rejection is the most common type in the transplant client. It is treated with increased immunosuppressive therapy and can be reversible. Rejection can be diagnosed by clinical manifestations, a renal scan, and renal biopsy. Table 72-12 summarizes the characteristics of the three types of rejection; Chapter 20 discusses their pathophysiology and treatment.

ACUTE TUBULAR NECROSIS. Prolonged preservation of cadaveric kidneys before transplantation can result in ischemic damage that is manifested as acute tubular necrosis (ATN). These clients usually need to be dialyzed until urine output becomes sufficient and the blood urea nitrogen (BUN) and creatinine normalize. Because ATN is often difficult to distinguish from acute rejection, clients need to undergo weekly biopsies to assess the need for further immunosuppression if rejection is occurring.

THROMBOSIS. Thrombosis may occur during the first 2 to 3 days following transplantation. A sudden decrease in

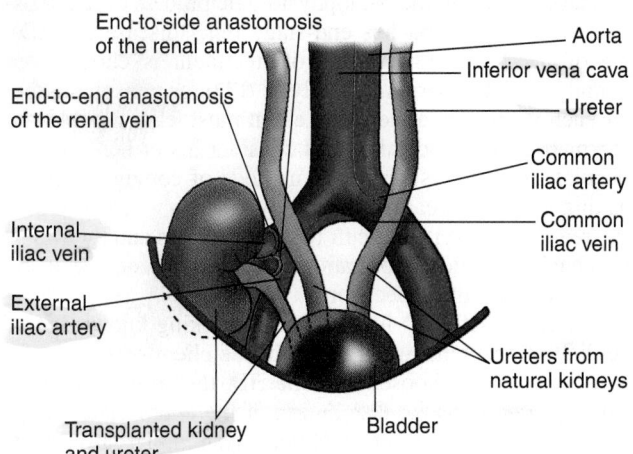

Figure 72-9 ● Placement of a transplanted kidney in the right iliac fossa.

TABLE 72-12 • A COMPARISON OF HYPERACUTE, ACUTE, AND CHRONIC POST-TRANSPLANT REJECTION

Hyperacute Rejection	Acute Rejection	Chronic Rejection
ONSET		
Within 48 hr after surgery	1 wk to 2 yr postoperatively (most common in first 2 wk)	Occurs gradually during a period of months to years
CLINICAL MANIFESTATIONS		
Increased temperature	Oliguria or anuria	Gradual increase in BUN and serum creatinine
Increased blood pressure	Temperature over 100° F (37.8° C)	levels
Pain at transplant site	Increased blood pressure	Fluid retention
	Enlarged, tender kidney	Changes in serum electrolyte levels
	Lethargy	Fatigue
	Elevated serum creatinine, BUN, potassium levels	
	Fluid retention	
TREATMENT		
Immediate removal of the transplanted kidney	Increased doses of immunosuppressive drugs	Conservative management until dialysis is required

BUN, Blood urea nitrogen.

urine production or output may signal impaired perfusion resulting from thrombosis. Ultrasound examination of the kidney will reveal decreased or absent blood supply, and emergency surgery is required to prevent further ischemic damage or loss of the graft (Bartucci, 1999).

RENAL ARTERY STENOSIS. Stenosis of the renal artery is detected by identification of hypertension, a bruit over the artery anastomosis site, and decreased renal function. The involved artery must be surgically resected and the kidney anastomosed to another artery. Clients with vascular complications nearly always require surgical intervention. Other vascular problems include vascular leakage or thrombosis, both of which require an emergency transplant nephrectomy.

OTHER COMPLICATIONS. Other complications may involve the wound or genitourinary tract. Wound complications, such as hematomas, abscesses, and lymphoceles, can become a medium for infection and can place external pressure on the new kidney. Infection is a significant cause of morbidity and mortality in the transplant recipient. Prevention of infection is paramount. Strict aseptic technique and handwashing must be rigorously enforced. Because of immunosuppression, transplant recipients may not present with typical signs of infection. Low-grade fevers, mental status changes, and vague complaints of discomfort may be present before sepsis. Nurses play a pivotal role in the early detection of infection.

Genitourinary tract complications include ureteral leakage, fistula, or obstruction; calculus formation; bladder neck contracture; scrotal swelling; and graft rupture. Surgical intervention may be required.

IMMUNOSUPPRESSIVE DRUG THERAPY. The success of renal transplantation depends on changing the client's immunologic response so that the new kidney is not rejected as a foreign organ. The nurse administers and is aware of the immunosuppressive drugs that protect the transplanted organ. These drugs include corticosteroids, antilymphocyte preparations, monoclonal antibodies, and cyclosporine (Cyclosporin A). Chapter 20 discusses the mechanisms of action for these agents and the associated client responses. Clients who must take immunosuppressant medications are vulnerable to infection secondary to myelosuppression. Clients are at risk for developing a number of fatal viral, fungal, bacterial, or protozoal infections (Giuliano & Sims, 1999).

● Community-Based Care

■ HOME CARE MANAGEMENT

Because of the complex nature of chronic renal failure (CRF), its progressive course, and multiple treatment modalities, a case manager may be useful in the planning, coordination, and evaluation of care. As the renal disease progresses, the client is seen by a physician or nurse practitioner regularly and may have frequent hospitalizations. The nurse, in conjunction with the dietitian and social worker, evaluates the home environment and determines special equipment needs before discharge. Once the client is discharged, home care nurses may direct care and monitor progress Chart 72-12 provides a focused assessment guideline for the client after renal transplantation.

The nurse provides ongoing health teaching about the diet in renal disease and the pathophysiologic process of renal disease. As CRF approaches end-stage renal disease (ESRD), one of the following courses of treatment is chosen: hemodialysis (HD), peritoneal dialysis (PD), or transplantation. For each form of treatment, the client must learn the relevant information and procedures and consider his or her personal lifestyle, support systems, and methods of coping. Decision making about the treatment modality, or even whether to pursue treatment, is very difficult for many clients and their families. Nurses provide information and emotional support to assist clients with these decisions.

Treatment with HD necessitates a working knowledge of the dialysis machine and the care of the client's vascular access. If the client chooses in-home HD, the home care nurse makes preparations for installation of the appropriate equipment, including a water treatment system. Regardless of whether the treatment is provided at home or in a center, the nurse provides ongoing physical assessment and health teaching to promote maximal independence at home.

CHART 72-12

FOCUSED ASSESSMENT *of*
Home Care Clients with Chronic Renal Failure

Assess cardiovascular and respiratory status, including:
- Vital signs, with special attention to blood pressure
- Presence of S$_3$ and/or pericardial friction rub
- Presence of chest pain
- Presence of edema (periorbital, pretibial, sacral)
- Jugular vein distention
- Presence of dyspnea
- Presence of crackles, beginning at the bases and extending upward

Assess nutritional status, including:
- Weight gain or loss
- Presence of anorexia, nausea, or vomiting

Assess renal status, including:
- Amount, frequency, and appearance of urine (in non-anuric clients)
- Presence of bone pain
- Presence of hyperglycemia secondary to diabetes

Assess hematologic status, including:
- Presence of petechiae, purpura, ecchymoses
- Presence of fatigue or shortness of breath

Assess gastrointestinal status, including:
- Presence of stomatitis
- Presence of melena

Assess integumentary status, including:
- Skin integrity
- Presence of pruritus
- Presence of skin discoloration

Assess neurologic status, including:
- Changes in mental status
- Presence of seizure activity
- Presence of sensory changes
- Presence of lower extremity weakness

Assess laboratory data, including:
- BUN
- Serum creatinine
- Creatinine clearance
- CBC
- Electrolytes

Assess psychosocial status, including:
- Presence of anxiety
- Presence of maladaptive behavior

BUN, Blood urea nitrogen; *CBC*, complete blood count.

The client receiving PD needs extensive training in the procedure. The client also needs assistance in obtaining equipment and the numerous supplies involved. Home care nurses perform physical assessments, monitor vital signs, assess compliance with drug and diet regimens, and carefully monitor for signs and symptoms of peritonitis.

The nurse plays a vital role in the long-term care of the client with a renal transplant. This client is usually discharged 3 to 4 weeks after surgery. Meticulous maintenance of prescribed immunosuppressive drug therapy is essential for the survival of the renal graft. Thus the nurse facilitates acceptance and understanding of this regimen as a part of daily life. The nurse also carefully monitors for signs of graft rejection and for complications, such as infection.

■ HEALTH TEACHING

Health teaching is a primary function of nurses caring for clients with any form of renal disease. The home care nurse collaborates with other members of the health care team, especially the dietitian, pharmacist, and physician, to instruct clients and family members or significant others in all aspects of diet therapy, necessary drug therapy, and associated renal pathologic changes. Clients and family members are taught to report signs and symptoms of complications, such as fluid overload and infection. When a client requires a more advanced form of therapy, such as dialysis or transplantation, the teaching focuses on the chosen therapeutic intervention.

HD is the most complex form of therapy for the client and family to understand. Even if clients receive HD in a dialysis center instead of at home, they are usually expected to have some knowledge of the HD machine. The client or a family member or other caregiver must be taught to care for the vascular access and to report signs of infection and stenosis. The client who plans to have in-home HD will need a partner. Both the client and the partner must be completely educated in the entire process of HD and must be able to perform it independently before the client is discharged from the HD center or hospital HD unit.

PD involves extensive health teaching. This instruction can be given to the client alone or to the client and a family member or other caregiver if the client cannot perform the procedure. The nurse emphasizes sterile technique because peritonitis is the most common complication of PD performed at home. The nurse instructs clients to report the signs and symptoms associated with peritonitis. They should report the presence of cloudy effluent and abdominal pain, especially when accompanied by rebound tenderness. Clients are taught that cloudy effluent needs to be analyzed promptly. A specimen is sent by the home care nurse for culture and sensitivity, cell count, and Gram stain to identify the causative organism. Clients are taught that peritonitis is treated with antimicrobial therapy, usually given by the intraperitoneal (IP) route. To prevent peritonitis, they are taught how breaks in aseptic technique can occur, resulting in peritonitis. In addition, to eradicate the infection, nurses must educate clients about the importance of completing the antibiotic regimen. Nurses need to teach that repeated episodes of peritonitis can result in diminished ultrafiltration capability, which may necessitate transfer to HD.

The client receiving a renal transplant also needs extensive health teaching. The nurse provides instruction about drug regimens, home monitoring, immunosuppression, signs and symptoms of rejection, infection, and prescribed changes in the diet and activity level.

■ PSYCHOSOCIAL PREPARATION

The nurse provides psychologic support for the client and family or significant others. The nurse facilitates the client's adjustment to the diagnosis of renal failure and eventual acceptance of the treatment regimens.

For many clients, the reduction of uremic symptoms in the initial weeks and months of dialysis treatment creates a sense of euphoria and well-being (the "honeymoon" period). They feel better physically, their mood may be happy and hopeful, and they tend to overlook the inconvenience and discomfort of frequent dialysis treatments. The nurse realizes that this mood is temporary and uses the time to initiate health care teaching. The nurse stresses that although the client's uremic symptoms have diminished, the client will not return completely to the previous state of well-being. The client and the family may have looked on dialysis as a cure instead of a required lifelong treatment.

Many clients enter a phase of discouragement and disillusionment sometime during the first year of treatment; this may last a few months to a year or longer. The difficulties of incorporating dialysis into daily life are staggering, and clients often become disappointed and depressed as the problems become apparent. During this time, they may struggle against the idea of having to be permanently dependent on a disruptive therapy. The fear of rejection by health staff and family members or significant others reinforces feelings of helplessness and dependence. Some people retreat into complete or partial denial of the disease and the need for treatment. They may deny the need for dialysis or may not comply with medication administration and dietary restrictions. Nurses who work with these clients need to monitor any maladaptive behaviors that may contribute to non-compliance and suggest psychiatric referrals. Nurses and family members should focus on the positive aspects of the treatments. The nurse continues health care education with clients as active participants and decision makers.

Most clients with chronic renal failure (CRF) eventually enter a phase of acceptance or, at least, resolution. The prospect of a chronic illness may be devastating for some people, and each person reacts differently. To make this long-term adaptation, the client must adjust to continuous change, but specific concerns depend on the current physical status and particular treatment method.

After clients have accepted or become resigned to the chronicity of their disease, they usually attempt to return to their previous activities. Resuming the previous level of activity, however, may not be possible. The nurse and other health care professionals can help clients to establish realistic goals that allow them to lead active, productive lives.

■ HEALTH CARE RESOURCES

Professionals from various disciplines are valuable resources for the client with renal failure. Home care nurses are often required to monitor the client's status and evaluate maintenance of the prescribed treatment regimen (HD or PD). A client with advanced renal failure may need the assistance of a home care aide in performing the activities of daily living. Social services personnel are usually involved because of the complex process of applying for financial aid to pay for the required medical care (see the Cost of Care box above). To increase the functional capacity of the client, a physical therapist may be beneficial. Consultation with a dietitian will assist the client and family members in understanding the special dietary needs. A psychiatric evaluation may be needed to assist with depressive symptoms and maladjustment. Clergy and pastoral care specialists offer spiritual support.

Clients with CRF are routinely observed by a physician, usually a nephrologist. Such organizations as the National Kidney Foundation (NKF), the American Kidney Fund, and the National Association of Patients on Hemodialysis and Transplantation (NAPHT) may be helpful to clients and families.

● Evaluation: Outcomes

NOC The nurse evaluates the care of the client with chronic renal failure (CRF) on the basis of the identified nursing diagnoses and collaborative problems. The expected outcomes are that the client will:
- Achieve and maintain appropriate fluid volume
- Maintain serum electrolyte levels in expected ranges

COST OF CARE
IMPLICATIONS FOR NURSING

ECONOMIC COST OF END-STAGE RENAL DISEASE

Cost of Care
- Public and private funds totaling $15.6 billion were spent in the treatment of ESRD in 1997.
- Payments to skilled nursing facilities, home care, and hospice for the care of individuals with ESRD account for 6.3% of total costs.
- Medicare spending for the care of individuals with ESRD from 1993 to 1997 totaled $44.93 billion.
- Medicare payments for kidney donor acquisitions are estimated to be $25,000 per acquisition.
- Health maintenance organizations (HMO) payments for the treatment of clients with ESRD average approximately $1438 to $2040 per month.

Implications for Nursing
ESRD has increased steadily since 1993. The chronic nature of the disease, with its relatively high morbidity and mortality rates, suggests a role for nurses in the prevention of renal impairment through rigorous teaching and follow-up of clients with diabetes and hypertension. Teaching efforts by nurses should also target those already diagnosed with the disease to prevent further decline to kidney function.

Data from U.S. Renal Data Systems. (1999). *USRDS 1999 annual data report.* Bethesda, MD: National Institutes of Health, National Institute of Diabetes and Digestive and Kidney Diseases.
ESRD, End-stage renal disease.

- Maintain heart rate and blood pressure in expected ranges
- Comply with the prescribed dietary regimen
- Maintain an adequate nutritional status
- Seek information to reduce anxiety
- Use effective coping strategies
- Report an absence of physical manifestations of anxiety

ONLINE RESOURCES

For suggested readings and Internet resources, go to http://www.wbsaunders.com/SIMON/Iggy/.

SELECTED BIBLIOGRAPHY

Asterisk indicates a classic or definitive work on this subject.

Baer, C. (1998). Care of the critically ill chronic renal failure patient: Crisis, challenges and choices. *Critical Care Nursing Clinics of North America, 10*(4), 433-448.

Baker, J., & Thomas, A. (2001). Progressive renal insufficiency program planning: A technique for evaluation and improvement. *Nephrology Nursing Journal, 28*(1), 13-18.

Bartucci, M.R. (1999). Kidney transplantation: State of the art. *AACN Clinical Issues: Advanced Practice in Acute and Critical Care, 10*(2), 153-163.

Behrens, J. (2001). Assessing anemia secondary to hemolysis in hemodialysis patients. *Nephrology Nursing Journal, 28*(2), 253-258.

Bonventre, J. (1998). Ischemic acute renal failure. In J.L. Jameson (Ed.), *Principles of molecular medicine* (pp. 651-657). Totowa, N.J.: Humana Press.

Brundage, D., & Linton, A.D. (1997). Age-related changes in the genitourinary system. In M.A. Matteson, E.S. McConnell, & A.D. Linton (Eds.), *Gerontological nursing: Concepts and practice* (2nd ed., pp. 342-343). Philadelphia: W.B. Saunders.

Craig, M. (1998). Continuous venous to venous hemofiltration. Implementing and maintaining a program: Examples and alternatives. *Critical Care Clinics of North America, 10*(2), 219-233.

Curtin, R.B., Svarstad, B., & Keller, T. (1999). Hemodialysis patients' noncompliance with oral medications. *ANNA Journal, 26*(3), 307-316.

Giuliano, K., & Pysznik, E. (1998). Renal replacement therapy in critical care: Implementation of a unit-based continuous venovenous hemodialysis program. *Critical Care Nurse, 18*(1), 40-51.

Giuliano, K., & Sims, T.W. (1999). Transplant issues: Infections and immunosuppressant drugs. *Dimensions of Critical Care Nursing, 18*(2), 16-19.

Hayes, D. (2000). Caring for your patient with a permanent renal dialysis access. *Nursing2000, 30*(3), 41-46.

Johnson, C., et al. (1998). Racial and gender differences in quality of life following kidney transplantation. *Image: The Journal of Nursing Scholarship, 30*(2), 125-130.

Johnson, J., & Lalonde, R. (1997). Congestive heart failure. In J.T. Dipiro et al. (Eds.), *Pharmacotherapy: A pathophysiologic approach* (3rd ed., pp. 219-256). New York: McGraw-Hill.

Kearney, K. (2000). Dialysis disequilibrium syndrome. *American Journal of Nursing, 100*(2), 53-54.

Kellum, J. (2000). An evaluation of pharmacological strategies for the prevention and treatment of acute renal failure. *Drugs, 59*(1), 79-91.

Kelly, M. (1997). Acute renal failure. *American Journal of Nursing, 97*(3), 32-34.

King, B. (2000). Meds and the dialysis patient. *RN, 63*(7), 54-59.

Kuhlmann, M.K., Schmidt, F., & Kohler, H. (1999). High protein/energy vs. standard protein: Energy nutritional regimen in the treatment of malnourished hemodialysis patients. *Mineral and Electrolyte Metabolism, 25*(4-6), 306-310.

Levine, D.Z. (1997). *Caring for the renal patient* (3rd ed.). Philadelphia: W.B. Saunders.

McAlpine, L. (1998a). CAVH: Principles and practical applications. *Critical Care Nursing Clinics of North America, 10*(2), 179-189.

McAlpine, L. (1998b). CAVHD: Transitioning from CAVH. *Critical Care Nursing Clinics of North America, 10*(2), 191-195.

Mehrotra, R., & Nolph, K.D. (1999). Low protein diets are not needed in chronic renal failure. *Mineral and Electrolyte Metabolism, 25*(4-6), 311-316.

Mehta, R., & Letteri, J. (1997). Current status of renal replacement therapy for acute renal failure: A survey of US nephrologists. The National Kidney Foundation Council on Dialysis. *American Journal of Nephrology, 19*(3), 377-382.

Orias, M., Mahnensmith, R., & Perazella, M. (1999). Extreme hyperphosphatemia and acute renal failure after a phosphorus-containing bowel regimen. *American Journal of Nephrology, 19*(1), 60-63.

Politoski, G., et al. (1998). Continuous renal replacement therapy, *Critical Care Nursing Clinics of North America, 10*(2), 171-177.

Ray, T. (2000). Chronic and acute renal failure: Primary care issues. *ADVANCE for Nurse Practitioners, 8*(8), 69-72.

Sehgal, A.R. (2000). Outcomes of renal replacement therapy among blacks and women. *American Journal of Kidney Diseases, 35*(4 Suppl. 1), S148-S152.

Sosa-Guerrero, S., & Gomez, N. (1997). Dealing with end-stage renal disease. *American Journal of Nursing, 97*(10), 44-50.

Stark, J. (1998a). Acute renal failure: Focus on advances in acute tubular necrosis. *Critical Care Nursing Clinics of North America, 10*(2), 159-170.

Stark, J. (1998b). The interrelationship between renal and cardiac function. *Critical Care Clinics of North America, 10*(4), 411-419.

Thamer, M., et al. (1999). Unequal access to cadaveric kidney transplantation in California based on insurance status. *Health Services Research, 34*(4), 879-900.

Tran, M., & Rutecki, G. (2000). Renal disease: Tips on prevention and early recognition. *Consultant, 40*(2), 222-229.

United Network for Organ Sharing online. (2001). http://www.unos.org.

U.S. Renal Data Systems. (1999). *USRDS 1999 annual data report.* Bethesda, MD: National Institutes of Health, National Institute of Diabetes and Digestive and Kidney Diseases.

Wade-Elliott, R. (1999). Caring for the elderly with renal failure: Gastrointestinal changes. *ANNA Journal, 26*(6), 563-569.

White, V. (1997). Hyperkalemia. *American Journal of Nursing, 97*(6), 35.

Zellner, K. (1999). Acute tubular necrosis. *RN, 62*(2), 42-45.

PROBLEMS OF REPRODUCTION

Management of Clients with Problems of the Reproductive System

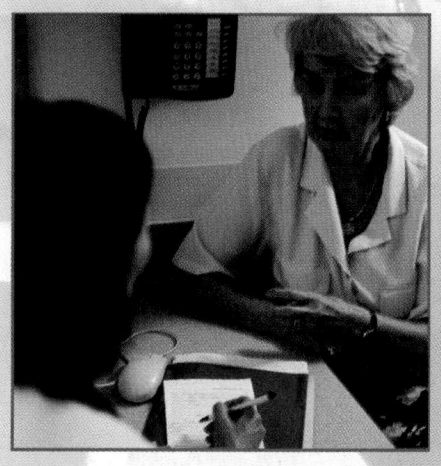

UNIT 16 PROBLEMS OF REPRODUCTION ■ Core Concepts Grid

Anatomy	Physiology	Pathophysiology	History	Physical Exam	Diagnostic Tests	Interventions	Pharmacology
• **Female** Ovaries Fallopian tubes Uterus Vagina • **Male** Penis Scrotum Testes Ducts • **Breasts**	• Procreation • Nurturing • Sexual pleasure • Urinary elimination	• Infection • Obstruction • Inflammation • Tumors	• **Client history** Past problems Contraceptives Obstetric history Self-examination Breast Testes Difficult/painful urination Menstrual history Erectile dysfunction Renal/endocrine dysfunction Hypertension • **Family history** Cancer Thyroid Diabetes • **Social history** Sexual history Alcohol use Smoking Exposure to sexually transmitted dis- ease (STDs) Age Race	• **Skin/hair** **distribution** • **Skin ulceration/** **rashes/color** • **Discharge** Vagina Penis Nipple • **Hernia** • **Breasts** Size Shape Masses	• Mammography • Ultrasonography • Pap smear • Estrogen levels • Androgen levels • Venereal Disease Research Labora- tory (VDRL) test • Fluorescent Tre- ponemal Antibody Absorption (FTA- ABS) test • Gram stain • Acid phosphate • Prostate-specific antigen (PSA) • Carcinoembryonic antigen (CEA)	• Radiation therapy • Client education Self-examination Breast Testes Safer sex Hormone replace- ment therapy (HRT) Kegel exercises • Bladder irrigations • Urinary catheter care Foley (3-way) Suprapubic • Penile implants • Postoperative care and monitor- ing for complica- tions (e.g., hemmorrhage) • Sperm banking • Emotional support • Health teaching	• Antibiotics • Antivirals • Antiprotozoals • Antifungals • Hormone replacement therapy • Anti-impotence agents • Chemothera- peutic agents

Assessment of the Reproductive System

DEITRA L. LOWDERMILK

Learning Objectives

After studying this chapter, you should be able to:

1. Review the anatomy and physiology of the reproductive system.
2. Discuss the components of a health history for reproductive health problems using Gordon's Functional Health Patterns.
3. Interpret common reproductive diagnostic tests.
4. Describe the client preparation for common reproductive diagnostic tests.
5. Develop a teaching plan for clients undergoing endoscopic studies for reproductive health problems.
6. Explain the importance of selected reproductive tests in promoting and maintaining health (e.g., mammogram).

SIMON

Go to http://www.wbsaunders.com/SIMON/Iggy/ for self-assessment questions related to these Learning Objectives.

The nurse is often the first health care professional to assess the client with a reproductive system disorder. Basic assessment of the male and female reproductive systems should be part of every complete physical examination. The nurse should be comfortable with his or her sexuality and be nonjudgmental about variations in sexual practices.

This chapter describes basic reproductive system assessment. Chapters 74 and 76 provide additional assessment data. The student is also referred to a fundamentals or basic nursing text for information on human sexuality.

ANATOMY AND PHYSIOLOGY REVIEW
Structure and Function of the Female Reproductive System

Females begin to develop secondary sex characteristics at a wide range of ages. The average age for a girl to begin pubertal development is 11 years. Delayed puberty may be caused by the following:

- A familial history of late growth
- A low percentage of body fat
- Abnormalities of the pituitary gland, ovaries, or hypothalamus
- Congenital structural abnormalities

■ EXTERNAL GENITALIA

The external female genitalia, or **vulva,** extends from the mons pubis to the anal opening. The mons pubis is a fat pad that covers the symphysis pubis and protects it during coitus (sexual intercourse). The mons becomes prominent and covered with hair during puberty.

The **labia majora** are two vertical folds of adipose tissue that extend posteriorly from the mons pubis to the perineum. Because fatty tissue deposits vary among individuals, the size of the labia majora varies. The skin over the labia majora is usually darker than the surrounding skin and is highly vascular. The labia become prominent during puberty and develop hair on the outer surfaces. The labia majora protect inner vulval structures and enhance sexual arousal.

The labia majora surround two thinner, vertical folds of reddish epithelium called the **labia minora.** The labia minora are highly vascular and have a rich nerve supply. Emotional or physical stimulation produces marked swelling and sensitivity. Numerous sebaceous glands in the labia minora lubricate the entrance to the vagina.

Anteriorly, the labia minora form the prepuce (the hood of the clitoris) and the frenulum (a fold connecting the undersurface of the clitoris with the labia minora). Posteriorly, the labia minora join to form a thin, flat tissue called the fourchette. The clitoris is a small, cylindric organ located beneath the prepuce that is composed of erectile tissue with a high concentration of sensory nerve endings. During sexual arousal, the clitoris becomes larger and increases sexual sensation.

The vestibule is a longitudinal area between the labia minora, the clitoris, and the fourchette. This area contains Bartholin's glands and the openings of the urethra, Skene's glands (paraurethral glands), and vagina. The two Bartholin's glands, located deeply posterior on both sides of the vaginal opening, secrete lubrication fluid during sexual excitement. Their ductal openings are usually not visible.

The connective tissue that partly or wholly occludes the vaginal opening in the vestibule is called the hymen. The hymen can tear during strenuous exercise, masturbation, coitus, or tampon insertion.

The area between the fourchette and the anus is the perineum. The skin of the perineum covers the muscles, fascia, and ligaments that support the pelvic structures and provide voluntary control of the vagina and of the urinary and anal sphincters.

INTERNAL GENITALIA

The internal female genitalia are shown in Figure 73-1.

Vagina

The **vagina** is a collapsible hollow tube that extends from the vestibule to the uterus. In addition to being the channel for the passage of the menstrual flow, the vagina allows reception of the penis during intercourse and passage of the fetus during a vaginal birth. Squamous epithelium and abundant blood vessels line the thin, muscular vaginal walls of the vagina that lie in transverse folds (rugae) during the reproductive years and are highly distensible (stretchable). Estrogen deprivation occurring during postpartum periods, lactation, and menopause causes the vaginal wall to become dry and thinner and the rugae to become smoother. There are few sensory nerve endings in the lower vaginal segment.

The amounts of glycogen and lubricating fluid secreted by the vaginal epithelium are influenced by ovarian hormones.

Döderlein's bacilli, the normal vaginal flora, interact with the secreted glycogen to produce lactic acid and maintain an acidic pH (4 to 5) in the vagina. This acidity reduces the vagina's susceptibility to infection.

At the upper end of the vagina, the uterine cervix projects into a cup-shaped vault of thin vaginal tissue. The recessed pockets around the cervix (the fornices) permit palpation of the internal pelvic organs. The posterior area is clinically significant because it provides access into the peritoneal cavity (through Douglas' cul-de-sac) for diagnostic or surgical purposes.

Uterus

The **uterus** is a thick-walled, muscular organ attached to the upper end of the vagina. This inverted pear–shaped organ is located within the true pelvis, between the bladder and the rectum. The uterus is composed of the corpus (body) and the cervix; these areas are separated by a constricted region called the isthmus. Functionally, the uterus responds to hormonal stimulation and prepares to receive, nurture and, finally, expel the products of conception.

The size of the uterus depends on the woman's developmental stage and obstetric history. In women who have never been pregnant, the average uterine dimensions are $3\frac{1}{2}$ inches × 2 inches × 1 inch (7.5 cm × 5 cm × 2.5 cm).

CORPUS

The upper segment of the uterine body, between the insertion sites of the fallopian tubes, is referred to as the fundus. Although the uterus is a hollow organ, its walls are in such close proximity in the nonpregnant state that its cavity is merely a

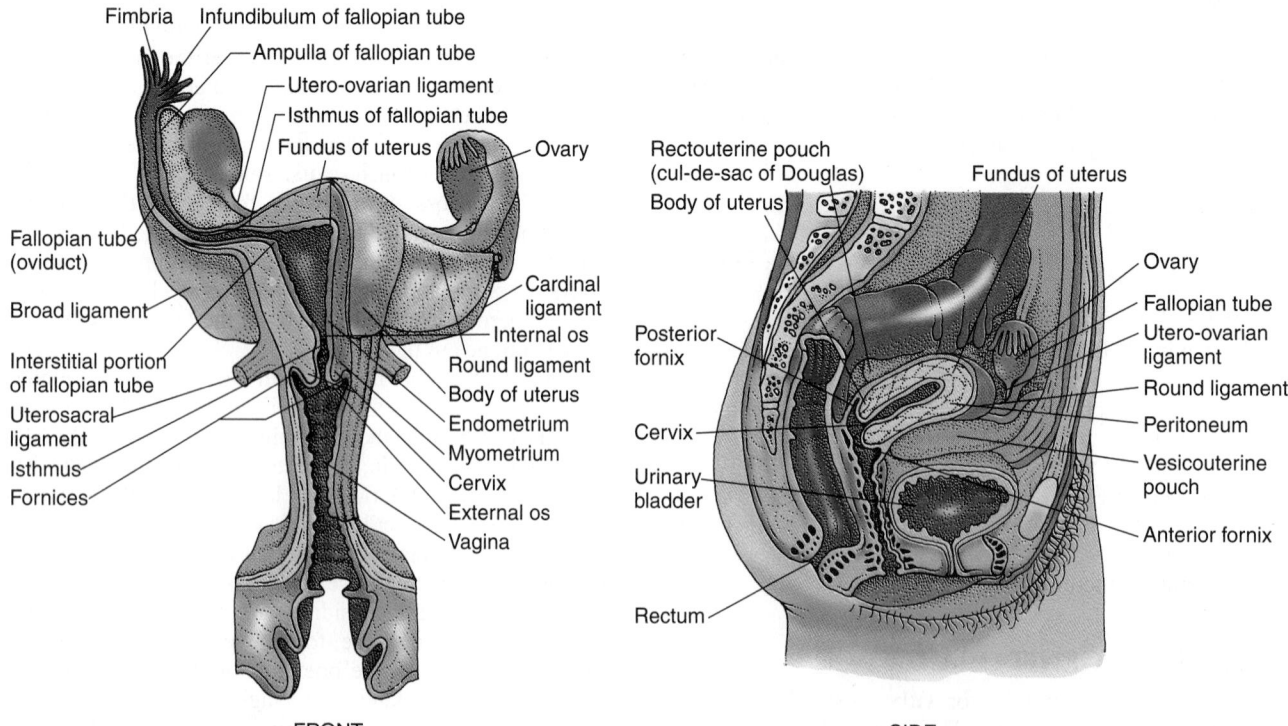

FRONT

SIDE

Figure 73-1 ● Internal female genitalia.

slit. The uterine walls are composed of three layers: the peritoneum, the myometrium, and the endometrium.

The peritoneum is the outer layer that separates the uterus from the abdominal cavity. The pouch formed by the peritoneum, where it lines the anterior uterus and extends to the top of the bladder, is called the vesicouterine pouch. The rectouterine pouch (also referred to as Douglas' cul-de-sac or the posterior cul-de-sac) is the posterior peritoneal pocket, between the rectum and the posterior uterine and vaginal walls.

The myometrium is the thick middle layer of the body of the uterus and is made up of three layers of smooth muscle fibers. These muscle fibers are arranged in opposing directions and are interlaced with blood vessels. Contraction of these muscle fibers can expel the products of conception and can constrict the blood vessels to control bleeding after childbirth.

The inner mucosal layer of the uterine body is the endometrium. The cyclic activity of estrogen and progesterone produces great variation in the thickness of this tissue (from 0.5 to 5 mm). The endometrium consists of a single layer of epithelial cells that cover tubular uterine glands, a spongy stroma (connective tissue framework), and a vascular network. The uterine glands secrete an alkaline fluid that keeps the cavity moist. All but the deepest layer of endometrium is shed during menses and after the delivery of a fetus.

CERVIX

The **cervix** lies below the isthmus of the uterus and extends into the vagina. The cervix provides a canal for the entry of sperm into the uterus and for the passage of menstrual flow, secretes mucus; it also provides a barrier to ascending vaginal bacteria. In addition, sphincter-like fibers that comprise the cervix hold the products of conception in the uterine cavity or stretch to permit vaginal birth.

The cervical portion of the uterus is approximately 1 inch (2.5 cm) long. The upper boundary is the internal os. The lower boundary, the external os, projects into the vaginal fornix. In the nonpregnant woman, the cervix around the external os is usually smooth, firm, and pink. A woman who has borne a child has a small, transverse, slitlike external os. A woman who has not had a child has a circular os. The endocervical canal connects the internal os with the external os and provides access from the vagina to the uterine cavity.

The outer cervix is covered with squamous epithelium, whereas the inner cervix is covered with columnar epithelium. These two types of cells meet at the squamocolumnar junction, which is usually located inside the cervical os. This is the site for Papanicolaou testing (see the later discussion on p. 1721).

CONNECTIVE TISSUE SUPPORT

The uterus is supported by the broad, round, uterosacral, and cardinal ligaments and by the muscles of the pelvic floor (see Figure 73-1).

Fallopian Tubes

The **fallopian tubes** (uterine tubes) insert into the fundus of the uterus and extend laterally to a site near the ovaries. Functionally, the uterine tubes provide a duct between the ovaries and the uterus for the passage of ova and sperm. In most cases, the ovum is fertilized in these tubes.

Each tube is about $3\frac{1}{8}$ to $5\frac{1}{2}$ inches (8 to 14 cm) long and is covered by one of the peritoneal folds of the broad ligament. The tubes are lined with longitudinal folds of ciliated and secretory columnar epithelial cells. Rhythmic contractions of the musculature of the tubes vary in response to the ovarian cycle. The tubal contractions and the current produced by the movement of cilia transport the ovum to the uterus.

The uterine tubes are divided into four anatomic sections (see Figure 73-1). The interstitial portion is the most proximal to the uterus, the isthmus and the ampulla are the middle segments, and the infundibulum is the most distal portion.

The fimbriated ends of the infundibulum extend almost to each ovary and facilitate the capture of a released ovum during ovulation.

Ovaries

The **ovaries** are a pair of almond-shaped organs situated near the lateral walls of the upper pelvic cavity. They are approximately $\frac{1}{8}$ inch x $\frac{7}{8}$ inch x $\frac{3}{8}$ inch (0.3 cm x 2 cm x 1 cm) but are significantly smaller after menopause. Functionally, these small organs develop and release ova. The cyclic maturation of a dominant follicle (the graafian follicle) and the subsequent release of the ovum is referred to as ovulation. The ovaries also produce the sex steroid hormones (estrogen, progesterone, androgen, and relaxin). Adequate amounts of these steroidal sex hormones are necessary for normal female growth and development and for the maintenance of a pregnancy.

Breasts

The female breasts are a pair of mammary glands that develop in response to secretions from the hypothalamus, pituitary gland, and ovaries. Functionally, the breasts are an accessory of the reproductive system meant to nourish the infant after birth. They also function as an organ for sexual arousal in the mature adult.

The breasts are located between the second and sixth ribs, between the edge of the sternum and the midaxillary line. About two thirds of the breast diameter is over the greater pectoral muscle, and one third is superficial to the anterior serratus muscle.

STRUCTURE

The structure of a mature female breast is shown in Figure 73-2. The nipple rises from the center of the pigmented areola, which is usually located slightly lateral to the midline of each breast. Montgomery's glands are small, round sebaceous glands that appear as elevations on the areola. These glands are thought to secrete a fatty substance that protects the nipple during breastfeeding.

Breast tissue is composed of a network of glandular and ductal tissue, fibrous tissue, and fat. The proportion of each component of breast tissue depends on genetic factors, nutrition, age, and obstetric history. The breast is supported by Cooper's suspensory ligaments that are attached to underlying muscles.

The breasts may not develop symmetrically during puberty but are usually symmetric in size and contour by adulthood. It is not unusual for the breast on the woman's dominant side (on

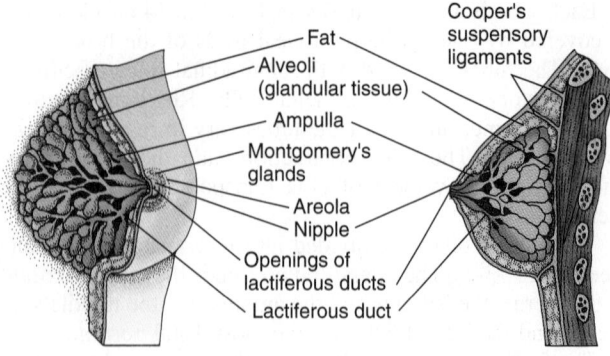

Figure 73-2 ● Structure of the mature female breast.

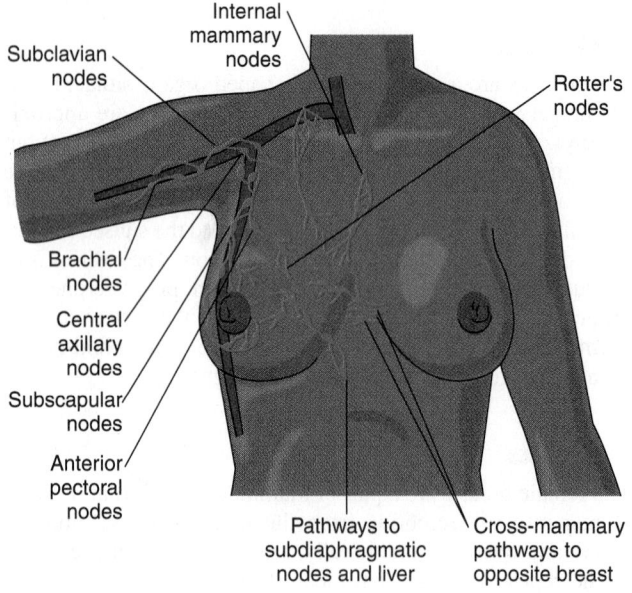

Figure 73-3 ● Lymphatic drainage of the female breast.

the basis of right-handedness or left-handedness) to appear larger because of the more developed pectoral muscle base.

In many women the breasts become slightly larger and tender during the premenstrual period. The tissue may also feel nodular at this time. Increasing levels of estrogen and progesterone 3 to 4 days before menses affect the breasts by increasing vascularity, inducing the growth of the ducts and alveoli, and promoting water retention.

▓ BLOOD SUPPLY

The abundant blood supply to the breasts comes from branches of the internal mammary and lateral thoracic arteries. The veins of the breast connect with the superior vena cava. Much of the lymph drains through an extensive network that is radial to the axilla (Figure 73-3).

Menstruation and Menopause

▓ NORMAL MENSTRUAL CYCLE

Menstruation is the cyclic shedding of the endometrial lining of the uterus. The term *menarche* refers specifically to the female's first menstruation and is one sign of puberty. Most girls begin to menstruate between 10 and 16 years of age.

The occurrence of cyclic menstruation and reproduction depends on maturation of the hypothalamic-pituitary-ovarian-uterine axis. Normally this cycle is not achieved for the first 1 to 2 years after menarche. The first menstrual cycles are typically anovulatory and irregular.

The menstrual cycle is under a feedback control system of three interrelated cycles:

- The hypothalamic-pituitary cycle
- The ovarian cycle
- The uterine (or endometrial) cycle

The relationship of these cycles is illustrated in Figure 73-4.

The idealized menstrual cycle is 28 days, but variations are normal. The first day of the menstrual cycle is calculated as the first day of monthly menstrual bleeding. The menstrual flow is referred to as the menses. Ovulation occurs approximately 14 days before the beginning of the next menstrual cycle. Regular menstrual cycles indicate normal sex hormone production and the occurrence of ovulation. Variations in the length of the menstrual cycle occur in response to variations in the length of the preovulatory stage compared with the postovulatory stage.

▓ MENOPAUSE AND THE CLIMACTERIC
▓ Natural Menopause

Menopause is the biologic end of reproductive ability, but the term applies to only the last menstrual period. The actual date of menopause cannot be determined until at least 1 year has passed without menses. The phase of a woman's life from the initial decline in the amount of estrogen produced by the ovaries to the cessation of symptoms produced by this phenomenon is called the *climacteric*. Lay terminology for this phase is "the change of life." Menopause is only one sign of the climacteric.

The follicles in the ovary atrophy continuously during a woman's life span. The progressive decline in the number of follicles that can produce estrogen in response to pituitary hormones causes the woman (usually between 40 and 50 years of age) to begin to notice physical changes in her body. Levels of estrogen and progesterone diminish gradually until the effect of these hormones on the endometrial lining of the uterus ceases. At the same time, the low levels of the ovarian hormones continue to stimulate the hypothalamic-pituitary axis. The anterior pituitary secretes high levels of follicle-stimulating hormone (FSH) and luteinizing hormone (LH) after menopause.

For a time, the inner core of the ovary produces androstenedione (a weak male hormone) and testosterone. Eighty percent of the androstenedione is produced by the adrenal glands. When the ovarian core ceases to function, the adrenal cortices are the only source of steroids. The production of androstenedione is significant, especially after menopause, because it is converted to a form of estrogen (estrone) in body fat. Consequently, women with a greater percentage of body fat have higher estrone levels after menopause.

During the climacteric, a woman experiences irregular menstrual and ovarian cycles. Ovulation often fails to occur. The menstrual flow may be lighter or heavier during these irregular cycles.

Decreased amounts of estrogen affect sites in the body other than the reproductive system, such as bone density and cardiovascular function. The uterus, cervix, ovaries, labia, and

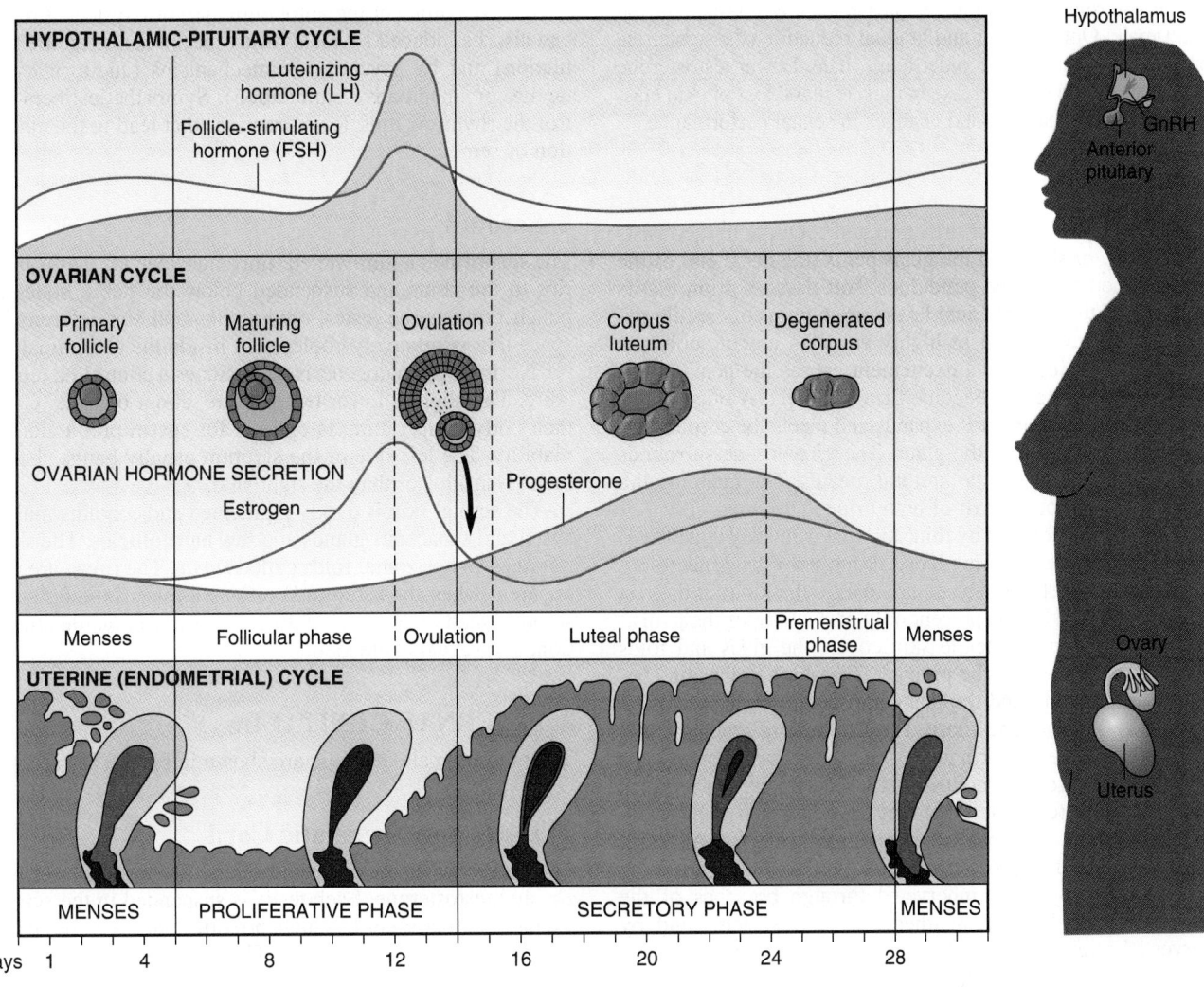

HYPOTHALAMIC-PITUITARY CYCLE

Luteinizing hormone (LH)

Follicle-stimulating hormone (FSH)

OVARIAN CYCLE

| Primary follicle | Maturing follicle | Ovulation | Corpus luteum | Degenerated corpus |

OVARIAN HORMONE SECRETION

Progesterone

Estrogen

| Menses | Follicular phase | Ovulation | Luteal phase | Premenstrual phase | Menses |

UTERINE (ENDOMETRIAL) CYCLE

| MENSES | PROLIFERATIVE PHASE | SECRETORY PHASE | MENSES |

Days   1   4   8   12   16   20   24   28

Hypothalamus

GnRH
Anterior pituitary

Ovary

Uterus

Figure 73-4 ● Interrelationships of the events of the menstrual cycle. (*GnRH*, Gonadotropin-releasing hormone.)

clitoris shrink in size. The low estrogen levels cause the vagina to narrow and shorten. The vaginal mucosa becomes thin and dry, which makes intercourse uncomfortable. The muscular support to the pelvis becomes more relaxed. The loss of tone also affects bladder support.

Bone density is a concern after estrogen production decreases. Estrogen is needed by bone tissue for calcium uptake. It also increases the metabolism of vitamin D, which is needed for the absorption of calcium from the intestines. Bone density decreases in clients with decreased calcium uptake. The reduction in the amount of bone mass is called **osteoporosis** (see Chapter 51).

One of the most common symptoms that occur during the climacteric are hot flashes, which are caused by vasomotor instability. Their cause is not clear, but it is thought that surges of FSH and LH on the hypothalamus cause vasodilation and increased heat production (Fogel, 2000). In addition to physical changes during the climacteric, the woman may also experience emotional changes (including mood changes) and fatigue.

Artificial Menopause

Menopause may occur for reasons other than the natural physiologic changes of the climacteric. Artificial menopause

is the cessation of menstruation by some artificial means, such as an oophorectomy (surgical removal of the ovaries) or radiation to the ovaries. A premenopausal woman who experiences artificial menopause from removal of her ovaries may need estrogen and progesterone therapy.

Structure and Function of the Male Reproductive System

EXTERNAL GENITALIA

The external male genitalia undergo multiple changes during puberty. The first visible sign of pubescence is enlargement of the scrotum and testes, which typically occurs between 11 and 13½ years of age.

These changes occur in response to an increase in testosterone production at puberty. The release of gonadotropin-releasing hormone (GnRH) from the male's hypothalamus stimulates the anterior pituitary to secrete LH and FSH. As the levels of the gonadotropins increase, the amount of testosterone significantly increases. Other signs of puberty that relate to testosterone production are the growth of axillary hair, lengthening and thickening of the vocal cords, increased sebaceous gland activity, and a general increase in muscle mass and body size.

Testosterone production remains relatively constant in the adult male. Only a slight and gradual reduction of testosterone production occurs in the older adult male. Lower testosterone levels contribute to a decrease in muscle mass, loss of skin elasticity, postural changes, and changes in sexual performance.

Penis

The **penis** is an organ for urination and copulation. It consists of the body or shaft and the glans penis (the distal end of the penis). The body is the pendulous, soft-tissue portion that is made up of three cylindrical layers or columns of erectile tissue. Engorgement of these highly vascular, erectile columns with blood during sexual excitement causes the penis to expand and elongate and become firm and erect. A ridge of tissue forms where the glans expands and meets the corpus; this is called the corona of the glans. The glans tissue surrounds the slitlike opening of the urethral meatus. The male urethra is the pathway for the exit of both urine and semen.

The penis is covered by thin skin that is loosely attached to the underlying fascia. This loose skin allows the penis to enlarge during erections. The skin is darker than that of the rest of the body, and hair is present only at the base of the penis.

A continuation of penile skin covers the glans and folds back on itself to form the prepuce (foreskin). Adhesions between the foreskin and the glans normally prevent retraction of the foreskin in the newborn. These adhesions gradually disintegrate, and the foreskin can usually be retracted by 3 years of age (the range is 4 months to 13 years). Surgical removal of the prepuce (circumcision) may be performed in the newborn period for religious or sociocultural reasons. An adult male may also undergo a circumcision.

The penis is richly innervated through branches of the sympathetic and parasympathetic nervous systems and by nerves of cerebral origin. Penile erection is under the control of these divisions of the autonomic nervous system. Erection can also be induced by local reflex mechanisms (tactile stimulation) and by psychogenic mechanisms (auditory, visual, tactile, or imaginative stimulation). Sympathetic fibers control the rhythmic muscle contractions that lead to the ejaculation of semen.

Scrotum

The **scrotum** is a thin-walled, fibromuscular sac that is posterior to the penis and suspended below the pubic bone. The pouch protects the testes, epididymis, and vas deferens in a space that is relatively cooler than inside the abdominal cavity. Normal spermatogenesis necessitates a controlled temperature. The slightly lower temperature, about 6° F (2° C) less than body temperature, is optimal for sperm production and viability. The left side of the scrotum usually hangs about ⅜ inch (1 cm) lower than the right side.

The scrotal skin is darkly pigmented and contains multiple sweat and sebaceous glands and few hair follicles. The skin is arranged in horizontal folds called *rugae*. The rugae are more apparent when the scrotum is retracted toward the body. The scrotum readily contracts with cold, exercise, tactile stimulation, and sexual excitement.

INTERNAL GENITALIA

The internal male genitalia are shown in Figure 73-5.

Testes and Spermatic Cord

The **testes** are a pair of ovoid organs that produce spermatozoa and testosterone. Each testis is suspended in the scrotum by the spermatic cord, which provides vascular, lymphatic, and nerve supply to the testis. The cord also covers the epi-

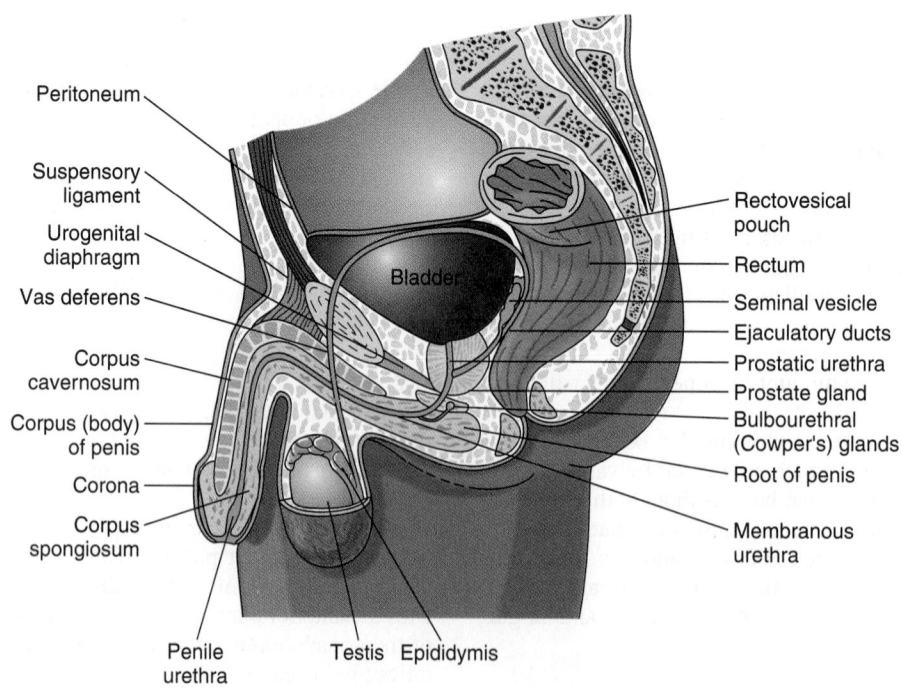

Figure 73-5 ● Internal male genitalia.

didymis and a portion of the vas deferens. The cord and testes are encircled by layers of spermatic fascia and cremaster muscle. Sympathetic nerve fibers are located on the arteries in the cord, and sympathetic and parasympathetic fibers are on the vas deferens. When the testes sustain a trauma, these autonomic nerve fibers transmit excruciating pain and a nauseating sensation.

■ EPIDIDYMIS

The epididymis is the first portion of a ductal system that transports sperm from the ductules of the testes to the urethra; it also aids in maturation of the sperm. The epididymis is comma shaped, lies posterolateral to one side of each testis, and is divided into a head, body, and tail.

The head of the epididymis attaches to the posterior aspect of the testis. The body descends against the lateral wall of the testis. At the lower border of the testis, the tail folds back over on itself and ascends toward the spermatic cord. The tail merges gradually into the vas deferens and provides storage for maturing sperm.

■ VAS DEFERENS

The vas deferens, or ductus deferens, is a firm, muscular tube about 17¾ inches (45 cm) long that continues from the tail of each epididymis. The terminal end of each vas deferens is a major reservoir for sperm and tubular fluids. They merge with ducts from the seminal vesicle to form the ejaculatory ducts at the base of the prostate gland. Sperm from the vas deferens and nutritive secretions from the seminal vesicles are transported through the ejaculatory duct to mix with prostatic fluids in the prostatic urethra.

Although the vas deferens secretes a small amount of fluid to support the sperm, its main function is to transport sperm from the epididymis to the ejaculatory ducts. In contrast to the movement of sperm through the epididymis by ciliary action, transport of sperm through the vas deferens occurs by means of peristaltic contractions of the ducts. A vasectomy, the surgical procedure for male sterilization, prevents only the passage of sperm to the ejaculatory ducts. It does not prevent the production of sperm, does not limit the erection of the penis, and does not greatly decrease the total amount of semen. Unexpelled sperm degenerate and are reabsorbed within the epididymis and the distal portion of the vas deferens.

■ Seminal Vesicles and Ejaculatory Ducts

The seminal vesicles are paired glands that secrete a major portion of the volume of the ejaculate. They are located behind the bladder near the prostate gland and are separated from the rectum by the rectovesical pouch. Each vesicle ends in a small duct that joins that of the ampulla of the vas deferens to form an ejaculatory duct. The two ejaculatory ducts are slender tubes that descend through the prostate gland; they end in slitlike openings in the prostatic urethra.

■ Prostate Gland

The **prostate gland** is the largest accessory gland of the male reproductive system. It is a chestnut-shaped, glandular, and fi-

bromuscular organ. Functionally, it secretes a milky alkaline fluid that adds bulk to the semen, enhances sperm motility, and neutralizes acidic vaginal secretions.

During emission, the first stage of the male orgasm, the smooth muscle of the prostate gland contracts and secretes its fluid at the same time as the vas deferens. Fluid from the prostate gland contributes 20% to 30% of the total ejaculate. The average pH of the combined secretions of semen is approximately 7.5, whereas secretions from the vagina normally have a pH of 3.5 to 4. Sperm need a surrounding fluid pH of 6 to 6.5 before they become optimally motile.

The prostate gland is approximately the size of an adult testis. It is situated between the neck of the bladder and the urogenital diaphragm. The prostate gland is separated from the anterior wall of the rectum by a thin fascial sheath that is part of the rectovesical septum. The prostate gland can be palpated through the rectum and should not project more than ⅜ inch (1 cm) into the rectal lumen.

As men age, the prostate gland becomes clinically significant. The gland is small at birth, but during puberty it rapidly enlarges to its normal adult size. By age 50 or 60 years, about 80% of men have an enlarged prostate (benign prostatic hyperplasia), which can cause urinary problems (Barkauskas et al., 1998).

Prostatic function depends on adequate levels of testosterone. As men age, testicular production of testosterone decreases.

■ Bulbourethral (Cowper's) Glands

Semen is ejaculated through the prostatic urethra, membranous urethra, and penile urethra. The bulbourethral glands are two yellow, pea-sized glands located posterior to the membranous urethra and connected to the penile portion of the urethra by ducts. The bulbourethral glands secrete an alkaline mucus into the penile urethra during emission. The mucus mixes with the sperm and other glandular secretions to form the semen. The bulbourethral glands contribute about 5% to 6% of the total ejaculate. The alkalinity of the mucus further protects the sperm against the relative acidity within the urethra.

Reproductive Changes Associated with Aging

Age affects the function of both the male and the female reproductive systems. After puberty, hormones produced by the gonads affect the normal functioning of many body systems. Many changes in the reproductive system are evident in older adults (Chart 73-1).

ASSESSMENT TECHNIQUES
History
■ DEMOGRAPHIC DATA

The nurse uses data about the client's age, sex, and culture to assess the risk for certain diseases. The nurse considers the client's age in evaluating the reproductive system. The age at which secondary sex characteristics developed in the client are compared with the established normal ranges for males or females.

CHART 73-1

NURSING FOCUS *on the* **OLDER ADULT**
Changes in the Reproductive System Related to Aging

Physiologic Change	Nursing Implications	Rationale
WOMEN		
Graying and thinning of the pubic hair	Discuss changes with the client (applies to all structures for both women and men).	Education helps prevent problems with body image (applies to all structures for both women and men).
Decreased size of the labia majora and clitoris		
Drying, smoothing, and thinning of the vaginal walls	Provide information about estrogen replacement therapy and water-soluble lubricants.	Education enables the client to make informed decisions about the treatment of vaginal dryness, which can cause painful intercourse.
Decreased size of the uterus	Provide information about Kegel exercises to strengthen pelvic muscles. Urinary incontinence can be a major problem.	Strengthening exercises may prevent or reduce pelvic relaxation and urinary incontinence.
Atrophy of the endometrium		
Decreased size and marked convolution of the ovaries		
Loss of tone and elasticity of the pelvic ligaments and connective tissue		
Increased flabbiness and fibrosity of the breasts, which hang lower on the chest wall; decreased erection of the nipples	Teach or reinforce the importance of breast self-examination (BSE).	BSE may detect lumps or other changes that may indicate the presence of cancer.
MEN		
Graying and thinning of the pubic hair	Teach or reinforce the importance of testicular self-examination (TSE).	TSE may detect changes that may indicate cancer.
Increased pedulousness of the scrotum and loss of rugae		
Prostate enlargement, with an increased likelihood of urethral obstruction	Teach the client the signs of urethral obstruction and the importance of prostate cancer screening.	Education helps the client detect enlargement or obstruction, which may indicate the presence of cancer.

CULTURAL CONSIDERATIONS

Cultural influences and expectations account for variations in acceptable gender-related and sexual identity. A child's attitude and behavior about the meaning and use of the genitals begin in infancy and are modeled on the behavior of significant adults. Religious dictates often parallel those of a specific culture and strongly affect sexual activity. A person's religious beliefs often influence specific sexual practices, the acceptable number of partners, contraceptive use, and specific treatments to terminate a pregnancy, end fertility, or remove barriers to infertility (Geissler, 1999).

Ethnicity often has an epidemiologic influence on particular diseases. For instance, the incidence of cancer of the reproductive system (excluding breast cancer) and associated death rates are higher for African Americans than for Caucasians (American Cancer Society [ACS], 1999).

PERSONAL AND FAMILY HISTORY
Personal History

The nurse assesses the client's health habits, such as diet, sleep, and exercise patterns. Low levels of body fat may be related to ovarian dysfunction. The nurse also determines the client's alcohol, tobacco, and drug use because libido, spermatogenesis, and potency can be affected by such substances (Nichols & Lowdermilk, 2000).

The client's personal medical history provides data about his or her general health. Certain childhood illnesses can have an effect on the reproductive system. Females need to be screened for sufficient rubella titers and should be treated, if necessary, to prevent possible teratogenic effects on their un-

born children if they get rubella during the first trimester of pregnancy. Mumps or smallpox in the postpubertal male may cause orchitis (painful inflammation and swelling of the testes) and occasionally leads to testicular atrophy and sterility.

The nurse also assesses for a history of major adult illnesses or chronic illnesses that may severely affect reproductive function. Endocrine disorders may affect the hypothalamic-pituitary-gonadal axis of the male or female. Almost any disease that disturbs a woman's metabolism or nutrition can depress ovarian function and cause amenorrhea. A history of infertility and failure of ovulation is associated with a greater risk for endometrial cancer. Clients with diabetes mellitus may experience physiologic changes such as vaginal dryness or impotence.

Some pre-existing cancers increase a woman's risk for developing other reproductive system cancers. Chronic disorders of the nervous system, respiratory system, or cardiovascular system can alter the sexual response. Some drugs (antihypertensives, opioids, monoamine oxidase inhibitors, histamine antagonists) may impair fertility (Nichols & Lowdermilk, 2000).

Reproductive system dysfunction can also result from irradiation, prolonged use of corticosteroids, exogenous estrogen or testosterone use, and chemotherapeutic agents.

In addition, past severe infections can alter a person's reproductive ability. For example, pelvic inflammatory disease or a ruptured appendix followed by peritonitis can cause strictures or adhesions in the fallopian tubes and pelvic scarring. Salpingitis (tubal infection) is most often caused by *Neisseria gonorrhoeae* infection and often results in female infertility. Infections or prolonged fever in males may damage sperm production or cause obstruction of the seminal tract, which leads to infertility. The nurse explores the client's history of surgeries, serious injuries, current medications, and allergies; each of these can affect reproductive structure or function.

Genitoreproductive History

The nurse completes a genitoreproductive history for both male and female clients. Chart 73-2 describes assessment data using Gordon's Functional Health Patterns.

FEMALE CLIENT

The nurse asks the female client about her menses, including age of menarche, cycle frequency and duration, amount of flow, spotting between periods, dysmenorrhea (painful menstrual periods), and premenstrual symptoms.

If the client is of menopausal age, the nurse determines the date of her last menstrual period, the presence of climacteric symptoms, and any medications or alternative therapies used for these symptoms. The nurse asks all women about the presence of vaginal discharge, a history and treatment of sexually transmitted diseases, the date and the result of her last Papanicolaou (Pap) test, breast self-examination practices, and vulvar self-examination practices.

The nurse also obtains an obstetric history. Women who have never had children have higher rates of ovarian, endometrial, and breast cancer than do multiparous women. If the woman has ever been pregnant, the nurse asks about the outcome of the pregnancies. In addition, the nurse collects information about the date and mode of deliveries or termination of the pregnancy; complications during pregnancy, labor, and delivery; birth weight and gestational age of the infants; and the condition of the infants at birth and at present.

The nurse also collects data about sexual activity. Heterosexual activity should not be assumed. Gay issues are often not assessed by the nurse or discussed by the client. The nurse explores information about sexual practices in a nonjudgmental manner.

An early age at first intercourse and multiple sex partners are associated with an increased risk of cervical cancer. The client is asked about satisfaction with sexual response, any pain or bleeding with sexual intercourse, and contraceptive use. Religious beliefs or type of sex (oral, anal, or vaginal) may dictate the contraceptive practices for a couple. Assessment for abuse may also be included at this point of the interview.

MALE CLIENT

The nurse asks the male client about testicular changes and self-examination practices, problems with urination, discharge from the penis, rectal problems, history and treatment of sexually transmitted diseases, and symptoms related to hernias.

The nurse also inquires about sexual functioning. Reproductive history and contraceptive use; current problems or changes in sexual response; any difficulty with erection, ejaculation, or infertility; and the use of medications or treatments also direct the physical assessment. The type of sex practiced also allows the nurse to focus on the body area involved.

Family History

The family history, including that of the parents, grandparents, siblings, and spouse, helps to determine the client's risk

---

CHART 73-2

REPRODUCTIVE ASSESSMENT
Using Gordon's Functional Health Patterns

Health Perception/Health Management Pattern
Has anyone in your family had cancer of the breast or reproductive organs? Who and what type of cancer?
If you engage in sexual activities, do you practice "safer" sex?
What do you do to keep healthy—regular health checkups, self-examination (breast, genital [vulvar, testicular]), healthy diet, exercise, use of medications or alternative therapies, use of alcohol, tobacco, or street drugs?

Sexuality-Reproductive Pattern
Male and Female: Are you sexually active? Do you find your sexual relationship satisfying? Have there been any changes in your relationship? Are you having any problems in your sexual relationship?
Do you use contraceptives? If so, do you have any problems with the method of contraception?
Have you had any sexually transmitted diseases? If yes, when, and what type did you have?
Female: When did you first start menstruating? When was your last menstrual period? Do you have any menstrual problems?
Have you ever been pregnant? If so, how many times, and what were the outcomes?
Have you had any symptoms of menopause?
Male: Do you have any problems with getting and maintaining an erection, or do you have difficulty with ejaculation?
Have you ever had a hernia or pain in the groin?

Self-Perception/Self-Concept Pattern
How would you describe yourself? Do you feel good or not so good about yourself?
Have you experienced changes in your body appearance or function? If so, are these problematic for you? Have you felt anxious, fearful, or depressed about these changes?

Based on Gordon, M. (2000). *Manual of nursing diagnosis* (9th ed.). St Louis: Mosby.

---

for conditions that affect reproductive system functioning. A delayed or early development of secondary sex characteristics may be a familial pattern.

The current age and state of health of the living members of the extended family are of interest. The cause of and age at death of specific family members may also be important. Evidence of serious diseases in family members (e.g., diabetes, cardiovascular disease, hypertension, renal disease, cancer, and complications of pregnancy) allows the nurse to better interpret the client's presenting symptoms. For example, daughters of women who were given diethylstilbestrol (DES) to control bleeding during pregnancy have an increased risk for infertility and reproductive tract carcinomas.

DIET HISTORY

A diet history is often critical for the correct interpretation of presenting symptoms of the reproductive system. For instance, fatigue and a lack of sexual interest may be associated with poor diet and anemia. Obesity raises the risk for uterine cancer. High-fat diets may increase the risk for cancer of the breast, ovary, and prostate gland (ACS, 1999). The nurse asks the client to recall his or her dietary intake for a recent 24-hour period to estimate the quality of the diet.

The nurse compares the client's height, weight, and body mass index with the dietary recall. The client may be hesitant to divulge practices such as bingeing, purging, anorexic behaviors, or excessive exercise; however, these practices may affect the reproductive system. A certain level of body fat and weight is necessary for the onset of menses and the maintenance of regular menstrual cycles. A decreased amount of body fat is associated with insufficient estrogen levels for the maintenance of normal ovulatory cycles.

Women have special dietary needs. The diet of women who use oral contraceptives should reflect increased sources of folic acid and vitamins B_6, B_{12}, and C. Heavy menstrual bleeding, particularly in women who have intrauterine devices, may necessitate oral iron supplements. All women need to be aware of their body's need for calcium. Although adequate calcium intake throughout life is optimal, it is especially important during the premenopausal and postmenopausal periods. A woman's bone density decreases because of the decreased production of estrogen during the climacteric, and this predisposes her to osteoporosis and fractures (see Chapter 51).

SOCIOECONOMIC STATUS

The social history of the client provides insight into the whole person, including stressors, job history, education, and support systems. The nurse asks about smoking and the use of substances such as alcohol and drugs. All of these factors can influence the health of the reproductive system.

Stressors

Stress has long been associated with menstrual and ovulatory irregularities. The nurse asks about leisure time activities that pose a high risk of injury to the reproductive system. For example, men who lounge for long periods in hot tubs or saunas may experience decreased sperm production. Women who exercise or train vigorously have reduced percentages of body fat and a higher degree of menstrual irregularities (West, 1998).

Occupation

The client's work may directly affect the reproductive system. Routine occupational exposure to potential teratogenic substances (agents capable of producing birth defects in offspring) results in a higher incidence of abnormal sperm cellular features and low sperm counts in men or miscarriages in women. People who work around certain chemicals, radiation, and heavy metals are at risk. Trauma and exposure to extremely high temperatures in the workplace are potential causes of male infertility. Exposure to some industrial agents, such as cadmium, may be related to the development of carcinomas of the reproductive system.

Education

The nurse assesses the educational level of the client to individualize health teaching. Lay language for body parts and functions is commonly used when discussing the reproductive system. The nurse must be familiar with such terms and be comfortable in their use. Clients may try to evoke a particular response in the nurse by using certain words, or they may have no other terminology to express the problem. The nurse who responds with shock or disdain displays a judgmental attitude that hinders successful data gathering. Health care pro-

fessionals can use teaching opportunities to provide more appropriate terminology.

Support Systems

The client's general satisfaction with life and the support systems available can directly relate to the current health problem. Questions designed to elicit information about daily routines often give insight into the client's perception of the quality of life and outlook for the future.

CURRENT HEALTH PROBLEM

If a client seeks medical attention for a problem related to the reproductive system, the nurse asks additional questions to explore the chief complaint. Most complaints concern pain, bleeding, discharge, masses, and reproductive functioning (Chart 73-3).

Pain

Pain related to reproductive system disorders may be confused with that associated with gastrointestinal or urinary tract problems. The client needs to describe the nature of the pain, including its type, intensity, timing and location, duration, and relationship to menstrual, sexual, urinary, or gastrointestinal function. Factors that exacerbate or give relief are also assessed.

Reproductive system disorders can be multifaceted; the nurse should not assume that the initial medical diagnosis is conclusive.

Bleeding

Heavy bleeding or a lack of bleeding may concern the client. The possibility of pregnancy is considered in any sexually ac-

---

CHART 73-3

**BEST PRACTICE *for*
Client Complaints Related to the Reproductive System**

COMPLAINT	NURSING ASSESSMENT
Pain	Type and intensity of pain
	Location and duration of pain
	Factors that relieve or worsen pain
	Relationship to menstrual, sexual, urinary, or gastrointestinal function
	Medications
Bleeding	Presence or absence of bleeding
	Character and amount of bleeding
	Relationship of bleeding to events or other factors (e.g., menstrual cycle)
	Onset and duration of bleeding
	Presence of associated symptoms, such as pain
Discharge	Amount and character of discharge
	Presence of genital lesions, bleeding, itching, or pain
	Presence of symptoms or discharge in sexual partner
Masses	Location and characteristics of mass
	Presence of associated symptoms, such as pain
	Relationship to menstrual cycle

tive woman with amenorrhea. Any postmenopausal bleeding needs to be evaluated. The nurse asks the client to describe the amount and character of abnormal bleeding from the vagina or penis. The nurse asks when the bleeding occurs in relation to certain events, such as the menstrual cycle or menopause, intercourse, trauma, and strenuous exercise. In addition, the nurse notes the presence of associated symptoms, such as pain, cramping or abdominal fullness, a change in bowel habits, urinary difficulties, and weight changes. Many factors can cause bleeding, and therefore the nurse considers sources other than the genital tract.

■ Discharge

Discharge from either the male or female reproductive tract can cause severe irritation of the surrounding tissues, itching, pain, embarrassment, and anxiety.

The nurse asks about the amount, color, consistency, odor, and chronicity of the discharge. Medications (e.g., antibiotics) and clothing (e.g., tight jeans and noncotton underwear) may also initiate or exacerbate genital discharge. Many types of discharge are caused by sexually transmitted diseases. The localization of these infections in the body depends on the client's sexual practices. The nurse questions the client about lesions, bleeding, itching, pain related to the genitals and orifices used during sexual activity, and the presence of symptoms in the sexual partner.

■ Masses

Any reported masses in the breasts, testes, or inguinal area need to be evaluated. Some masses change in character or size, and the client can often relate these changes to menstrual cycles, heavy lifting, straining, or trauma. The nurse inquires about associated symptoms such as tenderness, heaviness, pain, dimpling, and tender lymph nodes.

> **CRITICAL THINKING CHALLENGE**
> An 18-year-old woman has come to the clinic with a complaint of menstrual problems. A 47-year-old woman has also visited the clinic because she thinks she is going through menopause.
> * What assessment questions would be the same for these clients?
> * What assessment questions would be different for these clients?
>
> For suggested answer guidelines, go to SIMON http://www.wbsaunders.com/SIMON/Iggy/.

Physical Assessment
■ ASSESSMENT OF THE FEMALE REPRODUCTIVE SYSTEM

Examination of the breasts, axillae, and lymph nodes often precedes that of the anterior thorax in a complete physical examination. Inspection of the female genitalia and the pelvic examination are usually performed at the end of the physical examination. The client is often more apprehensive about these portions of the examination than about any other segment. Pain or lack of privacy during previous pelvic or breast examinations may prevent the client from relaxing.

The nurse can show the equipment to be used, along with three-dimensional models to demonstrate the assessment procedures. Relaxation and breathing techniques can be taught to enhance the client's sense of control. The nurse informs the client about what is going to be done and what she may feel as the examination proceeds. This information allows the client to incorporate learned coping mechanisms more successfully than if she were not expecting any discomfort. If the client displays signs of pain or exceptional concern during the procedures, the nurse should stop and make adjustments in the assessment plan or techniques. For example, clients who have been sexually abused may become upset during pelvic examinations (Heritage, 1998). The presence of a support person may also be of benefit to the client during the examination.

A pelvic examination is recommended every 1 to 3 years for women older than 18 years and for younger, sexually active adolescents (U.S. Department of Health and Human Services, 1997). A pelvic examination is indicated to assess the following:
* Menstrual irregularities
* Unexplained abdominal pain
* Vaginal discharge or infection
* Appropriateness of a desired contraceptive
* Rape trauma
* Physical changes in the vagina, cervix, uterus, and adnexa
* Infertility

The woman should not douche for at least 24 hours before the pelvic examination, because doing so may prevent an accurate evaluation of smears, cultures, and cytologic data.

Before the pelvic and breast examinations, the nurse asks the client to empty her bladder and to undress completely. The woman is adequately draped to protect modesty throughout the examination. If she is not wearing a gown, a small towel can be placed over the breasts under the larger drape. Drapes are removed only over the region being examined and are replaced when that area has been examined. Drapes that prevent eye contact between the examiner and the client dehumanize the client and prevent successful assessment of comfort during the examination. Mirrors can be used to facilitate teaching if the client so desires. The examination is performed in a room with adequate lighting for body inspection, a comfortable temperature, and the assurance of privacy.

■ Breast Examination

The physical examination of the reproductive system often includes the breasts (see Chapter 74).

■ Abdominal Examination

After the breast examination, the examiner generally completes the thoracic and cardiovascular examinations and then inspects, auscultates, and palpates the abdomen. The client's arms should be at her sides or over her chest to allow better relaxation of the abdominal muscles. During the gynecologic examination, the health care provider palpates for symptomatic and asymptomatic abdominopelvic masses. A mass can be of reproductive, gastrointestinal, or urinary tract origin. Careful history taking combined with the physical examination can usually determine the origin of a mass. Gynecologic masses, such as ovarian and adnexal masses, can be further differentiated from lesions on the body of the uterus during the bimanual portion of the pelvic examination.

Examination of the External Genitalia

After the abdominal examination, the nurse prepares the client for the inspection of the external genitalia and the pelvic examination. The nurse assists the woman into the lithotomy position and asks her to place her arms at her sides or over her chest. The client's buttocks extend slightly beyond the edge of the table, and her thighs are abducted. The nurse prepares all equipment for the vaginal and speculum examination and cytologic studies. The examiner wears gloves to protect against possible disease and potential cross-contamination from other clients. The client is informed that the genitalia will be touched and separated.

The initial inspection and palpation of the external genitalia provide an assessment of age-appropriate development. Hair color and distribution over the symphysis pubis and vulva suggest the woman's age and hormonal functioning. The pubic hair is inspected for the presence of lice or scabies. The skin and mucosa of the vulva are inspected in a systematic pattern from anterior to posterior for signs of inflammation, infestation, swelling, lesions, and discharge.

The paraurethral glands (Skene's glands) are barely visible on either side of the urethral meatus. If infection is suspected, the urethra should be gently "milked" by inserting the index finger into the vagina and gently pressing its pad against the anterior vaginal wall as the finger is being withdrawn. This procedure usually produces no pain or discharge unless there is inflammation or infection. The openings of the ducts from the Bartholin's glands cannot be visualized. The examiner carefully palpates the area just outside the lower vaginal orifice to assess for inflammation, tenderness, or swelling. Any discharge elicited from these ducts is cultured, because these structures are often involved in gonorrheal infections.

The examination of the external female genitalia is an excellent time for teaching about **vulvar self-examination (VSE).** The incidence of precancerous conditions and infectious diseases of the vulva is increasing, especially in young women (Lowdermilk, 2000). VSE can easily be taught and can lead to early diagnosis of vulvar conditions (Chart 73-4).

Perineal support and the strength of the vaginal walls are assessed by asking the woman to squeeze the vaginal opening closed after the examiner has inserted two fingers. The client is then asked to strain downward while the examiner assesses for urinary incontinence or any bulging of the anterior or posterior vaginal walls that would indicate a cystocele or rectocele, respectively.

Pelvic Examination

EXAMINATION WITH A SPECULUM

After the correct speculum size is selected, the speculum may be warmed and lubricated with warm water. Lubricant should not be used if cytologic studies are to be collected because it interferes with specimen analysis. The woman should be told when the speculum is going to be inserted. The examiner's fingers can ease insertion of the speculum by pressing down on the perineal body just inside of the vaginal orifice (Figure 73-6, step 1). The woman can also be asked to breathe slowly and to bear down. The examiner inserts the closed speculum in an

---

CHART 73-4

CLIENT EDUCATION GUIDE
Vulvar Self-Examination

- Perform a vulvar self-examination monthly between menstrual periods if you are older than 18 years or if you are sexually active.
- Sit in a well-lighted area on a soft surface (bed or carpeted floor).
- Use a handheld mirror to visualize your external genitalia.
- Examine the area around the vaginal opening from the mons pubis to the perianal area.
- Feel and visually inspect the area.
- Report to your health care provider new nodes, warts, growths of any type, ulcers, sores, blisters, change in skin color, painful areas, areas of itching or inflammation, or any change in vaginal discharge.

---

oblique position, with the pressure exerted toward the posterior vaginal wall. The examiner removes his or her fingers. The examiner then rotates the closed blades of the speculum to a horizontal position while inserting the speculum to its full length (see Figure 73-6, step 2). The blades are opened, and the speculum is maneuvered to enable visualization of the cervix. The examiner locks the blades in place by tightening the thumbscrew of the speculum (see Figure 73-6, step 3).

The examiner inspects the cervix for color, shape, and dilation of the os; erosions; nodules; masses; discharge; and bleeding.

Herpes simplex, syphilis, and carcinomas can produce characteristic lesions on the cervix. Specimens are obtained from the cervix, endocervix, and vaginal pool for cytologic studies (see Microscopic Studies, p. 1722). After completion of the cervical examination, the examiner loosens the thumbscrew of the speculum to close the blades and slowly rotates the speculum to a vertical position as it is withdrawn. The examiner inspects the vaginal tissue for lesions or inflammation during withdrawal.

BIMANUAL EXAMINATION

After withdrawing the speculum, the examiner proceeds with the bimanual examination. Using a new glove and lubricant, the examiner stands and inserts one or two fingers of one hand into the client's vagina (Figure 73-7). The examiner palpates the posterior vaginal wall and checks for masses or tenderness. The cervix and fornix around the cervix are identified. The examiner places the opposite hand on the client's abdomen—between her umbilicus and symphysis pubis—and presses downward. The examiner lifts the cervix and uterus with the pelvic hand toward the abdominal hand to trap the uterus and adnexa for assessment by palpation. The examiner assesses the size, shape, consistency, location, and mobility of the uterus and for any tenderness or masses. To palpate each ovary and tube, the examiner presses the abdominal hand into the right or left lower quadrant. The fingers in the fornix are used to palpate the ovaries and adnexa against the opposite hand.

Obesity or tense abdominal muscles may prevent the examiner from locating the ovaries. If palpable, the ovaries are 3 cm long, 2 cm wide, and 1 cm thick; they are ovoid, feel firm and smooth, and may feel somewhat tender. The uterine tubes are not usually palpable. Ovarian cysts may be painful

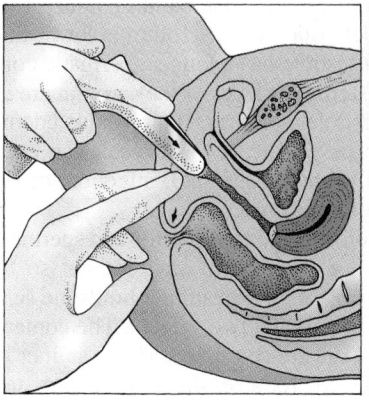 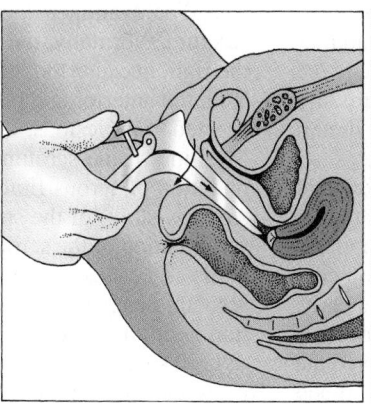 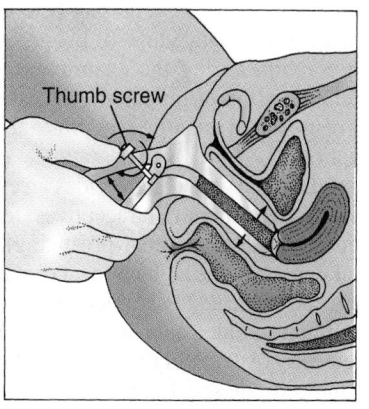 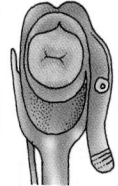

1. With the speculum blades positioned vertically, the nurse presses down on the perineal body just inside the vagina as the speculum is inserted.

2. The nurse removes the fingers from the vagina while continuing to insert the closed blades of the speculum to their full length and rotating them into a horizontal position.

3. The nurse opens the blades and maneuvers the speculum for optimal visualization of the cervix, then tightens the thumb screw to lock the blades in place.

View of the cervix through the speculum

Figure 73-6 ● Internal examination of the cervix.

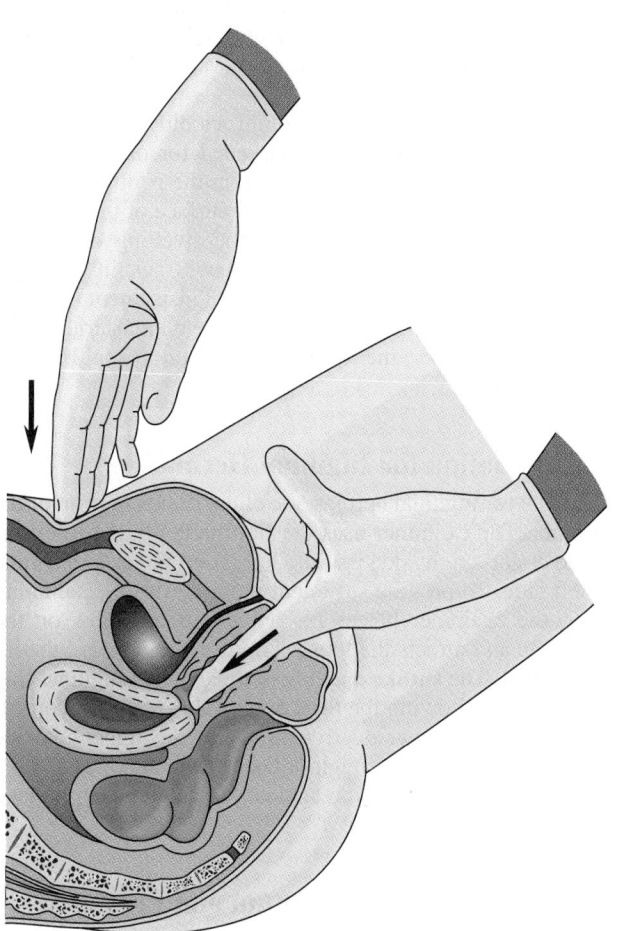

Figure 73-7 ● Technique of bimanual pelvic examination.

and recurrent in premenopausal women. An ovarian cyst smaller than 2 inches (5 cm) in diameter is usually functional and responds to hormonal influence. Cysts larger than 2⅜ inches (6 cm) in diameter are possible neoplasms. The ovaries are normally atrophied and not palpable 3 to 5 years after menopause; therefore any palpable structure in the adnexa of postmenopausal women suggest cancer.

▦ RECTOVAGINAL EXAMINATION

The rectovaginal and rectal examination is the last segment of the pelvic examination. The examiner changes and lubricates the glove and places the middle finger in the rectum and the index finger in the vagina. Insertion of the rectal finger is facilitated if the client strains and relaxes the anal sphincter. The procedure for the bimanual examination is repeated. The posterior vaginal and uterine walls are palpated through the rectal mucosa. This examination is especially helpful in assessing a retroflexed or retroverted uterus. The examiner can assess the tissue structure between the vagina and the rectum by palpating between the two fingers. The vaginal finger is removed and folded into the palm. The rectal finger is rotated as it is withdrawn; any fecal material that remains on the glove may be tested for occult blood.

After the examination, the foot of the examining table is raised. The client's feet are lowered from the stirrups at the same time to reduce strain on the perineal muscles and lumbosacral ligaments. Nurses should be aware that some clients experience orthostatic (postural) hypotension if they sit up too quickly. The nurse evaluates the client for signs of dizziness before letting her get off the examining table. The nurse provides appropriate supplies, such as perineal wipes and perineal napkins or minipads. The nurse allows the client privacy for dressing and is available to answer questions and provide support.

▦ ASSESSMENT OF THE MALE REPRODUCTIVE SYSTEM

Unless a male client seeks health care for a genital tract problem, inspection and palpation of the male genitalia and rectum may not be performed during physical examinations, depending on the health care setting and the age of the client. Male clients are often embarrassed and anxious when the reproductive system is assessed. This concern may be compounded when the examiner is a woman. The client may be concerned about discomfort, the developmental stage of his genitalia, or the likelihood of an erection during the examination. If the client does have an erection, the examiner should assure him that this is a normal response to a tactile stimulus and should continue the examination.

The examination of the male genitalia provides an excellent opportunity to teach the client about contraceptives, testicular self-examination, and the need for regular prostate gland examinations. Testicular cancer is one of the most common cancers in young men and can be treated effectively if found early. Prostate cancer is common in older men, and the prognosis is favorable if diagnosed early. Annual digital rectal and prostate gland examinations and prostate specific antigen (PSA) blood tests are recommended for men older than 50 years with a life expectancy of at least 10 years (ACS, 1999).

The examiner wears gloves to protect against possible infection. The examination room should offer the client privacy and a comfortable temperature. Proper light sources are mandatory for the inspection. The client undresses completely but should be given a gown to wear because the genitalia and buttocks need to be exposed. As with examinations of other body systems, the examiner explains each step of the assessment procedure before performing it. The client needs to be reassured that the examiner will stop and change the assessment plan or technique if the client perceives pain during the examination. Relaxation techniques and support during the examination can increase the tolerance of minimal discomfort.

▪ Examination of the External Genitalia

The client may be in a lying or a standing position for inspection and palpation of the external genitalia. The examiner is seated on a chair in front of the client. A general observation is made of the secondary sex characteristics. The examiner notes the age appropriateness of the developmental stage, including the distribution pattern of the pubic hair, the descent and size of the testes, and the size of the scrotum and penis. Pubic hair is inspected for the presence of lice or scabies.

The examiner inspects the skin of the penis for intactness; the dorsal vein should be apparent. Any lesions or ulcers on the penis are noted, and a specimen may be scraped for cytologic study. If the client has not been circumcised, he is asked to retract the foreskin. This should be accomplished easily unless the client has phimosis (a tight prepuce that cannot be retracted). The examiner inspects the glans penis for possible inflammation, fungal infection, syphilitic chancres, and carcinomas. Smegma, a white, cheesy secretion from the sebaceous glands in the glans, may accumulate under the prepuce. This secretion is not present in the circumcised male.

The glans is also inspected for placement of the urinary meatus. Positions other than at the distal end of the glans are abnormal. By compressing the glans between the thumb and index finger, the examiner separates the meatus and can determine whether any discharge is present. Urethral discharge is not normal, and a specimen should be obtained for culture. The foreskin is replaced if it has been retracted. The body of the penis is palpated between the examiner's thumb and first two fingers; the examiner notes tenderness, hard areas under the skin, and signs of inflammation.

Inspection of the scrotum and inguinal areas is best accomplished by having the client hold the penis up and to the side. The examiner documents the shape and contour of the scrotum. Normally, the left side of the scrotum is lower than the right because the left testicle has a longer spermatic cord. Both the anterior and posterior surfaces of the scrotum are inspected for lesions, nodules, rashes, pain, and edema. Swelling of the scrotum may indicate a hydrocele (an accumulation of serous fluid in the scrotal sac), infection, or torsion (twisting) of the spermatic cord.

Palpation of the scrotum, testes, epididymis, and spermatic cords is best accomplished in a warm environment so the scrotum hangs low and relaxed. The examiner holds the scrotum gently between the thumb and two fingers. The contents of each side of the scrotal sac are compared. The examiner locates and examines each testis for size, shape, symmetry, tenderness, nodules, and consistency.

The normal testis has smooth borders, is somewhat sensitive to light palpation, and feels rubbery. The epididymis can be palpated on the posterior surface of the testis. It is examined for size, shape, and tenderness. In clients with infection of the epididymis, its outline is indistinguishable from that of the testis. The examiner palpates the spermatic cord along its length between the epididymis and the superficial inguinal ring; nodules and swelling are noted and further evaluated. Varicose veins of the spermatic cord (varicocele) feel like a "bag of worms" above the testis.

Any swollen area of the scrotum should be transilluminated. The examining room is darkened for this procedure, and the examiner directs the beam from the penlight through the scrotal swelling from the posterior surface of the scrotum. The light transmits a red glow if the swelling contains a serous fluid. Blood and solid tissue do not transmit the light.

The inner thigh is stroked with a blunt instrument (e.g., the handle of the reflex hammer) to elicit the cremasteric reflex. If the reflex is intact, the testicle and scrotum should rise on the stroked side.

▪ Examination for Inguinal Hernia

To palpate for inguinal hernias, the client stands in front of the examiner. The examiner uses the right index finger to examine the client's right side and the left index finger to examine the left side. To provide sufficient mobility of the examining finger, the examiner places his or her fingertip low on the scrotal sac and directs the loose skin of the sac toward the inguinal canal. The slitlike opening of the external inguinal ring is located by following the direction of the spermatic cord. If possible, the examiner gently introduces the finger into the canal, asks the client to cough or bear down, and is alert for a tapping or pushing sensation against the finger—a sign that a hernia may be present.

▪ Examination of the Rectum and Prostate

The final assessment of the male reproductive system includes an examination of the rectum and the prostate gland. This examination can be performed with the client in a knee-chest position, in a lithotomy position, in a left lateral with knees flexed position, or standing and leaning over the examining table with the feet turned inward to relax the buttocks.

Proper lighting is necessary for visualization of the anus and surrounding tissue. The examiner notes any lesions, ulcerations, masses, or fissures.

To assess the prostate gland, the examiner presses the pad of a well-lubricated, gloved index finger against the anus. As the sphincter relaxes, the finger is slowly inserted in the direction of the umbilicus and is rotated to palpate the anterior rectal wall. The posterior surface of the prostate gland is felt extending less than ⅜ inch (1 cm) into the rectum. The client is informed that he may feel an urge to urinate as the prostate is being examined but that he will not do so. The examiner notes the size of the lateral prostate lobes and their contour and consistency. The prostate should feel firm (the consistency has been equated to that of a pencil eraser), smooth, and slightly mobile. It should be nontender across its diameter.

The examiner extends the finger further to attempt to palpate the seminal vesicles, which are palpable only if they are inflamed. If any discharge is secreted from the penis during palpation of the prostate gland and seminal vesicles, specimens are obtained for culture and microscopic examination. The examining finger is withdrawn, and any fecal material may be tested for occult blood.

Psychosocial Assessment

The psychosocial assessment may suggest some contributory factors to the client's illness. During the social history, the nurse asks about the client's sources of support, strengths, and likely reactions to illness or dysfunction.

A client's personal history or beliefs may negatively influence his or her ability to enjoy a satisfactory sexual life. These factors may include the following:

- Sexual trauma or abuse inflicted during childhood or adulthood
- Punishment or reproach for masturbation
- Psychologic trauma
- Cultural influences, such as the idea of female passivity during intercourse
- Concerns about sexual partners or sexual lifestyle
- Use of alcohol or street drugs

Fears may affect the client's satisfaction with sexuality or body image. He or she may also be concerned about the potential or actual reaction of family members to reproductive health problems (see Chart 73-2).

Diagnostic Assessment
■ LABORATORY TESTS
■ Papanicolaou Test

The **Papanicolaou test,** or **Pap smear,** is a cytologic study that is effective in detecting precancerous and cancerous cells from the cervix. Health care providers vary in their recommendations for the frequency of routine Pap tests. The American Cancer Society (ACS) advises all asymptomatic women who have been or are sexually active to have an annual Pap test. After three or more consecutive negative test results, Pap tests may be performed less frequently (ACS, 1999). However, many clinicians continue to suggest that the test be performed annually during routine physical examinations.

Cytologic examinations can also detect viral, fungal, and parasitic disorders. Examination of cells from the vaginal walls can evaluate the function of steroid hormones.

CLIENT PREPARATION. The Pap test should be scheduled between the client's menstrual periods so that the menstrual flow does not interfere with the test interpretation. The woman should not douche, use vaginal medications or deodorants, or have sexual intercourse for at least 24 hours before the test.

The nurse assists the woman into the lithotomy position. Relaxation techniques, including concentrating on breathing patterns or a visual focal point, may be valuable for the apprehensive client. All steps of the examination are explained to the client before they are performed.

PROCEDURE. The examiner first inserts a speculum into the vagina. For the conventional Pap smear, the cervix is visualized and then scraped with one of the various sampling tools available, such as a cytology brush, cotton-tipped applicator, endocervical aspirator, or wooden or plastic spatula. The use of brushes improves the quality of cells obtained for analysis (Seidel, 1999).

The examiner takes one sample from the endocervical canal and a second from the ectocervical and squamocolumnar junction (Figure 73-8). Both specimens are immediately transferred to glass slides and are either sprayed with or immersed in a fixative solution. If the smear is allowed to dry on the slide before the fixative is applied, the diagnosis will be inaccurate. The slides are sent to a laboratory for interpretation.

The ThinPrep Pap Test is an improved method of preserving the sample. After the sample has been obtained, the health care provider rinses the cells into a vial filled with a preserving solution. The vial is sent to the laboratory, where an automated instrument gently separates the cells from blood and mucus. The thinner layer of cells can then be better visualized under a microscope, which improves the accuracy of the test.

FOLLOW-UP CARE. The nurse can provide the client with a perineal pad after the procedure to protect her clothes from any bleeding from the cervix. The test results are shared with the client in person, by telephone, or by letter. If a woman's smear has demonstrated atypical cells, she is encouraged to have follow-up testing.

■ Blood Studies
■ PITUITARY GONADOTROPIN

Determinations of the quantitative levels of follicle-stimulating hormone (FSH), luteinizing hormone (LH), and prolactin are helpful in the diagnosis of male and female reproductive tract disorders. The serum levels are measured by the radioimmunoassay method. No dietary restrictions are necessary before the test. Chart 73-5 gives the normal values and the significance of abnormal findings.

■ STEROID HORMONES

The radioimmunoassay technique can detect estrogen, progesterone, and testosterone levels in adult men and women.

■ SEROLOGIC TESTS

Serologic blood studies detect antigen-antibody reactions that occur in response to foreign organisms. This form of diagnostic testing is beneficial only after an infection has be-

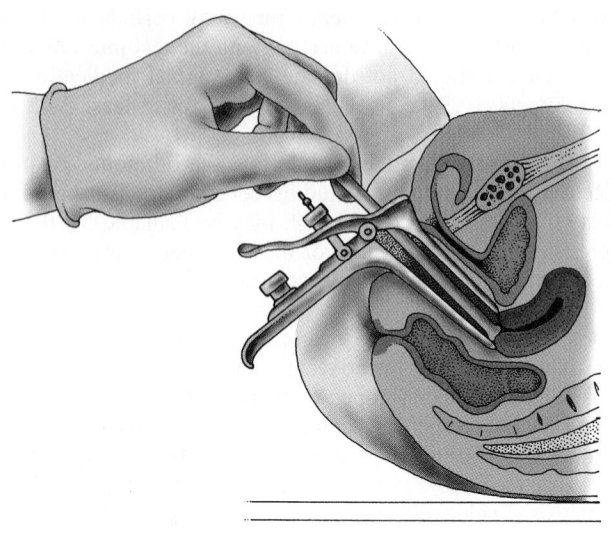
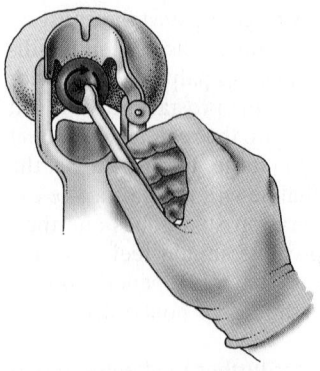
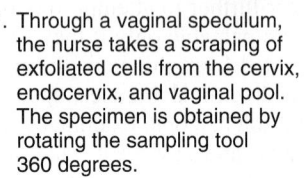
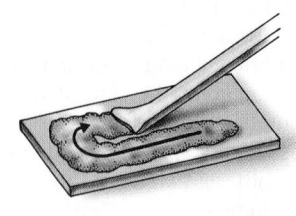

1. Through a vaginal speculum, the nurse takes a scraping of exfoliated cells from the cervix, endocervix, and vaginal pool. The specimen is obtained by rotating the sampling tool 360 degrees.

2. The nurse immediately transfers the specimens to a glass slide and applies a fixative solution.

Figure 73-8 ● Procedure for obtaining a cervical smear (Pap test).

come well established. Serologic testing can be used in the evaluation of exposure to organisms causing syphilis and rubella and to herpes simplex virus type 2 (HSV2). Results may be read as nonreactive, weakly reactive, or reactive. A single titer is not as revealing as serial titers, which can detect the rise in antibody reactions as the body continues to fight the intruder.

■ SYPHILIS DETECTION

The VDRL (Venereal Disease Research Laboratory) test, Serologic Test for Syphilis (STS), and the Rapid Plasma Reagin Test (RPR) are serologic tests used to detect, confirm, and monitor cases of syphilis. These tests are recommended for all pregnant women and persons at high risk for syphilis (Centers for Disease Control and Prevention [CDC], 1998). These nontreponemal antigen tests are used to screen for the presence of nonspecific reagin antibodies that appear and increase in titer after infection. They are not absolutely specific or sensitive for syphilis, but they are economical and highly diagnostic. Some acute and chronic conditions that cause false-positive results are the following:

- Tuberculosis
- Infectious mononucleosis
- Recent smallpox vaccination
- Rheumatoid arthritis
- Systemic lupus erythematosus
- Subacute bacterial endocarditis
- Hepatitis
- Recent ingestion of alcohol

Test results vary with the stage of syphilis. The serologic test result is usually positive about 2 weeks after the client has become infected. If the primary syphilis is treated, the serologic titers almost always return to nonreactive levels within 4 months.

If the VDRL or RPR test is positive, the diagnosis must be confirmed by a more specific test for *Treponema pallidum,* such as the fluorescent treponemal antibody absorption test (FTA-ABS). This expensive and time-consuming test be-

comes positive 4 to 6 weeks after infection. Most positive test results for *Treponema pallidum* remain positive for the rest of the infected person's life.

■ PROSTATE-SPECIFIC ANTIGEN

The prostate-specific antigen (PSA) test is used to screen for prostate cancer and to monitor the disease after treatment. PSA levels of <4 ng/mL are normal; elevated PSA levels are associated with prostate cancer. If combined with a digital rectal examination, almost 90% of all prostate cancers can be detected (Pagana & Pagana, 1998).

■ Urinalysis for Steroid Hormones

The health care provider may order 24-hour urine samples for levels of total estrogens and pregnanediol (a urinary byproduct of progesterone) to detect ovulation.

■ Microscopic Studies

■ WET PREPARATION (WET SMEARS)

The examiner can obtain secretions from the vaginal pool at the beginning of a speculum examination. Specimens can also be obtained from the vaginal walls, labia, or vulva during the examination. The specimens are placed on glass slides and are treated with a wet preparation such as saline and potassium hydroxide (KOH). The slides are examined under a microscope to confirm or rule out the presence of a pathogen. Table 73-1 presents the common types of wet preparations used to diagnose selected vaginal problems.

■ CULTURES

Cultures identify pathogenic organisms and are used to determine the appropriate antibiotic therapy. The examiner obtains specimens for culture analysis from any discharge or orifice of the male or female reproductive system. The health care provider orders routine bacteriologic cultures and antibiotic

CHART 73-5

LABORATORY PROFILE
Reproductive Assessment

Test	Normal Range for Adults	Significance of Abnormal Findings
SERUM STUDIES		
Follicle-stimulating hormone (FSH) (Follitropin)	*Men:* 1.42-15.4 mIU/mL *Women:* follicular phase, 1.37-9.9 mIU/mL; midcycle, 6.17-17.2 mIU/mL; luteal phase, 1.09-9.2 mIU/mL; postmenopause, 19.3-100.6 mIU/mL	Decreased levels indicate possible infertility, anorexia nervosa, neoplasm Elevations indicate possible Turner's syndrome
Luteinizing hormone (LH) (Lutropin)	*Men:* 1.24-7.8 mIU/mL *Women:* follicular phase, 1.68-15 mIU/mL; midcycle, 21.9-56.6 mIU/mL; luteal phase, 0.61-16.3 mIU/mL; postmenopause, 14.2-52.3 mIU/mL	Decreased levels indicate possible infertility, anovulation Elevations indicate possible ovarian failure, Turner's syndrome
Prolactin	*Men:* 0-20 ng/mL *Women:* 0-20 ng/mL *Pregnant women:* 20-400 ng/mL	Elevations indicate possible galactorrhea (breast discharge), pituitary tumor, disease of hypothalamus or pituitary gland, hypothyroidism
Estradiol	*Men:* 10-50 pg/mL *Women:* follicular phase, 20-350 pg/mL; midcycle, 150-750 pg/mL; luteal phase, 30-450 pg/mL; postmenopause, ≤20 pg/mL	Elevations of estradiol, total estrogens, and estriol in men indicate possible gynecomastia, decreased body hair, increased fat deposits, feminization
Total estrogens	*Men:* 20-80 pg/mL *Women:* follicular phase, 60-200 pg/mL; luteal phase, 160-400 pg/mL; postmenopause, <130 pg/mL	Elevations of estradiol, total estrogens, and estriol in women indicate possible uterine cancer, precocious puberty, cystic breast disease, corpus luteum cysts
Estriol	*Men and nonpregnant women:* <2.0 ng/dL	Decreased levels of estradiol, total estrogens, and estriol in women indicate possible amenorrhea, climacteric, impending abortion, hypothalamic disorders
Progesterone	*Men:* 10-50 ng/dL *Women:* follicular phase, <50 ng/dL; luteal phase, 300-2500 ng/dL	Decreased levels in women indicate possible inadequate luteal phase, amenorrhea Elevations in women indicate possible ovarian luteal cysts
Testosterone	*Men:* 280-1100 ng/dL *Women:* 15-70 ng/dL	Decreased levels in men indicate possible hypogonadism, Klinefelter's syndrome, hypopituitarism, orchidectomy Elevations in women indicate possible adrenal neoplasm, polycystic ovaries, ovarian tumors
URINE STUDIES		
Total estrogens	Men: 4-23 µg/24 hr *Women:* follicular phase, 7-65 µg/24 hr; luteal phase, 8-135 µg/24 hr; postmenopause, 0-10 µg/24 hr	Elevations indicate possible testicular tumors, adrenal tumors, ovarian tumors, pregnancy Decreased levels indicate possible ovarian dysfunction, intrauterine death, menopause
Pregnanediol	*Men:* 0-1.9 mg/24 hr *Women:* follicular phase, <2.6 mg/24 hr; luteal phase, 2.6-10.6 mg/24 hr	Elevations indicate possible luteal ovarian cysts, ovarian neoplasms, adrenal disorders Decreased levels indicate possible amenorrhea
17-Ketosteroids	*Men (20-50 yr):* 7-25 mg/24 hr *Women (20-50 yr):* 4-15 mg/24 hr Values decrease with age	Elevations indicate possible Cushing's syndrome, increased androgen or cortisol production, severe stress Decreased levels indicate possible Addison's disease, hypopituitarism

Data from Pagana, K.D., & Pagana, T.J. (1998). *Mosby's manual of diagnostic and laboratory tests.* St. Louis: Mosby.
mIU/mL, IU/L; *1 ng,* 1 nanogram or 1 billionth of a gram; *1 pg,* 1 picogram or 1 trillionth of a gram; *µg,* 1 microgram or 1 millionth of a gram.

sensitivity studies when a nonspecific bacterial infection is suspected.

The culture to detect *Neisseria gonorrhoeae* is one of the most important in evaluating the reproductive system. This culture is the only means of confirming a diagnosis of gonorrhea in asymptomatic women. Specimens from male clients can be taken directly from any penile discharge. In women, cervical cultures can be taken after the Pap test is obtained. Additional specimens from males or females can also be ob-

tained from the urethra, rectum, and oropharynx. The swab is then placed in a culture tube and sent to the laboratory for incubation and analysis.

Cultures to detect *Chlamydia trachomatis* use antigen detection methods. Tissue cultures are the most accurate but take several days for results. Less expensive and more widely available are a direct immunofluorescent test and an enzyme-linked immunosorbent assay (ELISA) (Pagana & Pagana, 1998). Nucleic acid amplification tests can be used to detect

TABLE 73-1 • WET PREPARATIONS USED FOR THE DIAGNOSIS OF COMMON VAGINAL PROBLEMS	
Wet Preparation	**Problems**
Normal saline	Cervicitis Trichomoniasis Bacterial vaginosis Atrophic vaginitis
Potassium hydroxide (KOH)	Candidiasis (Candida albicans, Monilia) Bacterial vaginosis
Gram stain	Mucopurulent cervicitis

 CRITICAL THINKING CHALLENGE

• What laboratory or diagnostic tests would be useful in evaluating a young adult's complaint of menstrual irregularity?
• What laboratory or diagnostic tests would be useful in evaluating a client experiencing menopausal symptoms?

For suggested answer guidelines, go to SIMON http://www.wbsaunders.com/SIMON/Iggy/.

N. gonorrhoeae and *C. trachomatis* in first-voided urine specimens or in specimens collected from the cervix (CDC, 1998).

RADIOGRAPHIC EXAMINATIONS

General X-ray Studies

A kidney, ureter, and bladder (KUB) study is an x-ray study of the abdomen that shows these structures and is used in the assessment of disorders of either the male or female reproductive system. Pelvic masses, calcified tumors or fibroids, dermoid cysts, and metastatic bone changes may be evident. Urologic studies may enhance the film by the use of contrast media. No specific client preparation is needed.

Bone scans, intravenous (IV) pyelograms, barium enema studies, and chest films are also included in the workup of the client with suspected metastatic cancer. They help to determine the extent of the metastasis and obstruction or displacement of the organs. These tests are discussed elsewhere in this text.

Computed Tomography

Computed tomography (CT) scans for reproductive system disorders primarily involve the abdomen and the pelvis. They can detect and evaluate masses and lymphatic enlargement from metastasis. This scan can differentiate solid tissue masses from cystic or hemorrhagic structures.

Hysterosalpingography

A **hysterosalpingogram** is an x-ray study of the cervix, uterus, and fallopian tubes and is performed after the injection of a contrast medium. This test is used in infertility workups to evaluate tubal anatomy and patency and uterine abnormalities such as fibroids, tumors, and fistulas. The study should not be attempted for at least 6 weeks after abortion, delivery, or dilation and curettage. Other contraindications include reproductive tract infection or uterine bleeding.

CLIENT PREPARATION. The examination should be scheduled in a radiology department 2 to 5 days after the end of the client's normal menses. The scheduling is important to prevent the accidental flushing of a fertilized ovum from the fallopian tube or the exposure of a fetus to radiation.

The client is usually instructed to take a laxative the evening before the test, followed by an enema or rectal suppository on the morning of the examination. These procedures reduce the distortion of the x-rays by gas shadows.

On the day of the examination, the date of the client's last menstrual period is confirmed and recorded in the medical record. The woman is assessed for an allergy to iodine dye or shellfish. She signs a consent form for the procedure. Because discomfort is anticipated during the examination, she may be premedicated with analgesics or nonsteroidal anti-inflammatory drugs. She should be informed that she may experience some nausea and vomiting, abdominal cramping, or faintness. The nurse provides support and assistance with relaxation techniques.

PROCEDURE. The client is placed in the lithotomy position. A speculum is inserted, and the cervix is visualized. Radiopaque oil or water-soluble dye is injected through the cervix to fill and highlight the interior of the cervix, uterus, and fallopian tubes. If the fallopian tubes are patent, the contrast material spills into the peritoneal cavity. Usually, only two or three films are taken to show the path and distribution of the contrast medium.

FOLLOW-UP CARE. The client may experience pelvic pain after the study and should receive medications accordingly. She may also experience referred shoulder pain because of irritation of the phrenic nerve caused by the dye. The nurse provides a perineal pad after the test to prevent the soiling of clothes as the dye drains from the cervix. The woman is instructed to contact her health care provider if bloody discharge continues for 4 days or longer and to report any signs of infection, such as lower quadrant pain, fever, malodorous discharge, and tachycardia.

Mammography

Mammography is an x-ray study of the soft tissue of the breast. Mammograms assess differences in the density of breast tissue. They are especially helpful in evaluating poorly defined masses, multiple masses or nodules, nipple changes or discharge, skin changes, and pain.

Mammography can detect many cancers that are not palpable by physical examination; however, some actual cancers are shown as benign by mammography.

In young women's breasts there is little difference in the density between normal glandular tissue and malignant tumors, which makes the mammogram less useful for the discovery and diagnosis of breast masses in these women. For that reason, annual screening mammograms are not recommended for women under 40 years of age (ACS, 1999). In older women, the percentage of fatty tissue is higher and the fatty tissue appears lighter than neoplasms. Cancer and cysts may have the same density. However, cysts usually have smooth borders, and neoplasms often have starburst-shaped margins.

CLIENT PREPARATION. No dietary restrictions are necessary before the mammogram. The woman is asked not to use creams, powders, or deodorant on the breasts or underarm areas before the study, because aluminum chlorhydrate can mimic calcium clusters. If there is any possibility that the client is pregnant, the test should be rescheduled. The purpose of the examination and its anticipated discomforts should be explained. A cover gown and adequate privacy for the client to undress above the waist are provided. The client also needs appropriate support and may need time to express her concerns about the mammogram and the presence of any lumps. Because this is a time when the client is anxious about the health of her breasts, it is an excellent opportunity to teach or reinforce the importance of breast self-examination.

PROCEDURE. The technician positions the client next to the x-ray machine with one breast exposed. A film plate and the platform of the machine are placed on opposite sides of the breast to be examined. The technician includes as much breast tissue as possible between the plates. The woman may experience some temporary discomfort when the breast is compressed during the positioning and the test. The test takes approximately 15 minutes, but the client is usually asked to wait until the films are developed in case a view needs to be repeated. Mammography usually necessitates two low-dose x-ray views of each breast: a view from the side and a view from above.

FOLLOW-UP CARE. If the results are not communicated at the time of the mammogram, the woman should know when to expect the report. She should be assessed for her knowledge of breast self-examination and given instructions if needed.

OTHER DIAGNOSTIC TESTS
Ultrasonography

Ultrasonography is a nonradiographic diagnostic technique that is routinely used to assess reproductive problems such as uterine fibroids, ovarian cysts, and pelvic masses. It can be used to locate intrauterine devices and to monitor the progress of tumor regression after medical treatment. Ultrasonography is also useful in differentiating solid tumors from cysts in breast examinations (Pagana & Pagana, 1998).

No specific preparations are necessary for this study. The client should have a full bladder to enable visualization of the uterus and to make the location of other structures more distinct with abdominal ultrasonography; a full bladder is not necessary for transvaginal scans.

For an abdominal or breast scan, the technician exposes the area and applies oil or gel to the area to be scanned. These substances provide better transmission of sound waves from the transducer through the client's skin. The transducer is moved in a linear pattern across the abdomen to outline and define soft-tissue masses and to differentiate tumor types, ascites, and encapsulated fluid.

For a transvaginal scan, the transducer is covered with a condom or vinyl glove into which transmission gel has been placed. The transducer is then inserted in the vagina. The client is often interested in the oscilloscope screen and appreciates a brief explanation of the landmarks and structures visualized. There is no special follow-up care for the client after this procedure except to provide wipes to remove the gel.

EVIDENCE-BASED PRACTICE FOR NURSING

Mailing informational handouts before colposcopy can increase knowledge

Tomaino-Brunner, C., et al. (1998). Can precolposcopy education increase knowledge and decrease anxiety? *Journal of Obstetric, Gynecologic, and Neonatal Nursing, 27*(6), 636-645.

Referral for colposcopy is the usual follow-up for women with abnormal Papanicolaou (Pap) tests. Previous studies have found that women expressed little understanding of the procedure before the appointment.

This randomized, controlled study investigated the impact of an informational handout about colposcopy on knowledge and anxiety levels. This handout was mailed to inner-city women scheduled for the procedure. The sample included 58 women in the intervention group and 55 women in the control group who did not receive the mailing. Knowledge was measured by content analysis of interviews held at the clinic at the time of the colposcopy; anxiety was measured using the Spielberger State/Trait Anxiety Inventory. Results indicated that 72% of the intervention group understood what a colposcopy was compared to 42% of the control group. No significant differences were found in mean anxiety scores between the groups.

Critique. This experimental, randomized controlled study of a small sample of inner city women did not include a pretest-posttest design, and therefore the knowledge and anxiety levels of the women before the intervention are not known. Further study is needed to understand what interventions can decrease anxiety about colposcopy.

Implications for Nursing. This study has implications for client education. Mailing a handout on colposcopy or other procedures shortly before the appointment is a simple yet effective method of providing information to clients. Because client education is an important nursing function, nurses need to be able to use a variety of methods to meet individual client needs.

Magnetic Resonance Imaging

Magnetic resonance imaging (MRI) uses a magnetic field and radiofrequency energy to scan for pelvic tumors. This scan effectively distinguishes between normal and malignant tissues. MRIs are also being investigated for use in the diagnosis of breast cancer (Mishell et al., 1997).

Endoscopic Studies
COLPOSCOPY

The colposcope allows three-dimensional magnification and intense illumination of epithelium with suspected disease. **Colposcopy** is suited for inspection of the cervical epithelium, vagina, and vulvar epithelium. This procedure can locate the exact site of precancerous and malignant lesions for biopsy.

CLIENT PREPARATION. The woman is placed in the lithotomy position and provided the same support as for a pelvic examination. The client should not douche or use vaginal preparations for 24 to 48 hours before the examination. This relatively painless procedure is usually better tolerated if it is explained in advance and if the instrument is shown to the client (see the Evidence-Based Practice for Nursing box above).

A colposcopy provides accurate site selection for tissue biopsy, and therefore the client should also be prepared for a biopsy. Materials necessary for cytologic studies and biopsy should be readily available.

PROCEDURE. The physician locates the cervix, or vaginal site, through a speculum examination. Lubricants other than water should not be used. Cells in the area may be stained or left unstained to enhance visualization. The physician cleans the cervix of secretions and moistens the cervix with normal saline. This allows for better visualization of vascular patterns and the junction between the columnar epithelium and the squamous epithelium. Acetic acid, 3%, applied to the cervix acts as a mucolytic agent to draw moisture from the tissue and to accentuate important morphologic features. The physician then uses a colposcope or colpomicroscope to inspect the area in question. A biopsy may also be taken if abnormal cells are seen (see discussion on cervical biopsy on p. 1727).

FOLLOW-UP CARE. After the procedure, the nurse assists the woman as for a pelvic examination and provides supplies to clean the perineum. The nurse also gives her a perineal pad to absorb any dye or discharge. If procedures other than direct visualization were performed, follow-up care needs to be revised appropriately.

■ LAPAROSCOPY

Laparoscopy is a highly accurate diagnostic tool for exploring the pelvic cavity. This procedure can rule out an ectopic pregnancy, evaluate ovarian disorders and pelvic masses, and aid in the diagnosis of infertility and unexplained pelvic pain. Laparoscopy is also used during surgical procedures such as the following:

- Tubal sterilization
- Ovarian biopsy
- Cyst or graafian follicle aspiration (to retrieve ova for in vitro fertilization)
- Lysis of adhesions around the fallopian tubes
- Retrieval of "lost" intrauterine devices

A **laparoscopy** is preferable to a laparotomy for minor surgical procedures because it necessitates only a small infraumbilical incision, involves less discomfort, and does not require hospitalization.

CLIENT PREPARATION. The physician explains the procedure, risks (complications associated with the use of general anesthesia, postoperative shoulder pain, and the rare occurrence of infection or electric burns), and anticipated discomforts and obtains the client's consent. The procedure can be performed with either a regional or general anesthetic. Clients should expect mild discomfort from the incision site and may experience referred shoulder pain from phrenic nerve irritation (Nichols & Lowdermilk, 2000).

PROCEDURE. The client is anesthetized and placed in the lithotomy position. A urinary catheter is inserted to drain the bladder. The operating table is placed in a slight Trendelenburg position to cause the intestines to fall away from the pelvis. The cervix is held with a cannula to allow movement of the uterus during laparoscopy (Figure 73-9). The surgeon inserts a needle below the umbilicus to infuse carbon dioxide into the pelvic cavity; this distends the abdomen and permits better visualization of the organs. The surgeon inserts a trocar and a cannula into an infraumbilical incision. After the trocar and cannula are in place in the abdominal cavity, the surgeon removes the trocar and inserts the laparoscope. The surgeon can thus visualize the pelvic cavity and reproductive organs. Further instrumentation is possible through a second small incision. The laparoscope is removed at the end of the procedure, and the abdomen is deflated. The physician usually closes the incision with absorbable sutures and dresses the area with an adhesive bandage.

FOLLOW-UP CARE. The client requires postoperative care similar to that for other clients after general anesthesia but is usually discharged on the day of the surgery. Discomfort from the incision is usually alleviated by the administration of oral analgesics. The greatest discomfort is due to referred shoulder pain caused by residual gas in the peritoneal cavity. Most of these sensations disappear within 48 hours. Clients are instructed to change the small adhesive bandage as needed and to observe the incision for signs of infection or hematoma. The client should avoid strenuous activity for the first week after the procedure.

■ HYSTEROSCOPY

Hysteroscopy is an endoscopic examination that permits visualization of the interior of the uterus and the cervical canal. The hysteroscope includes a lens with fiberoptic lighting; an aqueous solution of carbon dioxide is the medium used to distend the uterus. Hysteroscopy can be used for the removal of intrauterine devices and as a complement to other diagnostic tests for infertility and unexplained bleeding.

CLIENT PREPARATION. The surgeon informs the client of all aspects of the procedure and obtains consent. The client receives the same preparation as for a pelvic examination. The procedure is best performed 5 days after menses have ceased to eliminate the possibility of pregnancy. The

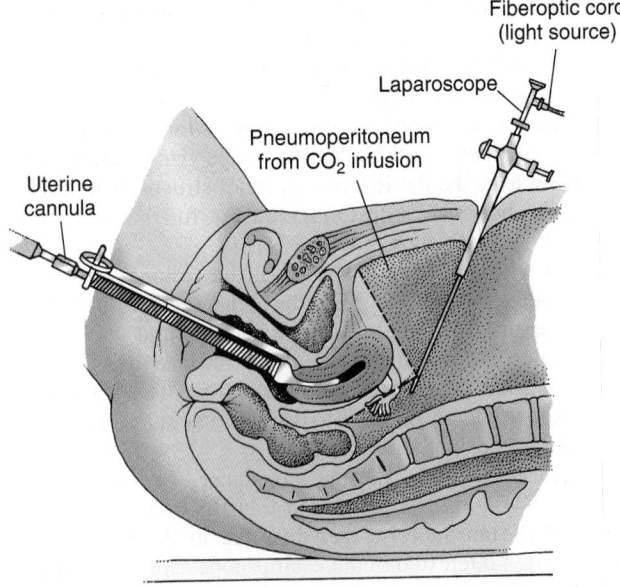

Figure 73-9 ● Laparoscopy.

client is placed in the lithotomy position and is usually anesthetized with a pericervical or other regional block.

PROCEDURE. After the client is anesthetized, the cervix is dilated. The physician inserts the hysteroscope through the cervix. Because a medium distends the uterus, cells can be pushed through the fallopian tubes and into the pelvic cavity. Therefore hysteroscopy is contraindicated in clients with suspected cervical or endometrial cancer, in clients with infection of the upper reproductive tract, and in pregnant clients.

FOLLOW-UP CARE. Care is the same as that after a pelvic examination. Analgesics may be ordered if the client experiences cervical and uterine cramping. Shoulder pain may be present for up to 24 hours if carbon dioxide was used to distend the uterus during the procedure.

Biopsy Studies

CERVICAL BIOPSY

In a cervical biopsy, cervical tissue is removed for additional cytologic study. A biopsy is definitely indicated in a client with an identifiable cervical lesion, regardless of the cytologic findings. The physician usually performs a biopsy in conjunction with colposcopy as a follow-up to a suspicious Pap test finding. This procedure may be performed in the health care provider's office.

Several techniques can be used for a cervical biopsy. If a lesion is clearly visible, an endocervical curettage can be performed as an outpatient procedure and with little or no anesthetic. Conization (removal of a cone-shaped sample of tissue) and loop electrosurgical excision procedures (LEEP) are usually not done unless the cervical biopsy is positive or the results of the colposcopy are unsatisfactory (Lowdermilk, 2000). Conization, if performed, can be done as a cold-knife procedure, a laser excision, or an electrosurgical incision.

CLIENT PREPARATION. The client should be scheduled for the biopsy in the early proliferative phase of the menstrual cycle, when the cervix is least vascular. The selected procedure should be explained to the client. Because a biopsy evaluates potentially malignant cells, most women become anxious and need time to discuss their feelings and fears. The use of relaxation techniques may facilitate comfort. The nurse assists the client into the lithotomy position and prepares her in the same way as for a pelvic examination. Further preparation depends on the type of procedure to be performed.

PROCEDURE. The physician may anesthetize the client according to the needs of the chosen procedure. The physician visualizes the cervix and obtains the tissue sample. All specimens are immediately placed into a formalin solution.

FOLLOW-UP CARE. The type of anesthetic used for the procedure determines the type of immediate postoperative care provided by the nurse. Discharge instructions are listed in Chart 73-6.

ENDOMETRIAL BIOPSY AND ASPIRATION

Both endometrial biopsy and aspiration are used to obtain cells directly from the lining of the uterus in women at risk for cancer of the endometrium. Endometrial biopsy is also valuable for assessing functional menstrual disturbances (especially anovulatory bleeding) and infertility (corpus luteum dysfunction).

When menstrual disturbances are being evaluated, the biopsy is generally done in the immediate premenstrual period to serve as an index of progesterone influence and ovulation. A biopsy performed in the second half of the menstrual cycle (approximately days 21 and 22) evaluates corpus luteum function and the presence or absence of a persistent secretory endometrium. Postmenopausal women may undergo biopsies at any time.

CLIENT PREPARATION. Menstrual data are obtained from the client and included on the specimen slip for the pathologist. The client is given the same preparation as for a pelvic examination. The nurse advises her that she may experience some cramping when the cervix is dilated. Analgesia before the procedure and relaxation and breathing techniques during the procedure are often of value.

PROCEDURE. An endometrial biopsy is often performed as an office procedure with or without anesthesia. After the uterus is sounded (measured) and the cervix sufficiently dilated, the physician inserts the curette or intrauterine cannula into the uterus. The physician withdraws a portion of the endometrium either with the cuplike end of the curette or with suction aspiration equipment. The client experiences moderate cramping. The specimens are placed in a formalin solution and sent for histologic examination.

FOLLOW-UP CARE. The client is allowed to rest on the examining table until the cramping has subsided. A perineal pad and a wipe to clean the perineum are provided. Spotting may be present for 1 to 2 days, but any signs of infection or excessive bleeding should be reported to the physician. The client is informed to refrain from intercourse or douching until all discharge has ceased. Results of the biopsy are usually available within 72 hours.

BREAST BIOPSY AND ASPIRATION

An incisional biopsy is the surgical removal of tissue from a breast mass. An excisional biopsy removes the mass itself for histologic (cellular) evaluation. Aspiration biopsy is the removal of fluid or tissue from the breast mass through a large-

---

CHART 73-6

CLIENT EDUCATION GUIDE
The Client Recovering from Cervical Biopsy

- Do not lift any heavy objects until the site is healed (about 2 weeks).
- Rest for 24 hours after the procedure.
- Report any excessive bleeding (more than that of a normal menstrual period) to your health care provider.
- Report signs of infection to your health care provider.
- Do not douche, use tampons, or have vaginal intercourse until the site is healed (about 2 weeks).
- Keep the perineum clean and dry by using antiseptic solution rinses (as directed by your health care provider) and changing pads frequently.

bore needle. Figure 73-10 shows these three types of breast biopsy.

Any breast mass needs to be evaluated further for the possibility of cancer. Fibrocystic lesions, fibroadenomas, and intraductal papillomas can be differentiated by biopsy. Any discharge from the breasts is examined histologically.

CLIENT PREPARATION. The instructions to the client depend on the type of biopsy and the type of anesthesia. The woman is told to expect pulling or probing sensations during the procedure.

PROCEDURE. Aspiration biopsy is often performed in an outpatient setting without an anesthetic. The mass is located by palpation of the breast. The surgeon then directs the needle into the lump and aspirates the contents into the syringe. The contents are placed on a slide for Pap evaluation. Fluid from benign cysts may appear clear to dark green-brown; bloody fluid suggests cancer. If no fluid is aspirated, the tumor should be examined by incisional biopsy.

Incisional or excisional biopsies are typically performed as same-day procedures with local or general anesthesia. The tumor specimen is evaluated by the frozen section technique. If cancer is found, the physician sends the tissue to the laboratory for estrogen receptor analysis.

FOLLOW-UP CARE. Postoperative discomfort is usually mild and is controlled with analgesic administration or the use of a heating pad. The client is taught how to assess the incisional site for bleeding and edema. A properly supportive

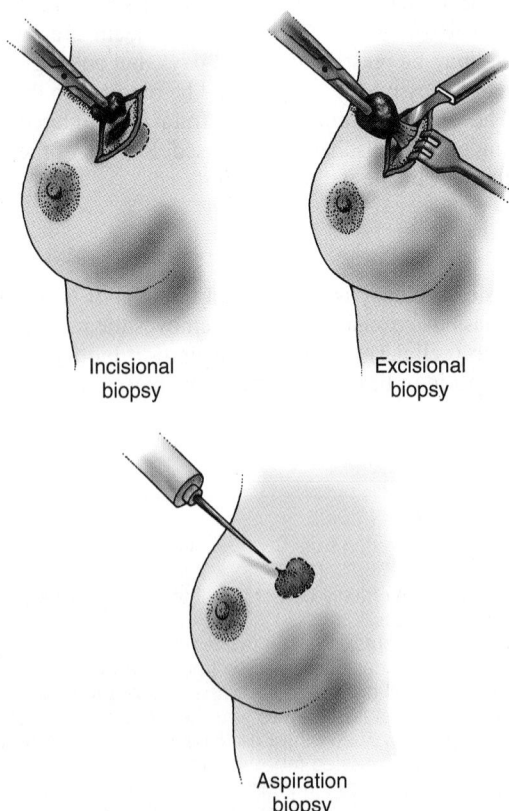

Figure 73-10 ● Breast biopsy techniques.

bra should be worn continuously by the woman for 1 week postoperatively. The woman should avoid cold temperatures to prevent nipple contractions that can cause stress on the incision. Numbness around the biopsy site may last 2 to 3 months. The woman should also be assessed about her knowledge of breast self-examination and given instructions if needed. If a malignancy is identified, the woman will need emotional support as well as information about follow-up treatment alternatives.

NEEDLE BIOPSY OF THE PROSTATE

When prostate cancer is suspected, the physician performs a needle aspiration biopsy of the prostate gland to retrieve cells for histologic study. This procedure is often performed at the same time as cystoscopy, with the client under anesthesia. The physician can perform needle biopsies without anesthesia or with the client under local anesthesia.

CLIENT PREPARATION. Preparation for the procedure depends on the technique used to puncture the gland. The nurse provides data on the expected discomforts. The nurse can also teach breathing and relaxation techniques for use during the examination. Because the purpose of this procedure is to evaluate prostate cells for potential malignancy, the man needs support and time to discuss his fears. Preparation for a transrectal biopsy involves the use of cleansing enemas and the administration of prophylactic antibiotics to reduce the risk of bacterial contamination of the bloodstream or prostate tissue. Local anesthesia is used at the site of transperineal biopsy.

PROCEDURE. The nurse places the client in the same position as for a rectal examination. After injecting a local anesthetic for the transperineal biopsy, the physician places a finger in the rectum to help guide the needle to the prostate. For the transrectal biopsy, the physician places the needle against the examining finger and then inserts it into the rectum to the prostate. From this site, the needle is advanced through the rectal mucosa and into the prostate gland. The aspiration may be repeated several times to obtain a satisfactory specimen.

FOLLOW-UP CARE. Sepsis is a potentially life-threatening complication of transrectal biopsy. Any signs of infection or septic shock must be reported immediately. Prophylactic antibiotics are usually prescribed.

ONLINE RESOURCES

For suggested readings and Internet resources, go to http://www.wbsaunders.com/SIMON/Iggy/.

SELECTED BIBLIOGRAPHY

Asterisk indicates a classic or definitive work on this subject.

American Cancer Society. (1999). *Cancer facts and figures, 1999.* New York: Author.

American College of Obstetricians and Gynecologists. (1997). *Committee opinion: Routine cancer screening.* Washington, D.C.: Author.

Angard, N. (1999). Diagnosis infertility. *AWHONN's Lifelines, 3*(3), 22-29.

Apgar, B. (1997). Dysmenorrhea and dysfunctional bleeding. *Primary Care, 24*(1), 161-168.

Barkauskas, V., et al. (1998). *Health and physical assessment* (2nd ed.). St. Louis: Mosby.

Centers for Disease Control and Prevention. (1998). Guidelines for the treatment of sexually transmitted diseases. *Morbidity & Mortality Weekly Report, 47*(RR-1), 1-116.

*Cook, M. (1994). Nursing assessment for the older woman. *RN, 57*(9), 40-43.

DiSaia, P., & Creasman, W. (1997). *Clinical gynecologic oncology* (5th ed.). St. Louis: Mosby.

Fernandez, M., Tortolero-Luna, G., & Gold, R. (1998). Mammography and Pap test screening among low-income foreign-born Hispanic women in the USA. *Cadernas de Saude Publica, 14*(Suppl. 3), 133-147.

Fishwick, N. (1998). Assessment of women for partner abuse. *Journal of Obstetric, Gynecologic, and Neonatal Nursing, 27*(6), 661-670.

Fogel, C. (2000). Common reproductive concerns. In D. Lowdermilk, S. Perry, & I. Bobak (Eds.), *Maternity and women's health care* (7th ed., pp. 115-143). St. Louis: Mosby.

Fogel, C., & Woods, N. (in press). *Women's health care: A comprehensive handbook* (2nd ed.). Thousand Oaks, CA: Sage.

*Geissler, E. (1999). *Pocket guide to cultural assessment* 2nd ed. St. Louis: Mosby.

Gordon, M. (2000). *Manual of nursing diagnosis* (9th ed.). St. Louis: Mosby.

Heritage, C. (1998). Working with childhood sexual abuse survivors during pregnancy, labor, and birth. *Journal of Obstetric, Gynecologic, and Neonatal Nursing, 27*(6), 671-677.

Higgins, P., & Smith, P. (1997). Assessing cervical cancer risks. *AWHONN's Lifelines, 1*(6), 43-47.

Lawson, E. (1998). A narrative analysis: A black woman's perception of breast cancer risks and early breast cancer detection. *Cancer Nursing, 21*(6), 421-429.

Lowdermilk, D. (1997). Caring for women with sexual and reproductive system disorders. In J. Luckmann (Ed.). *Saunders manual of nursing care.* (pp. 1441-1495). Philadelphia: W.B. Saunders.

Lowdermilk, D. (2000). Structural disorders and neoplasms of the reproductive system. In D. Lowdermilk, S. Perry, & I. Bobak (Eds.), *Maternity and women's health care* (7th ed., pp. 268-302). St. Louis: Mosby.

Lowdermilk, D. (in press). Reproductive surgery. In C. Fogel, & N. Woods (Eds.), *Women's health care: A comprehensive handbook* (2nd ed.). Thousand Oaks, CA: Sage.

Mishell, D., et al. (1997). *Comprehensive gynecology.* (3rd ed.). St. Louis: Mosby.

Morrell, V. (1997). Basic infertility assessment. *Primary Care, 21*(1), 195-204.

National Women's Health Resource Center. (1999). Breast health. *National Women's Health Report, 17*(5), 1-11.

Nichols, A., & Lowdermilk, D. (2000). Infertility. In D. Lowdermilk, S. Perry, & I. Bobak (Eds.), *Maternity and women's health care* (7th ed., pp. 206-224). St. Louis: Mosby.

Pagana, K.D., & Pagana, T.J. (1998). *Mosby's manual of diagnostic and laboratory tests.* St. Louis: Mosby.

Plourd, D. (1997). Practical guide to diagnosing and treating vaginitis. *Medscape Women's Health, 2*(2), 2.

Sampselle, C., et al. (1999). Continence for women: Evidence-based practice. *Journal of Obstetric, Gynecologic, and Neonatal Nurses, 28*(6 Suppl. 1), 25-33.

Schweitzer, M., et al. (1998). Cost-effectiveness of detecting breast cancer in lower socioeconomic status African-American and Hispanic women through mobile mammogram services. *Medical Care Research and Review, 55*(1), 99-115.

Seidel, H.M., et al. (1999). *Mosby's guide to physical examination* (4th ed.). St. Louis: Mosby.

Sinclair, B. (2000). Health promotion and prevention. In D. Lowdermilk, S. Perry, & I. Bobak (Eds.), *Maternity and women's health care* (7th ed., pp. 68-87). St. Louis: Mosby.

Snell, L. (2000). Problems of the breast. In D. Lowdermilk, S. Perry, & I. Bobak (Eds.), *Maternity and women's health care* (7th ed., pp. 247-266). St. Louis: Mosby.

Tomaino-Brunner, C., et al. (1998). Can precopolscopy education increase knowledge and decrease anxiety? *Journal of Obstetric, Gynecologic, and Neonatal Nursing, 27*(6), 636-645.

U.S. Department of Health and Human Services, Public Health Service. (1997). *Clinician's handbook of preventive medicine.* Washington, D.C.: U.S. Government Printing Office.

West, R. (1998). The female athlete: Disordered eating, amenorrhea, and osteoporosis. *Sports Medicine, 26*(2), 63-71.

Youngkin, E., & Davis, M. (1998). *Women's health: A primary care clinical guide* (2nd ed.). Stamford, CT: Appleton & Lange.

Zdanuk, J. (2000). Assessment of women. In D. Lowdermilk, S. Perry, & I. Bobak (Eds.), *Maternity and women's health care* (7th ed., pp. 88-114). St. Louis: Mosby.

Interventions for Clients with Breast Disorders

  >AMY NICHOLS • DONNA D. IGNATAVICIUS

Learning Objectives

After studying this chapter, you should be able to:

1. Describe the three-pronged approach to early detection of breast masses: mammography, clinical breast examination, and breast self-examination (BSE).
2. Teach a client how to do BSE.
3. Explain the options available to a woman at high genetic risk for breast cancer.
4. Compare and contrast assessment findings associated with benign and malignant breast lesions.
5. Analyze assessment data to determine priority nursing diagnoses and collaborative problems for a woman with breast cancer.
6. Develop a plan of care for a client with breast cancer.
7. Discuss the psychosocial aspects related to having breast cancer and undergoing surgery for breast cancer.
8. Formulate a community-based teaching plan for clients undergoing surgery for breast cancer.

Go to http://www.wbsaunders.com/SIMON/Iggy/ for self-assessment questions related to these Learning Objectives.

Breast cancer is the most commonly diagnosed cancer in women in the Western world, with more than 180,000 new cases identified annually and more than 40,000 deaths in the United States alone (Nass & Davidson, 1999). Although breast disorders affect both men and women, women are most often affected. The most common sign or symptom associated with a breast disorder is a palpable mass. The discovery of a mass in a woman's breast, whether the discovery is by the woman herself, her partner, or a health care provider, is a frightening experience. Even if the woman is aware that 90% of all breast lumps are benign, she may fear that the lump is cancerous. This fearful reaction accompanies the woman through the period of diagnosis, decision making, and treatment. Regardless of the severity of the diagnosis, the nurse must incorporate the physiologic and emotional factors involved to provide effective nursing care.

PREVENTION AND EARLY DETECTION OF BREAST MASSES

Early detection by screening for breast masses involves a three-pronged approach: mammography, breast self-examination, and clinical breast examination.

Mammography

The American Cancer Society (ACS), the National Cancer Institute (NCI), the National Comprehensive Cancer Network (NCCN), the American College of Radiology (ACR), and the American College of Physicians (ACP) have established guidelines for breast cancer screening. Most recommend a baseline screening **mammogram** (x-ray examination of the breast) at the age of 40 years and yearly screening for women beginning between the ages of 40 and 50 (Table 74-1).

Evidence-based data support a significant reduction in breast cancer mortality as a result of annual or biennial mammography and clinical breast examination (CBE) for asymptomatic women between the ages of 50 and 69 years. Champion (1995) conducted a study to determine what influences mammogram compliance and how compliance rates can be improved. Barriers to mammography may include fear of radiation, fear of results, concern about pain, and knowledge deficit. Compliance with mammogram guidelines has been significantly associated with health care provider recommendations for mammography (Champion, 1995).

Other factors influencing whether women have screening mammograms include accessibility and client cost. Not all health insurers pay for mammography. The Breast and Cervical Cancer Mortality Prevention Act of 1990 was established to provide screening services to medically underserved women after a 1992 National Health Interview Survey indicated that only 35% of women older than age 50 years had received a screening mammogram during the previous year. Currently, a number of state and federal programs that target low-income women are available in many areas of the United States.

Breast Self-Examination

Breast self-examination (BSE) is an inexpensive means for detecting breast cancer that has been encouraged by health

TABLE 74-1 • BREAST CANCER SCREENING GUIDELINES FOR ASYMPTOMATIC WOMEN AGE 40 YEARS OR OLDER

Screening Modality	ACS, ACR	NCI	NCCN	ACP
Two-view mammography	Annual Begin at age 40 yr No upper age	Biennial Begin at age 40 yr Upper age, 69 yr	Biennial Begin at age 40 yr No upper age	Annual Begin at age 50 yr Upper age, 74 yr
Clinical breast examination	Annual	Encourage	Annual	Encourage
Breast self-examination	Monthly	Encourage	Encourage	Encourage

From Overmoyer, B. (1999). Breast cancer screening. *Medical Clinics of North America, 83*(6), 1143-1460.
ACS, American Cancer Society; *ACR,* American College of Radiology; *NCI,* National Cancer Institute; *NCCN,* National Comprehensive Cancer Network; and *ACP,* American College of Physicians.

EVIDENCE-BASED PRACTICE FOR NURSING

Does special training improve the proficiency of breast self-examination?

Bragg Leight, S., et al. (2000). The effect of structured training on breast self-examination search behaviors as measured using biomedical instrumentation. *Nursing Research, 49*(5), 283-289.

Although breast self-examination (BSE) has been recommended for many years as a complement to the professional examination and mammography, only a small percentage of women in the United States report doing monthly BSE. The authors describe a study in which they asked 41 young women to participate in a structured training protocol for BSE instruction. Using biomedical instrumentation, the researchers evaluated the depth of breast palpation and the duration of the examination. The results showed that with individualized instruction, the examination was much more thorough for both palpation and duration.

Critique. This study was a small descriptive study that cannot be generalized to the female population. However, it demonstrates that individualized education may make a difference in compliance and thoroughness of the examination. Since the study subjects were young, the study should be replicated to represent a better cross-section of ages and cultures.

Implications for Nursing. Nurses are in a unique position to provide individualized instruction to their clients of any age in any setting. One-on-one training with follow-up may be the most successful way to increase participation in this very important health promotion practice.

CONSIDERATIONS FOR OLDER ADULTS

With the projected increase in the older adult population, especially women, during the next half-century, breast cancer will be an even greater health concern. The current recommendation is BSE monthly, CBE yearly, and mammography every 1 to 2 years for women age 65 years and older. Older women may be more resistant to practicing BSE if they have yearly CBE performed by their health care provider. Health teaching to promote compliance and competence in BSE is extremely important in this soon-to-be high-risk group.

CULTURAL CONSIDERATIONS

One of the national health objectives for the year 2010 is the prevention of cancer in minority ethnic populations. Some progress has been made in the area of research to examine the variables associated with BSE in minority women. Research results from one study population of Chinese-American women indicated that only 15% of the women studied practiced BSE monthly, and 48% reported never having done BSE. Although the majority of these women recognized the efficacy of BSE, perceived competency in the technique was the variable that most influenced whether they regularly performed BSE (Lu, 1995). A more recent study by Facione et al. (2000) found that Chinese-American women believe that they are not likely to get breast cancer and that cancer is linked to tragic luck. If they have symptoms suggestive of breast cancer, they are likely to delay Western treatment in favor of Chinese medicine to conserve money and modesty.

In similar studies of African-American women, 63% were found to practice BSE monthly and 76% had yearly CBE; however, only 20% had a mammogram according to age-related guidelines (Phillips & Wilbur, 1995). Like Chinese-American women, African-American women believe in chance and doubt the value of early diagnosis and treatment (Barroso et al., 2000). Culturally sensitive strategies need to be used to increase breast cancer awareness and screening practices among these culturally diverse groups (see Chapter 6).

care providers for decades. The goal of screening for breast cancer is *early detection.* Detection of breast cancer before axillary node invasion increases the chance of survival. BSE, used in conjunction with mammography and CBE, is extremely effective in detecting early breast cancer and reducing mortality rates. BSE *alone* as a screening technique has not been of equal value. The American Cancer Society recommends that all women older than age 20 years practice BSE monthly. Most women have heard of BSE, but many do not practice it regularly or proficiently (see the Evidence-Based Practice for Nursing box above). The reasons for nonpractice of BSE and the best methods for teaching BSE continue to be researched.

Whether the client seeks health care because she has found a breast lump, because she needs a routine physical examination, or because she has an unrelated health problem, the nurse's encounter with her provides an excellent opportunity to teach BSE. Health care providers must not assume that women who practice BSE do so competently and regularly. Also, most women prefer individualized instruction to learning from pamphlets and magazines. Women who are taught

by a health care provider on an individual or group basis practice BSE more often, more proficiently, and more confidently.

PREPARATION FOR TEACHING BREAST SELF-EXAMINATION

Before teaching BSE, the nurse assesses the psychologic factors influencing the client's motivation to practice BSE. Lack of knowledge about the technique and the benefits of early detection, uneasiness about self-assessment, and lack of confidence in self-assessment may be reasons why women fail to perform BSE regularly. The nurse stresses that treatment for breast cancer is more successful the earlier the disease is detected. It is also important for the client to develop confidence in her ability to detect breast changes. It should be emphasized to the client that a yearly breast examination by a health care provider cannot substitute for BSE.

BSE is used as an assessment tool for detecting cancer but does nothing to prevent breast cancer. Therefore the asymptomatic woman, when choosing whether to practice BSE, may think, "What's the use? It won't keep me from getting breast cancer." Again, the nurse can emphasize the advantages of early detection in terms of outcome and help the client to review risk factors to determine her risk of developing breast cancer. Women must believe that there are benefits to practicing BSE and that the barriers to practicing it are minimal. Addressing these issues will increase the client's knowledge and practice of BSE.

Discussing the client's fears, beliefs, and concerns about breast disease and BSE with her is an important step. Assessment for the presence of risk factors for breast cancer and a history of previous breast problems is essential. Proper timing for BSE should also be discussed. Premenopausal women should examine their breasts 1 week after the menstrual period. At this time, hormonal influence on breast tissue is minimal, so that fluid retention and tenderness are reduced. For these same reasons, if possible, the best time of the month to schedule a mammogram is also 1 week after the menstrual period. Women whose breast tissue is no longer influenced by hormonal fluctuations, such as after a hysterectomy or menopause, should pick a day each month when they will do BSE, such as the first day of the month. Clients who verbalize the need for monthly BSE, the need for yearly CBE, and the mammogram recommendations appropriate for their age demonstrate that client education has been successful.

TEACHING BREAST SELF-EXAMINATION

The setting in which BSE is demonstrated should be private and comfortable. The woman is asked to undress from the waist up and provided with a gown and sheet. Before teaching the technique of breast palpation, the nurse assesses the client's technique by asking her to demonstrate her own method. If the woman is unsure or has not performed BSE before, the nurse can slowly lead her through the examination while explaining the rationale for the technique and answering questions. It is also helpful for the nurse to point out different findings at this time, especially those that the client might perceive as abnormal. For example, nodular breast tissue may normally feel lumpy, which conjures up visions of widespread cancer in the unknowledgeable woman. Placing the client's hand directly on the involved area and showing her precisely what is normal for her can build self-confidence.

The nurse points out the inframammary ridge, the area of the breast where the skin folds under the breast. This thickened area may be perceived as a lump instead of a normal finding. In thin or small-breasted women, the ribs may be mistaken for masses. The nurse shows the client how to follow the rib to the sternum to be sure that what she is feeling is bone and not breast tissue. The client is taught to stand in front of a mirror to inspect the breast for abnormalities. She should raise her arms above her head and press her hands on her hips to emphasize any changes in the shape of the breasts. The breasts are examined in a lying position and while bathing or showering.

The nurse also demonstrates two other aspects of the examination: the amount of pressure needed and the correct position of the hands. The finger pads, which are more sensitive than the fingertips, are used when palpating the breasts. The finger pads should press firmly enough to detect the underlying tissue. However, the client should be instructed not to compress the tissue on the ribs, since this may falsely feel like a mass.

Use of teaching models of normal and abnormal breasts is helpful when teaching BSE. The nurse demonstrates the correct technique of examining the breasts with the arm overhead while lying down instead of having the arm by the side. Showing the difference in the two techniques, especially in large-breasted women, reveals the advantage of using the correct method, which spreads the tissue over the chest wall for more effective palpation.

Clinical Breast Examination

Clinical breast examination (CBE) is typically performed by advanced-practice nurses and physicians. However, nurses in general practice who are skilled in the technique can perform this examination. The examination can be done before, after, or during the teaching session. The same guidelines of providing a private and comfortable setting, maintaining dignity, and allowing time for discussion apply.

Taking a breast history is vital. Results may be recorded on a breast evaluation form, which is a part of the client's record (Figure 74-1). This record helps the nurse establish the relative risk for breast disease and the need for follow-up diagnostic tests, such as mammograms, and teaching.

The physical assessment begins with inspection. The woman undresses from the waist up and first sits or stands with her hands by her sides. The examiner inspects the breasts for symmetry and size, contour, skin changes (color, texture, and venous patterns), nipple changes, and lesions.

One breast may be larger than the other, and inverted nipples are not uncommon. The nurse asks the client whether these findings are normal for her. Any change in symmetry may indicate a problem. The contour should be even, and the skin should have a smooth texture. Venous patterns may be visible but should be similar bilaterally. The nipples and areola should be equal or nearly equal in size and should be a similar color. The nipples may be wrinkled or smooth, and Montgomery's tubercles on the areola are normal. Supernumerary nipples (extra nipples), although rare, are also normal. If a mass is palpated, the examiner notes its position by visualizing the breast as a clock face and noting the "area of the clock" where the mass is located. If it is necessary to move the arms away from the body, the woman should rest her arm on the examiner's to prevent flexion of the underlying muscles. While the arms are by the side and relaxed, the axillae can be palpated. The examiner palpates the axilla and the area above and below the clavicle for enlarged lymph nodes. The woman is then asked to raise her arms over her head, which exposes the sides and underneath portions of the breast for inspection. Finally, she is asked to place her hands on her hips and press, thus flexing the pectoral muscles. This action accentuates skin dimpling, retractions, or masses.

CLIENT'S NAME _____ Sex _____ Race _____ Age _____

Weight _____ Ideal Weight _____ Marital Status _____

HISTORY	Yes	No	Comments

Family history of breast cancer

Personal history of breast cancer

Previous mammograms

Previous biopsy (findings)

Nipple discharge

Hormone use (specify)

BSE Practice

High-fat diet

ETOH/smoking

Current medications (list)

Age at menses _____ Age at menopause _____

COMMENTS

_____

_____

_____

PHYSICAL FINDINGS

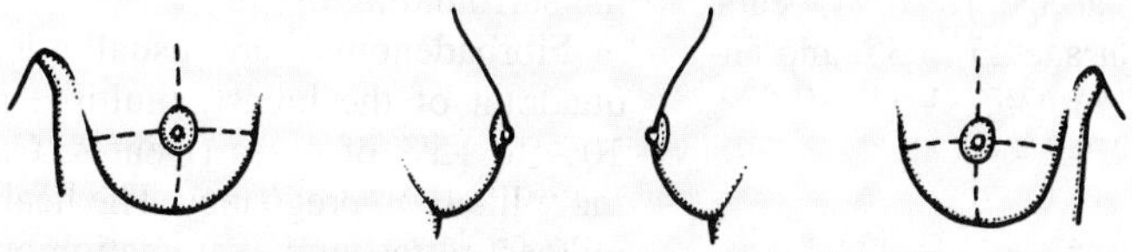

Mammogram Report _____

Biopsy/Cytology Results _____

BSE Return Demonstration _____

Plan _____

_____

CLIENT EDUCATION _____

Figure 74-1 ● A breast evaluation form.

The remainder of the examination is done with the client lying supine. The examiner places a pillow or rolled sheet under the client's shoulder, and the arm on that side is raised above the head. Each breast is palpated separately while the other breast remains covered. If the woman has identified a problem in one breast, the other, "normal" breast is examined first to establish a baseline for comparison.

The examiner palpates in a vertical pattern, in a horizontal pattern, or in concentric circles, covering every inch of the breast tissue, including the tail of Spence, which extends from the upper outer quadrant of the breast into the axilla. Supraclavicular lymph nodes are palpated for the presence of enlarged nodes by hooking the fingers over the clavicle.

Finally, the nipple is gently compressed to detect the presence of a discharge. If a discharge is produced, the examiner notes the "area of the clock" where the breast was compressed when the discharge was released. If there is a history of discharge, the client may be able to express the discharge more successfully than the examiner can and may be asked to do so.

Discovery of a suspicious lesion or discharge during the examination requires consultation or referral to a health care provider who specializes in caring for breast disorders. Follow-up usually involves mammography and possibly ultrasound. If there is a dominant mass or a suspicious clinical picture, the woman should be referred for biopsy even if the mammogram is negative.

CONSIDERATIONS FOR OLDER ADULTS

As women age, the breast tissue becomes flattened and elongated and is suspended loosely from the chest wall. On palpation the breast tissue of the older woman will have a finer, more granular feel than the lobular feel in a younger woman. The inframammary ridge may be more prominent as a result of atrophy of the breast tissue. Breast examination in older clients may be easier because of tissue atrophy and relaxation of the suspensory ligaments (Cooper's ligaments).

WOMEN AT HIGH GENETIC RISK FOR BREAST CANCER

A woman is considered to be at high genetic risk for breast cancer if her family history suggests a predisposition to the disease. Family history includes multiple relatives with breast cancer, early age at diagnosis, and in some families, ovarian cancer. Currently, inherited mutations in several genes are known to be manifested in hereditary patterns of breast cancer. The most common genes tested for breast cancer are BRCA1 and BRCA2. Mutations in these genes could account for 40% to 50% of hereditary breast cancers in the United States (Couch, DeShano, & Blackwood, 1997; Couch & Hartmann, 1998; Frank, Manley, & Olopade, 1998).

Cancer Surveillance

Cancer surveillance is currently the prevention option preferred by most high-risk women. Cancer surveillance is also referred to as "secondary prevention" and is used to detect cancer early in the initial stages. For breast cancer surveillance in high-risk women, the same combination of breast self-examination (BSE), clinical breast examination (CBE), and mammography are recommended as in the asymptomatic population. The difference for high-risk women is in the timing of examinations and starting age of mammography. The Cancer Genetics Studies Consortium, organized by the National Human Genome Research Institute, convened a task force to make recommendations for the management of women with BRCA1 and BRCA2 mutations (Burke, Daly, & Garber, 1997). The recommendations include monthly BSE beginning at age 18 to 21 years, CBE every 6 to 12 months beginning at age 25 to 35, and annual mammography beginning at age 25 to 35.

Prophylactic Mastectomy

Prophylactic **mastectomy** (surgical breast removal) is another option for reducing the risk of breast cancer. Although prophylactic mastectomy has been an option for decades, little information has been available until now regarding the long-term outcome of women who have elected to undergo this procedure (American Society of Clinical Oncology, 1998; Burke et al., 1997). Even though a woman may elect to undergo a prophylactic mastectomy, there is a small risk that breast cancer will develop in residual breast glandular tissue, because no mastectomy reliably removes all mammary tissue (Hartmann et al., 1999).

Chemoprevention

The third management option for women at high risk for breast cancer is **chemoprevention** with the prophylactic use of the drug known as tamoxifen citrate (Nolvadex, Tamofen✿, Tamone✿). In three clinical trials in which tamoxifen was introduced as a breast cancer chemopreventive, tamoxifen citrate was indicated to reduce the incidence of breast cancer in women at high risk for breast cancer (Fisher, Costantino, & Wickerman, 1998; Veronesi et al., 1998). Al-

though the drug treatment was successful, there were drawbacks. Women who were treated with tamoxifen complained of many serious side effects, and the medication treatment is very expensive (Fisher, Costantino, & Wickerman, 1998).

BENIGN BREAST DISORDERS

Most breast lumps are benign. Because the incidence of breast disease is related to age, breast disorders are described in an age-related order (Table 74-2).

Fibroadenoma

Fibroadenomas are the most common cause of breast masses during adolescence, although they may occur into the 30s. A fibroadenoma is a solid, slowly enlarging, benign mass of connective tissue that is unattached to the surrounding breast tissue and is typically discovered by the client herself. Although the immediate fear is that of breast cancer, only 0.9% of these masses are malignant. The mass is usually round, firm, easily movable, nontender, and clearly delineated from the surrounding tissue.

Fibroadenomas are usually located in the upper outer quadrant of the breast; multiple masses may be present in 10% to 15% of cases (Dent & Cant, 1999). Enlargement is more likely in pregnancy. The health care provider may order a breast ultrasound examination or may perform a needle aspiration to establish whether the lump is cystic or solid. If the lesion is solid, outpatient excision using local anesthesia is the treatment of choice.

> **CULTURAL CONSIDERATIONS**
> Fibroadenomas are most common in African-American women and tend to occur at an earlier age in African-American women than in women of other ethnic backgrounds (Tierney et al., 1995).

Fibrocystic Breast Disease

■ OVERVIEW

Fibrocystic changes, or physiologic nodularity of the breast, often referred to as **fibrocystic breast disease (FBD),** are the most common breast problem of women between the ages of 20 and 30 years. Over the life span, approximately 90% of women will have fibrocystic changes. Fibrocystic changes may proceed through several clinical stages or may present in only one form.

TABLE 74-2 • TYPICAL PRESENTATION OF BENIGN BREAST DISORDERS

Breast Disorder	Description	Incidence
Fibroadenoma	Most common benign lesion; solid mass of connective tissue that is unattached to the surrounding tissue	During teenage years into the 30s
Fibrocystic breast disease (FBD)	*First stage:* Characterized by premenstrual bilateral fullness and tenderness *Second stage:* Presence of bilateral, multicentric nodules *Third stage:* Presence of microscopic and macroscopic cysts	Late teens and 20s
Ductal ectasia	Hard, irregular mass or masses with nipple discharge, enlarged axillary nodes, redness, and edema; difficult to distinguish from cancer	Women approaching menopause
Intraductal ectasia	Mass in duct that results in nipple discharge; mass is usually not palpable	Women ages 40 to 55 yr

Data from National Cancer Institute.

The first stage commonly occurs between the late teens and early 20s. Premenstrual bilateral fullness and tenderness are present, especially in the outer upper quadrant. Symptoms usually resolve after menstruation and then recur before the next menstrual period in a cyclic fashion.

The second stage usually occurs in the late 20s and throughout the 30s. Bilateral multicentric nodular areas that feel like small marbles can be felt and accompany the fullness and soreness.

The third stage generally occurs between the ages of 35 and 55 years. Microscopic or macroscopic cysts generally appear suddenly and are associated with pain, tenderness, or burning. They are usually three-dimensional, smooth, mobile, and well delineated. Although the cysts may recede somewhat before menstruation, they do not disappear completely. Mammography is generally indicated, and fine-needle aspiration may be performed. Older clients receiving hormone replacement therapy may develop painful, fluid-filled cysts. Biopsy is indicated in the following situations:

* The aspirated fluid is bloody.
* No fluid is aspirated.
* The mammogram shows suspicious findings.
* A mass remains palpable after aspiration.
* The cytologic study of the aspirated fluid reveals malignant cells.

Although the cause of fibrocystic breast changes is unknown, the condition seems to be related to normal fluctuations in estrogen levels during the menstrual cycle. Symptoms usually resolve after menopause in the absence of estrogen supplementation.

► COLLABORATIVE MANAGEMENT

Medical management of FBD is generally symptomatic. Hormonal manipulation has been the primary means of pharmacologic intervention. Oral contraceptives can suppress oversecretion of estrogen, and progestins may be used to correct luteal insufficiency. Danazol (Danocrine, Cyclomen✤) suppresses ovarian function and estrogen stimulation of breast tissue. However, because hormonal therapy with danazol will not cure FBD, and because its side effects are undesirable, it is generally used only in clients with recurrent and unusually severe fibrocystic disease.

Medical management may also include the use of vitamins C, E, and B complex. The health care provider may prescribe diuretics to decrease premenstrual breast engorgement. Clients are counseled to avoid the use of caffeine; however, the role of caffeine in FBD is controversial.

The client is encouraged to continue prescribed medical interventions and monitors the effectiveness of these interventions. The nurse suggests supportive measures, such as the use of mild analgesics or limiting salt intake before menses, to help decrease swelling. The client may want to wear (both day and night) a well-padded, supportive brassiere to decrease tension on ligaments. Local application of ice or heat may provide temporary relief of pain. The nurse promotes the practice of BSE and teaches the procedure when necessary.

Ductal Ectasia

Ductal ectasia is a benign breast problem that is usually seen in women approaching menopause. The disease is caused by dilation and thickening of the collecting ducts in the subareo-

lar area. These ducts become distended and filled with cellular debris, which activates an inflammatory response. Two clinical signs result from these changes:

* A mass develops that feels hard, has irregular borders, and may be tender.
* A greenish brown nipple discharge, enlarged axillary nodes, and redness and edema over the site of the mass are noted.

These masses are often difficult to distinguish from breast cancer. Because the risk for breast cancer is increased in the menopause age-group, accurate diagnosis is vital. A microscopic examination of the nipple discharge is performed to detect any atypical or malignant cells, and the affected area is excised. Nursing care is directed at alleviating the anxiety associated with the threat of breast cancer and at supporting the woman through the diagnostic and treatment procedures.

Intraductal Papilloma

Intraductal papilloma, like ductal ectasia and breast cancer, occurs primarily in women ages 40 to 55 years. A benign process in the epithelial lining of the duct forms a papilloma, or pedunculated outgrowth of tissue. As the papilloma grows, trauma and erosion within the duct result in a serosanguineous or serous nipple discharge. A mass is rarely palpable.

Diagnosis is aimed first at ruling out breast cancer. Microscopic examination of the nipple discharge and surgical excision of the mass and ductal area are usually indicated.

Issues of Large-Breasted Women

Although Western society emphasizes large breasts as positive attributes, women with excessive breast tissue experience difficulties and discomfort. For instance, because fashion is directed at the small-breasted figure, a woman with large breasts may have difficulty finding clothes that fit well and in which she feels attractive. The breast size may be disproportionate to the rest of the body, which adds to the problem of finding clothes that fit. Brassieres are expensive and may have to be specially ordered, and the straps create large dents in the shoulders. In addition, many large-breasted women experience fungal infections under the breasts because it is difficult to keep this area dry and exposed to air.

Backaches from the added weight are also common. The only alternative for this condition, if well-fitting brassieres do not help and obesity is not part of the problem, may be breast reduction surgery. The surgeon removes excess breast tissue, repositions the nipple, and repositions the resultant skin flaps to produce the optimal cosmetic effect. This operation is a major surgical procedure and is termed a **reduction mammoplasty.**

The decision to undergo the procedure is usually made after years of living with the discomfort of excessive breast size. The nurse may be involved in the decision-making stage by listening to the client verbalize her feelings and providing information as appropriate. The postoperative diagnoses and goals are consistent with those for the woman undergoing reconstructive surgery (see Breast Reconstruction, p. 1744).

Gynecomastia

Gynecomastia literally means "female breasts" and is a symptom rather than a disease. It is usually a benign condition of breast enlargement in *men* (Figure 74-2). However, gynecomastia can be a result of a primary cancer such as lung cancer. The enlargement is usually bilateral, but enlargement is asymmetric in about 10% of cases. The condition is caused by proliferation of the glandular tissue, including the mammary ducts and ductal stroma. In many instances, it is difficult to distinguish gynecomastia from breast enlargement related to excess adipose tissue. Etiologic factors of gynecomastia include drugs; aging; obesity; underlying diseases causing estrogen excess, such as malnutrition, liver disease, or hyperthyroidism; and androgen deficiency states, such as age or chronic renal failure.

Although gynecomastia is not common, men with abnormal breast findings, especially a breast mass, are carefully evaluated for breast cancer.

BREAST CANCER

OVERVIEW

Breast cancer is the most commonly diagnosed cancer in women and is currently a leading cause of cancer mortality in women, second only to lung cancer. The ultimate goal of early diagnosis is to reduce mortality by identifying women at risk for breast cancer and predicting the prognosis and response to different therapies. Many of the current therapies for breast cancer are standard cytotoxic agents that treat all types of cancer; however, the increased use of the antiestrogen medication tamoxifen has been shown to be effective in the battle against breast cancer. Because of the high incidence of the disease, almost every woman has had a close personal association with another woman with the disease. Thus most women have strong reactions to the threat of breast cancer. These reactions greatly influence a woman's health habits, including breast self-examination (BSE) and her readiness to seek care when a suspicious area is discovered.

Until prevention becomes a viable option, early detection is the key to better treatment and survival. Statistics support

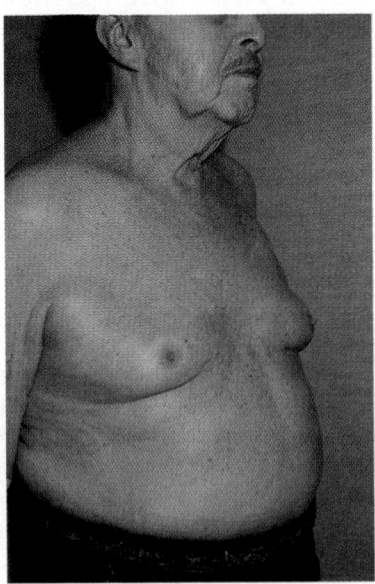

Figure 74-2 ● Gynecomastia. (From Swartz, M.H. [1998]. *Textbook of physical diagnosis: History and examination* [3rd ed.]. Philadelphia: W.B. Saunders.)

the advantages of early detection and treatment. The most reliable indicator of prognosis is related to the stage of the breast cancer at the time of diagnosis. Localized breast cancer with no regional spread is associated with a clinical cure rate of 75% to 90%. If the woman has a small tumor with no evidence of axillary node involvement, the 5-year survival rate is 90%. The 5-year survival rate drops to 40% to 50%, with a 10-year survival rate of 25%, when the axillary lymph nodes are involved (Tierney et al., 1995). Breast cancer is the second leading cause of cancer deaths in women in the United States and is the leading cause of cancer deaths in the 35- to 54-year-old age-group.

◼ Pathophysiology

◼ TYPES OF BREAST CANCER

There are many pathologic types of breast cancer, but the most common, accounting for more than 80% of cases, is *infiltrating ductal carcinoma*. As the name implies, the disease originates in the mammary ducts and specifically grows in the epithelial cells lining these ducts. The rate of cancer growth varies and partially depends on hormonal influences. It takes an estimated 5 to 9 years for a cancer cell to divide and result in a lesion large enough to be clinically palpable.

As long as the cancer remains within the duct, it is considered **noninvasive.** The cancer is classified as **invasive** when it penetrates the tissue surrounding the duct. Most breast cancers arise from the intermediate ducts and are invasive. Once invasive, the cancer grows into the tissue around it in an irregular pattern; for this reason, once the lesion is palpable, it is felt as an irregular, poorly defined mass.

As the tumor continues to grow, fibrosis develops around the cancer. This fibrosis may cause shortening of Cooper's ligaments and the resulting characteristic skin dimpling that is seen with more advanced disease.

◼ COMPLICATIONS OF BREAST CANCER

The tumor also invades the lymphatic channels, blocking skin drainage and causing skin edema and an orange peel appearance of the skin **(peau d'orange).** Invasion of the lymphatic channels carries tumor cells to the lymphatic nodes, including those in the axillary region. For this reason, pathologic examination of the axillary nodes is imperative for staging the disease. The tumor eventually replaces the skin itself, and ulceration of the overlying skin occurs. Metastases result from seeding of the cancer cells into the blood and lymph systems, which permits spread of these cells to distant sites. The most common sites of metastatic disease from breast cancer are bone, lungs, brain, and liver.

The course of metastatic breast cancer is related to the site affected and to the function impaired. The pathophysiologic process of cancer is further described in Chapter 25.

◼ BREAST CANCER IN MEN

About 1% of all cases of breast cancer occur in men. The average age of onset is 60 years. Men usually present with a hard, nonpainful, subareolar mass, and gynecomastia may be present. Occasionally the man may present with a nipple discharge, retraction, erosion, or ulceration. Although nipple discharge is not a common presenting symptom, about 75% of the men who present with nipple discharge are diagnosed with breast carcinoma. Breast cancer in men is staged the same as in women. However, the prognosis even for stage I breast cancer is worse for men. Five-year survival rates for stage I breast cancer in men are 58%; 5-year survival rates decrease to 38% for stage II disease (Tierney et al., 1995). Breast cancer in men is often a disseminated disease, which accounts for lower survival rates. Treatment of men with breast cancer parallels that of women at a similar stage of disease.

■ Etiology

There is no single known etiologic agent for breast cancer. Breast cancer can be attributed to multiple factors (Table 74-3).

Women with a familial history of breast cancer, particularly a history of a first-degree relative (mother, sister, or daughter) with premenopausal breast cancer, have a threefold risk increase. This risk is further increased if the relative had breast cancer bilaterally or before age 50 years. Ninety percent of clients with breast cancer have no familial history. Seventy percent of women over the age of 50 who are diagnosed with breast cancer have no identifiable risk factor for the development of the disease other than age and gender (Shapiro & Clark, 1995). Family history includes multiple relatives with breast cancer, early age at diagnosis, and in some families, ovarian cancer.

As discussed earlier, inherited mutations in several genes are known to be manifested in hereditary patterns of breast cancer. Breast cancer, however, is not an exclusively inherited, genetic disease. Exposure to high-dose ionizing radiation (especially before the age of 20 years), early menarche (before age 12), and late menopause (after age 50) are associated with an increased risk of breast cancer. A history of previous breast cancer, nulliparity (no pregnancies), and first birth after age 30 years are also considered to heighten risk.

Questionable risk factors include a diet high in animal fats, a diet low in fiber, alcohol consumption, and long-term estrogen replacement therapy (Leslie, 1995). Studies have shown a small increase in the risk of breast cancer in perimenopausal women receiving hormone replacement therapy (HRT) after 5 or more years of use. The risks of HRT must be weighed against the benefits. The benefits of HRT are a decreased risk of heart disease and osteoporosis and the control of menopausal symptoms. Decisions related to the use of HRT must be individualized on the basis of the client's risk profile.

TABLE 74-3 · RISK FACTORS FOR BREAST CANCER

Factor	Degree of Risk	Comments
Female gender	Increased	99% of all breast cancers occur in women.
History of a previous breast cancer	Increased	The risk of developing a cancer in the opposite breast is 5 times greater than for the average population at risk.
Age >40 yr	Increased	Incidence increases with age and peaks in the fifth decade.
Menstrual history Early menarche or late menopause or both	Increased	The risk of breast cancer rises as the interval between menarche and menopause increases; shortening the interval by mastectomy reduces the risk, especially if performed in women younger than age 35 yr.
Reproductive history Nulliparity First child born after age 30 yr	Increased	Childless women have an increased risk, as do women who bear their first child near or after age 30 yr.
Family history Mother or sister or both	Increased	Risk increases 2 to 3 times if the mother or a sister has had breast cancer and is further increased if the relative was diagnosed during the premenopausal state and if the cancer was bilateral.
Diet	Controversial	Animal data and descriptive epidemiology of breast cancer incidence strongly suggest an association of dietary factors, specifically a high-fat diet, with an increased risk of breast cancer. The National Academy of Science recommends decreasing total fat intake to 30% of available calories.
Alcohol	Unknown	A suggested small increase in risk with moderate alcohol consumption has been reported, although limitations in methodology have been cited and results require confirmation.
Obesity	Controversial	Weight, height, obesity, and increased body mass have been reported to be associated with an increased risk of breast cancer.
Ionizing radiation	Increased	Three groups of women who received low-level radiation exposure demonstrated an increased breast cancer risk, which was particularly notable if the exposure occurred in the early years (before age 30 yr).
Benign breast disease	None	Fibrocystic breast disease is not associated with breast cancer. However, biopsy-proven atypical hyperplasia is associated with an increased risk.
Oral contraceptives	None	There is no evidence yet to suggest a causal relationship between oral contraceptives and the incidence of and survival from breast cancer.
Exogenous hormones	Controversial	Several studies report no link with replacement hormones and breast cancer, and those that do appear to identify only subsets of clients at risk: those who have taken replacement estrogens for more than 5 yr and those who have taken large cumulative doses.

Modified from McCorkle, R., et al. (1996). *Cancer nursing: A comprehensive textbook* (2nd ed.). Philadelphia: W.B. Saunders.

TABLE 74-4 • AGE-RELATED RISK FOR BREAST CANCER	
Age (yr)	**Breast Cancer Risk**
25	1 in 19,608
30	1 in 2525
35	1 in 622
40	1 in 217
45	1 in 93
50	1 in 50
55	1 in 33
60	1 in 24
65	1 in 17
70	1 in 14
75	1 in 11
80	1 in 10
85	1 in 11
In a lifetime	1 in 8

Data from National Cancer Institute.

Being an older woman is the primary risk factor, although some women are at higher risk than others. As age increases, so does risk. More than 85% of clients are diagnosed after age 45 years. Obesity may be a factor associated with the development of breast cancer in postmenopausal women. Other genetic and environmental risk factors are listed in Table 74-3.

Incidence/Prevalence

Each year an estimated 184,000 women and 1400 men are diagnosed with breast cancer in the United States. Of these, approximately 46,000 women and 400 men die of the disease (Wingo et al., 1995). Although these numbers are staggering, there is a trend toward earlier diagnosis. In 1993, 75% of newly diagnosed breast cancers were stage I or II; in addition, negative nodes were found in one third of all breast cancers (Moore & Kinne, 1995). Breast cancer accounts for 1 in 4 cancers in women. It occurs most commonly in older adults, and its prevalence increases with age. With the aging female population, health care researchers are predicting a rise in the incidence of breast cancer in women over 67 years of age. By age 85 years, each American woman faces a 1-in-9 risk of being diagnosed with breast cancer. One of every eight American women will develop breast cancer in her lifetime (Table 74-4).

CULTURAL CONSIDERATIONS

The mortality rate of breast cancer is higher in African-American women. Overall, cancer remains a major public health problem for African Americans despite decreases in mortality for specific cancers. Although the incidence of breast cancer is lower in African Americans than in Caucasians, death rates are higher for African-American women at every stage of the disease. The 5-year survival rate for African Americans is 62% as compared with 79% for Caucasians (Allen & Phillips, 1997). Research suggests that poverty, less education, and inadequate access to screening are related to higher cancer morbidity and mortality rates in African Americans (Wingo et al., 1996).

Like the African-American female population, Latino and Hispanic women have a lower incidence of breast cancer than Caucasians but a higher death rate. The differences in survival rates reflect the stage at which the cancer is diagnosed. Breast cancer is the most common cancer in Asian and Pacific Island women; the death rates are higher for Hawaiian women than for all other ethnic groups (Allen & Phillips, 1997).

► COLLABORATIVE MANAGEMENT

● Assessment

■ HISTORY

The initial history may be taken after a mass has been discovered but before definitive diagnosis has been made, or the history may be obtained at the time the woman is seen for treatment of an identified cancer. The history should focus on three major areas: risk factors, the breast mass, and health maintenance practices.

RISK FACTORS. In the first area of assessment, the nurse records age, gender, marital status, weight, and height. Marital status and identification of the client's primary support person provide information about those to be included in the woman's care, teaching, and support. The nurse obtains specific information on personal and family histories of breast cancer. In addition to increasing the woman's own risk, these factors also affect any sister's or daughter's risk and should be incorporated into later counseling.

The gynecologic/obstetric history includes the following:
- Age at menarche
- Age at menopause
- Symptoms of menopause
- Age at first child's birth
- Number of children

Prolonged hormonal stimulation (e.g., early menses and/or late menopause) increases a woman's risk, as does birth of the first child after age 30 years and nulliparity.

HISTORY OF THE BREAST MASS. The second area of assessment focuses on the history of the breast mass. The history reveals not only the course of the disease but also data related to health care–seeking practices and health-promoting behaviors.

Knowledge of how, when, and by whom the mass was discovered and the interval between discovery and seeking care is crucial. If the woman found the mass, was it discovered through breast self-examination (BSE) or by accident? The answer to this question might alert the nurse to the need for discussion and teaching about BSE regardless of whether the mass proves to be malignant. What was the time interval between discovery and seeing the health care provider? If there was a delay, what caused it? These questions are linked to the psychosocial assessment but also reveal the length of time that the tumor has been present. The nurse notes procedures directed at diagnosing this problem and others in the past. Finally, a review of systems focusing on the most common areas for metastases is made.

HEALTH MAINTENANCE PRACTICES. The third area of assessment includes health maintenance practices. In addition to questioning the client about the knowledge, practice, and regularity of BSE, the nurse takes a mammographic history. The existence of previous mammograms allows the health care provider to compare current mammograms with past ones to facilitate diagnosis.

A brief diet history, in which the client is asked to recall a typical day's menu and alcoholic intake per week, reveals the usual intake of fat and alcohol. A high alcohol and fat intake *may* increase the risk of breast cancer.

The nurse asks the client what types of medications she uses, specifically, hormonal supplements, such as estrogen. Estrogen can be administered orally, intravaginally, or via a transdermal patch. The nurse documents the type and form of hormones (birth control pills, supplements) and length of use. Postmenopausal use of estrogen creams intravaginally is not uncommon and should be considered a major source of estrogen.

PHYSICAL ASSESSMENT/CLINICAL MANIFESTATIONS

The approach to physical assessment is discussed earlier under Breast Self-Examination (p. 1730) and under Clinical Breast Examination (p. 1732). The nurse notes specific information about the breast mass (Chart 74-1). The mass is described in the chart in terms of location (using the "face of the clock" method), shape, size, consistency, and fixation to the surrounding tissues.

Any skin change, such as **peau d'orange** (dimpling, orange peel appearance), increased vascularity, nipple retraction, or ulceration, can indicate advanced disease and needs to be documented. The nurse examines the axillary and supraclavicular areas thoroughly by palpating deeply for enlarged lymph nodes and noting their presence and location in the client's record. The presence of pain or soreness in the affected breast is evaluated. After gathering this information, the nurse draws a diagram on the chart (see Figure 74-1) that will be helpful for others involved in the client's care.

PSYCHOSOCIAL ASSESSMENT

The client with potential or diagnosed breast cancer faces three major issues: the fear of cancer; threats to body image, sexuality, intimate relationships, and survival; and decisional conflict related to treatment options.

The woman will need information about how advanced the disease is, the likelihood of cure, treatment options and side effects, how treatment will affect her life and self-image, how her family or significant others will be affected, and home self-care. A woman's previous experience with cancer, and especially with other women with breast cancer, influences her reactions to the disease. The client is asked whether she has known anyone with breast cancer and what types of experiences she has had with breast disease and cancer in general. The nurse explores the woman's feelings about the disease because her choices of treatment, her recovery, and her ability to learn are greatly influenced by these emotions. The client's and family's knowledge of breast cancer, the stage of the disease, and treatment options

are assessed. The client's level of education is a significant influencing factor in her treatment choices for stage I breast cancer. Her perception of her situation is often influenced by outdated information. Perhaps she knew someone who had a Halsted radical mastectomy 30 years ago and associates breast surgery with the chest deformity and lymphedema experienced by that woman. Dispelling misconceptions by providing current information can affect her attitude in a positive way.

The nurse may also assess the client with breast cancer for problems related to sexuality. Three critical areas of distress—psychologic, physiologic, and relational—contribute to the psychosexual morbidity of these clients. The nurse should inquire about the frequency of, and the client's satisfaction with, sexual relations with her partner. The client should reflect on the relationship with the partner and be asked if and how the breast cancer has changed the intimate relations with, sexual function of, or types of touch by the partner.

The need for additional resources is also evaluated at this time. Will extra psychologic counseling be needed? Are there financial concerns that need to be discussed with social services? Will the client's spouse, family, or friends support her throughout this period? How much support and teaching do they need? When does the client expect to hear about her pathology results, and whom would she like to have with her when she hears the results? Answers to these types of questions provide guidelines in establishing expected outcomes and in planning nursing care.

LABORATORY ASSESSMENT

The diagnosis of breast cancer relies primarily on pathologic examination of tissue from the breast mass. Serum-based laboratory tests are not used routinely to aid in this diagnosis; however, radioimmunoassay (RIA) is being used in research to detect and monitor breast cancer. Studies to identify breast cancer tumor markers are currently being conducted. One breast cancer tumor marker is 5-hydroxymethyl-2-deoxyuridine (Djuric et al., 1996).

After the presence of cancer is established, laboratory tests, including pathologic examination of the lymph nodes, help detect possible metastases. Elevated liver enzyme levels indicate possible liver metastases, and increased serum calcium and alkaline phosphatase levels suggest bone metastases.

RADIOGRAPHIC ASSESSMENT

Mammography is the most sensitive screening tool for breast cancer. However, it must be combined with BSE for optimal early detection and with clinical breast examination (CBE) for full interpretation of the findings. These three methods together are effective in detecting breast cancer as early as possible. The uniqueness of mammography results from its ability to reveal preclinical lesions (masses too small to be palpated manually). Client preparation and the procedure for mammography are discussed in Chapter 73.

Other radiographic procedures may be used preoperatively to rule out metastases. A chest x-ray examination to screen for lung metastases is routine. Bone, liver, and brain scans and computed tomography (CT) scans of the chest and abdomen can reveal distant metastases.

CHART 74-1

BEST PRACTICE *for*
Assessing a Breast Mass

- Identify the location of the mass by using the "face of the clock" method.
- Describe the shape, size, and consistency of the mass.
- Assess whether the mass is fixed or movable.
- Note any skin changes around the mass, such as dimpling (*peau d'orange*), increased vascularity, nipple retraction, and ulceration.
- Assess the adjacent lymph nodes, both axillary and supraclavicular nodes.
- Ask the client if she experiences pain or soreness in the area around the mass.

■ OTHER DIAGNOSTIC ASSESSMENT

Ultrasonography of the breast is an additional diagnostic tool used to clarify findings on mammography. If the mammogram reveals a lesion, ultrasonography is helpful in differentiating a fluid-filled cyst from a solid mass.

Postoperative pathologic examination of the breast tissue, or **breast biopsy,** is the key to diagnosis of breast cancer. It is estimated that as many as 1.8 million breast biopsies are performed each year (Shapiro & Clark, 1995). Breast tissue is obtained by one of several types of biopsies (see Chapter 73).

Several other tests are useful for establishing the stage of disease and prognosis after the diagnosis is made. These tests include a pathologic examination of the lymph nodes on the affected side. Other prognostic factors include the following (Donegan & Spratt, 1995):

- Estrogen and progesterone receptors
- S-phase index, or growth rate (done by flow-cytometric determinations of the S-phase fraction)
- DNA ploidy (the amount of DNA in a tumor cell as compared with a normal cell)
- Histologic or nuclear grade

Estrogen and progesterone receptors are cytoplasmic proteins present in and on the surface of breast cancer cells that bind to estrogen and progesterone. When estrogen and progesterone bind to the cell, the cell's activity is thought to change. A tumor that contains receptors capable of binding with circulating hormones, specifically estrogen and progesterone, is estrogen receptor (ER) positive. More post-menopausal women than premenopausal women are ER positive. Women with ER-positive tumors respond better to adjuvant therapy and usually survive longer.

The receptor status also predicts which women will respond to hormonal manipulation as a treatment. Thymidine labeling index, ploidy factor (deoxyribonucleic acid [DNA] content), and calculation of the number of cells in S phase by flow cytometry can reveal the growth rate of cells. Tumors with a high growth rate index and altered DNA content are associated with a worse prognosis (Donegan & Spratt, 1995).

Tumor cells are also examined for specialization or differentiation. Because well-differentiated tumors tend to be less aggressive than poorly differentiated ones, a woman with a well-differentiated breast cancer has a better prognosis than the woman with a poorly differentiated tumor.

As mentioned earlier, several procedures related to specific sites of possible metastases also help establish the stage or progression of the breast cancer. Figure 74-3 illustrates the four stages of breast cancer.

▶ Analysis

■ COMMON NURSING DIAGNOSES AND COLLABORATIVE PROBLEMS

A common nursing diagnosis for clients with breast cancer is Anxiety related to the diagnosis of cancer.

A common collaborative problem is Potential for Metastasis.

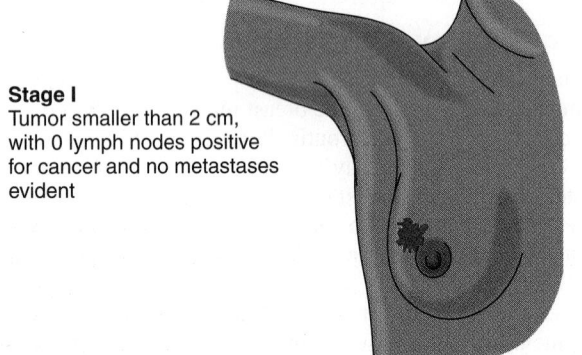

Stage I
Tumor smaller than 2 cm, with 0 lymph nodes positive for cancer and no metastases evident

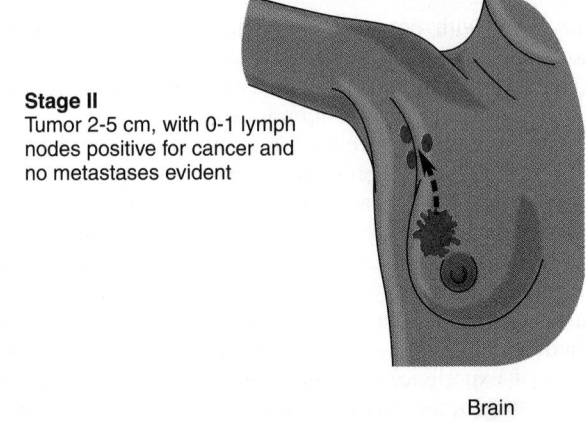

Stage II
Tumor 2-5 cm, with 0-1 lymph nodes positive for cancer and no metastases evident

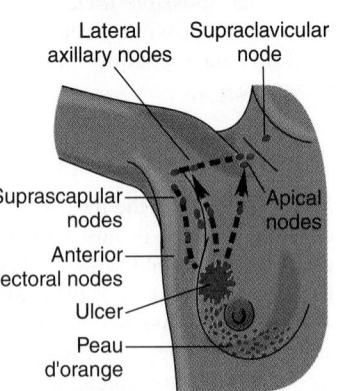

Stage III
Tumor larger than 5 cm, with 0 lymph nodes positive for cancer and no metastases evident

Tumor smaller than 2 cm, with axillary lymph nodes positive for cancer cells and no metastases evident

Tumor 2-5 cm, with axillary lymph nodes positive for cancer cells and no metastases evident

Lateral axillary nodes
Supraclavicular node
Suprascapular nodes
Apical nodes
Anterior pectoral nodes
Ulcer
Peau d'orange

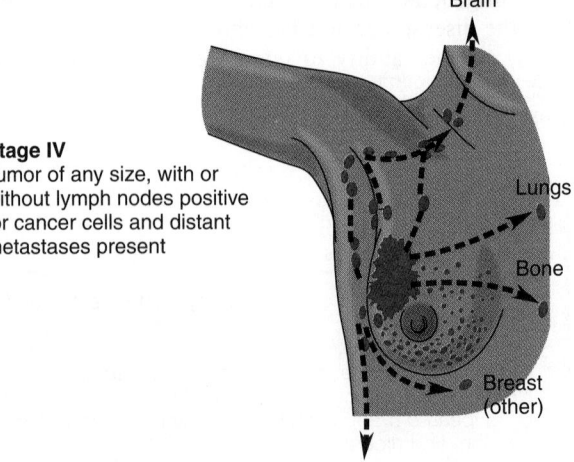

Stage IV
Tumor of any size, with or without lymph nodes positive for cancer cells and distant metastases present

Brain
Lungs
Bone
Breast (other)
Liver

Figure 74-3 ● Staging of breast cancer.

ADDITIONAL NURSING DIAGNOSES AND COLLABORATIVE PROBLEMS

In addition to the common nursing diagnoses and collaborative problems, clients with breast cancer (particularly advanced breast cancer) may have one or more of the following:

- Anticipatory Grieving related to loss and possible or impending death
- Acute Pain related to tumor compression on nerve endings
- Disturbed Sleep Pattern related to pain and anxiety
- Disturbed Body Image related to loss of a body part
- Sexual Dysfunction related to body image or self-esteem disturbance

Planning and Implementation

ANXIETY

NOC PLANNING: EXPECTED OUTCOMES. The client with breast cancer is expected to seek information to reduce anxiety, control anxiety responses, and use effective coping strategies throughout the treatment period by participating in decision making, discussing concerns, and learning self-care measures.

INTERVENTIONS. The woman with breast cancer is usually admitted to the health care facility with a definitive diagnosis established through an outpatient biopsy of the mass. The practice of admitting a woman with a suspicious lesion and using general anesthesia for a biopsy, frozen section, and possible mastectomy has largely been abandoned. Women who have an interval between the biopsy and treatment, during which they actively participate in the choice of treatment, cope more effectively after surgery, no matter which treatment is chosen.

NIC ANXIETY REDUCTION. The anxiety for the woman with breast cancer begins the moment the lump is discovered. The level of anxiety may be related to past experiences and personal associations with the disease. Many women also have an intuitive feeling about the diagnosis even before it has been established. The clinical likelihood that the lesion is or is not cancer is irrelevant to the level of fear. The client's perceptions of her own situation and personal level of anxiety are assessed. The nurse allows the client to ventilate these feelings even if a diagnosis has not been established (Chart 74-2).

CHART 74-2

NIC INTERVENTION ACTIVITIES for
The Client with Breast Cancer

Anxiety Reduction: *Minimizing apprehension, dread, foreboding, or uneasiness related to an unidentified source of anticipated danger*
- Listen attentively.
- Use calm, reassuring approach.
- Provide factual information concerning diagnosis, treatment, and prognosis.
- Encourage verbalization of feelings, perceptions, and fears.
- Identify when level of anxiety changes.
- Support the use of appropriate defense mechanisms.
- Determine client's decision-making ability.

If the mass has been diagnosed as cancer, many women feel a partial sense of relief to be dealing with a known entity. A feeling of shock or disbelief may predominate. It is difficult to accept a diagnosis of cancer when one feels basically well. Clients and their families or significant others deal in individual ways with the mix of feelings, which include shock, disbelief, and grief. Some may want to read and discuss any available information. Others may want to know as little as possible and resent attempts at teaching. Although one woman may want to talk at length about her concerns, another may want to be alone. Flexibility is the key to nursing care; the nurse adjusts the approach to care as the client's emotional state changes. An integral part of the plan to meet these emotional needs is the use of outside resources. Most health care providers view such groups as the American Cancer Society's Reach to Recovery as a source of support in the postoperative period, but the nurse can suggest these groups in the preoperative phase.

Health care providers working with breast cancer clients may know other clients willing to make a preoperative visit. These resource people may be chosen on the basis of the client's concerns. The woman who is worried in particular about the side effects of radiation therapy may benefit more from talking to someone who has undergone radiation than from talking to the nurse about secondhand experiences.

In addition to Reach to Recovery, formal and informal community support groups, such as ENCORE (Encouragement, Normalcy, Counseling, Opportunity, Reaching Out, and Energies Revived), may be available. These groups can be reached through the health care provider or by word of mouth.

POTENTIAL FOR METASTASIS

PLANNING: EXPECTED OUTCOMES. The client with breast cancer is expected to remain free of metastases or recurrence of disease.

INTERVENTIONS. There has been significant controversy in the past about the treatment of breast cancer. Until about 1950 the Halsted radical mastectomy was considered the treatment of choice. Gradually the modified radical mastectomy became popular. More recently, evidence has been presented that supports less traumatic procedures as having comparable survival rates. Because of the various options, the woman with breast cancer often faces difficult decisions.

Although most women with metastatic breast cancer eventually succumb to the disease, chemotherapy, hormonal therapy, radiotherapy, and limited surgery are all effective treatment modalities for palliative care, improvement in quality of life, and prolongation of life (Hortobagyi, 1998). Once cancer is found, the extent and location of metastases determine the overall therapeutic strategy. Treatment should be tailored specifically to each client, taking into account other comorbidities and the client's ability to tolerate a particular therapy. Most important, the nurse should thoroughly understand an individual's specific goals and the particular outcome she seeks from therapy.

NONSURGICAL MANAGEMENT. For clients with late-stage breast cancer, nonsurgical treatment may be the only alternative. If the disease is in a late stage, such as stage IV, with the presence of confirmed metastasis, or if the client cannot withstand a major surgical procedure, the tumor may be removed with a local anesthetic. Follow-up treatment may include hormonal therapy, chemotherapy, and sometimes radiation. If the tumor is attached to the skin or the underlying muscle, resection may be impossible. Follow-up therapy involves radiation, usually in conjunction with chemotherapy. Chapter 25 describes the nursing care associated with chemotherapy and radiation.

SURGICAL MANAGEMENT. The most common types of breast surgery are illustrated in Figure 74-4. Although controversy exists concerning the best treatment for a malignant mass, many experts agree that the mass itself should be removed to reduce the risk of local recurrence. Removal of the axillary lymph nodes for staging purposes may also be recommended. Axillary lymph node dissection (ALND) is usually performed for clients with palpable axillary lymph nodes;

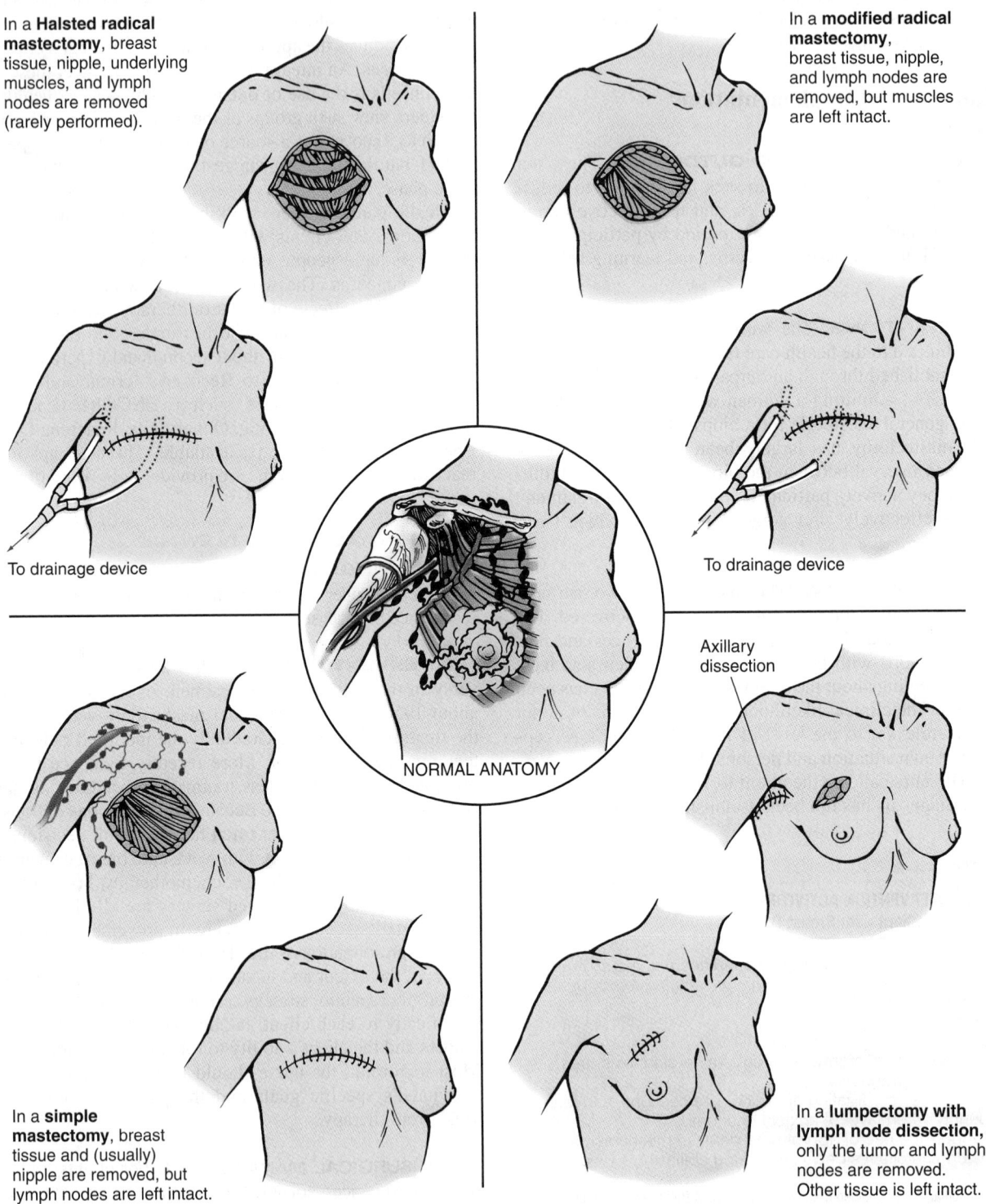

In a **Halsted radical mastectomy**, breast tissue, nipple, underlying muscles, and lymph nodes are removed (rarely performed).

In a **modified radical mastectomy**, breast tissue, nipple, and lymph nodes are removed, but muscles are left intact.

To drainage device

To drainage device

NORMAL ANATOMY

Axillary dissection

In a **simple mastectomy**, breast tissue and (usually) nipple are removed, but lymph nodes are left intact.

In a **lumpectomy with lymph node dissection**, only the tumor and lymph nodes are removed. Other tissue is left intact.

Figure 74-4 ● Surgical management of breast cancer.

it is unclear if clients with nonpalpable nodes should also have ALND.

PREOPERATIVE CARE. Care of the woman facing surgery for breast cancer focuses on psychologic preparation and preoperative teaching. The issues related to anxiety and lack of knowledge are primary. Efforts are directed toward educating the client, including the husband or significant other, who may be experiencing similar stress and confusion.

The type of procedure is reviewed. Open-ended questions (e.g., "What type of surgery are you having? Can you explain what will happen?") are used. This questioning helps the nurse assess the client's level of knowledge and allows for additional explanations as needed. The client should be knowledgeable about the type of procedure. Specific postoperative information, such as the following, is also provided:

* The need for a drainage tube
* The location of the incision
* Mobility restrictions
* The length of the hospital stay (if any)
* The possibility of additional medical therapy
* Basic preoperative and postoperative information needed by any surgical client (see Chapters 17 and 19)

Because of short hospital stays or same-day surgery procedures, preoperative teaching should be supplemented with written materials for the client and family to take home as references and should include who to call should there be any complications. The nurse helps the client address body image issues before surgery to correct misconceptions about postoperative appearance and to begin adjusting to changes after surgery. If available, clients and their caregivers may attend preoperative classes in an ambulatory care setting, such as a surgical clinic, to promote successful early discharge from the hospital. Preoperative programs that provide emotional support, information, and opportunities for discussion related to sexuality, body image, preoperative instructions, and postoperative care enhance the care of the short-stay mastectomy client.

OPERATIVE PROCEDURES. During **breast-conserving surgery,** the surgeon removes the bulk of the tumor; typically, radiation therapy follows to eradicate residual tumor cells. Radiation therapy plays a critical role in the therapeutic regimen and is effective treatment for nearly all sites where breast cancer can metastasize. The most common site for metastasis is to bone tissue.

The following types of breast-conserving surgery are used as primary treatment for stage I and stage II breast cancer:

* **Lumpectomy,** also known as tylectomy or local excision, is gross resection of the tumor.
* **Partial mastectomy,** which includes wide excision, quadrantectomy, or segmental mastectomy, is removal of the portion of the breast that contains the tumor.

Breast-conserving procedures are usually performed in same-day surgical settings. The breast-conserving approach offers 5- and 10-year survival and local recurrence rates at least equivalent to those of the modified radical mastectomy. The cosmetic results have been good to excellent, and other long-term problems are comparable to those of more radical procedures. For many women, the psychologic benefits of avoiding breast removal are significant and lead them to choose this option.

The **modified radical mastectomy** does *not* conserve the breast; the affected breast is completely removed. This procedure differs from the older Halsted radical mastectomy in that the surgeon leaves the pectoral muscles and nerves intact. Thus the breast tissue and skin and the axillary nodes are removed, and the underlying muscles are left in place. The typical incision is a 5- to 6-inch-long elliptic incision from the midchest to the axilla (see Figure 74-4). If reconstruction is to follow the procedure, the plastic surgeon may recommend a different location for the incision. When reconstruction is to be performed at the same time as the mastectomy, less invasive techniques, such as incising a 1.5-inch flap of skin around the nipple (excising the same amount of breast tissue as with conventional mastectomy), may be performed. Skin flaps or implants may be used to create a breast mound at the time of the original procedure.

The use of carbon dioxide laser procedures in place of cutting and cauterizing for mastectomies is an option that is becoming more available. Advantages of laser procedures include less blood loss and faster recovery.

POSTOPERATIVE CARE. Postoperative and home care of the woman undergoing a modified radical mastectomy or breast-conserving surgery is provided in the Client Care Plan on pp. 1744 and 1745. Before the woman returns from surgery, the nurse places a sign over the client's bed to warn nurses and other personnel to avoid using the affected arm for taking blood pressure measurements, giving injections, or drawing blood. The woman returns from the postanesthesia care unit (PACU) as soon as vital signs return to baseline levels and if no complications have occurred. On the client's return, the nurse focuses on maintaining physiologic stability and comfort. Vital signs are usually assessed on a schedule of decreasing frequency, such as every 30 minutes for two times, every hour for two times, and then every 4 hours. During these checks, the nurse or assistive nursing personnel assesses the dressing for bleeding.

Care of Drainage Tubes. During a modified radical mastectomy, the surgeon places one or two drainage tubes, usually Jackson-Pratt drains, under the skin flaps and attached to a small collection chamber. Gentle suction is exerted, and fluid that would accumulate under the flaps and delay healing is collected. Various drains are available, but all allow the drainage to be seen and measured. When taking vital signs, the nurse or assistive nursing personnel monitors the drain for the amount and color of drainage and adds this information to the intake and output record. Clients undergoing a lumpectomy may also have drainage tubes (usually Jackson-Pratt drains) placed if the lump is large or if axillary node dissection is performed.

The nurse or assistive nursing personnel continues to measure the amount of wound drainage, although measurements of general fluid intake and output are usually discontinued by the first postoperative day. The nurse observes the wound for signs of swelling and infection throughout the client's recovery. Drainage tubes are removed by the surgeon when drainage is less than 50 mL in 24 hours. With short hospital stays, drainage tubes are usually removed about 1 week after hospital discharge, when the client returns for her first postoperative office visit. The nurse informs the client that although these tubes lie just under the skin, removal may be painful.

$\mathscr{C}$LIENT $\mathscr{C}$ARE $\mathscr{P}$LAN • CARE OF THE CLIENT AFTER MASTECTOMY OR BREAST-CONSERVING SURGERY

NURSING DIAGNOSIS NO. 1 • Acute Pain related to tissue trauma from surgery

Expected Outcomes	Nursing Interventions	Rationale
The client will experience no pain or unnecessary discomfort.	Assess for pain and identify possible causes. Assess for sensation changes in the arm and the incision.	Thorough assessment allows identification of and appropriate intervention for the specific cause of pain.
	Reduce anxiety by reorienting the client to surroundings and explaining procedures, dressings, drains, and other equipment. **D**	Anxiety and fear of the unknown decrease the pain threshold.
	Medicate as appropriate with analgesics, as ordered.	Pain medications decrease the perception of pain.
	Position the client on the back or the unaffected side, with the arm on the affected side elevated on a pillow. **D**	Elevation of the arm decreases swelling, which might cause discomfort.
	Check drains and dressings for constriction, position, and functioning.	Impeded circulation or swelling under the skin flap caused by obstruction of the drain causes pain.
	Explain the potential for phantom sensations of the missing breast.	Previous knowledge of the event decreases anxiety when the event occurs.
	Explain the potential for numbness in the arm and in the incision.	

NURSING DIAGNOSIS NO. 2 • Risk for Ineffective Tissue Perfusion related to edema or bleeding

Expected Outcomes	Nursing Interventions	Rationale
The client will maintain adequate tissue perfusion.	Assess the client for signs of shock (decreased blood pressure, increased pulse, decreased urine output, confusion).	These signs indicate shock.
	Check the dressing and the sheet under the client for bleeding.	Bleeding may stain the dressing or seep under the dressing and be unnoticed unless the bed is checked.
	Empty and record the drainage in the drainage container. Report excessive amounts of and changes in drainage.	Excessive drainage indicates hemorrhage.
	Assess the operative site for swelling or the presence of fluid collection under the skin flaps.	Collection of fluid under the skin flaps disrupts healing and may indicate a malfunctioning drainage device or bleeding.

D indicates tasks that can be delegated to assistive nursing personnel.

Comfort Measures. The nurse or assistive nursing personnel assesses the client's position to ensure that the drainage tubes or collection device will not be pulled or kinked. The client should sit with the head of the bed up at least 30 degrees, with the affected arm (the arm on the same side as the axillary dissection) elevated on a pillow, while awake. Keeping the affected arm elevated promotes lymphatic fluid return after removal of axillary lymph nodes and channels. Other basic comfort measures, such as repositioning and pain medications, as prescribed, are provided on a regular basis until pain ceases.

Mobility and Diet. The hospital stay after a modified radical mastectomy is short—typically same-day or overnight—and recovery is usually not complicated. Because some managed care companies will not authorize an overnight stay in the hospital following a mastectomy, several states have enacted legislation mandating inpatient benefits. The client who chooses an early discharge should have a home care visit within 24 hours of the discharge.

Ambulation and a regular diet are resumed by the day after surgery. While the client is in an upright position, the arm on the affected side may need to be supported at first. Gradually the arm should be allowed to hang straight by the side while the client is walking. The nurse teaches the client to avoid the hunched-back position with the arm flexed because of the risk of elbow contractures. Beginning exercises that do not stress the incision can usually be started on the first postoperative day. These exercises include squeezing the affected hand around a soft, round object (a ball or rolled washcloth) and flexion/extension of the elbow. The progression to more strenuous exercises depends on the subsequent procedures planned (such as reconstruction) and the surgeon's orders.

As soon as the woman is fully ambulatory and eating well and her postoperative pain is under control, she is discharged to continue recuperation at home. Typical instructions for postmastectomy exercises are provided in Chart 74-3.

BREAST RECONSTRUCTION. Breast reconstruction has undergone a dramatic evolution in the last 20 years with substantial improvement in the quality, predictability, and complication rate of the procedures used to reconstruct the breast. Clients now present to the reconstructive surgeon with definite ideas regarding the type of reconstruction, timing of the procedure, and technique desired. With this trend, more women want immediate breast reconstruction using their own tissue (autogenous reconstruction). In addition, instantaneous

Client Care Plan • CARE OF THE CLIENT AFTER MASTECTOMY OR BREAST-CONSERVING SURGERY—cont'd

NURSING DIAGNOSIS NO. 3 • Impaired Physical Mobility related to pain and tissue trauma

Expected Outcomes	Nursing Interventions	Rationale
The client will experience a return of mobility to her preoperative level.	Tell the client that flexion and extension of the fingers and wrist can begin immediately postoperatively. Encourage gentle use of the arm for activities of daily living. Limited exercises include: Range of motion for the hand, wrist, and elbow Squeezing a ball Flexing the fingers Touching the hand to the shoulder and circular wrist motion	Early use of the hand and arm muscles and joints prevents muscle atrophy and contractures and enhances fluid return.
	Teach appropriate exercises, and ask the client to begin performing exercises 1 week after surgery or when sutures and drains are removed.	Active range-of-motion exercises preserve the range of motion in the client's arm in which axillary dissection was done.
	Inform the client about Reach to Recovery or a similar organization, and contact the organization with the client's permission to arrange a home visit.	Reach to Recovery provides volunteers and written materials on exercises that are safe to perform at home.
	Encourage the client to use an upright posture with the shoulders held back and the arm by the side while walking and standing. **D**	The tendency is to hold the arm bent across the waist and to stoop over, which results in elbow and shoulder contractures.

NURSING DIAGNOSIS NO. 4 • Risk for Infection related to disruption in skin integrity

The client will have an incision that remains free of infection.	Assess for signs of infection and swelling.	Infection and collection of serosanguineous fluid delay wound healing and disrupt adhesion of the skin flaps.
	Teach the client measures to reduce the risk of infection: Avoid taking blood pressure, drawing blood, and giving injections in the operative arm. Avoid injury to the arm, such as burns, scratches, insect bites, and scrapes. Treat injuries immediately to avoid infection.	Injury and infection in the operative arm increase the risk of lymphedema related to removal of lymph nodes.
	Encourage the client to look at the incision before discharge from the hospital, and explain signs of infection, including redness, heat, swelling, and wound discharge.	Discharge usually occurs before complete healing. The client or some other responsible person must monitor wound healing.
	Instruct the client to notify the physician if swelling, redness, or pain occurs.	Early intervention may prevent disruption of the skin flaps.

D indicates tasks that can be delegated to assistive nursing personnel.

breast reconstruction, both autogenous and prosthetic, has been shown to lessen the psychologic strain associated with undergoing a mastectomy.

The surgeon should offer the option of breast reconstruction before surgery is performed. If the client does not choose immediate reconstructive surgery, a temporary prosthesis is given to the client. Some surgeons allow women to use a temporary prosthesis in the immediate postoperative period as a component of the postoperative dressing. If this is the case, the client returns from surgery with a surgical brassiere and temporary sterile prosthesis in place. The nurse or social worker can refer the client to the American Cancer Society's Reach to Recovery program. In this program, a volunteer who has had breast cancer surgery visits the client at home, offering information on breast forms, clothing, coping with breast cancer, and possible reconstructive options. For this intervention to be as therapeutic as possible, the volunteer should be about the same age as the client and have experienced the same surgical procedure.

The client's level of satisfaction with her prosthesis is evaluated several weeks postoperatively. The nurse assesses the client's attitude by asking about plans for restoring appearance postoperatively. Although reconstruction is not appropriate for some clients and others may not be interested in it, the surgeon should discuss the indications and contraindications, advantages and disadvantages, and typical postoperative recovery. If immediate reconstruction is chosen, the surgeon should be aware of this preoperatively so that the surgeon's plans can be coordinated with those of the plastic surgeon.

Several procedures are available for restoring the appearance of the breast (Table 74-5). Reconstruction may begin during the original operative procedure or later in one to several stages. The following are some of the more common techniques:

- Use of a flap of skin and muscle from the abdomen, back, or hip to create a breast mound
- Placement of a saline- or gel-filled prosthesis
- Use of progressive tissue expanders to slowly create a pocket under the mastectomy site for placement of a permanent implant

Reconstruction of the nipple-areola complex is the last stage in the reconstruction of the breast. If necessary, a new

---

CHART 74-3

CLIENT EDUCATION GUIDE
Postmastectomy Exercises

Hand Wall Climbing
- Face the wall, and put the palms of your hands flat against the wall at shoulder level.
- Flex your fingers so that your hands slowly "walk" up the wall.
- Stop when your arms are fully extended.
- Slowly "walk" your hands back down the wall until they return to shoulder level.

Pulley Exercise
- Drape a 6-foot-long rope over a shower curtain rod or over the top of a door. If you use a door for this exercise, have someone put a nail or hook at the top of the door so that the rope does not slip off.
- Grab the ends of the rope, one in each hand, and extend your arms out to your sides until they are straight.
- Keeping your arms straight, pull down with your left arm to raise your right arm as high as you can.
- Pull down with your right arm to raise your left arm as high as you can.

Rope Turning
- Tie a rope to the knob of a closed door.
- Hold the other end of the rope and step back from the door until your arm is almost straight out in front of you.
- Swing the rope in a circle. Start with small circles and gradually increase to larger circles as you become more flexible.

---

nipple may be created with tissue from the other nipple or from other body tissue, such as the labia or inner thigh. In some cases, the client's natural nipple can be reattached to another part of the body if the reconstruction is planned for a later date.

In June 1992, the Food and Drug Administration (FDA) restricted the use of silicone gel implants to women in FDA-approved safety studies. The studies were open to women seeking implants after breast cancer surgery or traumatic injury (MacMahon, 1992). The restriction of silicone implants resulted from complaints that silicone leakage caused clients to experience connective tissue diseases, such as systemic lupus erythematosus, or other vague physical symptoms. In mid-1994, silicone gel implants were once again permitted for use in breast reconstruction, but not in breast augmentation (enlargement) (Corral & Mustoe, 1996).

The transverse rectus abdominis myocutaneous (TRAM) flap, a commonly used method of reconstruction, provides women with naturally appearing breasts without the risks associated with the silicone gel implant. This procedure has largely replaced the prosthetic implant as the first choice for breast reconstruction and can be combined with tissue expanders and implants to obtain symmetry (Moran et al., 2000). Postoperative nursing care of the woman who has undergone breast reconstruction is outlined in Chart 74-4.

ADJUVANT THERAPY. The decision to follow the original surgical procedure with chemotherapy, radiation, or hormonal therapy is based on the following:
- The stage of the disease
- The client's age and menopausal status
- Client preferences
- Pathologic examination
- Hormone receptor status

The purpose of adjuvant therapy is to decrease the risk of recurrence for the client who has no evidence of but is at risk for metastasis or to prolong survival after metastasis occurs. Adjuvant therapy for stage I and stage II (early-stage) breast cancer consists of breast-conserving surgery and postoperative radiotherapy or modified radical mastectomy. Women who have estrogen receptor (ER)–positive tumors are given tamoxifen (Nolvadex, Tamofen✦). This estrogen antagonist blocks the estrogen receptor sites in the tumor cells, thereby inhibiting growth. When this therapy is appropriate, the response rate is 50% to 60%.

Therapy for stage III, or locally advanced, breast cancer is still controversial. Treatment usually includes surgery (if the tumor is operable) and chemotherapy with or without radiotherapy. Although chemotherapeutic regimens differ among treatment centers, multiple-agent combinations are used. A common example of such a combination is cyclophosphamide (Cytoxan, Neosar, Procytox✦), methotrexate (Folex, Mexate), and fluorouracil (5-FU, Adrucil). The length of treatment may also vary. Autologous and allogeneic bone marrow transplantation (stem cell transplantation) and preoperative chemotherapy are being investigated as early treatment for women who have a high risk for recurrence or advanced disease (Smith, 1996). Autologous bone marrow transplantation (taken from the client's bone marrow), peripheral blood stem cell transplantation (taken from the client's circulating blood), or allogeneic bone marrow transplantation (taken from a healthy donor's bone marrow or peripheral blood) may be performed as a means of rescue following very high doses of chemotherapy or radiation. These procedures decrease the expected morbidity and mortality related to adjuvant therapy.

Before planning care and teaching for the breast cancer client undergoing chemotherapy, the nurse knows the specific agents to be used and their properties. A discussion of the care of the client undergoing chemotherapy and a discussion of the care of the client undergoing bone marrow transplantation are given in Chapter 25.

● Community-Based Care

▆ HOME CARE MANAGEMENT

Home care preparation should be initiated when the decision to have surgical therapy is made. Referral to a case manager can ensure that the educational needs of the client are met early in the perioperative period. The preadmission testing center or the surgeon could make referrals. Preoperative teaching and arrangements for home care management and referrals (Reach to Recovery, social services, home care) can be initiated before hospitalization. Planning ahead for the client's discharge needs facilitates discharge.

The client who has undergone breast surgery can be discharged to the home setting unless other physical disabilities exist. Some are discharged 1 to 2 days after surgery, with Jackson-Pratt or other types of drains in place. The current trend, however, is to be discharged to home on the same day that surgery is performed. These clients need assistance at home with drain care, dressings, and activities of daily living because of pain and impaired range of motion of the affected arm. Summaries of discharge instructions are given in Charts 74-5 and 74-6.

It is not necessary to modify the home for the client after breast surgery. Activities involving stretching or reaching for

TABLE 74-5 • EXAMPLES OF BREAST RECONSTRUCTION PROCEDURES

Procedure	Description	Procedure	Description
Implantation	An implant matching the size of the other breast is placed under the muscle on the operative side to create a breast mound.	Myocutaneous flaps	A flap of skin, fat, and muscle is transferred from the donor site to the operative area. The flap contains an appropriate amount of fat to match the other breast and is similar in appearance to breast tissue. A blood supply is established by reanastomosis of vessels from the operative area to those with the flap when possible. A new nipple may be created with tissue from the other nipple, labia, or thigh. Nipples can also be created by tattooing.

Latissimus dorsi musculocutaneous flap

Abdominal myocutaneous flap

Procedure	Description
Tissue expansion	A tissue expander is placed under the muscle and gradually expanded with saline to stretch the overlying skin and create a pocket. After several weeks, the tissue expander is exchanged for an implant.

heavy objects should be avoided. This restriction can be discussed with a family member or significant other who can perform these tasks or place the objects within easy reach of the client.

■ HEALTH TEACHING

The teaching plan for the client after surgery includes the following:

- Measures to optimize a positive body image
- Information to enhance interpersonal relationships and roles
- Exercises to regain full range of motion
- Measures to prevent infection of the incision

- Measures to avoid injury, infection, and subsequent swelling of the affected arm
- Care of the incision and drainage device

PHYSICAL CARE. The nurse has the opportunity to explain incisional care. The client may wear a light dressing to prevent irritation. The nurse explains that no lotions or ointments should be used on the area and that the use of deodorant under the affected arm should be delayed until healing is complete. Although swelling and redness of the scar itself are normal for the first few weeks, swelling, redness, increased heat, and tenderness of the surrounding area indicate infection and should be reported to the surgeon. If a lymph node dissection was performed, the client should elevate the affected

CHART 74-4
BEST PRACTICE *for*   **Postoperative Care of the Client After Breast Reconstruction**
• Assess the incision and flap for signs of infection (excessive redness, drainage, odor) during dressing changes.   • Assess the incision and flap for signs of poor tissue perfusion (duskiness, decreased capillary refill) during dressing changes.   • Avoid pressure on the flap and suture lines by positioning the client on her nonoperative side and avoiding tight clothing.   • Monitor and measure drainage in collection devices, such as Jackson-Pratt drains.   • Teach the client to return to her usual activity level gradually and to avoid heavy lifting.   • Avoid sleeping in the prone position.   • Avoid participation in contact sports or other activities that could cause trauma to the chest.   • Minimize pressure on the breast during sexual activity.   • Refrain from driving until advised by the physician.   • Remind the client to ask at the 6-week postoperative visit when full activity can be resumed.   • Reassure the client that optimal appearance may not occur for 3 to 6 months postoperatively.   • If implants have been inserted, teach the proper method of breast massage to enhance expansion and prevent capsule formation (consult with the physician).   • Review the breast self-examination procedure and the need to continue this practice monthly.   • Remind the client that mammograms should be scheduled at least yearly for the rest of her life.

CHART 74-5
CLIENT EDUCATION GUIDE   **Recovery from Breast Cancer Surgery**
• There may be a dry gauze dressing over the incision when you leave the hospital. You may change this dressing if it becomes soiled.   • A small, dry dressing will be around the site where a drain is placed. Often there is some leakage of fluid around the drain. Check the gauze dressing for drainage, and change it if it becomes soiled. Some leakage is normal, but if the dressing becomes soaked more than once a day, call your health care provider.   • Your nurse has shown you how to empty the reservoir from your drain and how to measure the volume of drainage. You should empty the drain twice a day and record the measurements.   • Drains are generally removed when drainage is less than 50 mL in 24 hours.   • Drains are often removed at the same time as the stitches or staples, generally 7 to 10 days after surgery.   • You may take sponge baths or tub baths, making certain that the area of the drain and incision stays dry. You may shower after the stitches and drains are removed.   • You can begin using your arm for normal activities, such as eating or combing your hair. Exercises involving the wrist, hand, and elbow, such as flexing your fingers, circular wrist motions, and touching your hand to your shoulder, are very good. You can usually resume more strenuous exercises after the drains have been removed.   • You can expect some discomfort or mild pain after surgery, but within 4 to 5 days most women have no need for pain medication or require medication only at bedtime.   • Numbness in the area of the surgery and along the inner side of the arm from the armpit to the elbow occurs in virtually all women. It is the injury to the nerves that causes sensation to the skin in those areas. Women have described sensations of heaviness, pain, tingling, burning, and "pins and needles." These sensations change over the months and usually resolve by 1 year.   • Pamphlets on exercises, hand and arm care, and general facts about breast cancer are available from your nurse or volunteer visitor. The American Cancer Society has volunteers who have had surgery similar to yours and are available to visit you.

Modified from McCorkle, R., Baird, S., & Grant, M. (1996). *Cancer nursing: A comprehensive approach* (2nd ed.). Philadelphia: W.B. Saunders.

arm on a pillow for at least 30 minutes a day for the first 6 months. The client should have someone bring a loose-fitting, nonwired brassiere or camisole for her to try before discharge with a soft cotton-filled or polyester fiber–filled form supplied by the hospital or by Reach to Recovery. The client wears this form until the incision is completely healed and the health care provider approves the fitting of a more sophisticated prosthesis, usually 6 to 8 weeks after discharge. After going home, the client should be encouraged to dress in loose-fitting street clothes, not pajamas, to further enhance a positive self-image.

Exercises that began in the hospital should continue at home. Active range-of-motion exercises should begin 1 week after surgery or when sutures and drains are removed. The nurse emphasizes that reaching and stretching exercises should continue only to the point of pain or pulling, never beyond that. ENCORE, a YWCA program, is appropriate for women as early as 3 weeks postoperatively and includes exercise to music, exercise in water, and psychologic support. Before discharge, the surgeon may prescribe precautions or limitations specific to plans for future procedures, such as reconstruction.

The nurse provides information needed to help the client avoid infection and subsequent lymphedema of the affected arm after the mastectomy. The client should avoid having blood pressure measurements taken on, having injections in, and having blood drawn from the arm on the side of the mastectomy. The client should wear a mitt when using the oven, wear gloves when gardening, and treat cuts and scrapes appropriately. If lymphedema occurs, the arm should be elevated when possible and special attention paid to the above-mentioned warnings. In addition, if lymphedema occurs, it can be managed with the use of an arm sleeve (similar to a Ted or Jobst stocking) or a sequential compression device. Management of lymphedema is directed toward measures that promote drainage of the affected arm; however, prevention is the best cure.

PSYCHOSOCIAL MANAGEMENT. Concerns about appearance after surgery are common and are often a threat to the client's self-concept as a woman. Before breast surgery, the woman and her partner can benefit from an explanation of the expected postoperative appearance. After a modified radical mastectomy, the chest wall is fairly smooth and has a horizontal incision from the axilla to the midchest area. After breast-conserving surgery, scars vary according to the amount of breast tissue removed. Scars may be red and raised at first, but these characteristics diminish in the first few months. After surgery, the nurse encourages the woman to look at her incision before she goes home and offers to be present when she does so.

Much of one's body image is a reflection of how others respond. Therefore the response of the client's family or partner to

CHART 74-6

FOCUSED ASSESSMENT *of*
Home Care Clients Recovering from Breast Cancer Surgery

Assess cardiovascular, respiratory, and urinary status, including:
- Vital signs
- Lung sounds
- Urine output patterns

Assess for pain and effectiveness of analgesics.

Assess dressing and incision site for:
- Excess drainage
- Signs and symptoms of infection
- Wound healing
- Intact staples

Assess drain and site for:
- Drainage around drain site and in drain
- Color and amount of drainage
- Signs and symptoms of infection

Review client's recordings of drainage.

Evaluate ability to care for and empty drain.

Assess status of affected extremity, including:
- Range of motion
- Ability to perform exercise regimen
- Lymphedema

Assess nutritional status, including:
- Food and fluid intake
- Presence of nausea and vomiting
- Bowel sounds

Assess functional ability, including:
- Activities of daily living
- Mobility and ambulation

Assess home environment, including:
- Safety
- Structural barriers

Assess client's compliance and knowledge of illness and treatment plan, including:
- Follow-up appointment with surgeon
- Signs and symptoms to report to health care provider
- Hand and arm care guidelines
- Referral to Reach to Recovery

Assess client and caregiver coping skills:
- Determine if client has looked at incision site
- Assess client's reaction to incision site

---

the surgery is crucial in determining the effect on self-concept. These people may also need the support of the nurse. They may have concerns about their ability to accept the changes and need to discuss these feelings with an objective listener. They may also need help with communicating their feelings, both negative and positive, with their loved one. Involving them in teaching may also help reinforce learning and increase retention.

Sexual concerns should be discussed before discharge. Sexual intercourse can be resumed whenever the client is comfortable. Clients may prefer to lay a pillow over the surgical site or wear a bra or camisole to prevent contact with the surgical site during intercourse. The client may be embarrassed to broach the topic, and the nurse should be sensitive to possible concerns and approach the subject first.

For women of childbearing age (approximately 25% of breast cancer clients), issues related to childbearing may be a concern. Some providers believe that the woman who has had breast cancer should wait 2 to 3 years after completing treatment to attempt pregnancy. Others, however, suggest no waiting period, since recurrences could happen at any time (Shapiro & Clark, 1995). Chemotherapy and radiation are considered serious **teratogenic** (birth defect–causing) agents, and sexually active clients receiving chemotherapy or radiotherapy

must use birth control during therapy. The method and length of birth control is discussed with the health care provider.

■ HEALTH CARE RESOURCES

Resources available to the client after discharge include personal support and community programs. After discharge, the spouse or significant other may need help in planning support for home responsibilities. For example, a partner who may be assuming additional duties at home and work may feel stressed. Exploring temporary relief resources for child care, cleaning, or cooking may be helpful until the woman regains her previous energy level. Discussing the need for ongoing emotional support is also beneficial to both the client and her partner. Leaving the hospital and appearing normal do not end the anxiety and fear. Identifying a support person with whom the client or couple can explore these feelings and discussing the need to ventilate feelings enhance personal and family recovery.

As mentioned, Reach to Recovery and ENCORE are two community resources for women with breast cancer. Reach to Recovery provides a volunteer who visits the client in the hospital or at home. She brings a personal message of hope, informational materials on breast cancer recovery, and a soft, temporary breast form. Some communities offer additional resources such as support groups and exercise classes.

▶ Evaluation: Outcomes

NOC The nurse evaluates the care of the client with breast cancer on the basis of the identified nursing diagnoses and collaborative problems. The expected outcomes include that the client will:

- Demonstrate the correct method of breast self-examination (BSE) and practice BSE on a monthly basis
- Comply with guidelines for mammography and professional examination
- Be able to cope with the diagnosis, as shown by her use of social support, use of information to deal with uncertainty, absence of physical signs of anxiety, and verbal confirmation of feeling calm
- State that she feels positive about her self-image
- Regain full range of motion of the affected arm
- Remain free from lymphedema or infection

ONLINE RESOURCES

For suggested readings and Internet resources, go to http://www.wbsaunders.com/SIMON/Iggy/.

SELECTED BIBLIOGRAPHY

Asterisk indicates a classic or definitive work on this subject.

Allen, K.M., & Phillips, J.M. (1997). *Women's health across the lifespan.* Philadelphia: J.B. Lippincott.

American Society of Clinical Oncology. (1998). *American Society of Clinical Oncology curriculum: Cancer genetics and cancer predisposition testing.* Alexandria, VA: Author.

*Baron, R.H., & Walsh, A. (1995). Nine facts everyone should know about breast cancer. *American Journal of Nursing, 95*(7), 29-33.

Barroso, J., et al. (2000). Comparison between African-American and white women in their beliefs about breast cancer and their health locus of control. *Cancer Nursing, 23*(4), 268-276.

*Bostwick, J. (1995). Breast reconstruction following mastectomy. *CA: A Cancer Journal for Clinicians, 45*(5), 289-303.

Bragg Leight, S., et al. (2000). The effect of structured training on breast self-examination search behaviors as measured using biomedical instrumentation. *Nursing Research, 49*(5), 283-289.

Burke, W., et al. (1997). Recommendations for follow-up care of individuals with an inherited predisposition to cancer: BRCA1 and BRCA2. *JAMA, 227*(12), 997-1003.

Cha, C., Kennedy, G., & Niederhuber, J. (1999). Metastatic breast cancer. *Surgical Clinics of North America, 79*(5), 1117-1136.

*Champion, V. (1995). Development of a benefits and barriers scale for mammography utilization. *Cancer Nursing, 18*(1), 53-59.

*Corral, C., & Mustoe, T. (1996). Controversy in breast reconstruction. *Surgical Clinics of North America, 76*(2), 310-312.

Couch, F.J., & Hartmann, L.C. (1998). BRCA1 testing advances and retreats. *Journal of the American Medical Association, 279*(12), 955-956.

Couch, F.J., et al. (1997). BRCA1 mutations in women attending clinics that evaluate the risk of breast cancer. *New England Journal of Medicine, 336*(20), 1409-1415.

Dent, D.M., & Cant, P.F. (1999). Fibroadenoma. *World Journal of Surgery, 13*(6), 706-710.

*Djuric, Z., et al. (1996). Levels of 5-hydroxymethyl-2-deoxyuridine in DNA from blood as a marker of breast cancer. *Cancer, 77*(4), 691-696.

*Donegan, W.L., & Spratt, J.S. (1995). *Cancer of the breast* (4th ed.). Philadelphia: W.B. Saunders.

Facione, N.C., et al. (2000). Perceived risk and help-seeking behavior for breast cancer: A Chinese-American perspective. *Cancer Nursing, 23*(4), 258-267.

Fisher, B., et al. (1998). Tamoxifen for prevention of breast cancer: Report of the National Surgical Adjuvant Breast and Bowel Project P-1 Study. *Journal of the National Cancer Institute, 90*(18), 1371-1388.

Frank, T.S., et al. (1998). Sequence analysis of BRCA1 and BRCA2: Correlation of mutations with family history and ovarian cancer risk. *Journal of Clinical Oncology 16*(7), 2417-2425.

Gaston-Johansson, F., et al. (2000). The effectiveness of the comprehensive coping strategy on clinical outcomes in breast cancer autologous bone marrow transplantation. *Cancer Nursing, 23*(4), 277-285.

*Giomuso, C.B., & Suster, V. (1994). Free flap breast reconstruction. *MEDSURG Nursing, 3*(1), 9-22.

*Gould, K., Gates, M.L., & Miaskowski, C. (1995). Breast cancer prevention: A summary of the chemoprevention trial with tamoxifen. *Oncology Nursing Forum, 21*(5), 835-840.

Hansen, N., & Morrow, M. (1998). Breast disease. *Medical Clinics of North America, 82*(2), 203-222.

Hartmann, L., et al. (1999a). Clinical options for women at high risk for breast cancer. *Surgical Clinics of North America, 79*(5), 1189-1204.

Hartmann, L., et al. (1999b). Efficacy of bilateral prophylactic mastectomy in women with a family history of breast cancer. *New England Journal of Medicine, 340*(2), 77-84.

Hilton, B.A., et al. (2000). Men's perspectives on individual and family coping with their wives' breast cancer and chemotherapy. *Western Journal of Nursing Research, 22*(4), 438-459.

Horden, A. (2000). Intimacy and sexuality for the woman with breast cancer. *Cancer Nursing, 23*(3), 230-236.

Hortobagyi, G. (1998). Treatment of breast cancer, *New England Journal of Medicine, 339*(4), 974-984.

*Hoskins, K.F., et al. (1996). Assessment and counseling for women with a family history of breast cancer: A guide for clinicians. *Journal of the American Medical Association, 273*(7), 577-585.

Jeffries, E. (1997). Home healthcare for patients receiving one-day mastectomy. *Home Healthcare Nurse, 115*(1), 31-37.

Kimmick, G., & Balducci, L. (2000). Breast cancer and aging. *Hematology/Oncology Clinics of North America, 14*(1) 213-234.

Kraus, P.L. (1999). Body image, decision making, and breast cancer treatment. *Cancer Nursing, 22*(6), 421-427.

Landis, S.H., et al. (1999). Cancer statistics. *CA: A Cancer Journal for Clinicians, 49*(1), 8-31.

Leitch, A.M., et al. (1997). American Cancer Society guidelines for the early detection of breast cancer: Update 1997, *CA: A Cancer Journal for Clinicians, 47*(3), 150-153.

*Leslie, N.S. (1995). Role of the nurse practitioner in breast and cervical cancer prevention. *Cancer Nursing, 18*(4), 251-257.

Lessick, M., Wickham, R., & Rehwaldt, M. (1997). Breast and ovarian cancer: Genetic update and implications for nursing. *MEDSURG Nursing 6*(6), 341-349.

*Lu, Z.J. (1995). Variables associated with breast self-examination among Chinese women. *Cancer Nursing, 18*(1), 29-34.

*Luker, K.A., et al. (1996). Information needs and sources of information for women with breast cancer: A follow up study. *Journal of Advanced Nursing, 23*(3), 487-495.

*MacMahon, A.T. (1992). FDA limits access to breast implants. *NAACOG Newsletter, 19*(6), 3.

Malone, K., et al. (1998). BRCA1 mutations and breast cancer in the general population: Analyses in women before age 35 years and in women before age 45 years with first-degree family history. *Journal of the American Medical Association, 279*(12), 922-929.

*Moore, M.P., & Kinne, D. (1995). The surgical management of primary invasive breast cancer. *CA: A Cancer Journal for Clinicians, 45*(5), 278-288.

Moran, S.L., et al. (2000). TRAM flap breast reconstruction with expanders and implants. *AORN Journal, 71*(2), 354-362.

Mushin, A.I., & Fintor, L. (1997). Is screening for breast cancer cost-effective? *Cancer, 69*(12), 1957-1962.

Nass, S., & Davidson, N. (1999). The biology of breast cancer. *Hematology/Oncology Clinics of North America, 17*(2), 311-327.

NCCN practice guidelines: Screening for and evaluation of suspicious breast lesions. (1998). *Oncology, 12*(2), 89-138.

Nogueira, S.M., & Appling, S.E. (2000). Breast cancer: Genetics, risks, and strategies. *Nursing Clinics of North America, 35*(3), 663-669.

Overmoyer, B. (1999). Breast cancer screening. *Medical Clinics of North America, 83*(6), 1143-1460.

*Phillips, J.M., & Wilbur, J. (1995). Adherence to breast cancer screening guidelines among African-American women of differing employment status. *Cancer Nursing, 18*(4), 258-269.

*Shapiro, T., & Clark, P. (1995). Breast cancer: What the primary care provider needs to know. *Nurse Practitioner, 20*(3), 39-40, 42.

*Smith, R.J. (1996). Buying more time in less time: Case management and bone marrow transplantation. *Case Manager, 7*(1), 77-83.

Templeman, C., & Hertweck, S. (2000). Breast disorders in the pediatric and adolescent patient. *Obstetric and Gynecology Clinics, 27*(1), 19-31.

*Tierney, L., et al. (1995). *Current medical diagnosis and treatment.* Norwalk, CT: Appleton & Lange.

Veronesi, U., et al. (1998). Prevention of breast cancer with tamoxifen. *Lancet 352*(9122), 93-97.

*Walkenstein, M. (1995). Surgical clinical nurse specialist facilitates discharge of patients undergoing breast surgery. *Oncology Nursing Forum, 22*(1), 147-148.

Weber, E.S. (1997). Questions and answers about breast cancer diagnosis. *American Journal of Nursing, 97*(10), 34-38.

*Wingo, P.A., et al. (1995). Cancer statistics, 1995. *CA: A Cancer Journal for Clinicians, 45*(1), 8-30.

*Wingo, P.A., et al. (1996). Cancer statistics for African Americans, 1996. *CA: A Cancer Journal for Clinicians, 46*(2), 113-125.

Interventions for Clients with Gynecologic Problems

AMY NICHOLS • DONNA D. IGNATAVICIUS

Learning Objectives

After studying this chapter, you should be able to:

1. Compare and contrast common menstrual cycle disorders.
2. Discuss common assessment findings associated with menopause.
3. Develop a teaching plan for a client with a vaginal inflammation or infection.
4. Prioritize postoperative care for the client undergoing an anterior and/or posterior repair.
5. Analyze assessment data for clients with leiomyomas to determine nursing diagnoses and collaborative problems.
6. Formulate a plan of care for a client undergoing a hysterectomy.
7. Identify the risk factors for gynecologic cancers.
8. Discuss the psychosocial issues associated with gynecologic cancers.
9. Explain the purpose of radiation and chemotherapy for clients with gynecologic cancers.
10. Develop a community-based plan of care for clients with gynecologic cancers.

SIMON

Go to http://www.wbsaunders.com/SIMON/Iggy/ for self-assessment questions related to these Learning Objectives.

The most common reasons for seeking gynecologic care are pain, vaginal discharge, and bleeding. Nurses can play an important role in assessing gynecologic disorders by being knowledgeable about disease presentation, being sensitive to the client's complaints, and encouraging discussion about menstrual or other reproductive problems. Educating women about their bodies, helping them to recognize when professional help should be sought, and teaching them how to make informed decisions about treatments are major goals for nurses working with female clients in any setting. Nurses also need to assess the effects of gynecologic problems on sexual health.

MENSTRUAL CYCLE DISORDERS

Primary Dysmenorrhea

OVERVIEW

Dysmenorrhea, or painful menstrual flow, is one of the most common gynecologic problems, occurring most often in women in their teens and early 20s. More than 50% of all women report some degree of dysmenorrhea, but only a small percentage are not able to function. Primary dysmenorrhea is not associated with pelvic pathologic changes, whereas secondary dysmenorrhea usually begins with an underlying disease condition.

Primary dysmenorrhea usually occurs after ovulation is established. Dysmenorrhea is painful uterine cramping characterized by spasmodic lower abdominal pain that begins with the onset of menstrual flow, and lasts 12 to 48 hours. The pain often radiates to the lower back and thighs; nausea and vomiting, fatigue, and nervousness may accompany the pain. Less common clinical manifestations include headache, syncope, diarrhea, bloating, and breast tenderness.

Most researchers believe that the cause of primary dysmenorrhea is increased production and release of uterine prostaglandins. Prostaglandins are produced by the endometrium during the luteal phase of the menstrual cycle, and the levels peak at the onset of menses. Excessive prostaglandin levels stimulate the myometrium and cause severe spasms, which constrict uterine blood flow, resulting in ischemia and pain.

▶ COLLABORATIVE MANAGEMENT

● Assessment

A thorough history of the client includes the following:
* The age at menarche (onset of menstruation)
* Characteristics of menstruation
* Obstetric history
* Contraceptive history
* The type of pain
* Previous therapy
* The need for contraception

The client is asked whether she has any conditions suggestive of pelvic problems. To plan care, the nurse assesses emotional factors, such as the individual woman's response to dysmenorrhea, her attitudes about menstruation, and the extent to which dysmenorrhea is perceived to disrupt her life.

Interventions

Interventions for primary dysmenorrhea include prevention, education, support, and therapeutic measures that are tailored to each woman's needs. Prostaglandin synthetase inhibitors (nonsteroidal anti-inflammatory drugs [NSAIDs]), such as ibuprofen (Motrin, Apo-Ibuprofen✤) and naproxen sodium (Anaprox, Naprosyn), are currently recommended for pain relief. In addition, numerous over-the-counter ibuprofen products, such as Advil and Nuprin, provide pain relief for many clients with primary dysmenorrhea. Aspirin is a mild prostaglandin synthetase inhibitor and may relieve mild dysmenorrhea. All of these drugs can cause gastrointestinal (GI) distress and should therefore be taken with meals or milk.

Before treatment, the health care provider must assess the client's contraception needs. When contraception is not needed, prostaglandin synthetase inhibitors are the treatment of choice because they are required only for the duration of symptoms. If contraception is a consideration, ovulation suppression with oral contraceptives is the treatment of choice.

COMPLEMENTARY AND ALTERNATIVE THERAPIES.
Complementary therapies that may alleviate or prevent pain include acupressure, aerobic exercise, swimming, yoga or other meditation, application of heat or cold, massage, biofeedback, and relaxation techniques. Dietary measures for the prevention of pain may include increasing the intake of vitamin B_6, calcium, magnesium, and protein and reducing the intake of sodium to reduce fluid retention.

Premenstrual Syndrome

OVERVIEW

The syndrome experienced by menstruating women in which adverse symptoms recur regularly in the luteal phase of each menstrual cycle has been recognized as **premenstrual syndrome (PMS).** Approximately 5% of menstruating women experience severe premenstrual symptoms; many more have moderate symptoms. Fortunately, because considerable progress has been made in understanding PMS, most affected women can be helped.

PMS is a collection of symptoms that are cyclic in nature. These symptoms are followed by relief with menses and a symptom-free phase. PMS affects women of all races, socioeconomic levels, and educational levels. It seems to be more prevalent in women 30 to 40 years old. The severity increases with aging until menopause. Women are at greater risk for PMS after pregnancy, childbirth, and tubal ligation; during the perimenopausal years; and during major life stresses.

Currently, there is no agreement on a single set of diagnostic criteria for PMS. Three elements are found in defining PMS: symptoms, severity level, and timing. Many women report experiencing six or more symptoms across emotional, physical, and cognitive categories.

Emotional symptoms include irritability, easily precipitated crying spells, low self-esteem, anxiety, and depression. Somatic or physical symptoms include breast tenderness, bloating, fluid retention, increased appetite and food cravings, insomnia, fatigue, hot flashes, headaches, and musculoskeletal discomfort. Cognitive problems include short-term memory problems, difficulty concentrating, and unclear thinking.

➤ COLLABORATIVE MANAGEMENT

Assessment

There is no reported objective means of diagnosing PMS. Some researchers have attempted to differentiate premenstrual patterns. Determining the timing of the symptoms is as critical as noting the type of symptoms. The most effective and readily available assessment tool is a menstrual chart. The nurse instructs the client to keep a chart for at least three consecutive cycles, showing the length of the menstrual cycle, the duration of bleeding, and the occurrence of symptoms. If the woman has PMS, the symptoms recur during the luteal phase (from ovulation to menstruation), which is followed by a symptom-free period (at least 7 days). When taking a menstrual history, the nurse also assesses to what extent the woman believes that her activities of daily living (ADLs) are disrupted by the symptoms. Often reassurance that the symptoms are legitimate and that other women share these problems can help the client learn more about PMS. Clinical manifestations vary greatly among women and affect many body systems (Chart 75-1).

Interventions

Management of PMS focuses on eliminating the uncomfortable symptoms. The syndrome is highly individualized; however, one of the most important interventions is education.

CHART 75-1

KEY FEATURES *of*
Premenstrual Syndrome

Dermatologic Manifestations
- Acne
- Urticaria
- Herpes

Respiratory Manifestations
- Sinusitis
- Asthma
- Rhinitis
- Colds

Urologic Manifestations
- Oliguria
- Cystitis
- Enuresis
- Urethritis

Ophthalmologic Manifestations
- Conjunctivitis
- Styes
- Glaucoma

Neurologic Manifestations
- Headaches
- Migraine
- Syncope
- Vertigo
- Numbness of hands and feet
- Epilepsy (if susceptible)

Metabolic Manifestations
- Edema
- Breast tenderness

Emotional or Psychologic Manifestations
- Depression
- Irritability
- Tension
- Panic attacks
- Change in libido
- Mood swings
- Anxiety

Behavioral Manifestations
- Lowered work performance
- Food cravings
- Alcohol and drug overindulgence
- Confusion
- Sleeplessness
- Lack of coordination
- Suicide
- Lethargy
- Child abuse
- Assaultive behavior

Other Manifestations
- Allergies
- Hypoglycemia
- Joint pain
- Backache
- Palpitations
- Water retention

Each woman needs information about her body, especially the menstrual cycle, so that she can begin to understand the physiologic basis of PMS.

Women may need to express their feelings and discuss their experiences with PMS. Self-help groups and support groups are helpful resources. These groups also encourage significant others to participate, because PMS usually affects not only the woman but also her family and friends. For example, increased family conflict, communication problems with family and friends, and decreased family cohesion occur. Other coping strategies for the woman with PMS may include spiritual support, especially participating in religious services and seeking advice from spiritual leaders.

DIET THERAPY. Diet and nutrition are also important in managing PMS. If hypoglycemia (low blood glucose) occurs, the nurse instructs the woman to eat six small meals a day and to limit her intake of sugar, red meat, alcohol, coffee, tea, and chocolate.

Eliminating caffeine may help reduce irritability. Salt and sodium intake should be limited if edema occurs. Calcium, magnesium, and vitamins A, B_6, and C have also been used for relief of PMS.

DRUG THERAPY. Drug therapy remains controversial, but some treatments have been effective. Mild potassium-sparing diuretics taken for 10 days before menstruation can provide relief for some women. Women may need to increase their intake of potassium-containing foods if they are receiving this therapy.

Progesterone may relieve physical and psychologic symptoms. Natural progesterone is preferable to synthetic progesterone, even though the drug must be specially made by a pharmacist at the time prescribed. The daily dosage is 50 to 100 mg IM from ovulation to menstruation. Long-term side effects are unknown.

Bromocriptine mesylate (Parlodel) 2.5 mg two or three times a day with meals during the luteal phase can relieve breast symptoms. The side effects (lightheadedness and hypotension) may not be well tolerated. Other drugs for PMS that have been used include birth control pills, gonadotropin-releasing hormone (GnRH) agonists, antidepressants, and prostaglandin inhibitors, such as nonsteroidal anti-inflammatory drugs (NSAIDs).

Amenorrhea
OVERVIEW

Amenorrhea (the absence of menstrual periods) can be either primary (menstruation that has failed to occur by age 16 years) or secondary (menstruation that has started but has since stopped and has not recurred for at least 3 months). Primary amenorrhea is often associated with anomalies of the reproductive tract, and the prognosis for fertility is usually poor. Secondary amenorrhea is probably due to a functional disorder, and the prognosis for fertility is better. Amenorrhea can cause a woman much distress and concern.

Menstruation is a complex series of events that rely on the interplay of the hypothalamic, pituitary, ovarian, and endometrial functions. Dysfunction related to any of these four factors may cause amenorrhea (Table 75-1). Primary amenorrhea is relatively uncommon. Congenital factors are re-

sponsible for about two thirds of cases, and the remaining one third of cases are caused by ovarian, pituitary, or hypothalamic disease. Pregnancy, lactation (breastfeeding), and menopause are the most common physiologic causes of secondary amenorrhea.

➤ COLLABORATIVE MANAGEMENT
Assessment

The nurse assesses both the menstrual history and the obstetric history and asks about possible sexual activity and symptoms of pregnancy. A medical history may identify a systemic disease as a cause of amenorrhea. The nurse asks about current eating habits and any history of dieting because both obesity and starvation (e.g., anorexia nervosa) can contribute to amenorrhea. Strenuous exercise associated with competitive athletics, such as long-distance running, can cause stress or a reduction in body fat, resulting in amenorrhea. The nurse assesses hormone deficiencies, such as those associated with menopause that can cause hot flashes and vaginal dryness. Women should be questioned about their ingestion of drugs (e.g., oral contraceptives, phenothiazines, and antihypertensives) and recent stressors. The nurse is also alert for signs of **galactorrhea** (watery or milky breast secretions in nonbreastfeeding or women who have not been pregnant and **hirsutism** (unusual hair growth in women), both of which are related to polycystic ovary disease and subsequent amenorrhea.

Interventions

The nurse's primary roles in implementing care are to explain amenorrhea in easily understandable terms and to answer questions about tests and treatments. Counseling and emo-

TABLE 75-1 • COMMON CAUSES OF AMENORRHEA

PRIMARY
- Congenital anomalies
- Hypothalamic and pituitary disorders, such as delayed puberty
- Systemic disease
  - Thyroid and adrenal dysfunction
  - Diabetes mellitus
  - Extreme malnutrition
- Ovarian disease
- Malformations of the reproductive tract

SECONDARY
- Pregnancy
- Menopause
- Lactation
- Cervical stenosis
- Polycystic ovary disease
- Pituitary tumor or insufficiency
- Psychogenic stress
- Excessive physical activities
- Medications
  - Antihypertensive agents
  - Birth control pills
  - Phenothiazines
- Nutritional disorders
  - Obesity
  - Anorexia nervosa
  - Sudden weight loss
- Ovarian disease, failure, or destruction

tional support must be provided. Amenorrhea may be a threat to a woman's self-concept; she usually needs to ventilate her feelings about sexuality or fertility.

Interventions for specific causes of amenorrhea are based on each woman's needs. Medical and surgical management of amenorrhea is directed at the underlying causes. Treatment includes hormone replacement, ovulation stimulation, and periodic progesterone withdrawal.

Postmenopausal Bleeding

OVERVIEW

Postmenopausal bleeding (vaginal bleeding occurring after a 12-month cessation of menses after the onset of menopause) is a symptom rather than a medical diagnosis. Bleeding is considered serious and should be evaluated. Gynecologic cancer occurs in 20% to 40% of women who experience postmenopausal bleeding.

Postmenopausal bleeding can be caused by numerous benign and malignant conditions (Table 75-2). The three most common causes are atrophic vaginitis, cervical polyps, and endometrial hyperplasia.

In a client with **atrophic vaginitis,** the vaginal mucosa is thin and dry and is easily traumatized by sexual intercourse and infection, causing spotting. Cervical polyps are usually soft, red, oval tissue masses that appear within the cervical canal, and they may bleed spontaneously or after intercourse.

The most serious cause of postmenopausal bleeding is **endometrial hyperplasia** (tissue overgrowth), a precursor of endometrial cancer. Bleeding is caused by declining ovarian function that leads to prolonged estrogen stimulation, producing the hyperplasia that eventually breaks down and bleeds. Estrogen stimulation can also be caused by estrogen replacement therapy (ERT).

Because many women who report postmenopausal bleeding need medical or surgical interventions, assessment is the major focus. The nurse assesses the menstrual history and family history initially, including the following:

* The client's age at menopause
* The frequency and amount of bleeding
* Previous bleeding episodes
* Use of medications (especially estrogen-only [unopposed estrogen] replacement therapy [ERT])
* Gastrointestinal (GI) or genitourinary symptoms

The nurse also identifies women who are at high risk for endometrial cancer (e.g., women who are obese, hypertensive, or diabetic or who have never had children).

Urine and stool specimens can be collected and tested for blood to differentiate other sources of bleeding. Blood specimens may be drawn for hemoglobin or hematocrit determinations, because clients are often anemic as a result of excessive bleeding. The nurse can prepare the woman for physical and pelvic examinations, including obtaining a specimen for a Papanicolaou (Pap) test, or smear, to evaluate the cause of bleeding.

▶ COLLABORATIVE MANAGEMENT

Nursing interventions focus on providing information and support for diagnostic and treatment procedures directed at the specific causes of bleeding. An endometrial biopsy can evaluate the presence of malignancy. A diagnostic dilation and curettage (D&C) procedure can be used to determine malignancy (see Dysfunctional Uterine Bleeding, p. 1756). Atypical hyperplasia is often treated with a hysterectomy (see Uterine Leiomyomas, p. 1764). Malignancy is usually treated with a combination of surgery, radiation therapy, and chemotherapy (see Endometrial Cancer, p. 1769).

The medical treatment of a woman receiving unopposed estrogen therapy may include the monthly administration of progesterone daily for the last 10 days of the estrogen therapy (days 16 to 25) or a once-per-month intramuscular (IM) progesterone injection. This treatment can reduce the abnormal endometrial proliferation and is suggested for the prevention of endometrial and breast cancer.

Atrophic vaginitis is managed by the administration of estrogen via the vaginal, oral, transdermal, or subdermal route. The nurse teaches the client about ERT (Chart 75-2). Women who use vaginal estrogen cream need to be aware that it can cause systemic effects. Women who take estrogen may be at risk for gallbladder disease, hypertension, breast cancer, endometrial cancer, and coronary artery disease.

CHART 75-2

CLIENT EDUCATION GUIDE
Estrogen Replacement Therapy

For All Types of Estrogen Replacement Therapy
* Call your health care provider if you have pain in your calves or groin, if you suddenly become short of breath, if you have abnormal vaginal bleeding, if you feel a lump in your breast, if you have a severe headache, or if you feel weak or numb in your arms or legs.
* Use sunscreen if you are in the sun for a prolonged period.
* Keep appointments for checkups.
* If your health care provider has prescribed progesterone to decrease your risk of endometrial cancer, take it as prescribed.

For Oral Therapy
* Take 1 pill a day for the first 25 days each month.
* If you feel nauseated or have intestinal upset, take your medication with food.

For Transdermal or Subdermal Administration
* Rotate the sites for the patches or injections to avoid skin irritation.
* Change the patches twice a week or according to your prescribed schedule.

For Vaginal Therapy
* Use an applicator to insert the suppository or cream daily as prescribed.
* You may need to wear a minipad to protect your clothing from soiling or staining by the drug.

TABLE 75-2 • COMMON CAUSES OF POSTMENOPAUSAL BLEEDING	
BENIGN	**MALIGNANT**
• Atrophic vaginitis	• Endometrial cancer
• Cervical polyps	• Cervical cancer
• Endometrial hyperplasia	• Ovarian cancer
• Uterine fibroids	• Vaginal cancer
• Cervical erosion	• Tubal cancer
• Estrogen therapy	

Endometriosis

OVERVIEW

Endometriosis is usually a benign disease characterized by implantation of endometrial tissue outside the uterine cavity. The tissue typically appears on the ovaries and the cul-de-sac and less commonly on other pelvic organs and structures (Figure 75-1). A "chocolate" cyst is an area of endometriosis inside an ovary.

Endometrial tissue located outside the endometrium responds similarly to the endometrium to hormonal stimulation and goes through the same cyclic changes. Bleeding occurs at the site of implantation, and the blood is trapped in the tissues; scarring and adhesions result as the blood is reabsorbed. Endometriosis progresses slowly. It regresses during pregnancy and at menopause. Rarely does endometriosis become a malignant disease.

The cause of endometriosis is unknown. The most accepted theories of causation are transportation and formation. There are two transportation theories: (1) implantation and (2) vascular and lymphatic dissemination. The implantation theory holds that endometrial tissue flows back through the fallopian tubes during menstruation and then implants on pelvic structures. Proponents of the vascular and lymphatic dissemination theory advocate that endometrial glands are transported through the vascular and lymphatic system to foreign locations. This latter theory may explain implantation in areas outside the pelvis, such as the lungs and the kidneys. Formation theories propose that endometrial tissue develops spontaneously outside the uterus.

Endometriosis occurs most often in women in their 30s and 40s; rarely does it appear before age 20. It is most common in women who have not been pregnant and in those whose mothers had endometriosis.

► COLLABORATIVE MANAGEMENT

Assessment

The nursing assessment should be as detailed as possible and include the client's menstrual history, her sexual history, and the characteristics of bleeding. Pain is the most common symptom of endometriosis. The pain usually peaks just before the menstrual flow. Pain is usually located in the lower abdomen, causing many women to feel a sense of rectal pressure. The degree of pain is not related to the extent of the endometriosis but is related to the site. Often women with minimal disease have more severe pain than do women with extensive disease. Other clinical manifestations include dyspareunia (painful sexual intercourse), painful defecation, sacral backache, hypermenorrhea (excessive, prolonged, or frequent bleeding), and infertility.

A pelvic examination may reveal pelvic tenderness, nodular uterosacral ligaments, and fixed or limited movement of the uterus. Psychosocial assessment may reveal anxiety because of uncertainty about the diagnosis. The woman may also have concerns about her self-concept if she is infertile and wants to become pregnant.

Diagnostic studies include blood tests (erythrocyte sedimentation rate [ESR] and white blood cell [WBC] count) to rule out pelvic inflammatory disease (PID). Ultrasonography is used to confirm or delineate pelvic masses that might be mistaken for endometriosis. Laparoscopy is the key diagnostic procedure for pelvic endometriosis. Examination of tissue specimens obtained during laparoscopy can confirm the diagnosis.

Interventions

Medical (hormonal) and surgical management may be used, depending on the symptoms, the extent of disease, and the client's desire for childbearing. Nursing management is aimed at the following:

* Reducing pain
* Restoring sexual function that was impaired by **dyspareunia** (painful sexual intercourse)
* Alleviating anxiety related to the clinical manifestations of the disease and the uncertainty of the diagnosis
* Eliminating the client's knowledge deficit about the disease or its treatment
* Alleviating fear related to the possibility of laparoscopy or surgery
* Preventing self-esteem disturbance related to infertility

Several organizations, including the Endometriosis Society and RESOLVE (an organization for infertile couples), offer additional information on endometriosis that may be helpful in planning care.

NONSURGICAL MANAGEMENT. Nonsurgical management involves the use of mild analgesics or nonsteroidal anti-inflammatory drugs (NSAIDs) for pain relief. The health care provider also uses hormonal therapies to relieve pain by suppressing ovulation. The hormonal therapies produce pseudo-pregnancy, pseudomenopause, or medical oophorectomy.

Pseudopregnancy is induced with oral contraceptives or progesterone. The health care provider usually prescribes a 6-month course of a low-dose estrogen oral contraceptive, followed by cyclic oral contraceptive use or therapy with progesterone alone.

The second hormonal treatment causes ovarian suppression, or pseudomenopause, by the use of danazol (Danocrine, Cyclomen✤), an antigonadotropin testosterone derivative. This therapeutic approach is the current choice of many health care providers, but it is expensive ($120 to $180 per month) and may cause undesirable side effects, including acne, hirsutism (abnormal hair growth in unwanted areas), weight gain, decreased breast size, and hot flashes.

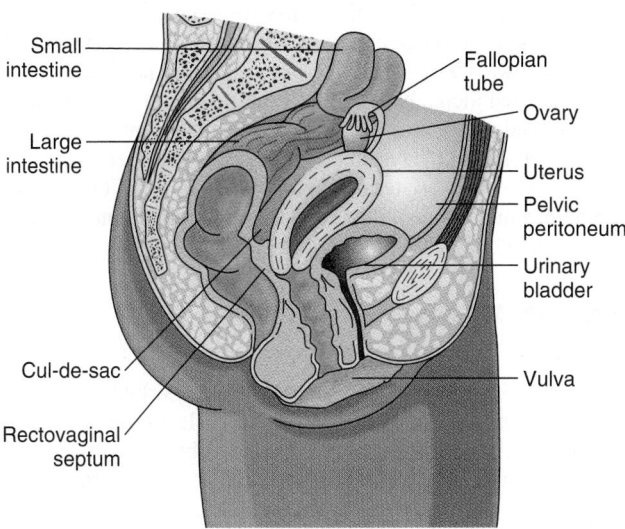

Small intestine
Large intestine
Cul-de-sac
Rectovaginal septum
Fallopian tube
Ovary
Uterus
Pelvic peritoneum
Urinary bladder
Vulva

Figure 75-1 ● Common sites of endometriosis.

The third hormonal treatment is the use of gonadotropin-releasing hormone (GnRH) agonists to produce a reversible medical oophorectomy. The drug can be administered by IM or subcutaneous injection or by nasal spray. Side effects include hot flashes, vaginal dryness, and insomnia.

COMPLEMENTARY AND ALTERNATIVE THERAPIES. Therapies that can relieve pain include the application of a heating pad to the abdomen or sacrum, relaxation techniques, yoga, and biofeedback. These approaches may decrease muscle tissue hypoxia and hypertonicity and relieve ischemia by increasing blood flow to the affected areas.

SURGICAL MANAGEMENT. Surgical management of endometriosis for a woman who wants to remain fertile is conservative and involves removal of endometrial implants and adhesions. The surgeon may use a carbon dioxide laser to treat endometriosis by vaporizing adhesions and endometrial implants. If the client does not wish to have children, the uterus and ovaries may be removed.

Dysfunctional Uterine Bleeding

OVERVIEW

Dysfunctional uterine bleeding (DUB), a nonspecific diagnostic term, is bleeding that is excessive or abnormal in amount or frequency without predisposing anatomic or systemic conditions. DUB occurs most often at either end of the span of a woman's reproductive years—when ovulation is becoming established or when it is becoming irregular at menopause.

Normally, the menstrual cycle represents a series of complex hormonal events related to balanced hypothalamic, pituitary, ovarian, and uterine functions. Menses, the sloughing of the endometrial lining, is an expected result. DUB occurs when there is a breakdown of these functions, causing hormonal imbalance.

The mechanism of DUB is unknown, but several theories have linked it with endometrial or myometrial dysfunction. Excessive fibrinolytic activity in the endometrium and changes in prostaglandin production in the uterus may also cause DUB.

Generally, DUB occurs in the absence of ovulation when the absence is associated with ovarian dysfunction. Estrogen stimulation of the endometrium is prolonged, and the endometrium grows past its hormonal support, causing bleeding and desquamation (shedding of uterine lining).

Anovulatory DUB during the reproductive years is associated with the following:
- Polycystic ovary disease
- Stress
- Extreme weight changes
- Long-term drug use (e.g., anticholinergics, morphine, or oral contraceptives)

Ovulatory causes of DUB are uncommon and are related to a dysfunctional corpus luteum, irregular maturation, and shedding of the endometrium.

► COLLABORATIVE MANAGEMENT

Assessment

When interviewing a woman with DUB, the nurse takes a complete menstrual history. The client is also asked about illnesses, variations in weight or diet, exercise, drug ingestion, and whether she has pain.

During the physical assessment, the nurse observes for symptoms of anemia or systemic disease, such as the following:
- Renal or hepatic disease
- Obesity
- Undernutrition
- Abnormal hair growth related to hormonal dysfunction
- Evidence of abdominal pain or masses

An examination that includes inspection of the external genitalia and a bimanual pelvic and rectal examination is essential to identify lesions or tenderness. A physician, a nurse practitioner, or a nurse midwife performs the internal pelvic examination.

Pelvic ultrasonography and hysteroscopy may be performed. In addition, the surgeon usually does an endometrial biopsy by suction aspiration or dilation and curettage (D&C). These are important procedures for women older than 40 years of age, who are at greater risk for endometrial cancer.

Interventions

NONSURGICAL MANAGEMENT. Nonsurgical management is usually the treatment of choice, although surgery may be needed to treat DUB. Most women can be treated successfully with hormonal manipulation. For those with anovulatory DUB, the health care provider typically prescribes medroxyprogesterone acetate (Depo-Provera) or combination oral contraceptives. If the client takes oral contraceptives, she should take 1 pill a day for 21 or 28 days, beginning on the first day of the menstrual cycle. Medroxyprogesterone is taken on days 16 to 25 of each month. Monthly withdrawal bleeding is expected with both therapies.

Women with ovulatory DUB may be treated with progestins during the luteal phase, oral contraceptives, prostaglandin inhibitors, or danazol. The nurse explains the desired and side effects of these drugs and evaluates the woman's knowledge of the effects, dosage, and administration schedule.

SURGICAL MANAGEMENT. Surgical management includes D&C, laser or balloon endometrial ablation, and hysterectomy. A D&C is usually used to treat an acute episode of bleeding, but the problem often returns. Laser or balloon endometrial ablation is a safe alternative for women who do not respond to medical management or who do not need a hysterectomy (Barrow, 1999). A hysterectomy is usually performed only after other treatments have failed. Table 75-3 compares the preoperative and postoperative care of clients undergoing a D&C or endometrial ablation. Hysterectomy is discussed later under Operative Procedures (Uterine Leiomyomas), p. 1766. If the woman has undergone a D&C or laser ablation, the nurse gives her postoperative instructions (Chart 75-3).

Menopause

OVERVIEW

Menopause is a normal biologic event marked for most women by the end of menstrual periods. It signifies the depletion of estradiol, a hormone produced by the ovaries. Although the meaning of menopause is the last menstrual period, the more clinically relevant perspective is to look at the months or years surrounding this event.

During the past decade there has been an explosion of interest among health care providers about all aspects of

TABLE 75-3 • NURSING CARE OF CLIENTS UNDERGOING SURGERY FOR DYSFUNCTIONAL UTERINE BLEEDING

	Dilation and Curettage (D&C)	Endometrial Ablation
Usual site	Outpatient	Outpatient
Anesthesia	Local, regional, general	Regional, general
Procedure	The cervical os is dilated; the endometrium is scraped.	The laser fiber is passed into the uterus through a hysteroscope; the endometrium is destroyed by laser energy, and tissues are removed by irrigating the uterine cavity with saline.
Preoperative care	Assess the client's knowledge of the procedure. The client is NPO after midnight. Teach postoperative expectations.	Same as for D&C. The client may be given danazol or GnRH agonist for 1 month before surgery to decrease endometrial thickness. Counsel the client about the likelihood of sterility as a result of uterine scarring.
Postoperative care	Monitor vital signs every 15 min until they are stable. Assess the need for pain relief. Assess for vaginal bleeding. Expect discharge when the client is stable.	Same as for D&C. Same as for D&C. Assess for spotting and vaginal drainage. Same as for D&C.

GnRH, Gonadotropin-releasing hormone.

CHART 75-3

CLIENT EDUCATION GUIDE
Endometrial Ablation and Dilation and Curettage

Endometrial Ablation
* Spotting and vaginal drainage are normal for several days after the procedure.
* If you have abdominal cramping, take mild analgesics, such acetaminophen (Tylenol, Atasol✦), or prostaglandin inhibitors, such as ibuprofen (Motrin).
* You can return to your normal activities within 2 or 3 days.
* You will probably be sterile because of uterine scarring.

Dilation and Curettage
* Take your temperature once a day for the next 2 days. If your oral temperature is more than 100° F (38° C), call the clinic or your doctor.
* Avoid sexual intercourse, tub bathing, and the use of tampons for 2 weeks to allow healing and prevent infection.
* Slight bleeding is normal. However, if bleeding is as heavy as during your normal menstrual period or if bleeding lasts longer than 2 weeks, call the clinic or health care provider.
* You can use a heating pad or hot water bottle to relieve abdominal cramping if it occurs.
* You can take mild analgesics, such as acetaminophen, for pain.

---

menopause—endocrinologic, metabolic, pathologic, sociocultural, and psychologic. Of particular interest for clinicians is the role of hormone replacement therapy (HRT) in the management of symptoms.

Much present-day interest in menopause is directed at the postmenopausal period and the medical illnesses common to postmenopausal women that may be affected by hormonal change. The most commonly discussed conditions are osteoporosis, coronary heart disease, and breast and endometrial cancer; interest in the effects of hormones on Alzheimer's disease has also emerged.

Women experience menopause as individuals, and care should be taken not to make generalizations. Women become menopausal in a variety of ways, including through surgery when the uterus and ovaries are removed and through medical

treatment for cancer. Natural menopause is experienced across a wide age range, occasionally as early as the 30s or 40s or as late as the 60s. The average age at which women experience their last menstrual period is between 50 and 52 years. All women under 40 who experience an early menopause, regardless of cause, are at higher than average risk for osteoporosis and osteoporosis-related fractures and may be at higher risk for cardiovascular disease. HRT is therefore particularly important in this group.

Several factors have been identified that may affect the timing of menopause. These include the following:
* Genetic influence
* Early **menarche** (beginning of menses)
* Hysterectomy
* Smoking
* Cancer treatment (chemotherapy or radiation)

► COLLABORATIVE MANAGEMENT
▶ Assessment

Menopause transition, or **perimenopause,** refers to the changes in spontaneous ovarian function that precede the last menstrual period and occur gradually. Common clinical characteristics of the transition are a change in the woman's usual menstrual periods and the beginning of vasomotor symptoms, such as hot flashes and night sweats. These symptoms may disturb the woman's usual sleep pattern. Vaginal dryness and mood changes may also occur. The nurse asks the client about these changes and reassures her that they are normal during perimenopause.

The most common early change in the bleeding pattern is a shortening of the time between menstrual periods, which is sometimes accompanied by an increase in menstrual flow. As the transition evolves, approximately 70% of women find that their periods become lighter and farther apart until they finally stop.

Some women simply stop menstruating without further change. The remaining women experience heavier bleeding, which can be either regularly timed or unpredictable. In addition, abnormal bleeding in this age-group can be caused by endometrial cancer, endometrial polyps, or uterine leiomyomas (tumors).

Most women pass through the menopause transition and into the postmenopause phase with minimal symptoms and never seek treatment for menopause-related problems. Approximately 20% of women, however, seek care for one or more of the symptoms discussed in this section, which are directly related to menopause.

● Interventions

Hormone replacement therapy (HRT), a combination of estrogen and progestin (progesterone), is the primary medical intervention for menopause. Estrogen given alone can cause gynecologic cancers and thromboembolitic conditions, such as deep vein thrombosis.

Estrogen is available as oral, transdermal, intravaginal, and intramuscular preparations. The oral estrogens have generally equivalent effects on symptoms and equivalent medical risk factors, so the choice of preparation for most women can be based on cost and individual side effect experience (Johnson, 1998). Transdermal estrogen offers a useful alternative route of administration for women who prefer not to take pills, who cannot tolerate oral therapy because of gastrointestinal (GI) side effects, or who have liver function test abnormalities, elevated triglycerides, or other conditions in which a first-pass hepatic effect is best avoided (Johnson, 1998). Side effects of estrogen occur and persist in approximately 10% of women.

The most common complaints are bloating, nausea, and breast tenderness. These symptoms often resolve after a few months of estrogen use.

CRITICAL THINKING CHALLENGE

As you are admitting a middle-aged woman to your hospital unit for cellulitis, she mentions that she thinks she is going through menopause. She complains that she gets hot flashes, is very moody, and cries a lot. She has been hesitant to tell her physician because she kept hoping that the symptoms would cease.
* How should you respond to the woman at this time?
* What other data should you obtain during the nursing history?
* What options will the health care provider have in treating the client's symptoms?

For suggested answer guidelines, go to SIMON http://www.wbsaunders.com/SIMON/Iggy/.

INFLAMMATIONS AND INFECTIONS

Vaginal discharge and itching are two of the most common complaints of female clients. Women may need information from their health care provider about the normal vaginal physiology, causes of symptoms, and methods of treatment. The nurse must be well informed about these topics to provide comprehensive care to clients with vaginal infections.

Vaginal infections are sometimes considered sexually transmitted diseases (STDs) because their causative organisms may be transmitted to sexual partners. However, infections can develop without sexual contact, and sexual partners do not always become infected. True STDs, such as gonorrhea, syphilis, chlamydial infection, and herpes simplex virus

infection, are discussed in Chapter 77. Acquired immunodeficiency syndrome (AIDS) is covered in Chapter 23.

Simple Vaginitis

■ OVERVIEW

Vaginitis can develop whenever there is a disturbance of the balance of hormones and bacterial interaction in the vagina as a result of one or more of the following:
* Changes in the normal flora
* Alkaline pH
* Insertion of foreign bodies, such as tampons and condoms
* Chemical irritations, such as from douches or sprays
* Medications, especially antibiotics

Vaginitis is an inflammation of the lower genital tract. The nurse completes the assessment of vaginitis by asking questions about the symptoms, assisting with a pelvic examination, and obtaining vaginal smears for laboratory testing (Chart 75-4). The nurse is nonjudgmental and reassuring during the assessment because the client may be embarrassed or afraid to discuss her symptoms.

► COLLABORATIVE MANAGEMENT

Interventions for vaginitis depend on the causes and the specific vaginal infection (Table 75-4). A woman's proper health habits can be beneficial to treatment. Therefore she should get enough rest and sleep, observe good dietary habits, get regular exercise, and use good personal hygiene. Popular, but not scientifically tested, hygiene practices to prevent vaginitis include the following:
* Perineal cleaning (wiping front to back) after urinating or defecating
* Wearing cotton underwear
* Avoiding strong douches and feminine hygiene sprays
* Avoiding tight-fitting pants

If antibiotics are prescribed, eating yogurt or taking *Lactobacillus* culture (Lactinex) tablets may help restore the natu-

---

CHART 75-4

BEST PRACTICE *for*
Care of the Client with Simple Vaginitis

In taking a client history, ask about:
* Onset of symptoms
* Characteristics of the discharge, especially the color and odor
* Associated symptoms such as itching and dysuria
* Types of contraceptives used
* Recent use of antibiotics
* Client's sexual activity
* Any history of vaginal infection
* Client's hygiene practices: douching and using tampons

In performing a physical examination:
* Palpate the abdomen for tenderness or pain.
* Inspect the external genitalia for erythema, edema, excoriation, odor, and discharge.
* If you are qualified, perform a speculum examination to visualize the vagina and cervix, and note the source of any discharge or inflammation.

If you are qualified, perform the following laboratory tests, as ordered: a saline or potassium hydroxide wet smear and a nitrazine paper test of vaginal pH.

TABLE 75-4 • COMMON VAGINAL INFECTIONS

Sexual Transmission	Assessment		Drug Therapy
	Physical Findings	Laboratory Findings	
CANDIDA ALBICANS INFECTION			
Unlikely	Odorless, white, curdlike discharge Patches on vaginal walls and cervix Inflamed vaginal walls and cervix Itching	Hyphae and spores visible on potassium hydroxide wet slide Vaginal pH 4.5 or less	Miconazole nitrate (Monistat), clotrimazone (Gyne-Lotrimin), or nystatin (Mycostatin) vaginal creams or suppositories for 7 days Terconazole (Terazol) cream or suppositories for 7 days or double strength for 3 days Tioconazole (Vagistat) single-dose vaginal application
TRICHOMONAS VAGINADIS INFECTION			
Yes	None or fishy Itching Strawberry spot on vaginal surface and cervix	Flagellated, pear-shaped protozoa on saline wet slide Vaginal pH 6-7	Oral metronidazole (Flagyl), single 2-g dose for client and sexual partners
BACTERIAL VAGINOSIS/GARDNERELLA VAGINALIS INFECTION			
Yes	Gray-white or green discharge Fishy odor Itching Normal vaginal mucosa 10%-40% asymptomatic	"Clue" cells on examination of saline wet slide Positive "whiff" test finding Vaginal pH 5-6	Oral metronidazole 500 mg qid for 7 days, or ampicillin or tetracycline Clindamycin 450 mg qid for 7 days
CERVICITIS			
Yes	Mucopurulent discharge from endocervix Pelvic pain, postcoital and intermenstrual bleeding The cervix may be inflamed and bleed when touched	Need to rule out herpes, gonorrhea, and chlamydial infection Vaginal pH 4.5 or less	Depends on diagnosis
ATROPHIC VAGINITIS			
No	Pale, thin, dry mucosa Itching No odor Scant white, yellow, gray, or green discharge Dyspareunia, postcoital bleeding	Parabasal cells Leukocyte predominance Vaginal pH 6	Topical conjugated estrogen cream $1/_2$ to 1 application at night for 7 nights, then twice weekly

ral flora (Döderlein's bacilli) of the vagina. Education of the client focuses on preventive measures and on information about infection transmission (Chart 75-5).

Vulvitis

◼ OVERVIEW

Vulvitis is an inflammatory condition of the vulva that is associated with symptoms of pruritus (itching) and a burning sensation. The vulvar skin is sensitive to hormonal, metabolic, and allergic influences. Symptoms can be caused by systemic conditions, direct contact with irritants, and extension of infection from the vagina.

The most common skin disease affecting the vulva is contact dermatitis, which can be caused by an irritant, such as feminine hygiene sprays, fabric dyes, soaps and detergents, or allergens. Primary infections that affect the vulva include herpes genitalis and condylomata acuminata (venereal warts) (see Chapter 77). Secondary infections of the vulva are caused by organisms responsible for the numerous types of vaginitis, including candidiasis in diabetic women. Pediculosis pubis (crab lice infestation) and scabies (itch mite infestation) are common parasitic infestations of the skin of the vulva. Other causes of vulvitis include the following:

* Atrophic vaginitis
* Vulvar kraurosis (postmenopausal disorder causing dryness and atrophy)
* Vulvar leukoplakia (postmenopausal atrophy and thickening of vulvar tissues)
* Cancer
* Urinary incontinence

▶ COLLABORATIVE MANAGEMENT

Assessment of the woman usually identifies symptoms of itching and burning sensation. Erythema (redness), edema, and superficial skin ulcers also may be present. Some women may have an itch-scratch-itch cycle, in which the itching

---

CHART 75-5

CLIENT EDUCATION GUIDE
Vaginal Infections

* Your risk of getting vaginal infections increases if you have sex with more than one person.
* When you have a vaginal infection, do not have sexual intercourse, or at least make sure that your partner wears a condom.
* Sexual partners may need to be treated for infection.
* The only way to identify what infection you have is to be examined by a health care provider and to get the results of laboratory tests.
* Take your medicine as prescribed, not just until your symptoms go away.

CHART 75-6

BEST PRACTICE *for*
Prevention of Vulvitis

* Wear cotton underwear.
* Avoid wearing tight clothing, such as pantyhose or tight jeans, because they can cause chafing. You can also get hot and sweaty, which can cause an infection.
* Always wipe front to back after having a bowel movement or urinating.
* Do not douche or use feminine hygiene sprays.
* If your sexual partner has an infection of his sex organs, do not have intercourse with him until he has been treated.
* You are more likely to get an infection if you are pregnant, have diabetes, take oral contraceptive drugs, or are menopausal.
* Practice vulvar self-examination monthly (see Chapter 73).

---

leads to scratching, which causes excoriation that then must heal. As healing takes place, itching occurs again, which leads to further scratching. If the cycle is not interrupted, the condition may become chronic, causing the vulvar skin to become white and thickened (leathery). This skin is dry and scaly and cracks easily, increasing the woman's chances of infection.

Medical treatment of clients with vulvitis depends on the cause. Nursing interventions to relieve itching include applying wet compresses, sitz baths for 30 minutes several times a day, and the application of prescribed topical medications, such as hydrocortisone and fluorinated corticosteroids (betamethasone valerate [Valisone, Betaderm♣] or fluocinolone acetonide [Synalar, Fluoderm]).

The health care provider prescribes oral antibiotics if infection is the underlying cause. Removal of any irritant or allergen, such as by changing detergents, should be encouraged. Treatment of pediculosis and scabies is instituted if needed and includes applying lindane (1% gamma benzene hexachloride [Kwell, Kwellada♣]) lotion, shampoo, or cream to the affected area as directed; cleaning affected clothes, bedding, and towels; and disinfecting the home environment (lice cannot live for more than 24 hours away from the body).

If the vulvitis is chronic or severe, laser therapy (see p. 1774) or a "skinning" vulvectomy (see p. 1779) may be performed. Preventive measures that may be helpful for vulvitis are listed in Chart 75-6.

Toxic Shock Syndrome
OVERVIEW

Toxic shock syndrome (TSS) was not commonly recognized by health care providers until 1980, when it was found to be related to menstruation and tampon use. Other conditions that have been associated with TSS include surgical wound infection, nonsurgical focal infections, postpartum conditions, and nonmenstrual vaginal conditions. Use of the diaphragm, cervical cap, and vaginal contraceptive sponge has also been linked to TSS.

The pathophysiology of TSS is not clearly understood. Certain strains of *Staphylococcus aureus* produce a toxin that has been associated with the symptoms of TSS. Numerous theories have been reported to explain the mechanism of *S. aureus* absorption in TSS. The vagina may be highly susceptible to the toxin released by *S. aureus*.

In menstrually related TSS, the theories about the mechanisms of absorption focus on tampon use. Risk for TSS is related to the degree of absorbency of the tampon. The following are possible explanations:

* Toxins readily cross the vaginal mucosa.
* Highly absorbent tampons rub the vaginal walls and cause ulceration, which allows transport of the toxins.
* Prolonged or continued tampon use can cause chronic vaginal ulcerations through which *S. aureus* is absorbed.
* Plastic tampon inserters can cause ulceration through which toxins are transported.
* Toxin producing *S. aureus* has a growth requirement for magnesium (some tampons contain magnesium).

► COLLABORATIVE MANAGEMENT

Influenza-like symptoms for the first 24 hours are common. The abrupt onset of a high temperature associated with a headache, sore throat, vomiting, diarrhea, generalized rash, and hypotension are often present. The most common clinical manifestations are skin changes (initially a rash resembling a severe sunburn that changes to a macular erythema similar to a drug-related rash). Because not all women experience all of these clinical manifestations, the criteria established by the U.S. Centers for Disease Control and Prevention (CDC) are used in epidemiologic studies to verify cases of TSS (Chart 75-7).

Management in the primary care setting focuses on client education and prevention. The nurse instructs the client on the prevention of TSS related to the use of tampons, vaginal sponges, and diaphragms (Chart 75-8).

Primary treatment in the acute care setting includes fluid replacement because dehydration and electrolyte imbalance result from vomiting and diarrhea. The health care provider also prescribes antibiotics if the penicillin-resistant strain of *S. aureus* is the cause of TSS. Other measures may include administering transfusions to reverse low platelet counts, corticosteroids to treat skin changes, and drugs to treat hypotension.

PELVIC STRUCTURE SUPPORT PROBLEMS
Uterine Prolapse
OVERVIEW

Three stages of **uterine prolapse** have been described according to the degree of descent of the uterus (Figure 75-2). Prolapse of the uterus can be caused by congenital defects, persistent high levels of intra-abdominal pressure related to

CHART 75-7

KEY FEATURES *of*
Toxic Shock Syndrome

- Fever (temperature > 102° F [38.9° C])
- Diffuse rash resembling sunburn
- Peeling of skin—primarily the soles of the feet and the palms of the hands—1 to 2 weeks after the onset of the illness
- Hypotension (systolic blood pressure <90 mm Hg or orthostatic syncope)
- Involvement of three or more of the following:
    Gastrointestinal system: vomiting, diarrhea at the onset of the syndrome
    Musculoskeletal system: severe aching or a serum creatinine phosphatase level twice the normal level
    Respiratory system: acute respiratory distress syndrome (ARDS)
    Renal/urinary system: decreased urine output, pyuria
    Cardiovascular system: decreased left ventrical contractility; ischemic changes shown on the electrocardiogram
    Liver: total bilirubin, aspartate aminotransferase (serum glutamic-oxaloacetic transaminase), and alanine aminotransferase (serum glutamic-pyruvic transaminase) levels elevated; jaundice; disseminated intravascular coagulation (DIC)
    Hematologic system: platelet levels below normal
    Central nervous system: disorientation, altered consciousness in the absence of fever or hypertension
    Mucous membranes: hyperemia of the vaginal walls, the throat, or the conjunctiva of the eye
- Negative results for the following: Rocky Mountain spotted fever, measles, scarlet fever, and throat, blood, and cerebrospinal fluid cultures
- Positive culture for *Staphylococcus aureus* from blood, urine, or stool

CHART 75-8

CLIENT EDUCATION GUIDE
Prevention of Toxic Shock Syndrome

Tampon Use
- Wash your hands before inserting a tampon.
- Do not use a tampon if it is dirty.
- Insert the tampon carefully to avoid injuring the delicate tissue in your vagina.
- Change your tampon every 3 to 6 hours.
- Do not use superabsorbent tampons.
- Use sanitary napkins at night.
- Call your health care provider if you suddenly experience a high temperature, vomiting, or diarrhea.
- Do not use tampons at all if you have had toxic shock syndrome.
- Not using tampons almost guarantees that you will not get toxic shock syndrome.

Vaginal Sponge Use
- Wash your hands before inserting a vaginal sponge.
- Use only clean water to wet the sponge.
- Do not use the sponge if it is dirty.
- Do not use the sponge for more than 30 hours at a time.
- Call your health care provider if you have two or more symptoms of toxic shock syndrome.

Diaphragm Use
- Wash your hands and the diaphragm before insertion.
- Remove the diaphragm within 24 hours after intercourse.
- Do not use the diaphragm during your menstrual period.
- After you take out the diaphragm, wash it with mild soap, rinse it, and dry it. Coating the diaphragm with a small amount of cornstarch will absorb any excess water and prevent damage to the latex rubber. Store it in a clean, dry place.

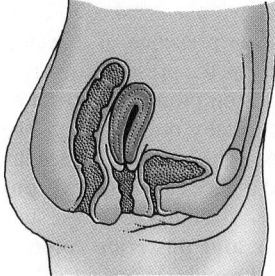

In **grade I uterine prolapse**, the uterus bulges into the vagina, but the cervix does not protrude through the entrance to the vagina.

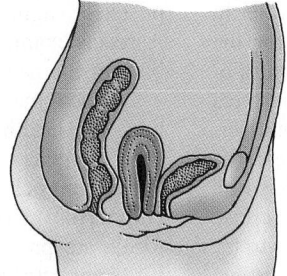

In **grade II uterine prolapse**, the uterus bulges farther into the vagina, and the cervix protrudes through the entrance to the vagina.

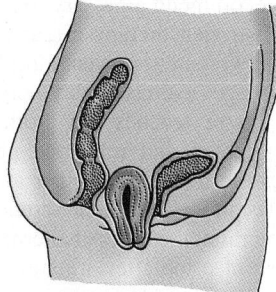

In **grade III uterine prolapse**, the body of the uterus and the cervix protrude through the entrance to the vagina. The vagina is turned inside out.

Figure 75-2   ●   Types of uterine prolapse.

heavy physical labor or exertion, or any other event that weakens the pelvic supports.

❀ CONSIDERATIONS FOR OLDER ADULTS
Prolapse is often a complication of childbirth injuries and repetitive stresses occurring many years later, but it also occurs in older adults who have never had children. The pelvic floor that supports the uterus is weakened by aging.

➤ COLLABORATIVE MANAGEMENT

Assessment findings include the client's verbalization of feeling as if "something is in my vagina," dyspareunia (painful sexual intercourse), backache, a feeling of heaviness or pressure in the pelvis, and bowel or bladder problems (if cystocele or rectocele is also present). A pelvic examination may reveal a protrusion of the cervix when the woman is asked to bear down.

Interventions are based on the degree of prolapse. Conservative treatment, such as the use of pessaries, is preferred over surgical treatment when possible. Vaginal hysterectomy with repair is the usual surgical procedure (see Operative Procedures [Uterine Leiomyomas], p. 1766). Before surgical intervention, the nurse questions the woman about her desire for future childbearing (surgery may be delayed) and her desire for sexual intercourse. Surgery usually shortens and narrows the vagina, possibly causing painful intercourse.

Whenever the uterus is displaced, other structures, such as the bladder, rectum, and small intestine, are affected and can protrude through the vaginal walls.

Cystocele

▌ OVERVIEW

A **cystocele** is a protrusion of the bladder through the vaginal wall (Figure 75-3). It is due to weakened pelvic structures. This protrusion can be caused by obesity, advanced age, childbearing, or genetic predisposition. The development of a cystocele is more noticeable in the postmenopausal years, when estrogen loss also weakens tissue supports and can cause relaxation of the supports.

➤ COLLABORATIVE MANAGEMENT

Assessment findings may include the following:
- Difficulty in emptying the bladder
- Urinary frequency and urgency
- Urinary tract infection
- Stress urinary incontinence (loss of urine during stressful activities such as laughing, coughing, sneezing, or lifting heavy objects)

A pelvic examination reveals a significant bulge of the anterior vaginal wall when the woman is asked to bear down. Diagnostic tests that may be ordered include cystography (to show the presence of bladder herniation), measurement of residual urine by catheterization, and urine culture and sensitivity testing (which may reveal infection caused by urinary retention).

If the client is asymptomatic or has mild symptoms, medical management is usually conservative. The health care provider may recommend a pessary to support the bladder in some clients. Estrogen therapy might be prescribed for the postmenopausal woman to prevent atrophy and weakening of vaginal walls. Kegel exercises may help strengthen perineal muscles. The nurse teaches the woman Kegel exercises, telling her to tighten and relax the perineal muscles; the woman presses the buttocks together and holds the position for at least 5 seconds. The client should repeat the exercise frequently throughout the day. An alternative exercise is to try to stop the flow of urine after urination has started and then hold the position for a few seconds before letting the urine flow again.

The health care provider may recommend surgery for severe symptoms. An **anterior colporrhaphy** (anterior repair) tightens the pelvic muscles for better bladder support. A vaginal surgical approach is used. Nursing care of a woman undergoing an anterior repair is similar to that for a woman undergoing a vaginal hysterectomy (see Operative Procedures [Uterine Leiomyomas], p. 1766).

Postoperatively, the nurse instructs the client to limit her activities, not lift anything heavier than 5 pounds, avoid strenuous exercises, and avoid sexual intercourse for 6 weeks. The woman should notify her health care provider if she has signs of infection, such as fever, persistent pain, or purulent, foul-smelling discharge. The client should keep her follow-up appointment after surgery.

Rectocele

▌ OVERVIEW

A **rectocele** is a protrusion of the rectum through a weakened vaginal wall (see Figure 75-3). This usually results from the pressure of a baby's head during a difficult delivery, a traumatic forceps delivery, or a congenital defect of the supporting tissues. Symptoms do not typically appear until the woman is older than 35 years of age.

➤ COLLABORATIVE MANAGEMENT

The woman's history may reveal symptoms of constipation, hemorrhoids, fecal impaction, and feelings of rectal or vaginal fullness. A pelvic examination may show a bulge of the posterior vaginal wall when the woman is asked to bear down. A rectal examination reveals the presence of a rectocele. A barium enema study also confirms the presence of a rectocele.

Medical management focuses on promoting bowel elimination. The health care provider usually orders a high-fiber diet, stool softeners, and laxatives. The surgical procedure that strengthens pelvic supports and reduces the bulging is **posterior colporrhaphy** (posterior repair). If both a cystocele and a rectocele are present, an **anterior and posterior colporrhaphy (anterior and posterior [A&P] repair)** is performed.

Cystocele

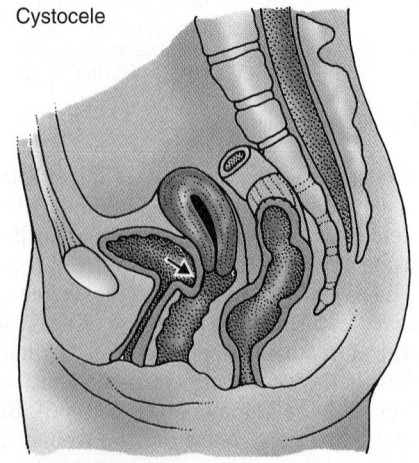

Rectocele

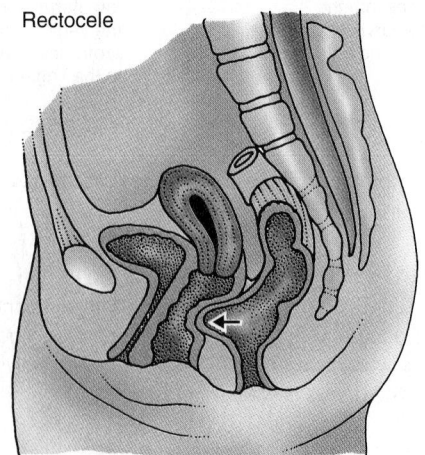

Figure 75-3 ● In cystocele, the urinary bladder is displaced downward, causing bulging of the anterior vaginal wall. In rectocele, the rectum is displaced, causing bulging of the posterior vaginal wall.

The nursing care after a posterior repair is similar to that after any rectal surgery. Postoperatively, the woman is usually given a low-residue diet to prevent bowel movements and allow time for the incision to heal. The woman is told not to strain when she does have a bowel movement so that she does not put pressure on the suture line. Bowel movements are often painful, and the client may need pain medication before having a bowel movement. Sitz baths may relieve discomfort. Postoperative instructions for the client undergoing a posterior repair are similar to those for an anterior repair.

Fistulas

■ OVERVIEW

Fistulas are abnormal openings between two adjacent organs or structures. Vaginal fistulas can occur between the vagina and the urethra (urethrovaginal), the vagina and the bladder (vesicovaginal), or the vagina and the rectum (rectovaginal). Trauma is the primary cause of fistulas, although they can result from complications of surgery, vaginal delivery complications, malignancy, or radiation therapy for cancer.

▶ COLLABORATIVE MANAGEMENT

Symptoms depend on the location of the fistula. A fistula should be considered as a possible cause if a woman's history includes the following complaints:

* Leakage of urine, flatus, or feces into the vagina
* Irritation or excoriation of the vulva and vaginal tissues
* An unpleasant odor (fecal or urine) in the vagina
* A feeling of wetness or dribbling in the vagina

Women who have fistulas may be embarrassed to seek help until symptoms are severe. The client may withdraw from social activities or from relationships with significant others as the symptoms become more difficult to manage.

Management depends on the fistula's location. Surgery is not recommended if infection or inflammation is present. Surgery may not be successful. Nursing care focuses on assisting the woman with the frequent and time-consuming perineal hygiene, including sitz baths; perineal cleaning with mild, unscented soap and water; and low-pressure douching with commercial deodorizing solutions or homemade solutions (1 teaspoon [5 mL] of nonchlorine household bleach to 1 quart [approximately 1 L] of water). The woman may need to wear sanitary napkins or disposable undergarments (such as Depends) if there is leakage of urine or feces. Other beneficial treatments may include the application of A and D ointment to excoriated tissues.

If the fistula is repaired surgically, nursing care focuses on preventing infection and avoiding stress on the repaired area (low-residue diet and administration of stool softeners for 2 weeks after rectovaginal fistula repair). Nursing care and postoperative teaching are similar to the care and teaching of the client who has a cystocele or rectocele repair (see p. 1762).

BENIGN NEOPLASMS
Functional Ovarian Cysts

Functional **ovarian cysts** can occur in a woman of any age but are rare after menopause.

■ FOLLICULAR CYSTS

Follicular cysts usually occur in young, menstruating females. These cysts are nonneoplastic and do not grow without hormonal influences. A cyst can develop when a mature follicle fails to rupture or an immature follicle fails to reabsorb follicular fluid during the second half of the menstrual cycle. The cyst is usually small (2.4 to 3.2 inches [6 to 8 cm]) and may be asymptomatic unless it ruptures. Rupture of a follicular cyst or torsion (twisting) may cause acute, severe pelvic pain. The pain usually resolves after several days of bedrest and the administration of mild analgesics. If the cyst does not rupture, it usually disappears within two or three menstrual cycles without medical intervention. If the cyst does not shrink, the health care provider may prescribe oral contraceptive pills for one or two menstrual cycles to depress ovulation. When the cyst is managed conservatively, follow-up care is necessary to confirm that it has disappeared.

If the cyst is larger than 6 to 8 cm, a neoplasm may be suspected, and further evaluation by ultrasonography or laparoscopy is necessary. Larger cysts are often associated with menstrual irregularities.

Surgery is recommended only before puberty, after menopause, or when cysts are larger than 3.2 inches (8 cm). A cystectomy (removal of the cyst) is recommended instead of an oophorectomy (removal of the ovary).

■ CORPUS LUTEUM CYSTS

Corpus luteum cysts occur after ovulation and are often associated with increased secretion of progesterone. The cysts are usually small, averaging 1.5 inches (4 cm). They are purplish red as a result of hemorrhage within the corpus luteum. Corpus luteum cysts are associated with a delay in the onset of menses and irregular or prolonged flow. They may be accompanied by unilateral low abdominal or pelvic pain that is usually described as dull or aching. If the cyst ruptures, intraperitoneal hemorrhage can occur.

Corpus luteum cysts may disappear in one or two menstrual cycles or with suppression of ovulation. The treatment is the same as that for follicular cysts.

■ THECA-LUTEIN CYSTS

Theca-lutein cysts are the least common of the functional cysts. They are associated with hydatidiform mole (molar pregnancy), occurring in 50% of these complicated pregnancies. Theca-lutein cysts develop as a result of prolonged stimulation of the ovaries by excessive amounts of human chorionic gonadotropin (hCG).

Theca-lutein cysts regress spontaneously within 3 months with the removal of the molar pregnancy or the source of excessive hCG. No other treatment is usually necessary.

■ POLYCYSTIC OVARY

Polycystic ovary, or Stein-Leventhal syndrome, results when elevated levels of luteinizing hormone (LH) cause hyperstimulation of the ovaries, which produces multiple cysts on one or both ovaries. High levels of estrogen are produced by these cysts and are unopposed by postovulatory progesterone. Endometrial hyperplasia (tissue overgrowth) or even carcinoma may result.

A typical client is obese, is hirsute (hairy), has irregular menses, and may be infertile because of lack of ovulation. Treatment depends on which disorder is of greatest concern to the woman. The best treatment is the administration of oral contraceptives because they inhibit LH production. The health care provider may advise a woman who is older than 35 years of age and no longer desires childbearing to undergo a **bilateral salpingo-oophorectomy (BSO)** (removal of both tubes and ovaries) and **hysterectomy** (removal of the uterus and cervix). Women who desire fertility can be treated with drugs such as clomiphene citrate (Clomid) to stimulate ovulation.

Other Benign Ovarian Cysts and Tumors
■ DERMOID CYSTS

Dermoid cysts are the most common germ cell tumors and are benign in more than 99% of cases. These cysts are the most common ovarian tumors of childhood, although they can develop in a female of any age.

Dermoid cysts may contain hair, sebaceous material, teeth, and other calcifications. They are usually asymptomatic unless they grow large and put pressure on other organs, such as the bladder and the bowel. The cysts develop bilaterally in some cases. They are often attached to the ovary by a pedicle (stalk).

Management of dermoid cysts is by surgical removal (cystectomy). If the cysts are not removed, they usually continue to grow and rupture, causing hemorrhage and infection.

■ OVARIAN FIBROMAS

Fibromas are the most common benign, solid ovarian neoplasms. These pearly white tumors of connective tissue origin have a low potential for becoming malignant. Fibromas can range in size from a small nodule to a mass weighing more than 50 pounds (22.7 kg). The average size is 2.4 inches (6 cm) in diameter, slightly smaller than a tennis ball. Ninety percent of fibromas are unilateral. On examination, they feel firm, have a slightly irregular contour, and are mobile. Fibromas greater than 6 cm in diameter may be associated with ascites and may cause feelings of pelvic pressure or abdominal enlargement. Unless rupture or torsion occurs, the neoplasm is usually asymptomatic. Fibromas often occur postmenopausally.

Solid ovarian neoplasms are surgically removed. The surgeon may perform an oophorectomy for borderline tumors (when there is a question of possible malignancy). Nursing care of a woman undergoing an oophorectomy is similar to that for a woman undergoing a tubal ligation. When both ovaries are removed, surgery-induced menopause occurs in a premenopausal women. As a result, a woman often experiences decreased vaginal lubrication, hot flashes, and atrophy of the vaginal epithelium. These symptoms may be treated with estrogen replacement therapy (ERT) (see Chart 75-2).

■ EPITHELIAL OVARIAN TUMORS

Epithelial ovarian tumors, serous and mucinous cystadenomas, occur in women between the ages of 30 and 50 years. Serous cystadenomas usually occur bilaterally and are more likely to become malignant than mucinous cystadenomas. Both tumors can be irregular and smooth, but mucinous cystadenomas tend to grow large, some to more than 100 pounds (45 kg).

Management of cystadenomas is usually by unilateral salpingo-oophorectomy (surgical removal of a fallopian tube and ovary), because it is often impossible to tell whether the tumor is benign or malignant. Small cystadenomas may be removed by cystectomy, but the larger ones are difficult to resect from the ovary.

Uterine Leiomyomas
■ OVERVIEW

Leiomyomas, also called **myomas** and **fibroids,** are the most commonly occurring pelvic tumors. They are benign, slow-growing solid tumors of the uterus.

■ Pathophysiology

Leiomyomas initially develop from the uterine myometrium. As they grow, fibroids stay attached to the myometrium by means of a pedicle. Leiomyomas are classified according to their position in the layers of the uterus and their anatomic position. The most common types of leiomyomas are intramural, submucosal, and subserosal (Figure 75-4).

Intramural leiomyomas are contained in the uterine wall within the myometrium. Submucosal leiomyomas protrude into the cavity of the uterus. Subserosal leiomyomas protrude through the outer surface of the uterine wall. Subserosal leiomyomas may grow laterally and extend to the broad ligament.

Although most fibroids develop within the uterine wall, about 5% may appear in the cervix. Rarely, a fibroid breaks off the pedicle and attaches to other tissues (parasitic fibroid).

■ Etiology

The cause of leiomyomas is not precisely known. Leiomyomas usually result from a localized proliferation of smooth muscle cells in their initial stages. The stimulus for proliferation may be physical or mechanical and may operate at points of maximal stress within the myometrial layer of the uterine wall. Because there are multiple points of stress caused by the contractions of the uterine muscle, multiple fibroids develop. The growth of leiomyomas may be related to estrogen stimulation; fibroids often enlarge during pregnancy and diminish in size after menopause.

■ Incidence/Prevalence

Leiomyomas occur in approximately 20% to 30% of women older than age 30. The rationale for why leiomyomas develop in some women and not in others is not known.

➤ COLLABORATIVE MANAGEMENT
● Assessment
■ HISTORY

Although most women with uterine leiomyomas are asymptomatic, abnormal bleeding is the most common complaint. Because African-American women and premenopausal women are at greatest risk for leiomyomas, any presence of

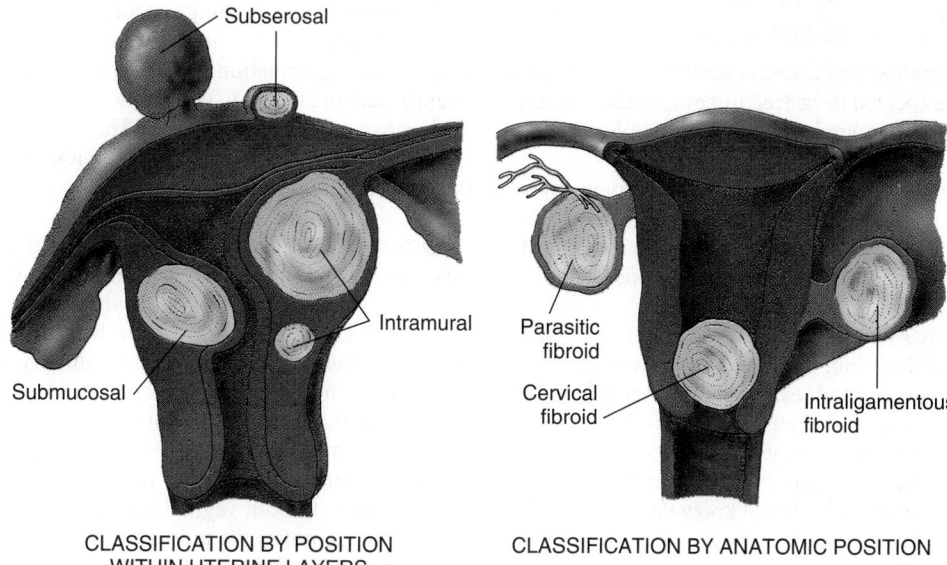

Subserosal

Intramural

Submucosal

Parasitic fibroid

Cervical fibroid

Intraligamentous fibroid

CLASSIFICATION BY POSITION
WITHIN UTERINE LAYERS

CLASSIFICATION BY ANATOMIC POSITION

Figure 75-4 ● Classification of uterine leiomyomas.

abnormal bleeding should be discussed. There may be an increase in menstrual bleeding **(menorrhagia),** the bleeding may occur between menstrual periods **(metrorrhagia),** or it may be continuous.

■ PHYSICAL ASSESSMENT/CLINICAL MANIFESTATIONS

Women with fibroids do not usually complain of pain, although acute pain may occur with torsion (twisting) of the fibroid on the pedicle. A woman may report a feeling of pelvic pressure, constipation, or urinary frequency or retention. These symptoms result when an enlarged fibroid presses on other organs. The client may also notice that her abdomen has increased in size with or without noticeable weight gain. Dyspareunia (painful sexual intercourse) and infertility have also been associated with leiomyomas.

Abdominal, vaginal, and rectal examinations usually establish the presence of a uterine enlargement that may indicate a leiomyoma. However, other diagnostic procedures may be ordered to differentiate benign lesions from malignant ones.

■ PSYCHOSOCIAL ASSESSMENT

A woman who is symptomatic may fear that she has a malignancy. She may be anxious about abnormal bleeding or her failure to conceive. She may also be concerned if surgical procedures are recommended. The nurse assesses the woman's feelings and concerns about her symptoms and fears of the unknown. If surgery is recommended, the significance of the loss of the uterus for the woman is explored.

■ LABORATORY ASSESSMENT

A complete blood count identifies iron deficiency anemia (related to bleeding). A pregnancy test may be done to determine whether pregnancy is the cause of the uterine enlargement. An endometrial biopsy may be performed to determine whether the lesion is malignant.

■ RADIOGRAPHIC ASSESSMENT

Computed tomography (CT) may be of some value. However, CT scans do not differentiate between benign and malignant myomas.

■ OTHER DIAGNOSTIC ASSESSMENT

Ultrasonography may be useful in differentiating other causes of pelvic masses, including ovarian masses and pregnancy. Culdoscopy or laparoscopy may also be of value in differentiating a uterine fibroid from an ovarian mass. These tests are described in Chapter 73.

▶ Analysis

■ COMMON NURSING DIAGNOSES AND COLLABORATIVE PROBLEMS

The most common collaborative problem for clients with leiomyomas is Potential for Hemorrhage.

■ ADDITIONAL NURSING DIAGNOSES AND COLLABORATIVE PROBLEMS

In addition to the common collaborative problems, clients with leiomyomas may have one or more of the following:
- Fear and Anxiety related to an uncertain diagnosis and potential surgical treatment
- Acute Pain related to pressure from tumors
- Anticipatory Grieving or Dysfunctional Grieving related to perceived or actual loss of the uterus or reproductive function
- Sexual Dysfunction related to dyspareunia
- Ineffective Coping related to depression as a response to treatment

● Planning and Implementation
■ POTENTIAL FOR HEMORRHAGE

PLANNING: EXPECTED OUTCOMES. The client with leiomyomas is expected to be free of complications such as hemorrhage and severe anemia from abnormal bleeding.

INTERVENTIONS. Observation of the leiomyomas over time, myomectomy, and hysterectomy are the methods of management. The choice depends on the size and symptoms of the fibroids and the woman's desire for future childbearing.

NONSURGICAL MANAGEMENT. If the client is asymptomatic or desires childbearing, the health care provider typically suggests observation and examination every 4 to 6 months. If the woman is menopausal, the fibroids usually shrink, and surgical intervention may not be necessary. However, a client who is receiving estrogen replacement therapy (ERT) for menopausal symptoms should know that the fibroids may continue to grow because of the estrogen stimulation.

SURGICAL MANAGEMENT. The treatment of leiomyomas depends on whether future childbearing is desired, the age of the woman, the size of the fibroids, and the clinical manifestations. If the woman desires childbearing, the surgeon may perform a **myomectomy** (the removal of leiomyomas with preservation of the uterus) regardless of the size, number, or location of the fibroids. The surgeon may use a laser to remove the tumors. Myomectomy is usually performed in the proliferative phase of the menstrual cycle to minimize blood loss and to avoid the possibility of interrupting an unsuspected pregnancy. A small percentage of leiomyomas that are removed recur. Nursing care is similar to that of a woman undergoing a hysterectomy, as described later in this section under Operative Procedures.

> **CONSIDERATIONS FOR OLDER ADULTS**
> Hysterectomy is the usual surgical management in the older woman who has multiple symptomatic leiomyomas. (The care of a woman undergoing a traditional total abdominal hysterectomy is described in the Clinical Pathway on pp. 1853-1854.)

PREOPERATIVE CARE. Preoperative teaching by the physician begins in his or her office. The physician's office nurse makes sure that the client can describe all of the options for surgery, the advantages and risks of surgery, preoperative and postoperative procedures, and recovery needs. With this information, the woman can make an informed consent to surgery.

Preoperative teaching is usually done on an individual basis. The nurse should explain routine preoperative procedures, including laboratory tests for baseline data and the administration of medications such as prophylactic antibiotics.

The client will need preparation for postoperative measures, including turning, coughing, deep breathing exercises (TCDB), and incentive spirometry; early ambulation; and the need for pain relief. Psychologic assessment is essential. The nurse first explores the significance of the loss of the uterus for the client. She may feel a great loss if she wishes to retain her childbearing ability, relates her uterus to her self-image and femininity, or believes that her sexual function is related to her uterus. Often a woman has misconceptions about the

effects of hysterectomy (e.g., associating it with masculinization and weight gain). The nurse identifies misconceptions so that correct information can be provided and assesses the client's support system. The client may fear rejection by her husband or other sexual partner. The nurse encourages inclusion of the partner in all teaching sessions unless this practice is not culturally acceptable.

OPERATIVE PROCEDURES. A **total abdominal hysterectomy (TAH)** is usually performed for leiomyomas larger than the gestational size of a 12-week pregnancy. The uterus and cervix are removed through a horizontal incision (traditional approach) or via laparoscopic surgery, which requires a very small umbilical incision.

A uterus that has smaller fibroids may be removed via a **total vaginal hysterectomy (TVH)**. The surgeon removes the uterus and cervix through the vagina without an external surgical incision. In both vaginal and abdominal hysterectomies, the surgeon removes the uterus from the five supporting ligaments, which are then attached to the vaginal cuff so that normal depth of the vagina is maintained (Table 75-5).

In some cases (e.g., treatment of submucous fibroids and menorrhagia), hysterectomy has been replaced by minimally invasive uterine surgery such as a **transcervical endometrial resection (TCER)**. A hysteroscope is inserted into the uterus, and the endometrium is destroyed, usually with a diathermy resectoscope (similar to the scope used with prostate surgery). Complications specific to hysteroscopic surgery include the following:

- Fluid overload (fluid used to distend the uterine cavity can be absorbed)
- Embolism
- Hemorrhage
- Perforation of the uterus, bowel, or bladder and ureter injury
- Persistent increased menstrual bleeding
- Incomplete suppression of menstruation

These complications occur less commonly when the procedure is performed by an experienced surgeon. In addition, there is a small risk of subsequent pregnancy and the possibility of cancer developing in the scar. Hysterectomy is still

---

TABLE 75-5 • COMMON GYNECOLOGIC SURGERIES

TOTAL HYSTERECTOMY
All of the uterus, including the cervix, is removed. The procedure may be vaginal abdominal or laparoscopic.

SUBTOTAL HYSTERECTOMY
All of the uterus, except the cervix, is removed. This procedure is rarely performed.

BILATERAL SALPINGO-OOPHORECTOMY
Fallopian tubes and ovaries are removed.

PANHYSTERECTOMY
Total abdominal hysterectomy and bilateral salpingo-oophorectomy. The uterus, ovaries, and fallopian tubes are removed adominally.

RADICAL HYSTERECTOMY
All of the uterus is removed abdominally. The lymph nodes, the upper third of the vagina, and the surrounding tissues (parametrium) are also removed.

the procedure of choice for women who have coexisting problems, especially those with malignancy or symptomatic uterovaginal prolapse.

POSTOPERATIVE CARE. Postoperative care of the woman who has undergone a TAH is similar to that of any client who has undergone abdominal surgery (see Chapter 19). For clients who have undergone an abdominal hysterectomy, the nurse (Chart 75-9):

- Assesses vaginal bleeding (there should be less than one saturated perineal pad in 4 hours)
- Assesses abdominal bleeding at the incision site (a small amount is normal)
- Checks the incision for intactness
- Maintains the urethral catheter (Foley catheter), if placed, usually for 24 hours or less for a traditional surgical approach
- Offers pain medications as ordered for the abdominal pain

Specific interventions for a vaginal hysterectomy include the following:

- Assessment of vaginal bleeding (there should be less than one saturated pad in 4 hours)
- Foley catheter care
- Perineal care (sitz baths or ice packs)

The surgeon usually removes the abdominal sutures or clips at the time of the first postoperative visit, whereas vaginal sutures are usually absorbed. The nurse recognizes and monitors for complications associated with hysterectomies (Table 75-6).

CHART 75-9

FOCUSED ASSESSMENT *of*
The Client After Total Abdominal Hysterectomy

Assess cardiovascular, respiratory, renal, and gastrointestinal status, including:
- Vital signs
- Heart, lung, and bowel sounds
- Urine output
- Temperature and color of the skin
- Red blood cell, hemoglobin, and hematocrit levels
- Activity tolerance
- Dressing and drains for color and amount of drainage
- Peripads for vaginal bleeding and clots
- Fluid intake (IVs until bowel sounds return and client is tolerating oral intake)
- Signs of thrombophlebitis

Use the following interventions to prevent postoperative complications:
- Cough and deep breathing exercises
- Incentive spirometry
- Sequential compression devices
- Ambulation
- Avoidance of heavy lifting or strenuous activity

Assess the home care teaching needs of the client related to the illness and surgery, including:
- Physiologic effects of the surgery
- Signs of symptoms to report
- Side or toxic effects of medications
- Activity limitations related to driving and use of stairs
- Follow-up care
- Postoperative restrictions related to sexual activity, use of tampons, and bathing
- Care of wound and/or drains

Assess the client's coping skills and reaction to the diagnosis and surgical procedure.

CRITICAL THINKING CHALLENGE

You are a nurse in the postanesthesia care unit (PACU) assigned to the care of an older adult who has undergone a total abdominal hysterectomy and bilateral salpingo-oophorectomy via a horizontal abdominal incision. On initial assessment, you note that her vital signs are within baseline, the dressing is dry and intact, and she has a scant amount of blood on her perineal pad. Immediately before she is to be transferred to the surgical unit, you find that her blood pressure has dropped from 124/78 to 108/60. Her pulse has increased from 80 to 96 within the past hour.
- Should you continue with plans to transfer the client to the surgical unit, since her vital signs are still within normal limits? Why or why not?
- What other assessments should you perform at this time?
- What might explain the change in her vital signs?

For suggested answer guidelines, go to SIMON http://www.wbsaunders.com/SIMON/Iggy/.

CONSIDERATIONS FOR OLDER ADULTS

Older women are more at risk for all complications, particularly pulmonary embolism. Obese women are more at risk for thromboembolism. Psychologic complications can occur with both abdominal and vaginal procedures. Depression is the most frequent reaction reported. Other reactions are perceived loss of femininity and decreased libido. Loss of femininity may be the problem if a woman was interested in her appearance before surgery but afterward has no interest, even when she is feeling better. Decreased sexual desire is often temporary, if it occurs, and is usually related to discomfort.

Community-Based Care

The client with uterine leiomyomas is managed on an ambulatory care basis unless surgical intervention is required. After hospital discharge, the client typically returns to her home.

HOME CARE MANAGEMENT

Planning for home care management begins at the time of admission. The woman is usually discharged to the home setting 1 to 2 days after a traditional TAH, depending on the age and

---

TABLE 75-6 •	COMMON POSTOPERATIVE COMPLICATIONS OF TRADITIONAL ABDOMINAL AND VAGINAL HYSTERECTOMIES

TRADITIONAL ABDOMINAL HYSTERECTOMY
- Intestinal obstruction (paralytic ileus)
- Thromboembolism
- Atelectasis
- Pneumonia
- Wound dehiscence (especially in obese clients)
- Urinary retention

VAGINAL HYSTERECTOMY
- Hemorrhage
- Urinary tract complications, especially infection or retention
- Wound infection
- Urinary retention

general health of the client. TVH, laparoscopic surgery, or TCER may be performed as same-day surgery in an ambulatory setting. The client undergoing a hysterectomy should be told to avoid or limit stair climbing for 1 month. She is advised to avoid tub baths (which may promote infection) and sitting for long periods (which causes pooling of blood in the pelvic vessels). The nurse also teaches the client to avoid engaging in strenuous activity or lifting anything weighing more than 5 pounds (2.3 kg). Some health care providers also restrict driving for 4 to 6 weeks.

■ HEALTH TEACHING

The nurse teaches the woman who has undergone a hysterectomy about the following (see Chart 75-9):
* The physical changes to be expected
* Exercise and activities
* Diet
* Sexual activity
* Wound care (if any)
* Complications
* Follow-up care

The physical changes include cessation of menses, inability to become pregnant, weakness and fatigue during convalescence (may last 2 to 3 months), and absence of menopausal symptoms unless the ovaries are also removed. Moderate exercise, such as walking, is encouraged, but active sports, such as jogging and aerobic exercise, should be avoided for at least 1 month.

The nurse teaches the client to consume foods that aid in healing tissues, such as foods high in protein, iron, and vitamin C. The nurse also reminds her to avoid sexual intercourse for 4 to 6 weeks. The first coital activity may cause some tenderness or pain because the vaginal walls are tight and need to be stretched. Water-soluble lubricants can decrease discomfort. The client should be taught the signs of complications, particularly infection. An appointment for follow-up medical care is scheduled for 1 week postoperatively.

Women who have undergone a hysterectomy need information about possible emotional reactions. Generally, women adjust well to surgery if they:
* Have completed childbearing
* Work
* Have interests outside the home
* Have no misconceptions about the effects of hysterectomy
* Have support from the family, especially the husband or their sexual partner

Reactions may be different after vaginal and abdominal procedures, because women who have undergone a vaginal hysterectomy have no external focus (no obvious change in body image) for their feelings. Psychologic reactions can occur 3 months to 3 years after surgery. Women identified as being at high risk for psychologic problems may need long-term follow-up care or referral. Women may need to be counseled about signs of depression. Intermittent sadness is normal, but continued feelings of low self-esteem or loss of interest or pleasure in usual activities and pastimes is not normal and should be evaluated. The incidence of psychologic reactions often decreases after the nurse provides written materials and discusses the positive forces in the client's life with her and her family or significant others.

■ HEALTH CARE RESOURCES

Usually no special home equipment is needed for a woman who has undergone a hysterectomy. A home care nurse may be needed to assess and monitor the older client's postoperative progress if other conditions (e.g., uncontrolled diabetes) are present. Financial assistance may be needed, and referral to the hospital's department of social services or case management department may be indicated if the woman has no insurance coverage. The nurse can provide a referral for psychologic or sexual counseling if potential problems are identified before discharge.

● Evaluation: Outcomes

NOC The nurse evaluates the care of the client who has undergone surgery for leiomyomas on the basis of the identified nursing diagnoses and collaborative problems. The expected outcomes include that the client will:
* Be free of hemorrhage
* State the role of the reproductive system and the changes that occur after a hysterectomy (without misconceptions)
* Recover from surgery without complications
* Demonstrate a positive psychologic adjustment to surgery as evidenced by the absence of depression and the presence of a positive self-concept
* Resume sexual activities at her previous level of satisfaction

Bartholin's Cysts

■ OVERVIEW

Bartholin's cysts are one of the most common disorders of the vulva. The cysts result from obstruction of a duct. The secretory function of the gland continues, and the fluid fills up the obstructed duct. The cause of the obstruction may be infection, congenital stenosis or atresia, thickened mucus near the ductal opening, or mechanical trauma, such as lacerations or episiotomy.

▶ COLLABORATIVE MANAGEMENT

● Assessment

The client may be asymptomatic if the cyst is small, but a history may reveal complaints of dyspareunia, inadequate genital lubrication, or a mass in the perineal area. A large cyst usually causes constant localized pain and may cause difficulty walking or sitting. Physical examination of the vulva reveals a swelling immediately beneath the skin in the posterior portion of the vulva. The cyst may appear brown or sanguineous, depending on its contents. Usually the cyst is unilateral and ranges from $3/8$ to 4 inches (1 to 10 cm) in size.

If the cyst is draining, the health care provider usually requests that the fluid be sent to the laboratory for culture (for gonorrhea and aerobic and anaerobic organisms) and sensitivity testing. If the woman is older than 40 years of age, a specimen of the cyst should be sent for pathologic examination to determine whether the lesion is benign or malignant.

● Interventions

If the woman is asymptomatic, no interventions are necessary. If the cysts are symptomatic, simple incision and drainage

(I&D) may provide temporary relief; however, cysts tend to recur as the opening of the duct becomes obstructed again. Usually the health care provider establishes a permanent opening for drainage. Marsupialization (formation of a pouch that is a new duct opening) is accomplished using local, regional, or general anesthesia. Any postoperative discomfort may be relieved by the administration of analgesics and sitz baths. The health care provider may prescribe prophylactic antibiotics.

Bartholin's cysts may become infected. Abscesses are formed when bacteria, such as *Escherichia coli* or *Staphylococcus aureus*, enter the duct, resulting in infection that closes the duct. An abscess usually ruptures spontaneously within 72 hours of formation. Interventions for the woman with an abscess include the administration of analgesics and application of moist heat (sitz baths or hot wet packs) to the vulva. The health care provider usually orders broad-spectrum antibiotics to treat the infection. I&D of the abscess may provide temporary relief.

The health care provider may totally excise the Bartholin's glands in women older than 40 years of age when cancer is suspected or if repeated infections with abscess formation occur. Postoperative interventions include the following:

- Application of ice packs or sitz baths several times a day for comfort and promotion of healing
- Administration of analgesics for pain, if needed
- Prophylactic administration of antibiotics
- Assessment of the incision for signs of healing or infection

Cervical Polyps

Cervical polyps are pedunculated (on stalks) tumors arising from the mucosa and extending to the opening of the cervical os. The cause is unknown, although polyps result from a hyperplastic condition of the endocervical epithelium. They may also be due to inflammation. Polyps are the most common benign neoplastic growth of the cervix. Cervical polyps are most common in multiparous women older than 40 years of age.

A woman may be asymptomatic, or a history may reveal complaints of premenstrual or postmenstrual bleeding or bleeding after coitus. A speculum examination may reveal small ($\frac{3}{8}$ to $1\frac{1}{2}$-inch [1- to 4-cm]) single or multiple polyps. They are bright red; have a soft, fragile consistency; and may bleed when touched.

Polyp removal is easily accomplished as an office procedure. The base of the polyp can be grasped with a clamp, and the polyp can be twisted off and sent to the pathology laboratory for evaluation. Electrocautery or chemical cautery usually stops any bleeding at the site of removal. After the procedure, the nurse may instruct the client to avoid tampon use, douches, and sexual intercourse for a week or until healing has taken place.

MALIGNANT NEOPLASMS
Endometrial Cancer
◼ OVERVIEW

Endometrial cancer (cancer of the uterus) is one of the most commonly occurring reproductive cancers (American Cancer Society, 2000). This type of cancer is asymptomatic in its early development and has a good prognosis in 80% to 90% of cases.

> ### ✤ CONSIDERATIONS FOR OLDER ADULTS
> Endometrial cancer is a slow-growing tumor primarily occurring in postmenopausal women. The average age at onset is 61 years. The incidence declines after the age of 70 years (DeStefano & Bertin-Matson, 1996).

◼ Pathophysiology

Adenocarcinoma of the endometrium accounts for 75% to 80% of all endometrial cancers. It arises from the glandular component of the endometrial mucosa and may be preceded by endometrial hyperplasia (tissue overgrowth). The initial growth of the cancer is within the uterine cavity, followed by extension into the myometrium and the cervix. Spread outside the uterus occurs as follows:

- Through lymphatic spread to the ovaries and parametrial, pelvic, inguinal, and para-aortic lymph nodes
- By hematogenous metastasis (spread by blood) to the lungs, liver, or bone
- By transtubal or intra-abdominal spread to the peritoneal cavity

◼ Etiology

Risk factors associated with endometrial cancer include obesity, diabetes mellitus, hypertension, a history of uterine polyps, a history of infertility, nulliparity and polycystic ovary disease. Estrogen stimulation, including unopposed menopausal estrogen replacement therapy (ERT), late menopause (after age 52 years), postmenopausal bleeding, and a family history of uterine cancer also predispose a woman to endometrial cancer. Table 75-7 compares the risk factors for endometrial cancer with those for other female reproductive cancers.

◼ Incidence/Prevalence

The National Cancer Institute (NCI) estimates that more than 35,000 new cases of endometrial cancer occur annually in the United States (American Cancer Society, 2000). Thus about 1 of every 100 women in the United States has endometrial cancer.

> ### 〰 CULTURAL CONSIDERATIONS
> Endometrial cancer occurs more often in Caucasian women than in African-American women and typically in postmenopausal women ages 50 to 65 years. Survival rates differ between Caucasian and African-American women with endometrial cancer; Caucasian women have higher survival rates (American Cancer Society, 2000). The difference in survival rates appears to be related to the occurrence of higher-grade lesions and more aggressive cell types in African-American women.

▶ COLLABORATIVE MANAGEMENT
◗ Assessment

The primary symptom of endometrial cancer is postmenopausal bleeding. In addition, the woman may complain of a watery, serosanguineous vaginal discharge, low back or

TABLE 75-7 • RISK FACTORS FOR CANCERS OF THE REPRODUCTIVE SYSTEM

Risk Factor	Endometrial Cancer	Cervical Cancer	Ovarian Cancer	Vulvar Cancer	Vaginal Cancer	Fallopian Tube Cancer	Gestational Trophoblastic Disease
Age	50-65 yr of age	CIS: 30-40 yr of age; Invasive: 40-60 yr of age	Infrequent before 35 yr of age; range usually is 40-65 yr of age	After 40 yr of age; peak is 60-70 yr of age	Most after 50 yr of age; adenocarcinoma: 14-30 yr of age	After 50 yr of age; range is 18-80 yr of age	After 40 yr of age; before 20 yr of age
Family history	Increased risk	—	Increased risk	—	DES exposure in utero	—	—
Personal history	Diabetes, hypertension	—	Breast, bowel, or endometrial cancer	Cervical cancer, diabetes, vulvar disease	Vulvar or cervical cancer	Ovarian or uterine cancer, infertility	Previous molar pregnancy (3%-5%)
Race	Caucasians	African Americans, Native Americans	Caucasians	—	—	—	Asian-Americans; Mexican-Americans
Mother's age at birth	—	<18 yr	>30 yr	—	—	—	—
Body size	Obesity	—	—	Possibly obesity	—	—	—
Parity	Nulliparity	Multiparity	Nulliparity	—	Multiparity	Nulliparity	—
Estrogen use	Prolonged use; >3 yr menopausally	Possibly long-term birth control pill use	—	—	—	—	—
Smoking	Possibly increased risk	Possibly double the risk	—	—	—	—	—
Infection (STD)	—	Possibly STD (herpes simplex virus type 2 or papillomavirus infection)	—	Possibly STD (papillomavirus infection)	STD (herpes simplex virus type 2 or papillomavirus infection)	PID, chronic salpingitis	Exposure to infectious agents

CIS, Carcinoma in situ; *DES*, diethylstilbestrol; *PID*, pelvic inflammatory disease; *STD*, sexually transmitted disease.

abdominal pain, and low pelvic pain (caused by pressure of the enlarged uterus). A pelvic examination may reveal the presence of a palpable uterine mass or uterine polyp. The uterus is enlarged if the cancer is in an advanced stage.

Before a diagnosis is made, the client may deny that the symptoms are related to cancer. During the diagnostic phase, the woman may express fears and concerns about having a malignancy. After the diagnosis is confirmed, she may express disbelief, anger, depression, anxiety, or withdrawal behaviors.

The health care provider orders basic diagnostic tests to determine the client's overall status. The results of the tests may also indicate the presence of metastasis. These tests include the following:

- Chest x-ray examination to detect metastasis
- Intravenous pyelography (IVP), or excretory urography, to assess renal function and to assess for renal metastasis
- Barium enema study to assess for intestinal metastasis
- Computed tomography (CT) of the pelvis to identify the origin and spread of the tumor
- Lymphangiography to assess for lymph node metastasis
- Liver and bone scans to assess for distant metastasis

Fractional dilation and curettage (D&C [scraping individual sections of the uterus]) and endometrial biopsy are the definitive diagnostic procedures for endometrial cancer. Other tests that may be useful for some clients include proctosigmoidoscopy, ultrasonography, and hysteroscopy (examination of the uterus via an endoscope).

Interventions

Nonsurgical interventions (radiation therapy and chemotherapy) and surgery may be used alone or in combination, depending on the stage of the cancer.

NONSURGICAL MANAGEMENT. Radiation therapy and chemotherapy are the two major nonsurgical methods used to treat endometrial cancer.

RADIATION THERAPY. The health care provider orders radiation therapy (external and internal) if the stage of cancer is hard to determine and if surgery is planned for stage II and III cancers. Clients usually receive radiation therapy for 6 weeks preoperatively to destroy cancer cells in the pericervical lymphatics and to inhibit recurrence.

Intracavitary Radiation. If intracavitary radiation therapy (IRT [brachytherapy]) is selected, the radiologist places an applicator within the woman's uterus through the vagina while she is anesthetized. After the correct position of the applicator is confirmed by x-ray examination, the client is taken to the hospital room and a radiologist places a radioactive isotope in the applicator, which remains for 1 to 3 days. Before the procedure, the nurse instructs the client on postprocedure activities, such as deep breathing and leg exercises. While the radioactive implant is in place, the woman is strictly isolated, usually in a private room. The nurse informs the client that she is restricted to bedrest on her back with the head of the bed flat or slightly elevated (20 degrees or less). Movement in bed is restricted to prevent dislodgment of the radioactive source.

A Foley catheter is inserted into the bladder to prevent dislodgment of the implant, which can be caused by a full bladder or attempts to void. The nurse carefully assesses the skin for breakdown over bony pressure points during the activity restriction period. The client is usually placed on a low-residue diet (to prevent bowel movements that might dislodge the implant), and fluid intake is encouraged (to prevent stasis of urine and possible infection). The health care provider usually prescribes the following:

- Antiemetics
- Broad-spectrum antibiotics (to prevent bladder infections)
- Tranquilizers (to help the client relax)
- Analgesics
- Heparin or Lovenox (to prevent thromboembolism)
- Antidiarrheal medications (to prevent bowel movements)

Radiation precautions are practiced while the implant is in place. The nurse organizes care so that minimal time is spent at the bedside. Care is given as far away from the radioactive source as possible and behind lead shields when possible. Nurses who are pregnant or attempting to become pregnant should not be assigned to these clients. Visitors are restricted to brief visits, and pregnant women and children younger than 18 years should not be allowed to visit.

External Radiation. External radiation therapy may be used to treat all stages of endometrial cancer. It is usually used in combination with surgery, preoperatively or postoperatively. Depending on the extent of the tumor, external radiation is given on an ambulatory care basis for 4 to 6 weeks. The lateral extensions of the tumor in the parametrium and pelvic wall nodes are irradiated (see also Chapter 25). Specific instructions for the woman undergoing external radiation for endometrial cancer include monitoring for signs of skin breakdown, especially in the perineal area, no sunbathing, and no bathing over the markings outlining the treatment site. The nurse informs the client that cystitis and diarrhea are common complications, as are nutritional problems that result from anorexia.

CHEMOTHERAPY. Chemotherapy is used as a palliative treatment in advanced and recurrent disease. Chemotherapeutic agents used for palliative treatment of endometrial cancer include doxorubicin (Adriamycin), cisplatin, and cyclophosphamide (Cytoxan, Procytox✦). These agents are used as single agents or in combination, and the length of treatment and dosage are determined by the woman's response to treatment. Chapter 25 discusses nursing interventions for clients receiving chemotherapy.

OTHER DRUG THERAPY. The health care provider may choose progestational therapy for stage I and II cancers that are estrogen dependent and for palliative treatment of stage IV cancer. The hormones commonly prescribed are medroxyprogesterone acetate (Depo-Provera) and megestrol acetate (Megace). Tamoxifen citrate (Nolvadex✦, Tamofen✦), an antiestrogen, is also used. The progestational agents do not cause acute side effects, but nausea and vomiting and hot flashes are associated with tamoxifen.

SURGICAL MANAGEMENT. The surgeon typically performs a total abdominal hysterectomy (removal of the uterus and cervix) and bilateral salpingo-oophorectomy (removal of both tubes and ovaries) for stage I tumors without cervical involvement. A radical hysterectomy (see Table 75-5) with bilateral pelvic lymph node dissection is performed for stage II cancer. Nursing care for a radical hysterectomy is essentially the same as that for a total abdominal hysterectomy except that the woman's hospitalization is usually longer and her convalescence may be extended.

PSYCHOSOCIAL SUPPORT. Women need to discuss their concerns about the presence of cancer and the potential for recurrence. The nurse provides emotional support and tries to create an atmosphere that encourages the woman to ask questions or express her fears and concerns. Family members or significant others are included in discussions when possible.

Reactions to radiation therapy vary. Some women may feel radioactive or "unclean" after treatments and may exhibit withdrawal behaviors. The nurse needs to correct such misconceptions.

Women who have chemotherapy may be upset if alopecia (hair loss) occurs. The nurse warns the client of this possibility before treatment starts. Wigs, scarves, or turbans can be worn until regrowth occurs.

● Community-Based Care

The client with endometrial cancer is managed at home unless surgery is indicated. After surgery, the client is usually discharged to her home.

■ HOME CARE MANAGEMENT

Home care after surgery for endometrial cancer is the same as that after a hysterectomy (see Operative Procedures [Uterine Leiomyomas], p. 1766). Women who are receiving chemotherapy or external radiation therapy are usually treated on an ambulatory care basis, which may mean that the woman and her family have to plan daily activities around trips to the clinic or the health care provider's office. If the tumor recurs and cure is not likely, the client and her family need to think about hospice care and whether the woman can be cared for in the home.

■ HEALTH TEACHING

For the woman who has undergone a hysterectomy for endometrial cancer, the teaching plan is the same as that for the woman who has undergone a hysterectomy for uterine leiomyomas (see Postoperative Care, p. 1767). Side effects to report to the health care provider include vaginal or rectal bleeding, foul-smelling discharge, abdominal pain or distention, and hematuria.

The high dose of radiation causes sterility, and vaginal shrinkage can occur. Vaginal dilators can be used with water-soluble lubricants for 10 min/day until sexual activity resumes (in 10 days to 6 weeks). The woman is not radioactive, and her partner will not "catch" cancer from engaging in sexual intercourse. A normal diet may be resumed.

All prescribed medications are reviewed, including the dosage and schedule of administration, therapeutic effects, and side effects. The nurse also emphasizes the importance of keeping appointments for follow-up care.

Often women experience emotional crises because of the physical effects of cancer treatments. Radical hysterectomy may be seen as mutilating, and chemotherapy may affect the woman's body image if hair loss occurs. A woman may exhibit a grief reaction to this perceived change in body image.

The feelings of loss depend on the visibility of the loss, the function of the loss, and the amount of emotional investment. The nurse may need to help the woman adapt to the body changes. One way to do this is to encourage self-care as soon as the woman's condition is stable. A calm, accepting attitude may also be helpful.

Death can occur with or without treatment. Women and their families or significant others have concerns about recurrence. All want to pass the 5-year survival mark without a recurrence. If there is a recurrence, the woman may be hostile and may exhibit characteristics of a grief reaction. The nurse encourages clients to ventilate their feelings. Response to loss and grieving are discussed in Chapter 9.

■ HEALTH CARE RESOURCES

In the United States, local American Cancer Society chapters provide written materials about endometrial cancer, as well as information about local support groups. If the client is in the terminal stages of cancer, hospice care may be appropriate (see Chapter 9). If nursing care is needed at home, the hospital nurse or case manager refers the client and her family to a community health or home care agency. A referral to a social services agency may be needed if the woman is unable to meet the financial demands of treatment and long-term follow-up.

Cervical Cancer

■ OVERVIEW

Cervical cancer is one of the most common reproductive cancers among women in the United States. Cervical cancer is also the third most common cause of death related to reproductive cancers (American Cancer Society, 2000). Death rates for cervical cancer have dropped 50% in the past two decades, primarily because of the availability of Pap tests for screening of premalignant cervical changes. However, among some ethnic/racial groups, Pap smears are not common as a screening test for cervical cancer. For example, in a study by Kim et al. (1999), only 34% of Korean-American women in the sample reported having a Pap smear (see the Evidence-Based Practice for Nursing box on p. 1773).

■ Pathophysiology

Cervical cancer may be described as preinvasive or invasive. Preinvasive cancer is limited to the cervix; invasive cancer is in the cervix and other pelvic structures. Preinvasive lesions usually originate in the area called the *transformation zone* (Figure 75-5). This area includes the squamocolumnar junction, which is located near the external cervical os, where changes in the squamous and columnar (glandular) epithelium normally occur. Abnormal squamous epithelium can also be found in this zone. These cells can develop into invasive carcinoma.

These premalignant changes can be described on a continuum from dysplasia—the earliest premalignant change—to carcinoma in situ (CIS), the most advanced premalignant change. Preinvasive cancers can also be designated by the term *cervical intraepithelial neoplasia (CIN)* and classified according to severity:

- CIN I: mild
- CIN II: moderate
- CIN III: severe to carcinoma in situ

Squamous cell cancers spread by direct extension to the vaginal mucosa, lower uterine segment, parametrium, pelvic wall, bladder, and bowel. Metastasis is usually confined to the pelvis, but distant metastases can occur through lymphatic spread and, rarely, via the circulatory system to the liver, lungs, or bones. Table 75-8 shows the clinical stages of cancer of the cervix.

Etiology

The exact cause of squamous cell cervical cancer is unknown, but numerous factors may be involved. An association has been identified with early and frequent sexual contact and with viral infections of the cervix, such as herpes simplex virus type 2, cytomegalovirus, and papillomavirus.

Risk factors associated with cervical cancer include low socioeconomic status, early age at first sexual contact or first pregnancy, multiple sexual partners, and intrauterine exposure to diethylstilbestrol (DES). Other possible risk factors include sexual intercourse with men whose previous sexual partners had cervical cancer, use of oral contraceptives, cigarette smoking, and vitamin A and C deficiencies. Nulliparity and diabetes mellitus are also associated with adenocarcinoma of the cervix.

EVIDENCE-BASED PRACTICE FOR NURSING

Do Korean-American women have Pap smears for screening of cervical cancer?

Kim, K., et al. (1999). Cervical cancer screening knowledge and practices among Korean-American women. *Cancer Nursing, 22*(4), 297-302.

The nursing researchers in this study surveyed 159 Korean-American women between 40 and 69 years of age to determine if they knew what a Pap smear was and if they had ever had one. The 1987 Cancer Control Supplement questionnaire was translated into Korean and used to collect the data. Twenty-six respondents had never heard of the Pap smear, and only 34% reported ever having one. The most commonly cited reason for not having a Pap test was the absence of disease symptoms.

Critique. The researchers undertook a study to examine possible differences among a group of non-Caucasian women. Although this was a descriptive study, it paves the way for further study of other non-Caucasian health practices.

Implications for Nursing. The findings of this study have implications for nurses who work with this population and other culturally diverse groups. Health education about Pap smears is crucial if cervical cancer is to be found in its earliest stage to ensure a positive outcome. Some subjects thought that the Pap smear was appropriate as a treatment rather than a health promotion/illness prevention intervention.

CULTURAL CONSIDERATIONS

The rate of cervical cancer is twice as high for African-American women as for Caucasian women. The mortality rate is more than twice as high for African-American women as for Caucasian women (American Cancer Society, 2000).

Incidence/Prevalence

The National Cancer Institute (NCI) estimates that there are more than 14,000 new cases of cervical cancer (excluding CIS) and more than 4400 deaths in the United States annually. Although the rate of invasive cervical cancer has decreased over the last several decades, it has increased in recent years in women younger than 50 years of age (American Cancer Society, 2000).

CIN occurs mainly in young women; the peak incidence of dysplasia occurs in clients in their mid-20s. CIS occurs in

---

TABLE 75-8 • CLINICAL STAGES OF CANCER OF THE CERVIX

Stage	Characteristics
I	Carcinoma is strictly confined to cervix (extension to corpus should be disregarded)
Ia	Preclinical carcinoma
Ia1	Minimal microscopically evident stromal invasion
Ia2	Microscopic lesions no more than 5-mm depth measured from base of epithelium surface or glandular surface from which it originates, and horizontal spread not to exceed 7 mm
Ib	All other cases of stage I; occult cancer should be marked "occ"
II	Carcinoma extends beyond cervix but has not extended to pelvic wall; it involves vagina, but not as far as lower third
IIa	No obvious parametrial involvement
IIb	Obvious parametrial involvement
III	Carcinoma has extended to pelvic wall; on rectal examination, there is no cancer-free space between tumor and pelvic wall; tumor involves lower third of vagina; all cases with hydronephrosis or nonfunctioning kidney should be included unless they are known to be due to another cause
IIIa	No extension to pelvic wall, but involvement of lower third of vagina
IIIb	Extension to pelvic wall, or hydronephrosis or nonfunctioning kidney due to tumor
IV	Carcinoma has extended beyond true pelvis or has clinically involved mucosa of bladder or rectum
IVa	Spread of growth to adjacent pelvic organs
IVb	Spread to distant organs

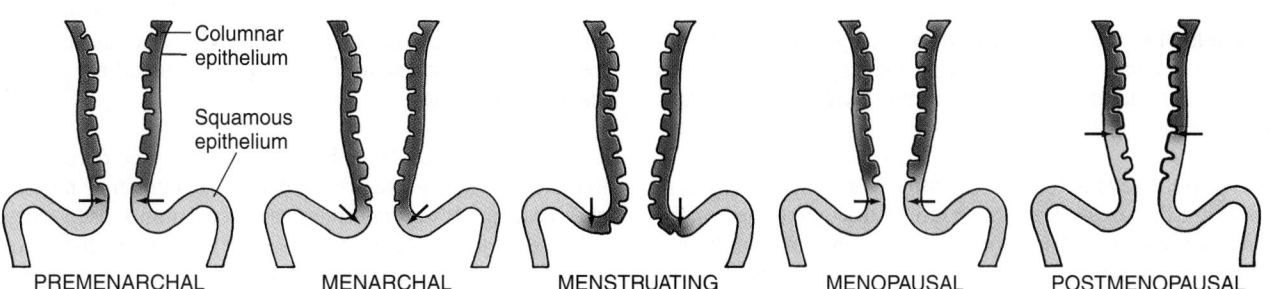

PREMENARCHAL   MENARCHAL   MENSTRUATING   MENOPAUSAL   POSTMENOPAUSAL

Columnar epithelium
Squamous epithelium

Figure 75-5 ● The location of the transformation zone at various stages of adult development.

women about 30 years old, and invasive cancer occurs most commonly in the late 40s.

► COLLABORATIVE MANAGEMENT

▶ Assessment

The woman who has preinvasive cancer is often asymptomatic. The classic symptom of invasive cancer is painless vaginal bleeding. The bleeding may start as spotting between menstrual periods or after coitus or douching. As the malignancy grows, the bleeding increases in frequency, duration, and amount. It may become continuous.

The woman may also complain of a watery, blood-tinged vaginal discharge that may become dark and foul smelling as the disease progresses. Leg pain (along the sciatic nerve) or unilateral swelling of a leg may be a late symptom or may indicate recurrent disease. Other signs of recurrence or metastasis (spread) may include unexplained weight loss, pelvic pain (caused by pressure of the tumor on the bladder or the bowel), dysuria (painful urination), hematuria (bloody urine), rectal bleeding, chest pain, and coughing. A physical examination may not reveal any abnormalities in early preinvasive cervical cancer; the internal pelvic examination may identify late-stage disease.

Laboratory assessment of the woman begins with a Pap smear. If the results are abnormal, the smear is repeated before further studies are done. If abnormal tissue is detected on a subsequent Pap test, further testing is done. If invasive cervical cancer is diagnosed, laboratory tests such as those described earlier for the investigation of endometrial cancer are performed (see Assessment, p. 1769).

The health care provider may perform a colposcopic examination to view the transformation zone, where dysplasia, cervical intraepithelial neoplasia (CIN), and carcinoma in situ (CIS) usually originate. If abnormal tissue is recognized, multiple biopsies of the cervical tissue are performed (see Chapter 73).

The health care provider usually performs an endocervical curettage (scraping of the endocervix from the internal to the external os) as well. Because this procedure is uncomfortable, the nurse may need to encourage the woman to use relaxation or breathing exercises to cope with the cramping and pain. A small amount of bleeding is expected and may occur for up to 2 weeks after the biopsies.

▶ Interventions

Nursing care of the client with cervical cancer is similar to that for endometrial cancer. The only interventions discussed here are those that differ from those for the client with endometrial cancer.

NONSURGICAL MANAGEMENT. Nonsurgical interventions for cervical cancer depend on the stage of disease and may include laser therapy, cryosurgery, radiation therapy, chemotherapy, or hysterectomy.

LASER THERAPY. Laser therapy is an ambulatory care procedure that is used whenever all of the boundaries of the lesion are visible under colposcopic examination and the endocervical curettage findings are normal. In laser therapy, the invisible beam is directed to the abnormal tissues, where en-

ergy from the beam is absorbed by the fluid in the tissues, causing them to vaporize. There is usually a small amount of bleeding associated with the procedure. The woman may have a slight vaginal discharge, and healing occurs in 6 to 12 weeks.

CRYOSURGERY. Cryosurgery is another common treatment for CIN. A probe is placed against the cervix to cause freezing of the tissues and subsequent necrosis. Although this treatment can also be considered a type of surgery, no anesthesia is required. After the procedure, the client may experience slight cramping. The woman has a heavy watery discharge for several weeks after the procedure; she should avoid sexual intercourse and the use of tampons while discharge is present because the cervix is friable and these precautions will decrease the risk of infection.

RADIATION THERAPY. Most women with invasive cervical cancer are treated with radiation. For cancer that has extended beyond the cervix but not to the pelvic wall, radiation therapy is as effective as a radical hysterectomy. Intracavitary and external radiation therapies are used in combination, depending on the extent and location of the lesion. Intracavitary implants (brachytherapy) are usually used for lesions that have extended beyond the pelvic wall. External therapy is often given first to shrink the tumor and increase the effectiveness of the implant. Nursing care related to radiation therapy is presented in the earlier discussion of endometrial cancer (see p. 1771) and in Chapter 25.

CHEMOTHERAPY. Chemotherapeutic agents have generally performed poorly in the treatment of cervical cancer. These agents are usually reserved for unresectable recurrent tumors or disseminated metastatic disease (DeStefano & Bertin-Matson, 1996). Two drugs that have shown some response are cisplatin and 5-fluorouracil (5-FU).

SURGICAL MANAGEMENT. The surgical procedure for cervical cancer depends on the extent of the disease and whether the client wants to have children.

CONIZATION. Conization is the definitive treatment for clients with microinvasive cervical cancer. This procedure is done when the lesion cannot be visualized by colposcopic examination. A cone-shaped area of cervix is removed surgically and sent to the laboratory to determine the extent of the malignancy. Potential complications associated with conization include hemorrhage, uterine perforation, incompetent cervix, cervical stenosis (hardening), and preterm labor for future pregnancies.

Conization may be used therapeutically for women with CIN who desire further childbearing or less extensive surgical treatment. Long-term follow-up care is needed because new lesions can develop.

HYSTERECTOMY. A hysterectomy may be performed as treatment of microinvasive cancer if the client does not desire childbearing. A vaginal approach is commonly used. A radical hysterectomy and bilateral pelvic lymph node dissection is as effective as radiation for treating clients with cancer that has extended beyond the cervix but not to the pelvic wall. Information about hysterectomy is found under Operative Procedures (Uterine Leiomyomas), p. 1766.

PELVIC EXENTERATION. One of the most radical surgical procedures is **pelvic exenteration.** It is performed for recurrent cancers if there is no evidence of tumor outside the pelvis and no lymph node involvement.

Preoperative Care. Nursing care of the woman scheduled for exenteration includes assessment of preoperative anxiety, concerns about the impact on sexual function, and the ability to adjust to her altered body image. The nurse involves family members or significant others in discussions about postoperative expectations. Physical preparation includes selection of stoma sites, extensive bowel preparation, and extensive radiographic and laboratory tests to assess for spread of cancer outside the pelvis. The nurse teaches the client about the following:

* Postoperative recovery in a critical care unit
* Pain management
* Presence of numerous intravenous (IV) and arterial catheters
* Nasogastric suction
* Colostomy and/or urinary diversion (e.g., ileal conduit, Kock ileal urinary pouch)

Operative Procedures. There are three types of exenteration: anterior, posterior, and total (Figure 75-6). Anterior exenteration is the removal of the uterus, cervix, ovaries, fallopian tubes, vagina, bladder, urethra, and pelvic lymph nodes. Posterior exenteration is the removal of the uterus, cervix, ovaries, fallopian tubes, descending colon, rectum, and anal canal. Total exenteration is a combination of anterior and posterior procedures. When the bladder is removed, urine is diverted through a urinary diversion (e.g., ileal conduit or Kock ileal urinary pouch). When the colon, rectum, and anal canal are removed, a colostomy is created for passage of feces. The stomas are located on the abdomen—the colostomy on the left and the ileal conduit on the right.

Postoperative Care. After surgery, the client often is admitted to a critical care unit for the first 1 to 2 days because of the high risk for complications resulting from the massive tissue resection. The nurse assesses for the following:

* Cardiovascular complications such as hemorrhage and shock
* Pulmonary complications such as atelectasis and pneumonia
* Fluid and electrolyte imbalances such as metabolic acidosis or alkalosis and dehydration
* Renal or urinary complications
* Pain

The nurse or assistive nursing personnel also assists with deep breathing and coughing hourly, monitors urine output and specific gravity, monitors parenteral nutrition, and provides colostomy and urinary diversion care.

Once the client's condition is stable, she returns to the regular postoperative unit. The nurse continues postoperative interventions. During the recovery period, the nurse assesses for the following:

* Late cardiovascular complications such as deep vein thrombosis and pulmonary emboli
* Gastrointestinal (GI) complications such as paralytic ileus
* Wound infections
* Wound dehiscence or evisceration
* Pain

The nurse administers prophylactic heparin or low–molecular weight heparin (enoxaparin [Lovenox]) and maintains the use of antiembolism stockings or sequential compression devices (SCDs) for the prevention of thrombosis, as ordered. The nurse also auscultates the lungs frequently, assesses for the presence of bowel sounds and wound infection, administers antibiotics as prescribed, and manages pain with a gradual withdrawal of opioid analgesics.

After the surgeon removes the operative dressings, perineal irrigations may be implemented. Irrigation is usually done with normal saline solution applied with an Asepto syringe. This is followed by drying of the perineum with a heat lamp (25 W at a distance of 18 inches [45 cm]) or a hair dryer (using warm air). Care must be taken to avoid burning the

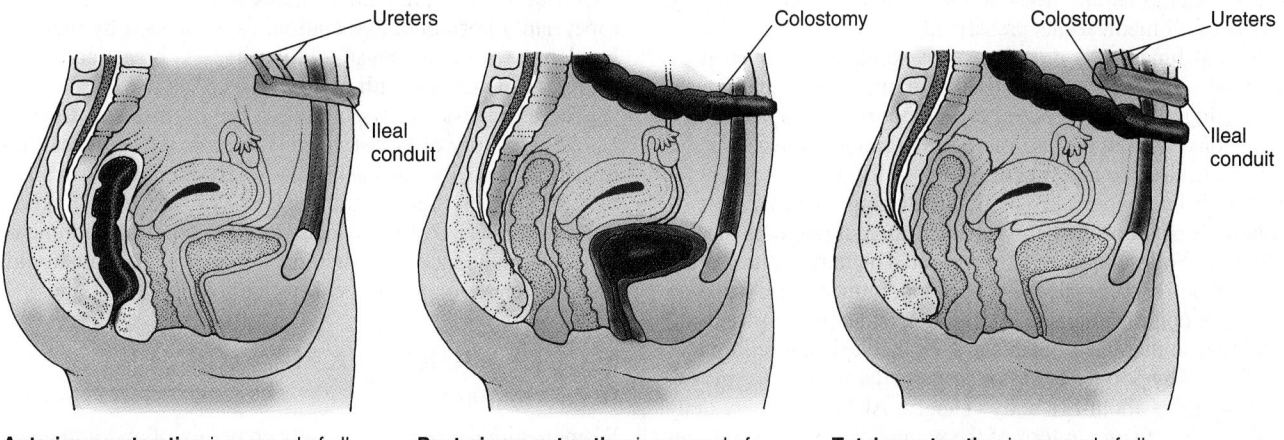

Anterior exenteration is removal of all pelvic organs except the descending colon, rectum, and anal canal. Urine can be diverted into an ileal conduit or urinary Kock pouch.

Posterior exenteration is removal of all pelvic organs except the bladder. A colostomy is created for the passage of feces.

Total exenteration is removal of all pelvic organs with creation of an ileal conduit or urinary Kock pouch and a colostomy.

Figure 75-6 ● Pelvic exenteration.

client. Sitz baths may be ordered as tolerated. (Postoperative care of clients with colostomies and urinary diversions is discussed elsewhere in this text).

● Community-Based Care

If the client has undergone a hysterectomy, the discharge planning is similar to that described for endometrial cancer. For the client who has undergone a pelvic exenteration, the discharge planning is more involved.

▓ HOME CARE MANAGEMENT

The client who has undergone a pelvic exenteration is usually in the hospital for at least 1 week postoperatively. She may be discharged to a skilled nursing facility or subacute unit for continued recovery and care or may be discharged directly to home. When the client returns home, she needs assistance. She is not able to engage in strenuous activities associated with most household work for up to 6 months. The family may need to consider outside help if there is no one in the family who can assume household responsibilities.

No special equipment is needed in the home, although a convoluted foam mattress or other special pressure-relieving device may be placed on the bed to prevent skin breakdown and to increase comfort. Colostomy and ureterostomy pouches and equipment for changing the pouches can be purchased in local pharmacies.

▓ HEALTH TEACHING

The nurse teaches the woman who has undergone a pelvic exenteration how to manage new functions with equipment (colostomy and urinary diversion) and to perform activities of daily living (ADLs) and self-care. The perineal opening may drain mucus for several months to a year. The client can wear sanitary napkins (minipads or maxipads) if they are beltless (so as not to interfere with the stomas). The woman may need help in adjusting her diet to maintain high nutritional requirements for healing while selecting foods that are tolerated. The woman should be able to state the effects, dosages, and side effects of all medications prescribed.

Sexual function is different after exenteration (even if an artificial vagina is constructed), and the couple may need counseling about alternatives to intercourse. Even with vaginal reconstruction, the use of vaginal dilators is necessary to achieve desired sexual function.

Physical activities may be limited during convalescence. If walking is not permitted, the nurse encourages range-of-motion exercises. Follow-up care is important. The nurse counsels the client about keeping all follow-up appointments. Information about late complications (e.g., infection and bowel obstruction) is needed so that the woman can seek medical care promptly.

Usually by 3 to 5 days after surgery, the woman begins expressing grief about her body changes. At first she may deny changes by refusing to look at the wound or stoma sites. Later she may become depressed or withdrawn or even angry or hostile. She may then move to reality testing by asking questions about her care, watching the nurses do wound care, and becoming actively involved in self-care.

The woman may have mood swings, and the nurse is alert when the woman becomes depressed so that interventions can be implemented. The woman needs intense emotional support if she is to adapt to her altered body image and functions.

Unless the woman has vaginal reconstruction after anterior or total pelvic exenteration, she is not able to have vaginal intercourse. The nurse must assess the need for sexual counseling by listening for cues about altered perceptions of body image and anxiety about her sexual partner's response. Further sexual counseling may be needed to provide information on alternative methods of sexual gratification.

▓ HEALTH CARE RESOURCES

Resources for the woman who has cervical cancer are similar to those for the woman with endometrial cancer.

Ovarian Cancer

▓ OVERVIEW

Ovarian cancer is the leading cause of death from female reproductive malignancies. Death rates have risen during the past four decades, and it is projected that 1 of every 70 women will develop ovarian cancer sometime in her life (American Cancer Society, 2000). Survival rates continue to be low because ovarian cancer is poorly detected in its early stages.

Of all ovarian cancers, 85% are epithelial tumors; the most common type is serous adenocarcinoma. These tumors grow rapidly, spread quickly, and are often bilateral. Of all epithelial tumors, ovarian tumors are associated with the worst prognosis.

The cancer spreads by several mechanisms:
* Direct spread to other organs in the pelvis that are in close proximity to the ovary (e.g., uterus, bladder, and colon)
* Distal spread through lymphatic drainage (via para-aortic and iliac lymph nodes to the rest of the pelvis, abdomen or liver, lung, or bones)
* Peritoneal seeding (malignant spread of free-floating cells, usually after the development of ascites)

The cause of ovarian cancer is not precisely known. Suggested etiologic theories include a familial association; an environmental association related to products of industry in countries such as the United States and those of western Europe; and a hormonal association, as evidenced by increased incidence with menopause, nulliparity, and breast cancer and decreased incidence with oral contraceptive use.

Therefore risk factors include a family history of ovarian cancer; a history of breast, bowel, or endometrial cancer; nulliparity; infertility; and a history of dysmenorrhea or heavy bleeding. Diets high in animal fat have also been linked to ovarian cancer. Ovarian cancer ranks second to endometrial cancer in incidence. The incidence increases in women older than 40 years of age and peaks at 50 to 55 years of age.

► COLLABORATIVE MANAGEMENT
● Assessment

Women with ovarian cancer may complain of abdominal pain or swelling or have vague symptoms of abdominal discomfort, such as dyspepsia, indigestion, gas and distention, and other mild gastrointestinal (GI) disturbances. The woman may have a history of ovarian imbalance, such as evidenced by premenstrual tension, heavy menstrual flow, or dysfunctional bleeding.

The only sign may be an abdominal mass, which may be noticed only after it reaches a size of 6 inches (15 cm). Most pelvic examinations do not identify abnormalities. However, an enlarged ovary found postmenopausally should be evaluated as though it were malignant.

The woman with ovarian cancer has concerns similar to those described for the woman with endometrial cancer. Because the malignancy is usually diagnosed in an advanced stage, fears of death and dying are common and may be more of a concern than the proposed treatments.

Cytologic examination has limited application because a Pap smear is abnormal in only 20% to 30% of women with ovarian cancer, even in advanced cases. Diagnosis depends on surgical exploration. Usually a complete laboratory workup is done before exploratory surgery, including a complete blood count, urinalysis, and liver studies if ascites occurs.

The level of ovarian antibody designated as CA-125 may be elevated if ovarian cancer is present. This test may be useful to monitor a woman's progress after treatment but may not be as useful for diagnostic purposes.

Ultrasonography, intravenous pyelography (IVP), computed tomography (CT), and radiography are used in detecting ovarian tumors. In addition, a barium enema study and an upper GI radiographic series can be performed to rule out tumor in the adjacent structures.

Exploratory laparotomy is performed to diagnose and stage ovarian tumors. Ovarian cancer is the only neoplasm that is staged when it is removed (Table 75-9).

● Interventions

Nursing care of the woman with ovarian cancer is similar to that of the woman with endometrial or cervical cancer. The options for treatment depend on the extent of the cancer and include chemotherapy (systemic or intraperitoneal), immunotherapy, radiation therapy (external or intraperitoneal), and surgery.

NONSURGICAL MANAGEMENT. Chemotherapy and radiation therapy are the two most common nonsurgical options for ovarian cancer.

CHEMOTHERAPY. The health care provider usually prescribes chemotherapeutic agents postoperatively for all stages of ovarian cancer, although their purpose is usually palliative for stage IV tumors. Cisplatin, carboplatin, paclitaxel (Taxol), isofamide, doxorubicin (Adriamycin), hexamethylmelamine, methotrexate, and 5-fluorouracil (5-FU) have been used as single agents for treating ovarian cancer (DeStefano & Bertin-Matson, 1996). Combinations of agents seem to obtain higher response rates, especially if cisplatin is one of the drugs used.

Chemotherapy is usually administered every 3 to 4 weeks for 1 week and can be administered on an inpatient or an ambulatory basis. Intraperitoneal chemotherapy is the instillation of chemotherapeutic agents into the abdominal cavity. With the use of this method, it is believed that the cytotoxic effects of the drugs on the tumor are increased. Immunotherapy is also used to treat ovarian cancer. It alters the immunologic response of the ovary and promotes tumor resistance.

RADIATION THERAPY. External radiation therapy is used postoperatively if tumors have invaded other organs. It

Stage	Characteristics
I	Growth limited to ovaries
Ia	Growth limited to one ovary; no ascites; no tumor on external surface; capsule intact
Ib	Growth limited to both ovaries; no ascites; no tumor on external surfaces; capsules intact
Ic	Tumor either stage Ia or Ib, but with tumor on surface of one or both ovaries, or with capsule ruptured, or with ascites present containing malignant cells, or with positive peritoneal washings
II	Growth involving one or both ovaries with pelvic extension
IIa	Extension and/or metastases to uterus and/or tubes
IIb	Extension to other pelvic tissues
IIc	Tumor either stage IIa or IIb, but with tumor on surface of one or both ovaries, or with capsule(s) ruptured, or with ascites present containing malignant cells or with positive peritoneal washings
III	Tumor involving one or both ovaries with peritoneal implants outside pelvis and/or positive retroperitoneal or inguinal nodes; superficial liver metastasis but with histologically proven malignant extension to small bowel or omentum
IIIa	Tumor grossly limited to true pelvis with negative nodes but with histologically confirmed microscopic seeding of abdominal peritoneal surfaces
IIIb	Tumor of one or both ovaries with histologically confirmed implants of abdominal peritoneal surfaces, none exceeding 2 cm in diameter; nodes are negative
IIIc	Abdominal implants greater than 2 cm in diameter and/or positive retroperitoneal inguinal nodes
IV	Growth involving one or both ovaries with distant metastases; if pleural effusion is present, there must be positive cytologic findings to allot a case to stage IV; Parenchymal liver metastasis equals stage IV

TABLE 75-9 · STAGING CLASSIFICATION OF OVARIAN CANCER

may be given with chemotherapy or alone (see Chapter 25). Radioactive colloids have also been injected into the abdomen to increase survival rates. A primary beta-emitter, ^{32}P, is injected through a catheter placed during surgery. After instillation, the woman is asked to turn frequently for 1½ to 2 hours to facilitate the distribution of the radioactive colloids throughout the peritoneal cavity (e.g., turning to the right, to the left, head down, feet down, prone, and supine).

SURGICAL MANAGEMENT. Total abdominal hysterectomy and bilateral salpingo-oophorectomy is the surgical procedure for all stages of ovarian cancer. In clients with stage III or IV cancer, the goal is to remove as much of the cancer as possible because it has spread to adjacent organs. Nursing care of the woman is similar to that of the woman undergoing a hysterectomy for uterine leiomyomas.

A second-look procedure (laparoscopy or laparotomy) is performed, usually after 1 year of chemotherapy, to confirm the absence or presence of tumor and to remove any new or residual tumor if it was too large to be removed at the first operation. Nursing care is similar to that of the client after any major abdominal surgery.

The woman who is faced with the diagnosis of advanced ovarian cancer may be concerned about dying. She needs to be encouraged to ventilate her feelings about her diagnosis. Realistic assurance, as well as accurate information about treatments, can be provided. Often providing the woman with information about ovarian cancer and its treatment decreases her fears. Providing continuity of care, with at least one regular caregiver, may be helpful. The nurse encourages the client to use her support system, including family members, friends, and a spiritual leader, such as a rabbi or other clergy member. A visit from another woman who has survived a similar disease may decrease fears.

If there is recurrence, the woman may deny symptoms at first or express feelings of anger and grief. The family is often fearful of the outcome. The nurse needs to provide encouragement and support during this difficult time and help the woman and her family or significant others work through their grief and prepare for death.

Vulvar Cancer
■ OVERVIEW

Vulvar cancer represents only 4% of all gynecologic malignancies, even though it ranks fourth in occurrence. Vulvar cancer is slow growing, stays localized for a long time, and metastasizes late. Vulvar cancer occurs most commonly in women 50 to 70 years of age. More than 50% of the cases of vulvar cancer occur in women older than 60 years of age. Of all vulvar cancers, 90% are squamous cell carcinomas. The other 10% consist of adenocarcinomas, sarcomas, and Paget's disease. Most vulvar cancers develop in the absence of premalignant changes in the epithelium, but occasionally they develop and spread similarly to cancer of the cervix.

The first change is usually vulvar atypia or mild dysplasia (vulvar intraepithelial neoplasia [VIN] I), followed by moderate dysplasia (VIN II) and then severe dysplasia or carcinoma in situ (VIN III) until the lesion becomes invasive. Vulvar cancer can spread directly to the urethra, the vagina, or the anus and through the lymphatic system to the inguinal, femoral, and deep iliac pelvic nodes.

The cause of vulvar cancer is unknown. There is no proven relationship with sexually transmitted diseases (STDs), although a history of condylomata acuminata (venereal warts) may be present. A strong relationship exists between vulvar cancer and herpes simplex type II, human papillomavirus, and capsid antigen. Obesity, hypertension, diabetes, smoking, and granulomatous disease of the vulva have been suggested as possible causes, but no scientific data support these suggestions.

Vulvar cancer seldom occurs before age 40 years, although studies have found premalignant changes in women in their 20s and 30s. This increase may be linked to the increase in sexually transmitted infections.

The prognosis for vulvar cancer is related to the stage of the cancer and whether cancer is present in the lymph nodes. Guidelines for the early detection and prevention of vulvar cancer include performing monthly vulvar self-examination, having an annual pelvic examination, and practicing "safe sex."

➤ COLLABORATIVE MANAGEMENT
● Assessment

Women with vulvar lesions are likely to report irritation or itching in their perineal area. Sometimes they describe a "sore that will not heal." Bleeding is a late symptom. Women usu-

ally try to treat themselves before seeking medical help. Often a lesion has been present for months. Embarrassment has been suggested as the reason why older women delay seeking medical attention.

Pelvic examinations usually reveal multifocal lesions, the majority of which develop on the labia. The lesions may be whitish or reddish, and the vulvar skin may be excoriated as a result of irritation.

The woman may be anxious or fearful about the diagnosis of cancer. She may have fears that her partner will reject her because of the diagnosis, or she may worry about disfigurement related to surgery. The nurse needs to assess the woman's past experiences in coping with stressful situations and whether she has the psychologic resources to cope with the present crisis.

A Pap smear and colposcopic examination of the vulva (see Assessment [Cervical Cancer], p. 1774) may aid in diagnosis. A toluidine blue test may be used to identify abnormal cells for biopsy. A 1% aqueous solution of toluidine blue is applied to the vulva and allowed to dry. Then a 1% acetic acid solution is applied. Biopsy of the areas that remain blue is performed. The test chemical stains nuclei in the superficial epithelium, where cells do not normally contain nuclei. An abnormal finding does not necessarily indicate malignancy, because ulcerations also stain.

A biopsy of the lesion is necessary for diagnosis. This is easily accomplished with a Keyes dermal punch (a device that removes a disk of tissue). Depending on the site of the lesion, one or more biopsy specimens may be taken.

● Interventions

Nursing care of the client with vulvar cancer is similar to that for endometrial cancer; only the interventions that differ are discussed.

NONSURGICAL MANAGEMENT. Nonsurgical management of vulvar cancer depends on the extent of the spread and may include laser therapy, chemotherapy, and radiation therapy.

LASER THERAPY. If a woman has premalignant vulvar lesions, laser therapy may be used (see p. 1774). The treatment is usually done on an outpatient basis; local, regional, or general anesthesia is used. Healing occurs over a period of several weeks, and usually the lesions are removed without scarring.

CHEMOTHERAPY. Chemotherapy in the form of a topical application of 5-FU has been used to treat carcinoma in situ successfully. However, the treatment causes severe vulvar edema and pain and is not often used.

RADIATION THERAPY. External radiation therapy to the deep pelvic nodes may be used postoperatively (see earlier discussion of endometrial cancer [p. 1771] and Chapter 25). Radiation treatments cause ulceration and dermatitis, which can be uncomfortable for the woman.

SURGICAL MANAGEMENT. The surgeon performs a vulvectomy to remove the cancerous vulvar lesions.

PREOPERATIVE CARE. The woman needs a complete explanation of the extent of the surgical procedure to be performed and information about preoperative and postoperative procedures (see Chapters 17 and 19). Specific preoperative care for a vulvectomy may include an abdominal or perineal shave, an enema, douching, and insertion of an indwelling catheter into the bladder.

OPERATIVE PROCEDURES. Several surgical procedures are effective for the treatment of vulvar cancer. A local wide excision may be used to remove the abnormal area (for carcinoma in situ [CIS]). A simple vulvectomy (removal of the vulva, the labia majora, the labia minora, and possibly the clitoris) may also be performed for CIS, but this disfiguring surgery is used less often today. Instead, a **skinning vulvectomy**—the removal of superficial vulvar skin (without removal of the clitoris) and replacement of removed skin with split-thickness grafts—is performed (Figure 75-7). Sexual function is less affected, and the appearance of the vulva is less changed.

For invasive cancer, the surgery most often recommended is the modified radical or **radical vulvectomy** (removal of the entire vulva—skin, labia, clitoris, subcutaneous tissues, and possibly inguinal and femoral node dissection), depending on node involvement (see Figure 75-7).

POSTOPERATIVE CARE. Postoperatively, the woman can expect to have multiple suction drains (Hemovac or Jackson-Pratt drains) in the inguinal or vulvar areas for

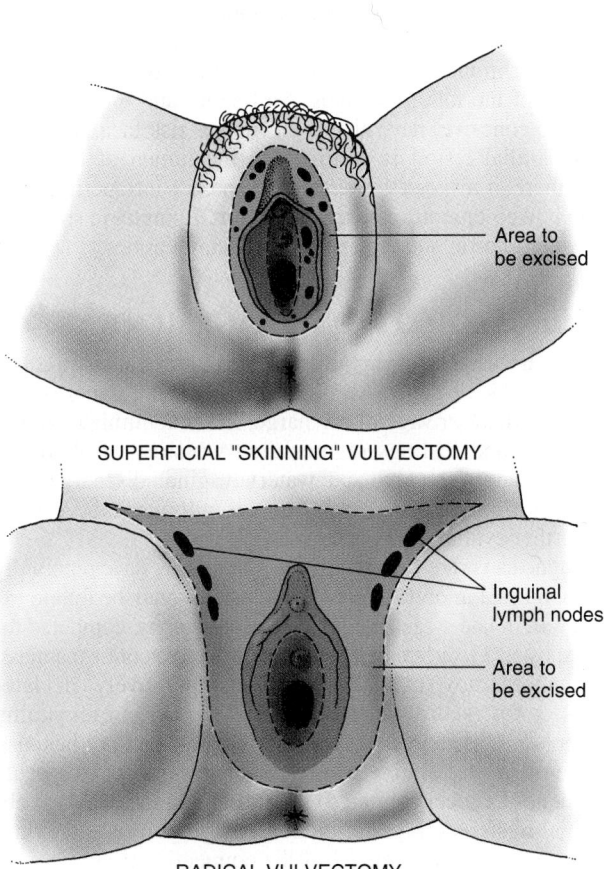

SUPERFICIAL "SKINNING" VULVECTOMY

RADICAL VULVECTOMY

Figure 75-7 ● Vulvectomy.

wound drainage for 7 to 10 days. A pressure-reducing mattress may be placed on the bed to prevent pressure ulcers and increase comfort. A bed cradle may be used to keep linens off the incision site. The client usually wears antiembolism stockings or sequential compression devices to prevent thromboembolism and leg edema.

Providing Wound Care. The major focus of nursing care is wound healing. The nurse changes the dressings over the incision frequently because of the amount of wound drainage and the risk of infection. Wound complications, such as infection and dehiscence, often occur after vulvectomies; subsequently, the healing process may take up to 6 months. Meticulous wound care is necessary and usually involves debridement. The nurse typically uses normal saline solution, which may be applied with an Asepto bulb syringe or a water pick (on low speed). The wound is then dried with a heat lamp or air dried with a hair dryer (using warm air). Wound care is usually done three or four times a day.

Diet in the postoperative period should include foods rich in vitamin C, iron, and protein to promote wound healing.

Promoting Urinary and Bowel Elimination. The Foley catheter remains in the bladder for 7 to 10 days to prevent ureteral stenosis and incontinence. After the catheter is removed, the urine stream may be deflected down the leg as a result of edema or even may be uncontrolled. Having the woman stand while voiding may decrease the incidence of these annoying problems. Antiperistaltic medications are usually given for 7 to 10 days to prevent defecation and decrease the risk of wound infection. Then stool softeners may be given to prevent straining and decrease discomfort related to bowel movements. Perineal care or sitz baths after voidings or bowel movements may prevent contamination of the incision site.

Managing Pain. Postoperative discomfort is usually controlled with analgesics during the first couple of days after surgery. Medicating for pain before wound care may help the woman relax and tolerate the procedure with less distress.

Addressing Sexuality. The woman needs complete explanations of the changes that occur as a result of surgery. If a radical vulvectomy is done, the clitoris is removed and loss of orgasm usually occurs. Dyspareunia may result from any of the surgical procedures. Vaginal dilators may be useful to stretch the remaining vaginal tissues. Discomfort can also be reduced during sexual intercourse by having the couple use water-soluble lubricants or a side-lying position. The couple may need counseling about alternatives to vaginal intercourse. The woman may need to be encouraged to express feelings of grief related to her loss of normal sexual function.

A vulvectomy can be devastating to a woman's self-concept. She often has a grief reaction related to the loss of the vulva and subsequent disfigurement. She may fear rejection from her sexual partner or significant others and may be reluctant to make herself vulnerable by getting involved in any relationship. Fears of recurrence or metastasis may be present. The nurse's role is one of support. The woman needs encouragement to vent her feelings and concerns about her perceived or actual losses and body changes. Family members or significant others should be encouraged to share their feelings and concerns with the woman. A visit by a woman who has successfully recovered from similar surgery could be beneficial.

Vaginal Cancer

OVERVIEW

Primary invasive vaginal cancer is rare, accounting for less than 2% of all gynecologic cancers. Usually vaginal cancer is an extension of cervical, endometrial, or vulvar cancers. Most vaginal cancers are squamous cell carcinomas that develop in the upper one third of the vagina. They occur most often in women older than 50 years of age; 90% of cases are found postmenopausally. Adenocarcinoma of the vagina is found in females between the ages of 14 and 30 years and is associated with intrauterine exposure to diethylstilbestrol (DES) as a result of maternal ingestion during pregnancy.

The cause of vaginal cancer is unknown. Predisposing factors include repeated pregnancies; vaginal trauma; sexually transmitted diseases (STDs), especially syphilis and herpes simplex virus type 2 and papillomavirus infections; and prior radiation.

The spread of vaginal cancer depends on the location of the tumor. Upper vaginal lesions spread in the same manner as cervical cancer, whereas lower lesions spread similarly to vulvar cancer. Because of the rich lymphatic drainage in the vaginal area, metastasis can occur early.

➤ COLLABORATIVE MANAGEMENT

● Assessment

Premalignant lesions (vaginal intraepithelial neoplasia) are usually asymptomatic. An abnormal Pap smear is the most common presenting problem. Uncommon or late symptoms include pain, foul-smelling vaginal discharge, painless vaginal bleeding, pruritus, and urinary symptoms attributable to the pressure of the lesion on the bladder.

A pelvic examination may reveal a lesion. Premalignant changes are diagnosed through colposcopic examination and biopsy.

● Interventions

Both nonsurgical and surgical interventions may be used to treat women with vaginal cancer.

NONSURGICAL MANAGEMENT. Noninvasive malignancy and early-stage vaginal cancers may be treated nonsurgically with a variety of techniques. Laser therapy (see p. 1774) may be used. The health care provider stains the abnormal tissues with an iodine solution to identify the area for treatment. A vaginal discharge may be present for several days after treatment, and healing normally takes a few weeks. Close follow-up is necessary and includes a Pap smear and colposcopic examination every 4 months for 1 year and then every 6 to 12 months.

Local application of 5-fluorouracil (5-FU) cream to the vagina daily for 1 week is another treatment option. This chemotherapeutic agent is irritating to the skin, and often zinc oxide ointment is recommended for application to the vulvar area. The treatment is repeated in 3 to 4 weeks, and follow-up is the same as that for laser therapy.

Radiation therapy can be used for all stages of vaginal cancer. Intracavitary radiation therapy (IRT, brachytherapy) is usually used alone for the treatment of cancer limited to the vaginal wall, and external radiation therapy is combined with IRT for the treatment of cancer that extends beyond the vaginal wall. Complications of radiation therapy include vaginal stenosis, adhesions, and discharge. Women need to use vaginal dilators after treatment, and assessment for sexual dysfunction is suggested.

Chemotherapy may be used for recurrent disease, although there is no effective therapy.

SURGICAL MANAGEMENT. A local wide excision may be performed for localized lesions. A partial or total **vaginectomy** (removal of part or all of the vagina) may be done for invasive disease. Vaginectomy affects sexual function. Without surgical reconstruction, vaginal intercourse is impossible. The woman and her sexual partner need counseling about alternative activities for achieving sexual satisfaction. A radical hysterectomy or pelvic exenteration may also be performed, depending on the extent of the cancer.

Preventive and early detection measures for vaginal cancer are to avoid taking DES during pregnancy (to prevent one's daughter from developing cancer) and to continue to have Pap screening and pelvic examinations after menopause on a regular basis.

Fallopian Tube Cancer

OVERVIEW

Fallopian tube cancer is the rarest of gynecologic cancers; it is associated with an incidence of less than 1%. It occurs in women older than 50 years of age; 80% to 90% of cases result from metastasis from ovarian and endometrial cancers.

The cause of squamous cell fallopian tube cancer is unknown. It has been suggested that pelvic inflammatory disease (PID) and chronic salpingitis may be associated with adenocarcinomas of the fallopian tubes. Nulliparity and infertility (inability to conceive) have also been cited as risk factors.

The initial lesion is confined to the lumen of the tube. From there, it invades the serosa and spreads intraperitoneally to the bowel, omentum, and peritoneum. Lymphatic spread is to the para-aortic and retroperitoneal lymph nodes.

➤ COLLABORATIVE MANAGEMENT

Women are usually asymptomatic until the tumor is in a late stage. In 50% of the cases, bleeding is present. Other symptoms include clear vaginal discharge, lower abdominal pain or distention, and feelings of pressure. A history of abnormal bleeding, adnexal pain, and watery vaginal discharge in a postmenopausal woman may suggest fallopian tube cancer, and further evaluation is needed.

Diagnosis is rare preoperatively. Pap smears have reportedly been abnormal in only 10% of cases. A mass may be felt on examination in late stages. Vaginal ultrasonography, computed tomography (CT), or laparoscopy may be used to confirm a mass.

Chemotherapy may be used postoperatively in later stages or for recurrence. The lesions respond to alkylating agents (see Chapter 25). External radiation therapy has also been used postoperatively for late-stage tumors. The usual treatment of cancer limited to the fallopian tube is a total abdominal hysterectomy and bilateral salpingo-oophorectomy with omentectomy (removal of the connective tissues covering these organs). Care of the woman with fallopian tube cancer is similar to that described earlier for cancer of the ovary (see Interventions [Ovarian Cancer], p. 1777).

ONLINE RESOURCES

For suggested readings and Internet resources, go to http://www.wbsaunders.com/SIMON/Iggy/.

SELECTED BIBLIOGRAPHY

Asterisk indicates a classic or definitive work on this subject.

American Cancer Society. (2000). *Cancer facts and figures—2000.* Report No. 00-300M-No. 5008.00. Atlanta: Author.

*Baird, G. (1996). Advances in gynaecology. *The Practitioner, 240,* 90-95.

*Barrett, R.J., et al. (1995). Endometrial cancer: Stage at diagnosis and associated factors in black and white patients. *American Journal of Obstetrics and Gynecology, 173*(2), 414-422.

Barrow, C. (1999). Balloon endometrial ablation as a safe alternative to hysterectomy. *AORN Journal, 70*(1), 80, 83-86, 89-90.

*Chuong, C.J., Pearsall-Otey, L.R., & Rosenfeld, B.L. (1995). A practical guide to relieving PMS. *Contemporary Nurse Practitioner, 1*(3), 31-37.

*DeStefano, M.S., & Bertin-Matson, K. (1996). Gynecologic cancers. In R. McCorkle et al. (Eds.), *Cancer nursing: A comprehensive textbook* (2nd ed., pp. 698-727). Philadelphia: W.B. Saunders.

*Jarrett, M., et al. (1996). Relationship between gastrointestinal and dysmenorrheic symptoms at menses. *Research in Nursing and Health, 19*(1), 45-51.

Jennings-Dozier, K. (1999). Predicting intentions to obtain a Pap smear among African American and Latina women: Testing the theory of planned behavior. *Nursing Research, 48*(4), 198-205.

Johnson, S. (1998). Menopause and hormone replacement therapy. *Medical Clinics of North America, 82*(2), 297-320.

Kim, K., et al. (1999). Cervical cancer screening knowledge and practices among Korean-American women. *Cancer Nursing, 22*(4), 297-302.

Lessick, M., Wickham, R., & Rehwaldt, M. (1997). Breast and ovarian cancer: Genetic update and implications for nursing. *MEDSURG Nursing, 6*(6), 341-349.

*Lowdermilk, D.L. (1995). Reproductive surgery. In C.I. Fogel & N.F. Woods (Eds.), *Women's health care* (pp. 629-650). Springhouse, PA: Springhouse.

Mazmanian, C.M. (1999). Hysterectomy: Holistic care is key. *RN, 62*(6), 32-35.

McCance, K.L., & Huether, S.E. (1998). *Pathophysiology: The biological basis for disease in adults and children* (3rd ed.). St. Louis: Mosby.

Pearl, M.L., et al. (1999). Transcutaneous electrical nerve stimulation as an adjunct for controlling chemotherapy-induced nausea and vomiting in gynecologic oncology. *Cancer Nursing, 22*(4), 307-311.

*Rose, P.G. (1996). Endometrial carcinoma. *New England Journal of Medicine, 335*(9), 640-649.

Scura, K.W., & Whipple, B. (1997). How to provide better care for the postmenopausal woman. *American Journal of Nursing, 97*(4), 36-44.

Shurpin, K. (1997). Clinical snapshot: Ovarian cancer. *American Journal of Nursing, 97*(4), 34-35.

Taylor, L.K., et al. (1998). The effect of music in the postanesthesia care unit on pain levels in women who have had abdominal hysterectomies. *Journal of Perianesthesia Nursing, 13*(2), 88-94.

Wade, J., et al. (2000). Hysterectomy: What do women need and want to know? *Journal of Obstetric, Gynecologic, and Neonatal Nursing, 29*(1), 33-42.

76

Interventions for Male Clients with Reproductive Problems

LORI KLINGMAN

Learning Objectives

After studying this chapter, you should be able to:

1. Describe common physical assessment findings for the client with benign prostatic hyperplasia (BPH).
2. Discuss options for nonsurgical and surgical management of the client with BPH.
3. Develop a postoperative plan of care for a client undergoing a transurethral resection of the prostate (TURP).
4. Identify the procedures for prostate cancer screening.
5. Explain the role of hormonal therapy in treating prostate cancer.
6. Describe the options for treating erectile dysfunction.
7. Discuss the cultural considerations related to male reproductive problems.
8. Analyze assessment data to determine priority nursing diagnoses and collaborative problems for a man with testicular cancer.
9. Develop a plan of care for a client with testicular cancer.
10. Formulate a community-based teaching plan for continuing care of clients with testicular cancer.
11. Compare and contrast hydrocele, spermatocele, and varicocele.
12. Discuss issues related to sexuality and body image for a man experiencing male reproductive health problems.

Go to http://www.wbsaunders.com/SIMON/Iggy/ for self-assessment questions related to these Learning Objectives.

Nurses need to know about the anatomy and physiology of male reproductive functions so that they can instruct clients about the impact of a disease process or treatment on their reproductive ability. The nurse includes the client and his spouse, sexual partner, or significant other in the decision-making process and works with members of the interdisciplinary team in providing collaborative care.

BENIGN PROSTATIC HYPERPLASIA

■ OVERVIEW

The prostate gland is the major accessory sex gland of the male. It is often a site of infection and benign and malignant neoplasms, all of which can affect urinary elimination.

■ Pathophysiology

In a young adult male, the prostatic capsule is thin and is attached to the underlying tissue. As the man ages, the glandular units in the prostate begin to undergo tissue **hyperplasia** (an abnormal increase in the number of cells), resulting in prostatic **hypertrophy** (enlargement). Although benign prostatic hypertrophy is the more common term used to describe this phenomenon, **benign prostatic hyperplasia (BPH)** is the correct term for the pathologic process.

When the prostate gland enlarges, it extends upward, into the bladder, and inward, narrowing the prostatic urethral channel, and obstructs the outflow of urine by encroaching on the bladder opening (Figure 76-1). In response to this outlet resistance, the bladder is affected in several ways (Figure 76-2). First, it may become hyperirritable, which produces urgency and frequency. As the bladder tries to compensate for its increased workload, muscles in the bladder wall hypertrophy and may develop cellules and diverticula. If allowed to continue, this obstruction of urine flow can cause a gradual dilation of the ureters **(hydroureter)** and kidneys **(hydronephrosis).** The enlarged prostate may also obstruct the bladder neck or the prostatic urethra, leading to urinary retention or incomplete bladder emptying. Overflow urinary incontinence is common; the urine "leaks" around the enlarged prostate, causing dribbling. Urinary stasis can result in urinary tract infections.

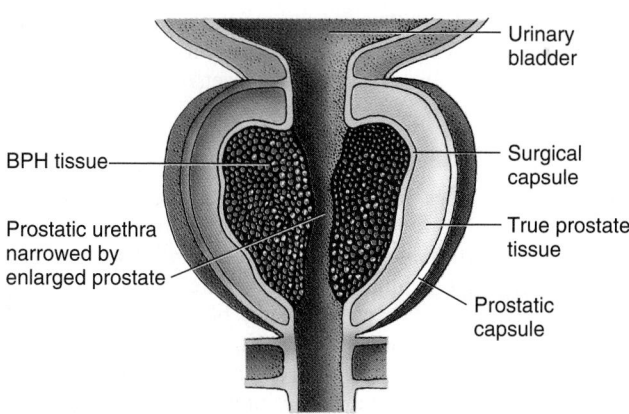

Figure 76-1 ● Benign prostatic hyperplasia (BPH) grows inward, causing narrowing of the urethra.

Etiology

The exact cause of BPH remains unknown. Because the development of BPH is almost universal in older men, several theories have been examined:

- The effect of chronic inflammation of the prostate gland
- The role of general metabolic and nutritional factors (diet)
- The possible contribution of atherosclerosis

Demographic data (such as race) and social factors (such as socioeconomic status and heredity) have been examined as predictors for the development of BPH. Although these theories continue to be investigated, it is thought that BPH results from a systemic hormonal alteration. Support for this theory is based on the observations that aging is the major contributing factor and that another factor is the presence of testicular androgen. BPH does not occur in men who have been castrated before puberty (testicular androgen is absent). Men with BPH experience a regression of BPH after a bilateral orchiectomy (testicular androgen is removed).

Incidence/Prevalence

> ### CONSIDERATIONS FOR OLDER ADULTS
> The incidence of BPH consistently increases with age. Characteristically, BPH is a disease of men older than 40 years of age, with an increase in incidence occurring with each decade of life. By age 50, at least 50% of all men have some degree of BPH, although not all are symptomatic (Matteson, McConnell, & Linton, 1997).

➤ COLLABORATIVE MANAGEMENT

◗ Assessment

◗ HISTORY

The nurse pays particular attention to the client's report of his urinary pattern. Commonly, the client complains of frequency, **nocturia** (voiding at night), and other symptoms of bladder neck obstruction known as **lower urinary tract symptoms (LUTS)** (Holtgrave, 1998). The symptoms of LUTS include hesitancy, intermittency, diminished force and caliber of the urinary stream, a sensation of incomplete bladder emptying, and postvoid dribbling. If frequency and nocturia are not accompanied by symptoms of restricted flow, the

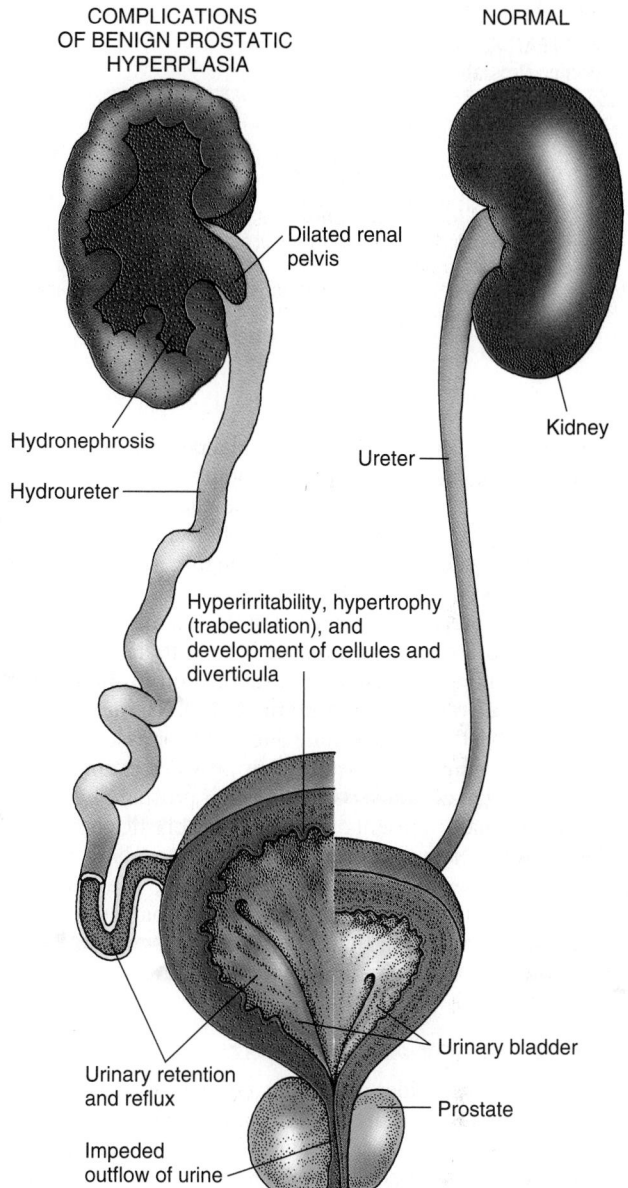

Figure 76-2 ● Potential complications of benign prostatic hyperplasia. The right side of the illustration shows a normal male urologic system. The left side shows potential complications.

possibility of a nonobstructive etiology, such as infection, is considered.

The nurse questions whether the client has experienced any **hematuria** (blood in the urine) when initiating or at the end of urination. BPH is a common cause of hematuria in men older than 60 years of age.

◗ PHYSICAL ASSESSMENT/CLINICAL MANIFESTATIONS

The client is instructed to void before the physical assessment. The nurse inspects, palpates, and percusses the abdomen for any evidence of a distended bladder. Normally, the bladder must contain 150 mL of urine to allow its palpation and percussion. A bladder with a larger amount of urine may

---

CHART 76-1

KEY FEATURES *of*
Benign Prostatic Hyperplasia

- Urinary frequency
- Nocturia
- Urinary hesitancy, particularly on initiation of voiding
- Hematuria
- Diminished force of the urinary stream
- Postvoid dribbling (overflow incontinence)
- Bladder distention
- Possible evidence of renal insufficiency, including edema, pallor, and pruritus
- A uniform, elastic, nontender palpable prostate

---

be visible on inspection. An enlarged bladder may be palpated as a mass in the lower abdomen. If suprapubic pressure on the mass results in a feeling of urgency, the nurse may be able to ascertain that the mass is a distended bladder. The bladder of an obese client is best identified through percussion rather than inspection or palpation.

The nurse prepares the client for the examination of the prostate gland. Because the prostate is close to the rectal wall, the easiest and most satisfactory examination of the prostate is by a **digital rectal examination (DRE).** The nurse helps the client to bend over the examination table or assume a side-lying fetal position. The health care provider examines the prostate for size and consistency. Benign prostatic hyperplasia (BPH) usually presents as a uniform, elastic, nontender enlargement, whereas cancer of the prostate gland usually presents as a stony-hard nodule (Chart 76-1). The nurse advises the client that after the prostate gland is palpated, it may be massaged to obtain a fluid sample for examination to rule out **prostatitis** (inflammation of the prostate).

■ LABORATORY ASSESSMENT

The health care provider may order a urinalysis and obtains a urine specimen for culture to detect any urinary abnormality or evidence of urinary tract infection. Urinalysis includes tests for glucose, protein, occult blood, and pH levels. If an infection is present, the specimen may contain white blood cells (WBCs) (pus) or red blood cells (RBCs).

Blood studies that may be performed at the initial evaluation, depending on the client's condition and third-party payer, include the following:

- A complete blood count (CBC) to evaluate any evidence of infection or anemia
- Blood urea nitrogen (BUN) and serum creatinine determinations to evaluate renal function
- A prostate-specific antigen (PSA) and a serum acid phosphatase measurement if a prostatic malignancy is suspected (see Prostate Cancer Screening, p. 1790).

If the health care provider expresses prostatic fluid during the examination, the fluid is sent to the laboratory for microscopic examination and cultures.

■ RADIOGRAPHIC ASSESSMENT

Radiologic studies that may be conducted in the workup of the client with suspected BPH include x-ray studies of the kidneys, ureters, and bladder (KUB) and intravenous pyelography (IVP).

The KUB outlines the structure of the urinary tract in the abdomen. The IVP is particularly useful in revealing the structure and function of the urinary tract.

■ OTHER DIAGNOSTIC ASSESSMENT

Urodynamic studies are very important in the diagnosis and evaluation of clients with bladder neck obstruction. Urodynamic flow studies include flow rate analysis **(flowmetry)** and assessment of residual urine. Flow rate analysis is simply a way of assessing the activity of the bladder and the outlet during the emptying phase of micturition.

During a cystourethroscopic examination, the physician uses a cystoscope to visualize the interior of the bladder, the bladder neck, and the urethra. This examination is necessary to study the presence and effect of bladder neck obstruction. The procedure is usually done in an ambulatory care setting.

Residual urine may be determined by catheterizing the client immediately after he voids. As an alternative, because the client always voids before cystourethroscopy, residual urine may be measured at that time.

▶ Interventions

Traditionally, the only effective treatment for the relief of the symptoms caused by BPH has been surgical, although some clients can be managed without surgery.

NONSURGICAL MANAGEMENT. Medical management of BPH includes drug therapy and other measures to minimize obstruction.

DRUG THERAPY. The health care provider may prescribe finasteride (Proscar) to shrink the prostate gland and improve urine flow. Finasteride lowers the level of **dihydrotestosterone (DHT),** a major cause of prostate growth. In some men, decreasing the DHT levels can shrink the enlarged prostate. The client may need to take the drug for as long as 6 months before any improvement occurs. The major side effects of the drug are erectile dysfunction (ED) and decreased libido, although these effects are not common.

The presence of alpha-adrenergic receptors in the prostatic smooth muscle makes it treatable by alpha-blocking agents, such as terazosin (Hytrin), doxazosin (Cardura), and tamsulosin (Flomax). When alpha-blocking agents are given, the prostate gland constricts, thereby reducing urethral pressure, improving urine flow, and decreasing residual mass. A variety of hormonal agents, including estrogens and androgens, alone or in combination, also have been used in attempts to alter BPH and its effects on voiding. This type of hormonal manipulation has usually not been successful.

COMPLEMENTARY AND ALTERNATIVE THERAPIES. Health care providers in Europe have successfully treated benign BPH with saw palmetto extract, a natural herb, for many years. In the United States most health care providers have been reluctant to recommend the herb because of lack of adequate clinical research on its effectiveness. Despite this trend, many men with early to moderate BPH believe that saw palmetto has relieved their symptoms and prefer this treatment over prescription drugs or surgery. A study in the United States by Marks at al. (2000) found that a saw palmetto herbal blend was a safe, highly desirable option for men with BPH. The herb caused epithelial tissue contraction in the prostate gland.

OTHER MEASURES. Some nonsurgical measures seem to minimize obstructive symptoms, including those that cause the release of prostatic fluid, such as prostatic massage, frequent sexual intercourse, and masturbation. These measures are very helpful for the client whose urinary obstructive symptoms have resulted from an enlarged prostate with a large amount of retained prostatic fluid. The nurse instructs the client to avoid drinking large amounts of fluid in a short time; to avoid alcohol, diuretics, and caffeine; and to void as soon as the urge is felt. These measures are aimed at preventing overdistention of the bladder, which may result in loss of detrusor muscle tone. Clients should also avoid any medications that can cause urinary retention, especially anticholinergics, antihistamines, and decongestants. The nurse emphasizes the importance of telling the health care provider about the diagnosis of BPH so that these drugs will not be prescribed.

SURGICAL MANAGEMENT. Because most older men have some evidence of BPH, the mere presence of the condition does not mean that the client requires surgical intervention. Some or all of the following criteria are typically present when surgical intervention is considered necessary:

- Acute urinary retention
- Chronic urinary tract infections secondary to residual urine in the bladder
- Hematuria
- Hydronephrosis
- Bladder neck obstruction symptoms that are worrisome to the client, such as urinary frequency and nocturia

The goals of surgical intervention are to relieve the symptoms associated with bladder neck obstruction and to improve the quality of the client's life by allowing him to void at normal intervals while retaining adequate urinary control and normal sexual functioning.

PREOPERATIVE CARE. When planning surgical interventions, the physician considers the client's general physical condition, the size of the prostate gland, and the client's preference.

> ### ✤ CONSIDERATIONS FOR OLDER ADULTS
> The client is thoroughly evaluated for any other diseases that are common in older persons, such as cardiovascular disease, chronic pulmonary disease, diabetes mellitus, or renal disease. If the client has renal disease, the nurse or physician may insert a Foley catheter. The client's intake, output, and serum electrolyte and creatinine levels are closely monitored until renal status has improved. In some cases, a thorough workup and evaluation of the client's medical condition may indicate that surgery would be too risky. In such cases, bladder neck obstruction may be relieved by permanent Foley drainage. The physician also assesses for the presence of urinary tract infection and treats any infection before performing surgery.

Preoperatively, the client may have many fears and misconceptions about prostatic surgery, such as automatic loss of sexual functioning or permanent incontinence. The nurse assesses the client's anxiety, corrects any misconceptions about

the surgery, and provides accurate information to him and his family or significant others. Regardless of the type of surgery to be performed, the nurse provides information about anesthesia (see Chapter 19). The client may have concurrent medical problems that put him at risk for complications of general anesthesia and may be advised to have epidural anesthesia. Epidural anesthesia may be used for any of the procedures and is the most commonly used type of anesthesia for a transurethral resection of the prostate. Because the client is awake, it is easier to assess for hyponatremia, fluid overload, and water intoxication.

The nurse also includes the topic of urinary catheters in the preoperative teaching plan. After prostatic surgery, all clients have an indwelling urethral (Foley) catheter for at least a day. The nurse instructs the client that he may also have continuous bladder irrigation (CBI) and traction on the catheter, but this may not be known until the client returns from the postanesthesia care unit (PACU). The nurse also explains before surgery that it is normal postoperatively for the urine to be blood tinged. Small blood clots and tissue debris may pass while the catheter is in place and immediately after it is removed.

OPERATIVE PROCEDURES. Several surgical procedures are possible for removing the hypertrophied portion of the prostate gland (Figure 76-3). In all approaches, the surgeon removes the hyperplastic tissue and leaves the prostatic capsule.

In the last few years, a variety of less invasive surgical procedures for BPH have emerged. These procedures include transurethral thermotherapy, transurethral needle ablation, visual laser ablation, and electrovaporization (using electrocautery) of the prostate. The advantages of these minimally invasive procedures are that the client can be discharged from the hospital within 24 hours with a Foley catheter because there is minimal postoperative bleeding. Postoperatively, the nurse teaches the client to monitor for catheter patency, hematuria, and infection. Clients and their caregivers should also be told that delayed hematuria and urinary retention may occur days to weeks after the electrovaporization procedure (Gray & Allensworth, 1999).

Transurethral Resection of the Prostate. The traditional **transurethral resection of the prostate (TURP)** is a "closed" surgical procedure and is still commonly performed. The prostate may also be removed using an "open" procedure because of the need for a surgical incision. The choice of procedure depends on the following:

- The size of the prostate gland
- The location of the enlargement
- Whether surgery on the bladder is also needed
- The client's age and physical condition

To perform the TURP procedure, the most common type of prostatic surgery, the surgeon inserts a resectoscope (an instrument similar to a cystoscope, but with a cutting and cauterizing loop) through the urethra. The enlarged portion of the prostate gland is then resected in small pieces (prostate chips).

The surgeon chooses this procedure when the major enlargement exists in the medial lobe of the prostate that directly surrounds the urethra and when the amount of tissue to be removed is relatively small. A TURP is safer for the client who is at high risk for open surgery because a surgical incision is not necessary. Hospitalization and convalescence are shorter than with any other type of **prostatectomy** (prostate removal).

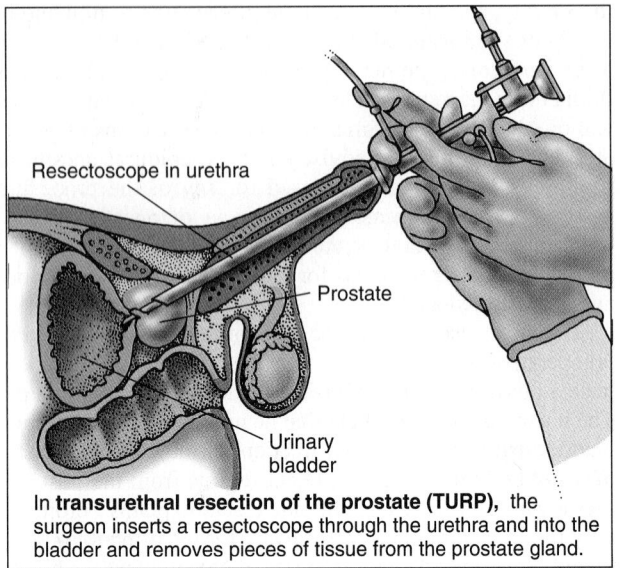

In **transurethral resection of the prostate (TURP),** the surgeon inserts a resectoscope through the urethra and into the bladder and removes pieces of tissue from the prostate gland.

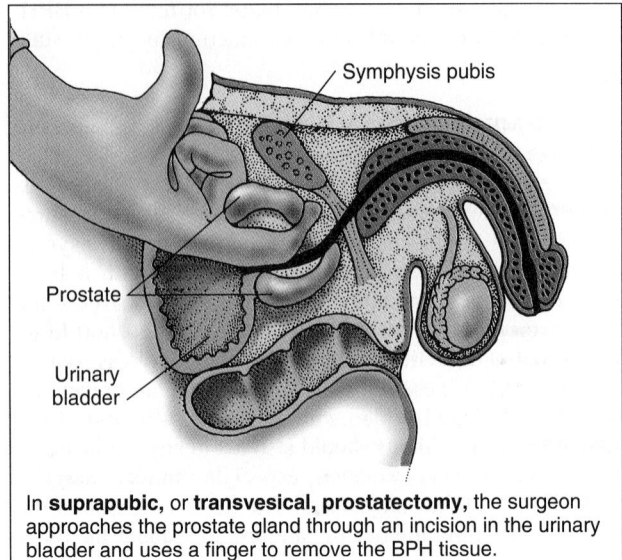

In **suprapubic,** or **transvesical, prostatectomy,** the surgeon approaches the prostate gland through an incision in the urinary bladder and uses a finger to remove the BPH tissue.

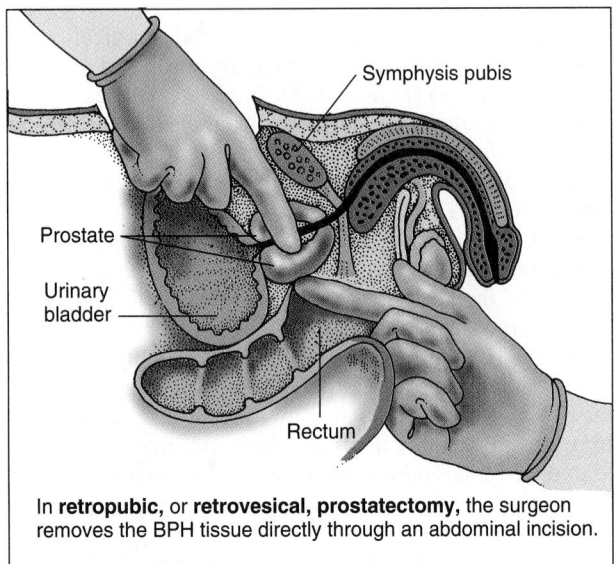

In **retropubic,** or **retrovesical, prostatectomy,** the surgeon removes the BPH tissue directly through an abdominal incision.

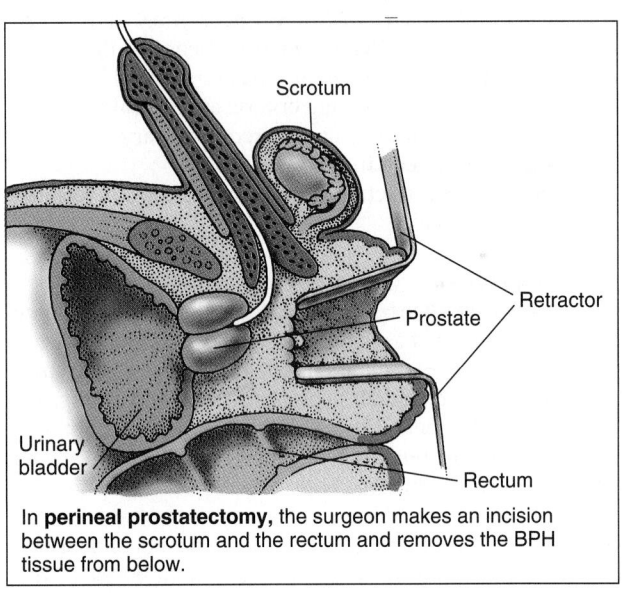

In **perineal prostatectomy,** the surgeon makes an incision between the scrotum and the rectum and removes the BPH tissue from below.

Figure 76-3 ● Prostatectomy procedures. (*BPH,* Benign prostatic hyperplasia.)

The disadvantage of a TURP is that because only small pieces of the gland are removed, prostatic tissue may grow back, resulting in recurrent urinary obstruction and necessitating additional TURPs. There is also the possibility of urethral trauma from the resectoscope, with resultant urethral strictures.

Suprapubic Prostatectomy. **Suprapubic,** or transvesical, **prostatectomy** is performed when the prostate is larger than the surgeon believes can be removed transurethrally and if the client has any coexisting bladder abnormalities that can be treated concurrently.

The surgeon makes a low, horizontal abdominal incision just above the symphysis pubis and exposes the bladder. The bladder is then distended with fluid, and a small incision is made in the bladder wall. The prostate gland is removed through the bladder cavity, and any bladder disease is treated at this time.

The ability to treat bladder problems is the major advantage of suprapubic prostatectomy because an incision is made into the bladder to reach the prostate. The following are disadvantages:

* An abdominal incision and an incision into the bladder are necessary.
* The client has a suprapubic tube in place postoperatively.
* There is an increased risk of urinary tract infection, incontinence, bladder spasms, and hemorrhage.
* The surgery is more painful.
* Convalescence is longer than with a TURP.

Retropubic Prostatectomy. **Retropubic,** or extravesical, **prostatectomy** may be selected when the prostate is too large to be resected via the transurethral approach but no coexisting bladder abnormalities have been identified. The surgeon makes an abdominal incision above the symphysis pubis to expose the prostate gland. A small incision is made in the prostate gland, and the gland is removed. The difference between the suprapubic and the retropubic approaches is the bladder incision.

Perineal Prostatectomy. Perineal prostatectomy is performed primarily to:

* Remove an enlarged prostate gland that is filled with calculi (stones)
* Treat prostatic abscesses that have not responded to conservative treatment
* Repair complications, such as lacerations in the prostatic capsule, that may have occurred during a different type of prostatectomy
* Treat clients who are poor surgical risks

The client is placed in an exaggerated lithotomy position, and the knees are positioned on the chest. The surgeon makes a U-shaped incision between the ischial tuberosities, the scrotum, and the rectum. The prostatic capsule is then opened and enucleated. This type of prostatectomy provides a direct anatomic approach to the prostate gland.

The major disadvantage of this procedure is the loss of sexual potency resulting from damage to the pudendal nerve. Clients with peripheral vascular disease or chronic pulmonary problems cannot tolerate the exaggerated lithotomy position and are not candidates for a perineal prostatectomy. Other disadvantages of this procedure include a greater risk for infection, the possibility of damage to the rectum and anal sphincter, and the possibility of urinary incontinence. For these reasons, this surgical approach is not commonly used.

POSTOPERATIVE CARE. The general postoperative care for the client who has undergone prostatic surgery is similar regardless of the type of procedure done and the type of anesthesia used (see Chapter 19). However, the nurse is aware of several differences as they affect nursing care.

Nursing Care After a Transurethral Resection of the Prostate. After a TURP, the surgeon inserts a three-way Foley catheter with a 30- to 45-mL retention balloon through the urethra into the bladder (Figure 76-4). The catheter is pulled down into the prostatic fossa to help prevent bleeding. The surgeon often applies traction on the catheter by pulling it taut and taping it to the client's abdomen or thigh.

Catheter Care and Continuous Bladder Irrigation. If the catheter is taped to the client's thigh, the nurse instructs him to keep his leg straight. The surgeon determines when the traction should be removed; usually it is removed on the first postoperative day.

The nurse explains that because of the Foley catheter's large diameter and the pressure of the retention balloon on the internal sphincter of the bladder, the client will continually feel the urge to void. This is a normal sensation and not a surgical complication. The nurse advises the client not to try to void around the catheter, which causes the bladder muscles to contract and may result in painful bladder spasms. He is reassured that an antispasmodic medication can be given to keep him comfortable.

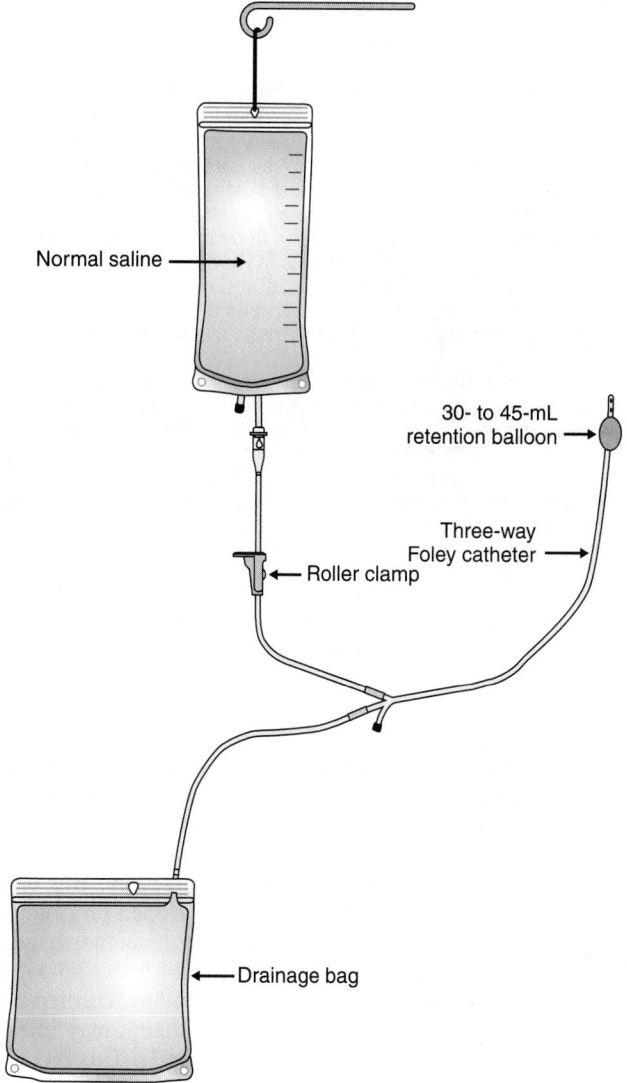

Figure 76-4 ● Continuous bladder irrigation.

Normal saline

30- to 45-mL retention balloon →

Three-way Foley catheter →

← Roller clamp

← Drainage bag

Continuous bladder irrigation (CBI) with normal saline or other solution, as ordered by the physician, may keep the catheter free of obstruction and facilitates detection of obstruction or other complications. The nurse adjusts the irrigation fluid rate to maintain a colorless or light pink drainage return. (For the nursing care of the client undergoing CBI, see Chart 76-3.) The continuous irrigation is usually discontinued 24 hours after a TURP. The Foley catheter is usually removed when CBI is discontinued.

Postcatheterization Care. When the Foley catheter is removed, the client may experience some burning on urination, as well as some urinary frequency, dribbling, and leakage. The nurse reassures the client that these symptoms are normal and will subside. The client may also pass small clots and tissue debris for several days after the TURP. The nurse instructs him to increase fluid intake to a minimum of 2000 to 2500 mL/day, which helps to decrease the dysuria and to keep the urine clear. An older client who has renal disease or who is susceptible to congestive heart failure may not be able to tolerate this much fluid. By the time of discharge (usually

---

⚕ CONSIDERATIONS FOR OLDER ADULTS

When caring for older men who may become confused after surgery, the nurse reorients them frequently and reminds them not to pull on the catheter (Chart 76-2). If the client is restless or "picks" at tubes, the nurse may provide a familiar object, such as a family picture, for him to hold on to for distraction and a feeling of security. If possible, the client should not be restrained; other alternatives should be tried first.

CHART 76-2

NURSING FOCUS on the OLDER ADULT
Prostate Surgery

- Monitor the client closely for signs of infection. Older clients undergoing prostate surgery often also have underlying chronic diseases (such as cardiovascular disease, chronic lung disease, or diabetes) and multiple invasive lines that predispose them to infections.
- Help the client out of bed to the chair as soon as permitted to prevent complications of immobility. Older clients may need assistance because of underlying changes in the musculoskeletal system, such as decreased range of motion and stiffness in joints. These clients are at *high risk* for falls.
- Encourage the client to turn, cough, and deep breathe and to use the incentive spirometer every 2 hours to prevent atelectasis and pneumonia. Older adults are at risk for pneumonia because of the decreases in lung elasticity and vital capacity associated with aging.
- Assess the client's pain every 2 to 3 hours, and administer pain medication as needed.
- Provide a safe environment for the client. Anticipate a temporary change in mental status in the immediate postoperative period as a result of anesthetics and unfamiliar surroundings. Reorient the client frequently. Keep IV lines and catheter tubes secure.

CHART 76-3

BEST PRACTICE for
Care of the Client with Continuous Bladder Irrigation

- Use normal saline solution for the bladder irrigant unless otherwise ordered by the physician. Normal saline solution is isotonic.
- Adjust the rate of the irrigation solution to the physician's specifications. The physician may order a solution rate that keeps the output clear and free of clots.
- Monitor the color, consistency, and amount of urine output.
- Check the drainage tubing frequently for external obstructions (such as kinks) and internal obstructions (such as blood clots and decreased output).
- Assess the client for complaints of bladder spasms, which may indicate obstruction.
- If the urinary catheter is obstructed, turn off the continuous bladder irrigation (CBI) and irrigate the catheter with 30 to 50 mL of normal saline solution using a large piston syringe.
- Notify the physician immediately if the obstruction does not resolve by hand irrigation or if the urinary return becomes "ketchupy."

---

2 days postoperatively), he should be voiding 150 to 200 mL of clear yellow urine every 3 to 4 hours. By discharge, postoperative pain is minimal, and analgesics may not be required.

Complications of Transurethral Resection of the Prostate. Clients who undergo a TURP or open prostatectomy are at risk for postoperative bleeding or hemorrhage. Bleeding is most common within the first 24 hours postoperatively and may not occur until the client has returned to his hospital room. Bladder spasms or movement may initiate bleeding from previously controlled vessels. This bleeding may be arterial or venous, but venous bleeding is more common.

The nurse or assistive nursing personnel monitors the client's urine output every 2 hours and vital signs every 4 hours. If the bleeding is arterial, the nurse will notice that the urinary drainage is bright red or ketchup-like with numerous clots. If arterial bleeding occurs, the nurse notifies the surgeon immediately and increases the CBI rate or intermittently irrigates the catheter with normal saline solution. The surgeon may order aminocaproic acid (Amicar) to control bleeding. The nurse keeps in mind that if the medication does not work, surgical intervention may be necessary to clear the bladder of clots and to stop the arterial bleeding.

If the bleeding is venous, the urine output will be burgundy, with or without any change in vital signs. The nurse informs the client's surgeon of any of the signs and symptoms of bleeding. The surgeon may apply traction on the catheter for a few hours, which may control venous bleeding. The nurse assesses the success of this procedure in stopping the bleeding and is aware that the traction on the catheter is quite uncomfortable and increases the risk of bladder spasms. The physician usually orders analgesics or antispasmodics, such as dicyclomine hydrochloride (Bentyl, Antispas, Formulex ✤, Lomine ✤), oxybutynin (Ditropan), or bel-

ladonna and opium (B&O) suppositories, to decrease painful bladder spasms.

The nurse closely monitors the client's hemoglobin (Hgb) and hematocrit (Hct) levels for anemia as a result of blood loss. Some clients may require blood transfusions to return the Hgb and Hct values to baseline levels.

Nursing Care After Suprapubic Prostatectomy. If the client has undergone a suprapubic prostatectomy, a **suprapubic catheter,** in addition to a Foley catheter, will be in place. Each catheter is connected to a separate closed drainage system and drains the bladder via gravity. The nurse is aware that catheter traction is not effective for the client who experiences postoperative bleeding after a suprapubic prostatectomy. Such a client needs brisk CBI via the catheter. If the CBI does not control the postoperative bleeding, the client needs surgical intervention.

If the client has an suprapubic catheter in place, the Foley catheter is generally removed on the second postoperative day. After the Foley catheter is removed, the nurse clamps the suprapubic catheter and the client attempts to void. After the client has urinated, the nurse checks the residual urine in the bladder by unclamping the suprapubic tube. The client may be discharged from the hospital with a suprapubic catheter in place. When the client consistently empties his bladder and the residual urine in the bladder is 75 mL or less, the suprapubic catheter is then removed. An antimicrobial ointment may be applied daily to the site, depending on hospital policy or the physician's order.

The client with a suprapubic catheter in place is at increased risk for bladder spasms. The incision dressing for these clients should be observed and changed more frequently than for clients who do not have an incision drain, because the dressing becomes saturated with urine until the incision heals. If the suprapubic drain is not connected to gravity drainage, the nurse may enclose the drain with an ostomy bag to measure the output accurately and to prevent any skin problems or breakdown.

Nursing Care After Retropubic Prostatectomy. After a retropubic prostatectomy, the urinary sphincter muscles are seldom damaged, the bladder is not entered, and no urinary drainage should be seen on the abdominal dressing. The nurse notifies the client's surgeon of any urinary or purulent drainage, fever, or increased pain because these symptoms indicate a serious complication such as a deep wound infection or pelvic abscess.

Nursing Care After Perineal Prostatectomy. After the perineal approach to prostatectomy, the client has an incision dressing and may or may not have an incision drain. The use of rectal thermometers and rectal tubes and enemas are contraindicated because they may cause trauma or bleeding.

⊚ CRITICAL THINKING CHALLENGE

You are caring for a man who has just been admitted to your surgical unit after a TURP. The nurse from the postanesthesia care unit (PACU) reported that the urine that was draining was pinkish and that he was undergoing CBI. When you check his urine output, you notice that his Foley catheter is not draining and that there are several large, bright red blood clots in his drainage bag.

- What other assessments should you make at this time?
- What action should you take as soon as possible?

For suggested answer guidelines, go to SIMON http://www.wbsaunders.com/SIMON/Iggy/.

● Community-Based Care

The client with benign prostatic hyperplasia (BPH) is typically managed at home. Clients who have surgery are also discharged to their home.

▨ HEALTH TEACHING

After any type of prostatectomy, some clients, and especially those who have undergone a transurethral resection of the prostate (TURP), may experience some temporary loss of control of urination or a dribbling of the urine. The client is reassured that these symptoms are almost always temporary and will resolve. The nurse assists the client and his family or significant others in devising ways to keep his clothing dry until sphincter control returns. He is instructed to contract and relax his sphincter frequently to re-establish urinary control (Kegel exercises). External urinary (condom or Texas) catheters are not used except in extreme cases, because they may give the client a false sense of security and delay his urinary control.

The nurse provides specific instructions for each client on the basis of the type of surgical procedure performed and any further interventions he may need in the future. Discharge instructions for a client undergoing surgery of the prostate gland are listed in Chart 76-4.

The client who undergoes prostatic surgery usually needs emotional support. The client who undergoes a perineal prostatectomy is at risk for permanent sexual dysfunction. The nurse informs the client of the options, such as a penile prosthesis, that are available to treat erectile dysfunction (ED) (see Interventions [Erectile Dysfunction], p. 1794).

Other surgical procedures for prostate removal should not cause physiologic ED. However, some clients may have functional ED for a short time after surgery during the recovery phase.

CHART 76-4

⊙ CLIENT EDUCATION GUIDE
Care After a Transurethral Resection of the Prostate

- Drink 12 to 14 glasses of water each day, preferably before 8 PM, *unless otherwise contraindicated.*
- Use alcohol, caffeinated beverages, and spicy foods in moderation to avoid overstimulation of your bladder.
- If your urine becomes bloody, rest quietly and increase your fluid intake. If the bleeding does not subside shortly, contact your doctor.
- Avoid strenuous activities, such as driving and working, during the first 2 to 3 weeks after surgery.
- Schedule a follow-up appointment with your doctor after you leave the hospital.

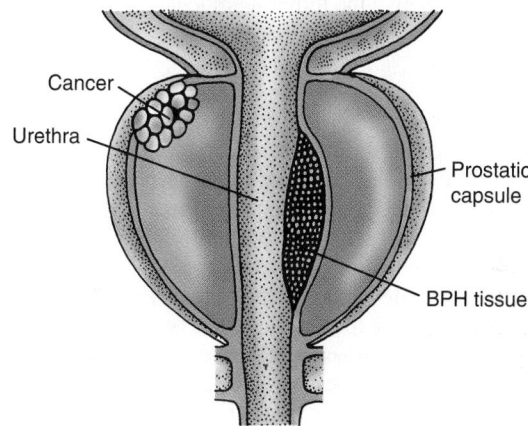

Figure 76-5 ⊙ The prostate gland with cancer and benign prostatic hyperplasia (BPH). Note that cancer normally arises in the periphery of the gland, whereas BPH occurs in the center of the gland.

▨ HOME CARE MANAGEMENT

Unless there is a complication of surgery, such as a wound infection or an unusual problem with voiding, the client does not have a dressing or indwelling catheter at the time of discharge. In some cases, the suprapubic tube may remain in place for several weeks after discharge.

PROSTATE CANCER

▮ OVERVIEW

Prostate cancer is the most common cancer among American men, other than skin cancer, and follows lung cancer as the second leading cause of cancer deaths in this group (American Cancer Society, 2000).

▮ Pathophysiology

Of all cancers of the prostate, 95% are adenocarcinomas. These adenocarcinomas arise from the epithelial cells of the prostate and are usually located in the posterior lobe or outer portion of the gland (Figure 76-5). The remaining types of prostatic neoplasms are classified as *nonepithelial* carcinomas and include ductal carcinomas, transitional cell carcinomas, squamous cell carcinomas, and sarcomas.

Of all malignancies, prostate cancer is one of the slowest growing and metastasizes in a fairly predictable pattern. The most common sites of metastatic spread are the prostatic and perivesicular lymph nodes, the pelvic lymph nodes, bone marrow, and the bones of the pelvis, sacrum, and lumbar spine.

Metastatic involvement of the visceral organs tends to occur late in the natural history of the disease. The most common sites for metastatic prostate cancer are the lungs, liver, adrenals, and kidneys.

Tumor grade is an important variable in the management of prostate cancer. Grading is the pathologist's interpretation of the aggressiveness of the cancer. Usually the Gleason grading system is used. Normal prostate tissue cells are given a score of 1 (best), and abnormal cells are given a score of 5 (worst). The scores of the two most common cell types found in the specimen are added to give the tumor a grade between 2 and 10.

Etiology

Although the cause of prostate cancer remains unclear, two factors influence its development. First, an intact hypothalamic-pituitary-testicular pathway must be present. Men who have been castrated before puberty are at little risk for prostate cancer. Second, the advancing age of the client increases his risk of prostate cancer.

Other contributing factors include a family history of prostate cancer, heavy metal exposure, and a history of vasectomy or sexually transmitted disease (STD). Several viruses, including cytomegalovirus and herpesvirus type 2, are present more commonly in cancerous prostatic tissue than in noncancerous tissue.

The relationship between benign prostatic hyperplasia (BPH) and cancer of the prostate is controversial. Although some researchers say that BPH and cancer of the prostate are unrelated diseases, others suggest that cancer is more likely to occur within or adjacent to any proliferative cell population (Haas & Sakr, 1997).

Incidence/Prevalence

Prostate cancer is the sixth most common cancer in the world and the fourth most common in men. Incidence rates have been influenced by the diagnosis of latent cancers found during screening of asymptomatic men. Developing countries in Africa, South America, and the Caribbean have a very high incidence of the disease. In contrast, the rate is low in Asian countries.

In the United States the introduction of screening with prostate-specific antigen (PSA) has resulted in the doubling of cases diagnosed between 1984 and 1992. If the rate continues to increase, almost 1 million new cases per year could be expected by 2010 (Parkin et al., 1999).

> **CONSIDERATIONS FOR OLDER ADULTS**
> The incidence of prostate cancer increases with age. More than 75% of all prostate cancers are diagnosed in men over 65 years of age (American Cancer Society, 2000).

> **CULTURAL CONSIDERATIONS**
> African-American men have the highest prostate cancer incidence rates in the world. Associated mortality rates are twice those of Caucasian men (von Eschenbach et al., 1997).

African-American men tend to be affected at an earlier age and have more advanced disease at the time of diagnosis. Lack of cancer awareness has been identified as a cause of increased mortality rates (Collins, 1997). Prostate cancer also occurs more often in Scandinavians than in Caucasians.

Hispanic and Asian-American men have lower rates of prostate cancer than Caucasian men and lower mortality rates, implying cultural, genetic, or lifestyle variables (Huff & Kline, 1999).

▶ COLLABORATIVE MANAGEMENT
● Assessment

As with any cancer, accurate staging is necessary for treatment planning and for monitoring the clinical course of the disease. As in BPH, the first symptoms that the client may experience are related to bladder neck obstruction, such as difficulty in initiating urination, recurrent bladder infections, and urinary retention. Gross, painless hematuria is the most common presenting clinical manifestation.

At times, a client may be undergoing intervention for BPH and is discovered to have cancer of the prostate. Bone pain is a symptom of a more advanced stage of prostate cancer. The client who has symptoms of urinary obstruction (urinary hesitancy, back pain) and bone pain is most likely to have metastatic disease at diagnosis.

■ PROSTATE CANCER SCREENING

The most effective procedures for screening for cancer of the prostate are the **digital rectal examination (DRE)** and the PSA test. In 1997 the American Cancer Society updated its guidelines for cancer screening (Chart 76-5). Beginning at age 50 years, all men should have an annual DRE and PSA test (Mettlin, 1997). Men at high risk for prostate cancer, including African Americans or men with a history of prostate cancer in first-degree relatives, should consider screening at an earlier age. On rectal examination, a prostate that is found to be stony hard and with palpable irregularities or indurations is suspected to be malignant.

Prostate-specific antigen (PSA) is a highly immunogenic glycoprotein produced solely by the prostate. The normal

---

CHART 76-5

CLIENT EDUCATION GUIDE
1997 American Cancer Society Prostate Screening and Detection Guidelines

- An annual digital rectal examination (DRE) and prostate-specific antigen (PSA) test should be offered to:
    Men beginning at age 50 years
    Men who have a life expectancy of at least 10 years
    Younger men who are at high risk (at least by age 45 years)
- Men at high risk include those with a strong familial predisposition (e.g., two or more first-degree relatives with prostate cancer) and African-American men.
- DRE should be performed by health care professionals skilled in recognizing subtle prostate abnormalities.
- DRE is less effective than PSA in detecting prostate cancer. An abnormal PSA test result is a value above 4.0 ng/mL.

level of PSA established by the American Cancer Society is a value of less than 4 ng/mL. PSA levels are elevated in clients with increased prostatic tissue as a result of various conditions, including carcinoma of the prostate, benign prostatic hyperplasia (BPH), prostatic infarction, and prostatitis.

PSA blood levels should never be used as a screening test without a physical examination of the prostate. The PSA serum level was never meant to replace the DRE, but to be used in conjunction with it. Twenty-five percent of clients with prostate cancer have PSA levels less than 4 ng/mL (Mettlin, 1997).

PSA is not elevated in healthy men or in men with carcinomas other than prostate carcinoma. However, the normal PSA level is slightly higher in older adults and in African Americans. An elevated PSA level should decrease a few days after a prostatectomy. An increase in the PSA level at postoperative visits usually indicates that the disease has recurred.

CULTURAL CONSIDERATIONS

The participation rate of African-American men in prostate cancer screening programs remains very low. A nursing study by Collins (1997) showed that educational intervention had a positive effect on short-term knowledge and awareness of prostate cancer by African-American men (see the Evidence-Based Practice for Nursing box below).

After screening by DRE and PSA, some clients undergo a **transrectal ultrasound** study of the prostate, although its effectiveness is controversial. The urologist inserts a small probe into the rectum and obtains an ultrasonogram of the prostate. A specimen for biopsy may also be obtained with the rectal probe.

When the diagnosis of prostatic cancer is suspected, a biopsy is necessary for confirmation. Prostatic ultrasonography may be performed to isolate the area of the prostate for biopsy. One of several procedures may be used to obtain the biopsy specimen. The most common procedure is the needle-core or aspiration biopsy.

EVIDENCE-BASED PRACTICE FOR NURSING

Educating African-American men about early detection of cancer

Collins, M. (1997). Increasing prostate cancer awareness in African American men. *Oncology Nursing Forum, 24*(1), 91-95.

The intent of this study was to assess the effect of an educational program about prostate cancer on the knowledge level of African-American men. A convenience sample of 75 men between the ages of 23 and 83 years completed a preintervention and postintervention questionnaire. The findings were positive in that test scores improved after the educational session.

Critique. Although a convenience sample was used, the researcher addressed a major health concern (i.e., the lack of knowledge and participation of African-American men in prostate screening programs). Unfortunately, only short-term retention was evaluated. A follow-up test weeks or months later could determine the lasting effects of education. The sample could also be followed to see if they participated in prostate screening as a result of learning more about prostate cancer.

Implications for Nursing. Nurses have to continue their efforts to educate the public, especially high-risk groups, about the need for prevention and early detection of all types of cancers. African-American men are at the highest risk for prostate cancer.

After the diagnosis of prostate cancer is made, the client undergoes radiographic and blood studies to ascertain the extent of the disease. Common tests include computed tomography (CT) of the pelvis and abdomen and magnetic resonance imaging (MRI) to assess the status of the pelvic and para-aortic lymph nodes. A bone scan is performed to find any evidence of metastatic disease. Hepatomegaly or abnormal results of liver function studies indicate a need for further evaluation for the presence of liver metastases.

Most clients with advanced prostate cancer also have elevated levels of **serum acid phosphatase.** Approximately 90% of clients with prostate cancer metastatic to the bone have elevated **serum alkaline phosphatase** levels.

● Interventions

Management of the client with prostate cancer includes surgery, radiation therapy, and drug therapy. Management is based on the extent of the disease and the client's physical condition. The client may undergo surgery for a tumor biopsy, staging and removal of the tumor, or palliation to control the spread of disease or relieve distressing symptoms. The health care provider and client must weigh the benefits of treatment against potential adverse effects such as incontinence and erectile dysfunction (ED).

SURGICAL MANAGEMENT. Because as many as 30% of localized prostate cancers are resistant to radiation, surgery is the standard treatment and is therefore presented first. The surgical approaches for prostatectomy in the client with prostate cancer are similar to those for BPH (see Surgical Management [Benign Prostatic Hyperplasia], p. 1785). In most cases, however, the surgical procedure is much more extensive and includes a **pelvic lymphadenectomy** (removal of pelvic lymph nodes).

Clients who have stage 0 cancer of the prostate require only close follow-up by their health care provider. If obstruction recurs, repeated needle biopsies or transurethral resections of the prostate (TURPs) should be part of the screening.

RADICAL PROSTATECTOMY. Clients with more severe disease typically undergo a radical prostatectomy via a retropubic, perineal, or suprapubic approach. In the radical prostatectomy, instead of removing only the prostate gland, as in the procedure for BPH, the surgeon removes the entire gland along with the prostatic capsule, the cuff at the bladder neck, the seminal vesicles, and the regional lymph nodes. The remaining urethra is anastomosed to the bladder neck. The removal of tissue at the bladder neck allows the seminal fluid to travel upward into the bladder rather than down the urethral tract, resulting in retrograde ejaculations. The client is sterile, but his ability to have an erection and an orgasm should not be permanently impaired.

Sexual Dysfunction. The surgeon advises clients who are undergoing radical perineal prostatectomy that they may have ED after the surgery. This consequence is directly related to any damage done to the pudendal nerve (which is necessary for erection and orgasm) during the surgery.

The surgeon may perform a nerve-sparing prostatectomy in the following cases:

- There is no evidence of disease in adjacent lymph nodes.
- Serum acid phosphatase levels are not elevated.
- There is no clinical evidence of cancer extension beyond the prostate gland.

As the name of the procedure implies, the surgeon keeps the nerves responsible for penile erection intact. After surgery, the client may experience temporary ED, but normal function usually returns in 3 to 12 months.

Urinary Incontinence. Because the internal and external sphincters of the bladder lie close to the prostate gland, urinary incontinence can be another complication of a radical prostatectomy. The nurse teaches the client perineal exercises to help facilitate the return of urinary continence after surgery or after removal of the Foley catheter. To perform the exercises, the client contracts and relaxes the perineal and gluteal muscles in several ways. For one of the exercises, the nurse teaches the client to:

1. Tighten the perineal muscles for 3 to 5 seconds as if to prevent voiding, then relax
2. Bear down as if having a bowel movement
3. Relax and repeat the exercise

The nurse shows the client how to inhale through pursed lips while tightening the perineal muscles and how to exhale when he relaxes. To regain urinary control, the client can also practice holding an object, such as a pencil, in the fold between the buttock and the thigh. He may also sit on the toilet with his knees apart while voiding and start and stop his stream several times. Chart 76-6 summarizes the most important aspects of postoperative nursing care for the client who has undergone a radical prostatectomy.

Complementary and Alternative Therapies for Incontinence. Biofeedback has been successfully used as a noninvasive treatment for incontinence after radical prostatectomy. In a nursing study by Jackson et al. (1996), 27 postoperative radical prostatectomy clients were treated by biofeedback for urinary incontinence. Forty-eight percent of the sample had complete success, 26% had significant improvement but were not completely dry, and 26% experienced failure. The authors concluded that biofeedback training can work as a first-line option for most clients if they are motivated to decrease their incontinence.

Other Measures for Incontinence. If the client cannot recover urinary continence, an artificial urinary sphincter may be surgically implanted (Figure 76-6). Artificial sphincters have been more successful in males than in females, possibly because of the difference in urethral length.

After the sphincter has been implanted, the nurse instructs the client to report any complications, such as fever, pain on inflation of the device, edema or cellulitis in the genitalia, or recurrence of incontinence, indicating a possible mechanical malfunction in the system.

CRYOSURGICAL ABLATION. A newer, minimally invasive procedure that is becoming more popular as an alternative to radical prostatectomy is cryosurgical ablation of the prostate. During surgery, the client is placed in the lithotomy position to facilitate placement of the transrectal ultrasound probe. The probe helps determine the size of the prostate and the subsequent number of small cryoprobes that are positioned around the prostate gland. Liquid nitrogen freezes the gland, whose dead cells are then absorbed by the body.

The primary advantages of this procedure are minimal blood loss, minimal postoperative pain, decreased risk for postoperative urinary incontinence, and a short hospital stay. Most clients are permitted to return to their usual activity level in about 1 week after surgery. The procedure can be repeated if necessary (Schmidt et al., 1998).

BILATERAL ORCHIECTOMY. Unlike radical prostatectomy, **bilateral orchiectomy** (removal of both testes) is palliative

---

CHART 76-6

BEST PRACTICE *for*
Care of the Client After a Radical 794

- Encourage the client to use patient-controlled analgesia (PCA) as needed. The PCA device may be used through the second postoperative day.
- Keep the client on bedrest on the day of surgery. Help the client to get out of bed and ambulate for a short distance by the first postoperative day.
- Maintain the sequential compression device until the client begins to ambulate. Apply antiembolic stockings until discharge.
- Monitor the client for deep vein thrombosis and pulmonary embolus.
- Keep an accurate record of intake and output, including Jackson-Pratt or other drainage device drainage.
- Keep the urinary meatus clean using soap and water.
- Avoid rectal procedures or treatments.
- Teach the client how to care for the urinary catheter because he will be discharged with the catheter in place.
- Teach the client how to use a leg bag.
- Emphasize the importance of not straining during bowel movement. Advise the client to avoid suppositories or enemas.
- Remind the client about the importance of follow-up appointments with the physician to monitor progress.

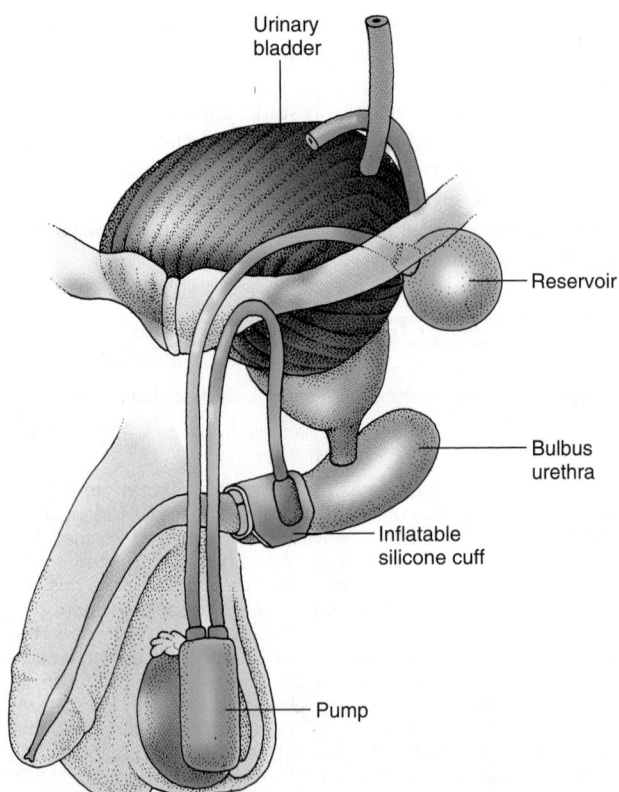

Urinary bladder

Reservoir

Bulbus urethra

Inflatable silicone cuff

Pump

Figure 76-6 ● An artificial urinary sphincter is a fluid-filled system with a silicone cuff that surrounds the urethra and functions as a urinary sphincter. A pump is placed in the scrotum, and a fluid reservoir is placed in the abdomen. When the pump is squeezed, fluid leaves the urethral cuff and flows into the reservoir, allowing the client to empty his bladder.

surgery. The intent of the surgery is not to cure the disease but to arrest its spread by removing testosterone. This procedure is described later in this chapter under Testicular Cancer, p. 1798.

NONSURGICAL MANAGEMENT. Nonsurgical management is usually done as an adjunct to surgery but may be done as an alternative intervention. Modalities include radiation therapy and drug therapy.

RADIATION THERAPY. External beam radiation therapy is important in the treatment of prostate cancer. It is performed for the following purposes:
- As an alternative curative treatment to surgery for locally contained tumors
- As an adjunct to radical prostatectomy when surgical margins or regional lymph nodes show malignancy postoperatively
- For palliation of the client's symptoms

Palliative radiation therapy alleviates pain caused by skeletal metastases and relieves ureteral or bladder neck obstruction.

Another popular treatment is ultrasonically guided iodine-125 or pallidium-103 **interstitial brachytherapy** (radiation therapy) or radioactive **seed implantation.** These procedures are done on an ambulatory care basis and are the most cost-effective treatment for early-stage prostate cancer. The client is reassured that these treatments are safe and well tolerated with minimal complications.

DRUG THERAPY. Drug therapy may consist of either hormonal therapy or chemotherapy. A vaccine to prevent prostate cancer is also being investigated (Tjoa et al., 1999).

Hormonal Therapy. Because prostate cancer is hormone dependent, clients with extensive tumors or those with metastatic disease are usually managed by androgen deprivation. Manipulating the hormonal environment in the client may be accomplished in two ways:
- The testosterone influence can be removed by a bilateral orchiectomy.
- Estrogens or gonadotropin-releasing hormone (GnRH) agonist analogs can be administered (Chart 76-7).

Estrogens such as diethylstilbestrol (DES) inhibit the release of luteinizing hormone (LH) from the pituitary gland. Clients with significant cardiovascular disease may not be candidates for estrogen therapy because of the side effects of estrogens,

such as sodium and water retention and thromboembolic episodes. Other hormonal drugs, such as megestrol (Megace) and medroxyprogesterone (Depo-Provera), are sometimes used if first-line hormonal treatments lose their effectiveness.

Leuprolide acetate (Lupron), a GnRH agonist analog (which suppresses LH release by the pituitary), also reduces serum testosterone levels without any of the estrogenic side effects of DES. Flutamide (Eulexin, Euflex✤), an oral androgen-blocking agent, inhibits tumor progression by blocking the uptake of testicular and adrenal androgens at the prostate tumor site.

The health care provider may prescribe goserelin acetate (Zoladex), a potent GnRH agonist analog, for palliation of advanced prostatic carcinoma. This drug is an alternative treatment when orchiectomy or estrogen administration is neither acceptable nor indicated for the client.

Chemotherapy. Systemic cytotoxic chemotherapy has not proved effective in the treatment of prostate cancer. It is used for the client who fails to respond to hormonal manipulation. Unfortunately, only a small percentage of clients respond to cytotoxic chemotherapy with a partial shrinkage of their tumors, and the response usually lasts only a few months. (See Chapter 25 for a discussion of chemotherapy.)

● Community-Based Care

Nursing management of the client with prostate cancer always includes his spouse or sexual partner. Clients with prostate cancer may require nursing interventions in a wide variety of settings—at the hospital, the radiation therapy department, the oncologist's office, or home—and at any stage of the disease process. Ongoing care of the client undergoing surgery is similar to that described under Community-Based Care for benign prostatic hyperplasia, p. 1789. Major quality-of-life issues facing the client with prostate cancer include body image, sexuality, and the impact of the cancer diagnosis on his life.

ERECTILE DYSFUNCTION

▌ OVERVIEW

Erectile dysfunction (ED), previously known as **impotence,** is the inability to achieve or maintain an erection for sexual intercourse. It affects approximately 10 to 20 million

---

CHART 76-7

DRUG THERAPY *for* **Prostate Cancer: Commonly Used Drugs**

Drug	Usual Dosage	Nursing Interventions
Leuprolide acetate (Lupron)	7.5 mg q mo IM	Use at least a 22-gauge needle. Mix the solution well; it is a milky suspension. Observe for side effects, including "hot flashes" and sweating. Be aware that the client's symptoms may temporarily worsen, caused by a temporary testosterone increase.
Flutamide (Eulexin, Euflex✤)	750 mg in 3 daily divided doses PO	Teach the client that side effects include "hot flashes," loss of libido, and impotence. Diarrhea and nausea with vomiting are less common.
Goserelin acetate (Zoladex)	3.6 mg every 28 days SC	The prefilled syringe cannot be aspirated. If a blood vessel is damaged, blood will enter the syringe. Teach the client that side effects include "hot flashes," sexual dysfunction, and decreased erections.

men in the United States (Colpo, 1998). During the last decade, there has been a major change in the management of men with ED as a result of increased understanding of the physiology of erectile function and the development of new, effective therapies. There are two classes of ED: organic and functional.

Organic Erectile Dysfunction

Organic ED is characterized by a gradual deterioration of function. The man first notices diminishing firmness and a decrease in frequency of erections. Causes include the following:

- Inflammation of the prostate, urethra, or seminole vesicles
- Surgical procedures such as prostatectomy
- Pelvic fractures
- Lumbosacral injuries
- Vascular disease, including hypertension
- Chronic neurologic conditions, such as Parkinson's disease or multiple sclerosis
- Endocrine disorders, such as diabetes mellitus or thyroid disorders
- Smoking and alcohol consumption
- Medications
- Poor overall health that prevents sexual intercourse

Functional Erectile Dysfunction

If the client has episodes of ED, it usually has a functional (psychologic) cause. Men with **functional ED** have normal nocturnal (nighttime) and morning erections. Presentation of symptoms is usually sudden and preceded by a period of high stress.

▶ COLLABORATIVE MANAGEMENT

● Assessment

For a man to have an erection, he must have normal innervation and a normal **libido** (sex drive). Therefore a medical, social, and sexual history along with a complete physical examination is necessary. The first step is to determine if there is an organic cause. Diagnostic testing is done to rule out possible organic causes, as described in the preceding section.

If test results are negative, then the diagnostic evaluation focuses on the specific causes that may have been indicated in the health care provider's medical history. For example, hormone testing is used for clients who have a poor libido, small testicles, or a diminished beard growth. Serum levels of testosterone and gonadotropins are also measured.

Duplex Doppler ultrasonography is another test to evaluate ED. It provides information about arterial and venous blood flow to the penis. It can also be used to determine the best treatment for ED. A **nocturnal penile tumescence test** that measures nighttime erections is done in a sleep laboratory. Usually an erection is expected with each rapid eye movement (REM) episode. This study can determine if ED is caused by an organic or functional problem. If the man has nocturnal erections, the ED is functional. Sexual counseling is needed in this case, and the client is referred to a certified sexual therapist.

● Interventions

Current methods of treatment include vacuum devices, intracorporal injections, intraurethral applications, prostheses, and oral medications.

VACUUM DEVICES. **Vacuum devices** have been used for many years. The basic design of any model is a cylinder that fits over the penis and sits firmly against the body. Using a pump, a vacuum is created to draw blood into the penis to maintain an erection. The cylinder is then removed. The advantage of this procedure is that the device is easy and safe to use. The disadvantage is its clumsiness and lack of spontaneity. In addition, the man may experience pain from the rubber ring or from pumping the device too quickly. The ring should be removed after an hour, or tissue damage may occur. Most insurance companies pay for this device, which typically costs between $350 and $500.

INTRACORPORAL INJECTIONS. In the 1980s it was discovered that injecting the penis with vasoconstrictive drugs would make the penis erect. The most common agents used for this purpose today are papaverine and phentolamine (Regitine). These drugs may be used alone but are most often given in combination. Adverse effects include priapism (prolonged erection), penile scarring, bleeding, bruising at the injection site, pain, and infection.

INTRAURETHRAL APPLICATIONS. In a single-use urethral suppository, alprostadil (Muse) is self-administered with an applicator. The drug is absorbed into the corpora, which causes an erection in about 10 minutes. Advantages include the simplicity of the procedure and noninvasiveness. Disadvantages are a decrease in spontaneity, burning of the urethra, syncope ("blackout") after the application, and cost.

PROSTHESES. **Penile implants** have been used for more than 20 years and are still used when other modalities fail. The three-piece inflatable device is the most commonly implanted prosthesis. This surgical procedure is performed on an ambulatory basis. To inflate the prosthesis, the man squeezes the pump located in the scrotum. To deflate the prosthesis, a release button is activated. Advantages include the man's ability to control his erections. The major disadvantage is that the device is permanent.

Postoperatively, the nurse gives the client instructions for home care. These instructions are similar to postoperative instructions for any client, including observation for bleeding and infection.

ORAL THERAPIES. The most promising oral medication to treat ED is sildenafil (Viagra), used to treat both types of the problem. Clients are instructed to take the pill 1 hour before sexual intercourse. Sexual stimulation is needed within a half hour to 1 hour to promote the erection. Because the erection occurs more naturally when compared with other treatment options, most men and their partners prefer this option.

Clients should abstain from alcohol before sexual intercourse because it may impair the ability to have an erection. Common side effects of the drug include headaches, facial flushing, and diarrhea. If more than 1 pill a day is being taken, leg and back cramps, nausea, and vomiting may be added to the more common side effects. Men who take nitrates should not take Viagra because of vasodilation effects.

TESTICULAR CANCER

■ OVERVIEW

Although malignant tumors of the testis are rare and represent less than 2% of all cancers in men, testicular cancer is the most common malignancy in males ages 15 to 35 years (American Cancer Society, 2000). Testicular cancer strikes young men at a productive time of life and thus has significant economic, social, and psychologic impact on the client and his family or significant others. However, with the advent of combination chemotherapy and earlier detection by testicular self-examination (TSE) (Chart 76-8), this form of cancer can be one of the most curable solid neoplasms.

■ Pathophysiology

Primary testicular cancers fall into two major groups:
- Germinal tumors arising from the sperm-producing germ cells
- Nongerminal tumors arising from the other structures in the testes

Germinal tumors are the most common type of testicular tumors, accounting for more than 95% of cases.

■ GERMINAL TUMORS

Germinal tumors of the testis are classified into two broad categories: seminomas and nonseminomas (Table 76-1).

SEMINOMAS. The most common type of testicular tumor is **seminoma.** Clients with pure seminomatous tumors have the most favorable prognoses because the tumors generally remain localized and metastasize late. In most clients with seminomatous testicular tumors, seminomas are diagnosed when they are confined to the testicles and retroperitoneal lymph nodes. These tumors also respond extremely well to radiation therapy. Clients with early-stage seminomas have about a 95% 5-year survival rate with surgery (orchiectomy) and radiation therapy (American Cancer Society, 2000).

NONSEMINOMAS. Nonseminomatous germ cell tumors include three types: embryonal carcinoma, teratoma, and choriocarcinoma.

These tumors are made up of cells that are not as sensitive to treatment with radiation therapy. They are treated with surgery or chemotherapy, depending on the extent of the disease at presentation.

Pure embryonal carcinomas are common in young men between the ages of 19 and 26 years. Embryonal carcinomas tend to spread earlier than seminomas and usually first affect the retroperitoneal lymph nodes. This type of tumor may also spread via the bloodstream to other sites in the body, such as the lung or the liver. Pure teratomas rarely occur. They are usually found mixed with other types of testicular tumors. Choriocarcinoma is a lethal type of nonseminomatous cancer, which spreads rapidly throughout the body. Clients with choriocarcinomas almost always have metastatic disease at the initial diagnosis because choriocarcinoma spreads via the hematogenous route rather than via the lymphatic system.

MIXED CELL TYPES. Testicular cancers with a mixture of cell types are also common. Almost any combination of germ cell tumors is possible, but the most common combination is embryonal carcinoma and teratoma *(teratocarcinoma).* About 25% of all testicular cancers are teratocarcinomas.

■ NONGERMINAL TUMORS

The remaining 5% of testicular tumors arise from the nongerminal elements in the testes, such as the interstitial cells or cells that make up fibrous or vascular networks. Nongerminal testicular neoplasms are classified as either *interstitial cell tumors* or *androblastomas* (testicular adenomas).

Interstitial cell tumors arise from the Leydig cells, which secrete testosterone into the bloodstream. These tumors are rare and usually benign. They may secrete an excessive amount of androgenic hormones, which cause young boys with such tumors to undergo early puberty.

Androblastomas are also rare and usually benign. They sometimes secrete estrogen, which accounts for the feminization and gynecomastia (breast enlargement) occasionally seen in these clients.

CHART 76-8

CLIENT EDUCATION GUIDE
Testicular Self-Examination

- Examine your testicles monthly immediately after a bath or a shower, when your scrotal skin is relaxed.
- Examine each testicle by gently rolling it between your thumbs and fingers. Testicular tumors tend to appear deep in the center of the testicle.
- Report any lump or swelling to your doctor as soon as possible.

TABLE 76-1 • CLASSIFICATION OF TESTICULAR TUMORS

GERMINAL (GERM CELL) TUMORS
- Seminoma
- Nonseminoma
  Embryonal carcinoma
  Teratoma
  Choriocarcinoma

NONGERMINAL (NON–GERM CELL) TUMORS
- Intestinal cell tumor
- Androblastoma

■ Etiology

The cause of testicular cancer is unknown. The risk for testicular tumors is reported to be higher in males who have an undescended testis (**cryptorchidism**). In males with cryptorchidism, the testicular cancer usually develops in the undescended testis (80%), and there is a 25% chance of cancer developing in the normally descended testis. Seminoma is the most common type of testicular cancer associated with cryptorchidism. The undescended testis undergoes gradual involution and degeneration over time, which may contribute to tumor development. It is not known why the normally descended testis is at risk for cancer. Brothers and close male relatives of clients with testicular cancer have a slightly greater risk of testicular cancer than the general population.

Although a history of trauma or infection is common in clients with testicular cancer, neither has been established as a cause of testicular cancer and may be coincidental findings at the time of the testicular examination. The client with a history of trauma or infection should be examined by a health care provider after the acute episode subsides to rule out the existence of a tumor.

Testicular cancer is rarely bilateral. There is only a minute chance that a client with a tumor in one testis will have another primary testicular tumor in the other testis. In rare instances, leukemias, lymphomas, plasmacytomas, and metastatic carcinomas may involve the testes. A client with bilateral testicular tumors is more likely to have metastatic disease to the testes than bilateral primary testicular tumors.

Incidence/Prevalence

In the United States it is estimated that 7400 new cases of testicular cancer will be diagnosed each year, and an estimated 300 men will die of the disease. This cancer is the most common solid tumor diagnosed in men between the ages of 15 and 40 years. Testicular cancer can occur during infancy and middle age (after age 50); however, the peak incidence is between the ages of 18 and 40 years (American Cancer Society, 2000).

> **CULTURAL CONSIDERATIONS**
> Testicular cancer occurs most often in Caucasians and is rare in African Americans (American Cancer Society, 2000).

▶ COLLABORATIVE MANAGEMENT

Activity Link

● Assessment

■ HISTORY

When taking a history from a client with a suspected testicular tumor, the nurse keeps the risk factors in mind. Basic but important data to collect are age and race, because the disease occurs most often in young Caucasian males. The nurse is also alert to other risk factors, including a history or presence of an undescended testis and a family history of testicular cancer.

The nurse then assesses the client's family situation. Is the client married? Does he have children? Does he want children in the future? Depending on the treatment plan chosen, would he be interested in sperm storage in a sperm bank?

If the client has one healthy testis, he can function sexually and may not have any reproductive dysfunction. If the client undergoes a retroperitoneal lymph node dissection or chemotherapy, he may become sterile because of treatment effects on the sperm-producing cells or surgical trauma to the sympathetic nervous system, resulting in retrograde ejaculations.

■ PHYSICAL ASSESSMENT/CLINICAL MANIFESTATIONS

The testes, lymph nodes, and abdomen are thoroughly examined. The health care provider or generalist nurse palpates the testes for lumps or swelling (Chart 76-9). The presence of any palpable lymphadenopathy, abdominal masses, or gy-

---

CHART 76-9

FOCUSED ASSESSMENT *of*
A Male Client with a Testicular Lump

Obtain a medical history from the client:
- When was the lump discovered?
- Are there any other symptoms (sensation of heaviness, dragging in testicle, pain, discharge from penis)?
- Is there a history of cryptorchidism?

Assess the genital system. Always wear gloves during the examination of the male genitalia.
- Inspect and palpate the scrotal contents. Have the client perform a Valsalva maneuver, and palpate for a varicocele.
- Any lump or enlargement that does not transilluminate should be suspected as malignant.

Palpate for any enlarged lymph nodes. Most common lymphadenopathy is in the inguinal or supraclavicular regions.
Assess the abdomen for a possible mass or hepatomegaly.

---

necomastia (enlarged breasts) usually indicates metastatic disease.

■ PSYCHOSOCIAL ASSESSMENT

Because the diagnosis of testicular cancer usually occurs in the young adult, the nurse pays close attention to the psychosocial ramifications of the disease. Even if the cancer is detected at an early stage and the client is cured after orchiectomy, he may be afraid that he will be sexually handicapped. Even if the client's disease is arrested with surgery, radiation, or chemotherapy, he may think of himself as less than a whole man. These fears can disrupt the psychosocial and sexual development of the young male and can threaten the identity of adult males. The client may be afraid that he will not be able to perform sexually, will no longer be sexually attractive or desirable, and will face rejection. Feelings of sexual inadequacy may be denied, repressed, or displaced, causing increased stress on the man's personal and work relationships.

The nurse performs a psychosocial assessment of these clients on a routine basis because problems may arise at any time. The nurse also makes referrals to other resources as appropriate.

■ LABORATORY ASSESSMENT

An important diagnostic indicator for the client with a testicular mass is the presence of any serum or urinary marker proteins (tumor markers) that are often produced by testicular cancers. Benign testicular tumors *never* cause an elevation in the levels of any of these marker proteins.

The primary tumor markers for testicular cancer are **alpha-fetoprotein (AFP)** and the beta subunit of human chorionic gonadotropin (hCG). Approximately 90% of clients with nonseminomatous testicular tumors (embryonal carcinoma, teratoma, or choriocarcinoma) initially have elevated serum levels of AFP, hCG, or both. Clients with a pure seminoma do not have an elevated AFP level, and only 10% have a slightly elevated hCG level. This level resolves after orchiectomy.

If a client has a diagnosis of seminoma and also has an elevated AFP level, the tumor specimen must be re-examined for evidence of a component of nonseminomatous cancer. This step is necessary because the treatments differ for seminomatous and nonseminomatous tumors.

AFP and hCG determinations are also used to evaluate responses to therapy for testicular cancer and to document the presence of residual or recurrent disease. With effective treatment, the levels of abnormal markers fall. The persistence of elevated levels of markers after orchiectomy is substantive evidence that the client has metastatic disease, even if results of clinical staging procedures (x-ray studies and scans) are normal. The reappearance of the tumor markers heralds a recurrence of the cancer. Therefore marker levels must be monitored regularly during the follow-up of clients treated for testicular cancer.

OTHER DIAGNOSTIC ASSESSMENT

After the diagnosis of testicular cancer, the client should have a computed tomography (CT) scan of the abdomen and the chest, or chest tomograms, to identify any small lesions not apparent on conventional x-ray films or physical assessment.

Magnetic resonance imaging (MRI) is used to detect enlarged lymph nodes and abnormal nodules in certain organs that may indicate metastasis from the testicles. Chest x-ray studies and bone scans may also be performed if metastasis is suspected.

Clients with a pure seminoma may undergo bipedal lymphangiography as part of the staging workup to assess for any evidence of retroperitoneal lymph node involvement. Lymphangiograms are also valuable in determining the extent of radiation therapy fields.

Analysis

COMMON NURSING DIAGNOSES AND COLLABORATIVE PROBLEMS

A common nursing diagnosis in clients with testicular cancer is Risk for Sexual Dysfunction related to disease or treatment. A common collaborative problem is Potential for Metastasis.

ADDITIONAL NURSING DIAGNOSES AND COLLABORATIVE PROBLEMS

In addition to the common nursing diagnoses and collaborative problems, clients with testicular cancer may have one or more of the following:

- Dysfunctional Grieving or Anticipatory Grieving related to loss of a body part or changes in body function
- Disturbed Body Image related to the diagnosis of cancer and its treatment
- Acute or Chronic Pain related to tumor compression or effects of metastasis
- Anxiety related to the diagnosis of cancer

Planning and Implementation

RISK FOR SEXUAL DYSFUNCTION

NOC **PLANNING: EXPECTED OUTCOMES.** The client with testicular cancer is expected to identify potential or actual alterations in reproductive function and identify alternative methods of meeting reproductive needs if necessary.

INTERVENTIONS. At the time of diagnosis, the incidence of **oligospermia** (low sperm count) and **azoospermia** (minimal sperm) is increased in clients with testicular cancer.

> **CHART 76-10**
>
> **CLIENT EDUCATION GUIDE**
> **Sperm Banking**
>
> - You may want to investigate sperm storage in a sperm bank as a way to preserve your sperm for future use.
> - No one knows how long sperm can be stored successfully, but pregnancies have resulted from sperm stored for longer than 10 years.
> - Check with the sperm bank to see how much it charges to process and store your sperm and to see whether you must pay when the service is provided.
> - Investigate whether your health insurance company will reimburse you for sperm collection and storage.

This finding may be due to the disease process itself and to stress, but the exact reasons are unknown. The client may not discover that he is oligospermic or azoospermic until he has a presurgery sperm count.

Male cancer clients who are not candidates for sperm storage in a sperm bank may select from other options such as donor insemination, adoption, or not fathering children. The nurse initiates health teaching about reproduction, fertility, and sexuality in the pretreatment phase. Normal reproductive function is reviewed, as well as the possible effects of cancer and its treatment on reproductive function. The nurse explains various reproductive options (e.g., sperm banks and artificial insemination) (Chart 76-10). The sperm bank facility provides comprehensive information on semen collection, storage of semen, the storage contract, costs, and the insemination process.

When preparing the client for the collection and storage of sperm, the nurse assumes the role of client advocate and keeps in mind the effect of the cancer diagnosis on the client. The psychologic benefit of having stored sperm may be important for the client and may influence his response to treatment. Knowing that the potential for being a father still exists may help the client cope with other assaults to his masculinity, such as alopecia or erectile dysfunction (ED).

The client should arrange for semen storage as soon as possible after diagnosis. Sperm collection should be completed *before* he begins radiation therapy or chemotherapy or undergoes a radical retroperitoneal lymph node dissection. After radiation therapy or chemotherapy has been implemented, the client may be at increased risk for producing mutagenic sperm, which may not be viable or may result in fetal abnormalities.

The recommended number of samples to optimize the chances of later fertilization is three to six ejaculates, collected 2 to 4 days apart. The process of sperm collection can delay treatment for as long as 1 month, especially if the client is still recovering from surgery and multiple procedures or tests. The client's diagnosis (e.g., acute leukemia, sarcoma, advanced lymphoma, or testicular cancer) and his physical condition may not allow treatment to be postponed, thus making sperm storage an unfeasible reproductive option.

POTENTIAL FOR METASTASIS

PLANNING: EXPECTED OUTCOMES. The client with testicular cancer is expected not to experience complications of the tumor, including metastasis or recurrence of disease.

INTERVENTIONS. A combination of nonsurgical and surgical management is often necessary to prevent metastatic disease (or to alleviate symptoms associated with it) and to bring about tumor regression. The nurse explains the interventions for treating testicular cancer.

NONSURGICAL MANAGEMENT. Chemotherapy and radiation therapy are indicated for nonsurgical management of clients at high risk for metastatic disease or those with metastatic disease.

CHEMOTHERAPY. Combination chemotherapy may be used as adjuvant therapy for *nonseminomatous* testicular tumors or as primary treatment when there is evidence of metastatic disease. Combination chemotherapy is dramatically effective in treating nonseminomatous testicular cancer, particularly if cisplatin (Platinol) is used. This agent is necessary in any successful combination chemotherapy regimen for treating testicular cancer.

The following are other drugs commonly used in combination with cisplatin:

- Bleomycin sulfate (Blenoxane)
- Vinblastine sulfate (Velban, Velbe✤)
- Etoposide (VP-16, VePesid)
- Dactinomycin (Cosmegen)
- Cyclophosphamide (Cytoxan, Procytox✤)
- Doxorubicin (Adriamycin)

The specific combination of drugs, the route of administration, and the frequency, cycling, and duration of treatment can vary considerably from client to client, depending on the extent of the disease and the protocol being followed by the health care provider. Chapter 25 discusses the nursing care of the client receiving chemotherapy.

RADIATION THERAPY. After orchiectomy (removal of one or both testes), external beam radiation therapy is the treatment of choice for clients with pure seminomatous testicular cancer because of the marked radiosensitivity of this type of testicular cancer. If radiation therapy is administered, a staging lymphangiogram is used to determine the treatment portals. An advantage of using radiation therapy instead of radical lymph node dissection is that reproductive function is preserved because surgical dissection of the sympathetic ganglia is avoided.

For the client undergoing radiation therapy to the retroperitoneal lymph nodes, the remaining testis is shielded with a lead cup to preserve reproductive function. Yet, even with these precautions, the client may have transient oligospermia (a decreased sperm count) as a result of radiation scatter. Normally, the sperm count returns to the pretreatment level within 24 to 30 months after the radiation treatment is completed. If metastases develop outside the lymphatic system, the client may still be cured with radiation therapy if the area of involvement is limited. If lymphatic involvement is extensive, or if the visceral organs are involved, the health care provider uses combination chemotherapy similar to that for nonseminomatous testicular cancer.

STEM CELL TRANSPLANTATION. Studies are being conducted to explore whether high-dose chemotherapy with stem cell transplantation may be valuable in treating men with advanced germ cell cancer. In this procedure, the client's blood-forming stem cells are removed from the bone marrow and preserved by freezing while the client receives high-dose chemotherapy. Once the chemotherapy is completed, the stem cells are returned to the client. This procedure helps to prevent the infection and anemia that accompany chemotherapeutic drug use.

SURGICAL MANAGEMENT. The physician performs a unilateral orchiectomy for diagnosis and uses primary surgical management. Clients with testicular cancer may also undergo a radical retroperitoneal lymph node dissection. Using this procedure, the physician can accurately stage the disease and debulk (reduce) the tumor volume so that chemotherapy or radiation therapy is more effective.

PREOPERATIVE CARE. Like most clients with cancer, the client with testicular cancer is usually apprehensive. The nurse offers support and reinforces the teaching provided by the surgeon.

The client's postoperative needs should be anticipated and planned for before surgery. The physician's office nurse or case manager informs the client and his family or significant others about what to expect after surgery. The surgical incision for a retroperitoneal lymph node dissection is extensive. Depending on the extent of the dissection and the need for surgical exploration, the surgeon might make not only a midline incision but also a transthoracic incision or a combination of the two incisions (thoracoabdominal).

The nurse informs the client that radical retroperitoneal lymph node dissections are relatively long operations, lasting 6 to 12 hours. These clients need close and frequent observation, which may be done by nurses in a critical care unit.

OPERATIVE PROCEDURES. To perform a radical retroperitoneal lymph node dissection, the surgeon removes the retroperitoneal nodes in the iliac and lumbar regions. Because the blood supply and the lymphatic vessels of the testes and kidneys are directly related, an extensive midline incision from the xiphoid process to the pubis is necessary. After mobilization of the colon, the surgeon removes the perinephric nodes along with the nodes near the aorta and both renal hila. The node dissection also includes the inguinal area on the affected side. During the lymphadenectomy, the sympathetic ganglia around the lower lumbar lymphatics are dissected. The removal of the sympathetic ganglia abolishes peristalsis in the ductus deferens and contractions of the seminal vesicles. This disruption results in sterility because the client's ejaculate no longer contains sperm. The surgery, however, usually does not interfere with the client's ability to have a normal erection and does not affect his ability to experience orgasm.

A gel-filled silicone prosthesis can usually be surgically implanted into the scrotum at the time of the orchiectomy or later, if the client desires. The nurse reassures the client that this procedure does not impair fertility or sexual function; the client cosmetically appears to have two testes.

POSTOPERATIVE CARE. Because of the length of the surgery, the manipulation of the abdominal and retroperitoneal viscera, and the loss of a major part of the lymphatic fluid, nodes, and channels, the nurse observes and assesses the client for any of the complications of major abdominal surgery. The nurse intervenes for any of the following expected problems:

- Pain from surgical incisions
- Immobility related to prolonged maintenance of surgical positioning and postoperative pain
- Injuries related to any invasive catheters or tubes

The client is usually hospitalized for 3 to 4 days after a radical retroperitoneal lymph node dissection. During this time, the nurse explains care after discharge.

CRITICAL THINKING CHALLENGE

While visiting your sister, she confides that her husband has just been diagnosed with early-stage testicular cancer. She wants to have children and is very concerned about her husband's future and the possibility of starting a family. She was told by the physician that there are several options for treatment and having a family, but she is confused and scared.

- What reassurance can you give your sister at this time?
- How will they be able to have children if he is treated for cancer?
- What options will your brother-in-law have to treat his cancer?

For suggested answer guidelines, go to [SIMON] http://www.wbsaunders.com/SIMON/Iggy/.

• Community-Based Care

After an orchiectomy, the client is typically hospitalized for 1 to 2 days. This period may need to be extended if he must undergo additional surgery or chemotherapy. Because it may not be known until after the orchiectomy whether the client has cancer, what type of testicular cancer he has, or if he needs additional surgery or treatment with radiation therapy or chemotherapy, specific discharge planning may need to be deferred until the postoperative period.

■ HEALTH TEACHING

For the client who has undergone testicular surgery, the nurse emphasizes the importance of scheduling a follow-up visit with the physician, who will examine the incision for healing and complications. The nurse instructs the client to notify the physician if any of the following symptoms occurs before the scheduled appointment: chills, fever, increasing tenderness or pain around the incision, drainage, or dehiscence of the incision.

These symptoms may indicate the presence of an infection for which medical attention is needed. The nurse instructs the client that he will be able to resume most of his usual activities within 1 week after discharge, except for lifting heavy objects (objects weighing 20 pounds [9.1 kg]) or stair climbing. The nurse also reminds him to ask his physician when strenuous activities may be resumed.

The client who has undergone an orchiectomy is informed that he may make arrangements with his physician to have a silicone prosthesis inserted into the scrotum if a prosthesis was not inserted during the orchiectomy.

The nurse also explains the importance of performing monthly testicular self-examination (TSE) on the remaining testis and scheduling follow-up examinations with the physician. The client who has had testicular cancer should schedule determinations of urinary and serum levels of tumor markers and computed tomography (CT) or magnetic resonance imaging (MRI) studies as part of his routine follow-up for a minimum of 3 years.

Depending on the pathologic findings and the stage of the cancer, the client may need further treatment. This information may not be available at the time of discharge. If it is known that the client needs further surgery, he and his family need information about the future surgery. If it is known that he must

undergo radiation therapy or chemotherapy, he needs education about a radiation therapy and chemotherapy regimen.

The client who undergoes treatment for testicular cancer may need emotional support. If permanent sterility occurs and sperm storage has not been feasible, the man may need counseling about other reproductive options.

■ HOME CARE MANAGEMENT

After a unilateral orchiectomy, unless the client has a wound complication, he is discharged without a dressing on the inguinal incision. The client may want to wear a dressing to prevent his clothing from rubbing on the sutures and producing irritation. Because his sutures are intact at the time of discharge, he is told that they will be removed in the physician's office 7 to 10 days postoperatively.

■ HEALTH CARE RESOURCES

The client may be referred to agencies or support groups such as the American Fertility Society or RESOLVE (an organization for infertile couples).

• Evaluation: Outcomes

NOC The nurse evaluates the care of the client who has been treated for testicular cancer on the basis of the identified nursing diagnoses and collaborative problems. The expected outcomes include that the client will:

- Not experience a recurrence of cancer or metastases
- Accept body image changes and show adaptation to his altered self-concept
- Verbalize feelings of grief
- Recover from surgery, chemotherapy, or radiation therapy without complications
- Verbalize an understanding of the effects of surgery or radiation therapy on sexual function and identify alternative methods of meeting reproductive needs

OTHER COMMON PROBLEMS AFFECTING THE TESTES AND ADJACENT STRUCTURES

Problems that develop inside the scrotum usually occur as a mass or as scrotal edema. Some problems produce pain, but others do not. Figure 76-7 shows some of the most common conditions found in the male, including hydrocele, spermatocele, varicocele, and scrotal trauma.

Hydrocele
■ OVERVIEW

A **hydrocele** is a cystic mass, usually filled with straw-colored fluid, that forms around the testis (see Figure 76-7). It results from a disorder in the lymphatic drainage of the scrotum, causing a swelling of the tunica vaginalis, which surrounds the testes. Unless the swelling becomes large and uncomfortable or begins to compromise the circulation to the testis, no treatment is necessary.

▶ COLLABORATIVE MANAGEMENT

A hydrocele may be aspirated via a needle and syringe, or it may be removed surgically. To correct a hydrocele surgically,

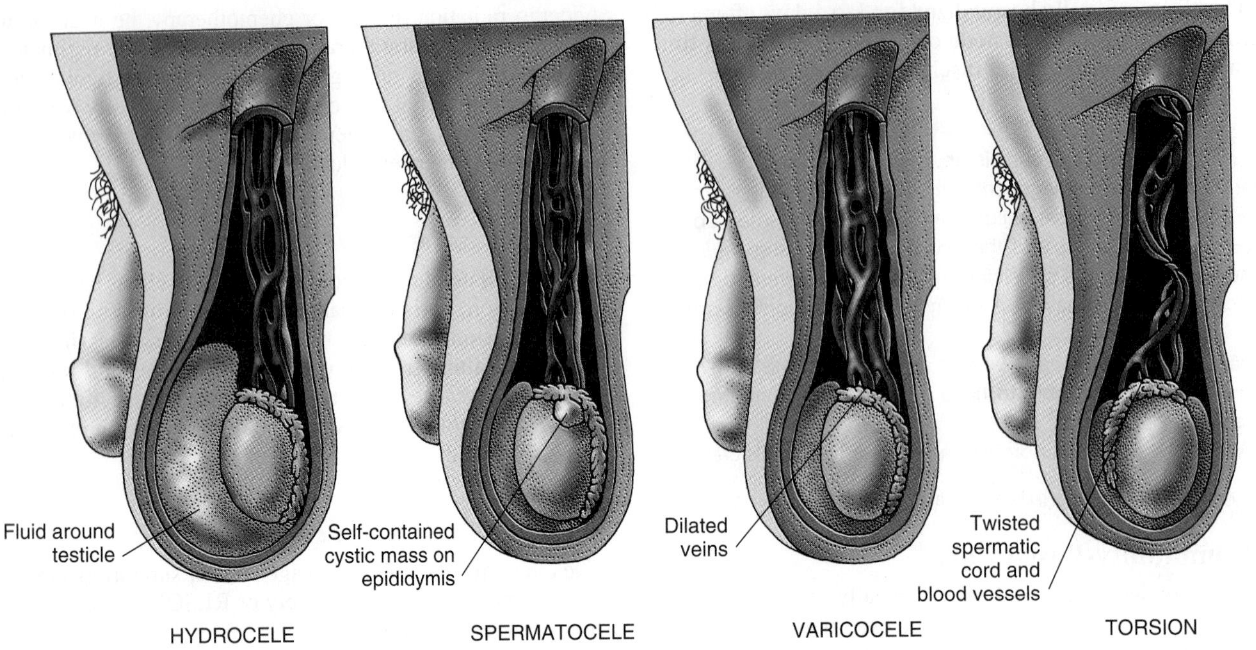

Figure 76-7 ● Common problems affecting the testes and adjacent structures.

the physician makes an incision in the scrotum and removes the hydrocele. The client may or may not return from the operating suite with a drain at the incision site. Typically, hydrocelectomies are performed on an outpatient basis; if the client requires hospitalization, it is for only 1 or 2 days. The nurse instructs the client that if an incision drain is present, there may be some serosanguineous drainage for the first 24 to 48 hours after surgery. The nurse also explains the importance of wearing a scrotal support. The scrotal support keeps the scrotal dressing in place and keeps the scrotum elevated, which helps to prevent edema.

Clients vary considerably in the degree of pain that they experience with this surgery. The nurse assesses and observes the client for pain every 2 to 3 hours in the immediate postoperative period. Moderate incision pain is expected for approximately 24 hours after surgery and should markedly decrease within 1 or 2 days. If the client's pain does not resolve within this time, the nurse is alert to the possible development of wound complications.

The client is instructed to schedule a follow-up visit with the surgeon to have the wound evaluated for healing. The nurse stresses the importance of continuing to wear a scrotal support to promote drainage and comfort. The scrotum can remain swollen from residual inflammation and edema for as long as several weeks. The client is reassured that this swelling is normal and eventually subsides.

Spermatocele

A **spermatocele** is a sperm-containing cystic mass that develops on the epididymis alongside the testicle (see Figure 76-7). Normally, spermatoceles remain small and asymptomatic, and no interventions are necessary. If the spermatocele becomes large enough to cause discomfort to the client, a spermatocelectomy is performed. In this simple procedure, the spermatocele is excised through a small scrotal incision. Routinely, no incision drain is used because drainage and swelling are minimal.

Varicocele

◼ OVERVIEW

A **varicocele** is a cluster of dilated veins posterior to and above the testis (see Figure 76-7). The diagnosis is made by scrotal palpation, particularly when the client performs a Valsalva maneuver. The scrotum feels "wormlike" when palpated. Varicoceles can be either unilateral or bilateral, but most are unilateral and on the left side of the scrotum. In many cases, varicoceles are asymptomatic, with no treatment required. In a few men, varicoceles are painful and must be removed surgically.

Varicoceles can also cause infertility. It is thought that the increase in scrotal temperature resulting from the venous stasis near the testis is the cause of the altered spermatogenesis.

▶ COLLABORATIVE MANAGEMENT

A **varicocelectomy** (surgical removal of the varicocele) is usually performed through an inguinal incision, in which the spermatic veins are ligated in the cord, or through an incision adjacent to the superior iliac spine, in which the spermatic veins are ligated in the retroperitoneal space. A varicocelectomy may be done on an ambulatory care basis, or the client may be hospitalized overnight.

Before surgery, the nurse explains to the client that persistent venous congestion of the scrotum is common after this type of surgery because of the changed circulation in the area. To promote drainage of the scrotum, a rolled towel is placed under the scrotum while the client is in bed. The nurse may also apply ice to the scrotum if necessary. Any intervention that facilitates drainage and decreases swelling from the area promotes relief. The nurse instructs the client about the importance of wearing a scrotal support while ambulating.

At the time of discharge, the nurse instructs the client to make a follow-up appointment with the surgeon to have the sutures removed. The nurse also reminds him to notify the physician of any increasing discomfort at the incision site or in the scrotum, which might indicate an infection. Increasing scrotal discomfort can mean that the circulation to the testis has been impaired. Testicular atrophy, a rare complication of a varicocelectomy, may occur if the blood supply to the testis becomes insufficient.

Scrotal Trauma

Because of the mobility of the scrotum, scrotal injuries are relatively rare. Torsion of the testes involves the twisting of the spermatic cord and occurs most often during puberty (see Figure 76-7). Torsion may occur after strenuous exercise or trauma, or it may develop spontaneously. Because the testes are sensitive to any decrease in blood flow, torsion of the testis is considered a surgical emergency. The client experiences pain, which does not subside with scrotal elevation. In addition to pain, he usually complains of nausea and vomiting.

In addition to caring for the client's physical needs, the nurse is also attuned to his psychosexual needs. Of primary concern to the male client with an injury to his external genitalia are his masculinity and sexuality. The nurse is prepared to use crisis intervention techniques and is knowledgeable about sexuality in order to help the client adjust to an injury in the genital area.

At discharge, the nurse instructs the client to maintain ice to the scrotum for at least 72 hours and elevate the scrotum to minimize edema. The client should avoid lifting heavy objects for 4 to 6 weeks, limit stair climbing, and suspend strenuous physical activity for 1 month. The client is also reminded to wear a scrotal support for at least 3 weeks (Miller, 1999).

Cryptorchidism

An undescended testis, or **cryptorchidism,** is mainly a pediatric problem. Three percent of full-term male infants and 20% of premature infants have an undescended testis. In 80% of cases, the undescended testis descends spontaneously during the infant's first year. If an adult has cryptorchidism, an **orchidopexy** (surgical placement of the testicle into the scrotum) may be performed for cosmetic and psychosexual reasons. The surgery may also prevent the adverse effect of body temperature on spermatogenesis and reduce the risk of testicular cancer. As an alternative, an orchiectomy of the cryptorchid testicle may be recommended.

During an orchidopexy, the client is placed in a supine position. The surgeon makes an inguinal incision, and the spermatic cord is released from the surrounding fascia to obtain maximal length. The surgeon then creates a dartos pouch and places the testis between the skin and the dartos muscle of the scrotum. The tunica albuginea of the testis is sutured to the dartos muscle of the scrotum. The inguinal incision and the scrotal incision (if there is one) are then closed, and a dressing is applied. If there is an incision in the scrotum, it is also covered with a dressing and the client is instructed to wear a scrotal support.

Cancer of the Penis
▌ OVERVIEW

Cancer of the penis represents less than 1% of all malignancies in men in the United States.

CULTURAL CONSIDERATIONS
Epidermoid carcinoma is the most common cancer of the penis. In countries where circumcision is not practiced, such as India, China, and Africa, this type of cancer represents 12% of all cancers (American Cancer Society, 2000).

► COLLABORATIVE MANAGEMENT
▶ Assessment

Carcinoma of the penis usually occurs as a painless, wartlike growth or ulcer on the glans under the prepuce (foreskin) and may initially be mistaken for a venereal wart. A penile carcinoma may also appear as a reddened lesion with plaque.

▶ Interventions

Small lesions involving only the skin may be controlled by excisional biopsy. When the lesion is not curable by excisional biopsy or radiation therapy, a **penectomy** (partial or total removal of the penis) may be required.

PARTIAL PENECTOMY. When the lesion is limited to the glans, a partial penectomy is performed. The client is placed in the lithotomy position, and a tourniquet is applied around the penis. The surgeon makes an incision to amputate a portion of the corpus cavernosum and the corpus spongiosum. The urethra is anastomosed to the skin, and a dressing is applied. A Foley catheter is in place for 3 to 5 days after surgery until the edema surrounding the urethra subsides. The nurse assesses the dressing for drainage, which should be minimal. The catheter is checked for patency every 4 hours for the first postoperative day.

TOTAL PENECTOMY. A total penectomy is required when the lesion has penetrated the shaft of the penis or when the tumor has recurred after a partial penectomy or radiation therapy. The client is placed in the lithotomy position. The surgeon makes an incision from the pubic bone, which encircles the penis and extends into the perineum. The bases of both corpora cavernosa are exposed and excised, and the penis is amputated. The surgeon places an incision drain in the wound before it is sutured. Clients who undergo a total penectomy also have a perineal urethrotomy (anastomosis of the urethra to the skin in the perineum) for urinary drainage.

After a total penectomy, the nurse observes the incision dressing every 2 to 4 hours during the first 24 to 48 hours. There may be a moderate amount of serosanguineous drainage from the incision drains.

The nurse is aware that regardless of how accepting the client may appear preoperatively, he may experience severe emotional problems postoperatively. After a partial penectomy, the client must adjust to considerable changes in body image and sexuality. The nurse encourages him to verbalize his feelings about the loss of his penis. After a total penectomy, the client can no longer have penile-vaginal or penile-anal intercourse and cannot urinate in a standing position. It is difficult for most clients to accept the possibility that they might die because of a lesion on the penis, especially because they are rarely experiencing any systemic cancer symptoms and are otherwise healthy. The nurse helps the client realize that the removal of his penis may save his life. The nurse is aware of the possibility of suicide attempts, since the client's penis may be more important to him than his life. The nurse may be the one to detect the need for professional psychologic assistance for the client or his partner. Early interventions by the nurse can make a tremendous difference in the client's or partner's well-being.

Circumcision (the surgical removal of the prepuce from the penis) in infancy almost eliminates the possibility of penile cancer in that chronic irritation and inflammation of the glans penis predispose uncircumcised men to penile cancer. Because of the ongoing controversy about neonatal circumcision, the nurse teaches both men and new mothers of boys that strict personal hygiene is an important preventive measure against penile cancer.

Phimosis

In a man with **phimosis,** the prepuce is constricted so that it cannot be retracted over the glans. Because of the recent trend away from routine circumcision of newborns, the nurse instructs new mothers, male children, and adult men about the importance of cleaning the prepuce. Phimosis is corrected by circumcision.

Circumcision

■ OVERVIEW

Circumcision (the surgical removal of the prepuce or foreskin) in the adult male is usually done for medical reasons, such as to correct phimosis and to eliminate the infections that often result from this condition.

▶ COLLABORATIVE MANAGEMENT

Circumcision in the adult male is usually performed in a same-day surgical setting. If the client has a dressing, the nurse instructs him to soak in a warm bath that evening to allow the dressing to loosen. If the dressing falls off before the next day, the client is cautioned not to replace it. The nurse explains that the sutures will be absorbed and need not be removed. No residual or side effects result from this surgery, and the client should be able to resume his normal activities within 1 week; sexual intercourse may be resumed after 1 to 2 weeks.

The client may be discharged with a prescription for a barbiturate sleeping medication to be taken for several nights postoperatively. The nurse emphasizes that barbiturate sleeping medications suppress the rapid-eye-movement (REM) phase of sleep so that normal nocturnal erections do not occur. This prevents any tension on the sutures by an erection.

Nonbarbiturate sleeping medications do not inhibit the nocturnal erection pattern. The nurse explains the relationship between barbiturate sleeping medications and nocturnal erections because the client may not comply with the instructions to take the medication, especially if he is not having any difficulty sleeping.

The nurse advises the client to notify his physician if he has any wound complications, such as swelling at the incision area of drainage, and to schedule a postoperative office visit.

Priapism

■ OVERVIEW

Priapism is an uncontrolled and long-maintained erection without sexual desire, which causes the penis to become large, hard, and painful. Priapism affects the two corpora cavernosa; the corpus spongiosum and glans penis are not affected.

Priapism can occur from neural, vascular, or pharmacologic causes, including the following:

- Thrombosis of the veins of the corpora cavernosa (usually resulting from trauma)
- Leukemia
- Sickle cell anemia
- Diabetes
- Malignancies

Sickle cell disease causes priapism through the accumulation of erythrocytes within the corporal bodies. Leukemia may cause priapism because the increased number of white blood cells (WBCs) permits persistent engorgement of the corporal bodies. Malignancies may also infiltrate the corporal bodies, causing persistent engorgement. Priapism can also result from an abnormal neurogenic reflex, psychotropic medications, antidepressants, and antihypertensive medications.

▶ COLLABORATIVE MANAGEMENT

Priapism is considered a urologic emergency because the circulation to the penis may be compromised and the client may not be able to void with an erect penis. The goal of medical intervention is to improve the venous drainage of the corpora cavernosa. Conservative measures involve prostatic massage, sedation, and bedrest.

Meperidine (Demerol) is usually administered immediately because of its hypotensive effect. Warm enemas may be given to bring about venous dilation and thus increase the outflow of the trapped blood. Urinary catheterization is required if the client cannot void.

If conservative therapy is unsuccessful, treatment may proceed to aspiration of the corpora cavernosa with a large-bore needle or surgical intervention. The priapism should be resolved within the first 24 to 30 hours to prevent penile ischemia, gangrene, fibrosis, and impotence. If a cause of priapism is identified, treatment is directed toward that underlying cause.

The nurse who is caring for the client with priapism is sensitive to his emotional needs. The client may be uncomfortable and in crisis but at the same time embarrassed by his erection and loss of control. The nurse reassures the client that he or she understands that the client is not in control of his erection and provides him with privacy.

Prostatitis

■ OVERVIEW

A number of inflammatory conditions can affect the prostate gland, causing **prostatitis.** The most common is abacterial prostatitis.

■ Abacterial Prostatitis

Abacterial prostatitis can occur after a viral illness or may be associated with sexually transmitted diseases (STDs), especially in young males. In many instances, an exact cause of the perineal discomfort cannot be found. The prostatitis can be related to psychosexual problems. The term *prostatodynia* is sometimes used to described this condition.

■ Bacterial Prostatitis

Bacterial prostatitis is usually associated with urethritis or an infection of the lower urinary tract. Organisms may reach the prostate via the bloodstream or the urethra. The most common organisms are *Escherichia coli, Enterobacter, Proteus,* and group D streptococci. Acute bacterial prostatitis may be manifested by fever, chills, **dysuria** (painful urination), urethral discharge, and a boggy, tender prostate.

Gentle palpation of the prostate usually results in a urethral discharge, which is evidenced by white blood cells (WBCs) in the prostatic secretions.

➤ COLLABORATIVE MANAGEMENT

The client with chronic prostatitis usually complains of backache, perineal pain, mild dysuria, and urinary frequency; hematuria may be present. The prostate may feel irregularly enlarged, firm, and slightly tender when palpated. Complications of prostatitis are epididymitis (inflammation of the epididymis) and cystitis (inflammation of the bladder). A rare complication is a prostatic abscess. The client with either acute or chronic bacterial prostatitis is likely to experience urinary tract infections. Sexual functioning may be diminished because of discomfort.

Early diagnosis and treatment of prostatitis with antimicrobials, such as carbenicillin indanyl sodium (Geocillin, Geopen Oral), or fluoroquinolones (ciprofloxacin [Cipro]), can help prevent an abscess. The nurse emphasizes the importance of comfort measures, such as sitz baths, and taking prescribed antibiotics on schedule. The physician orders stool softeners to prevent straining and rectal irritation of the prostate during a bowel movement. Analgesics may be used for symptomatic relief.

The nurse instructs the client with chronic prostatitis about the long-term nature of the problem. Because prostatitis can cause other urinary tract infections, the nurse explains the importance of increasing fluid intake and long-term antibiotic therapy (therapy lasting 30 days). Because trimethoprim (Bactrim✚, Septra) diffuses into the prostatic fluid, it is the antibiotic of choice. The nurse instructs the client about activities that drain the prostate (sexual intercourse, masturbation, and prostatic massage), which may help in the management of chronic prostatitis.

Epididymitis
▮ OVERVIEW

Epididymitis, an infection of the epididymis, may result from an infection of the prostate. It used to be a frequent complication of gonorrhea. Although not common, epididymitis can also be a complication of long-term use of an indwelling Foley catheter, prostatic surgery, or a cystoscopic examination.

In men younger than 35 years of age, the major causative organism in epididymitis is *Chlamydia trachomatis,* which is transmitted sexually (see Chapter 77). The infective organism passes upward through the urethra and the ejaculatory duct, then along the vas deferens to the epididymis.

The client with epididymitis usually complains of pain along the inguinal canal and along the vas deferens, followed by pain and swelling in the scrotum and the groin. If epididymitis is untreated, the epididymis becomes swollen and painful, and the client's temperature may become elevated. Pyuria and bacteriuria may develop, with resultant chills and fever. An abscess may form, necessitating an orchiectomy (removal of one or both testes).

➤ COLLABORATIVE MANAGEMENT

The nurse instructs the client with epididymitis to remain in bed with his scrotum elevated on a towel to prevent traction on the spermatic cord, to facilitate venous drainage, and to relieve pain. The client may be given antibiotics until all acute symptoms of inflammation are gone. If the epididymitis is chlamydial or gonorrheal in origin, the client's sexual partners are also treated with antibiotics.

The client may find other comfort measures effective, such as applying cold compresses or ice to the scrotum intermittently and taking sitz baths. The nurse advises him to avoid lifting, straining, or sexual activity until the infection is under control (which may take as long as 4 weeks).

In clients with epididymitis, there must always be the suspicion of a testicular tumor, especially if the condition does not resolve in a week or two. Ultrasound study is often done to rule out an abscess or tumor. Clients with recurrent or chronic painful conditions may require an epididymectomy (excision of the epididymis from the testicle).

Orchitis

Orchitis, or acute testicular inflammation, may result from trauma or infection. The infection may be caused by the direct spread of bacteria through the urethra or by an infection elsewhere in the body, such as pneumonia, tuberculosis, gonorrhea, syphilis, or mumps. It is rare that the testes alone are involved; usually both the testes and the epididymis are involved (epididymo-orchitis).

Orchitis may be unilateral or bilateral. If the orchitis is bilateral, the client is at increased risk for sterility because of the testicular atrophy and fibrosis that occur during healing.

The signs and symptoms of orchitis are the same as those of epididymitis (scrotal pain and edema). In addition, the client may experience nausea and vomiting and pain radiating to the inguinal canal.

The treatment of orchitis is the same as for epididymitis and includes the following:
- Bedrest with scrotal elevation
- Application of ice
- Administration of analgesics and antibiotics

Mumps orchitis, which occurs in approximately 20% of males who have mumps after puberty, is usually bilateral, and orchitis symptoms develop 4 to 6 days after the parotitis. Any postpubertal male who has not had mumps and is exposed to or contracts mumps is usually given gamma globulin. Although gamma globulin does not prevent mumps, the clinical course of the disease is likely to be less severe, with fewer complications. Childhood vaccination against mumps is an important preventive measure.

ONLINE RESOURCES

For suggested readings and Internet resources, go to http://www.wbsaunders.com/SIMON/Iggy/.

SELECTED BIBLIOGRAPHY

Asterisk indicates a classic or definitive work on this subject.
American Cancer Society. (2000). *Cancer facts and figures—2000.* Report No. 00-300M-No. 5008.00. Atlanta: Author.
Collins, M. (1997). Increasing prostate cancer awareness in African American men. *Oncology Nursing Forum, 24*(1), 91-95.

Colpo, L. (1998). Evaluation, treatment, and management of erectile dysfunction: An overview. *Urologic Nursing, 18*(2), 100-106.

Gray, M., & Allensworth, D. (1999). Electrovaporization of the prostate: Initial experiences and nursing management. *Urology Nursing, 19*(1), 25-31.

Haas, G.P., & Sakr, W. (1997). Epidemiology of prostate cancer. *CA: A Cancer Journal for Clinicians, 47*(5), 273-285.

Holtgrave, H. (1998). Current trends in management of men with lower urinary tract symptoms and benign prostatic hyperplasia. *Urology, 51* (Suppl. 4A), 1-7.

Huff, R., & Kline, M. (1999). *Promoting health in multicultural populations.* London: Sage.

*Jackson, J., et al. (1996). Biofeedback: A noninvasive treatment for incontinence after radical prostatectomy. *Urology Nursing, 16*(2), 50-54.

Klingman, L. (1999). Assessing the male genitalia. *American Journal of Nursing, 99*(7), 47-50.

Marks, L.S., et al. (2000). Effects of a saw palmetto herbal blend in men with symptomatic benign prostatic hyperplasia. *Journal of Urology, 163*(5), 1451-1456.

Matteson, M.A., McConnell, E.S., & Linton, A.D. (1997). *Gerontological nursing: Concepts and practices* (2nd ed.). Philadelphia: W.B. Saunders.

Mettlin, C. (1997). The American Cancer Society National Prostate Cancer Detection Project and national patterns of prostate cancer detection and treatment. *CA: A Cancer Journal for Clinicians, 47*(5), 265-272.

Miller, K. (1999). Emergency! Testicular torsion: A surgical emergency primarily affecting young men. *American Journal of Nursing, 99*(6), 33.

Parkin, D., et al. (1999). Global cancer statistics. *CA: A Cancer Journal for Clinicians, 49*(1), 33-64.

Pickett, M., et al. (2000). Prostate cancer elder alert: Living with treatment choices and outcomes. *Journal of Gerontological Nursing, 26*(2), 22-34.

Redmond, M.C. (1998). Ultrasonically guided interstitial brachytherapy for prostate cancer: Care of the patient in ambulatory surgery. *Journal of Perianesthesia Nursing, 13*(3), 156-164.

Schmidt, J., Doyle, J., & Larison, S. (1998). Prostate cryoablation: Update 1998. *CA: A Cancer Journal for Clinicians, 48*(4), 239-253.

Tingen, M., et al. (1998). Perceived benefits: A predictor of participation in prostate cancer screening. *Cancer Nursing, 21*(5), 349-357.

Tjoa, B., et al. (1999). Dendritic cell-based immunotherapy for prostate cancer. *CA: A Cancer Journal for Clinicians, 49*(2), 117-128.

von Eschenbach, A., et al. (1997). American Cancer Society guideline for the early detection of prostate cancer: Update 1997. *CA: A Cancer Journal for Clinicians, 47,* 261-264.

Weinrish, S.P., et al. (2000). Barriers to prostate screening. *Cancer Nursing, 23,* 117-121.

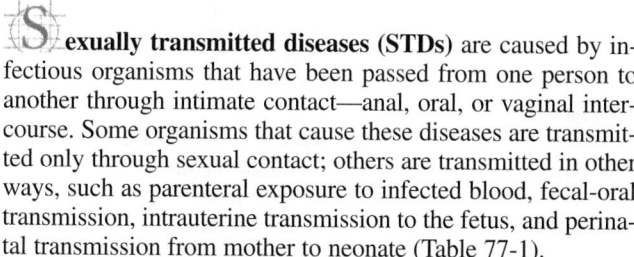

CHAPTER 77

Interventions for Clients with Sexually Transmitted Diseases

SHIRLEY E. VAN ZANDT

Learning Objectives

After studying this chapter, you should be able to:

1. Explain how sexually transmitted diseases (STDs) can be prevented.
2. Compare and contrast the stages of syphilis.
3. Prioritize nursing care for the client with syphilis at each stage.
4. Identify the role of drug therapy in managing clients with genital herpes.
5. Discuss the psychosocial effects of having an STD.
6. Develop a teaching plan for clients diagnosed with gonorrhea.
7. Describe the assessment findings that are typical in clients with *Chlamydia trachomatis* infection.
8. Analyze assessment data to determine common nursing diagnoses for women with pelvic inflammatory disease (PID).
9. Formulate a collaborative plan of care for a client with PID.
10. Develop a community-based teaching plan for clients with PID.
11. Evaluate care for a client with PID.
12. Identify common causes of vaginal infections.

Go to http://www.wbsaunders.com/SIMON/Iggy/ for self-assessment questions related to these Learning Objectives.

Sexually transmitted diseases (STDs) are caused by infectious organisms that have been passed from one person to another through intimate contact—anal, oral, or vaginal intercourse. Some organisms that cause these diseases are transmitted only through sexual contact; others are transmitted in other ways, such as parenteral exposure to infected blood, fecal-oral transmission, intrauterine transmission to the fetus, and perinatal transmission from mother to neonate (Table 77-1).

The list of STDs continues to grow because of improved diagnostic techniques, an increased number of organisms and systemic diseases that can be sexually transmitted, and sexual attitudes and practices. In the United States, sexual issues are often controversial. The nurse must respect the choices that clients make, and provide confidentiality (see the Legal/Ethical Issues in Health Care box on p. 1806).

The prevalence of STDs is a major health concern worldwide. Increasing population, cultural factors (e.g., later marriages), political and economic policies, and human physiology patterns such as earlier menarche affect the prevalence of STDs in any given geographic area. Sexual attitudes and behaviors and access to care play a major role in the risk of acquiring an STD (Amaral, 1998). STDs also cause complications that can contribute to severe physical and emotional

suffering, including infertility, ectopic pregnancy, cancer, and death. Some of the most common complications caused by sexually transmitted organisms are listed in Table 77-2.

STDs and acquired immunodeficiency syndrome (AIDS) are reportable to local health authorities in every state. Some STDs, such as genital herpes, may or may not be reported, depending on local legal requirements. Chlamydial infection is now reportable in most states (Centers for Disease Control and Prevention [CDC], 1998). Rigorous reporting and follow-up efforts by federal and local public health departments and health care providers is one intervention for decreasing the incidence of STDs.

Nurses in a variety of community settings are responsible for identifying clients at risk for STDs, caring for clients with diagnosed STDs, and preventing further cases through education and case finding. Nurses in secondary and tertiary care settings, such as hospitals, also have a responsibility to recognize clients who are at risk for or who have symptoms of STDs. Nurses also need to be aware of the individual and societal costs of the care of clients with STDs (see the Cost of Care box on p. 1807).

The Centers for Disease Control and Prevention (CDC) regularly updates its guidelines for treatment of STDs. The 1998

TABLE 77-1 • SEXUALLY TRANSMITTED DISEASES

- Human immunodeficiency virus infection
- Chancroid
- Syphilis
- Lymphogranuloma venereum
- Genital herpes simplex virus infection
- Genital warts
- Gonococcal infection
- Chlamydial infection
- Nongonococcal urethritis
- Mucopurulent cervicitis
- Epididymitis
- Pelvic inflammatory disease
- Sexually transmitted enteritis
- Sexually transmitted proctitis
- Trichomoniasis
- Candidal infection
- Bacterial vaginosis
- Viral hepatitis
- Cytomegalovirus infection
- Ectoparasitic infection
  - Pediculosis pubis
  - Scabies

From Centers for Disease Control and Prevention. (1998). 1998 guidelines for treatment of sexually transmitted diseases. *Morbidity and Mortality Weekly Report, 47*(No. RR-1), 1-103.

LEGAL/ETHICAL ISSUES IN HEALTH CARE

SEXUAL DECISION MAKING AND CONFIDENTIALITY FOR CLIENTS WITH SEXUALLY TRANSMITTED DISEASES

Sexual issues are surrounded with much controversy in the United States. Personal values, cultural mores, and public health standards often collide as clients make decisions about their sexual health. Americans hold strongly to the principle of autonomy. Autonomy in sexual decision making (e.g., about whether to be sexually active, how to choose sexual partners, and the type of sexual behavior that is appropriate) is held as a high value. The parental right to know about a minor's sexual activity is debated as one challenge to this principle of autonomy. The standard of confidentiality protects this principle of autonomy in some clinical situations and under some state laws.

As nurses aim to respect this principle of autonomy about sexual decision making and confidentiality, they can be challenged by the public health concerns of protecting the health of the entire community versus the autonomy of the individual to make his or her own decisions. Increasing rates of chlamydial infection, especially in the teenage population, with the costly risk of infertility complications, make this notion of autonomy in sexual decision making more problematic. Clients who refuse to discuss their sexually transmitted disease with their partners, or partners who choose not to get tested or treated pose additional challenges to our respect for autonomy in light of the overwhelming public health concerns. Nurses are conflicted in their commitment to both confidentiality (autonomy) and promotion of the public's health (beneficence).

TABLE 77-2 • COMPLICATIONS CAUSED BY SEXUALLY TRANSMITTED ORGANISMS

Complication	Causative Organisms
Salpingitis, infertility, and ectopic pregnancy	*Neisseria gonorrhoeae* *Chlamydia trachomatis* *Mycoplasma hominis* *Ureaplasma urealyticum*
Reproductive loss (abortion/miscarriage)	*N. gonorrhoeae* *C. trachomatis* Herpes simplex virus *M. hominis* *U. urealyticum* *Treponema pallidum*
Puerperal infection	*N. gonorrhoeae* *C. trachomatis*
Perinatal infection	Hepatitis B virus Human immunodeficiency virus Human papillomavirus *N. gonorrhoeae* *C. trachomatis* Herpes simplex virus *T. pallidum* Cytomegalovirus Group B streptococcus
Cancer of genital area	*C. trachomatis* Herpes simplex virus Human papillomavirus
Male urethritis	*M. hominis* Herpes simplex virus *N. gonorrhoeae* *C. trachomatis* *U. urealyticum*
Vulvovaginitis	Herpes simplex virus *Trichomonas vaginalis* Bacteria causing vaginosis *Candida albicans*
Cervicitis	*N. gonorrhoeae* *C. trachomatis* Herpes simplex virus
Proctitis	*N. gonorrhoeae* *C. trachomatis* Herpes simplex virus *Campylobacter jejuni* *Shigella* species *Entamoeba histolytica*
Hepatitis	*T. pallidum* Hepatitis A, B, and C virus
Dermatitis	*Sarcoptes scabiei* *Phthirus pubis*
Genital ulceration or warts	*C. trachomatis* Herpes simplex virus Human papillomavirus *T. pallidum* *Haemophilus ducreyi* *Calymmatobacterium granulomatis*

COST OF CARE
IMPLICATIONS FOR NURSING

SEXUALLY TRANSMITTED DISEASES

Cost of Care

- Estimates of annual direct and indirect costs for sexually transmitted diseases (STDs) and their complications in 1994 were $9.9 billion as compared with the national public investment of $231 million in STD prevention (Hein, 1998).
- The Institute of Medicine has estimated that the sequelae of *Chlamydia trachomatis* infections in women (i.e., PID, infertility, and ectopic pregnancy) result in an estimated $4 billion in health care costs per year (Stamm, 1999).
- Approximately $5.5 billion is spent on PID and its sequelae a year (Paavonen, 1998).
- Managed care poses some new obstacles to prevention of STDs. An emphasis on short-term cost savings, differences in technical capabilities for diagnosis and treatment, and challenges to reliable follow-up because partners of those infected may not be members of the same health plan may undermine public health strategies of the past.
- Costs of individual antibiotics used to treat STDs may be a hindrance to proper treatment, especially for the rapidly increasing uninsured segment of the U.S. population.

Costs (Wholesale) of Oral Medications*

ORAL DRUGS	APPROXIMATE COST OF DRUG PER DOSE	APPROXIMATE COST FOR COURSE OF TREATMENT
Acyclovir 200 mg 5 times/day for 10 days	$1.14	$57.00
Azithromycin 1 g once (4 tablets, 250 mg each)	$24.80	$24.80
Cefixime 400 mg once	$6.90	$6.90
Ciprofloxacin 500 mg once	$3.74	$3.74
Clindamycin 450 mg qid for 14 days	$1.56	$87.36
Doxycycline 100 mg bid for 7 days	$0.11	$1.54
Famciclovir 125 mg bid for 5 days	$1.59	$15.90
Metronidazole 500 mg bid for 14 days	$0.06	$1.68
Ofloxacin 400 mg once	$4.34	$4.34
Valacyclovir 500 mg bid for 5 days	$2.82	$28.20

Implications for Nursing

Nurses have a unique role in the prevention and early detection of STDs. Their role has high potential for decreasing the cost of disease to the nation and individuals. Ongoing education with clients about their risk of contracting or transmitting a disease and methods of prevention is essential. Discussing the cost, both financial and emotional, of STDs, including the cost of unintended infertility, is part of the nurse's teaching to clients. Nurses include thorough health histories in their assessment of clients. This information may be more revealing in terms of the client's ability to prevent or treat disease than what other members of the health care team have been able to elicit.

Since most clients are treated for STDs as outpatients, assessing the client's ability to pay for medication and access and pay for follow-up care is a significant part of the nurse's assessment and intervention.

*Modified from Bartlett, J.G. (1998). *Pocket book of infectious disease therapy.* Baltimore: Williams & Wilkins

WOMEN'S HEALTH CONSIDERATIONS

Women are at the greatest risk for health problems caused by STDs. Pregnancy and adolescence substantially increase the risk of transmission and complications. Because of differences in the physiology of reproductive structures, women have greater rates of transmission of STDs if exposed. Adolescence tends to be a time of risk taking. Young women who are sexually active have more frequent unprotected sexual intercourse than their older counterparts because of the following:

- Lack of knowledge about the risk of disease
- Their belief that they are not vulnerable to disease
- Alcohol consumption, which promotes risky sexual behavior

The rates of many STDs are highest among adolescents, more frequently in adolescent females (CDC, 1998). Postmenopausal women also may be at high risk for STDs, since many do not use barrier protection because of age-related infertility. Mucosal tears from vaginal atrophy in postmenopausal women may also place them at greater risk (Rosen & Brown, 1998b).

Women have more asymptomatic infections that may delay diagnosis and treatment. This delay increases the likelihood of more serious problems, including irreversible damage to reproductive organs and systemic illness. Embarrassment, denial, or fear about STDs may further delay treatment, increasing the potential for serious complications.

guidelines provide information, treatment standards, and counseling advice to help decrease the spread of STDs (CDC, 1998).

ACQUIRED IMMUNODEFICIENCY SYNDROME

Acquired immunodeficiency syndrome (AIDS), a disease caused by infection with the human immunodeficiency virus (HIV), is a disorder of immunosuppression affecting the body's ability to fight disease. HIV is transmitted through infected body fluids (e.g., semen, vaginal secretions, blood and blood products, breast milk) infected with HIV. People at high risk include the following (Youngkin & Davis, 1998):

- People who engage in anal sexual activity
- People who share needles
- People who have unprotected sexual intercourse with multiple partners
- People who have unprotected sexual intercourse with partners infected with HIV
- Infants born to women who are infected with HIV
- People who have hemophilia or other clotting disorders
- People who used untested blood and blood products before 1985
- Health care workers
- Sexual partners of anyone at risk for HIV (of both sexes)

Because HIV affects the immune system and can be transmitted in ways other than by sexual contact, it is discussed in detail in Chapter 22.

INFECTIONS ASSOCIATED WITH ULCERS
Syphilis
OVERVIEW

Syphilis is a complex sexually transmitted disease (STD) that can become systemic and cause serious complications and even death. Before penicillin was available in the 1940s, syphilis af-

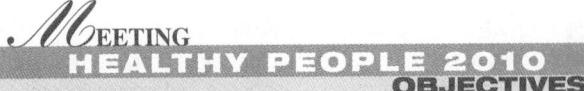

fected nearly 25% of the U.S. population. Between 1958 and 1990 there was no appreciable change or improvement in the rates of syphilis despite successful treatment. However, in 1990 the number of cases increased to a post–World War II peak of over 50,000. Since 1990 there has been a steady *decrease* in cases, with only 6993 primary and secondary cases reported in 1998 (CDC, 1999). One of the Healthy People 2010 objectives is to eliminate syphilis in the United States (see the Meeting Healthy People 2010 Objectives box above).

The causative organism of syphilis is *Treponema pallidum,* a spirochete with a slender, spiral shape that resembles a corkscrew. Nonpathogenic *Treponema* species are found in the mouth, intestinal tract, and genital areas of people and animals. Although the organism can be seen only with a dark-field microscope, several serologic tests may be used to screen for the presence of syphilis antigen/antibody. *T. pallidum* is susceptible to dry air or any known disinfectant. The organisms die within hours at temperatures of 105.8° to 107.6° F (41° to 42° C) and are not airborne. The infection is usually transmitted by sexual contact, but transmission can occur through close body contact and kissing.

Syphilis progresses through stages: primary, secondary, latency, and tertiary.

▮ Primary Syphilis

The appearance of an ulcer, called a **chancre,** is the first sign of syphilis. The chancre develops at the site of inoculation, or entry, of the organism from 10 to 90 days after exposure (3 weeks is average). Chancres may be found on any area of the skin or mucous membranes but most frequently occur on the genitalia, lips, nipples, and hands and in the oral cavity, anus, and rectum.

During this highly infectious stage, the chancre begins as a small papule. Within 3 to 7 days, it breaks down into its characteristic appearance: a painless, indurated, smooth weeping lesion. Regional lymph nodes enlarge, feel firm, and are not painful. Without treatment, the chancre usually disappears within 6 weeks. However, the organism spreads throughout the body, and the client is still considered infectious.

▮ Secondary Syphilis

Secondary syphilis develops 6 weeks to 6 months after the onset of primary syphilis. Secondary syphilis is a systemic disease, since the spirochetes circulate throughout the bloodstream. Clinical manifestations include malaise, low-grade fever, headache, muscular aches and pains, and sometimes a sore throat.

These symptoms are frequently mistaken for those of influenza. A generalized rash develops, which involves the palms and soles of the feet. Although there is no typical appearance of the rash, it tends to evolve sequentially from papules to squamous papules to pustules. Other skin lesions can include psoriasis-like rashes, wartlike lesions (condyloma lata), and mucous patches. The lesions are highly contagious and should not be touched without gloves. The rash subsides spontaneously in 4 to 12 weeks.

▮ Early and Late Latent Syphilis

After the second stage of syphilis, there is a period of latency. *Early* latent syphilis occurs during the first year after infection, and infectious lesions can recur. *Late* latent syphilis is a disease of more than 1 year's duration after infection. This stage is noninfectious except to the fetus of a pregnant woman. Clients with latent syphilis may or may not have reactive serologic test findings.

▮ Tertiary Syphilis

Tertiary, or late, syphilis occurs after a highly variable period, from 4 to 20 years. This stage develops in untreated cases and can mimic almost any pathologic condition, since virtually any organ system can be affected. The following are manifestations of late syphilis:

- Benign lesions (gummas) of the skin, mucous membranes, and bones
- Cardiovascular syphilis, usually in the form of aortic valvular disease and aortic aneurysms
- Neurosyphilis, which includes central nervous system involvement (e.g., meningitis, sensorineural hearing loss, generalized paresis)

> **CULTURAL CONSIDERATIONS**
>
> Specific ethnic groups in the United States seem to be more affected by syphilis than Caucasians. Primary and secondary syphilis rates of African Americans are nearly 60 times those of Caucasians, and the rates of Hispanics are 4 times those of Caucasians (Rosen & Brown, 1998a).

▶ COLLABORATIVE MANAGEMENT
● Assessment

Assessment of the client presenting with symptoms of syphilis begins with a history to gather information about the lesions or rash noticed. The history should include a risk assessment and sexual history and whether previous testing or treatment for syphilis or other STDs has ever been done (Chart 77-1). The nurse asks about allergic reactions to drugs, especially penicillin. A woman may present with complaints of inguinal lymph node enlargement, the location that drains the area of the vagina and cervix. She may state a history of sexual contact with a male partner who had an ulcer that she

CHART 77-1

FOCUSED ASSESSMENT *of*
The Client with a Sexually Transmitted Disease

Assess history of present illness:
- Chief complaint
- Symptoms by quality and quantity, precipitating and palliative factors
- Any treatments taken (self-prescribed or over-the-counter products)

Assess past medical history:
- Major health problems—including any history of STDs/PID
- Surgeries—obstetric and gynecologic

Assess current health status:
- Menstrual history for irregularities
- Sexual history
    - Type and frequency of sexual activity
    - Number of sexual contacts
    - Sexual orientation
- Contraceptive history
- Medications
- Allergies
- Lifestyle risks—drugs, alcohol, tobacco

Assess preventive health care practices:
- Having Pap smears
- Regular STD screening
- Use of barrier contraceptives to prevent STDs and pregnancy

Assess physical examination findings:
- Vital signs
- Oropharyngeal findings
- Abdominal findings
- Genital or pelvic findings
- Anorectal findings

Assess laboratory data:
- Urinalysis
- Hematology
- Cervical and/or urethral, oral, rectal specimens
- Lesion samples for microbiology/virology
- Pregnancy testing

STDs, Sexually transmitted diseases; *PID*, pelvic inflammatory disease.

noticed during the encounter. Men usually discover the chancre on the penis or scrotum.

A physical examination, including inspection and palpation, is then conducted to identify manifestations of syphilis. Gloves should be worn while palpating any lesions because of the highly contagious treponemes that are present. Women frequently have the chancre on areas that are not easily visible to them, such as the vagina or cervix. Rashes of any type should be noted because of the variable presentation of secondary syphilis

After the physical examination, the physician, nurse practitioner, or nurse-midwife obtains a specimen of the chancre for examination under a darkfield microscope. Diagnosis of primary or secondary syphilis is confirmed if *T. pallidum,* the characteristic spirochete, is present. If the first slide is negative for *T. pallidum,* the procedure should be repeated in 3 days because many conditions can cause a false-negative result.

Blood tests are also used to diagnose syphilis. The usual screening test is the Venereal Disease Research Laboratory (VDRL) serum test. This test is based on an antibody-antigen reaction that determines both the presence and the amount of antibodies produced by the body in response to an infection by *T. pallidum.* The VDRL test becomes reactive 2 to 6 weeks after infection. VDRL titers are also used to monitor the ef-

fectiveness of treatment. The antibodies are not specific to *T. pallidum,* and false-positive reactions can occur frequently from such conditions as drug addiction, cancer, hepatitis, some viral diseases, and systemic lupus erythematosus (SLE).

If a positive VDRL result is obtained, the health care provider orders a more specific test, such as the *fluorescent treponemal antibody absorption (FTA-ABS)* test or the *microhemagglutination assay for T. palladium* (MHA-TP), to confirm the infection. These tests are more sensitive for all stages of syphilis, although false-positive results may still occur.

● Interventions

The health care provider prescribes antibiotic therapy for the client with syphilis. The drug therapy of choice is benzathine penicillin G. Allergic reactions to the antibiotic occur frequently, and the nurse monitors for these signs and symptoms. Penicillin desensitization is recommended for penicillin-allergic clients. The client who has never had penicillin previously should have a skin test before receiving a penicillin injection. All clients who have received injections of antibiotics should remain at the health care agency for at least 30 minutes so that signs of a severe and immediate allergic reaction can be detected. If an allergic reaction does occur, treatment can begin immediately. The most severe reaction is anaphylaxis. All nurses working in clinics or physicians' offices where injections of penicillin are given should be familiar with the symptoms and treatment of anaphylaxis.

The **Jarisch-Herxheimer reaction** may also follow antibiotic therapy for syphilis. This reaction is due to the rapid release of products from the disruption of the cells of the organism. Onset occurs within 2 hours after therapy, with a peak at 4 to 8 hours. Symptoms include generalized aches and pain at the injection site, vasodilation and hypotension, and a rise in temperature. These symptoms do not always occur and generally are benign. This reaction may be treated symptomatically with analgesics and antipyretics.

Nursing interventions are based on information gained during the history and physical assessment. Common nursing diagnoses for clients with syphilis, as well as STDs in general, are listed in Table 77-3.

The nurse reinforces the information provided to the client about the cause of infection (sexual transmission); treatment, including side effects, possible complications of untreated or incompletely treated disease; and the need for follow-up care. All sexual partners must be adequately treated as soon as possible. Sensitive discussion with the client about the importance of partner notification and treatment should include the risk of reinfection if the partner goes untreated. The nurse informs the client that the disease must be reported to the local health authority and that all information will be held in strict confidence. The client must be encouraged to provide accurate information for this follow-up to ensure that all at-risk partners are treated appropriately. The nurse provides a setting that offers privacy and encourages open discussion.

The client is urged to comply with the treatment regimen, which includes follow-up visits. Sexual abstinence until the treatment is completed is urged. Prevention of infection with other STDs must be frankly discussed.

The emotional responses to syphilis vary and may include feelings of fear, depression, guilt, and anxiety. Clients may experience guilt if they have infected others or anger if they

TABLE 77-3 • SELECTED NURSING DIAGNOSES FOR CLIENTS WITH SEXUALLY TRANSMITTED DISEASES

- Risk for Injury related to the disease process
- Ineffective Coping related to fear, guilt, or anger
- Noncompliance related to treatment and/or partner follow-up
- Sexual Dysfunction related to fear of transmission
- Impaired Skin Integrity related to the presence of genital ulcers, warts, or rash
- Ineffective Health Maintenance related to Deficient Knowledge about the mode of transmission, disease process, or need for treatment
- Impaired Social Interaction related to social stigma
- Acute Pain related to the infection process
- Anxiety related to possible infertility as a result of having an STD
- Chronic Low Self-Esteem/Situational Low Self-Esteem related to the effects of having an STD

CHART 77-2

BEST PRACTICE *for*
Care of the Client with Genital Herpes

- Administer oral analgesics as prescribed.
- Apply local anesthetic sprays or ointments as prescribed.
- Apply ice packs or warm compresses to the client's lesions.
- Administer sitz baths three or four times a day.
- Encourage an increase in fluid intake.
- Encourage frequent urination.
- Pour water over the client's genitalia while the client is voiding, or encourage voiding while the client is sitting in a tub of water or standing in a shower.
- Catheterize the client as necessary.
- Encourage genital hygiene, and encourage keeping the skin clean and dry.
- Wash hands thoroughly after contact with lesions, and launder towels that have had direct contact with lesions.
- Wear gloves when applying ointments.
- Advise the client to avoid sexual activity when lesions are present.
- Advise the client to use latex or polyurethane condoms during all sexual exposures.
- Instruct the client in the use, side effects, and risks versus benefits of antiviral agents.

have been infected by a partner. If further psychosocial interventions are necessary, the nurse encourages the client to discuss these feelings or refers him or her to other resources such as psychotherapy groups, self-help support groups, or STD clinics.

Genital Herpes

OVERVIEW

Genital herpes (GH) is an acute, recurring, incurable viral disease. Two serotypes of herpes simplex virus (HSV) affect the genitalia: type 1 (HSV-1) and type 2 (HSV-2). Most nongenital lesions, such as cold sores, are caused by HSV-1; HSV-2 causes most of the genital lesions. However, this differentiation is academic, since the transmission, symptoms, diagnosis, and treatment are identical for the two types. Either type can produce oral or genital lesions through oral-genital contact with an infected person.

On the basis of serologic studies, not symptoms, 45 million persons in the United States may have HSV-2 (CDC, 1998). HSV-2 is believed to cause 70% to 95% of the primary episodes of GH and recurs more frequently than HSV-1. Approximately 32% of the U.S. population was reported to have acquired HSV-2 by the early 1990s (Schaffer, 1998). Most people infected with HSV have not received a diagnosis because they have mild symptoms and shed virus intermittently.

The incubation period is 2 to 20 days, with the average period being 1 week. Many people are asymptomatic during the primary infection, but symptoms, if they occur, are usually most severe during this first infection and infrequently require hospitalization.

Itching or a tingling sensation may be felt in the skin 1 to 2 days before an outbreak. These sensations are followed by the appearance of vesicles (blisters) in a characteristic cluster on the penis, scrotum, vulva, perineum, vagina, cervix, or perianal region. The vesicles rupture spontaneously in a couple of days and leave painful erosions. These lesions can become extensive, and other symptoms, such as headaches, fever, general malaise, and inguinal lymphadenopathy, may be present. Urination may be painful, and clients with urinary retention may require catheterization. Lesions resolve within 2 to 6 weeks.

After the lesions heal, the virus remains in a dormant state in the nerve ganglia (specifically, in the sacral ganglia). Peri-

odically, the virus may activate, and symptoms recur. These recurrences may be stimulated by many factors, including stress, fever, sunburn, poor nutrition, menses, and sexual activity.

Recurrences are not caused by reinfection. Recurrent episodes are usually less severe and of shorter duration than the primary infection; there may not even be symptoms at all. Occasionally, HSV infection may become active without producing apparent clinical manifestations. However, there is viral shedding, and the client is infectious. Long-term complications of GH include the risk of neonatal transmission and an increased risk of acquiring HIV infections. The risk of transmission to the neonate is greater in a pregnant woman who has a primary infection than in one who has a recurrence.

► COLLABORATIVE MANAGEMENT

● Assessment

The diagnosis of GH is usually based on the client's history and physical examination and is confirmed through a viral culture (see Chart 77-1). Cultures are most accurate if specimens are obtained within 48 hours of the first outbreak of the blisters. Fluid from inside the vesicle should be obtained to ensure a correct diagnosis. GH is frequently diagnosed presumptively by the health care provider if the presenting signs and symptoms are classic.

● Interventions

Treatment of HSV-infected clients is usually symptomatic. The goals of collaborative management are to decrease the discomfort from painful ulcerations, to promote healing without secondary infection, to decrease viral shedding, and to prevent transmission of the infection (Chart 77-2).

DRUG THERAPY. Antiviral drugs are used to treat GH. The drugs do not cure the infection but do decrease the severity, accelerate the healing, and decrease the frequency of re-

CHART 77-3

DRUG THERAPY *for* Genital Herpes: First Clinical Episode of Genital Herpes

Drug	Dosage	Nursing Interventions	Rationale
Acyclovir (Zovirax, Avirax✦)	400 mg tid PO for 7-10 days *Or* 200 mg 5 times/day PO for 7-10 days	Instruct client that nausea and vomiting may occur when taking the drug. Same as above.	The client is prepared for possible side effect. Same as above.
Famciclovir (Famvir)	250 mg tid PO for 7-10 days	Instruct client that the drug is most effective if started within the first 48 hours of symptoms.	Efficacy has not been established for the first dose started more than 72 hours after the onset of symptoms.
Valacyclovir (Valtrex)	1 g bid PO for 7-10 days	Observe for side effects, including gastrointestinal disturbances, headaches, and dizziness.	The client is prepared for possible side effects.

current outbreaks. Topical therapy is not as effective as oral therapy. Acyclovir (Zovirax, Avirax✦), famciclovir (Famvir), or valacyclovir (Valtrex) may be used. The differences in these drugs are primarily in cost and frequency of use. Dosage and length of treatment differ for primary outbreaks (lasting 7 to 10 days) and recurrent outbreaks (lasting 5 days) (Chart 77-3). Mild recurrent episodes do not benefit appreciably from antiviral treatment, and their cost seems to outweigh their benefit. Therapy for severe recurrent outbreaks may be beneficial if it is started within 2 days of the appearance of lesions.

Clients who have frequent recurrences (more than six in a year) may benefit from daily suppressive treatment with any of the antivirals mentioned. Long-term safety and efficacy has been established for up to 6 years with acyclovir and for 1 year with valacyclovir and famciclovir. Clients receiving continuous therapy should stop after 1 year for reassessment of recurrences.

The cost of care for clients with GH is enormous, making it a major public health problem with a large economic burden. In 1999 the direct medical costs in the United States were estimated at $207 million. Of that amount, health care provider visits accounted for 36%, and drug therapy accounted for 64% (Tao et al., 2000).

NURSING MANAGEMENT. Nursing management includes client counseling and education about the infection, the potential for recurrent episodes, viral shedding even when clients are asymptomatic, and sexual transmission. Discussion about sexual activity is extremely important. The nurse reminds clients to abstain from sexual activity while lesions are present. Condom use during all sexual exposures is urged because of the increased risk of HSV transmission, since viral shedding can occur even when lesions are not present. The nurse teaches the client about how and when to use condoms (Chart 77-4).

The nurse also emphasizes the risk of fetal infection to all clients, both male and female. Women and men who have genital herpes need to inform the maternity care provider of their history during future pregnancies.

The nurse also assesses the client's psychologic responses to the diagnosis of genital herpes. Many clients are initially shocked and need reassurance that they can manage the disease. Infected clients have reported feelings of disbelief, uncleanness, isolation, and loneliness. They have also reported

CHART 77-4

CLIENT EDUCATION GUIDE
Use of Condoms

- Use latex or polyurethane condoms rather than natural membrane condoms.
- Use a condom with every sexual encounter.
- Female condoms—polyurethane sheaths in the vagina—are effective in preventing transmission of viruses, including HIV.
- Condoms infrequently (2 per 100) break during sexual intercourse, unless used incorrectly.
- Keep condoms (especially latex) in a cool, dry place, out of direct sunlight.
- Do not use condoms that are in damaged packages or that are brittle or discolored.
- Always handle a condom with care to avoid damaging it with fingernails, teeth, or other sharp objects.
- Put condoms on before any genital contact. Hold the condom by the tip and unroll it on the penis. Leave a space at the tip to collect semen.
- If you use a lubricant with condoms, make sure that the lubricant is water based and washes away with water. Oil-based products may damage latex condoms.
- Use of spermicide with condoms, either lubricated condoms or vaginal application, has not been proved to be more or less effective against STDs than use without spermicide. Spermicide does provide added protection against pregnancy. Spermicide-coated condoms have been associated with *Escherichia coli* urinary tract infections in women.
- If a condom breaks, replace it immediately.
- After ejaculation, withdraw the erect penis carefully, holding the condom at the base of the penis to prevent the condom from slipping off.
- Never use a condom more than once.

Modified from Centers for Disease Control and Prevention. (1998). 1998 guidelines for treatment of sexually transmitted diseases. *Morbidity and Mortality Weekly Report, 47*(No. RR-1), 1-103.

anger at their partners for transmitting the infection or fear of rejection by partners because they have the infection. The nurse helps clients cope with the diagnosis by being sensitive and supportive during assessments and interventions. Social supports should be encouraged, and referrals to support groups such as HELP (local support groups of the National Herpes Resource Center) may be beneficial. Symptomatic care may include oral analgesics, topical anesthetics, sitz baths, and increased oral fluid intake.

Lymphogranuloma Venereum

■ OVERVIEW

Lymphogranuloma venereum (LGV) is the result of genital inoculation with one of three serotypes of *Chlamydia trachomatis,* which is spread systemically until it localizes in the genital or rectal lymph nodes. The incubation period is 3 to 30 days. The primary lesion, at the point of inoculation, is transient and painless and is not usually noticed by the client. The lesion usually appears on the penis in men and on the vaginal wall in women; however, sores may also be located in the mouth and rectum. Five times as many men are diagnosed with this disease as women.

Lesions vary in form from herpes-like blisters (vesicles), to ulcers, papules, or pustules. Within 1 to 2 weeks after the appearance of the primary lesion, secondary signs of infection appear. Lymphadenopathy (primarily inguinal) is present, and symptoms of headache, malaise, arthralgia, and anorexia may occur. Most clients seek care at this point. Lymphadenopathy can recede or develop into abscesses. When the abscesses rupture, healing occurs slowly. Sinus tracts, formed as a result of the infection, drain thick, viscous pus for several weeks, leaving behind deep scars.

Complications of the infection can be chronic lymphadenopathy, fistulas, rectal strictures, and proctitis. Systemic involvement can also cause carditis, arthritis, and pneumonia.

> **CULTURAL CONSIDERATIONS**
> LVG has a worldwide distribution, but it occurs primarily in South America, Southeast Asia, India, and East and West Africa and rarely in the United States. Cases in the United States usually occur in clients who have visited these countries or had sexual contact with someone who is from or has traveled to or from these areas (Kellock et al., 1997).

▶ COLLABORATIVE MANAGEMENT

The diagnosis of LGV is usually made on physical examination and serologic testing. The serologic test, an antibody complement fixation test (LGV-CF), is considered diagnostic if the titer is higher than 1:64. Cultures from the enlarged lymph nodes, although technically difficult and expensive, are considered the "gold standard" if the organism can be isolated, which occurs only 50% of the time (Rosen & Brown, 1998).

The health care provider prescribes doxycycline (Monodox, Doxy-Caps, Doxycin✿) 100 mg twice a day orally or tetracycline (Tetracyn, Tetram, Nu-Tetra✿, Apo-Tetra✿) 500 mg four times a day orally for 21 days. Antibiotic treatment cures the infection and prevents further tissue damage. Infected lymph nodes may be aspirated by needle or incised and drained to prevent ulcer formation. Surgical intervention may be required for late complications, such as perianal or perirectal strictures and fistulas. Nursing management and client education is similar to that for syphilis. Sexual partners should be tested for cervical or urethral chlamydial infection and treated if they had sexual contact with the client during the 30 days before the client's onset of symptoms.

Chancroid

■ OVERVIEW

Painful genital ulcerations characterize **chancroid.** Genital lesions and inguinal lymphadenopathy without systemic illness are the usual presentation. Although chancroid has a worldwide distribution, it is most common in developing tropical and subtropical countries, such as Africa, the West Indies, and Asia, but is endemic in parts of the United States. Chancroid is a cofactor for HIV transmission, leading to high rates of HIV infection of those with chancroid. Estimates of 10% of clients with chancroid being co-infected with syphilis and herpes simplex virus have been made. This co-infection appears to be the result of the open genital lesions. Uncircumcised men may be at greater risk for infection than circumcised men.

The incubation period for chancroid varies from 3 to 10 days. A tender papule appears at the site of inoculation. This lesion rapidly breaks down to form an irregularly shaped, deep ulcer that has a purulent discharge and bleeds easily.

Complications include inguinal adenitis, balanitis, phimosis, and urethral fistulas. Chancroids differ from chancres caused by syphilis in that chancroids are soft and painful. Transmission of the disease is through contact with the ulcer or with the discharge from the infected local lymph glands during sexual activity.

▶ COLLABORATIVE MANAGEMENT

Cultures from the ulcers can isolate the *Haemophilus ducreyi* organism. Gram staining of the exudate from the ulcer can be difficult because of polymicrobial contamination, but the gram-negative rods may be seen. Usually the diagnosis is based on clinical signs, the exclusion of syphilis and herpes by appropriate testing, and a positive culture.

Management for chancroid consists of azithromycin (Zithromax) 1 g in a single dose orally, ceftriaxone (Rocephin) 250 mg in a single dose intramuscularly, ciprofloxacin (Cipro) 500 mg twice a day orally for 3 days, or erythromycin (E-Mycin, Apo-Erythro✿) 500 mg four times a day orally for 7 days. These antibiotics cure the infection, resolve the symptoms, and prevent further transmission. Clients should be observed periodically by a physician or nurse practitioner until ulcers heal, usually in 7 days. Client education is similar to that for syphilis. Sexual contacts must be located and treated whether or not they are symptomatic. The nurse's responsibility in management of the client with chancroid is similar to that for other sexually transmitted diseases (STDs).

Granuloma Inguinale

■ OVERVIEW

The causative organism of granuloma inguinale, or donovanosis, is *Calymmatobacterium granulomatis.* A nodule appears at the site of inoculation after 1 to 12 weeks. This lesion ulcerates, and others are formed; they grow together, becoming a spreading ulcer on the genitalia. Left untreated, these lesions can be mutilating. Regional lymphadenopathy does not occur. The ulcerated lesions bleed easily on contact.

> **CULTURAL CONSIDERATIONS**
> Granuloma inguinale is endemic in parts of Australia (among the central aborigines) and common in Africa, Southeast Asia, southern India, and New Guinea. Occurrence in the United States, Japan, and Europe is rare.

▶ COLLABORATIVE MANAGEMENT

Biopsy and cytologic smears from the ulcers are the only conclusive methods for diagnosis. Definitive diagnosis depends on finding characteristic Donovan bodies in these samples. This can be difficult, and frequently treatment will be given empirically before results of these tests are available.

Granuloma inguinale is treated with 1 tablet of trimethoprim/sulfamethoxazole (Bactrim✤, Septra) double strength twice a day orally or doxycycline 100 mg twice a day orally for a minimum of 3 weeks. Treatment needs to continue until all the lesions are completely healed. Relapse can occur within 6 to 18 months, even after successful initial treatment.

Sexual contacts within 60 days of the onset of symptoms or those displaying any signs or symptoms should be treated.

The nurse's responsibility in management of the client with granuloma inguinale is similar to that for other STDs. A thorough history that includes sexual contacts, travel abroad, and contact with partners who may have traveled to or are from endemic areas is taken (see Chart 77-1). Collecting the history about genital lesions that may have disappeared or changed is essential diagnostic information that can be used in collaboration with the health care provider.

The nurse explains cultures, biopsies, or other diagnostic tests that will be done to make a correct diagnosis. Comfort measures and emotional support need to be provided, since some procedures may be invasive or painful. The nurse teaches the client about the diagnosis, the risk for complications if granuloma inguinale is left untreated or incompletely treated, and the antibiotics prescribed.

The client should be encouraged to provide the names of sexual contacts for follow-up and treatment. Concerns about coping with the disease may arise; the nurse encourages the client to verbalize concerns and/or refers him or her for further counseling. Because these infections are relatively rare, the client may experience the added discomfort and inconvenience of being evaluated by specialists to get a correct diagnosis, which may contribute to his or her anxiety.

INFECTIONS OF THE EPITHELIAL STRUCTURES
Condylomata Acuminata
▮ OVERVIEW

Condylomata acuminata (also known as genital *warts*) are caused by certain types of human papillomavirus (HPV). At least 6 of the approximately 70 HPV genotypes are found on the skin of the genitalia. Some of these are considered high risk in their association with genital cancers. Genital warts are the most common sexually transmitted viral disease and are often seen with other infections. Approximately 20% to 40% of the sexually active population in the United States is thought to be infected with HPV (Beutner et al., 1999). Sites commonly affected include the urinary meatus, labia, vagina, cervix, penis, scrotum, anus, and perineal area. Pregnancy seems to lead to increased growth of the lesions. The incubation period is usually 2 to 3 months.

The genital warts are initially single, small papillary growths that may grow into large cauliflower-like masses. Bleeding may occur if the wart is disrupted. Warts may regress spontaneously without treatment.

HPV infection is strongly associated with genital dysplasia and cervical carcinoma. A Pap smear is useful in the isolation and diagnosis of HPV from the cervix. HPV can also be detected in genital swab specimens using a more sensitive polymerase chain reaction (PCR) assay. A specimen for biopsy is obtained from any atypical, pigmented, or persistent warts.

➤ COLLABORATIVE MANAGEMENT
● Assessment

The diagnosis of condylomata acuminata is made by examination of the lesions, which appear wartlike. To rule out the presence of other infections, a VDRL test and cultures for chlamydial infection and gonorrhea are obtained. A Pap smear is obtained to assess for cervical dysplasia (abnormal tissue growth). If lesions bleed easily or appear to be infected, a biopsy may be done to rule out other pathologic conditions. Colposcopy with biopsies is recommended for assessment of lesions that appear atypical, lesions that do not respond to treatment, and any lesions on the cervix.

● Interventions

The goals of management are to remove the warts, treat the symptoms, and prevent progression of neoplasias. No therapy has been shown to eradicate HPV; therefore recurrences after treatment are likely.

The treatment options for external warts are client applied or provider applied. Clients may apply podofilox 0.5% solution or gel twice a day for 3 days with no treatment for the next 4 days. This regimen should be repeated for four cycles. Another option is imiquimod 5% cream applied topically at bedtime three times a week for up to 16 weeks.

Cryotherapy, podophyllin, and trichloroacetic acid (TCA) are relatively inexpensive provider-applied treatments. Cryotherapy (freezing), usually with liquid nitrogen, can be used every 1 to 2 weeks until lesions are resolved. Podophyllin resin 10% to 25% in a compound of tincture of benzoin can be applied weekly but needs to be washed off 1 to 4 hours after application. Trichloroacetic acid (80% to 90%) can be applied weekly. Extensive warts have been treated with the carbon dioxide laser or by surgical removal.

For effective management of condylomata acuminata, sexual partners must also be treated. Clients should avoid intimate sexual contact until external lesions are healed.

Nursing management focuses on client education about the mode of transmission, incubation period, treatment, and complications. Reinforcing instructions about local care of the lesions or patient-applied treatment is essential. After treatment with cryotherapy, podophyllin, or TCA, clients may experience discomfort, bleeding or discharge from the site, or sloughing of parts of warts. The nurse instructs the client to keep the area clean (shower or bath) and dry, and to be alert for any signs or symptoms of infection or side effects of the treatment.

Condoms are recommended to help reduce transmission (see Chart 77-4). Clients need to know that recurrence is likely and that repeated treatments may be necessary. The nurse encourages women who have had condylomata acuminata to have an annual Pap smear. As with other STDs, emotional support is needed, and a referral for counseling may help.

Gonorrhea
▮ OVERVIEW

Gonorrhea continues to be the most reported communicable disease in the United States and may be on the rise. An estimated 600,000 new infections occur each year. The incidence is highest in sexually active people between the ages of 15 and 19 years. This bacterial infection occurs in men and women, and infants can be infected during childbirth. The causative organism is *Neisseria gonorrhoeae*, a gram-negative intracellular diplococcus. *N. gonorrhoeae* is transmitted by direct sexual contact with mucosal surfaces (vaginal intercourse, orogenital or anogenital contact) or, in the neonate, through an infected birth canal). Although the organism has been found on inanimate surfaces where it has been artificially inoculated, there is no evidence that transmission occurs naturally in this manner.

The initial symptoms of gonorrhea may appear 3 to 10 days after sexual contact with an infected person. The infection can be asymptomatic in both men and women, but women have asymptomatic, or silent, infections more often than men do. If symptoms are present, men most likely notice dysuria and a penile discharge that can be either profuse yellowish green fluid or scant clear fluid. The urethra is the site most commonly affected, but infection can extend to the prostate, the seminal vesicles, and the epididymis. Men seek curative treatment sooner, usually because they are symptomatic, and thereby avoid some of the serious complications. Women may report a change in vaginal discharge (yellow, green, profuse, odorous), urinary frequency, or dysuria. The cervix and urethra are the most common sites of infection. Gonorrhea can sit asymptomatically in the cervix and be transmitted or progress without warning. Ascending spread of the gonococci can cause pelvic infection (pelvic inflammatory disease [PID]), endometritis (endometrial infection), salpingitis (fallopian tube infection), and/or pelvic peritonitis. Both symptomatic and asymptomatic infections can lead to PID and tubal scarring. Rare sequelae of gonorrhea include arthritis, meningitis, perihepatitis, and disseminated infection. Neonates contacting the infection at birth can develop conjunctivitis and blindness.

Anal manifestations may include anal itching and irritation, rectal bleeding or diarrhea, and painful defecation. Oral manifestations are related to pharyngeal infection. Symptoms are seldom noted but may include a sore throat, ulcerated lips, tender gingivae, and vesicles in the oropharynx. Figure 77-1 shows common sites of gonococcal infections.

Asymptomatic clients may be found to have positive cultures for gonorrhea when they present to a health care facility for routine physical examination, for hospital admission, or for preoperative assessments. Others may present to the

THROAT

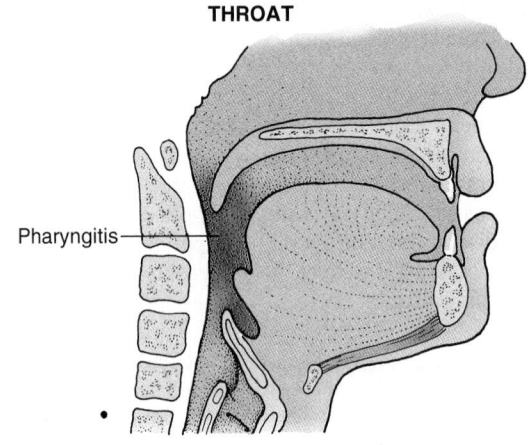

PELVIC/GENITAL

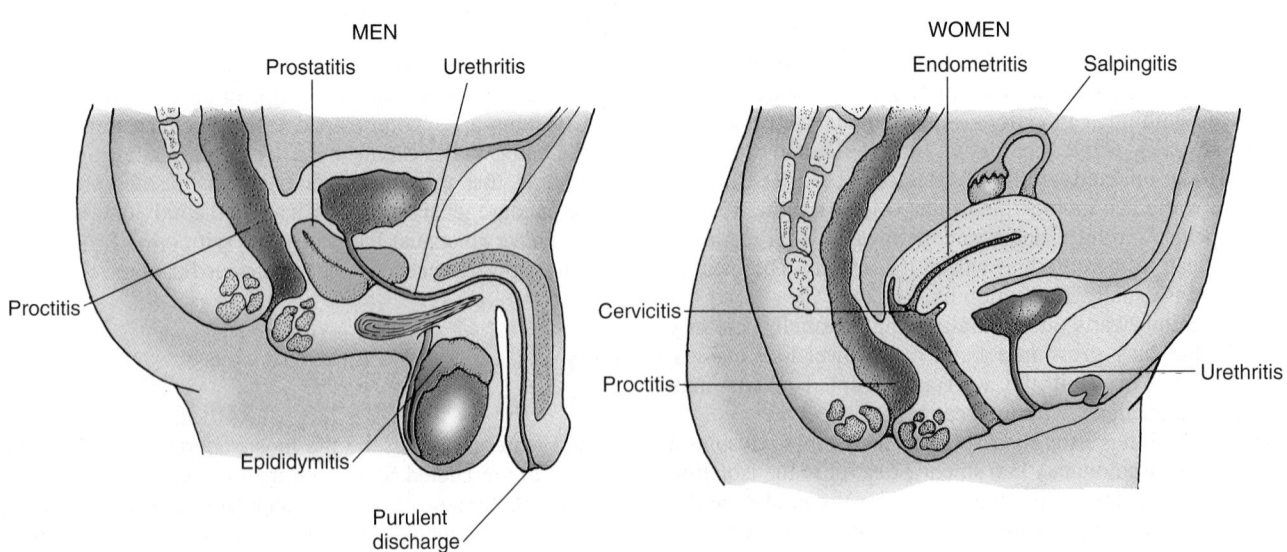

Figure 77-1 ● Some areas of involvement with gonorrhea in men and women.

health care agency because the sexual partner has been diagnosed with the infection. Screening all sexually active men and women for gonorrhea is a useful public health tool to avoid spread of asymptomatic infection.

> ### CULTURAL CONSIDERATIONS
> In 1998 in the United States, African Americans had 61% of the reported cases of gonorrhea, Caucasians had 11%, and Hispanics had 5%, with rates in women nearly equal to those of men (CDC, 1999).

➤ COLLABORATIVE MANAGEMENT

● Assessment

A complete history includes reviewing possible symptoms of gonorrhea, taking a sexual history that includes sexual orientation and sites of intercourse, and assessing for allergies to antibiotics (see Chart 77-1). The nurse's nonjudgmental approach helps elicit appropriate and complete information. These techniques may decrease the client's anxiety and fear about having a sexually transmitted disease (STD).

Physical assessment includes inspection for discharge from the urethra, cervix, and rectum. Palpation of the lower abdomen may reveal tenderness. Fever may be present, especially in complicated infections.

Definitive diagnosis involves laboratory testing. Identification of gonorrhea in men can be made with smears of the discharge that has been swabbed onto a glass slide, dried, and Gram stained. The presence of gram-negative diplococci is diagnostic for gonococcal urethritis. Gram stains are 50% to 70% sensitive and 97% specific for gonorrhea. Gram staining allows for immediate diagnosis and earlier treatment.

Smears do not confirm the diagnosis in women, because the female genital tract normally harbors organisms that resemble *N. gonorrhoeae*. Cultures provide a more definitive diagnosis and are the most reliable method of confirming a diagnosis for men and women. The sensitivity of cultures is 80% to 90%.

A specimen is obtained from the male urethra or the female cervix and inoculated onto Thayer-Martin (chocolate agar) culture medium. The medium must be placed in a carbon dioxide–rich environment for the organism to grow. Depending on the history given by the client, culture specimens may also be obtained from the throat and rectum. After 24 to 48 hours, the culture is examined for the presence of gram-negative diplococci.

Direct fluorescent antibody tests, collected on a swab as with cultures, are available and are very sensitive and specific. First-voided urine specimens tested by the multiplex PCR methodology are an additional highly sensitive and specific method for screening and diagnosing *N. gonorrhoeae* (and *Ureaplasma urealyticum, Chlamydia trachomatis,* and *Mycoplasma genitalium* all in one specimen) (Mahoney et al., 1997).

All clients with gonorrhea should be tested for syphilis, chlamydial infection, hepatitis B and C, and HIV infection because they may have been exposed to these STDs as well. Sexual partners who have been exposed in the last 30 days should be examined, and specimens for culture should be obtained.

● Interventions

The health care provider treats uncomplicated gonorrhea with antibiotics. Treatment has changed because of penicillin-resistant strains and now quinolone-resistant strains of *N. gonorrhoeae*. Chlamydial infections are frequently found in clients with gonorrhea. Management for gonorrhea includes medications that also eradicate *Chlamydia*.

DRUG THERAPY. Drug therapy recommended by the Centers for Disease Control and Prevention (CDC) is cefixime (Suprax) 400 mg orally, ceftriaxone (Rocephin) 125 mg intramuscularly, ciprofloxacin (Cipro) 500 mg orally, *or* ofloxacin (Floxin) 400 mg orally, *each* in a single dose *plus* azithromycin (Zithromax) 1 g in a single dose orally *or* doxycycline (Monodox, Doxy-Caps, Doxycin✦) 100 mg twice a day orally for 1 week. The quinolones (ciprofloxacin, ofloxacin) are contraindicated in clients younger than 18 years of age. These combinations seem to be effective for all mucosal gonorrheal infections; treatment failure is rare. Sexual partners must be treated as well. A test of cure is not required, but the client is advised to return for a follow-up examination if symptoms persist after treatment. Reinfection is frequently the cause of these symptoms and indicates a need for more education of the client and sexual partner.

Gonorrheal infections that have become systemic may develop abruptly. Symptoms of disseminated gonococcal infection (DGI) may include fever, chills, skin lesions on distal parts of extremities, and asymmetric arthralgias with or without joint swelling, heat, or erythema. Treatment includes intravenous (IV) or intramuscular antibiotic therapy (ceftriaxone 1 g every 24 hours). If symptoms resolve within 24 to 48 hours, the client may be discharged to home to continue oral antibiotic therapy for at least 1 week.

Meningitis and endocarditis occur rarely. Hospitalization for these clients is recommended for the initial treatment, especially if endocarditis or meningitis is suspected. Treatment is with IV antibiotic therapy, usually ceftriaxone 1 to 2 g every 12 hours. If meningitis or endocarditis is present, therapy should be continued for 10 to 14 days for meningitis and at least 4 weeks for endocarditis. Infectious disease specialists are consulted for management of these infections.

HEALTH TEACHING. Nursing interventions focus on health teaching about transmission and treatment of gonorrhea. Clients must understand why medications should be taken for the prescribed time for maximal effectiveness. The nurse discusses the possibility of reinfection. Clients should avoid sexual activity until the antibiotic therapy is completed and they no longer have symptoms. Men and women are urged to use condoms, especially if abstinence is not possible. The nurse explains that gonorrhea is a reportable disease. All sexual contacts need to be examined and treated for both gonorrhea and chlamydial infection.

When a diagnosis of gonorrhea is made, clients may have feelings of fear or guilt. They may be concerned that they have contracted other STDs or see the disease as a punishment for promiscuity or "unnatural" sex acts. They may believe that acquiring gonorrhea (or any STD) is a risk that they must take to pursue their desired lifestyle. Such feelings can impair relationships with sexual partners. The nurse encourages expression of feelings during assessments and teaching sessions. Privacy for client teaching and maintenance of confidentiality of medical records are important nursing interventions in meeting the client's psychosocial needs.

> **CRITICAL THINKING CHALLENGE**
>
> A middle-aged woman visits her gynecologist with complaints of a greenish yellow, odorous vaginal discharge that is very irritating and itchy. On examination, the physician suspects gonorrhea and asks her about sexual activity. She states that she has been married for 32 years and has never had sexual intercourse with any man other than her husband. Laboratory tests confirm the STD diagnosis.
> - What questions will you need to ask the client at this time?
> - How do you think she became infected with the disease?
> - What emotional support will she need as she begins treatment for gonorrhea?

For suggested answer guidelines, go to [SIMON] http://www.wbsaunders.com/SIMON/Iggy/.

Chlamydial Infection

▌ OVERVIEW

Chlamydia trachomatis is the most common sexually transmitted infection in the United States. The disease is now reportable to local health departments in almost all states. More than 500,000 acute infections are reported annually, but estimates of 3 million genital infections per year have been made (Groseclose et al., 1999). Asymptomatic infections, perhaps in up to 80% of women infected with *C. trachomatis,* account for most of this difference. In men, about 10% to 20% of the cases of nongonococcal urethritis are caused by *C. trachomatis.* In women, 20% to 40% of those infected with *C. trachomatis* develop pelvic inflammatory disease (PID), discussed on pp. 1817-1823. Transmission to the newborn can occur during vaginal delivery, with resultant neonatal eye infections and pneumonia.

C. trachomatis invades the columnar epithelial tissues in the reproductive tract and causes clinical manifestations similar to those of gonorrheal infections. The incubation period ranges from 1 to 3 weeks, but the pathogen may be present in the genital tract for months without producing symptoms. The average duration of infection before diagnosis has been estimated to be about 1 year in women and 5 months in men because of its frequent asymptomatic status (Groseclose et al., 1999).

In men, the primary symptom is nongonococcal urethritis, accompanied by dysuria, frequent urination, and a mucoid discharge that is more watery and less copious than a gonorrheal discharge. Some men have the discharge only in the morning on arising. Complications include epididymitis, prostatitis, infertility, and Reiter's syndrome, a type of connective tissue disease (see Chapter 21).

In contrast, up to 80% of women may have no symptoms. Women with symptoms have a mucopurulent cervicitis that presents with a change in vaginal discharge, easily induced cervical bleeding, urinary frequency, and abdominal discomfort or pain. The vaginal discharge typically becomes yellow and more opaque (Sellors et al., 2000). Complications of infection with *C. trachomatis* include salpingitis, PID, ectopic pregnancy, and infertility.

➤ COLLABORATIVE MANAGEMENT

▌● Assessment

A complete history, including medical, menstrual, and sexual history is obtained from the client (see Chart 77-1). The nurse asks about the following:
- Presence of symptoms

- Any history of sexually transmitted diseases (STDs)
- Whether sexual partners have had symptoms or have a history of STDs

The nurse understands that many women with chlamydial infections are asymptomatic and that a history may reveal only risk factors associated with *C. trachomatis.* These factors include pregnancy, age younger than 20 years, being unmarried, nulliparity, having a higher number of sexual partners or a new sexual partner, use of a nonbarrier method of birth control (hormonal, intrauterine device [IUD]), and concurrent gonorrhea. As with all interviews concerning sexual behavior, the nurse uses a nonjudgmental approach and provides privacy and confidentiality.

Diagnosis of chlamydial infections is made by sampling cells from the endocervix and/or urethra. Since chlamydiae are obligate intracellular pathogens, host cells that harbor the organism (or parts of it) are required in the sample. Gram staining of urethral or cervical samples can help exclude gonorrhea. The presence of polymorphonuclear leukocytes and the absence of gram-negative intracellular diplococci (suggestive of gonorrhea) points to a chlamydial infection. Absolute diagnosis of chlamydial infection is made with a tissue culture. Culture for *Chlamydia,* which detects 70% to 80% of cervical infections with *C. trachomatis,* has been the "gold standard." Special transport medium is required.

Two enzyme immunoassay tests can be performed easily, less expensively, and more quickly than cultures: the Chlamydiazyme, an enzyme-linked immunoassay (ELISA), and the MicroTrak, a direct fluorescent antibody test (DFA); these tests detect about 60% to 90% of infections.

DNA probe (GenProbe) testing also detects 60% to 90% of infections. Newer genetic amplification tests or DNA amplification tests (ligase chain reaction [LCR] and polymerized chain reaction [PCR]) appear able to detect more than 90% to 95% of infections and can be done additionally on urine but are more expensive (Mahoney et al., 1997). If affordable, these tests are the best choice. Specimens with cervical or urethral secretions, obtained with swabs, are used.

Screening asymptomatic women who may have risk factors for having chlamydial infections is strongly encouraged. Screening adolescents every 6 months regardless of other risk factors is now being recommended by some experts (see Evidence-Based Practice for Nursing box on p. 1817).

▌● Interventions

The treatment of choice for chlamydial infections is azithromycin (Zithromax) 1 g in a single dose or doxycycline (Monodox, Doxy-Caps, Doxycin✤) 100 mg twice a day for 7 days. The one-dose course, although more expensive, is preferred because of the ease in completing the treatment. Administering the drug while in the health care facility helps ensure compliance. Sexual partners should be tested and treated if at all possible.

Client education is an important nursing intervention. The nurse explains the following:
- The mode of disease transmission
- The incubation period
- Signs and symptoms, including the possibility of asymptomatic infections
- Medical treatment

Sexually active adolescent females are recommended to have screening for *Chlamydia* every 6 months regardless of other risk factors

Burnstein, G.R., et al. (1998). Incident *Chlamydia trachomatis* infections among inner-city adolescent females. *Journal of the American Medical Association,* 280(6), 521-526.

Adolescents are at highest risk for *Chlamydia trachomatis* infection for multiple reasons. Chlamydial infection is an important preventable cause of pelvic inflammatory disease (PID) and subsequent infertility. Since sexually transmitted disease (STD) prevention and screening are the responsibility of those providing care in many settings, identifying adolescent females at risk for infection is an important practice issue.

A consecutive convenience sample of 3202 sexually active females, 12 to 19 years old, who were seen at an urban health department family planning or STD clinic or school-based clinic, were screened. Specimens (cervical or urine) for *Chlamydia* testing were obtained as part of the standard care after informed consent was received. Demographic and behavioral data were collected that included age, race or ethnicity, reason for testing or examination (e.g., STD contact, STD symptoms, asymptomatic screening), and prior STD history. The adolescents were asked about sexually risky behaviors in the previous 90 days (i.e., new or multiple partners, inconsistent condom use). They were tested again on repeat visits, which ranged from 1 to 9 visits per woman. The median time between visits was 4 months.

Twenty-nine percent of all adolescent females tested were positive for *Chlamydia,* which is a higher percentage than in other populations of adolescent women that have been studied. Fourteen-year-olds had the highest proportion of positive test results; 24% tested positive on their first visit, and 14% tested positive on a repeat visit. This study confirmed that risk factors failed to identify a high-risk subgroup needing targeted screening. For adolescents who had initially had a negative test, the mean time until they had a positive result was 7.2 months. For those with a previous positive test result, the median time until a repeat positive test was 4.1 months. The researchers therefore recommend screening all sexually active adolescent females every 6 months regardless of their risk.

Critique. This well-designed study demonstrates that previous recommendations for *Chlamydia* screening based on risk factors may not be appropriate for the adolescent female population. A limitation of the study is that the study sample was racially and socioeconomically homogeneous. More study needs to be done with ethnically diverse populations using the newer, more sensitive nucleic acid amplification tests used in this study.

Implications for Nursing. Nurses educating clients about STD risk and need for screening have new data on which to base their recommendations. Adolescent females are at greatest risk for acquiring chlamydial infections. Nurses in every setting should view this age-group as a high-risk subset that needs additional education on STD prevention, as well as screening every 6 months.

- The need for abstinence from sexual intercourse until the client and partner(s) have completed treatment (7 days from the start of treatment, including a single-dose regimen)
- The fact that no test of cure is required
- The need to return for evaluation if symptoms recur or new symptoms develop
- Possible complications of untreated or inadequately treated infection

Psychosocial support is similar to that discussed in the previous section on gonorrhea.

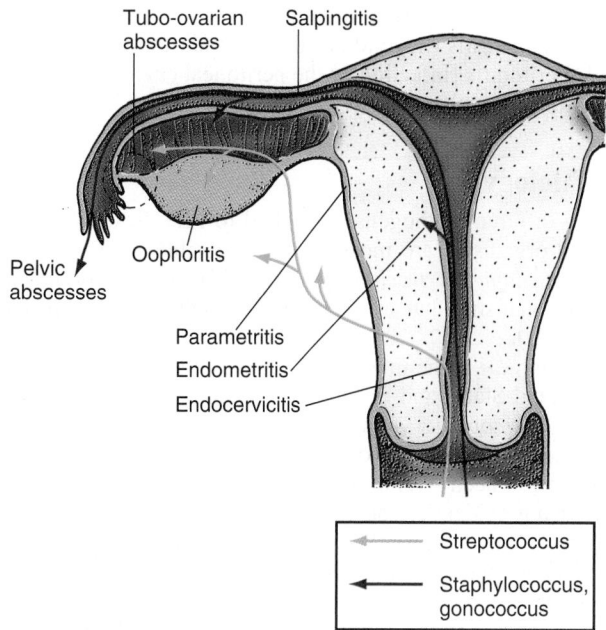

Figure 77-2 ● The spread of pelvic inflammatory disease.

OTHER GYNECOLOGIC CONDITIONS
Pelvic Inflammatory Disease
■ OVERVIEW

Pelvic inflammatory disease (PID) is considered a costly gynecologic health problem in the United States, affecting over 1 million women annually (see the Cost of Care box on p. 1807). It is an infectious process that may involve one or more pelvic structures, including the uterus, fallopian tubes, and adjacent pelvic structures. The most common site is the fallopian tube.

Many practitioners use the terms *PID* and *salpingitis* synonymously for acute infections. PID is one of the leading causes of infertility and is related to the rise in the number of ectopic pregnancies reported in the United States. PID is generally viewed as an acute syndrome resulting in tenderness in the tubes and ovaries (adnexa) and low, dull abdominal pain. However, many women experience only mild discomfort or menstrual irregularity; others experience no symptoms at all—so-called silent or subclinical PID. Diagnosis and treatment of PID in these women is a challenge to health care providers. Irreversible scarring or stricture, causing sterility, may occur before PID is diagnosed.

■ Pathophysiology

PID is a complex process in which organisms from the lower genital tract migrate from the endocervix upward through the endometrial cavity to the fallopian tubes. The spread of infection to other organs of the upper genital tract occurs by way of direct contact with mucosal surfaces or through the fimbriated ends of the tubes to the ovaries, parametrium, and peritoneal cavity (Figure 77-2). Resultant infections include the following:

- Endometritis (infection of the endometrial cavity)
- Salpingitis (inflammation of the fallopian tubes)

- Oophoritis (ovarian infection)
- Parametritis (infection of the parametrium)
- Peritonitis (infection of the peritoneal cavity)
- Tubal or tubo-ovarian abscess

■ Etiology

Many different pathogens are linked to PID. Sexually transmitted organisms are most often responsible for PID, especially *Chlamydia trachomatis* and *Neisseria gonorrhoeae*. Microorganisms that are part of the vaginal flora can also cause PID.

Chlamydia is the most common causative agent of PID in the United States and Europe. In addition, *Gardnerella vaginalis, Haemophilus influenzae, Staphylococcus, Streptococcus, Escherichia coli,* and other aerobic and anaerobic organisms have been identified in clients with PID. There is increasing evidence that the anaerobes involved in bacterial vaginosis may have a role in the development of PID (Peipert, 1997; Winefield & Murphy, 1998). The infectious organisms most likely invade the pelvis from an infection ascending from the vagina or cervix. Infections have been spread during sexual intercourse, during childbirth (including the postpartum period), and after abortion. Rarely do infections result from transperitoneal spread from a ruptured appendix or intra-abdominal abscess.

■ Incidence/Prevalence

The incidence of PID is on the rise. Accurate rates are unavailable because PID is not a reportable disease. Many of the same factors that place women at risk for STDs also place them at risk for PID.

Risk factors for sexually active women include the following:

- Age less than 20 years
- Multiple sexual partners
- Intrauterine device (IUD) in place
- Use of vaginal douches
- Smoking
- Chlamydial or gonococcal infection; bacterial vaginosis
- A history of sexually transmitted diseases (STDs)
- A history of PID

► COLLABORATIVE MANAGEMENT

Activity Link

● Assessment

■ HISTORY

The nurse obtains a complete medical, family, menstrual, obstetric, and sexual history, including a history of previous episodes of pelvic inflammatory disease (PID) or other sexually transmitted infections (see Chart 77-1). The nurse also assesses for contraceptive use (especially the intrauterine device), a history of reproductive surgery, and other risk factors previously identified. The possibility of sexual abuse should be raised.

One of the most frequent symptoms of PID is lower abdominal pain. Other symptoms include menstrual irregularities or abnormal vaginal bleeding, dysuria, an increase or change in vaginal discharge, dyspareunia, malaise, fever, and chills.

■ PHYSICAL ASSESSMENT/CLINICAL MANIFESTATIONS

On physical assessment, the nurse may observe the client's discomfort with movement. Often the client will have a hunched-over gait that she uses to intuitively protect her abdomen. She may find it difficult to independently get on the examination table or stretcher. She may be fatigued, diaphoretic, and hyperthermic.

On abdominal assessment, the nurse notes lower abdominal tenderness, possibly with rigidity or rebound tenderness. A pelvic examination by the health care provider may reveal yellow or green cervical discharge and a reddened or friable cervix (a cervix that bleeds easily). On bimanual examination, uterine or cervical tenderness with motion and tender adnexa (tubes and ovaries) are typically present. If the client is using an IUD for contraception, the device should be removed at the time of the examination if possible. Ectopic pregnancy and appendicitis must be ruled out as potential causes of the pain.

■ PSYCHOSOCIAL ASSESSMENT

The woman who presents with symptoms of PID is usually anxious and fearful of the examination and unknown diagnosis. She may need much reassurance and support during the physical examination because the abdomen is likely to be quite tender and she may wish to avoid further pain. An explanation of what is taking place often helps promote cooperation during the examination.

Because PID is most frequently associated with an STD, the woman may feel embarrassed or uncomfortable discussing her symptoms or history. The nurse uses a nonjudgmental approach and encourages the client to express her feelings and concerns. The client's ability to follow through with the treatment plan (taking antibiotics, resting, returning for follow-up evaluation in 48 hours) is essential in deciding if ambulatory care treatment is appropriate.

■ LABORATORY ASSESSMENT

The health care provider typically obtains cultures of the cervix, urethra, and rectum to determine the presence of *N. gonorrhoeae* or *C. trachomatis*. The white blood cell (WBC) count and erythrocyte sedimentation rate (ESR) may be elevated but are not sensitive enough by themselves for diagnosis of PID. Gram stains of endocervical secretions may show the presence of *N. gonorrhoeae*. A sensitive test that detects human chorionic gonadotropin in urine or blood should be performed to determine if the client is pregnant. Microscopic examination of vaginal discharge should be done to evaluate for signs of infection. The presence of more than 10 WBCs/HPF (high-power field) in vaginal discharge correlates with infection. Bacterial vaginosis can be found by observing the diagnostic clue cells.

OTHER DIAGNOSTIC ASSESSMENT

Abdominal ultrasonography is not helpful in establishing the diagnosis of PID, since it is usually normal. Sonography has been found to be useful in the diagnosis of appendicitis and tubo-ovarian abscesses that need to be ruled out when the diagnosis of PID is made. Transvaginal ultrasound has been used in some cases to detect tubal enlargement and tubal wall thickening associated with PID.

Laparoscopy, although expensive, invasive, and requiring anesthesia, is most definitive, giving an immediate, accurate diagnosis through direct inspection of the tubes and ovaries. Magnetic resonance imaging (MRI) and endometrial biopsy have been used to increase the accuracy of the diagnosis.

Because of great variations in client signs and symptoms, the diagnosis of acute PID is difficult. Because women may display subtle symptoms not typical of PID, delay in diagnosis and treatment may add to the sequelae of PID in the upper genital tract. Laparoscopy is considered the definitive diagnostic tool for PID but is not usually feasible. Therefore PID is diagnosed on the basis of clinical signs and symptoms. The Centers for Disease Control and Prevention (CDC) has set minimum criteria for the diagnosis of PID, but there are no laboratory or physical examination techniques that alone are both sensitive and specific for the diagnosis of acute PID. The CDC recommends empiric treatment of PID with antibiotics if all of the minimum criteria have been met and no other causes of illness can be found (Table 77-4).

CRITICAL THINKING CHALLENGE

On your initial physical assessment, you find that the 28-year-old married client has an oral temperature of 100.2° F (37.9° C). The abdominal assessment is significant for grimacing and holding the abdomen as the woman moves onto the examination table. Her abdomen is tender in the suprapubic and right lower quadrant areas. The nurse practitioner plans to perform the pelvic examination.

- What further physical assessment and laboratory data should be obtained?
- When she learns that she has PID, the woman begins to cry and then yells, "I can't have that. Only loose women have that!" How would you respond to this statement?

For suggested answer guidelines, go to SIMON http://www.wbsaunders.com/SIMON/Iggy/.

● Analysis

COMMON NURSING DIAGNOSES AND COLLABORATIVE PROBLEMS

The primary collaborative problem for clients with pelvic inflammatory disease (PID) is Infection related to invasion of pelvic organs by pathogens.

The following are common nursing diagnoses for clients with PID:

1. Acute Pain related to the effects of the infectious process
2. Anxiety related to possible infertility as a result of infection

---

TABLE 77-4 • DIAGNOSTIC CRITERIA FOR PELVIC INFLAMMATORY DISEASE

MINIMUM CRITERIA FOR INITIATING EMPIRIC TREATMENT FOR PELVIC INFLAMMATORY DISEASE
- Lower abdominal tenderness *and*
- Adnexal tenderness *and*
- Cervical motion tenderness (chandelier sign)

ADDITIONAL CRITERIA TO INCREASE THE SPECIFICITY OF THE DIAGNOSIS OF PID
- Oral temperature >101° F (>38.3° C)
- Abnormal cervical or vaginal discharge
- Elevated erythrocyte sedimentation rate
- Elevated C-reactive protein
- Laboratory documentation of cervical infection with *Neisseria gonorrhoeae* or *Chlamydia trachomatis*

DEFINITIVE CRITERIA FOR DIAGNOSING PID, WARRANTED IN SELECTED CASES
- Histopathologic evidence of endometritis on endometrial biopsy
- Transvaginal sonography or other imaging techniques showing thickened fluid-filled tubes with or without free pelvic fluid or tubo-ovarian complex
- Laparoscopic abnormalities consistent with PID

Modified from Centers for Disease Control and Prevention. (1998). 1998 guidelines for treatment of sexually transmitted diseases. *Morbidity and Mortality Weekly Report, 47*(No. RR-1), 1-103.
PID, Pelvic inflammatory disease.

ADDITIONAL NURSING DIAGNOSES AND COLLABORATIVE PROBLEMS

In addition to the common nursing diagnoses and collaborative problems, clients with PID may have one or more of the following:

- Altered Health Maintenance related to knowledge deficit about risks, prevention, symptoms, treatment, and effects of PID
- Chronic Pain related to recurrent PID episodes
- Sexual Dysfunction related to the effects of the infectious process
- Situational Low Self-Esteem/Chronic Low Self-Esteem related to feeling guilty for having PID (associated with sexual transmission)

● Planning and Implementation

INFECTION

PLANNING: EXPECTED OUTCOMES. The client with PID is expected to have her infection resolve as evidenced by (1) a decrease in pain and tenderness of the pelvis, (2) being afebrile, and (3) resolution of other associated symptoms (vaginal discharge, positive cultures).

INTERVENTIONS. Infection control is accomplished by the administration of antibiotics, self-care measures, and surgical intervention if needed (Chart 77-5).

INFECTION CONTROL. Uncomplicated PID is usually treated on an ambulatory care basis. The CDC recommends hospitalization for PID if the client:

- Has appendicitis, ectopic pregnancy, or other surgical emergency that has not been excluded

---

CHART 77-5

NIC **INTERVENTION ACTIVITIES** *for*
The Client with Pelvic Inflammatory Disease

Infection Control: *Minimizing the acquisition and transmission of infectious agents*
- Encourage rest.
- Encourage fluid intake, as appropriate.
- Administer antibiotic therapy, as appropriate. *Or*
- Instruct client to take antibiotics, as prescribed.
- Promote appropriate nutritional intake.
- Teach client and family about signs and symptoms of infection and when to report them to the health care provider.
- Teach client and family members how to avoid infections.

Anxiety Reduction: *Minimizing apprehension, dread, foreboding, or uneasiness related to an unidentified source of anticipated danger*
- Create an atmosphere to facilitate trust.
- Listen attentively.
- Encourage verbalization of feelings, perceptions, and fears.
- Provide factual information concerning diagnosis, treatment, and prognosis.
- Instruct client on the use of relaxation techniques.

NIC intervention activities selected from McCloskey, J.C., & Bulechek, G.M. (2000). *Nursing interventions classification (NIC)* (3rd ed.). St. Louis: Mosby. No part of this work is to be altered without prior written permission from the Publisher.

- Is pregnant
- Does not respond clinically to oral antibiotic therapy
- Is unable to follow or tolerate an outpatient regimen
- Has severe illness, nausea and vomiting, or high fever
- Has a tubo-ovarian abscess
- Is immunodeficient (e.g., has HIV infection with low CD4 counts, is taking immunosuppressive therapy, or has another disease)

Drug therapy consists of oral and possibly intramuscular or IV antibiotics (Chart 77-6). Oral treatment lasts for 14 days. All clients should be re-evaluated 48 to 72 hours after antibiotic therapy is started. If the infection has not responded to treatment, the client may need to be hospitalized for IV antibiotic therapy and further evaluation.

Inpatient therapy initially involves a combination of several IV antibiotics until the client has shown signs of clinical improvement, such as decreased abdominal tenderness, for at least 24 hours. Then oral antibiotics can be continued until the course of treatment has lasted 14 days.

When a client is treated as an outpatient, she should be encouraged to rest, abstain from sexual intercourse, and check her temperature twice a day. She will need to be seen by the health care provider 48 to 72 hours from starting the antibiotics and then 1 and 2 weeks from the time of the initial diagnosis.

In a small number of clients, the pain and tenderness may not be relieved by antibiotic therapy. The surgeon may perform a laparotomy to remove an abscess or a pelvic mass through a subumbilical incision that is several inches long to provide better access to the fallopian tubes. Preoperatively, the nurse provides information about hospital routines and procedures. General preoperative care is described in Chapter 17.

The postoperative care of the woman with PID is similar to that of any client after abdominal surgery. One difference is that the client with PID may have a wound drain in place for drainage of abscess fluid that may not have been completely removed during surgery. The nurse observes, measures, and records wound drainage every 4 to 8 hours as ordered.

ACUTE PAIN

NOC **PLANNING: EXPECTED OUTCOMES.** The client with PID is expected to report or demonstrate reduced pain and increased comfort as indicated by decreased restlessness; decreased blood pressure, heart rate, and respiratory rate; and decreased facial expressions of pain.

INTERVENTIONS. Pain management of PID begins with treatment of the infection. Antibiotic treatment relieves pain. If the client is ill enough to be hospitalized, parenteral antibiotic administration is usually chosen. Oral therapy can begin once the client's clinical status has shown improvement for at least 24 hours. Doxycycline (Monodox, Doxy-Caps, Doxycin✦) is usually given orally because of the pain associated with parenteral administration but is given as part of a parenteral inpatient regimen.

Other pain relief measures include taking analgesics or sitz baths and applying heat to the lower abdomen or back. Bedrest in a semi-Fowler's position promotes gravity drainage and consolidation of the infection that may relieve pain as well.

ANXIETY

NOC **PLANNING: EXPECTED OUTCOMES.** The client with PID is expected to take actions to reduce anxiety about infertility as indicated by identifying effective coping patterns, verbalizing a sense of control, using available social support, using effective coping strategies, and seeking professional help as appropriate.

INTERVENTIONS. Infertility is the most common complication of PID and affects at least 15% to 25% of women who have had at least one episode of PID. Nursing interventions are aimed at seeking to understand the client's perspective on the diagnosis and future complications.

NIC **ANXIETY REDUCTION.** If the client has anxiety, the nurse tries to provide an atmosphere in which she feels comfortable expressing her feelings and asking questions. The nurse provides information about the diagnosis, treatment, and prognosis. Providing information about the advantages of early diagnosis and treatment (possibly limiting damage to one area of the pelvis) and the advances in treatments for infertility may reassure the client. The nurse helps the client assess the emotional support available from family members or significant others. Relaxation techniques may be useful to decrease the anxiety (see Chart 77-5).

Community-Based Care

The client with pelvic inflammatory disease (PID) needs to have regular follow-up with her health care provider to assess for complications and ensure that the infection has resolved. The ongoing role of the nurse is to vigilantly assess for any continued risk of contracting PID again, signs of persistent or recurrent infection, and ongoing education to prevent expo-

CHART 77-6

DRUG THERAPY *for* Acute Pelvic Inflammatory Disease

Drug	Dosage	Nursing Interventions	Rationale
PARENTERAL TREATMENT			
Regimen A			
Cefotetan (Cefotan)	2 g every 12 hr IV, which can be changed to oral therapy after 24 hr of clinical improvement	Assess the client for rash, itching, and hypotension.	Assessment detects adverse reactions.
Or			
Cefoxitin (Mefoxin)	2 g IV every 6 hr, which can be changed to oral therapy after 24 hr of clinical improvement	Assess the client for rash, itching, and hypotension. Observe the IV site for signs of redness, heat, and tenderness.	Assessment detects adverse reactions. Phlebitis can be detected.
Plus			
Doxycycline (Monodox, Doxy-Caps, Doxycin✤)	100 mg every 12 hr IV or PO for 14 days. (Orally is preferred because of the pain associated with infusion.)	Assess the client for rash, nausea, and diarrhea. Encourage fluid intake. Instruct the client about possible photosensitivity. Instruct the client that it is beneficial to take the drug with food.	Assessment detects drug side effects. Fluid intake decreases esophageal irritation. This precaution prevents sunburning by limiting the client's exposure to the sun. Food decreases gastrointestinal upset.
Regimen B			
Clindamycin (Cleocin)	900 mg every 8 hr IV	Observe the client for rash and urticaria. Observe the client for hypotension, dyspnea, and restlessness. Observe the client for diarrhea. Observe the IV site for redness, heat, and tenderness.	Adverse reactions are detected. Anaphylactic reaction is detected. This precaution avoids pseudomembranous colitis. Phlebitis can be detected.
Plus			
Gentamicin (Garamycin IV)	2 mg/kg once IV or IM followed by 1.5 mg/kg every 8 hr IV or IM until there have been signs of clinical improvement for 24 hr	Encourage oral intake of fluids. Observe the IV site for redness, heat, and tenderness. Measure fluid intake and output. Observe the client for hearing loss, fever, or decreased renal function. Draw serum for peak and trough levels.	Fluid intake prevents irritation to renal tubules. Phlebitis can be detected. Oliguria or anuria can be detected. Ototoxicity, nephrotoxicity, and fever are known side effects. Serum levels can vary, and drug has low threshold for toxic level.
Then			
Doxycycline (Monodox, Doxy-Caps, Doxycin✤)	100 mg bid PO to complete a total of 14 days of treatment	See above for doxycycline.	See above for doxycycline.
Or			
Clindamycin (Cleocin)	450 mg qid PO to complete a total of 14 days of treatment	Give with 8 oz of water. See above for clindamycin.	Water decreases esophageal irritation. See above for clindamycin.

Modified from Centers for Disease Control and Prevention (1998). 1998 guidelines for treatment of sexually transmitted diseases. *Morbidity and Mortality Weekly Report, 47*(No. RR-1), 1-103.

Continued

CHART 77-6

DRUG THERAPY *for* Acute Pelvic Inflammatory Disease—cont'd

Drug	Dosage	Nursing Interventions	Rationale
ORAL TREATMENT			
Regimen A			
Ofloxacin (Floxin)	400 mg bid PO for 14 days	Monitor the serum level if the client is taking theophylline.	This drug raises the serum level of theophylline.
		Do not administer this drug to clients <18 yr of age.	The safety of this drug has not been established in clients <18 yr of age.
		Administer or instruct the client to take this drug on an empty stomach.	Food decreases this drug's absorption.
Plus			
Metronidazole (Flagyl, Novonidazol✤)	500 mg bid PO for 14 days	Monitor the serum level if the client is taking lithium.	This drug raises the serum level of lithium.
		Avoid alcohol within 24 hr of use.	Avoids disulfiram (Antabuse)–like effect.
Regimen B			
Ceftriaxone (Rocephin)	250 mg once IM	Give deep IM injection in the outer upper quadrant of the gluteus maximus.	Local irritation is avoided, and drug absorption is increased.
		Watch for fever, chills, and nausea.	Allergic reactions can be detected.
		Tell the client that the injection may be painful.	The client is prepared for discomfort related to the inflammatory reaction.
Or			
Cefoxitin (Mefoxin)	2 g once IM	Give deep IM injection in the outer upper quadrant of the gluteus maximus.	Local irritation is avoided, and drug absorption is increased.
		Watch for fever, chills, and nausea.	Allergic reactions can be detected.
		Tell the client that the injection may be painful.	The client is prepared for discomfort related to the inflammatory reaction.
Plus			
Probenecid (Benemid, Benuryl✤)	1 g once PO concurrently	Give with food.	Taking the medication with food avoids gastrointestinal upset.
		Encourage fluid intake (10 glasses a day).	Fluid intake prevents formation of kidney stones.
Or			
Other parenteral third-generation cephalosporin (e.g., ceftizoxime or cefotaxime)			
Plus			
Doxycycline (for all of the above regimens)	100 mg bid PO for 14 days	See above for doxycycline.	See above for doxycycline.

Modified from Centers for Disease Control and Prevention (1998). 1998 guidelines for treatment of sexually transmitted diseases. *Morbidity and Mortality Weekly Report, 47*(No. RR-1), 1-103.

sure to and infection with all STDs (e.g., a decrease in the number of partners, consistent condom use). The nurse establishes an atmosphere of trust that encourages the client to return frequently, if needed, for education or reassurance.

■ **HEALTH TEACHING**

Client teaching focuses on providing information about PID, identifying recurrences (persistent pain, dysmenorrhea, low backache, fever), and urging early treatment to prevent complications. The nurse also reviews teaching for oral antibiotic therapy (Chart 77-7).

The client needs to be counseled to contact her sexual partner(s) for examination and treatment. The partner is usually given treatment for gonorrhea and chlamydial infection. The nurse reminds her client about follow-up care and counsels her about the complications that can occur after an episode of PID, including increased risk for recurrence of PID, increased risk for ectopic pregnancy, increased risk for infertility, and chronic pelvic pain.

CHART 77-7

CLIENT EDUCATION GUIDE
Oral Antibiotic Therapy for Sexually Transmitted Diseases

- Take your medicine for the number of times a day it is prescribed and until it is completed.
- Your sexual partner must be tested and may need to be treated.
- Be sure to return for your follow-up appointment after completing your antibiotic treatment.
- Call if you have any questions or concerns.
- Do not have sex until after you complete your antibiotic therapy. If your partner is being treated, you can go back to having sex together 48 hours after he or she starts taking antibiotics if you use a condom.
- Drink at least 8 to 10 glasses of fluid a day while taking your antibiotics.
- Do not take antacids containing calcium, magnesium, or aluminum, such as Tums, Maalox, or Mylanta, with your antibiotics. They may decrease the effectiveness of the antibiotic.
- Take your antibiotics on an empty stomach unless your health care provider instructs you to take them with food.

If the client desires contraception, the nurse discusses methods that may decrease the risk of future episodes of PID, such as oral contraceptive pills, barrier methods in combination with spermicides containing nonoxynol 9, and tubal ligation.

Counseling is also given to help the client understand lifestyle factors that heighten the risk for recurrent episodes of PID, including sexual intercourse with multiple partners and vaginal douching.

Psychosocial concerns may require teaching and counseling as well. A client who has PID may exhibit a variety of feelings (guilt, disgust, anger) about having a condition that may have been transmitted to her sexually. These feelings may affect her relationship with significant others and future sexual relationships. She may also have concerns about future fertility if PID has caused damage or scarring of the fallopian tubes and other reproductive organs. The nurse provides emotional support and allows time for the client to express her feelings.

■ HOME CARE MANAGEMENT

Parenteral antibiotic therapy may be administered at home, but usually the health care provider changes the treatment regimen to oral antibiotics before hospital discharge (see Planning and Implementation, p. 1819).

■ HEALTH CARE RESOURCES

If infertility is a result of PID, the client may need referral to a clinic specializing in infertility treatment and counseling. The client can also contact support groups for infertile couples; such groups exist in many local communities.

The costs of antibiotics for care of clients with PID and other STDs may be a concern for those who are uninsured or underinsured. The case manager, social worker, or ambulatory care nurse seeks community resources for free or discounted medications for clients with financial limitations.

▶ Evaluation: Outcomes

NOC The nurse evaluates the care of the client with PID on the basis of the identified nursing diagnoses and collaborative problems. The expected outcomes include that the client will:

- Show evidence that the infection has resolved by (1) a decrease in pain and tenderness of the pelvis, (2) being afebrile, and (3) resolution of other associated symptoms (vaginal discharge, positive cultures)
- Report or demonstrate that pain is relieved or reduced and that she feels more comfortable
- Take action to manage anxiety about future infertility
- Describe the risk factors, signs and symptoms, management, and effects of PID
- Resume usual sexual activities without discomfort
- Express her feelings about having an infection that was probably caused by a sexually transmitted organism

SEXUALLY TRANSMITTED VAGINAL INFECTIONS

Vaginal infections, which are associated with discharge and vaginal irritation, are frequent and recurring problems for sexually active women. The following are common causes of vaginal infection:

- *Trichomonas vaginalis*
- *Candida,* primarily *C. albicans*
- Bacteria that produce bacterial vaginosis, including *Gardnerella vaginalis* and anaerobes

These infections can be spread by sexual contact. Men can also acquire these infections but are not always symptomatic. Several studies have shown that *T. vaginalis* is common in men, especially those who have other STDs, such as *Chlamydia trachomatis* (Bachmann et al., 2000; Joyner et al., 2000). However, because most of these infections are usually seen more commonly in women, assessments and interventions are discussed with other causes of vaginitis in Chapter 75.

Trichomoniasis and candidal infections are limited to the vagina. They can be very irritating and bothersome but will not cause any long-term sequela. The partner must also be treated for trichomoniasis if the infection is to be resolved. Candidiasis does not usually require partner treatment, but if the male partner is symptomatic (irritation of the genital skin), then treatment is indicated.

Bacterial vaginosis (BV) has been implicated in upper genital tract infections. Women undergoing surgery of the upper genital tract should be evaluated and treated if BV is found (Peipert et al., 1997). There has also been evidence that BV in pregnancy can lead to preterm labor and premature delivery. This has been controversial, but evaluation for BV during pregnancy has been suggested.

HEPATITIS B AND C

In the United States, 30% to 60% of the new cases of hepatitis B and in 15% to 20% of the new cases of hepatitis C are transmitted sexually. Each year an estimated 240,000 new cases of hepatitis B virus (HBV) and 36,000 new cases of hepatitis C (HCV) occur. Of those infected as adults, 1% to 6% of those with HBV and 75% to 85% of those with HCV develop chronic hepatitis, which can lead to cirrhosis and primary hepatocellular carcinoma. Each year approximately

6000 people die from HBV and 8000 to 10,000 die from HCV (CDC, 1998a; CDC, 1998b). Hepatitis is discussed further in Chapter 59.

Prevention of sexually transmitted diseases (STDs) should include educating clients about the risks of contracting hepatitis B and C. Screening for STDs should include serum evaluation for hepatitis B and C. Hepatitis B vaccine, a series of three injections over a period of 6 months, is now recommended for all newborns, children 11 to 12 years of age if they have not already received the vaccine, and adolescents and adults at high risk for STDs.

ONLINE RESOURCES

For suggested readings and Internet resources, go to http://www.wbsaunders.com/SIMON/Iggy/.

SELECTED BIBLIOGRAPHY

Asterisk indicates a classic or definitive work on this subject.

Amaral, E. (1998). Current approaches to STD management in women. *International Journal of Gynecology and Obstetrics, 63*(Suppl. 1), S183-S189.

Bachmann, L.H., et al. (2000). Risk and prevalence of treatable sexually transmitted diseases at a Birmingham substance abuse treatment facility. *American Journal of Public Health, 90*(10), 1615-1618.

Bartlett, J.G. (1998). *Pocket book of infectious disease therapy.* Baltimore: Williams & Wilkins.

Barton, S.E. (1998). Herpes management and prophylaxis. *Dermatologic Clinics, 16*(4), 799-803.

Beutner, K.R., et al. (1999). Genital warts and their treatment. *Clinical Infectious Diseases, 28*(Suppl. 1), S37-S56.

Black, C.M. (1997). Current methods of laboratory diagnosis of *Chlamydia trachomatis* infections. *Clinical Microbiology Review, 10*(1), 160-184.

Bob, P.S.S., & Famolare, N.E. (1998). Teaching and communication strategies: Working with the hospitalized adolescent with pelvic inflammatory disease. *Pediatric Nursing, 24*(1), 17-20, 29-30.

Burnstein, G.R., et al. (1998). Incident *Chlamydia trachomatis* infections among inner-city adolescent females. *Journal of the American Medical Association,, 280*(6), 521-526.

Carrico, C.W. (1999). Impact of sonography on the diagnosis and treatment of acute lower abdominal pain in children and young adults. *American Journal of Roentgenology, 172*(2), 513-516.

Centers for Disease Control and Prevention. (1997). *Chlamydia trachomatis* genital infections—United States, 1995. *Journal of the American Medical Association, 277*(12):952-953.

Centers for Disease Control and Prevention. (1998a). 1998 guidelines for treatment of sexually transmitted diseases. *Morbidity and Mortality Weekly Report, 47*(RR-1), 1-103.

Centers for Disease Control and Prevention. (1998b). Recommendations for prevention and control of hepatitis C virus (HCV) infection and HCV-related chronic disease. *Morbidity and Mortality Weekly Report, 47*(RR-19), 1, 7-8.

Centers for Disease Control and Prevention. (1999). Primary and secondary syphilis—United States, 1998. *Morbidity and Mortality Weekly Report, 48*(39), 873-878.

Centers for Disease Control and Prevention. (2001). Tracking the hidden epidemic: Trends in STDs in the United States 2000; www.cdc.gov/nchstp/dstd/Stats_Trends/Trends2000.pdf.

Cohen, C.R., & Brunham, R.C. (1999). Pathogenesis of chlamydia induced pelvic inflammatory disease. *Sexually Transmitted Infections, 75*(1), 21-24.

Daley, E.M. (1998). Clinical update on the role of HPV and cervical cancer. *Cancer Nursing, 21*(1), 31-35.

Faro, S. (1998). Sepsis in obstetric and gynecologic patients. *Current Clinical Topics in Infectious Disease, 19,* 60-82.

Groseclose, S.L., et al. (1999). Estimated incidence and prevalence of genital *Chlamydia trachomatis* infections in the United States, 1996. *Sexually Transmitted Diseases, 26*(6), 339-344.

Hein, K. (1998). Health policy implications of emerging infections. *Emerging Infectious Diseases, 4*(3), 1-5.

Joyner, J.L., et al. (2000). Comparative prevalence of infection with *Trichomonas vaginalis* among men attending a sexually transmitted disease clinic. *Sexually Transmitted Diseases, 27*(4), 236-240.

Kellock, D.J., et al. (1997). Biopsy, serology, and molecular biology, *Genitourinary Medicine, 73*(5): 399-401.

Mahoney, J.B., et al. (1997). Detection of Chlamydia trachomatis, Neisseria gonorrhoeae, Ureaplasma urealyticum, and Mycoplasma genitalium in first-void urine specimens by multiplex polymerase chain reaction. *Molecular Diagnosis, 2*(3), 161-168.

Marr, L. (1998). *Sexually transmitted diseases: A physician tells you what you need to know.* Baltimore: Johns Hopkins University Press.

McOwan, A.G., Broughton, C., & Robinson, A.J. (1999). Advising patients with genital warts: A consensus approach. *International Journal of STD and AIDS, 10*(9), 619-622.

*Morse, S.A., Moreland, A.A., & Holmes, K.K. (1996). *Atlas of sexually transmitted diseases and AIDS* (2nd ed.). London: Mosby-Wolfe.

Norton, N.J. (1998). Coping with HPV: How to help a patient diagnosed with this sexually transmitted disease. *Nursing98, 28*(9), 73-74.

Paavonen, J. (1998). Pelvic inflammatory disease: from diagnosis to prevention. *Dermatologic Clinics, 16*(4), 747-756.

Peipert, J.F., et al. (1997). Bacterial vaginosis as a risk factor for upper genital tract infection. *American Journal of Obstetrics and Gynecology, 177*(5), 1184-1187.

Rosen, T., & Brown, T.J. (1998a). Cutaneous manifestations of sexually transmitted diseases, *Medical Clinics of North America, 82*(5), 1081-1104.

Rosen, T., & Brown, T.J. (1998b). Genital ulcers—Evaluation and treatment. *Dermatologic Clinics, 16*(4), 673-685.

Schaffer, S.D. (1998). Vaginitis and sexually transmitted diseases. In E.Q. Youngkin & M.S. Davis (Eds.), *Women's health care: A primary care clinical guide* (2nd ed., pp. 265-299). Stamford, CT: Appleton & Lange.

Schmid, G.P. (1999). Treatment of chancroid. *Clinical Infectious Diseases, 28*(Suppl. 1), S14-S20.

Sedlacek, T.V. (1999). Advances in the diagnosis and treatment of human papillomavirus infections. *Clinical Obstetrics and Gynecology, 42*(2), 206-220.

Sellors, J.W., et al. (2000). A new visual indicator of chlamydial cervicitis? *Sexually Transmitted Infections, 76*(1), 46-48.

Stamm, W.E. (1999). Chlamydia trachomatis infections: Progress and problems. *Journal of Infectious Diseases, 179*(Suppl. 2), S380-383.

Stanberry, L.R. (1998). Control of STDs: The role of prophylactic vaccines against herpes simplex virus. *Sexually Transmitted Infections, 74*(6), 391-394.

Tao, G., et al. (2000). Medical care expenditures for genital herpes in the United States. *Sexually Transmitted Diseases, 27*(1), 32-38.

Winefield, A.D., & Murphy, S.A. (1998). Bacterial vaginosis: A review. *Clinical Excellence for Nurse Practitioners, 2*(4), 212-217.

Youngkin, E.Q., & Davis, M.S. (1998). *Women's health care: A primary care clinical guide* (2nd ed.), 1998, Stamford, CT: Appleton & Lange.

APPENDIXES

Abbreviations

AAA	abdominal aortic aneurysm
AACN	American Association of Critical Care Nurses
AAKP	American Association of Kidney Patients
ABC	airway, breathing, and circulation
ABG	arterial blood gas
ABI	ankle-brachial index
ABPM	ambulatory blood pressure monitoring
ABVD	Adriamycin, bleomycin, vinblastine, dacarbazine
AC	assist-control; alternating current
ACE	angiotensin-converting enzyme
ACh	acetylcholine
AChRAb	acetylcholine receptor antibody
ACL	anterior cruciate ligament
ACLS	advanced cardiac life support
ACS	acute compartment syndrome; American Cancer Society
ACTH	adrenocorticotropic hormone
ADC	AIDS dementia complex
ADH	antidiuretic hormone
ADL	activities of daily living
ADP	adenosine diphosphate
ADPKD	autosomal-dominant polycystic kidney disease
AED	automatic external defibrillation
aFP	alpha-fetoprotein
AGC	absolute granulocyte count
AGN	acute glomerulonephritis
AGR	abdominal/gluteal ratio
AHA	American Heart Association
AHRQ	Agency for Healthcare Research and Quality
AIDS	acquired immunodeficiency syndrome
AIVR	accelerated idioventricular rhythm
AJCC	American Joint Committee on Cancer
AKA	above-knee amputation
AL	ascending limb
ALA	American Lung Association
ALG	antilymphocyte globulin
ALL	acute lymphocytic leukemia
ALP	alkaline phosphatase
ALS	amyotrophic lateral sclerosis
AMI	antibody-mediated immunity
AML	acute myelocytic leukemia
AMSN	Academy of Medical-Surgical Nurses
ANA	American Nurses' Association; anti-nuclear antibody
ANC	absolute neutrophil count
ANOVA	analysis of variance
ANP	atrial natriuretic peptide
ANS	autonomic nervous system
AORN	Association of periOperative Room Nurses
AP	anteroposterior
APSAC	anisoylated plasminogen streptokinase activator complex
APSGN	acute poststreptococcal glomerulonephritis
aPTT	activated partial thromboplastin time
ara-A	adenine arabinoside
ARDS	acute respiratory distress syndrome
ARF	acute renal failure
ASA	acetylsalicylic acid
ASPEN	American Society of Parenteral and Enteral Nutrition
AST	aspartate aminotransferase
ATG	antithymocyte globulin
ATN	acute tubular necrosis
ATP	adenosine triphosphate
ATPase	adenosine triphosphatase
AV	atrioventricular, arteriovenous
AVM	arteriovenous malformation
AVN	avascular necrosis
AZA	azathioprine
AZT	azidothymidine (zidovudine)
BBIAT	Baird Body Image Assessment Tool
BC	Bowman's capsule
BCG	bacille Calmette-Guérin
BCNU	carmustine
BCS	Body Cathexis Scale
BE	barium enema
BGMS	blood glucose monitoring strip
bid	*bis in die* (twice a day)
BKA	below-knee amputation
BMI	body mass index
BMT	bone marrow transplantation
BP	blood pressure
BPEG	British Pacing and Electrophysiology Group
BPH	benign prostatic hyperplasia (hypertrophy)
BPM	breaths per minute; beats per minute
BRM	biologic response modifier
BSE	breast self-examination
BSI	body substance isolation
BSO	bilateral salpingo-oophorectomy
BUN	blood urea nitrogen
c	cup(s)
C&S	culture and sensitivity
CABG	coronary artery bypass graft
CAD	computer-assisted design; coronary artery disease
CAH	chronic active hepatitis
CAL	chronic airflow limitation
CALLA	common acute lymphoblastic leukemia antigen
CAM	complementary and alternative medicine
cAMP	cyclic adenosine monophosphate
CAPD	continuous ambulatory peritoneal dialysis
CAVH	continuous arteriovenous hemofiltration
CAVHD	continuous arteriovenous hemofiltration and dialysis
CBC	complete blood count
CBD	common bile duct
CBE	charting by exception
CBI	continuous bladder irrigation
CBS	chronic brain syndrome
CCA	circumflex coronary artery
CCP	critical closing pressure
CCPD	continuous-cycle peritoneal dialysis
CD	Cotrel-Dubousset; collecting duct

CD4	cluster of differentiation 4	DIC	disseminated intravascular coagulation
CDC	Centers for Disease Control and Prevention; chenodeoxycholic acid	DIP	distal interphalangeal joint
		DJD	degenerative joint disease
CEA	carcinoembryonic antigen	dL	deciliter(s)
CFU	colony-forming unit	DL	descending limb
CGN	chronic glomerulonephritis	DLCO	diffusion capacity for carbon monoxide
CHF	congestive heart failure	DLE	discoid lupus erythematosus
CIC	Certified in Infection Control	DNA	deoxyribonucleic acid
CIN	cervical intraepithelial neoplasia	DNP	dinitrophenol
CIS	carcinoma in situ	DNR	do not resuscitate
CK	creatine kinase	DOE	dyspnea on exertion
CLE	centrilobular emphysema	DP	dopamine
CLL	chronic lymphocytic leukemia	DPOA	durable power of attorney
cm	centimeter(s)	DRE	digital rectal examination
CMG	cystometrogram	DRG	diagnosis-related group
CMI	cell-mediated immunity	DS	double-strength
CML	chronic myelocytic leukemia	DSA	digital subtraction angiography
CMS	circulation, movement, sensation	DTIC	dacarbazine
CMV	cisplatin, methotrexate, vinblastine; cytomegalovirus	DTR	deep tendon reflex
		DUB	dysfunctional uterine bleeding
CNS	central nervous system	DVT	deep vein thrombosis
CO	cardiac output	EAT	Eating Attitudes Test
COHb	carboxyhemoglobin	EBL	estimated blood loss
COLD	chronic obstructive lung disease	EBV	Epstein-Barr virus
COPD	chronic obstructive pulmonary disease	ECCC	Emergency Cardiac Care Committee
COPES	Family Crisis-Oriented Personal Evaluation Scale	ECCE	extracapsular cataract extraction
		ECF	extracellular fluid
CPAP	continuous positive airway pressure	ECG	electrocardiogram
CPB	cardiopulmonary bypass	EDI	Eating Disorder Inventory
CPK	creatine phosphokinase	EGD	esophagogastroduodenoscopy
CPM	continuous passive motion	EHDP	etidronate disodium
CPN	chronic pyelonephritis	EIA	enzyme immunoassay
CPO	certified prosthetist-orthotist	ELISA	enzyme-linked immunosorbent assay
CPP	cerebral perfusion pressure	EMD	electromechanical dissociation
CPR	cardiopulmonary resuscitation	EMG	electromyography
cps	cycles per second	EMS	emergency medical services
CQI	continuous quality improvement	EMT	Emergency Medical Technician
CREST	calcinosis, Raynaud's phenomenon, esophageal dysfunction sclerodactyly, telangiectasia	ENCORE	encouragement, normalcy, counseling, opportunity, reaching out, revived energies
CRF	chronic renal failure	ENG	electronystagmography
CRH	corticotropin-releasing hormone	ENT	ear, nose, and throat
CRI	chronic renal insufficiency	EOM	extraocular movement
CRNA	Certified Registered Nurse Anesthetist	EPO	erythropoietin
CS	crush syndrome	EPS	electrophysiologic study
CSA	cyclosporine A	ER	estrogen receptor
CSF	cerebrospinal fluid	ERCP	endoscopic retrograde cholangiopancreatography
CST	Certified Surgical Technologist		
CT	computed tomography	ERS	endoscopic retrograde sphincterotomy
CTD	connective tissue disease	ERT	estrogen replacement therapy
CTS	carpal tunnel syndrome	ESR	erythrocyte sedimentation rate
CVA	cerebrovascular accident (stroke); costovertebral angle	ESRD	end-stage renal disease
		ET	Enterostomal Therapist; endotracheal tube
CVC	central venous catheter	ETDR	early treatment diabetic retinopathy
CVP	central venous pressure	ETT	exercise tolerance test
D&C	dilation and curettage	EVS	early vitrectomy study
DARE	Drug Awareness Resistance Education	FACT	fruits, animals, colors, and towns
dB	decibel(s)	FAM	fluorouracil, Adriamycin, and mitomycin C
DCCT	Diabetes Control and Complications Trial	FANA	fluorescent antinuclear antibody
DCM	dilated cardiomyopathy	FAST	fluoroallergosorbent test
DCT	distal convoluted tubule	FBD	fibrocystic breast disease
DDAVP	desmopressin acetate	FBSS	failed back surgery syndrome
ddI	dideoxyinosine (didanosine)	FDA	(US) Food and Drug Administration
DDS	dapsone	FEF	forced expiratory flow
DES	diethylstilbestrol	FES	fat embolism syndrome
DHE	dihydroergotamine	FEV	forced expiratory volume
DHHS	(US) Department of Health and Human Services	FEV_1	forced expiratory volume in one second
DHT	dihydrotestosterone	FEV_1/FVC	ratio of expiratory volume in one second to forced vital capacity
DI	diabetes insipidus		

FFP	fresh frozen plasma
FIM	Functional Independence Measure
F$_{IO_2}$	fraction of inspired oxygen
FNB	Food and Nutrition Board
FNCR	Family Nursing Chart Review
FOBT	fecal occult blood test
FR	flutter rate
Fr	French
FRC	functional residual capacity
FS	full-strength
FSBS	fingerstick blood sugar
FSH	follicle-stimulating hormone
ft	foot (feet)
FTA-ABS	fluorescent treponemal antibody absorption test
5-FU	5-fluorouracil
FUDR	floxuridine
FVC	forced vital capacity
FWB	full weight-bearing
g/day	gram(s) per day
g	gram(s)
G6PD	glucose-6-phosphate dehydrogenase
GABA	gamma-aminobutyric acid
GAS	general adaptation syndrome
GB	gallbladder
GBS	Guillain-Barré syndrome
GCS	Glasgow Coma Scale
GCSF	granulocyte colony-stimulating factor
GDM	gestational diabetes mellitus
GE	gastroenteritis
GF	glomerular filtrate
GFR	glomerular filtration rate
GH	growth hormone
GH-IH	growth hormone–inhibiting hormone
GH-RH	growth hormone–releasing hormone
GI	gastrointestinal
GM-CSF	granulocyte-macrophage colony-stimulating factor
Gn-RH	gonadotropin-releasing hormone
GSW	gunshot wound
GVHD	graft-versus-host disease
Gy	Gray(s)
h	hour(s)
HAT	hearing assessment test
Hb	hemoglobin
HBIG	hepatitis B immunoglobulin
HBO	hyperbaric oxygen
HBV	hepatitis B virus
hCG	human chorionic gonadotropin
HCM	hypertrophic cardiomyopathy
Hct	hematocrit
HCV	hepatitis C virus
HD	hemodialysis
HDL	high-density lipoprotein
HDV	hepatitis delta virus
HEPA	high-efficiency particulate air
HEV	hepatitis E virus
Hgb	hemoglobin
HIDA	hepatobiliary iminodiacetic acid analog (radionuclide labeled with technetium-99m)
HIP	Help for Incontinent Persons
HITT	heparin-induced thrombocytopenia/thrombosis
HLA	human leukocyte antigen
HMO	health maintenance organization
HPA	hypothalamic-pituitary-adrenal
HPV	human papillomavirus
HR	heart rate
HSV	herpes simplex virus
5-HT	5-hydroxytryptamine (serotonin)
HTLV	human T-cell lymphotropic virus
Hz	Hertz
I&D	incision and drainage
IABP	intra-aortic balloon pumping
IBS	irritable bowel syndrome
IBW	ideal body weight
ICD	implantable cardioverter-defibrillator
ICE	Institutional Ethics Committee
ICF	intracellular fluid
ICHD	Intersociety Commission for Heart Disease
ICP	intracranial pressure
ICS	intercostal space
ICU	intensive care unit
IF	interstitial fluid
Ig	immunoglobulin
IHSS	idiopathic hypertrophic subaortic stenosis
IL	interleukin
IL-2	interleukin-2
IL-3	interleukin-3
IL-4	interleukin-4
IL-5	interleukin-5
IL-8	interleukin-8
IM	intramedullary rod; intramuscular
IMF	intermaxillary fixation
IMV	intermittent mandatory ventilation
INF	interferon
INR	International Normalized Ratio
IOL	intraocular lens
IOP	intraocular pressure
IP	intraperitoneal
IPD	intermittent peritoneal dialysis
IPG	impedance plethysmography
IRT	intracavitary radiation therapy
IS	incentive spirometer
ITH	idiosyncratic toxic hepatitis
ITP	idiopathic thrombocytopenic purpura
IU	International Unit(s)
IUD	intrauterine device
IU/L	International Unit(s) per liter
IV	intravenous
IVC	inferior vena cava
IVP	intravenous pyelography
JCAHO	Joint Commission on the Accreditation of Healthcare Organizations
JGC	juxtaglomerular cell
JVD	jugular-venous distention
JVP	jugular venous pressure
KCS	keratoconjunctivitis sicca
kg	kilogram(s)
kJ	kilojoule(s)
KS	Kaposi's sarcoma
KUB	kidneys, ureters, and bladder
KW	Keith-Wagner classification
LAC	long arm cast
LAD	left anterior descending
LAK	lymphokine-activated killer (cell)
LAP	leukocyte alkaline phosphatase
LAS	localized adaptation syndrome
LATS	long-acting thyroid stimulator
LBP	low back pain
LCA	left coronary artery
LDH	lactate dehydrogenase
LDL	low-density lipoprotein
LE	lupus erythematosus; lower extremity
LES	lower esophageal sphincter
LGV	lymphogranuloma venereum
LH	luteinizing hormone
LL	left lateral

LLC	long leg cast	MTP	metatarsophalangeal
LLQ	left lower quadrant	MTX	methotrexate
LMN	lower motor neuron	mU	milliunit(s)
LOA	leave of absence	mU/mL	milliunit(s) per milliliter
LOC	level of consciousness	MUGA	multigated angiography
LORS	Level of Rehabilitation Scale	mV	millivolt(s)
LP	lumbar puncture, light perception	MVA	motor vehicle accident
LPS	lipopolysaccharide	MVAC	methotrexate, vinblastine, Adriamycin, cisplatin
LR	lactated Ringer's (solution)	NANDA	North American Nursing Diagnosis Association
LRD	living related donor	NAON	National Association of Orthopaedic Nurses
LTC	long-term care	NAPHT	National Association of Patients on Hemodialysis and Transplantation
LUQ	left upper quadrant		
LVD	left ventricular dysfunction	NASPE	North American Society for Pacing and Electrophysiology
LVEDP	left ventricular end-diastolic pressure		
mA	milliampere(s)	NCI	National Cancer Institute
MAC	*Mycobacterium avium* complex	NE	norepinephrine
MAO	monoamine oxidase	ng	nanogram(s)
MAP	mean arterial pressure	NG	nasogastric
MAST	military antishock trousers	NHANES	National Health and Nutrition Examination Survey
MAT	multifocal atrial tachycardia		
MB-CAPD	multiple-bag continuous ambulatory peritoneal dialysis	NHIF	National Head Injury Foundation
		NIC	Nursing Interventions Classification
MCA	middle cerebral artery	NK	natural killer (cell)
MCH	mean corpuscular hemoglobin	NKF	National Kidney Foundation
MCHC	mean corpuscular hemoglobin concentration	NLN	National League for Nursing
MCL	modified chest lead	NRC/NAS	National Research Council/National Academy of Sciences
MCP	metacarpophalangeal		
M-CSF	monocyte-macrophage colony-stimulating factor	NS	nephrotic syndrome; normal saline
MCV	mean corpuscular volume	NSAID	nonsteroidal anti-inflammatory drug
MD	muscular dystrophy	NSNA	National Student Nurse Association
MDF	myocardial depressant factor	NSR	normal sinus rhythm
MDI	metered-dose inhaler	NTP	noninvasive temporary pacing
MEN	multiple endocrine neoplasia	NWB	non-weight-bearing
mEq	milliequivalent(s)	NYHA	New York Heart Association
mEq/L	milliequivalent(s) per liter	OA	osteoarthritis
MFH	malignant firous histiocytoma	OBS	organic brain syndrome
μg	microgram(s)	OCG	oral cholecystogram
mg	milligram(s)	OD	oculus dexter (right eye)
MG	myasthenia gravis	OFP	Optimal Functioning Plan
mg/dL	milligram(s) per deciliter	OI	osteogenesis imperfecta
MH	malignant hyperthermia	OR	operating room
MHAUS	Malignant Hyperthermia Association of the United States	ORIF	open reduction, internal fixation
		ORT	oral rehydration therapy; operating room technician
MHC	major histocompatibility complex		
MI	myocardial infarction	OS	oculus sinister (left eye)
MICU	medical intensive care unit	OSHA	(US) Occupational Safety and Health Administration
MIH	melanocyte-inhibiting hormone		
min	minute(s)	OT	occupational therapist
mL	milliliter(s)	OTC	over-the-counter
mL/kg	milliliter(s) per kilogram	oz	ounce(s)
mm	millimeter(s)	PA	posteroanterior; physician's assistant
mm Hg	millimeter(s) of mercury	PAB	prealbumin
mmol	millimole(s)	PAC	premature atrial complex
mmol/L	millimoles per liter	$Paco_2$	partial pressure of arterial carbon dioxide
MMPI	Minnesota Multiphasic Personality Inventory	PACU	postanesthesia care unit
MMSE	Mini-Mental State Examination	Pao_2	partial pressure of arterial oxygen
MMV	maximum mandatory ventilation	Pap	Papanicolaou (test, smear)
MODY	maturity-onset diabetes of the young	PAP	pulmonary artery pressure
MOPP	mechlorethamine, Oncovin, procarbazine, prednisone	PASG	pneumatic antishock garment
		PAT	paroxysmal atrial tachycardia
mOsm	milliosmole(s)	PAWP	pulmonary artery wedge pressure
mOsm/L	milliosmole(s) per liter	PCA	patient-controlled analgesia; patient care assistant
MRB	manual resuscitation bag	PCAC	Patient Care Advisory Committee
MRC	Medical Research Council	PCM	protein-calorie malnutrition
MRI	magnetic resonance imaging	PCN	penicillin
MS	multiple sclerosis; morphine sulfate	PCP	*Pneumocystis carinii* pneumonia
msec	millisecond(s)	PCR	polymerase chain reaction
MSH	melanocyte-stimulating hormone	PCT	proximal convoluted tubule

PD	peritoneal dialysis	PV	polycythemia vera
PE	pulmonary embolism; pharyngoesophageal	PVC	premature ventricular contraction
PEA	pulseless electrical activity	PVD	peripheral vascular disease
PEEP	positive end-expiratory pressure	PVR	postvoiding residual
PERRLA	pupils equal, round, and reactive to light and accommodation	PVS	persistent vegetative state
		PWB	partial weight-bearing
PES	problem, etiology, symptoms	q	*quaque* (every)
PES-EO-IO	problem, etiology, signs and symptoms; expected outcome, interventions, outcome	qd	*quaque die* (every day)
		qid	*quater in die* (four times a day)
PET	positron emission tomography	qod	every other day
PFT	pulmonary function test	QOL	quality of life
PGE$_2$	prostaglandin E$_2$	QOLY	Quality of Life Year(s)
PGI$_2$	prostaglandin I$_2$ (prostacyclin)	RA	rheumatoid arthritis
pH	the negative logarithm of the hydrogen ion concentration	rad	radiation absorbed dose
		RAI	radioactive iodine
PHP	plasma hydrostatic pressure	RAIU	radioactive iodine uptake
PHS	Public Health Service	RAS	reticular activating system
PICC	peripherally inserted central catheter	RBC	red blood cell
PID	pelvic inflammatory disease	RCA	right coronary artery
PIE	plan, interventions, evaluation	RDA	recommended daily allowance; recommended dietary allowance
PIH	prolactin-inhibiting hormone		
PIP	proximal interphalangeal; peak inspiratory pressure	REM	rapid eye movement
		RFUT	radiofibrinogen uptake test
PJC	premature junctional complex	RIA	radioimmunoassay
PJT	premature junctional tachycardia	RIND	reversible ischemic neurologic deficit
PKD	polycystic kidney disease	RL	right lateral
PLE	panlobular emphysema	RLQ	right lower quadrant
PLP	phantom limb pain	RNA	ribonucleic acid
PMI	point of maximal impact	RNI	Recommended Nutrient Intake
PMN	polymorphonuclear cell	ROM	range of motion
PMR	progressive muscle relaxation; polymyalgia rheumatica	RPGN	rapidly progressive glomerulonephritis
		RSD	reflex sympathetic dystrophy
PMS	premenstrual syndrome	RTA	renal tubular acidosis
PMT	premenstrual tension	RUQ	right upper quadrant
PND	paroxysmal nocturnal dyspnea	RV	residual volume
PNS	parasympathetic nervous system; peripheral nervous system	SA	sinoatrial
		SAC	short arm cast
PO	*per os* (by mouth)	SAECG	signal-averaged electrocardiography
POAG	primary open-angle glaucoma	SAM	smoking-attributable mortality
POC	point-of-care	Sao$_2$	saturation of arterial oxygen
POR	problem-oriented record	SBE	subacute bacterial endocarditis
PPD	purified protein derivative	SBFT	small bowel follow-through
ppm	parts per million	SC	subcutaneous
PPM	pulses per minute	SCD	sequential compression device
PPN	partial parenteral nutrition	SCI	spinal cord injury
PPS	post-polio sequelae (syndrome)	SCID	severe combined immunodeficiency
PRL	prolactin	SCS	Self-Cathexis Scale
PRN	*pro re nata* (as needed)	SDA	same-day admission
PSA	prostate-specific antigen	SDAT	senile dementia Alzheimer's type
PSE	portal-systemic encephalopathy	SDS	same-day surgery
PSS	progressive systemic sclerosis	SEAPort	side-entry access port
PSV	pressure support ventilation	sec	second(s)
PSVT	paroxysmal supraventricular tachycardia	SEP	somatosensory evoked potential
PT	physical therapy; physical therapist; prothrombin time	SF6	sulfahexafluoride
		SFA	superficial femoral artery
PTA	percutaneous transluminal angioplasty; peritonsillar abscess	SGOT	serum glutamic-oxaloacetic transaminase
		SI	Système International d'Unites
PTC	peritubular capillary	SIADH	syndrome of inappropriate antidiuretic hormone
PTCA	percutaneous transluminal coronary angioplasty	SIMV	synchronized intermittent mandatory ventilation
PTFE	polytetrafluoroethylene	SLC	short leg cast
PTH	parathyroid hormone (parathormone)	SLE	systemic lupus erythematosus
PTT	partial thromboplastin time	SLP	speech/language pathologist
PTU	propylthiouracil	SLR	straight-leg raise
PUD	peptic ulcer disease	SMI	sustained minimal inspiration; self-management inventory
PULSES	physical condition, upper limb function, lower limb function, sensory components, excretory function, support factors		
		SMR	submucous resection
		SMX	sulfamethoxazole
PUVA	psoralen and ultraviolet A	SNF	skilled nursing facility

SNS	sympathetic nervous system
SOAP	subjective data, objective data, analysis, plan
SOAPIER	subjective data, objective data, analysis, plan, interventions, evaluation, revision of plan
SP	suprapubic
SPD	supply processing and distribution
SPECT	single photon emission computed tomography
SPEP	serum protein electrophoresis
SPF	suntan photoprotection factor
SSKI	saturated solution of potassium iodide
STA	superficial temporal artery
STD	sexually transmitted disease
STS	serologic test for syphilis
STSG	split-thickness skin graft
SV	stroke volume
SVC	superior vena cava
T&A	tonsillectomy and adenoidectomy
T_3	triiodothyronine
T_3RU	triiodothyronine resin uptake
T_4	thyroxine
TAF	tumor angiogenesis factor
TAH	total abdominal hysterectomy
TB	tuberculosis
TBI	total body irradiation
TBSA	total body surface area
tbsp	tablespoon(s)
TCDB	turn, cough, and deep breathe
TCT	thyrocalcitonin
TDT	terminal deoxynucleotidyl transferase
TED	thromboembolic device
TEE	transesophageal echocardiography
TEF	tracheoesophageal fistula
TEN	toxic epidermal necrolysis
TENS	transcutaneous electrical nerve stimulation
THA	tetrahydroaminoacridine
THP	tissue hydrostatic pressure
THR	total hip replacement
TIA	transient ischemic attack
TIBC	total iron-binding capacity
tid	*ter in die* (three times a day)
TJR	total joint replacement
TKR	total knee replacement
TLC	total lung capacity; total lymphocyte count
TLS	tumor lysis syndrome
TLSO	thoracic lumbar sacral orthosis (thoracolumbosacral orthosis)
TMJ	temporomandibular joint
TMP	trimethroprim
TNF	tumor necrosis factor
TNM	tumor, node, metastasis
TOP	tissue osmotic pressure
TOPS	Take Off Pounds Sensibly

t-PA	tissue plasminogen activator
TPI	treponemal immobilization (test)
TPN	total parenteral nutrition
TQM	total quality management
TRH	thyrotropin-releasing hormone
TSE	testicular self-examination
TSH	thyroid-stimulating hormone
TSI	thyroid-stimulating immunoglobulin
TSM	transparent semipermeable membrane
tsp	teaspoon(s)
TSS	toxic shock syndrome
TTD	transtelephonic defibrillation/monitoring
TTO	transtracheal oxygen
TTP	thrombotic thrombocytopenic purpura
TURBT	transurethral resection of bladder tumor
TURP	transurethral resection of the prostate
TVH	total vaginal hysterectomy
UGI	upper gastrointestinal
UMN	upper motor neuron
UPJ	ureteropelvic junction
UPP	urethral pressure profilometry
US	ultrasonography
USDA	United States Department of Agriculture
UTI	urinary tract infection
UV	ultraviolet
UVA	ultraviolet A
UVB	ultraviolet B
UVJ	ureterovesical junction
VAD	venous access device
VADS	Visual Analog Dyspnea Scale
VAS	visual analog scale
VC	vital capacity
VCUG	voiding cystourethrogram
VDRL	Venereal Disease Research Laboratory (test)
VEP	visual evoked potential
VF	ventricular fibrillation
VLS	vascular leak syndrome
VMA	vanillylmandelic acid
$\dot{V}_{O_2}$	oxygen consumption
VOD	veno-occlusive disease
VPB	ventricular premature beat
$\dot{V}/\dot{Q}$	ventilation-perfusion
VR	vasa recta
VSE	vulvar self-examination
VT	ventricular tachycardia
V_T	tidal volume
VZV	varicella-zoster virus
WAIS	Wechsler Adult Intelligence Scale
WBC	white blood cell
WHO	World Health Organization
WHR	waist-to-hip ratio

Screening Guidelines for Secondary Prevention of Selected Cancers in Asymptomatic People

Cancer	Screening Test*
Breast cancer	Breast self-examination (monthly) Clinical examination (yearly) Mammography (baseline at age 35, every 2 years for ages 40-49, yearly after age 50)
Cervical cancer	Papanicolaou test and pelvic examination (yearly for sexually active women)
Ovarian cancer	Pelvic examination (yearly for women over age 40) Pelvic ultrasonography and blood test for CA-125 (yearly for women at high-risk)
Prostate cancer	Digital rectal examination and blood test for prostate-specific antigen (yearly starting at age 40)
Testicular cancer	Testicular self-examination (monthly after puberty) Clinical examination (yearly)
Colorectal cancer	Digital rectal examination and stool blood test (yearly starting at age 40) Colonoscopy (yearly starting at age 50)
Skin cancer	Visual self-examination of skin lesions (monthly for all ages) Clinical examination (yearly)

*Recommended frequency of screening tests varies by agency, preference of the health care provider, and individual client risk.

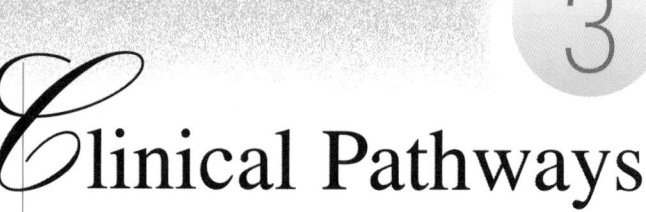

Clinical Pathways

Clinical Pathway ■ **ANKLE SPRAIN CONTINUUM OF CARE**

This pathway is designed to help you understand how to care for your ankle sprain during the initial healing phase and the rehabilitation phase. It is important for you to understand what to expect and to be able to participate actively in your recovery.

	Initial Healing Phase	Rehabilitation Phase
PAIN MANAGEMENT	Swelling increases the amount of pain in the ankle. Keep swelling down to reduce your pain. Use pain medicine prescribed by your doctor.	Ask your doctor about medicine you may buy without a prescription for pain management.
SWELLING	**RICE** **Rest** the ankle; use crutches if directed by your doctor. Limit walking to activity that is absolutely necessary. **Ice** the ankle for the first 24 hr after injury. Then use ice on the ankle 3-4 times a day for 20 min until swelling is no longer a problem. *Caution: Do not place ice directly on skin; always place towel between ice and skin.* **Compression** on the ankle with an elastic wrap or a brace if ordered by your doctor. *Caution: If the foot or toes become numb, call your doctor.* **Elevate** your ankle above your heart whenever possible (ankle above knee, knee above heart).	Swelling may occur after exercise or after standing or walking long distances. Continue to use ice and elevation after long periods of standing or walking to reduce swelling.
WALKING	Walk only when absolutely necessary. Use crutches or a cane if prescribed by your doctor. Use crutches properly, with weight on the ankle only as prescribed by your doctor. Use a brace only if prescribed by your doctor.	Walking on flat, level surfaces decreases the chance of reinjuring the ankle. Use a brace only if prescribed by your doctor.
DAILY ACTIVITIES	You may be limited in the distance you can walk because of pain or difficulty in walking with crutches. Plan your activities with frequent rest periods. Plan times for elevation of your ankle throughout the day.	Perform strengthening exercises as directed by your doctor or therapist. Return to normal walking pattern (avoid limping) as pain and swelling disappear.
PREVENTION		Prevent injury by avoiding potholes and uneven walking surfaces.

From Maher, A.B., Salmond, S.W., & Pellino, T. (1998). *Orthopaedic nursing* (2nd ed.). Philadelphia, W.B. Saunders.

CATHOLIC MEDICAL CENTER—MANCHESTER, NH.

Clinical Pathway ■ Coronary Artery Bypass

Name: _____

Admission date: _____ Admitting diagnosis: _____

Significant other: _____ Can be reached at: home # _____ other # _____

DISCHARGE GOAL ☐ HOME ☐ SNF/REHAB

Allergies: _____

Addressograph

Day Prior to Surgery

Outcome	Standard	Completed date/time/initial	Misc. Information.
Appropriate lab/diagnostic testing is completed with results available on chart	If not done in the preceeding 15 days: CBC, chemistry group (CGR), U/A, PT, PTT, ECG, chest PA and lateral	_____	BUN: _____ Creatinine: _____
Blood products are available as ordered for surgery	Day prior to surgery: type and crossmatch ____ units of PRBCs or type and screen ____ units of PRBCs		Hgb: ____ Hct: ____ Potassium: ____
Risk of stroke is reduced	Carotid ultrasound studies to be done on all clients 60 years or older ☐ done ☐ N/A ☐ report on chart for OR		Ejection fraction _____
Client is educated to enhance understanding of surgery and the immediate postoperative period prior to discharge	Consult Cardiac Health and Wellness for preop teaching Preop teaching is completed prior to surgery, including significant others whenever possible	_____	Past medical history:
IS goal: ____ mL IS achieved: ____ mL	Consult respiratory therapy for IS teaching Respiratory therapist completes instruction with client able to return demonstration	_____	
Discharge planning starts on admission to the hospital; clients' needs are identified at the earliest possible date Spiritual needs are assessed on admission	Diabetics will be referred to the Diabetic Institute ☐ done ☐ N/A Social Service is consulted for all clients who will require SNF or VNA service or those with financial concerns ☐ done ☐ N/A Pastoral Care is consulted to meet spiritual needs ☐ done ☐ N/A	_____	Current problem list:
Nursing history and physical exam is completed within 4 hours	Nursing assessment and history is completed; abnormal findings are communicated to the physician; appropriate interventions occur Current medications needing to be resumed after surgery include:	_____	
pHisoHex scrub and shower to entire body is completed evening before surgery and after prep AM of surgery	pHisoHex scrub and ☐ shower or ☐ bed bath is done evening prior to surgery pHisoHex scrub and ☐ shower or ☐ bed bath is done AM of surgery after prep	_____	Medication list from home:
Prep of lower neck, chest, pubic area, groin, both wrists, and both legs to below ankle	Each client will be prepped for surgery as close to surgery as possible; standard prep will be done as a wet prep with a razor Physician is notified of any skin/skin integrity issues Area prepped/abnormal skin findings are documented in this space	_____	

Courtesy of Catholic Medical Center, Manchester NH.

Preoperative Check List

Yes	No	N/A	
			Permits signed ☐ Operative ☐ Anesthesia ☐ Blood
			☐ ID bracelet on ☐ Blood band on Blood available ☐ yes ☐ no _____ units _____ T&S
			Allergies (including dyes, latex, tape, prep solutions)
			Medex, Addressograph card, operating note, and anesthesia record on chart
			Significant medical history (diabetic, cardiac, seizures, pulmonary, ETOH, renal)
			Sensory/motor impairment noted; include inability to stand, speak, hear, see, decreased level of awareness
			Permanent pacemaker/AICD
			Client NPO after midnight
			Rings, hairpins, accessories, makeup, and nail polish removed
			Eyeglasses/contact lenses/dentures removed
			Current blood work U/A, ECG, chest x-ray reports, history and physical, and consults on chart Glucose-AccuChek if diabetic
			Height _____ Weight _____
			Pre-op medications given, vital signs taken and recorded
			T _____ P _____ R _____ BP _____
			Old records with chart
			Skin breakdown present? If yes, location:
			Shave prep completed and checked
			Foley drainage bag emptied
			Client had pHisoHex scrub and shower or bed bath evening before and AM of surgery
			Chest x-rays brought by client sent to OR with client chart
			Cath report on chart
			Carotid ultrasounds report on chart

Nurses signature: _____ Date _____

DATE: _____ ROOM FROM: _____ TO: _____

MEDS: CASSETTE: _____ REFRIG: _____ OWN: _____

DENTURES: _____

PROSTHESIS: _____

GLASSES: _____ WATCH: _____

HEARING AID: _____ RINGS: _____

JEWELRY: _____

OTHER: _____

Transferring Unit Sig: _____

Receiving Unit Sig: _____

Messenger Sig: _____

DATE: _____ ROOM FROM: _____ TO: _____

MEDS: CASSETTE: _____ REFRIG: _____ OWN: _____

DENTURES: _____

PROSTHESIS: _____

GLASSES: _____ WATCH: _____

HEARING AID: _____ RINGS: _____

JEWELRY: _____

OTHER: _____

Transferring Unit Sig: _____

Receiving Unit Sig: _____

Messenger Sig: _____

The following items have been sent home with:

Print name: _____ Telephone # _____

Signature: _____

Witness: _____ Date _____

CVSPCU Clinical Pathway for the CABG

Outcomes	Interventions	Surgical Day	POD 1	POD 2	POD 3	Day
Client is hemodynamically stable as evidenced by SBP 90-150; DBP 50-90, HR 60-100 beats/min and stable rhythm, temp 99° F	1. Cardiac monitor/assess pattern q4h × 48 hr 2. Assessment q4h × 48 hr then q shift until discharge 3. Obtain CSP on POD 2 4. D/C pacing wires on POD 3					
Respirations are 12-22/min at rest with regular rhythm and clean lung sounds	1. Cont. resp. care postextubation cardiac surgery protocol orders 2. O_2 as ordered 3. Assess lung sounds and obtain O_2 sats q4h × 48 hr then q shift 4. IS/CDB qh WA 5. If wheezes or rales present, refer to respiratory protocol 6. Obtain CXR on POD 2					
Client returns to baseline neuro status	1. Assess q4h × 48 hr then q shift till discharge					
Client will indicate adequate pain relief	1. Assess for pain q2-4h 2. MSO_4 SC for pain × 24 hr then PO analgesia through discharge and document effect					
Chest tube drainage will be <50 mL/hr Maintain Hct >24	1. CT to 20 cm H_2O seal suction 2. Check patency q1-2h 3. Measure and document drainage q1-2h 4. Consider removal when drainage ____ mL/hr or less					
Wound drainage within normal limits	1. Assess drainage q4h and change dressings prn 2. Remove dressings on POD 2 3. Apply TEDS on POD 2					
Client tolerates diet as ordered Client is free of nausea/vomiting after appropriate medication Client will have BM prior to discharge	1. Assess bowel sounds q4h × 48 hr then q shift 2. Clear liquid/diet as tolerated 3. Stool softeners/consider laxatives					
Client tolerates progressive activity Client remains free from injury	1. Phase I activity 2. Ambulate 50-500 feet tid 3. Stairs if able					
Client will maintain adequate urine output as evidenced by I&O balance Fluid restriction maintained as ordered	1. I&O q4h 2. Daily weights 3. D/C Foley POD # 4. 2000 mL/24 hr fluid restriction					
Client/SO demonstrates understanding of procedures, CV surgical routine, and plan of care	1. Review plan of care with client/SO 2. Review meds with client/SO 3. Client/SO attends discharge/dietary classes 4. Client receives diabetic teaching if indicated					

Client/SO demonstrates effective coping mechanism and verbalizes a discharge plan	1. Psychologic assessment
	2. Review discharge plan
	3. Review referral needs daily:
	  Social Service
	  Case Manager
	  Diabetic
	  Dietary
	  Pastoral
	  PT
	  OT					

Courtesy of Catholic Medical Center, Manchester NH.

Coronary Artery Bypass Pathway Day of Surgery

Date: _____

Admit time: _____ Extubation time: _____ Discharge time: _____

☐ Hour 1 / ☐ Hour 0 through 4

HEMODYNAMICS
Management of hemodynamic parameters ☐
- Protocol(s) initiated to achieve hemodynamic stability

RESPIRATORY
Extubation protocol initiated ☐

LABS AND DIAGNOSTICS
Appropriate labs/diagnostics obtained ☐
- Follow labs and diagnostic protocol

METABOLIC
K repletion ☐
- K⁺ replacement protocol initiated
Rewarming ☐
- Protocol for management of hypothermia initiated

PAIN MANAGEMENT
Pain protocol initiated ☐

MISC
Significant other contact/visit ☐
Safety protocol initiated ☐
Follow standards of care ☐

☐ Hour 2 through 4 / ☐ Hour 5 through 12

HEMODYNAMICS
Wean vasoactive meds ☐
- Follow inotrope, vasoactive, pacing, and volume protocols

RESPIRATORY
Weaning from ventilator ☐
- Follow extubation protocol

LABS AND DIAGNOSTICS
Appropriate labs/diagnostics obtained ☐
- Follow labs and diagnostic protocol

METABOLIC
Return to baseline neuro status ☐
Temp ≥36° C ☐
- Continue with hypothermia protocol

PAIN MANAGEMENT
Pain controlled by meds ☐
- Continue pain protocol

☐ Hour 4 through 8 / ☐ Hour 13 through 18

HEMODYNAMICS
Hemodynamics stable rhythm with HR producing
SBP ≥90, DBP 45-90 ☐
- Wean vasoactive meds
Pacer thresholds determined ☐
- Follow standards of care

RESPIRATORY
Extubated: Spo2 ≥92% on Fio₂ ≤60% and RR < 25 beats/min and unlabored ☐
- Follow extubation protocol
- Initiate postextubation cardiac surgery treatment protocol ☐

METABOLIC
K⁺ ≥ 4.0 ☐
- Follow K⁺ replacement protocol

PAIN MANAGEMENT
Pain controlled by meds ☐
- Continue pain protocol

MOBILITY
Dangled ☐

MISC
Clear liquids tolerated ☐

☐ Hour 8 through 12 / ☐ Hour 19 through 24

HEMODYNAMICS
Hemodynamics stable rhythm with HR producing
SBP ≥ 90, DBP 45-90 ☐
- Off vasoactive medications
- A line D/C according to protocol
- PA line D/C according to protocol

PAIN MANAGEMENT
Pain controlled by meds ☐

MOBILITY
Up to chair ☐

MISC
Ready for transfer ☐
- Documentation completed
- Referrals initiated
- Family/significant others notified
- Report called to receiving RN

Clinical Pathway ■ Endovascular Stent Graft

TIME FRAME / LOCATION	Hospital Day *Day of Procedure*	Hospital Day *POD 1*	Hospital Day *POD 2*	Hospital Day *POD 3*
Client Satisfaction	"What can we do to enhance your stay with us?"	"What can we do to enhance your stay with us?"	"What can we do to enhance your stay with us?"	"What can we do to enhance your stay with us?"
Discharge Planning	Assess discharge needs Assess need for social worker or case manager Identify caregiver	Determine discharge plans and confirm with client and caregiver		
Client Education	Assess client and caregiver learning needs	Provide discharge instructions Instruct no lifting or straining at stools Review risk factors; offer smoking cessation information if smoker	Reinforce discharge instructions	
Tests/Procedures/ Consults	CBC, BMP, ECG, KUB in PACU	CBC, BMP, ABI, ultrasound of abdomen, spiral CT Test all stools for blood	CBC, BMP Test all stools for blood	
Allied Health Interventions		PT/OT consult for mobility Consult nutritional therapy if needed Consult respiratory therapy if needed		
Nursing/Medical Interventions	PACU 4 to 6 hr Bedrest with head of bed elevated Vital signs every 1/2 hr times 4 and then every hr until discharge to regular nursing unit Check bilateral groin/angioplasty site every 1/2 hr times 4 and then every hr until discharge to regular nursing unit Check peripheral pulses every 4 hr NPO, IV/Fluid for hydration, I&O Foley catheter Assess skin integrity Neurologic checks every 2 hr Pressure dressings to bleeding sites Assess pain every 4 hr and maintain pain level <5 on pain scale (1 to 10) with analgesics Encourage coughing and deep breathing every 1 hr while awake DVT prophylaxis, pneumatic antiembolism sleeves to the legs, SC heparin	Vital signs every shift Check bilateral groin/angioplasty site every shift Check peripheral pulses every shift Discontinue IV fluids and foley catheter Remain NPO until spiral CT and ultrasound of abdomen complete, then advance diet as tolerated Assess skin integrity Assess pain every 4 hr and maintain pain level <5 on pain scale (1 to 10) with analgesics Encourage coughing and deep breathing every 1 hr while awake Ambulate tid	Vital signs every shift Assess peripheral pulses and angioplasty site every shift Return to pre-op diet Activity up ad lib DVT prophylaxis Discontinue saline lock when client is discharged to home	
Outcome Criteria	Client/family satisfaction addressed PACU discharge criteria met Hemodynamically stable Bleeding controlled, pain controlled Maintain urine output >240 mL for 8 hr	Client/family satisfaction addressed Vital signs stable Pain controlled Tolerates diet Tolerates activity Fluid/electrolyte balanced	Client/family satisfaction addressed Discharge criteria for home met	Client/family satisfaction addressed

University of Maryland Medical System

CLINICAL PATHWAY :
Ischemic Cerebral Infarction (Mild, moderate)
[Page 2; 1/00 Revision]

Day #1 Neuro IMC/Gudelsky 5   Targeted LOS ≤ 5 days VARIANCE AND ACTIONS   DATE:____

Addressograph

TESTS CD, and transthoracic echo within 24 hours of admission
TCD if indicated

ASSESSMENT Weight on admission   VS & neuro checks q1-2h
EKG monitoring for arrhythmias   Pulse oximetry
I & O   Assess voiding
Fingersticks q6h if diabetic   Heme test all stools for patients
Assess chronic med regimen (MD/Pharmacist)   on thrombolytics
Preliminary swallow assessment by nursing; **if swallowing problems identified, request swallow eval**

TREATMENTS ○Aspiration precautions until swallowing cleared
NGT if fail swallowing eval or if otherwise warranted Saline lock or IV
Venodynes   Fall precautions
Soft care mattress if indicated

MEDS ○Resume chronic meds, except for BP & DM: list to right
○**Thrombolytic or Neuroprotective agents as per standing order sets** *(list drugs given to right)*
○Aspirin, ticlopidine, IV heparin, & warfarin on hold for 24 hrs after thrombolytic therapy or study drug infusion
○Heparin at _____units/hr (15 units/kg, starting dose; see dosing card)
○Warfarin____mg po qhs *or*   ○IV labetalol/hydralazine prn
○Aspirin___mg po___ *or*   ○Other HTN agents as prescribed (list to right)
○Ticlopidine 250 mg po bid *or* ○Lipid lowering agent as prescribed
○Clopidogrel 75 mg qd   ○IV fluids if indicated
○Saline lock flush   ○Insulin sliding scale, if applicable
○Sucralfate 1 gm po ac & hs *or* ○Antacid:_____(list)
○Nizatidine 150 mg po bid   ○Colace 100 mg po bid
○MOM 10 ml q pm prn   ○Tylenol po/pr/NG q4h prn
○Heparin 5000U subq bid for DVT prophylaxis if not on heparin IV
○Diphenhydramine 12.5-25 mg po/NG in pm for sleep

DIET NPO until preliminary swallowing assessment

ACTIVITY Bedrest except for PT eval

TEACHING ○Orientation to unit   ○Advance directives
○Diagnostic tests: TCD & CD, TTE   ○Request family to bring in list of meds
○Passive ROM exercises with patient/family
○Anticipated LOS & DC plng process (review pathway as appropriate)
○Review content of handouts: ○Krames booklet pp. 1-4 on coping, recovery, and stroke affects, ○Stroke a Med Emergency, ○Warning Signs
○Include note "see pathway" on Multidiscip Educ Summary Form

DISCHARGE PLANNING RN completion of intake/triage form
○Case manager initiation of discharge planning within 48° of admission

EXPECTED OUTCOMES □Neuro status stable
□Vital signs stable   □Free from aspiration
□Voiding spontaneously   □Controlled fingersticks, if applicable
□No evidence of DVT or PE   □Free from falls
□No evidence of bleeding   □PTT approaching therapeutic goal if on IV heparin
□Completes TCD, CD, and TTE within 24 hours of admission
□Verbalizes understanding of diagnostic tests; □explains stroke effects and warning signs
□Returns demonstration of ROM exercises

DAILY EVALUATION: **Did patient meet expected outcomes?**
YES__ NO__ (If NO, document under `variance and action')
YES__ NO__

Admitted from: _____
Date and time of symptom onset: _____

Rxs/drug study prior to inpatient admission:
__ IV rt-PA (0-3 hr)___ Citicoline
__ BMS 204352   __ Other:_____

Neuro deficits present on admission:

If foley catheter inserted, document need for insertion:

SIGNATURES: (RNs/PT/OT/Speech/Nutrition/SW/Case Manager)
7A-7P_____ /Date:____
7P-7A_____ /Date:____
Team_____ /Date:____

UNIVERSITY OF MARYLAND MEDICAL SYSTEM

CLINICAL PATHWAY:
Ischemic Cerebral Infarction (Mild, moderate)
[Page 3, 1/00 Revision]

Addressograph

Day #2 Neuro Stepdown/Gudelsky 5

VARIANCE AND ACTIONS DATE:__

TESTS Fasting lipid panel

PTT q6h after any heparin dose change   INR qd in am if on warfarin
If no etiology established, proceed to MRI/A, TEE, and/or further lab testing as indicated (list
tests ordered/requested to right)

ASSESSMENT Social Work assessment completed

OT, PT, Speech and language assessments initiated if patient stable or improving
Nutrition screening   Neuropsych consult if indicated
VS & neuro checks q2h   I&O; assess voiding
EKG monitoring   Pulse oximetry
Heme test stools if on heparin   Fingersticks q6h if diabetic, ac & hs if eating
Assess for orthostatic changes if OOB   Continued need for monitored bed documented (MD)

TREATMENTS Venodynes   Fall precautions: Level I/II

Soft care mattress if indicated   Saline lock
Passive ROM exercises by patient/family

MEDS ○Resume chronic meds: list to right

○Resume po BP meds if tolerates po well: list to right
○Heparin at _____units/hr as per protocol; see dosing card
○Warfarin_____mg po qhs *or*   ○IV Labetalol/hydralazine prn
 ○Aspirin____mg po___ *or*   ○Other HTN agents (list to right)
 ○Ticlopidine 250 mg po bid c food *or*   ○Lipid lowering agent as prescribed
 ○Clopidogrel 75 mg po qd   ○IV fluids if indicated or ○Saline lock flush
○Sucralfate 1 gm po ac & hs *or* ○Antacid:_____(list)
 ○Nizatidine 150 mg po bid   ○Colace 100 mg po bid
○MOM 10 ml q pm prn   ○Tylenol po/pr/NG q4h prn
○Heparin 5000U subq bid or DVT prophylaxis if not on heparin IV
○Insulin sliding scale, if applicable
○Diphenhydramine 12.5-25 mg po/NG in pm for sleep

DIET Cardiac diet unless otherwise ordered/recommended by Nutrition &/or Speech

ACTIVITY Progress with activity as ordered (with supervision) *or OOB in chair unless
medically contraindicated*

TEACHING   ○Diagnostics--MRI/A if test ordered

○Review content of handouts: ○Krames' Brain Attack brochure pp 5-9,
○Antiplatelet/anticoagulation therapy (AHA ho), ○Nutrition tips, ○MRI

DISCHARGE PLANNING

On-going discharge planning with case manager
Transfer to floor if medically stable

EXPECTED OUTCOMES   □Neuro status stable

□Vital signs stable   □Free from aspiration
□Voiding spontaneously   □No evidence of DVT or PE
□Controlled fingersticks, if applicable   □Tolerates being OOB
□Free from falls   □No evidence of bleeding
□PTT within desired therapeutic range if on IV heparin
□Successfully completes MRI/A if ordered
□PT, OT, Speech evaluations initiated for stable/improving cases
□Patient/family describe □purpose of antiplatelet/anticoagulation therapy and □stroke affects on
speech/language, swallow, and motor function

DAILY EVALUATION: Did patient meet expected outcomes?
YES__ NO__ (If NO, document under `variance and action')
YES__ NO__

Neuro deficits:

SIGNATURES: (RNs/PT/OT/Speech/Nutrition/SW/Case Manager)
7A-7P_____ /Date:
7P-7A_____ /Date:
Team _____ /Date:

UNIVERSITY OF MARYLAND MEDICAL SYSTEM

CLINICAL PATHWAY:
Ischemic Cerebral Infarction (Mild, moderate)
[Page 4, 1/00 Revision]

Addressograph

Day #3 Gudelsky 5

VARIANCE AND ACTIONS

TESTS

○During resident rounds, review diagnostic test results & probable etiology; develop plans for further stroke workup (TEE, angio etc) and therapy (medications, diet, surgery)

PTT q6h after any heparin dose change

INR qd if on warfarin

ASSESSMENT OOT/OPT/OSpeech evaluations completed

VS & neuro checks q2-8h	I&O if still indicated
Fingersticks ac & hs if diabetic and eating	Heme test stools if on heparin
Assess for orthostatic changes when OOB	Nutrition screening completed
Consultation for carotid endarterectomy if indicated	

TREATMENTS Venodynes

Fall precautions

Soft care mattress

OOT/OPT/OSpeech/lang Rx initiated if applicable

MEDS ○Chronic meds: list to right (if different than previous page)

○Resume po BP meds if tolerates po well: list to right

○Heparin at _____units/hr as per protocol; see dosing card

○Warfarin_____mg po qhs *or*	○IV Labetalol/hydralazine prn
○Aspirin___mg po___ *or*	○Other HTN agents (list to right)
○Ticlopidine 250 mg po bid c food	○Lipid lowering agent as prescribed
○Clopidogrel 75 mg po qd	○IV fluids if indicated/○Saline lock flush
○Sucralfate 1 gm po ac & hs* *or*	○Antacid:_____(list)*
○Nizatidine 150 mg po bid*	○Colace 100 mg po bid
○MOM 10 ml q pm prn	○Tylenol po/pr/NG q4h prn

○Heparin 5000U subq bid or DVT prophylaxis if not on heparin IV

○Insulin sliding scale, if applicable

○Diphenhydramine 12.5-25 mg po/NG in pm for sleep   ***DC if tolerates po well**

DIET Cardiac diet unless otherwise ordered

ACTIVITY OOB with supervision

TEACHING ○Review content in the following handouts: ○Krames' Brain

Attack brochure pp. 10-13, ○cholesterol, ○cholesterol lowering, ○BP

○Any further diagnostic tests (TEE etc)

○Nutrition education, if appropriate (consult)

DISCHARGE PLANNING

On-going discharge planning with case manager; identify discharge disposition

Discuss anticipated discharge date/location with resident/attending and family members

EXPECTED OUTCOMES

☐Probable stroke etiology established and stroke prophylaxis initiated

☐Neuro status stable or improving	☐Vital signs stable
☐Voiding spontaneously	☐No evidence of DVT or PE
☐Free from aspiration	☐Tolerates increased activity
☐Controlled fingersticks, if applicable	☐Free from falls

☐PTT within therapeutic range if on heparin

☐BM every 3rd day

☐OT/PT/Speech evaluations completed

☐Patient/family describe purpose of lipid lowering agents and importance of HTN control

Neuro deficits:

DAILY EVALUATION: **Did patient meet expected outcomes?**

YES__ NO__ (If NO, document under `variance and action')

YES__ NO__

SIGNATURES: (RNs/PT/OT/Speech/Nutrition/SW/Case Manager)

7A-7P_____/Date:_____

7P-7A_____/Date:_____

Team _____/Date:_____

UNIVERSITY OF MARYLAND MEDICAL SYSTEM

CLINICAL PATHWAY:
Ischemic Cerebral Infarction (Mild, moderate)
[Page 5, 1/00 Revision]

Addressograph

Day #4 Gudelsky 5

VARIANCE AND ACTIONS DATE:_____

TESTS PTT q6h after any heparin dose change INR qd in am in on warfarin	Neuro deficits:

ASSESSMENT VS & neuro checks q4-8h

Fingersticks ac & hs if diabetic & eating
Heme test stools if on IV heparin therapy
Check for orthostatic changes when OOB

TREATMENTS IV > saline lock if po intake adequate

Venodynes if still indicated   Fall precautions
Soft care mattress if indicated   OPT Rx
OOT Rx   OST Rx

MEDS OChronic meds: list to right if different than previous page

OAntihypertensive po as ordered: list to right
OHeparin at _____units/hr as per protocol; see dosing card
OWarfarin_____mg po qhs or OAspirin___mg po___ or OTiclopidine 250 mg po
bid c food or Clopidogrel 75 mg po qd
OIV fluids if indicated   OSaline lock flush
OSucralfate 1 gm po ac & hs* or   OAntacid:_____(list)*
 ONizatidine 150 mg po bid*   OColace 100 mg po bid
OMOM 10 ml q pm prn   OTylenol po/pr/NG q4h prn
OLipid lowering agent as prescribed
OHeparin 5000U subq bid or DVT prophylaxis if not on heparin IV
OInsulin sliding scale, if applicable
ODiphenhydramine 12.5-25 mg po/NG in pm for sleep

                                        *DC if tolerates po well

DIET Cardiac diet unless otherwise ordered

ACTIVITY OOB as tolerated

TEACHING OComplete teaching from Krames' brochure, pp. 14-16

OCheck with MD regarding meds patient to continue on after discharge
ODiscuss content of specific med handouts for stroke prophylaxis and lipid lowering
agents to be discharged on; assess patient/family ability to read handouts
OSmoking cessation handout if applicable
OLevel of supervision needed in the home

DISCHARGE PLANNING

On-going discharge planning with case manager
Home Health assessment for patients being discharged home
Discuss anticipated discharge date and time with pt/family

EXPECTED OUTCOMES

☐Stroke etiology established (MD)   ☐Neuro status stable or improving
☐Vital signs stable   ☐Voiding spontaneously
☐No evidence of DVT or PE   ☐Free from aspiration
☐No evidence of bleeding   ☐Free from infection
☐Controlled fingersticks, if applicable   ☐Free from falls
☐PTT within desired range, INR 2-3 if on warfarin
☐Patient/family state name, dosage, frequency, purpose, possible side effects, and lab
monitoring needs of/for prescribed medications incl those for stroke prophylaxis and
lipid lowering

DAILY EVALUATION: **Did patient meet expected outcomes?**
YES___ NO___ (If NO, document under `variance and action')
YES___ NO___

SIGNATURES: (RNs/PT/OT/Speech/Nutrition/SW/Case Manager)
7A-7P_____ /Date:
7P-7A_____ /Date:
Team _____ /Date:

UNIVERSITY OF MARYLAND MEDICAL SYSTEM

CLINICAL PATHWAY:
Ischemic Cerebral Infarction (Mild, Moderate)
[Page 6, 1/00 Revision]

Addressograph

Day #5 Gudelsky 5

VARIANCE AND ACTIONS DATE:___

TESTS CBC if on ticlopidine   INR qd in am if on warfarin

Determine if any other labs needed prior to discharge

ASSESSMENT VS & neuro checks q8h

Assessment and documentation of patient ability to sit in chair at least 1 hr (if patient going to inpatient rehab)

TREATMENTS Safety evaluations by therapies as indicated

Venodynes	Fall precautions	Soft care mattress
PT Rx	OT Rx	ST Rx

MEDS ○Chronic meds: list to right if different than previous pages

○Antihypertensive po as ordered: list to right
○Heparin at _____units/hr as per protocol; see dosing card
○Warfarin_____mg po qhs *or* ○Aspirin____mg po___ *or* ○Ticlopidine 250 mg po bid with food *or* ○Clopidogrel 75 mg po qd

○IV fluids if indicated	○Saline lock flush
○Colace 100 mg po bid	○MOM 10 ml q pm prn
○Tylenol po/pr/NG q4h prn	○Insulin sliding scale, if applicable

○Lipid lowering agent as prescribed
○Heparin 5000U subq bid or DVT prophylaxis if not on heparin IV
○Diphenhydramine 12.5-25 mg po/NG in pm for sleep

DIET Cardiac diet unless otherwise ordered

ACTIVITY OOB as tolerated

TEACHING ○Evaluate patient/family understanding of content in Krames brochure on Brain Attack and prescribed medications; reinforce as necessary
○Discuss plans for medical follow-up
Include note "see pathway" on Multidiscip Educ Summary Form

DISCHARGE PLANNING On-going discharge planning with case manager

○Final arrangements with Home Health/Rehab facility if indicated
○Insurance coverage for rehab/home health services reviewed with
pt/family if indicated
○Arrange outpatient therapy if needed
○Discuss planned time of discharge with family; ○give prescriptions to family member
○Schedule follow up appointments, including Neuro Ambul Center
If dc'd on ticlopidine, arrange follow-up CBCs and make application to Roche-Centex for financial support if indicated
If dc'd home on warfarin, referral form completed and faxed to AC clinic and follow-up appointment made for labs unless being done by home health
MD & RN discharge summaries

EXPECTED OUTCOMES

□Neuro status stable or improving	□Vital signs stable
□Voiding spontaneously	□BM every 3rd day
□No evidence of DVT or PE	□Free from aspiration
□Controlled fingersticks, if applicable	□Free from falls

□PTT within desired range, INR 2-3 if on warfarin
□Increased participation in ADLs
□Patient/family verbalize understanding of discharge instructions & medication
counselling, & plans for further testing & follow-up
□Pt aware of insurance benefits for ongoing care needs
□Referrals made to hospital/community resources

Neuro deficits:

DAILY EVALUATION: **Did patient meet expected outcomes?**
YES__   NO__ (If NO, document under `variance and action')
YES__   NO__

SIGNATURES: (RNs/PT/OT/Speech/Nutrition/SW/Case Manager)
7A-7P_____/Date:_____ 7P-
7A_____/Date:
Team _____/Date:

UNIVERSITY OF MARYLAND MEDICAL SYSTEM

CLINICAL PATHWAY:
Ischemic Cerebral Infarction (Mild, moderate)

[Page 7, 1/00 Revision]

Discharge

VARIANCE AND ACTIONS   DATE:____

TESTS

If on Ticlopidine, CBC with diff arranged for every 2 weeks until the end of 3 months of therapy
If on warfarin and INR not stable at discharge, INR scheduled twice weekly x 2; then every week x 3; then every 3-4 weeks
If on warfarin and INR is stable at discharge, INR scheduled every 5-6 weeks

ASSESSMENT

VS and neuro checks prior to discharge
Assessment of home health needs by liaison RN

Neuro deficits remaining at discharge:

TREATMENTS

Fall precautions
Seizure precautions, if indicated
Continuing PT/OT/Speech after discharge if indicated

MEDS ○Chronic meds

○Antihypertensive po as ordered: list to right
○Saline lock flush
○Warfarin ___mg po qhs *or* ○Aspirin____ mg po___ *or* ○Ticlopidine 250 mg po bid c meals *or* ○Clopidogrel 75 mg po qd
○Lipid lowering agent as prescribed
○Colace 100 mg po bid   ○MOM 10 ml q pm prn
○Dulcolax supp prn   ○Tylenol prn
○Insulin sliding scale,
  if applicable

Medications at discharge (list):

DIET As recommended by Nutrition &/or Speech

ACTIVITY OOB as tolerated

TEACHING Reinforce discharge instructions as needed

Level of supervision needed in home

DISCHARGE PLANNING

Home Health referral if not being discharged to transitional or acute rehab, or skilled facility
Discharge summary completed and chart dictated
○Clerk to set follow-up appointment at Neuro Ambul Center (fax request after hours)

Appointments scheduled for: Neuro Ambulatory Center __, AC Clinic __, Internal Med/Fam Practice __, Hypertension Clinic __, Diabetes Clinic __, PT __, OT __, Speech __, Other (please list):

Discharge date and time: (goal < 12 N)_____
Discharge location and level of care (acute rehab, transitional/subacute rehab): _____
_____

EXPECTED OUTCOMES

☐Neuro status stable   ☐BP controlled
☐Maximum participation in ADLs   ☐Free from falls
☐Free from aspiration
☐Controlled fingersticks, if applicable
☐Patient/family understands discharge instructions, including plans for
  follow-up and further testing if indicated
☐WBC > 4.2 X 10^3/mm^3 with neutrophils > 1200/mm^3 if on Ticlopidine
☐INR 2-3 if on warfarin

DAILY EVALUATION: **Did patient meet expected outcomes?**
YES__ NO__ (If NO, document under `variance and action')
YES__ NO__

SIGNATURES:
7A-7P_____
7P-7A_____

NOTE: FAX this page at time of patient discharge to Neuro Ambul Center, 8-1149, ATTN: J. Valino, RN

NOTE: Send/keep copy of pathway on C5 upon patient's discharge

UNIVERSITY OF MARYLAND MEDICAL SYSTEM

CLINICAL PATHWAY:
Ischemic Cerebral Infarction (Mild, moderate)

[Page 8, 1/00 Revision]

Home Home Health/Rehab   VARIANCE AND ACTIONS   DATE:_____

TESTS
If on ticlopidine, CBC with diff arranged for every 2 weeks until the end of 3 months of therapy
If on warfarin and INR not stable at discharge, INR twice weekly x 2; then every week x 3; then every 3-4 weeks
If on warfarin and INR is stable at discharge, INR every 5-6 weeks
INR results to be sent STAT to neuro attending/primary care MD as arranged prior to discharge

ASSESSMENT
O Home Health RN assessment for neuro worsening, blood pressure and blood sugar stability, home environment (incl. function and safety in home and supports available), any needs for durable medical equipment, safety or adaptive devices, compliance with diet and medication regimen, sufficiency of intake & output, therapeutic blood levels if applicable
Primary Care and Neuro Ambul Center follow-up visits
Nutrition, DM, and HTN follow-up visits as indicated
Screen for depression
Driving evaluation, if indicated
Social Work referrral if indicated
Transportation needs for health care follow-up assessed

TREATMENTS PT, OT, Speech therapies as indicated
Institute treatment of depression if indicated

MEDS O All meds, list to right:

DIET Cardiac diet

ACTIVITY Increasing activity as tolerated

TEACHING Needs for medical follow-up
Results of lab tests and any necessary medication adjustments
Activity prescription
Safety and ADL adaptation in home
Driving and return to work status

DISCHARGE PLANNING
Home Health follow-up after discharge if not being transferred to transitional or acute rehab, or skilled facility
Summary note from home health/rehab to Neuro Ambul Center/attending MD
Vocational rehab referral, if indicated

EXPECTED OUTCOMES
☐ Neuro status stable ☐ Maximum participation in ADLs
☐ Free from falls   ☐ Tolerating medication therapy
☐ WBC > $4.2 \times 10^3/mm^3$ with neutrophils > $1200/mm^3$, if on Ticlopidine
☐ INR 2-3 if on warfarin
☐ Treatment for depression begun (if indicated) and patient free from adverse side effects
☐ Patient medical follow-up appointment date and transportation arranged

EVALUATION: **Did patient meet expected outcomes?**
YES__   NO__   (If NO, document under `variance and action')

SIGNATURES:
_____
_____

NOTE: At completion of home health visits/rehab stay, FAX copy of summary note of outcomes achieved and plans for follow-up to Neuro Ambulatory Center, ATTN: J. Valino, RN at 328-1149.

UNIVERSITY OF MARYLAND MEDICAL SYSTEM

CLINICAL PATHWAY:

Ischemic Cerebral Infarction (Mild, Moderate)
[Page __, 1/00 Revision]

Extended Stay

Addressograph

Day #___ Gudelsky 5

VARIANCE AND ACTIONS DATE:___

TESTS CBC if on ticlopidine INR qd in am if on warfarin Determine if any other labs needed prior to discharge	****Note reason(s) for extended stay and actions being taken to address variances** (use back of form if necessary)

ASSESSMENT VS & neuro checks q8h

Heme test stools if on IV heparin

TREATMENTS Safety evaluations by therapies as indicated

Venodynes	Fall precautions	Soft care mattress
PT Rx	OT Rx	ST Rx

MEDS ○Chronic meds: list to right if different than previous pages

○Heparin at _____units/hr as per protocol

○Warfarin_____mg po qhs *or*	○IV Labetalol/hydralazine prn
○ASA____mg po___ *or*	○Other HTN agents (list to right)
○Ticlopidine 250 mg po bid c food *or*	○Lipid lowering agent as prescribed
○Clopidogrel 75 mg po qd	○IV fluids if indicated/○Saline lock flush
○Heparin 5000U subq bid	○Insulin sliding scale,
if not on Heparin IV if applicable	
○Sucralfate 1 gm po ac & hs or ○Antacid:_____(list)	
○Nizatidine 150 mg po bid	○Colace 100 mg po bid
○MOM 10 ml q pm prn	○Tylenol po/pr/NG prn
○Diphenhydramine 12.5-25 mg po/NG in pm for sleep	

DIET As recommended by Nutrition &/or Speech

ACTIVITY OOB as tolerated

TEACHING ○Complete review of Krames' Brain Attack brochure with patient and family
Other (list):

DISCHARGE PLANNING

○**Family/team meeting as needed to discuss discharge plans**
○Final arrangements with rehab facility if indicated
○Insurance coverage for rehab/home health services reviewed with pt/family if indicated
○Arrange outpatient therapy if needed
○Prescriptions to family member
Schedule follow up appointments, including Neuro Ambulatory Center
If on Ticlopidine or Warfarin, arrange appointment for blood work
MD & RN discharge summaries

EXPECTED OUTCOMES

☐Neuro status stable or improving	☐Vital signs stable
☐Voiding spontaneously	☐BM every 3rd day
☐No evidence of DVT or PE	☐Free from aspiration
☐Controlled fingersticks, if applicable	☐Free from falls

☐PTT within desired range, INR 2-3 if on warfarin
☐Increased participation in ADLs
☐Demonstrates understanding of discharge instructions & medication counselling, & plans for further testing & follow-up
☐Pt aware of insurance benefits for ongoing care needs
☐Referrals made to hospital/community resources

DAILY EVALUATION: **Did patient meet expected outcomes?** YES__ NO__ (If NO, document under `variance and action') YES__ NO__	**SIGNATURES:** (RNs/PT/OT/Speech/Nutrition/SW/Case Manager) _____ _____

This clinical pathway is intended as a general guideline. Patient care continues to require individualization based on patient needs and responses. 4/95, rev. 12/98

Addressograph

CLINICAL PATHWAY: Mild/moderate ischemic cerebral infarction

Date/Time	VARIANCE NOTES
	Signature:_____
	Signature:_____

University Hospitals of Cleveland

CARE PATH NAME: KIDNEY TRANSPLANT
DRG: ELOS: 7 Days
Expected Disposition: Home
Surgery Date: ___/___/___
Pre-Op Dry Weight: _____ Kg

Collaborative Problem List
1. Impaired Home Maintenance Management
2. Potential for Infection
3. Knowledge Deficit
4. Fluid and Electrolyte Imbalance
5. Plan Management
6.
7.

Focus	Pre-Op Date: __/__/__	Day of Surgery Date: __/__/__	Post-Op to Day 1 Date: __/__/__	Post-Op to Day 2 Date: __/__/__	Post-Op to Day 3 Date: __/__/__	Post-Op to Day 4 Date: __/__/__
Laboratory Tests/ Procedures	• Chem 23 • CBC + Diff • PT/PTT • Urine C&S • T&C 2u PRBC • Check CMV status • Chemstick of diabetic • CMV IgG quantitative	• Immediately post-op: Chem 7, CBC • 8 hours post-op: Chem 7, CBC • CXR on arrival to PACU	• CBC + Diff • Chem 23 • CD3 level if on OKT3 • CXR • Ultrasound as indicated per protocol	• Chem 7 • Urine for bacteria/fungus • CBC (Diff if on OKT3) • CD3 level if on OKT3 • CYA level starting day 2 of therapy		• Chem 23
Consults/ Referrals			• Consider PT Consult • Dietary screen and evaluation			
Physical Assessment	• VS q 4 h • Weight • Baseline skin assessment • Renal assessment regarding need for dialysis	• BP, AP, Rq 1/2 h until stable then q 2 h-q 4 h then q 4 h prn • Temp. immediately and q 2 h x 16 h then q 4 h • CVP q 2-4 x 16 h then q 4 h • Pulse ox baseline and prn • Urine output q 1 h x 24 h then q 4 h x 24 then qs	• VS q 4 h with CVP • Urine output q 4 h weight • Bowel sounds	• VS q 4 h • I&O q shift • Weight • Pulse ox x 2	• VS q shift	
Activity	• Up ad lib	• Bed rest	• Out of bed → chair		• Out of bed ad lib	
Treatments	• Fleets enemas x 2 • Hibiclens shower • SCDs with patient to OR • Apply Teds pre-op	• O2 per order, wean as tolerated • CVP dressing • JP dressing • Incision dressing • Incentive spirometry q 1 h W/A • Foley care • Guaiac stools • SCDs and Teds	• D/C O2 if RA pulse ox > 92% • Incision care	• Up with assistance • CVP dressing • D/C JP if output < 30 cc • Remove incision dressing	• Incentive spirometry q 2 h W/A	• CVP dressing • D/C Foley
Diet	• NPO	• NPO, ice chips • Advance as tolerated	• Diabetic/or any other diet restrictions as indicated			
Medications	• On call to OR: Antibiotic Solumedrol 250 mg IV Imuran 5 mg/kg IV maximum dose — 500 mg • Induction options: OKT3, ATG, Cyclosporine, MMF, Neoral	• Solumedrol 60 mg q 6 IV • Antibiotic • Fluid replacements	• Imuran or Mycophenolate • OKT3, ATG, Cyclosporine, Neoral • Gancyclovir 2.5 mg/kg qd if CMV (+) or CMV (−) receiving (+) organ • MSO4 PRN	• Solumedrol 60 mg IV q 8 h • OKT3, ATG, Cyclosporine, Neoral • Gancyclovir • Bactrim ss or Trimethoprim qd • Colace • Clotrimazole • Acyclovir • Zantac	• Solumedrol 60 mg IV q 12 h • Tylenol #3 • CytoGam if donor CMV (+) and recipient (−)	• Prednisone 1 mg/kg/day • OKT3, CYA, or ATG • Tylenol or Darvon

Courtesy University Hospitals of Cleveland.

Focus	Pre-Op Date: __/__/__	Day of Surgery Date: __/__/__	Post-Op to Day 1 Date: __/__/__	Post-Op to Day 2 Date: __/__/__	Post-Op to Day 3 Date: __/__/__	Post-Op to Day 4 Date: __/__/__
Patient/ Family Teaching	• View pre-op transplant video • Orient to Tower 9		• Give teaching materials to patient • Renal transplant booklet • Preprinted cards • I&O sheet • Outcome criteria form	• Review of meds and teaching material with patient/family ⟶	⟶	• Continued review and if ready, take test
Discharge Planning		• Social Worker review notes from information appointments	• Review chart, interview RN and patient • Collect psychosocial data (insurance, financial issues discharge needs)	• Psychosocial assessment, support and education/ information ⟶	• Initial note in chart • Discuss prescription plan	• Arrange financial applications • Begin arranging prescription plans • Meet/talk with family prn • Consult/refer to other disciplines prn • For patients using mail order program, arrange forms with physicians
Intermediate Outcomes	1. Viewed video 2. Negative crossmatch	1. Hemodynamically stable 2. CVP 10–12 3. Euvolemic with fluid replacements 4. Vital signs returned to baseline 5. K + < 6.0 6. Equal and clear breath sounds 7. Pain controlled	1. Hemodynamically stable 2. CVP 10–12 3. Euvolemic with or without fluid replacements 4. Vital signs at baseline 5. Decrease in BUN and Cr from pre-op 6. Equal and clear breath sounds 7. Pain controlled 8. Teaching material given to patient/family 9. Immunosuppression dosages adjusted	1. Hemodynamically stable 2. Euvolemic without fluid replacements 3. Decrease in BUN and Cr 4. Electrolytes WNL 5. Equal and clear breath sounds 6. Pain controlled 7. Ambulating 8. Tolerating oral meds and diet 9. Teaching begun 10. JP removed if drainage is < 30 cc for 24 h 11. Immunosuppression dosages adjusted 12. Wound dry and approximated	1. Hemodynamically stable 2. Euvolemic 3. Decrease in BUN and Cr 4. Electrolytes WNL 5. Equal and clear breath sounds 6. Pain controlled 7. Actively participates in ADLs 8. Ambulates at baseline 9. Has bowel movement 10. Initial Social Worker note in chart 11. Teaching continues 12. JP removed if drainage is < 30 cc for 24 h 13. Immunosuppression dosages adjusted 14. Wound dry and approximated	1. Hemodynamically stable 2. Euvolemic 3. Decrease in BUN and Cr 4. Electrolytes WNL 5. Equal and clear breath sounds 6. Actively participates in ADLs 7. Pain controlled 8. Ambulates at baseline 9. Has bowel movement 10. Teaching continues 11. Foley discontinued 12. JP removed if drainage is < 30 cc for 24 h 13. Immunosuppression dosages adjusted 14. Wound dry and approximated 15. Financial and prescription arrangements made
Intermediate Outcomes RN Signature Days	☐ Met ☐ Not Met (see notes) #s not met _____ Signature _____	☐ Met ☐ Not Met (see notes) #s not met _____ Signature _____	☐ Met ☐ Not Met (see notes) #s not met _____ Signature _____	☐ Met ☐ Not Met (see notes) #s not met _____ Signature _____	☐ Met ☐ Not Met (see notes) #s not met _____ Signature _____	☐ Met ☐ Not Met (see notes) #s not met _____ Signature _____
Intermediate Outcomes RN Signature Evenings	☐ Met ☐ Not Met (see notes) #s not met _____ Signature _____	☐ Met ☐ Not Met (see notes) #s not met _____ Signature _____	☐ Met ☐ Not Met (see notes) #s not met _____ Signature _____	☐ Met ☐ Not Met (see notes) #s not met _____ Signature _____	☐ Met ☐ Not Met (see notes) #s not met _____ Signature _____	☐ Met ☐ Not Met (see notes) #s not met _____ Signature _____
Intermediate Outcomes RN Signature Nights	☐ Met ☐ Not Met (see notes) #s not met _____ Signature _____	☐ Met ☐ Not Met (see notes) #s not met _____ Signature _____	☐ Met ☐ Not Met (see notes) #s not met _____ Signature _____	☐ Met ☐ Not Met (see notes) #s not met _____ Signature _____	☐ Met ☐ Not Met (see notes) #s not met _____ Signature _____	☐ Met ☐ Not Met (see notes) #s not met _____ Signature _____

University Hospital's carepaths have been developed to assist clinicians in patient management and clinical decision-making. The carepaths are intended to meet the needs of patients in most circumstances. They are not intended to replace a clinician's judgment or establish a protocol for all patients with this diagnosis.

SP-9601 (01/05/96)

Focus	Post-Op Day 5 Date: __/__/__	Post-Op Day 6 Date: __/__/__	Post-Op Day 7 Date: __/__/__
Laboratory/ Tests/ Procedures	• CBC (Diff on OKT3) • Chem 7 • CD3 level if on OKT3 • CYA level		↑ ↑ ↑ ↑
Consults/ Referrals	• Consider Home Team referral		
Physical Assessment	• VS qs • I&O qs • Weight		↑ ↑ ↑
Activity	• OOB ad lib		↑
Treatments	• Guaiac stools • Incentive spirometry q 2 h W/A	• CVP dressing	• D/C central line ↑
Diet	• Diabetic or any other diet restriction as indicated		↑
Medications	• Prednisone — taper as indicated • Imuran or Mycophenolate • OKT3, ATG, Neoral, or Cyclosporine • Gancyclovir • Bactrim • Colace • Clotrimazole • Acyclovir • T3 or Darvon • Zantac		• D/C Ganciclovir • Acyclovir **SrCr** **Dosage** < 1.4 800 mg po q 6 h 1.5-2.5 800 mg po q 8 h 2.6-4.5 800 mg po q 12 h > 4.5 800 mg po q 24 h HD 800 mg po q 48 h

Courtesy University Hospitals of Cleveland.

Focus	Post-Op Day 5 Date: __/__/__	Post-Op Day 6 Date: __/__/__	Post-Op Day 7 Date: __/__/__
Patient/ Family Teaching	• Take test • Diet teaching prn	• Review material as needed and retake test if needed	• Review homegoing med dosages, clinic and lab test follow-up appointments
Discharge Planning	• Arrange financial applications • Arrange prescription plans • Meet/talk with family prn • Consult/refer to other disciplines prn • Other D/C plans • Psychosocial assessment, support, and education/information	• Transportation arrangements prn • Other D/C plans carried out prn • Final note in chart with D/C plan • Psychosocial assessment, support, and education/information	
Homegoing Medications	• Mail order prescription forms completed and faxed by 2:00 PM. (If weekend/ holiday D/C anticipated must do this by 2:00 PM, Friday)	• Delivery of medications prn	
Intermediate Outcomes	1. Hemodynamically stable 2. Euvolemic 3. Electrolytes WNL 4. Independent in ADLs and ambulation 5. Has bowel movement 6. Test taken and passed with 90% or continue med review 7. Scale and thermometer arranged for home 8. JP removed if drainage is < 30 cc for 24 h 9. Immunosuppression dosage assessed 10. Financial and prescription plans arranged 11. Cyclosporine levels assessed and adjusted	1. Therapeutic cyclosporine level 2. Homegoing meds obtained 3. Test taken and passed with 90%	1. D/C to home with written instructions 2. Medications available to take at home 3. Refer to discharge order form
Intermediate Outcomes RN Signature Days	☐ Met ☐ Not Met (see notes) #s not met _____ Signature _____	☐ Met ☐ Not Met (see notes) #s not met _____ Signature _____	☐ Met ☐ Not Met (see notes) #s not met _____ Signature _____
Intermediate Outcomes RN Signature Evenings	☐ Met ☐ Not Met (see notes) #s not met _____ Signature _____	☐ Met ☐ Not Met (see notes) #s not met _____ Signature _____	☐ Met ☐ Not Met (see notes) #s not met _____ Signature _____
Intermediate Outcomes RN Signature Nights	☐ Met ☐ Not Met (see notes) #s not met _____ Signature _____	☐ Met ☐ Not Met (see notes) #s not met _____ Signature _____	☐ Met ☐ Not Met (see notes) #s not met _____ Signature _____

University Hospital's carepaths have been developed to assist clinicians in patient management and clinical decision-making. The carepaths are intended to meet the needs of patients in most circumstances. They are not intended to replace a clinician's judgment or establish a protocol for all patients with this diagnosis.

SP-9601 (01/05/96)

Clinical Pathway ■ LAPAROSCOPIC CHOLECYSTECTOMY

Aspect of Care	Preadmission/Preoperative	Preoperative/DOS	Postoperative
ASSESSMENT	Physician assessment	Preoperative check, nursing assessment, psychosocial assessment	Vital signs, intake and output; assess abdomen, bowel sounds, pain, breath sounds, incisions
TEACHING	Education by physician; review clinical pathway with client and family	Teach/demonstrate turning, coughing, and deep breathing	Review discharge information: pain control, activity, wound care, complications
CONSULTS	Anesthesia if indicated; social worker, dietitian, spiritual guide		
LABORATORY TESTS AND DIAGNOSTIC TESTS	CBC, ECG if age >40 yr; liver/pancreas screen		If indicated: CBC, H&H
MEDICATIONS	Assess allergies; identify home medications	Preoperative medications taken at home; IVF antibiotic per hospital protocol	Analgesic, antiemetic
TREATMENT/ INTERVENTIONS	NPO after midnight		Elevate head of bed; Band-Aids, turning, coughing, and deep breathing; emotional support Encourage fluids, solid food per client choice
ACTIVITY	Activity ad lib		Progressive ambulation
DISCHARGE PLANNING	Determine needs: transportation, financial, home care		Arrangements made on basis of preoperative assessment needs; follow-up appointment with physician

Modified from *Clinical path: Outpatient laparoscopic cholecystectomy.* (1995). Asheville, NC: Saint Joseph's Hospital; and Ignatavicius, D.D., & Hausman, K.A. (1995). *Clinical pathways for collaborative practice.* Philadelphia: W.B. Saunders.

Clinical Pathway ■ CARE PATH NAME: TOTAL ABDOMINAL HYSTERECTOMY

□ With Burch   □ Without Burch

DRG: 353-358   ELOS: 2 Days
Expected Disposition: Home

Collaborative Problem List
1. Discharge Planning
2. Pain/Comfort Management
3. Coping Response to Surgery/Diagnosis
4. _____

Focus	Preadmission	Day of Surgery	Post-Op Day 1	Post-Op Day 2
LABORATORY/ TESTS/ PROCEDURES	□ Blood work □ <40 years Hct □ >40 years SMA 6, CBC □ EKG if >40 years □ CXR if >60 years □ Type and screen		□ CBC	□ CBC
CONSULTS/ REFERRALS/	□ Anesthesia Consult □ Nursing Consult		□ Primary RN	
PHYSICAL ASSESSMENT	□ H & P obtained	□ VS per post-op routine □ Routine post-op assessment □ I/O	□ VS Q shift □ Q shift assessment □ I/O □ Weight □ Fever assessment (if temp >39° C)	□ VS Q shift □ Q shift assessment □ I/O □ Weight □ Fever assessment (if temp >38.5° C)
DIAGNOSIS:			□ Exam □ Cultures of surgical area □ CBC with diff □ Blood cultures	□ Exam □ Cultures of surgical area □ CBC with diff □ Blood cultures
ACTIVITY	□ Ad lib	□ Dangle at bedside or OOB to chair	□ OOB to chair	□ Ambulate QID
TREATMENTS	□ Instruction on IS □ Review of procedure	□ IS/C&DB Q 1 h WA □ Foley □ SCD's □ Drains: **BURCH ONLY:** □ Suprapubic Catheter	□ IS/C&DB Q 1 h WA □ D/C Foley □ SCD's **BURCH ONLY:** □ Suprapubic Catheter	□ IS/C&DB Q 1 h □ D/C Drains: **BURCH ONLY:** □ Suprapubic Catheter □ Monitor postvoid residuals □ Begin clamp routine 24 h after surgery if no hematuria
DIET	□ NPO pre-op	□ Ice chips □ Clear liquids	□ Advanced as tolerated	□ House diet
MEDICATIONS		□ PCA protocol □ Epidural protocol □ IV pain meds □ IV antibiotics: □ IVF:	□ D/C PCA at 08:00 □ D/C Epidural □ IV pain meds to PO □ IVF: □ Heplock when taking PO	□ PO meds □ D/C HL

Clinical Pathway ■ Care Path Name: Total Abdominal Hysterectomy (Continued)

☐ With Burch   ☐ Without Burch

DRG: 353-358   ELOS: 2 Days
Expected Disposition: Home

Collaborative Problem List
1. Discharge Planning
2. Pain/Comfort Management
3. Coping Response to Surgery/Diagnosis
4. _____

Focus	Preadmission	Day of Surgery	Post-Op Day 1	Post-Op Day 2
DISCHARGE PLANNING/ TEACHING	☐ Discharge Planning Review: ☐ Pre-op checklist ☐ Advanced directives ☐ Client care path pamphlet ☐ Determine services needed ☐ Client lives alone ☐ Client lives with others ☐ Support person: Phone number:	☐ Client lives alone ☐ Client lives with others Support person: Phone Number:	☐ Provide Homegoing Instructions: ☐ Hysterectomy PI-128 ☐ "Women and AIDS" pamphlet ☐ Breast self exam pamphlet ☐ Hormone replacement therapy ☐ Instruct on pericare **BURCH ONLY:** ☐ Clamp Routine PI Sheets	☐ Review home-going instructions.
INDIVIDUALIZED CARE FOCUS				
INTERMEDIATE OUTCOMES	☐ Client able to explain home-going plan ☐ Client able to describe procedure(s) to be performed ☐ Client states she has participated in decision making and plan	☐ Afebrile ☐ Client states pain is adequately controlled ☐ Client shows no evidence of post-op complications	☐ Able to void without difficulty ☐ Afebrile or temp <38° with normal WBC ☐ Tolerating PO fluids ☐ Ambulates with assistance ☐ Client states pain is adequately controlled with PO pain medication	☐ Ambulates independently ☐ Has had a bowel movement and/or passed flatus ☐ Tolerates house diet ☐ Client able to describe procedure(s) performed ☐ Client able to describe pericare ☐ Client able to explain all discharge instructions **BURCH ONLY:** ☐ Able to measure and record postvoid residuals

	Met	Not Met	Comments	Dat/Initials

Discharge Outcomes:

1. Abdominal incision approximated and healing
2. Has minimal, odorless vaginal discharge
3. Able to describe/perform pericare
4. Has functional pattern for bladder and bowel
5. Maintains adequate nutritional intake
6. Pain controlled by oral medication
7. States use of homegoing medications
8. Describes plan for follow-up care
9. Describes feeling about effects of surgery on health and sexuality
10. Identifies support systems and resources available to her after discharge
11. Afebrile or Temp <38° C with normal WBC
12. **BURCH ONLY:** Able to demonstrate clamp routine

Clinical Pathway ■ **VENTILATOR-DEPENDENT CLIENTS WITH A TRACHEOSTOMY OR ENDOTRACHEAL TUBE**

Phase I Acute Ventilatory Support	Phase II Ventilatory Support	Phase III Weaning	Phase IV Resolution
DIAGNOSTIC TESTS, LABORATORY VALUES, AND PROCEDURES			

ABG analysis   Pulse oximetry
CXR   CBC
SMA-7   SMA-12
ECG
 	
Sputum culture and sensitivity after 72 hr ETT
Blood cultures as needed
Phosphorus 4 times daily if on TF or TPN for
  first week
Prealbumin prn
	Pulmonary mechanics
	ECG prn CBC CXR
	SMA-7 SMA-12 weekly
	ABG prn Pulse oximetry
	24-hr urine urea nitrogen prn (if no renal
	  failure)
	Prealbumin prn
		Pulmonary mechanics
		ECG prn CXR
		SMA-7 SMA-12 weekly
		ABG prn Pulse oximetry
		24-hr urine urea nitrogen prn (if no renal
		  failure)
		Prealbumin prn
			Pulmonary mechanics
			Pulse oximetry prn

CONSULTS			

Pulmonologist consultation if intubated after 72
  hr or if reintubation is required
Assess need for swallow/speech consultation
Nutritional support dietitian
Respiratory care clinician
Social worker: Supportive counseling/crisis
  intervention
	Physical medicine and rehabilitation
	Physical therapy
	Occupational therapy
	Swallow/speech consultation
	Social worker: Supportive counseling/
	  crisis intervention
	Social worker assesses client's and fam-
	  ily's resource needs
		Physical medicine and rehabilitation
		Social worker: Supportive counseling
		Social worker to evaluate client for
		  placement options	

TREATMENTS			
SvO₂ prn Mechanical ventilation Respiratory treatments Secretion management Tracheostomy after ETT in place × 7 days GI protection (histamine blockers/carafate) Sedation prn IV medications Diuretics prn Packed cells prn Vasopressors Antibiotics prn Vasoactive infusions Paralytics prn Daily weight I&O hourly Special bed prn Suction prn Foley Swallowed/dysphagia assessment	Respiratory treatments Packed cells prn Secretion management Antibiotic prn Sedation prn Diuretics prn Tracheostomy care Daily weight Suction prn I&O Foley Evaluate need for permanent IV access	Respiratory treatments Packed cells prn Secretion management Antibiotic prn Diuretics prn Tracheostomy care Daily weight Suction prn I&O D/C Foley prn If prolonged TFs, evaluate need for PEG Evaluate continued need for IV access	Tracheostomy collar Decannulator Extubator Continue vent and slow wean Daily weight I & O every 8 hr Suction prn

Clinical Pathway ◼ **Ventilator-Dependent Clients with a Tracheostomy or Endotracheal Tube (Continued)**

Phase I Acute Ventilatory Support	Phase II Ventilatory Support	Phase III Weaning	Phase IV Resolution
DIET Nutritional assessment TPN/TF TF preferred	If on TPN, transition to TF Reassess nutritional status every 10 days	Transition to PO diet if no dysphagia Reassess nutritional status every 10 days	Continue PO diet or TF
ACTIVITY Bedrest Passive range of motion every 4 hr Increase activity as tolerated	Up on side of bed with assistance Foot support Up in chair if tolerated Active range of motion	Up in chair 3 times daily Increase ambulation	Up in chair 3 times daily for increased time Increased ambulation Increased client involvement in self-care activities
TREATMENT Establish a communication mode with the client Orient client to environment Orient family to environment, procedures, client's current condition and prognosis, care needs, and hospital policy	Keep client and family updated about client's condition, new and continuing procedures, treatment plans, and changes in care needs	Teach client and family about weaning procedures and expected responses	Keep client and family informed regarding progress, changes in treatment plan, expected responses, new equipment or personnel
DISCHARGE PLANNING Family members and social worker Assessment of resources and a discharge plan appropriate and individualized to the expected outcomes for the ventilator-dependent client	Inform social worker of client's progress Social worker to assess client's and family's resource needs; explore rehabilitation and long-term insurance coverage	Keep social worker updated about client's progress Social worker to evaluate client for placement options Social worker to initiate referrals	Social worker to finalize client's transportation and disposition Social worker to finalize arrangements for needed equipment, home health services, and follow-up care

INDEX

b indicates boxed material, *c* indicates charts,
f indicates illustrations, and *t* indicates tables.

Esophageal cancer
  assessment of, 1205-1206
  client teaching, 1211-1212
  cultural considerations, 1205b
  description of, 1204
  etiology of, 1205
  gastroesophageal reflux disease and, 1205
  health care resources, 1212
  health teaching, 1211-1212
  home care management of, 1211
  incidence of, 1204, 1205
  interventions for
    chemotherapy, 1208
    esophagectomy, 1208-1211
    nutritional, 1207
    photodynamic therapy, 1208
    prosthesis, 1208
    radiation therapy, 1207-1208
    surgical, 1208-1211
    swallowing therapy, 1207, 1207c
  nursing diagnoses, 1206-1207
  pathophysiology of, 1205
  prevalence of, 1205
Esophageal reflux. *See* Gastroesophageal
    reflux disease.
Esophageal sphincter, 1192
Esophagectomy
  complications of, 1208
  nutritional support after, 1210-1211
  operative procedure, 1209, 1210f
  postoperative care, 1209-1211
  preoperative preparations, 1209
Esophagitis
  in acquired immunodeficiency
    syndrome, 373
  in progressive systemic sclerosis,
    357, 357c
Esophagogastric balloon tamponade,
    1308-1309, 1309c
Esophagogastroduodenoscopy
  esophageal cancer evaluations, 1206
  gastritis evaluations, 1217
  gastrointestinal evaluations, 1174, 1175f
  peptic ulcer disease evaluations, 1223
Esophagogastrostomy
  complications of, 1208
  nutritional support after, 1210-1211
  operative procedure, 1209, 1210f
  postoperative care, 1209-1211
  preoperative preparations, 1209
Esophagomyotomy, 1204
Esophagus
  anatomy of, 1161, 1192
  Barrett's, 1193
  cancer of. *See* Esophageal cancer.
  dilation of
    for achalasia, 1204, 1204f
    for esophageal cancer, 1208
  diverticula of, 1212
  perforation of, 1212t
  trauma, 1212-1213
  tumors of. *See* Esophageal cancer.

Esophagus—cont'd
  varices
    characteristics of, 1299-1300
    endoscopic ligation of, 1310
    injection sclerotherapy for, 1309-1310
    recurrent, 1311
Estrace. *See* Estrogen replacement therapy.
Estraderm. *See* Estrogen replacement
    therapy.
Estradiol, 1723c
Estramustine, 431t
Estriol, 1723c
Estrogen
  bone growth and metabolism effects,
    1082-1083
  bone resorption inhibition by, 187c
  menopausal effects, 1710-1711
  urinary incontinence treated using, 1627c
Estrogen replacement therapy
  breast cancer and, 1737, 1737t
  cardiovascular conditions and, 627
  client education, 1754c
  osteoporosis management using,
    1098-1099, 1100c
Etanercept, 349
Ethacrynic acid
  for hypertension, 739c
  ototoxicity of, 1052t
  urine output increased by, 1655c
Ethambutol
  for opportunistic infections, 379t
  for pneumonia, 587t
Ethics, 58-59
Ethmozine. *See* Moricizine hydrochloride.
Ethosuximide, 902c
Ethrane. *See* Enflurane.
Etibi. *See* Ethambutol.
Etidronate, 1107
Etodolac, 75t, 82t, 91b
Etoposide, 431t, 563t
ets, 417t
Euflex. *See* Flutamide.
Euglobin lysis time, 832t
Eulexin. *See* Flutamide.
Euthanasia, 114-115
Eversion, 1087f
Evil eye, 56
Evisceration of wound, 291, 291f, 296, 296c
Evista. *See* Raloxifene.
Ewing's sarcoma, 1112-1113
Exchange system, 1466, 1467t
Excitability, 654
Excretory urogram. *See* Intravenous
    urography.
Exercise
  assessment of, 629-630
  asthma managed using, 538
  atherosclerosis prevention, 732
  back pain managed using, 927, 928c
  cholesterol reductions, 812, 813c
  client teaching, 1468, 1469c
  diabetes mellitus managed using, 1468-1469

Exercise—cont'd
  hypertension reductions, 738
  hypoglycemia and, 1480
  in heart failure, 710
  older adults, 38-39, 1469b
  osteoporosis prevention and management
    by, 1101-1102
  Parkinson's disease management, 911
  peripheral arterial disease managed
    using, 746
  recommendations, 629
  respiratory conditioning, 547
  stress incontinence managed using, 1626
  urge incontinence managed using, 1628
Exercise electrocardiography, 646-647
Exercise testing
  characteristics of, 483-484, 485t
  coronary artery disease assessments, 795
  peripheral arterial disease assessments,
    746
  valvular heart disease assessments, 714
Exophthalmos, 1016, 1424, 1425f
Exotoxins, 446
Exploratory laparotomy
  for intestinal obstruction, 1258-1259
  for peritonitis, 1270
Extension, 1087f
External fixation, for fractures, 1138f,
    1138-1139
External otitis
  characteristics of, 1061-1062
  malignant, 1108b
Extracellular fluid
  acid-base regulatory mechanisms, 218-220
  calcium concentrations, 152
  definition of, 140t, 143
  distribution of, 148
  pH, 220
  phosphorus levels in, 153
  potassium movement from, 180
  sodium transport, 144
Extracorporeal shock wave lithotripsy, 1336,
    1336f, 1635
Extravasation, 433, 433c
Extremities
  amputation of. *See* Amputation.
  ankle brachial index for assessing, 635
  assessment of, 633-634, 1087, 1087f
  blood flow assessments, 1148
  casts for, 1135t
  clubbing of, 633, 633f
  nutritional deficiency manifestations,
    1366t
  pain, 632
Eye(s)
  age-related changes, 1014c, 1014-1015
  anatomy of, 1011-1013
  assessment of
    computed tomography, 1019
    corneal staining, 1019
    electroretinography, 1022
    fluorescein angiography, 1022

Communication Quick Reference for Spanish-Speaking Clients

THE BODY • EL CUERPO (ehl KWEHR-poh)

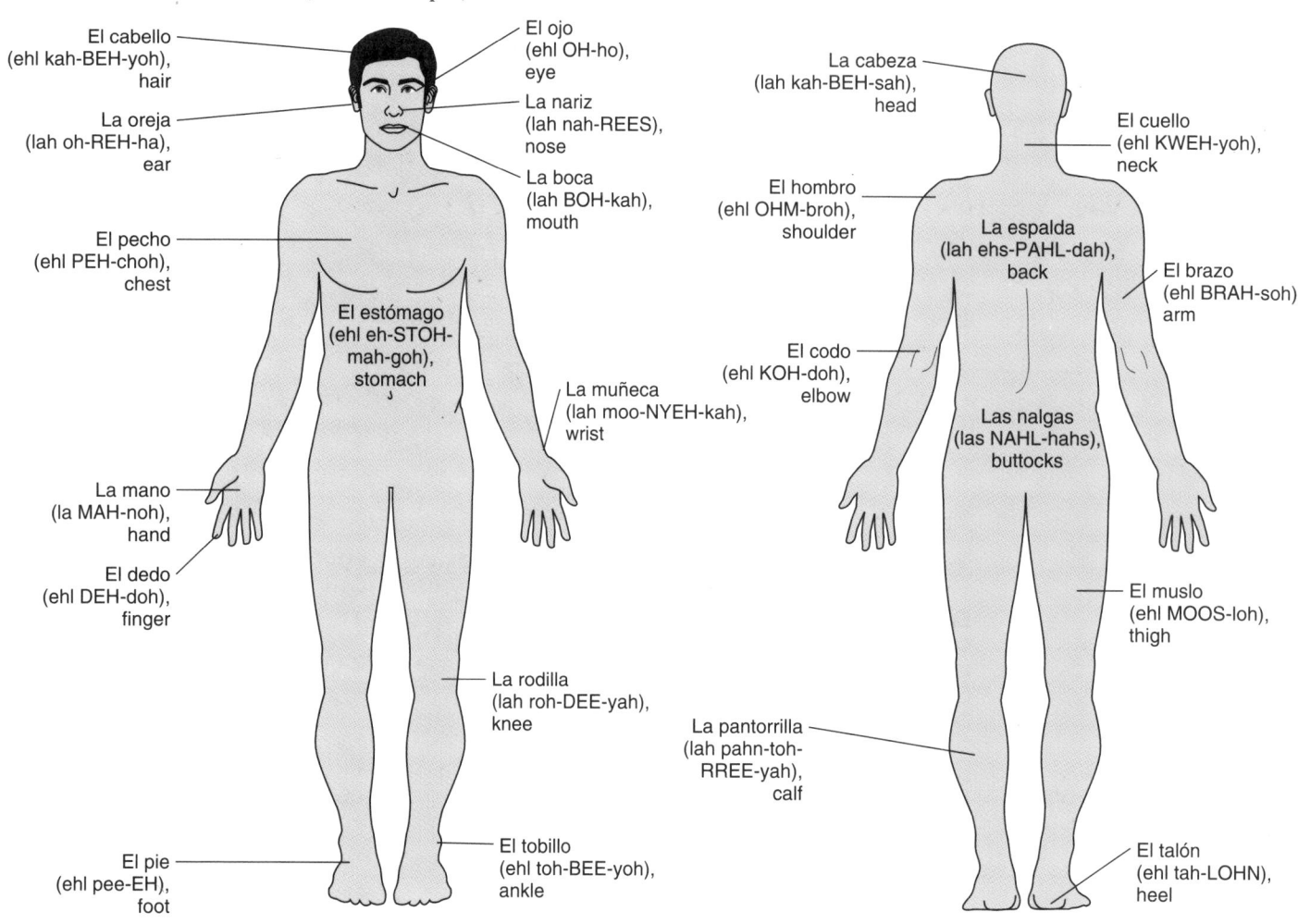

El cabello (ehl kah-BEH-yoh), hair

El ojo (ehl OH-ho), eye

La oreja (lah oh-REH-ha), ear

La nariz (lah nah-REES), nose

La boca (lah BOH-kah), mouth

El pecho (ehl PEH-choh), chest

El estómago (ehl eh-STOH-mah-goh), stomach

La muñeca (lah moo-NYEH-kah), wrist

La mano (la MAH-noh), hand

El dedo (ehl DEH-doh), finger

La rodilla (lah roh-DEE-yah), knee

El pie (ehl pee-EH), foot

El tobillo (ehl toh-BEE-yoh), ankle

La cabeza (lah kah-BEH-sah), head

El cuello (ehl KWEH-yoh), neck

El hombro (ehl OHM-broh), shoulder

La espalda (lah ehs-PAHL-dah), back

El brazo (ehl BRAH-soh), arm

El codo (ehl KOH-doh), elbow

Las nalgas (las NAHL-hahs), buttocks

El muslo (ehl MOOS-loh), thigh

La pantorrilla (lah pahn-toh-RREE-yah), calf

El talón (ehl tah-LOHN), heel

COMMON INSTRUCTIONS TO BE USED WITH THE BODY PARTS

Move the, Mueva (*mooh-EH-bah*)   Touch the, Toque (*TOH-keh*)   Point to the, Señale (*seh-NYAH-leh*)

MORE PARTS OF THE BODY

Armpit, la axila (*lah ahk-SEE-lah*)
Breasts, los senos (*lohs SEH-nohs*)
Collarbone, la clavícula (*lah klah-BEE-koo-lah*)
Diaphragm, el diafragma (*ehl dee-ah-FRAH-mah*)
Forearm, el antebrazo (*ehl ahn-teh-BRAH-soh*)

Groin, la ingle (*lah EEN-gleh*)
Hip, la cadera (*lah kah-DEH-rah*)
Kneecap, la rótula (*lah ROH-too-lah*)
Nail, la uña (*lah OON-yah*)
Pelvis, la pelvis (*lah PEHL-beece*)

Rectum, el recto (*ehl REHK-toh*)
Rib, la costilla (*lah koh-STEE-yah*)
Spine, el espinazo (*ehl ehs-pee-NAH-soh*)
Throat, la garganta (*lah gahr-GAHN-tah*)
Tongue, le lengua (*lah LEHN-gwah*)

ORGANS

Appendix, el apéndice (*ehl ah-PEHN-dee-seh*)
Bladder, la vejiga (*lah beh-HEE-gah*)
Brain, el cerebro (*ehl seh-REH-broh*)
Colon, el colon (*ehl KOH-lohn*)
Esophagus, el esófago (*ehl eh-SOH-fah-goh*)
Gallbladder, la vesícula biliar (*lah beh-SEE-koo-lah bee-lee-AHR*)
Genitals, los genitales (*lohs heh-nee-TAH-lehs*)

Heart, el corazón (*ehl koh-rah-SOHN*)
Kidney, el riñón (*ehl ree-NYOHN*)
Large intestine, el intestino grueso (*ehl een-tehs-TEE-noh groo-EH-so*)
Liver, el hígado (*ehl EE-gah-doh*)
Lungs, los pulmones (*lohs pool-MOH-nehs*)
Pancreas, el páncreas (*ehl PAHN-kreh-ahs*)

Small intestine, el intestino delgado (*ehl een-tehs-TEE-noh dehl-GAH-doh*)
Spleen, el bazo (*ehl BAH-soh*)
Thyroid gland, la tiroides (*lah tee-ROH-ee-dehs*)
Tonsils, las amígdalas (*lahs ah-MEEG-dah-lahs*)
Uterus, el útero (*ehl OO-teh-roh*)